# COMPREHENSIVE GYNECOLOGY

# COMPREHENSIVE GYNECOLOGY

*8th edition*

**David M. Gershenson, MD**
Professor
Gynecologic Oncology and Reproductive Medicine
University of Texas MD Anderson Cancer Center
Houston, Texas

**Gretchen M. Lentz, MD**
Professor, Obstetrics and Gynecology
Adjunct Professor, Urology
Division Director, Urogynecology
University of Washington Medical Center
Seattle, Washington

**Fidel A. Valea, MD**
Professor and Chair
Department of Obstetrics and Gynecology
Division of Gynecologic Oncology
Virginia Tech Carilion School of Medicine
Roanoke, Virginia

**Roger A. Lobo, MD**
Professor, Obstetrics and Gynecology
Division of Reproductive Endocrinology
Columbia University
New York, New York

ELSEVIER

Elsevier
1600 John F. Kennedy Blvd.
Ste 1800
Philadelphia, PA 19103-2899

COMPREHENSIVE GYNECOLOGY, EIGTH EDITION ISBN: 978-0-323-65399-2


Library of Congress Control Number: 2020951463

*Senior Content Strategist:* Nancy Duffy
*Director, Content Development:* Ellen Wurm-Cutter
*Senior Content Development Specialist:* Kathleen Nahm/Melissa Rawe
*Publishing Services Manager:* Shereen Jameel
*Project Manager:* Manikandan Chandrasekaran
*Cover Design and Design Direction:* Bridget Hoette/Ryan Cook

Printed in India

Last digit is the print number: 9 8 7 6 5 4 3 2 1

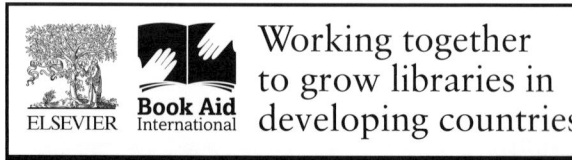

# List of Contributors

**Arnold P. Advincula, MD, FACOG, FACS**
Levine Family Professor of Women's Health
Vice-Chair, Department of Obstetrics & Gynecology
Chief of Gynecologic Specialty Surgery, Sloane Hospital for Women
Columbia University
New York, New York

**Jamie N. Bakkum-Gamez, MD**
Professor
Obstetrics and Gynecology
Mayo Clinic
Rochester, Minnesota

**Genevieve Bouchard-Fortier, MD, FRCSC, MSc**
Assistant Professor
University Health Network
Division of Gynecologic Oncology
Obstetrics and Gynecology University of Toronto
Toronto, Ontario, Canada

**Anne Burke, MD, MPH**
Associate Professor
Gynecology and Obstetrics
Johns Hopkins University
Baltimore, Maryland

**Leslie H. Clark, MD**
Assistant Professor
Obstetrics and Gynecology, Division of Gynecologic Oncology
University of North Carolina at Chapel Hill,
Chapel Hill, North Carolina

**Robert L. Coleman, MD**
Professor & Deputy Chair
Department of Gynecologic Oncology & Reproductive Medicine
University of Texas MD Anderson Cancer Center
Houston, Texas

**Allan Covens, MD, FRCSC**
Head
Sunnybrook Health Science Center;
Professor & Chair
Division of Gynecologic Oncology
Obstetrics and Gynecology University of Toronto
Toronto, Ontario, Canada

**Deborah S. Cowley, MD**
Professor
Psychiatry and Behavioral Sciences
University of Washington
Seattle, Washington

**Anne R. Davis, MD, MPH**
Wyeth Ayerst Professor
Obstetrics and Gynecology
Columbia University Irving Medical Center
New York, New York

**Mary Segars Dolan, MD, MPH**
Associate Professor
Gynecology and Obstetrics
Emory University
Atlanta, Georgia

**Sarah K. Dotters-Katz, MD, MMHPE**
Assistant Professor
Obstetrics and Gynecology
Duke University
Durham, North Carolina

**Nataki C. Douglas, MD, PhD**
Associate Professor
Department of Obstetrics, Gynecology and Women's Health
Rutgers–New Jersey Medical School
Newark, New Jersey

**Sean C. Dowdy, MD**
Professor
Obstetrics and Gynecology
Mayo Clinic
Rochester, Minnesota

**Linda O. Eckert, MD**
Professor
Department of Obstetrics and Gynecology;
Adjunct Professor
Department of Global Health
University of Washington
Seattle, Washington

**Michael Fialkow, MD, MPH**
Professor
Obstetrics and Gynecology
University of Washington School of Medicine
Seattle, Washington

**Eric J. Forman, MD, HCLD**
Medical and Laboratory Director
Department of Obstetrics and Gynecology
Columbia University Irving Medical Center
Division of Reproductive Endocrinology & Infertility
New York, New York

**Michael Frumovitz, MD, MPH**
Professor and Associate Chief Patient Experience Officer
Gynecologic Oncology and Reproductive Medicine
University of Texas MD Anderson Cancer Center
Houston, Texas

**Paola Alvarez Gehrig, MD**
Professor & Chief
Division of Gynecologic Oncology
University of North Carolina
Chapel Hill, North Carolina

**David M. Gershenson, MD**
Professor
Gynecologic Oncology and Reproductive Medicine
University of Texas MD Anderson Cancer Center
Houston, Texas

**Jennifer Bushman Gilner, MD, PhD**
Assistant Professor
Obstetrics and Gynecology
Duke University
Durham, North Carolina

**Laura J. Havrilesky, MD, MHSc**
Professor, Division of Gynecologic Oncology
Obstetrics and Gynecology
Duke University
Durham, North Carolina

**Cherie C. Hill, MD**
Assistant Professor
Gynecology and Obstetrics
Emory University School of Medicine
Atlanta, Georgia

**Hye-Chun Hur, MD, MPH**
Associate Professor
Minimally Invasive Gynecologic Surgery
Department of Obstetrics and Gynecology
Columbia University Irving Medical Center
New York, New York

**Anuja Jhingran, MD**
Professor
Radiation Oncology
University of Texas MD Anderson Cancer Center
Houston, Texas

**James M. Kelley III, BA, JD**
Managing Partner
Medical Malpractice
Elk & Elk Co Ltd
Cleveland, Ohio

**Anna C. Kirby, MD, MAS**
Assistant Professor
Obstetrics and Gynecology
University of Washington
Seattle, Washington

**Jeffrey A. Kuller, MD**
Professor of Obstetrics and Gynecology
Division of Maternal-Fetal Medicine
Duke University Medical Center
Durham, North Carolina

**Eduardo Lara-Torre, MD, FACOG**
Vice Chair, Department of OBGYN
Section Chief, Academic Specialists in General OBGYN
Carilion Clinic
Professor
Department of OBGYN and Pediatrics
Virginia Tech-Carilion School of Medicine
Roanoke, Virginia

**Gretchen M. Lentz, MD, FACOG**
Professor, Obstetrics and Gynecology
Adjunct Professor, Urology
Division Director, Urogynecology
University of Washington Medical Center
Seattle, Washington

**Roger A. Lobo, MD**
Professor, Obstetrics and Gynecology
Division of Reproductive Endocrinology
Columbia University
New York, New York

**Karen H. Lu, MD**
Chair and Professor
Gynecologic Oncology and Reproductive Medicine
University of Texas MD Anderson Cancer Center
Houston, Texas

**Vicki Mendiratta, MD**
Associate Professor
Obstetrics and Gynecology
University of Washington
Seattle, Washington

**Larissa A. Meyer, MD, MPH**
Associate Professor
Gynecologic Oncology and Reproductive Medicine
University of Texas MD Anderson Cancer Center
Houston, Texas

**Jane L. Miller, MD**
Associate Professor
Urology
University of Washington
Seattle, Washington

**Andra Nica, MD, MSc, FRCSC**
Clinical Fellow
Obstetrics and Gynaecology
Division of Gynecologic Oncology
University of Toronto
Toronto, Ontario, Canada

**Jaclyn D. Nunziato, MD, MS**
Assistant Professor of Obstetrics and Gynecology
Department Obstetrics and Gynecology
Virginia Tech Carilion School of Medicine Roanoke, Virginia
Roanoke, Virginia

**James W. Orr, Jr., MD, FACS, FACOG**
Clinical Professor, Florida State College of Medicine
Medical Director, Regional Cancer Center Lee Health
Chief of Surgical Oncology, GenesisCare
Tallahassee, Florida

**Amanda Padro, MS, CGC**
Prenatal Genetic Counselor
MFM OB/GYN
Duke University
Raleigh, North Carolina

**Natacha Phoolcharoen, MD**
Lecturer
Obstetrics and Gynecology
Faculty of Medicine, Chulalongkorn University Bangkok
Thailand;
Visiting Scientist
Gynecologic Oncology and Reproductive Medicine
University of Texas MD Anderson Cancer Center
Houston, Texas

**Thomas M. Price, MD**
Professor
Obstetrics and Gynecology
Duke University
Durham, North Carolina

**Beth W. Rackow, MD**
Associate Professor
Obstetrics & Gynecology and Pediatrics
Columbia University Medical Center
New York, New York

**Pedro T. Ramirez, MD**
Professor
Gynecologic Oncology & Reproductive Medicine
University of Texas MD Anderson Cancer Center;
Director
Minimally Invasive Surgical Research & Education
University of Texas MD Anderson Cancer Center
Houston, Texas;
Editor in Chief
International Journal of Gynecological Cancer

**Licia Raymond, MD**
Clinical Assistant Professor
Obstetrics-Gynecology
University of Washington
Seattle, Washington

**Eleanor H. J. Rhee, MD**
Assistant Professor
Division of Maternal Fetal Medicine
Obstetrics and Gynecology
Duke University

**Katherine Rivlin, MD, MSc**
Assistant Professor
Obstetrics and Gynecology
The Ohio State University Wexner School of Medicine
Columbus, Ohio

**David T. Rock, MD**
Director of Breast Surgery Fellowship
21st Century Oncology;
Breast Surgeon
Regional Breast Care
Fort Myers, Florida

**Timothy Ryntz, MD**
Assistant Professor
Obstetrics and Gynecology
Columbia University School of Medicine
New York, New York

**Mila Pontremoli Salcedo, MD, PhD**
Associate Professor
The Department of Obstetrics & Gynecology
Federal University of Health Sciences/ Irmandade Santa Casa de Misericordia de Porto Alegre, Porto Alegre, Brazil;
Visiting Assistant Professor
The Department of Gynecologic Oncology and Reproductive Medicine
University of Texas MD Anderson Cancer Center
Houston, Texas

**Gloria Salvo, MD**
Medical Research
Gynecologic Oncology and Reproductive Medicine
University of Texas MD Anderson Cancer Center
Houston, Texas

**Samith Sandadi, MD, MSc**
Gynecologic Oncologist
Breast Surgeon
Clinical Assistant Professor
Florida State School of Medicine
Florida Gynecologic Oncology
21st Century Oncology
Fort Myers, Florida

**Kathleen M. Schmeler, MD**
Professor
Department of Gynecologic Oncology & Reproductive Medicine
The University of Texas MD Anderson Cancer Center
Houston, Texas

**Judith A. Smith, BS, PharmD**
Associate Professor
Obstetrics, Gynecology and Reproductive Sciences
UTHealth-McGovern Medical School
Houston , Texas;
Oncology Clinical Pharmacy Specialist
Pharmacy
Memorial Hermann Hospital Cancer Center
Houston, Texas

**Pamela T. Soliman, MD, MPH**
Professor
Gynecologic Oncology and Reproductive Medicine
University of Texas MD Anderson Cancer Center
Houston, Texas

**Anil K. Sood, MD**
Professor and Vice Chair
Gynecologic Oncology & Reproductive Medicine
University of Texas MD Anderson Cancer Center
Houston, Texas

**Premal H. Thaker, MD, MSc**
Professor and Director of Gynecologic Oncology Clinical Research
Department of Obstetrics and Gynecology
Washington University School of Medicine
St. Louis, Missouri

**Mireille Truong, MD**
Assistant Professor
Program Director, Fellowship in Minimally Invasive Gynecologic Surgery
Cedars-Sinai Medical Center

**Jenna Turocy, MD**
Reproductive Endocrinology and Infertility Fellow
Obstetrics and Gynecology
Columbia University
New York, New York

**Fidel A. Valea, MD**
Professor and Chair
Department of Obstetrics and Gynecology
Division of Gynecologic Oncology
Virginia Tech Carilion School of Medicine
Roanoke, Virginia

**Catherine H. Watson, MD**
Gynecologic Oncology Fellow
Obstetrics and Gynecology
Duke University
Durham, North Carolina

**Shannon N. Westin, MD, MPH**
Associate Professor
Gynecologic Oncology and Reproductive Medicine
University of Texas MD Anderson Cancer Center
Houston, Texas

**Zev Williams, MD, PhD**
Associate Professor and Division Chief
Department of Obstetrics and Gynecology
Division of Reproductive Endocrinology & Infertility
Columbia University Irving Medical Center
New York, New York

# Preface

*"Wisdom is not a product of schooling but of the lifelong attempt to acquire it."*

**Albert Einstein**

Having first been published in 1987, *Comprehensive Gynecology* is now in its eighth edition. And once again, it is appropriate to pay tribute to the legacy of the original editors—Drs. William Droegmueller, Arthur L. Herbst, Daniel R. Mishell, Jr., and Morton A. Stenchever—each of whom was a giant within our discipline and who had the wisdom and foresight to create a textbook that has guided generations of gynecologists to make a difference in the lives of women.

At this writing, we are in the midst of the 2020 COVID-19 pandemic. "The Great Influenza" pandemic occurred a little over a century ago, and one of the scientists in that fight was Simon Flexner, first Director of the Rockefeller Institute and brother of Abraham Flexner, author of the 1910 *Flexner Report*, which examined the state of American medical education. Thinking about Flexner's emphasis on medical education reform, Einstein's advice about the acquisition of wisdom, and the current attention to lifelong learning and self-assessment by the American Board of Obstetrics and Gynecology, it is appropriate to introduce this latest edition of *Comprehensive Gynecology*, with the hope that it will be of value to practicing gynecologists, trainees in obstetrics and gynecology, and subspecialists alike.

The doubling time of medical knowledge was estimated to be 50 years in 1950, 7 years in 1980, and 3.5 years in 2010. In 2020, it is projected to be 0.2 years (73 days). Certainly, the field of gynecology is no exception. Mastering complex surgical procedures, keeping abreast of the latest medical therapies for gynecologic conditions, grasping the advances and nuances of the electronic medical record, and understanding the rapidly expanding field of molecular biology and genetics as it relates to our specialty is challenging.

Despite the doubling time of medical information, the contributors and editors have made every effort to deliver the most updated and relevant content. In this edition, we have maintained the same chapters, although in two instances we have consolidated chapters, combining vulvar and vaginal cancers, as well as combining fallopian tube and peritoneal cancers with ovarian cancer. As in the previous two editions, we have added several new coauthors to continue to enhance the expertise necessary to maintain the book's high quality. Importantly, each of the chapters has been significantly updated.

We have provided the most important references in the body of the chapter, allowing the reader to have immediate access to the source, rather than having to search for the reference. In addition, we have maintained a limited number of Key References at the end of each chapter and Suggested Readings, which are available online.

As in the prior edition, we have provided video content to provide a more visual experience for the reader. New and better illustrations have also been added to assist in visual learning.

Nearly every chapter has key points, which have been bundled together in an online synopsis of the entire book. This will allow rapid assessment of the content of each chapter for more in-depth reading of areas of greater interest, as well as provide key learning facts in all areas of gynecology.

We hope readers will enjoy this edition and learn as much as they can from this ever-evolving field in order to provide better health care for women.

We would like to extend our gratitude to the Elsevier staff—Sarah Barth, Senior Content Strategist; and Melissa Rawe, Content Development Specialist—who have shepherded this entire process with extraordinary professionalism.

We would also like to thank our families, without whose support, patience, and encouragement this project could not have been accomplished.

**David M. Gershenson, MD**
**Gretchen M. Lentz, MD**
**Fidel A. Valea, MD**
**Roger A. Lobo, MD**

# Contents


## PART I
## Basic Science

1 Fertilization and Embryogenesis, 1
*Thomas M. Price, Fidel A. Valea*

2 Reproductive Genetics, 21
*Jennifer Bushman Gilner, Eleanor H. J. Rhee, Amanda Padro, Jeffrey A. Kuller*

3 Reproductive Anatomy, 47
*Jaclyn D. Nunziato, Fidel A. Valea*

4 Reproductive Endocrinology, 76
*Nataki C. Douglas, Roger A. Lobo*

5 Evidence-Based Medicine and Clinical Epidemiology, 106
*Catherine H. Watson, Fidel A. Valea, Laura J. Havrilesky*

6 Medical-Legal Risk Management, 116
*James M. Kelley III, Gretchen M. Lentz*

## PART II
## Comprehensive Evaluation of the Women

7 History, Physical Examination, and Preventive Health Care, 127
*Vicki Mendiratta, Gretchen M. Lentz*

8 Interaction of Medical Diseases and Female Physiology, 140
*Sarah K. Dotters-Katz, Fidel A. Valea*

9 Additional Considerations in Gynecologic Care, 148
*Deborah S. Cowley, Anne Burke, Gretchen M. Lentz*

10 Endoscopy in Minimally Invasive Gynecologic Surgery, 188
*Licia Raymond, Gretchen M. Lentz*

## PART III
## General Gynecology

11 Congenital Abnormalities of the Female Reproductive Tract, 207
*Beth W. Rackow, Roger A. Lobo, Gretchen M. Lentz*

12 Pediatric and Adolescent Gynecology, 221
*Eduardo Lara-Torre, Fidel A. Valea*

13 Contraception and Abortion, 238
*Katherine Rivlin, Anne R. Davis*

14 Menopause and Care of the Mature Woman, 255
*Roger A. Lobo*

15 Breast Diseases, 289
*Samith Sandadi, David T. Rock, James W. Orr Jr., Fidel A. Valea*

16 Early and Recurrent Pregnancy Loss, 323
*Jenna Turocy, Zev Williams*

17 Ectopic Pregnancy, 342
*Hye-Chun Hur, Roger A. Lobo*

18 Benign Gynecologic Lesions, 362
*Mary Segars Dolan, Cherie C. Hill, Fidel A. Valea*

19 Endometriosis, 409
*Arnold P. Advincula, Mireille Truong, Roger A. Lobo*

20 Pelvic Organ Prolapse, Abdominal Hernias, and Inguinal Hernias, 428
*Anna C. Kirby, Gretchen M. Lentz*

21 Lower Urinary Tract Function and Disorders, 461
*Gretchen M. Lentz, Jane L. Miller*

22 Anal Incontinence, 495
*Gretchen M. Lentz, Michael Fialkow*

23 Genital Tract Infections, 515
*Linda O. Eckert, Gretchen M. Lentz*

24 Preoperative Counseling and Management, 543
*Jamie N. Bakkum-Gamez, Sean C. Dowdy, Fidel A. Valea*

25 Perioperative Management of Complications, 559
*Leslie H. Clark, Paola Alvarez Gehrig, Fidel A. Valea*

26 Abnormal Uterine Bleeding, 594
*Timothy Ryntz, Roger A. Lobo*

## PART IV
## Gynecologic Oncology

27 Molecular Oncology in Gynecologic Cancer, 606
*Premal H. Thaker, Anil K. Sood*

28 Principles of Radiation Therapy and Chemotherapy in Gynecologic Cancer, 618
*Judith A. Smith, Anuja Jhingran*

29 Intraepithelial Neoplasia of the Lower Genital Tract (Cervix, Vagina, Vulva), 637
*Mila Pontremoli Salcedo, Natacha Phoolcharoen, Kathleen M. Schmeler*

30 Neoplastic Diseases of the Vulva and Vagina, 648
*Michael Frumovitz*

31 Malignant Diseases of the Cervix, 674
*Anuja Jhingran, Larissa A. Meyer*

32 Malignant Diseases of the Uterus, 691
*Pamela T. Soliman, Karen H. Lu*

33 Malignant Diseases of the Ovary, Fallopian Tube, and Peritoneum, 707
*Robert L. Coleman, Shannon N. Westin, Pedro T. Ramirez, Gloria Salvo, David M. Gershenson*

34 Gestational Trophoblastic Disease, 754
*Andra Nica, Geneviève Bouchard-Fortier, Allan Covens*

## PART V
## Reproductive Endocrinology and Infertility

35 Primary and Secondary Dysmenorrhea, Premenstrual Syndrome, and Premenstrual Dysphoric Disorder, 768
*Vicki Mendiratta, Gretchen M. Lentz*

36 Primary and Secondary Amenorrhea and Precocious Puberty, 781
*Roger A. Lobo*

37 Hyperprolactinemia: Evaluation and Management, 801
*Roger A. Lobo*

38 Androgen Excess in Women, 810
*Roger A. Lobo*

39 Polycystic Ovary Syndrome, 824
*Roger A. Lobo*

40 Infertility, 838
*Roger A. Lobo*

41 In Vitro Fertilization, 861
*Eric J. Forman, Roger A. Lobo*

Index, 873

# Video Contents


1 Fertilization and Embryogenesis
*Thomas M. Price, Fidel A. Valea*

**1.1** Embryo Biopsy and Cell Extrusion

3 Reproductive Anatomy
*Jaclyn D. Nunziato, Fidel A. Valea*

**3.1** Uterine Artery Dissection

**3.2** Anatomy of Uterosacral Ligaments

**3.3** Identification of the Course of the Ureter

10 Endoscopy in Minimally Invasive Gynecologic Surgery
*Licia Raymond, Gretchen M. Lentz*

**10.1** Transection of the Round Ligament and Dissection of the Broad Ligament

# PART I Basic Science

# 1 Fertilization and Embryogenesis

*Thomas M. Price, Fidel A. Valea*

## KEY POINTS

- Oocyte meiosis is arrested in prophase I from the fetal period until a luteinizing surge (LH) preceding ovulation. With the LH surge, the oocyte completes meiosis I associated with a decrease to 23 chromosomes with diploid (2*N*) DNA quantity and extrusion of the first polar body. With fertilization, meiosis II is completed with separation of sister chromatids resulting in 23 chromosomes with haploid (1*N*) DNA content and extrusion of the second polar body.
- Implantation is a complex process necessitating hormones of estrogen and progesterone, cytokines such as growth factors and interleukins along with prostaglandins. During implantation extravillous trophoblast invade the endometrium to anchor the pregnancy and to remodel the spiral arteries to make the placenta a high-flow, low-resistance organ. Villous trophoblast are in contact with maternal blood in the intervillous space for gas and nutrient transfer.
- Human chorionic gonadotropin (hCG) is secreted by syncytiotrophoblast and functions to maintain steroid production by the corpus luteum through interaction with the LH receptor. Other functions may include promotion of angiogenesis in the uterus, myometrial relaxation, inhibition of immune interaction at the uteroplacental interface, stimulation of fetal testosterone production and mediation of hyperemesis through receptors in the brain.
- Genetic sex is determined at the time of conception. Male differentiation is determined by expression of the *SRY* (sex-determining region Y) gene found on the short arm of the Y chromosome. SRY protein is a transcription factor and expression is unique to the Sertoli cell of the developing testis. SRY induces expression of another transcription factor, SOX9, which is also obligatory for male sex differentiation. A loss of function mutation of either *SRY* or *SOX9* results in XY sex reversal in which genetic men are phenotypic women. Several genes regulate SRY/SOX9 expression including *WT1* (Wilms' tumor suppressor 1) and *SF1* (steroidogenic factor 1). Although ovarian formation can only occur in the absence of *SRY/SOX9*, there are unique genes necessary for development. *FOXL2* encodes a transcription factor necessary for granulosa cell expansion. *BMP15*, located on the X chromosome, and *GDF9* on chromosome 5 encode growth factors expressed in oocytes required for granulosa cell proliferation.
- Renal and internal genital development are closely related. Under the influence of testosterone, the primordial renal mesonephros (wolffian ducts) differentiate into the vas deferens, epididymis, and seminal vesicles, while the paramesonephric ducts (müllerian ducts) are suppressed because of the secretion and action of antimüllerian hormone (AMH), also known as *müllerian Inhibitory Substance (MIS)*, by Sertoli cells. In the absence of MIS, the wolffian ducts regress and the müllerian ducts differentiate into the fallopian tubes, uterus, and cervix.

**Accompanying video for this chapter is available on ExpertConsult.com.**

## MEIOSIS, FERTILIZATION, IMPLANTATION, EMBRYONIC DEVELOPMENT, AND SEXUAL DIFFERENTIATION

Several areas of medical investigation have brought increased attention to the processes of **fertilization** and embryonic development, including teratology, stem cell research, immunogenetics, and assisted reproductive technology (ART). The preimplantation, **implantation,** and embryonic stages of development in the human can now be studied because of the development of newer techniques and areas of research. This chapter considers the processes of oocyte meiosis, fertilization and early **cleavage,** implantation, development of the genitourinary system, and sex differentiation.

## THE OOCYTE AND MEIOSIS

The oocyte is a unique and extremely specialized cell. The primordial germ cells in both males and females are large eosinophilic cells derived from endoderm in the wall of the yolk sac. These 700 to 1300 cells migrate to the germinal ridge by way of the dorsal mesentery of the hindgut by ameboid action by 5 to 6 weeks. **Oogenesis** begins with the replication of the diploid oogonia through mitosis to produce primary oocytes, reaching a peak number of 600,000 (confidence interval [CI]: 70,000 to 5,000,000) at 18 to 22 weeks of gestation. Through apoptosis, the numbers decline to about 360,000 (CI: 42,000 to 3,000,000) at menarche (Wallace, 2010). As can be seen, there is a large variance among individuals and a direct correlation between the number of fetal oocytes and the age of menopause. The maximum rate of fetal apoptosis occurs between 14 and 28 weeks gestation. Accelerated apoptosis is seen in Turner syndrome resulting in few oocytes at birth.

**The meiotic process actually begins at 10 to 12 weeks gestation** and is the mechanism by which diploid organisms reduce their gametes to a haploid state so that they can recombine again during fertilization to become diploid organisms. In humans this process reduces 46 chromosomes to 23 chromosome structures in the gamete. The haploid gamete contains only one chromosome for each homologous pair of chromosomes, so that it has either the maternal or paternal chromosome for each pair, but not both. Meiosis is also the mechanism by which genetic exchange is completed through **chiasma**

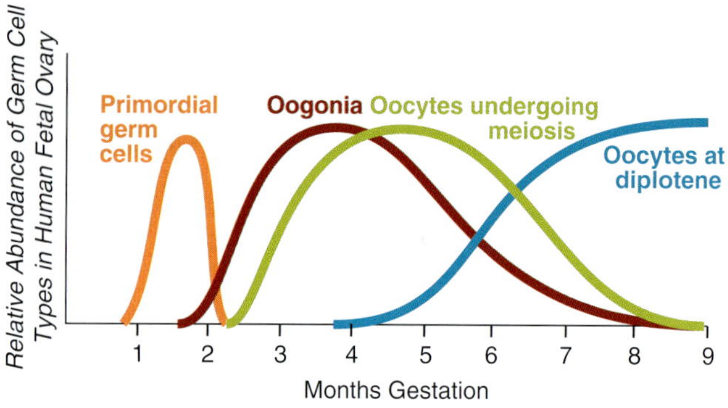


**Fig. 1.1** Diagram of the different meiotic cell types and their proportions in the ovaries during fetal life. (Courtesy Edith Cheng, MD.)

formation and crossing over (**recombination**) between homologous chromosome pairs. Two meiotic cell divisions are required to produce haploid gametes. In the human female, oogonia enter meiosis in "waves" (Fig. 1.1), that is, not all oogonia enter meiosis at the same time.

Meiosis initiation is dependent on mesonephric-produced retinoic acid (Childs, 2011). Oocytes in the first substage of prophase, leptotene, are found in the human fetal ovaries as early as 10 weeks' gestation. With increasing gestational age, greater proportions of oocytes in later stages of meiosis may be observed, and by the end of the second trimester of pregnancy, the majority of oocytes in the fetal ovaries have cytologic characteristics that are consistent with the diplotene/dictyotene substages of prophase I of meiosis I (the stage at which the oocytes are arrested until ovulation) (Fig. 1.2).

Meiosis is preceded by interphase I during which DNA replication occurs, thus transforming the diploid oogonia with a DNA content of $2N$ to an oocyte with a DNA content of $4N$. Meiosis is defined in two stages. The first, known as the *reduction division* (division I, or meiosis I), initiates in the fetal ovaries but is then arrested and completed at the time of ovulation.

Meiosis I starts with prophase I (prophase includes leptotene, zygotene, pachytene, and diplotene), which occurs exclusively during fetal life and sets the stage for genetic exchange that ensures genetic variation in our species (Fig. 1.3). More oocytes are found in the leptotene stage of prophase then in the other three stages of zygotene, pachytene, and diplotene in the fetal ovary. Leptotene is proportionately the most abundant of all the prophase I substages in early gestation. Cells in this meiotic phase are characterized by a large nucleus with fine, diffuse, string-like chromatin evenly distributed within the nucleus (Fig. 1.3A). Chromatin of homologous pairs occupies "domains" and does not occur as distinct linear strands of chromosomes. The zygotene substage is defined by the initiation of pairing, which is characterized by the striking appearance of the synaptonemal complex formation in some of the chromosomes (Fig. 1.3B). There is cytologic evidence of chromosome condensation and linearization, and the chromatin is seen as a fine, stringlike structure. The

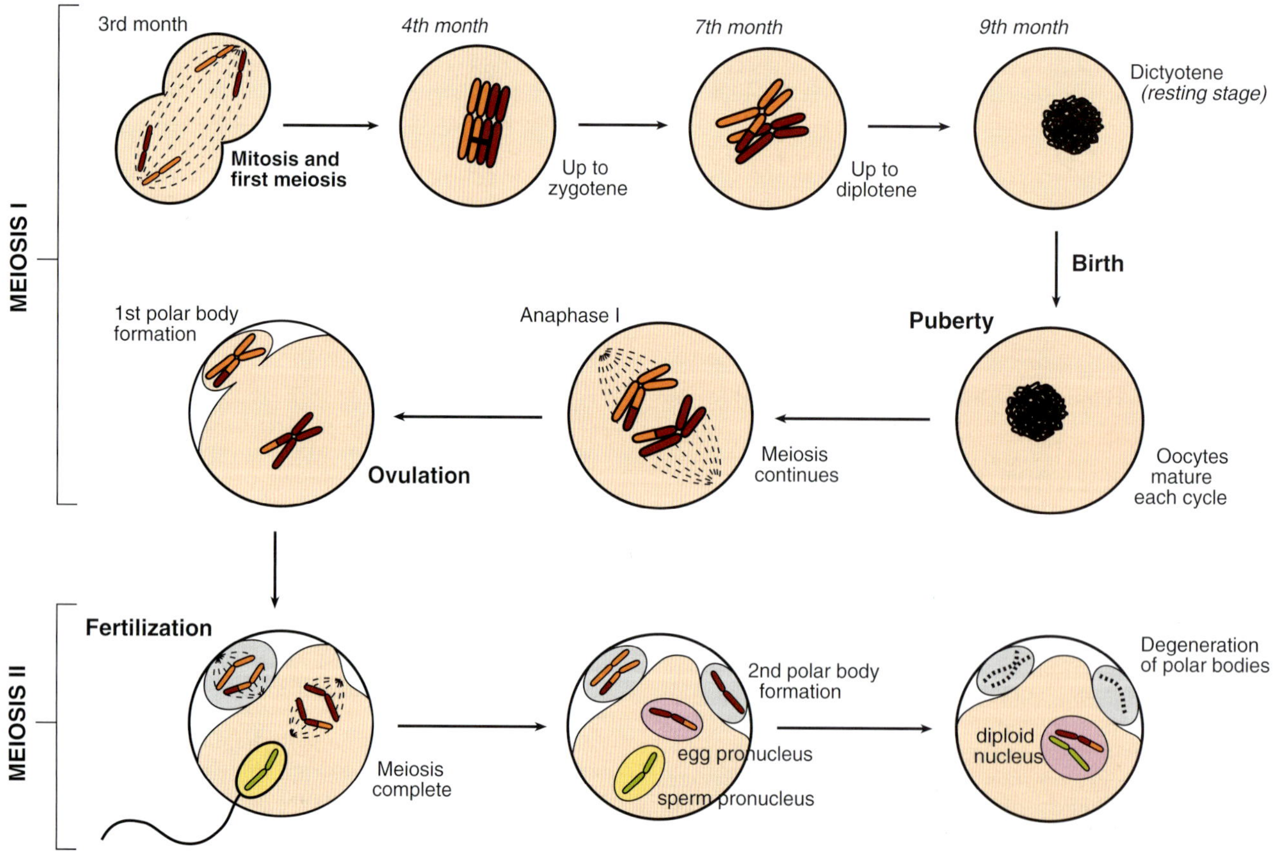


**Fig. 1.2** Diagram of oocyte meiosis. For simplicity, only one pair of chromosomes is depicted. Prophase stages of the first meiotic division occur in the female during fetal life. The meiotic process is arrested at the diplotene stage ("first meiotic arrest"), and the oocyte enters the dictyotene stages. Meiosis I resumes at puberty and is completed at the time of ovulation. The second meiotic division takes place over several hours in the oviduct only after sperm penetration. (Courtesy Edith Cheng, MD.)

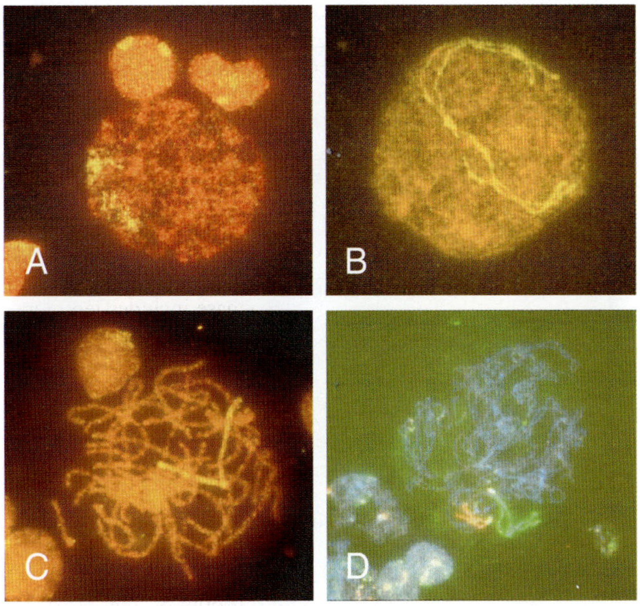


**Fig. 1.3** Fetal ovary with fluorescent in situ hybridization. The first three images are meiotic cells from a 21-week fetal ovary. **A,** Fluorescent in situ hybridization (FISH) with a whole chromosome probe for chromosome X was completed to visualize the pairing characteristics of the X chromosome during leptotene. **B,** Zygotene. **C,** Pachytene. **D,** Image of a meiotic cell from a 34-week fetal ovary that underwent dual FISH with probes for chromosomes 13 (*green signal*) and 21 (*red signal*) to illustrate the pairing characteristics of this substage of prophase in meiosis I. (Courtesy Edith Cheng, MD.)

pachytene substage is the most easily recognizable period of the prophase and is characterized by clearly defined chromosomes that appear as continuous ribbons of thick beadlike chromatin (Fig. 1.3C). By definition, this is the substage in which all homologues have paired. In this substage the paired homologues are structurally composed of four closely opposed chromatids and are known as a *tetrad.* The frequency of oocytes in pachytene increases with gestational age and peaks in the mid-second trimester of pregnancy (about 20 to 25 weeks' gestation). The diplotene substage is a stage of desynapsis that occurs as the synaptonemal complex dissolves and the two homologous chromosomes pull away from each other. However, these **bivalents**, which are composed of a maternally and a paternally derived chromosome, are held together at the centromere and at sites of chiasma formation that represent sites where crossing over has occurred (Fig. 1.3D). In general, chiasma formation occurs only between chromatids of homologous pairs and not between sister chromatids. Usually, one to three chiasma occur for each chromosome arm. Oocytes at this stage of prophase I constitute the majority of third-trimester fetal and newborn ovaries. Diplotene merges with diakinesis, the last substage of meiosis I, and is a stage of transition to metaphase, lasting many years in the humans.

During puberty, folliculogenesis includes progression of the follicle, consisting of the oocyte and granulosa cells from primordial to antral, which is characterized by granulosa cell proliferation, development of gonadotropin receptors, and expression of enzymes for sex steroid production (Baerwald, 2012). It takes approximate 85 days for a follicle to mature to the point of ovulation. There is no change in the chromosome stage during folliculogenesis.

**Meiosis I resumes with the surge of luteinizing hormone** before ovulation completing metaphase, anaphase, and telophase. The result is two daughter cells, which are diploid (2*N*) in DNA content but contain 23 chromosome structures, each containing two closely held sister chromatids. One daughter cell, the oocyte, receives the majority of the cytoplasm, and the other becomes the first **polar body.** The polar body is located in the perivitelline space between the surface of the oocyte (oolemma) and the zona pellucida (ZP).

Meiosis II is rapid, with the oocyte advancing immediately to metaphase II, where the sister chromatids for each chromosome are aligned at the equatorial plate, held together by spindle fibers at the centromere. **With sperm penetration, meiosis II is completed with extrusion of the second polar body yielding a haploid oocyte (1N) that is entered by a haploid (1N) sperm** (Fig. 1.4).

## Crossover and Female Aneuploidy

Aneuploidy in embryos is the most common cause of miscarriage and certain chromosomal abnormalities in live births, including Down syndrome (trisomy 21). The majority of the time these originate from an abnormal oocyte, increasing with age, and are more likely to affect chromosomes with short p arms (acrocentric). These chromosome segregation errors occur predominantly during meiosis I and are more common in the oocyte compared with the sperm. This is associated with deficient formation of chiasma between homologous chromosomes associated with DNA crossover (recombination) sites. Defective sites lead to less tension between homologous chromosomes, making segregation errors more likely as the spindles (microtubules) attached to the kinetochore protein complex adjacent to the centromere pull chromosomes toward the centrioles (Wang, 2017).

### Oocyte Cryopreservation

The clinical importance of meiotic spindle integrity was evident during the development of oocyte cryopreservation. Oocyte freezing is becoming more common for fertility preservation in women with medical conditions, such as cancer, for which chemotherapy and/or radiation therapy may result in ovarian failure, and in women of increasing reproductive age. The original technique for oocyte freezing was referred to as *slow freezing*, which was subsequently replaced by vitrification. Freezing involves removal of intracellular water so that ice crystals will not form during freezing, which may disrupt organelles. With slow freezing, cryoprotectants such as dimethyl sulfoxide (DMSO) and ethylene glycol are allowed to permeate the cell, replacing the water, as the oocyte is slowly cooled at 1°C to 2°C/min to −196°C and stored in liquid nitrogen. In contrast, vitrification involves the use of higher concentrations of cryoprotectant and very rapid cooling at 15,000°C to 30,000°C/min. With slow freezing there is a slow change from liquid to solid, whereas vitrification consists of immediate solidification of the cryoprotectant into a glasslike consistency. With human oocytes, vitrification causes much less spindle damage, resulting in higher oocyte survival rates.

## FERTILIZATION AND EARLY CLEAVAGE

In most mammals, including humans, **the egg is released from an ovary in the metaphase II stage** (Fig. 1.5). When the egg enters the fallopian tube, it is surrounded by a cumulus of granulosa cells (cumulus oophorus) and intimately surrounded by a clear ZP. Within the ZP are both the egg and the first polar body. Meanwhile, spermatozoa are transported through the cervical mucus and the uterus and into the fallopian tubes.

Although 20 to 200 million sperm may enter the vagina during intercourse, only 1 in 25,000 will make it to the fallopian tubes (Williams, 1993). This journey involves processes of **capacitation, chemotaxis, hyperactivated motility,** and **acrosome reaction**

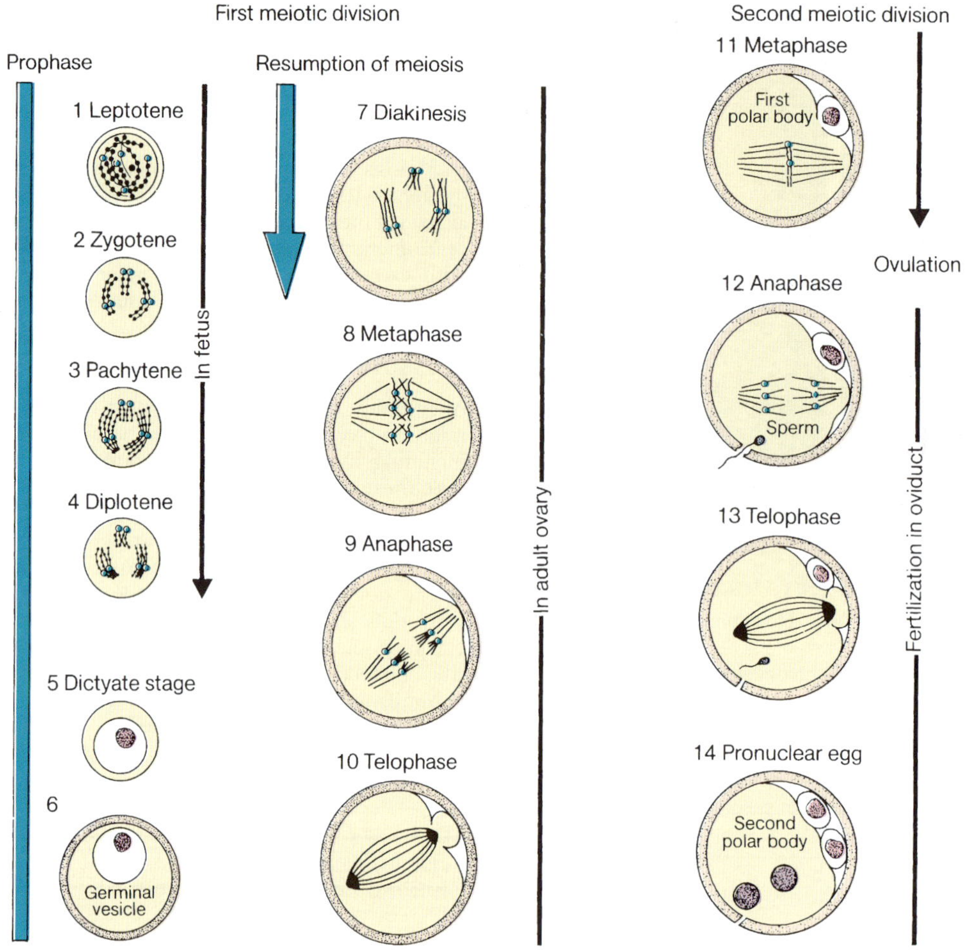


**Fig. 1.4** Diagram of oocyte meiosis. For simplicity, only three pairs of chromosomes are depicted (*1 to 4*). Prophase stages of the first meiotic division, which occur in most mammals during fetal life. The meiotic process is arrested at the diplotene stage ("first meiotic arrest"), and the oocyte enters the dictyate stages (*5 to 6*). When meiosis is resumed, the first maturation division is completed (*7 to 11*). Ovulation occurs usually at the metaphase II stage (*11*), and the second meiotic division (*12 to 14*) takes place in the oviduct only after sperm penetration. (From Tsafriri A. Oocyte maturation in mammals. In Jones RE, ed. *The Vertebrate Ovary.* New York: Plenum; 1978. With permission of Springer Science and Business Media.)

(Fig. 1.6). Capacitation precedes all other changes and involves initial removal of cholesterol from the plasma membrane altering the permeability and fluidity. This allows influx of calcium and bicarbonate, with many downstream effects, such as increased cyclic adenosine monophosphate (cAMP), protein tyrosine phosphorylation, and activation of protein kinases. A function of capacitation is to allow localization of protein complexes in the head of the sperm that will subsequently bind the ZP. Chemotaxis is shown by a greater number of sperm in the ampullary portion of the fallopian tube containing a cumulus-oocyte complex (COC) compared with the side lacking a COC. In vitro, follicular fluid acts as a chemoattractant, possibly because of progesterone, but the exact responsible constituents of the fluid continue to be debated (Eisenbach, 1999). Hyperactivated motility involves increased vigorous movement of the sperm to penetrate the cumulus (granulosa) cells surrounding the oocyte and is most likely caused by progesterone. A major action of progesterone is to increase calcium influx into the sperm, with multiple downstream effects. Likely the progesterone concentration increases as the sperm approaches the egg, resulting in more aggressive motility. **When the egg is reached, receptor complexes on the outer most plasma membrane bind to specific ZP glycoprotein receptors (primarily ZP 3).** These interactions are very species specific. Human sperm can only bind to the ZP of human, baboon, and gibbon oocytes. Binding results in fenestrations forming between the plasma membrane and the underlying acrosome membrane, releasing enzymes, including acrosin (a serine protease), to locally degrade the ZP.

Because many sperm may initially bind the ZP, a mechanism must be in place to prevent fertilization by more than one sperm (polyspermia). With initial binding of the sperm membrane to the oolemma, a calcium-dependent release of cortical granules occurs. Cortical granules are vesicles containing protein made during oogenesis and located in the periphery of the cell. Contents are released into the perivitelline space and modify ZP proteins and enlarge the perivitelline space to prevent sperm entry. **With sperm entry, the oocyte completes its second meiotic division, casting off the second polar body into the perivitelline space.**

The majority of a single sperm enters the oocyte, and this is indeed the case during intracytoplasmic sperm injection (ICSI) for infertility. Only the centrioles and the nucleus survive, whereas

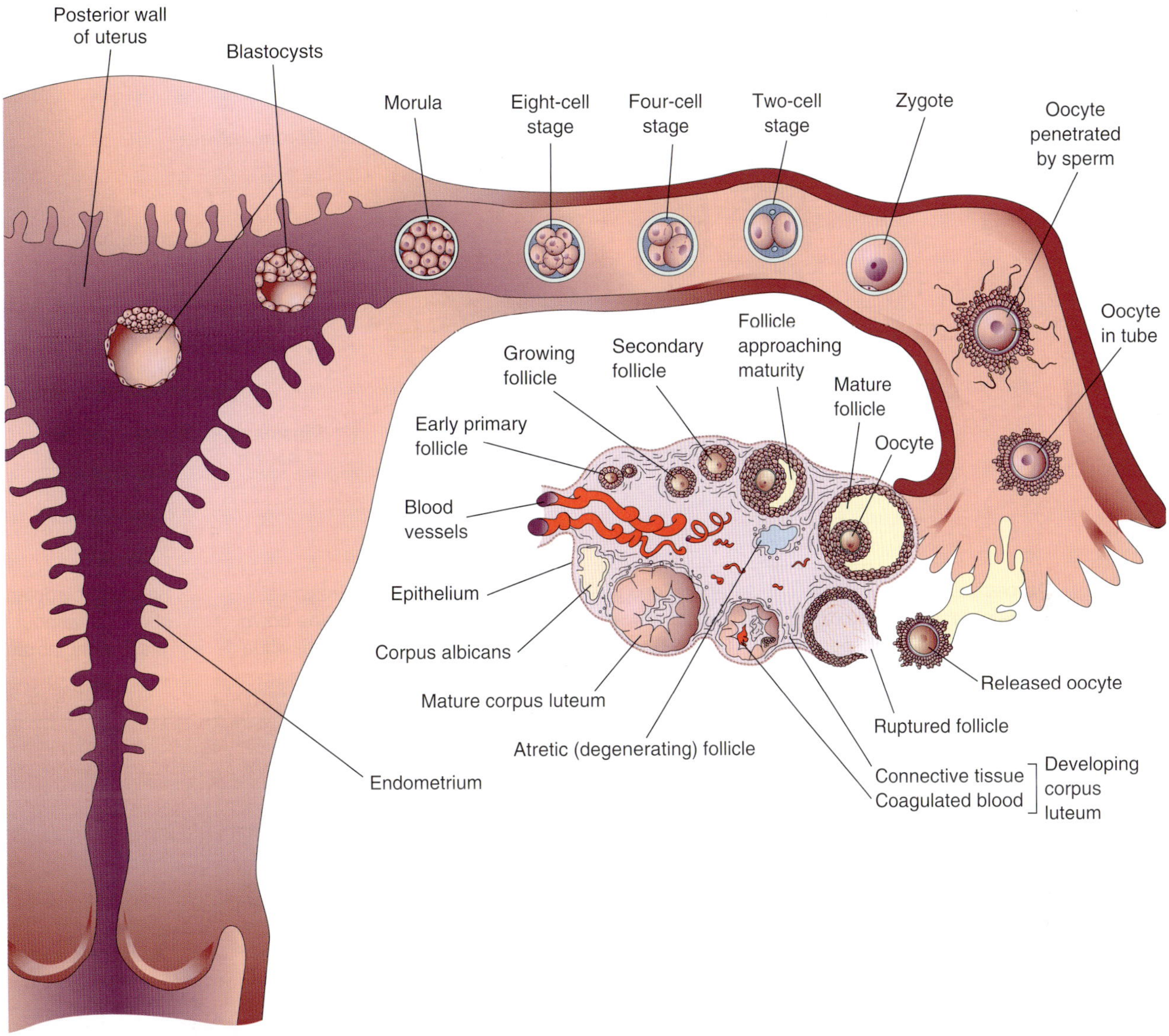


**Fig. 1.5** Summary of the ovarian cycle, fertilization, and human development during the first week. Stage 1 of development begins with fertilization in the uterine tube and ends when the zygote forms. Stage 2 (days 2 to 3) comprises the early stages of cleavage (from 2 to approximately 32 cells, the **morula**). Stage 3 (days 4 to 5) consists of the free (unattached) blastocyst. Stage 4 (days 5 to 6) is represented by the blastocyst attaching to the posterior wall of the uterus, the usual site of implantation. The blastocysts have been sectioned to show their internal structure. (From Moore KL, Persaud TVN. *The Developing Human: Clinically Oriented Embryology.* 7th ed. Philadelphia: WB Saunders; 2003.)

mitochondria in the midpiece and tail are destroyed. The sperm centrioles interact with α-tubulin from the oocyte to form a microtubule network for migration of pronuclei and subsequent separation of chromosomes during the first mitosis (Schatten, 2009). Thus mitochondria are of maternal origin and centrioles are paternal.

Early cell division (cleavage) is not synchronous and varies in time (Fig. 1.7). Time intervals from two pronuclei to two cells, two cells to three cells, three cells to four cells, and four cells to five cells are 26 hours, 12 hours, 0.8 hours, and 14 hours, respectively, as determined with time-lapse photography during in vitro fertilization (IVF) (Meseguer, 2011). A significant number of fertilized oocytes do not complete cleavage for a number of reasons, including failure of appropriate chromosome arrangement on the spindle, specific gene defects that prevent the formation of the spindle, and environmental factors. Importantly, **teratogens** acting at this point are usually either completely destructive or cause little or no effect. Twinning may occur by the separation of the two cells produced by cleavage, each of which has the potential to develop into a separate embryo. Twinning may occur at any stage until the formation of the blastocyst (blast) because each cell is totipotent. Both genetic and environmental factors are probably involved in the causation of twinning.

## Morula and Blastula Stage: Early Differentiation

After fertilization the zygote (term for a fertilized egg) has a diameter of 83 to 105 μm and undergoes rapid mitotic division to reach the next stage of approximately 16 cells called a *morula*. The cells of the zygote and early cleavage embryo are considered **totipotent**

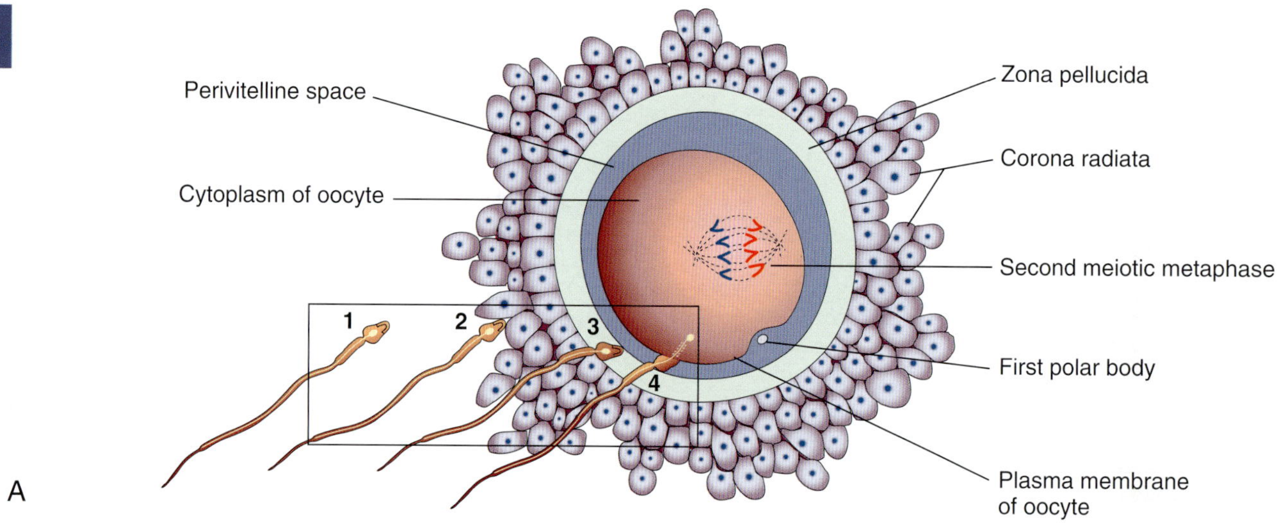


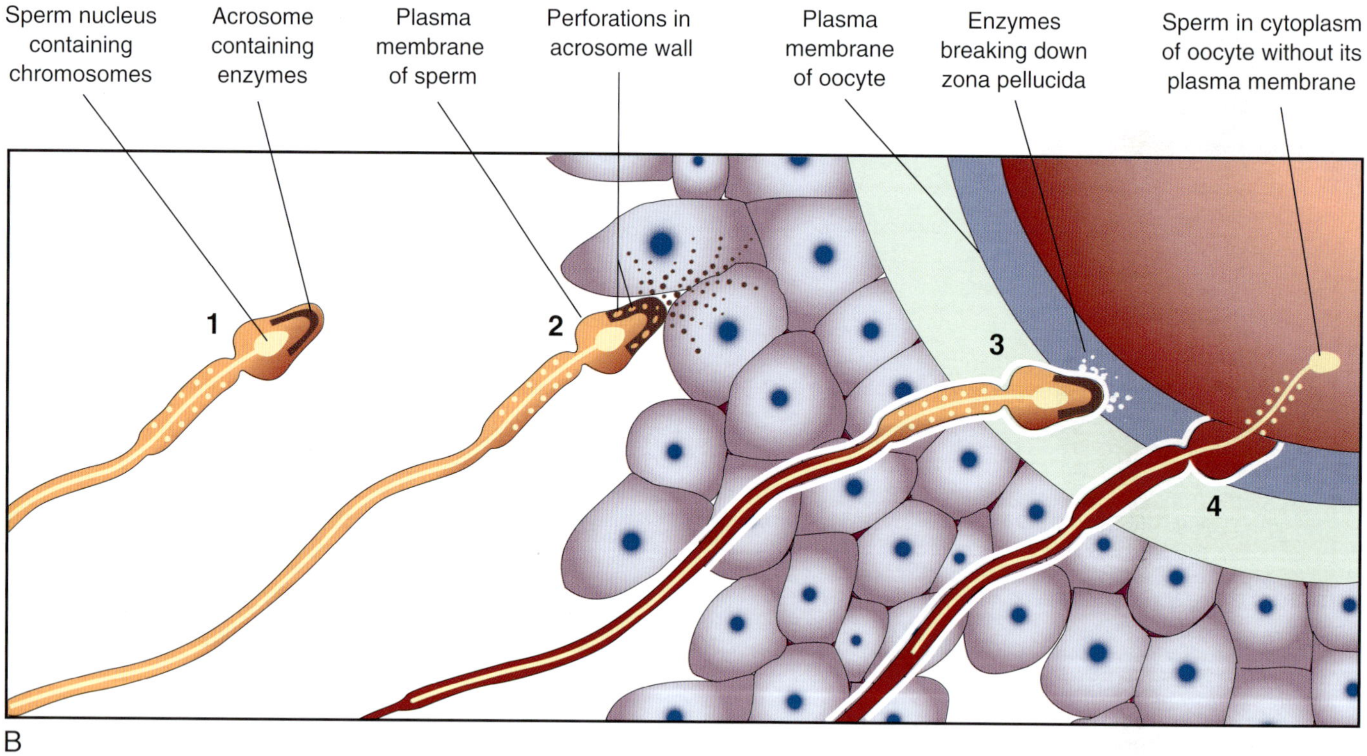


**Fig. 1.6** Acrosome reaction and a sperm penetrating an oocyte. The detail of the area outlined in **A** is given in **B**. *1,* Sperm during capacitation, a period of conditioning that occurs in the female reproductive tract. *2,* Sperm undergoing the acrosome reaction, during which perforations form in the acrosome. *3,* Sperm digesting a path through the zona pellucida by the action of enzymes released from the acrosome. *4,* Sperm after entering the cytoplasm of the oocyte. Note that the plasma membranes of the sperm and oocyte have fused and that the head and tail of the sperm enter the oocyte, leaving the sperm's plasma membrane attached to the oocyte's plasma membrane. (From Moore KL, Persaud TVN: The Developing Human: Clinically Oriented Embryology, 7th ed. Philadelphia, WB Saunders, 2003.)

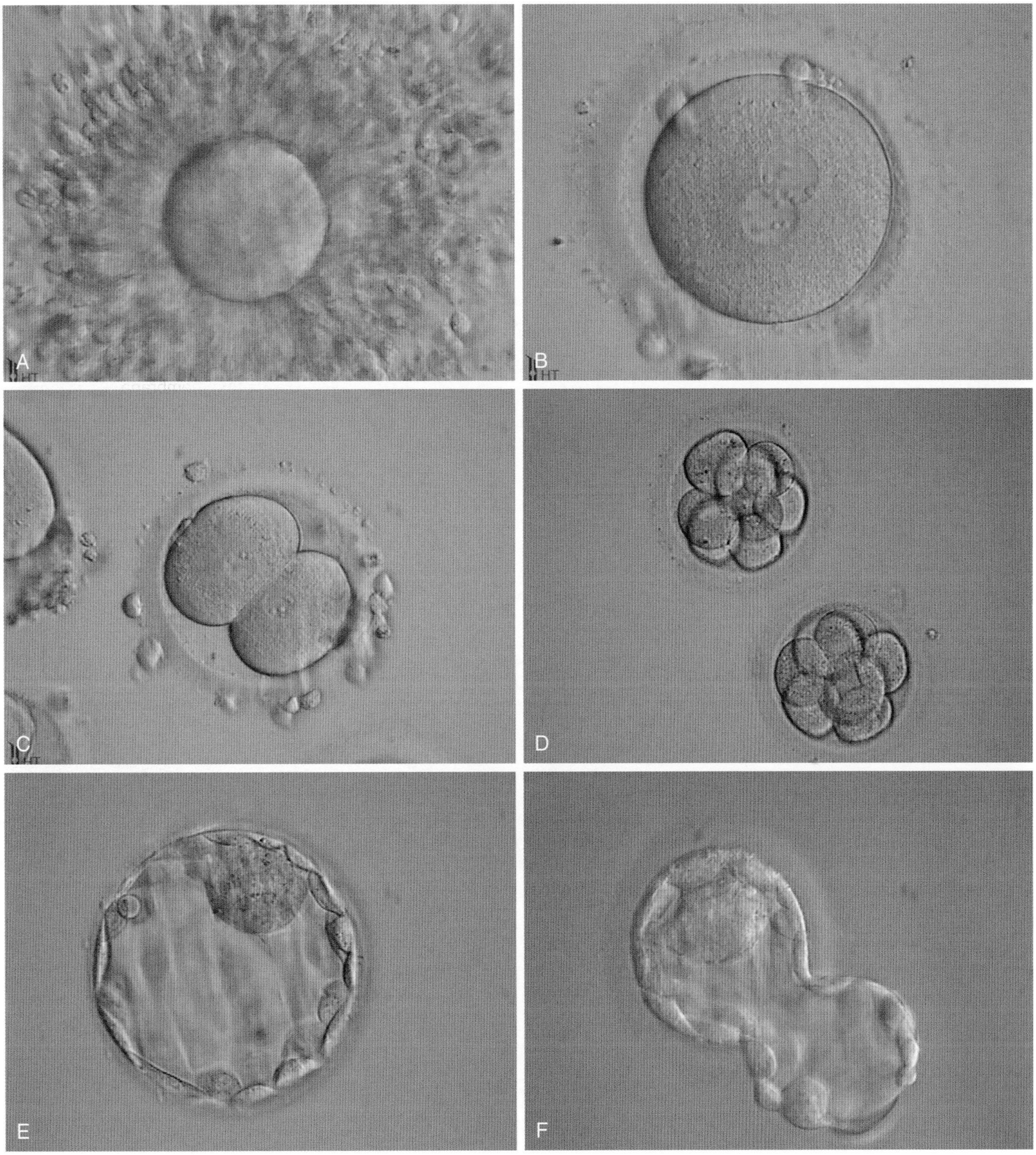


**Fig. 1.7** Six photomicrographs of fresh, unmounted human eggs and embryos. **A,** Recently retrieved human oocyte surrounded by cumulus cells. **B,** Fertilized oocyte demonstrating male and female pronuclei and both polar bodies at approximately 11 and 12 o'clock position. **C,** Two-cell zygote with scattered cumulus cells remaining attached to the zone pellucida. **D,** Eight-cell zygotes. **E,** Blastocyst with the inner cell mass seen at 12 o'clock. **F,** A hatching blastocyst in which a portion of the trophectoderm has extruded from the zona pellucida at the 4 o'clock position. (Photos Courtesy Douglas Raburn, PhD.)

because they are capable of producing all human tissue types (embryonic and extraembryonic). **After 4 to 5 days traversing the fallopian tube, the embryo arrives in the uterine cavity at the blastocyst (blast) stage.** The blast is characterized by a cavity (blastocoele) and differentiation of cells into the trophectoderm (TE), which will ultimately produce the fetal membranes and placenta, and the inner cell mass (ICM) that will produce the fetus. The cells in the blastocyst are referred to as **pluripotent,** meaning cells have differentiated into a group that can only yield embryonic cells and a group that can only yield extraembryonic cells. During IVF the blast forms 5 days after fertilization with a diameter of 155 to 265 μm consisting of about 40 TE cells and 20 ICM cells. In the human, implantation generally takes place 3 days after the embryo enters the uterus. The development of the blast with the separation of the ICM from the developing TE together make up the first stage of differentiation in the embryo. Differentiation within the ICM proceeds fairly rapidly, and if separation of cells and twinning occur at this point, the twins may be conjoined in some fashion.

Advances in ART and genetics now provide practitioners assess to the early embryo for **preimplantation genetic testing (PGT).** This includes PGT for monogenic/single-gene disorders (PGT-M), testing for aneuploidy (PGT-A), and testing for chromosome structural rearrangements (PGT-SR) such as translocations (Fig. 1.8). This technique involves removal of up to 10 (typically 5 to 10) TE cells from the day 5 blast for analysis. For PGT-M of single-gene disorders, DNA is extracted from the cells and the mutation analyzed by polymerase chain reaction (PCR) amplification or single nucleotide polymorphism (SNP) microarray. For PGT-A and PGT-SR, analysis of DNA is performed with comparative genomic hybridization (CGH) array or partial genomic sequencing (next generation sequencing).

## IMPLANTATION

Implantation consists of **apposition, attachment,** and **invasion.** This very complex process has redundancy and involves multiple factors, including ovarian hormones, cytokines, transcription factors, growth factors, and extracellular matrix proteins (ECM) (Table 1.1). These factors are produced by both the endometrium and the embryo. Communication between the embryo and the

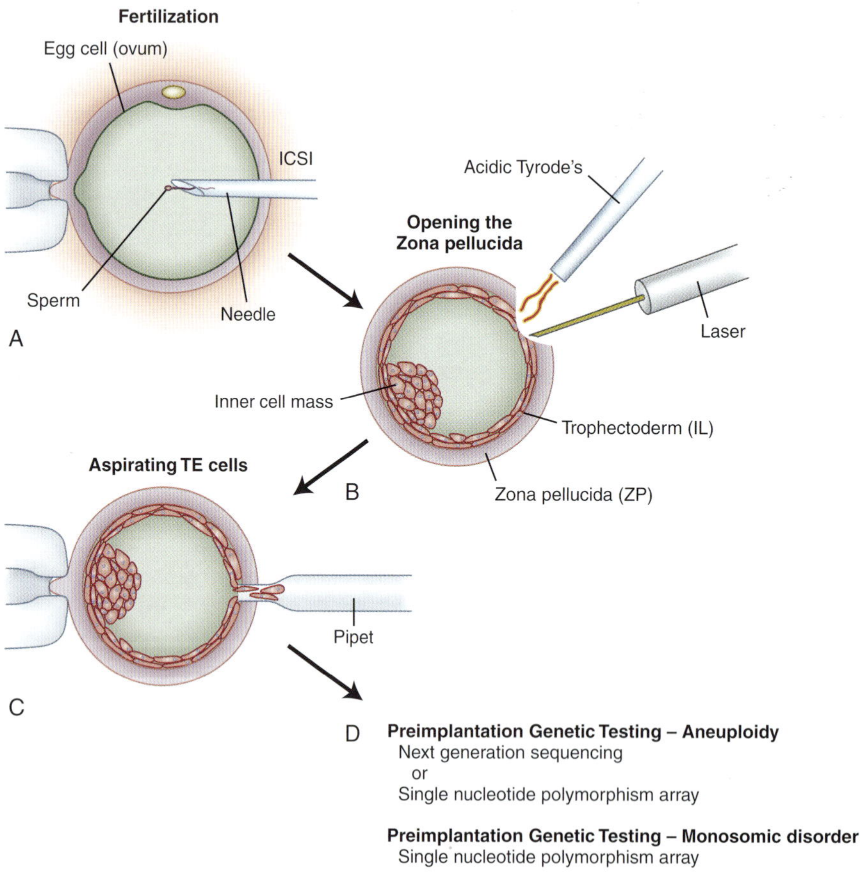


**Fig. 1.8** Schematic of preimplantation testing. **A,** Commonly the oocyte is fertilized with a single sperm using the technique of intracytoplasmic sperm injection (ICSI). This precludes the possibility of contamination from sperm remaining attached to the outside of the embryo during embryo biopsy. **B,** On day 3 of culture, when the embryo has cleaved to about eight cells, a small opening is made in the zona pellucida (ZP) with either a laser or through brief exposure to an acid solution. **C,** By day 5 of culture the embryo has progressed to the blastocyst stage and a portion of the trophectoderm (TE) cells have prolapsed out the opening in the ZP. These cells are removed for subsequent DNA isolation. **D,** DNA from TE cells is used to determine chromosome number and insertions and deletions for preimplantation genetic screening using techniques of array comparative genomic hybridization or next generation sequencing. DNA may also be used to detect single-gene abnormalities for different diseases using single nucleotide polymorphism microarray or polymerase chain reaction amplification in the process of preimplantation genetic diagnosis.

TABLE 1.1 Events of Implantation

| Event | Days After Ovulation |
|---|---|
| Zona pellucida disappears | 4-5 |
| Blastocyst attaches to epithelial surface of endometrium | 6 |
| Trophoblast erodes into endometrial stroma | 7 |
| Trophoblast differentiates into cytotrophoblastic and syncytial trophoblastic layers | 7-8 |
| Lacunae appear around trophoblast | 8-9 |
| Blastocyst burrows beneath endometrial surface | 9-10 |
| Lacunar network forms | 10-11 |
| Trophoblast invades endometrial sinusoids, establishing a uteroplacental circulation | 11-12 |
| Endometrial epithelium completely covers blastocyst | 12-13 |
| Strong decidual reaction occurs in stroma | 13-14 |

endometrium is key. Implantation occurs 7 to 10 days after ovulation, corresponding to cycle days 21 to 24 of an idyllic 28-day cycle with ovulation on day 14. During apposition the human embryo is oriented with the ICM and polar TE (the TE next to the ICM) adjacent to the endometrium.

For attachment to the endometrium, the embryonic cells must first be expelled from the surrounding ZP during the process of "hatching." **Hatching involves the rupture of the ZP in one small area as opposed to a general dissolution of the entire ZP.** This may involve both hydrostatic pressure from inside the ZP and from zonalytic proteases produced by the TE and endometrium. These cysteine proteases, named cathepsins, are essential for hatching. Attachment of the embryonic cells to the endometrial cells involves cell adhesion proteins, integrins, and ECM proteins such as fibronectin, laminin, and collagen. Integrins are cell surface proteins that bind extracellular matrix proteins and are expressed on both the luminal epithelium and TE.

Next, invasion of TE cells occurs by penetration between the luminal epithelial cells, through the basement membrane and into the stroma of the endometrium. These initial TE cells form the **extravillous trophoblasts (EVTs),** which invade the inner third of the myometrium for anchoring and into the spiral arteries for remodeling. During spiral artery remodeling, endovascular EVT disorganize and partially replace the smooth muscle wall and the vascular endothelial cells. Proliferation of endovascular EVT leads to plugging and obstruction of the decidual spiral arteries, resulting in a decrease in blood flow and oxygen tension. A low oxygen setting promotes proliferation and transformation of cytotrophoblast to syncytiotrophoblast. Before 8 weeks' gestation, nutrition to the embryo is derived from endometrial gland secretion and plasma seeping through the obstructed spiral arteries into the intervillous space. With continued remodeling of the spiral arteries, patency is reestablished and maternal blood cells enter the intervillous space around 9 weeks' gestation with a rise in oxygen tension. **Lack of adequate EVT invasion and spiral artery remodeling is a key feature in preeclampsia, intrauterine growth restriction, and stillbirths.**

The idea of low oxygen tension during early embryo development has been explored with IVF. With a limited number of trials, culturing embryos in 5% oxygen as opposed to 20% oxygen results in a modest increase in implantation rate (Bontekoe, 2012).

**Villous trophoblast form fingerlike projections extending into the intervillous space and that are surrounded by maternal blood.** Syncytiotrophoblast form the outer layer with an underlying layer of precursor cytotrophoblast surrounding matrix containing capillaries, fibroblasts, and macrophages (Hofbauer cells). Cytotrophoblast become less numerous as pregnancy progresses.

Blood levels of the pregnancy hormone human chorionic gonadotropin (hCG) can be detected within 48 hours of implantation. Regular hCG is produced by the syncytiotrophoblast of placental villi. Blood levels peak at 56 to 68 days, reach a nadir at 18 weeks, and then remain fairly consistent until delivery. Gonadotropin-releasing hormone (GnRH) produced in the cytotrophoblast induces expression of hCG. In spontaneous pregnancies hCG can be detected 9 days after follicle rupture observed by ultrasound. In IVF pregnancies the hormone can be found 8 days after embryo transfer. The hCG levels rise exponentially up to 8 weeks from the last menstrual period (LMP), but the doubling time increases as the level increases. For example, in a conception cycle with ovulation on cycle day 14, the doubling time from cycle days 25 to 37 for hCG is 1.6 days and from days 38 to 44 is 2.3 days (Zegers-Hochschild, 1994). The doubling time is independent of the number of gestations, although the absolute hCG level is higher for multiple pregnancies.

**The classic action of regular hCG is maintenance of the corpus luteum (CL) by binding the luteinizing hormone (LH) receptor** for continued estrogen and progesterone production. Yet other identified actions include promotion of angiogenesis in the uterus, myometrial relaxation, inhibition of immune interaction at the uteroplacental interface, stimulation of fetal testosterone production, and mediation of hyperemesis through receptors in the brain.

**Hyperglycosylated hCG (H-hCG) is produced by EVT.** H-hCG is key in promoting angiogenesis and cell invasion and correspondingly is found in the early first trimester. The protein does not activate the LH receptor and does not preserve CL function. Instead it appears to function via the transforming growth factor beta (TGF-β) receptor. Low levels of H-hCG indicate poor EVT development and are associated with spontaneous abortion and early preeclampsia (Fournier, 2015).

## Decidualization

Progesterone is responsible for "decidualization" of the endometrium. This refers to morphologic and functional changes in stromal cells. In humans, stromal cells close to the spiral arteries undergo progesterone-induced decidual changes in the late secretory phase and this process progresses throughout the stroma with implantation and hCG production. HCG derived from a pregnancy within the uterus is not required, as decidualization is a common finding with ectopic pregnancies. Decidual cells show morphologic changes of increased size with increased glycogen and lipid accumulation. During pregnancy the endometrium is now referred to as the *decidua*, separated into areas of the decidua basalis or placentalis, which interact with the TE (area of mature placenta), the decidua vera or parietalis (decidua distant from implantation site), and the decidua capsularis (surrounding the embryo on the side opposite the placenta).

Another classic histologic change seen in early pregnancy is the Arias-Stella reaction (Fig. 1.9). This occurs in the glandular cells with a hallmark of nuclear enlargement. These cells may be misinterpreted as atypical or malignant. In the presence of hCG the Arias-Stella reaction may be seen in extrauterine tissues such as endometriosis, vaginal adenosis, paraovarian cysts, and mucinous cystadenomas (Arias-Stella, 2002).

Morphologically, luminal epithelial cells develop extensions of the plasma membrane called *pinopods* (also called *uterodomes*)

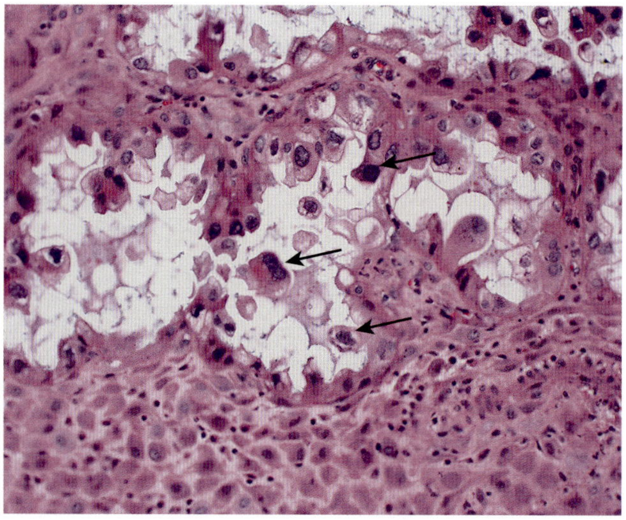

Fig. 1.9 Photomicrograph of the Arias-Stella reaction. The hCG action results in nuclear enlargement in endometrial glandular cells (*arrows*) resulting in visual characteristics of malignant cells. Magnification ×200. (Courtesy Rex Bentley, MD, and Stanley Robboy, MD, Duke University.)

during the window of receptivity. Pinopods release key proteins, including leukemia inhibitory factor (LIF), through exocytosis and apocrine secretion (Kabir-Salmani, 2005).

Downstream effects of progesterone-dependent decidualization have not been completely elucidated, but loss of function studies show the necessity of transcription factors including CCAAT/enhancer binding protein beta (C/EBPβ), homeobox A10 (Hoxa10), forkhead/winged helix protein (Fox01) and chicken ovalbumin upstream-promoter (COUP-TFII). A functional progesterone receptor requires interaction with chaperone proteins. In mice one of these proteins, named FK506 binding protein 52 (FKBP52), is expressed in the endometrium during the window of receptivity, and a loss of function mutation disrupts decidualization.

LIF is a cytokine produced by endometrial glandular cells around the time of implantation. LIF acts on EVT to increase fibronectin production necessary for embryo attachment and invasion. Mice lacking expression of LIF (knockout mice) have both failure of decidualization and implantation.

Indian hedgehog (*Ihh*) protein is a morphogen produced by luminal epithelial cells under the control of progesterone. Morphogens are signaling proteins that diffuse throughout the decidua yielding a concentration gradient. Signaling is dependent on the concentration in a given area. *Ihh* knockout mice fail to decidualize or implant (Ramathal, 2010).

## Embryo-Endometrial Communication

Implantation involves molecular interactions between the embryo and the adjacent endometrium. For example, the embryo produces heparin-binding epidermal growth factor-like growth factor (HB-EGF), which is both found on the cell membrane and is released from the cell (soluble). HB-EGF induces expression of itself in the adjacent endometrial cells (auto-induction loop). HB-EGF on the endometrial cells then acts to attach the embryo via EGF receptors expressed on the embryo (Lim, 2009). Additionally, the soluble HB-EGF from the embryo induces expression of cyclooxygenase to increase prostacyclin ($PGI_2$) in the endometrium, resulting in enhanced endometrial vascular permeability to help with embryo invasion.

## Immunology of Implantation

The paternal contribution to the embryo results in the mother being exposed to allogenic cells. Although villous trophoblast do not express major human leukocyte antigens (HLAs), the EVT express HLA-C, -E, and -G, which may be recognized by the maternal immune system. Thus the maternal immune system must be locally suppressed to prevent rejection.

The majority of immune cells in the decidua are uterine natural killer (uNK) cells. These cells are present in the secretory endometrium, under the control of progesterone, and increase in number with pregnancy to form an infiltrate around the invading EVT. These cells start to dissipate in the second trimester. uNK cells are not cytotoxic to trophoblast cells and in fact appear to be supportive. A low number of uNK cells in the decidua of early pregnancy is associated with poor invasion of the EVT. Cytokines such as interferon gamma and angiogenic factors secreted by uNK cells are key to proper EVT development and function.

T-helper (Th) cells are also found in the decidua and are functionally classified as Th1 (cellular immunity), Th2 (humoral immunity), Th3 (production of transforming growth factor beta for immunosuppression), and Tr1 (production of interleukin 10 for immunosuppression). In early pregnancy there is an increase in the percentage of decidual Th2 and Th3 cells.

T-regulatory (Treg) cells function in antigen recognition for future immune tolerance. Mice lacking Treg cells experience abortion when mated with an allogenic male but not when mated with a syngenic male (Darasse-Jèze, 2006). These cells are key in developing tolerance to male antigens. Development of immunity to specific paternal antigens may explain observations including lower preeclampsia rates in women exposed to their partner's semen before pregnancy compared with women conceiving with donor insemination (Salha, 1999) and the lower preeclampsia rate in the second pregnancy with the same partner as opposed to a new partner.

## Early Organogenesis in the Embryonic Period

During the third week after fertilization, the primitive streak forms in the caudal portion of the embryonic disk, and the embryonic disk begins to grow and change from a circular to a pear-shaped configuration. At that point the epithelium superiorly is considered ectoderm and will eventually give rise to the developing central nervous system, and the epithelium facing downward toward the yolk sac is endoderm. During this week the neuroplate develops with its associated notochordal process. By the sixteenth day after conception the third primitive germ layer, the intraembryonic mesoderm, begins to form between the ectoderm and endoderm. Early mesoderm migrates cranially, passing on either side of the notochordal process to meet in front in the formation of the cardiogenic area. The heart soon develops from this area. Later in the third week extraembryonic mesoderm joins with the yolk sac and the developing amnion to contribute to the developing membranes.

An intraembryonic mesoderm develops on each side of the notochord and neural tube to form longitudinal columns, the paraxial mesoderm. Each paraxial column thins laterally into the lateral plate mesoderm, which is continuous with the extraembryonic mesoderm of the yolk sac and the amnion. The lateral plate mesoderm is separated from the paraxial mesoderm by a continuous tract of mesoderm called the *intermediate mesoderm.* By the twentieth day, paraxial mesoderm begins to divide into paired linear bodies known as *somites.* About 38 pairs of somites form during the next 10 days. Eventually a total of 42 to 44 pairs will develop, and these will give rise to body musculature.

Angiogenesis, or blood vessel formation, can be seen in the extraembryonic mesoderm of the yolk sac by day 15 or 16. Embryonic vessels can be seen about 2 days later and develop when mesenchymal cells known as *angioblasts* aggregate to form masses and cords called *blood islands*. Spaces then appear within these islands, and the angioblasts arrange themselves around these spaces to form primitive endothelium. Isolated vessels form channels and then grow into adjacent areas by endothelial budding. Primitive blood cells develop from endothelial cells as the vessels develop on the yolk sac and allantois. However, blood formation does not begin within the embryo until the second month of gestation, occurring first in the developing liver and later in the spleen, bone marrow, and lymph nodes. Separate mesenchymal cells surrounding the primitive endothelial vessels differentiate into muscular and connective tissue elements. The primitive heart forms in a similar manner from mesenchymal cells in the cardiogenic area. Paired endothelial channels, called *heart tubes*, develop by the end of the third week and fuse to form the primitive heart. By the twenty-first day, this primitive heart has linked up with blood vessels of the embryo, forming a primitive cardiovascular system. Blood circulation starts about this time, and the cardiovascular system becomes the first functioning organ system within the embryo (Clark, 1987). All the organ systems form between the fourth week and seventh week of gestation.

A teratogenic event that takes place during the embryonic period gives rise to a constellation of malformations related to the organ systems that are actively developing at that particular time. Thus cardiovascular malformations tend to occur because of teratogenic events early in the embryonic period, whereas genitourinary abnormalities tend to result from later events. Teratogenic effects before implantation often cause loss of the embryo but not malformations. The effects of a particular teratogen depend on the individual's genetic makeup, other environmental factors in play at the time, the embryonic developmental stage during which the teratogenic exposure occurred, and in some cases the dose of the teratogen and the duration of exposure. Some teratogens in and of themselves are actually harmless, but their metabolites cause the damage. Teratogens may be chemical substances and their by-products, or they may be physical phenomena, such as temperature elevation and irradiation. The embryo is most sensitive to teratogens during organogenesis of the embryonic period from 18 to 56 days after conception. Before day 18, exposure is most likely to either result in embryo death with miscarriage or no effect because the majority of cells are pluripotent. Teratogen exposure after the embryonic period of development may injure or kill the embryo or cause developmental and growth retardation but usually will not be responsible for specific malformations. The period of embryonic development is said to be complete at 56 days (8 weeks) from fertilization or 70 days (10 weeks) from the LMP followed by the fetal stage.

## DEVELOPMENT OF THE GENITOURINARY SYSTEM

The development of the genital organs is intimately involved with the development of the renal system.

### Renal Development

Nephrogenic cords develop from the intermediate mesoderm as early as the 2-mm embryo stage, beginning in the more cephalad portions of the embryo. Three sets of excretory ducts and tubules develop bilaterally (Little, 2010). The first, the pronephros, with its pronephric ducts, forms in the most cranial portion of the embryo at about the beginning of the fourth week after conception. The tubules associated with the duct probably have no excretory function in the human, but the caudal end will form the adrenal gland. Late in the fourth week, a second set of tubules, the mesonephric tubules, and their accompanying mesonephric ducts begin to develop. These are associated with tufts of capillaries, or glomeruli, and tubules for excretory purposes. Thus the **mesonephros** functions as a fetal kidney, producing urine for about 2 or 3 weeks. As new tubules develop, those derived from the more cephalad tubules degenerate. Usually about 40 mesonephric tubules function on either side of the embryo at any given time. The gonads arise from the central region of the mesonephros. The **metanephros**, or permanent kidney, begins its development early in the fifth week of gestation and starts to function late in the seventh or early in the eighth week. The metanephros develops both from the metanephrogenic mass of mesoderm, which is the most caudal portion of the nephrogenic cord, and from its duct system, which is derived from the metanephric diverticulum (ureteric bud). It is a cranially growing outpouching of the mesonephric duct close to where it enters the cloaca. The metanephric duct system gives rise to the ureter, the renal pelvis, the calyces, and the collecting tubules of the adult kidney. A critical process in the development of the kidney requires that the cranially growing metanephric diverticulum meets and fuses with the metanephrogenic mass of mesoderm so that formation of the kidney can take place. Originally the metanephric kidney is a pelvic organ, but by differential growth it becomes located in the lumbar region.

The fetus produces urine starting at 8 weeks' gestation (Underwood, 2005). Starting in the second trimester, fetal urine is a major contributor to amniotic fluid volume. The fetus may swallow the amniotic fluid and recirculate it through the digestive system. Congenital abnormalities that impair normal development or function of the fetal kidneys generally result in little or no amniotic fluid (oligohydramnios or anhydramnios), whereas structural abnormalities of the gastrointestinal tract or neuromuscular conditions that prevent the fetus from swallowing can lead to excess amniotic fluid (polyhydramnios).

### Bladder and Urethra

The embryonic cloaca is divided by the urorectal septum into a dorsal rectum and a ventral urogenital sinus. The urogenital sinus, in turn, is divided into three parts: the cranial portion (the vesicourethral canal), which is continuous with the allantois; a middle pelvic portion; and a caudal urogenital sinus portion, which is covered externally by the urogenital membrane. The epithelium of the developing bladder is derived from the endoderm of the vesicourethral canal. The muscular layers and serosa of the bladder develop from adjacent splanchnic mesenchyme. As the bladder develops, the caudal portion of the mesonephric ducts is incorporated into its dorsal wall. The portion of the mesonephric duct distal to the points where the metanephric duct is taken up into the bladder becomes the trigone of the bladder. Although this portion is from the mesoderm, it probably is epithelialized by endodermal epithelium from the urogenital sinus. In this way the ureters, derived from the metanephric duct, come to open directly into the bladder.

In the male the mesonephric ducts open into the urethra as the ejaculatory ducts. Also in the male, mesenchymal tissue surrounding the developing urethra where it exits the bladder develops into the prostate gland, through which the ejaculatory ducts traverse. Fig. 1.10 demonstrates graphically the development of the male and female urinary systems.

The epithelium of the female urethra is derived from endoderm of the vesicourethral canal. The urethral sphincter develops from a mesenchymal condensation around the urethra after the division of the cloaca in the 12- to 15-mm embryo. After the opening of the anal membrane at the 20- to 30-mm stage, the puborectalis muscle appears. At 15 weeks' gestation, striated muscle can be seen and a smooth muscle layer thickens at the level of the developing bladder neck, forming the inner part of the urethral musculature. Thus the urethral sphincter is composed of both central smooth muscle and peripheral striated muscle. The sphincter develops primarily in the anterior wall of the urethra in a horseshoe or omega shape.

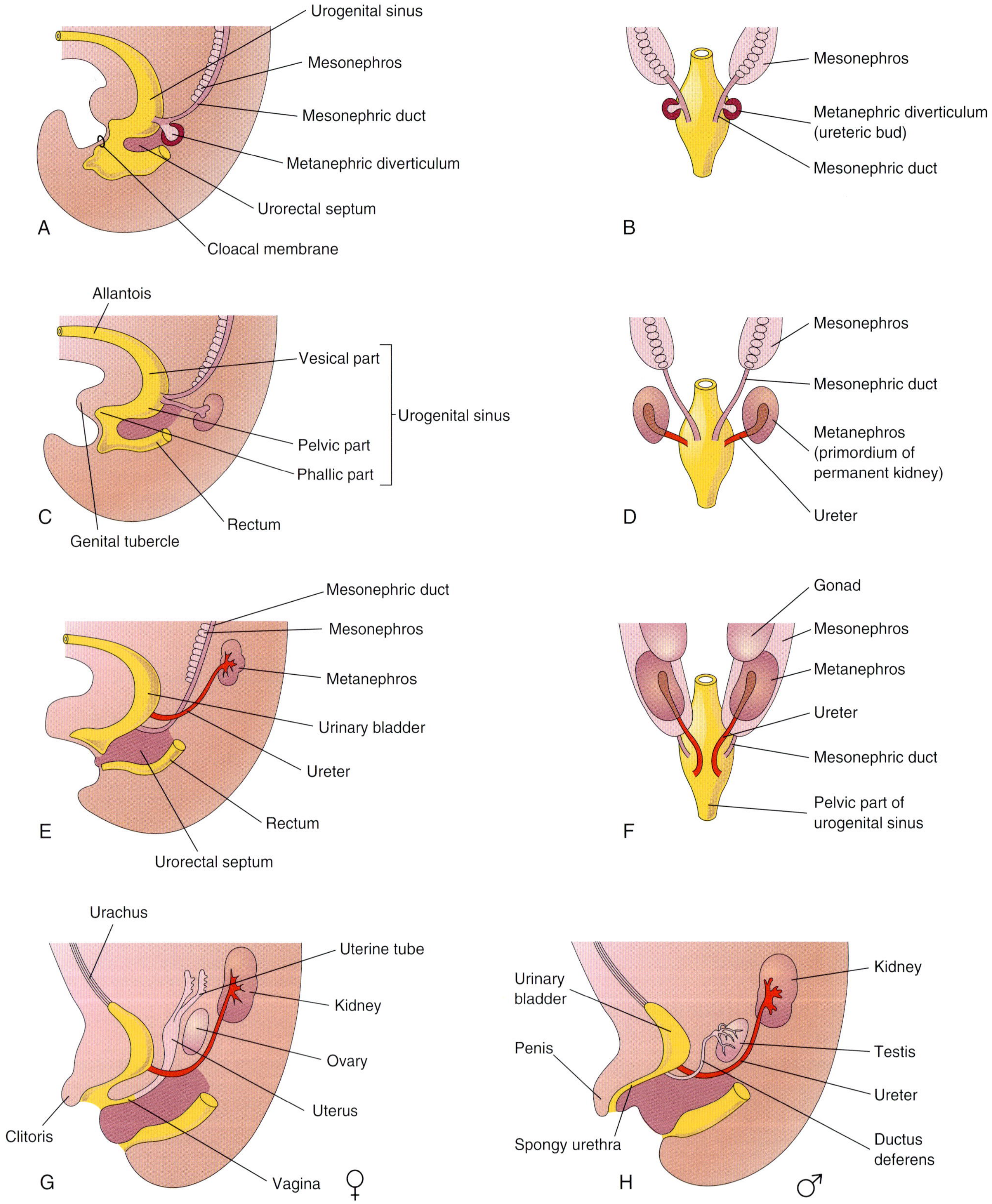


**Fig. 1.10** Diagrams showing division of the cloaca into the urogenital sinus and rectum; absorption of the mesonephric ducts; development of the urinary bladder, urethra, and urachus; and changes in the location of the ureters. **A**, Lateral view of the caudal half of a 5-week embryo. **B, D,** and **F,** Dorsal views. **C, E, G,** and **H,** Lateral views. The stages shown in **G** and **H** are reached by the twelfth week. (From Moore KL, Persaud TVN. *The Developing Human: Clinically Oriented Embryology.* 7th ed. Philadelphia: WB Saunders; 2003.)

## MOLECULAR BASIS OF SEX DIFFERENTIATION

Genetic sex is determined at the time of conception. A Y chromosome is necessary for the development of the testes, and the testes are responsible for the organization of the sexual duct system into a male configuration and for the suppression of the **paramesonephric (müllerian) system** of the female. In the absence of a Y chromosome or in the absence of a gonad, development will be female in nature. Male differentiation is determined by expression of the *SRY* gene found on the short arm of the Y chromosome. SRY protein is a transcription factor and expression is unique to the Sertoli cell of the developing testis. SRY induces expression of another transcription factor, SOX9, which is also obligatory for male sex differentiation. A loss of function mutation of either *SRY* or *SOX9* results in XY sex reversal in which genetic males are phenotypic females. Several genes regulate *SRY/SOX9* expression, including Wilms' tumor suppressor 1 (*WT1*) and steroidogenic factor 1 (*SF1*). *WT1* is a transcription factor expressed in both urinary tract and gonadal tissue. A loss of function mutation results in glomerulosclerosis and gonadal dysgenesis. *SF1* encodes a nuclear receptor necessary for steroidogenesis, gonadal differentiation and adrenal formation. A loss of function mutation is associated with adrenal failure and XY sex reversal (Ozisik, 2003).

Although ovarian formation can only occur in the absence of *SRY/SOX9*, there are unique genes necessary for development. *FOXL2* encodes a transcription factor necessary for granulosa cell expansion. A loss of function mutation causes ovarian failure with other associated abnormalities found in blepharophimosis-ptosis-epicanthus inversus syndrome (BPES) (De Baere, 2001). *BMP15*, located on the X chromosome, and *GDF9* on chromosome 5 encode growth factors expressed in oocytes required for granulosa cell proliferation. A heterozygous loss of function mutation results in ovarian failure (Di Pasquale, 2004).

The understanding of the molecular basis of sex determination continues to expand with more than 25 genes so far identified in the process (Wilhelm, 2007).

### Genital Development

Male gonadal development precedes female development (Fig. 1.11). During the fifth week after conception, coelomic epithelium, later known as *germinal epithelium*, thickens in the area of the medial aspect of the mesonephros. As germinal epithelial cells proliferate, they invade the underlying mesenchyme, producing a prominence known as the *gonadal ridge*. In the sixth week the primordial germ cells (PGCs), which have formed at about week 4 in the wall of the yolk sac, migrate up the dorsal mesentery of the hindgut and enter the undifferentiated gonad. The somatic cells of the primitive gonadal ridge then differentiate into interstitial cells (Leydig cells) and Sertoli cells. As they do the PGCs and Sertoli cells become enclosed within seminiferous tubules, and the interstitial cells remain outside these tubules. Sertoli cells are encased in the seminiferous tubules in the seventh and eighth weeks. In the eighth week Leydig cells differentiate and begin to produce testosterone. At this point the mesonephric (wolffian) duct differentiates into the vas deferens, epididymis, and seminal vesicles, whereas the paramesonephric duct (müllerian duct) is suppressed because of the secretion and action of antimüllerian hormone (AMH), also known as *müllerian inhibitory substance (MIS)*, by Sertoli cells.

Primary sex cords, meanwhile, have condensed and extended to the medullary portion of the developing testes. They branch and join to form the rete testis. The testes therefore is primarily a medullary organ, and eventually the rete testis connects with the tubules of the mesonephric system and joins the developing epididymal duct.

Development of the ovaries occurs at about the eleventh or twelfth week, although the PGCs have migrated several weeks

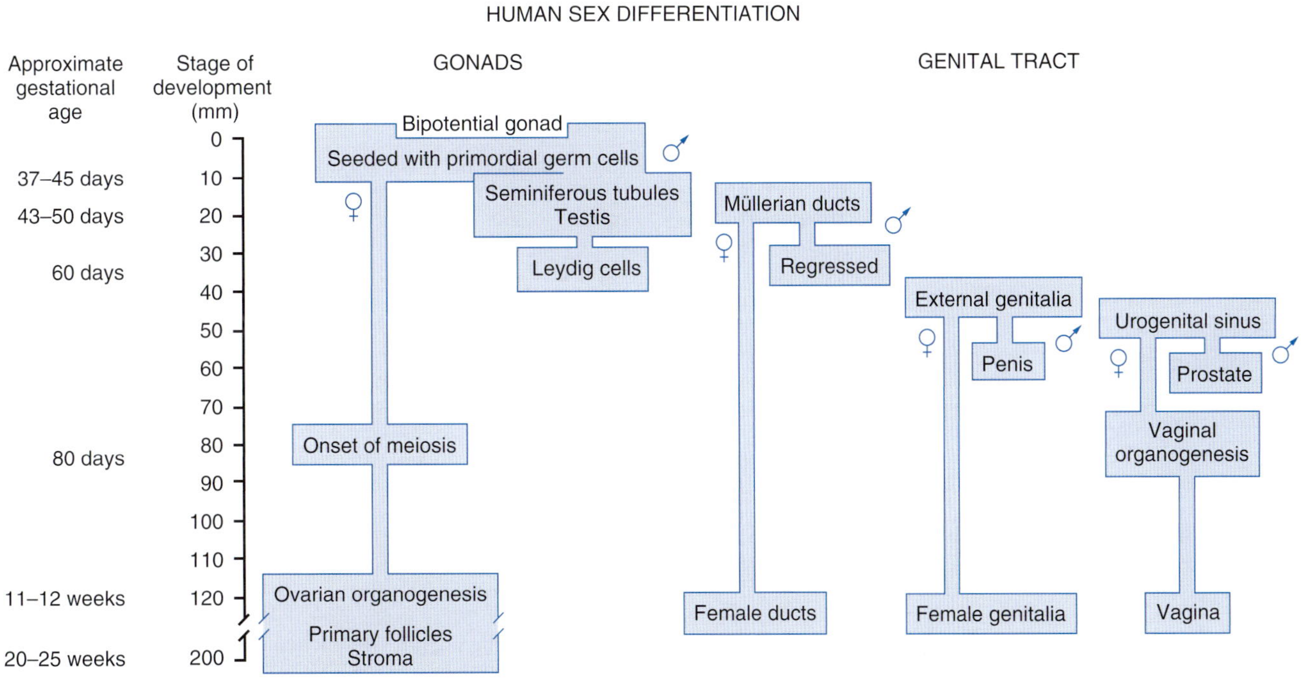


**Fig. 1.11** Development of sexual differentiation in the human. Note the lag from male to female development. (Modified from Grumbach MM, Hughes IA, Conte FA. Disorders of sex differentiation. In Larsen PR, Kronenberg HM, Melmed S, Polonsky KS, eds. *Williams Textbook of Endocrinology.* 10th ed. Philadelphia: WB Saunders; 2003:870.)

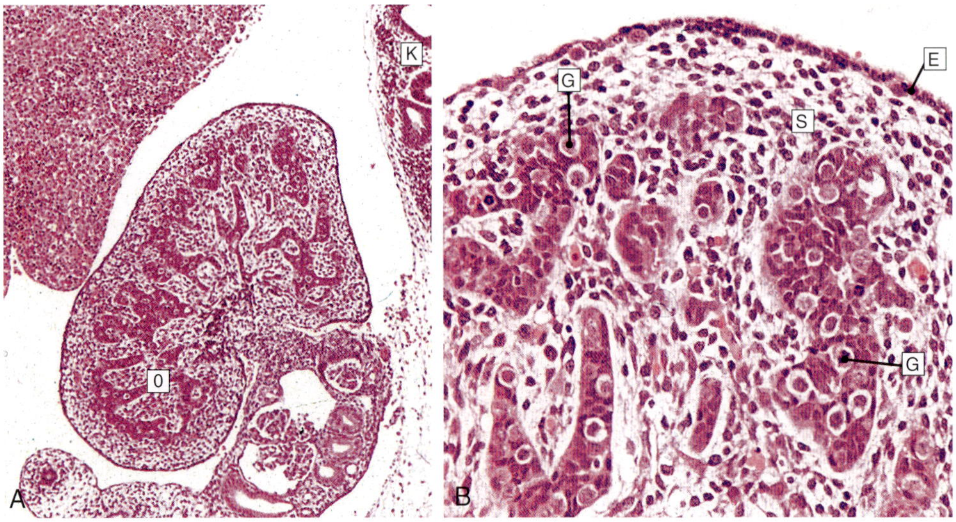


**Fig. 1.12** Ovary in embryo. **A**, A developing ovary (*O*) in a 9-week-old embryo is shown close to the developing kidney (*K*). **B,** At this stage of development, the columns of primordial germ cells (*G*) are embedded in a mesenchymal stroma (*S*) covered by a layer of cuboidal surface cells (*E*). (From Stevens A, Lowe J. *Human Histology.* 3rd ed. Philadelphia: Elsevier Mosby; 2005:357.)

earlier to the germinal ridge (Fig. 1.12). Two functional X chromosomes are necessary for optimal development of the ovaries. Deletion of either the short arm or the long arm of a single X chromosome precludes normal ovarian function, with the former being associated with Turner syndrome. The processes of gonadal development are schematically summarized in Fig. 1.13.

## Genital Duct System

Early in embryonic life, two sets of paired genital ducts develop in each sex: the mesonephric (wolffian) ducts and the paramesonephric (müllerian) ducts. The mesonephric duct development precedes the paramesonephric duct development. The paramesonephric ducts develop on each side of the mesonephric ducts from the evaginations of the coelomic epithelium. The more cephalad ends of the ducts open directly into the peritoneal cavity, and the distal ends grow caudally, fusing in the lower midline to form the uterovaginal **primordium**. This tubular structure joins the dorsal wall of the urogenital sinus and produces an elevation, the müllerian tubercle. The mesonephric ducts enter the urogenital sinus on either side of the tubercle.

### Male Genital Ducts

Seminiferous tubules are produced in the fetal testes during the seventh and eighth weeks after conception. During the eighth week, interstitial (Leydig) cells differentiate and begin to produce testosterone. Male internal genital development is mainly dependent on testosterone, whereas external genitalia development is dependent on 5α-dihydrotestosterone (DHT). Testosterone produced by the Leydig cells stimulates growth and development of the wolffian duct structures of the vas deferens, epididymis, and seminal vesicles. DHT formed in target tissues by the enzyme type 2 5α-reductase is responsible for formation of the prostate, scrotum, and penis.

Maternal hCG production may be key to male genital development. The maximum serum level of hCG at approximately 8 weeks after conception or 10 menstrual weeks correlates with the timing of male genital formation, and the highest fetal testosterone levels are seen at 11 to 17 weeks with a subsequent decline. hCG acting via the LH receptor is responsible for stimulating Leydig cell testosterone production.

The bulbourethral glands, which are small structures that develop from outgrowths of endodermal tissue from the membranous portion of the urethra, incorporate stroma from the adjacent mesenchyme. The most distal portion of the paramesonephric duct remains, in the male, as the appendix of the testes. The most proximal end of the paramesonephric duct remains as a small outpouching within the body of the prostate gland, known as the *prostatic utricle.* Rarely, the prostatic utricle is developed to the point where it will excrete a small amount of blood and cause hematuria in adult life (Schuhrke, 1978).

### Female Genital Ducts

In the absence of AMH, the mesonephric ducts regress and the paramesonephric ducts develop into the female genital tract. This process begins at about 6 weeks and proceeds in a cephalad to caudal fashion. The more cephalad portions of the paramesonephric ducts, which open directly into the peritoneal cavity, form the fallopian tubes. The fused portion, or uterovaginal primordium, gives rise to the epithelium and glands of the uterus and cervix. Endometrial stroma and myometrium are derived from adjacent mesenchyme. Failure of development of the paramesonephric ducts leads to agenesis of the cervix and the uterus, referred to as *müllerian agenesis* or *Mayer-Rokitansky-Kuster-Hauser syndrome* (Langman, 1982). Failure of fusion of the caudal portion of these ducts may lead to a variety of uterine anomalies, including complete duplication of the uterus and cervix or partial duplication of a variety of types, which are outlined in Chapter 11 (Congenital Anomalies of the Female Reproductive Tract). Peritoneal reflections in the area adjacent to the fusion of the two paramesonephric ducts give rise to the formation of the broad ligaments. Mesenchymal tissue here develops into the parametrium.

Development of the uterine ligaments includes the round ligament at the eighth week, the cardinal ligaments at the tenth week, and the broad ligament at week 19. The round ligament (ligament teres) is analogous to the male gubernaculum. It extends from the uterine body through the broad ligament and

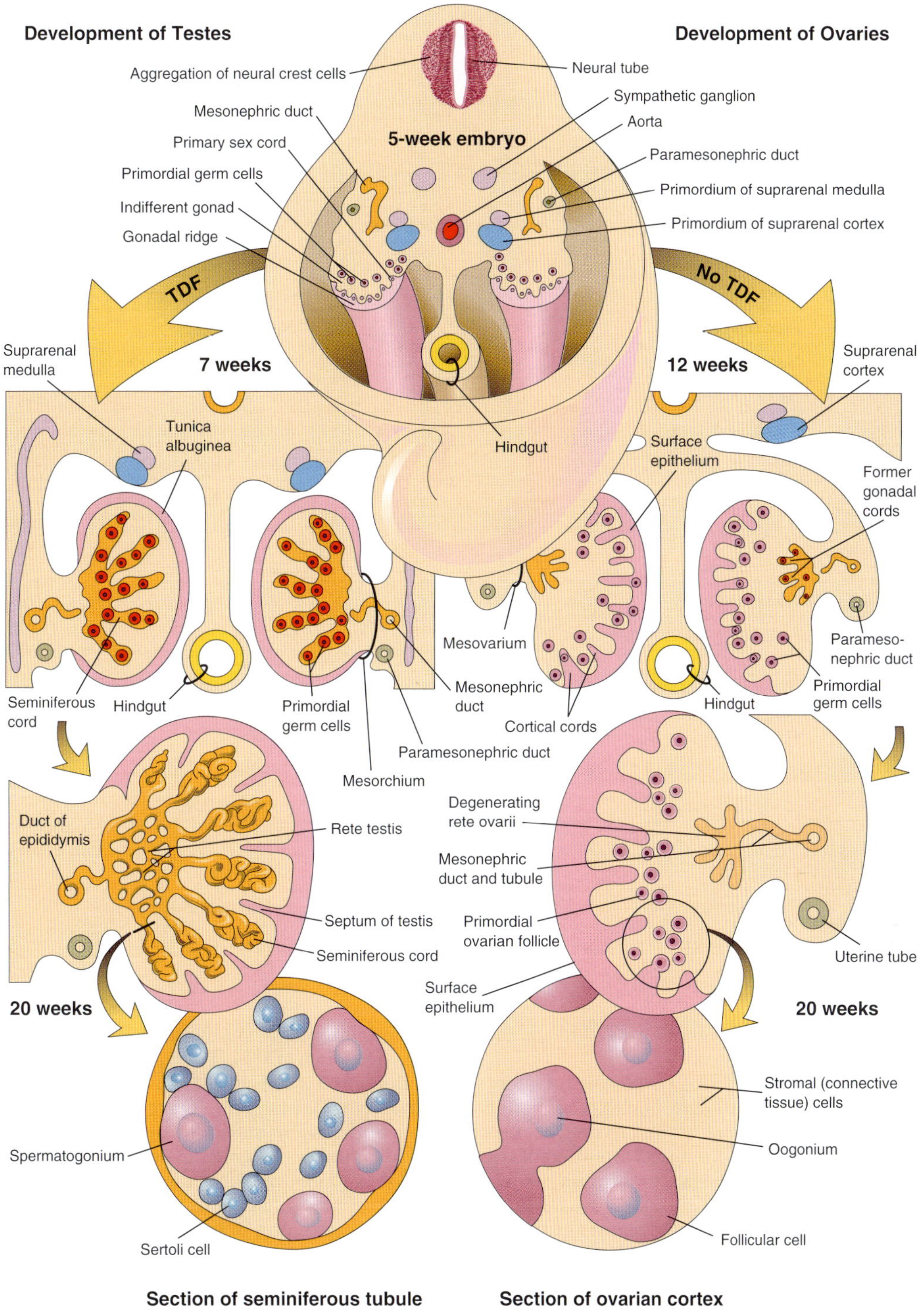


**Fig. 1.13** Schematic illustration showing differentiation of the indifferent gonads of a 5-week embryo *(top)* into ovaries or testes. Left side shows the development of testes resulting from the effects of the testis-determining factor (TDF), also called the *SRY* gene, located on the Y chromosome. Note that the gonadal cords become seminiferous cords, the primordium of the seminiferous tubules. The parts of the gonadal cords that enter the medulla of the testis form the rete testis. In the section of the testis at the bottom left, observe that there are two kinds of cells: spermatogonia derived from the primordial germ cells and sustentacular (Sertoli) cells derived from mesenchyme. Right side shows the development of ovaries in the absence of TDF. Cortical cords have extended from the surface epithelium of the gonad, and primordial cells have entered them. They are the primordia of the oogonia. Follicular cells are derived from the surface epithelium of the ovaries. (From Moore KL, Persaud TVN. *The Developing Human: Clinically Oriented Embryology.* 7th ed. Philadelphia: WB Saunders; 2003.)

**TABLE 1.2** Male and Female Derivatives of Embryonic Urogenital Structures

| | Derivatives | |
|---|---|---|
| **Embryonic Structure** | **Male** | **Female** |
| Labioscrotal swellings | Scrotum | Labia majora |
| Urogenital folds | Ventral portion of penis | Labia minora |
| Phallus | Penis | Clitoris |
| | Glans, corpora cavernosa penis, and corpus spongiosum | Glans, corpora cavernosa, bulb of the vestibule |
| Urogenital sinus | Urinary bladder | Urinary bladder |
| | Prostate gland | Urethral and paraurethral glands |
| | Prostatic utricle | Vagina |
| | Bulbourethral glands | Greater vestibular glands |
| | Seminal colliculus | Hymen |
| Paramesonephric duct | Appendix of testes | Hydatid of Morgagni |
| | | Uterus and cervix |
| | | Fallopian tubes |
| Mesonephric duct | Appendix of epididymis | Appendix vesiculosa |
| | Ductus of epididymis | Duct of epoophoron |
| | Ductus deferens | Gartner duct |
| | Ejaculatory duct and seminal vesicle | — |
| Metanephric duct | Ureters, renal pelvis, calyces, and collecting system | Ureters, renal pelvis, calyces, and collecting system |
| Mesonephric tubules | Ductuli efferentes | Epoophoron |
| | Paradidymis | Paroöphoron |
| Undifferentiated gonad | Testis | Ovaries |
| Cortex | Seminiferous tubules | Ovarian follicles |
| Medulla | — | Medulla |
| | Rete testis | Rete ovarii |
| Gubernaculum | Gubernaculum testis | Round ligament of uterus |

peritoneum exists the pelvis via the internal ring through the inguinal canal ending in the labia majora.

The vagina develops from paired solid outgrowths of endoderm of the urogenital sinus—the sinovaginal bulbs. These grow caudally as a solid core toward the end of the uterovaginal primordium. This core constitutes the fibromuscular portion of the vagina. The sinovaginal bulbs then canalize to form the vagina. Abnormalities in this process may lead to either transverse or horizontal vaginal septa. The junction of the sinovaginal bulbs with the urogenital sinus remains as the vaginal plate, which forms the hymen. This remains imperforate until late in embryonic life, although occasionally perforation does not take place completely (imperforate hymen). Failure of the sinovaginal bulbs to form leads to agenesis of the vagina. Auxiliary genital glands in the female form from buds that grow out of the urethra. The buds derive contributions from the surrounding mesenchyme and form the urethral glands and the paraurethral glands (Skene glands). These glands correspond to the prostate gland in males. Similar outgrowths of the urogenital sinus form the vestibular glands (Bartholin glands), which are homologous to the bulbourethral glands in the male. The remnants of the mesonephric duct in the female include a small structure called the *appendix vesiculosa*, a few blind tubules in the broad ligaments (the epoophoron), and a few blind tubules adjacent to the uterus (collectively called the *paroöphoron*). Remnants of the mesonephric duct system are often present in the broad ligaments or may be present adjacent to the uterus or the vagina as **Gartner duct** cysts (Deppisch, 1975). The epoophoron or paroöphoron may develop into cysts. Cysts of the epoophoron are known as *paraovarian cysts* (Chapter 18, Benign Gynecologic Lesions). Remnants of the paramesonephric duct in the female may be seen as a small, blind cystic structure attached by a pedicle to the distal end of the fallopian tube: the hydatid of Morgagni. Table 1.2 categorizes the adult derivatives and residual remnants of the urogenital structures in both the male and the female. Fig. 1.14 outlines schematically the development of the internal sexual organs in both sexes.

## External Genitalia

In the fourth week after fertilization, the genital tubercle develops at the ventral tip of the cloacal membrane. Two sets of lateral bodies, the labioscrotal swellings and urogenital folds, develop soon after on either side of the cloacal membrane. The genital tubercle then elongates to form a phallus in both males and females. By the end of the sixth week, the cloacal membrane is joined by the urorectal septum. The septum separates the cloaca into the urogenital sinus ventrally and the anal canal and rectum dorsally. The point on the cloacal membrane where the urorectal septum fuses becomes the location of the perineal body in later development. The cloacal membrane is then divided into the ventral urogenital membrane and the dorsal anal membrane.

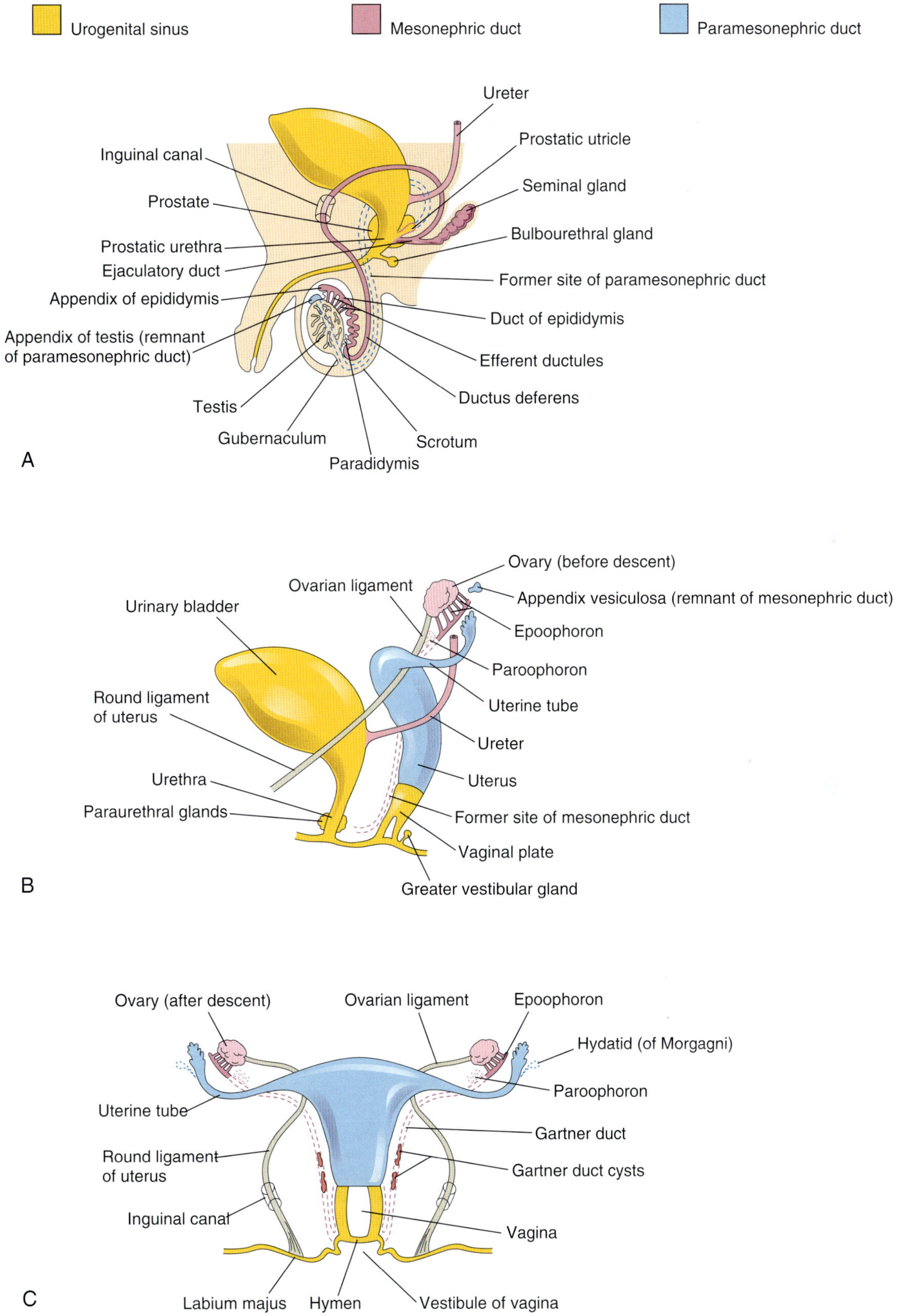


**Fig. 1.14** Schematic drawings illustrating development of the male and female reproductive systems from the genital ducts and urogenital sinus. Vestigial structures are also shown. **A,** Reproductive system in a newborn male. **B,** Female reproductive system in a 12-week fetus. **C,** Reproductive system in a newborn female. (From Moore KL, Persaud TVN. *The Developing Human: Clinically Oriented Embryology.* 7th ed. Philadelphia: WB Saunders; 2003.)

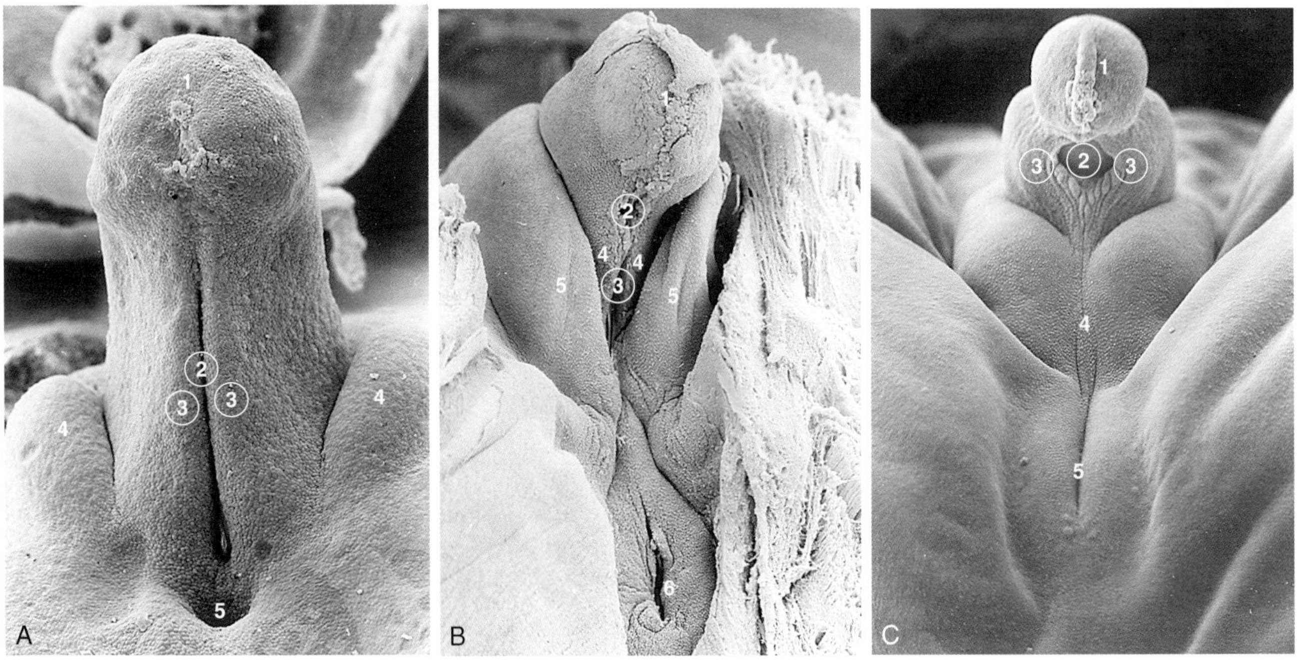


**Fig. 1.15** Scanning electron micrographs (SEMs) of the developing male external genitalia. **A,** SEM of the perineum during the indifferent state of a 17-mm, 7-week embryo (×100). *1,* Developing glans of penis with the ectodermal cord. *2,* Urethral groove continuous with the urogenital sinus. *3,* Urogenital folds. *4,* Labioscrotal swellings. *5,* Anus. **B,** External genitalia of a 7.2-cm, 10-week female fetus (×45). *1,* Glans of clitoris. *2,* External urethral orifice. *3,* Opening into urogenital sinus. *4,* Urogenital folds (labia minora). *5,* Labioscrotal swelling (labia majora). *6,* Anus. **C,** SEM of the external genitalia of a 5.5-cm, 10-week male fetus (×40). *1,* Glans of penis with ectodermal cord. *2,* Remains of urethral groove. 3, Urogenital folds in the process of closing. *4,* Labioscrotal swelling fusing to form the raphe of the scrotum. *5,* Anus. (From Moore KL, Persaud TVN. *The Developing Human: Clinically Oriented Embryology.* 7th ed. Philadelphia: WB Saunders; 2003.)

These membranes then open, yielding the vulva and the anal canal. Failure of the anal membrane to open gives rise to an imperforate anus. With the opening of the urogenital membrane, a urethral groove forms on the undersurface of the phallus, completing the undifferentiated portion of external genital development. Differences between male and female embryos can be noted as early as the ninth week, but the distinct final forms are not noted until 12 weeks' gestation (Fig. 1.15).

The phallus grows in length to form a penis, and the urogenital folds are pulled forward to form the lateral walls of the urethral groove on the undersurface of the penis. These folds then fuse to form the penile urethra. Defects in fusion of various amounts give rise to various degrees of hypospadias. The skin at the distal margin of the penis grows over the glans to form the prepuce (foreskin). The vascular portion of the penis (corpora cavernosa penis and corpus cavernosum urethrae) arises from the mesenchymal tissue of the phallus. Finally, the labioscrotal swellings grow toward each other and fuse in the midline to form the scrotum. Later in embryonic life, usually at about the twenty-eighth week, the testes descend through the inguinal canal guided by the gubernaculum (Frey, 1984).

Feminization of the undifferentiated external genitalia occurs in the absence of androgen stimulation. The embryonic phallus does not demonstrate rapid growth and becomes the clitoris. Urogenital folds do not fuse except in front of the anus. The unfused urogenital folds form the labia minora. The labioscrotal folds fuse posteriorly in the area of the perineal body but laterally remain as the labia majora. Beyond 12 weeks' gestation, the labioscrotal folds will not fuse if the fetus is exposed to androgens, though masculinization may occur in other organs of the external genitalia such as growth of the clitoris. The labioscrotal folds fuse anteriorly to form the mons pubis. A portion of the urogenital sinus between the level of the hymen and the labia develops into the vestibule of the vagina, into which the urethra, the vagina, and the ducts of Bartholin glands enter. Female external genitalia are intensely estrogen receptor positive compared with the genitalia of the male. These receptors may be seen primarily in the stroma of the labia minora and in the periphery of the glans and interprepuce (Kalloo, 1993). The presence of such receptors suggests that there may be a direct role of maternal estrogens in the development of female external genitalia. Virilization (masculinization) of a female (karyotype XX) fetus may occur from exposure to androgens, either from the mother or through fetal androgens as a result of genetic deficiencies in the steroid biosynthetic pathway such as occurs in congenital adrenal hyperplasia.

The ovaries do not descend into the labioscrotal folds. A structure similar to the gubernaculum develops in the inguinal canal, giving rise to the round ligaments, which suspend the uterus in the adult. Fig. 1.16 summarizes the development of the external genitalia in each sex.

## Acknowledgments

The authors wish to acknowledge previous authors and contributors who laid the foundation for this chapter. With each edition, the chapter has been revised and expanded to include new information gained from expanding scientific capabilities and applications of new discoveries to patient care.

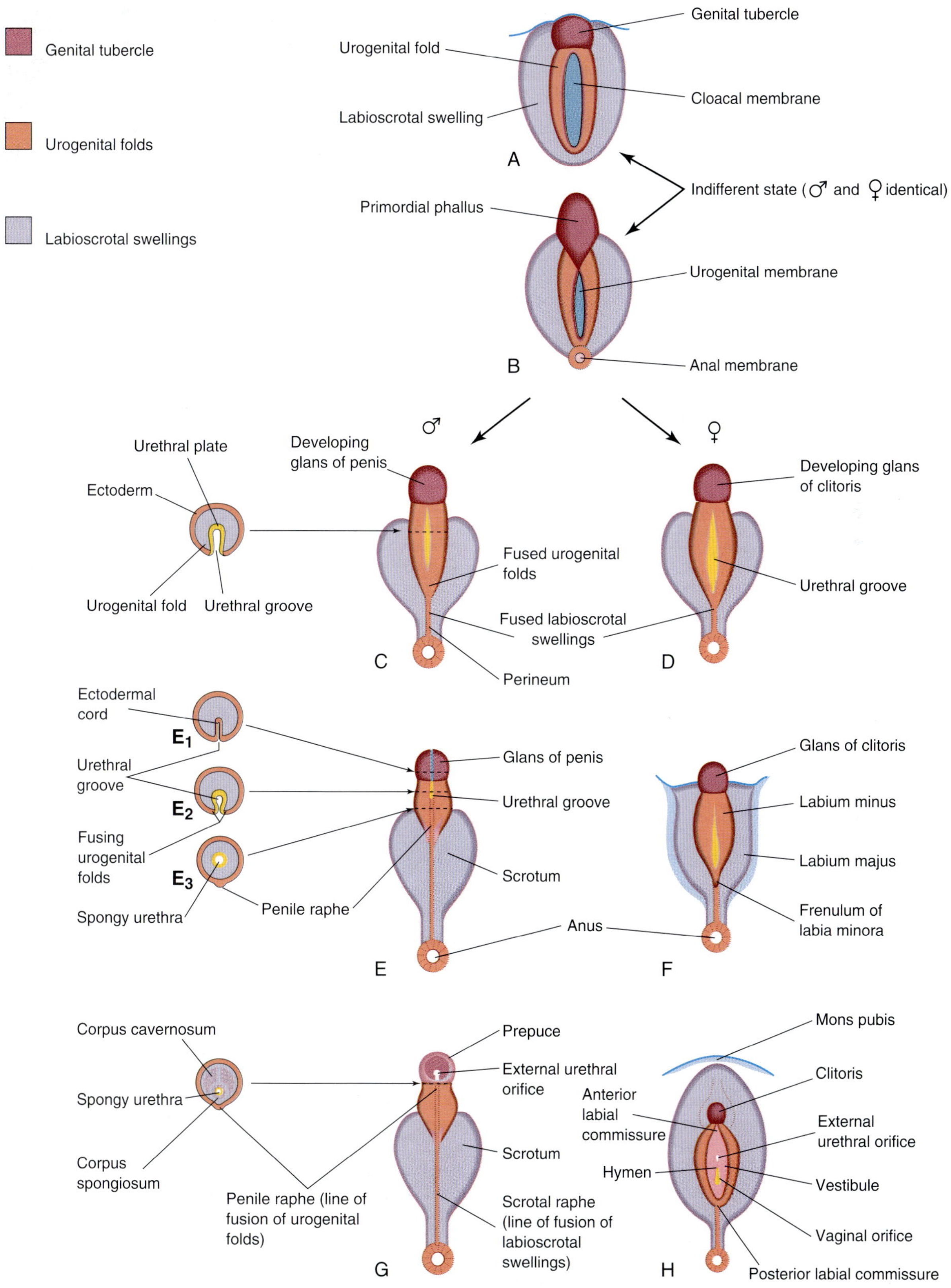


**Fig. 1.16** Development of the external genitalia. **A** and **B,** Diagrams illustrating the appearance of the genitalia during the indifferent state (fourth to seventh weeks). **C, E,** and **G,** Stages in the development of male external genitalia at 9, 11, and 12 weeks, respectively. To the left are schematic transverse sections of the developing penis, illustrating formation of the spongy urethra. **D, F,** and **H**, Stages in the development of female genitalia at 9, 11, and 12 weeks, respectively. (From Moore KL, Persaud TVN: *The Developing Human: Clinically Oriented Embryology.* 7th ed. Philadelphia: WB Saunders; 2003.)

## REFERENCES


Arias-Stella J. The Arias-Stella reaction: facts and fancies four decades after. *Adv Anat Pathol.* 2002;9(1):12–23.

Baerwald AR, Adams GP, Pierson RA. Ovarian antral folliculogenesis during the human menstrual cycle: a review. *Hum Reprod Update.* 2012;18(1):73–91.

Bontekoe S, Mantikou E, van Wely M, Seshadri S, Repping S, Mastenbroek S. Low oxygen concentrations for embryo culture in assisted reproductive technologies. *Cochrane Database Syst Rev.* 2012;11(7):CD008950.

Childs AJ, Cowan G, Kinnell HL, Anderson RA, Saunders PTK. Retinoic acid signalling and the control of meiotic entry in the human fetal gonad. *PLoS One.* 2011;6(6):e20249.

Clark E. Mechanisms in the pathogenesis of congenital cardiac malformations. In: Pierpont M, Moller J, eds. *The Genetics of Cardiovascular Disease.* New York: Springer; 1987:3–11.

Darasse-Jèze G, Klatzmann D, Charlotte F, Salomon BL, Cohen JL. CD4+CD25+ regulatory/suppressor T cells prevent allogeneic fetus rejection in mice. *Immunol Lett.* 2006;102(1):106–109.

De Baere E, Dixon MJ, Small KW, et al. Spectrum of FOXL2 gene mutations in blepharophimosis-ptosis-epicanthus inversus (BPES) families demonstrates a genotype–phenotype correlation. *Hum Mol Genet.* 2001;10(15):1591–1600.

Deppisch LM. Cysts of the vagina: classification and clinical correlations. *Obstet Gynecol.* 1975;45(6):632–637.

Di Pasquale E, Beck-Peccoz P, Persani L. Hypergonadotropic ovarian failure associated with an inherited mutation of human Bone Morphogenetic Protein-15 (BMP15) Gene. *Am J Hum Genet.* 2004;75(1):106–111.

Eisenbach M, Tur-Kaspa I. Do human eggs attract spermatozoa? *Bioessays.* 1999;21:203–210.

Fournier T, Guibourdenche J, Evain-Brion D. Review: hCGs: different sources of production, different glycoforms and functions. *Placenta.* 2015;36(Suppl 1):S60–S65.

Frey H, Rajfer J. Role of the gubernaculum and intraabdominal pressure in the process of testicular descent. *J Urol.* 1984;131(3):574–579.

Kabir-Salmani M, Nikzad H, Shiokawa S, Akimoto Y, Iwashita M. Secretory role for human uterodomes (pinopods): secretion of LIF. *Mol Hum Reprod.* 2005;11(8):553–559.

Kalloo NB, Gearhart JP, Barrack ER. Sexually dimorphic expression of estrogen receptors, but not of androgen receptors in human fetal external genitalia. *J Clin Endocrinol Metab.* 1993;77(3):692–698.

Langman J, Wilson D. Embryology and congenital malformations of the female genital tract. In: Blaustein A, ed. *Pathology of the Female Genital Tract.* New York: Springer; 1982:1–12.

Lim HJ, Dey SK. HB-EGF: A unique mediator of embryo-uterine interactions during implantation. *Exp Cell Res.* 2009;315(4):619–626.

Little M, Georgas K, Pennisi D, Wilkinson L. Chapter Five - Kidney development: two tales of tubulogenesis. In: Peter K, ed. *Current Topics in Developmental Biology.* Vol 90. Academic Press; 2010:193–229.

Meseguer M, Herrero J, Tejera A, Hilligsøe KM, Ramsing NB, Remohí J. The use of morphokinetics as a predictor of embryo implantation. *Hum Reprod.* 2011;26(10):2658–2671.

Ozisik G, Achermann JC, Meeks JJ, Jameson JL. SF1 in the development of the adrenal gland and gonads. *Horm Res Paediatr.* 2003;59(Suppl 1):94–98.

Ramathal CY, Bagchi IC, Taylor RN, Bagchi MK. Endometrial decidualization: Of mice and men. *Semin Reprod Med.* 2010;28(1):17–26.

Salha O, Sharma V, Dada T, et al. The influence of donated gametes on the incidence of hypertensive disorders of pregnancy. *Hum Reprod.* 1999;14(9):2268–2273.

Schatten H, Sun Q. The identity of zona pellucida receptor on spermatozoa: an unresolved issue in developmental biology. *Mol Hum Reprod.* 2009;15(9):531–538.

Schuhrke T, Kaplan G. Prostatic utricle cysts (mullerian duct cysts). *J Urol.* 1978;119(6):765–767.

Underwood MA, Gilbert WM, Sherman MP. Amniotic fluid: not just fetal urine anymore. *J Perinatol.* 2005;25(5):341–348.

Wallace WH, Kelsey TW. Human ovarian reserve from conception to the menopause. *PLoS One.* 2010;5(1):e8772.

Wang S, Hassold T, Hunt P, et al. Inefficient crossover maturation underlies elevated aneuploidy in human female meiosis. *Cell.* 2017;168(6):977–989.e917.

Wilhelm D, Palmer S, Koopman P. Sex determination and gonadal development in mammals. *Physiol Rev.* 2007;87:1–28.

Williams M, Hill CJ, Scudamore I, Dunphy B, Cooke ID, Barratt CLR. Physiology: sperm numbers and distribution within the human Fallopian tube around ovulation. *Hum Reprod.* 1993;8(12):2019–2026.

Zegers-Hochschild F, Altieri E, Fabres C, Fernandez E, Mackenna A, Orihuela P. Predictive value of human chorionic gonadotropin in the outcome of early pregnancy after in-vitro fertilization and spontaneous conception. *Hum Reprod.* 1994;9(8):1550–1555.

# 2 Reproductive Genetics

Jennifer Bushman Gilner, Eleanor H. J. Rhee, Amanda Padro, Jeffrey A. Kuller

## KEY POINTS

- Virtually all human diseases have an underlying genetic component. All health care professionals need a basic level of familiarity with genetics and genomics because it is an integral part of mainstream medicine.
- Genetic variation between healthy individuals exists in the form of single nucleotide polymorphisms (SNPs) and copy number variants (CNVs) providing different "doses" of a large repeated DNA sequence at a given genetic locus or of alterations in three-dimensional DNA structures called *epigenetic modification.*
- Naturally occurring variations in genetic sequence, such as SNPs, may mediate an individual's susceptibility to disease or responsiveness to a particular medication.
- The human genome contains about 3 billion base pairs, of which only about 1.5% makes up the exome, or protein-coding portion. The remaining 98.5% of the human genetic sequence encodes biologically active nucleic acid molecules, which are an active area of molecular biology research.
- Genetic pathology can arise from alteration in the sequence of a gene, changes in the normal amount of a gene product, or sequence changes in regulatory regions that prevent the cell from expressing the intended gene product. The old term *mutation* has been replaced by *variant,* which is further classified as benign, likely benign, of unknown significance, likely pathogenic, or pathogenic.
- When a heterozygous individual who has an autosomal dominant trait mates with a normal individual, 50% of their offspring will have the trait.
- When two individuals who carry an autosomal recessive trait mate, 25% of their offspring will have the trait and 50% will be carriers.
- X-linked recessive characteristics are transmitted from maternal carriers to male offspring and will affect 50% of the male offspring.
- The mechanism of trinucleotide repeat disorders is DNA misalignment during meiosis, which leads to unstable dynamic expansion of the number of three-nucleotide repeats within the gene as it is passed from generation to generation, causing progressively more severe manifestations of disease.
- Prader-Willi and Angelman syndromes demonstrate the concept that certain regions of genetic material are imprinted and depend on dose and inheritance from two separate gametes for normal function.
- The phenotype and severity of disorders that affect the mitochondria are determined by the source of the genetic material (nuclear or mitochondrial DNA), the proportion of affected mitochondria inherited by the cell, and the threshold for energy production needed in the affected cell.
- In general, if a couple produces an offspring with a multifactorial defect and the problem has never occurred in the family, it can be expected to be repeated in 2% to 5% of subsequent pregnancies.
- Individuals who carry balanced rearrangements of genetic material are phenotypically normal, but their gametes are at risk for unbalanced genetic content, which may lead to infertility or recurrent pregnancy loss.
- Nondisjunctional events have been described in every autosome except chromosomes 1 and 17. Live births can result from nondisjunctional events involving chromosomes 21, 18, 13, or 22, and these occur more commonly with advancing maternal age.
- Screening and diagnostic tests are available for prenatal diagnosis of a large number of genetic diseases and syndromes. Indications for testing may include family history of a specific disease or recurrent clinical phenotype, ethnic background with increased carrier frequency of a certain disease, poor obstetric outcome history, increased maternal age, or population-based prevalence risk.
- In genetic counseling the role of the care providers (genetic counselors and physicians) is to conduct nondirectional counseling of screening and diagnostic options to provide prospective parents with information to optimize pregnancy outcomes based on their personal values and preferences. Before screening or testing, the patient needs to understand the options that may result from a positive test result.
- If an individual proceeds with carrier screening and is found to be a carrier of an autosomal recessive genetic condition, screening should be offered to his or her reproductive partner to assess the risk of disease in any of their children. Screening should also be offered to family members of the known carrier, who may also be an increased risk of carrying the same variant.
- Current recommendations state that all women who are considering pregnancy or are currently pregnant should be offered carrier screening for cystic fibrosis and spinal muscular atrophy, regardless of family history or reported ethnic background.
- Genetic screening based on cell-free DNA may be pursued by any patient regardless of risk.
- Definitive diagnosis of a genetic disease in the prenatal period requires tissue diagnosis obtained through invasive testing methods such as preimplantation genetic diagnosis, chorionic villus sampling, or amniocentesis.
- Aneuploidy screening and confirmatory prenatal diagnostic testing should still be offered to all women with pregnancies achieved via in vitro fertilization with preimplantation genetic testing because testing does not eliminate risk of genetic disorders and is not 100% accurate.
- With next-generation sequencing, it is possible to determine the complete sequence data for an individual exome (protein-coding region) or genome (complete genetic material). However, accurate interpretation of these data is limited by unknown functions of natural genetic variation and noncoding DNA regions, which make up the majority of the sequence.
- All cancer is genetic. However, most cancer is not inherited. For a normal cell line to be transformed into a malignant cell line, several genetic pathogenic variants in that somatic cell line must occur that alter cell growth and differentiation.
- In 5% to 10% of families with a history of cancer, a germline (inherited) pathogenic variant is present that predisposes certain tissues to become malignant.
- Types of genes and genetic mechanisms involved in malignancy may be grouped into four categories: oncogenes, tumor suppressor genes, DNA repair genes, and epigenetic mechanisms of aberrant DNA packaging.
- Oncogenes (gain of function) behave as growth-promoting genes, and they act in a genetically dominant manner. In other words,

*Continued*

KEY POINTS—cont'd

only one abnormal copy of the gene is needed to produce a clinically relevant phenotype because of increased gene function.
- Tumor suppressor genes restrain cell growth in damaged cells; therefore loss of the tumor suppressor gene through introduction of a pathogenic variant leads to increased cell proliferation of abnormal cells and thus to cancer development. They account for the majority of autosomal dominant cancer syndromes.
- DNA repair genes identify and mend DNA replication errors made during replication. When they are nonfunctional, replication errors can lead to cancer development.
- Epigenetic mechanisms involve alterations in patterns of DNA methylation or DNA packaging (3D structure determined by histone interaction and nucleosome positioning).
- Lynch syndrome has a prevalence of 3% to 5% in all patients with newly diagnosed endometrial cancer.
- In patients with endometrial cancer, the actual tumor tissue can be screened for Lynch syndrome using immunohistochemical analysis for the four mismatch repair proteins (MLH1, MSH2, MSH6, and PMS2), microsatellite instability analysis, and MLH1 hypermethylation testing.

## GENETIC BASIS OF DISEASE

Medical research and medical care have been profoundly influenced by the advancement of science that resulted in sequencing the human genome, allowing scientists to concentrate on translating this genomic text to meaningful prose. As the code is deciphered with increasing resolution, it is apparent that **virtually all human diseases have an underlying genetic component, although the conversion from genotype to ultimate clinical phenotype is not always easily understood**.

The overarching goals of medical care have not changed: diagnose, treat, and focus on disease prevention. The new promise of medicine in the postgenomic era is to individualize these goals, such that lifestyle interventions, screening modalities, and pharmaceuticals ultimately can be tailored to each person based on his or her unique genomic sequence. These goals have begun to materialize through examples such as detailed breast cancer screening for women in families with known *BRCA1* or *BRCA2* variants and tailored chemotherapeutic regimens based on molecular testing of an individual tumor. Furthermore, there is unprecedented public accessibility to the genomic screening technology and application of genetic information to medical treatment. Since completion of the Human Genome Project in April 2003, technology has advanced at an extraordinary pace to allow *high-throughput* data generation at an increasingly reasonable cost. High-throughput methods involve automation of experiments or assays to allow for simultaneous large-scale repetition. Over the first postgenomic decade, the time to prepare and sequence a complete human genome plummeted from 13 years to a matter of 3 to 4 days, and the cost dropped from a bit less than $30 million to around $1000 (Topol, 2014).

As a result, genetics is a field with which all health care professionals, not just subspecialists, need a basic level of familiarity. **Genetics, genomics, and the technology to interpret the information are now integral parts of mainstream medicine** (Table 2.1). The obstetrician/gynecologist is often the first-line provider helping patients navigate this complicated landscape. This chapter focuses on developing a basic understanding of genetic makeup, heritability, and the most commonly used tools for detecting genetic disorders in patients and their offspring.

## BUILDING BLOCKS OF GENETICS

### Molecular Building Blocks

Genetic information is encoded in **deoxyribonucleic acid (DNA)** in the nucleus of each cell of the body. DNA molecules are made up of two complementary linear sequences of nucleotides intertwined together as a double helix. **The backbone of the linear DNA molecule is composed of a phosphate and a pentose sugar (deoxyribose) to which is attached a nitrogen base. Four such bases are found in a DNA molecule: two purines (adenine [A] and guanine [G]) and two pyrimidines (thymine [T] and cytosine [C])**. Purine and pyrimidine occur in equal amounts; A is always paired with T in the two strands of the double helix, and G is always paired with C. The order of bases along the molecule is the genetic **sequence**, and the complete sequence of all 6 billion bases in an individual cell nucleus (3 billion paired bases, arranged in linear antisense strands) makes up the **human genome**.

The Central Dogma published by Francis Crick in 1970 remains at the heart of molecular biology (Crick, 1970). The DNA is transcribed to a complementary **ribonucleic acid (RNA)** molecule (messenger RNA), which may be modified by regulatory sequences or three-dimensional (3D) structure. Three-base **codons** are read and translated to amino acids, which are linked to form a protein with some function within the cell or organism (Fig. 2.1). The traditional concept of a **gene** refers to a unit of DNA sequence that codes for production of a protein. Surprisingly, with completion of the Human Genome Project, this gene-centric view of biology turned out to be only the tip of the iceberg in understanding the complex manner in which the genetic sequence translates to human life. **Of the 3 billion base pairs that make up the genome, only about 1.5% of the assembled sequence codes for proteins.** This coding portion, or **exome** contains about 20,000 to 25,000 genes, which is only a fraction of previous estimates that were predicated based on gene numbers correlating with complexity of the species (Gerstein, 2007). There is now significant interest in the remaining 98.5% of the genome and how it carries out the blueprint of life. There is a growing field of discovery in the regulatory function of specialized noncoding RNA molecules, called **microRNA (miRNA)**, which appear to be the gatekeepers of many biologic processes (Pritchard, 2012).

### Mitosis/Meiosis

The full genome consists of two copies of the total DNA sequence, packaged into two homologous sets of 23 separate **chromosomes** (22 autosome pairs and 1 allosome, or sex chromosome pair). During cell division, an exact replica of this biologic blueprint is passed to each daughter cell through the process of mitosis. The formation of gametes requires even distribution of the chromosomes to the progeny through the process of meiosis, as described in Chapter 1. On fertilization, the zygote regains a full diploid complement of genetic material, equally derived from each parent. This process of replicating, packaging, and passing on genetic material from generation to generation forms the basis of heredity. Furthermore, errors in these processes can cause sequence changes or rearrangement of larger portions of DNA, introducing genetic variation or pathology, depending on the location of the change.

**TABLE 2.1** Publicly Available Online Resources for Human Genomic Information

| | | |
|---|---|---|
| **General Reference** | | |
| National Human Genome Research Institute (NHGRI) | | www.genome.gov |
| **Sequence Databases** | | |
| GenBank: Collection of all publicly available DNA sequences | National Institutes of Health (NIH) | www.ncbi.nlm.nih.gov/genbank |
| Genome Reference Consortium: Maintains responsibility for the human reference genome | Members: The Genome Center at Washington University, Wellcome Trust Sanger Institute, European Bioinformatics Institute (EBI), and National Center for Biotechnology Information (NCBI) | www.ncbi.nlm.nih.gov/grc |
| SNPedia: Wiki investigating human genetics | River Road Bio, LLC (Cariaso, 2012) | www.SNPedia.com |
| ISGR: The International Genome Sample Resource | EMBL-EBI and the Wellcome Trust: Maintain and build upon the *1000 genomes* reference data, the largest public catalogue of human variation and genotype data | www.1000genomes.org |
| ENCyclopedia Of DNA Elements (ENCODE) | International consortium to annotate functional elements in the genome (Davis, 2018) | www.encodeproject.org |
| Database of Genomic Structural Variation (dbVar) | NCBI database of human genomic structural variation | www.ncbi.nlm.nih.gov/dbvar |
| **Genotype/Phenotype Correlation** | | |
| Database of Genotypes and Phenotypes (dbGaP): Description and results of studies investigating interaction of genotype and phenotype | NCBI archive and distribution center | www.ncbi.nlm.nih.gov/gap/ |
| Online Mendelian Inheritance in Man (OMIM) | McKusick-Nathans Institute of Genetic Medicine, Johns Hopkins University School of Medicine (Amberger, 2015) | omim.org |
| Genome-Wide Association Study (GWAS) Central | (Beck, 2014) | www.gwascentral.org |
| **Genome Browsers** | | |
| Ensembl | Wellcome Trust, Sanger Institute, European Bioinformatics Institute | www.ensembl.org |
| University of California Santa Cruz (UCSC) Genome Bioinformatics | University of California at Santa Cruz | genome.ucsc.edu |
| NCBI | National Center for Biotechnology Information | www.ncbi.nlm.nih.gov/genome |

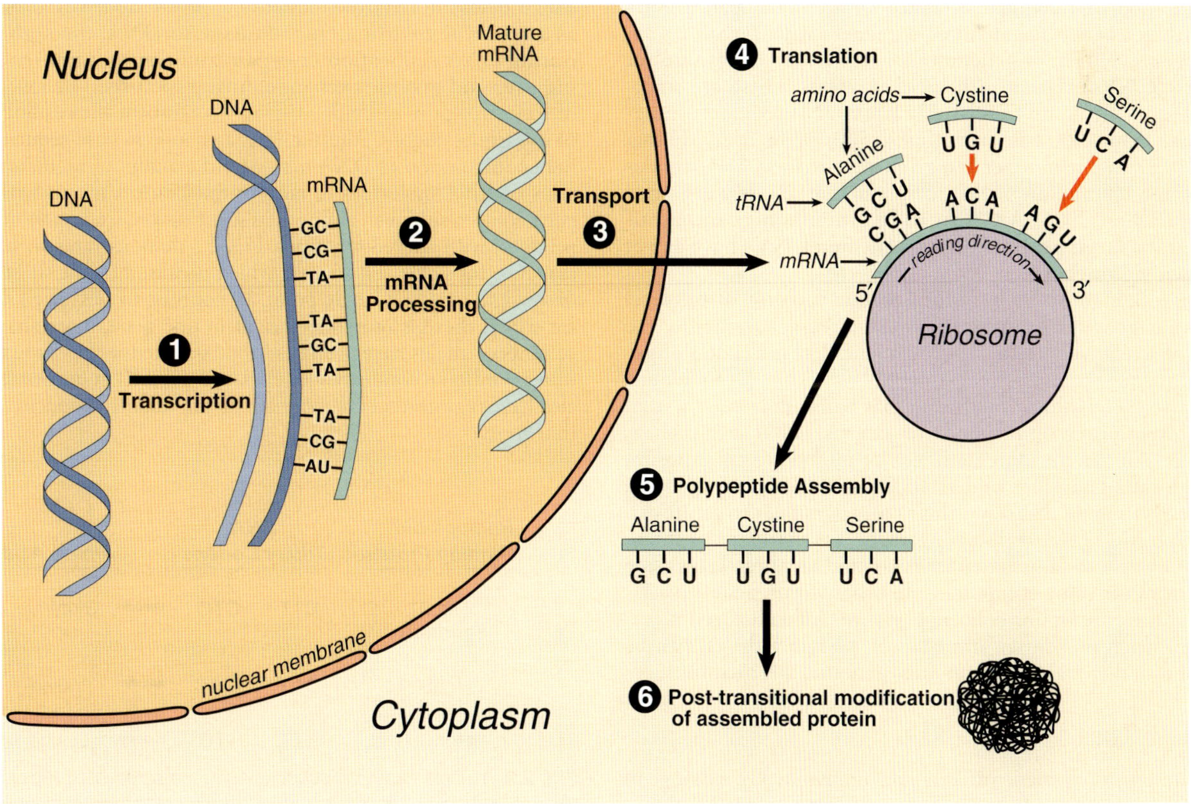


**Fig. 2.1** Schematic representation of polypeptide production from genetic message to final product. (Courtesy Edith Cheng, MD.)

## Genomic Variation

### Genetic Variation

On April 14, 2003, the Human Genome Project was declared complete, with successful sequencing of the full human genome. Initial interpretation of the sequence result claimed 99.9% similarity between healthy individuals at the DNA sequence level, leaving only 0.1% of the genome sequence to account for individual differences in phenotype (Lee, 2007). **Each alternative form of genetic code at any given locus is referred to as an allele.** An individual inherits two alleles of every genetic locus, one from each parent. If both inherited alleles have the same sequence, the individual is **homozygous** for the given locus. If the alleles are different, the individual is **heterozygous**. The allelic options at any given genetic locus derive from single nucleotide substitutions within the DNA sequence. Population sampling has demonstrated that among healthy individuals, the genetic sequence differs at around 10 million points (out of 3.2 billion DNA base pairs). These naturally occurring differences are called **single nucleotide polymorphisms**, or SNPs. To be classified as an SNP, two or more versions of nucleotide sequence must be present in at least 1% of the general population. **The term SNP is used to describe genetic variation of healthy individuals because no disease-causing nucleotide change is this common.** An example of an SNP known to mediate susceptibility to disease is the delta 32 allele of the beta-chemokine receptor 5, or CCR5. Individuals carrying one copy of the delta 32 allele are somewhat resistant to infection by human immunodeficiency virus (HIV), the virus that causes acquired immunodeficiency syndrome (AIDS), and individuals with two copies (delta 32 homozygotes, ~1% of the white population) are almost completely immune to infection by HIV (Huang, 1996). Thus the genetic variant is not the cause of disease (HIV) but is importantly associated with the manifestation of disease in humans.

In addition to individual sequence variation, comparative genome studies between individual sequences have revealed a far more pervasive form of genetic variation, termed **copy number variants (CNVs)** (Iafrate, 2004; Sebat, 2004). These are structural variants, made up of relatively large DNA segments (ranging in size from 1000 base pairs [bp] to 500,000 bp or more) that appear in a variable number at a given genetic locus and cumulatively affect 360 million nucleotides, or about 12% of the human genome (Redon, 2006). **A CNV can be either benign or pathogenic, and a large proportion of identified CNVs have as yet unknown significance.**

Thus although SNPs introduce genetic variation at the level of individual base substitutions, CNVs represent variation in the "dose" of a relatively large DNA segment. The collection of genetic sequence variants (SNPs) or CNVs within an individual forms a sort of biologic landscape that will influence how that person experiences or responds to external influences such as challenge from an invading pathogen or ultraviolet ray exposure from the sun. Therefore understanding genetic variation in the form of SNPs and CNVs and their biologic influence can reveal a predisposition toward disease, variable susceptibility to infections, or diverse responses to pharmacologic agents as well as side effects from the same compounds. In other words, genetic variation is at the core of our collective goal of "individualized medicine," in which preventive strategies or "designer drugs" can be tailored to individuals based on one's genomic information.

### Epigenetic Variation

There are forms of genetic variation that do not involve a change in nucleotide sequence. Instead, persistent alterations in three-dimensional DNA structure can change the expression pattern of a gene. Covalent modification of histones to alter **chromatin** structure and the covalent addition of methyl groups to cytosine residues in the DNA are the most common three-dimensional DNA alterations. These patterns of **epigenetic** modification of genes are replicated through successive cell divisions despite unchanged DNA sequence and have the potential to be heritable (Portela, 2010).

**Two well-studied mechanisms of epigenetic modification influencing disease phenotype include genomic imprinting and CpG island methylation patterns.** Genomic imprinting is a process by which hypermethylation of a specific parental allele causes that allele of the gene to be silenced, and disease may arise if the remaining allele is abnormal. Variable methylation of CpG islands in cancer cells can promote tumorigenesis through loss of proliferative supervision of the cell. Epigenetics is a growing field enhancing our understanding of complex genotype-phenotype interactions. Epigenetic mechanisms such as methylation have been shown to play a role in multiple other human disease types beyond cancer, including neurodevelopmental disorders, neurodegenerative and neurologic diseases, and autoimmune diseases (Portela, 2010).

## GENETIC PATHOLOGY

High-frequency sequence variants, CNV, and epigenetic modifications are part of the normal backdrop of the human genome, providing variation within the species without negative consequences. Overt genetic pathologic change, in contrast, usually arises from genetic variants that disrupt the normal expression or function of one or more genes. **The old term mutation has been replaced by variant, which is further classified as benign, likely benign, of unknown significance, likely pathogenic, or pathogenic.** The latter two categories refer to changes in the genetic code that lead to altered function and clinical consequences based on consistent human case reports, identification of the type of variant, and verification by functional studies and/or animal models. The variant may involve changing a single base or a larger segment, in which bases are removed, duplicated, or inserted. **Variants occur as a result of environmental damage to DNA, through errors during DNA replication or repair, and through uneven crossing over and genetic exchange during meiosis.** The loss or gain of bases in a protein-coding region may disrupt the reading frame of the triplet codons. Alternatively, a change in base sequence in a noncoding region of DNA may alter the ability of regulatory proteins or RNA molecules to bind to the DNA. Variants within the gene could result in an amino acid substitution, leading to different products with altered functions. Fig. 2.2 demonstrates such an occurrence for sickle cell anemia, which is caused by the substitution of a single base at a single point. In contrast to sickle cell anemia, for which there is only one variant in one gene, more than 1000 variants or alleles have been described to date for the cystic fibrosis transmembrane conductance regulator (CFTR) gene. Some genes also have regions that are more at risk for variant-producing events (hot spots).

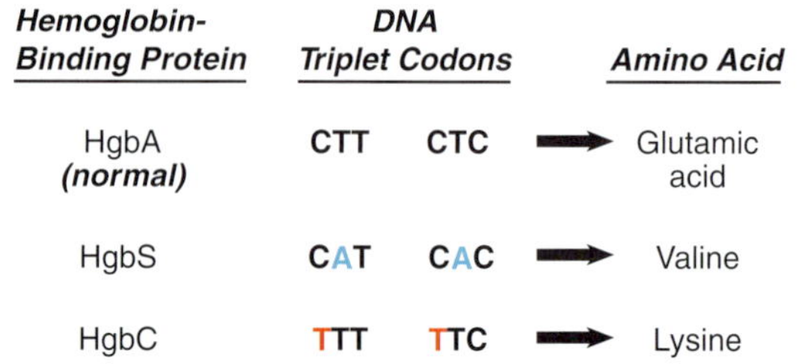

Hemoglobin-Binding Protein
DNA Triplet Codons
Amino Acid
HgbA (normal)
CTT CTC
Glutamic acid
HgbS
CAT CAC
Valine
HgbC
TTT TTC
Lysine


**Fig. 2.2** A single base pair substitution in the same DNA triplet codon for glutamic acid at amino acid position 6 for normal hemoglobin results in hemoglobin S (valine in sickle cell disease) or hemoglobin C (lysine in HgbC disease). (Courtesy Edith Cheng, MD.)

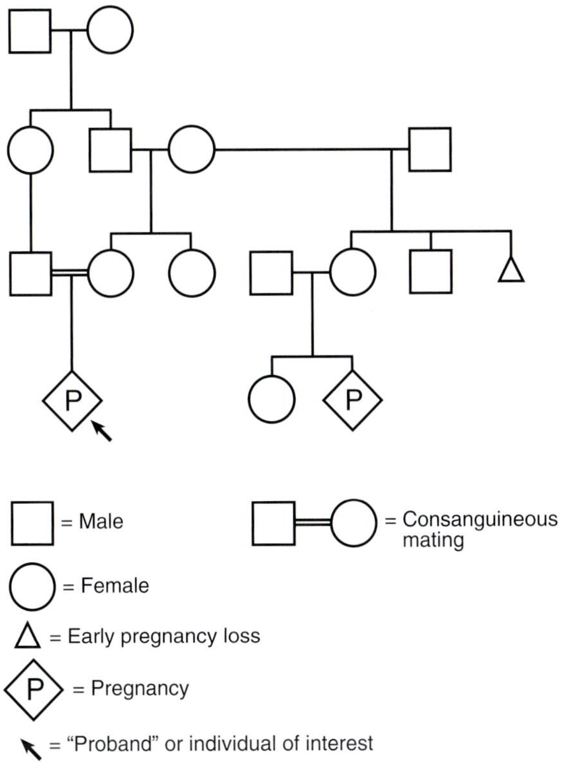


**Fig. 2.3** Standard figures and nomenclature for a pedigree. (Courtesy Edith Cheng, MD.)

## Single Gene Disorders

Disease-causing genetic alterations are categorized by patterns of familial segregation. Any evaluation of the segregation pattern of a trait or disease in a family requires the development of a three-generation **pedigree** (Fig. 2.3). This graphic representation of family history data assists in determining the transmission pattern of the gene and predicting the risk of recurrence. In some conditions the pattern of transmission and the constellation of clinical characteristics of affected individuals in the pedigree provide the diagnosis, which otherwise would not be evident if only one individual were evaluated.

### Mendelian Inheritance Patterns

#### Autosomal Dominant

**In an autosomal dominant mode of inheritance, only one copy of the variant gene is required for expression of the trait, and the individual is said to be heterozygous for the trait.** There are more than 4000 known autosomal dominant conditions, and most occur in the heterozygous form in affected individuals. With a few exceptions, autosomal dominant conditions occurring in the homozygous form (two copies of the affected gene) are rare, the phenotype is more severe, and the conditions are often lethal. An example is achondroplasia, in which two copies of the variant gene result in a lethal condition.

The general characteristics of autosomal dominant inheritance are illustrated in Fig. 2.4 and summarized as follows:

1. Every affected individual has an affected parent (unless this is a new pathogenic variant—to be discussed later). The inheritance pattern is vertical.
2. If reproductively fit, the affected person has a 50% risk of transmitting the gene with each pregnancy.
3. The sexes are affected equally.

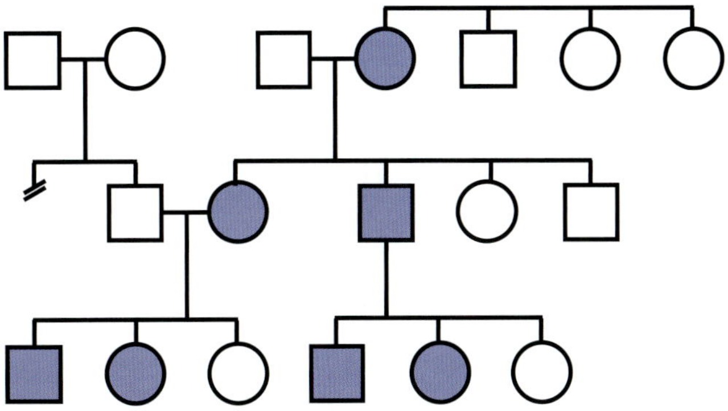

**Fig. 2.4** Example of autosomal dominant inheritance. (Courtesy Edith Cheng, MD.)

4. There is father-to-son transmission.
5. An individual who does not carry the pathogenic variant will have no risk of transmission to his or her offspring.

**Three additional properties associated with, but not exclusive to, autosomal dominant traits are variable expressivity, penetrance, and new pathogenic variants. Variable expressivity** describes the severity of the phenotype in individuals who have the pathogenic variant. Some autosomal dominant conditions have a clear clinical demarcation between affected and unaffected individuals. However, some conditions express the clinical consequences of the pathogenic variant in varying degrees among members of the same family and between different families. These differences in expression are modified by age, the sex of the affected individual, the individual's genetic background, and the environment. Variable expression of a condition can lead to difficulties in diagnosis and interpretation of inheritance pattern. **Penetrance** refers to the probability that a gene will have any clinical manifestation at all in a person known to have the pathogenic variant. A condition is 100% penetrant if all individuals with the pathogenic variant have any clinical feature of the disease (no matter how minor). A number of autosomal dominant conditions are the result of **new pathogenic variants.** For example, about 70% of achondroplasia cases occur as new variants. Because this condition has 100% penetrance, the recurrence risk in subsequent pregnancies in the normal parents of an affected child is extremely low, but the risk to the offspring of the affected is 50%. If an autosomal dominant condition is associated with poor reproductive fitness, then the likelihood that the cases occurred because of a new pathogenic variant is greater.

#### Autosomal Recessive

**Autosomal recessive conditions are rare and require the affected individual to have two copies of the pathogenic variant allele (homozygous) to manifest the condition.** In the heterozygote carrier, the product of the normal allele is generally able to compensate for the pathogenic variant allele and prevent occurrence of the disease. Fig. 2.5 is a typical pedigree illustrating autosomal recessive inheritance. The following general statements can be made about an autosomal recessive trait:

1. The characteristic will occur equally in both sexes.
2. For an offspring to be at risk, both parents must have at least one copy of the pathogenic variant.
3. If both parents are heterozygous (carriers) for the condition, on average 25% of the offspring will be homozygous for the pathogenic variant and will manifest the condition and 50% will be carriers and will be unaffected. The remaining 25% will not have inherited the variant at all, will be unaffected, and will not be at risk of transmitting the variant to any offspring.
4. Consanguinity is often present in families demonstrating rare autosomal recessive conditions.

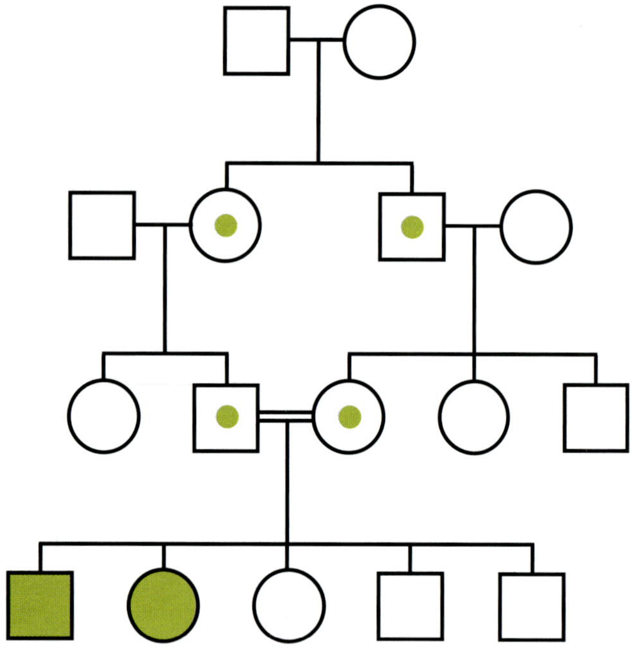

**Fig. 2.5** Pedigree illustrating autosomal recessive inheritance. Here the parents of the affected children are first cousins, as denoted by the double line connecting them. (Courtesy Edith Cheng, MD.)

**TABLE 2.2** Carrier Frequencies for Cystic Fibrosis in Different Populations

| Ethnicity | Chance of Being Carrier | Chance Both Carriers* |
|---|---|---|
| European descent | 1 in 29 | 1 in 841 |
| Hispanic American | 1 in 46 | 1 in 2116 |
| African American | 1 in 65 | 1 in 4225 |
| Asian American | 1 in 90 | 1 in 8100 |

*The chance of an affected child being born to these couples is the chance that both are carriers multiplied by 0.25.

5. If the disease is relatively rare, it will be clustered among the siblings and will not be seen among other family members such as ancestors, cousins, aunts, and uncles.

Because autosomal recessive conditions require two copies of the pathogenic variant allele, and because most matings are not consanguineous, **counseling couples about the risk for an autosomal recessive condition requires knowledge of the carrier frequency of the condition in the general population**. Cystic fibrosis exemplifies the importance of knowing the population in which screening or counseling is being provided (Table 2.2). Depending on the ethnic group of the mother and father, the risk for a child having cystic fibrosis could be as high as 1 in 1936 (1/22 × 1/22 × 1/4) if they are of Northern European descent or considerably less so if they are of Asian descent.

### X-linked Trait

The human X chromosome is quite large, containing about 160 million bps, or about 5% of the nuclear DNA. Of the 500 genes that have been mapped to the X chromosome, 70% are known to be associated with disease phenotypes. **Diseases caused by genes on the X chromosome are said to be X linked, and most are recessive.** In contrast, the Y chromosome is quite small, about 70 million bps, and contains only a few genes.

The expression of genes located on the X chromosome demonstrate a unique characteristic known as dosage compensation, a concept that was described by Mary Lyon in the 1960s to explain the equalization of X-linked gene products in men and women (Lyon, 1961). Achievement of dosage compensation is through the principles of X inactivation, also known as the **Lyon hypothesis**. The tenets of the Lyon hypothesis are as follows:

1. One X chromosome in each cell is randomly inactivated in the early female embryo (soon after fertilization).
2. The inactivation process is random: Either the paternally or maternally derived X chromosome is chosen. The woman is thus a mosaic for genes located on the X chromosome.
3. All descendants of the cell will have the same inactive X chromosome.

The Lyon hypothesis is supported by clinical evidence derived from animal and human observations of traits located on the X chromosome, such as the calico cat pattern of red and black patches of fur on female cats but not on male cats. In humans, men and women have equal quantities of the enzyme glucose-6-phosphate dehydrogenase (G6PD), which is encoded by a gene on the X chromosome. The mechanism for X inactivation is unknown at this time but clearly requires the presence of the X inactivation center, which has been mapped to the proximal end of the long arm of the X chromosome (Xq). This center contains an unusual gene called the **X-inactive specific transcript (XIST), which seems to control X inactivation, a process that cannot occur in its absence.**

The principles of the Lyon hypothesis remain true for the majority of genes located on the X chromosome. The silencing of these genes appears to occur as a function of DNA methylation at the promoter regions of these genes. However, several regions remain genetically active on both chromosomes. They include the **pseudoautosomal regions located at the tips of the long and short arms**, which are the regions that contain the genes for steroid sulfatase, the Xg blood group, and Kallmann syndrome (hypogonadism and anosmia). **The pseudoautosomal region on the short arm shares extensive homology with the Y chromosome and is the region involved in the pairing of the X and Y chromosome at meiosis.**

Another exception to the Lyon hypothesis is that one X chromosome is nonrandomly, preferentially inactivated. This is observed for most cases of **translocations** between an X chromosome and an autosome. If the translocation is balanced, the structurally normal X chromosome is preferentially inactivated. If the translocation is unbalanced, then the structurally normal X chromosome is always active. These nonrandom patterns of inactivation functionally minimize the clinical consequences of the chromosomal rearrangement. Studies can be done to look at patterns of inactivation, as in the case of prenatal diagnosis, to predict the clinical consequences of a de novo X/autosome translocation in the fetus.

**Random inactivation confers a mosaic state for the female carrier.** The normal allele is able to compensate for the abnormal allele (as in autosomal recessive traits), and female carriers of X-linked recessive conditions usually do not have clinical manifestations of the disease. Occasionally, however, there is a skewed, or less than 50/50, chance of inactivation such that the X chromosome carrying the normal allele is inactivated more frequently. In such cases, female carriers display some features of the condition and are referred to as **manifesting heterozygotes**. Manifesting heterozygotes have been described for hemophilia A, Duchenne muscular dystrophy, ornithine transcarbamylase deficiency, and X-linked color blindness. **Genetic counseling of recurrence risks for an X-linked recessive condition depends on the sex of the affected parent and of the offspring.** Fig. 2.6 is a pedigree illustrating X-linked recessive inheritance, the characteristics of which are the following:

1. Affected individuals are usually male unless X-chromosome activation is skewed in the female carrier or the individual is homozygous for the trait.

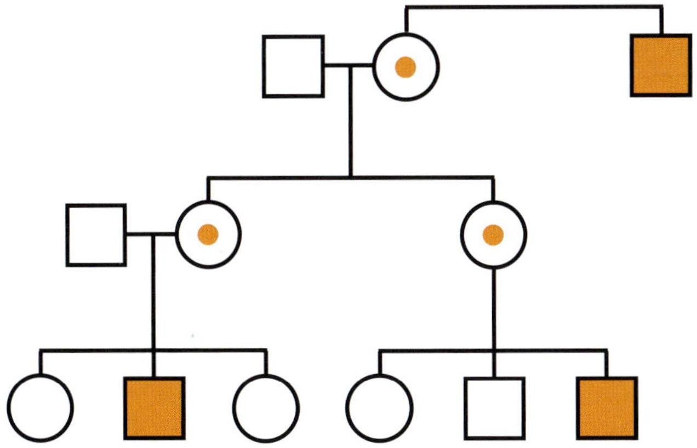

**Fig. 2.6** Pedigree illustrating X-linked recessive condition. (Courtesy Edith Cheng, MD.)

2. The affected men in a kindred are related through women.
3. The gene is not transmitted from father to son.
4. All daughters of affected men will be carriers.
5. Daughters of female carriers have a 50% chance of being carriers; sons of female carriers have a 50% chance of being affected.

### X-linked Dominant Inheritance

**The major feature of X-linked dominant inheritance is that all heterozygotes, both male and female, manifest the condition.** Although the pedigree may resemble autosomal dominant inheritance, the distinguishing feature is that affected men never have affected sons, and all daughters of affected men are affected. There are usually more affected women than men, and the majority of the women are heterozygotes. Examples of diseases with this mode of inheritance are hypophosphatemic rickets and Rett syndrome.

## Nonmendelian Inheritance Patterns (Complex Traits)

### Trinucleotide-Repeat Disorders: Unstable Repeated Sequence Variants

In the early 1990s a new class of genetic conditions was recognized as being caused by unstable dynamic variants in a gene. In classic genetic inheritance the diseases and their inheritance patterns are due to pathogenic variants that are passed on from generation to generation in a stable form. That is, all affected members in a family have the identical inherited variant. In 1991, however, a number of reports began to describe a new class of genetic condition in which the gene sequence variation was dynamic and changed with different affected individuals within a family. The most common group of disorders is known as *triplet,* or **trinucleotide repeat, disorders**. More than a dozen diseases are now known to be associated with unstable trinucleotide repeats (Table 2.3) (Cummings, 2000).

**These conditions are characterized by an expansion of variable size, within the affected gene, of a segment of DNA that contains a repeat of three nucleotides such as CAGCAGCAG (CAG)n, or CCGCCG (CCG)n.** These triplet repeats are unstable in that they tend to expand as the gene is passed on from generation to generation. The molecular mechanism is most likely misalignment at the time of meiosis. The result of increasing triplet expansion is progressively earlier onset and/or more severe manifestation of disease with each successive generation. This phenomenon is known as *anticipation.*

The commonality of this group of genetic conditions stops at the shared molecular mechanism. Each disease, otherwise, has its own features. Some, such as myotonic dystrophy, are inherited in an autosomal dominant pattern, but others, such as Friedrich ataxia, are autosomal recessive conditions. The susceptibility of the triplet repeat to expansion also may depend on the parent of origin: It is typically more severe with paternal inheritance in Huntington disease and exclusively maternal in fragile X syndrome.

### Fragile X Syndrome

Fragile X syndrome, a disease within the unstable triplet repeat disorder group, is the most common heritable form of moderate intellectual disabilities and is second to Down syndrome among causes of intellectual disabilities in men. The affected gene (fragile X mental retardation 1, *FMR1*) is located on the X chromosome at Xq27.3, and triplet repeat expansion in the gene causes a pattern of abnormalities, including intellectual disabilities, characteristic facial features, and autistic behaviors. Disease frequency is approximately 1 in 4000 men and 1 in 8000 women. The condition is due to an expansion of the triplet repeat CGG located in the untranslated region of the first exon of the gene. The triplet expansion blocks normal function of the *FMR1* gene, thus causing the syndrome. **Fragile X is associated with maternal anticipation, meaning female carriers are at increased risk of passing on expanded repeated sequence variants to their children, whereas the repeated sequence variants in male carriers will not typically expand when passed on to their daughters.** Risk of expansion may also be associated with the original size of the repeated sequence variant and the presence or absence of AGG repeats within the CGG expanded region (Latham, 2014).

Individuals with normal X chromosome alleles have CGG repeats in the 6 to 44 range, whereas affected individuals have expanded "full mutations" of 200 to more than 1000 repeats. Individuals with 55 to 200 repeats are known as **premutation carriers**. Men are more likely to be affected with fragile X than women, and features of the condition tend to be milder in women than men. Individuals with 45 to 54 CGG repeats are known as intermediate carriers. Intermediate carriers are not at an increased chance to

**TABLE 2.3** Some Commonly Known Disorders Associated with Unstable Triplet Repeats

| | | | | Repeat Number | | |
|---|---|---|---|---|---|---|
| **Disease** | **Inheritance Pattern** | **Triplet Repeat** | **Location of Expansion** | **Normal** | **Unstable** | **Affected** |
| Huntington disease | Autosomal dominant | CAG | Exon coding region | <36 | 29-35 | >35 |
| Fragile X | X-linked | CGG | 5′ untranslated region | <45* | 56-200 | >200 |
| Myotonic dystrophy | Autosomal dominant | GTG | 3′ untranslated region | <35 | 50-100 | >100 |
| Spinal cerebellar ataxias† | Autosomal dominant | CAG | Exon | <40 | Different for each subtype | >40 |
| Friedrich ataxia | Autosomal recessive | GAA | Intron of gene | <33 | 34-65 | >65 |

*Fragile X intermediate mutations (45-54 CGG repeats) may expand to premutations but not full mutations
†Spinal cerebellar ataxias are a heterogeneous group of conditions, all of which appear to be associated with a CAG repeat. Each subtype has its own specific range of normal, unstable, and affected repeat sizes.

have children affected with fragile X syndrome. However, female intermediate carriers are at an increased chance to have children who are premutation carriers (14% risk of expansion). Premutation carriers are not usually affected with features of fragile X syndrome, but they are at increased risk for having affected children or descendants if the premutation expands to a full mutation in successive generations. Conversely, intermediate and premutation alleles can be passed on without expanding, and in rare instances, expanded alleles may even contract when inherited.

Long-term follow-up of premutation carriers has revealed that these individuals are at increased risk for certain adult-onset conditions separate from the fragile X syndrome. **Male premutation carriers are at increased risk for fragile X–associated tremor/ataxia syndrome (FXTAS) later in life** (Hagerman, 2004). FXTAS may also occur in female premutation carriers, though more rarely. **Female premutation carriers are also at increased risk for premature ovarian insufficiency (POI), which is the cessation of menses before age 40.** In contrast, intermediate carriers are not at any increased risk to develop FXTAS or POI (Finucane, 2012).

Although the unstable triplet is transmitted in an X-linked pattern, the probabilities of the different phenotypes are far from traditional X-linked inheritance. Understanding the features of fragile X syndrome is crucial for genetic counseling and assessment of recurrence risks. The possible outcomes of the offspring of a premutation female carrier are the following:

1. Male offspring—three possibilities:
   a. Unaffected: does not inherit the X chromosome with the premutation.
   b. Unaffected: inherits the X chromosome with the premutation that did *not* expand. At risk for FXTAS *and* at risk for passing the premutation to daughters, who in turn will be at risk for having children who are premutation carriers or affected.
   c. Affected: inherits an expanded full mutation.
2. Female offspring—four possibilities:
   a. Unaffected: does not inherit the X chromosome with the premutation.
   b. Unaffected: inherits the X chromosome with the premutation that did *not* expand to a full mutation. At risk for POI and FXTAS *and* at risk for having children who are premutation carriers or affected.
   c. Unaffected: inherits the X chromosome with an expanded full mutation; about 50% of women with a full mutation appear to be clinically unaffected.
   d. Affected: inherits the X chromosome with an expanded full mutation.

### Genomic Imprinting and Uniparental Disomy

**Genomic imprinting and uniparental disomy refers to the differential activation or expression of genes depending on the parent of origin.** In contrast to Mendel's hypothesis that the phenotype of a gene is no different if inherited from the mother or the father, we now understand that there is a group of diseases in which the parent of origin of a gene or chromosome plays a role in the phenotype of the affected individual. The best-studied examples of this mechanism are **Prader-Willi syndrome (PWS) and Angelman syndrome (AS). Both diseases arise from loss of function of the same gene on chromosome 15, but two different disease phenotypes arise depending on which parental allele is affected.** PWS is characterized by obesity, hyperphagia, small hands and feet, hypogonadism, and mental retardation (Jones, 2006). In about 70% of cases, cytogenetic deletion of the proximal arm of the paternally inherited chromosome 15 is observable (15q11-q13). In contrast, the same deletion of the maternally inherited chromosome 15 results in the Angelman phenotype of severe mental retardation, short stature, spasticity, and seizures (Jones, 2006). Interestingly, 30% of subjects with PWS do not have a cytogenetic deletion but rather inherit two intact chromosomes 15 from the mother. No genetic information on chromosome 15 is inherited from the father. This is referred to as **maternal uniparental disomy**. Individuals with Angelman syndrome without a cytogenetic deletion have two copies of the paternally derived chromosome 15 and no chromosome 15 from the mother, a condition termed **paternal uniparental disomy**. These findings indicate that for the region of 15q11-q13, the expression of the PWS phenotype is brought on by the absence of a paternal contribution of the genes in this region. Likewise, the expression of Angelman syndrome is due to the absence of the maternal contribution of genes located at 15q11-q13. The genes in this region are said to be "imprinted" because their parent of origin has been "marked."

Many regions of the human genome have now demonstrated evidence of imprinting. Knowledge of diseases that occur as a result of imprinting are important for clinical care because they have implications for prenatal diagnosis, especially when mosaicism is encountered.

### Germline Mosaicism

**Mosaicism is defined as the presence of two or more genetically different cell lines in the same individual or in tissue derived from a single zygote.** All women, because of X inactivation, are mosaics for genes on the X chromosome. Mosaicism, however, is not necessarily evenly or randomly distributed throughout the body. In other words, using the entire body as the whole organism, an individual is mosaic either because different organs or tissues have genetically different cells but each organ or tissue has the same cell line or because the genetically different cell lines are dispersed throughout many tissues in the body. The distinction between these two types of mosaicism is particularly important in making a prenatal diagnosis in cases in which mosaicism is identified in amniotic fluid cells. For instance, one cannot be confident that a fetus identified as having trisomy 21 mosaicism would necessarily have a less severe mental retardation phenotype because of mosaicism. The brain cells could potentially all contain full trisomy 21, but the cells of the skin could all be normal diploid. **In germline mosaicism, the implication is that the pathogenic variant is present in only one parent and arose during embryogenesis in all or some of the germ line cells but few or none of the somatic cells of the embryo.** This concept was developed to explain **recurrence of a genetic condition in a sibship** (usually autosomal dominant) in which incorrect diagnosis, autosomal recessive inheritance, reduced penetrance, or variable expression could not be the reason for the recurrence. The best example of germline mosaicism is osteogenesis imperfecta type II (lethal form). At the molecular level, the pathogenic variant causing the condition is dominant—that is, only one copy of the abnormal gene is necessary to cause this perinatal lethal condition. Yet there are families in which multiple affected pregnancies are seen in the same couple or one parent has recurrences with different partners. If the spontaneous pathogenic variant rate for an autosomal dominant variant is 1 chance in $10^5$, then the probability of two independent spontaneous variants for the same lethal autosomal dominant condition is $(1/10^5)^2$, a highly unlikely event. Germline mosaicism is now well documented for about 6% of cases of osteogenesis imperfecta type II (Zlotogora, 1998). Unfortunately, the exact recurrence risk in an individual family is difficult to assess because the proportion of gametes containing the pathogenic variant is unknowable.

### Mitochondrial Inheritance: Maternal Inheritance

Most inherited conditions occur as a result of variants in the DNA of the nucleus (nuclear genome). However, **mitochondria have their own DNA molecules, which contain a small fraction of genes whose products are vital to the function of the cell.** Mitochondrial DNA (mtDNA), which was completely sequenced in 1981, is small, about 16.5 kilobase pairs (kb), and is packaged as a circular chromosome located in the mitochondria. A growing number of conditions resulting from abnormalities of the mitochondria have now been identified. Because the mitochondrial apparatus and its function are under the control of both nuclear and mitochondrial genes, many diseases affecting the mitochondria do not follow the typical Mendelian pattern of inheritance. Each human cell contains a population of several hundred or more mitochondria in its cytoplasm. Most of the subunits that make up the mitochondrial apparatus are encoded by the nuclear genome.

Because the primary function of the mitochondria is to provide energy for the cell in the form of adenosine triphosphate (ATP), genetic variants that affect the genes that code for oxidative phosphorylation will likely result in cell dysfunction and death. The organs most affected would be those that depend heavily on mitochondria. **The diseases that result are generally neuromuscular in nature, such as encephalopathies, myopathies, ataxias, and retinal degeneration, but the genetic variants have pleiotropic effects, meaning multiple different clinical traits are caused by a single gene defect** (Johns, 1995).

The most significant characteristic of mitochondrial diseases caused by pathogenic variants in mtDNA is that **they are all maternally inherited**. This is because the cytoplasm of the ovum is abundant with mitochondria, but the sperm contain very few mitochondria. Therefore an individual's mitochondria (and mtDNA) are essentially all inherited from the mother. If the mother has a mtDNA pathogenic variant, then all of her children will inherit that variant. When a pathogenic variant arises in the DNA of a mitochondrion in the cytoplasm of the ovum, it begins as one variant in one mitochondrion. However, as replication and division of this variant mitochondrion occur, they become randomly distributed among the normal mitochondria and between the daughter cells. One daughter cell by chance may contain a large population of mitochondria with the pathogenic variant, but the other may have none or very little. Fertilization of the egg with a large proportion of mitochondria containing the variant would result in an offspring at risk for manifesting a mitochondrial disease. Leber hereditary optic neuropathy (LHON) is a well-known mitochondrial disease in which rapid, bilateral loss of central vision occurs as a result of a pathogenic variant in mitochondrial DNA. Men and women are affected equally, and all affected individuals are related through maternal lineage.

A second feature of mitochondrial diseases is that of variable expression. Within each cell and tissue, there is a threshold for energy production below which the cells will degenerate and die. **Organ systems with large energy requirements are most susceptible to mitochondrial abnormalities.** Thus if an mtDNA pathogenic variant is present, the severity of the mitochondrial disease will depend on the proportion of mitochondria with the variant that the individual inherited from his or her mother and the susceptibility of different tissues to altered ATP metabolism.

In contrast, abnormalities of mitochondrial function caused by pathogenic variants of genes encoded in the nuclear genome will exhibit traditional Mendelian inheritance patterns; autosomal dominant, autosomal recessive, and X-linked patterns of mitochondrial disorders have been observed. A few mitochondrial diseases occur as sporadic somatic pathogenic variants and have little or no recurrence risk. Table 2.4 lists some of the known diseases of mitochondrial function and their inheritance patterns.

## Multifactorial Inheritance

**Multifactorial inheritance is defined as traits or characteristics produced by the action of several genes, with or without the interplay of environmental factors.** A number of structural abnormalities occurring as isolated defects and not part of a syndrome, such as cleft lip with or without cleft palate, open neural tube defects (including anencephaly and spina bifida), and cardiac defects, are examples of such conditions. **When both parents are normal and an affected child is conceived, the chance of recurrence is generally between 2% and 5% for any given pregnancy.**

**TABLE 2.4** Features of Some Disorders of Mitochondrial Function

| Disease | Features | Genetics | Inheritance Pattern |
|---|---|---|---|
| Barth syndrome | Dilated cardiomyopathy, cyclic neutropenia, skeletal myopathy, growth deficiency, abnormal mitochondria | Nuclear DNA encoding mitochondrial protein tafazzin (*TAZ* gene) | X linked |
| Friedreich ataxia | Limb movement abnormalities, dysarthria, absent tendon reflexes | Nuclear DNA encoding mitochondrial protein frataxin (*FXN* gene, triplet repeat) | Autosomal recessive |
| Leber hereditary optic neuropathy (LHON) | Blindness, rapid optic nerve death in young adulthood | Mitochondrial DNA | Maternal |
| Leigh disease (subacute necrotizing encephalomyelopathy) | Infant-onset progressive psychomotor regression after viral illness, hypotonia, peripheral neuropathy, lactic acidosis | Many genes: 20%-25% mitochondrial DNA (includes neuropathy, ataxia, and retinitis pigmentosa [NARP]) | Mitochondrial DNA: maternal |
| | | 75%-80% nuclear DNA | Nuclear DNA: autosomal recessive or X linked |
| MERRF | Myotonic epilepsy, ragged red fibers in muscle, ataxia, sensorineural deafness | Mitochondrial DNA | Maternal |
| MELAS | Mitochondrial encephalopathy, lactic acidosis, strokelike episodes, sensorineural deafness | Mitochondrial DNA | Maternal |
| MIDD | Maternally inherited diabetes and deafness | Mitochondrial DNA | Maternal |
| MNGIE | Mitochondrial neurogastrointestinal encephalopathy, childhood-onset gastrointestinal dysmotility, peripheral neuropathy | Nuclear DNA (*TYMP* gene) causes destabilization of mitochondrial DNA | Autosomal recessive |

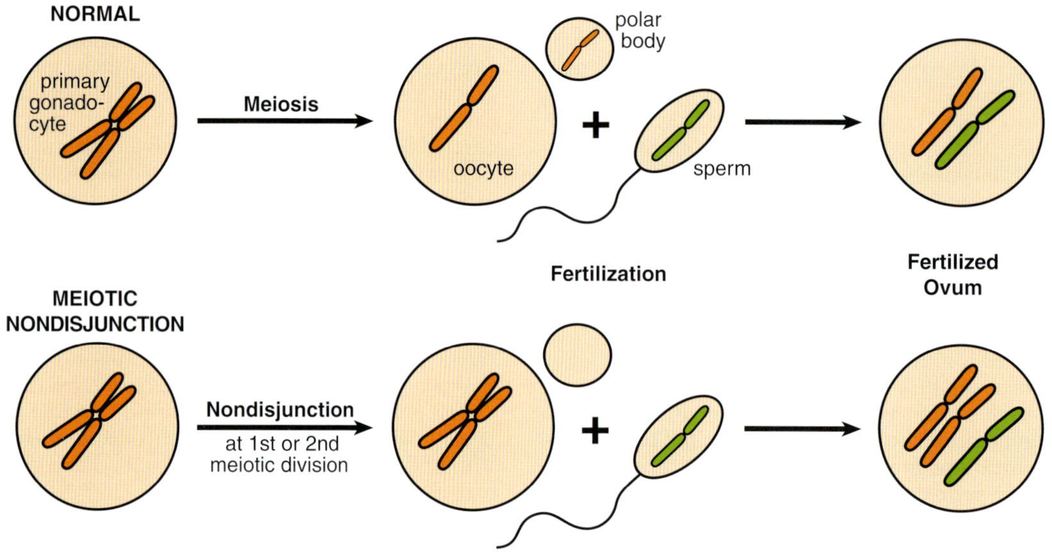


**Fig. 2.7** Graphic representation of meiotic nondisjunction. (Courtesy Edith Cheng, MD.)

Because the underlying mechanisms by which the genes and the environment interact to cause these conditions are largely unknown, genetic counseling of recurrence risks must measure the observed recurrence risks in collections of families to generate a population-based empiric risk. These risk rates, however, are modified by many factors, including ethnicity, the sex of the affected parent and at-risk offspring, the presence of the defect in one or both parents, the number of affected family members, and consanguineous parentage (Kuller, 1996).

## Chromosomal Abnormalities

In general, genetic replication machinery of the cell is astonishingly accurate, and the cell uses many repair mechanisms to maintain the fidelity of DNA copies. Thus the incidence of any given single gene disorder, even in high-prevalence populations, is relatively low. In contrast, the distribution of genetic material during cell division by mitosis or meiosis is far more at risk for mistakes, so that **on a population level the risk of chromosome-level genetic rearrangements occurs at least 100 times more often than single-gene disorders**. Consider the rate of 1 in 2500 for white children affected by cystic fibrosis (the most common inherited disease in this population) compared with the estimation that an abnormal chromosome complement occurs in up to 4% of clinically recognized pregnancies (Creasy, 2014).

A variety of chromosome abnormalities may occur during meiosis or mitosis (see Chapter 1) leading to an abnormal **karyotype**, or chromosome complement. Chromosome abnormalities fall into several general categories, and many clinical conditions are associated with each type.

### Numerical Chromosomal Abnormalities

Two terms are used to describe numerical chromosomal abnormalities: **Aneuploidy refers to an extra or missing chromosome**, such as in trisomy 21 (Down syndrome) or monosomy X (Turner syndrome), respectively; **polyploidy refers to numerical chromosome abnormalities in which there is an addition of an entire complement of haploid chromosomes**, such as in triploidy, in which three haploid sets occur (69,XXX, 69,XXY, or 69,XYY). Numerical or aneuploid chromosome abnormalities involve either autosomes or sex chromosomes. Most occur as the result of **nondisjunction during meiosis or mitosis in which homologous chromosome pairs fail to disjoin**. The result in meiosis is that one daughter cell receives two copies of the homologues and the other receives none. Fertilization with a gamete containing a normal chromosome complement results in a zygote that is either trisomic or monosomic (Fig. 2.7). Nondisjunctional events during mitosis in the early embryo (after fertilization) produce individuals with cell populations containing different chromosome numbers. This condition, known as **mosaicism**, may involve the autosomes or the sex chromosomes. The actual phenotype depends on the proportion of aneuploid and euploid cells in the embryo and in the specific organs or tissues involved.

The majority of trisomic conceptions are nonviable, and autosomal trisomies have been seen in abortus material in all but chromosomes 1 and 17. However, **trisomies 21, 18, 13, and 22 can result in live births and are associated with advanced maternal age** (Fig. 2.8). Trisomy 13 (Patau syndrome) occurs in approximately 1 in 10,000 live births. The syndrome is characterized by prenatal growth restriction and multiple severe structural defects involving the midline (holoprosencephaly, cleft lip and/or palate, cardiac defects), and postaxial polydactyly. Trisomy 18 (Edwards syndrome) is found in 1 in 6000 live births and is associated with prenatal growth restriction, rocker bottom feet, and cardiac and renal defects. Trisomy 21 is the most common viable autosomal trisomy and has an incidence of 1 in 800 live births. The majority (95%) of individuals with Down syndrome have complete trisomy 21—that is, three separate copies of chromosome 21 because of maternal nondisjunction. However, about 2% to 3% of individuals with clinical Down syndrome have a structural rearrangement (Robertsonian translocation—to be discussed in the next section), and another 1% to 3% are mosaic for trisomy 21 (Jones, 2006). Trisomy 22 has been seen in a few live-born individuals and is associated with severe neurologic impairment. Monosomic states involving autosomes are extremely rare and generally lethal.

Sex chromosome aneuploidy usually occurs in the trisomic state. Monosomy Y is lethal and has never been seen in a clinical situation or even in an abortus. In contrast, **monosomy of the X chromosome (known as Turner syndrome) is the most common chromosomal abnormality found in first trimester abortuses**. Because most 45,X conceptions are lethal, the actual incidence of live female births is about 1 in 5000. At birth, Turner syndrome is characterized by lymphedema, hypotonia, and a webbed neck. Girls with Turner syndrome have short stature, a broad chest with widely spaced nipples, cubitus valgus (widened carrying angle of the arms), and gonadal dysgenesis resulting in a lack of secondary sex characteristics, amenorrhea, and infertility

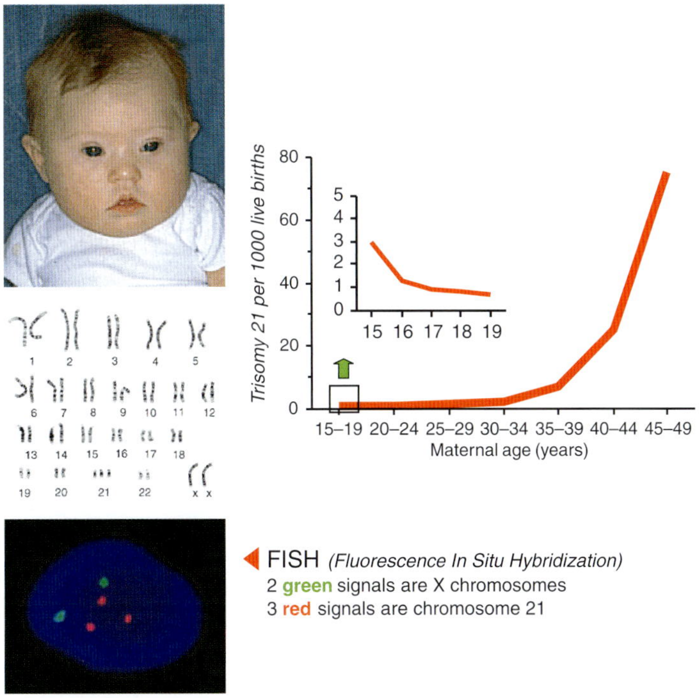


**Fig. 2.8** Trisomy 21 infant with karyotype demonstrating three separate chromosomes 21. Interphase fluorescence in situ hybridization (FISH) illustration of screening for trisomy 21. Graph illustrating the maternal age association and increasing risk for aneuploidy. Note that there is an increased risk at the peripubertal ages as well. (Courtesy Edith Cheng, MD.)

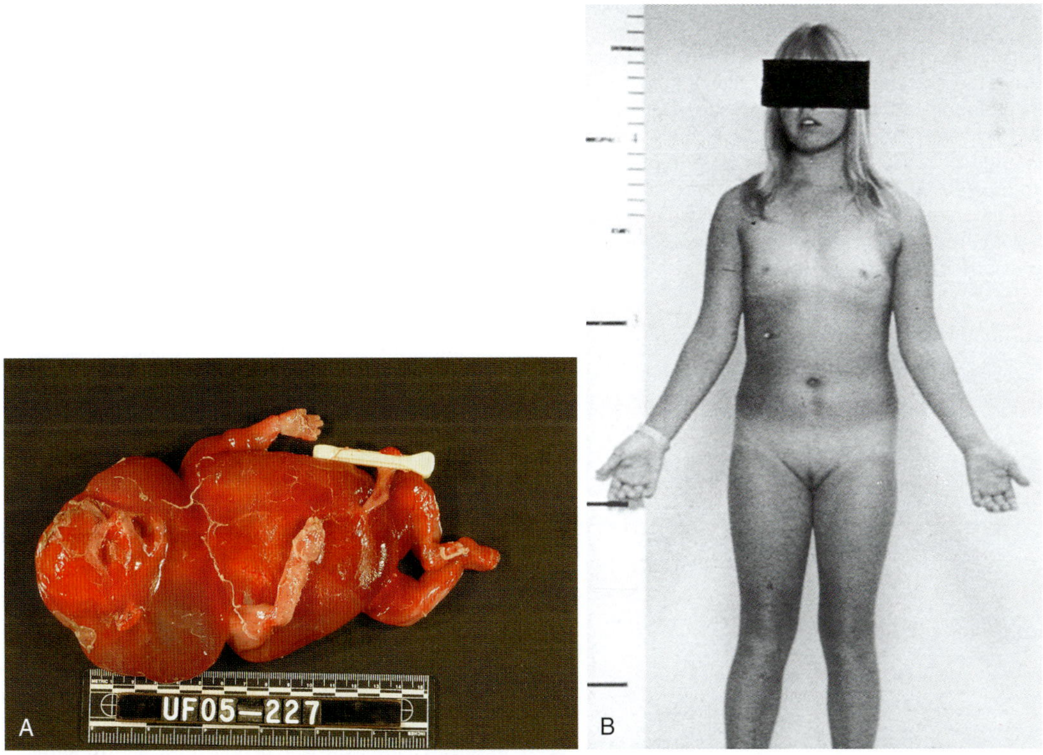


**Fig. 2.9** **A**, Photo of a 20-week fetus with Turner syndrome, 45,X. This fetus was diagnosed during a routine 20-week ultrasound for anatomy and growth and was found to have a large cystic hygroma and hydrops. The autopsy revealed a complex cardiac defect, abnormal kidneys, streaked ovaries, and malrotation of the gut with the appendix in the left lower quadrant. **B**, A 17-year-old girl with Turner syndrome. Note the short stature, poor sexual development, and increased carrying angles at elbows; webbing of the neck is present as well. (**A,** Courtesy Drs. W. Tony Parks and Corrine Fligner, Department of Pathology, University of Washington.)

(Fig. 2.9). Other features include congenital heart disease (coarctation of the aorta is the most common), kidney abnormalities, and hypertension in later life. Intelligence is generally normal although spatial perception abnormalities are common (Jones, 2006). Hormonal supplementation during puberty allows girls with Turner syndrome to develop secondary sex characteristics.

**Unlike autosomal trisomies in which the majority of cases are maternally derived, the risk 45,X karyotype occurs through paternal nondisjunction and is not associated with advanced maternal or paternal age.** There is no increased recurrence risk for 45,X, which accounts for 50% of women with Turner syndrome. Another 30% to 40% of individuals with Turner syndrome are mosaic for the 45,X cell line and another cell line (usually 46,XX) because of postzygotic nondisjunction during mitosis. The clinical features of these women vary depending on the proportion of normal 46,XX cell lines present. However, **women who are mosaic with a 45,X/46,XY karyotype are at an increased risk for gonadoblastoma. Therefore women suspected of having Turner syndrome should have a chromosomal analysis, not only for diagnosis but for exclusion of mosaicism for a 46,XY cell line.** The remaining 10% to 20% of individuals with Turner syndrome have a structural abnormality of the X chromosome such as a ring chromosome (Table 2.5).

Other trisomies involving the sex chromosomes include 47,XXX, 47,XXY (Klinefelter syndrome), and 47,XYY karyotypes. Karyotype 47,XXX results from maternal nondisjunction associated with increasing maternal age; the incidence is approximately 1 in 1000 live female births. Most women with 47,XXX are phenotypically normal with the exception of possible mild developmental delay; fertility is normal, and there may be a slightly increased risk for offspring with aneuploidy involving the sex chromosomes and autosomes. **Klinefelter syndrome, 47,XXY, is a common sex chromosome abnormality associated with maternal age and occurs in 1 in 1000 live male births.** Clinical features include tall gynecoid stature, gynecomastia (with an increased risk for breast cancer), and testicular atrophy. Mental retardation is not a typical feature, but affected individuals may have IQ scores that are lower than those of their siblings. Nondisjunction during spermatogenesis involving the Y chromosome leads to 47,XYY. These men may be taller than average, but they are otherwise phenotypically normal. Contrary to previous and outdated observational studies, this sex chromosome aneuploidy is not associated with an increased disposition to violent crime. However, behavioral problems such as attention deficit disorder may be observed.

## Structural Chromosome Abnormalities

Chromosome breaks and rearrangements may lead to no obvious phenotypic consequences (genetically balanced), loss or gain of chromosomal material (genetically imbalanced) that produces abnormalities, or abnormalities resulting from the interruption of a critical gene at the breakpoint site on the chromosome. **Types of structural rearrangements include translocations (reciprocal and Robertsonian), insertions, inversions, isochromosomes, duplications, and deletions.** The rate of formation of balanced rearrangements is generally very low, $1.6 \times 10^{-4}$, although some chromosomal segments (hot spots) are more at risk for breakage than others.

**TABLE 2.5** Karyotypes Discovered in Subjects with Phenotypic Characteristics of Turner Syndrome

| Karyotype | Error |
|---|---|
| 45,X | Deletion X |
| 45,Xi(Xq) | Deletion Xp, Isochromosome Xq |
| 45,X,Xq | Deletion Xp |
| 45,X/46,XX | Mosaicism |
| 45,X/46,XX/47,XXX | Mosaicism |
| 45,X/46,XY | Mosaicism |
| 45,X/46,XY/47,XYY | Mosaicism |
| 45,XringX | Ring chromosome |
| 46,XX | Phenotype with normal karyotype |

### Balanced Reciprocal Translocations

**Translocations occur as a result of a mutual and physical exchange of chromosomal (genetic) material between nonhomologous chromosomes, or chromosomes that are not part of an identical matched pair.** There are two main types of translocations, reciprocal and Robertsonian. Balanced reciprocal translocations are found in about 1 in 11,000 newborns. Fig. 2.10 is an example of a hypothetical balanced translocation between the short arms (p arms) of two chromosomes. The carrier of a reciprocal balanced translocation is usually phenotypically normal. However, the carrier is at an increased risk for producing offspring who are chromosomally abnormal. The viability of the genetically unbalanced gametes is highly dependent on the location and amount of involved DNA. In general, however, the recurrence for an unbalanced conception is 3% to 5% for male carriers and 10% to 15% for female carriers of reciprocal balanced translocations. Recurrence risks depend on the chromosomes involved and the size of the translocated segments.

A second type of translocation is the **Robertsonian translocation. This is a structural rearrangement between the acrocentric chromosomes: chromosome pairs 13, 14, 15, 21, and 22.** These chromosomes have a centromere that is severely offset from the center such that the short arm (p arm) contains minimal genetic material, which can be lost with little or no functional consequence. In this structural rearrangement, the short arms (p arms) of two nonhomologous chromosomes are lost, and the long arms fuse at the **centromere**, forming a single chromosome structure. Fig. 2.11 is an example of a Robertsonian translocation involving chromosomes 14 and 21. The phenotypically normal carrier of a Robertsonian translocation has 45 chromosomes in each cell because the two acrocentric chromosomes involved in the translocation have formed into one chromosome structure. This Robertsonian translocation carrier is genetically balanced—that is, he or she has two copies of each chromosome. However, the gametes are at risk to be unbalanced.

One important exception in translocation Down syndrome is associated with a 21q21q translocation. In this situation two chromosomes 21 are present. Although this chromosome rearrangement is extremely rare, this translocation confers a 100% risk that the carrier will have abnormal gametes and 100% of viable gametes will result in a conception with Down syndrome. The only other possible outcome is monosomy 21, a complement that results in early miscarriage.

**Chromosome inversions occur when two breaks on a chromosome are followed by a 180-degree turn of the segment and reinsertion at its original breakpoints.** If the centromere is included in the inverted segment, it is called a **pericentric inversion**. If the centromere is not involved, the inversion is called a **paracentric inversion**. Chromosome inversions are generally considered balanced and usually do not confer an abnormal phenotype unless one of the breakpoints disrupts a critical gene. Inversions, however, do interfere with pairing at meiosis and can result in gametes with chromosome abnormalities.

**Isochromosomes occur as a result of the chromosome dividing along the horizontal axis rather than the longitudinal axis at the centromere.** The result is a chromosome that has two copies of one arm (p or q) and no copies of the other. Isochromosomes involving autosomes are generally lethal because the resultant conception will be both trisomic and monosomic for genetic

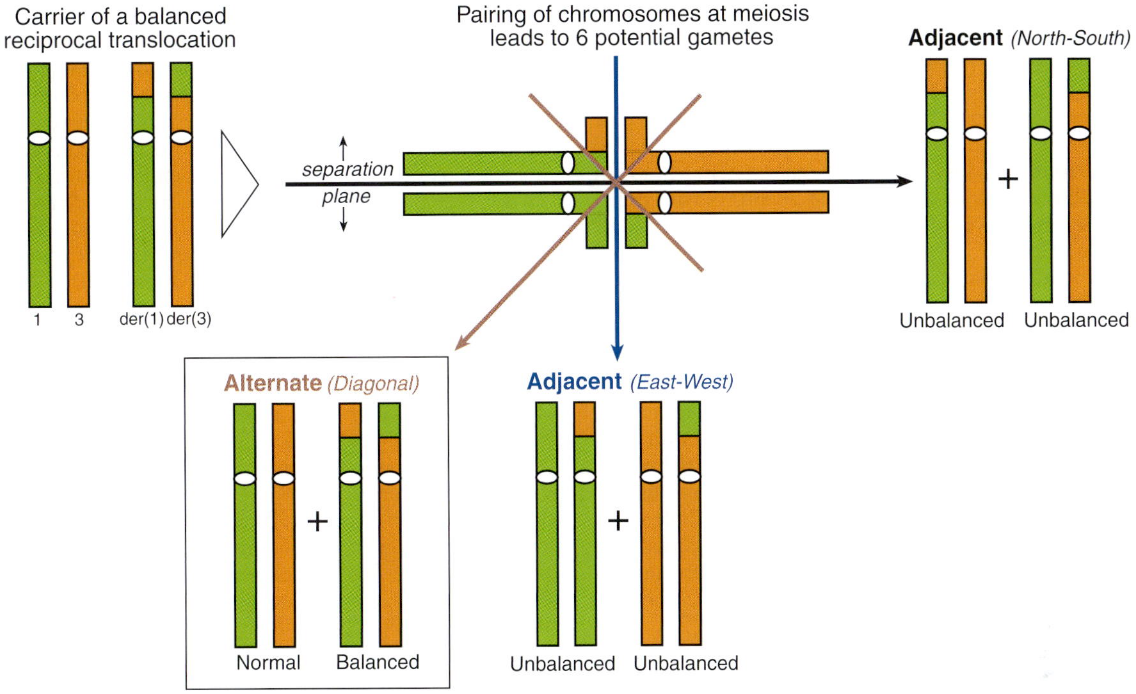


**Fig. 2.10** Schematic representation of segregation patterns of a diploid gamete with a reciprocal balanced translocation. Here, exchanges have occurred between the short arms of chromosomes 1 and 3. The two pairs of chromosomes pair in a quadriradial fashion. There are three potential axes in which the cell can divide. Only two of the six potential gametes will be genetically balanced. (Courtesy Edith Cheng, MD.)

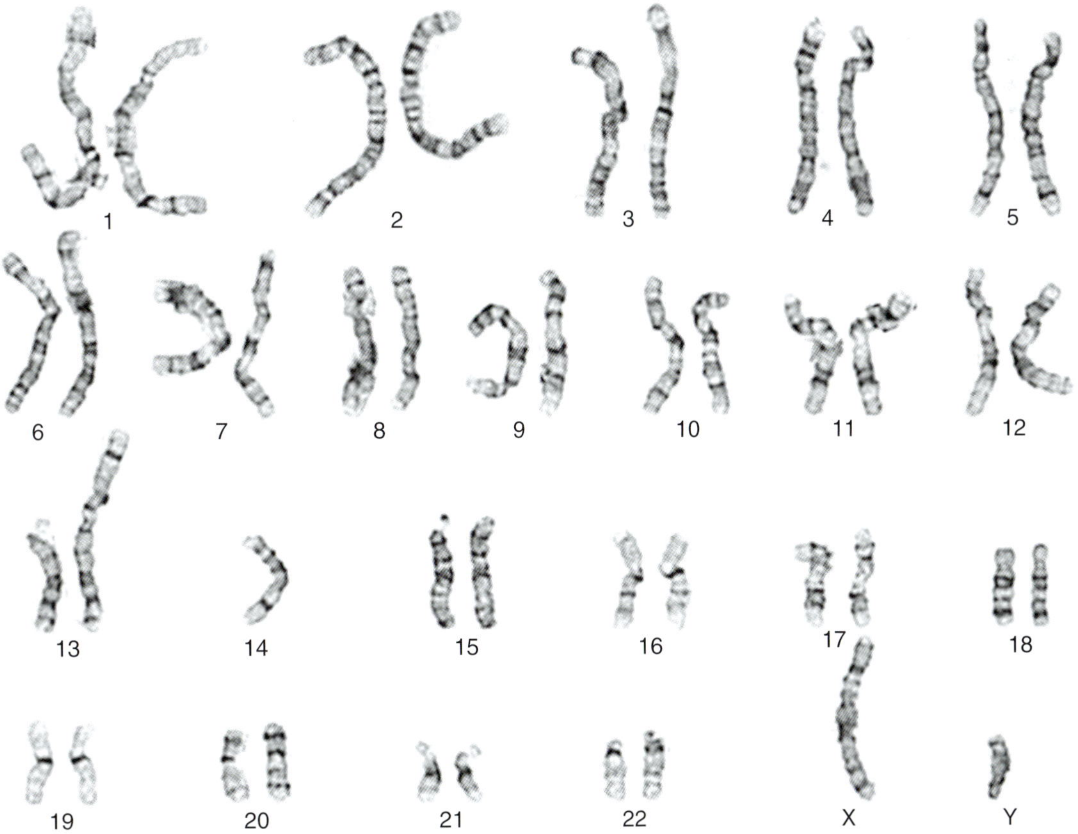


**Fig. 2.11** Karyotype demonstrating a Robertsonian translocation between chromosomes 13 and 14. Notice that there are only 45 chromosome structures, but this man is genetically diploid. (Courtesy Edith Cheng, MD.)

information. However, an isochromosome involving the long arm of the X chromosome (iso Xq) is compatible with life.

Finally, deletions and duplications of chromosome segments arise from unequal crossing over at meiosis or from crossing over during pairing of inversions or reciprocal translocations. Breaks resulting in loss of chromosome material at the tip are called **terminal deletions**, and loss of chromosome material between two breaks within a chromosome is called an **interstitial deletion**. There are several well-documented terminal deletion syndromes. Cri du chat (5p−) syndrome, a well-described terminal deletion syndrome, is characterized by microcephaly, profound mental retardation, growth retardation, a unique facial appearance, and a distinctive catlike cry.

For each of the previously described structural chromosome rearrangements, counseling and prognosis in the prenatal diagnostic setting are critically dependent on comparison with parental karyotypes. Phenotype correlations, particularly with balanced translocations and inversions, may be highly variable and dependent on whether the chromosomal break points disrupt critical genes. If the rearrangement found in a fetal sample is inherited from one of the parents, there is a higher likelihood of a normal phenotype, whereas de novo structural rearrangements have an increased risk of microscopic missing genetic material with phenotypic consequences.

### Microdeletion/Duplication or Contiguous Gene Syndromes

The discussion in the previous section described only phenotypes associated with chromosomal abnormalities visible with traditional cytogenetic techniques and light microscopy, which implies involvement of large segments of chromosomes containing a large number (hundreds) of genes. High-resolution chromosome banding and advances in molecular cytogenetic technology have revealed a new class of chromosomal syndromes known as **microdeletions**. These are **contiguous gene syndromes** in which the involved chromosome regions are submicroscopic and so small that a molecular cytogenetic technique such as targeted fluorescence in situ hybridization (FISH) or some form of **sequence analysis is necessary to localize the affected region**. Table 2.6 lists some of the more commonly recognized syndromes, most of which are due to deletions; however, some duplication syndromes have now been identified. **The phenotypes of these conditions are due to the absence (or duplication) of multiple contiguous genes within the involved region**. Fine mapping of the breakpoints in some of these conditions has implicated unequal or abnormal recombination between low-copy repetitive DNA sequences in the area of the deleted or duplicated regions. The discovery of microdeletion/microduplication or contiguous gene syndromes has been important in clinical genetics and genetic counseling in that it finally provides a diagnosis, recurrence risk, and prenatal diagnosis for a large group of syndromes that previously had no cytogenetic confirmation. Moreover, these "naturally occurring" sequestered small regions of contiguous genes have provided a powerful tool for developmental geneticists to decipher the critical genes for normal human development. A common example of this concept is the 22q11 region, which appears to be rich in genes responsible for specific congenital heart defects and craniofacial anomalies. Importantly, **microdeletions and microduplications have no age-associated risk of occurrence** (Wapner, 2012).

## Chromosome Abnormalities and Pregnancy Outcome

The incidences and types of chromosomal abnormalities differ among spontaneous abortions, stillbirths, and live births. Experience from pregnancies achieved by assisted reproductive technology indicates that 15% of fertilized ova fail to divide. Another 15% fail to implant, and 25% to 30% are aborted spontaneously before formation of villi. Of the roughly 40% of fertilized ova that survive the first missed menstrual period, as many as one-fourth are aborted spontaneously, so only about 30% to 35% of fertilized ova actually result in live-born infants. Chromosomal and lethal genetic abnormalities play a major role in early losses (Zinaman, 1996). This topic is discussed further in Chapter 16. In continuing pregnancies, chromosomal abnormalities occur in 1 out of every 154 live births (0.6% overall incidence). The breakdown by the type of abnormality is as follows: 22% autosomal trisomy (most commonly trisomy 21, followed by a much lower incidence of trisomy 18 and trisomy 13), 37% sex chromosome aneuploidy, and 41% structural abnormalities (including translocations, insertions, inversions, isochromosomes, duplications, and deletions). **Trisomy 21 is the most commonly occurring singular genetic abnormality in live births,** occurring at a rate of 1 in 830 live births (0.1%) (Creasy, 2014).

# PERINATAL GENETICS

Technology is available to detect a wide range of the previously described genetic and biochemical abnormalities in a developing fetus. As a result, the indications to pursue screening or diagnostic testing for a patient who is pregnant or considering pregnancy include each of the following: known family history of a specific disease, family history suggestive of hereditary neurodevelopmental or cognitive disorders, ethnic background with increased carrier frequency of certain diseases, personal history of miscarriage or infertility, increased risk of aneuploidy related to maternal age

**TABLE 2.6** Common Microdeletion/Contiguous Gene Syndromes

| | | Chromosome | | |
|---|---|---|---|---|
| **Syndrome** | **Incidence** | **Location** | **Abnormality** | **Size (Mb)** |
| Sotos | Rare | 5q35 | Deletion | 2.2 |
| Smith-Magenis | 1/25,000 | 17p11.2 | Deletion and duplication | 4 |
| Williams-Beuren | 1/20,000-1/50,000 | 7q11.23 | Deletion | 1.5-1.8 |
| Charcot-Marie-Tooth type Ia/HNPP | 1/10,000 | 17p12 | Duplication and deletion | 1.5 |
| DiGeorge/velocardiofacial | 1/4,000 | 22q11.21-q11.23 | Deletion | 1.5 |
| Cat's eye | Rare | 22q11 | Duplication | 3 |
| der(22) Emanuel | Rare | | Duplication | 3 |
| Neurofibromatosis | 1/40,000-1/80,000 | 17q11 | Deletion | 1.5 |

*HNPP,* Hereditary neuropathy with liability to pressure palsies.

or previous aneuploidy, or an identified carrier couple based on genetic carrier screening.

## Genetic Counseling and Risk Assessment

Ordering and sending a genetic test is simple, but the counseling time to ensure appropriate interpretation of the results (positive or negative) is crucial and often time consuming. **The role of the care providers (genetic counselors and physicians) is to conduct nondirectional counseling of screening and diagnostic options to provide prospective parents with information to optimize pregnancy outcomes based on their personal values and preferences.**

All patients considering genetic screening or testing should have the opportunity to meet with providers who can perform formal pedigrees, conduct patient education and counseling on advantages and disadvantages of testing, and discuss the availability of screening and invasive diagnostic testing when needed. **Before screening or testing, the patient needs to understand the options that may ensue from a positive test result.**

Information regarding genetic carrier screening should be provided to all women considering pregnancy or currently pregnant. After counseling and consideration, screening may be accepted or declined. **The ideal time to consider carrier screening is before pregnancy**, so couples at increased risk for a genetic condition may incorporate the information into family planning, including consideration of whether to have children, available assistive reproductive techniques (in vitro fertilization [IVF] with preimplantation genetic diagnosis [PGD]) to minimize risk of disease in offspring, and prenatal diagnostic testing of at-risk pregnancies. **If an individual proceeds with carrier screening and is found to be a carrier of an autosomal recessive genetic condition, screening should be offered to the reproductive partner** as well to determine the risk of disease in any of their children. Screening should also be offered to family members of the known carrier, who may also be an increased risk of carrying the same variant. Individuals or reproductive couples who screen positive for genetic conditions should be referred for genetic counseling.

Diseases that should be included in carrier screening are determined by general population guidelines, patient autonomy, family history, and ethnic background (Table 2.7). Obtaining the family history of a reproductive couple may identify specific genetic conditions for screening recommendation. Screening may also be facilitated on patient request for conditions not recommended by other guidelines, as long as the patient has been properly counseled regarding the benefits, risks, and limitations of such screening. Recommendations state that all women who are considering pregnancy or who are pregnant should be offered carrier screening for cystic fibrosis and spinal muscular atrophy, regardless of family history or reported ethnic background.

## Common Diseases Included in Carrier Screening

Cystic fibrosis (CF) is an autosomal recessive genetic disease typically affecting pulmonary, pancreatic, and gastrointestinal systems; cognitive functions are not affected. Given advances in treatment, the average life expectancy for individuals affected with CF is now in the 40s. CF occurs in 1 in 2500 individuals in the non-Hispanic Caucasian population, with disease incidence being considerably less in other ethnicities. **More than 1700 pathogenic variants have been identified as causative for CF in the CFTR gene on chromosome 7, and a minimum panel of the 23 most common pathogenic variants developed by the American College of Medical Genetics and Genomics (ACMG) is recommended for general carrier screening.** DNA sequencing of the entire *CFTR* gene is not recommended for routine carrier screening, though it may be appropriate for consideration in specific situations in consultation with a genetics counselor or geneticist.

Spinal muscular atrophy (SMA) is an autosomal recessive genetic disease characterized by progressive degeneration of spinal cord motor neurons leading to atrophy of skeletal muscles and weakness. Genotype may not be predictive of the severity of phenotypes for this condition, though the most common form of SMA (accounting for 60% to 70% of patients with SMA), type 1 (Werdnig-Hoffman), is also the most severe, with symptom onset by 6 months of life and a life expectancy less than 2 years. There are at least three other subtypes of SMA with less severe phenotypes. SMA occurs in 1 in 6000 to 1 in 10,000 live births, with carrier frequency in the non-Hispanic Caucasian population

**TABLE 2.7** Common Autosomal Recessive Disorders in Ethnic Groups: Carrier Screening Recommended

| Ethnic Group | Genetic Disorder | Carrier Frequency in Ethnic Group | Frequency of Carrier Couples | Screening Test Available? | Detection Rate (%) |
|---|---|---|---|---|---|
| African ancestry | Sickle cell disease (HbS and C) | HbS, 1:10<br>HBC, 1:20 | 1:130 | Hb electrophoresis | 100 |
| | Sickle cell S–β-thalassemia | | | MCV, Hb electrophoresis | |
| | α-Thalassemia | | | MCV, DNA | |
| Ashkenazi Jews (and Jewish people of unknown descent) | Tay-Sachs disease | 1:30 | 1:150 | Hexosaminidase A level | 98 |
| | Canavan disease | 1:40 | 1:1600 | DNA pathogenic variant | |
| | Familial dysautonomia | 1/32 | 1:32 | DNA pathogenic variant | 99 |
| Chinese | α-Thalassemia | | 1:625 | MCV | |
| French Canadian, Cajun | Tay-Sachs disease | | | Hexosaminidase A level | |
| Mediterranean (Italian/Greek/ Turkish/ Spanish) | β-Thalassemia | | 1:900 | MCV | |
| All patients seeking preconception counseling (especially white patients of European origin) | Cystic fibrosis<br>Spinal Muscular Atrophy | 1:25-29<br>1:35-40 | 1:625 | DNA pathogenic variant | 80* |

From Creasy RK, Resnik R, Greene MF, et al. *Creasy and Resnik's Maternal-Fetal Medicine Principles and Practice*. 7th ed. Philadelphia: Elsevier; 2014.
*Hb*, Hemoglobin; *MCV*, mean corpuscular volume.
*Depends on ethnic group: 70% for southern European descent, 90% for northern European descent.

of 1 in 35 to 1 in 40. Disease frequency is less common in other ethnicities. **SMA is caused by pathogenic variants in the survival motor neuron gene (SMN1), and severity of the disease may be mitigated by higher number of SMN2 gene copies, though the exact phenotype cannot be predicted.** Most healthy noncarrier individuals have one *SMN1* gene on each chromosome 5, though a small number of individuals have two copies on the same chromosome and no copies on the other, making carrier detection more difficult. **Deletion of both SMN1 genes is causative for SMA in 95% of affected individuals**, though pathogenic variants within the gene may also be associated with disease. Approximately 2% of SMA cases are caused by one inherited pathogenic variant and one de novo pathogenic variant. Advances in treatment of SMA focus on delay of symptom onset and slowing disease progression, though the effectiveness of these treatments is still being researched and no curative treatments are available.

**Fragile X screening should be offered to all women with a family history of fragile X–associated disorders or intellectual disability or features associated with fragile X of unknown cause.** All women with unexplained ovarian insufficiency or elevated follicle-stimulating hormone levels when younger than age 40 should also be offered fragile X screening. Individuals who screen positive for fragile X intermediate or premutation alleles should be referred for genetic counseling. Universal screening for fragile X in individuals not at risk is not recommended by any organization, including the American College of Obstetricians and Gynecologists (ACOG) and ACMG, although it may be included as part of an expanded carrier screening panel.

A complete blood cell count with red blood cell indices should be performed on all women considering pregnancy or currently pregnant to assess for risk of both anemia and hemoglobinopathy. A hemoglobin electrophoresis should also be performed for women who report certain ethnic backgrounds (African, Mediterranean, Middle Eastern, Southeast Asian, or West Indian), given the known increased incidence of hemoglobinopathies in these populations. If red blood cell indices are microcytic, indicated by low mean corpuscular hemoglobin or low mean corpuscular volume, ferritin studies and hemoglobin electrophoresis should be performed to differentiate between iron deficiency anemias and hemoglobinopathies. **The most common hemoglobinopathies include sickle cell anemia, alpha-thalassemia and beta-thalassemia, all of which are autosomal recessive genetic conditions affecting the structure and function of hemoglobin in red blood cells.** Given the complexity of these conditions and the possible variations of hemolytic disease, individuals who screen positive for a hemoglobinopathy should be referred for genetic counseling.

**Individuals who report Eastern, Central European, or unspecified Jewish descent should be offered genetic carrier screening for a number of autosomal recessive genetic conditions with higher disease incidence in the Ashkenazi Jewish population.** Genetic screening panels including cystic fibrosis, Tay-Sachs disease, Canavan disease, and familial dysautonomia should be offered to anyone reporting Jewish ancestry. More comprehensive panels for individuals reporting Ashkenazi Jewish ancestry may include additional conditions, such as Bloom syndrome, familial hyperinsulinism, Fanconi anemia, Gaucher disease, Glycogen storage disease type 1, Joubert syndrome, maple syrup urine disease, mucolipidosis type IV, Niemann-Pick disease, and Usher syndrome, though this list is not comprehensive. When only one partner of a reproductive couple reports Jewish ancestry, that partner should be offered carrier screening first. If that partner is found to be a carrier of the condition, then the other partner should be offered screening for the condition, though detection rates for many of these conditions in non-Jewish ethnic groups is unknown, so residual risk assessment of disease may be difficult.

Tay-Sachs disease is an autosomal recessive genetic lysosomal storage disease characterized by severe, progressive neurodegeneration. Deficiency in the enzyme hexosaminidase A leads to accumulation of GM2 gangliosides throughout the body, and damage in the central nervous system results in early childhood death in affected individuals. Approximately 1 in 30 individuals in the Ashkenazi Jewish population are carriers of Tay-Sachs disease. Three pathogenic variants in the *HEXA* gene on chromosome 15 account for 98% of carriers of Tay-Sachs disease in the Ashkenazi Jewish population. Individuals reporting French Canadian or Cajun ancestry also have a carrier frequency higher than the general population (1 in 30 to 1 in 50), and should also be offered screening for Tay-Sachs, with deletions accounting for a greater percent of carriers. The carrier rate for Tay-Sachs in the general population is estimated to be approximately 1 in 300. Carrier testing for Tay-Sachs can be performed via DNA variant analysis or hexosaminidase enzymatic activity testing on serum or leukocytes. Enzyme testing should be performed on leukocytes in pregnant women and women taking oral contraceptives, given a known increased false positive rate associated with serum testing in these populations. The enzyme assay will detect 98% of all carriers, regardless of ethnicity. In comparison, targeted molecular genetic testing is highly effective in groups at the highest risk but may be less effective in the general population.

**Testing for a specific disease may be warranted by family history or ethnic background, and prenatal diagnosis may potentially allow interventions before the disease would have been detected in the child clinically.** In some rare cases, diagnosis in utero may allow the opportunity to preclude irreversible changes in early development. However, the provider must relay the **scope** and **accuracy** of available testing modalities. For instance, a test that detects a phenotypic manifestation of disease (such as biochemical screening of hexosaminidase activity to assess for Tay-Sachs disease) is more sensitive for detecting an affected fetus than a genetic sequence panel that may include only a subset of the pathogenic variants. Alternatively, combination testing panels may be available that allow assessment for multiple diseases at once, but all tests are based on the same molecular methods, such as DNA sequence or SNP analysis, so sensitivity of detection for specific diseases may be sacrificed. The increasing availability of these "expanded carrier screening panels" has prompted ACOG to issue guidelines for patient consent before offering expanded screening (Edwards, 2015):

1. Carrier screening of any nature is voluntary, and it is reasonable to accept or decline.
2. Results of genetic testing are confidential and protected in health insurance and employment by the Genetic Information Non-Discrimination Act of 2008.
3. Conditions included on expanded carrier screening panels vary in severity. Many are associated with significant adverse outcomes such as cognitive impairment, decreased life expectancy, and need for medical or surgical intervention.
4. Pregnancy risk assessment depends on accurate knowledge of paternity. If the biologic father is not available for carrier screening, accurate risk assessment for recessive conditions is not possible.
5. A negative screen does not eliminate risk to offspring.
6. Because expanded carrier screening includes a large number of disorders, it is common to identify carriers for one or more conditions. In most cases, being a carrier of an autosomal recessive condition has no clinical consequences for the individual carrier. If each partner is identified as a carrier of a different autosomal recessive condition, offspring are not likely to be affected.
7. In some instances, individuals may learn that they have two pathogenic variants for a condition (homozygous or compound heterozygous) and thus learn through carrier screening that they have an autosomal recessive condition that could affect their personal health. Some expanded screening panels

screen for selected autosomal dominant and X-linked conditions, and likewise individuals may learn that they have one of these conditions that might affect their health. Referral to an appropriate specialist for medical management and genetic counseling is indicated in such circumstances to review the inheritance patterns, recurrence risks, and clinical features.

## Genetic Testing

Although genetic assessment in some form has become commonplace, it is critically important that providers and patients carefully consider the objectives and potential results of the individual testing options before selecting a test. In the case of aneuploidy screening, the assayed markers only pertain to a **subset** of genetic material (usually the most common trisomies, affecting chromosomes 21, 13, 18, and possibly sex chromosomes), and abnormal results require follow up before any diagnosis can be made. Measuring the value of screening tests is traditionally based on sensitivity (detection rate), false-positive rate, and positive predictive value within a population. **The predictive value of these tests, or the chance that a positive or negative result is a true positive or true negative, is highly dependent on the prevalence of the disease in the population.**

### Biochemical and Sonographic Screening

Multiple screening options are available for detecting fetuses at risk for the most common aneuploidy syndromes, namely trisomies 21, 18, and 13. The choice of test depends on the gestational age at presentation, number of fetuses, obstetric history, family history, availability of sonologists or sonographers certified to detect or measure test parameters, and options or preferences for pregnancy termination.

**First-trimester aneuploidy screening typically consists of serum measurement of pregnancy-associated plasma protein A (PAPP-A) and either free or total beta human chorionic gonadotropin (b-hCG) combined with sonographic measurement of the fluid collection at the back of the fetal neck** called the **nuchal translucency** (the three measurements together are called **combined first-trimester screening**). The inclusion of additional analytes (e.g., alpha-fetoprotein [AFP]) and fetal nasal bone assessment with first-trimester screening can increase detection rates for Down syndrome. Nuchal translucency measurements are performed from 10 0/7 weeks to 13 6/7 weeks as determined by crown-rump length measurements between 45 to 84 mm. Guidelines for measurement are standardized and must be followed for the test to maintain published detection rates. A risk estimate for fetal aneuploidy is then generated using these results, as well as information regarding maternal age, weight, race, history of aneuploidy, and number of fetuses. A nuchal translucency measurement less than 3 mm is considered normal (Malone, 2005). The primary advantage of first-trimester screening is earlier results, which allow for greater privacy and broader options of diagnostic testing and reproductive choices.

**Second-trimester biochemical screening for aneuploidy** (available between about 15 0/7 weeks and 22 6/7 weeks' gestation) **combines measurement of maternal serum AFP (msAFP), hCG, and unconjugated estriol (to make up the "triple screen"), and it may include dimeric inhibin A (called a quad screen)**. These analytes, in addition to maternal factors such as age, weight, race, presence of diabetes, and fetal number, are used to calculate a risk estimate. In addition, msAFP can be obtained for the detection of neural tube defects when measured between 16 to 18 weeks' gestation. Various iterations of screening tests are available that combine elements of both first- and second-trimester screening measurements, and the performance statistics of these methods depend on the specific analytes included, whether the measurements are independent of one another, and the timing of risk calculation. **The most favorable performance statistics are achieved with the "integrated screening" approach, which combines first-trimester PAPP-A and nuchal translucency with quad markers in the second trimester, and results are not reported until all measurements are obtained.** This method has a Down syndrome detection rate of 94% to 96% with a false-positive rate of 5%; however, the advantage of an early result is lost if first-trimester screening results are withheld until second-trimester screening results have been obtained (Malone, 2005), and most patients do not wish to have their first-trimester results held until second-trimester screening is completed.

**Abnormal results of some of the individual elements assayed in aneuploidy screening are also predictive of adverse pregnancy outcomes.** Maternal serum levels of PAPP-A in the first trimester that are less than the 5% are associated with increased risks for fetal growth restriction, preeclampsia, placental abruption, preterm delivery, and spontaneous fetal or neonatal loss (Dugoff, 2004). Elevated hCG, AFP, or dimeric inhibin A in the second trimester, without structural anomalies seen on ultrasound, are associated with fetal growth restriction, intrauterine fetal demise, and preeclampsia (Chandra, 2003; Dugoff, 2005). Additionally, low estriol has been associated with Smith-Lemli-Opitz and X-linked ichthyosis. However, the follow-up for patients with these abnormal analytes remains variable and institutionally dependent, and it is unclear if outcomes are affected by antenatal fetal testing or follow-up ultrasound examinations.

### Cell-Free DNA Screening

Prenatal screening for fetal aneuploidy has evolved rapidly, with cell-free DNA (cfDNA) serving as an example of testing's quick integration into prenatal care. Initially described in 1997 (Lo, 1997), cfDNA is a technology to assess single-gene disorders for which the abnormal DNA sequence is known in the family, or for determination of fetal gender in cases of families carrying traits for X-linked recessive diseases. Early attempts at noninvasive genetically based prenatal screening were focused on isolation of intact fetal cells within the maternal circulation. To date, this technology has been unsuitable for clinical application because of multiple technologic obstacles such as limited numbers of fetal cells, unreliable recovery of fetal cells, and evidence that the cells persist long after pregnancy, thus complicating specificity in the setting of subsequent pregnancies (Bianchi, 2002). In contrast, the development of methods to identify fetal-derived cfDNA in maternal plasma has been more successful. In 2011 cfDNA aneuploidy screening had its clinical introduction in the United States and Asia, followed by Canada and Europe in 2012.

**In maternal plasma, cfDNA consists of small fragments of maternal and fetal DNA. The fetal component is primarily derived from placental cells undergoing apoptosis or programmed cell death** (Ashoor, 2013). It may be detected as early as 4 weeks' gestation, continues to increase throughout gestation, and is cleared within hours after childbirth (Lo, 1997). The amount of fetal cfDNA to maternal cfDNA is referred to as the fetal fraction. **Studies suggest that a fetal fraction of at least 4% is necessary for a reliable result with cfDNA testing, and testing can generally be performed as early as 9 to 10 weeks' gestation** (Norton, 2012).

**The cfDNA testing is widely used to screen for trisomy 21, trisomy 18, trisomy 13, and sex chromosome aneuploidy.** Other potential applications include assessing for fetal Rh determination, microdeletions, and other single-gene disorders. Screening with cfDNA has higher sensitivities and lower false positive rates than other screening modalities, and these detection rates and false positive rates do not differ with maternal age. However, positive predictive values of cfDNA results increase with maternal age given the increased prevalence of aneuploidy associated with advanced maternal age (Table 2.8).

TABLE 2.8 Cell-free DNA Screening Performance Characteristics

| Chromosomal Abnormality | Number of Affected Cases | Detection Rate % (95% CI) | False-Positive Rate % (95% CI) | Positive Predictive Value* 25-Year- Old | Positive Predictive Value* 40-Year- Old |
|---|---|---|---|---|---|
| Trisomy 21 | 1963 | 99.7 (99.1-99.9) | 0.04 (0.02-0.07) | 51% | 93% |
| Trisomy 18 | 563 | 97.9 ( 94.9-99.1) | 0.04 (0.03-0.07) | 15% | 69% |
| Trisomy 13 | 119 | 99.0 (65.8-100.0) | 0.04 (0.02-0.07) | 7% | 50% |
| Monosomy X | 36 | 95.8 (70.3-99.5) | 0.14 (0.05-0.38) | 41% | 41% |
| 47,XXY | 17† | 100.0 (83.6-97.8)† | 0.004 (0.0-0.08)† | 29% | 52% |
| 47,XYY | | | | 25% | 25% |
| 47,XXX | | | | 27% | 45% |

*Positive predictive values (PPVs) obtained using PPV calculator from https://www.perinatalquality.org/Vendors/NSGC/NIPT/.
†Pooled for 47,XXY; 47,XYY; and 47,XXX.
*CI*, Confidence interval.

**All women with a positive result or test failure should be offered genetic counseling and confirmatory diagnostic testing, given risk for false positives.** Diagnostic confirmation should always be obtained before irreversible action such as pregnancy termination. Causes of discrepant results include low fetal fraction of DNA, confined placental mosaicism, true fetal mosaicism, maternal sex chromosome abnormality, organ transplant, co-twin demise, maternal chromosome deletion, maternal tumor, and laboratory error. A "no-call" result may be due to low fetal fraction, assay failure, uninformative DNA pattern, or sampling/collection errors and occurs in 0.03% to 12.2% of samples. The incidence of these "no-call" rates is higher for sex chromosome aneuploidies than the trisomies, and low fetal fraction may account for 0.1% to 6.1% of "no calls." Increased chance of a "no-call" result because of low fetal fraction has been associated with elevated body mass index (BMI), early gestational age, fetal aneuploidy, or treatment with low-molecular-weight heparin (Burns, 2017).

Several testing platforms are available for fetal cfDNA analysis using next-generation sequencing technology, including whole-genome sequencing (massively parallel sequencing), sequencing of select chromosome regions (targeted sequencing), and SNP analysis. These varying modalities all have similar sensitivities and specificities regarding aneuploidy screening. However, the different methodologies allow for different applications because of varying strengths and limitations.

Until recently, guidelines from multiple U.S. and international professional societies recommended the use of cfDNA screening be limited to women with increased risk of fetal aneuploidy. Women at increased risk of fetal aneuploidy include women of advanced maternal age (older than 35 years at delivery); women with ultrasound findings indicating increased risk of trisomy 13, 18, or 21; pregnancy history of a fetus with trisomy 13, 18, or 21; biochemical screening result positive for increased risk of aneuploidy; and a known parental balanced Robertsonian translocation with increased risk of trisomy 13 or 21. The relatively lower contribution of Down syndrome to all congenital anomalies in a low-risk cohort argues for the use of a screening tool with a broader scope. **cfDNA is the most sensitive and specific screening test for the common aneuploidies. ACOG states that all prenatal genetic screening and testing options should be discussed and offered to all patients regardless of maternal age or risk of chromosomal abnormality.** After review and discussion, every patient has the right to pursue or decline prenatal screening and diagnostic testing (ACOG, 2020). cfDNA screening can be used in multiple gestations but is limited in that results do not distinguish if one fetus is euploid and the other is aneuploid and data are lacking regarding diagnostic accuracy. Women with positive conventional screening test results may elect to have cfDNA screening before diagnostic testing; however, they should be counseled regarding a 2% residual risk of fetal aneuploidy with a normal cfDNA result (ACOG, 2019). It has been reported that when abnormal traditional aneuploidy screening results lead to abnormal results on invasive diagnostic testing, 17% of those fetal chromosomal abnormalities would not have been detected by cfDNA screening. Such aneuploidies include mosaic cases of trisomy 21, 18, or 13; mosaic sex chromosome aneuploidies; balanced and unbalanced rearrangements; other trisomies, insertions, and deletions; and triploidy, tetraploidy, and extrastructurally abnormal chromosomes (Norton, 2014).

Some laboratories have extended their cfDNA screening panels to include microdeletion syndromes such as 22q11.2 (DiGeorge), 5p deletion (Cri du chat), 4p deletion (Wolf-Hirschhorn), 1p36 deletion syndrome, and Prader-Willi and Angelman syndromes. Microdeletions are a significant cause of neurocognitive abnormalities; thus validation of microdeletion testing form cfDNA samples could significantly expand the utility of cfDNA in the obstetric population. Because of the low prevalence of these syndromes, it is difficult to provide validation for microdeletion screening using cfDNA, and therefore ACOG and SMFM do not support routine cfDNA screening for these microdeletion syndromes. **Invasive diagnostic testing via chorionic villus sampling (CVS) and amniocentesis with microarray analysis is the current recommendation for women who desire testing for microdeletions.**

Applications beyond aneuploidy for cfDNA testing also include screening pregnancies for single-gene disorders, which may arise as a result of advanced paternal age or de novo autosomal dominant conditions. Clinical testing via cfDNA is available for such disorders, including Noonan syndrome, achondroplasia, osteogenesis imperfecta, neurofibromatosis, craniosynostosis syndromes, congenital adrenal hyperplasia, and many others. However, there are not sufficient data regarding the accuracy and positive and negative predictive values in the general population. Thus single-gene cfDNA screening to test for such conditions in pregnancy is not recommended (ACOG, 2019).

## Diagnostic Techniques for Genetic Abnormalities

### Invasive Prenatal Diagnostic Tests

For the goal of prenatal **diagnosis**, the most commonly employed forms of genetic testing are chorionic villus sampling and amniocentesis to obtain cellular samples from pregnancy tissue for cytogenetic analysis.

In the early days of prenatal diagnosis, invasive testing options were offered to women with a high age-related risk of aneuploidy. However, ACOG recommendations now are that **all women,**

**regardless of age or risk, be offered biochemical or ultrasound screening and invasive testing** (ACOG, 2020). The decision to pursue invasive testing must incorporate considerations of level of risk that the fetus is affected, level of risk associated with the procedure, and the patient's personal impression of the impact of having an affected child. Of note, the risks involved with invasive testing may be much lower than estimates that have been quoted since the advent of invasive testing in the 1970s. Results of a meta-analysis that included only contemporary large studies (published after the year 2000, reporting on more than 1000 procedures) demonstrated no significant difference in the risk of miscarriage before 24 weeks' gestation for women undergoing amniocentesis or CVS compared with those who do not have invasive testing (Akolekar, 2015). Procedure-related risk of miscarriage for amniocentesis was 0.5%, and for CVS it was 1.0%. Studies suggest that the risk of amniocentesis is more likely to be approximately 0.1% and for CVS approximately 0.2% for complications that could lead to miscarriage (ACOG, 2009).

Nevertheless, rates of performance of these invasive procedures are significantly declining as screening tests with higher detection rates and lower false-positive rates have become available (e.g., cfDNA screening). It is important to note that **the range of abnormalities that can be detected is far greater with invasive testing than with any available noninvasive screening tests.**

**CVS** can be performed early in pregnancy (10 0/7 to 13 6/7 weeks' gestation); in this case **a biopsy specimen of cytotrophoblast tissue is obtained via ultrasound-guided transabdominal or transcervical route.** The patient should be aware of a small rate (1.1%) of indicated follow-up testing to resolve issues of maternal cell contamination or placental mosaicism, but overall cytogenetic diagnosis is successful in 99.7% of those tested (Ledbetter, 1990).

**Amniocentesis, generally performed after 15 completed weeks of pregnancy, involves ultrasound-guided transabdominal collection of amniotic fluid containing sloughed fetal cells from skin, gastrointestinal tract, amnion, and genitourinary tract.**

CVS or amniocentesis samples are predominately used for cytogenetic karyotype analysis. Cells can be analyzed directly or after about a week of cell culture to synchronize cells in metaphase for chromosomal Giemsa staining, or G-banding. With this type of staining, each chromosome has a unique pattern. The stained chromosomes are visualized under light microscopy, and large deletions or rearrangements can be detected (resolution on the order of 5 to 10 million bp, or Mb). Higher resolution or more specific testing for known disease-causing chromosome regions such as 22q11 requires molecular cytogenetic technology. The most widely used procedure is FISH, which takes advantage of the complementary nature of DNA. In this approach, denatured DNA sequences labeled with a fluorescent dye are hybridized onto denatured chromosomes that have been immobilized on a slide. The chromosomes are then viewed with a wavelength of light that excites the fluorescent dye (Fig. 2.12). **FISH is a powerful tool to confirm or diagnose syndromes caused by microdeletions of segments of chromosomal material** (Fig. 2.13).

At the individual gene level, disease-specific testing for families that carry known genetic variants may be performed on cells from either of these invasive methods using polymerase chain reaction (PCR)–based methods (discussed later). An updated list of relatively common genetic conditions for which DNA-based prenatal diagnosis is available is kept on the Genetic Testing Registry website (www.ncbi.nlm.nih.gov/gtr).

Another powerful diagnostic and investigational tool for human chromosome analysis directly expanded from FISH technology is comparative genome hybridization (CGH). **CGH is used to measure differences in copy number or dosage of a particular chromosome segment.** Its initial application was in the study of gene dosage in normal and cancer cell lines (Fig. 2.14). This technology has since come into widespread use because of the development of automated platforms that allow

WCP: Chromosomes 1 and 4

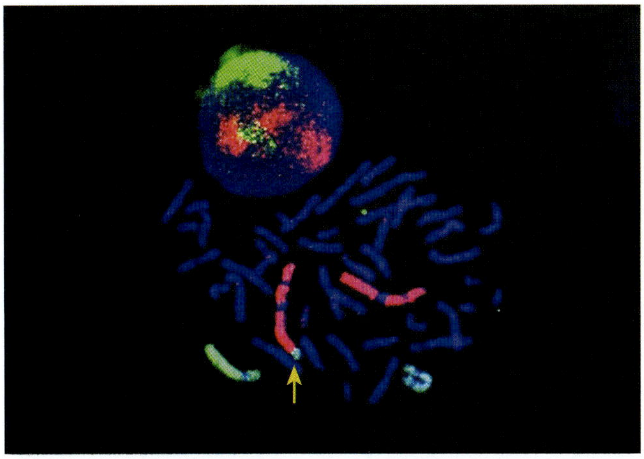

**Fig. 2.12** Example of fluorescence in situ hybridization (FISH) with whole-chromosome DNA (whole-chromosome paint [WCP]) from chromosomes 1 (red signal) and 4 (green signal) hybridized onto a metaphase nucleus containing all 46 chromosomes. This FISH study revealed a translocation of a piece of material from chromosome 4 onto chromosome 1. (Courtesy Lisa Shaffer, PhD, Washington State University.)

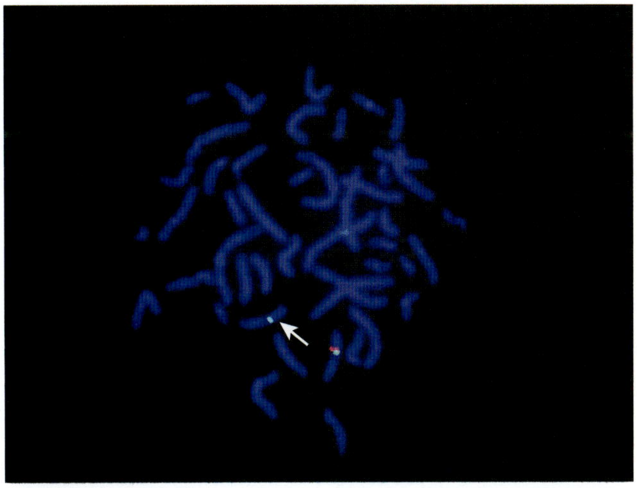

Deletion of 11p

**Fig. 2.13** Example of fluorescence in situ hybridization (FISH) technology in the diagnosis of microdeletion syndromes. Here, standard karyotyping appears to be normal. However, using FISH microdeletion probes, this child was discovered to have a submicroscopic deletion *(arrow)* of the terminal section of the long arm of chromosome 1. The other chromosome containing the red signal is the normal chromosome. (Courtesy Lisa Shaffer, PhD, Washington State University.)

for the assessment of thousands or even millions of DNA molecules at once at a rapidly decreasing cost.

## Molecular Genetic Analysis Techniques

### Polymerase Chain Reaction, Southern Blot, Restriction Fragment Length Polymorphism, Linkage

The use of PCR permits rapid, simultaneous amplification of a sequence of DNA or multiple different sequences for analysis. This is essentially a form of cloning because **PCR can selectively amplify a single sequence of DNA or RNA several billion fold in only a few hours.** By taking advantage of the double-stranded

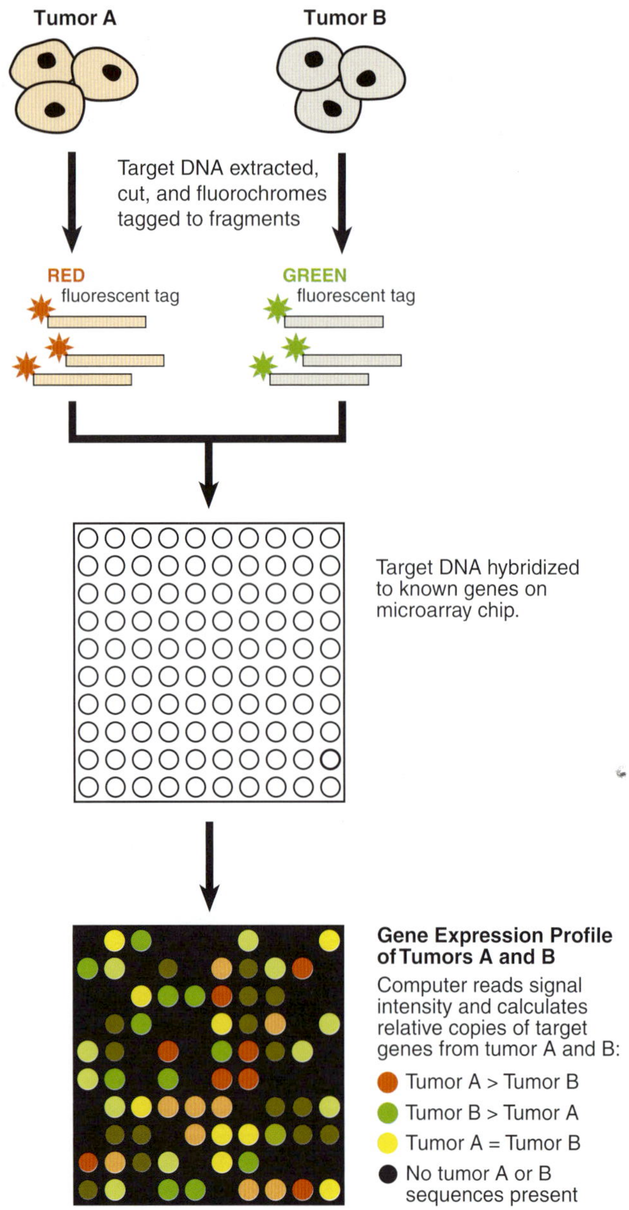


**Fig. 2.14** Schematic example of how microarray technology can be used to study or compare gene expression patterns from different sources. Here it is used to compare the gene expression profiles of two different tumors. However, one can easily substitute DNA from two individuals with diabetes. (Courtesy Edith Cheng, MD.)

complementary pairing characteristics of DNA, the PCR reaction separates (denatures) the two strands and uses each strand as a template to synthesize two more copies (Fig. 2.15). Target sequences of DNA flanked by primers undergo repeated cycles of heat penetration, hybridization with primers, and DNA synthesis, resulting in an exponential amplification of the target DNA sequence. The amplified DNA sequences can then be "cut" by bacterial enzymes, called **restriction endonucleases**, which recognize and cut specific nucleotide sequences (restriction sites) in the double-stranded DNA molecule. Each enzyme recognizes a unique sequence of nucleotides, usually a palindrome 4 to 8 bp long. Because of this sequence specificity, the pattern of DNA fragments resulting from restriction endonuclease digestion are unique to each gene sequence. The resulting fragments are separated by gel electrophoresis, transferred (blotted) onto a membrane, and hybridized with a radioactively labeled probe with a known sequence. This method, known as **Southern blotting**, permits identification of specific DNA fragments of interest and, in some cases, the number of copies of the fragment. Fig. 2.16 is an example of how Southern blotting is used to detect the sickle cell gene. Variants within a gene or near a gene can also alter the recognition sites of restriction endonucleases, which will generate an altered length of DNA fragment containing the gene of interest. These restriction fragment length polymorphisms (RFLPs) can be used to follow the transmission of a gene in a family.

When direct testing is not possible, as is the case when the disease-causing gene has not been isolated, when the gene is too large to sequence, or when a variant cannot be directly found, **indirect testing using linkage analysis is the alternative strategy**. The simplest explanation for the concept of linkage is that DNA markers located (or tightly linked) to the presumptive disease-causing gene or variant are used as road maps to identify the travel or passage of the gene from an affected parent to an at-risk offspring. This strategy requires that the affected individual has markers that are informative—in other words, unique or distinctive from markers of the nonaffected individual. Multiple family members, both affected and unaffected, must have DNA available for linkage analysis for this approach to be informative. The "markers" are often RFLPs. Fig. 2.17 uses autosomal dominant breast cancer as an example of how linkage studies are used to predict the inheritance of a gene for which direct variant analysis is not possible.

## Chromosomal Microarray

**Chromosomal microarray (CMA) is a high-throughput technique to detect the relative "dose" of genetic material by comparison with a reference standard.** A microarray generally consists of a thin slice of glass or silicon about the size of a postage stamp on which threads of synthetic nucleic acids are arrayed. Sample probes are added to the chip, and matches are read by an electronic scanner. **The resolution of CMA is on the order of 10 to 400 kb, or more than 100-fold greater resolution than traditional G-banding karyotyping.**

There are two general platforms in common use for genome assessment. The first is a form of comparative genomic hybridization, or "array CGH." In brief, two genomic libraries are mixed and hybridized to a panel of reference sequences such that relative "doses" of hybridized sequence can be quantitated. Using this platform, a patient's genome is compared with a normal control, and a readout is expressed by comparative intensity between the patient and the control (Snijders, 2001).

The second popular platform is an SNP array. In an SNP array, probes are chosen from DNA locations known to vary by a single base pair. A patient's DNA is hybridized to the array (note that this platform does not require a normal standard), and readout is by absolute intensity of signal from bound DNA fragments. This method can detect more abnormalities than just copy number variants or deletions and duplications, such as uniparental disomy, zygosity, consanguinity, parent of origin for a given variant, and maternal cell contamination (Beaudet, 2008). A comparison of the various techniques can be seen in Table 2.9.

**In neonatal and pediatric studies, microarray results have revealed underlying genetic causes for 15% to 20% of cases with previously unexplained developmental delay, intellectual disability, or congenital anomalies.** Only about 3% of these cases would have been diagnosed by traditional karyotyping (Miller, 2010). Notably, the rate of pathogenic CNVs is higher than the risk of Down syndrome in women younger than age 36 years, and the risk of pathogenic CNV is four times higher than the risk of trisomy 21 in women younger than age 30.

In contrast to neonatal studies, which have the advantage of correlating genomic findings with complete physical examination

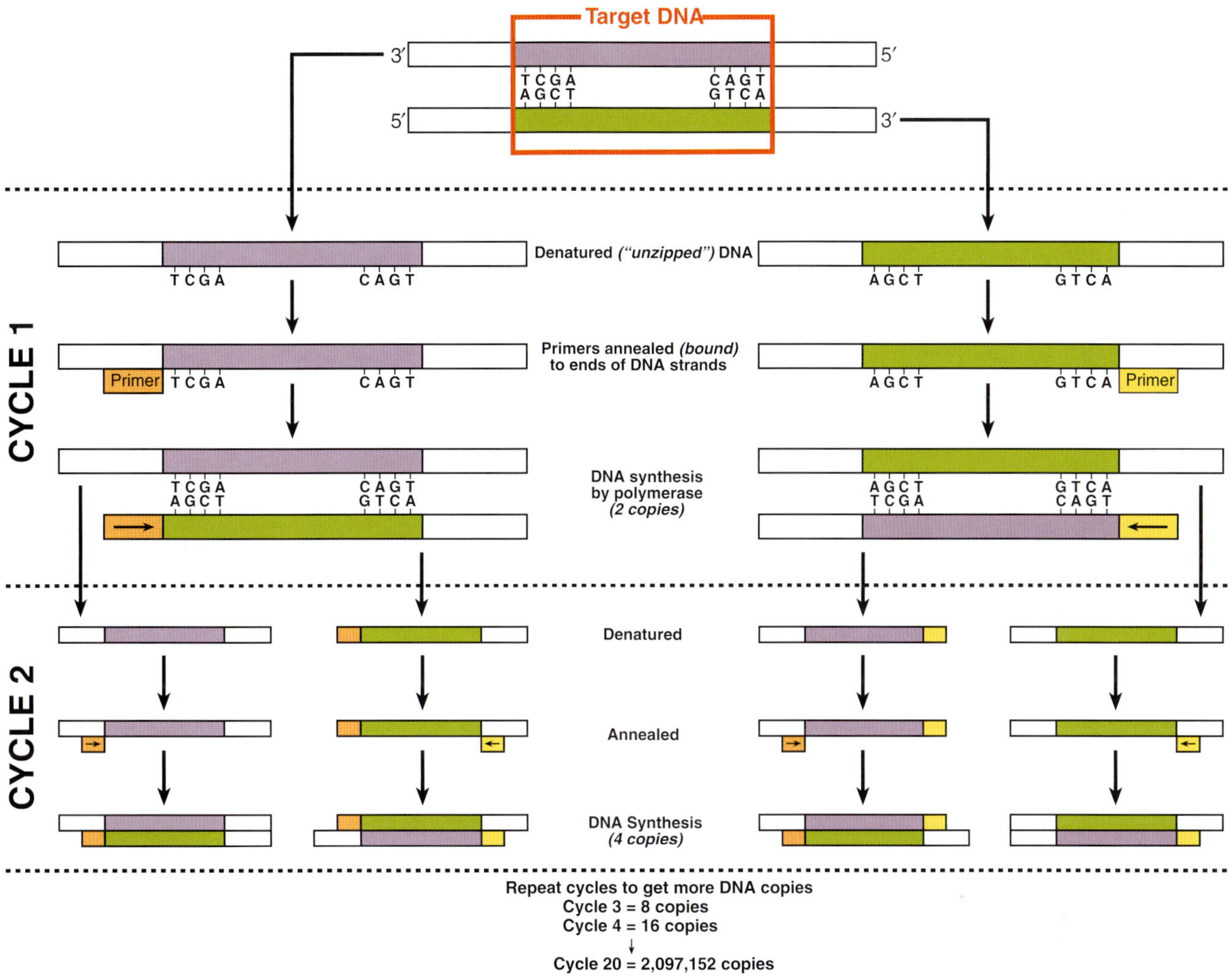


**Fig. 2.15** Schematic representation of the polymerase chain reaction. (Courtesy Edith Cheng, MD.)

results and behavioral phenotyping, prenatal applications are limited to phenotypic findings that can be detected by ultrasound. Several studies have demonstrated the incremental diagnostic utility of CMA analysis in the setting of a fetus with one or more anomalies on ultrasound but a normal karyotype. A prospective National Institute of Child Health and Human Development (NICHD) study identified clinically relevant copy number variants by microarray in 6% of anomalous fetuses with a normal karyotype and 1% to 1.7% of fetuses with a normal karyotype and normal anatomy on prenatal ultrasound examination (Wapner, 2012). Furthermore, the likelihood of identifying either pathogenic CNVs or CNVs of uncertain significance was more likely in fetuses with multiple anomalies, whereas for isolated findings, the greatest yield was in cardiac and renal anomalies (Donnelly, 2014). **CMA is considered the first-line test for an individual with unexplained birth defects or intellectual disabilities or in cases of unexplained fetal demise** (Hillman, 2015). In 2013 ACOG and SMFM jointly recommended that CMA should replace or supplement karyotyping in the evaluation of a fetus with anomalies. CMA should also be made available to any patient electing prenatal diagnostic testing. However, **despite the rise of CMA as first-line testing for fetal abnormalities, it is important to note that it cannot detect balanced translocations or inversions and, importantly, it cannot detect single-gene disorders such as cystic fibrosis and skeletal dysplasias**. Other logistic considerations that may ultimately affect a patient's choice of diagnostic testing include cost, insurance coverage, turnaround time for results, and gestational age.

Clinicians and genetic counselors must continue to exercise reasonable caution when interpreting results of microarray findings. Accurate genotype-phenotype correlations will require ongoing expansion of CNV databases. Many CNVs may have dose-dependent phenotypic effects or may be modified by the presence of other genotypic variants.

Traditionally, screening modalities focused on diseases that significantly affect quality of life and have a fetal, neonatal, or early childhood onset and well-defined phenotype. In the postgenome era with high-throughput microarray technology, the identification of molecular alterations in DNA may reveal previously unrecognized genetic variants associated with disease. Yet variant recognition still outstrips our ability to interpret these alterations. Previously unreported and relatively rare variants with unknown phenotypes will be identified, which requires skilled counseling and interpretation to help patients decide what to do with this information. **Informing patients of variants of uncertain significance (VUS) may generate significant anxiety and negative anticipation.** Learning that one's fetus has a potential abnormality with unquantifiable risks of consequences naturally fosters apprehension, may lead to ambiguity about continuing the pregnancy, and has the potential to cast a shadow of worry in the parents' minds throughout the life of the child.

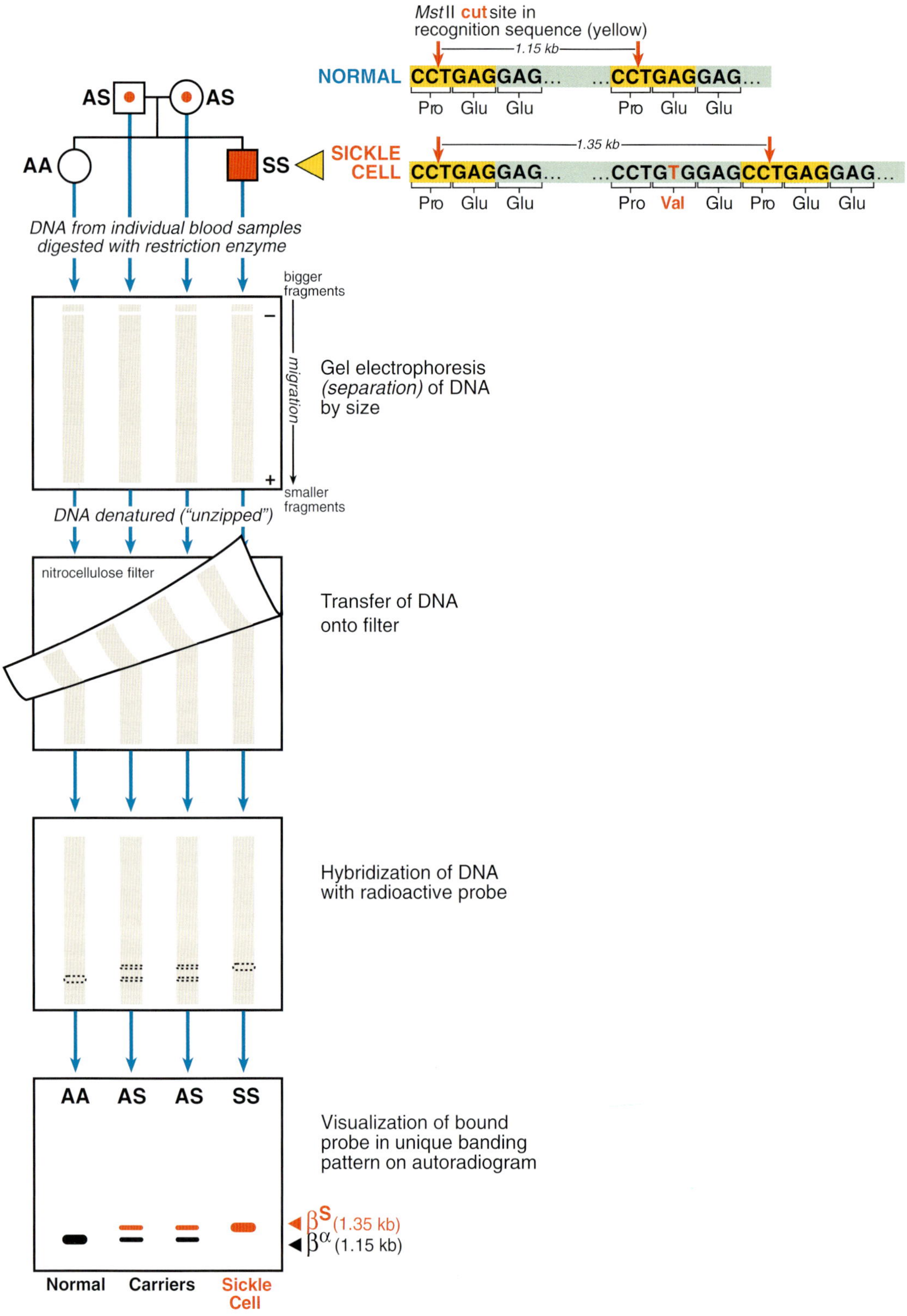


**Fig. 2.16** Schematic representation of the Southern blot procedure—in this case, for diagnosis of sickle cell disease. Genomic DNA from the carrier parents, an unaffected daughter, and the affected son is extracted from a sample of peripheral blood. The DNA samples are digested with restriction enzymes and fragmented into smaller pieces. In this case the restriction enzyme MstII is used specifically because it recognizes the normal sequences that encompass the codons for glutamic acid at position 6 of the hemoglobin A polypeptide. The DNA fragments are separated based on size by gel electrophoresis, then they are transferred (blotted) onto a nitrocellulose filter. The DNA of the filter paper is then hybridized with a specifically labeled DNA probe containing the sequences of interest. The fluorescent or radioactive probe is visualized as bands at sites where the genomic DNA has hybridized with the labeled DNA. *AA,* normal *AS,* carrier *SS,* sickle cell disease (Courtesy Edith Cheng, MD.)

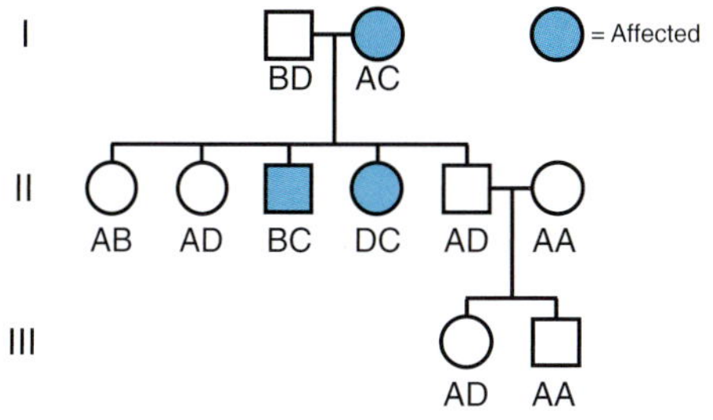


**Fig. 2.17** Hypothetical autosomal dominant condition illustrating the principle of indirect variant analysis. Genetic markers A, B, C, and D are used. In this pedigree, it appears that the condition segregates (travels) with marker C. Therefore the man and woman in generation III, who did not inherit marker C, are not expected to manifest the condition. (Courtesy Edith Cheng, MD.)

## Preimplantation Genetic Testing

**Preimplantation genetic diagnosis** once referred to single-cell extraction and genetic analysis from either an embryo or the polar body from an oocyte during the process of IVF (see Chapter 1). The initial impetus was to decrease the chances of propagating known genetic disorders in a family. The earliest application was in the setting of a patient known to carry an X-linked recessive gene, so only female embryos (by definition unaffected by the disease of interest) were transferred to the uterus. Since that time, the timing of cellular biopsy and options for genetic analysis have changed. Contemporary terminology is **preimplantation genetic testing (PGT) which consists of trophectoderm biopsy of the 5- to 6-day blastocyst, with amplification of DNA from 4 to 10 cells for analysis.** PGT-M (monogenic) and PGT-SR (chromosomal structural rearrangements) have become readily available for diagnosis of translocations, single-gene disorders, and inherited pathogenic variants that are known to cause cancer susceptibility syndromes. Preimplantation genetic testing for aneuploidy (PGT-A) is also available to screen for euploid embryos to increase the likelihood of positive pregnancy outcomes for certain clinical indications; however, it is not yet recommended for all IVF patients (ASRM, 2018). **Aneuploidy screening and confirmatory prenatal diagnostic testing should still be offered to all women with pregnancies achieved via IVF with PGT because testing does not eliminate risk of genetic disorders and is not 100% accurate.**

## Sequencing

**Sequencing determines the complete nucleotide sequence, or specific order of nucleotides in a gene.** By listing the full code, variations from an accepted "normal" (reference or consensus sequence) may be discovered. This has the potential to uncover pathogenic and benign variants and, given our limited understanding of how the genome is translated, will certainly identify variants of unknown significance to clinical phenotype.

**Clinical use of sequence data from the whole exome (the protein-coding region of DNA), or ultimately the whole genome, is considered the next frontier in genetic diagnostic techniques.** Whole-exome sequencing continues to raise the bar of expectation for molecular diagnosis with genetic analysis methods. The first large series of clinically applied whole-exome analysis touted a 25% molecular diagnosis rate among all patients referred for phenotypes suggesting a potential genetic component, and among patients in the study with a neurologic phenotype, molecular diagnosis was as high as 33% (Yang, 2013).

Goals of this magnitude have come within reach through development of **next-generation sequencing**. The original technique of sequencing, called **Sanger sequencing**, involves synthesizing multiple copies of DNA that is complementary to a single-stranded template of interest using nucleotide-specific chain terminators. This generates synthesized fragments of varying length that can be arranged by size, and the reactions containing each terminating base (A, T, G, or C) are kept separated. Then, by "reading" the terminating base of the synthesized copies from smallest to largest, the sequence of the original single-stranded template is revealed. This molecular method was revolutionary but very time consuming, labor intensive, and limited to relatively short DNA sequences. The quest to uncover the sequence of all 3 billion bases in the human genome propelled extraordinary improvements in scale, speed, and data management. Next-generation sequencing involves preparation of a full DNA library (no longer one small segment at a time) by amplifying (making many copies) and fragmenting the DNA source of interest (genomic DNA, coding DNA). The DNA library now consists of thousands or even millions of small overlapping DNA copy fragments, which are physically bound to a solid surface (platform specific, often beads or glass slides). The fragments are loaded into specialized multiplex machines for parallel sequencing; in other words, the sequence of every fragment on the surface can be assayed simultaneously. Individual sequence readings are subsequently aligned (recall the expected overlap as a result of random fragmentation of many identical copies of DNA) using various bioinformatics platforms for comparison with a reference sequence. The full set of aligned readings reveals the entire sequence of the starting DNA product. **Thus next-generation sequencing can apply the concept of Sanger sequencing to an entire genome with results produced in a matter of hours.**

At present, the practical clinical application of sequencing is to search one or many genes (or the whole genome) for a causative variant in the setting of a recognized abnormal phenotype. Particularly in pediatric literature, sequencing has been reported

**TABLE 2.9** Comparison of Detection of Diagnostic Technologies.

| Technology | Aneuploidy | Balanced Translocations and Inversions | Unbalanced Translocations | Triploidy | Long Contiguous Stretch of Homozygosity, Consanguinity, Zygosity, and Parentage | Copy Number Variants | Culture Required |
|---|---|---|---|---|---|---|---|
| G-banded karyotype | Yes | Yes | Yes | Yes | No | No | Yes |
| Comparative genomic hybridization array | Yes | No | Yes | No | No | Yes | No |
| SNP array | Yes | No | Yes | Yes | Yes | Yes | No |

From Norton M, Kuller J, Dugoff L, eds. *Perinatal Genetics*. St. Louis: Elsevier; 2019.
*SNP*, Single nucleotide polymorphism.

to identify the genetic cause in cases of rare malformation syndromes and previously unexplained neurodevelopmental morbidity. Sequencing can be useful in prenatal counseling or diagnosis if the specific pathogenic variant can be identified for a previous child affected by a genetic disorder. Consider, for example, a family with a child diagnosed with cystic fibrosis, but only one parent has one of the known CF pathogenic variants. Sequencing of the CF gene in the **proband,** or first affected child, may reveal the previously unrecognized causative pathogenic variant in that family.

Data generated from sequencing methods are vast. **The primary limitation of both whole-exome sequencing (WES) and whole-genome sequencing (WGS) is that accurate interpretation lags behind the ability to generate sequence data because although sequencing is high throughput, there are no similar high-throughput assays that assess putative pathologic sequence findings.** There is enough natural variation in the human genome that any putative finding requires rigorous validation at the level of sequence, molecular function, and interaction within the full biologic system. Many interrogation tools are available to assess protein-coding portions of the genome. However, the comprehension of the remaining 98.5% of the DNA sequence is relatively nascent, with no way to assay functional loss or gain from these regions (Goldstein, 2013). Therefore routine use of WES as a prenatal diagnostic test is not recommended because of insufficient validation (Best, 2017).

However, WES may have clinical utility in certain scenarios. WES may be offered in consultation with genetic specialists, often in a research setting, when standard genetic testing (karyotype or chromosomal microarray) is normal or uninformative, in the case of a fetus with multiple anomalies or a major structural anomaly, or in the case of a family history of recurrent fetal abnormalities or fetal loss with similar phenotypes (ISPD, 2018). A combination of trio analysis, in which fetal and both parental samples are sequenced and analyzed concurrently, focusing on multiple fetal anomalies, and cataloging variants increases the likelihood for timeliness and being able to offer an interpretation of the results. Data collection and sharing of results among laboratories, patients, and clinicians will also be imperative for the reinterpretation of older tests and developing a diagnosis. **Pretest counseling, obtaining informed consent, and results disclosure with posttest counseling should be performed by a multidisciplinary team with genetic expertise.** The ability to prenatally diagnose the cause of genetic disorders continues to grow and evolve with WES and WGS but is currently limited by cost, the invasive means necessary to obtain a sample, and genomic knowledge.

## GENETICS OF REPRODUCTIVE MALIGNANCIES

**All cancer is genetic. However, most cancer is not inherited.** For a normal cell line to be transformed into a malignant cell line, several genetic variants in that somatic cell line must occur that alter cell growth and differentiation. **All cells have mechanisms to either repair a pathogenic variant or inhibit growth and replication if errors in DNA occur. Thus before malignancy can arise, most cancer cells have to "escape" those repair functions.** The first pathogenic variants must occur in either DNA repair genes or genes that suppress growth of abnormal cells (the genes that maintain the integrity of the genome). Subsequent variants are then passed on to daughter cells. Increasing cell replications occur, and as pathogenic variants build up, some will allow the cell line to grow abnormally and often confer biologic advantages over surrounding normal cells. **When "enough" DNA change occurs, the resulting abnormal cells are capable of metastasizing, thereby usurping resources of vital organs and, without treatment, eventually may lead to death.** This process of the development of multiple sequential pathogenic variants is called the **multistep process of cancer.** In 5% to 10% of families with cancer, a germline (inherited) pathogenic variant is present that predisposes certain tissues to begin to move through the multistep series of variants more easily. More than 50 inherited cancer syndromes have been described, although the majority of these are inherited through highly penetrant pathogenic variants in a dominant fashion. These inherited cancer genes do not cause cancer; rather they allow cancer to "happen more easily." Inherited cancer syndromes that affect female organs are listed in (Table 2.10).

Carefully regulated cellular processes, such as differentiation, proliferation, and programmed cell death, are altered in cancer cells. The stages of carcinogenesis are termed **initiation** (single initial proliferative cell), **promotion** (acquired selective growth advantage), **progression** (tumor characteristics become irreversible), and **metastasis** (process by which cells are displaced). **The types of genes and genetic mechanisms involved in malignancy may be grouped into four categories: oncogenes, tumor suppressor genes, DNA repair genes, and epigenetic mechanisms.**

Oncogenes (gain of function) behave as growth-promoting genes, and they act in a genetically dominant manner. In other words, only one abnormal copy of the gene will produce a clinically relevant phenotype because of increased gene function. They originate from normal cellular genes called **proto-oncogenes.**

**TABLE 2.10** Inherited Cancer Syndromes Affecting Gynecologic Organ Systems

| Body Part | Cancer Syndrome | Gene Name/ Location |
|---|---|---|
| Breast | Inherited breast and ovarian cancer (autosomal dominant; tumor suppressor gene, involved in the maintenance of genomic stability) | *BRCA1,* 17q21 |
| | Inherited breast and ovarian cancer (autosomal dominant; tumor suppressor gene, involved in the maintenance of genomic stability) | *BRCA2,* 13q12.3 |
| | Li-Fraumeni (autosomal dominant; regulates the cell-cycle arrest that is required to permit repair of DNA damage) | *p53,* 17p13.1 |
| | Cowden | *PTEN,* 10q23.31 |
| | Peutz-Jeghers | *LKB1,* 19p13.3 |
| | $p16^{INK4a}$ | *CDKN2A,* 9p21.3 |
| | $p14^{arf}$ | *CDKN2A,* 9p21.3 |
| Endometrium | Chordoma | |
| | Cowden | |
| | Lynch syndrome (HNPCC) | |
| | Peutz-Jeghers | |
| Fallopian tube | Inherited breast and ovarian cancer | *BRCA1* |
| | Inherited breast and ovarian cancer | *BRCA2* |
| Ovarian | Basal cell nevus | |
| | Inherited breast and ovarian cancer | *BRCA1* |
| | Inherited breast and ovarian cancer | *BRCA2* |
| | Lynch syndrome (HNPCC) | |
| | Peutz-Jeghers | |
| Vulva | Fanconi | |

*HNPCC,* Hereditary nonpolyposis colorectal cancer.

The **proto-oncogenes have normal functions within a cell to control and enhance cell growth.** Oncogene activation (through introduction of pathogenic variants) can lead to either increased expression of proteins or changes in structure and function of a proto-oncogene's product. For example, the HER2/neu receptor may be overexpressed by an oncogene. Only a few inherited cancer syndromes involve oncogenes. Examples include the *RET*, *CDK4*, and *KIT* oncogenes. The *RET* oncogene is the underlying cause of multiple endocrine neoplasia (MEN type 2). These individuals have an increased risk of developing endocrine tumors.

**Tumor suppressor genes restrain cell growth in damaged cells**; therefore loss of the tumor suppressor gene through introduction of a pathogenic variant leads to increased cell proliferation of abnormal cells and cancer development. They account for the majority of autosomal dominant cancer syndromes. Some examples include *BRCA1* and *BRCA2* genes and the *P53* gene (Li-Fraumeni syndrome). Tumor suppressor genes are dominantly inherited. However, on the cellular level, they are recessive. In other words, a cell must have two genetic hits (one hit to each copy of the gene in question) before the cell can head down the multistep process to cancer. The first hit is inherited, and the second hit is acquired.

**DNA repair genes identify and mend DNA replication errors made during replication.** When they are nonfunctional, replication errors can lead to cancer development. Lynch syndrome (hereditary nonpolyposis colorectal cancer [HNPCC]) has at least four mismatch repair genes (*MLH1*, *MSH2*, *MSH6*, and *PMS2*) that predispose an individual to colon cancer and uterine cancer. One could imagine these genes as editors that find and correct spelling errors. Loss of their function allows pathogenic variants to accumulate and leads the daughter cells down the path of the multistep process of cancer. Other genes concentrate on repairing DNA sequences that were damaged by an external source such as radiation. Fanconi anemia, Bloom syndrome, ataxia-telangiectasia, and xeroderma pigmentosum are the few cancer syndromes that follow an autosomal recessive pattern of inheritance.

Epigenetic mechanisms, as discussed previously, involve alterations in patterns of DNA methylation or DNA packaging (a 3D structure determined by histone interaction and nucleosome positioning). **Cancer cells are often characterized by global loss of DNA methylation with paradoxical hypermethylation at CpG islands of certain promoters.** Coupled with aberrant packaging that may expose inappropriate genetic areas to allow transcription, the overall consequence is abnormal gene expression, either increased or decreased. One can use this clinically to try to identify the 3% to 5% of patients with endometrial cancer who have Lynch syndrome. **Lynch syndrome differs from other hereditary cancer syndromes in that the actual tumor tissue can be screened for Lynch syndrome using immunohistochemistry (IHC) for the four mismatch repair proteins (MLH1, MSH2, MSH6, PMS2), microsatellite instability (MSI) analysis, and MLH1 hypermethylation testing.** Positive tests require confirmatory diagnostic testing, but they help guide germline genetic testing. In an attempt to identify Lynch syndrome in women with endometrial cancer, the Society of Gynecologic Oncology Clinical Practice Statement on Screening for Lynch Syndrome in Endometrial Cancer recommends that **all women who are diagnosed with endometrial cancer should undergo systematic clinical screening for Lynch syndrome** (review of personal and family history) or molecular screening. Molecular screening of endometrial cancers for Lynch syndrome is the preferred strategy when resources are available (SGO, 2014).

When considering a family history of cancer, one should first obtain a complete history, including who has and who has not had cancer in the family. This information will help determine to which group the family likely belongs: **average risk** (sporadic—somatic cell changes), **moderate risk** (common exposures—somatic cell changes or low penetrance genes), or **high risk** (inherited cancer genes—germline pathogenic variants). For certain cancer syndromes, computer models are available to help determine the chance that a family has an inherited cancer syndrome. It is important to note that taking a detailed family history involves more than asking who has had cancer. One important factor to be cognizant of is the difference between primary cancers, recurrences, and metastatic disease. Patients rarely understand the subtleties of these important distinctions and inadvertently report inaccurate information. It is common for a woman to tell her physician about a family member who was treated for uterine cancer; however, on detailed history taking the physician finds that the woman had a procedure for cervical dysplasia. This type of information is critical to sort this out to provide a risk estimate. Once it is determined to which group the person belongs, an estimation of that person's risk to develop cancer can be determined, and, finally, an individualized cancer screening recommendations can be agreed on. Generally, at-risk patients should be referred to genetic counselors or medical geneticists with particular expertise in cancer genetics.

## CANCER GENOME SEQUENCING

With the advent of next-generation sequencing, several commercial entities are available to provide fast and relatively inexpensive tumor DNA sequencing, which has not only revolutionized genetic research on cancer but also created potentially new therapeutic opportunities as well. **Tumor specimens can be tested for a "panel" of genes with a known association to cancer, specifically looking for genetic variants that are "actionable" variants, in that pharmacologic agents exist that target these pathogenic variants.** Different tumor types can have genetic features in common, making them treatable with the same drugs aimed at the genetic defect. Consider trastuzumab (Herceptin), the first cancer drug approved for use with a DNA test to determine who should receive it (now there is also a protein-based test). The U.S. Food and Drug Administration (FDA) cleared it in 1998 to target breast cancers that overexpress the *HER2* gene, a change that drives the cancer cells to multiply. The same pathogenic variant has been found in gastric, ovarian, and other cancers. As a result of testing, the drug was approved in 2010 to treat patients with gastric cancers that overexpress the *HER2* gene. The potential application of the next-generation sequencing technology is vast but still must be subjected to scientific scrutiny before it replaces more standard treatment options. Even with the great advances in targeted therapies, personalized chemotherapeutic regimens, and immunotherapy, primary prevention and risk reduction strategies for the hereditary cancers, rather than treatment, should still be the gold standard of care.

## ETHICAL CONSIDERATIONS OF GENETIC DIAGNOSIS

Commonly identified pitfalls of identifying genetic anomalies that lead to formidable counseling challenges include VUS, identification of adult-onset disease or parental presymptomatic disorders, revelation of nonpaternity, unsuspected consanguinity, findings linked to diseases with variable expressivity, and microdeletions involving a gene linked to cancer development or progression. There are also growing concerns that complete sequence data may lead to overstated associations of disease with findings of genetic variation.

Prenatal genetic discovery, whether through cfDNA screening or direct analysis techniques such as CMA or exome sequencing, may have especially precarious consequences. **There is a relative paucity of information when basing disease prediction on genetic information alone.** Because of variations in the strength of association with a given phenotype, differences in penetrance, and the potential influence of other genetic or environmental factors on disease phenotype, the weight of the evidence for the reported finding must be carefully considered before irrevocable action such as pregnancy termination or fetal treatment is undertaken.

The potential impact even goes beyond the possibility of pregnancy termination. Consider the effect of incidental findings such as Mendelian diseases with **adult-onset symptoms or inherited pathogenic variants of cancer-associated genes**. This raises the risk of labeling the unborn child and the parents or extended family with a predestined illness. Furthermore, these findings may cause considerable unfounded anxiety throughout pregnancy and into childhood, depending on the strength of disease association.

Within the world of IVF, PGT has been used to identify unaffected embryos and to improve implantation and take-home pregnancy rates. In this quest for better clinical outcomes, **genome editing and modification** came into being, with the removal of harmful variants and easy insertion of other viable nucleotide variants into mammalian embryos. However, the risks of mosaicism and the uncertainty regarding what some of the modifications may bring created concern over the possible outcomes. **Transfer of mtDNA** is another area of ethical concern, with difficulties in how to police the efforts to remove pathogenic variants from maternal mtDNA and reduce the transmission of defective genes and disorders. **Amid the fears of unmonitored genetic engineering and the recognition of the importance of these technologies lies a balance between continued research and limiting the implantation in human embryos**.

At the outset of the Human Genome Project in 1990, the National Human Genome Research Institute established the Ethical, Legal, and Social Implications (ELSI) Program, a component of the extramural genomics research program of the National Institutes of Health (NIH) (McEwen, 2014). This program has focused on four high-priority areas: the use and interpretation of genetic information, clinical integration of genetic technology, issues surrounding genetics research, and public and professional education about these issues. Research such as the programs funded under ELSI are essential to establish basic guidelines; however, the uses and influence of genetic/genomic diagnosis are vast, and ultimately the individual provider must assume responsibility for pursuing and interpreting the information conscientiously.

## KEY REFERENCES


Akolekar R, Beta J, Picciarelli G, et al. Procedure-related risk of miscarriage following amniocentesis and chorionic villus sampling: a systematic review and meta-analysis. *Ultrasound Obstet Gynecol.* 2015;45(1):16-26.

Amberger JS, Bocchini CA, Schiettecatte F, et al. OMIM.org: Online Mendelian Inheritance in Man (OMIM®), an online catalog of human genes and genetic disorders. *Nucleic Acids Res.* 2015;43(Database issue):D789-D798.

American College of Obstetricians and Gynecologists (ACOG). Screening for fetal chromosomal abnormalities: ACOG Practice Bulletin, Number 226. *Obstet Gynecol.* 2020;136(4):e48-e69.

American College of Obstetricians and Gynecologists (ACOG). ACOG Practice Advisory: cell free DNA to screen for single-gene disorders. *Obstet Gynecol.* 2019. https://www.acog.org/clinical/clinical-guidance/practice-advisory/articles/2019/02/cell-free-dna-to-screen-for-single-gene-disorders

American College of Obstetricians and Gynecologists (ACOG). ACOG Committee Opinion No. 430: preimplantation genetic screening for aneuploidy. *Obstet Gynecol.* 2009;113(3):766-767.

American Society for Reproductive Medicine (ASRM), Practice Committees of the American Society for Reproductive Medicine and the Society for Assisted Reproductive Technology. The use of preimplantation genetic testing for aneuploidy (PGT-A): a committee opinion. *Fertil Steril.* 2018;109(3):429-436.

Ashoor G, Syngelaski A, Poon LC, Rezende JC, Nicolaides, KH. Fetal fraction in maternal plasmacell-free DNA at 11-13 weeks' gestation: relation to maternal and fetal characteristics. *Ultrasound Obstet Gynecol.* 2013;41:26-32.

Beaudet AL, Belmont JW. Array-based DNA diagnostics: let the revolution begin. *Annu Rev Med.* 2008;59:113-129.

Beck T, Hastings RK, Gollapudi S, et al. GWAS Central: a comprehensive resource for the comparison and interrogation of genome-wide association studies. *Eur J Hum Genet.* 2014;22(7):949-952.

Best S. Wou K, Vora N, et al. Promises, pitfalls and practicalities of prenatal whole exome sequencing. Prenat Diagn. 2017;38(1):10-19.

Bianchi DW, Simpson JL, Jackson LG, et al. Fetal gender and aneuploidy detection using fetal cells in maternal blood: analysis of NIFTY I data. National Institute of Child Health and Development Fetal Cell Isolation Study. *Prenat Diagn.* 2002;22(7):609-615.

Burns W, Koelper N, Barberio A, et al. The association between anticoagulation therapy, maternal characteristics, and a failed cfDNA test due to low fetal fraction. *Prenat Diagn.* 2017; 37:1125-1129.

Cariaso M, Lennon G. SNPedia: a wiki supporting personal genome annotation, interpretation and analysis. *Nucleic Acids Res.* 2012;40 (Database issue):D1308-D1312.

Chandra S, Scott H, Dodds L, et al. Unexplained elevated maternal serum alpha-fetoprotein and/or human chorionic gonadotropin and the risk of adverse outcomes. *Am J Obstet Gynecol.* 2003;189:775-781.

Creasy RK, Resnik R, Greene MF, et al. *Creasy and Resnik's* Maternal-Fetal Medicine Principles and Practice. 7th ed. Philadelphia: Elsevier; 2014.

Crick F. Central dogma of molecular biology. *Nature.* 1970;227(5258): 561-563.

Cummings CJ, Zoghbi HY. Fourteen and counting: unraveling trinucleotide repeat diseases. *Hum Mol Genet.* 2000;9(6):909-916.

Donnelly JC, Platt LD, Rebarber A, et al. Association of copy number variants with specific ultrasonographically detected fetal anomalies. *Obstet Gynecol.* 2014;124(1):83-90.

Davis CA, Hitz BC, Sloan CA et al. The Encyclopedia of DNA elements (ENCODE): data portal update. *Nucleic Acids Res.* 2018;46(D1): D794-D801.

Dugoff L, Hobbins JC, Malone FD, et al. First-trimester maternal serum PAPP-A and free-beta subunit human chorionic gonadotropin concentrations and nuchal translucency are associated with obstetric complications: a population-based screening study (the FASTER Trial). *Am J Obstet Gynecol.* 2004;191(4):1446-1451.

Dugoff L, Hobbins JC, Malone FD, et al. Quad screen as a predictor of adverse pregnancy outcome. FASTER Trial Research Consortium. *Obstet Gynecol.* 2005;106:260-267.

Edwards JG, Feldman G, Goldberg J, et al. Expanded carrier screening in reproductive medicine-points to consider: a joint statement of the American College of Medical Genetics and Genomics, American College of Obstetricians and Gynecologists, National Society of Genetic Counselors, Perinatal Quality Foundation, and Society for Maternal-Fetal Medicine. *Obstet Gynecol.* 2015;125(3):653-662.

Finucane B, Abrams L, Cronister A, Archibald AD, Bennett RL, McConkie-Rosell A. Genetic counseling and testing for FMR1 gene mutations: practice guidelines of the national society of genetic counselors. *J Genet Couns.* 2012;21:752-760.

Gerstein MB, Bruce C, Rozowsky JS, et al. What is a gene, post-ENCODE? History and updated definition. *Genome Res.* 2007;17(6):669-681.

Goldstein DB, Allen A, Keebler J, et al. Sequencing studies in human genetics: design and interpretation. *Nat Rev Genet.* 2013;14(7):460-470.

Hagerman PJ, Hagerman RJ. The fragile-X premutation: a maturing perspective. *Am J Hum Genet.* 2004;74(5):805-816.

Hillman SC, Willams D, Carss KJ, et al. Prenatal exome sequencing for fetuses with structural abnormalities: the next step. *Ultrasound Obstet Gynecol.* 2015;45(1):4-9.

Huang Y, Paxton WA, Wolinsky SM, et al. The role of a mutant CCR5 allele in HIV-1 transmission and disease progression. *Nat Med.* 1996;2(11):1240-1243.

Iafrate AJ, Feuk L, Rivera MN, et al. Detection of large-scale variation in the human genome. *Nat Genet.* 2004;36(9):949-951.

International Society for Prenatal Diagnosis. Joint Position Statement from the International Society for Prenatal Diagnosis (ISPD), the Society for Maternal Fetal Medicine (SMFM) and the Perinatal Quality Foundation (PQF) on the use of genome-wide sequencing for fetal diagnosis. *Prenat Diagn.* 2018;38(1):6-9.


**Full references and Suggested readings for this chapter can be found on ExpertConsult.com.**

# 3 Reproductive Anatomy

## Gross and Microscopic Clinical Correlations

*Jaclyn D. Nunziato, Fidel A. Valea*

### KEY POINTS

- The labia majora are homologous to the scrotum in the man. The labia minora are homologous to the penile urethra and a portion of the skin of the penis in men.
- The clitoris complex is composed of both erectile and nonerectile tissue and includes the glans, prepuce, body, crura, bulbs, suspensory ligament, and the root.
- The clitoral complex is the female homologue of the penis in the man and is a critical organ responsible for sexual arousal, function, and sexual health.
- The female urethra measures 3.5 to 5 cm long. The mucosa of the proximal two-thirds of the urethra is composed of stratified transitional epithelium, and the distal one-third is stratified squamous epithelium.
- When a woman is standing, the axis of the upper portion of the vagina lies close to the horizontal plane, with the upper portion of the vagina curving toward the hollow of the sacrum.
- The vaginal length increases with weight and height, and it decreases with age.
- The lower third of the vagina is in close anatomic relationship with the urogenital and pelvic diaphragms.
- The middle third of the vagina is supported by the levator ani muscles and the lower portion of the cardinal ligaments.
- The primary lymphatic drainage of the upper third of the vagina is to the external iliac nodes, the middle third of the vagina drains to the common and internal iliac nodes, and the lower third has a wide lymphatic distribution, including the common iliac, superficial inguinal, and perirectal nodes.
- Descriptive terms for pelvic organs are derived from the Latin root, whereas terms relating to surgical procedures are derived from the Greek root.
- The length and width of the endocervical canal vary. The width of the canal varies with the parity of the woman and changing hormonal levels. It is usually 2.5 to 3 cm long and 7 to 8 mm at its widest point.
- The fibromuscular cervical stroma is composed primarily of collagenous connective tissue and ground substance. The connective tissue contains approximately 15% smooth muscle cells and a small amount of elastic tissue.
- The major arterial supply to the cervix is located in the lateral cervical walls at the 3 and 9 o'clock positions.
- The pain fibers from the cervix accompany the parasympathetic fibers to the second, third, and fourth sacral segments.
- The transformation zone of the cervix encompasses the border of the squamous epithelium and columnar epithelium. The location of the transformation zone changes on the cervix depending on a woman's hormonal status.
- The uterus of a nulliparous woman is approximately 8 cm long, 5 cm wide, and 2.5 cm thick and weighs 40 to 50 g. In contrast, in a multiparous woman each measurement is approximately 1.2 cm larger and normal uterine weight is 20 to 30 g heavier. The maximal weight of a normal uterus is 110 g.
- In the majority of women the long axis of the uterus is both anteverted in respect to the long axis of the vagina and anteflexed in relation to the long axis of the cervix. However, a retroflexed uterus is a normal variant found in approximately 25% of women.
- The uterine and ovarian arteries provide the arterial blood supply of the uterus. The uterine arteries are large branches of the anterior division of the hypogastric arteries, whereas the ovarian arteries originate directly from the aorta.
- Afferent nerve fibers from the uterus enter the spinal cord at the eleventh and twelfth thoracic segments.
- The fallopian tubes are 10 to 14 cm long and are composed of four anatomic sections. Closest to the uterine cavity is the interstitial segment, followed by the narrow isthmic segment, then the wider ampullary segment, and distally the trumpet-shaped infundibular segment.
- The right fallopian tube and appendix are often anatomically adjacent. Clinically it may be difficult to differentiate inflammation of the upper portion of the genital tract and acute appendicitis.
- During the reproductive years, the ovaries measure approximately 1.5 cm × 2.5 cm × 4 cm.
- The ovary in nulliparous women rests in a depression of peritoneum named the *fossa ovarica.* Immediately adjacent to the ovarian fossa are the external iliac vessels, the ureter, and the obturator vessels and nerves.
- Three prominent ligaments determine the anatomic mobility of the ovary: the mesovarian, the ovarian ligament, and the infundibulopelvic ligament.
- The arterial supply of the pelvis is paired, bilateral, and has multiple collaterals and numerous anastomoses.
- The extent of collateral circulation after hypogastric artery ligation depends on the site of ligation and may be divided into three groups: branches from the aorta, branches from the external iliac arteries, and branches from the femoral arteries.
- The internal iliac nodes are found in an anatomic triangle whose sides are composed of the external iliac artery, the hypogastric artery, and the pelvic sidewall. This rich collection of nodes receives channels from every internal pelvic organ and the vulva, including the clitoris and urethra.
- The femoral triangle is the anatomic space lying immediately distal to the fold of the groin. The boundaries of the femoral triangle are the sartorius and adductor longus muscles and the inguinal ligament.
- The pudendal nerve and its branches supply the majority of both motor and sensory fibers to the muscles and skin of the vulvar region.
- The femoral nerve may be compromised by pressure on the psoas muscle during abdominal surgery and by hyperflexion of the leg during vaginal surgery.

*Continued*

**KEY POINTS—cont'd**

- The pelvic diaphragm is important in supporting both abdominal and pelvic viscera and facilitates equal distribution of intraabdominal pressure during activities such as coughing. The levator ani muscles constitute the greatest bulk of the pelvic diaphragm.
- The major function of the urogenital diaphragm is to support the urethra and maintain the urethrovesical junction.
- Contained within the broad ligaments are the following structures: oviducts, ovarian and round ligaments, ureters, ovarian and uterine arteries and veins, parametrial tissue, embryonic remnants of the mesonephric duct and Wolffian body, and two secondary ligaments.
- The cardinal ligaments provide the major support to the uterus.
- A congenital anomaly of a double, or bifid, ureter occurs in 1% to 4% of women.
- When the urinary bladder is empty, the ureteral orifices are approximately 2.5 cm apart. This distance increases to 5 cm when the bladder is distended.
- The distal ureter enters into the cardinal ligament. In this location the ureter is approximately 1 to 2 cm lateral to the uterine cervix and is surrounded by a plexus of veins. In approximately 12% of women, the cervix will be less than 0.5 cm from the cervix.
- Two ways of distinguishing the ureter from pelvic vessels are (1) identification of peristalsis after stimulation with a surgical instrument and (2) identification of Auerbach plexuses.
- Surgical compromise of the ureters may occur during clamping or ligating of the infundibulopelvic vessels, clamping or ligating of the cardinal ligaments, or wide suturing in the endopelvic fascia during an anterior repair.
- The following three important axioms should be in the forefront of decision making during difficult gynecologic surgery: (1) Do not assume that the anatomy of the left and right side of the pelvis are invariably identical mirror images; (2) during difficult operations with multiple adhesions, operate from known anatomic areas into the unknown; and (3) from the sage advice of a distinguished Canadian gynecologist, Dr. Henry McDuff: "If the disease be rampant and the anatomy obscure, and the plans of dissection not pristine and pure, do not be afraid, nor faint of heart, try the retroperitoneum, it's a great place to start."

**Accompanying videos for this chapter are available on ExpertConsult.com.**

The organs of the female reproductive tract are classically divided into the external and the internal genitalia. The external genital organs are present in the perineal area and include the mons pubis, clitoris, urinary meatus, labia majora, labia minora, vestibule, Bartholin glands, and periurethral glands. The internal genital organs are located in the true pelvis and include the vagina, uterus, cervix, oviducts, ovaries, and surrounding supporting structures. This chapter integrates the basic anatomy of the female pelvis with clinical situations.

Embryologically, the urinary, reproductive, and gastrointestinal tracts develop in close proximity. This relationship continues throughout a woman's life span. In adults the reproductive organs are in intimate contact with the lower urinary tract and large intestines. Because of the anatomic proximity of the genital and urinary systems, altered pathophysiology in one organ often produces symptoms in an adjacent organ. **The gynecologic surgeon should master the intricacy of these anatomic relationships to avoid surgical complications. The clinician must also appreciate that wide individual differences in anatomic detail exist among patients.** Understanding these variations is one of the greatest challenges of clinical medicine.

This chapter focuses on the norms of human anatomy; it does not duplicate the completeness of an anatomic text or surgical atlas.

## EXTERNAL GENITALIA

### Vulva

The *vulva*, or *pudendum*, is a collective term for the external genital organs that are visible in the perineal area. The vulva consists of the following: the mons pubis, labia majora, labia minora, hymen, clitoris, vestibule, urethra, Skene glands, Bartholin glands, and vestibular bulbs (Fig. 3.1).

The boundaries of the vulva extend from the mons pubis anteriorly to the rectum posteriorly and from one lateral genitocrural fold to the other. The entire vulvar area is covered by **keratinized**, stratified squamous epithelium. The skin becomes thicker, more pigmented, and more keratinized as the distance from the vagina increases.

### Mons Pubis

The mons pubis is a fatty, rounded eminence that develops hair after puberty. It is directly anterior and superior to the symphysis pubis. The hair pattern, or **escutcheon**, of most women is triangular. Genetic and racial differences produce a variety of normal hair patterns, with approximately one in four women having a modified escutcheon that has a diamond (male-like) pattern.

### Labia Majora

The labia majora are two large, longitudinal, cutaneous folds of adipose and fibrous tissue. Each labium majus is approximately 7 to 8 cm long and 2 to 3 cm wide. The labia majora are homologous to the scrotum in the man. The labia extend from the mons pubis anteriorly to become lost in the skin between the vagina and the anus in the area of the posterior fourchette. The skin of the outer convex surface of the labia majora is pigmented and covered with hair follicles. The thin skin of the inner surface does not have hair follicles but has many sebaceous glands, making this area at risk for sebaceous cysts. Histologically the labia majora have both sweat and sebaceous glands (Fig. 3.2). Abundant apocrine glands are present in the vulvar area and secrete sweat directly into the hair follicles before the follicle opens onto the skin surface in a similar fashion to those of the breast and axillary areas. The size and contour of the labia are related to fat content. During menopause the labia atrophies as a result of a lack of estrogen, which is no longer produced by the ovary.

The clinical significance of the hair-bearing areas of the vulva is that conditions that involve the skin, such as **vulvar intraepithelial neoplasia (VIN)**, may be found as deep as 3 mm below the surface because they can involve the skin down into the hair shafts. That is not the case in the non–hair-bearing areas, such as the labia minora, where the full thickness of the epidermis is usually no more than 1 mm. Hence, treatment of the non–hair-bearing areas does not have to be any deeper than 1 mm to be effective, whereas treatment of the hair-bearing areas must to be at least 3 mm in depth to cover the potentially deeper skin down the hair shafts.

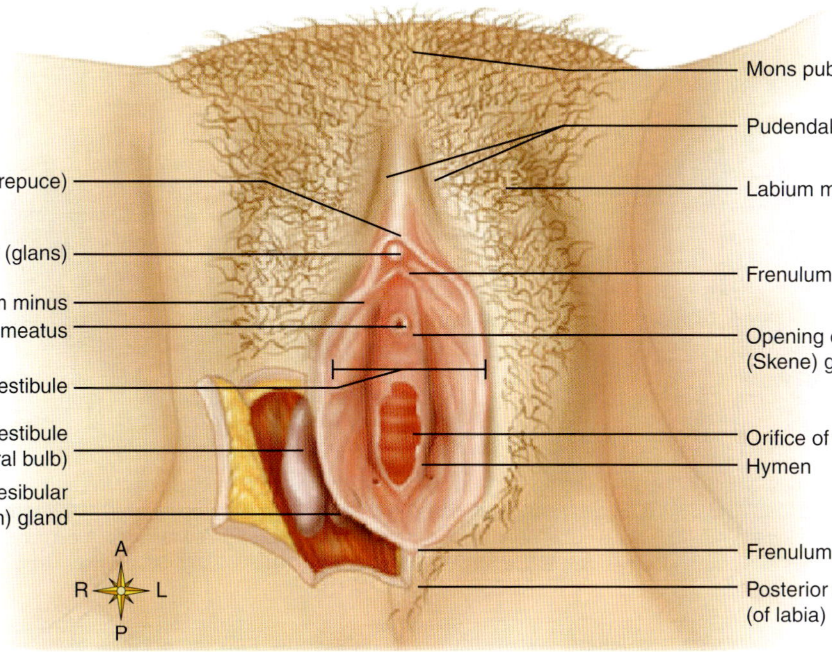


**Fig. 3.1** The structures of the external genitalia that are collectively called the *vulva.* (From Thibodeau, GA, Patton KT. *Anatomy and Physiology.* 6th ed. St. Louis: Elsevier; 2006.)

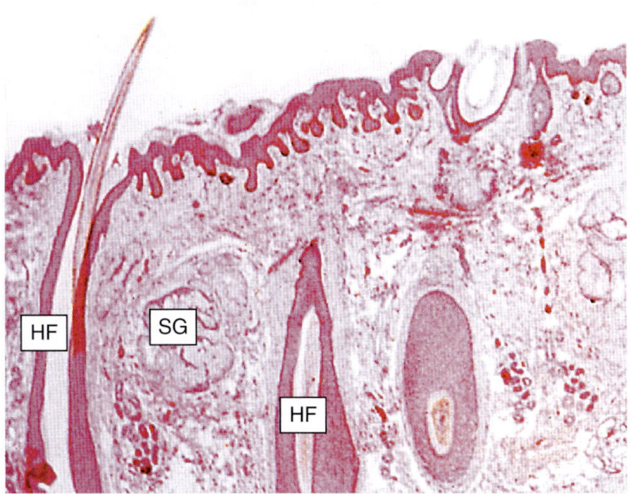


**Fig. 3.2** Histologic section from the labia majora. Note the eccrine glands and ducts. *HF,* Hair follicles; *SG,* sebaceous glands. (From Stevens A, Lowe J. *Human Histology.* 3rd ed. Philadelphia: Elsevier; 2002:346.)

## Labia Minora

The labia minora, or **nymphae**, are two small, red cutaneous folds situated between the labia majora and the vaginal orifice. They are more delicate, shorter, and thinner than the labia majora. Anteriorly they divide at the clitoris to form superiorly the prepuce and inferiorly the frenulum of the clitoris. Histologically they are composed of dense connective tissue with erectile tissue and elastic fibers, rather than adipose tissue. The skin of the labia minora is less cornified and has many sebaceous glands but no hair follicles or sweat glands. The labia minora and the breasts are the only areas of the body rich in **sebaceous glands** but without hair follicles. Among women of reproductive age, there is considerable variation in the size of the labia minora, and they are relatively more prominent in children and postmenopausal women. The labia minora are homologous to the penile urethra and part of the skin of the penis in men.

## Hymen

The hymen is a thin, usually perforated membrane at the entrance of the vagina. There are many anatomic variations in the structure and shape of the hymen that require surgical resection. Please refer to Chapter 12 for examples of hymenal variants. The hymen histologically is covered by stratified squamous epithelium on both sides and consists of fibrous tissue with a few small blood vessels and lacks innervation. In newborns the hymen is annular in shape and vascular as a result of circulating maternal estrogen. In prepubertal girls the lack of estrogen results in atrophy of the hymen and it becomes friable until puberty, at which point the hormonal influences lead to increased elasticity. During pregnancy this tissue becomes thickened with glycogen. Small tags, or what appear to be nodules of firm fibrous material, termed **carunculae myrtiformes**, are the remnants of the hymen identified in adult women. The postmenopausal hymen is pale pink and thin from a lack of estrogen.

## Clitoris

The clitoris, better known now as the **clitoral complex**, is a multiplanar structure that contains both **erectile** and **nonerectile** tissue (Fig. 3.3).

It is located deep to the superficial structures of the vulva and attaches to the pubic arch with supporting tissue at the mons pubic and labia. The complex consists of the glans, prepuce, body, crura, bulbs, suspensory ligament, and root. The visible external portion of the clitoris is composed of nonerectile tissue, known as the glans, and its skin covering, called the **prepuce**. The average dimensions of the glans are 3.4 mm by 5.1 mm by 16 mm.

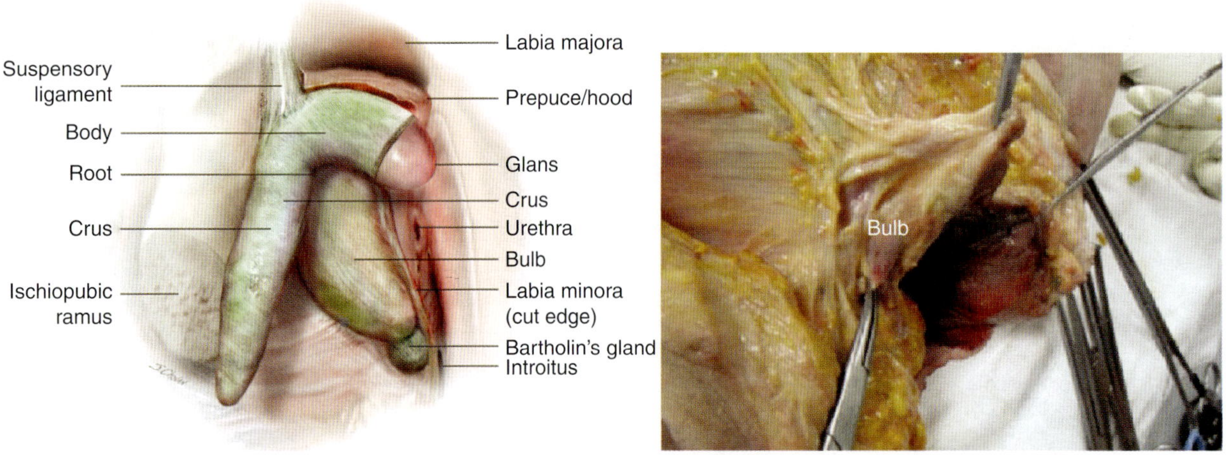


**Fig. 3.3 A,** Components of the clitoral complex. (From Pauls RN. Anatomy of the clitoris and the female sexual response. *Clin. Anat.* 2015;28(3):378, with permission. https://onlinelibrary.wiley.com/doi/epdf/10.1002/ca.22524). **B,** Cadaveric dissection of the clitoral bulb. (With permission from Mazloomdoost D, Pauls RN. A comprehensive review of clitoris and its role in female sexual function. *Sexual Med. Rev.* 2015;3(4);245-263. https://pubmed.ncbi.nlm.nih.gov/27784598/)

Parity has been associated with larger glans length and width. However, age, weight, and oral contraceptive use do not change the anatomic dimensions. The erectile portion of the clitoris is composed of paired bulbs, the crura and the body. The bulbs are 4 cm long when flaccid and can engorge up to 7 cm when erect.

The body of the clitoris (1 to 2 cm long) has two cylindrical corpora cavernosa composed of thin-walled tissue, which diverge to form the crura. The bilateral crura attaches to the periosteum of the symphysis pubis and surrounds the urethra. The **root** is the center of sexual arousal and stimulates the engorgement of the glans. It is in close proximity to the skin surface and the urethral opening and unifies all the erectile tissue essential to sexual function. The clitoral complex is innervated by the dorsal nerve of the clitoris, the pudendal nerve, and the cavernous nerves. The clitoral complex is the female homologue of the penis in the man.

## Vestibule

The vestibule is the lowest portion of the embryonic urogenital sinus. It is the cleft distal to the vagina between the labia minora that is visualized when the labia are held apart. The vestibule extends from the clitoris to the posterior fourchette. The orifices of the urethra and vagina and the ducts from the Bartholin glands open into the vestibule. Within the area of the vestibule are the remnants of the hymen and numerous small mucinous glands.

## Urethra

The urethra is a membranous conduit for urine from the urinary bladder to the vestibule. The female urethra measures 3.5 to 5 cm long. The mucosa of the proximal two-thirds of the urethra is composed of stratified transitional epithelium, whereas the distal one-third is stratified squamous epithelium. The distal orifice is 4 to 6 mm in diameter, and the mucosal edges grossly appear everted.

## Skene Glands

Skene glands, or **paraurethral glands**, are branched, tubular glands that are adjacent to the distal urethra. Usually Skene ducts run parallel to the long axis of the urethra for approximately 1 cm before opening into the distal urethra, but sometimes the ducts open into the area just outside the urethral orifice. Skene glands are the largest of the paraurethral glands; however, many smaller glands empty into the urethra. Skene glands are homologous to the prostate in the man, and the glands may be involved in sexual stimulation and lubrication for sexual intercourse.

## Bartholin Glands

Bartholin glands are vulvovaginal glands located immediately beneath the fascia at about 4 and 8 o'clock, respectively, on the posterolateral aspect of the vaginal orifice. Each lobulated, racemose gland is about the size of a pea. Histologically the gland is composed of cuboidal epithelium. The duct from each gland is lined by transitional epithelium and is approximately 2 cm long. Bartholin ducts open into a groove between the hymen and the labia minora. Bartholin glands are homologous to Cowper glands in the man (Fig. 3.4).

## Vestibular Bulbs

The vestibular bulbs are two elongated masses of erectile tissue situated on either side of the vaginal orifice. Each bulb is immediately below the bulbocavernosus muscle. The distal ends of the vestibular bulbs are adjacent to Bartholin glands. They are homologous to the bulb of the penis in the man.

# CLINICAL CORRELATIONS

The skin of the vulvar region is subject to both local and general dermatologic conditions. The intertriginous areas of the vulva remain moist, and obese women are particularly susceptible to chronic infection. The vulvar skin of a postmenopausal woman is sensitive to topical cortisone and testosterone but insensitive to topical estrogen. The most common large cystic structure of the vulva is a **Bartholin duct cyst** (Fig. 3.5). This condition may become painful if the cyst develops into an acute abscess. The management of Bartholin cysts includes sitz baths, incision and drainage, placement of a Word catheter, antibiotics, and possible marsupialization for chronic infections.

Chronic infections of the periurethral glands may result in one or more urethral diverticula. The most common symptoms of a urethral diverticulum are similar to the symptoms of a lower urinary tract infection: urinary frequency, urgency, and dysuria.

Vulvar trauma such as a straddle injury often results in large hematomas or profuse external hemorrhage. The richness of the vascular supply and the absence of valves in vulvar veins

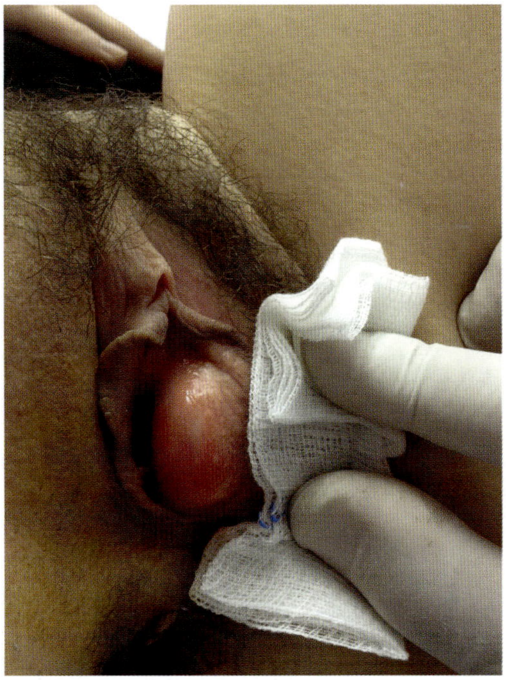

Fig. 3.4 Photograph of a left-sided Bartholin duct cyst. (From Di Donato V, Bellati F, Casorelli A, et al. $CO_2$ laser treatment for Bartholin gland abscess: ultrasound evaluation of risk recurrence. *J Minim Invasive Gynecol.* 2013;20(3):346-352.)

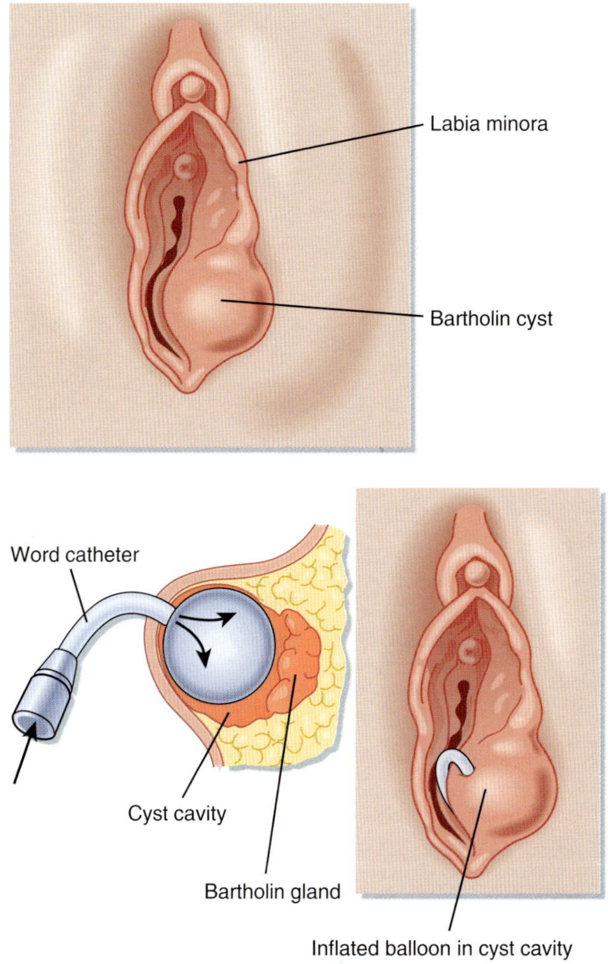


Fig. 3.5 A no. 11 scalpel incision is made inside the hymenal ring, making the opening just large enough to insert the Word catheter. The balloon is then inflated within the cavity of the cyst. (From Adams JG, et al. *Emergency Medicine: Clinical Essentials.* 2nd ed. Philadelphia: Saunders; 2013.)

contribute to this complication. The abundant vascularity of the region promotes rapid healing, with an associated low incidence of wound infection in episiotomies or obstetric tears of the vulva. The subcutaneous fatty tissue of the labia majora and mons pubis are in continuity with the fatty tissue of the anterior abdominal wall. When infections such as cellulitis and necrotizing fasciitis occur in this space, they are poorly contained and may rapidly extend in a cephalad direction.

## INTERNAL GENITALIA

### Vagina

The vagina is a thin-walled, distensible, fibromuscular tube that extends from the vestibule of the vulva to the uterus. The potential space of the vagina is larger in the middle and upper thirds. The walls of the vagina are normally in apposition and flattened in the anteroposterior diameter. Thus the vagina has the appearance of the letter H in cross section (Fig. 3.6).

The axis of the upper portion of the vagina lies fairly close to the horizontal plane when a woman is standing, with the upper portion of the vagina curving toward the hollow of the sacrum. In most women an angle of at least 90 degrees is formed between the axis of the vagina and the axis of the uterus (Fig. 3.7). The vagina is held in position by the surrounding endopelvic fascia and ligaments.

The lower third of the vagina is in close relationship with the urogenital and pelvic diaphragms. The middle third of the vagina is suspended by the lower portion of the cardinal ligaments and supported by the levator ani muscles. The upper third is suspended by the upper portions of the cardinal ligaments and the parametria. The vagina of reproductive-age women has numerous transverse folds, vaginal rugae. They help provide accordion-like distensibility and are more prominent in the lower third of the vagina. The cervix extends into the upper part of the vagina. The spaces between the cervix and attachment of the vagina are called **fornices**. The posterior fornix is considerably larger than the anterior fornix; thus the anterior vaginal length is approximately 6 to 9 cm compared with a posterior vaginal length of 8 to 12 cm. Vaginal length is increased slightly by a woman's weight and height. Age, conversely, leads to a shortening of the vagina. A study by Tan and colleagues noted a decrease of 0.08 cm per 10 years (Tan, 2006). The lack of estrogen during menopause also leads to loss of vaginal elasticity.

Histologically the vagina is composed of four distinct layers. The mucosa consists of a stratified, nonkeratinized squamous epithelium (Fig. 3.8). If the environment of the vaginal mucosa is modified, as in uterine prolapse, then the epithelium may become keratinized. The squamous epithelium is similar microscopically to the exocervix, although the vagina has larger and more frequent papillae that extend into the connective tissue. The normal vagina does not have glands. The next layer is the lamina propria, or tunica. It is composed of fibrous connective tissue. Throughout this layer of collagen and elastic tissue is a rich supply of vascular and lymphatic channels. The density of the connective tissue in the endopelvic fascia varies throughout the longitudinal axis of the vagina. The muscular layer has many interlacing fibers;

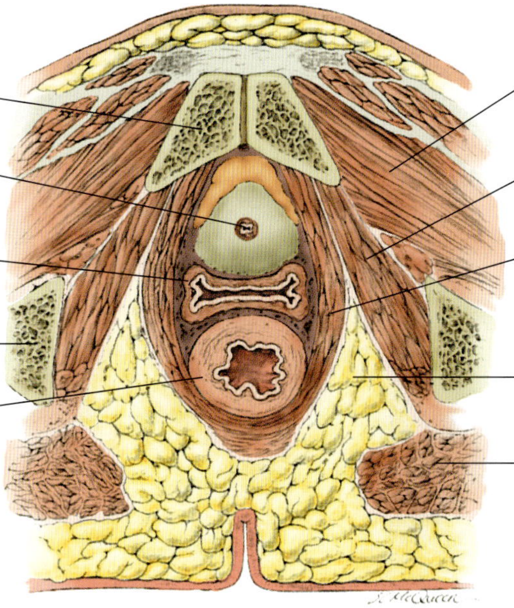

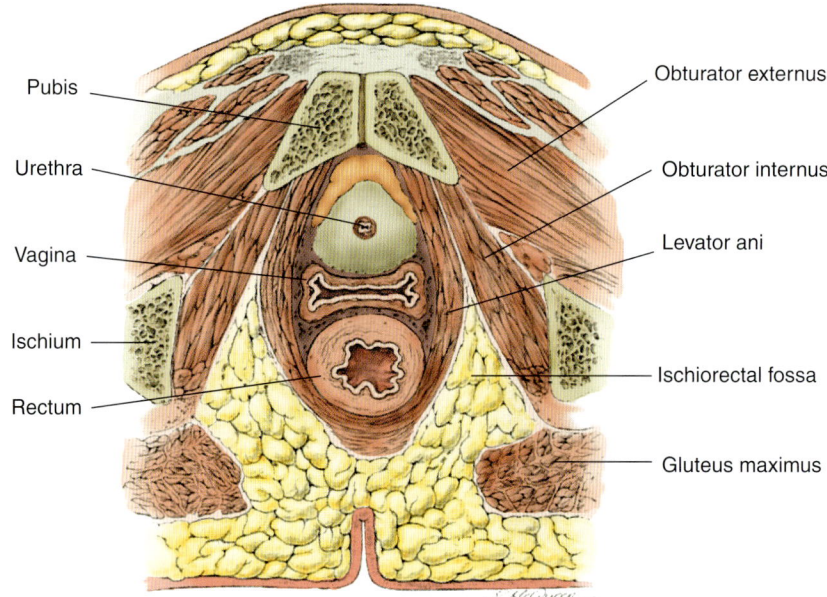

**Fig. 3.6** A schematic drawing of a cross section of the female pelvis, demonstrating the H shape of the vagina. Note the surrounding levator ani muscle. (Modified from Pritchard JA, MacDonald PC, Gant NF. *Williams' Obstetrics*. 17th ed. New York: Appleton-Century-Crofts; 1985:12.)

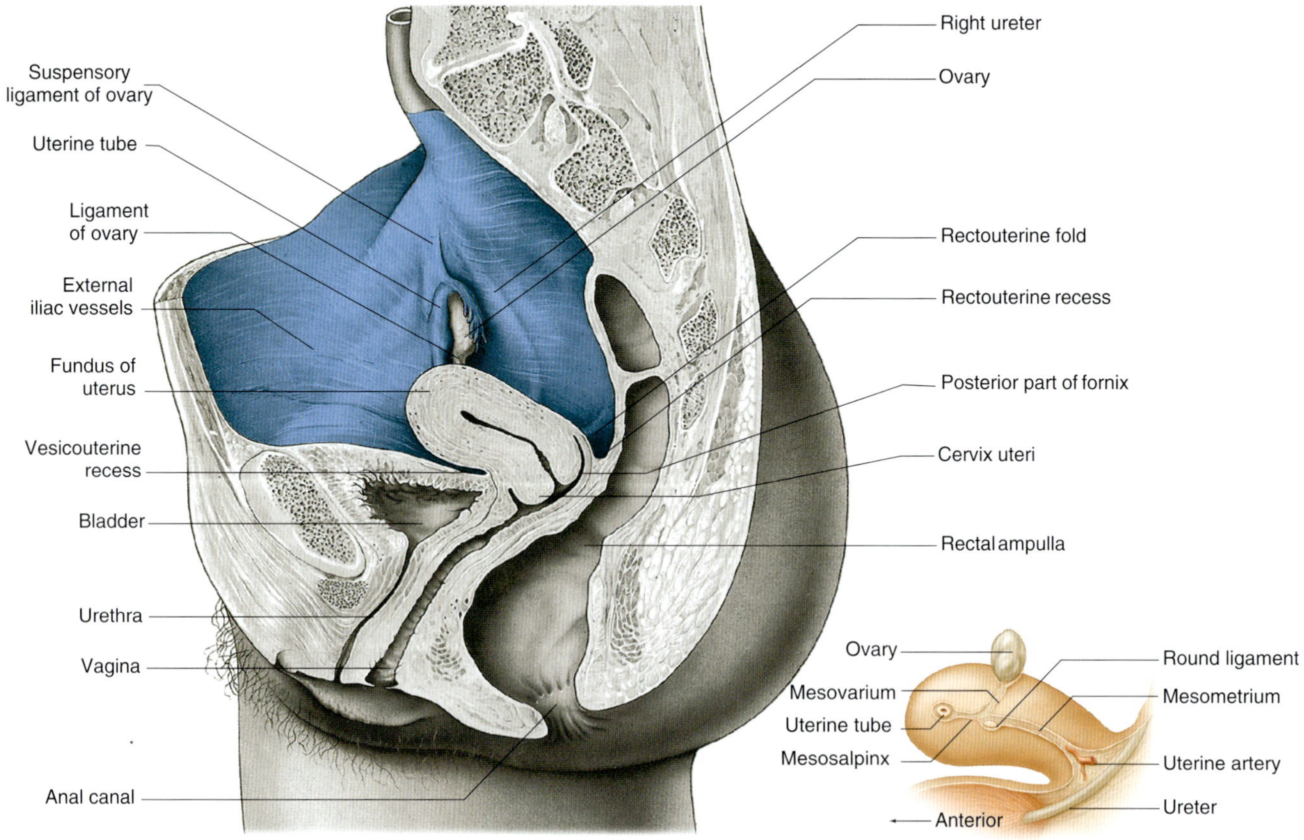


**Fig. 3.7** A median sagittal section through the pelvis. The peritoneum is shaded blue. Note the proximal vagina at a diagonal axis and in a near 90-degree juxtaposition to the uterus. In this woman the uterus is anteflexed. (From Standring S, ed. *Gray's Anatomy*. 39th ed. Edinburgh: Churchill Livingstone; 2005:1321.)

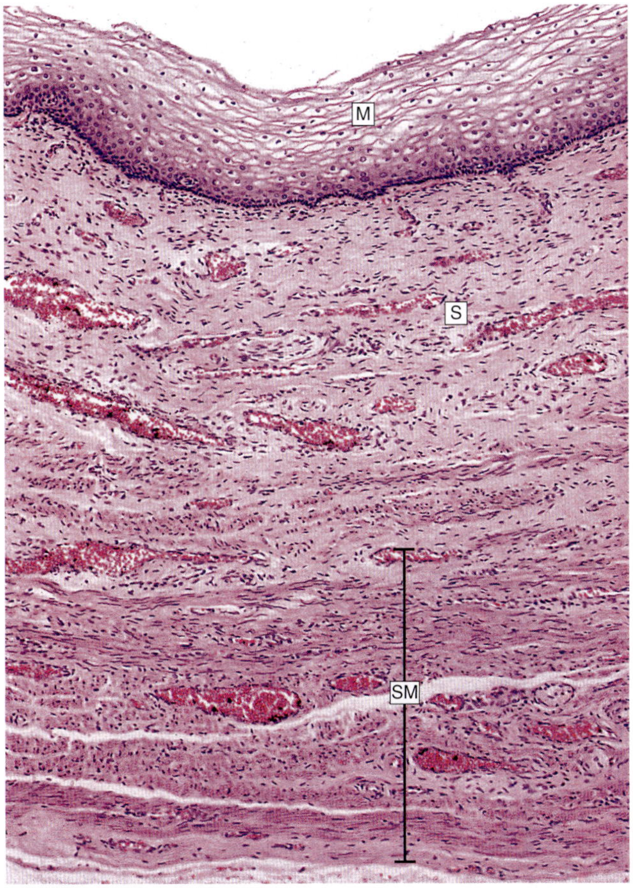


**Fig. 3.8** Histologic section of the vaginal squamous epithelium *(M)*. The submucosa *(S)* is well vascularized (lamina propria). *SM,* Smooth muscle. (From Stevens A, Lowe J. *Human Histology.* 3rd ed. Philadelphia: Elsevier; 2002:347.)

however, an inner circular layer and an outer longitudinal layer can be identified. The fourth layer consists of cellular areolar connective tissue containing a large plexus of blood vessels.

The vascular system of the vagina is generously supplied with an extensive anastomotic network throughout its length. The vaginal artery originates either directly from the uterine artery or as a branch of the internal iliac artery arising posterior to the origin of the uterine and inferior vesical arteries. Multiple vaginal arteries may be present on each side of the pelvis. There is an anastomosis with the cervical branch of the uterine artery to form the azygos arteries. Branches of the internal pudendal, inferior vesical, and middle hemorrhoidal arteries also contribute to the interconnecting network and the longitudinal azygos arteries.

The venous drainage is complex and accompanies the arterial system. Below the pelvic floor, the principal venous drainage occurs via the pudendal veins. The vaginal, uterine, and vesical veins, as well as those around the rectosigmoid, all provide venous drainage of the venous plexuses surrounding the middle and upper vagina.

The nerve supply of the vagina comes from the autonomic nervous system's vaginal plexus, and sensory fibers come from the pudendal nerve. Pain fibers enter the spinal cord in sacral segments two to four. There is a paucity of free nerve endings in the upper two-thirds of the vagina.

The lymphatic drainage is characterized by its wide distribution and frequent crossovers between the right and left sides of the pelvis. In general the primary lymphatic drainage of the upper third of the vagina is to the external iliac nodes; the middle third of the vagina drains to the common and internal iliac nodes; and the lower third has a complex and variable distribution, including the common iliac, superficial inguinal, and perirectal nodes.

## CLINICAL CORRELATIONS

In clinical practice, anatomic descriptions of pelvic organs are derived from Latin roots, such as the word **vagina**, which is derived from the Latin word for "sheath." In contrast, the names for surgical procedures of pelvic organs are derived from Greek roots. For instance, **colpectomy, colporrhaphy**, and **colposcopy** are derived from **kolpos** ("fold"), the Greek word for the **vagina**; another example is **hysterectomy** (Greek) versus *uterus* (Latin).

Clinicians should consider the H shape of the vagina when they insert a speculum and inspect the walls of the vagina. The posterior fornix is an important surgical landmark because it provides direct access to the cul-de-sac of Douglas. The distal course of the ureter is an essential consideration in vaginal surgery. Ureteral injury can result from vaginally placed sutures used to obtain hemostasis in patients with vaginal lacerations. The anatomic proximity and interrelationships of the vascular and lymphatic networks of the bladder and vagina are such that inflammation of one organ can produce symptoms in the other. For example, vaginitis sometimes produces urinary tract symptoms such as frequency and dysuria.

A **Gartner duct cyst** is a congenital abnormality caused by incomplete regression of the wolffian (mesonephric) duct (Fig. 3.9A). It is usually present on the lateral wall of the vagina. However, if encountered in the lower third of the vagina, these cysts are located anteriorly and may be difficult to distinguish from a large urethral diverticulum. Often these cysts remain small and require no treatment, but they may be excised surgically if they produce symptoms or interfere with sexual function. Before excision, magnetic resonance imaging (MRI) is often obtained to confirm the diagnosis (Fig. 3.9B).

An interesting phenomenon is the source of vaginal lubrication during intercourse. For years there was speculation on how an organ without glands is able to "secrete" fluid. Vaginal lubrication occurs from **a transudate** produced by engorgement of the vascular plexuses that encircle the vagina. This richness of vascularization allows many drugs to readily enter the systemic circulation when placed in the vagina. Medications that are absorbed vaginally go directly into the systemic circulation, bypassing the liver and its metabolism on the first round through the circulation.

The anatomic relationship between the long axis of the vagina and other pelvic organs may be altered by pelvic relaxation resulting primarily from the trauma of childbirth. Atrophy or weakness of the endopelvic fascia and muscles surrounding the vagina may result in the development of a **cystocele, rectocele, or enterocele**, all possibly contributing to a **vaginal vault prolapse**. One of many popular operations for vaginal vault prolapse is fixation of the vaginal apex to the sacrospinous ligament. A rare complication of this operation is massive hemorrhage, usually from the arterial or venous branches of the inferior gluteal or pudendal vasculature.

## Cervix

The lower, narrow portion of the uterus is the cervix. The word *cervix* originates from the Latin word for *neck*. The Greek word for *neck* is *trachelos*, and when the cervix is removed, the surgical procedure is termed a *trachelectomy*. The cervix may vary in shape from cylindric to conical. It consists of predominantly fibrous tissue, in contrast to the primarily muscular corpus of the uterus.

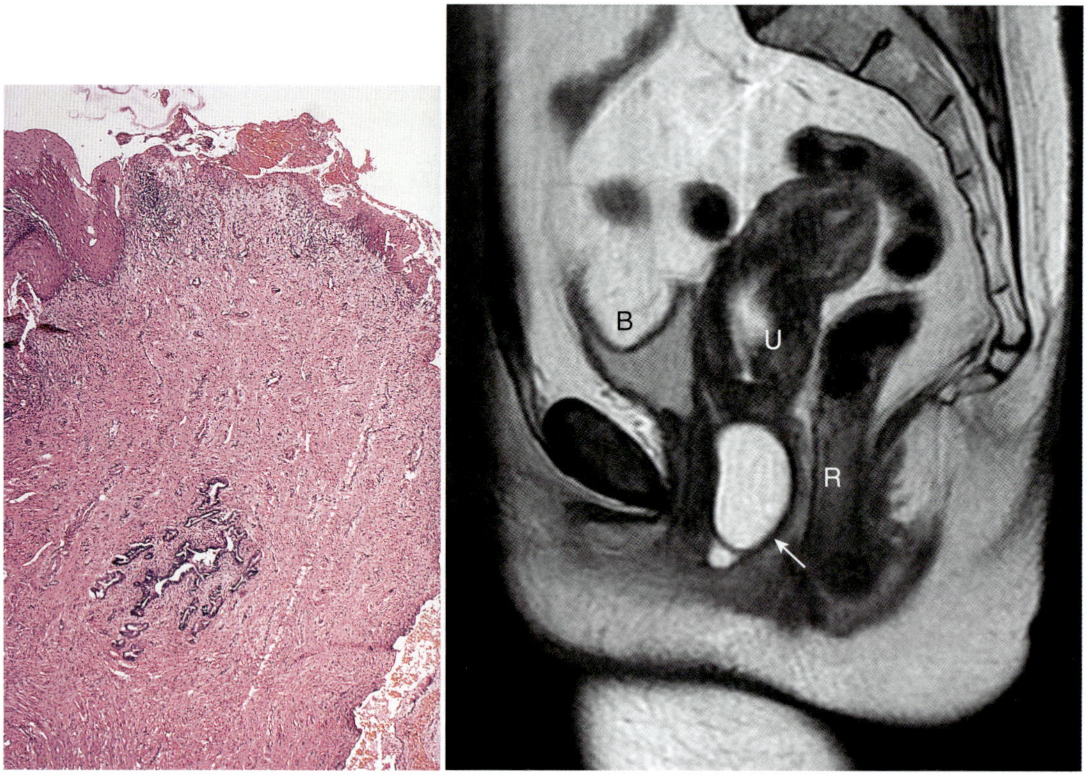


**Fig. 3.9 A,** Mesonephric duct remnant in the vaginal wall. (From Robboy SJ, Anderson MC, Russell P, eds. *Pathology of the Female Reproductive Tract.* Edinburgh: Churchill Livingstone; 2002:77.) **B,** T2-weighted image shows a cyst in the upper vagina and MRI confirms structure is separate from the ureter. The *arrow* points to the Gartner cyst representing a vestigial remnant of the mesonephric duct. *B,* Bladder; *R,* rectum; *U,* uterus. (From Brady C. The female genital tract. In Zagoria RJ, Dyer R, Brady C, eds. *Genitourinary Imaging: The Requisites.* 3rd ed. Philadelphia: Elsevier; 2016:248-308.)

The vagina is attached obliquely around the middle of the cervix; this attachment divides the cervix into an upper, supravaginal portion and a lower segment in the vagina called the *portio vaginalis* (Fig. 3.10). The supravaginal segment is covered by peritoneum posteriorly and is surrounded by loose, fatty connective tissue—**the parametrium**—anteriorly and laterally.

The canal of the cervix is fusiform, with the widest diameter in the middle. The length and width of the endocervical canal varies; it is usually 2.5 to 3 cm long and 7 to 8 mm at its widest point. The width of the canal varies with the parity of the woman and with changing hormonal levels. The cervical length increases in pregnancy, reaching maximal length in the second trimester. The cervical canal opens into the vagina at the external os of the cervix. In the majority of women the external os is in contact with the posterior vaginal wall. The external os is small and round in nulliparous women but is wider and gaping after vaginal delivery. Often, lateral or stellate scars, which are residual marks of previous cervical lacerations, are present.

The mucous lining of the endocervical canal of nulliparous women is arranged in longitudinal folds, called **plicae palmatae**, with secondary branching folds called the arbor vitae. These folds, which form a herringbone pattern, often disappear after vaginal delivery.

A single layer of columnar epithelium lines the endocervical canal and the underlying glandular structures. This specialized epithelium secretes mucus, which facilitates sperm transport. An abrupt transformation usually is seen at the junction of the columnar epithelium of the endocervix and the nonkeratinized stratified squamous epithelium of the portio vaginalis (Figs. 3.11 and 3.12). The stratified squamous epithelium of the exocervix is identical to the lining of the vagina.

The dense, fibromuscular cervical stroma is composed primarily of collagenous connective tissue and mucopolysaccharide ground substance. The collagen framework and ground substance are sensitive to hormonal effects. The connective tissue contains approximately 15% smooth muscle cells and a small amount of elastic tissue (Fig. 3.13). However, there are few muscle fibers in the distal portions of the cervix.

It is not surprising that the cervical and uterine vascular supplies are interrelated. The arterial supply of the cervix arises from the descending branch of the **uterine artery**. The cervical arteries run on the lateral side of the cervix and form the coronary artery, which encircles the cervix. The azygos arteries run longitudinally in the middle of the anterior and posterior aspects of the cervix and the vagina. There are numerous anastomoses between these vessels and the vaginal and middle hemorrhoidal arteries. The venous drainage accompanies these arteries. The lymphatic drainage of the cervix is complex, involving multiple chains of nodes. The principal regional lymph nodes are the obturator, common iliac, internal iliac, external iliac, and visceral nodes of the parametria. Other possible lymphatic drainage includes the following chains of nodes: superior and inferior gluteal, sacral, rectal, lumbar, aortic, and visceral nodes over the posterior surface of the urinary bladder. The stroma of the endocervix is rich in **free nerve endings**. Pain fibers accompany the parasympathetic fibers to the second, third, and fourth sacral segments.

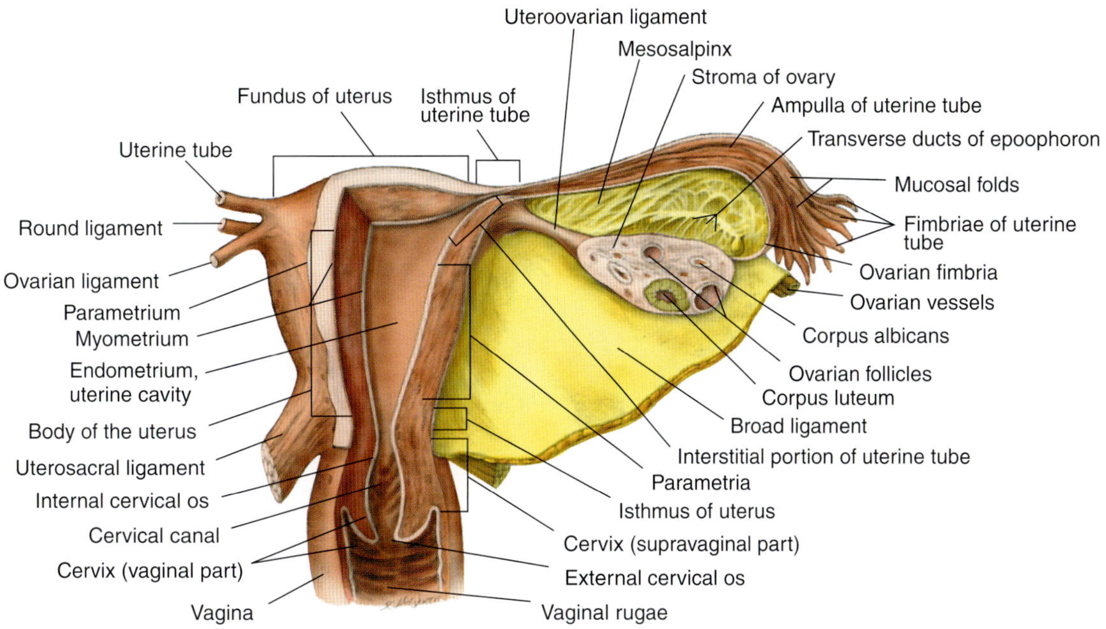


**Fig. 3.10** A schematic drawing of a posterior view of the cervix, uterus, fallopian tube, and ovary. Note that the cervix is divided by the vaginal attachment into an external portio segment and a supravaginal segment, and the uterus is composed of the dome-shaped fundus, the muscular body, and the narrow isthmus. Also note the fimbria ovarica, or ovarian fimbria, attaching the oviduct to the ovary. (Modified from Clemente CD. *Anatomy: A Regional Atlas of the Human Body.* 3rd ed. Baltimore-Munich: Urban & Schwarzenberg; 1987.)

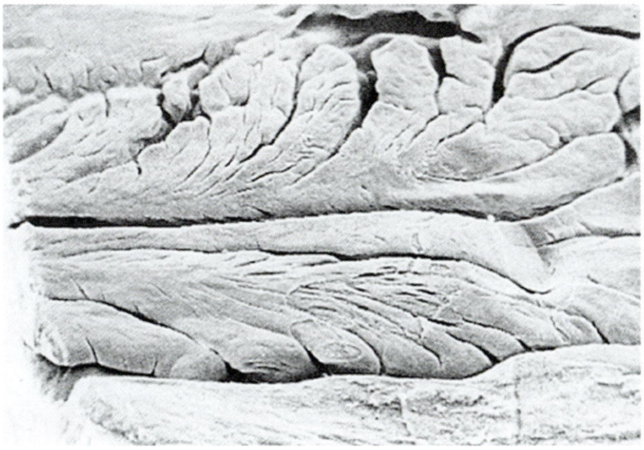

**Fig. 3.11** An electron micrograph of the endocervical canal, demonstrating the arbor vitae. These folds and crypts provide a reservoir for sperm. (From Singer A, Jordan JA. The anatomy of the cervix. In Jordan JA, Singer A, eds. *The Cervix.* Philadelphia: WB Saunders; 1976:18.)

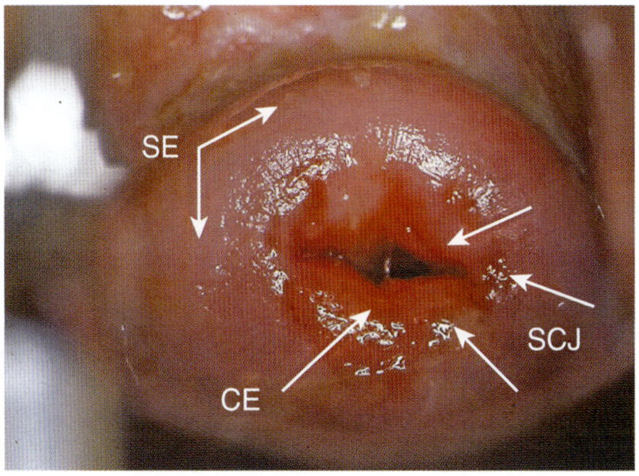


**Fig. 3.12** A histologic section through the squamocolumnar junction of the cervix. Note the abrupt transformation from squamous to columnar epithelium. *CE*, Columnar epithelium; *SCJ*, squamocolumnar junction; *SE*, squamous epithelium. (From Standring S, ed. *Gray's Anatomy.* 39th ed. Edinburgh: Churchill Livingstone; 2005:1335.)

## CLINICAL CORRELATIONS

The major arterial supply to the cervix is located on the lateral cervical walls at **the 3 and 9 o'clock positions,** respectively. Therefore a deep figure-of-eight suture through the vaginal mucosa and cervical stroma at 3 and 9 o'clock helps to reduce blood loss during procedures such as cone biopsy. If the gynecologist is overzealous in placing such a hemostatic suture high in the vaginal fornix, it is possible to compromise the course of the distal ureter just before it enters the bladder.

The transformation zone, also known as the **squamocolumnar junction (SCJ),** of the cervix is an important anatomic landmark for clinicians. This area encompasses the transition from stratified squamous epithelium to columnar epithelium. Most cases of cervical dysplasia develop within this **transformation zone** and are due to **human papillomavirus (HPV)** infections.

The position of a woman's transformation zone, in relation to the long axis of the cervix, depends on her age and hormonal status. When the woman is young, the transformation zone is located further out on the cervical portio. This is called an

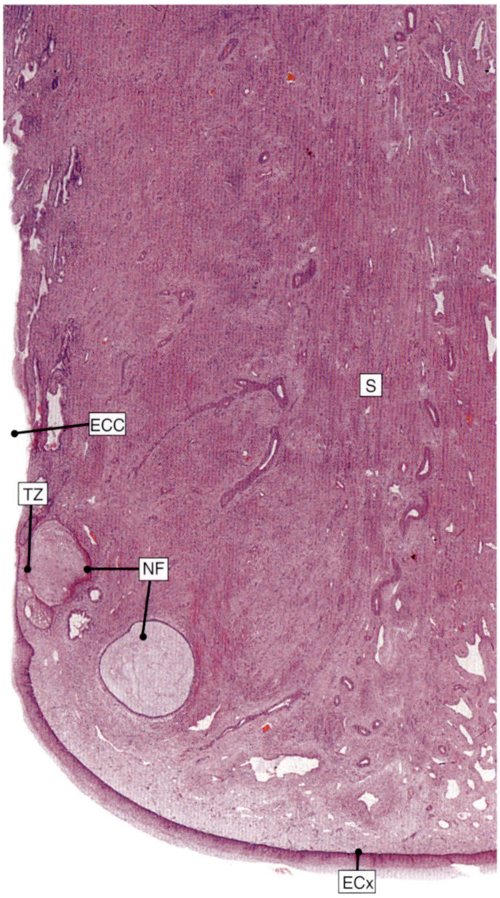


**Fig. 3.13** A low-power histologic section of the cervix. The stroma *(S)* has a small amount of smooth muscle. The ectocervix *(ECx)* is covered in stratified squamous epithelium. The endocervix *(ECC)* is lined by tall columnar cells. *NF,* Nabothian follicles (a normal finding); *TZ,* transformation zone. (From Stevens A, Lowe J. *Human Histology.* 3rd ed. Philadelphia: Elsevier; 2002:349.)

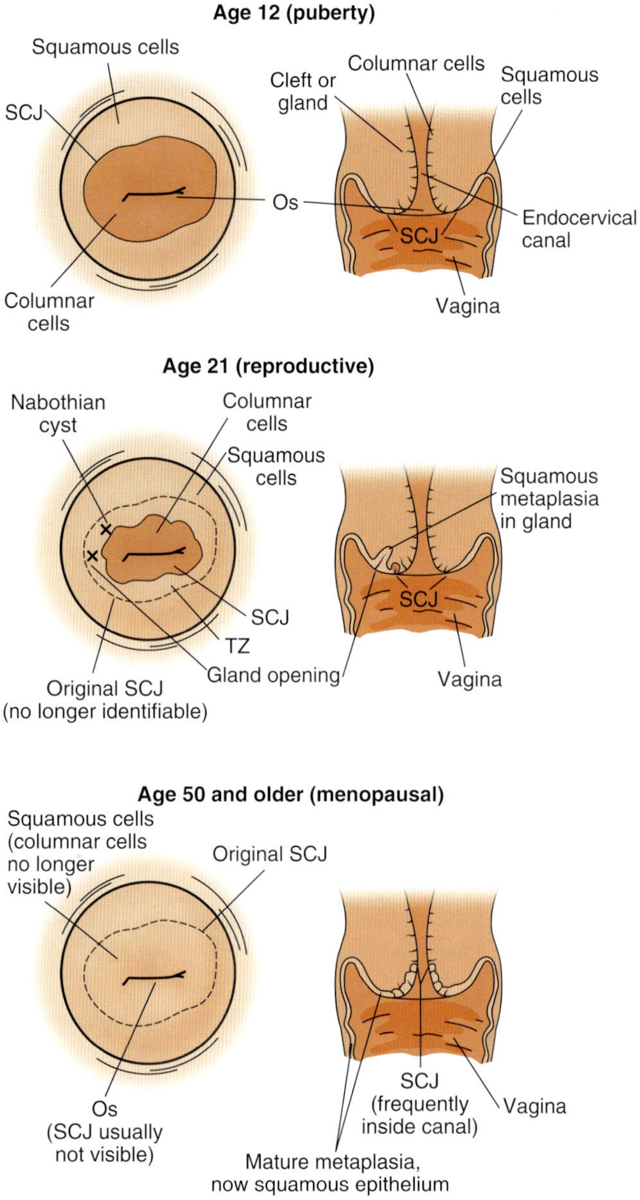


**Fig. 3.14** A schematic drawing showing the migration of the transformation zone as a women ages. The first schematic shows a larger more robust squamocolumnar junction (SCJ). During the reproductive years the glands open, the SCJ migrates slightly inward, and on examination Nabothian cysts may be seen. During menopause the lack of estrogen causes the transformation zone to migrate higher up the endocervical canal. The SCJ is often lost into the cervical canal during menopause. (From Newkirk GR. Pap smear and related techniques for cervical cancer screening. In Fowler G, ed. *Pfenninger and Fowler's Procedures for Primary Care.* 4th ed. St. Louis: Elsevier; 2020: 814-824.)

*ectropion* and is a normal finding, especially during pregnancy. As a woman ages, the transformation zone migrates higher up the endocervical canal (Fig. 3.14).

The endocervix is rich in free nerve endings. Occasionally, women experience a vasovagal response during transcervical instrumentation of the uterine cavity. Serial cardiac monitoring during insertion of intrauterine devices demonstrates a reflex bradycardia in some women. The sensory innervation of the exocervix is not as concentrated or sophisticated as that of the endocervix or external skin. Therefore usually the exocervix may be cauterized by either cold or heat without major discomfort to the patient.

The lymphatic drainage of the cervix is fairly organized, as described earlier. Similar to other disease sites, **sentinel lymph node (SLN) mapping** and biopsy for cervical cancer are replacing the more traditional full lymphadenectomies in favor of fewer complications, specifically lymphedema. Sentinel lymph node mapping in cervical cancer was first described in 1999 by Echt and coworkers when they injected 13 patients who had early-stage cervical cancer with a blue dye, lymphazurin, and identified SLNs in 15% (Echt, 1999). This technique has been refined over the years and is now performed using near-infrared fluorescence imaging and indocyanine green (ICG) and achieves detection of SLNs in 85% to 90% of cases.

## Uterus

The **uterus** is a thick-walled, hollow, muscular organ located centrally in the female pelvis. Adjacent to the uterus are the urinary bladder anteriorly, the rectum posteriorly, and the broad ligaments laterally (see Fig. 3.7). The uterus is globular and slightly flattened anteriorly; it has the general configuration of an inverted pear. The short area of constriction in the lower uterine segment is termed the *isthmus* (Fig. 3.15). The dome-shaped top of the uterus is termed the *fundus.* The lower edge of the fundus

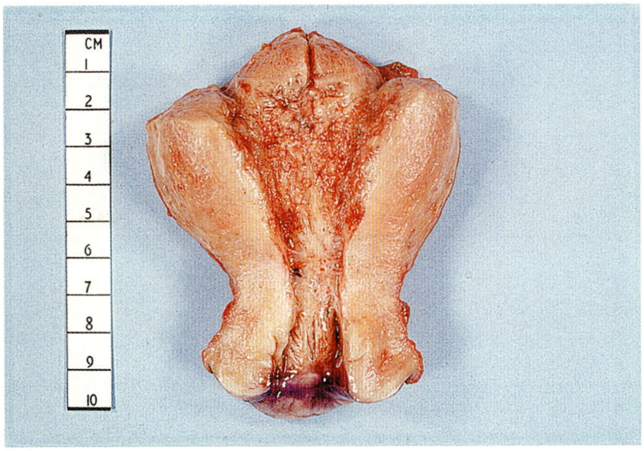


**Fig. 3.15** A surgical specimen of a uterus that has been opened. (From Robboy SJ, Anderson MC, Russell P, eds. *Pathology of the Female Reproductive Tract.* Edinburgh: Churchill Livingstone; 2002:241.)

is described by an imaginary line drawn between the site of entrance of each oviduct. The size and weight of the normal uterus depend on previous pregnancies and the hormonal status of the individual. The uterus of a nulliparous woman is approximately 8 cm long, 5 cm wide, and 2.5 cm thick and weighs 40 to 50 g. In contrast, in a multiparous woman the uterus on average is 9 to 10 cm long, 6 to 7 cm wide, and 4 cm thick and normally weighs approximately 80 to 110 g. The capacity of the uterus to enlarge during pregnancy results in **a 10- to 20-fold increase** in weight at term. This growth is accompanied by an increase of blood flow to approximately 10% of cardiac output at term. After menopause the uterus atrophies and the measurements vary depending on years since menopause.

The cavity of the uterus is flattened and triangular. The oviducts enter the uterine cavity at the superolateral aspects of the cavity in the areas designated the cornua. In the majority of women, the long axis of the uterus is both anteverted in respect to the long axis of the vagina and anteflexed in relation to the long axis of the cervix. However, a retroflexed uterus is a normal variant found in approximately **25% of women** (Fig. 3.16).

The uterus has three layers, similar to other hollow abdominal and pelvic organs. The thin, external serosal layer makes up the visceral peritoneum. The peritoneum is firmly attached to the uterus in all areas except anteriorly at the level of the internal os of the cervix, where it is only loosely attached. The wide middle muscular layer is composed of three indistinct layers of smooth muscle. The outer longitudinal layer is contiguous with the muscle layers of the oviduct and vagina. The middle layer has interlacing oblique, spiral bundles of smooth muscle and large venous plexuses. The inner muscular layer is also longitudinal. The endometrium is a reddish mucous membrane that varies from 1 to 6 mm in thickness, depending on hormonal stimulation (Fig. 3.17).

The uterine glands are tubular and composed of tall columnar epithelium. The cells of the endometrial stroma resemble embryonic connective tissue with scant cytoplasm and large nuclei. The endometrium may be divided into an inner stratum basale and an outer stratum functionale. The stratum functionale may be further subdivided into an inner compact stratum and a more

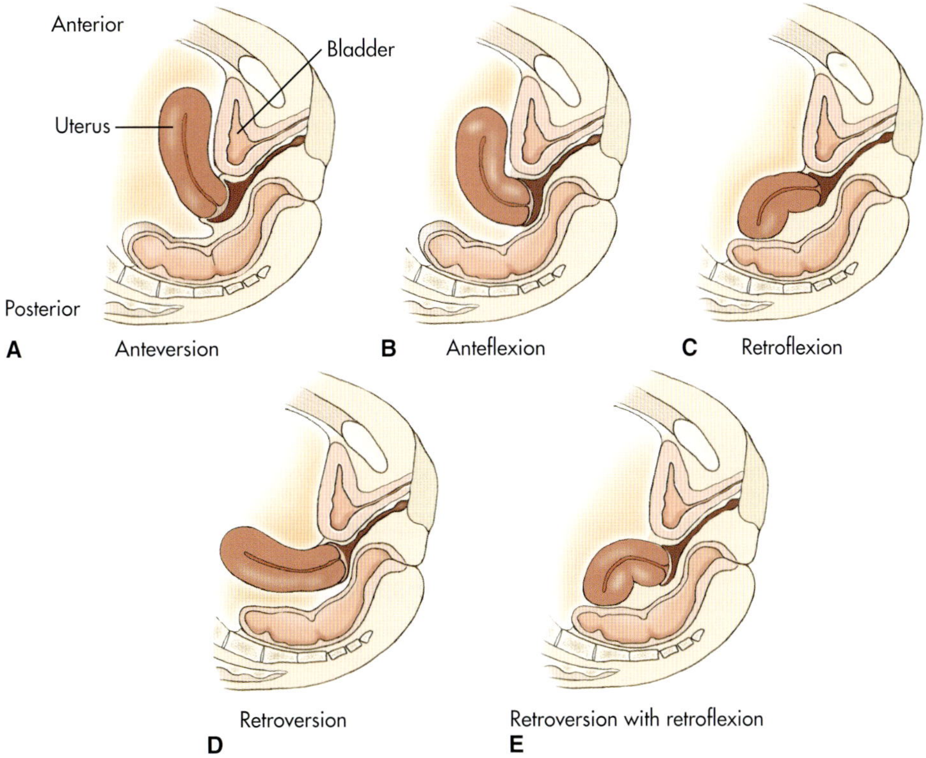


**Fig. 3.16** A schematic view of the variations in the position of the uterus in relations to the cervix. **A-E** are all normal variants, but the most common variant is retroflexion, (C) which is palpable in more than 25% of patients and may make visualization of the cervix challenging during a speculum examination. (From Goldstein C. Normal anatomy and physiology of the female pelvis. In Hagen-Ansert SL, ed. *Textbook of Diagnostic Sonography.* 8th ed. St. Louis: Elsevier; 2018:1049-1065.)

| Day of Cycle | | Before 14 | 15-16 | 17 | 18 | 19-22 | 23 | 24-25 | 26-27 | 28+ |
|---|---|---|---|---|---|---|---|---|---|---|
| Post-ovulatory day | | - | 1-2 | 3 | 4 | 5-8 | 9 | 10-11 | 12-13 | 14+ |
| Cycle phases | | Proliferative | 'Interval' | Early secretory | | Mid-secretory | | | Late secretory | Menstrual |
| Key feature | | Mitoses | Mitoses and subnuclear vacuoles | Maximum subnuclear vacuoles | Subnuclear vacuoles present | Stromal edema | Focal decidua around spiral arteries | Patchy decidua | Extensive decidua | Stromal crumbling |
| Microscopic features of functional zone | Stroma | Loose stroma. Mitoses | Same as proliferative | Loose stroma, scanty mitoses | Loose stroma | Stromal edema | Focal decidua around spiral arteries. Edema prominent | Decidua throughout stroma. Some edema | Extensive decidua. Prominent granulated lymphocytes | Stromal crumbling. Hemorrhage |
| | Glands | Straight to tightly coiled tubules. Mitoses | Some subnuclear vacuoles, otherwise as proliferative | Extensive subnuclear vacuoles | Dilated glands. Some subnuclear vacuoles | Dilated glands with irregular outline. Luminal secretion | | "sawtooth" glands | Prominent "sawtooth" glands | Disrupted glands. Secretory exhaustion. Regenerating epithelium |
| Appearances | | 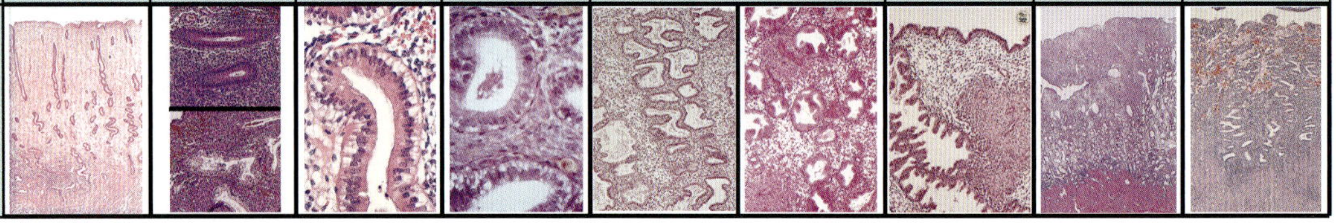 | | | | | | | | |

**Fig. 3.17** The endometrium is responsive to the hormonal changes of the menstrual cycle. Glands and stroma change activity and thus histologic appearance throughout the cycle. (From Robboy SJ, Anderson MC, Russell P, eds. *Pathology of the Female Reproductive Tract.* Edinburgh: Churchill Livingstone; 2002:248.)

superficial spongy stratum. Only the stratum functionale responds to fluctuating hormonal levels.

The uterine and ovarian arteries provide the arterial blood supply of the uterus. The uterine arteries are large branches of the hypogastric arteries, whereas the ovarian arteries originate directly from the **aorta**. The veins of the pelvic organs accompany the arteries. Therefore venous drainage from the fundus goes to the ovarian veins and blood from the corpus exits via the uterine veins into the iliac veins. The lymphatic drainage of the uterus is complex. The lymphatics from the fundus and the body of the uterus go to the aortic, lumbar, or pelvic nodes surrounding the iliac vessels, especially the internal iliac nodes. However, it is possible for metastatic disease from the uterus to be transported to the superior inguinal nodes via lymphatics in the round ligament or directly spread to the paraaortic nodes. Surprisingly, the lymphatic drainage of the uterus is not that different from the lymphatic drainage of the cervix.

In contrast to other pelvic organs, the **afferent sensory nerve** fibers from the uterus are in close proximity to the sympathetic nerves. Afferent nerve fibers from the uterus enter the spinal cord at the eleventh and twelfth thoracic segments. The sympathetic nerve supply to the uterus comes from the hypogastric and ovarian plexuses. The parasympathetic fibers are largely derived from the pelvic nerve and from the second, third, and fourth sacral segments.

## CLINICAL CORRELATIONS

Removal of the uterus is termed a *hysterectomy*, which is derived from the Greek word *hystera*, meaning "womb." The symptoms of primary dysmenorrhea are successfully treated in most women with the use of prostaglandin synthetase inhibitors such as **nonsteroidal anti-inflammatory drugs (NSAIDs)**. However, it is possible to alleviate uterine pain by cutting the sensory nerves that accompany the sympathetic nerves. This operation is termed a *presacral neurectomy*. During the operation the gynecologist must be careful to avoid injuring the ureters and also careful to control hemorrhage from vessels in the retroperitoneal space. This operation has lost popularity because of its association with autonomic dysfunction of the bladder and rectum presumed to be secondary to the inadvertent disruption of motor fibers.

The position of the fundus of the uterus in relation to the long axis of the vagina is quite variable (Fig. 3.16; see Fig. 3.7). Not only are there differences among individual women, but also in the same woman differences occur secondary to normal activity. In some women the uterus is anteflexed or anteverted, whereas in others the normal position is retroflexed or retroverted.

The arterial blood supply enters the uterus on its lateral margins. This relationship allows morcellation of an enlarged uterus to facilitate removal of multiple myomas without appreciably increasing blood loss during vaginal hysterectomy.

Similar to the lymphatic drainage of the cervix, the lymphatic drainage of the uterus has also been studied. Sentinel lymph nodes can be found on either side of the pelvis and paraaortic areas in 85% to 90% of cases using near-infrared fluorescence imaging and ICG (Abu-Rustum, 2014) (Fig. 3.18).

### Fallopian Tubes (Oviducts)

The paired uterine tubes, more commonly referred to as the *fallopian tubes* or *oviducts*, extend outward from the superolateral portion of the uterus and end by curling around the ovary. The oviducts are also referred to using the prefix *salpingo-*, from the Greek *salpinx*, meaning "tube." The tubes are contained in a free edge of the superior portion of the broad ligament. The mesentery of the tubes, the mesosalpinx, contains the blood supply and nerves. The uterine tubes connect the cornua of the uterine cavity and the peritoneal cavity. The ostia into the endometrial cavity are 1.5 mm in diameter, whereas the ostia into the abdominal cavity are approximately 3 mm in diameter.

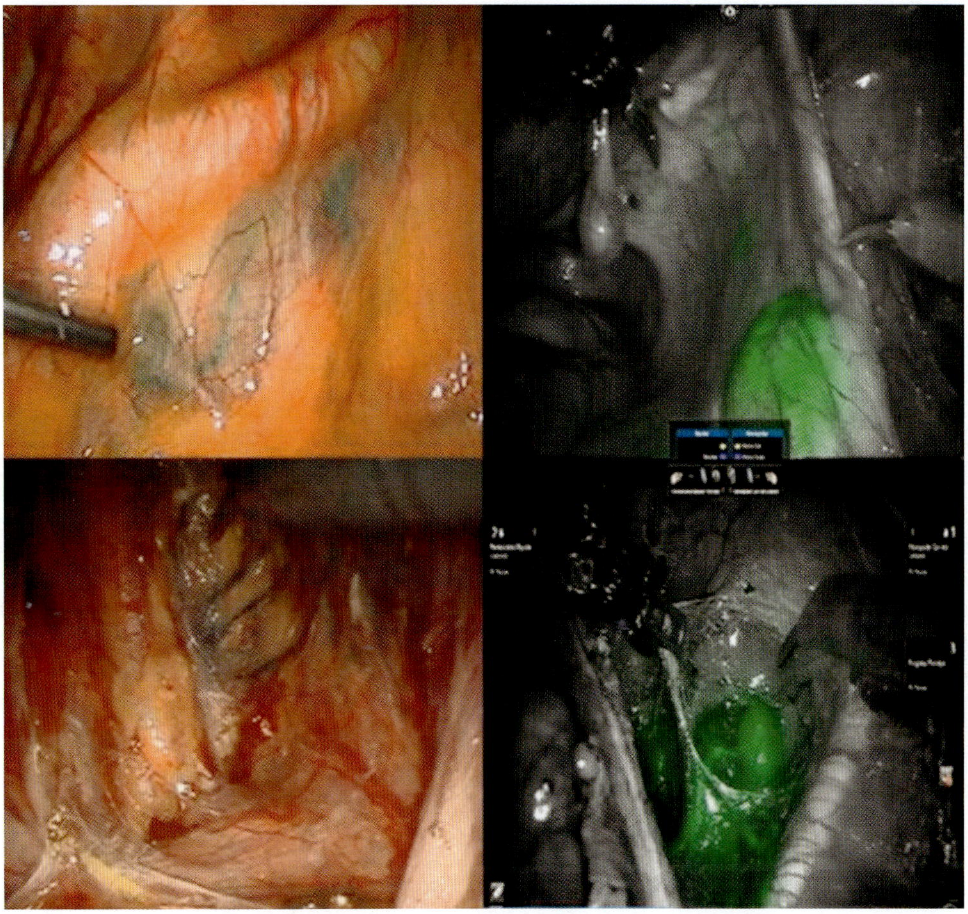

Fig. 3.18 Intraoperative view of sentinel lymph node mapping with isosulfan blue dye on the left and indocyanine green on the right. (From Sinno AK, Fader AN, Roche KL, et al. A comparison of colorimetric versus fluorometric sentinel lymph node mapping during robotic surgery for endometrial cancer. *Gynecol Oncol.* 2014;134(2):281-286.)

The **oviducts** are between 10 and 14 cm long and slightly less than 1 cm in external diameter. Each tube is divided into four anatomic sections. The uterine intramural, or interstitial, segment is 1 to 2 cm long and is surrounded by myometrium. The isthmic segment begins as the tube exits the uterus and is approximately 4 cm long, narrow, 1 to 2 mm in inside diameter, and straight; it has the most highly developed musculature. The ampullary segment is 4 to 6 cm long, approximately 6 mm in inside diameter, and is wider and more tortuous in its course than other segments. **Fertilization** normally occurs in the ampullary portion of the tube. The infundibulum is the distal trumpet-shaped portion of the oviduct. Approximately 20 to 25 irregular finger-like projections, termed *fimbriae*, surround the abdominal ostia of the tube. One of the largest fimbriae is attached to the ovary, the fimbria ovarica.

The tube contains numerous longitudinal folds, called *plicae*, of mucosa and underlying stroma. Plicae are most prominent in the ampullary segment (Fig. 3.19).

The mucosa of the oviduct has three different cell types. Columnar ciliated epithelial cells are most prominent near the ovarian end of the tube and make up 25% of the mucosal cells overall (Fig. 3.20).

Secretory cells, also columnar in shape, comprise 60% of the epithelial lining and are more prominent in the isthmic segment. Narrow peg cells are found between secretory and ciliated cells and are believed to be a morphologic variant of secretory cells. The stroma of the mucosa is sparse. However, there is a thick lamina propria with vascular channels between the epithelium and muscular layers. The smooth muscle of the tube is arranged into inner circular and outer longitudinal layers. Between the peritoneal surface of the tube and the muscular layer is an adventitial layer that contains blood vessels and nerves.

The arterial blood supply to the oviducts is derived from terminal branches of **the uterine and ovarian arteries**. The arteries anastomose in the mesosalpinx. Blood from the uterine artery supplies the medial two-thirds of each tube. The venous drainage runs parallel to the arterial supply. The lymphatic system is separate and distinct from the lymphatic drainage of the uterus. Lymphatic drainage includes the internal iliac nodes and the aortic nodes surrounding the aorta and the inferior vena cava at the level of the renal vessels. The tubes are innervated by both sympathetic and parasympathetic nerves from the uterine and ovarian plexuses. Sensory nerves are related to spinal cord segments T11, T12, and L1.

## CLINICAL CORRELATIONS

An ectopic pregnancy occurs when a fertilized ovum is implanted and develops outside the normal uterine cavity. The majority of ectopic pregnancies occur in the fallopian tube, with 70% found within the **ampulla** and 12% found in the isthmus of the fallopian tube. Quick evaluation and assessment are

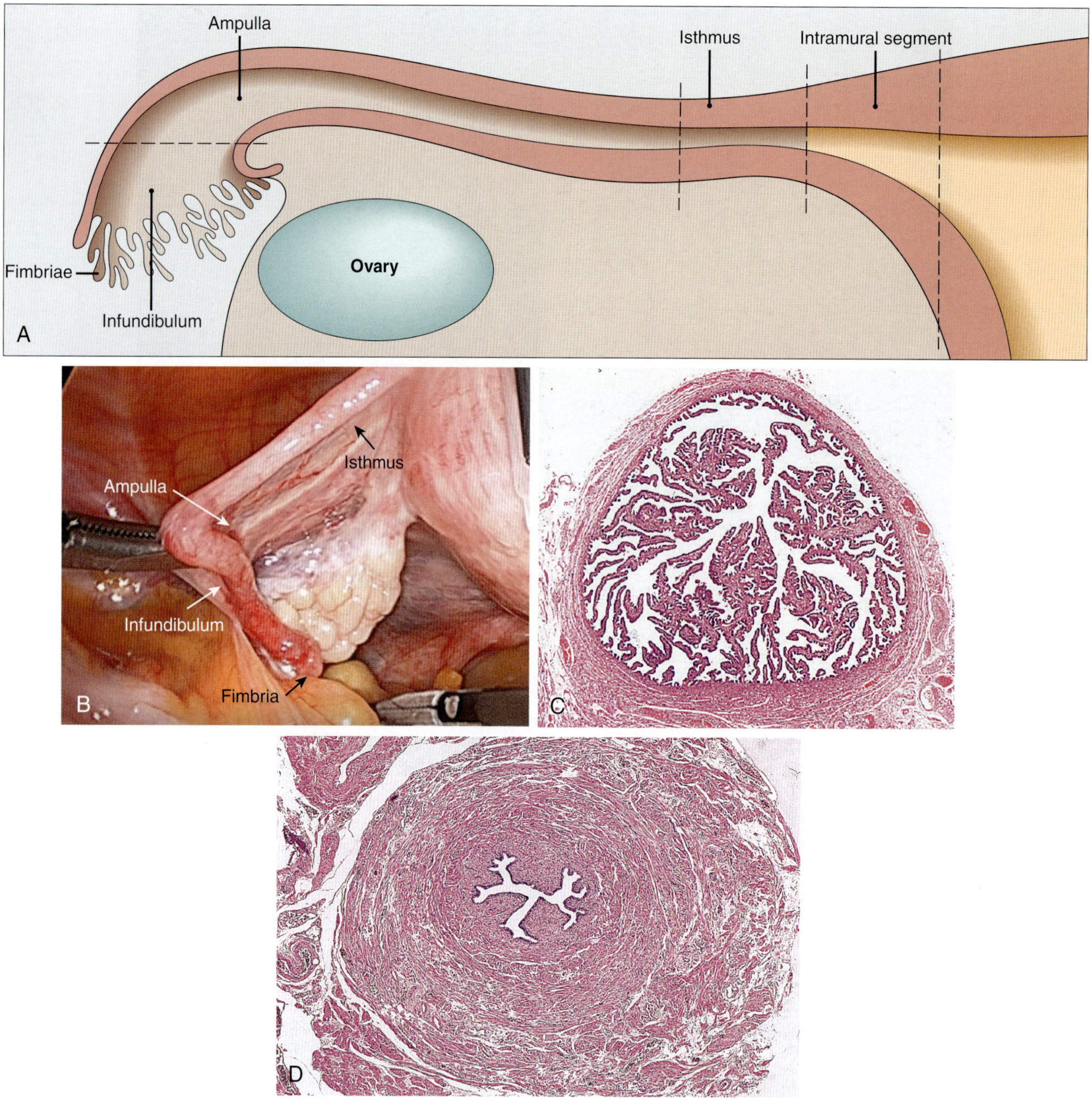


**Fig. 3.19** The fallopian tube. **A,** Schematic representation. Note that the intramural segment is within the uterine body. **B,** Intraoperative picture of the fallopian tube closely resembling the schematic view. **C,** Low-power histologic section from the ampulla. **D,** Section from the isthmus of the tube. Note the thick muscular wall. (**A** and **C,** From Stevens A, Lowe J. *Human Histology.* 3rd ed. Philadelphia: Elsevier; 2002:354; **D,** From Robboy SJ, Anderson MC, Russell P, eds. *Pathology of the Female Reproductive Tract.* Edinburgh: Churchill Livingstone; 2002:416. **B,** Courtesy Fidel A. Valea, MD.)

critical to this diagnosis and are often done in an emergency department setting. The most catastrophic bleeding associated with ectopic pregnancy occurs when the implantation site is in the intramural segment of the tube; many of these patients present with unstable vital signs and need to be taken the operating room emergently. The isthmic segment of the oviduct is the preferred site to apply an occlusive device, such a clip, or cauterization for female sterilization. The right oviduct and appendix are often adjacent. Clinically it may be difficult to differentiate inflammation of the tube from acute appendicitis. Accessory tubal ostia are discovered commonly and always connect with the lumen of the tube. These accessory ostia are usually found in the ampullary portion of the tube. The wide mesosalpinx of the ampullary segment of the tube allows torsion of the tube, which occasionally results in ischemic atrophy of the ampullary segment. Paratubal or paraovarian cysts can reach 5 to 10 cm in diameter and occasionally are confused with ovarian cysts before surgery.

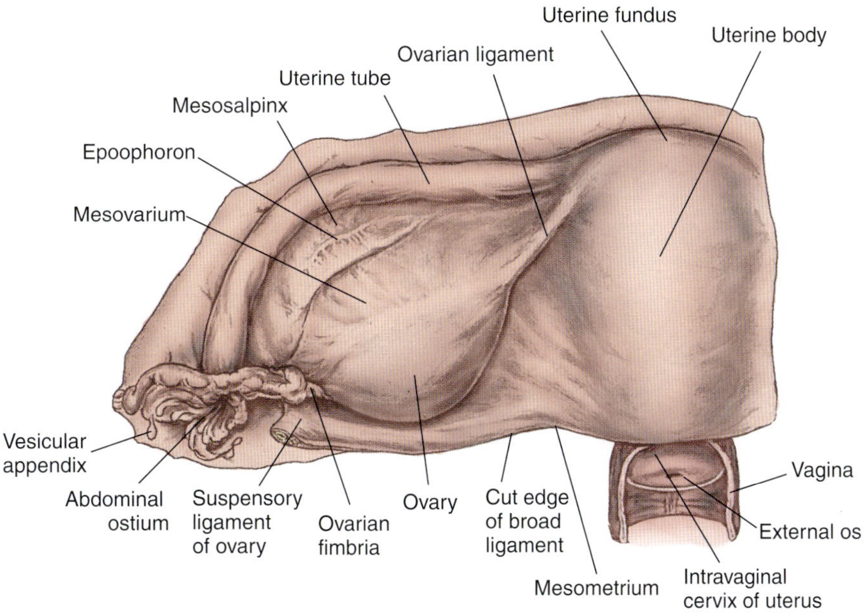


**Fig. 3.20** The posterior aspect of the broad ligament, spread out to demonstrate the ovary. (From Standring S, ed. *Gray's Anatomy.* 39th ed. Edinburgh: Churchill Livingstone; 2005:1322.)

## Ovaries

The paired ovaries are light gray, and each one is approximately the size and configuration of a large almond. The surface of the ovary of adult women is pitted and indented from previous ovulations. The ovaries contain approximately 1 to 2 million oocytes at birth. During a woman's reproductive lifetime, about 8000 follicles begin development. The growth of many follicles is blunted in various stages of development; however, approximately 300 ova eventually are released. The size and position of the ovary depend on the woman's age and parity. During the reproductive years, ovaries weigh 3 to 6 g and measure approximately 1.5 cm by 2.5 cm by 4 cm. As a woman ages, the ovaries become smaller and firmer. The long axis of the ovary is vertical in a nulliparous woman who is standing, and the ovary rests in a depression of peritoneum named the ovarian fossa. Immediately adjacent to the ovarian fossa are the external iliac vessels, the ureter, and the obturator vessels and nerves.

Three prominent ligaments determine the anatomic mobility of the ovary (Figs. 3.20 and 3.21).

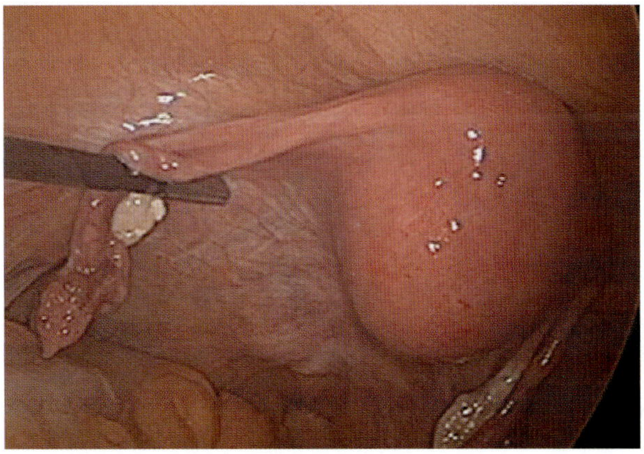

**Fig. 3.21** Intraoperative picture of the left broad ligament spread out to demonstrate the ovary. (Courtesy Fidel A. Valea, MD.)

The posterior portion of the broad ligament forms the mesovarium, which attaches to the anterior border of the ovary. The mesovarium contains the arterial anastomotic branches of the ovarian and uterine arteries, a plexus of veins, and the lateral end of the ovarian ligament. The ovarian ligament is a narrow, short, fibrous band that extends from the lower pole of the ovary to the uterus. The **infundibulopelvic ligament**, or suspensory ligament of the ovary, forms the superior and lateral aspect of the broad ligament. This ligament contains the ovarian artery, ovarian veins, and accompanying nerves and attaches the upper pole of the ovary to the lateral pelvic wall.

The ovary is subdivided histologically into an outer cortex and an inner medulla (Fig. 3.22). The ovarian surface is covered by a single layer of cuboidal epithelium, termed the *germinal epithelium.* This term is a misnomer because the cells are similar to those of the coelomic mesothelium, which forms the peritoneum, and because the germinal epithelium is not related to the histogenesis of graafian follicles. If the ovary is transected, numerous transparent, fluid-filled cysts are noted throughout the cortex. Microscopically these are graafian follicles in various stages of development, active or regressing corpus luteum, and atretic follicles. The stroma of the cortex is composed primarily of closely packed cells around the follicles. These specialized connective tissue cells form the theca. The medulla contains the ovarian vascular supply and a loose stroma. The specialized polyhedral hilar cells are similar to the interstitial cells of the testis.

Each of the ovarian arteries arises directly from the aorta just below the renal arteries. They descend in the retroperitoneal space, cross anterior to the psoas muscles and internal iliac vessels, and enter the infundibulopelvic ligaments, reaching the mesovarium in the broad ligament. The ovarian blood supply enters through the hilum of the ovary. The venous drainage of the ovary collects in the pampiniform plexus and consolidates into several large veins as it leaves the hilum of the ovary. The ovarian veins accompany the ovarian arteries, with the left ovarian vein draining into the left renal vein, whereas the right ovarian vein connects directly with the inferior vena cava.

The lymphatic drainage of the ovaries is primarily to the aortic nodes adjacent to the great vessels at the level of the renal

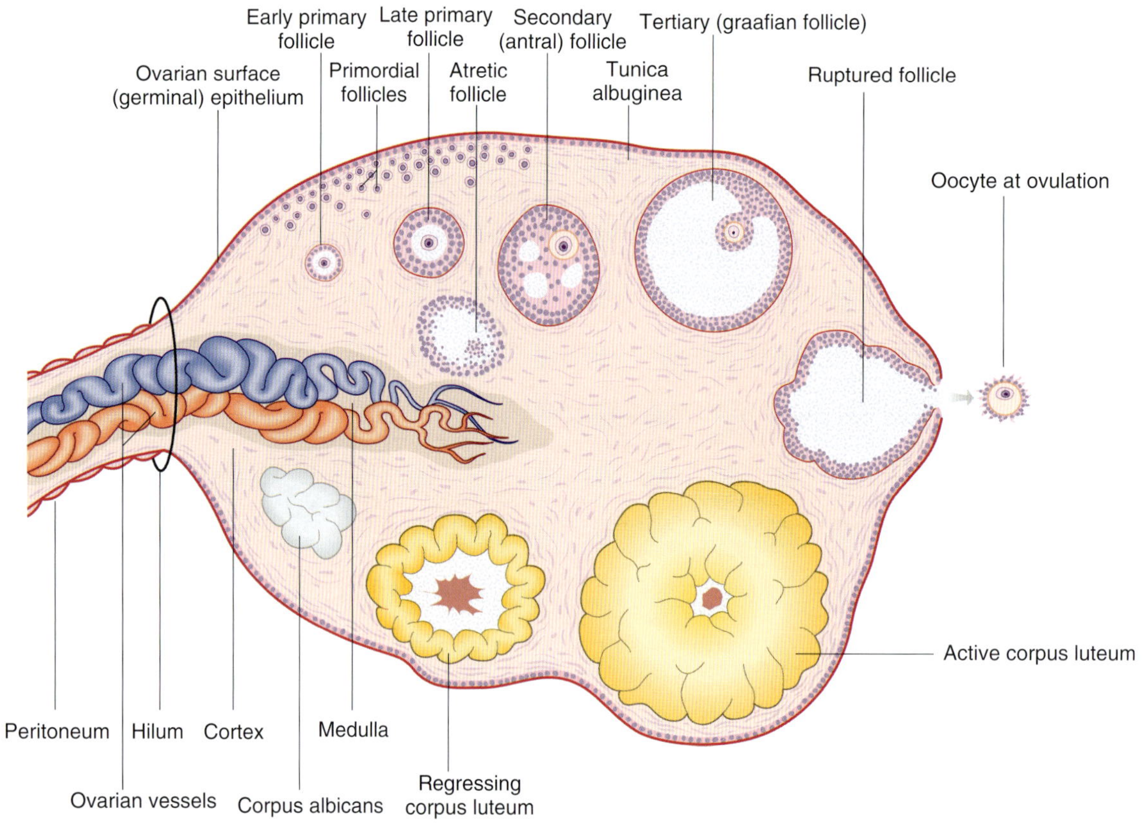


**Fig. 3.22** A schematic drawing of the ovary. Note the single layer of cuboidal epithelium called the *germinal epithelium.* Note the graafian follicles in different stages of development. (From Standring S, ed. *Gray's Anatomy.* 39th ed. Edinburgh: Churchill Livingstone; 2005:1324.)

veins. Metastatic disease from the ovary occasionally takes a shorter course to the iliac nodes. The autonomic and sensory nerve fibers accompany the ovarian vasculature in the infundibulopelvic ligament. They connect with the ovarian, hypogastric, and aortic plexuses.

## CLINICAL CORRELATIONS

The size of the "normal" ovary during the reproductive years and the postmenopausal period is important in clinical practice. Before menopause a normal ovary may be up to 5 cm long. Thus a small physiologic cyst may cause an ovary to be 6 to 7 cm in diameter. In contrast, the normal atrophic postmenopausal ovary usually cannot be palpated during pelvic examination and is often not visible by ultrasound imaging.

It is important to emphasize that the ovaries and surrounding peritoneum are not devoid of pain and pressure receptors. Therefore it is not unusual for a woman to experience discomfort when normal ovaries are palpated bimanually during a routine pelvic examination. Patients can present in an acute setting or during a routine office visit with complaints of pelvic pain.

The close anatomic proximity of the ovary, ovarian fossa, and ureter is emphasized in surgery to treat severe endometriosis or pelvic inflammatory disease. It is important to identify the course of the ureter to facilitate removal of all of the ovarian capsule that is adherent to the peritoneum and surrounding structures so as to avoid immediate ureteral injury and residual retroperitoneal ovarian remnants in the future. Prophylactic oophorectomy is performed at the time of pelvic operations in many postmenopausal women older than 65. Sometimes bilateral oophorectomy is technically more difficult when associated with a vaginal procedure in contrast to an abdominal or laparoscopic hysterectomy. Vaginal removal of the ovaries may be facilitated by identifying the anatomic landmarks, similar to the abdominal approach, and separately clamping the round ligaments and infundibulopelvic ligaments.

## VASCULAR SYSTEM OF THE PELVIS

Several generalizations can be made in describing the network of arteries that bring blood to the female reproductive organs. The arteries are paired, bilateral, and have multiple collaterals (Fig. 3.23).

The arteries enter their respective organs laterally and then unite with anastomotic vessels from the other side of the pelvis near the midline. There is a long-standing teaching generalization that the pelvic reproductive viscera lie within a loosely woven basket of large veins with numerous interconnecting venous plexuses. The arteries thread their way through this interwoven mesh of veins to reach the pelvic reproductive organs, giving off numerous branching arcades to provide a rich blood supply.

### Arteries

#### Inferior Mesenteric Artery

The inferior mesenteric artery, a single artery, arises from the aorta approximately 3 cm above the aortic bifurcation. It supplies part of the transverse, descending and sigmoid colon, as well as the rectum, and terminates as the superior hemorrhoidal artery.

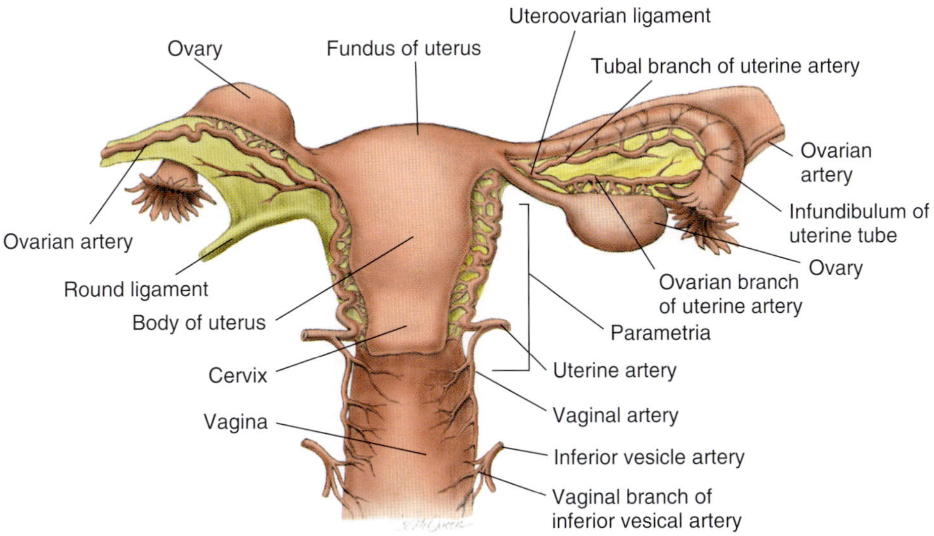


**Fig. 3.23** The arteries of the reproductive organs. Note the paired arteries entering laterally and freely anastomosing with each other. (Modified from Clemente CD. *Anatomy: A Regional Atlas of the Human Body.* 3rd ed. Baltimore-Munich: Urban & Schwarzenberg; 1987.)

The inferior mesenteric artery is occasionally torn during node dissections performed in staging operations for gynecologic cancer. Because of the rich collateral circulation from the middle and inferior hemorrhoidal arteries, as well as the marginal artery of Drummond, the inferior mesenteric artery can be ligated without compromise of the distal portion of the colon.

### Ovarian Artery

The ovarian arteries originate from the aorta just below the renal vessels. Each one courses in the retroperitoneal space, crosses anterior to the ureter, and enters the infundibulopelvic ligament. As the artery travels medially in the mesovarium, numerous small branches supply the ovary and oviduct. The ovarian artery unites with the ascending branch of the uterine artery in the mesovarium just under the suspensory ligament of the ovary.

### Common Iliac Artery

The bifurcation of the aorta occurs at the level of the fourth lumbar vertebra, forming the two common iliac arteries. Each common iliac artery is approximately 5 cm in length before the vessel divides into the external iliac and hypogastric arteries.

### Hypogastric Artery (Internal Iliac Artery)

The hypogastric arteries are short vessels, approximately 3 to 4 cm long. Throughout their course they are in close proximity to the ureters, which are anterior, and to the hypogastric veins, which are posterior. Most commonly (variations are frequent), each hypogastric artery branches into an anterior and a posterior division (or trunk). The branching is usually 2 cm from the common iliac. The posterior trunk gives off three parietal branches: the iliolumbar, lateral sacral, and superior gluteal arteries. The anterior trunk has nine branches. The three parietal branches are the obturator, internal pudendal, and inferior gluteal arteries. The six visceral branches include the umbilical, middle vesical, inferior vesical, middle hemorrhoidal, uterine, and vaginal arteries. The superior vesical artery usually arises from the umbilical artery. The individual branches of the hypogastric artery may vary from one woman to another.

### Uterine Artery

The uterine artery arises from the anterior division of the hypogastric artery and courses medially toward the isthmus of the uterus. Approximately 2 cm lateral to the endocervix, it crosses over the ureter and reaches the lateral side of the uterus. The ascending branch of the uterine artery courses in the broad ligament, running a tortuous route to finally anastomose with the ovarian artery in the mesovarium (Fig. 3.24).

Through its circuitous route in the parametrium, the uterine artery gives off numerous branches that unite with arcuate arteries from the other side. This series of arcuate arteries develops radial branches that supply the myometrium and the basalis layer of the endometrium. The arcuate arteries also form the spiral arteries of the functional layer of the endometrium. The descending branch of the uterine artery produces branches that supply both the cervix and the vagina. In each case the vessels enter the organ laterally and anastomose freely with vessels from the other side.

## Vaginal Artery

The vaginal artery may arise either from the anterior trunk of the hypogastric artery or from the uterine artery. It supplies blood to the vagina, bladder, and rectum. There are extensive anastomoses with the vaginal branches of the uterine artery to form the azygos arteries of the cervix and vagina.

### Internal Pudendal Artery

The internal pudendal artery is the terminal branch of the hypogastric artery. It supplies branches to the rectum, labia, clitoris, and perineum.

## Veins

The venous drainage of the pelvis begins in small sinusoids that drain to numerous venous plexuses contained within or immediately adjacent to the pelvic organs. Invariably there are numerous anastomoses between the parietal and visceral branches of the venous system. In general the veins of the female pelvis and perineum are thin walled and have few valves.

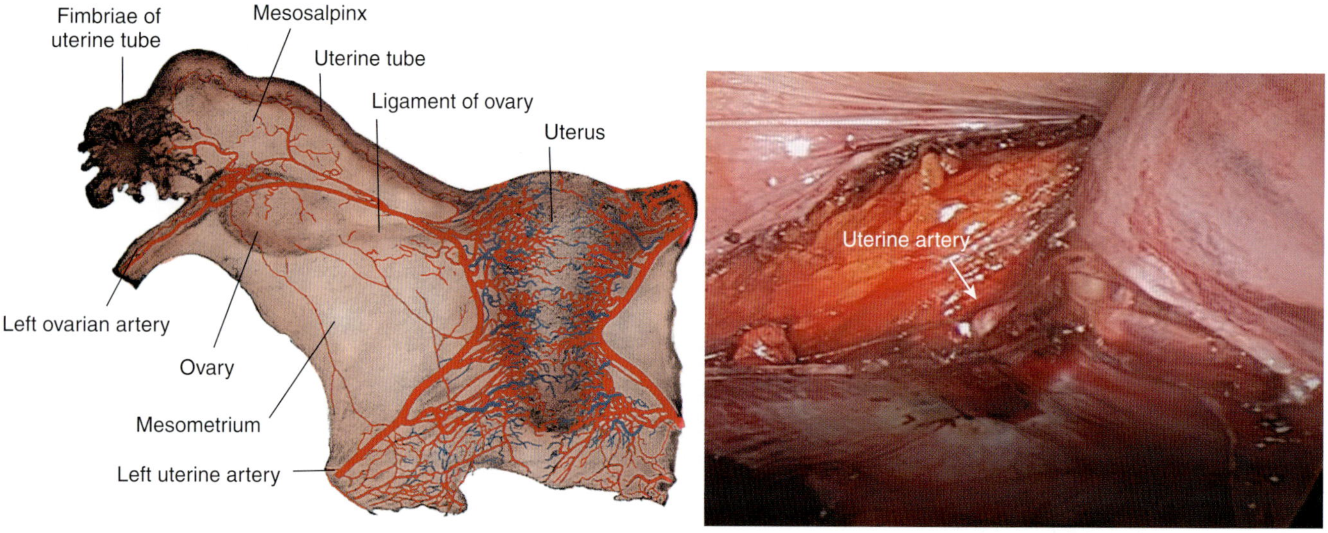


**Fig. 3.24 A,** Photograph of an injected specimen demonstrating the rich anastomoses of the uterine and ovarian arteries. (From Warwick R, Williams PL. *Gray's Anatomy.* 35th ed. Edinburgh: Churchill Livingstone; 1973:1361.) **B,** Intraoperative picture showing dissection of the uterine artery on patients left side. (Courtesy Fidel A. Valea, MD.)

The veins that drain the pelvic plexuses follow the course of the arterial supply. Their names are similar to those of the accompanying arteries. Often multiple veins run alongside a single artery. One special exception is the venous drainage of the ovaries. The left ovarian vein empties into the left renal vein, whereas the right ovarian vein connects directly with the inferior vena cava.

## CLINICAL CORRELATIONS

Although the external iliac artery and its branches do not supply blood directly to the pelvic viscera, they are important landmarks in surgical anatomy. The fact that the external iliac artery gives rise to **the obturator artery** in 15% to 20% of women must be considered in radical cancer operations with associated node dissections of the obturator fossa. The external iliac artery also gives rise to the inferior epigastric artery. The inferior epigastric artery should be avoided when performing laparoscopic operative procedures.

In certain clinical situations associated with profuse hemorrhage from the female pelvis, hypogastric artery ligation is performed. Because of the extensive collateral circulation, this operation does not produce hypoxia of the pelvic viscera but reduces hemorrhage by decreasing the arterial pulse pressure. The extent of collateral circulation after hypogastric artery ligation depends on the site of ligation and may be divided into three groups (Box 3.1).

In cases of intractable pelvic hemorrhage, it may be necessary to supplement the effects of bilateral hypogastric artery ligation with ligation of the anastomotic sites between the ovarian and uterine vessels. Ligation of the terminal end of the ovarian artery (utero-ovarian ligament) preserves the direct blood supply to the ovaries and minimizes the fear of subsequent cystic degeneration of the ovaries that may occur after ligation of the vessels in the infundibulopelvic ligaments. Arterial embolization provides an alternative approach to ligation. A catheter is advanced under fluoroscopic visualization, and small particulate material is injected to produce hemostasis in the bleeding vessels. This less invasive technique, when appropriate, may preserve fertility. A rare condition that presents an interesting challenge to the clinician is a congenital arteriovenous (AV) malformation in the female pelvis. Most of these AV fistulas are treated with preoperative embolism and subsequent operative ligation.

One of the treatments for repetitive embolization arising from thrombosis is the placement of a vascular umbrella into the inferior vena cava. Collateral circulation exists between the portal venous system of the gastrointestinal tract and the systemic venous circulation through anastomosis in the pelvis, especially in the hemorrhoidal plexus. The pelvic veins also anastomose with the presacral and lumbar veins. Thus, though rare, patients may develop trophoblastic emboli to the brain without the trophoblast being filtered by the capillary system in the lungs.

**BOX 3.1** Collateral Arterial Circulation of the Pelvis

**BRANCHES FROM AORTA**

*Ovarian artery*—anastomoses freely with uterine artery
*Inferior mesenteric artery*—continues as superior hemorrhoidal artery to anastomose with middle and inferior hemorrhoidal arteries from hypogastric and internal pudendal
*Lumbar and vertebral arteries*—anastomose with iliolumbar artery of hypogastric
*Middle sacral artery*—anastomoses with lateral sacral artery of hypogastric

**BRANCHES FROM EXTERNAL ILIAC ARTERY**

*Deep iliac circumflex artery*—anastomoses with iliolumbar and superior gluteal of hypogastric
*Inferior epigastric artery*—gives origin to obturator artery in 25% of cases, providing additional anastomoses of external iliac with medial femoral circumflex and communicating pelvic branches

**BRANCHES FROM FEMORAL ARTERY**

*Medial femoral circumflex artery*—anastomoses with obturator and inferior gluteal arteries from hypogastric
*Lateral femoral circumflex artery*—anastomoses with superior gluteal and iliolumbar arteries from hypogastric

From Mattingly RF, Thompson JD. *Te Linde's Operative Gynecology.* 6th ed. Philadelphia: JB Lippincott; 1985.

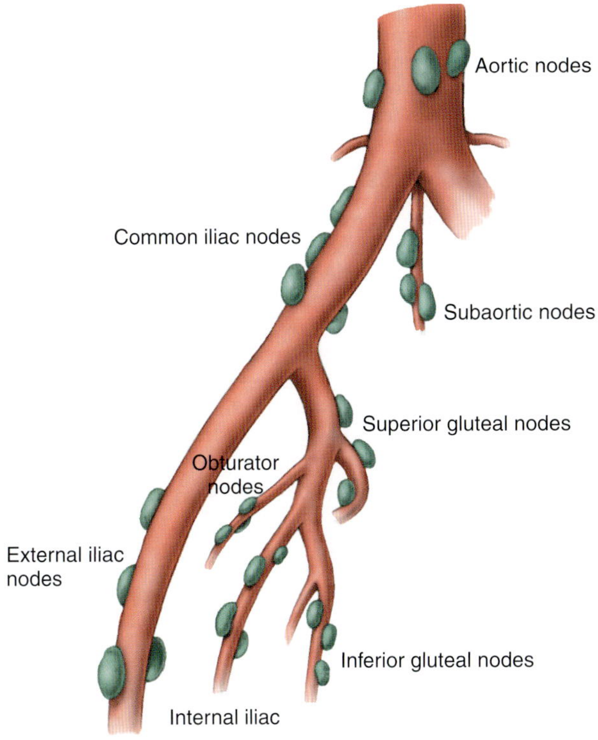


**Fig. 3.25** Schematic view of the pelvic lymph nodes. (From Plentl AA, Friedman EA. *Lymphatic System of the Female Genitalia.* Philadelphia: WB Saunders; 1971:13.)

## LYMPHATIC SYSTEM

### External Iliac Nodes

The external iliac nodes are immediately adjacent to the external iliac artery and vein (Figs. 3.25 and 3.26). There are two distinct groups, one situated lateral to the vessels and the other posterior to the psoas muscle. The distal portion of the posterior group is enclosed in the femoral sheath. Most of the lymphatic channels to this group of nodes originate from the vulva, but there are also channels from the cervix and lower portion of the uterus. The external iliac nodes receive secondary drainage from the femoral and internal iliac nodes.

### Internal Iliac Nodes

The internal iliac nodes are found in an anatomic triangle whose sides are composed of the external iliac artery, the hypogastric artery, and the pelvic sidewall. Included in this clinically important area are nodes with special designation, including the nodes of the femoral ring, the obturator nodes, and the nodes adjacent to the external iliac vessels. This rich collection of nodes receives channels from every internal pelvic organ and the vulva, including the clitoris and urethra. The sentinel lymph nodes from the cervix and uterus are often found within the internal iliac chain of nodes, most commonly inferior and medial to the bifurcation of iliac vein.

### Common Iliac Nodes

The common iliac nodes are a group of nodes located adjacent to the vessels that bear their name and are between the external iliac and aortic chains. Most of these nodes are found lateral to the vessels. To remove this chain, it is necessary to dissect the common iliac vessels away from their attachments to the psoas muscle, as well as the genitofemoral nerve, which is commonly encased in lymph nodes. This group receives lymphatics from the cervix, uterus, and ovary and the upper portion of the vagina. Secondary lymphatic drainage from the internal iliac, external iliac, superior gluteal, and inferior gluteal nodes flows to the common iliac nodes.

### Inferior Gluteal Nodes

A small group of lymph nodes, the inferior gluteal nodes, are located in anatomic proximity to the ischial spines and are adjacent to the sacral plexus of nodes. It is difficult to remove these nodes surgically. They receive lymphatic drainage from the

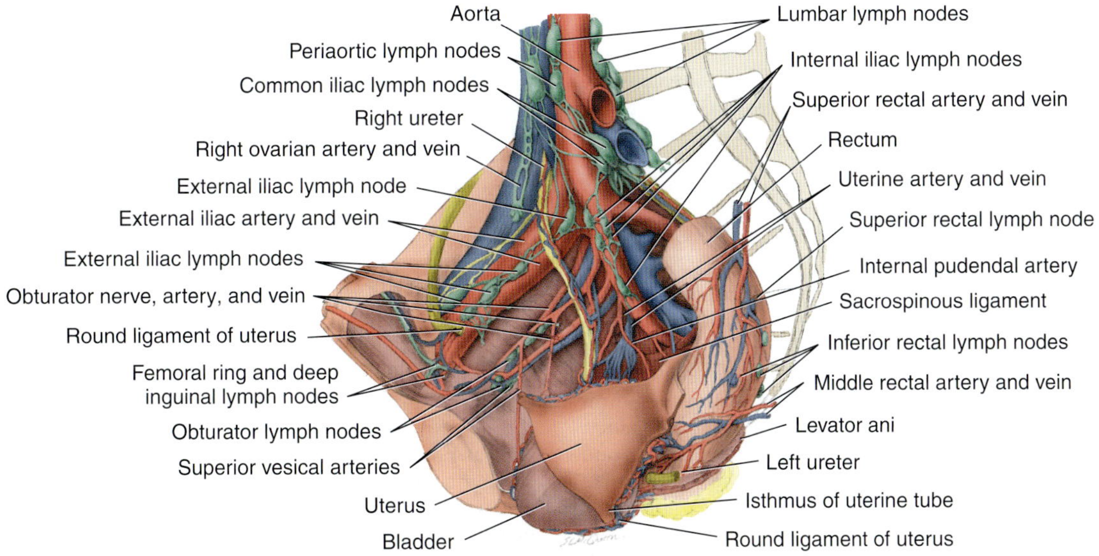


**Fig. 3.26** A lateral view of the female pelvis demonstrating the extensive lymphatic network. Note that most of the lymphatic channels follow the courses of the major vessels. (Modified from Clemente CD. *Anatomy: A Regional Atlas of the Human Body.* 3rd ed. Baltimore-Munich: Urban & Schwarzenberg; 1987.)

cervix, the lower portion of the vagina, and Bartholin glands and secondarily drain to the internal iliac, common iliac, superior gluteal, and subaortic nodes.

### Superior Gluteal Nodes

The superior gluteal nodes are a group of nodes found near the origin of the superior gluteal artery and adjacent to the medial and posterior aspects of the hypogastric vessels. The superior gluteal nodes receive primary lymphatic drainage from the cervix and the vagina. Efferent lymphatics from this chain drain to the common iliac, sacral, or subaortic nodes.

### Sacral Nodes

The sacral nodes are found over the middle of the sacrum in a space bounded laterally by the sacral foramina. These nodes receive lymphatic drainage from both the cervix and the vagina. Secondary drainage from these nodes runs in a cephalad direction to the subaortic nodes.

### Subaortic Nodes

The subaortic nodes are arranged in a chain and are located below the bifurcation of the aorta, immediately anterior to the most caudal portion of the inferior vena cava and over the fifth lumbar vertebra. The primary drainage to this chain of nodes is from the cervix, with a few lymphatics from the vagina. This group is the first secondary chain to receive the efferent lymphatics as lymph flow progresses in a cephalad direction from the majority of other pelvic nodes.

### Aortic Nodes

The many aortic nodes are immediately adjacent to the aorta on both its anterior and lateral aspects, predominantly in the furrow between the aorta and inferior vena cava. Primary lymphatics drain from all the major pelvic organs, including the cervix, uterus, oviducts, and especially the ovaries. The aortic chain receives secondary drainage from the **pelvic nodes**. In general, primary afferent lymphatics drain into the nodes over the anterior aspects of the aorta, whereas secondary efferent drainage from other pelvic nodes is found in those nodes situated lateral and posterior to the aorta.

### Rectal Nodes

The rectal nodes are found subfascially and in the loose connective tissue surrounding the rectum. Primary drainage from the cervix flows to the superior rectal nodes, and drainage from the vagina appears in the rectal nodes in the anorectal region. Secondary drainage from the rectal nodes goes to the subaortic and aortic groups.

### Parauterine Nodes

The number of lymph nodes in the group of parauterine nodes is small; most commonly there is a single node immediately lateral to each side of the cervix and adjacent to the pelvic course of the ureter. Though anatomists often do not comment about the parauterine nodes, the group receives special attention in radical surgical operations to treat uterine or cervical malignancy. Primary drainage to this node originates in the vagina, cervix, and uterus. Secondary drainage from this node is to the internal iliac nodes on the same side of the pelvis.

### Superficial Femoral Nodes

The superficial femoral nodes are a group of nodes found in the loose, fatty connective tissue of the femoral triangle between the superficial and deep fascial layers. These lymph nodes receive lymphatic drainage from the external genitalia of the vulvar region, the gluteal region, and the entire leg, including the foot. Efferent lymphatics from this group of nodes penetrate the fascia lata to enter the deep femoral nodes.

### Deep Femoral Nodes

The deep femoral nodes are located in the femoral sheath, adjacent to both the femoral artery and the vein within the femoral triangle. The femoral triangle is the anatomic space lying immediately distal to the fold of the groin. The boundaries of the femoral triangle are the sartorius and adductor longus muscles and the inguinal ligament. Each space contains, from medial to lateral, the femoral vein, artery, and nerve. This chain receives the primary lymphatics for the lower extremity and receives secondary efferent lymphatics from the superficial lymph nodes and thus the vulva. This group of lymph nodes is in direct continuity with the iliac and internal iliac chains.

## CLINICAL CORRELATIONS

A precise knowledge of pelvic lymphatics is important for the gynecologic oncologist who is surgically determining the extent of spread of a pelvic malignancy. Aortic and pelvic lymphadenectomy operations require precise knowledge of normal anatomy and possible anomalies in both the urinary and vascular systems. The fact that most lymphatic metastatic spread from ovarian carcinoma occurs in a **cephalad** direction should be emphasized. This explains the importance of sampling paraaortic nodes in staging operations for some ovarian and uterine malignancy. In carcinoma of the vulva, lymphatic drainage is usually unilateral for cancers that are clearly lateral to the midline but may drain to either side with midline or near midline lesions of the pelvis (Coleman, 2013). Thus bilateral node sampling is important for midline lesions, although most vulvar cancers less than 4 cm can be managed with SLN mapping and biopsy, limiting the extent of nodal dissection and hopefully limiting morbidity as well. In vulvar cancer surgery the SLN often can be found just inferior and lateral to the pubic tubercle (Figs. 3.27 and 3.28).

Pelvic hemorrhage, usually from venous bleeding, is the most common acute complication of a lymph node dissection because most pelvic lymph nodes are in anatomic proximity to major pelvic vessels. Lymphocysts in the retroperitoneal space are the most common chronic complication associated with radical node dissections.

For many years it was believed that all the superficial femoral nodes drained to a sentinel node called the *Cloquet node*. The Cloquet node, by the present classification system, would be one of the most distal and medial of the nodes in the external iliac chain. Now the node is only of historical interest because that assumption is neither anatomically nor clinically correct.

## INNERVATION OF THE PELVIS

### Internal Genitalia

The innervation of the internal genital organs is supplied primarily by the autonomic nervous system. The sympathetic portion of the autonomic nervous system originates in the thoracic and lumbar portions of the spinal cord, and sympathetic ganglia are located adjacent to the central nervous system. In contrast, the parasympathetic portion originates in cranial nerves and the middle three sacral segments of the cord, and the ganglia are located near the visceral organs. Although the fibers of both subdivisions of the autonomic nervous system often are intermingled in the same peripheral nerves, their physiologic actions are usually directly antagonistic. As a broad generalization, sympathetic

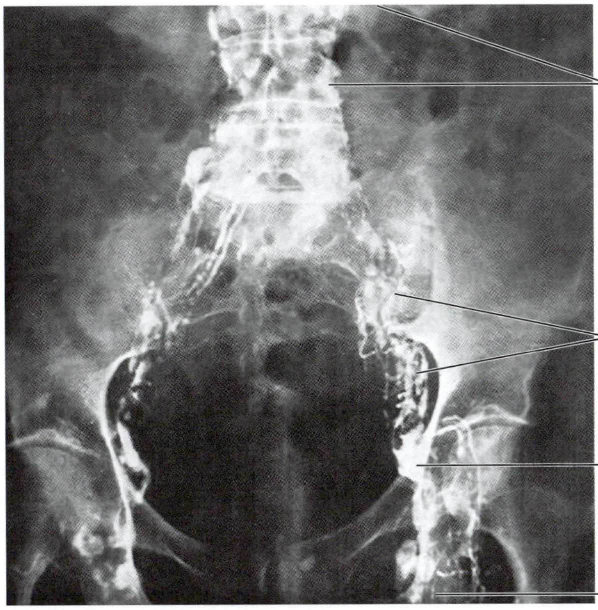


**Fig. 3.27** A lymphangiogram of the pelvis and lumbar areas. This radiograph shows the course of the lymphatics from the deep femoral nodes into the iliac nodes. Note the extensive network of nodes in the inguinal region. (From Clemente CD. *A Regional Atlas of the Human Body.* 3rd ed. Baltimore-Munich: Urban & Schwarzenberg; 1987.)

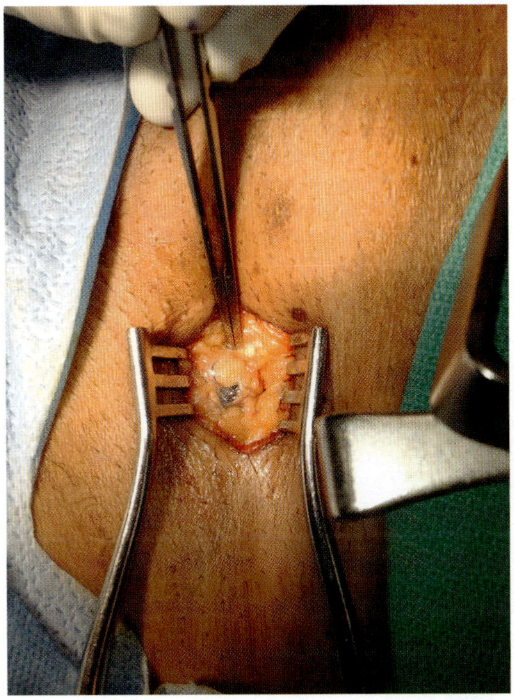

**Fig. 3.28** Photo of a blue vulvar sentinel lymph node with a blue lymphatic channel leading to the node. (Courtesy Fidel A. Valea, MD.)

fibers in the female pelvis produce muscular contractions and vasoconstriction, whereas parasympathetic fibers cause the opposite effect on muscles and vasodilation.

The semantics of pelvic innervation are confusing and imprecise. A *plexus* is a mixture of preganglionic and postganglionic fibers; small, inconsistently placed ganglia; and afferent (sensory) fibers. Throughout both the anatomic and surgical literature, a plexus may also be termed a *nerve.* For example, the superior hypogastric plexus is also called the *presacral nerve.*

Although autonomic nerve fibers enter the pelvis by several routes, most are contained in the superior hypogastric plexus, which is a caudal extension of the aortic and inferior mesenteric plexuses. The superior hypogastric plexus is found in the retroperitoneal connective tissue. It extends from the fourth lumbar vertebra to the hollow over the sacrum. In its lower portion the plexus divides to form the two hypogastric nerves, which run laterally and inferiorly. These nerves fan out to form the inferior hypogastric plexus in the area just below the bifurcation of the common iliac arteries. The nerve trunks descend farther into the base of the broad ligament, where they join with parasympathetic fibers to form the pelvic plexus. Both motor fibers and accompanying sensory fibers reach the pelvic plexus from S2, S3, and S4 via the pelvic nerves, or nervi erigentes. The pelvic plexus is found adjacent to the coccygeus muscle and sacrospinous ligaments. This complex is richly vascularized. The motor fibers to the levator ani (levator ani nerve) arise from the S2 to S4 nerve roots (primarily S3 and S4), traversing perpendicular to the muscle bundles and branching out to innervate the muscle fibers. The levator ani nerve does not innervate the anal sphincter, but the nerve is responsible for pelvic floor support. The pudendal nerve fibers also originate from the sacral plexus, with nerve fibers from S2 to S4. From the pelvic plexus, secondary plexuses are adjacent to all pelvic viscera—namely, the rectum, anus, urinary bladder, vagina, and Frankenhäuser plexus in the uterosacral ligaments.

The Frankenhäuser plexus is extensive and contains both myelinated and nonmyelinated fibers passing primarily to the uterus and cervix, with a few fibers passing to the urinary bladder and vagina. The ovarian plexus, like the blood supply to the ovaries, is not part of the hypogastric system; rather, it is a downward extension of the aortic and renal plexuses.

It is impossible to separate afferent sensory fibers from pelvic organs into morphologically independent tracts. Most fibers accompany the vascular system from the organ and then enter plexuses of the autonomic nervous system before eventually entering white rami communicates to the cell bodies in dorsal root ganglia of the spinal column. The major sensory fibers from the uterus accompany the sympathetic nerves, which enter the nerve roots of the spinal cord in segments **T11 and T12**. Thus referred uterine pain is often located in the lower abdomen. In contrast, afferents from the cervix enter the spinal cord in nerve roots of **S2, S3, and S4**. Referred pain from cervical inflammation and uterine irritation is characterized as low back pain in the lumbosacral region.

### External Genitalia

The **pudendal nerve** and its branches supply the majority of both motor and sensory fibers to the muscles and skin of the vulvar region. The pudendal nerve arises from the second, third, and fourth sacral roots. It has an interesting course in which it initially leaves the pelvis via the greater sciatic foramen. Next, it crosses beneath the ischial spine, running on the medial side of the internal pudendal artery. The pudendal nerve then reenters the pelvic cavity and travels in Alcock canal, which runs along the lateral aspects of the ischial rectal fossa. As the nerve reaches the urogenital diaphragm, it divides into three branches: the inferior hemorrhoidal, the deep perineal, and the superficial perineal (Fig. 3.29). The dorsal nerve of the clitoris is a terminal branch of the deep perineal nerve.

The skin of the anus, clitoris, and medial and inferior aspects of the vulva is supplied primarily by distal branches of the pudendal nerve. The vulvar region receives additional sensory fibers from three nerves: The anterior branch of the ilioinguinal nerve sends fibers to the mons pubis and the upper part of the labia majora; he genital femoral nerve supplies fibers to the labia majora; and the posterior femoral cutaneous nerve supplies fibers to the inferoposterior aspects of the vulva.

## CLINICAL CORRELATIONS

An unusual but troublesome postoperative complication of gynecologic surgery is injury to the femoral nerve. During abdominal hysterectomy, the femoral nerve may be compromised by pressure from the lateral blade of a self-retaining retractor in the area adjacent to where the femoral nerve penetrates the psoas muscle. During vaginal surgery, the femoral nerve may be injured from exaggerated hyperflexion of the legs in the lithotomy position because hyperflexion produces stretching and compression of the femoral nerve as it courses under the inguinal ligament.

Because of the low density of nerve endings in the upper two-thirds of the vagina, women are sometimes unable to determine the presence of a foreign body in this area. This explains how a "forgotten tampon" may remain unnoticed for several days in the upper part of the vagina until its presence results in a symptomatic discharge, abnormal bleeding, or odor. Infrequent but serious complications of pudendal nerve block are hematomas from trauma to the pudendal vessels and intravascular injection of anesthetic agents. The vessels and nerves are in close anatomic proximity to the ischial spine.

The **fallopian tube** is one of the most sensitive of the pelvic organs when crushed, cut, or distended, a fact that is appreciated in performing tubal ligations with the patient under local anesthesia. Damage to the obturator nerve during radical pelvic operations does not affect the pelvis directly. Although the nerve has an extensive pelvic course, its motor fibers supply the adductors of the thigh, and its sensory fibers innervate skin over the medial aspects of the thigh. Stitches placed during sacrospinous ligament fixation for pelvic support may interfere with neural roots S2 to S4 and the muscle pudendal and levator ani nerves.

## DIAPHRAGMS AND LIGAMENTS

### Pelvic Diaphragm

The pelvic diaphragm is a wide but thin muscular layer of tissue that forms the inferior border of the abdominopelvic cavity. Composed of a broad, funnel-shaped sling of fascia and muscle, it extends from the symphysis pubis to the coccyx and from one lateral sidewall to the other. The primary muscles of the pelvic diaphragm are the levator ani and the coccygeus (Fig. 3.30). This structure is the evolutionary remnant of the tail-wagging muscles in lower animals. *Endopelvic fascia* is another term often

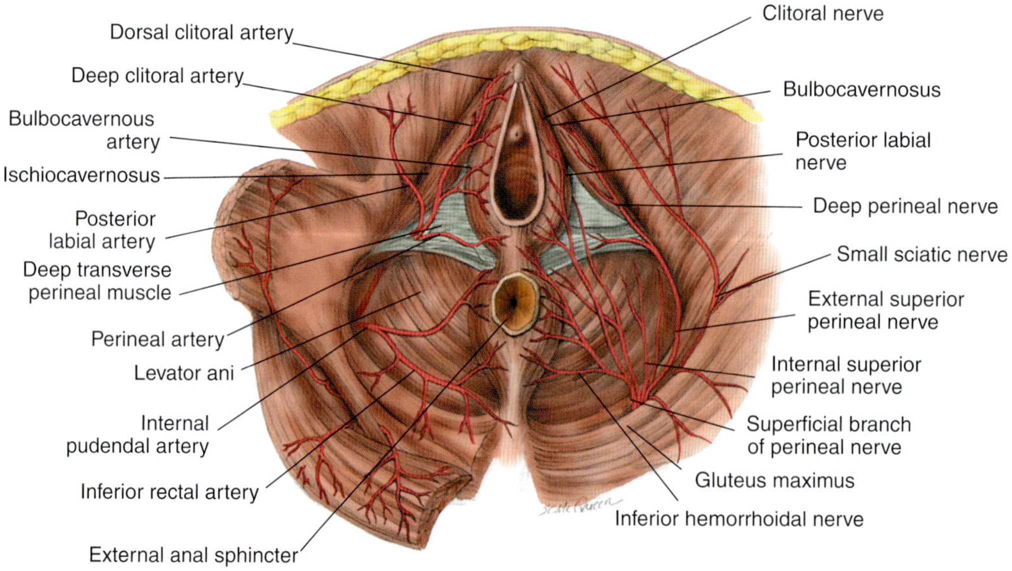


**Fig. 3.29** A posterior view of the female perineum demonstrating the pudendal nerve emerging externally. The nerve divides into three segments as it passes out of the pelvis: the inferior hemorrhoidal nerve and the deep and superficial perineal nerves. The clitoral nerve is the terminal branch of the deep perineal nerve. (Modified from Mattingly RF, Thompson JD. *Te Linde's Operative Gynecology.* 6th ed. Philadelphia: JB Lippincott; 1985:49.)

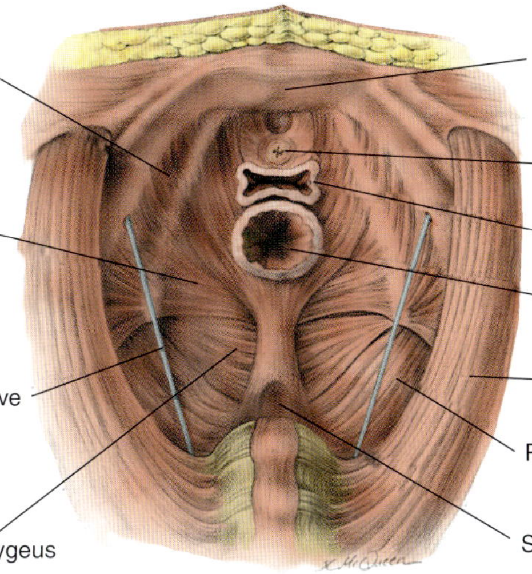


**Fig. 3.30** A superior view of the pelvic diaphragm and the pelvic floor. The primary muscles that compose this funnel-shaped sling are the coccygeus and the levator ani. (Modified from Mattingly RF, Thompson JD. *Te Linde's Operative Gynecology.* 6th ed. Philadelphia: Lippincott; 1985:41.)

used interchangeably with **pelvic diaphragm**, and both are terms used to characterize the connective tissue, the support for the pelvis, and the pelvic floor. The pelvic diaphragm is composed of collagen, elastic tissue, and muscle.

The muscles of the pelvic diaphragm are interwoven for strength, and a continuous muscle layer encircles the terminal portions of the urethra, vagina, and rectum. The levator ani muscles constitute the greatest bulk of the pelvic diaphragm and are divided into three components, which are named after their origin and insertion: pubococcygeus, puborectalis, and iliococcygeus. Studies using MRI and three-dimensional ultrasound validate the change in terminology from *pubococcygeus muscle* to a more accurate name, *puboviscera1 muscle*, and cadaveric dissection has validated the imaging studies. This intermediate component of the levator ani muscle lies posterior to the pubic bone and may be visualized as pubovaginalis, puboanalis, and puboperinealis muscle bundles. These three bundles constitute the pubovisceralis, or puboviscera1 muscle. The puborectalis component of the levator ani muscle is dorsal to the rectum and helps form the sling supporting the rectum. The coccygeus is a triangular muscle that occupies the area between the ischial spine and the coccyx.

The paired levator ani muscles act as a single muscle and functionally are important in the control of urination, in parturition, and in maintaining fecal continence. The pelvic diaphragm is important in supporting both abdominal and pelvic viscera and facilitates equal distribution of intraabdominal pressure during activities such as coughing.

## Urogenital Diaphragm

The **urogenital diaphragm**, also called the *triangular ligament*, is a strong, muscular membrane that occupies the area between the symphysis pubis and ischial tuberosities (Fig. 3.31) and stretches across the triangular anterior portion of the pelvic outlet. The urogenital diaphragm is external and inferior to the pelvic diaphragm. Anteriorly, the urethra is suspended from the pubic bone by continuations of the fascial layers of the urogenital diaphragm. The free edge of the diaphragm is strengthened by the superficial transverse perineal muscle. Posteriorly the urogenital diaphragm inserts into the central point of the perineum. Situated farther posteriorly is the ischiorectal fossa. Located more superficially are the bulbocavernosus and ischiocavernosus muscles.

The urogenital diaphragm has two layers that enfold and cover the striated, deep transverse perineal muscle. This muscle surrounds both the vagina and the urethra, which pierce the diaphragm. The pudendal vessels and nerves, the external sphincter of the membranous urethra, and the dorsal nerve to the clitoris are also found within the urogenital diaphragm. The deep transverse perineal muscle is innervated by branches of the pudendal nerve. The major function of the urogenital diaphragm is to support the urethra and maintain the urethrovesical junction.

## Ligaments

The pelvic ligaments are not classic ligaments but are thickenings of retroperitoneal fascia and consist primarily of blood and lymphatic vessels, nerves, and fatty connective tissue. Anatomists call the retroperitoneal fascia *subserous fascia*, whereas surgeons refer to this fascial layer as *endopelvic fascia*. The connective tissue is denser immediately adjacent to the lateral walls of the cervix and the vagina.

### Broad Ligaments

The **broad ligaments** are a thin, mesenteric-like double reflection of peritoneum stretching from the lateral pelvic sidewalls to the uterus (Fig. 3.32). They become contiguous with the uterine serosa, and thus the uterus is contained within two folds of peritoneum. These peritoneal folds enclose the loose, fatty connective tissue termed the *parametrium*. The broad ligaments afford minor support to the uterus but are conduits for important anatomic structures. Within the broad ligaments are found the following structures: oviducts; ovarian and round ligaments; ureters; ovarian and uterine arteries and veins; parametrial tissue; embryonic remnants of the mesonephric duct, wolffian body, and secondary two ligaments; the mesovarium; and the mesosalpinx. The round ligament is composed of fibrous tissue and muscle fibers. It attaches to the superoanterior aspect of the uterus, anterior and caudal to the oviduct, and runs via the broad ligament to the lateral pelvic wall. It, too, offers little support to the uterus. The round ligament crosses the external iliac vessels and enters

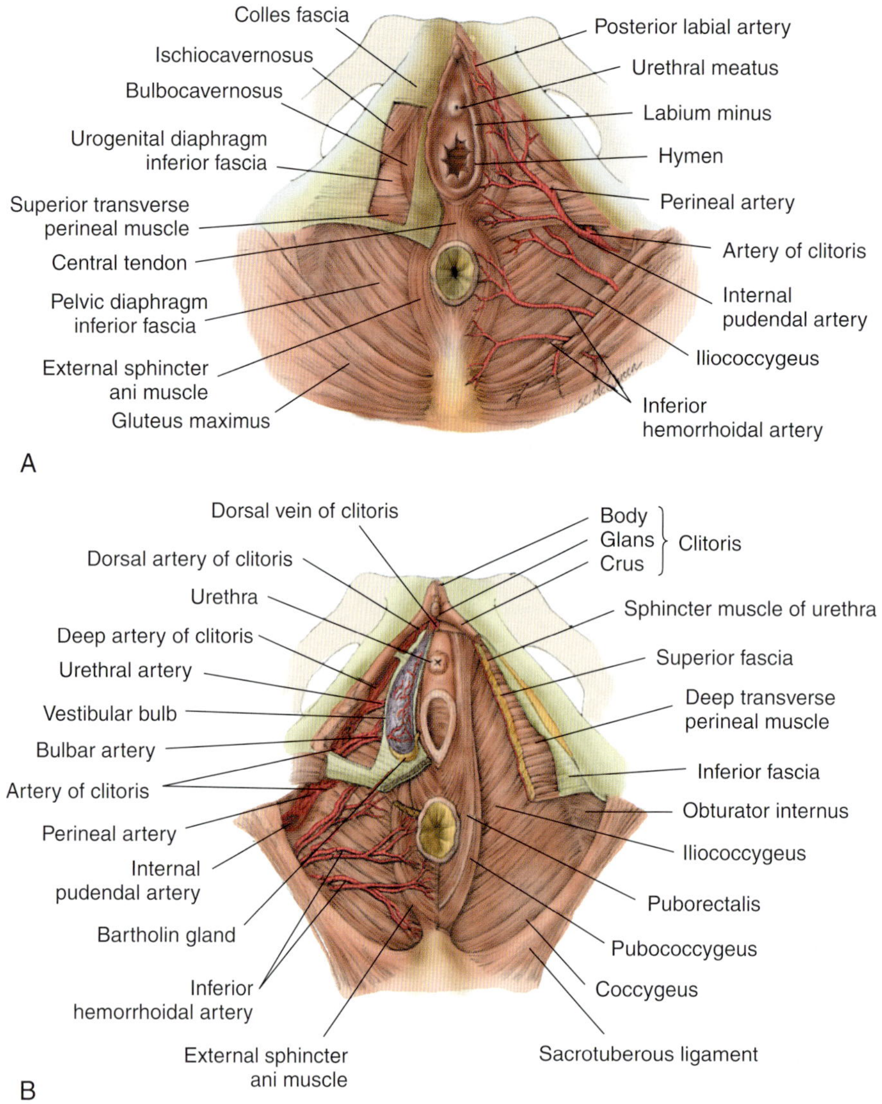


**Fig. 3.31** **A,** Schematic views of the perineum demonstrating superficial structures. Note the two layers of the urogenital diaphragm enfolding the deep transverse perineal muscle. **B,** Schematic views of the perineum demonstrating superficial structures and deeper structures. (Modified from Pritchard JA, MacDonald PC, Gant NF. *Williams' Obstetrics.* 17th ed. New York: Appleton-Century-Crofts; 1985:14.)

the inguinal canal, ending by inserting into the labia majora in a fan-like fashion. In the fetus a small, finger-like projection of the peritoneum, known as the *Nuck canal,* accompanies the round ligament into the inguinal canal. Generally the canal is obliterated in adult women.

## Cardinal Ligaments

The cardinal, or **Mackenrodt, ligaments** extend from the lateral aspects of the upper part of the cervix and the vagina to the pelvic wall. They are a thickened condensation of the subserosal fascia and parametria between the interior portion of the two folds of peritoneum. The cardinal ligaments form the base of the broad ligaments, laterally attaching to the fascia over the pelvic diaphragm and medially merging with fibers of the endopelvic fascia. Within these ligaments are blood vessels and smooth muscle. The cardinal ligaments help maintain the anatomic position of the cervix and the upper part of the vagina and provide the major support of the uterus and cervix.

## Uterosacral Ligaments

The uterosacral ligaments extend from the upper portion of the cervix posteriorly to the third sacral vertebra. They are thickened near the cervix and then run a curved course around each side of the rectum and subsequently thin out posteriorly. The external surface of the uterosacral ligaments is formed by an inferoposterior fold of peritoneum at the base of the broad ligaments. The middle of the uterosacral ligaments is composed primarily of nerve bundles. The uterosacral ligaments serve a role in the anatomic support of the cervix (Fig. 3.33).

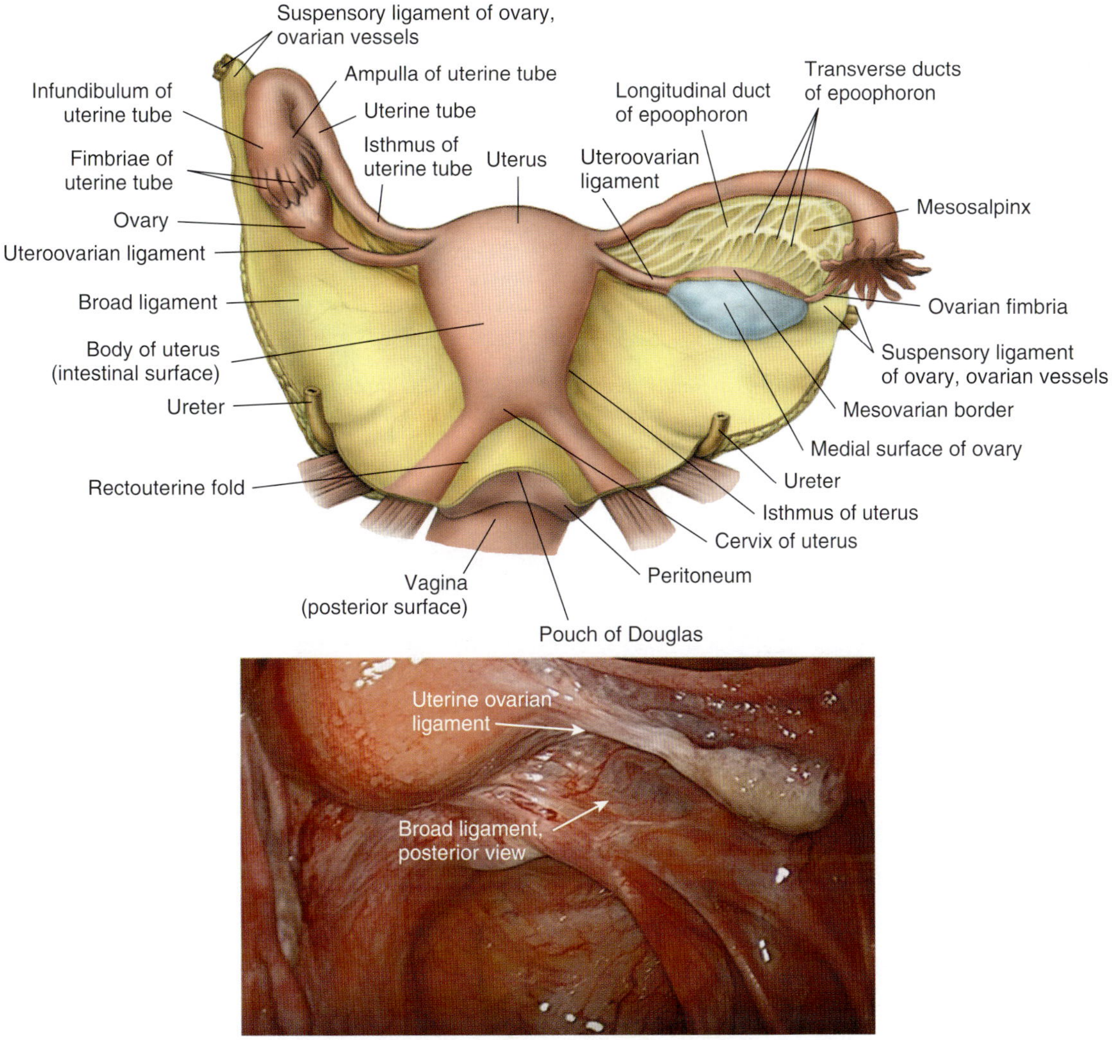


**Fig. 3.32** **A,** A schematic drawing of the broad ligament, posterior view. Note the many structures contained within the broad ligament. Also note the posterior aspect of the rectouterine fold, called the cul-de-sac, or pouch, of Douglas. (Modified from Clemente CD. *Anatomy: A Regional Atlas of the Human Body.* 3rd ed. Baltimore-Munich: Urban & Schwarzenberg; 1987.) **B,** Intraoperative picture of the broad ligament the posterior view. Note the location in relation to the uterine ovarian ligament. (Courtesy Fidel A. Valea, MD.)

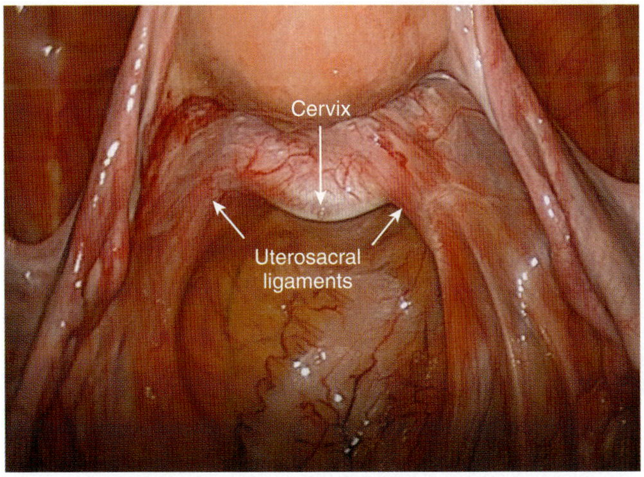


**Fig. 3.33** An intraoperative picture showing bilateral uterosacral ligaments in relation to the cervix. The uterosacral ligaments serve a role in anatomic support of the cervix.

## CLINICAL CORRELATIONS

The posterior fibers of the levator ani muscles encircle the rectum at its junction with the anal canal, thereby producing an abrupt angle that reinforces fecal continence. Surgical repair of a displacement or tear of the rectovaginal fascia and levator ani muscles resulting from childbirth is important during posterior colporrhaphy. Normal position of the female pelvic organs in the pelvis depends on mechanical support from both fascia and muscles. Vaginal delivery sometimes results in dysfunction of the anal sphincter. The cause of this problem may be direct injury to the **striated muscles** of the pelvic floor or damage to the pudendal and presacral nerves (levator ani nerves) during labor and delivery.

The round ligament is an important surgical landmark in making the initial incision into the parietal peritoneum to gain access to the retroperitoneal space. Direct visualization of the retroperitoneal course of the ureter is an important step in many pelvic operations, including dissections in women with endometriosis, pelvic inflammatory disease, large adnexal masses, broad ligament masses, and pelvic malignancies. A cyst of the Nuck canal may be confused with an indirect inguinal hernia. When a large amount of fluid is placed in the abdominal cavity, postoperative bilateral labial edema may develop in some women because of patency of the canal of Nuck.

During pelvic surgery, traction on the uterus makes the uterosacral and cardinal ligaments more prominent. There is a free space approximately 2 to 4 cm below the superior edge of the broad ligament. In this free space there are no blood vessels, and the two sides of the broad ligament are in close proximity. Often gynecologic surgeons use this area to facilitate clamping of the anastomosis between the uterine and ovarian arteries.

## NONGENITAL PELVIC ORGANS

### Ureters

The ureters are whitish, muscular tubes, 28 to 34 cm long, extending from the renal pelvis to the urinary bladder. The ureter is divided into **abdominal and pelvic** segments whose diameters vary. The abdominal segment is approximately 8 to 10 mm in diameter, whereas the pelvic segment is approximately 4 to 6 mm. A congenital anomaly resulting in a double, or bifid, ureter occurs in 1% to 4% of women. Ectopic ureteral orifices may occur in either the urethra or the vagina. The abdominal portion of the right ureter is lateral to the inferior vena cava. The course of the left ureter is similar to its counterpart on the right side in that it runs downward and medially along the anterior surface of the psoas major muscle.

The iliopectineal line serves as the marker for the pelvic portion of the ureter. The ureters run along the common iliac artery and then cross over the iliac vessels as they enter the pelvis (Fig. 3.34). There is a slight variation between the two sides of the female pelvis. The right ureter tends to cross at the bifurcation of the common iliac artery, whereas usually the left ureter crosses 1 to 2 cm above the bifurcation.

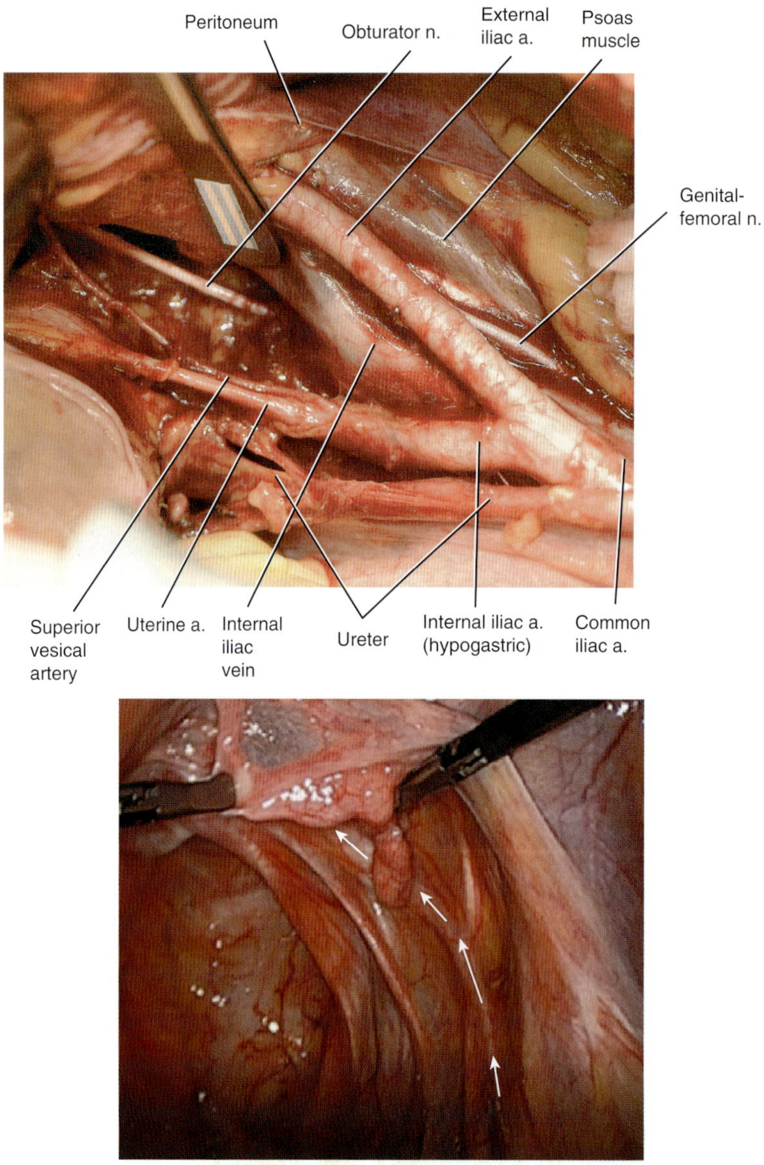


**Fig. 3.34 A,** A photograph taken during a dissection of the lateral pelvic wall at the time of a radical hysterectomy. Note the ureter coursing over the common iliac artery in close proximity to the bifurcation. The ureter then drops under and very close to the uterine artery. The retractor is lifting the internal iliac vein. (Courtesy Deborah Jean Dotters, MD, Eugene, OR.) **B,** The ureter can be found in the medial leaf of the broad ligament. *Arrows* indicate that the ureter enters into the cardinal ligament and is located 1 to 2 cm lateral to the uterine cervix. (Courtesy Fidel A. Valea, MD.)

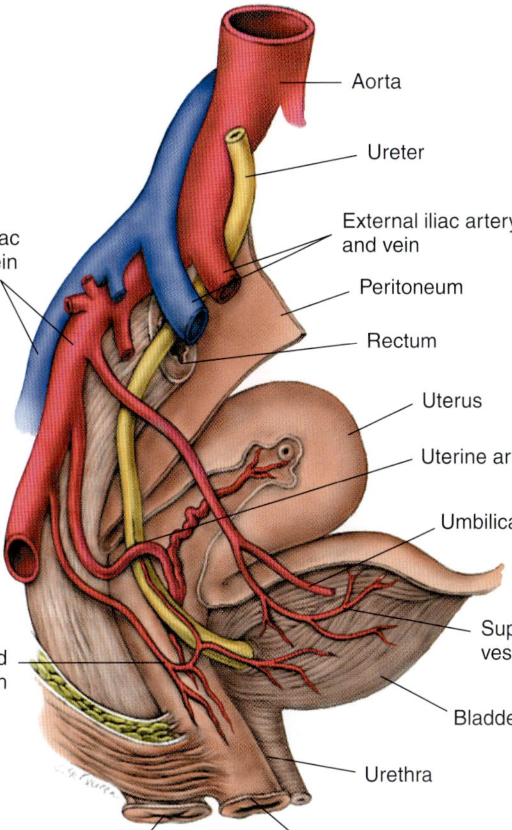


**Fig. 3.35** A schematic drawing of the female pelvis, lateral view, demonstrating the ureter's relation to the major arteries. Note the uterine artery crossing over the ureter. (From Buchsbaum HJ, Schmidt JD. *Gynecologic and Obstetric Urology.* Philadelphia: WB Saunders; 1978:24.)

The ureters follow the descending, convex curvature of the posterolateral pelvic wall toward the perineum. Throughout its course, the ureter is retroperitoneal in location. It can be found on the medial leaf of the parietal peritoneum and in close proximity to the ovarian, uterine, obturator, and superior vesical arteries (Fig. 3.35). The uterine artery lies on the anterolateral surface of the ureter for 2.5 to 3 cm. At approximately the level of the ischial spine, the ureter changes its course and runs forward and medially from the uterosacral ligaments to the base of the broad ligament. There the ureter enters into the cardinal ligaments. In this location the ureter is approximately **1 to 2 cm lateral to the uterine cervix** and is surrounded by a plexus of veins. A cross-sectional study by Hurd and colleagues, using computed tomography of women with normal anatomy, evaluated the distance from the ureter to the lateral aspect of the cervix. The measurement of the closest distance in any individual woman was 2.3 cm ± 0.8 cm (the median of all subjects) (Hurd, 2001). However, the authors noted that in 12% of women, the ureter was less than 0.5 cm from the cervix. This finding emphasizes the caution needed in surgery to prevent ureteral injury. This close proximity also underscores the fact that ureteral injury may be unavoidable in some women. The ureter then runs upward (ventral) and medially in the vesical uterine ligaments to obliquely pierce the bladder wall. Just before entering the base of the bladder, the ureter is in immediate contact with the anterior vaginal wall and the inferolateral aspect of the space of Retzius.

The ureter has a rich arterial supply with numerous anastomoses from many small vessels that form a longitudinal plexus in the adventitia of the ureter, commonly referred to as the *Waldeyer sheath*. The parent vessels that send branches to this arterial plexus surrounding the ureter include the renal, ovarian, common iliac, hypogastric, uterine, vaginal, vesical, middle hemorrhoidal, and superior gluteal arteries. The ureter is resistant to injury resulting from devascularization unless the surgeon strips the adventitia from the muscular conduit. In general the blood supply of the abdominal ureter comes from medial sources and the blood supply of the pelvic ureter originates from lateral sources.

## Urinary Bladder

The **urinary bladder** is a hollow muscular organ that lies between the symphysis pubis and the uterus. The size and shape of the bladder vary with the volume of urine it contains. Similarly, the anatomic proximity to other pelvic organs depends on whether the bladder is full or empty. The superior surface of the bladder is the only surface covered by peritoneum. The inferior portion is immediately adjacent to the uterus. The **urachus**, the adult remnant of the embryonic allantois, is a fibrous cord extending from the apex of the bladder to the umbilicus; it is occasionally patent for part of its length. The base of the bladder lies directly adjacent to the endopelvic fascia over the anterior vaginal wall. The bladder neck and connecting urethra are attached to the symphysis pubis by fibrous ligaments. The prevesical or retropubic space of Retzius is the area lying between the bladder and symphysis pubis and is bounded laterally by the obliterated hypogastric arteries. This space extends from the fascia covering the pelvic diaphragm to the umbilicus between the peritoneum and transversalis fascia.

The mucosa of the anterior surface of the bladder is light red and has numerous folds. The inferoposterior surface delineated by the two ureteral orifices and the urethral orifice is the trigone. The trigone is a darker red than the rest of the bladder mucosa and is free of folds. When the bladder is empty, the ureteral orifices are approximately 2.5 cm apart. This distance increases to 5 cm when the bladder is distended. The muscular wall of the bladder, the detrusor muscles, is arranged in three layers. The arterial supply of the bladder originates from branches of the hypogastric artery: the superior vesical, inferior vesical, and middle hemorrhoidal arteries. The nerve supply to the bladder includes sympathetic and parasympathetic fibers, with the external sphincter supplied by the pudendal nerve.

### Rectum

The rectum is the terminal 12 to 14 cm of the large intestine. It begins over the second or third sacral vertebra, where the sigmoid colon no longer has a mesentery. After the large intestine loses its mesentery, its anatomic posterior wall is in close proximity to the curvature of the sacrum. Anteriorly, peritoneum covers the upper and middle thirds of the rectum. The lowest one-third is below the peritoneal reflection and is in close proximity to the posterior wall of the vagina. The rectum empties into the anal canal, which is 2 to 4 cm long. The anal canal is fixed by the surrounding levator ani musculature of the pelvic diaphragm. The external sphincter of the anal canal is a circular band of striated muscle. Studies of the cross-sectional anatomy of the external anal sphincter by both ultrasound and MRI have identified two distinct layers of the external anal sphincter. Using MRI with three-dimensional reconstruction, Hsu and colleagues noted three separate components to the external sphincter: a main muscle body, a separate encircling subcutaneous band of muscles, and bilateral wing-shaped muscle bands that attach near the ischiopubis (Hsu, 2005). The rectum, unlike other areas of **the large intestine, does not have teniae** coli or appendices epiploicae. The arterial supply of the rectum is rich, originating from five arteries: the superior hemorrhoidal artery, which is a continuation of the inferior mesenteric; the two middle hemorrhoidal arteries; and the two inferior hemorrhoidal arteries. Approximately 10% of carcinomas of the large bowel occur within the rectum. Therefore during rectal examination special emphasis to palpate the entire circumference of the rectum, not just the area of the rectovaginal septum, is an important part of screening for colon cancer.

## CLINICAL CORRELATIONS

The anatomic proximity of the ureters, urinary bladder, and rectum to the female reproductive organs is a major consideration in most gynecologic operations. Surgical compromise of the ureter may occur during clamping or ligating of the infundibulopelvic vessels, clamping or ligating of the cardinal ligaments, or wide suturing in the endopelvic fascia during an anterior repair, even with apparent normal anatomy and utmost surgical care. Particular attention to the proximity of the distal ureter to the anterior vagina is very important. Operative injuries to the bladder or ureter occur in approximately 1 out of 100 major gynecologic operations. Bladder injuries are approximately **five times more common** than ureteral injuries. Two of the classic ways to differentiate a ureter from a pelvic vessel are (1) visualization of peristalsis after stimulation by a surgical instrument and (2) visualization of Auerbach plexuses, which are numerous, wavy, small vessels that anastomose over the surface of the ureter. Injury to the ureter or bladder during urethropexy operations for genuine stress incontinence is common. Therefore many surgeons routinely inject indigo carmine and either open the bladder or perform cystoscopy near the end of the operative procedure.

For years, gynecologic teachers have referred to the area in the base of the broad ligament near the cervix where the uterine artery crosses the ureter as the area where "water flows under the bridge."

The urinary bladder, if properly drained, will heal rapidly after a surgical insult if the blood supply to the bladder wall is not compromised. This capacity allows the gynecologist to use suprapubic cystostomy tube without fear of fistula formation.

There are many different surgical techniques for the repair of urinary stress incontinence. They usually involve either suspension of the periurethral tissues or bladder neck itself. Occasionally these surgical procedures are complicated by a significant amount of postoperative venous bleeding. A subfascial hematoma may extend as high as the umbilicus in the space of Retzius. One of the most common causes of female urinary incontinence is defective connective tissue, especially in the periurethral connective tissue, pubourethral ligaments, and pubococcygeus muscles.

Rectal injury may occur during vaginal hysterectomy with associated posterior colporrhaphy. In the middle third of the vagina, the distance between vaginal and rectal mucosa is only a few millimeters, and usually the connective tissue is densely adherent and should be separated by sharp dissection. The rectum bulges anteriorly into the vagina in this area, producing a further challenge during the operative procedure.

## OTHER STRUCTURES

### Cul-De-Sac of Douglas

The cul-de-sac of Douglas is a deep pouch formed by the most caudal extent of the parietal peritoneum. The cul-de-sac is a potential space and is also called the *rectouterine pouch* or *fold* (see Fig. 3.33). It is anterior to the rectum, separating the uterus from the large intestine. The parietal peritoneum of the cul-de-sac covers the cervix and upper part of the posterior vaginal wall, then reflects to cover the anterior wall of the rectum. The pouch is bounded on the lateral sides by the peritoneal folds covering the uterosacral ligaments.

### Parametria

The parametria are the coats of extraperitoneal fatty and fibrous connective tissues adjacent to the uterus; they lie between the leaves of the broad ligament and in the contiguous area anteriorly between the cervix and bladder. This connective tissue is thicker and denser adjacent to the cervix and vagina, where it becomes part of the connective tissue of the pelvic floor. The parametria may also thicken in response to radiation, pelvic cancer, infection, or endometriosis.

### Paravesical and Pararectal Spaces

The paravesical and pararectal spaces are actually potential spaces that become true spaces when developed by the surgeon. Development of these spaces is useful in pelvic lymph node dissection and in radical pelvic surgery because it makes the anatomic landmarks so clear. The paravesical space is bordered medially by the bladder and upper vagina and is contiguous with, but lateral to, **the space of Retzius**. Laterally it is bordered by the obturator fossa and the external iliac vessels; inferiorly it is bordered by the pubic ramus, and superiorly it is bordered by the cardinal ligament.

The pararectal space is developed by dissecting the adventitial tissue within the broad ligament, between the ureter (medially) and the internal iliac vessels (laterally). More deeply, the medial border is the rectum. Superiorly the pararectal space is limited by the sacral hollow. Inferiorly it is limited by the cardinal ligament, containing the uterine artery. The paravesical and pararectal spaces are actually potential spaces that become true spaces when developed by the surgeon. Development of these spaces is useful in pelvic lymph node dissection and in radical pelvic surgery because the anatomic landmarks become so clear.

## CLINICAL CORRELATIONS

The parametria and cul-de-sac of Douglas are important anatomic landmarks in advanced pelvic infection and neoplasia. Intrauterine infection, cervical carcinoma, and endometrial carcinoma may penetrate the endocervical stroma or the myometrium and secondarily may invade the loose connective tissue of the parametria.

The pouch of Douglas is easily accessible in performing transvaginal surgical procedures. Posterior colpotomy is often chosen for drainage of a pelvic abscess occurring in the cul-de-sac of Douglas.

When the paravesical and pararectal spaces have been developed and the uterus is held on traction medially, the pelvic anatomy, including the ureter, internal and external iliac vessels, obturator fossa, and cardinal ligament, with the uterine artery crossing the ureter, can be clearly and readily identified.

Many women with uterine prolapse have an associated enterocele, which is a hernia that protrudes between the uterosacral ligaments. Occasionally the cul-de-sac of Douglas is obliterated by the inflammatory process associated with either endometriosis or advanced malignancy.

## REFERENCES


Abu-Rustum N. Sentinel lymph node mapping for endometrial cancer: a modern approach to surgical staging. *J Natl Compr Canc Netw.* 2014;12:288-297.

Coleman RL, Ali S, Levenback CF, et al. Is bilateral lymphadenectomy for midline squamous carcinoma of the vulva always necessary? An analysis from Gynecologic Oncology Group (GOG) 173. *Gynecol Oncol.* 2013;128(2):155-159.

Echt ML, Finan MA, Hoffman MS, et al. Detection of sentinel lymph nodes with lymphazurin in cervical, uterine and vulvar malignancies. *South Med J.* 1999;92(2):204-208.

Hsu Y, Fenner DE, Weadock WJ, et al. Magnetic resonance imaging and 3-dimensional analysis of external anal sphincter anatomy. *Obstet Gynecol.* 2005;106(6):1259-1265.

Hurd WW, Chee SS, Gallagher KI, et al. Location of the ureters in relation to the uterine cervix by computed tomography. *Am J Obstet Gynecol.* 2001;184:336.


**Suggested readings for this chapter can be found on ExpertConsult.com.**

# 4 Reproductive Endocrinology

## Neuroendocrinology, Gonadotropins, Sex Steroids, Prostaglandins, Ovulation, Menstruation, and Hormone Assay

*Nataki C. Douglas, Roger A. Lobo*

### KEY POINTS

- Gonadotropin-releasing hormone (GnRH) analogs are synthesized by substitution of amino acids in the parent molecule at the 6 and 10 positions for GnRH agonists and at the 2 or 3 position for GnRH antagonists. The various analogs have greater potencies and longer half-lives than the parent GnRH and are used clinically for suppression.
- LH and FSH have the same α subunit as thyroid-stimulating hormone (TSH) and human chorionic gonadotropin (HCG). The β subunits of all these hormones have different amino acids and carbohydrates, which provide specific biologic activity.
- Kisspeptin (KISS1) plays a key role in the regulation of GnRH release.
- Ovulation occurs about 24 hours after the estradiol peak and 32 hours after the initial rise in LH, as well as about 12 to 16 hours after the peak of LH levels in serum. Serum progesterone is less than 1 ng/mL before ovulation and reaches midluteal levels of 10 to 20 ng/mL.
- Four characteristics of hormone assays establish their reliability: sensitivity, specificity, accuracy, and precision.

The endocrine regulation of the reproductive system is very complex. This chapter presents only the basic information required to understand this complex subject. More detailed and in-depth information is found in the several books that have been dedicated to this subject.

Successful function of the reproductive system requires the involvement of several organs, none of which acts independently. In this chapter we discuss the physiology of the hypothalamic-pituitary-ovarian (HPO) axis. For ease of understanding, each organ will be discussed first as an individual unit; information will include the central nervous system control of gonadotropin-releasing hormone (GnRH), the primary neurohormone controlling the whole reproductive endocrine axis; the GnRH action on the anterior pituitary and the resultant secretion of the gonadotropins; the gonadotropins' action on the ovaries and the release of gonadal steroids; and finally the action of these sex steroids on the uterus and cervix. Although it is fair to state that **the HPO axis is driven by the hypothalamus and its release of GnRH, it is important to point out that normal function of the HPO-endocrine axis requires a remarkable information flow and coordination between each of these organs, as exemplified by the existing inhibitory and stimulatory feedback loops.** Their relevance will become obvious in the discussion of the menstrual cycle, which closes the chapter.

## THE HYPOTHALAMUS AND GNRH

The reproductive process starts in the brain, through the activation of the initial hormonal signal that will release the gonadotropins from the pituitary gland. This hormone released by the hypothalamus is GnRH, a decapeptide (10 amino acids) (Fig. 4.1). The GnRH gene (GNRH1, situated on the short arm of chromosome 8) encodes for a 92 amino acids precursor molecule, composed of a signal peptide sequence, the GnRH sequence itself, a posttranscriptional processing signal (3 amino acids long), and a 56-amino acid peptide known as GnRH-associated peptide (GAP). (Several forms of the GnRH decapeptide have been identified, the principal of which is GnRH-2, which differs from GnRH by 3 amino acids. It is found in several areas of the body, where it may subserve functions unrelated to those of GnRH.) Its role in fertility, if any, remains to be determined.

### Anatomy

#### The Relationship of the Olfactory and GnRH Systems in Early Fetal Life

Surprisingly, GnRH-synthesizing neurons do not originate within the brain, like the majority of all neurons. Rather, GnRH neurons derive from progenitor cells in the embryonic olfactory placode where they develop. In a particular journey unique for a neuron, **GnRH neurons migrate toward the brain during early fetal life to reach the locations that they will occupy during adult life.** This migration of GnRH neurons over long distances and through changing molecular environments suggests that numerous factors, local and possibly external, influence this process at its different stages. Such factors play critical roles, such as mediating the adhesion of GnRH neurons to changing surfaces along their voyage, promoting cytoskeleton remodeling, and modulating axonal guidance.

Functional connections between GnRH neurons and the hypophyseal portal system that will transport GnRH to the anterior pituitary gland are established by about 16 weeks of fetal life. **Migration failure of GnRH neurons and the resultant lack of the establishment of functional connections are characteristic of patients with the Kallmann syndrome,** who show **hypogonadotropic hypogonadism** accompanied by anosmia (Tsai, 2006). In the 19-week-old fetus with X-linked Kallmann syndrome, the GnRH neurons accompanying the olfactory nerves have been shown to be arrested in their voyage within the meninges, and therefore contact with the brain and the hypophyseal portal system is not established.

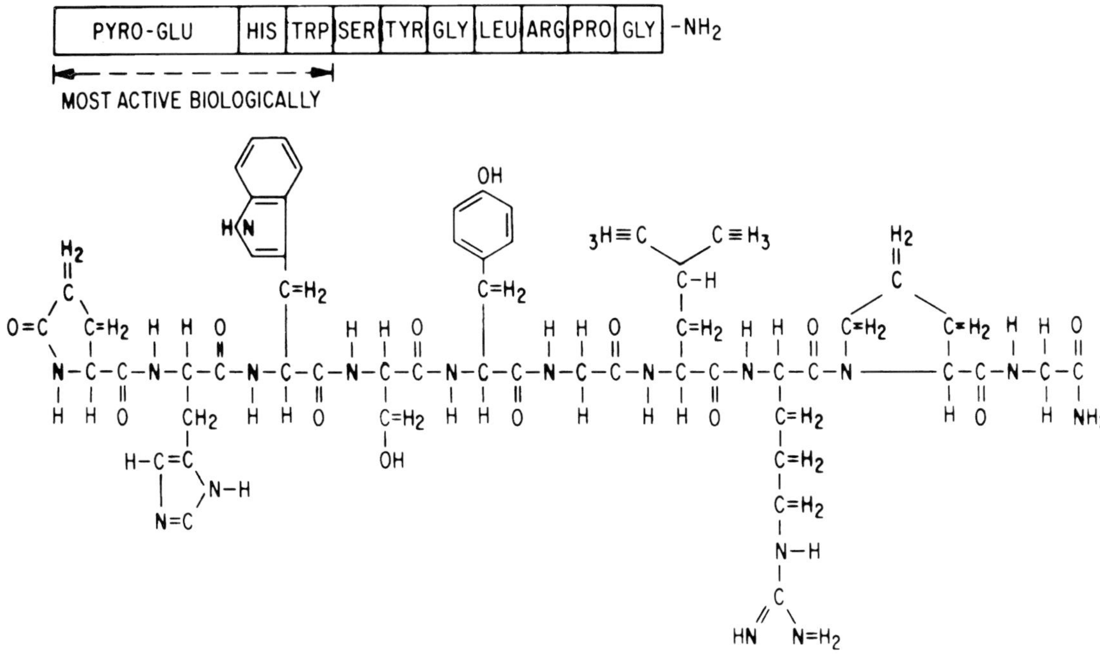


**Fig. 4.1** The 10-amino acid sequence of gonadotropin-releasing hormone (GnRH). (From Klerzky OA, Lobo RA: Reproductive neuroendocrinology. In Mishell DR, Davajan V, Lobo RA, eds. *Infertility, Contraception and Reproductive Endocrinology.* 3rd ed. Cambridge, MA: Blackwell Scientific; 1991.)

## The GnRH Neuronal System

In adults, neurons producing GnRH are present in several hypothalamic nuclei and other parts of the brain. However, the majority of GnRH neurons controlling the HPO axis are located within the anterior hypothalamus and primarily within the medial basal hypothalamus, with the greatest number in the primate within the **arcuate nucleus**. The 92 amino acid GnRH precursor is released into the axons of these neurons and cleaved during transport to yield GnRH and GAP. (The biologic function of GAP or fragments thereof remains to be clarified.)

A substantial number of GnRH axons terminate within the external zone of the **median eminence** (infundibulum) **where GnRH is released.** This area is the site of an important capillary plexus, with a fenestrated epithelium similar to that of peripheral capillaries, which allows passage of large molecules. (These capillaries differ from brain capillaries, which are not fenestrated. Thus the median eminence is viewed as an area outside the blood-brain barrier.) This pathway is the most relevant one in regard to the control of the pituitary-ovarian axis (Fig. 4.2, A). Another substantial projection of GnRH axons is through circumventricular organs, the major of which is the organum vasculosum of the lamina terminalis (OVLT). These areas are also outside the blood-brain barrier. (The function of GnRH release into these areas remains somewhat unknown. One role may be to enable the release of GnRH into cerebrospinal fluid [CSF], perhaps to facilitate actions of GnRH in other areas of the brain. GnRH levels have been found to be elevated in CSF as opposed to being minimal in peripheral blood.) Another possible route of GnRH release may involve specialized ependymal cells, referred to as **tanycytes**. These have been found to extend from the lumen of the third ventricle to the external zone of the median eminence.

## Transport of GnRH to the Anterior Pituitary

The capillary plexus of the external median eminence, into which GnRH is released, collects into several hypophyseal portal vessels, which descend along the pituitary stalk to terminate within another capillary plexus (hence the term *portal*) within the anterior lobe of the pituitary (see Fig. 4.2A). (Unlike the posterior lobe of the pituitary, also referred to as the neurohypophysis, the anterior lobe has no direct blood supply and receives all of its vascularization from this portal system.) The vascular arrangement whereby GnRH and other neurohormones reach the anterior pituitary is very important to the proper function of the endocrine system: It allows for the rapid (within minutes) and undiluted transport of relatively small amounts of neurohormones to the pituitary. This is especially crucial to GnRH because this neurohormone has a short half-life of about 2 to 4 minutes (it is rapidly degraded by peptidases in blood; as a consequence, GnRH is not measurable in peripheral blood) and because of its pulsatile mode of release (discussed later).

# Physiology

## The GnRH Pulse Generator

Studies have shown that GnRH is characteristically released intermittently, in a pulsatile fashion. From this comes the concept of the "GnRH pulse generator" responsible for the pulsatile release of the hormone (Herbison, 2018). GnRH pulses occur at about hourly intervals (Fig. 4.3). The rising edge of each GnRH pulse is abrupt, such that GnRH can increase by a factor of 50 within 1 minute. Each GnRH pulse is preceded by an increase in multiunit activity within the area of the arcuate nucleus.

## Mechanisms Responsible for GnRH Pulsatility

The cellular basis and the mechanisms that determine the timing of the increase in multiunit activity resulting in pulsatile GnRH activity are still under study. First, there is a growing consensus that pulsatile activity originates from an inherent pace-making

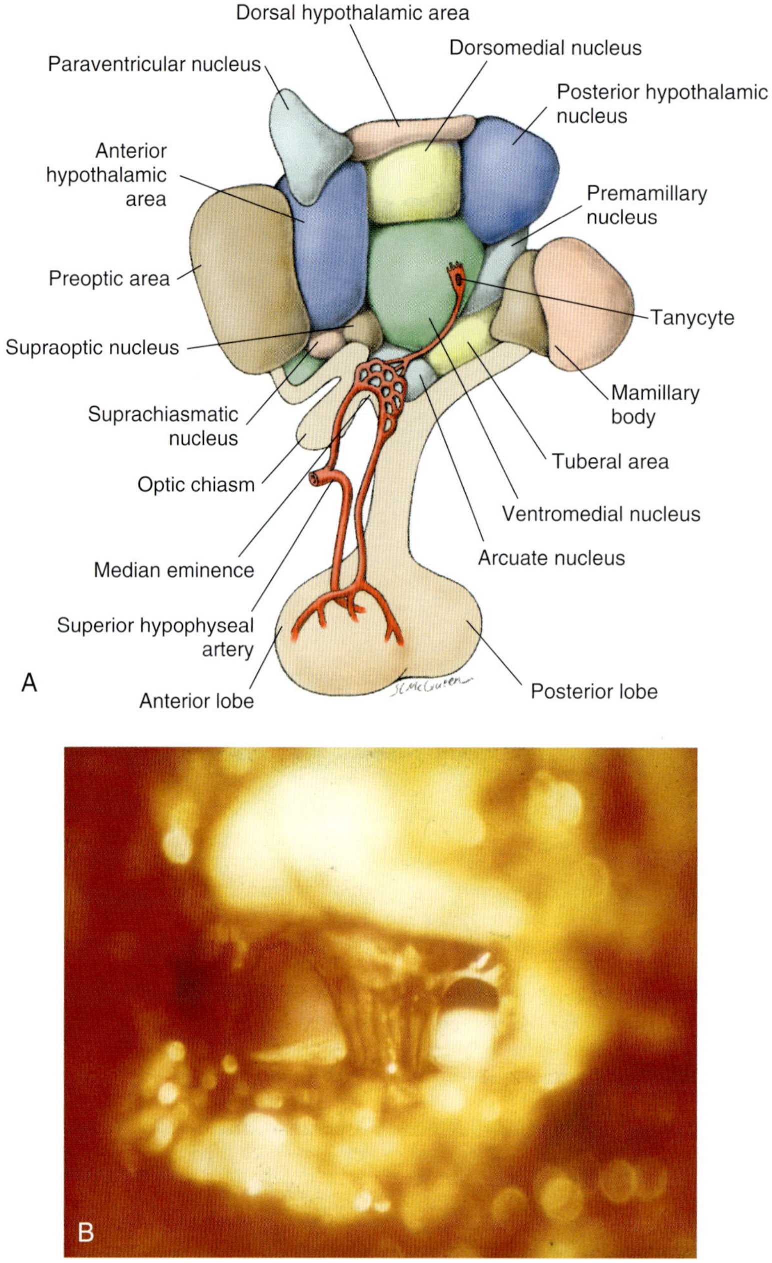


**Fig. 4.2 A,** Nuclear organization of the hypothalamus, shown diagrammatically in a sagittal plane as viewed from the third ventricle. Rostral area is to the left and caudal area is to the right. Fast transport of GnRH pulses released into the median eminence from axons originating from GnRH neurons in the arcuate nucleus occurs through the portal vessels derived from the capillary plexus in the median eminence. **B,** The pituitary stalk and several individual hypophyseal portal veins transporting hypothalamic neurohormones to the anterior pituitary in a nonhuman primate. *GnRH,* Gonadotropin-releasing hormone. (**A,** Redrawn from Moore RY: Neuroendocrine mechanisms: Cells and systems. In Yen SSC, Jaffe R, eds. *Reproductive Endocrinology: Physiology, Pathophysiology and Clinical Management.* Philadelphia, WB Saunders; 1986. **B,** Image courtesy Drs. Peter Carmel and Michel Ferin.)

activity of the GnRH neuron itself; in vitro data have shown that individual neurons have the capacity of spontaneous oscillations in activity. In this case such activity would also require a synchronized action from enough neurons to provide a discrete GnRH pulse. Intercommunication between GnRH neurons may occur through gap junctions between such neurons, which have been demonstrated, and through synaptic forms of interaction between cells. Second, **evidence identifies a key role of kisspeptin (KISS1), a product of the *KISS1* gene, and its receptor (GPR54 or KISS1R) in the regulation of GnRH release** (Skorupskaite, 2014). KISS1 neurons have been found to directly innervate and stimulate GnRH neurons. In humans, **mutations or targeted deletions of *KISS1* or of its receptor cause hypogonadotropic hypogonadism.** Patients with these mutations, however, do not have anosmia, unlike those with Kallmann syndrome, suggesting that there are no major deficits in

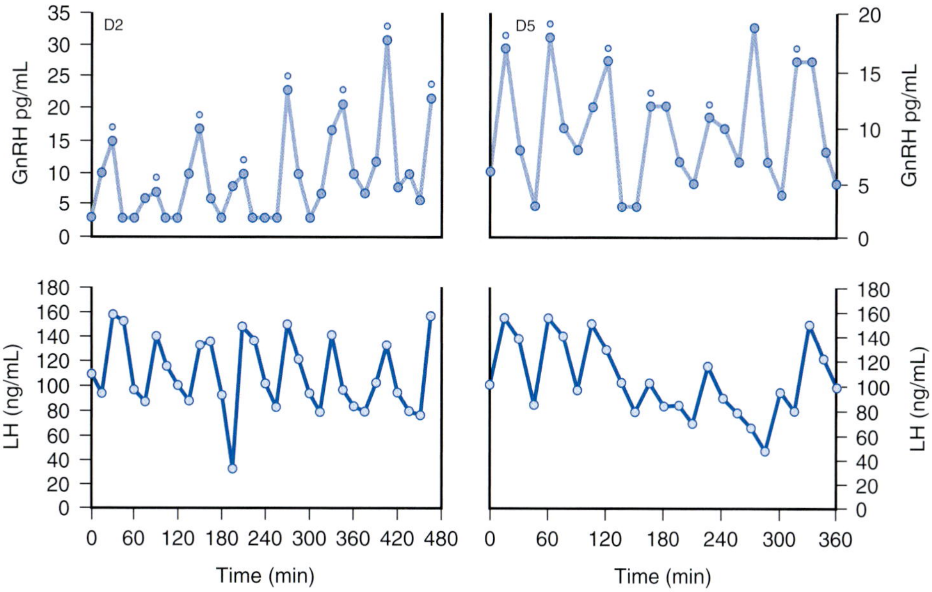


**Fig. 4.3** GnRH release by the hypothalamus is pulsatile. Shown in the *upper panel* are hourly GnRH pulses over an 8-hour period in an ovariectomized monkey in the absence of ovarian steroid modulation. Note the concordance of LH pulses *(lower panel). GnRH,* Gonadotropin-releasing hormone; *LH,* luteinizing hormone. (From Xia L, Van Vugt D, Alston EJ, et al. A surge of gonadotropin-releasing hormone accompanies the estradiol-induced gonadotropin surge in the rhesus monkey. *Endocrinology.* 1992;131:2812.)

the embryonic migration of olfactory or GnRH neurons. **KISS1 neurons within the arcuate nucleus (rodents) and infundibular nucleus (humans) express the estrogen, progesterone, and androgen receptors**, and KISS1 signaling in the brain is implicated in mediating sex steroids feedback loops, especially during the preovulatory GnRH/luteinizing hormone (LH) surge. Kisspeptin has been used to induce egg maturation in women undergoing in vitro fertilization therapy, with subsequent fertilization of the mature eggs, embryo transfer into the uterus and successful human pregnancy (Jayasena, 2014). There is the potential for routine use of kisspeptin to induce ovulation during fertility treatment cycles. **KISS1 has also been shown to play a role in the initiation of puberty**. A subpopulation of kisspeptin neurons in the human infundibular nucleus coexpress neuropeptides neurokinin B and dynorphin (an opioid inhibitor) (Skorupskaite, 2014). These **kisspeptin-neurokinin-dynorphin (KNDy) neurons express neurokinin B and dynorphin receptors, as well as estrogen and progesterone receptors**. KNDy neurons coordinate inputs, including sex steroid feedback, to regulate pulsatile kisspeptin secretion. The interaction of KISS1 neurons with other neurotransmitter systems is currently being studied. Fig. 4.4 **depicts the hypothalamic circuitry between the KNDy neurons and GnRH release, as well as the newly appreciated connections to the thermoregulatory areas in the hypothalamus** (Mittleman-Smith, 2012). Thus **blockade of the neurokinin (NK3) receptor with a specific antagonist** has been found to control hot flushes in postmenopausal women by blocking the pathways of the thermoregulatory center.

## Modulatory Influences on GnRH Pulsatility

The foremost modulatory influence on the frequency and amplitude of GnRH pulses is exerted by the ovarian steroid hormones through their feedback loop actions. In general, estradiol is known to decrease GnRH pulse amplitude, whereas progesterone decreases GnRH pulse frequency (see the discussion presented later for details).

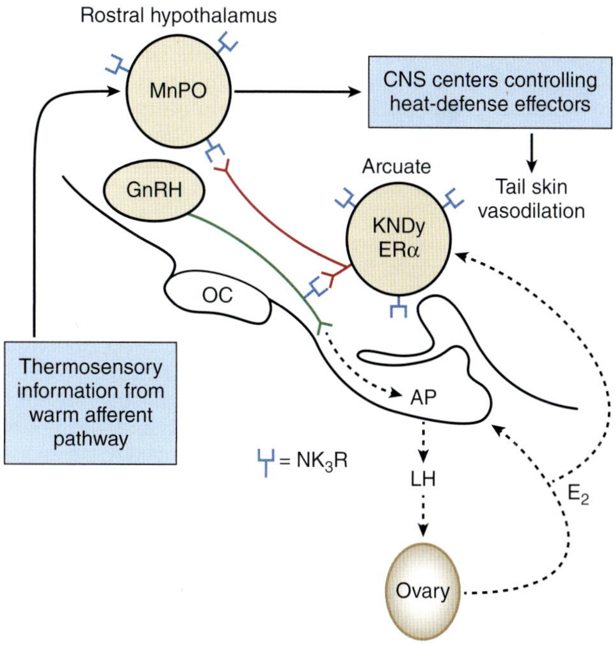


**Fig. 4.4** Diagrammatic depiction (in a rat model) of KNDy neurons in the hypothalamus, not only influencing GnRH pulses and gonadotropin secretion but interacting with thermoregulatory and heat regulatory centers in the brain. *AP,* Anterior pituitary; *CNS* central nervous system; $E_2$, estradiol; *ERα*, estrogen receptor alpha; *GnRH,* gonadotropin-releasing hormone; *KNDy,* kisspeptin, neurotensin, and dynorphin; *LH,* luteinizing hormone; *MnPO,* median preoptic nucleus; *NK*$_3$*R*, neurokinin receptor. (From Lobo RA: menopause and aging. In Strauss JF and Barbieri RL, eds. *Yen and Jaffe's Reproductive Endocrinology: Physiology, Pathophysiology and Clinical management.* 8th ed. Philadelphia: Elsevier; 2019.)

Numerous other studies suggest that the spontaneous activity of the GnRH pulse generator may also be modulated by a variety of additional stimulatory and inhibitory afferent neural signals. **Stimulatory inputs to GnRH release may originate from neurons using the biogenic amine neuroepinephrine (NE), the amino acid glutamate, and the peptide neuropeptide Y (NPY). Inhibitory inputs may come from the amino acid gamma-aminobutyric acid (GABA), the biogenic amine dopamine (DA), the endogenous opioid β-endorphin, and the neurosecretory peptide corticotropin-releasing hormone (CRH) neurons.** These systems may affect the GnRH pulse generator either *tonally* or *conditionally*.

In the first category we find, for example, NE as a potential tonal stimulator and GABA as a tonal inhibitor of GnRH release. Administration of alpha-adrenergic blockers has been shown to reduce pulse frequency in animals, in accord with the postulated tonal stimulatory role for NE. The role of GABA as a tonal inhibitor may be more prominent during the prepubertal period, at which time a diminishing inhibitory GABA tone may activate puberty and the resumption of GnRH pulsatile release. Glutamate's role is more uncertain, although it also is suspected in the initiation of pulses at puberty. Dopamine infusions in women are associated with a decrease in circulating LH and prolactin (dopamine is also known as the prolactin-inhibitory neurohormone). The effect on LH is thought to be mediated through GnRH because, in patients with hypothalamic amenorrhea in whom there appears to be an excess of dopaminergic tone, administration of a dopamine blocker may return the LH pulse frequency to normal. It should also be remembered that specific effects of neurotransmitters on GnRH neurons may be altered by the administration of certain drugs, which may interfere with the proper synthesis, binding, storage, or receptor function of these neurotransmitters. Thus **on treatment with such drugs (e.g., methyldopa; reserpine; tricyclic antidepressants such as propranolol, phentolamine, haloperidol, and cyproheptadine; selective serotonin reuptake inhibitors [SSRIs]; and serotonin-norepinephrine reuptake inhibitors [SNRIs]), patients may develop disorders such as oligomenorrhea or galactorrhea, the result of alterations in GnRH secretion or hyperprolactinemia**. Other studies also suggest that hypothalamic prostaglandins may also modulate the release of GnRH; for instance, the midcycle surge of LH (see The Menstrual Cycle later in this chapter) can be abolished in animals by the administration of aspirin or indomethacin, which blocks the synthesis of prostaglandins.

In the second category, other systems may affect the GnRH system only *conditionally*—that is, under specific hormonal or physiologic conditions. One example is the endogenous opioid β-endorphin, which exerts an inhibitory action on GnRH pulsatile activity that depends largely on the endogenous endocrine milieu. This is related to the fact that ovarian hormones control the release of β-endorphin within the brain, which is lowest in the absence of estradiol, such as in the ovariectomized nonhuman primate, and highest in the presence of both estradiol and progesterone, such as during the luteal phase of the menstrual cycle. Experimental administration of the opiate antagonist naloxone during the luteal phase increases GnRH/LH pulse frequency, significantly suggesting the reversal of a inhibitory action under the endocrine milieu that characterizes the luteal phase. No effect on LH pulsatility follows naloxone injection in postmenopausal or ovariectomized women, unless they are treated with an estrogen-progesterone therapy. **Another example is CRH, the main neuropeptide controlling the adrenal endocrine axis, which is released in greater amount during stress. In this condition, increased CRH release negatively affects the GnRH pulse generator, which results in a decrease in GnRH pulse frequency**. This action is indirect through the release of β-endorphin and is prevented by the administration of the opiate antagonist naloxone, as demonstrated in studies in nonhuman primates and in patients with hypothalamic amenorrhea, many of whom have elevated levels of cortisol.

## Metabolic Influences and GnRH Release

There is good clinical evidence linking energy homeostasis and reproductive function in the human. A functional reproductive system requires an accurate integration of energy balance, and a significant imbalance may lead to reproductive dysfunction and amenorrhea. **Nutritional deprivation and abnormal eating habits are known to interfere with the normal reproductive process. Anorexia nervosa** is a well-known and extreme example of how alteration in food intake can result in the suppression of the menstrual cycle. **Obesity** also may contribute to menstrual disorders.

Growing evidence indicates that complex and extensively integrated physiologic mechanisms connect an active reproductive axis to the metabolic state. The brain, and in particular the hypothalamus and the GnRH pulse generator, function as the center for the integrative metabolic response process. The nature of the afferent signals that provide information about energy metabolism to the reproductive axis is presently under intense study, and data have shown possible roles for several energy-related proteins.

One such example is **leptin, an anorexigenic protein that is the product of the *ob* gene and that is primarily produced by adipocytes** (Ahima, 2000). Leptin levels are reduced when body fat stores are decreased by fasting. Besides conveying metabolic information to several parts of the brain through its own receptors, leptin also appears to function as one of the metabolic cues regulating the GnRH pulse generator. **High leptin levels are interpreted as conducive to reproduction, and the administration of leptin stimulates the secretion of GnRH** and of the gonadotropins, with the effects most pronounced in individuals showing signs of reproductive impairment. Peripheral injections of leptin can prevent the reduction in GnRH/gonadotropins and the disturbances in cyclicity that accompany caloric reduction. *Ob/ob* mice, which are **leptin deficient because of a mutated leptin gene, besides exhibiting a pronounced obesity, show a complete failure to display normal estrous cycles because of absent GnRH secretion**. The latter can be reversed by leptin administration. Evidence suggests a role for kisspeptin in modulating metabolic leptin signals on the hypothalamus and pituitary (Skorupskaite, 2014). Forty percent of kisspeptin neurons in the mouse arcuate nucleus express leptin. Leptin-deficient mice show decreased expression of *Kiss1* messenger RNA (mRNA). However, leptin administration only partially restores *Kiss1* mRNA levels, indicating that other mediators are involved in inhibiting kisspeptin signaling in leptin deficiency (Smith, 2006). Another example is the **orexigenic peptide NPY**, which is synthesized in the arcuate nucleus. **During fasting, expression of NPY mRNA increases in this nucleus and intracerebroventricular injection of NPY stimulates food intake**. NPY has been shown to affect pulsatile GnRH/LH activity in the nonhuman primate, but this occurs in two apparently contradictory modes, one excitatory and one inhibitory. It was shown in the ovariectomized monkey and rodent that a pulsatile intracerebroventricular infusion of NPY stimulates GnRH release, whereas a continuous infusion clearly decreases the pulsatile electric activity of GnRH neurons, as well as pulsatile LH release. In accord with this observation of an inhibitory effect of NPY is that, whereas fasting decreases LH secretion in normal mice, fasting mice lacking NPY Y1 receptor have a higher pituitary LH content than wild-type ones. What these data suggest is that although a supportive effect of NPY on the GnRH pulse generator may occur within a limited window of normalcy (i.e., within a normal background of basic and pulsatile NPY release), in physiopathologic situations (i.e., in circumstances mimicking increased endogenous NPY activity such as in undernutrition) an inhibitory effect of NPY on the GnRH pulse generator can be observed. **Evidence suggests that kisspeptin neurons can sense and convey information about energy status to GnRH neurons.** In rodents, hypothalamic levels of *Kiss1* mRNA are reduced in metabolic conditions, such as undernutrition, uncontrolled diabetes, and immune/inflammatory challenge, which are associated with suppressed gonadotropins. Administration of kisspeptin in rodent models with disrupted metabolism and energy reserves restores gonadotropin secretion, suggesting a potentially important central role of KISS1 neurons in the regulation of reproduction by metabolic factors (Skorupskaite, 2014).

**Overall, in regard to the reproductive system, the GnRH pulse generator actually acts as the link between the environment, the internal milieu, and the reproductive axis.** Its overall activity most probably reflects the summation of simultaneous stimulatory and inhibitory inputs. It is evident that events, disorders, or drug administration may tip the physiologic balance, cause disruption or cessation of GnRH pulse activity, and lead to disruptions of the menstrual cycle and to reproductive disorders such as oligomenorrhea and hypothalamic amenorrhea.

# THE ANTERIOR PITUITARY GLAND AND THE GONADOTROPINS

## Anatomy

The anterior pituitary (also referred to as the **adenohypophysis**) derives from *Rathke's pouch*, a depression in the roof of the developing mouth in front of the buccopharyngeal membrane. It originates at about the third week of life. Origin of the adenohypophysis contrasts with that of the posterior pituitary *(neurohypophysis)*, which develops as a direct extension of the brain. It should also be noted that whereas the neurohypophysis receives a direct arterial blood supply from the hypophyseal arteries, the only vascularization to the adenohypophysis is through the hypothalamic-hypophyseal portal system (into which GnRH and several other neuropeptides are secreted; discussed earlier).

**The gonadotropes are the specialized cells within the adenohypophysis that produce the gonadotropins.** On stimulation of the gonadotropes by GnRH, two gonadotropins are released into the general circulation and regulate endocrine function in the ovaries and testes.

## Physiology

### The GnRH Receptor

Pulses of GnRH released by the GnRH neurons in the arcuate nucleus reach the gonadotropes in the anterior pituitary via the hypophyseal portal circulation. These GnRH pulses then act on GnRH receptors (GnRH-Rs) on the gonadotropes to stimulate both the synthesis and release of both gonadotropins, LH and follicle-stimulating hormone (FSH). Women with GnRH-R mutations typically present with incomplete or absent pubertal development and primary amenorrhea. Although reproductive function is compromised, conception may be successfully obtained after gonadotropin treatment.

On the cell membranes of the gonadotrope, GnRH interacts with high-affinity GnRH-Rs. The gene encoding the GnRH-R is located on chromosome 4q13.2-13.3, spanning 18.9 kb. This **receptor belongs to a large family of G protein–coupled receptors.** These contain seven transmembrane helices connected by six alternating intracellular and extracellular loops, with the amino-terminus located on the extracellular side. In contrast to other protein receptors (see Fig. 4.10, presented later in the chapter), the GnRH-R lacks a carboxy-terminus located on the intracellular site.

#### Activation of the GnRH Receptor

GnRH activation of the receptor requires the release of constraining intramolecular bonds, which maintain the receptor in an inactive configuration. Once activated, the GnRH-R stimulates cellular production of specific membrane-associated lipid-like diacylglycerols, which, acting as a second messenger, activate several cellular proteins. Among these are the enzyme **protein kinase C (PKC) and mitogen-activated protein kinase** (ERK; also called MAPK). Phosphorylated ERK activates transcription factors, the end result being gene transcription of gonadotropin subunits and the synthesis of both gonadotropins.

**Binding of GnRH to its receptor also rapidly mobilizes transient intracellular calcium,** which triggers a burst of exocytosis to rapidly release LH and FSH. It also provokes a rapid influx of $Ca^{+}+$ into the cell from the extracellular pool, which in turn activates calmodulin, a calcium-binding protein, maintaining gonadotropin release. Diacylglycerols amplify the action of $Ca^{+}+$-calmodulin, thereby synergistically enhancing the release of gonadotropins. Administration of a calmodulin antagonist has been shown to decrease GnRH-stimulated gonadotropin release.

#### Estrogens and the GnRH Receptor

Pulsatile GnRH increases GnRH-R gene expression and the number of GnRH-Rs on the gonadotrope's cell surface. The number of GnRH-Rs also varies with the hormonal environment, with highest number of receptors expressed when high concentrations of estrogens are present. This leads to an increase in the overall $Ca2^{+}+$ response and a significantly amplified gonadotropin response to a GnRH pulse. **This action explains the variations in the gonadotropin response to GnRH at various times of the menstrual cycle**: GnRH pulses of similar amplitude elicit greater gonadotropin responses during the late follicular phase and luteal phase when estradiol levels are highest, but the responses are lower during the early follicular phase when estradiol levels are lowest (Fig. 4.5).

#### GnRH Pulse Frequency and Gonadotropin Release

It is also important to note that varying frequencies of the GnRH pulse signal regulate gonadotropin subunit gene transcription differentially. Overall, **a low GnRH pulse frequency favors FSH synthesis, whereas a high GnRH pulse frequency favors LH synthesis.** This is well demonstrated experimentally where changing a pulsatile infusion from a high to a low pulse frequency results in a matter of days in an increase in the FSH/LH ratio (Fig. 4.6). This phenomenon may play a role during the luteal phase of the menstrual cycle and in the changing FSH/LH ratio that occurs during the passage from one menstrual cycle to another (see The Luteal Phase, discussed later). It is also reflected in **patients known to have a high GnRH pulse frequency, such as in women with the polycystic ovary syndrome, a high proportion of whom have a characteristically elevated LH:FSH ratio.**

#### GnRH Receptor Desensitization

Gonadotropin release after a GnRH pulse is rapid: Within minutes, both FSH and LH are released. It is important to recognize that the pulsatile release mode of GnRH is essential for the maintenance and control of normal gonadotropin secretion.

In contrast to the response to the normal pulsatile mode of GnRH release, sustained exposure of the GnRH-R to constant GnRH concentrations drastically reduces the response of the gonadotrope to subsequent stimulation with GnRH. This phenomenon is referred to as homologous desensitization or down-regulation of the receptor, which denotes a reduction in the

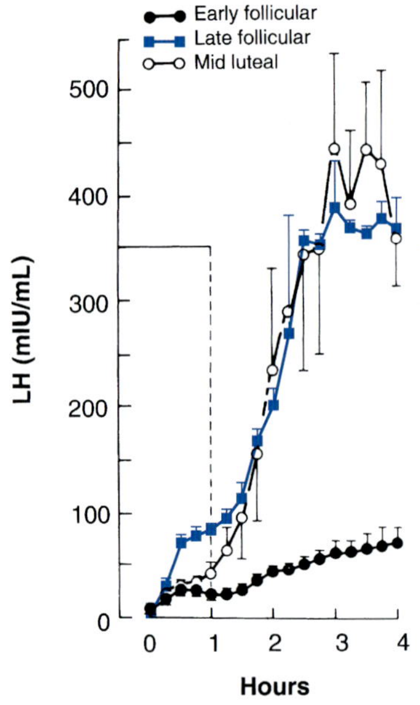


**Fig. 4.5** GnRH pulses of similar amplitude elicit greater overall gonadotropin responses during the late follicular phase and luteal phase when estradiol levels are highest, but they elicit lower responses during the early follicular phase when estradiol levels are lowest. Note also a greater early response in the late follicular phase, denoting greater LH reserves under the effect of estradiol. *GnRH,* Gonadotropin-releasing hormone; *LH,* luteinizing hormone. (From Hoff JD, Lasley BL, Wang CF, Yen SSC. The two pools of pituitary gonadotropins: regulation during the menstrual cycle. *J Clin Endocrinol Metab.* 1977;44:302.)

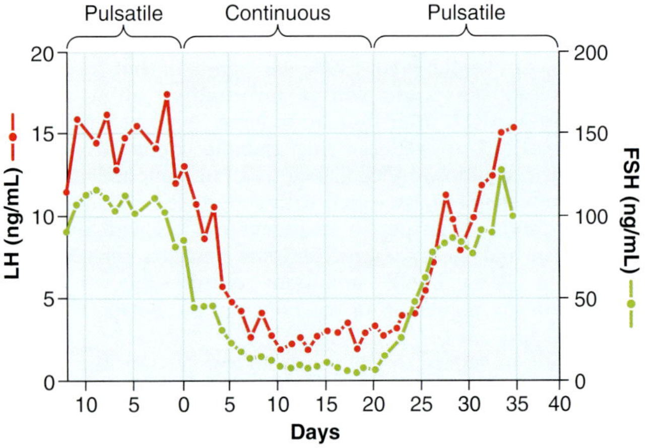


**Fig. 4.7** Gonadotropin-releasing hormone (GnRH) release in a pulsatile mode is required for a normal pituitary gonadotropin response. An experiment was performed in a monkey lacking endogenous GnRH and infused with hourly pulses of GnRH *(left and right panels)* or with a continuous GnRH infusion *(center panel). LH,* Luteinizing hormone. (From Belchetz PE, Plant TM, Nakai Y, et al. hypophyseal responses to continuous and intermittent delivery of hypothalamic gonadotropin-releasing hormone. *Science.* 1978;202:631-633.)

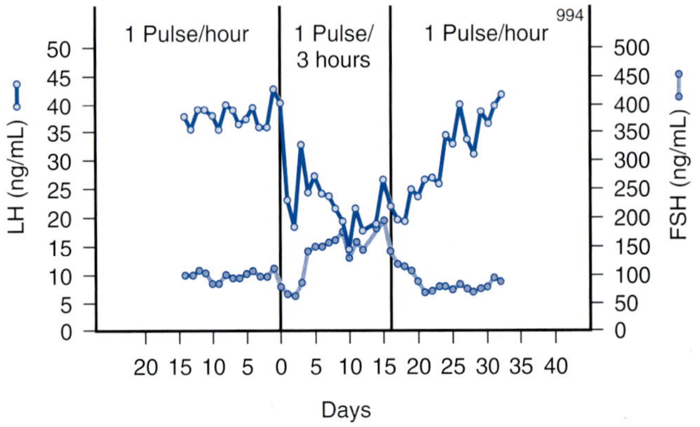


**Fig. 4.6** Increase in the FSH/LH ratio after a decrease in the gonadotropin-releasing hormone (GnRH) pulse frequency (from 1 pulse/hour; *left and right panels*) to 1 pulse/3 hour *(center panel).* Experiment was performed in a monkey lacking endogenous GnRH and infused with GnRH. *FSH,* Follicle-stimulating hormone; *LH,* luteinizing hormone. (From Wildt L, Hausler A, Marshall G, et al. Frequency and amplitude of gonadotropin-releasing hormone stimulation and gonadotropin secretion in the rhesus monkey. *Endocrinology.* 1981;109:376.)

ability of GnRH to elicit gonadotropin release after prior continuous exposure to GnRH. This phenomenon is well illustrated in a classic experiment in ovariectomized monkeys lacking endogenous GnRH secretion after lesion of the arcuate nucleus (Fig. 4.7). As illustrated, 6-minute pulses administered once an hour restored normal LH levels in these animals. In contrast, when a continuous mode of GnRH infusion was substituted to the pulsatile mode, a profound inhibition of LH concentrations occurred, which reflects desensitization of the GnRH-R. This phenomenon, which takes a few days to be established, may reflect a loss of active cell surface receptors and be maintained by a loss of functional $Ca^{++}$ channels. However, the mechanism of desensitization is still under investigation, and additional intermediary changes remain to be characterized.

## GnRH Analogs and the GnRH Receptor

The GnRH half-life in the peripheral circulation is very short because peptidases rapidly degrade naturally occurring GnRH by cleaving the decapeptide molecule at the $Gly^6$ to $Leu^7$ and at the $Pro^9$ to $Gly^{10}$ bonds. However, by substituting amino acid 6 in the natural GnRH molecule with a d-amino or replacing amino acid 10 with an N-methylamide (Na-CH2-CH3) or Aza-Gly (NHNHCO) moiety, GnRH analogs were synthesized and shown to have acquired a greater resistance to enzymatic proteolysis and hence a longer half-life (hours vs. 2 to 4 minutes). **After administration of these GnRH agonists, there is an initial stimulation of gonadotropin release (flare), followed by the process of desensitization blocking the releasing effect on the gonadotropins.** This observation has led to the clinical application of the functional desensitization property of GnRH:GnRH analogs; they have been used to induce a "medical castration" state by shutting down the pituitary-gonadal axis in a variety of clinical conditions. **In contrast to GnRH agonists, GnRH antagonists act by competing with GnRH for receptor sites and thereby never activating a stimulatory signal.** Many of these result from the substitution of amino acids at the 2 or 3 position. **Thus GnRH antagonists have the advantage over the GnRH agonists of a rapidly decreasing LH and FSH release, without the flare.** Clinical applications for both GnRH agonists and antagonists are listed in Box 4.1. Although GnRH agonists have been in use longer and have several Food and Drug Administration (FDA)–approved indications, the GnRH antagonists, though theoretically useful for the same conditions, are only approved for a few indications at present. **An orally active GnRH antagonist, elagolix (Orilissa),** is available in the United States and has been approved in two dosages, 150 and 200 mg twice daily, for the treatment of severe endometriosis.

**BOX 4.1 Clinical Applications of GnRH Agonists and Antagonists**

Activation of pituitary–gonadal function (GnRH)
Delayed puberty
Cryptorchidism
Functional hypothalamic amenorrhea
Hypogonadotropic hypogonadism (Kallmann syndrome)
Pituitary–gonadal inhibition (agonists)
Precocious puberty
Hormone-dependent tumors
Endometriosis
Uterine leiomyoma
Breast cancer
Prostatic cancer
Suppression of ovarian function in polycystic ovary syndrome and in vitro fertilization
Premenstrual syndrome
Abnormal uterine bleeding including clotting disorders
Contraception
Suppression of spermatogenesis
Ovulation inhibition

*GnRH,* Gonadotropin-releasing hormone.

### The Gonadotropins

There are two distinct gonadotropins: **LH** and **FSH** (Bousfield, 2006). (A third gonadotropin, human chorionic gonadotropin [HCG], is produced in the primate by the placenta.)

**Structure**
LH and FSH are glycoproteins of high molecular weight. **They are heterodimers, containing two monomeric units (subunits).** Both LH and FSH have a similar α-subunit, the structure (92 amino acids) of which is highly conserved. **(The same α-subunit is also shared with HCG and thyroid-stimulating hormone [TSH].)** However, β-subunits have different structures consisting of different amino acids and carbohydrates. These LH and FSH subunits are each encoded by a separate gene. (The HCG subunits are also different and encoded by six genes.)

The α- and β-subunits are joined by disulfide bonds, which are essential to maintain biologic activity. Reducing agents break the disulfides bounds and reduce or remove the biologic activity of the gonadotropin. Highly purified free subunits have little if any biologic activity relative to that of the intact hormone. However, **it is the β-subunit that confers the specific biologic activity of each hormone.** For instance, LH has a β-subunit of 121 amino acids, a structure that is responsible for the specificity of the interaction with the LH receptor. LH and FSH also differ in the composition of their sugar moieties. The different composition of several different oligosaccharides affects bioactivity and speed of degradation of each gonadotropin. For example, the biologic half-life of LH is 20 minutes, much shorter than that of FSH (3 to 4 hours). (The half-life of HCG is 24 hours.)

Although both gonadotropins act synergistically in women, FSH acts primarily on the granulosa cells of the ovarian follicles to stimulate follicular growth, whereas LH acts primarily on the theca cells of these follicles, as well as on the luteal cells to stimulate ovarian steroid hormone production (see the following discussion).

# THE OVARIES

## Anatomy

### Ovarian Gametogenesis (Oogenesis)

Oogenesis begins in fetal life when the *primordial* germ cells, or oogonia, migrate to the genital ridge. The number of oogonia increases dramatically from about 600,000 by the second month of fetal life to a maximum of about 7 million by the sixth to seventh month. The oogonia then begin meiotic division (they are now referred to as primary oocytes) until they reach the diplotene stage of the prophase (the germinal vesicular stage), in which they will remain until stimulation by gonadotropins in adulthood during the menstrual cycle (discussed later). However, by a process of apoptosis and atresia of the enveloping follicle, which starts prenatally and persists throughout childhood, the number of primary oocytes declines drastically from about 2 to 4 million at birth to become 90% depleted by puberty. Further depletion of the pool occurs throughout adulthood, so that by age 37 only about 25,000 and by age 50 only about 1000 oocytes remain.

In recent years, the traditional dogma that mammals have fixed, nonrenewable oocyte stores established before birth has been challenged. Some studies suggest that adult mammalian ovaries possess pluripotent germline stem cells (GSCs) that can differentiate into oocytes, as well as other cell types. Nonmammalian organisms, such as Drosophila, do possess ovarian GSCs. Whereas the existence of spermatogonial cells in the adult human testis that give rise to pluripotent GSCs is well accepted, there is considerable evidence that disputes the existence of mammalian adult ovarian GSCs. At this point, there is not sufficient evidence to prove that mammalian oogenesis occurs after birth (Hanna, 2014).

### Ovarian Folliculogenesis

The primary oocyte is surrounded by a single layer of flattened granulosa cells in a unit referred to as the **primordial follicle.** Even in the absence of stimulation by gonadotropins, some primordial follicles will develop into **primary** (or preantral) follicles, at which stage multiple layers of cuboidal granulosa cells surround them. Development of follicles to this stage appears to be relatively independent of pituitary control but is probably influenced by intraovarian, nonsteroidal processes that remain to be understood. Development to this stage occurs during the nonovulatory stages of childhood, pregnancy, and oral contraceptive use, as well as during ovulatory cycles.

With formation of an antrum (cavity), the follicle, now referred to as secondary or antral follicle, enters the final stages of folliculogenesis, characterized by the transition from intraovarian regulation to a major control by the hypothalamic-pituitary unit. This requires the presence of the characteristic increase in FSH that occurs in the early menstrual cycle (see The Menstrual Cycle, presented later).

The development process from primary follicle (preantral follicle) to secondary or antral follicle and to a mature preovulatory follicle, the latter during the follicular phase of the cycle, takes about 1 year to complete (Fig. 4.8). Only about 400 follicles complete this process, whereas the majority of follicles undergo programmed cell death. Although little is known about factors controlling growth during the earlier stages, more is known about the final stage of folliculogenesis during the follicular phase of the menstrual cycle (discussed later).

## Physiology

### The Gonadotropin Receptors

Although the two gonadotropins act synergistically in the woman, FSH acts primarily on the granulosa cells of the maturing antral

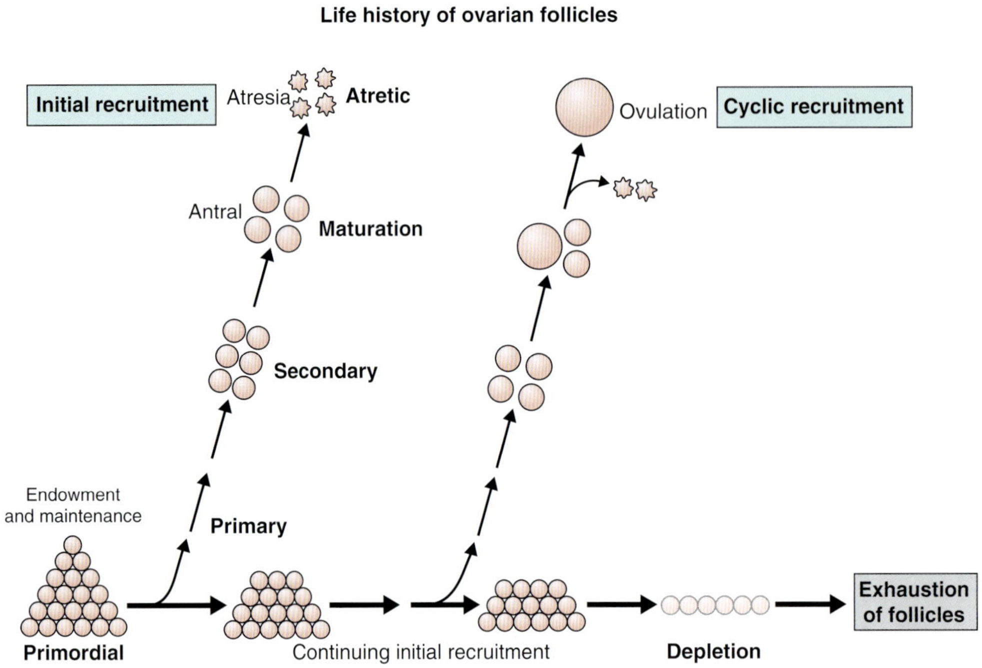


**Fig. 4.8** Life history of ovarian follicles: endowment, maintenance, initial recruitment, maturation, atresia or cyclic recruitment, ovulation, and exhaustion. A fixed number of primordial follicles are endowed during early life, and most of them are maintained in a resting state. Growth of some of these dormant follicles is initiated before and throughout reproductive life (initial recruitment). Follicles develop through primordial, primary, and secondary stages before acquiring an antral cavity. At the antral stage, most follicles undergo atresia; however, under the optimal gonadotropin stimulation that occurs after puberty, a few of them are rescued (cyclic recruitment) to reach the preovulatory stage. Eventually, depletion of the pool of resting follicles leads to ovarian follicle exhaustion and senescence. (From McGee EA, Hsueh AJW. Initial and cyclic recruitment of ovarian follicles. *Endocrine Rev.* 2000;21:200-214.)

follicle to stimulate follicular growth, whereas LH acts primarily on the theca cells of these follicles to induce steroidogenesis. Binding to and activation of their respective receptors at the cell surface membrane is the necessary first step in the hormonal function of both FSH and LH.

Gonadotropin receptors are transmembrane G protein–coupled receptors that possess seven membrane-spanning domains (Fig. 4.9). It is believed that the receptor molecule exists in a conformational equilibrium between active and inactive states, which is shifted by binding of LH or FSH. **On binding to the gonadotropin, the receptor shifts conformation and mechanically activates the G protein, which detaches from the receptor and activates cyclic adenosine monophosphate (cAMP)–dependent protein kinases.** These protein kinases are present as tetramers with two regulatory units and two catalytic units. On binding of cAMP to the regulatory units, the catalytic units are released and initiate the phosphorylation of proteins, which bind to DNA in the cell nucleus, resulting in the activation of genes and leading to the physiologic action (Fig. 4.10).

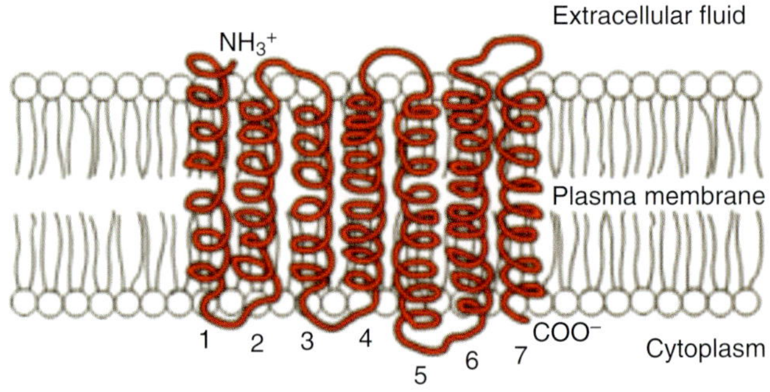


**Fig. 4.9** The seven transmembrane α-helix structure of a G protein–coupled receptor, such as that for LH or HCG. *GnRH,* Gonadotropin-releasing hormone; *HCG,* human chorionic gonadotropin; *LH,* luteinizing hormone. (The structure for the GnRH receptor is similar, except that the GnRH receptor lacks a carboxy-terminus on the intracellular site; see the preceding text "Physiology: The GnRH Receptor".) (From Wikipedia. Trans-membrane helix of G-protein coupled FSH receptor. https://commons.wikimedia.org/wiki/File:7TM_receptor.png)

## The Ovarian Steroids: Biosynthesis

One primary function of the ovary is the secretion of ovarian steroids, which occurs after binding of both FSH and LH to their respective receptors. The ovary secretes three primary hormones: **estradiol** (the primary estrogen), **progesterone,** and **androstenedione.** These hormones are the chief secretory products of the maturing follicle, the corpus luteum, and the ovarian stroma. The ovary also secretes, in varying amounts, estrone (a less potent estrogen), pregnenolone, 17-hydroxyprogesterone, testosterone, and dehydroepiandrosterone (DHEA). Because of the lack of the appropriate enzymes, the ovary does not synthesize mineralocorticoids or glucocorticoids.

Steroids are lipids that have a basic chemical structure or nucleus (Fig. 4.11). The nucleus consists of three six-carbon rings (A, B, and C) joined to a five-carbon atom (D) ring. The carbon atoms are numbered as shown in Fig. 4.11. Functional groups above the plane of the molecule are preceded by the $\beta$ symbol

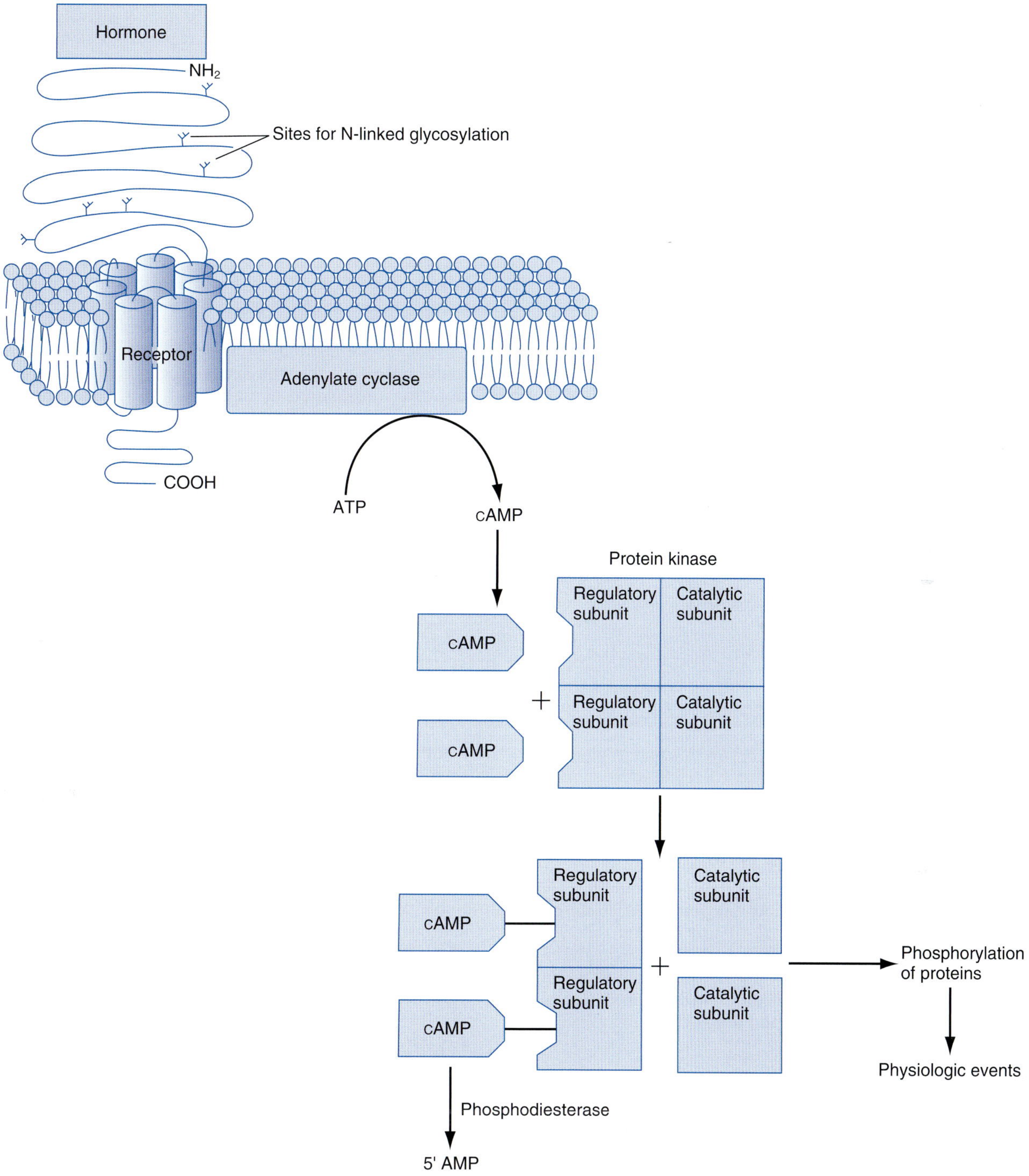


**Fig. 4.10** On binding to their receptor, the gonadotropins activate cAMP–dependent protein kinases (see text). *ATP,* Adenosine triphosphate; *cAMP,* cyclic adenosine monophosphate. (Adapted from Speroff L, Friz M, eds. *Clinical Gynecologic Endocrinology and Infertility.* New York: Lippincott Williams & Wilkins; 2005:71-72.)

and shown in the structural formula by a solid line, whereas those below the plane are indicated by an α symbol and a dotted line. All steroids, whether secreted by the ovary, testis, or adrenal, are derived from **acetate** (a 2-carbon compound), which, in a series of complex reactions, is transformed into **cholesterol** (a 27-carbon steroid) (Fig. 4.12).

The sex steroids (as well as the corticosteroids) are then derived from a stepwise transformation of the cholesterol molecule into steroids with 21 carbon atoms (the corticosteroids, pregnenolone, 17-hydroxypregnenolone, progesterone, and 17-hydroxyprogesterone), 19 carbon atoms (androgens such as DHEA, androstenedione, and testosterone), and 18 carbon atoms (estrogens such as estradiol and estrone). In the first step, cholesterol is transferred from the outer mitochondrial membrane to the inner membrane where cytochrome P450 enzyme is located. The latter will split off the cholesterol side chain, which is the first enzymatic step in steroid biosynthesis. Being lipophilic, cholesterol is unable to cross the aqueous phase between these

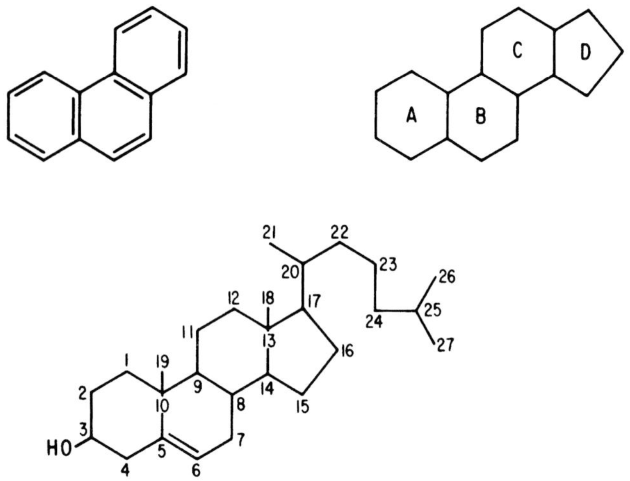


**Fig. 4.11** Phenanthrene *(top left).* Cyclopentanoperhydrophenanthrene nucleus *(top right),* which incorporates the three six-carbon rings of the phenanthrene ring system (**A, B**, and **C**) and a five-carbon ring **(D)**, which resembles cyclopentane. Cholesterol *(bottom)* is the common biosynthetic precursor of steroid hormones. Numbers *1* to *27* indicate the conventional numbering system of the carbon atoms in steroids. (From Stanczyk FZ. Steroid hormones. In Lobo RA, Mishell DR, Paulson RJ, Shoupe D, eds. *Mishell's Textbook of Infertility, Contraception and Reproductive Endocrinology.* 4th ed. Malden, MA: Blackwell Science; 1997.)

two membranes unassisted. It is now believed that steroidogenic acute regular protein (StAR) plays that role. The next steps in steroid biosynthesis require participation of a variety of enzymes, most of which are part of the cytochrome P450 superfamily of heme-based enzymes. First is the transformation of cholesterol into pregnenolone by hydroxylation of C-20 and C-22 and cleavage between these two atoms, reducing the C-27 cholesterol to the C-21 compound pregnenolone. At this point, ovarian steroid biosynthesis proceeds along two major pathways, controlled by specific enzymes at each step: (1) the $\Delta^5$ *pathway* through 17-hydroxypregnenolone and DHEA to $\Delta^5$ androstenediol and (2) the $\Delta^4$ *pathway* via progesterone and 17-hydroxyprogesterone to the androgens androstenedione and testosterone.

## The Aromatase Enzyme

**Androgens are converted to the estrogens estrone or estradiol by the enzyme aromatase,** through the loss of the C-19 methyl group and the transformation of the A-ring to an aromatic state (hence the enzyme's name) through oxidation and subsequent elimination of a methyl group. **The aromatic (or phenolic) ring is characteristic of the estrogens** (Fig. 4.13).

Aromatase is a complex enzyme comprising two proteins. The first, P450arom (also a member of the cytochrome P450 superfamily of genes), catalyzes the series of reactions required for the formation of the phenolic A ring. The second is reduced nicotinamide adenine dinucleotide phosphate (NADPH)–cytochrome P450 reductase, a ubiquitous protein required for transferring reducing equivalents from NADPH to any microsomal form of cytochrome P450 with which it comes into contact. (All microsomal P450 enzymes require this reductase for catalysis. Disruption of this reductase has lethal consequences, as shown in knockout mice.)

The aromatase enzyme is found in many tissues besides the gonads, such as the endometrium, brain, placenta, bone, skin, and other tissues, and has been found to play a significant role in endometriosis, where aromatase is expressed in endometriotic lesions. It is also particularly relevant to note that in humans, in contrast to other species, estrogens are also synthesized in adipose tissue, which in postmenopausal women becomes the major site of estrogen biosynthesis. The tissue-specific expression of the CYP19 aromatase gene is regulated by the use of different promoters. For instance, expression in the ovary uses a promoter element proximal to the start of translation, whereas expression in adipose tissue uses distal elements. Overall, the $C_{18}$ estrogen produced in different tissue sites of biosynthesis is rather specific and dependent on the nature of the $C_{19}$ steroid presented to the aromatase enzyme: In the ovary, the main androgen source is ovarian testosterone and thus the main estrogen product from the ovary is estradiol, whereas in adipose tissue the main androgen source is circulating androstenedione (produced by the adrenals) and hence the principal estrogen produced is estrone. (The greater the amount of fat present, the greater the amount of androstenedione that is converted to estrone.)

Mutation of the CYP19 aromatase gene leads to the **aromatase deficiency syndrome,** which is inherited in an autosomal recessive way (Morishima, 1995). In these female patients, accumulation of androgens during pregnancy may lead to virilization at birth. Individuals of both sexes have abnormal pubertal maturation and are tall because of the lack of estrogen to affect epiphyseal closure. Female patients have primary amenorrhea. Aromatase inhibition evidently leads to profound hypoestrogenism. Aromatase inhibitors have become useful in the management of patients with estrogen receptor positive tumors—for example, in breast cancer.

Interconversion between androstenedione and testosterone and estrone and estradiol can occur outside the ovaries. Oxidation of the latter to the former reduces biologic potency because both androstenedione and estrone have weaker biologic activity. Estrone is also converted to estrone sulfate, which has a longer half-life and is the largest component of the pool of circulating estrogens. Estrone sulfate is not biologically active; however, sulfatases in various tissues (such as breast and endometrium) can readily convert it to estrone, which in turn can be converted to the more biologically active estradiol. Steroids are, in general, insoluble in water but dissolve readily in organic solvents. In contrast, steroids that have a sulfate or glucuronide group attached (conjugated steroids)—such as, for example, estrone sulfate, dehydroepiandrosterone sulfate (DHEAS), or pregnanediol glucuronide—are water soluble.

## The Ovarian Steroids: Blood Transport and Metabolism

After release into the circulation, sex steroids bind to a steroid-specific transport protein, **sex hormone–binding globulin (SHBG)** (a $\beta$-globulin synthesized by the liver), to the non–steroid-specific albumin, or circulate in an unbound or "free" form. (There is a separate steroid specific protein, corticosteroid-binding protein [CBG; transcortin], which binds primarily adrenal steroids and to a lesser degree progesterone.) Both SHBG and CBG have a high affinity (by definition) but low capacity for steroids. Albumin, in contrast, has a high capacity but binds with low affinity; thus steroids can readily dissociate from its binding and enter target cells.

The free and loosely albumin-bound steroids are believed to be the most biologically important fractions because the steroid is free to diffuse or be actively transported through the capillary wall and bind to its receptor. (There is also evidence, however, that uptake of protein-bound hormone may also play a role.) SHBG binds primarily dihydrotestosterone, testosterone, and estradiol, in order of decreasing affinity. Thus in premenopausal women, 65% of testosterone is bound to SHBG, 30% to albumin, and 5% is free, whereas 60% of estradiol is bound to SHBG,

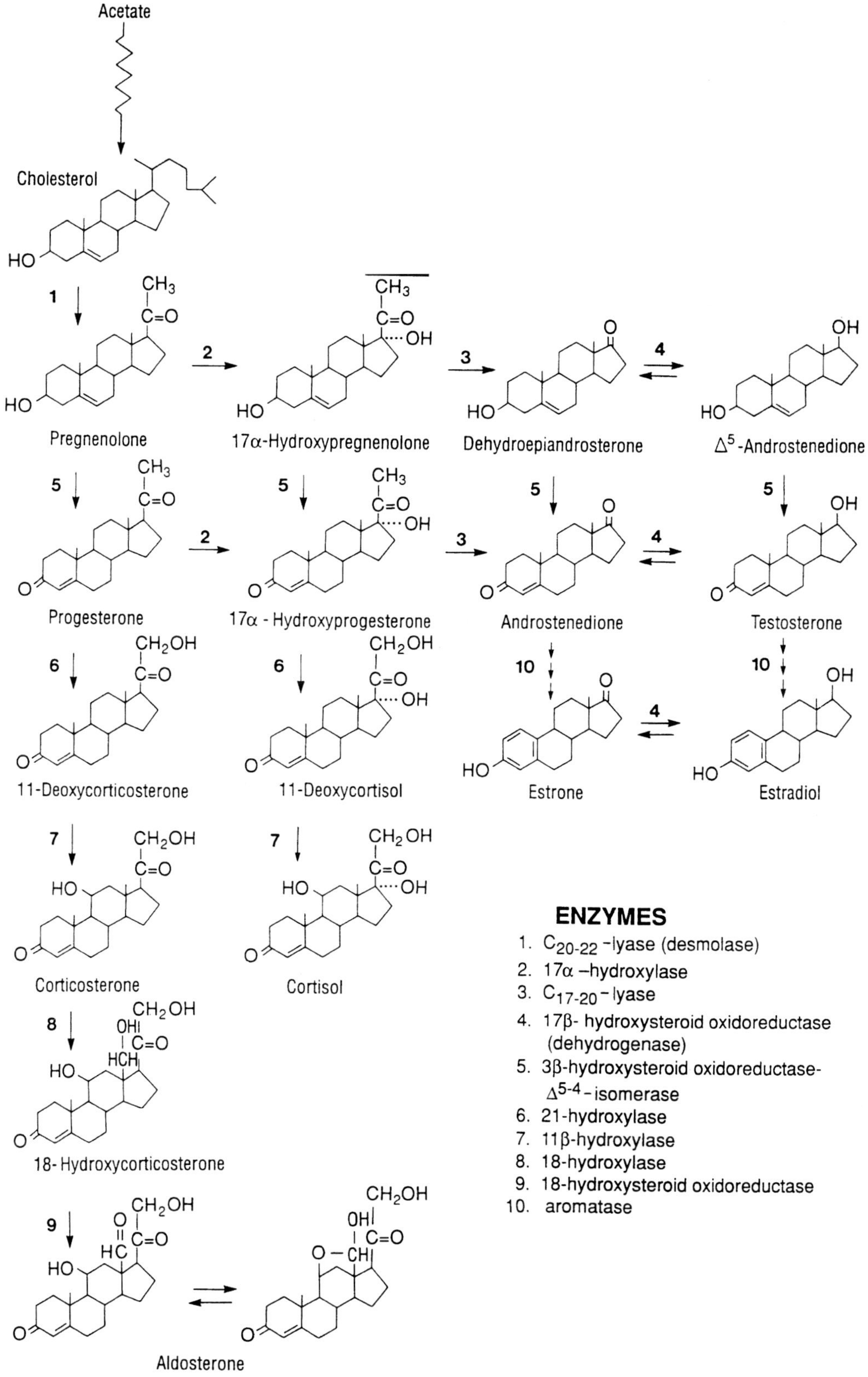


**Fig. 4.12** Biosynthesis of androgens, estrogens, and corticosteroids. (From Stanczyk FZ. Steroid hormones. In Lobo RA, Mishell DR, Paulson RJ, Shoupe D, eds. *Mishell's Textbook of Infertility, Contraception and Reproductive Endocrinology.* 4th ed. Malden, MA: Blackwell Science; 1997.)

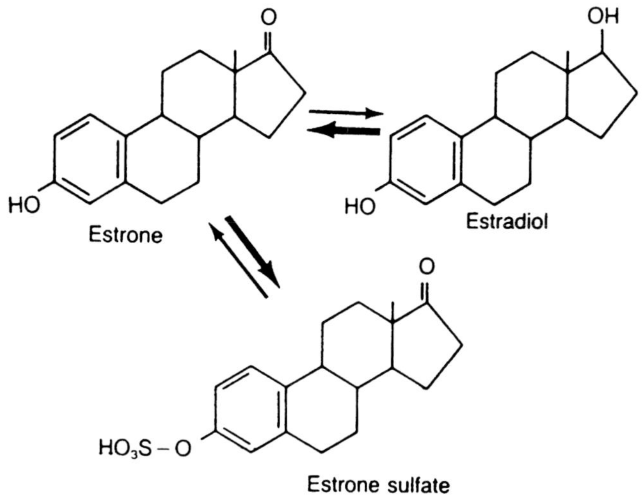


**Fig. 4.13** Interconversion of the three main circulating estrogens. (From Stanczyk FZ. Steroid hormones. In Lobo RA, Mishell DR, Paulson RJ, Shoupe D, eds. *Mishell's Textbook of Infertility, Contraception and Reproductive Endocrinology.* 4th ed. Malden, MA, Blackwell Science, 1997.)

38% to albumin, and 2% to 3% is free. The metabolic clearance rate of sex steroids is inversely related to their affinity to SHBG. It is thus important to remember that the level of SHBG, and therefore the level of free active hormone, may be influenced by various clinical conditions. For instance, circulating levels of SHBG are increased by estrogens (oral contraceptives, pregnancy) and by thyroid hormone (hyperthyroidism) and are lowered by androgens and in hypothyroidism.

The major sites of steroid metabolism are the liver and kidney. Steroids are mainly oxidized by cytochrome P450 oxidase enzymes through reactions that introduce oxygen into the steroid ring, allowing a breakdown by other enzymes to form bile acids as final products. These bile acids can then be eliminated through secretion from the liver. In another process, which involves conjugation, the steroids are transformed from lipophilic compounds, which are only sparingly soluble in water, into metabolites that are readily water soluble and can be eliminated in urine. Examples are estradiol-17 glucuronide, estrone sulfate, and pregnanediol-3-glucuronide (the major urinary metabolite of progesterone).

### Prostaglandins

Prostaglandins (a subclass of eicosanoids and prostanoids) are in general mediators of inflammatory and anaphylactic reactions. **Their most abundant precursor is arachidonic acid,** itself formed from linoleic acid supplied in the diet. Their biosynthesis can be inhibited by several groups of compounds, including the nonsteroidal antiinflammatory drugs (NSAIDs) type 1 (aspirin and indomethacin), which inhibit endoperoxide formation (the immediate precursor of eicosanoids), and type 2 (phenylbutazone), which inhibits the action of endoperoxidase isomerase and reductase. Corticosteroids also can inhibit prostaglandins synthesis.

In contrast to steroid hormones, which are stored and act at targets distant from their source, prostaglandins are produced intracellularly shortly before they are released and generally act locally. Specific prostanoids can have variable effects on different tissues and variable effects on the same organ, even when released at the same concentration, hence the difficulty of studying their actions. One important effect is their ability to modulate the responses of endogenous stimulators and inhibitors, such as ovarian stimulation by LH, which is modulated by prostaglandin F2α (PGF2α), which in turn regulates ovarian receptor availability.

Prostaglandins play an important role in ovarian physiology. They help control early follicular growth by increasing blood supply to certain follicles and inducing FSH receptors in granulosa cells of preovulatory follicles. Both PGF2α and PGE2 are concentrated in follicular fluid of preovulatory follicles and may assist in the process of follicular rupture by facilitating proteolytic enzyme activity in the follicular walls. Many prostanoids are produced in the endometrium. Concentrations of PGE2 and PGF2α increase progressively from the proliferative to the secretory phase of the cycle, with highest levels at menstruation. These prostaglandins may help regulate myometrial contractility and may also play a role in regulating the process of menstruation.

## COMMUNICATION WITHIN THE HYPOTHALAMIC-PITUITARY-OVARIAN ENDOCRINE AXIS

### The Steroid Receptors

Gonadal steroids are integrated into every aspect of reproduction, and disruption of their signaling pathways, which obviously require initial binding to their receptors, leads to reduced fecundity and aberrations in multiple organs systems. For the sex steroid feedback loops (discussed later) to be active, there must be steroid receptors in the appropriate regions of the hypothalamus and pituitary gland to respond to the ovarian signals.

As opposed to peptide or protein hormone receptors that reside on the cell membrane (discussed earlier), steroid receptors reside in the nucleus or in the cytoplasm, in between which they may shuttle in the absence of hormone (Fig. 4.14). The cytoplasmic receptor is sequestered (hence in an "inactive" state) within a multiprotein inhibitory complex that includes heat shock proteins. Hormone binding leads to dissociation from the heat shock proteins. The lipophilic steroids freely diffuse across the nuclear membrane to bind to their cognate receptor. This binding leads to conformational changes that transform the receptor into an "activated" state, which allows it to bind to a hormone responsive element (HRE), the specific DNA-binding site to which steroid receptors bind conferring hormone sensitivity within target gene promoters. Nuclear receptors can inhibit or enhance transcription by recruiting an array of coactivator or corepressor proteins to the transcription complex (Fig. 4.15) (Ellmann, 2009). mRNA is then generated from a segment of nuclear DNA in the process of transcription. Transcription is the most important process regulated by steroid hormones. All genes share a common basic design composed of a structural region in which the DNA encodes the specific amino acids of the protein and a regulatory region that interacts with various proteins to control the rate of transcription. Coactivators and corepressors modify the chromatin state and recruit/activate or hinder the basal transcriptional machinery. Members of the SRC family of coactivators, including SRC-1, SRC-2, and SRC-3, and the nuclear receptor corepressor (NCoR1) interact with both the estrogen and progesterone receptors (see Fig. 4.15) (Ellmann, 2009; Horwitz, 1996). The mRNA migrates into the cytoplasm, where it translates information to ribosomes to synthesize the required new protein.

Several alternative receptor mechanisms besides the classic one outlined previously appear to exist. Some are plasma membrane steroid signaling events that are mediated through various kinases and second messengers including cAMP. These are independent of nuclear interactions and do not involve direct steroid activation of gene transcription (nongenomic). As opposed to the longer time required by the genomic pathway (hours to days), these alternate mechanisms may be responsible for some of the very rapid effects of steroids—for instance, as activated by the

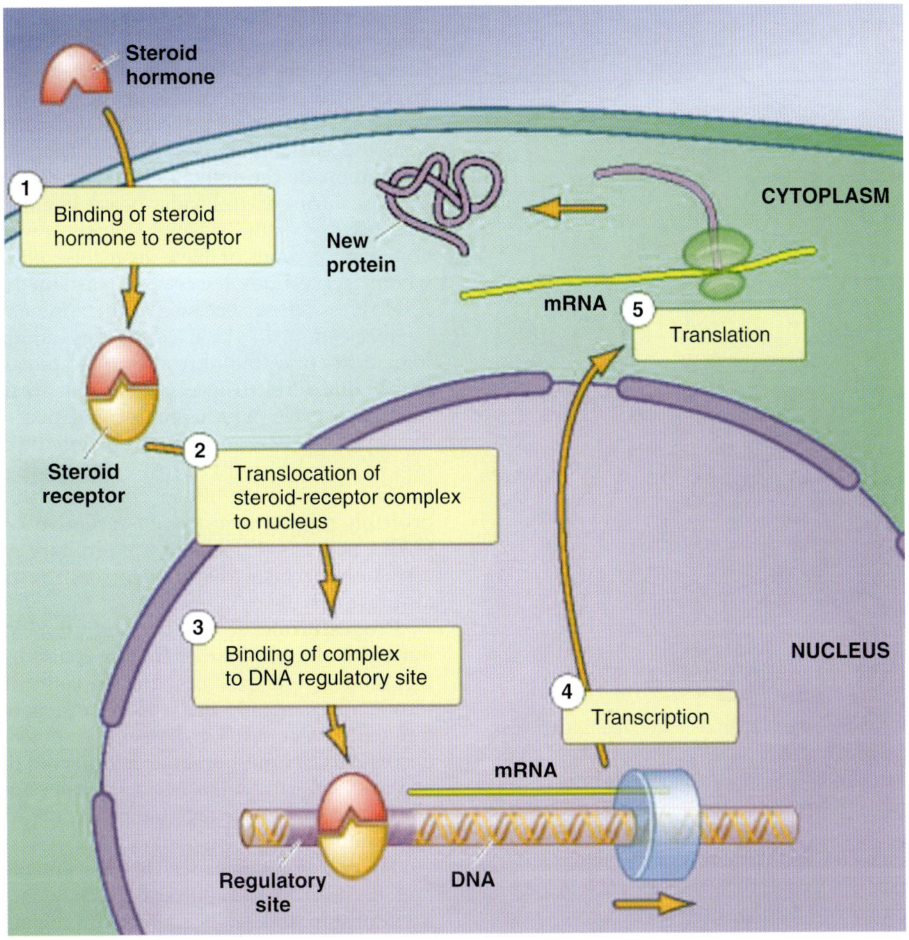


**Fig. 4.14** The steroid receptor activation process. As opposed to protein hormones receptors, which reside on the cell membrane, steroid receptors reside in the nucleus or in the cytoplasm. See the text for details. *mRNA,* Messenger RNA.

negative steroid feedback loop (discussed later), which occurs within minutes.

Members of the steroid receptor superfamily share amino acid homology and a common structure. They contain key structural elements that enable them to bind to their respective ligands with high affinity and specificity and to recognize and bind to discrete response elements within the DNA sequence of target genes with high affinity and specificity. For instance, estrogen receptors will bind natural and synthetic estrogens, but not androgens or progestins. The affinity of a receptor for a steroid also correlates with steroid potency; for example, the estrogen receptor has a greater affinity for estradiol than for estrone and estriol, which are much less potent than estradiol. Overall, the magnitude of the signal to the cell and of the cell response to the steroid depend on the concentration of the hormone and of the receptors, as well as on the affinity of the receptor to the hormone.

In humans there are actually two estrogen receptors, ER-$\alpha$ and ER-$\beta$, which are distinct receptor forms encoded by separate genes. There are also two forms of the progesterone receptor, but these are isoforms (differing only by minor structural differences), which are encoded by the same gene.

## The Ovarian-Hypothalamic-Pituitary Feedback Loops

FSH and LH act on the ovaries to induce morphologic changes and ovarian steroid secretion. Morphologic processes include folliculogenesis (i.e., the cyclic recruitment of a pool of follicles to produce a mature follicle ready for ovulation) and the formation of a corpus luteum. These processes occur in sequence, conferring a monthly rhythm to the reproductive cycle. Granulosa and theca cells within the follicle and luteal cells respond to LH by synthesizing and releasing ovarian steroids, mainly estradiol-17$\beta$ and progesterone. The type and amount of hormone released depend on the status of the follicle and the corpus luteum (see The Menstrual Cycle, presented later).

Feedback communication between the ovaries and the hypothalamic-pituitary unit is an essential component to the physiology of the reproductive cycle. It is important for the brain and pituitary gland to modulate their secretion in response to the minute-to-minute activity status of the ovary. Through their receptors, both in various areas of the hypothalamus and in the anterior pituitary gland, the two ovarian steroids, estradiol and progesterone, play a major role in these feedback communications. Evidence now shows that several nonsteroidal compounds are also involved in these feedbacks.

### The Negative Steroid Feedback Loop

As in other endocrine systems, the major ovarian to brain-pituitary feedback loop is inhibitory (the **negative feedback loop**), whereby the steroid secreted by the target organ (the ovary) regulates the hypothalamic-hypophyseal unit to adjust GnRH and gonadotropin secretion appropriately (Fig. 4.16).

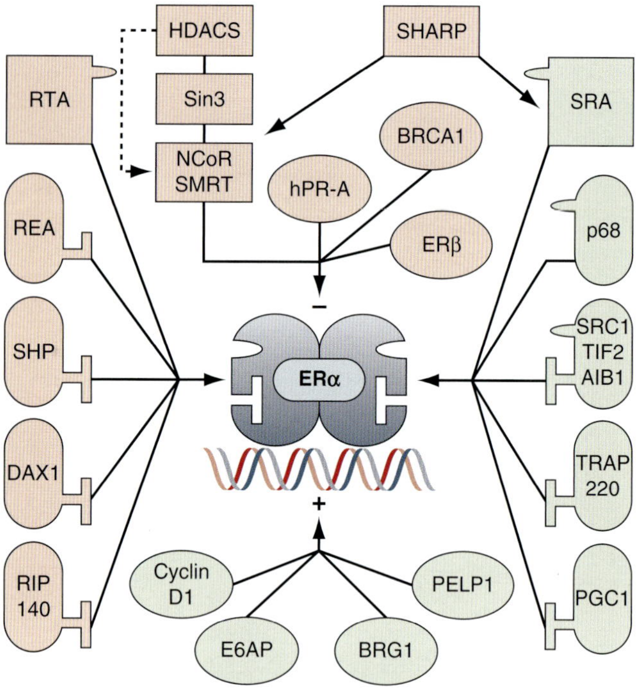


**Fig. 4.15** A connections map for the human estrogen receptor (ER). The ER interacts with a large number of proteins that can either positively or negatively regulate target gene transcription. ERα cofactors interact with different target proteins linking the receptor to other signal transduction pathways. Some of the key connections that positively (+) or negatively (–) regulate ERα transcriptional activity are shown. (From McDonnell DP, Norris JD. Connections and regulation of the human estrogen receptor. *Science.* 2002;296:1642.)

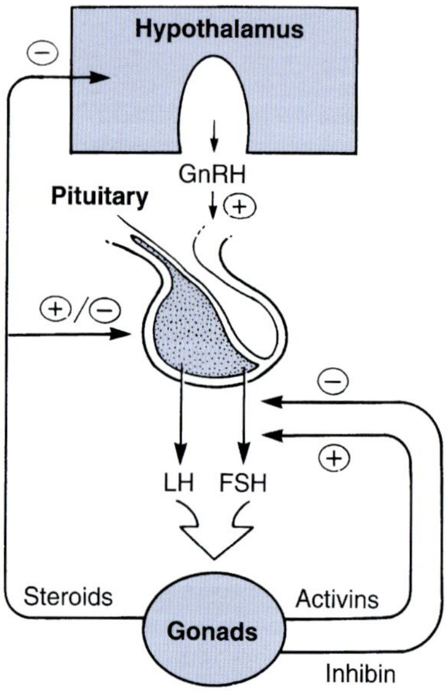


**Fig. 4.16** The rapidly acting negative feedback loop of steroids on GnRH and both gonadotropins' release is supplemented by a slower-acting negative feedback loop by the inhibins. *FSH,* Follicle-stimulating hormone; *GnRH,* gonadotropin-releasing hormone; *LH,* luteinizing hormone. (From Hylka VW, di Zerega GS. Reproductive hormones and their mechanisms of action. In Mishell DR Jr, Davajan V, Lobo RA, eds. *Infertility, Contraception and Reproductive Endocrinology.* 3rd ed. Cambridge, MA: Blackwell Scientific; 1991.)

Estradiol-17$\beta$ is a potent physiologic inhibitor of GnRH and of gonadotropin secretion. The threshold for the negative feedback action of estradiol is such that even small increases in the levels of the hormone induce a decrease in gonadotropins. Levels of LH and FSH during the follicular phase vary in accord with the changes in estradiol concentrations that accompany maturation of the follicle. Thus, as circulating estradiol levels increase during the follicular phase, gonadotropin concentrations decrease. In postmenopausal women or women who have undergone ovariectomy or have aromatase enzyme deficiency, all of whom lack estradiol secretion, sustained increases in LH and FSH release occur because of the absence of an active negative feedback loop. In these conditions, administration of physiologic doses of estradiol results in a rapid and sustained decrease in LH and FSH to levels equivalent to those seen during the menstrual cycle. The estradiol negative feedback loop acts to decrease LH secretion rapidly, mainly by controlling the *amplitude* of each LH pulse. Most evidence suggests that this action is secondary to inhibitory effects on the GnRH pulse, most probably relayed by estrogen-receptive kisspeptin and possibly GABA neurons. Effects on the pituitary gonadotrope, whereby estradiol decreases the gonadotropin response to GnRH, may also take place.

**Progesterone**, at high concentrations such as those observed during the luteal phase of the cycle, also exerts an inhibitory effect on gonadotropin secretion. In contrast to estradiol, progesterone affects mainly the GnRH pulse generator by slowing the frequency of pulses. This effect is responsible for the significant decrease in LH pulse frequency observed during the luteal phase of the cycle, when high levels of progesterone are present, and which becomes more pronounced as the luteal phase progresses (discussed later).

There is good evidence that the slowing action of progesterone on GnRH-LH pulse frequency is mediated by central $\beta$-endorphin. Indeed, brain levels of this opioid peptide, as measured in hypophyseal portal blood in the nonhuman primate, are elevated during the luteal phase (Fig. 4.17, *A*). Furthermore, administration of naloxone (an opiate antagonist) in women during the luteal phase results in a significant acceleration in pulse frequency (Fig. 4.17, *B*).

In view of these estradiol and progesterone inhibitory feedback loops, it is not surprising that the characteristics of pulsatile LH secretion vary greatly with the stage of the menstrual cycle. During the estrogenic stage or follicular phase, pulses of high frequency but low amplitude are seen, whereas during the progesterone stage or luteal phase, there is a progressive reduction in the frequency of the LH pulse, with pulse intervals reaching 200 minutes or more by the end of the luteal phase. This decreased pulse frequency is accompanied by a significant increase in pulse amplitude.

## The Positive Estradiol Feedback Loop

At higher physiologic concentrations, estradiol can also exert a separate stimulatory effect (positive feedback loop) on gonadotropin secretion. This positive feedback is dependent on rapidly rising estradiol levels, in combination with a small but significant progesterone rise, both produced by the mature dominant follicle and responsible for the generation of the preovulatory LH and FSH surge. The positive feedback loop is observed in many species: It serves as the critical signal to the hypothalamic-pituitary axis that the dominant follicle is ready to ovulate. In most species, a GnRH surge precedes the LH surge, suggesting that the positive feedback loop acts centrally. However, there is also ample evidence that high levels of estradiol can increase GnRH pituitary receptors and augment the

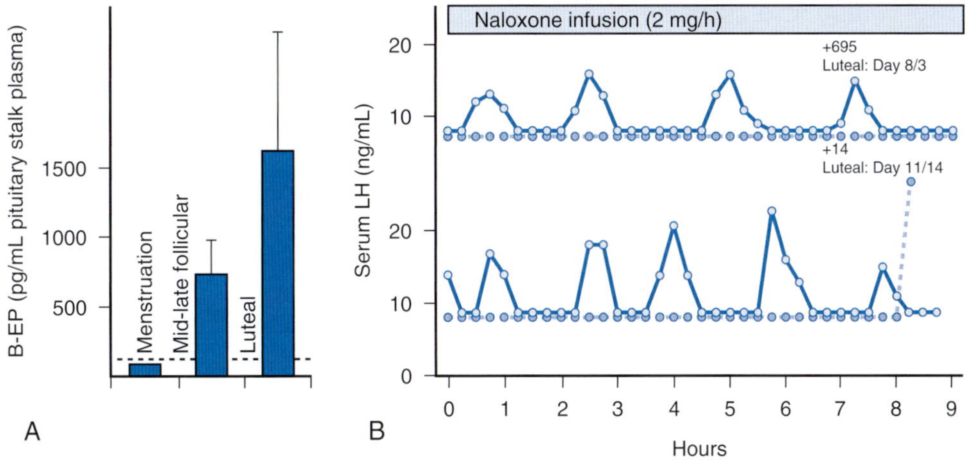


**Fig. 4.17** The endogenous opiates and the menstrual cycle. **A,** Changes in hypothalamic β-endorphin activity (as determined by its secretion into the pituitary stalk portal vasculature) during the menstrual cycle in the nonhuman primate. In the presence of low ovarian steroids, such as at menstruation, endorphin levels are lowest. They are highest in the presence of progesterone during the luteal phase. **B,** Role of β-endorphin in modulating the negative feedback action of progesterone during the luteal phase; note the dramatic increase in LH pulse frequency after endogenous opiate antagonism by naloxone *(closed circles)* compared with controls receiving saline *(open circles)*. *B-EP,* β-Endorphin; *LH,* luteinizing hormone. (**A,** Van Vugt DA, Lam NY, Ferin M. Reduced frequency of pulsatile luteinizing hormone secretion in the luteal phase of the rhesus monkey: involvement of endogenous opiates. *Endocrinology.* 1984;115:1095. **B,** Ferin M, Van Vugt D, Wardlaw S. The hypothalamic control of the menstrual cycle and the role of endogenous opioid peptides. *Rec Prog Horm Res.* 1984;40:441.)

pituitary response to GnRH, suggesting effects at the pituitary site as well.

Experimentally, late follicular phase estradiol levels infused during the early follicular phase are able to activate the positive feedback loop and release an LH surge, however inappropriate and untimely, because no mature follicle is present at the time (Fig. 4.18).

### Ovarian Peptides Feedback Loops

In addition to the negative steroid feedback loop, there is also evidence that nonsteroid ovarian factors exert negative feedback effects on the anterior pituitary. Such are the **inhibins,** which are a family of glycoproteins that consist of a dimer with two dissimilar α and β subunits (Stenvers, 2010). The two subunits are coded by different genes. **Two forms of the *β* subunit have been identified, and thus inhibin can exist as *α-β*A (inhibin A) and as *α-β*B** (inhibin B) (Fig. 4.19), both of which are detected in serum in women during the reproductive years. The ovaries are the only source of circulating dimeric inhibins.

The inhibins are characterized by their preferential inhibition of FSH over LH through their own negative feedback loop (see Fig. 4.16). This negative feedback loop, however, functions at a significantly slower rate (hours) than that of the steroid negative feedback loop (which is activated within minutes) and is directed mainly at the pituitary gland. It is believed that the decline in FSH after its peak in the early follicular phase of the normal cycle results from a negative feedback action of inhibin B at the pituitary level. At menopause or in premature ovarian failure, data show a decreased secretion of inhibin with reproductive aging, suggesting that inhibin B negative feedback may be an important factor controlling the early monotropic increase in FSH with aging (reflecting the decreasing number of small antral follicles recruited in each cycle and the consequent insufficient inhibin B production).

The circulating patterns of inhibin A and B during the menstrual cycle are different: Plasma concentrations of inhibin B rise rapidly on the day after the intercycle FSH rise (discussed later), remain elevated for a few days, then fall progressively during the remainder of the follicular phase. After a short-lived peak after the ovulatory gonadotropin surge, inhibin B falls to a low concentration during the luteal phase. In contrast, inhibin A concentrations rise only in the later part of the follicular phase and are maximal during the midluteal phase (Fig. 4.20). These different patterns of circulating inhibin B and inhibin A during the human menstrual cycle suggest different physiologic roles (discussed later).

Other dimers of the *β* subunit have also been described, such as activin A (A-*β*/ A-*β*), which in contrast to the inhibins stimulate FSH release from the pituitary (see Fig. 4.19). This effect is probably not very significant because of the irreversible binding of activin to follistatin, which neutralizes activin's bioactivity.

## THE MENSTRUAL CYCLE

The menstrual or ovulatory cycle involves a remarkable coordination of morphologic changes and hormonal secretion occurring not only at several levels of the HPO axis but also in organs outside of this main axis, such as the uterus and the cervix, and expressed in an orderly sequence of events (Ferin, 1996). The initial stimulus from the brain under the form of GnRH pulses is crucial to proper gonadotropin responses, which in turn instigate folliculogenesis, ovulation, and the formation of the corpus luteum. Essential to the coordination of these events is the communication between the ovaries and the hypothalamic-pituitary unit through the hormonal feedbacks, which provide continuous information of the ovarian status to the brain, which in turns responds with the proper pattern of GnRH pulses and of gonadotropin release. Humans are spontaneous ovulators (as opposed to light or seasonally related) in that the gonadotropin surge, the

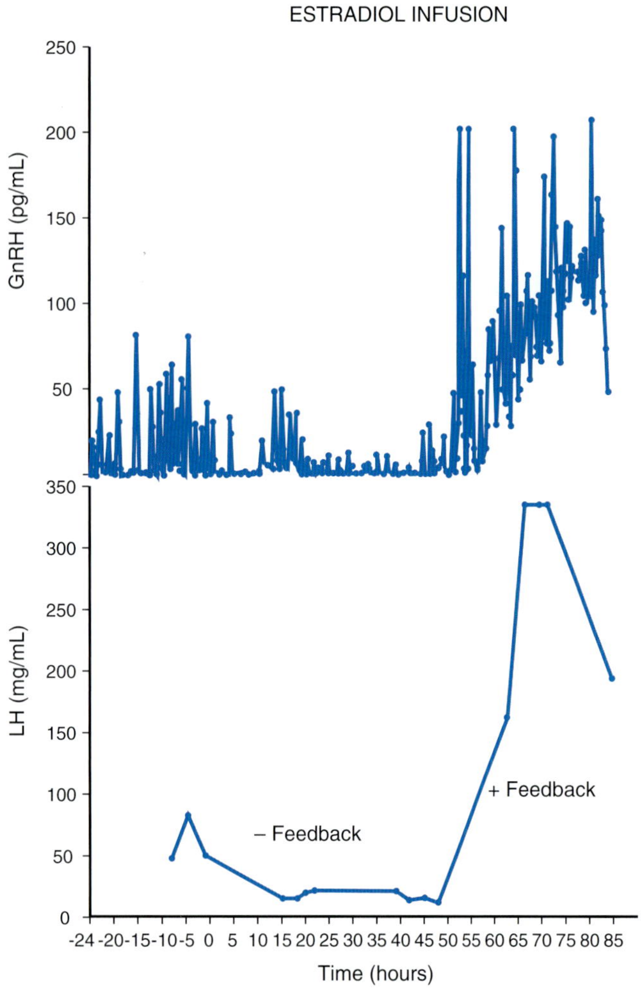


**Fig. 4.18** GnRH and LH responses to a 3.5-hour estradiol infusion mimicking late follicular phase estradiol levels. After a period of suppression (caused by the rapid estradiol negative feedback), note the large increase in both GnRH and LH (caused by the positive estradiol feedback). *GnRH,* gonadotropin-releasing hormone; *LH,* luteinizing hormone. (From Xia L, van Vugt D, Alston EJ, Luckhaus J, Ferin M. A surge of gonadotropin-releasing hormone accompanies the estradiol-induced gonadotropin surge in the rhesus monkey. *Endocrinology.* 1992;131:2812-2820.)

initiator of ovulation, is triggered by the endogenous changes in estradiol that accompany the maturation of the follicle.

This sequence of events is such that the reproductive process in the human occurs in a cyclic process at about monthly intervals. The primate menstrual cycle is divided into two phases: the follicular phase, followed by the luteal phase. These are separated by the ovulatory period. Mean duration of the menstrual cycle is 28 ± 7 days. **The length of the follicular phase is more variable, whereas the life span of the corpus luteum is about 14 days.** In many women older than 40, the **length of the follicular phase decreases from about 14 days to about 10 days.** However, menstrual cycle length also varies in an individual woman: It is most variable in the 2 years after menarche and preceding menopause, times of life during which anovulatory cycles are most frequent. The mean age of menarche (the first menstruation) occurs around age 12, and menopause (the end of the reproductive phase) usually occurs between ages 45 to 55. Endocrine changes during the menstrual cycle are illustrated in Fig. 4.20.

## The follicular phase

The follicular phase can be subdivided into three periods; these denote the successive recruitment of a cohort of antral follicles, the selection of a dominant follicle, and the growth of the selected dominant follicle.

### Recruitment of a Cohort of Antral Follicles

When cohorts of growing follicles reach the early antral stage (Fig. 4.21; see also Fig. 4.8), continuing growth requires a proper gonadotropin stimulatory action. **FSH** provides the critical signal for the recruitment of a **cohort** of preantral follicles. This FSH signal (cyclic recruitment) is the major survival factor that rescues the follicles from their programmed death (atresia) and allows them to start growing, increasing in size and beginning to synthesize steroids. In fact, the start of each follicular phase is characterized by a small but significant increase in the FSH/LH ratio (see Fig. 4.20), resulting in the recruitment of a cohort consisting of about three to seven secondary preantral follicles. (Only preantral follicles are able to respond to the FSH signal; follicles at an earlier stage of development lack an independent vascular system, so the signal does not reach them.)

*Ovarian reserve* is a term that is used to denote the number of antral follicles in the ovaries and therefore to determine the capacity of the ovary to provide oocytes that are capable of being fertilized. **The determination of the ovarian reserve is an important tool in the treatment of infertility.** It is primarily assessed by the following means: (1) measurement of **FSH** on day 2 to 3 of the cycle; higher FSH levels denote ovarian aging (resulting from a decreased activity of the estradiol negative feedback loop) and hence fewer recruitable follicles; (2) sonographic **antral follicle count**; (3) measurement of **inhibin B** on day 2 to 3 of the cycle, the recruitment of the follicle cohort being reflected by an increase in this hormone produced and secreted by these recruited follicles; thus inhibin B levels provide an early indicator of the number of recruited follicles and of their secretory activity (see Fig. 4.21); and (4) measurement of **anti-müllerian hormone (AMH)** (also called müllerian inhibiting substance [MIS]). AMH belongs to the transforming growth factor-β superfamily. It is a secretory product of granulosa cells in preantral and in small antral follicles. Together with other factors, AMH appears to inhibit the initiation of premature follicle growth. Data have indicated that in the treatment of infertility, **the measurement of AMH in conjunction with sonography offers a more useful assessment of ovarian reserve and a better correlation with the number of oocytes retrieved than that provided by FSH measurement.** Unlike FSH, AMH may be measured at any time of the menstrual cycle, with minimal variation, and AMH levels do not vary considerably between cycles. Serum AMH levels decline with age, in parallel with the reduced follicle pool, and become undetectable during the 3 to 5 years before the onset of menopause. It remains unclear whether low AMH levels are predictive of lower spontaneous fertility and whether AMH can be used to predict age of menopause onset. AMH is increasingly used in clinical practice to identify women with premature ovarian insufficiency or polycystic ovary syndrome; very high levels of AMH may reflect polycystic ovary syndrome (La Marca, 2009). Studies show significantly lower age-specific AMH levels in women currently using oral contraceptives, with an increase in AMH levels after discontinuation of oral contraceptives (Dolleman, 2013; van den Berg, 2010).

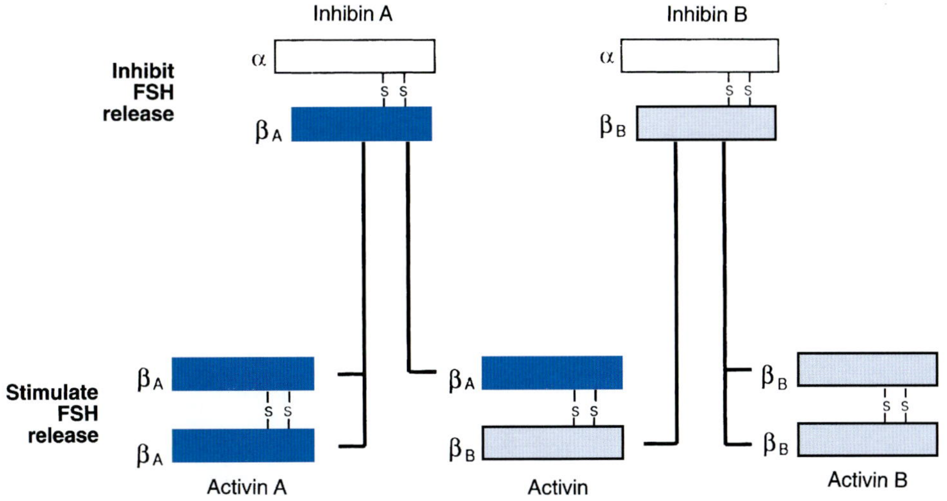


**Fig. 4.19** Chemical relationships of inhibins and activins. *FSH,* Follicle-stimulating hormone; *S,* disulfide bond. (From Hylka VW, Di Zerega GS. Reproductive hormones and their mechanisms of action. In Mishell DR, Davajan V, Lobo RA, eds. *Infertility, Contraception and Reproductive Endocrinology.* 3rd ed. Cambridge, MA: Blackwell Scientific; 1991.)

## Selection of a Dominant Follicle

Although several primary preantral follicles are recruited at the start of each cycle as part of a cohort, **in the primate usually only one (the dominant follicle) is selected to complete growth to maturity** (see Fig. 4.21), and the other follicles in the cohort become atretic. Although the process of selection is not well understood, it most probably reflects the competitive advantage of the dominant follicle, characterized by a well-vascularized theca layer allowing a better access of the gonadotropins to their target receptors. This results in a greater local estradiol secretion, which in turn increases the density of gonadotropin receptors and promotes cell multiplication.

At the same time, elevation of peripheral estradiol levels activates the negative estradiol feedback loop and results in a decrease in circulating FSH to a concentration insufficient to sustain growth in the other follicles of the cohort. Experimentally in the nonhuman primate, this process can be overridden by injecting antibodies to estradiol; this prevents the estradiol negative feedback loop from decreasing FSH secretion and results in the maturation of several follicles at the same time. In addition to estradiol, granulosa cells of the recruited follicles also secrete inhibin B (discussed earlier), the action of which selectively suppresses FSH secretion, further decreasing the stimulus to maturation. The dominant follicle, however, continues to grow because of its greater density of FSH receptors and greater vascularization of its theca cell layer, allowing more FSH to reach its receptors.

**The process of selection is completed by day 5 of the follicular phase.** At this point, if the dominant follicle is experimentally destroyed, no surrogate follicle is available to replace it during that cycle.

## Growth of the Dominant Follicle: The Maturing Secondary or Antral Follicle

GnRH pulse frequency at this time of the follicular phase is at its maximum, at about 1 GnRH pulse/90 minutes (Fig. 4.22). This is the optimal pulse frequency to activate the proper gonadotropin response to increase steroid biosynthesis and the production of estradiol within the ovary. The main role of the gonadotropins and of locally produced estradiol is to continue to stimulate growth of the dominant follicle during the remainder of the follicular phase.

Production of estradiol requires successive events within different locations in the growing follicle (Fig. 4.23). **FSH receptors** are located within the avascular **granulosa** cell layer of the antral follicle. Stimulation by FSH of its receptors activates production of the enzyme **aromatase** (responsible for the biosynthesis of estrogens) within these cells. An important change in the structure of maturing follicles is the acquisition of the **theca** cell layer, which surrounds the granulosa layer and rapidly differentiates into the theca interna and the theca externa. The theca layer rapidly becomes well vascularized (in contrast to the granulosa layer, which remains avascular) through an active angiogenesis process, characterized by the presence of several vascular growth-promoting proteins such as vascular endothelial growth factor (VEGF), which stimulates growth of new blood vessels. This allows access of blood, and the hormones and nutrients it carries, to reach the follicle and to diffuse through to the granulosa layer. Circulating FSH now stimulates **LH receptor** synthesis within stromal cells of the **theca interna**. LH, in turn, promotes steroid biosynthesis by theca cells and the production of **androgens**. These androgens, after diffusion into the granulosa layer where the enzyme aromatase is located, are then biotransformed into **estradiol**. This leads to an overall increase in estradiol production, increased intraovarian estradiol levels, and increased estradiol secretion into the peripheral circulation, which parallels follicular parameter (Fig. 4.24).

Thus **the growing dominant follicle generates its own estradiol microenvironment**. Estradiol, being a mitogenic hormone, in turn directly promotes its exponential growth. (Testosterone, on the other hand, increases follicular atresia in the absence of adequate aromatase activity, which converts it to estradiol.) Indirectly, estradiol also promotes follicular growth through the activation of several regulatory protein and peptide hormones, such as inhibins, activin, folliculostatins, insulin-like growth factors (IGFs), and others. For instance, various IGFs have been shown to stimulate granulosa cell proliferation and

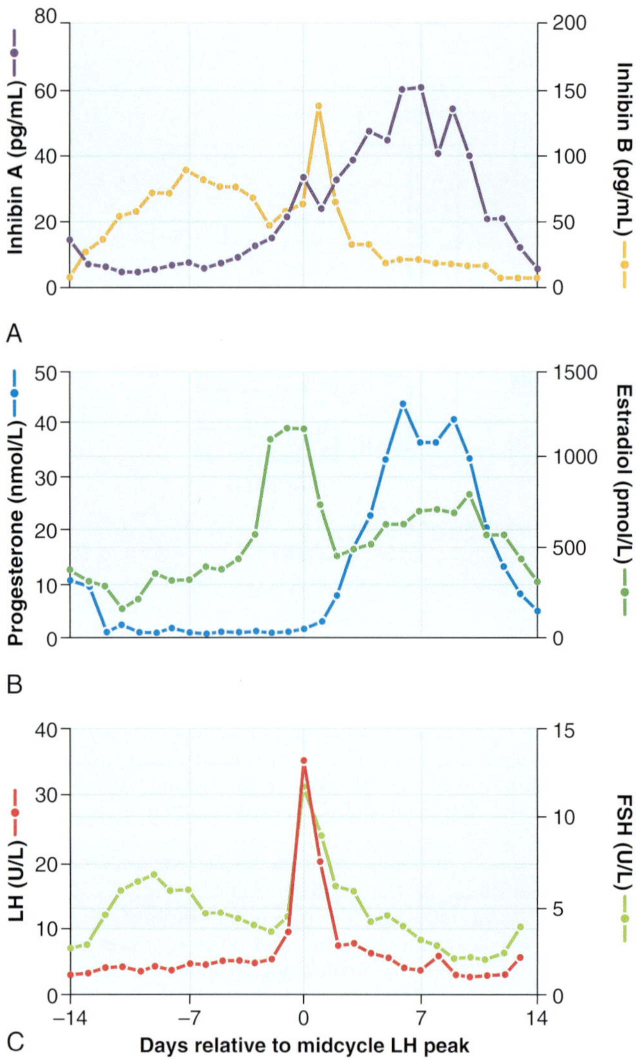


**Fig. 4.20** Mean plasma concentrations of inhibin A and inhibin B *(upper panel)* compared with estradiol and progesterone *(center panel)*, and LH and FSH *(lower panel)* during the menstrual cycle. Day 0 is the day of the LH surge. *FSH,* Follicle-stimulating hormone; *LH,* luteinizing hormone. (From Groome NP, Illingworth PJ, O'Brien M, et al. Measurement of dimeric inhibin B throughout the human menstrual cycle. *J Clin Endocrinol Metab.* 1996;81:1401-1405.)

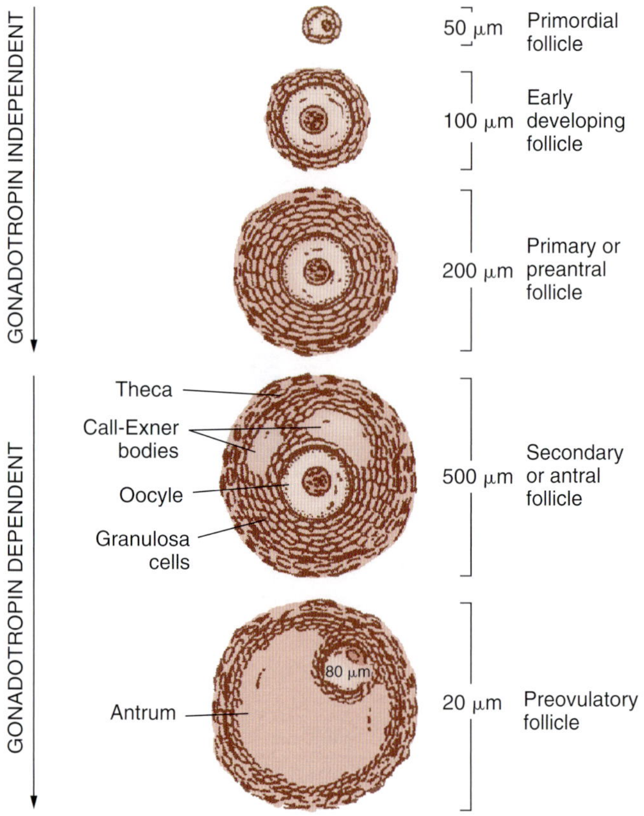


**Fig. 4.21** Follicle development. Note that progress beyond the primary or preantral follicle stage depends on follicle-stimulating hormone stimulation. (From Paulson RJ. Oocytes: from development to fertilization. In Mishell DR, Davajan V, Lobo RA, eds. ***Infertility, Contraception and Reproductive Endocrinology.*** 3rd ed. Cambridge, MA: Blackwell Scientific; 1991.)

aromatase activity. However, most actions of these factors remain to be elucidated in the primate. By the time the follicle reaches the preovulatory stage, the number of granulosa cells has increased from about 50 at the primordial stage to $5 \times 10^7$. This is accompanied by an exponential increase in peripheral estradiol levels (see Fig. 4.23).

As the dominant follicle grows, an **antrum** (cavity) forms into which follicular fluid accumulates. This fluid contains several steroids, peptide and protein hormones, and nutrients. The growth pattern of the dominant follicle can be documented by ultrasonography, which is well correlated with the endocrine pattern; indeed, increases in both follicle diameter and volume parallel the increase in estradiol levels in blood. At maturation, the dominant follicle reaches a mean diameter range of 18 to 25 mm.

Within the dominant follicle, the oocyte also develops and becomes surrounded by the **zona pellucida**. This is a mucopolysaccharide coat containing specific protein sites that later will allow only spermatozoa to penetrate and fertilize the ovum. Underneath the zona pellucida is the **vitelline membrane** that surrounds the ooplasm. At the end of the follicular phase, the antral follicle contains an oocyte that is fully grown but is unable to undergo normal activation if retrieved and fertilized in vitro. Activation will have to await the ovulatory LH surge.

## The Ovulatory Gonadotropin Surge and Ovulation

Maturation of the dominant follicle is marked by high blood levels of estradiol. When a threshold is reached, estradiol activates the positive feedback loop, thereby signaling to the hypothalamus and anterior pituitary gland that the follicle is ready for ovulation and that a large gonadotropin surge is to be released (see Fig. 4.18). (A small but significant increase in progesterone is also secreted by the follicle before the LH surge; because administration of a progesterone receptor antagonist delays the timing of the surge, it is thought that these low levels of progesterone help synchronize the surge.)

In the nonhuman primate, the gonadotropin surge has been shown to be preceded by a surge of GnRH, as measured centrally, suggesting a major hypothalamic site for the positive feedback loop. For reasons unknown, this **GnRH surge** significantly outlasts the LH surge. Because GnRH cannot be measured in the human in peripheral blood, the relative importance of the sites of action of estradiol during the spontaneous surge remains to be established. (Studies in GnRH-deficient women receiving

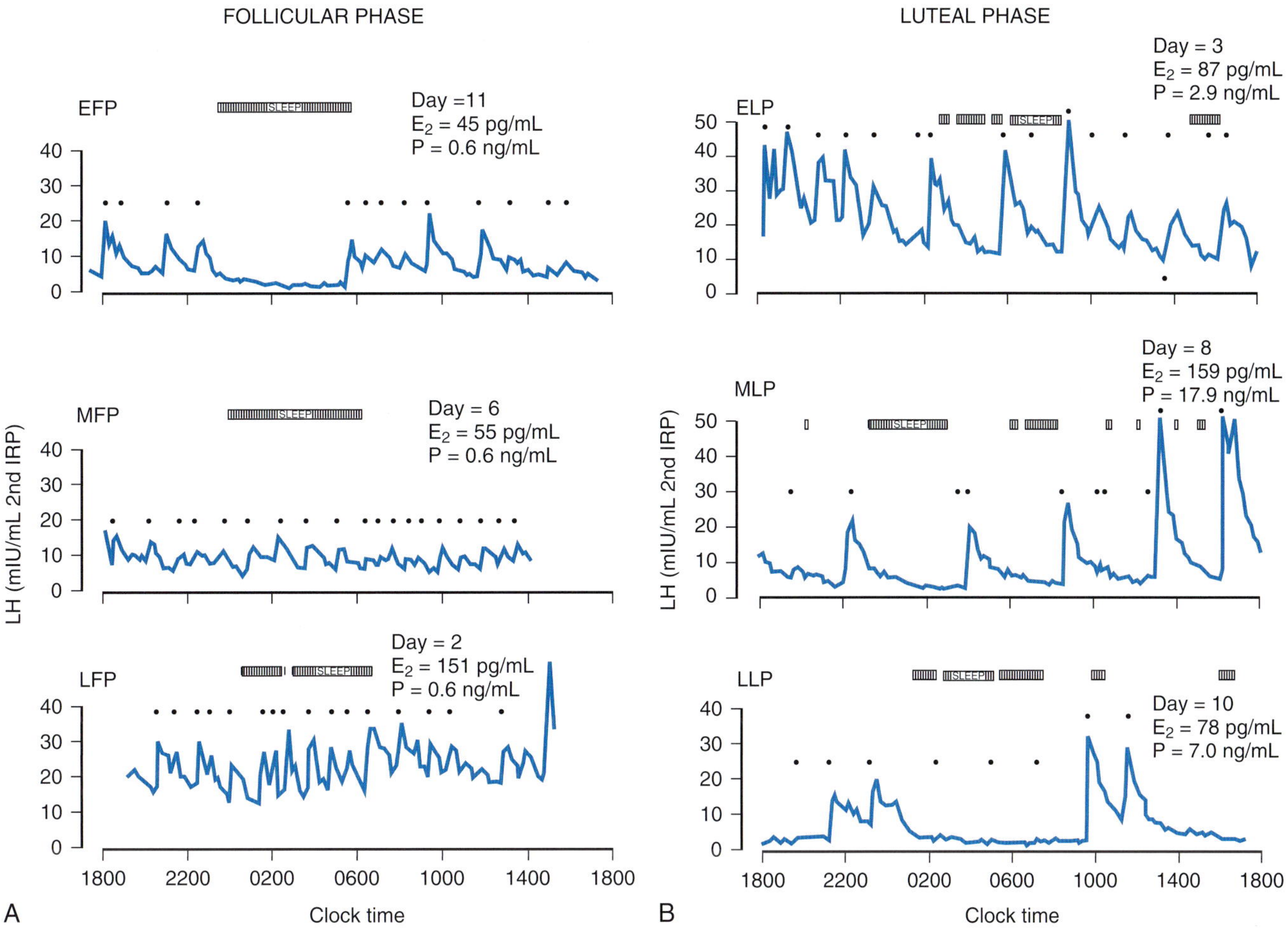


**Fig. 4.22** Contrasting patterns of pulsatile LH secretion throughout the follicular phase *(left panel)* and luteal phase *(right panel)* of the menstrual cycle. Representative examples of early *(EFP),* mid *(MFP),* and late *(LFP)* follicular phases are shown. LH pulses are indicated by *asterisks*. (Note that in about 20% of volunteers, there is a suppression of pulsatility during deep sleep in EFP. This does not appear to interfere with the normal cycle.) *$E_2$*, estradiol; *LH,* luteinizing hormone; *P,* progesterone. (From Filicori M, Santoro N, Merriam GR, et al. Characterization of the physiological pattern of episodic gonadotropin secretion throughout the menstrual cycle. *J Clin Endicrinol Metab.* 1986;62:1136.)

exogenous GnRH replacement in an unchanging 60-minute pulse frequency provide evidence for the relevance of pituitary sensitization to GnRH in the presence of high estradiol, as abrupt LH increases can be observed under this experimental protocol.)

During the ovulatory surge, LH levels increase 10-fold over a period of 2 to 3 days, whereas FSH levels increase about 4-fold. This gonadotropin surge is an absolute requirement for the final maturation of the oocyte and the initiation of the follicular rupture.

The LH surge initiates germinal vesicle (or nucleus) disruption, and the fully grown oocyte resumes meiosis (**meiotic maturation**). Thus it progresses from the diplotene stage of the first meiosis (which was initiated during fetal life; discussed earlier) to metaphase II of the second meiotic division. As the oocyte enters metaphase II, the first polar body appears. (Three haploid polar bodies are produced during the two-step meiosis process, at ovulation and fertilization.) To conserve nutrients, most of the cytoplasm is concentrated into the oocyte or egg. The polar bodies generated from the meiotic events contain relatively little cytoplasm, and the oocyte eventually discards them. At ovulation, meiosis is arrested again (the **second meiotic arrest**). The second meiotic division will only be completed at the time of fertilization. The oocyte's ability to be fertilized coincides with the completion of meiotic maturation and the associated increased secretion of specific proteins such as the $IP_3$ receptor, glutathione and calmodulin-dependent protein kinase II, and others.

Ovulation (follicle rupture) occurs about 32 hours after the initial rise of the LH surge and about 16 hours after its peak (Table 4.1). Ultrasonographic pictures of ovaries with antral follicles, a preovulatory follicle, and a hemorrhagic corpus luteum are shown in Fig. 4.25. The LH surge induces a cascade of molecular events and changes in the mature follicle that are associated with ovulation. Studies of these have been complex, with the result that the precise mechanisms underlying ovulation remain to be completely understood. It is postulated that the LH surge induces an acute inflammatory-like reaction; inflammatory cytokines, such as interleukins, and countless genes are also upregulated. An increase cyclooxygenase catalyzes the conversion of arachidonic acid into several prostanoids, which include the prostaglandins that are produced intracellularly. Prostaglandins then

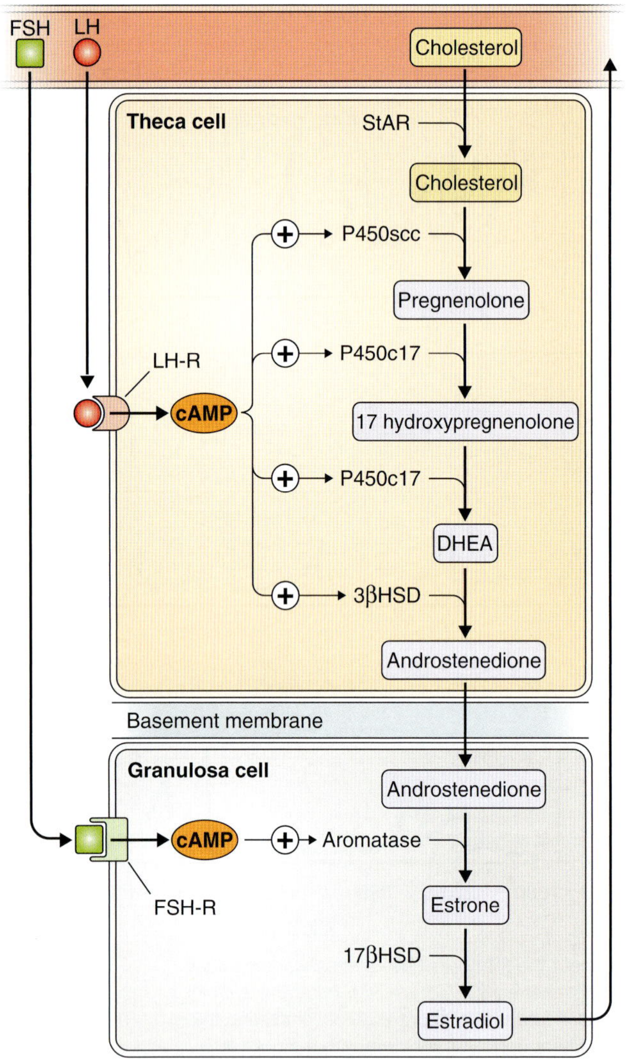


**Fig. 4.23** Production of estradiol within the growing dominant follicle requires successive events within different locations (see text). **FSH receptors** are located within the avascular **granulosa** cell layer, whereas synthesis of **LH receptors**, stimulated by FSH, occurs within stromal cells of the **theca interna.** The enzyme **aromatase** (responsible for the biosynthesis of estrogens) stimulated by FSH originates within the granulosa cells. LH, in turn, promotes steroid biosynthesis by theca cells and the production of **androgens**. These androgens, after diffusion into the granulosa layer where the enzyme aromatase is located, are then biotransformed into **estradiol**. *A,* androgen; *ATP,* adenosine triphosphate; *cAMP,* cyclic adenosine monophosphate, which mediates the action of each gonadotropin; *DHEA,* dehydroepiandrosterone; *FSH,* follicle-stimulating hormone; *R,* receptor.

act locally—for instance, to induce the hyperemia and edema seen in the first hours of the process of ovulation and that result from increased blood flow and vascular permeability. Intense protease activity is generated in the follicle. The resultant proteolytic cascade, which among others involves collagenases and plasminogen activator (which converts plasminogen into the proteolytic enzyme plasmin), leads to the degradation of the follicular layers and wall, which plays an essential role in follicle rupture. Plasmin helps in detaching the cumulus cell–enclosed oocyte from the granulosa cells, which initiates the process of extrusion of the oocyte and cumulus when the follicle ruptures. (It is worthwhile to point out that the LH surge paradoxically stimulates the expression of both proteolytic enzymes and their inhibitors. This allows for a tight regulation of proteolytic activity during both the follicle rupture process and the formation of the corpus luteum out of the remaining follicle.)

## The Luteal Phase

After the oocyte is extruded from the mature dominant follicle, the amount of follicular fluid is markedly reduced, the follicular wall becomes convoluted, and the follicular diameter and volume greatly decrease. As a result, a new ovarian structure evolves from the ovulated follicle, the **corpus luteum**.

The corpus luteum is the result of two important events initiated at ovulation. First, granulosa and theca cells hypertrophy, take up increasing amounts of lipids, and acquire organelles associated with steroidogenesis. Simultaneously, tissue-specific gene transcription results in the activation of new key steroidogenic enzymes; the hallmark of the human corpus luteum is its secretion primarily of **progesterone**. Although there is a significant drop in estradiol and androgen secretion at ovulation, 17-hydroxylase and aromatase are present in the corpus luteum, so that **it also secretes 17-hydroxyprogesterone and estradiol**. **Significant amounts of inhibin A are also produced.** Second, the basal lamina, which separated the granulosa and theca cell layers, is disrupted, and capillaries from the theca interna now invade the granulosa layer (which up to now had been avascular) to form an extensive capillary network. The result is that each steroidogenic cell within the corpus luteum is in close proximity to blood vessels.

Like the dominant follicle, growth and development of the corpus luteum occur rapidly. Vascular growth plays a central role in this process. Angiogenic factors, such as VEGF, are present in high quantity in the forming and developing corpus luteum. In nonhuman primates, experimental treatment that interferes with normal VEGF activity in the early and midluteal phase of the cycle suppresses vascular development and hence luteal growth; luteal function is compromised, as indicated by a marked fall in plasma progesterone levels.

### Endocrine Factors and the Corpus Luteum

Normal function of the corpus luteum depends primarily on LH stimulation throughout the luteal phase. This has been demonstrated in hypophysectomized women, in whom ovulation was induced by LH treatment. In these patients, continuing injections of small amounts of LH were essential to maintain the secretory viability of the corpus luteum. Other studies have shown that GnRH antagonist treatment (by interrupting LH secretion) readily disrupts luteal cell morphology and suppresses plasma progesterone levels.

Progesterone dominance in the luteal phase results in a significant activation of the **progesterone negative feedback loop** on the GnRH pulse generator, which acts to decrease GnRH pulse frequency. Thus during the luteal phase, there is progressive slowing down of LH pulse frequency, from 1 pulse/90 minute at the beginning of the luteal phase to 1 pulse/3 hours or even less toward the later luteal phase (see Fig. 4.22, *B*). This negative progesterone feedback effect is not directly exerted on the GnRH pulse generator as it is mediated by central **β-endorphin** (an endogenous opioid peptide). *β*-endorphin neurons are preferentially concentrated in the arcuate nucleus, in close proximity to GnRH neurons. Studies in the nonhuman primate have shown that *β*-endorphin release from the hypothalamus is significantly increased in the presence of progesterone, such as in the luteal phase, and lowest in its absence, such as after ovariectomy or at menstruation. Experimental administration of a competitive *β*-endorphin antagonist, such as naloxone, is particularly effective in accelerating LH pulse frequency when given in the luteal phase (see Fig. 4.17, *B*).

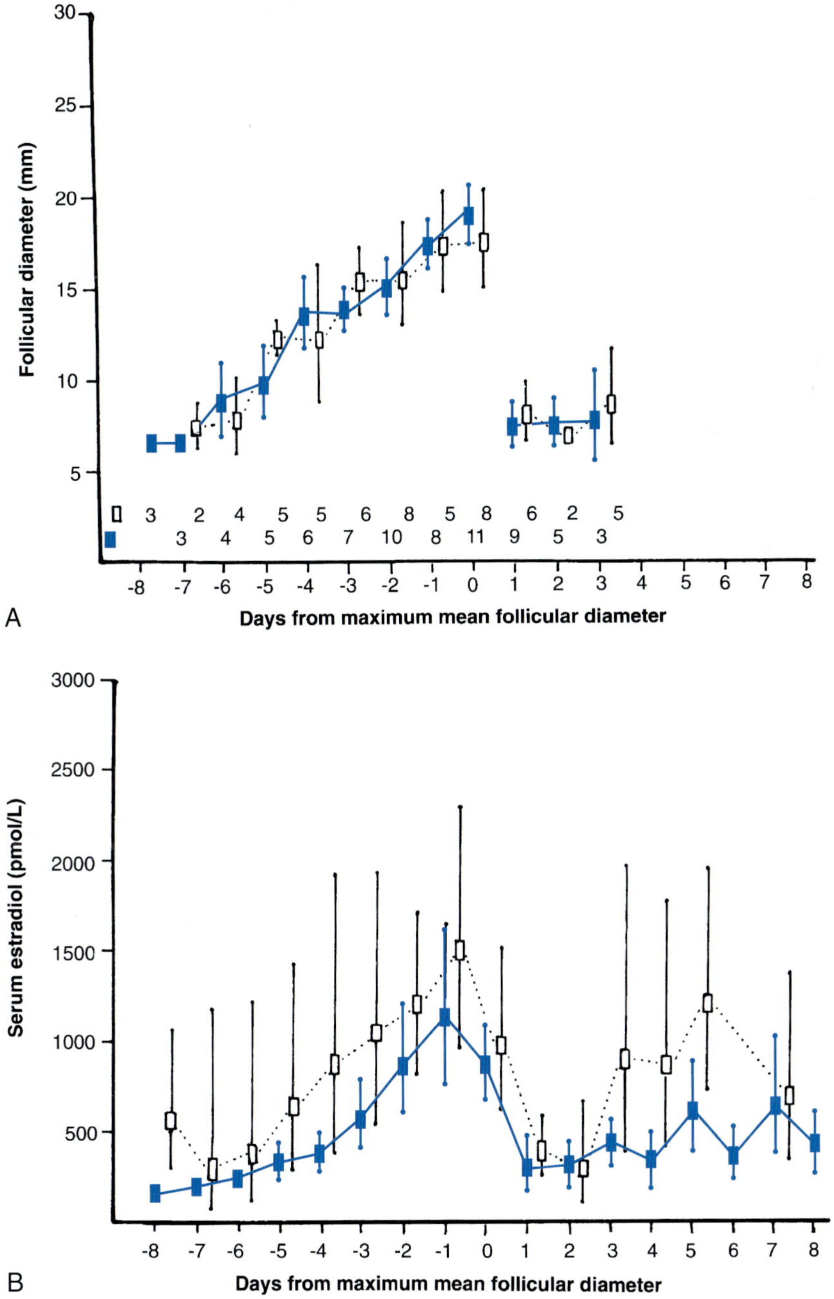


**Fig. 4.24** Correlation of follicular growth, as indicated by follicular diameter (**A**), with serum estradiol levels (**B**), in spontaneous *(black bars)* and induced conception *(blue bars)* cycles. (Adapted from Eissa MK, Obhrai MS, Docker MF, et al. Follicular growth and endocrine profiles in spontaneous and induced cycles. *Fertil Steril.* 1986;45:191.)

**TABLE 4.1** Range of Observed Times from Defined Hormonal Events and Time of Ovulation

| | Time of Ovulation (hr) from Rise to Peak | | | |
|---|---|---|---|---|
| | First Significant Rise | | Peak | |
| **Hormone** | **Median** | **Range** | **Median** | **Range** |
| 17$\beta$-Estradiol | 82.5 | 48-168 | 24.0 | 0-48 |
| LH | 32.0 | 24-56 | 16.5 | 0-48 |
| FSH | 21.1 | 8-24 | 15.3 | 8-40 |
| Progesterone | 7.8 | 0-32 | — | — |

From World Health Organization: Temporal relationships between ovulation and defined changes in the concentration of plasma estradiol-17 beta, luteinizing hormone, follicle-stimulating hormone, and progesterone. I. Probit analysis. World Health Organization, Task Force of Methods for the Determination of the Fertile Period, Special Programme of Research, Development and Research Training in Human Reproduction. *Am J Obstet Gynecol.* 1980;138:383-390.
*FSH,* Follicle-stimulating hormone; *LH,* luteinizing hormone.

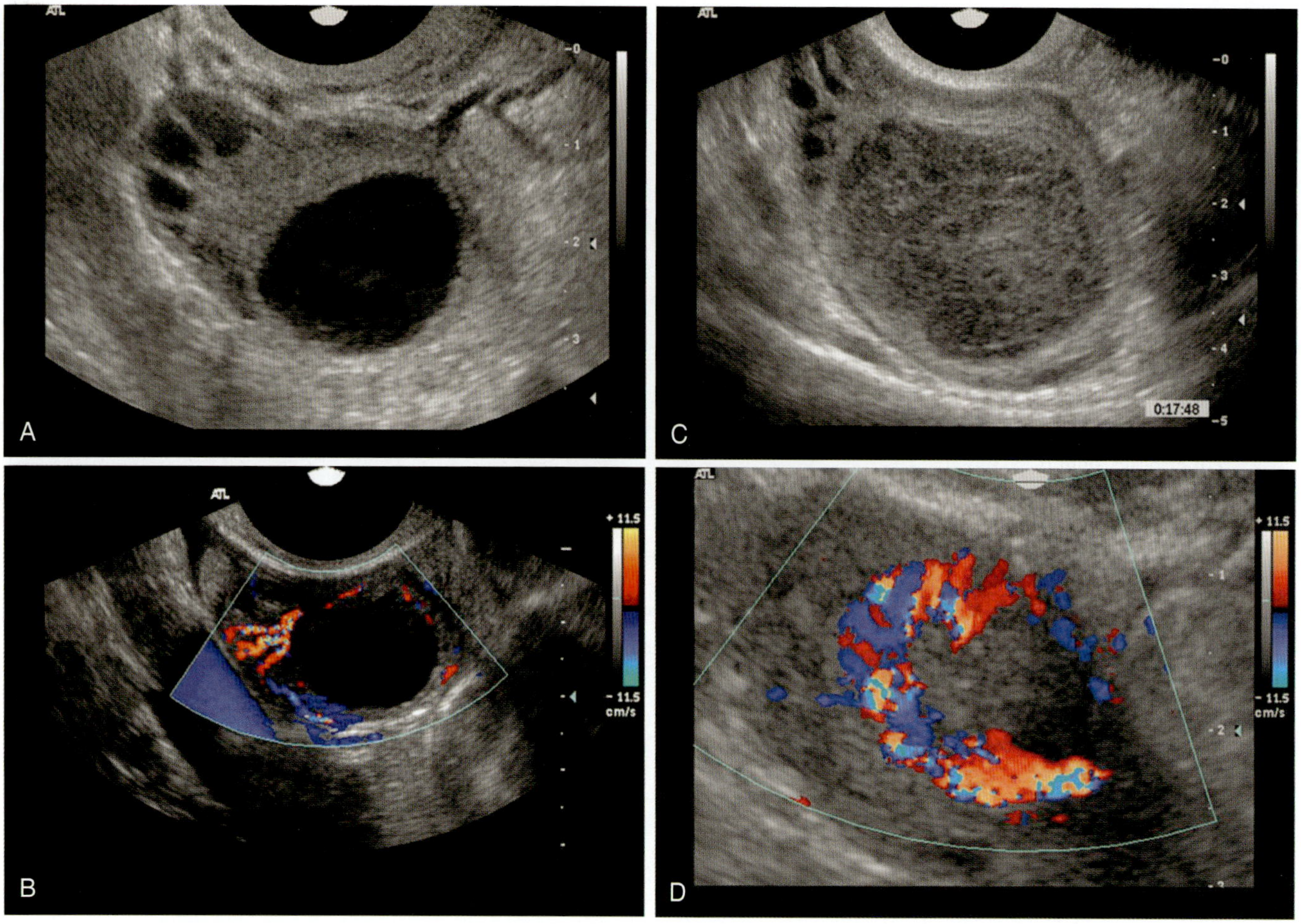


**Fig. 4.25** Ovary and corpus luteum during a natural menstrual cycle. **A,** On day 12 after menstruation, a dominant follicle is visualized in the central portion of the image and several subordinate follicles from the wave (2-5 mm) are observed in the left lateral aspect of the ovary. **B,** Color flow Doppler image demonstrating perifollicular vascularity around a preovulatory follicle. **C,** A blood-filled corpus luteum, called a corpus hemorrhagicum, demonstrating thick walls of peripheral luteal tissue and a central hemorrhagic clot with an interspersed fibrin network. **D,** Color flow Doppler image of a recently ovulated follicle/new luteal glands on the day of ovulation. (From Chizen D, Pierson R. Transvaginal ultrasonography and female infertility. *Glob Libr Womens Med.* 2010:10.3843/GLOWM.10326.)

Progesterone dominance during the luteal phase also affects the hypothalamic thermoregulatory center, such that a small increase in basal body temperature (BBT) reflects increased progesterone secretion during the luteal phase. Thus the typical BBT curve of the ovulatory menstrual cycle is biphasic (i.e., elevated during the duration of the luteal phase). **(This small temperature rise does not, however, reflect the quantity of progesterone increase in that it occurs when progesterone reaches the low threshold level of 2 to 3 ng/mL.)**

## Corpus Luteum Regression (Luteolysis)

In primates **the life span of the corpus luteum is limited to a period of about 14 days.** Histologically and biochemically, the corpus luteum reaches maturity 8 to 9 days after ovulation, after which time luteal cells start to degenerate and its secretory capability begins to decline (Stouffer, 1996). Thus after a progressive increase in progesterone, estradiol, and inhibin A levels in the first half of the luteal phase, the period after the midluteal peak is paralleled by a decline in these hormones. (Only rapidly rising concentrations of HCG [secreted by the syncytiotrophoblast] after conception can rescue the corpus luteum and maintain the production of progesterone.)

Structural luteolysis is a complex process responsible for the elimination of the corpus luteum, and little progress has been made in defining the factors responsible for luteolysis in the primate. Steroidogenic luteal cells undergo characteristic degenerative changes, with intense cytoplasmic vacuolization and invasion by macrophages. It has been postulated that regression of the corpus luteum may be related to an alteration in age-dependent luteal cell responsiveness to LH and is dictated by various luteotropic and luteolytic agents, the existence and dynamics of which remain to be investigated in the human. (Although uterine prostaglandin $F_2\alpha$ seems to be an important luteolytic signal in nonprimate species, the primate uterus is not the source of luteolytic agents because hysterectomy does not result in a prolonged luteal phase in humans.) Degradation of the luteal cells terminates in a perimenstrual apoptotic wave, and menstruation follows ovulation by 13 to 15 days, unless conception has occurred ("the missed menses").

## The Luteal-Follicular Transition

The end of the luteal phase is characterized by a dramatic decrease in progesterone, estradiol, and inhibin A. This is accompanied by a characteristic divergence in the FSH/LH ratio, now favoring a specific rise in FSH (see Fig. 4.20). The increase in the FSH/LH ratio heralds a new menstrual cycle and the recruitment of a new cohort of follicles.

The increase in the FSH/LH ratio most probably reflects the following interacting phenomena: (1) A rise in FSH may be the result of the rapid decline in estradiol accompanying the demise of the corpus luteum because FSH seems to be slightly more sensitive to the estradiol negative feedback loop than LH. (2) The end of the luteal phase is also characterized by a decline in inhibin A, a hormone that specifically suppresses FSH. (3) The rise in FSH also reflects the differential effects of GnRH pulse frequency on the synthesis of LH and FSH: The lower GnRH pulse frequency throughout the luteal phase favors FSH β-subunit synthesis over that of the LH β-subunit (discussed earlier), and thus a larger pituitary pool of FSH is available for release at the end of the luteal phase. The naturally occurring slowing of GnRH pulse frequency during the luteal phase is very relevant to a timely passage to a new cycle; indeed, imposed changes in the normal pulse frequency of this hypophysiotropic signal during the luteal phase results in significant disturbances in cyclicity.

The decrease in progesterone levels at the end of the cycle results in decreased activity in central β-endorphin, and consequently there is a resultant increase in GnRH pulse frequency. The return to a 1 pulse/90 minute frequency is essential to create the optimal conditions for the new menstrual cycle.

## THE MENSTRUAL CYCLE AND THE ENDOMETRIUM

Integration and synchronization between cyclic changes within the HPO axis and the endometrium is an essential prerequisite for viable reproduction. The primary goal is to ensure an appropriate environment for the implantation of the developing conceptus.

Human endometrium (the glandular part of the uterus) is made up of two major layers: (1) The stratum basale, which lies on top of the myometrium (the muscle part of the uterus), consists of primordial glands and densely cellular stroma, which change little during the menstrual cycle and do not desquamate at menstruation. (2) The stratum functionale, which lies between the basale and the lumen of the uterus, is composed of two layers. The superficial layer (stratum compactum) consists of the neck of the glands and densely populated stromal cells. The lower layer (stratum spongiosum) consists primarily of glands with less populated stroma and large amounts of interstitial tissue. Differences in structure in the two layers reflect different biologic functions; whereas the upper layer serves as the site of blastocyst implantation and provides the metabolic environment for it, the lower layer maintains the integrity of the mucosa. Changes in hormones during the menstrual cycle affect mainly the *stratum functionale.* A diagrammatic representation of endometrial changes during the menstrual cycle is presented in Fig. 4.26.

## The Endometrium in the Proliferative (Follicular) Phase

Immediately after menstruation, the endometrium is only 1 to 2 mm thick and consists mainly of the *stratum basale* and a few glands. As estradiol levels increase with the growth and maturation of the dominant follicle, the number of estradiol receptors in the endometrium increases and the *stratum functionale* proliferates greatly by multiplication of both glandular and stromal cells. Synthesis of DNA is increased, and mitoses are numerous. Toward the late follicular phase, the straight glands become progressively more voluminous and tortuous. At the time of onset of the LH surge and before ovulation, subnuclear vacuoles appear at the base of the cells lining the glands. This is the first indication of an effect by progesterone, reflecting the small but significant increase in progesterone seen at that time. Sonography during the follicular phase shows that endometrial thickness, including both anterior and posterior layers, increases from a

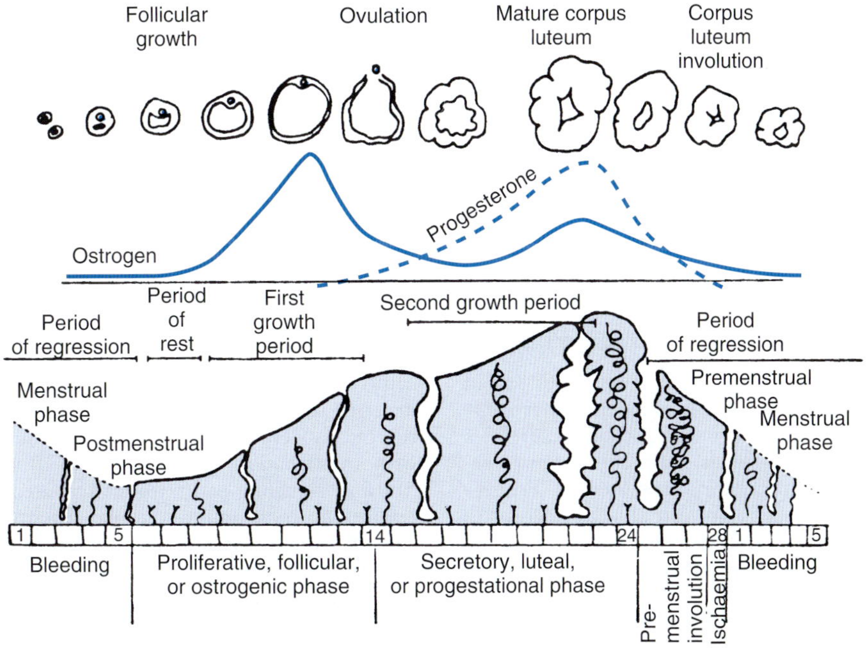


**Fig. 4.26** Diagram of changes in normal human ovarian and endometrial cycles. (From Shaw ST, Roche PC: Menstruation. In Finn CA, ed. *Oxford Review of Reproductive Endocrinology.* Vol. 2. London: Oxford University Press; 1980.)

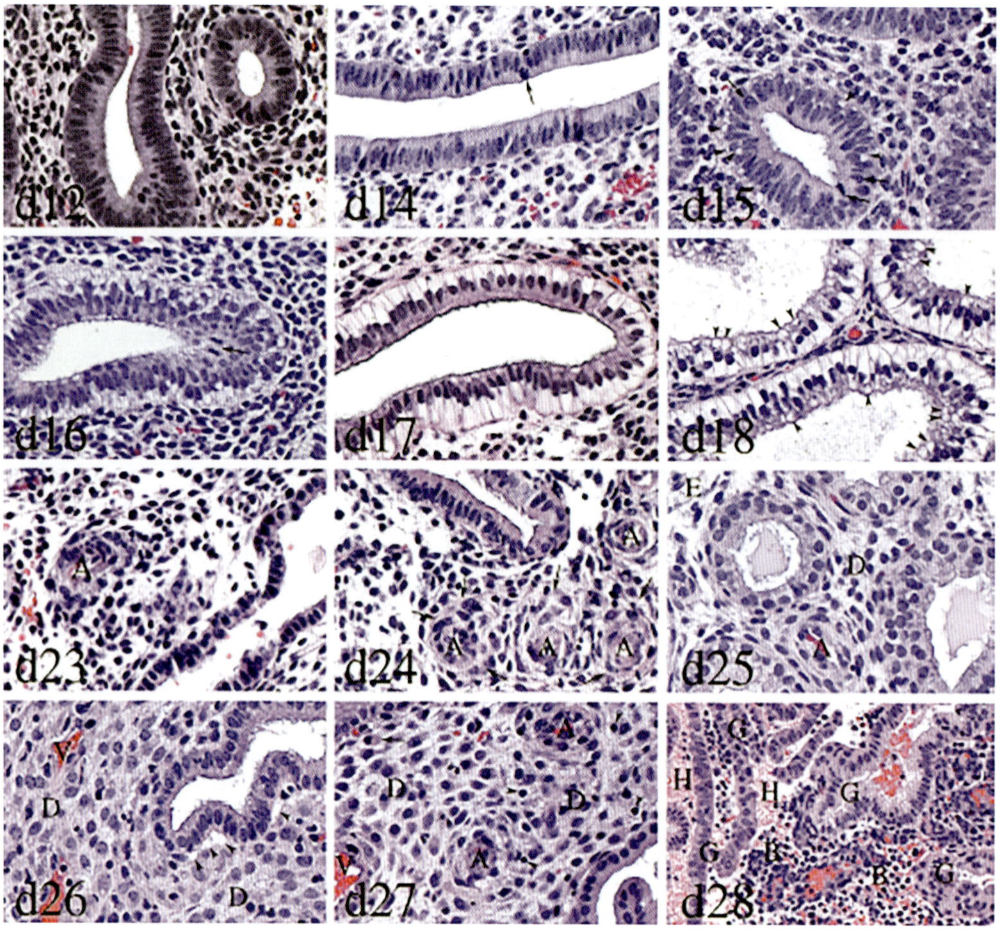


**Fig. 4.27** Histologic changes of the endometrium through an idealized 28-day menstrual cycle. *First row:* Cycle day *(d)* 12: Bent endometrial glands without evidence of secretions or mitotic figures. D14: On the day of ovulation, mitotic figures are noted and vacuoles are absent. D15: Mitotic figures are numerous and vacuoles are observed in more than 50% of the glands. *Second row:* D16: More than 50% of the glands exhibit vacuoles. D18: Vacuoles move to a luminal position and mitotic figures are rare. *Third row:* D23: Prominent spiral arterioles *(A)* are observed. D25: Edematous *(E)* and decidualized *(D)* stroma surround the spiral arterioles. *Fourth row:* D27: The stroma is completely decidualized, with interspersed spiral arterioles *(A)*, veins *(V)*, and lymphocytes. D28: The stroma has broken down *(B)*, with obvious areas of hemorrhage *(H)* and interspersed gland fragments *(G)*. (From Kliman H, Frankfurter D. Clinical approach to recurrent implantation failure: evidence-based evaluation of the endometrium. *Fertil Steril.* 2019;111:618-628.)

mean of about 4 mm in the early follicular phase to about 12 mm at the time of ovulation. Examples of structural changes of the endometrium during the menstrual cycle are shown in Fig. 4.27.

## The Endometrium in the Secretory (Luteal) Phase

After ovulation, the proliferative endometrium undergoes a rapid **secretory** differentiation: well-developed subnuclear glycogen-rich vacuoles appear in every cell of a given gland. This correlates with a total lack of mitoses in all glands. Both effects can be attributed to rising levels of postovulatory progesterone. Progesterone antagonizes the mitotic action of estradiol by decreasing estrogen receptors and by increasing the progesterone-specific enzyme 17 $\beta$-hydroxy dehydrogenase, which converts estradiol into the much less active estrone.

As progesterone levels increase during the first part of the luteal phase, the glycogen-containing vacuoles ascend progressively toward the gland lumen. Soon thereafter, the contents of the glands are released into the endometrial lumen. The peak of intraglandular content and its release into the lumen coincides well with the arrival of the free-floating blastocyst, which reaches the uterine cavity by about 3.5 days after fertilization. This release of glycogen-rich nutrients is crucial in that it provides energy to the energy-starved free-floating blastocyst.

Appropriately timed exposure to estrogen and progesterone alters gene transcription in the endometrium, resulting in a "receptive endometrium" that is prepared to engage in a molecular dialogue with the blastocyst. The window of implantation (WOI) is typically defined as days 20 to 24 of a 28-day menstrual cycle, with implantation occurring about 1 week after fertilization. Multiple signaling pathways are activated in the endometrium to ensure successful embryo implantation (Fig. 4.28) (Cha, 2012). Several proteins, including glycodelin, IGF binding protein 1 (IGFBP-1), homeobox A10, and leukemia inhibitory factor, are produced by secretory phase endometrium and may play integral roles in endometrial function (Douglas, 2013). Glycodelin is also known as PP14 or progestogen-associated endometrial protein. Although it has also been referred to as pregnancy-associated endometrial alpha-2-globulin, it is actually not a placental protein but rather a major secretory product of the glandular

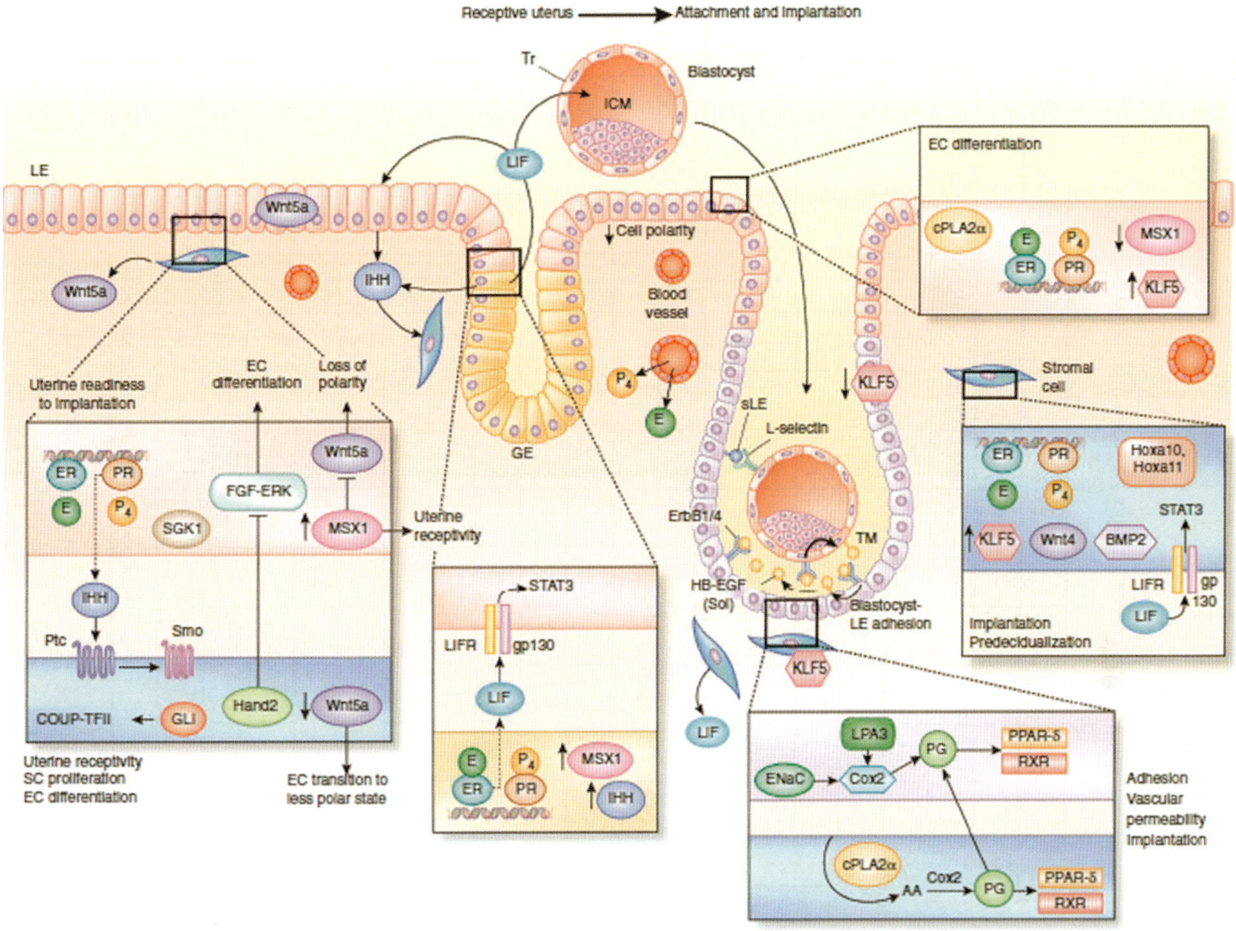


**Fig. 4.28** Signaling network for uterine receptivity and implantation. This is a hybrid cartoon based on mouse and human studies, portraying compartment- and cell type–specific expression of molecules and their potential functions necessary for uterine receptivity, implantation, and decidualization. *E,* estrogens; *EC,* epithelial cell (luminal and glandular epithelia); *ER,* estrogen receptor; *GLI,* glioblastoma; *HB-EGF,* heparin-binding epidermal growth factor-like growth factor; *ICM,* inner cell mass; *Tr,* trophectoderm; *P4,* progesterone; *PR,* progesterone receptor; *SC,* stromal cell. (From Cha J, Sun X, Dey SK. Mechanisms of implantation: strategies for successful pregnancy. *Nat Med.* 2012;18:1754.)

endometrial epithelium during the secretory phase. Circulating levels of glycodelin correlate well with serum progesterone levels. Glycodelin is a glycoprotein of which there are three distinct forms, with identical protein backbones but different glycosylation profiles. These glycoproteins appear to have essential roles in producing a uterine environment suitable for pregnancy and in the timing and occurrence of the appropriate sequence of events in the fertilization process.

After the first week of the luteal phase, changes in the stroma rather than in the glands become more important and relevant. The stroma becomes more edematous as a result of increased capillary permeability. Endothelial proliferation results in the coiling of capillaries and vessels, particularly in the upper functionale level producing vascular clusters. (These changes have been postulated to be mediated by PGF2α and PGE2, the production of which is stimulated by estradiol and progesterone.) These changes are essential in the steps that will lead to the predecidual transformation of stromal cells.

**Predecidual stromal cells** are precursor forms of gestational decidual cells. (These cells are not involved in the implantation process because they develop after implantation.) In the nongestational endometrium, predecidual cells are engaged in phagocytosis and digestion of extracellular collagen matrix. These cellular activities may contribute to the breakdown of the endometrium at menstruation. (Predecidual cells also have metabolic functions related to pregnancy; for example, they secrete prolactin, which is related to osmoregulation of amniotic fluid. These cells also play a supportive role to the endometrial mucosa and appear to control the invasive nature of the normal trophoblast. In their absence, the trophoblast may invade the myometrium leading to placenta accreta.) Decidualization succeeds predecidualization if pregnancy occurs.

Clinically the measurement of hormonal levels in parallel with the use of quantitative morphometric endometrial measurements produces a significant correlation with chronologic dating of the length of the luteal phase. Clinical dating of the endometrium, however, is somewhat subjective and is rarely carried out today. Sonography shows that endometrial thickness remains at the same level reached at ovulation (8 to 14 mm) throughout the luteal phase.

## Menstruation

If implantation of the blastocyst does not occur in the late luteal phase and HCG is not produced to maintain the corpus luteum, the endometrial glands begin to collapse and fragment.

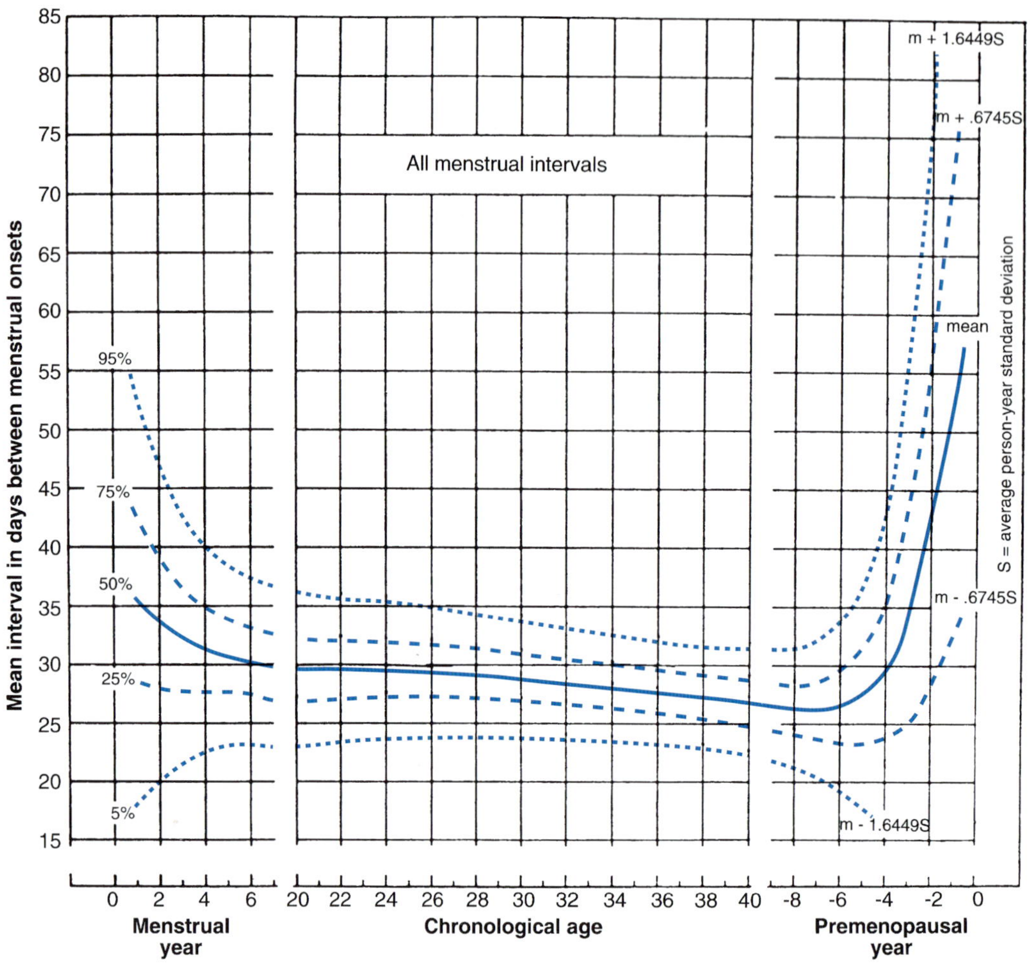


**Fig. 4.29** Normal curve contours for the distribution of menstrual intervals in three zones of menstrual life. (From Treloar AE, Boynton RE, Brown BW. Variation of the human menstrual cycle through reproductive life. *Int J Fert.* 1967;12:77.)

Subsequently, **polymorphonuclear leukocytes and monocytes infiltrate the glands and stroma, autolysis of the stratum functionale occurs, and desquamation begins.**

Data support the contention that cyclic elimination of the endometrium functional layer through menstrual bleeding results from intense tissue breakdown by proteolytic enzymes, mainly members of the matrix **metalloproteinase** (MMP) family, and that these enzymes are stimulated by the products of an inflammatory process. A number of MMPs, capable of degrading both interstitial matrix and basement membrane components, have been localized to perimenstrual endometrium, and the focal nature of their production suggests local regulation. There are probably important relationships between cells of the immune system (such as mast cells, eosinophils, neutrophils, and macrophages) and the local production and activation of MMPs.

The degrading actions by MMPs lead to the loss of integrity of blood vessels, destruction of endometrial interstitial matrix, and the resultant bleeding characteristic of menstruation. **Regular menstruation lasts for usually 3 to 5 days, but anywhere from 2 to 7 days is considered normal.** Menstrual intervals vary depending on age and time of initiation of the premenopause period (Fig. 4.29). **The average blood loss is 35 mL, with 10 to 80 mL considered within the normal range. A similar volume of nonhematogenous fluid is also shed during menstruation.** Many women also notice shedding of the endometrial lining, which appears as tissue mixed with the blood. (Sometimes this may be erroneously thought to indicate an early-term miscarriage of an embryo.) The enzyme plasmin tends to inhibit the blood from clotting. Because of the blood loss, premenopausal women have higher dietary requirements for iron to prevent iron deficiency.

## THE MENSTRUAL CYCLE AND THE CERVICAL GLANDS

The cervix plays a substantial role in fertility. Changes in the production and property of mucus secreted by the cervical glands are closely correlated to changes in estradiol and progesterone during the menstrual cycle. Enhanced production of cervical mucus and the presence of crypts within the endocervix serve to facilitate the transport and storage of spermatozoa around midcycle. Cervical mucus is produced in copious amounts in response to high estradiol levels at the end of the follicular phase. It has a clear, water-like appearance, which is acellular; takes the aspect of a "fern" when it dries as viewed under the microscope; and is "stringy," which is referred to as *spinnbarkeit* (i.e., cervical mucus that can stretch on a slide at least 6 cm). So characteristic are these findings that the appearance of this type of mucus signifies the fertile period in women practicing natural family planning methods. In contrast, one of the actions of progesterone (as seen after ovulation during the luteal phase or as used in the "minipill") is to thicken the cervical mucus, thereby making it less conducive for sperm transport, thus providing a contraceptive effect.

From a fertility testing perspective, postcoital tests examining spermatozoa within the cervical canal at midcycle to rule out a cervical factor are seldom used in today's practice. The subjective nature of this testing makes it not highly predictive of the ability to conceive.

## Hormone Assay Techniques: Immunoassays

No other method has had such an impact on the measurement of hormones as immunoassay methods (Wheeler, 2006). These techniques provide ways of measuring very small amounts of hormone in small quantities of serum or plasma rapidly and relatively specifically. The use of these techniques, pioneered by Yalow and Berson, has indeed increased the knowledge of reproductive endocrinology exponentially since the 1960s. Immunoassays and their variants have rapidly replaced previously used, cumbersome bioassays. They are comparatively much faster and much easier to perform, have a much enhanced sensitivity, and usually require far less than 1 mL of serum or plasma. **It should be kept in mind, however, that these techniques measure the immunologic property of a hormone, not its biologic activity (as tested by bioassays)**. These two effects may differ in magnitude under certain physiologic or pathologic conditions.

The basic principle of an immunoassay involves the competition between an unlabeled antigen (the hormone in the blood sample) and a labeled antigen, both of which are present in excess, for binding sites on a limited amount of antibody. The following is a brief description of the several steps required in the creation of such an assay. Even though the availability of commercial assays for many hormones has greatly facilitated the measurement of hormones, proper interpretation of the generated data requires a general knowledge of these steps.

### Preparation of Antibodies

The first step in setting up an immunoassay is the production or availability of an antibody to the analyte (here, the hormone) to be measured. Antibodies used in immunoassays are either polyclonal or monoclonal. **Polyclonal antibodies** are usually produced after the injection of the hormone in larger animals such as sheep or rabbits. For many **protein hormones**, this means injecting the purified hormone, which will be recognized by the host as foreign. In the natural immune reaction that follows, the host will produce polyclonal antibodies against the hormone. In contrast to protein hormones, **steroid hormones** are too small to produce an immune reaction on their own (haptens) and are not recognized as foreign because they are the same in most species. To become antigenic, they need to be attached to a carrier protein (usually bovine serum albumin). This conjugated compound is now perceived as a foreign body to the host animal and large enough to induce antibody formation.

Even with the injection of a purified antigen, polyclonal antibodies may "cross-react" with other closely related hormones and thus in some assays may lack specificity to the concerned hormone. To increase assay specificity, one may now choose to produce **monoclonal antibodies**, which provide unique specificity by recognizing only one epitope (antigenic determinant). These antibodies are produced by first injecting the antigen into a mouse to induce an immunogenic reaction in its spleen. The spleen cells are then screened to identify and separate those clones capable of secreting a single antibody type. These cells are then fused with a myeloma cell from the same species to form a hybrid cell (hybridoma), which can be maintained in culture. Because of its immortality, the hybridoma continues to produce homogenous antibodies as long as the culture is maintained.

### The Choice of Assay Markers

The second step in preparation for an immunoassay is the availability of a **labeled analyte** (hormone) in the competitive immunoassay or a **labeled second antibody** to the analyte in a reagent excess immunoassay. The choice of labels to be attached to the analyte or antibody is multiple.

In the initially developed radioimmunoassays, these labels were radioactive, such as iodine $I^{125}$. Although these assays were initially the norm, they mostly have been replaced by new types of immunoassays, which do not require the use of radioactive elements and thus avoid the attendant problems related to their use and to radioactivity disposal.

Major advances in the identification of nonradioactive labels and new measurement equipment to detect and quantitate these have occurred. Most assays now use nonradioactive labels. Enzyme immunoassays (enzyme-linked immunosorbent assays, or ELISA; immunometric assays) use enzymes as labels, such as, for example, horseradish peroxidase or alkaline phosphatase. Chemiluminescent immunoassays (CIA) use luminol. Fluorimetric immunoassays (FIA) use fluorescent compounds (e.g., fluorescein) as labels.

### The Separation of Bound and Unbound Antigen

The third step requires a method to separate antibody-bound antigen from unbound antigen to determine how much antigen is bound to the antibody. In commercial assays, antibodies can be attached to solid surfaces such as to plastic tubes, beads or plates, or cellulose particles. Separation can then be assured by washing off the unbound antigen.

Separation can also be performed by the use of a second antibody-label conjugate, which is directed against an antigenic site different from that recognized by the first antibody (see sandwich ELISA, discussed later).

### The Immunoassay Reaction

In step 1, a specific antibody (ab) to the hormone (which served as the antigen, ag) binds in the patient's blood sample to the antigen during a fixed period of incubation. A set amount of labeled form of the hormone ($ag^x$) is added to compete with the unlabeled hormone to bind to the antibody, resulting in the following reaction:

$$ab + ag + ag^x \rightleftharpoons ab.ag + ab.ag^x$$

In this competitive reaction, the amount of labeled antigen bound to the antibody will be inversely proportional to the amount of antigen (hormone) present in the blood sample. For measurement, the bound antigen is then separated for the free antigen by washing or other approaches.

Immunometric assays (also referred to as "sandwich assays") use a labeled second antibody, which is usually attached to a solid phase, such as the assay tube or assay plate, in the following reactions. The second antibody is directed against an antigenic site different from that recognized by the first antibody:

$$Ab1 + ag \rightleftharpoons ab1.ag$$
$$Ab1.ag + ab^x2 \rightleftharpoons ab1.ag.ab^x2$$

Because the sandwich assay depends on occupancy of the binding sites rather than competition for these sites, an excess of reagents is used.

### The Standard Curve

To allow for the actual measurement of the hormone levels in the blood sample, a standard curve must accompany each assay.

A standard preparation of the hormone to be measured is used at various increasing or decreasing concentrations, and each concentration is then processed as for the measurement of the sample with unknown concentrations. A standard curve is then constructed by plotting the measured end points. The result for each unknown sample is then located on the ordinate of the standard curve. By drawing a perpendicular line to the abscissa, the amount of hormone present in the unknown sample can be determined. These determinations are now rapidly computed.

Standard curves require varying amounts of pure preparations of hormone. This is no problem for steroid hormones, which are available in chemically pure preparations. Thus the amount added to construct the standard curve to determine the amount in the patient's sample can be expressed in terms of absolute mass or weight, such as nanograms (ng; $10^{-9}$ g) or picograms (pg; $10^{-12}$ g). Sometimes the results may be expressed in nanomoles (nmol). For most steroids, 1 ng/mL is equivalent to about 3 nmol/L.

Because proteins have higher molecular weights and are more complex, it is not always possible to obtain these in their pure form. In these cases the results are usually expressed in terms of the amounts of a standard reference preparation used for the standard curve. Standard preparations are obtained by extracting the hormone from large collections of blood, urine, or tissues (such as the pituitary gland for FSH and LH.) These protein standards are then most often an international reference preparation with the results expressed as international units. However, because of the use of different standard preparations, data obtained from different laboratories or assays may not agree. Thus clinicians should be aware of the normal levels reported by each laboratory reporting to them. Further complicating interpretation is the observation that protein hormones may also circulate in several forms, varying slightly by amino acid or carbohydrate content.

## ASSAY EVALUATION

When evaluating the value, accuracy, and relevance of an assay, four items must be examined:

1. **Sensitivity** measures the least hormone that can be measured with accuracy. This will set the lower limit of the assay.
2. **Specificity** is the ability of the assay to measure only the specific hormone of interest. Often with polyclonal antibodies, results may be altered by the presence of other cross-reacting substances also recognized by the antibody, although usually at lower levels of detection. This is important to know because cross-reaction may influence the precise measurement of the hormone of interest. In such instance, a preassay separation of the cross-reacting hormones may be necessary.
3. **Accuracy** is the ability to measure the exact amount of the hormone present in the sample. Controls containing varying low and high amounts of the hormone must be always assayed alongside the patient's samples in each assay.
4. **Precision** is the ability of the assay to consistently reproduce the same results. Precision is determined by two measurements. The first, the **intraassay coefficient of variation (intraassay CV)** measures the within assay variation. It is calculated by determining the results obtained from measuring a known sample in a number of replicates (usually 10) in the same assay. The second measurement is the **interassay coefficient of variation (interassay CV)**, which is calculated by measuring known samples in multiple assays.

### Mass Spectrometry Assays

There has been an increase in the use of mass spectrometry (MS) assays in both clinical and research laboratories. A particular strength of MS assays is the ability to measure large numbers of structurally similar compounds. MS assays have high specificity, sensitivity, and throughput (Xu, 2005), and MS is the most powerful assay method for defining defects in steroid hormone metabolism. **In larger reference laboratories, these assays have replaced the conventional radioimmunoassays**, which are cumbersome and time consuming, and direct immunoassays, which lack specificity and/or sensitivity. The MS technology has been implemented successfully for routine analysis of steroid hormones in major clinical diagnostic laboratories. Although the high cost of MS instrumentation, related operating costs, and requirement for technical expertise have prohibited smaller laboratories from using this instrumentation for routine testing of steroid hormones, this situation is changing and MS assays are becoming much more widely used.

### REFERENCES

Ahima RS, Flier JS. Leptin. *Annu Rev Physiol.* 2000;62:413.

Bousfield JR, Jia I, Ward, DN. Gonadotropins: chemistry and biosynthesis. In: Neill JD, ed. *Physiology of Reproduction.* Cambridge, MA: Elsevier-Academic Press; 2006:1581-1634.

Cha J, Sun X, Dey SK. Mechanisms of implantation: strategies for successful pregnancy. *Nat Med.* 2012;18:1754.

Dolleman M, Verschuren WM, Eijkemans MJ, et al. Reproductive and lifestyle determinants of anti-Mullerian hormone in a large population-based study. *J Clin Endocrinol Metab.* 2013;98:2106.

Douglas NC, Thornton II MH, Nurudeen SK, et al. Differential expression of serum glycodelin and insulin-like growth factor binding protein 1 in early pregnancy. *Reprod Sci.* 2013;20:1376.

Eissa MK, Obhrai MS, Docker MF, et al. Follicular growth and endocrine profiles in spontaneous and induced conception cycles. *Fertil Steril.* 1986;45:191.

Ellmann S, Sticht H, Thiel F, et al. Estrogen and progesterone receptors: from molecular structures to clinical targets. *Cell Mol Life Sci.* 2009;66:2405.

Ferin M. The menstrual cycle: an integrative view. In: Adashi EY, Rock JA, Rosenwaks Z, eds. *Reproductive Endocrinology, Surgery, and Technology.* New York: Raven Press; 1996:103.

Ferin M, Van Vugt D, Wardlaw S. The hypothalamic control of the menstrual cycle and the role of endogenous opioid peptides. *Recent Prog Horm Res.* 1984;40:441.

Filicori M, Santoro N, Merriam GR, et al. Characterization of the physiological pattern of episodic gonadotropin secretion throughout the human menstrual cycle. *J Clin Endocrinol Metab.* 1986;62:1136.

Hanna CB, Hennebold JD. Ovarian germline stem cells: an unlimited source of oocytes? *Fertil Steril.* 2014;101:20.

Herbison AE. The gonadotropin-releasing hormone pulse generator. *Endocrinology.* 2018;159:3723-3736.

Horwitz KB, Jackson TA, Bain DL, et al. Nuclear receptor coactivators and corepressors. *Mol Endocrinol.* 1996;10:167.

Jayasena CN, Abbara A, Comninos AN, et al. Kisspeptin-54 triggers egg maturation in women undergoing in vitro fertilization. *J Clin Invest.* 2014;124:3667.

La Marca A, Broekmans FJ, Volpe A, et al. Anti-Mullerian hormone (AMH): what do we still need to know? *Hum Reprod.* 2009;24:2264.

McGee EA, Hsueh AJ. Initial and cyclic recruitment of ovarian follicles. *Endocr Rev.* 2000;21:200.

Morishima A, Grumbach MM, Simpson ER, et al. Aromatase deficiency in male and female siblings caused by a novel mutation and the physiological role of estrogens. *J Clin Endocrinol Metab.* 1995;80:3689.

Skorupskaite K, George JT, Anderson, RA. The kisspeptin-GnRH pathway in human reproductive health and disease. *Hum Reprod Update.* 2014;20:485.

Stenvers KL, Findlay JK. Inhibins: from reproductive hormones to tumor suppressors. *Trends Endocrinol Metab.* 2010;21:174.

Stouffer RL. Corpus luteum formation and demise. In: Adashi EY, Rock JA, Rosenwaks Z, eds. *Reproductive Endocrinology, Surgery, and Technology.* Philadelphia: Lippincott-Raven; 1996:251.

Tsai PS, Gill JC. Mechanisms of disease: insights into X-linked and autosomal-dominant Kallmann syndrome. *Nat Clin Pract Endocrinol Metab.* 2006;2:160.

van den Berg MH, van Dulmen-den Broeder E, Overbeek A, et al. Comparison of ovarian function markers in users of hormonal contraceptives during the hormone-free interval and subsequent natural early follicular phases. *Hum Reprod.* 2010;25:1520.

Wheeler MJ. Immunoassay techniques. *Methods Mol Biol.* 2006;324:1.


**Suggested readings for this chapter can be found on ExpertConsult.com.**

# 5 Evidence-Based Medicine and Clinical Epidemiology

Catherine H. Watson, Fidel A. Valea, Laura J. Havrilesky

## KEY POINTS

- Evidence-based medicine (EBM) seeks to improve the care of patients and the delivery of care to patients.
- Descriptive-observational studies, including cross-sectional studies and case series, help generate hypotheses and characterize the context of disease.
- Case-control studies allow us to study rare diseases and evaluate for a wide range of exposures.
- Cohort studies allow us to study many outcomes over time.
- Randomized controlled trials (RCTs) are considered to be the gold standard of experimental clinical study design.
- Pragmatic clinical trials (PCTs) are designed to study the effectiveness of an intervention in the real world.
- Comparative effectiveness research (CER) encompasses patient-centered research, PCTs, meta-analyses, systematic reviews, evidence-based guidelines, and health services research (HSR) to study the benefits and harms of an intervention to improve patient care on the individual and population levels.
- Estimating the value of health care involves assessment of the quality and integration of care and the overall cost to provide all services included in that care.

Hippocrates, often hailed as the "father" of Western medicine, introduced the notion that an individual's disease originates from natural causes that can be observed and described within that person's environment. Although medicine has evolved in innumerable ways since the era of Hippocrates, the concept of disease as an observable entity related to an individual's environment is the foundation of evidence-based medicine. Basic and clinical sciences have built significantly on this foundation in the last 50 to 60 years, undergoing an exponential accumulation of research and advancement of knowledge. The main goal of this research is to gain knowledge of disease processes, identify causes and effects of disease states, and develop and assess the efficacy of treatments and interventions. The construction of a translational bridge from the laboratory to clinical practice presents a unique challenge to researchers and clinicians. Published results do not necessarily imply meaningful clinical utility and must often be evaluated in the context of the inherent constraints imposed by research study designs. This chapter discusses traditional clinical study designs and explores modern research constructs, comparative effectiveness research (CER), and health services research (HSR).

## INTRODUCTION TO EVIDENCE-BASED MEDICINE

The goal of evidence-based medicine is to guide clinical decision making using the full body of knowledge built from well-designed and well-conducted research. However, research evidence rarely applies directly to a particular individual or clinical problem. Clinical decisions must be formulated within the specific context of patient care by integrating it with clinical expertise that coincides with the values and goals of the individual patient. Clinical decision making must incorporate the most recent and valid information regarding disease prevention, diagnosis, prognosis, and treatment.

Epidemiologic studies form the foundation on which clinical evidence-based studies and the practice of evidence-based medicine are built. The World Health Organization (WHO) defines epidemiology as "the study of distribution and determinants of health-related states or events (including disease), and the application of this study to the control of disease and other health problems" (www.who.int). In simpler terms, epidemiology studies the cause and effect of a particular disease within a defined population in an attempt to assess association and/or causality between exposure and outcome.

One of the most influential studies in gynecology, the Women's Health Initiative, was designed after epidemiologic data indicated an association between the use of hormone replacement therapy (HRT) and the prevention of coronary heart disease and osteoporosis. The collection of this observational data led to the development of one of the largest randomized controlled trials and U.S. prevention studies ever published, with more than 160,000 postmenopausal women enrolled. Interestingly, this trial, rather than validating the observational finding of a cardioprotective effect of HRT, instead showed an increased risk of coronary heart disease. It also demonstrated an increased risk of venous thromboembolism, stroke, and breast cancer, which were unexpected results (Rossouw, 2002). This study is a good example both of the limitations of observational epidemiologic study design and of the importance of developing well-designed experimental clinical trials to test the validity, when plausible, of prior observations and associations.

Epidemiologic studies can be classified as either observational or experimental. The three most common types of observational epidemiologic studies are cohort, case-control, and cross-sectional studies. Case series can also be included among these, although their data is of lower quality. The gold standard of experimental study is the randomized controlled trial (RCT), in part because of its ability to control for confounding variables through the process of eligibility criteria and randomization. However, although the RCT is the traditionally heralded as the gold standard, it often does not directly represent the real-world therapeutic population.

In acknowledgment of these limitations, new fields of study design have been introduced and implemented, including CER and HSR. The primary objective of CER is to compare both clinical and public health interventions to determine which are most efficacious. CER is geared toward assisting "consumers, clinicians, purchasers, and policy makers to make informed decisions that will improve health care at both the individual and population levels" (Iglehart, 2009). The importance of this decision-making assistance has been increasingly recognized; 1.1 billion dollars of the American Recovery and Reinvestment stimulus package in 2009 was allocated specifically to CER. HSR, another emerging field, examines how patients get access to care, the cost and quality of that care, and ultimately the result of delivery of care. Health economic analysis is an emerging subgroup of HSR. There are several forms of economic analysis; the most common is cost-effectiveness analysis (CEA), which is used to compare the relative cost and effectiveness of alternative strategies, usually using a standard willingness-to-pay threshold.

In the following sections we review both traditional clinical study design and emerging clinical research methods.

## TRADITIONAL CLINICAL STUDY DESIGN

**Traditional clinical study designs are not created equal regarding the quality of evidence they produce.** Table 5.1 demonstrates a grading system that assesses clinical study design and evidence quality. Blinded RCTs offer the highest quality of evidence. Some authorities advocate that systematic reviews and meta-analyses of these types of trials produce an equal quality of evidence, although the validity of such studies relies on the quality and validity of the chosen articles (Grondin, 2011). The next level of evidence comes from cohort studies and case-control studies. The lowest-quality ranking is assigned to case series, case reports, and expert opinion. Table 5.2 compares advantages, limitations, and statistical considerations of each study design. Whether experimental or observational, these clinical studies are invaluable to modern medicine and affect patient care. In this section we discuss each clinical study design individually.

**TABLE 5.1** Levels of Evidence in Clinical Study Design

| Level | Evidence |
|---|---|
| 1a | Systematic review (with homogeneity) of randomized controlled trials |
| 1b | Individual randomized controlled trials |
| 2a | Systematic review (with homogeneity) of cohort studies |
| 2b | Individual cohort study |
| 2c | "Outcomes research" and ecological studies |
| 3a | Systematic review of case-control studies |
| 3b | Individual case-control study |
| 4 | Case series |
| 5 | Expert opinion without explicit critical appraisal, or based on physiology, bench research, or "first principles" |

Modified from Oxford Centre for Evidence Based Medicine. Levels of evidence; 2009. Available at www.cebm.net.

### Observational Studies

The term **observational study** describes a wide range of study designs. Observational studies can be classified as either analytical or descriptive. Analytical studies contain a control group for comparison, which includes nonrandomized prospective and retrospective cohort studies, case-control studies, and cross-sectional studies. Descriptive studies lack a control or comparison group and consist of case reports and case series. Observational studies play an important role in evidence-based medicine and are an important source of information when RCTs cannot be performed. The descriptive aspect of all observational studies is an invaluable attribute to clinical research, offering statistics about incidence, prevalence, and mortality rates of diseases in particular populations that provide clinicians with the context of a disease within a population. However, observational studies cannot determine causality, even if such associations appear highly plausible, and they are unfit to test hypotheses or answer etiologic questions. Despite these clear limitations, they still play an important role in generating new hypotheses to be tested by more formal, experimental study design.

#### Case Reports and Case Series

The basic element or unit of observational studies, as described by Grimes and Schulz, is the **case report** (Grimes, 2002). Case reports and case series are the least methodologically sound of all observational study designs, but this does not mean that they are not valuable contributors to the literature. Case reports often describe rare or new entities in medicine and offer an opportunity to describe characteristics about a disease and allow for postulation of hypotheses of pathophysiology. It was through case reports of unusual infections and disturbed immunity that acquired immunodeficiency syndrome (AIDS) was first described (CDC, 1981). Case reports can describe infrequent adverse

**TABLE 5.2** Comparison of Traditional Clinical Study Designs

| Study Design | Advantages | Limitations | Statistical Analysis |
|---|---|---|---|
| **Randomized controlled trials (RCTs)** | Gold standard; prospective; multiple study groups; randomization; can determine causality or a treatment advantage; time consuming; expensive; internal validity | Selection bias; confounding factors; performance bias; detection bias (RCT can control for confounding factors and biases with double-blinding and randomization); limited external validity | Relative risk (RR); absolute or attributable risk (AR); confidence interval (CI); number needed to treat (NNT) |
| **Cohort studies** | Prospective; can assess many outcomes over time | Take many years to complete; expensive; selection bias; confounding factors; patients can be lost to follow-up; changing exposure profile | Incidence; RR; AR |
| **Case-control studies** | Efficient; inexpensive; can study multiple exposures; can study rare disease | Retrospective; recall bias; sampling bias; confounding factors; good external validity | Odds ratio (OR) |
| **Cross-sectional studies** | Can determine the frequency of disease or outcomes; highlights possible associations; efficient | Capture one moment in time; cannot determine incidence or causality; sampling bias; participation bias; recall bias | Prevalence |
| **Case series** | Descriptive of rare or new entities; hypothesis generating | Lack of comparison group; no clinical conclusions | No statistical analysis |

events associated with medications and other treatments. The association of phocomelia with thalidomide, a drug used to treat pregnancy-associated nausea in the 1960s, was first published in the form of two case reports in 1962, resulting in the swift removal of the drug from the market (Coodin, 1962; Ward, 1962). Case reports can also describe the plausibility and early use of novel treatment methods or surgery. However, the scientific audience may use weaker objective landmarks, such as historical controls, when interpreting the meaning of noted observations. Case reports and case series should be considered no more than "the first step toward more sophisticated research" (Gehlbach, 2002).

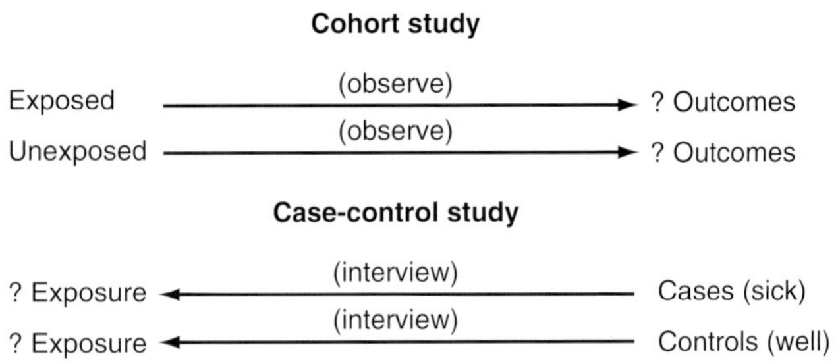

**Fig. 5.1** Schematic diagram of clinical study design comparing cohort studies and case-control studies.

## Cross-Sectional Studies

**Cross-sectional studies** are prevalence studies that examine the relationship between exposure and the outcomes of interest in a defined population at a single point in time. Prevalence is defined as the number of cases in a population at a given time. It is a ratio, or proportion, of affected individuals in relation to a pooled population. Cross-sectional studies cannot determine incidence, or the number of new cases in a population over time. Rather, they are snapshots of a disease in a specific population. With reference to only a designated moment in time, these studies are not able to provide causal evidence. Case reports and cross-sectional studies can highlight possible associations that deserve additional evaluation, but they cannot determine causality.

**One advantage of cross-sectional studies is efficiency.** Because the study population is examined at one moment in time, conclusions can be generated at the same time as data collection. However, cross-sectional studies are plagued by uncertain causality. **Population selection, participation bias, and recall bias are also possible limitations.** If a tertiary care center or major referral center is conducting a research study and the study population is taken from patients that present to these facilities, they are unlikely to accurately represent the general population or even a more specific population of patients with a particular disease undergoing therapy within the community. In 1990, Gayle et al. published data regarding the prevalence of human immunodeficiency virus (HIV) among university students, examining more than 17,000 specimens from 19 universities (Gayle, 1990). Thirty students, or 0.2%, had detectable HIV antibodies, which was higher than prior studies within the public. The media sensationalized these data, reporting that more than 25,000 college students across the nation might be infected with HIV. However, patient selection in this study was poor because specimens collected for examination were not random, but rather represented those students who presented to student health whose condition warranted a blood sample. Researchers must be careful that patients selected for cross-sectional studies are representative of the study population desired.

Participation bias arises when selected subjects do not participate, such as in survey studies. If 100,000 surveys are sent out but only 10,000 are completed, the study is likely affected by participation bias. The minority of patients who respond may not be representative of the desired study population. Recall bias becomes an issue when self-reporting, as in survey studies, is a part of study design. Patients often report inaccurate information regarding certain exposures or events. Despite these limitations, well-conducted cross-sectional studies have their place in evidence-based medicine. They are simply prevalence studies, which allow us to determine frequencies of disease or outcomes within particular populations or groups.

## Case-Control Studies

The purpose of a **case-control study** is to determine whether an exposure is associated with an outcome (e.g., a disease of interest). Study participants are selected on the basis of having or not having the outcome of interest (the case group versus the control group, respectively). Case-control studies are always retrospective because they start with an outcome and then evaluate previous exposures or habits. Fig. 5.1 illustrates the differences in methodologies between case-control studies compared with cohort studies. Participants in the case group need to be carefully defined and should include all cases of new-onset disease drawn from an identifiable population. Controls should be sampled from that same population. The purpose of the control group is to allow for comparison in frequencies of exposures of a case group with the outcome of interest versus the control group without that outcome. In 1971, Herbst et al. published a case-control study of 8 cases and 32 matched controls identifying a strong association between vaginal adenocarcinoma and in utero exposure to diethylstilbestrol (DES) (Herbst, 1971). Although further cohort studies were required to confirm causality, this case-control study allowed for identification of a suspected culprit (exposure) for the development of vaginal adenocarcinoma in young women (outcome of interest).

**Case-control studies offer the advantages of being relatively inexpensive, simple to conduct, and efficient.** They are retrospective and thus do not require a prolonged period of data collection. They can be used to study multiple exposures as they relate to a particular outcome of interest, and they offer the ability to study rare diseases. The quality of the results from these studies is dependent on meticulous selection of cases, control groups, and data collection among the groups. There are also disadvantages to case-control studies, including the risk of recall and sampling biases. **Recall bias is particularly problematic because cases and controls are likely to recount historical exposures differently.** Patients or families coping with an illness may recall in great detail all events they believe might be associated with the illness, whereas healthy controls may not remember similar exposures. The potential problematic power of recall bias was highlighted in the case-control studies that suggested a correlation between talcum powder use and epithelial ovarian cancer. Although significant legal claims were made concerning this correlation, no significant relationship was ever documented in a prospective study. In the case-control studies, talcum powder use was a solely subjective measure that could not be tracked by any method other than patient report; thus the potential for recall bias was great (Terry, 2013). Recall bias may also occur when information on the case group is obtained by chart review but information on the control group is obtained either by interview or mail survey. It may ultimately be impossible to eliminate recall bias.

**Sample selection, or sampling bias, arises if the cases selected do not appropriately represent a particular disease or outcome.** This is similar to sample selection issues in cross-sectional studies. Sampling bias can also occur within the control group if a representation of the desired general population either underestimates or overestimates exposures. Matching, or selecting control group participants similar in characteristics to the case group, helps to decrease bias in the selection of controls. Matching also helps to decrease possible confounding, which occurs when factors relate both to the measured outcome and measured exposures. As Stephen Gehlbach, a renowned epidemiologist, once wrote, "Confounding is the epidemiologist's eternal triangle...Are we seeing cause and effect, or is a confounding factor exerting its unappreciated influence?" (Gehlbach, 2002). Controlling sample selection and confounding factors allows for external validity, or the generalizability of the study to the desired population. Researchers can use statistical techniques such as multivariate analysis and logistic regression to help eliminate confounders.

Because case-control studies are retrospective by design, they are also limited in their statistical analysis. They cannot provide data on incidence, relative risks, or attributable risks between an exposure and a measured outcome. **Case-control study results are reported as odds ratios, which represent the odds that an individual affected by the specific disease being studied has been exposed to a particular risk factor (case group) divided by the odds that the control group has been exposed.** It is loosely considered a reasonable estimate of relative risk, but it is not a true calculation of relative risk.

### Cohort Studies

A **cohort study** selects a group of individuals at risk for an outcome of interest and divides them into subgroups based on the presence or absence of one or more exposures to be studied. Subgroups are then followed prospectively to evaluate the potential development of the outcome of interest. Cohort studies are unique in that the study participants select their exposure, as opposed to experimental research, in which the investigator selects, either knowingly or unknowingly, the exposure. Several types of comparisons can be made in a cohort study: An intervention or exposure can be compared with an alternate intervention or exposure, or it can be compared with no intervention. These comparisons can be made in general or restricted populations (Rochon, 2005).

An excellent example of a cohort study is the Nurses' Health Study (NHS). In 1976, the NHS began surveying more than 120,000 female nurses regarding medical history, hormone use, and many other points of interest. The investigators have updated the study every 2 years by mailing out questionnaires to the original enrolled patients. In 2001, Grodstein et al. published data regarding the use of postmenopausal hormone therapy and the secondary prevention of coronary events (Grodstein, 2001). The results demonstrated a short-term increased risk of coronary events in patients with a history of coronary disease but a decreased risk with long-term hormonal use.

A **strength of cohort studies is the possibility of assessing many different outcomes over time**. Also, although RCTs establish the outcomes of interest before study initiation, cohort study outcomes are more flexible and can be defined after the intervention. From a statistical standpoint, cohort studies also allow for the calculation of incidence rates, relative risks, and attributable risks. Incidence is defined as the number of new outcomes of interest in a given population over a set period. In cohort studies, incidence can be calculated for the population as a whole, but it is most often calculated for populations with and without an identifiable risk factor. **Relative risk (RR), or risk ratio, can be calculated from these incidence rates. RR should be thought of as a simple ratio of the probability of an outcome (disease) occurring within an exposed population compared with a nonexposed population.** It is calculated as the ratio of the incidence in a population exposed to the risk factor over the incidence in the unexposed population. Attributable risk (AR), or absolute risk, represents the absolute additional risk in the exposed population over what may be considered the baseline occurrence in the population. It is determined by calculating the difference between the incidence in the exposed population and the incidence of the unexposed population.

**Cohort studies also have disadvantages: They are often time consuming, take many years to complete, and can become costly.** The NHS is a clear example of the time and money it takes to complete a prospective cohort study. As with all analytic-observational studies, subject selection is important to control for selection bias and confounding factors. Matching of patients in control and study groups helps address these issues. To the extent that information is collected about known or suspected confounding factors, it is also possible to control for their effect in the statistical analysis using techniques such as regression and stratification (Normand, 2005). Adjustment techniques can work only for confounding variables that an investigator knows about and measures. Participants may also be lost to follow-up over the often years-long courses of these studies. Investigators must be diligent in keeping accurate follow-up records of each subject. In the same manner, researchers should be aware that patient habits may change over time, thus changing their exposure risks.

## Experimental Studies: Randomized Controlled Trials

**RCTs are considered the gold standard of clinical study design.** Within the constructs of epidemiologic studies, RCT is another type of analytical study. In cohort studies the patient controls the exposure to a factor of interest, whereas in RCTs the clinical investigator controls exposure to the factor of interest. RCTs are designed to establish evidence of causal associations. They are characterized by the prospective assignment of study participants to a study group (who receive the factor of interest, typically a new treatment) or a control group (placebo, no treatment, or standard care). Although there are often only two study arms or groups within an RCT, investigators can develop designs involving multiple study groups. These groups are followed over time to evaluate for differences in outcomes. Outcomes of interest may include prevention or cure of a disease, reduction in severity of a condition, or differences in costs, quality of life, or side effects between treatments. An example is the Women's Health Initiative already mentioned, which examined the use of HRT and the prevention of coronary heart disease, osteoporosis, and other conditions. The trial did not demonstrate a cardioprotective effect of HRT but instead showed an increased risk of coronary heart disease. Although it did demonstrate protection against osteoporosis and colon cancer, it showed an increased risk of venous thromboembolism, stroke, and breast cancer (Rossouw, 2002). Thus the results of this prospective randomized trial directly contradicted findings of previous observational studies.

RCTs are considered the gold standard because of several key design features. Perhaps the most important of these features is **randomization**, a process that eliminates selection bias and allows for better control of known and unknown confounding factors. Confounding factors can also be controlled by strict eligibility criteria, eliminating possible interference from any peripheral contributing factors. This technique is also called *internal validity*, or the ability to control for confounding factors to demonstrate a true causal association. An additional feature of most RCTs is **blinding**, which helps decrease both performance and detection bias. Performance bias is encountered when systemic differences exist in the care delivered to subjects. In other words, performance bias occurs when a patient receives less or more therapy based on knowing what particular group or treatment a patient is randomized to on trial. Detection bias occurs when patients are evaluated more intensely as a result of being in the study group of interest. The double-blinded RCT is a superior study design because the blinding of both subjects and investigators is preferred to control for any performance or detection bias while also controlling for selection bias and confounding factors.

Despite the theoretical design superiority of the RCT approach, these studies are not without limitations and provide the best evidence only if the study has been thoughtfully designed, implemented, analyzed, and reported. Both ethical and practical considerations may limit the use of RCT to answer clinical questions. It is clearly unethical to expose patients to potential disease-causing factors just to learn about their negative effects on a particular outcome of interest. Additional ethical concerns arise when designing treatment groups to be studied. A placebo control group is often most efficient to study the effect of a given treatment. However, if an effective treatment already exists, it is not ethical to use a placebo control group. The concept of *primum non nocere*, or "first, do no harm," also applies in clinical research, and harm can be caused by denying patients a known, effective treatment. If a condition is mild, the treatment period is brief, or effective treatment is not generally available, most investigators believe that a placebo control group is ethical. Most often in RCTs study groups will have similar, or at least balanced, benefits and harms. This leaves the researchers to instead investigate what treatment is preferred and if there is an advantage of one treatment over another. This uncertainty can be defined as therapeutic equipoise, or the general uncertainty of the benefits and harms of competing treatments. The assumption of therapeutic equipoise underlies many RCTs, providing patients with an equal chance to undergo at least standard-of-care treatment versus a possible improved treatment plan. Thus RCTs allow an unbiased assessment to assist in determining a preferred treatment. It should be noted that RCTs are ideal to study outcomes over short periods; RCTs intended to study long-term or rare outcomes are time consuming, cost prohibitive, and much more difficult to complete. As already discussed, cohort studies may be more appropriate to evaluate rare outcomes. Unfortunately, for many clinical questions, the time, effort, and expense involved in carrying out an RCT become prohibitive.

One further weakness of RCTs is the possibility that subjects and controls may be special populations whose results are not generalizable to the public, or even a specific subset of the public. In 1971, Cochrane noted this issue, stating "Between measurements based on RCTs and benefit…in the community there is a gulf which has been much under-estimated" (Cochrane, 1972). Although the RCT's strength of design is a strong internal validity, it often lacks strong external validity. External validity is the ability of a result to be generalizable in the real world. Often the more complex the study protocol, the greater the difference between RCT results and general clinical outcomes. RCTs also often use surrogate markers to substitute for clinical outcomes. A surrogate marker is defined as "an outcome measure that substitutes for a clinical event of true importance…an intermediate measure…commonly laboratory measurements or imaging studies thought to be involved in the causal pathway to a clinical event of interest" (Grimes, 2005). An ideal surrogate marker is a measurable event that is necessary along the pathway to the clinical endpoint. For example, Skaznik-Wikiel et al. demonstrated in a retrospective analysis of 124 women that normalization of CA-125 levels in ovarian cancer after three cycles of chemotherapy was associated with an improved overall survival (Skaznik-Wikiel, 2011). However, this was a retrospective analysis and there are no studies demonstrating an association between the response of CA-125 and overall survival. Researchers must be careful when using surrogate markers because they may not always equate with the disease process being assessed. For example, a medication that has the effect of lowering cholesterol does not necessarily prevent heart attacks; lipid levels therefore may be a flimsy surrogate marker if myocardial infarction is the actual clinical endpoint of interest. When interpreting randomized trials, surrogate markers must be used with caution. Grimes and Schulz have emphasized that surrogate markers should, among other characteristics, have similar confounders and influences, and they should show a near identical response to a treatment as the desired clinical endpoint. As an example they cite fluoride treatments, which improve bone mineral density (a surrogate marker) but increase fracture risk, which is the true clinical endpoint of interest. Occasionally authors use a combined outcome, which includes a surrogate marker and a valid clinical outcome. This combined outcome should be interpreted cautiously because the relative effect of treatments on the various components remains unknown.

Researchers may also report secondary outcomes, or subgroup analyses, within an RCT. These outcomes may or may not have similar validity as the set primary outcomes. RCTs are designed to test hypotheses on primary outcomes, controlling for confounding variables that affect the primary outcome. Often, secondary outcomes are not considered in the study design, and thus the study does not control for confounding factors affecting secondary outcomes. A subgroup exploratory analysis was conducted for ICON7, a large RCT that evaluated the addition of bevacizumab, a vascular endothelial growth factor inhibitor, to the traditional adjuvant treatment of ovarian cancer. Although the trial demonstrated an improvement in progression-free survival, there was no significant increase in overall survival for patients in the bevacizumab arm. However, a subgroup analysis performed during evaluation of the final survival results indicated a significant improvement in overall survival among subjects with the worst prognoses (Perren, 2011). Although such results may appear promising, it must be remembered that they are not the result of the initial study framework and therefore must be interpreted with caution in clinical settings unless the original study design included internal validity regarding these subgroups. This concern is particularly pertinent when secondary outcomes and subgroup analyses are incorporated into meta-analyses, which will be addressed later.

## Statistical Interpretation

Epidemiologic studies use a quantitative approach to describe both exposures and outcomes. Case-control studies, cohort studies, and RCTs all attempt to present their results as a single number, usually referred to as the point estimate, that quantifies the relationship between the exposure and the outcome. This number is an estimate of the truth rather than the truth itself because each study, however large, includes only a sample of all the people who are affected by the exposure-outcome relationship. The point estimate expresses the strength of the association between exposure and outcome. In an RCT or a cohort study the point estimate is the RR. Risk in the study subjects is the number of cases or outcomes that occur over time. The RR is simply the risk of disease (or other outcome) among the exposed or treated subjects divided by the risk in the unexposed subjects. As already discussed, case-control studies do not measure risk directly but instead report an odds ratio (OR), which is generally considered a rough estimate of RR.

Interpretations of RR and OR are similar. As the ratio approaches 1.0, there is little to no association. For both RRs and ORs, the further away the value is from 1.0, the stronger the relationship between the exposure and the outcome. Values less than 1.0 represent a negative association, or a decreased risk of an exposure-outcome relationship. Values greater than 1.0 represent a positive association, or a greater risk of an exposure-outcome relationship. A strong positive RR may be greater than 2.0 and a strong negative RR may be less than 0.5. Weaker associations can often be explained by confounding variables. However, enthusiastic investigators, worried patients, or sensationalistic media often overinterpret weak associations. One must also remember that an OR or RR is based on results of a specific study group and may not represent the general population. This possible difference is understood as a sampling error, or the possible difference in statistics of a study compared with the actual unknown statistics within a population. As a result, investigators will use a confidence interval (CI) to express the precision of a point estimate. **Researchers do not rely solely on the traditional *P* value to determine whether a study's findings are due to a chance occurrence, especially when discussing ratios and risks.** Confidence intervals represent with high probability (95%) the values within which the actual population point estimate would fall. A narrow CI indicates strong precision and is easier to achieve with larger studies or studies with very little variance. A wide CI indicates poor precision and may be representative of an underpowered study or considerable variance among results. It must be noted that CIs do not address uncertainty in the results caused by confounding factors or poor study quality. Furthermore, a wide CI is not definitive proof of a lack of association between the exposure and the outcome. CI is simply a measure of precision. Even an imprecise point estimate remains the best explanation of the relationship until a larger or better study is performed. CIs are most often graphically represented as a straight line around a point estimate to show the width of their range. However, a more accurate visualization of the concept is a bell-shaped curve centered around the point estimate value. Fig. 5.2 demonstrates examples of point estimates and their respective confidence intervals.

The calculation of RR does not take into account the incidence or the scale of the problem being evaluated. An RR of 4 says that the outcome increases 400% in exposed individuals compared with unexposed individuals. However, the RR must be interpreted in the context of the frequency of the outcome. For instance, the incidence of venous thromboembolism (VTE) in young women who do not use oral contraceptives is about 1 in 10,000, and the incidence while using oral contraceptives is 4 in 10,000; thus the RR is 4. However, the absolute risk of VTE is still low in both groups of women, with a difference in risk of 3 in 10,000. This difference in risk is considered the absolute risk, or AR. It is very helpful for putting large RRs into a clinically useful perspective. It can also be reported as the absolute risk reduction when a benefit is identified or the absolute risk increase when a harm is identified.

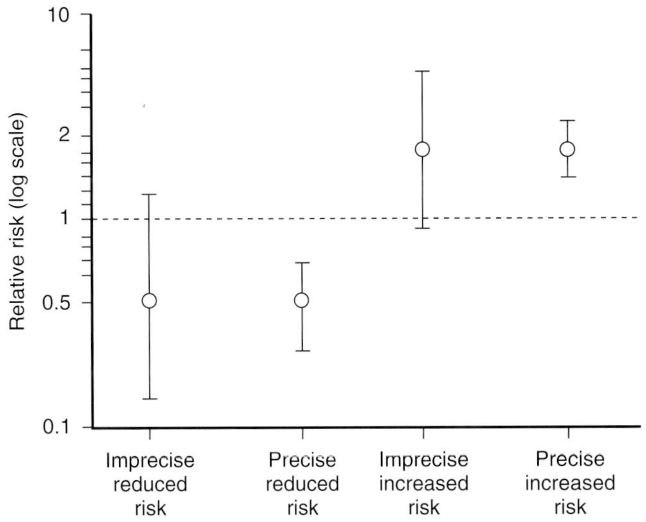


**Fig. 5.2** Schematic diagram of point estimates (*open circles*) with varying confidence intervals (*lines with crossbars*). X-axis represents interpretation of respective point estimate and confidence interval. If the confidence interval crosses 1.0, the change in risk is statistically insignificant.

An alternative calculation to AR looks at a complementary concept: How many patients need to be treated to observe one benefit or one adverse event? This concept is referred to as the number needed to treat (NNT), or the number of patients who need to be treated to achieve an additional positive outcome. It is the reciprocal of the absolute risk reduction (the risk difference for good outcomes). If the effect is dangerous, the value is called the number needed to harm (NNH). The number of patients who, if they received the treatment, would lead to one additional patient being harmed, compared with patients not receiving the treatment, is the reciprocal of the absolute risk increase (the risk difference for bad outcomes). Thus using the example of oral contraceptives, with an AR risk of VTE of 3 in 10,000, the NNH (i.e., to experience one extra VTE) is 3333. It is simply the reciprocal of 3 in 10,000. Calculations of NNT and NNH are essential to understanding the potential benefits and harms of therapies, preventive services, and screening tests. They also allow us to compare benefits and harms across different treatment strategies. It must be taken into consideration, however, that NNT and NNH may vary over time. The data from which an NNT is calculated are often specific and may not be generalizable to a person's lifetime or the course of a disease. NNT and NNH derived from meta-analysis should be viewed with caution. If the studies are from varied populations or used slightly different methods, the NNT and NNH may not always apply to an individual patient or be a simple arithmetic summation.

## COMPARATIVE EFFECTIVENESS RESEARCH

Pervasive problems in the quality of delivered care, a lack of high quality evidence to guide clinical practice and health policy, and concerns about health care spending led to the advent of a new research initiative called comparative effectiveness research. The National Academy of Medicine, formerly called the Institute of Medicine (IOM), has defined CER as "the generation and synthesis of evidence that compares the benefits and harms of alternative methods to prevent, diagnose, treat, and monitor a clinical condition or to improve the delivery of care. The purpose of CER is to assist consumers, clinicians, purchasers, and policy makers to make informed decisions that will improve health care at both the individual and population levels" (IOM, 2009). The formal process of developing a CER focus was initiated in the 2003 Medicare Modernization Act, which appropriated $50 million to conduct research that addresses the needs and priorities related to improve outcomes, clinical effectiveness, and appropriateness of certain services and treatments. Data from these earlier efforts was first integrated into coverage for these interventions in 2006, when the Centers for Medicare and Medicaid Services (CMS) provided support to the concept of inclusion of evidence-based decision making and research into coverage determination policies (Havrilesky, 2013a). Analysis of costs linked to health-related quality of life was later included as part of CER. The Congressional Budget Office (CBO) definition of CER in 2007 included costs as a factor relevant to comparison of different interventions but took a narrow view of interventions by focusing solely on treatment for individual medical conditions (CBO, 2007). **CER studies often incorporate different practice settings, a wide range of subgroups, and patient-reported outcomes.** Several aspects of CER are depicted in Fig. 5.3 and discussed in this section.

### Meta-Analyses, Systematic Reviews, and Evidence-Based Guideline Development

**Meta-analyses were developed in response to the problem of conflicting and inconclusive results of individual studies.** Uncommon diseases or conditions can be difficult to study because of the small numbers of those afflicted, leading to studies

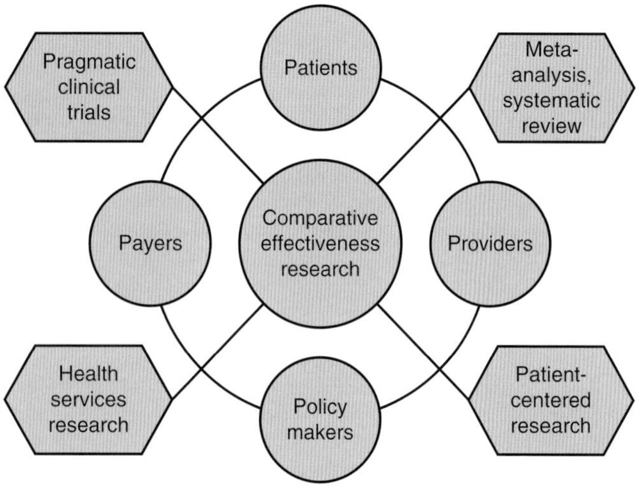


**Fig. 5.3** Schematic diagram of comparative effectiveness research.

that lack sufficient numbers of patients and therefore the power to report significant results. In a meta-analysis a researcher combines the results of multiple studies to enlarge the group of patients being studied. The ultimate goal of a meta-analysis is to produce a more precise result with a tighter confidence interval. However, not all meta-analyses are created equal. A meta-analysis involving well-constructed and well-performed RCTs is ideal. Meta-analyses of observational studies must be interpreted with extreme caution. Each individual study varies in population, entry criteria, and definitions of case and exposure. These disparities make the combination of data in observational studies problematic, particularly if the analysis uses data from published tables rather than combining the raw data from the original studies. In this way, meta-analyses differ from pooled analyses, which instead reexamine the original raw data from multiple individual studies for statistical consideration. If the results from individual studies differ drastically in direction or outcome, then a meta-analysis is not an appropriate tool to answer the question. A pooled analysis can control for heterogeneity by controlling for confounding factors in the original data. A meta-analysis can provide the same type of control by inclusion of similar, high-quality studies. Perhaps the main value of a meta-analysis is the rigorous approach to collecting and evaluating all the relevant data on a particular clinical problem from multiple sources, but a risk of meta-analysis is finding an inaccurate significant effect from the evaluation of multiple small studies. It has been have suggested that when multiple studies are analyzed together to produce a new finding, the results should be interpreted with caution and viewed only as hypothesis generating until an RCT with adequate power can be performed (Hennekens, 2009). This precaution is particularly true when the additional reported results are secondary outcomes. Neither meta-analyses nor pooled analyses are appropriate for conclusions regarding secondary outcomes, although meticulous examination of original raw data can generate associations for further study.

The clinical need for sound evidence and for more stringent and objective synthesis of evidence has led to the development of systematic approaches to reviewing evidence. Evidence-based systematic reviews include a comprehensive review and evaluation of the literature. A **systematic review is a review of a clearly formulated question that uses systematic and explicit methods to identify, select, and critically appraise relevant research and to collect and analyze data from the studies that are included in the review** (Higgins, 2011). Systematic reviews are reported using a standardized format that must include a detailed description of the search strategy used to identify the relevant literature and the results of the search. Systematic reviews also carry out critical appraisal of the studies they evaluate. Critical appraisal employs a rigid standardized assessment of the relevance and quality of each study. The goal of systematic reviews is to synthesize the literature regarding a specific clinical question and to use an approach that minimizes bias and random error. Systematic reviews are often performed in conjunction with a meta-analysis.

In 1996, to address the suboptimal reporting of meta-analyses, an international group of researchers released the QUOROM, or Quality of Reporting of Meta-analysis, statement, to improve standards. **In 2009, the guideline was updated to address several conceptual and practical advances in the science of systematic reviews and was renamed PRISMA (Preferred Reporting Items of Systematic reviews and Meta-Analyses).** PRISMA provides a 27-item checklist that describes the content of a systematic review, including the title, abstract, methods, results, discussion, and funding, as well as a flow diagram that represents the flow of information through the different phases of a systematic review. It characterizes information about the number of records identified in the literature searches, the number of studies included and excluded, and the reasons for exclusions (http://www.prisma-statement.org/statement.htm). For example, in 2013 Havrilesky et al. published a systemic review and meta-analysis of the use of oral contraceptive pills (OCP) as primary prevention for ovarian cancer (Havrilesky, 2013b). This study employed methodology that followed PRISMA guidelines. In a flow diagram the authors describe literature searches, abstract screening, number of studies included and excluded, and explanations for exclusions. It also illustrates the advantage of systemic review and meta-analysis, which is to provide an answer to focused research questions through a rigorous and transparent form of literature review. In this case the authors confirmed previous large studies demonstrating a duration-dependent protective effect of OCP use on the incidence of ovarian cancer.

The Cochrane Collaboration is a major source of systematic reviews (www.cochrane.org). This collaboration is an international organization that aims to help people make well-informed decisions about health care by preparing, maintaining, and promoting the accessibility of systematic reviews of the effects of health care interventions. The collaboration is funded by proceeds from the Cochrane Library and other Cochrane products, along with donations from national and international governments, private foundations, and private funders. Of note, they do not accept commercial donations to prevent undue influence.

The Agency for Healthcare Research and Quality (AHRQ) also works with a number of partners to publish systematic reviews. The AHRQ lists its mission as "producing evidence to make health care safer, higher quality, more accessible, equitable, and affordable, and to work within the U.S. Department of Health and Human Services and with other partners to make sure that the evidence is understood and used." The AHRQ also works in conjunction with the U.S. Preventive Services Task Force (USPSTF) to perform systematic reviews regarding clinical preventive services. These are published in both book and electronic forms. Many professional groups issue practice guidelines to help translate these often lengthy reviews into briefer, clinically useful documents. An electronic collection of such guidelines is now available at the National Guideline Clearinghouse (NGC; www.guideline.gov).

## Pragmatic Clinical Trials

As previously discussed, RCTs are the gold standard in evaluating the effects of treatment; however, they are often not generalizable because of the tightly controlled environment in which they are conducted. In recent years, clinicians and policymakers have made a concerted effort to distinguish between the *efficacy* and the *effectiveness* of an intervention. RCTs are efficacy trials (explanatory trials) that are designed to determine whether an intervention produces the expected result under ideal circumstances. On the other hand, **pragmatic clinical trials (PCTs) are effectiveness trials measuring the benefit of treatment under real-world circumstances or routine clinical practice**. In 1967, Schwartz defined a PCT as a trial "for which the hypothesis and study design are formulated based on information needed to make a decision" (Schwartz, 1967). They address real questions of cost, risk, and benefits that arise in everyday clinical practice in an attempt to provide direct, useful information to clinicians, patients, payers, and other decision makers (Roland, 1998). PCTs resemble RCTs in the use of randomization, but PCTs do not place strict constraints on the setting of the trial, target patients, or intervention delivery. Traditional RCT approaches prioritize internal validity and efficacy by testing whether the intervention has the intended effect in ideal, highly controlled settings. In contrast, PCTs prioritize external validity, or generalizability to the public, and thus have fewer selection criteria. Pragmatic trials test effectiveness, or the degree of beneficial effect in everyday clinical practice.

A document released by the AHRQ and the Patient-Centered Medical Home (PCMH), lists five ways in which PCTs differ from RCTs: **(1) comparison of clinically relevant alternatives; (2) enrollment of diverse study populations; (3) recruitment from a variety of practice settings; (4) measurement of a broad range of outcomes; and (5) adaptation of the intervention being tested to the local context.** However, PCTs also have disadvantages. The excellent external validity of PCTs comes at the cost of decreased internal validity. Effects of a particular treatment may be lessened or heightened because the results were obtained in a more real-world setting. It also may be more difficult to determine what component of an intervention is responsible for a certain outcome because the interventions can be heterogeneous. PCTs also require significant resources to keep meticulous records of implementation and to ensure rigor of the study design. Regardless, PCT is an excellent alternative to traditional RCT in certain clinical settings. An example of the benefits of this study design is the SAFETY trial, a study examining standard care of atrial fibrillation versus atrial fibrillation–specific management strategy. This trial was designed as a pragmatic RCT. The standard group received routine primary care and hospital discharge follow-up. The SAFETY group included a home visit, a Holter monitor for 1 to 2 weeks, prolonged follow-up by a specialized cardiac nurse, and multidisciplinary support as needed. The SAFETY group was associated with more days alive out of the hospital, but no significant change in prolonged event-free survival was found (Stewart, 2015). This trial demonstrates the nature of PCTs focusing on the generalizability of an intervention while still adhering to RCT study design. It also demonstrates the amount of planning and support that is required to conduct a PCT. As PCT designs become more commonly used, clinicians and researchers will have to discern what quality of evidence these trials represent.

### Patient-Centered Outcomes Research Institute

The Patient-Centered Outcomes Research Institute (PCORI) is an independent nonprofit, nongovernmental organization established by the 2010 Patient Protection and Affordable Care Act. PCORI's purpose is to assist patients and clinicians in making informed health decisions by advancing the quality and relevance of evidence concerning a broad range of health conditions. PCORI directs research to improve prevention, diagnosis, management, and monitoring of disease in varied patient subpopulations (Patient Protection and Affordable Care Act, 2010). Patient-centered outcomes research (PCOR) differs from CER in its primary target. The institution's primary goal is to inform individual patient decision making rather than targeting a wider range of audiences such as payers and policymakers. According to a working definition approved in March 2012 by the PCORI Board of Governors, the purpose of PCOR is to help patients and their providers communicate and make informed health care decisions, allowing the patient's voice to be heard in assessing the value of health care options. One way that PCORI operationalizes the focus on individuals is through examination of outcomes "that people notice and care about such as survival, function, symptoms, and health related quality of life" (D'Arcy, 2012). The mechanism by which PCORI aims to achieve this mission is by producing and promoting the use of high-integrity, evidence-based information stemming from research guided by patients, caregivers, and the broader health care community. PCORI funds comparative clinical effectiveness research and supports work that improves the methods used to conduct such studies. Hundreds of projects are currently funded by the PCORI, including many gynecologic initiatives, ranging from evaluation of hysteroscopic sterilization patient outcomes to contraceptive option education. In 2013 $20 million was given to researchers by PCORI in collaboration with AHRQ to compare patient-centered results for uterine fibroids (COMPARE-UF) (www.pcori.org/research-results).

## HEALTH SERVICES RESEARCH

The AHRQ defines health services research as a "multidisciplinary field of scientific investigation that studies how social factors, financing systems, organizational structures and processes, health technologies, and personal behaviors affect access to health care, the quality and cost of health care, and ultimately, our health and well-being." In 1993, the NIH Revitalization Act created a National Information Center on Health Services Research and Health Care Technology (NICHSR), with a goal "to make the results of health services research, including practice guidelines and technology assessments, readily available to health practitioners, health care administrators, health policy makers, payers, and the information professionals who serve these groups; to improve access to data and information needed by the creators of health services research; and to contribute to the information infrastructure needed to foster patient record systems that can produce useful health services research data as a by-product of providing health care" (https://www.nlm.nih.gov/hsrph/html). As the cost of health care in the United States continues to increase, amounting to almost $3 trillion in 2013, HSR has the ability to make major contributions to the future of medicine. Clinical research has long shaped the practice of medicine, but HSR looks to study the infrastructure of practicing medicine. The following sections contain examples of HSR.

### Data Registry Studies

Large national cancer registries and state cancer registries provide the patient health care data needed for HSR. In 1971 the National Cancer Act provided funding to the National Cancer Institute (NCI) to detect, treat, and perform research of cancers in the United States. In 1973, the Surveillance, Epidemiology, and End Results (SEER) Program of NCI was established as the first national cancer registry. The SEER registry "collects and publishes cancer incidence and survival data from population-based cancer registries…on patient demographics, primary tumor site, tumor morphology and stage at diagnosis, first course of treatment, and follow-up for vital status" (http://seer.cancer.gov). The SEER database is updated annually and provided to the public. Since 1998, the Centers for Disease Control and Prevention (CDC), the American Cancer Society (ACS), the NCI, and the North American Association of Central Cancer Registries have collaborated on the Annual Report to the Nation on the Status of Cancer. SEER data are used by countless researchers and clinicians, along with legislators and policymakers. SEER and CMS have also partnered to form the SEER-Medicare Linked Database. SEER continues to collect clinical and demographic information, and CMS provides Medicare claims for covered health care services of patients with Medicare eligibility until death. The linkage of these two data sources allows for a unique collaboration incorporating epidemiologic and health services research. Forde et al. (2015) used the SEER-Medicare database to examine the cost of treatment for elderly women with ovarian cancer in the Medicare population. Neoadjuvant chemotherapy (NACT) and primary debulking surgery (PDS) were compared for cost and effectiveness (Forde, 2015). NACT and PDS were comparable in stage IIIC disease, but PDS was associated with a 12% increase in cost in stage IV disease. In both groups, NACT was associated with a decreased 5-year overall survival (OS), with a hazard ratio (HR) of 1.27 and 1.19, respectively.

Although cancer registries have been mentioned here, a number of data registries exist for different patient populations in broader fields of medicine and across the disciplines of obstetrics and gynecology. The Pelvic Floor Disorders Registry (PFDR) is the national patient registry supported by the American Urogynecologic Society; it prospectively collects both patient and provider-reported outcomes of surgical and nonsurgical interventions for urogynecologic conditions (Weber, 2016). Although this database is fairly new, reproductive technology outcomes have been recorded extensively since 1985 in the Society for Assisted Reproductive Technology Clinic Outcome Reporting System (SART CORS). This database reports on more than 90% of in vitro fertilization (IVF) treatment cycles that are received in the United States, and the SART website currently lists 117 publications that have used its results (www.SART.org).

Registry studies are not without limitations, however. Certain variables—particularly patient-reported or quality-of-life–associated outcomes—are often not included. Furthermore, they contain only in-hospital data and are subject to possible coding bias. Despite these potential constraints, the construction and maintenance of these prospective registries help clinicians and patients evaluate realistic outcome data to help guide their decision making.

## Quality Improvement

**Quality improvement (QI) is a unique format of HSR, encompassing both research and QI program development to improve the quality of health care.** The National Academy of Medicine defines quality in health care as the direct correlation between the level of improved health services and the desired health outcomes of individuals and populations (https://nam.edu). QI projects can be developed and conducted within small practices, in large hospital systems, or on a much larger national and international scale. The Health Resources and Services Administration (HRSA), part of the U.S. Department of Health and Human Services, provides a toolkit to help develop and implement QI projects (www.hrsa.gov). There are numerous organizations and committees whose sole purpose is to examine the issue of health care quality. In 1990 the National Committee for Quality Assurance was founded as a not-for-profit organization to help build consensus around important health care quality issues. It has a simple formula: "Measure, Analyze, Improve, Repeat" (www.ncqa.org). The National Quality Forum (NQF) is a not-for-profit, nonpartisan, membership-based organization whose mission is to "lead national collaborations to improve health and health care quality through measurement" (qualityforum.org). Their vision is "to be the convener of key public and private sector leaders to establish national priorities and goals to achieve health care that is safe, effective, patient-centered, timely, efficient, and equitable." The American Medical Association (AMA) also convenes the Physician Consortium for Performance Improvement (PCPI). It is physician-led program with a mission "to align patient-centered care, performance measurement and quality improvement" (www.ama-assn.org).

The CMS Physician Quality Reporting System (PQRS) was the first quality reporting program to focus on the care given to Medicare beneficiaries. In 2015, the CMS began applying a negative payment adjustment to providers and groups who did not meet requirements of reporting data to PQRS. The CMS quality payment program has since transitioned to the merit-based incentive payment system (MIPS) and alternative payment model (APM) in an attempt to better correlate payments to both quality and cost of care. Under MIPS, clinicians report outcome data and are then evaluated according to quality of care, promoter interoperability, cost, and improvement activities. The last of these, improvement activities, is a marker for clinician quality improvement initiatives and highlights the important role of QI in new health care legislation, payment modeling, and clinical care.

The role of quality improvement is also felt heavily in surgical specialties. CMS and other payers are increasingly refusing to pay for complications of surgery deemed preventable. The American College of Surgeons National Surgical Quality Improvement Program (ACS NSQIP) helps surgeons and hospitals identify preventable surgical complications. Data are collected directly from patient's charts by a surgical clinical reviewer (SCR), rather than collecting data from billing codes. In 2009, Hall et al. published data on 118 hospitals nationally participating in ACS NSQIP from 2006 to 2007; they reported that 82% of hospitals had improved risk-adjusted complication rates and 66% of hospitals had improved risk-adjusted mortality compared with their own prior rates reported the year before (Hall, 2009). By the end of 2007, ACS NSQIP had enrolled 183 hospitals and reported that participating hospitals avoided an average of 52.5 complications per year. ACS NSQIP helps identify and rectify preventable surgical outcomes. QI projects are a necessity for all health care providers and health care institutions and have already made an impact on a variety of patient outcomes in gynecologic patients.

Perhaps the most studied and replicated QI initiative in gynecology to date is the Enhanced Recovery After Surgery (ERAS) protocol. The initial investigators of ERAS found that many common surgical practices, including delayed feeding and preoperative bowel preparation, may actually be detrimental to patient recovery. The goal of ERAS is to decrease patient length of stay and patient complications through the introduction of multimodal pain regimens; postoperative diet, fluid, and activity modifications; and antibiotic and venous thromboembolism prophylaxis. Although standardization of recommendations and full compliance with recommendations are often problematic in individual institutions' implementations of the ERAS system, QI efforts have been shown to reduce opioid use, improve postoperative pain, and decrease patient length of stay (Kalogera, 2013). In this and other aspects of patient care, QI initiatives are capable of systematically challenging non–evidence-based medicine, evaluating the quality of care delivered, and introducing novel action plans to improve patient outcomes.

## Cost-Effectiveness Analysis

The term *cost-effectiveness analysis* has become a catchall term referring to all health economic analyses. The cost of health care continues to rise in the United States and was expected to exceed $3.9 trillion in 2022. This exponential and unsustainable economic burden makes health economic analysis an increasingly relevant tool. **There are four methods of health economic analysis, although cost-effectiveness analysis (CEA) is the most commonly used method. The other three methods are cost-utility analysis (CUA), cost-minimization analysis (CMA), and cost-benefit analysis (CBA).** CEA compares relative costs and outcomes of varying treatments by measuring cost per unit of effectiveness (e.g., additional survival time, number of adverse events, etc.). It determines the incremental cost-effectiveness ratio (ICER), or the ratio of the difference in costs to the difference in effectiveness between two strategies. This value is often used when determining the allocation of resources for treatment or intervention. CUA instead takes into account the quality of life associated with each intervention by using quality-adjusted life-years (QALYs). This metric represents the differences in survival and quality of life among interventions. CUA is an important effectiveness measure when morbidity and mortality are affected by an intervention. CMA assumes comparable effectiveness among intervention strategies and is simply a comparison of the mean cost of each intervention. CBA incorporates not only the monetary expense of intervention but also the costs of the consequences of each intervention.

In CEA an intervention has traditionally been considered cost-effective if the ICER is less than $50,000 per QALY societal willingness to pay threshold, although this is defined with some leeway. It is important to understand that the term *cost-effective* does not represent an intervention's ability to save money; instead, it is a statement that the additional cost of that intervention is worthwhile based on the improved efficacy it achieves. This methodology often has been used in obstetric and gynecologic research. For example, a 2014 CEA compared conservative versus surgical management for the treatment of stress urinary incontinence. The estimated ICER for surgical management was $32,132 per QALY, which fell beneath the threshold of $50,000. Thus the authors concluded that surgical management was more cost-effective at 1 year compared with conservative management strategies (Richardson, 2014). Cost-effectiveness research is an integral part of understanding the costs and quality of health care, a dilemma that must be addressed as the cost of health care continues to rise.

## NEW HORIZONS: VALUE IN HEALTH CARE

The discussion of value in health care is gaining interest. Value in health care is defined as "the health outcomes achieved per dollar spent" (Porter, 2006). Outcomes are inherently linked to the medical condition of interest, whereas the "dollar spent" represents the total amount spent during a cycle of care, not the cost of individual service. Porter argues that "the proper unit for measuring value should encompass all services or activities that jointly determine success in meeting a set of patient needs. These needs are determined by the patient's medical condition, defined as an interrelated set of medical circumstances that are best addressed in an integrated way…and that value should be measured for everything included in that care" (Porter, 2010). Large clinical societies are also recognizing the importance of this field: The American Society of Clinical Oncology (ASCO) is developing a conceptual framework to assess the value of cancer treatment options, many of which are accompanied by a significant cost burden (Schnipper, 2015). Although the study of value in health care is in its infancy, it is increasingly recognized as a promising navigational tool in an era of ever-rising costs and growing complexity of patient care.

### Acknowledgment

The authors wish to acknowledge the contributions of Dr. Jonathan R. Foote, one of the authors of the previous edition of this chapter.

### KEY REFERENCES

Centers for Disease Control and Prevention (CDC). Pneumocystis pneumonia—Los Angeles. *MMWR.* 1981;30(21):250–252.

Cochrane et al. *Effectiveness and efficiency: random reflections on health services.* London: Nuffield Provincial Hospitals Trust; 1972.

Congressional Budget Office (CBO). *Research on the Comparative Effectiveness of Medical Treatments: Issues and Options for an Expanded Federal Role.* Washington, DC: CBO; 2007.

Coodin FJ, Uchida CM, Murphy CH. Phocomelia: report of three cases. *CMAJ.* 1962;87:735–739.

D'Arcy LP, Rich EC. From comparative effectiveness research to patient-centered outcomes research: policy history and future directions. *Neurosurg Focus.* 2012;33(1):E7.

Forde GK, Chang J, Ziogas A, et al. Costs of treatment for elderly women with advanced ovarian cancer in a Medicare population. *Gynecol Oncol.* 2015;137(3):479–484.

Gayle HD, Keeling RP, Garcia-Tunon M, et al. Prevalence of the human immunodeficiency virus among university students. *N Engl J Med.* 1990;323(22):1538–1541.

Gehlbach SH. *Interpreting the Medical Literature.* 4th ed. New York: McGraw-Hill; 2002.

Grimes DA, Schulz KF. Bias and causal associations in observational research. *Lancet.* 2002;359:248–252.

Grimes DA, Schulz KF. Surrogate end points in clinical research: hazardous to your health. *Obstet Gynecol.* 2005;105:1114–1118.

Grodstein F, Manson JE, Stampfer MJ. Postmenopausal hormone use and secondary prevention of coronary events in the Nurses Health Study. *Ann Intern Med.* 2001;135(1):1–8.

Grondin SC, Schieman C. Evidence-based medicine: levels of evidence and evaluation systems. In: *Difficult Decisions in Thoracic Surgery.* London: Springer-Verlag; 2011.

Hall BL, Hamilton BH, Richards K, et al. Does surgical quality improve in the American College of Surgeons National Surgical Quality Improvement Program: an evaluation of all participating hospitals. *Ann Surg.* 2009;250(3):363–376.

Havrilesky LH, et al. Comparative effectiveness research in gynecologic oncology. In: Barakat RR, Berchuck A, eds. *Principles and Practice of Gynecologic Oncology.* 6th ed. Philadelphia: Lippincott Williams & Wilkins; 2013a:501–521.

Havrilesky LJ, Moorman PG, Lowery WJ, et al. Oral contraceptive pills as primary prevention for ovarian cancer: a systematic review and meta-analysis. *Obstet Gynecol.* 2013b;122(1):139–147.

Hennekens CH, DeMets D. The need for large-scale randomized evidence without undue emphasis on small trials, meta-analyses, or subgroup analyses. *JAMA.* 2009;302:2361–2362.

Herbst AL, Ulfelder H, Poskanzer DC. Adenocarcinoma of the vagina: association of maternal stilbestrol therapy with tumor appearance in young women. *N Engl J Med.* 1971;284(16):878–881.

Higgins JPT, Green S, eds. *Cochrane Handbook for Systematic Reviews of Interventions* Version 5.1.0 [updated March 2011]. The Cochrane Collaboration; 2011. Available at https://training.cochrane.org/handbook/current.

Iglehart JK. Prioritzing comparative-effectiveness research—IOM recommendations. *N Engl J Med.* 2009;361(4):325–328.

Institute of Medicine (IOM). *Initial National Priorities for Comparative Effectiveness Research.* Washington, DC: National Academies Press; 2009.

Kalogera E, Bakkum-Gamez JN, Jankowski CJ, et al. Enhanced Recovery in gynecologic surgery. *Obstet Gynecol.* 2013;122:319–328.

Normand SL, Sykora K, Li P, et al. Readers guide to critical appraisal of cohort studies: 3. Analytical strategies to reduce confounding. *BMJ.* 2005;330:960–962.

Patient Protection and Affordable Care Act, 42 U.S.C. § 18001 (2010).

Perren et al. A phase 3 trial of bevacizumab in ovarian cancer. *NEJM* 2011;365:2484–2496.

Porter ME, Teisberg EO. *Redefining Health Care: Creating Value-Based Competition Based on Results.* Boston: Harvard Business School Press; 2006.

Porter ME. What is value in healthcare? *N Engl J Med.* 2010;363(26): 2477–2481.

Richardson, et al. A cost-effectiveness analysis of conservative versus surgical management for the initial treatment of stress urinary incontinence. Am J Obstet Gynecol 2014; 211(5): 565.e1–6.

Rochon PA, Gurwitz JH, Sykora K, et al. Reader's guide to critical appraisal of cohort studies: 1. Role and design. *BMJ.* 2005;330:895–897.

Rossouw JE, Anderson JL, Prentice RL, et al. Risks and benefits of estrogen plus progesterone in health postmenopausal women: principle results from the women's health initiative randomized controlled trial. *JAMA.* 2002;288(3):321–333.

Roland M, Torgerson DJ. What are pragmatic trials? *BMJ.* 1998; 316(7127):285.

**Full references and Suggested readings for this chapter can be found on ExpertConsult.com.**

# 6 Medical-Legal Risk Management

*James M. Kelley III, Gretchen M. Lentz*

## KEY POINTS

- Malpractice is patient injury secondary to failure to exercise that degree of care used by reasonably careful physician of like qualifications
- Negligence is failure to extend the degree of diligence and care that a reasonably and ordinarily prudent person would exercise
- Informed consent is the physician's fiduciary duty to give the patient all the information needed for the patient to make an intelligent decision about therapies offered.
- Communication is the cornerstone of good care-verbal and written
- CAP -communication, anticipation, preparation can help reduce medical errors, improve patient safety and reduce medical legal risk

The word *malpractice* evokes guttural responses in physicians and health care providers. This is perhaps most true in the areas of obstetrics and gynecology, where the physical damages are often catastrophic and the economic damages reach millions of dollars. The fear of being unjustly involved in litigation and judged by nonphysicians as liable, despite having provided reasonable and appropriate care, seems unavoidable to many conscientious health care providers. The little-known reality, however, is that the growing consensus of empirical data on outcomes of malpractice actions shows that the legal system actually works for the health care provider more often than it does not. Understanding how the system works and making minor practice modifications can greatly minimize the risk of legal exposure by avoiding claims and adverse outcomes.

**A medical negligence case is composed of three basic elements: a deviation from the standard of care, proximate causation, and damages. Each of these elements is required to be proved by way of "competent" expert testimony.** The definition of "competent" varies state to state, but all states are uniform in requiring a physician to agree that malpractice occurred and that it directly resulted in injury. **A deviation from the standard of care,** though a cumbersome legal phrase, **is simply a failure to act reasonably compared with another health care provider in the same or similar clinical circumstance.** A deviation from the standard of care can be an act (intraoperative bowel perforation, administration of the wrong medication, etc.) or an omission (failure to run the bowel intraoperatively if a bowel injury is possible or failure to review laboratory results in a timely manner).

Proximate causation is often a more medically complex component of a malpractice action. The law requires that the deviation from the standard of care be *a* direct, proximate cause of injury to the plaintiff. It is important to note that the deviation does not have to be *the* exclusive cause of injury, but rather need only be *a* direct proximate cause. **Proximate cause, legally, merely means that with appropriate or reasonable treatment, the injury would not have occurred.**

The final element of a malpractice claim is damages. **Damages can be both economic and noneconomic.** Economic damages include easily quantifiable losses such as past and future medical bills and past and future wage losses. Noneconomic damages include factors such as past and future physical pain, emotional suffering, and, in certain instances, wrongful death. To be successful, the plaintiff, through presentation of expert testimony, must prove each of these elements to a probability. A failure on any one of the elements will result in a verdict for the defendant.

As mentioned, many health care providers will be surprised to learn what the growing consensus of empirical data reflects regarding medical claims. A review of approximately 1400 closed malpractice claims from five different liability carriers showed that only 3% of claims filed had no verifiable medical injuries to justify a claim. Additionally, 37% of the 3% did not involve errors but rather would be what a physician would commonly refer to as "frivolous." Despite common perceptions about runaway juries and lottery verdicts levied against faultless physicians, the study demonstrated that 84% of the claims that did not involve errors nonetheless resulted in nonpayment. Conversely, approximately six times that rate of claims resulted in nonpayment to the plaintiff, despite the presence of medical errors and verifiable injuries (Studdert, 2006) (Box 6.1).

A 2017 study of 10,915 claims from the Physician Insurers' Association of America data-sharing project specifically presented data in malpractice claims for obstetrics and gynecology procedures (Glaser, 2017). Fig. 6.1 shows the percent of claims by method of resolution of all closed claims. The majority (59.5%) were dropped, withdrawn, or dismissed. Claims most often related to gynecologic surgery, but obstetric procedures were more expensive. They also reported a 55% decrease in paid claims from 1992 to 2014. On the flip side, the average payment per pain claim rose 16% and there was an increase in payments greater than $1 million. Fig. 6.2 shows the procedures most commonly associated with closed claims.

Although these data should be heartening for health care providers, they do little to eliminate burdens of excessive litigation costs, time away from practice and families, and the stress of participating in litigation. **The goal for conscientious providers must be one focused on risk management: balancing improved patient care and minimizing medical legal risk.**

A safe health care system must further incorporate efficient redundancies that promote safety without being cost prohibitive. **"Errors can be prevented by designing systems that make it hard for people to do the wrong thing and easy to do the right thing" (IOM, 2000).**

Realizing lawsuits will inevitably occur, what follows is a brief historical overview along with practical insights aimed at helping

**BOX 6.1** What Constitutes Medical Malpractice?

To successfully maintain a medical malpractice action, a plaintiff must be able to establish three distinct elements of his or her case by way of expert testimony:

1. *Deviation from the standard of care:* The health care provider deviated from what a reasonable provider would have done in the same or similar circumstances.
2. *Causation:* The deviation was a direct cause of the injury suffered.
3. *Damages:* Economic and noneconomic damages were suffered as result of the injury.

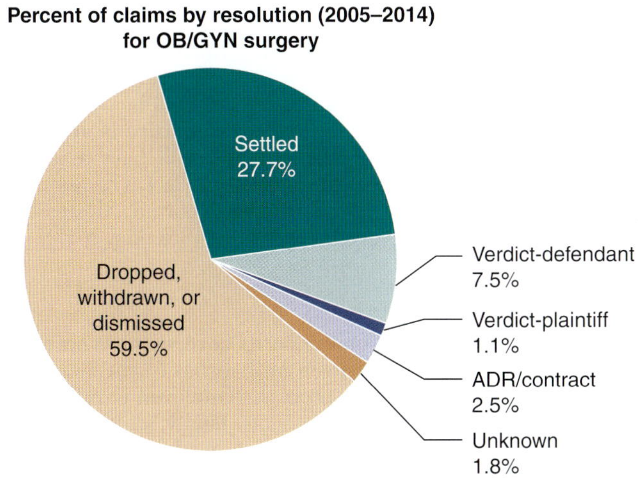


**Fig. 6.1** Method of resolution of all closed claims related to obstetric and gynecologic procedures. *ADR,* Alternative dispute resolution. (From Glaser LM, Alvi FA, Milan MP. Trends in malpractice claims for obstetric and gynecologic procedures, 2005 through 2014. *Am J Obstet Gynecol.* 2017;217:340.e1–6.)

one enhance patient care and communication, minimize the risk of involvement in meritless litigation, and provide the best defense in the event a claim is made.

## HISTORICAL PERSPECTIVE

*A doctor who knows nothing of the law and a lawyer who knows nothing of medicine are deficient in essential requisites of their professions.*

—**David Paul Brown, 1795–1872**

British North America inherited its law, as well as its language, from England. Most European countries originally occupied by the Romans adopted a form of law based on the Roman law codes. That law is called *civil law.* England's law, on the other hand, was based mainly on Scandinavian (Danish) law with a dose of folk law of undetermined origin thrown in. It was called the *common law.* One should not be deceived by its name. It was not law designed to protect the common man. It takes its name from the fact that it was the law that was common to all of England by about the year 1240. The two forms of law differ significantly.

**Civil law is a codified system of laws.** That is, the laws are spelled out in a series of written statutes adopted by the jurisdiction. Civil law therefore tends to be fairly static. **Common law is largely law made by judges.** It may incorporate some statutory elements on specific issues, but even statutes are subject to judicial interpretation. Judges in the civil law are academics specially trained for their positions and act as prosecutor, judge, and jury. Civil law is therefore inquisitorial in nature and heavily dependent on the written word. In contrast, common law is an adversarial system in which the oral argument between the parties plays a much larger role. Judges are chosen from the practicing bar and are not usually academics. The judge is essentially a referee and instructs the jury, which makes the ultimate decision on the merits of the case. In common law, the law is made by judges who hear a disputed case on appeal. Those decisions become precedent for future cases. However, higher appellate courts or

| 2010–2014 | | | | | |
|---|---|---|---|---|---|
| **Procedure** | **Closed claims** | Paid claims | **% Paid-to-closed** | **Total indemnity** | **Average indemnity** |
| Operative procedures on the uterus | 943 | 262 | 27.8 | $73,198,625 | $279,384 |
| Cesarean section deliveries | 879 | 287 | 32.7 | $158,741,223 | $553,105 |
| Manually assisted deliveries | 730 | 261 | 35.8 | $136,706,000 | $523,778 |
| Miscellaneous manual examinations and nonoperative procedures | 510 | 124 | 24.3 | $52,599,371 | $424,188 |
| Operative procedures on the fallopain tubes & ovaries, exclusive of sterilization | 278 | 96 | 34.5 | $27,728,721 | $288,841 |
| Diagnostic interview, evaluation, or consultation | 237 | 39 | 16.5 | $9,343,641 | $239,581 |
| No care rendered | 184 | 24 | 13.0 | $6,983,939 | $290,997 |
| Vacuum extraction | 145 | 69 | 47.6 | $30,536,872 | $442,563 |
| Prescription of medication | 114 | 33 | 28.9 | $19,011,375 | $576,102 |
| General physical examination | 101 | 28 | 27.7 | $9,530,500 | $340,375 |

**Fig. 6.2** Procedures most commonly associated with obstetrics and gynecology closed claims, 2010 to 2014. (From Glaser LM, Alvi FA, Milan MP. Trends in malpractice claims for obstetric and gynecologic procedures, 2005 through 2014. *Am J Obstet Gynecol.* 2017;217:340.e1–6.)

future appellate courts of the same level can overturn or overrule a prior decision if circumstances change or new information develops. Therefore change, albeit slow and irregular, is a constant element of the common law.

Under the early common law, to bring a civil action, a King's Writ was needed; therefore little attention was paid to compensating the individual for personal wrongs (tort law). Doctors were essentially immune from suit for malpractice. Technically some suits might have been pursued as contract suits, but written contracts were highly unusual between a physician and his patient, and without the written document such suits became almost impossible for the plaintiff to win.

In 1346, the bubonic plague arrived in Italy. It spread over Europe rapidly but did not reach England until 1348. The major effect of the epidemic occurred between 1348 and 1351, but the bubonic plague became endemic and continued more or less uninterrupted until 1381. It is estimated that between 1348 and 1351, 50% of the population died, and by 1381, two-thirds of the English population was decimated by the epidemic. (Because there was no accurate census at the time, such figures are estimates based on church records, burial records, tax rolls, and contemporary accounts.)

The loss of manpower was a major blow to the English economy. Overnight, people became as important as real property (land) and personal property (including livestock) in the English economy. Therefore a physician's mistake that deprived the economy of a worker became an important enough matter to be brought before the courts. Physicians suddenly lost their immunity for practice errors. Actually, it was an even worse scenario: The physician became strictly liable for an unfavorable outcome, and because there was no tort law (law compensating the individual for personal wrongs), the physician was prosecuted under the criminal law for mayhem. By 1364 it had become obvious that this was too draconian a remedy, and two property terms that had been previously used in livestock cases were introduced to permit civil malpractice cases. *Trespass* (trespass by force and arms) was charged for direct injury and *trespass on the case* for indirect injury.

These same concepts, refined over the centuries, were brought to the North American colonies and adopted almost entirely by the American court system after independence. In the early 1800s, the modern concept of negligence replaced trespass and trespass on the case. In the period of rapid industrialization after the Civil War, American courts refined these claims. **The four elements of a cause of action for medical negligence are as follows:**

1. **Duty:** The obligation created through physician patient relationship.
2. **Breach:** A deviation from the "standard of care" for a reasonable practitioner in the same clinical circumstance.
3. **Proximate causation:** A direct and foreseeable connection between breach and injury.
4. ***Damages:*** Economic (medical costs, wage loss, etc.) and noneconomic (physical and emotional pain and suffering).

**There is no greater asset in risk management for the clinician than a strong physician-patient relationship.** Patients are typically trusting and respectful of their providers, which gives the best opportunity to avoid litigation. The typical patient will become a plaintiff when he or she loses trust in the provider or fails to get understandable answers to the complex medical issues surrounding a less than optimal outcome. "I don't know or understand either what happened or how this happened" is the statement that begins nearly all inquiries into the quality of care. This chapter provides insights that will allow the physician to supply answers to the patient, to document appropriately, and to participate more functionally in a medical-legal claim while maintaining a high level of care and professionalism.

## REPRODUCTIVE MEDICINE AND THE COURTS

No area of medicine receives more court scrutiny, legal scholarly review, or social commentary (even including presidential directives) than the fields of obstetrics and gynecology. In addition, some of the most expensive categories of malpractice claims arise from the obstetrician/gynecologist's practice (pregnancy/birth claims, operative procedures on the uterus, prescription medication errors, and failure to diagnose breast cancer). Practically speaking, nearly every malpractice issue that has been litigated in American courts deserves a volume of its own to discuss and dissect adequately. Indeed, a single chapter in a general textbook of gynecology can do little but cover the generalities and touch on the more important issues the courts have addressed. Overall, applying the four elements noted previously to most claims, a malpractice case is typically a review of case facts applied to the "standard of care" and "proximate cause" through medical testimony to determine whether care was simply "reasonable." It is important to note that the care does not have to be perfect, nor do all decisions have to be correct. Instead, **if care is attentive and the decisions rational, the provider will have a strong defense position regardless of outcome. In** fact, a review of all paid claims for obstetrician/gynecologists reported a decrease in paid claims from 1992 compared with 2014 (Schaffer, 2017).

## PRACTICAL INSIGHT

**Medical-legal risk management, at its core, centers on communication in both the written and verbal form.** Awareness of the common pitfalls in the processes employed in communicating information to patients, patients' family, and concurrent and subsequent care providers will be invaluable if problems or litigation arise. The medical record, institutional policies and guidelines, and information communicated to patients (prospective plaintiffs) are the only information attorneys, claim representatives, and reviewing expert physicians have available to judge the validity of a potential malpractice claim. The following discussion examines good practices to improve communications with patients (both before and after treatment), improve the accuracy of the medical records, and provide useful information about navigating the litigation process to your best outcome.

### Communication With the Patient

Physicians well understand that the relationship with a patient is in large measure a relationship of trust. More often than not, a perceived breach of that trust is the impetus for a patient to seek the advice of an outsider for explanations about unfortunate medical outcomes. **It must become a routine practice for physicians to discuss potential problems with their patients thoroughly and carefully before treatment.** Taking the time necessary to assess a patient's understanding of the procedures and possible outcomes and answering all the patient's questions are critical to managing and controlling expectations. Concurrent notations in the record that you have in fact reviewed all risks and benefits of a potential treatment, thoroughly explained alternative treatments or procedures, and answered all patient questions provide important evidence of careful and appropriate treatment should it later become necessary to demonstrate this (Box 6.2).

**BOX 6.2** Practice Tip

**Sample Progress Note**

Risks/benefits/alternatives discussed with patient. All questions answered in full.

The 11 words in the sample progress note shown in Box 6.2 are an invaluable resource in the event of a complication or litigation. Although this is brief documentation, it does indicate the physician personally reviewed the critical elements mentioned earlier and allowed for questions. This note portrays the provider discussing the case with the patient, which will supplement the standard preprinted consent that is more "legalese" than substantive documentation.

## Informed Consent, Informed Refusal of Care, Surgical Documentation, and Postoperative Care

**Surgery in particular requires more discussion and documentation than office visits.** A thorough note tells a story of why a surgery is necessary or indicated:

1. Surgical indication (diagnosis and nature of condition or illness calling for intervention)
2. Supportive diagnostic testing
3. Correlation with proposed surgery and clinical symptoms
4. Conservative treatment course and failure
5. Impact of preoperative condition on the patient's activities and quality of life
6. Patient goals and concerns

**Informed consent is a process, not just a signed piece of paper. It is the conversation that occurred with the patient to review the details of the forms and documents:**

1. Alternatives to surgery (including the option of taking no action)
2. Benefits of surgery
3. Discussion of major risks
4. Probability of success (no result should ever be guaranteed)

Consider underlining or highlighting the major risk or risks listed on your consent form, such as bleeding, infection, and damage to nearby organs, nerves, and muscles. If you use an online version for informed consent, consider printing it out so you can add items in the lines provided and underline particular sections relevant to the patient's surgery. The form can be scanned in.

Many decision aids have been developed to help with patient education. The American College of Obstetricians and Gynecologists has partnered with the Choosing Wisely campaign. This program promotes conversations between clinicians and patients by helping patients choose care that is supported by evidence, not duplicative of other tests or procedures already received, free from harm, and truly necessary. There are specialty-specific lists of "Things Providers and Patients Should Question." This does not dictate care, but the patient-friendly materials are meant to spur conversation about what is appropriate and necessary treatment. Decision aids are interventions that support patients by making their decisions explicit, providing information about options and associated benefits and harms, and helping clarify congruence between decisions and personal values. Decision aids may be pamphlets, videos, or web-based tools. People can use decision aids when there is more than one option and neither is clearly better or when options have benefits and harms that people value differently. Compared with usual care across a wide variety of decision contexts, people exposed to decision aids felt more knowledgeable, better informed, and clearer about their values and had more accurate risk perception. The median effect of decision aids on length of consultation was 2.6 minutes longer (24 vs. 21; 7.5% increase) (Stacey, 2017). Patient decision aids are associated with improved decision quality and decision-making processes without worse patient or health system outcomes.

The electronic medical record can be helpful for documentation using smart phrases for the previously mentioned topics, as well as for documenting the following:

- Patient education materials given
- YouTube videos recommended
- Specific website recommendations
- Shared decision-making steps (Légaré, 2018)
- Questions answered and concerns addressed (Sepucha, 2016)
- Details of postoperative limitations regarding missing work or caring for children

Of course, any smart phrases must be edited for individual patient circumstances.

These steps will help anticipate what could go wrong and help mitigate risk by planning ahead.

**Patients can refuse medical treatment. Every reasonable effort should be made to protect the patient's health, but autonomy should be respected.** Document the need for a test, medication, intervention, or surgery. Explain the needed intervention in language the patient can understand. Explain the risks of not having the intervention so the patient can make a decision. In nonemergency situations, a patient may need to speak with other people. Keep the conversation open. In emergencies, document that the patient chose to leave against medical advice; that all the risks, benefits, and alternatives were discussed; and that the patient chose to leave. Consultation with others might be sought.

Detailed surgical templates can be helpful. However, using templates without adding important surgical details and findings for individual patients is careless and potentially dangerous. Document the following:

1. Patient consent
2. Intraoperative findings, especially unexpected findings
3. Equipment and devices used
4. Key events (e.g., how the ureter was identified)
5. Abandonment of or change in procedure and the reasons this occurred

**Postoperative care and examination is an area of concern because documentation of this phase of care is often lacking.** Postoperative pain level is important to attend to. You or a colleague needs to be available during the postoperative period to care for the patient and to answer patient, family and/or nursing questions. Be careful not to disregard questionable postoperative findings or laboratory results. However distressing it may be, do not delay a return to the operating room when necessary. Call for consultation when appropriate for potential urologic or bowel complications, serious infection concerns, or bleeding emergencies. Because most surgeries are performed on an outpatient basis now, a phone call the next day by the physician or nurse is not only appreciated but provides a chance to review medications and instructions.

Maintaining an adequate procedural volume and appropriate technical competence and judgment for procedures is likely necessary to avoid adverse outcomes and to avoid litigation risk.

## Poor Outcome

**In the unfortunate event of a poor outcome, it is imperative for the physician to communicate more, not less, with the patient or the patient's family where appropriate.** Health care providers often dramatically change, or end entirely, their relationship with patients after a maloccurrence. For example, in situations in which the patient may have ongoing care issues but is transferred to a tertiary center or a different specialist, there is often minimal or no ongoing relationship. Despite what may be the urge to distance yourself from an unpleasant or uncomfortable interaction, keep in mind that your patient and his or her family members will begin to assess whether you are forthcoming with them at this very time. If there is an attempt to avoid interaction it can, and likely will, be misperceived as an attempt to avoid explaining the cause or causes of the bad outcome. It is important that your trust relationship with the patient and the patient's family continues at this crucial time and that they feel you are willing to answer all questions.

**BOX 6.3** Practice Tip

Communication with the patient when a problem occurs is an opportunity to explain how, despite vigilance, the poor outcome happened. Patients will naturally have questions, and most who contact a malpractice attorney are doing so to get answers to questions they feel were not sufficiently answered by the health care provider.

When discussing the outcome or problem, revisit the discussion of risks and outcomes at the time of the informed consent. Reiterate the information you previously provided, and explain how this result is related to the risks previously discussed, if appropriate. Finally, it is also important that you are involved in establishing the plan for care going forward, even if it is outside your specialty. Remaining involved preserves the physician-patient relationship. Patients are far less likely to file claims against physicians with whom they have an ongoing, trusting relationship. It is therefore important to make yourself available as long as is necessary to assure the patient and his or her family that you are answering all their questions. Absence or avoidance will create suspicion by the patient or another family member and can ultimately lead them to seek answers to their questions from an outside source, most often an attorney.

Once again, it is imperative you write contemporaneous and accurate notes. The timing of such notes, combined with their detail and clarity, will begin to establish a good defense in the event the records are reviewed for a possible claim. It is easy to defend conscientious care, regardless of outcome, if the record supports you (Box 6.3).

When patients are lost to follow up after a complication, possibly when transferred to a tertiary medical center or another service, legal inquiries often start when the medical bills are turned over to collections. Do not pick a fight with a patient who had a poor outcome.

**Times are changing in regard to communication, disclosure, and apologies in medicine.** Some hospitals offer disclosure training to help with difficult discussions regarding poor outcomes (Shapiro, 2018). Each state may have different apology statutes, so always check with your risk management team and insurance carrier. However, clinicians should not under- or over-rely on each statute. A sincere, empathetic statement might be appreciated. For example:

"I am so sorry you are going through this."
"I am so sorry you suffered the complication."

These statements are very different from the message conveyed by a statement such as "I am sorry, this is my fault. I cut the ureter and did not recognize prior to closure."

The first two apologies show empathy without admitting fault. That is protected and maintains a relationship in this critical period. However, in some states the apology may not shield the provider from the factual admissions that follow. A recent study found almost three times as many participants receiving a full apology would (probably/definitely) recommend the hospital compared with those receiving no apology (34.1% vs 13.6% respectively [$p < 0.0001$]) (Fisher, 2020).

Managing a poor outcome well is critical and can require skills that are not taught in medical school (Slade, 2017).

## Cancellations and "No Shows"

Cancellations and "no shows" of patients' follow-up appointments are often ignored in the busy clinic or office; however, they commonly lead to subsequent malpractice suits. Each cancellation or no show should be documented in the chart. The treating physician should then review the chart, and, where appropriate, a letter or phone call should be made to the patient. All efforts to communicate with the patient should be documented.

## Coverage Arrangements

As mentioned earlier, improper coverage arrangements may lead to charges of abandonment. Poor communication among coverage groups often leads to offended patients and can be the first step on the path to a malpractice suit. **Developing thorough patient sign-out protocols can aid in transmitting important information during patient handoffs.** In a prospective resident handoff improvement program at nine hospitals with more than 10,740 patient admissions, the medical error rate decreased by 23% from the preintervention period to the postintervention period, and the rate of preventable adverse events decreased by 30% (Starmer, 2014).

## Medication Errors

About 1.5 million people are injured each year in the United States as a result of medication errors, according to a 2006 review of medication management in the U.S. health care system by the Institute of Medicine (now the National Academy of Medicine) (IOM, 2007). In a 2017 study of all medical specialties, medication errors and medication treatment made up a large share of medical malpractice cases (24.5%), although for obstetrician/gynecologists this was lower (8.8%). The results can range from minor allergic response to death. Medications pose a liability risk to both the institution and the provider.

The reasons for this include but are not limited to the frequency with which patients are being prescribed medication, the popularity of at-home prescription administration, and the many lookalike, sound-alike drugs. The Institute of Medicine report states, "The extra medical cost of treating drug-related injuries occurring in hospitals alone conservatively amounts to $3.5 billion a year, and this estimate does not take into account lost wages and productivity or additional health care costs" (IOM, 2007).

**Medication errors are always preventable through system and personal practice modifications.** Data show that 400,000 preventable drug-related injuries occur each year in hospitals (IOM, 2007). Another report states that adverse drug events cause more than 770,000 injuries and deaths each year and cost up to $5.6 million per hospital (AHRQ, 2015). Prescribing via the electronic medical record has reduced some errors and probably explains the drop in overall malpractice claims paid.

The National Coordinating Council for Medication Error and Prevention has approved the following definition of medication error:

> Any preventable event that may cause or lead to inappropriate medication use or patient harm, while the medication is in the control of the health care professional, patient, or consumer. Such events may be related to professional practice, health care products, procedures, and systems including: prescribing; order communication; product labeling, packaging and nomenclature; compounding; dispensing; distribution; administration; education; monitoring; and use. (FDA, 2016)

### Practical Tip

The reality of practice is that many orders are verbal, telephonic, or standing. **Verbal or telephonic orders should always be read back to the provider to verify drug, dosage, frequency, and method of administration**. This minimizes the likelihood of a communication lapse. Furthermore, telephonic orders are often signed after the medication is administered. Closely review these to be sure you are not validating the error as your own order. Litigation often occurs more than a year later, and remembering the details of a specific order will be difficult with an inconsistent record. If on review an error is noted, correct it in the record with a single line and the corrected information at the side. Note the time and date of your correction as well. Timely signing of electronic orders provides that date and time. Limiting verbal orders except in emergencies reduces errors.

Be aware of your orders and those of other providers as well, such as anesthesiologists, infectious disease specialists, and so on, to monitor for medication interactions. Standing orders often pose a risk in this circumstance.

## Communication through Medical Records

Once the litigation process has commenced, a plaintiff attorney's best friend is inaccurate or inconsistent documentation of the care provided. Inaccurate documentation can stem from a genuine standard-of-care issue; however, inaccuracies can also arise from use of inappropriate nomenclature. In either situation, the health care provider will be in the untenable position of attempting to defend a narrative note or deposition testimony that is factually inconsistent with literature, policies, or objective data in the medical record. Needless to say, in a courtroom, inconsistencies never favor the inconsistent party. **Careful attention to record keeping will not only demonstrate attentive care and rationally based treatment decisions but will ultimately become a provider's best defense in a courtroom.**

Within your hospital, facility, office, and charts, you must use nomenclature designed to standardize the verbiage used among providers. Unfortunately, despite the attempts at standardization, many health care providers have been slow to adapt. This is often based on variable levels of education by health care providers and is also generational. This increases not only the risk of inaccurate communication among health care providers but also the risk of a medical record replete with inconsistencies. Inconsistencies can be easily used to portray a provider as incompetent or disingenuous.

From a medicolegal risk management standpoint, it is critical to keep in mind that when a plaintiff's counsel attempts to determine whether medical malpractice may have occurred, the medical record is the primary (and often the only) source of information available to evaluate the potential claim. Any narrative notes supplied will be read against subsequent health care providers' notes and the objective data, such as laboratory results and imaging. As stated earlier, clearly noted and accurate recognition and description of reassuring and nonreassuring findings in the record will demonstrate attentive and competent care. However, inaccurate terminology, when read against the objective data, could result in the commencement of litigation.

The electronic medical record had introduced a new set of documentation problems. The following practices can help to avoid these problems:

- Avoid cutting and pasting from another patient's chart.
- Close notes in a timely fashion.
- Carrying forward notes from a past visit without carefully updating can lead to inaccuracies and potential fraudulent billing.

Many institutions have "open notes" where patients can read all of their chart notes now. This can be beneficial as patients may communicate errors that can be corrected.

Beyond the initial review phase of a potential claim, inconsistent and inaccurate nomenclature and record keeping will continue to present obstacles to a favorable resolution of the claim during the testimonial phase of trial. When a witness employs modified or nonstandardized nomenclature, other health care providers, including expert medical witnesses, do not necessarily understand the full extent of what is meant. This unclear communication can result in actual medical errors among providers or, at a minimum, the appearance of errors within a medical record (Box 6.4).

**BOX 6.4** Factual Scenario

In a previous deposition, a physician was questioned regarding a nursing narrative note:

A. Dr. Doe, do you expect the nurse to relay to you if there are any postoperative changes?
B. Any relevant postoperative changes should be relayed to me, particularly if there are more than one.
C. By relevant change, do you mean if any vital signs manifest persistent change?
D. I do not understand what that means. However, if a nurse sees vitals change, I want to know about it immediately, especially if it persists.

The narrative notes within the case included the nurse describing labile blood pressures. Using charting terminology such as *labile* created a scenario in which the physician had expectations of being told immediately and a medical record suggesting the call should have been made. Further testimony demonstrated that no information regarding these changes was relayed. The nurse testified as follows:

A. Did you relay to Dr. Doe that the blood pressures were labile?
B. No.
C. Why not?
D. Because I felt it was not necessarily significant and may be routine postop fluctuations.
E. So you felt it was unstable but not labile?
F. Yes.
G. So when you chart the word ***labile,*** you want the jury to believe it doesn't mean labile?
H. I guess.

**BOX 6.5** Practice Tip

The consistent use of appropriate nomenclature not only minimizes risk in the defense of a medicolegal action but also allows the physicians and nurses to communicate clearly by ensuring they are discussing the same findings and placing the same significance on those findings.

The example in Box 6.4 shows how the inappropriate and inconsistent nomenclature forced the physician to be critical of the nurse's actions, whereas the nurse attempted to separate herself from her own charting. This is not only a difficult posture to defend but also reflects poorly on the competency and truthfulness of the parties involved. Simply employing appropriate, consistent nomenclature would have provided an easy defense (Box 6.5).

## Alteration of Records

A medical malpractice case can go from defensible to indefensible immediately with an alteration of the record. An alteration is typically defined as an entry added to or redacted from the record to avoid culpability. In many states an alteration is a basis for punitive damages (noninsured). Furthermore, it may invalidate coverage under some professional policies. Most providers do not add for the purpose of deceit but to make the record more "complete" after an unfortunate outcome. Accordingly, it is not typical to chart after a shift has passed. In the event it is necessary, clearly note the entry as a "late entry" and date when it is entered and the date and time to which it refers. There is nothing wrong with a late entry if you accurately describe it as such. Today technology can, through impression, discern the sequence and time when notes were written and, using infrared light, whether the ink is the same. A record that can be alleged to be altered will cause a loss of credibility with any jury and may expose you to personal liability. Of course, electronic medical records are dated and timed and cannot be altered without a digital footprint.

## Responding to Patient Reviews

Your office should have a plan for dealing with patient reviews. They do affect business. Replies must be compliant with Health Insurance Portability and Accountability Act (HIPAA) regulations. A sample statement might be as follows:

> We appreciate your complaint and welcome the chance to discuss our position privately with. Your medical information is privileged, and we respect that privacy, so we cannot provide a detailed response here. Please contact us at your convenience so we can better understand your concern, and explain our strong belief in the care provided.

Your availability, responsiveness to complaints, and defense of service are opportunities to improve your care.

## Communication Consistent with Institutional Policies

Published institutional policies and procedures should be reviewed regularly and integrated into your daily practice. The purpose of the policies or protocols is not merely for The Joint Commission on Accreditation of Healthcare Organizations (JCAHO) or to fill shelf space but to effectuate patient care and create a consistent safe administration of medication and care to patients. However, each individual patient obviously deserves individual care and modifications to the policy or protocol as may be necessary. Policies and protocols relevant to the issues that are the bases of any litigation should be familiar to you *before* providing sworn testimony under oath. Because these written policies can form the basis of an accepted standard of care in your institution, any testimony or records inconsistent with these policies can be viewed by a jury as being outside the standard of care or negligent (Box 6.6).

In the example in Box 6.6, a lack of familiarity with the standard policy within the hospital created a scenario in which the physician and nurse were uncertain what the hospital expected. Compounding matters, the lack of familiarity with the policy and protocol before deposition created a scenario in which not only did the nurse provide testimony that she deviated from the policy but also she was forced to acknowledge a total lack of familiarity with the same. In short, **knowledge of and compliance with institutional policies, guidelines, and resources can demonstrate the implementation of appropriate care, and documentation can be the shield of your defense; conversely, ignorance of and deviation from such policies can provide a documented deviation from the standard of care that will be the sword of the plaintiff.** Reviewing, using, and incorporating professional guidelines into your patient discussions and charting can improve patient care and shield you in case of a lawsuit.

## When a Claim Is Made

The institution of a claim varies from state to state and is defined differently among various insurance policies. It is imperative that through your institution and insurance policy and within your state you have an understanding of what constitutes knowledge or notice of a claim. **When notice of a claim is received, it is imperative that you immediately notify your hospital or group administrator and your insurance company.** A failure to provide timely notification to relevant individuals can jeopardize insurance coverage or compromise your defense and, in a worst-case scenario, may potentially result in a default judgment for failure to timely respond. Although the legal system does move slowly, there are certain parameters, and timely responses are mandatory at the beginning of litigation.

Participation in a claim is aggravating, frightening, and an imposition on your professional or personal time. However, it is critical to avoid procrastination or deprioritization of the claim regardless of the level of merit or damages perceived by you. A lawsuit is typically commenced by the filing of a legal pleading known as a *complaint*. Thereafter, there will be a statutory amount of time for an *answer* to be filed on your behalf. The first portion of litigation is thereafter referred to as *discovery*. This is where each side exchanges information either through documents or sworn testimony between the sides—first regarding factual information and then regarding expert opinions in the claim. **A deposition is simply the opposing attorney's**

### BOX 6.6 Factual Scenario

Many gynecologic cases involve the failure to recognize postoperative bowel perforations or significant bleeding. Total abdominal hysterectomy usually carries with it a specific physician's postoperative orders or, more commonly, a hospital's postoperative policy or protocol. It is of critical importance that the nurse and physician both have an understanding of the specific details of the policy or protocol before executing care and before testifying regarding these issues. The following example highlights why this is important:

A. Are you aware as to whether or not there is a postoperative policy at this facility?
B. I don't know. I guess there probably is.
C. Do you agree that you, as a reasonable nurse, have a duty to follow the policy here at the facility?
D. I don't really know what the policy says, but I'm sure it's reasonable and yes I should probably follow it.
E. If you failed to follow the policy, can we agree that you would have been acting unreasonably and beneath the accepted standards of care?
F. I probably should follow a policy if it exists. I guess if I didn't, I was beneath the standard of care.

The nurse went on to define terms differently from the definition contained in the policy and testified that the physician with whom she was working was aware of her actions. When the physician was questioned, he testified as follows:

A. Do you expect the nurses to follow your specific orders and, when orders are not present specific to the chart, to follow policies or protocols that are in place for the delivery of health care to patients?
B. Absolutely.
C. For this patient, did you write a specific postoperative order?
D. No.
E. Your order says, "post total abdominal hysterectomy protocol"?
F. Yes.
G. Does that mean the nurse should follow the hospital's policy or protocol?
H. Absolutely.
I. Is a reasonable nurse allowed to deviate from that policy or protocol without calling you first?
J. No.

**opportunity to ask questions under oath that are reasonably calculated to lead to relevant discoverable evidence.**

Your deposition is an obligation, not an opportunity. In that regard it is critical that you meet with your attorney in advance of your deposition so that you can be prepared for the relevant issues. A critical review with your attorney of the care you provided is important so that you that can anticipate all areas of questioning and avoid surprise questioning under oath. The answers you give under oath are sworn testimony in the case, and often depositions circulate through the legal community even after the case closes. It is recommended that you meet at least 1 week in advance of your deposition with counsel for a preparatory session, which will allow you adequate time in the event your practice requires rescheduling that meeting, before you actually give your testimony at deposition. Additional preparation could include a mock deposition, or simulation in a question-and-answer format, with another attorney to give you a sense of the actual deposition. This can be very useful to isolate and review medically complex issues and to enhance your preparation for giving sworn testimony.

Your deposition testimony, along with that of the other factual witnesses, will supplement the medical record for the expert witnesses retained by all parties to litigation to use in formulating their opinions and testimony, all of which, in turn, will ultimately become the evidence jurors use to judge which positions they find most reasonable. **Accordingly, just as accurate, concise, and consistent communication in your medical record is a priority, so too should it be within your deposition.**

After discovery, cases are usually scheduled for jury trials based on individual court docket systems. You should plan on attending each day of your trial and participating in the trial all day and some evenings. Although it is no physician's desire to take time away from his or her practice to be in a courtroom, it is imperative that when you arrive you have an accurate medical record and deposition to support the reasonableness of the decisions you made at the time you made them (Box 6.7).

**BOX 6.7** Practice Tip

1. Secure and isolate the patient's complete medical record.
2. Make no additions, modifications, or alterations to that chart.
3. To preserve malpractice coverage, immediately notify either your institutional administrative or insurance representative of the claim.
4. Participate fully—and as a priority—in the defense of the quality of your care.

## Fraud and Abuse

In 1972, as part of the first amendments to the Medicaid and Medicare rules and regulations, Congress passed antifraud and abuse regulations. The first such laws were hardly more than a slap on the wrist. However, in 1977 Congress made those laws draconian. False statements include the following:

1. Knowingly and willfully making or causing to be made any false statement or representation of a material fact in seeking to obtain any benefit or payment
2. Fraudulently concealing or failing to disclose information affecting one's rights to a payment
3. Converting any benefit or payment rightfully belonging to another
4. Presenting or causing to be presented a claim for a physician's service knowing that the individual who furnished the service was not licensed as a physician

These also encompass false claims, bribes, kickbacks, rebates, or "any remuneration" and are felonies with a maximum penalty of 5 years in jail and a $25,000 fine possible for each such offense. (The law states that any provider who knowingly and willfully solicits, pays, offers, or receives any remuneration, in cash or in kind, directly or indirectly, overtly or covertly, to induce or in return for arranging for or ordering items or services that will be paid for by Medicare or Medicaid will be guilty of a felony.) These rules and regulations essentially made it impossible to practice without violating some aspect of the fraud and abuse laws. It was, however, 10 years before the laws were refined in the Medicaid-Medicare Patient Protection Act of 1987, which provided some safe harbors to free normal course-of-business procedures. Since 1987, the government has pursued fraud and abuse cases with ever-increasing vigor. In 2018 settlements in fraud and abuse cases netted the government more than $4.1 billion (U.S. Department of Justice, 2019). The real danger to the physician is not the fine that may force him or her into bankruptcy or the unusual imposition of jail time (to date, the government has seemed more interested in recovering cash and calling a halt to illegal practices than it has in jailing doctors), but the felony **conviction that may result in the automatic loss of the license to practice. Thus Medicare/Medicaid fraud and abuse is a far more dangerous hazard than is malpractice.**

### Practical Tip

Have your patients sign in regardless of whether they have come for an office visit or just a procedure. If you are worried about privacy issues, use a privacy sign-in sheet to prevent subsequent signers from seeing previous signers. (Colwell Publishing provides several styles of such sheets, and local firms likely supply them as well.)

Do not unbundle procedures that are supposed to be bundled on a physician's visit. Do not unbundle surgical procedures. Do not charge for procedures done by another licensed provider or charge for a physician's services if the physician is not physically present. Send your personnel to an accredited coding course, and make sure your coding is being done in an accurate manner. Do not be tempted to code up. Time studies and statistics are against you. Finally, beware of the "coding consultant" who promises to increase your accounts receivable.

## Laboratory Tests

In my experience, one of the most common reasons for malpractice suits is the unreported abnormal laboratory or x-ray finding. The usual story is that the pathologist or radiologist returns the report and the efficient clerk, receptionist, or nurse staples it in the medical record and files the record or scans it into the electronic medical record without notifying the provider. The alternative story is that the report is never sent and there is no follow-up. Of course, normal clerical errors do occur in any business; nevertheless, the physician's fiduciary duty extends to communicating the results and meanings of all abnormal tests to the patient. The electronic medical record can be helpful for reports generated within the institution, but for outside laboratories and reports, there must be a system to flag critical results and communicate with patients. The failure to communicate the results of an abnormal Papanicolaou (Pap) smear, glucose tolerance test, or mammogram to a patient can have disastrous legal consequences.

### Practical Tip

**An obstetrician/gynecologist must have a system to track and document all laboratory and diagnostic tests and imaging studies ordered.** There is no totally satisfactory way to do this. Old-fashioned "tickler" files are the least efficient, but they are better than nothing. Some office-generated computer programs have been highly successful, and some of the commercially available programs even generate an automatic notification letter. In any case, the physician must track all ordered tests and make every reasonable effort to notify the patient. The notification and follow-up must be documented. Telling the patient to call for the test results does not relieve the physician of his or her duty to notify. Finally, use the information you secure. Do not order laboratory or other diagnostic tests and then ignore or belittle those results.

## CAP STRATEGY

**CAP (communication, anticipation, and preparation) should be the cornerstone of simple practice philosophies that, when effectively put into practice by qualified, trained health care providers in a safe medical system, increase patient safety and thereby "cap" exposure to liability** (Fig. 6.3).

The optimal health system will assimilate CAP between and among the care providers within any given institution or health system. **Applying the principles of CAP will, by employing efficient written, verbal, and policy guidelines, ensure that the right health care providers have the correct information necessary to effectuate optimal care. There is no single greater way to reduce medical liability than to increase patient safety.**

Next we will review how these simple, sound, and commonsense approaches can be incorporated to increase patient safety. Errors will continue to occur in any system that involves people performing duties or tasks. "The most extensive study of adverse events is the Harvard medical practice study, a study of more than 30,000 randomly selected discharges from 51 randomly selected hospitals in New York State in 1984. Adverse events, manifested by prolonged hospitalization or disability at the time of discharge, or both occurred in 3.7% of the hospitalizations. The proportion of adverse events attributed to errors (i.e., preventable adverse events) was 58% and the proportion of adverse events due to negligence was 27.6%." These data were corroborated in the 1992 studies in Colorado, Utah, and New York state (IOM, 2000).

The American College of Obstetrics and Gynecology (ACOG) Committee Opinion 447 further placed patient safety in obstetrics and gynecology at the forefront (ACOG, 2009). The committee opinion set forth that a culture of safety should be the framework for any effort to reduce medical errors. Since then, extensive research has linked specific patient care initiatives to improved patient safety and mitigation of adverse events. Some examples include interprofessional communication training (Slade, 2017), quality improvement (Lefebvre, 2020), preprocedure huddles (http://www.ihi.org/resources/Pages/Tools/Huddles.aspx), time-out processes (Haynes, 2009), rapid response systems to rescue deteriorating patient situations before a code is needed, simulation-based teamwork interventions for improved team performance (Herzberg, 2019) and reduction in patient morbidity on labor and delivery (Wu, 2020) and patient safety bundles for preventing gynecologic surgical site infections (Pellegrini, 2017). Decreasing ambulatory safety risks has also been studied (Schiff, 2017). The goal is to encourage obstetricians and gynecologists to adopt and develop safe practices that will reduce the likelihood of system failures that can cause adverse outcomes in their patient populations.

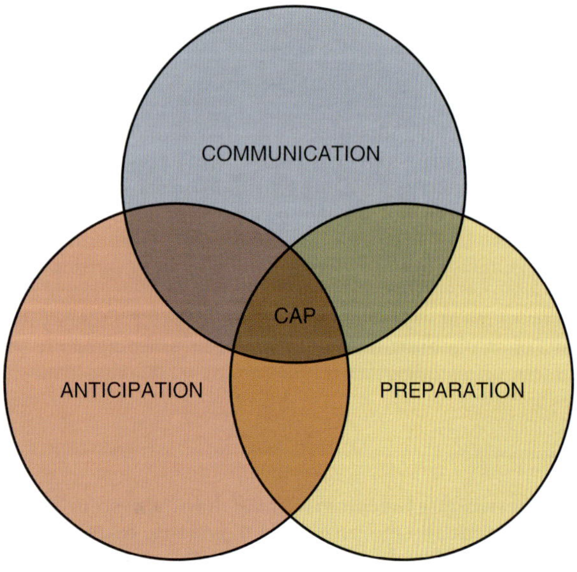


**Fig. 6.3** Communication + Anticipation + Preparation = Patient safety and reduced medicolegal risk.

## COMMUNICATION

As explained previously, communication is the bedrock of safety and efficiency in every high-risk organization. Health care communications can be written in the medical record, published as guidelines and literature, treated as verbal communications, and accepted as cultural norms within an institution. In its analysis of sentinel events, **The Joint Commission found that almost two thirds of the events involved communication failure as a root cause (TJC, 2004). By the time of their report in 2015, communication errors was still the third in most commonly identified root cause for sentinel events, barely behind human factors and leadership. Communication training is recognized as the cornerstone of any patient safety program.** AHRQ developed the TeamSTEPPS trademark program to address this issue (AHRQ, 2015). Obvious times for increased risk of communication slipping through the cracks include patient handoffs, patient transfers, and shift changes. ACOG found that an increased awareness of the importance of clear communication among all members of the health care team would measurably enhance the safety of the care delivered by obstetricians and gynecologists. Others are working on new apps to foster communication and patient safety in gynecology and obstetrics to lower the probability of adverse patient events (Lippke, 2019). Training around these issues for all health care providers is highly recommended.

Communication requires, first, a basic understanding of roles and responsibilities. Team members must be clearly trained in their roles and familiar with the appropriate policies, guidelines, or procedures for delivering routine and emergent care. Through enhanced and clear communication, medical errors can be avoided.

## ANTICIPATION

*Anticipation* is defined as an expectation or prediction. Within each patient's clinical presentation, a health care provider's ability to anticipate outcomes varies. **Anticipation assists in ensuring the right people and necessary equipment are in place to provide appropriate and safe care when needed. Anticipation requires an understanding of the patient's clinical presentation, hospital resources, and any likely encumbrance to the delivery of safe and effective care.** Of 62,966 paid malpractice claims, 13,682 (22%) were diagnosis-related. Inpatient diagnosis-related malpractice payments are common and more often associated with disability and death than other claim types. (Gupta, 2017). In another malpractice claims database, three diseases accounted for 74.1% of high-severity cases (vascular events 22.8%, infections 13.5%, and cancers 37.8%). Causes were disproportionately clinical judgment factors (85.7%). While neither of these two studies were specific to obstetrics and gynecology, they point to the provider needing to anticipate these problems with misdiagnoses and to act accordingly.

## PREPARATION

**The Joint Commission has recommended and mandated, at various levels, simulation programs or training.** Simulations are a way for institutional practices to be perfected before one's handling of life-threatening emergencies. The concept of a simulation, though basic and simple, requires more than just the simple actions that day. The preparation required includes appropriate staffing; reasonable, updated, and appropriately disseminated policies and guidelines that include definitions of roles and responsibilities; and planned simulations of foreseeable emergencies.

## CONCLUSION

In the broadest sense, medical malpractice is defined by whether or not conduct and decisions were reasonable. The fear of all physicians is that ultimately they will be judged by lesser-trained individuals who identify more with the patient than with the provider. The tests of reasonableness the jurors will use are often as simple as asking the question, based on the care and the testimony you provided, Would the jurors be comfortable being treated by you? If the answer to that question is yes, regardless of the complications, decision making, and outcomes, then the most likely jury verdict will be in favor of you, the defendant physician. However, if the care appears to be inattentive or inconsistent and the records or depositions are inaccurate, the chance to explain your decision and the reasonableness you feel is behind it may be lost through no one's fault but your own.

Breakdowns in the systems of communication—with patients and care providers or through the medical records—can create a host of problems for physicians, nurses, and health care institutions in the event of an unfavorable treatment outcome. **Many problems can be avoided or quickly resolved by focusing attentively on both system-wide and individual best practices for accurate and contemporaneous communications.** Awareness that your patients will have serious questions about unexpected, often life-altering, outcomes is integral to avoiding legal problems. Only when patients feel that they have not received satisfactory answers from their care providers will they seek those answers elsewhere—most likely from an attorney.

Focusing on communication, anticipation, and preparation will ensure the appropriate people are in the appropriate place with the appropriate information to deliver health care in a timely manner. The concept of capping one's liability is far too often looked at retrospectively through litigation or discussed after an error occurs. In reality **the best ways to cap liability are through enhanced communication and the development of a cohesive system of health care, which are both patient focused and health care provider friendly** (Box 6.8).

Balancing practice modifications that become oppressive or interfere with the delivery of reasonable and efficient health care can be challenging. However, ensuring adequate layers of redundancies and safeguards to make certain a single or perhaps even two human errors are offset by a well-designed cohesive system will prevent an undesirable outcome or patient harm (Fig. 6.4).

**BOX 6.8** Effective Communication Steps

- Establish a healthy rapport (communication is a two-way process).
- Respect the patient as a person and seek to understand her beliefs.
- Be honest and be an ally.
- Obtain an accurate record of symptoms and medical history.
- Disclose all relevant facts.
- Explain clearly any alternatives to care and reservations.
- Ask for comprehension from the patient and ensure that the patient understands the information, advice, and instructions.
- Answer all questions.
- Obtain valid informed consent.
- Follow-up questions, lab tests, imaging, etc.

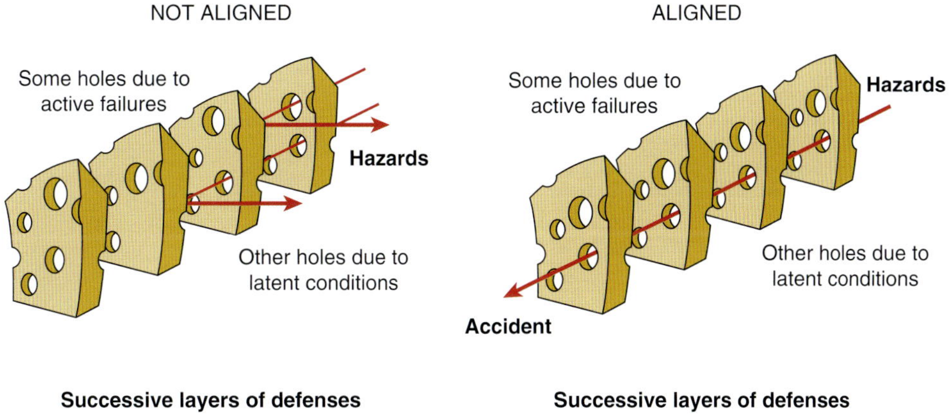


**Fig. 6.4** Swiss cheese model system errors and benefits of redundancies.

## REFERENCES


Agency for Healthcare Research and Quality (AHRQ). *TeamSTEPPS®: Strategies and Tools to Enhance Performance and Patient Safety.* Rockville, MD: AHRQ; 2015. Available at http://www.ahrq.gov/professionals/education/curriculum-tools/teamstepps/index.html.

American College of Obstetricians and Gynecologists (ACOG). ACOG Committee Opinion No. 792: clinical guidelines and standardization of practice to improve outcomes. September 2019.

American College of Obstetricians and Gynecologists. ACOG Committee opinion no. 551: coping with the stress of medical professional liability litigation. *Obstet Gynecol.* 2013 Jan;121(1):220–222. doi: 10.1097/01.aog.0000425665.64635.1c. PMID: 23262965.

American College of Obstetricians and Gynecologists (ACOG). ACOG Committee Opinion No. 447: Patient safety in obstetrics and gynecology. *Obstet Gynecol.* 2009;114(6):1424–1427. (Reaffirmed 2019).

American College of Obstetricians and Gynecologists (ACOG). ACOG Committee Opinion No. 621, Patient safety and health information technology. January 2015.

American College of Obstetricians and Gynecologists Committee on Patient Safety and Quality Improvement. ACOG Committee Opinion No. 400: Technologic advances to reduce medication-related errors. *Obstet Gynecol.* 2008 Mar;111(3):795–798. doi: 10.1097/AOG.0b013e318169f705. PMID: 18310390.

Fisher KA, Gallagher TH, Smith KM, Zhou Y, Crawford S, Amroze A, Mazor KM. Communicating with patients about breakdowns in care: a national randomised vignette-based survey. *BMJ Qual Saf.* 2020 Apr;29(4):313–319. doi: 10.1136/bmjqs-2019-009712. Epub 2019 Nov 13. PMID: 31723017; PMCID: PMC7170008.

Glaser LM, Alvi FA, Milan MP. Trends in malpractice claims for obstetric and gynecologic procedures, 2005 through 2014. *Am J Obstet Gynecol.* 2017;217:340.e1–6.

Gupta A, Snyder A, Kachalia A, et al. Malpractice claims related to diagnostic errors in the hospital. *BMJ Qual Saf.* 2017;27(1).

Haynes AB, Weiser TG, Berry WR, et al; Safe Surgery Saves Lives Study Group. A surgical safety checklist to reduce morbidity and mortality in a global population. *N Engl J Med.* 2009;360(5):491–499.

Herzberg S, Hansen M, Schoonover A, et al. Association between measured teamwork and medical errors: an observational study of prehospital care in the USA. *BMJ Open.* 2019;9(10):e025314.

Institute for Healthcare Improvement. *Huddles.* Available at http://www.ihi.org/resources/Pages/Tools/Huddles.aspx. Retrieved March 21, 2016.

Institute of Medicine (IOM). *To Err is Human: Building a Safer Health System.* Washington, DC: National Academies Press; 2000.

Institute of Medicine (IOM). *Preventing Medication Errors: Quality Chasm Series.* Washington, DC: National Academies Press; 2007. doi: 10317226-11623.

Joint Commission Online. *Sentinel Event Statistics Released for 2014.* April 29, 2015. Available at: https://www.jointcommission.org/assets/1/23/jconline_April_29_15.pdf.

Lefebvre G, Honey L, Hines K, et al. Implementing obstetrics quality improvement, driven by medico-legal risk, is associated with improved workplace culture. *J Obstet Gynaecol Can.* 2020;42(1):38–47.e5.

Légaré F, Adekpedjou R, Stacey D, et al. Interventions for increasing the use of shared decision making by healthcare professionals. *Cochrane Database Syst Rev.* 2018;7:CD006732.

Lippke S, Wienert J, Keller FM, et al. Communication and patient safety in gynecology and obstetrics—study protocol of an intervention study. *BMC Health Serv Res.* 2019;19(1):908.

Pellegrini JE, Toledo P, Soper DE, et al. consensus bundle on prevention of surgical site infections after major gynecologic surgery. *Obstet Gynecol.* 2017;129(1):50–61.

Professional Liability and Gynecology-Only Practice: ACOG COMMITTEE OPINION, Number 790. *Obstet Gynecol.* 2019 Oct;134(4):e115–e116. doi: 10.1097/AOG.0000000000003449. PMID: 31568366.

Schaffer AC, Jena AB, Seabury SA, et al. Rates and characteristics of paid malpractice claims among US physicians by specialty, 1992–2014. *JAMA Intern Med.* 2017;177(5):710–718.

Schiff GD, Reyes Nieva H, Griswold P, et al. Randomized trial of reducing ambulatory malpractice and safety risk: results of the Massachusetts PROMISES Project. *Med Care.* 2017;55(8):797–805.

Sepucha KR, Breslin M, Graffeo C, Carpenter CR, Hess EP. state of the science: tools and measurement for shared decision making. *Acad Emerg Med.* 2016;23(12):1325–1331.

Shapiro J, Robins L, Galowitz P, Gallagher TH, Bell S. Disclosure coaching: an Ask-Tell-Ask model to support clinicians in disclosure conversations. *J Patient Saf.* 2018.

Slade IR, Beck SJ, Kramer CB, et al. Communication training, adverse events, and quality measures: 2 retrospective database analyses in Washington State Hospitals. *J Patient Saf.* 2017.

Stacey D, Légaré F, Lewis KB. Patient decision aids to engage adults in treatment or screening decisions. *JAMA.* 2017;318(7):657–658.

Starmer AJ, Spector ND, Srivastava R, et al; I-PASS Study Group. Changes in medical errors after implementation of a handoff program. *N Engl J Med.* 2014;371(19):1803–1812.

Studdert DM, Mello MM, Gawande AA, et al. Claims, errors and compensation payments in medical malpractice litigation. *N Engl J Med.* 2006;354(19):2024–2033.

The Joint Commission (TJC). *Sentinel Event Alert, Issue 30: Preventing infant death and injury during delivery;* July 21, 2004. Available at http://www.jointcommission.org/assets/1/18/SEA_30.PDF.

The Joint Commission (TJC). *The Joint Commission's implementation guide for NPSG.07.05.01 on surgical site infections: the SSI change project.* Available at http://www.jointcommission.org/implementation_guide_for_npsg070501_ssi_change_project/. Retrieved March 25, 2016.

U.S. Food and Drug Administration (FDA). *Medication Errors;* 2016. Available at http://www.fda.gov/Drugs/DrugSafety/MedicationErrors/default.htm.

Wu M, Tang J, Etherington N, Walker M, Boet S. Interventions for improving teamwork in intrapartem care: a systematic review of randomised controlled trials. *BMJ Qual Saf.* 2020 Jan;29(1):77-85. doi: 10.1136/bmjqs-2019-009689. Epub 2019 Oct 10. PMID: 31601734.

Wu M, Tang J, Etherington N, Walker M, Boet S. Interventions for improving teamwork in intrapartem care: a systematic review of randomised controlled trials. *BMJ Qual Saf.* 2020;29(1):77–85.


**Suggested readings for this chapter can be found on ExpertConsult.com.**

# 7 History, Physical Examination, and Preventive Health Care

*Vicki Mendiratta, Gretchen M. Lentz*

**KEY POINTS**

- Strive to become a culturally sensitive and aware physician with a nonjudgmental approach to women regardless of race or ethnicity, age, faith, disabilities, profession, sexual orientation/identity, or activities.
- Goals of preventive medicine include maintaining good health and function and promoting high-quality longevity.
- A complete gynecologic evaluation should always include a review of menstruation, sexuality, contraception, pregnancies, gynecologic infections, gynecologic procedures, and any history of physical, emotional, or sexual abuse.
- The specific examination components of the annual well-woman visit are based on patient age, health concerns, and risk factors. Whether to perform breast or pelvic examinations is a joint decision between individual providers and their patients.
- Screenings, such as Papanicolaou smears, mammography, and sexually transmitted infection testing, should be in accordance with national recommendations.

The first contact a physician has with a patient is critical. **It allows an initial bond of trust to be developed on which the future relationship may be built.** The patient will share sensitive medical, reproductive, and psychosocial information. The physician will gain her confidence and establish rapport by the understanding and nonjudgmental manner in which he or she collects these data. Today's obstetrician/gynecologist (OB/GYN) will care for women from around the globe with varying cultural, social, and religious beliefs and values. Women will be of differing socioeconomic status, may have physical or mental disabilities, and may identify as lesbian, bisexual, transgender, or queer. Open communication, with an awareness of and sensitivity to the vast diversity of our patient population, will help create a collaborative environment in which to explore health issues.

The annual well-woman visit is a crucial part of general medical care. The purpose of this visit includes the following:

- Discussing healthy lifestyle and minimizing health risks
- Promoting preventive health practices
- Performing or providing age-specific screening, evaluation and counseling, and immunizations
- Taking a comprehensive history and vital signs (including body mass index [BMI])
- Performing indicated physical examinations

This chapter focuses on the appropriate manner that an OB/GYN should use to conduct a history and physical examination and discusses the appropriate ingredients of ongoing health maintenance.

## DIRECT OBSERVATIONS BEFORE SPEAKING TO THE PATIENT (NONVERBAL CLUES)

When meeting a patient, it is important to *look* at her even before speaking. Differing cultural backgrounds and belief systems may greatly affect the transfer of information and challenge effective communication. Addressing each patient by the patient's preferred pronoun, she, he, or they, is crucial to demonstrate respect and understanding of each individual patient's identity. The general demeanor of the patient should be evaluated. Many new patients are apprehensive about meeting a new physician and the potential for a pelvic examination. This apprehension may create barriers to an open and positive first encounter.

By observing nonverbal clues, such as eye contact, posture, facial expressions, and tone of voice, the physician can determine the appropriate approach for conducting the interview. The act of greeting the patient by name, making eye contact, and shaking hands is a formal but friendly start to the visit.

Four qualities have been recognized as potentially important in caring communication skills: comfort, acceptance, responsiveness, and empathy. Despite the busy demands of clinical practice, effective communication skills enhance patient satisfaction and patient safety and decrease the likelihood of medical liability litigation. Box 7.1 lists some components of effective physician communication.

## ESSENCE OF THE GYNECOLOGIC HISTORY

### Chief Complaint

The patient should be encouraged to tell the physician why she has sought care. The chief complaint is a concise statement describing the woman's concerns in her words. Questions such as "What is the nature of the concern that brought you to me?" or "How may I help you?" are appropriate.

### History of the Present Illness

The patient should be able to present her concern as she sees it, in her own words. During the interview the physician should ideally face the patient with direct eye contact and acknowledge important

**BOX 7.1 Components of Effective Physician Communication**

Be culturally sensitive.
Establish rapport.
Listen and respond to the woman's concerns (empathy).
Be nonjudgmental.
Include both verbal and nonverbal communication.
Engage the woman in discussion and treatment options (partnership).
Convey comfort in discussing sensitive topics.
Abandon stereotypes.
Check for understanding of your explanations.
Show support by helping the woman to overcome barriers to care and compliance with treatment.

points of the history. This approach allows the physician to be involved in the problem and demonstrates a degree of caring to the patient. Now that electronic medical records (EMRs) are almost universally used, the ability to sit and just listen to the patient and provide that direct eye contact can be challenging because providers are often documenting while the patient is sharing her story. When the patient has completed the history of the present illness (HPI) or a review of her overall health, pertinent open-ended questions should be asked with respect to specific points. This process allows the physician to develop a more detailed database. Directed questions may be asked where pertinent to clarify points. A general outline for a gynecologic and general history is given in Box 7.2.

## Pertinent Gynecologic History

**A pertinent gynecologic history can be divided into several parts. These include menstrual history, pregnancy history, history of gynecologic infections; history of cervical cancer screenings, history of contraceptive use, history of gynecologic surgical procedures, sexual history, and history of pelvic pain.**

### Menstrual History

A menstrual history should include the following:

- Age of menarche
- Interval between cycles
- Number of days bleeding
- Regularity of menstrual cycles.
- Intermenstrual or unexpected vaginal bleeding
- Date of last menstrual period
- Characteristics of the menstrual flow: the amount of flow, any clots, any accompanying symptoms, such as cramping, nausea, headache, or diarrhea

In general, menstruation that occurs monthly (range: 21 to 35 days), lasts 4 to 7 days, is bright red, and is often accompanied by cramping on the day preceding and the first day of the period is characteristic of an ovulatory cycle. Menstruation that is irregular, often dark colored, painless, and often short or very long may indicate lack of ovulation. Often adolescents or premenopausal women have anovulatory cycles with resultant irregular menstruation. For the postmenopausal woman, the age at last menses, history of hormone replacement therapy, and any postmenopausal bleeding should be noted.

### Pregnancy History

A pregnancy history should include the following:

- Chemical pregnancies
- Abortions: miscarriages and terminations and method of resolution (medical or surgical)

**BOX 7.2 History Outline**

I. Observation—nonverbal clues
II. Chief complaint
III. History of gynecologic issues/concerns(s)
  A. Menstrual history
  B. Pregnancy history
  C. Vaginal and pelvic infections
  D. Gynecologic surgical procedures
  E. Urologic history
  F. Pelvic pain
  G. Vaginal bleeding
  H. Sexual orientation, activity, concerns
  I. Contraceptive status
IV. Significant health issues
  A. Systemic illnesses
  B. Surgical procedures
  C. Other hospitalizations
V. Medications, habits, and allergies
  A. Medications
  B. Allergies
  C. Smoking history
  D. Alcohol usage
  E. Illicit drug usage
VI. Family history
  A. Illnesses and causes of death of close family
  B. Congenital malformations, mental retardation, and reproductive loss
VII. Occupational and avocational history
VIII. Social history, including current safety and any history abuse (physical, verbal, emotional, sexual)
IX. Review of systems
  A. Constitutional
  B. Head, eyes, ears, nose, mouth, throat
  C. Cardiovascular
  D. Respiratory
  E. Gastrointestinal
  F. Genitourinary
  G. Musculoskeletal
  H. Skin
  I. Neurologic
  J. Psychiatric—often using a depression questionnaire, such as the Patient Health Questionnaire (PHQ) 2 or PHQ-9
  K. Endocrine
  L. Hematologic
  M. Allergic/immunologic

- Molar or ectopic pregnancies and how they were managed (medically and/or surgically)
- Live births:
  - Year of birth
  - Gestational age at delivery
  - Type of delivery
  - Infant birth weight
  - Complications of pregnancy or delivery
- Infertility
- Future family planning goals

### Gynecologic Infections

A history of gynecologic infections should include the following:

- Specific infections, treatment received, and any complications
- Risk factors for infections such as human immunodeficiency virus (HIV) and hepatitis C:
  - Intravenous (IV) drug use or coitus with IV drug users
  - Unprotected sex

**TABLE 7.1** Initial HIV Screening Recommendations

| CDC, 2006 | ACP, 2009 | IDSA, 2009 | AAP, 2011 | AAFP, 2013 | USPSTF, 2013 | ACOG, 2014 |
|---|---|---|---|---|---|---|
| Initial screening age 13-64, regardless of risks | Initial screening age 13-64, regardless of risks | Screen all sexually active adults | Adolescents screened once by age 16-18 | Screen all individuals aged 18-65 | Initial screening age 15-65; however, optimum frequency of repeat screening unable to be determined | All women aged 13-64 screened at least once and annually based on risk factors |

*AAP,* American Academy of Pediatrics; *AAFP,* American Academy of Family Physicians; *ACP,* American College of Physicians; *ACOG,* American College of Obstetricians and Gynecologists; *CDC,* Centers for Disease Control and Prevention; *HIV,* human immunodeficiency virus; *IDSA,* Infectious Diseases Society of America; *USPSTF,* U.S. Preventive Services Task Force.

  - Sex with bisexual men
  - Being a commercial sex worker
  - History of blood transfusion between 1978 to 1985
- Sexual activity with partner with known HIV or hepatitis C infection

The 2013 U.S. Preventive Services Task Force (USPSTF) report states with "high certainty that the net benefit of screening for HIV infection in adolescents, adults and pregnant women is substantial" (Moyer, 2013). Part of this rationale stems from the fact that 20% to 25% of individuals living with HIV infection are unaware they are infected (Table 7.1).

### Cervical Cancer Screening

The physician should obtain a Papanicolaou (Pap) test screening history:

- Date of last Pap test
- Result of last Pap test, including if human papilloma virus (HPV) was concurrently checked (cotest)
- Frequency of screening
- Any abnormal tests and subsequent follow-up or treatment
- HPV vaccination status

### Contraception

Contraceptive history should be investigated:

- Specific methods used
- Duration of use
- Effectiveness of contraceptive method
- Complications or significant side effects

### Gynecologic Surgical Procedures

All gynecologic procedure should be noted, including office procedures, such as endometrial, vulvar, vaginal, or cervical biopsies, and their results. For any minor or major surgeries, such as laparoscopy or laparotomy, the following data should be collected:

- Dates
- Specific types of procedures
- Specific diagnoses, pathology reports
- Results of the surgery (e.g., resolution of pain or heavy bleeding)
- Significant complications

In cases where pertinent, operative and pathology reports should be obtained.

### Sexual History

A complete sexual history should be obtained (Box 7.3), and specific problems should be evaluated. The history should include whether the patient is currently sexually active or has been in the past. Patients should be asked if they have one or more current partners and if they have sex with men, women, or both. The provider should also inquire about any sexual dysfunction such as dyspareunia or anorgasmia.

**BOX 7.3** Important Points of Sexual History

1. Sexual activity (presence of)
2. Types of relationships
3. Individual(s) involved
4. Satisfaction? Orgasmic? Desire/interest?
5. Dyspareunia
6. Sexual dysfunction
    a. Patient
    b. Partner

### Pelvic Pain

Any current pelvic pain should be discussed fully. Six common questions should be asked about the pain:

- Location
- Timing
- Quality, such as throbbing, burning, or colicky
- Radiation to other body areas
- Intensity on a scale of 1 to 10, with 10 being the worse pain imaginable
- Duration of symptoms

Additional questions about what causes the pain to worsen or subside, the context of the pain symptoms, and associated triggers, signs, and symptoms may be helpful. The pain should be described, noting the presence or absence of a relationship to the menstrual cycle and its association with other events, such as coitus or bleeding and bladder and bowel symptoms.

## General Health History

**The woman should be asked to list any significant health problems that she has had during her lifetime, including all hospitalizations and operative procedures.** It is reasonable for the physician to ask about specific illnesses, such as diabetes, hypertension, or heart disease, that seem likely based on what is known about the woman or about her family history. Many physicians use a history checklist of the most common conditions.

All medications, including over-the-counter drugs and complementary and alternative medicines, being used and reasons for doing so should be noted. In addition, a careful review of medication allergies or reactions is essential.

A history of smoking should be obtained in detail, including amount, length of time she has smoked, and attempts at smoking cessation. She should be questioned about the use of illicit drugs, including heroin, methamphetamines, and cocaine, as well as prescription opioids. Any affirmative answers should be followed by specific questions concerning length of use, types of drugs used, and side effects that may have been noticed. Her use of alcohol should be detailed carefully, including the number of drinks per day and any history of binge drinking or previous therapy for alcoholism. Vaping and marijuana use should be assessed.

## Family History

A detailed family history of first- and second-degree relatives (parents, siblings, children, aunts, uncles, and grandparents) should be taken and a family tree constructed if relevant (Fig. 7.1). Serious illnesses or causes of death for each individual should be noted. If the patient desires fertility now or in the future, an inquiry should be made about any congenital malformations, mental retardation, or pregnancy loss in either the patient's or her spouse's family. Such information may offer clues to hereditarily determined causes of reproductive problems.

### Occupational and Social History

The patient should be asked to detail her occupation. A nonjudgmental way to approach this could be to ask if she is currently working outside the home. It is very important to determine whether she is currently exercising, what type of activity she engages in, and the frequency of exercise.

Additional information that may be relevant include hobbies and other avocations that may affect health or reproductive capacity, where and with whom the woman lives, other individuals in the household, areas of the world where the woman has lived or traveled, and unusual experiences that may affect her health. The physician should discuss possible stressors in the patient's life, such as her relationship with her partner and other family members, her satisfaction or dissatisfaction with her job, and other social problems that she may be experiencing.

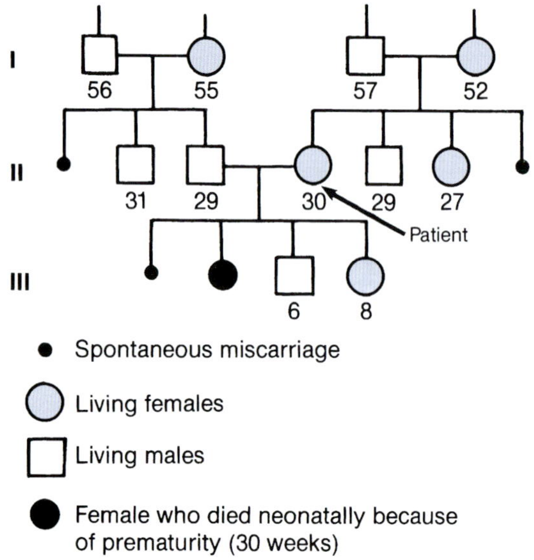


**Fig. 7.1** Family tree of typical gynecologic patient.

## Safety Issues

The patient should be questioned about safety. She should be asked about the use of seat belts and helmets where applicable. She should be asked whether there are firearms in her household and, if so, whether appropriate safety precautions are taken. **A question about intimate partner violence is crucial and can be asked in a nonthreatening manner, such as "Has anyone threatened or physically hurt you?" Sexual violence is a widespread problem, and as more is being learned about prevention, providers should be knowledgeable about resources** (Senn, 2015).

## Nutritional and Dietary Assessment

It is important to inquire about dietary choices that our patients make. Assessment of folic acid is important in reproductive-aged women. Asking about fruits and vegetables, as well as calcium-containing foods should be standard. Vegetarians and vegans may need additional discussion about adequate protein and vitamin and mineral intake. A referral to a certified nutritionist may be a valuable addition to routine preventive health care.

## Review of Systems

A complete review of systems (ROS) should be obtained and documented. (See Box 7.2 for comprehensive ROS and some relevant examples.)

# COMPONENTS OF THE PHYSICAL EXAMINATION

The scope of services and examination provided by an OB/GYN in the ambulatory setting vary from practice to practice. **In 2018 the American College of Obstetricians and Gynecologists (ACOG) recommended that the annual well-woman visit include obtaining a comprehensive history and vital signs, including body mass index (BMI) (ACOG, 2018). However, they stated that the physical examination may not be required at a well-woman visit and that engaging patients in shared decision making is key in determining which, if any, examinations to perform.** The extent to which additional examinations are performed is based on many factors, such as age, patient concerns, family history, and whether the patient has a primary care provider whom she also sees for routine and concern-driven care. Not all women will require a clinical breast or pelvic examination at each yearly visit. Significant controversy exists regarding recommendations for screening breast and pelvic examinations. Refer to Tables 7.2 through 7.4 for contemporary recommendations from national organizations such as the American College of Physicians and USPSTF.

## Physical Examination

The patient should disrobe completely and cover herself with a hospital gown that ensures warmth and modesty. During each step of the examination she should be allowed to maintain personal control by being offered options whenever possible. These options begin with the presence or absence of a chaperone. The chaperone, a third party, usually a woman, serves a variety of purposes. She may offer warmth, compassion, and support to the patient during uncomfortable or potentially embarrassing portions of the examination. She may help the physician to carry out procedures and in some cases act as a witness to the doctor-patient interaction. Although the presence of a chaperone is not imperative in every physician-patient relationship, one should be immediately available for any encounter (ACOG, 2020).

TABLE 7.2 Examination, Screening, and Immunization Recommendations for the Annual Health Maintenance Visit

| | Age (Years) | | |
|---|---|---|---|
| | 19-39 | 40-64 | 65+ |
| Vital signs | Ht, Wt, BMI, BP | Ht, Wt, BMI, BP | Ht, Wt, BMI, BP |
| Chlamydia/gonorrhea | <26 and sexually active, yearly | As indicated | As indicated |
| Diabetes testing | As indicated based on personal or family history | 45+, every 3 years | Every 3 years |
| Lipids | If indicated | 45+, every 5 years | Every 5 years |
| Thyroid-stimulating hormone | If indicated | 50+, every 5 years | Every 5 years |
| Bone mineral density | | If indicated | Every 2+ years |
| Immunizations | HPV, Tdap once, TD q 10 years; influenza yearly | Tdap once, TD q 10 years; influenza yearly; herpes zoster twice (50+) | Influenza yearly; Tdap once, TD every 10 years; pneumococcus once |

Additional data from American the Congress of Obstetricians and Gynecologists (ACOG). Well-woman care: assessment and recommendations. Available at: http://www.acog.org/wellwoman.
These are general recommendations for low-risk populations. High-risk populations may have more recommended vaccines.
High-risk groups based on lifestyle, concurrent medical conditions, and family history may have other testing or intervals for testing. Chart represents recommendations for the general populations.
*ACS,* American Cancer Society; *BMI,* body mass index; *BP,* blood pressure; *CDC,* Centers for Disease Control and Prevention; *HIV,* human immunodeficiency virus; *HPV,* human papillomavirus; *Ht,* height; *TD,* booster tetanus and diphtheria; *Tdap,* tetanus, diphtheria, and pertussis; *Wt,* weight.

TABLE 7.3 Recommendations for Screening Breast Examination (BE)

| Organization | Recommendations |
|---|---|
| USPSTF, 2009 | Insufficient evidence to recommend screening BE |
| ACS, 2015 | No screening BE for average risk women of any age |
| AAFP, 2016 | Current evidence is insufficient to assess the benefits and harms of clinical breast examination for women aged 40+ years |
| NCCN, 2016 | Recommends BE: age 25-39, every 1-3 years; age 40+, yearly |
| ACOG, 2017 | Recommends BE: age 25-39, every 1-3 years; age 40+, yearly |

*AAFP,* American Academy of Family Physicians; *ACOG,* American College of Obstetricians and Gynecologists; *ACP,* American College of Physicians; *NCCN,* National Comprehensive Cancer Network; *USPSTF,* U.S. Preventive Services Task Force.

TABLE 7.4 Recommendations for Screening Pelvic Examination (PE)

| Organization | Recommendations |
|---|---|
| ACP, 2014 | Recommends against screening PE in asymptomatic, nonpregnant, adult women |
| SGO, 2016 | Offer PE to every woman, in context of a balanced discussion of risks/benefits |
| USPSTF, 2017 | Insufficient evidence to recommend screening PE for asymptomatic, nonpregnant women |
| AAFP, 2017 | Recommends against screening PE in asymptomatic women |
| ACOG, 2018 | No evidence supports or refutes the annual PE, speculum, bimanual exam for low-risk, asymptomatic patients. Discussion: benefits, harms, lack of data. Shared decision making. |

*AAFP,* American Academy of Family Physicians; *ACOG,* American College of Obstetricians and Gynecologists; *ACP,* American College of Physicians; *SGO,* Society of Gynecologic Oncology; *USPSTF,* U.S. Preventive Services Task Force.

The examination should begin with a general evaluation of the patient's appearance and affect. Her weight, height, and blood pressure should be taken initially. A BMI should be calculated and is an important "vital sign" to track over time. Most EMRs will automatically calculate BMI when height and weight data are entered. Postmenopausal women should have their height measured routinely to document evidence of osteoporosis, which causes loss of height from vertebral compression fractures. Some institutions require pain scale reporting at each visit and consider it a fourth vital sign.

Most gynecologists will not perform a comprehensive screening head, eye, ears, neck, and throat (HEENT) examination. The American Academy of Ophthalmology (AAO) recommends that adults with no signs or risk factors for eye disease should receive a baseline comprehensive eye evaluation at age 40 and then every 2 to 4 years until age 55; every 1 to 3 years through age 64: and yearly to every other year for individuals 65 years old or older (AAO, 2015).

If indicated, the thyroid gland should be palpated for irregularities or increase in size (goiter). Discrete areas of enlargement, hardness, and tenderness should be described, and the patient's neck should be palpated for evidence of adenopathy along the supraclavicular and posterior auricular chains.

In a comprehensive preventive health examination, both the chest and cardiac systems should be evaluated. Whether this is necessary in an annual well-woman visit for a healthy woman is at the discretion of the provider. A nongynecologic primary care provider or subspecialist will primarily care for women with medical conditions such as hypertension or diabetes. If performing, the components of the chest and cardiac examination include the following:

- Inspection for symmetry of movement of the diaphragm
- Respiratory effort
- Palpation
- Percussion
- Auscultation (heart sounds and rhythm, neck auscultation for vascular bruits in older women)
- Peripheral pulses

## Breast Examination

A systematic approach is indicated if performing a clinical screening breast examination. For a summary of a detailed clinical breast

**BOX 7.4 Clinical Breast Examination Elements**

1. With the patient sitting up, position her hands at her hips and ask her to gently push inward. Visualize for symmetry. Ask the patient to put her hands together above her head and press inward. Visualize for symmetry. With her arms at her side, palpate axilla bilaterally, feeling for lymph nodes.
2. In the supine position, ask the patient to place her arms above her head. Pay attention to the entire breast tissue from midsternum to the posterior axillary line and from the inframammary crease to the clavicle.
3. Perform inspection and palpation. A variety of palpation techniques exist to examine for the following:
   - Skin flattening or dimpling
   - Skin erythema
   - Skin edema
   - Nipple retraction
   - Nipple eczema
   - Nipple discharge
   - Breast fixation
   - Tissue thickening
   - Palpable masses
   - Tenderness

examination, refer to Box 7.4. Research has shown that the following factors are associated with a high-quality breast examination: longer duration, thorough coverage of the breast, a consistent examination pattern, use of variable pressure with the finger pads, and use of the three middle fingers. **ACOG, the American Cancer Society (ACS), and the National Comprehensive Cancer Network (NCCN) all recommend the teaching of breast self-awareness.** Women are no longer instructed to examine their own breasts monthly but rather if they feel or see any concerning symptom or abnormality such as redness, pain, skin changes, or a mass.

## Abdominal Examination

If performed as part of the well-woman visit, an abdominal examination should include the following:

- Inspection for symmetry, scars, masses, distention, visible organomegaly or hernia, and hair pattern. The typical female escutcheon is that of an inverted triangle over the mons pubis. A male escutcheon involves hair growth between the area of the mons pubis and the umbilicus, also known as a *diamond pattern*, and may indicate excessive androgen activity in the patient (Fig. 7.2).
- Auscultation for bowel sounds. Hypoactive or absent bowel sounds may imply an ileus caused by peritoneal irritation of the bowel. Hyperactive bowel sounds may imply intrinsic irritation of the bowel or partial or complete bowel obstruction.
- Percussion to differentiate fluid waves and outline solid organs and masses. Localized percussion tenderness may suggest peritoneal inflammation.
- Palpation for organomegaly, presence of fluid wave, rigidity, rebound tenderness, and trigger points. The groin should be palpated for adenopathy and inguinal hernias.

## Pelvic Examination

After careful review of the patient's history and any concerns and after shared decision making, a comprehensive pelvic examination may be indicated. The pelvic examination is conducted with the patient lying supine on the examining table with her legs in stirrups and a sheet draped across her.

### Inspection

The vulva, perineum, and introitus should be carefully inspected. The inspection should include the following:

- Quality and pattern of the hair on the mons and the labia majora
- Evidence of body lice (pediculosis)
- Presence of any erythema, excoriation, discoloration, loss of pigment, vesicles, ulcerations, pustules, warty growths, or neoplastic growths
- Presence of pigmented nevi, other pigmented lesions, or varicose veins
- Presence of skin scars

Next, the specific structures of the vulva should be systematically evaluated as follows (Fig. 7.3):

- Clitoris. The size and shape should be described. Normally it is 1 to 1.5 cm in length.
- Labia minora/majora. Any irregularities or abnormalities of the labia majora or minora should be noted and carefully described. At times these areas are injured by trauma related to coitus, accident, or childbearing. The patient should be questioned about evidence of trauma when appropriate.
- Introitus. Evaluate if the hymen is intact, imperforate, or open and whether the perineum gapes or remains closed in the usual lithotomy position.
- Perineal body
- Perianal area. Examine for hemorrhoids, sphincter injury, warts, and other lesions.

### Palpation

The next step of the pelvic examination involves palpation. The labia minora are gently separated, the urethra is inspected, and

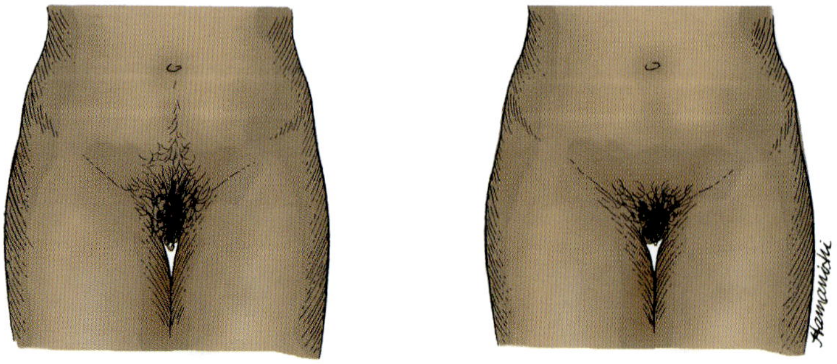

**Fig. 7.2** Normal female pubic hair pattern *(right)* and hair pattern of female showing male (androgenized) pattern *(left)*.

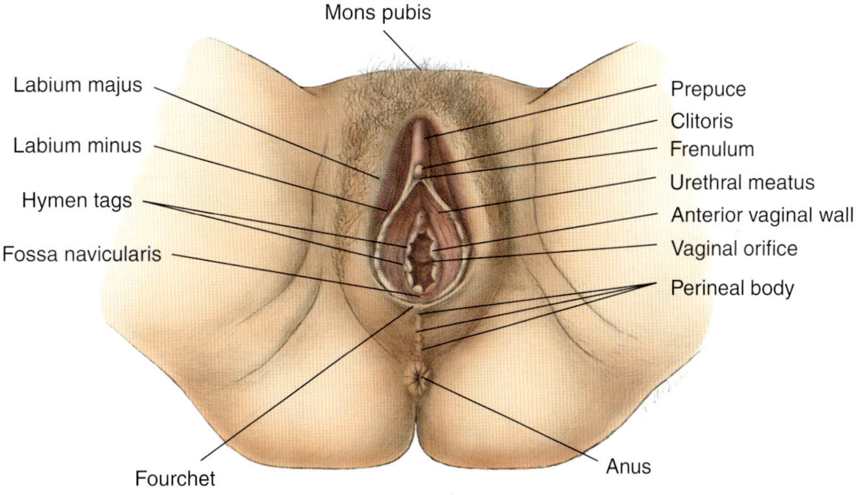


**Fig. 7.3** Normal female perineum. (Modified from Krantz KE. Anatomy of the female reproductive system. In: Benson RC, ed. *Current Obstetric and Gynecologic Diagnosis and Treatment.* 5th ed. Los Altos, CA: Lange Medical; 1984.)

the length of the urethra is palpated and "milked" with the middle finger. In this way, irregularities and inflammation of Skene glands (periurethral glands), expressed pus or mucus, or a suburethral diverticulum can be noted. Any pus expressed from the urethra should be submitted for pathologic testing with culture and Gram staining because it is occasionally found to contain gonococci. Next, the area of the posterior third of the labia majora is palpated by placing the index finger inside the introitus and the thumb on the outside of the labium. In this way, enlargements or cysts of Bartholin glands are noted. This examination should be performed on each side.

The opening of the vagina should be inspected. The presence of a cystocele or a cystourethrocele should be noted. This would be seen as a bulging of vaginal mucosa downward from the anterior wall of the vagina. The presence of this abnormality may be noted either by simply observing or by asking the patient to bear down (Fig. 7.4). Likewise, the posterior wall should be observed for a bulging upward, which would represent a rectocele (Fig. 7.5). A cystic bulge in the cul-de-sac may represent an enterocele (Fig. 7.6). Also, with the patient bearing down, the cervix

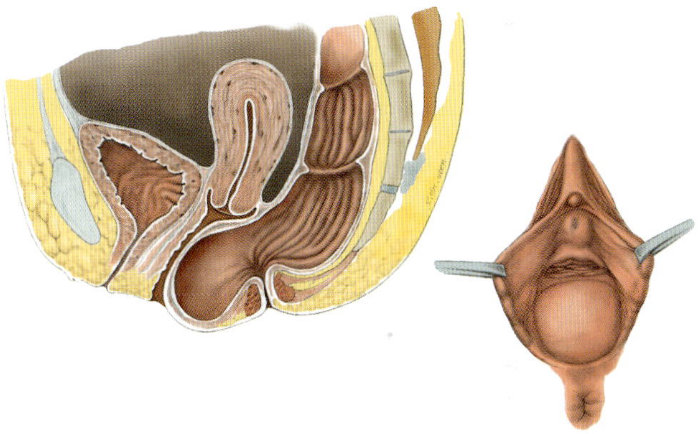

**Fig. 7.5** Side and direct views of rectocele. (Modified from Symmonds RE: Relaxations of pelvic supports. In: Benson RC, ed. *Current Obstetric and Gynecologic Diagnosis and Treatment.* 5th ed. Los Altos, CA: Lange Medical; 1984.)

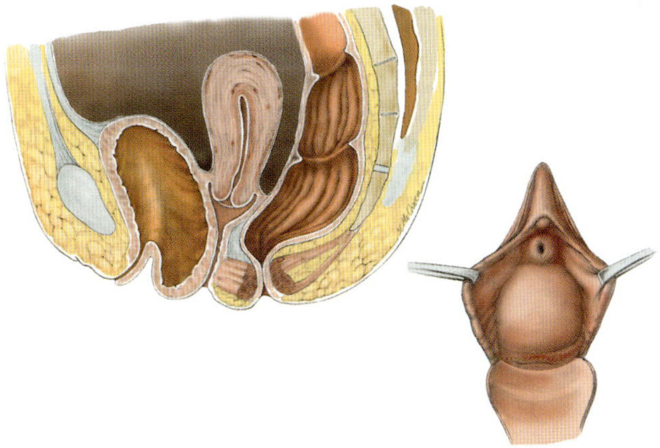

**Fig. 7.4** Side and direct views of cystocele. (Modified from Symmonds RE. Anatomy of the female reproductive system. In: Benson RC, ed. *Current Obstetric and Gynecologic Diagnosis and Treatment.* 5th ed. Los Altos, CA: Lange Medical; 1984.)

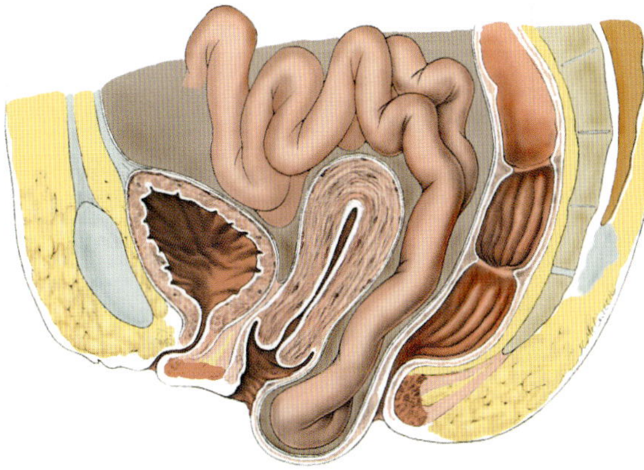

**Fig. 7.6** Lateral view of enterocele. (Modified from Symmonds RE: Relaxations of pelvic supports. In: Benson RC, ed. *Current Obstetric and Gynecologic Diagnosis and Treatment.* 5th ed. Los Altos, CA: Lange Medical; 1984.)

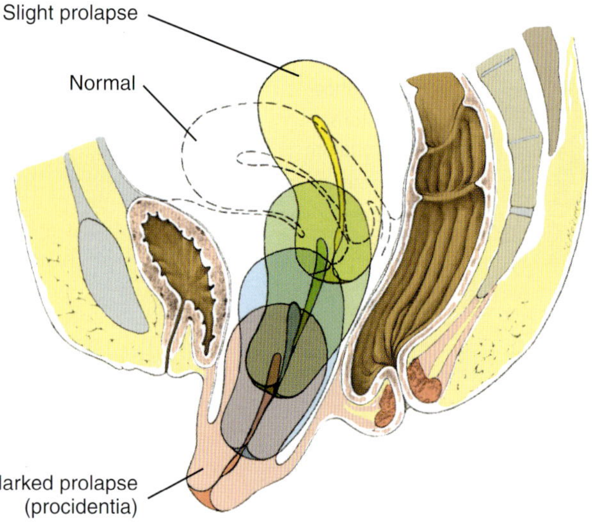


**Fig. 7.7** Depiction of prolapse of uterus. (Modified from Symmonds RE: Relaxations of pelvic supports. In: Benson RC, ed. *Current Obstetric and Gynecologic Diagnosis and Treatment.* 5th ed. Los Altos, CA: Lange Medical; 1984.)

may become visible, indicating prolapse of the uterus (Fig. 7.7). Each of these observations is evidence for relaxation of the pelvic supports. Accurate evaluation of pelvic organ prolapse is improved by examining the woman while she is standing with her legs spread apart and while performing a Valsalva maneuver. Pelvic organ prolapse and pelvic floor dysfunction are defined and extensively discussed in Chapter 20.

## Speculum Examination

After palpation, the physician chooses the appropriate speculum for the patient. The most commonly used are the Grave and the Pederson specula. The Pederson speculum is narrower and may be more appropriate for virginal or nulligravid women; women with a history of sexual abuse, vaginal pain, or dyspareunia; or postmenopausal women. Each is available in several sizes corresponding to length of the blades (small, medium, large, and extra-large) (Fig. 7.8).

The speculum should be warmed, either by a warming device or by being placed in warm water, and then touched to the patient's leg to determine that she feels the temperature is appropriate and comfortable. Judicious use of a water-based or Pap-specific lubricant can facilitate a more comfortable examination for the patient. The speculum is then inserted by placing the transverse diameter of the blades in the anteroposterior position and guiding the blades through the introitus in a downward motion with the tips pointing toward the rectum. Because the anterior wall of the vagina is backed by the pubic symphysis, which is rigid, pressure upward causes the patient discomfort. This is avoided by following the described method of introducing the speculum. Also, in the resting state the vagina lies on the rectum and actually extends posteriorly from the introitus. Placing two fingers into the introitus and pressing down may facilitate the procedure.

Once the speculum is fully inserted to its full length and then opened, the physician should inspect the entire vagina and cervix. If the cervix cannot be visualized with repositioning of the speculum, the physician should digitally palpate for the position of the cervix and then reinsert the speculum accordingly.

The vaginal canal is then inspected during the insertion of the speculum and on its removal. The vaginal epithelium should be noted for evidence of the following:

- Erythema
- Lesions, such as areas of adenosis (see Chapter 11), clear cystic structures (Gartner cysts), or inclusion cysts on the lines of scars or episiotomy incisions
- Abnormal discharge

Any discharge identified can then be collected for a wet mount and potential cultures. Saline wet mount allows for visualization of normal vaginal epithelial cells and any abnormal findings such as motile trichomonads, clue cells (vaginal epithelial cells studded with adherent coccobacilli, indicative of bacterial vaginosis), or polymorphonuclear leukocytes (indicative of inflammation). A potassium hydroxide wet mount includes the whiff-amine test, which, if positive for a distinct fishy odor, may indicate bacterial vaginosis. In addition, inspection of the slide may reveal hyphae and budding yeast, indicative of *Candida* vaginitis.

In many instances, particularly with women younger than 26 years, it is appropriate to screen for chlamydia and gonorrhea using swabs that sample secretions from the endocervical canal or the vagina. The gold standard is nucleic acid amplification testing (NAAT) of the urine or vaginal or cervical discharge, rather than a culture. Yearly chlamydia testing is recommended for all sexually active women up to age 25 (LeFevre, U.S. Preventive Services Task Force, 2014).

Next the cervix is inspected. It should be pink and without lesions. In a nulliparous individual, the external os should be round. When a woman is parous, the external os takes on a slitlike appearance, and if there have been cervical lacerations, healed stellate lacerations may be noted (Fig. 7.9). In premenopausal women the transformation zone (i.e., the junction of squamous and columnar epithelia) is visible at the level of the external os. Occasionally, glandular epithelium may be present on the portio vaginalis, moving the transformation zone onto the portio. This is common in adolescent girls, women who have been exposed to diethylstilbestrol (DES) in utero, some women with vaginitis, and women immediately postpartum or postabortion. Generally this

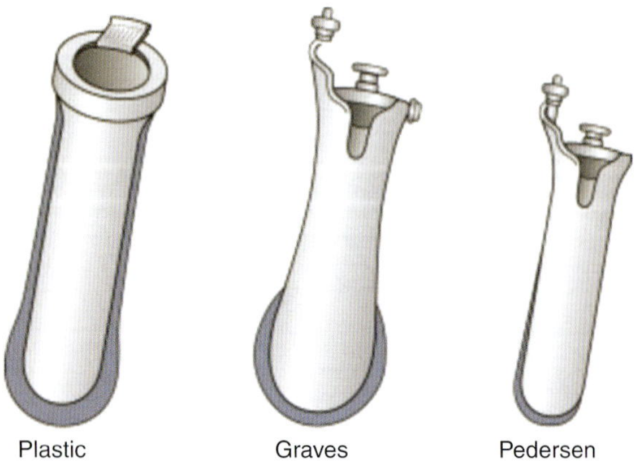


**Fig. 7.8** Graves *(left)* and Pederson *(right)* specula.

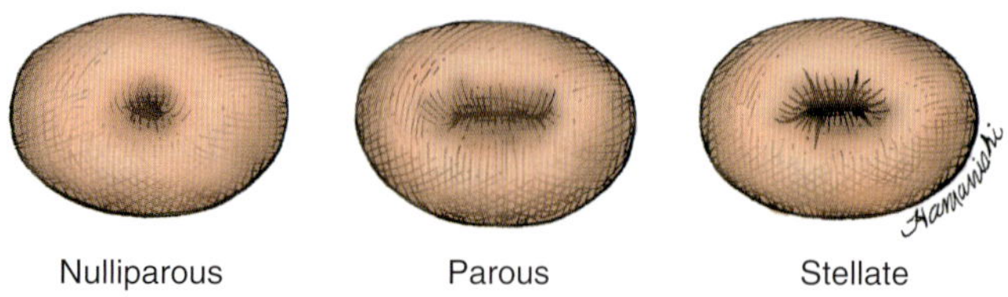


**Fig. 7.9** Nulliparous, parous, and stellate lacerations of cervix.

is cleared by a process of metaplasia, in which squamous epithelium covers the columnar epithelium. This process, however, may leave small areas of irregularities and inclusion cysts, called *nabothian cysts*, which may be seen in various sizes and shapes. They are typically translucent and range from a few millimeters to up to 3 cm in size. These cysts are common benign findings and require no additional evaluation or treatment.

Cervical ectropion occurs when the endocervical epithelium is exposed to the vaginal environment and takes on a reddish appearance, similar to granulation tissue. This ectropion is not a pathologic condition.

Any lesions of the cervix should be noted and, where appropriate, a biopsy should be performed. In a patient with acute herpes simplex, vesicles or ulcers may be noted. In a patient infected with human papillomavirus (HPV), warts (condylomata acuminata) on the cervix may also be observed.

## Papanicolaou Smear

At this point in the examination cervical cancer screening test is usually taken, if indicated. In 1943 Papanicolaou and Trout published their now classic monograph demonstrating the value of vaginal and cervical cytologic examination as a screening tool for cervical neoplasm. With the use of the Pap smear in screening programs, the incidence of invasive cervical cancer has been reduced by 50%. Table 7.5 shows the current recommendations for initiation of screening, options for screening (Pap, cotest, or primary HPV), and frequency of screening. Exceptions to the screening frequency illustrated in Table 7.5 include women who are HIV seropositive or immunosuppressed and women exposed to DES in utero, all of whom should be screened annually (Saslow, 2012). It is crucial to educate women that this extended interval shown in Table 7.5 between Pap smears is based on long-term, excellent analysis of the existing data. However, the **importance of this cancer screening should continue to be highlighted during annual preventive visits because we know that 50% of cervical cancer cases develop in women who have never had a Pap test, and an additional 10% occur in women who have been underscreened** (Saslow, 2012). No Pap smear screening is necessary after a complete hysterectomy done for benign conditions. However, if a supracervical hysterectomy was performed, the same screening guidelines pertain as if there had been no hysterectomy because the cervix remains in situ. In 2020, the American Cancer Society (ACS) updated their guidance for cervical cancer screening. This guidance is based on large clinical data sets that reveal "consistent low cervical cancer incidence and mortality among women aged <25 years, the high incidence of transient infections, the risk of adverse obstetric outcomes of treatment, and the decision analysis demonstrating a favorable benefit-to-harm balance for beginning screening at age 25 years." Other organizations such as ASCCP, ACOG, and USPSTF have not changed their screening guidelines, however. ACS is recommending the following:

- cervical cancer screening be initiated at age 25, rather than age 21;
- screening should be performed with primary HPV, where available, not pap smear or co-test;
- follow-up screening with HPV should be every 5 years (Fontham, 2020).

The goal of the Pap smear is to collect cells from the transformation zone of the cervix. The presence of adequate endo- and ectocervical cells ensures that this area is captured in the specimen. After excess mucus is gently removed (routine swabbing may cause insufficient cells to be sampled), the endocervical canal is sampled with a Cytobrush, which is placed into the canal and rotated. A spatula is then used to collect ectocervical cells (Figs. 7.10 and 7.11). A single broomlike sampling device can also be used to collect both populations of cells in a single step. The collected material is placed in the liquid preservative solution. HPV testing can be concurrently ordered from the collected sample, as indicated.

Chapter 28 discusses cervical dysplasia, classifications of abnormalities, surveillance, and treatment options.

## Bimanual Examination

**The bimanual examination allows the physician to palpate the uterus and the adnexa.** The lubricated index and middle fingers of the dominant hand are placed within the vagina, and the thumb is folded under so as not to cause the patient distress in the area of the mons pubis, clitoris, and pubic symphysis. The fingers are inserted deeply into the vagina so that they rest beneath the cervix in the posterior fornix. The opposite hand is placed on the patient's abdomen above the pubic symphysis. The flat of the fingers are used for palpation. The physician then elevates the uterus by pressing up on the cervix and delivering the uterus to the abdominal hand so that the uterus may be placed between the two hands, thereby identifying its position, size, shape, consistency, and mobility. In the normal and nonpregnant state, the uterus is approximately 6 cm × 4 cm and weighs approximately 60 g. It may be somewhat larger in a woman who has had children (Fig. 7.12).

Enlargement of the uterus should be described in detail. Size may be estimated in centimeters or by comparing with weeks of normal gestational age. The position of the uterus should be noted:

**TABLE 7.5** Cervical Cancer Screening Recommendations

| Age/Status | ASCCP/ACS/ASCP | USPSTF | Comments |
|---|---|---|---|
| <21 | No screening | No screening | |
| 21-29 | • Cytologic testing every 3 years<br>• Optional HPV primary screen (age 25+) | Cytologic testing every 3 years | |
| 30-65 | • HPV/Pap (cotest) every 5 years<br>• Pap every 3 years | • Pap every 3 years<br>• HPV primary every 5 years<br>• Cotest every 5 years | |
| 66+ | No screening after adequate negative prior screening | No screening after adequate negative prior screening | If CIN2+, should screen for at least 20 years |
| After hysterectomy | No screening | No screening | With a history of normal screening or >20 years since CIN2+, no cancer diagnosis |

*ACS*, American Cancer Society; *ASCCP*, American Society for Colposcopy and Cervical Pathology; *ASCP*, American Society for Clinical Pathology; *CIN*, cervical intraepithelial neoplasia; *HPV*, human papillomavirus; *Pap*, Papanicolaou test; *USPSTF*, U.S. Preventive Services Task Force.

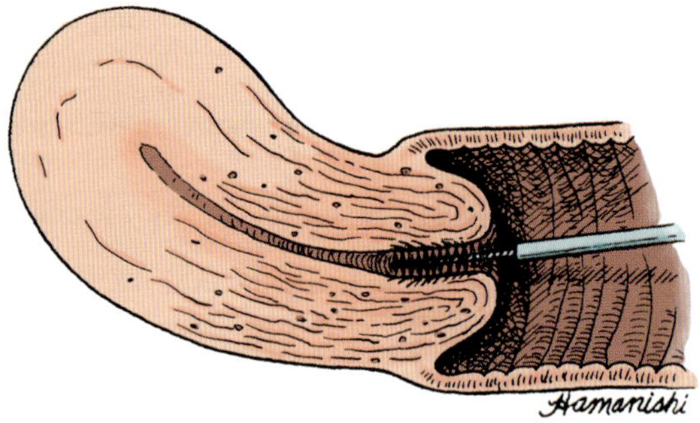


Fig. 7.10 Obtaining cells from endocervix using a Cytobrush.

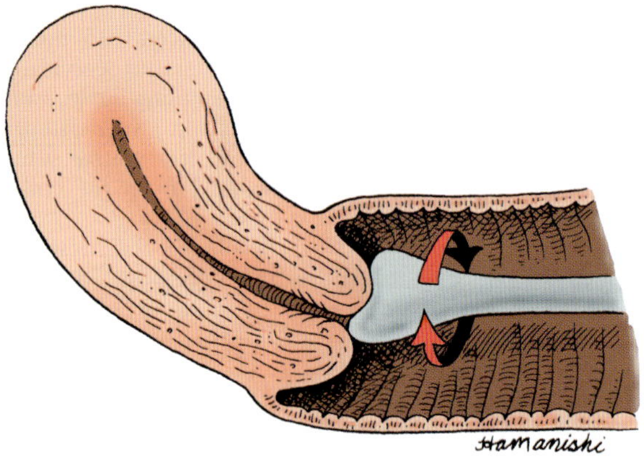


Fig. 7.11 Obtaining cells from transformation zone using Ayers spatula.

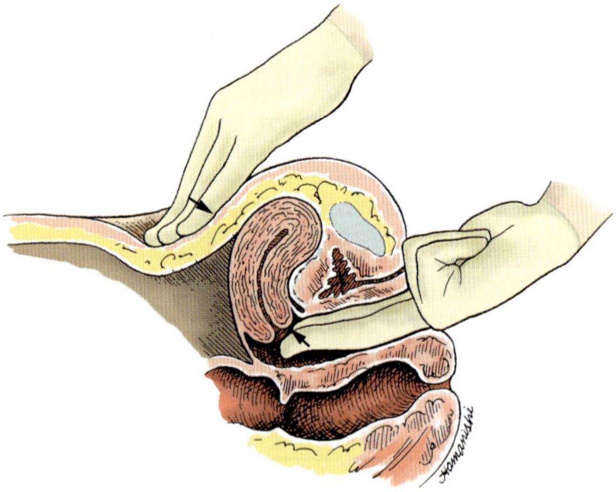


Fig. 7.12 Bimanual examination of uterus.

- Anteverted: The uterus is tipped forward toward the symphysis pubis.
- Anteflexed uterus: The fundus points anteriorly as well.
- Retroverted: The uterus tips posteriorly.
- Retroflexed: The fundus points posteriorly as well.
- Midposition or neutral: The uterus is positioned in a straight line with the vagina.

A markedly retroverted uterus that cannot be brought forward by manipulation is best inspected by rectovaginal examination, which is described later in the chapter. The general shape of the uterus is that of a pear, with the broadest portion at the upper pole of the fundus. Generally the uterus is mobile, and if it fails to move,

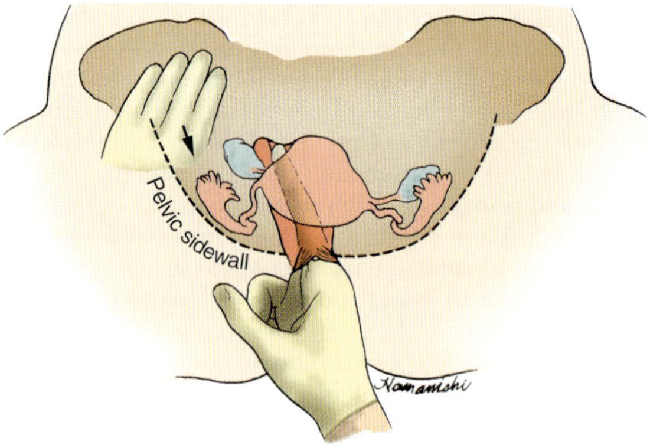


Fig. 7.13 Bimanual examination of adnexa.

it may be fixed by adhesions. The surface should be smooth; irregularities may indicate the presence of uterine leiomyomas (fibroids).

The shape of the uterus should also be described in detail. The consistency of the uterus is generally firm but not rock hard, and this should be noted in the examination. Any undue tenderness caused by palpation or movement of the uterus should be noted because it may imply an inflammatory process.

Attention is then turned to examination of the adnexa. If the right hand is the pelvic hand, the first two fingers of the right hand are then moved into the right vaginal fornix as deeply as they can be inserted. The abdominal hand is placed just medial to the anterior superior iliac spine on the right, the two hands are brought as close together as possible, and with a sliding motion from the area of the anterior superior iliac spine to the introitus, the fingers are swept downward, allowing for the adnexa to be palpated between them. A normal ovary is approximately 3 × 2 cm (about the size of a walnut) and will sweep between the two fingers with ease unless it is fixed in an abnormal position by adhesions. When the adnexa are palpated, its size, mobility, and consistency should be described. When the right adnexa has been palpated, the left adnexa should be palpated in a similar fashion by turning the vaginal hand to the left vaginal fornix and repeating the exercise on the left side (Fig. 7.13). Adnexa are usually not palpable in postmenopausal women because of involution and retraction of the ovary to a position higher in the pelvis. A palpable organ in such an individual may need further investigation for ovarian pathologic changes if enlarged, although they are mostly benign, or no disease is found.

## Rectovaginal Examination

Historically, the rectovaginal (RV) examination has been a part of the annual examination. In fact, however, the **sensitivity of the RV examination in detecting pathologic conditions is very low, limiting its capacity as a screening test. The RV examination should therefore only be performed as indicated based on patient symptoms or complaints or based on findings from the pelvic examination**.

After completing the vaginal portion of the bimanual examination, the middle finger is relubricated with a water-soluble lubricant and placed into the rectum. The index finger is reinserted into the vagina. In this fashion the rectovaginal septum is palpated between the two fingers, and any thickness or mass is noted. The finger should also attempt to identify the uterosacral ligaments, which extend from the posterior wall of the cervix posteriorly and laterally toward the sacrum. Any thickening or nodularity of these structures may imply an inflammatory reaction or endometriosis. If the uterus is retroverted, that organ should be outlined for size, shape, and consistency at this point. It may be examined appropriately using the fingers inserted into the vagina and the rectum, as well as using the abdominal hand (Fig. 7.14).

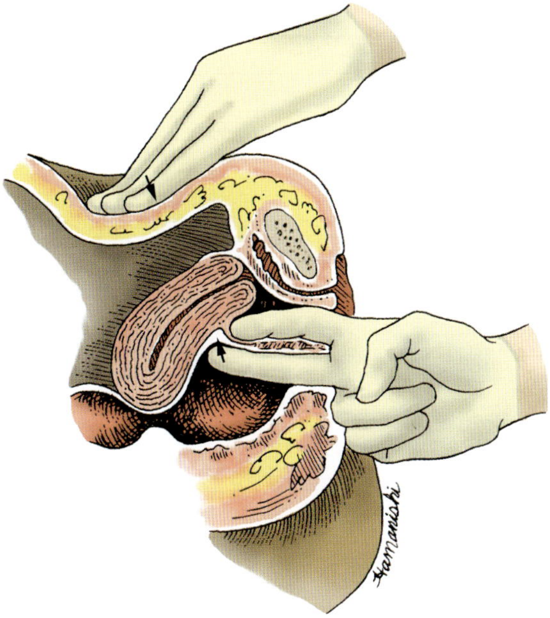

**Fig. 7.14** Rectovaginal examination.

## Rectal Examination

**The USPSTF and the ACS find that a digital rectal examination, by itself, is not adequate screening for colorectal cancer.** Furthermore, testing a single stool specimen for fecal occult blood is also inadequate. Therefore routine assessment of the rectum is not recommended during female pelvic examinations. Colon cancer screening recommendations are described later in this chapter.

Like the RV examination, a rectal examination should only be performed based on patient symptoms, concerns, or findings on the pelvic examination. As noted earlier, simple inspection of the perianal area can reveal abnormalities such as genital warts, hemorrhoids, or skin lesions.

The rectum is then palpated in all dimensions with the rectal examining finger. It should be possible to palpate as many as 70% of distal bowel lesions with the rectal finger. The physician should also note the tone of the anal sphincter and any other anal abnormalities, such as hemorrhoids, fissures, or masses. At the end of the examination the physician should give the patient some tissue or a washcloth so that she may remove the lubricating gel from her perineum before she dresses.

It is important that each step of the examination be explained to the patient and that she is reassured about all normal findings. Wherever possible, abnormal findings should be pointed out to the patient either by allowing her to palpate the location of the pathologic condition or by demonstrating it to her using a hand mirror. The physician can use the examination as a vehicle for teaching the patient about her body.

# ADVOCACY, SCREENING, INTERVENTIONS, AND REFERRAL

Once a comprehensive history and any relevant physical examination are completed, the provider now has not only the opportunity but also the responsibility to advocate for the patient's health. **The annual visit is important for both health maintenance and preventive medicine reasons. Although the visit varies in emphasis depending on the patient's age, the long-term goals should be to maintain the woman in the best health and functional status possible, to promote high-quality longevity, and to aid in early detection of disease.** Long-term continuity of care may improve health status. Major preventable problems must be discussed because patient behavior can make a difference. Various medical groups update recommendations for primary and preventive screening services regularly. Much of this chapter uses guidelines from the USPSTF, ACOG, and Centers for Disease Control and Prevention (CDC); the CDC's *Morbidity and Mortality Weekly Report (MMWR)*; and the Agency for Healthcare Research and Quality. The latter is a clearinghouse of evidence-based guidelines that allows comparison of differing recommendations because many societies do not always agree on these guidelines. Their websites can be checked for updates.

According to the CDC (https://www.cdc.gov/heartdisease/women.htm) cardiovascular disease is the number one cause of death among U.S. women, with cancer being the second leading cause. Tobacco use, inactivity, poor nutrition, and ever-increasing rates of obesity all contribute to both cardiovascular illness and to malignancies. Obviously, patients taking an active role in changing their behavior can alter many of these factors, and direct physician recommendations may promote wellness activities. **Although the gynecologist may or may not function as the sole primary care provider for women, the annual visit is an opportunity to discuss patient choices, lifestyle, and habits. It offers a perfect environment to provide education about healthy lifestyle and prevention strategies to reduce harm and improve health.**

At each checkup the physician should also encourage the patient to develop an exercise program appropriate for her abilities and taking into account her overall health status and recommendations from any other health care providers. Table 7.6 presents the CDC recommendations for types and duration of exercise by age group.

For patients who smoke, benefits of reduction and cessation should be addressed and resources provided. Tobacco use is a leading preventable cause of death in the United States. More intensive options to aid in smoking cessation include pharmacotherapy with nicotine replacement, bupropion, or varenicline. Appropriate referrals to specialists and support groups are indicated.

Any alcohol or drug use and potential abuse should also be discussed. Short alcohol use screening questionnaires such as the CAGE questionnaire are used in many primary and specialty care clinics. Women with substance use disorders can then be appropriately referred for ongoing care.

With an updated list of all medications and supplements, the physician should review indications for their use and also potential adverse drug interactions.

The annual visit is an opportunity for the physician to screen for a variety of illnesses affecting not only the reproductive organs but also all the organ systems. **In addition to the clinical breast and pelvic examinations and cervical cancer screening, in 2013 ACOG published online Well-Woman Care: Assessments & Recommendations, which recommended screening examinations, immunizations, and laboratory tests for the annual visit for women in different age groups (see Table 7.2).** Women with concurrent medical conditions such as obesity or hypertension, women with certain lifestyle choices such as tobacco use, and women with certain family histories should be directed to screening that may be sooner or more frequent than that recommended for the general population.

Recommendations for screening mammography have evolved substantially in the past several years. Three different ages of mammography initiation and varying frequency recommendations concurrently exist in the United States (Table 7.7). **A thorough discussion between patient and provider will allow patient-centered decision making in regard to when to start mammography screenings and the interval for follow-up screening. This approach takes into consideration the woman's actual risks, tolerance for risk, and preferences.**

**TABLE 7.6** CDC Exercise Recommendations

| | Minimum Exercise | | |
|---|---|---|---|
| **Age (Years)** | **Option 1** | **Option 2** | **Option 3** |
| 18-64 | 2.5 hours moderate-intensity aerobic activity/week* and muscle-strengthening† activities 2+ days/week | 75 minutes vigorous-intensity aerobic activity/week‡ and muscle-strengthening activities 2+ days/week | Equivalent mix of moderate and vigorous aerobic activity and muscle-strengthening‡ activities 2+ days/week |
| 65+ | 2.5 hours moderate-intensity aerobic activity/week* and muscle-strengthening† activities 2+ days/week | 75 minutes vigorous-intensity aerobic activity/week‡ and muscle-strengthening activities 2+ days/week | Equivalent mix of moderate and vigorous aerobic activity and muscle-strengthening‡ activities 2+ days/week |

Data from Centers for Disease Control and Prevention (CDC). Physical activity basics. How much physical activity do adults need? 2015. Available at http://www.cdc.gov/physicalactivity/basics/adults/index.htm; and Centers for Disease Control and Prevention (CDC): Physical Activity Basics. How much physical activity do older adults need? 2015. Available at http://www.cdc.gov/physicalactivity/everyone/guidelines/olderadults.html.
*Moderate-intensity aerobic activity: brisk walking, water aerobics, pushing lawn mower.
†Muscle-strengthening activities: weightlifting, resistance bands, pushups, heavy gardening, yoga. Older adults need to adjust both type and intensity of exercise. Increasing overall time of aerobic exercise beyond the minimal recommendations further increases health benefits.
‡Vigorous-intensity aerobic activity: running, swimming laps, basketball.

**TABLE 7.7** Mammography Guidelines: Recommendations for Women at Average Risk

| Patient Age | ACS, 2015 | ACP, 2015 | ACOG/NCI/ACR, 2016 | USPSTF, 2016 | AAFP, 2016 |
|---|---|---|---|---|---|
| 40-44 | Shared decision making (SDM) | SDM, biennial | Annual | SDM | SDM, biennial |
| 45-49 | Annual | SDM, biennial | Annual | SDM | SDM, biennial |
| 50-74 | Annual, biennial, SDM | Biennial | Annual | Biennial | biennial |
| 75+ | SDM | No | SDM | No | SDM |

*AAFP,* American Academy of Family Physicians; *ACOG;* American College of Obstetricians and Gynecologists; *ACP* American College of Physicians; *ACR,* American College of Radiology; *ACS,* American Cancer Society; *NCI,* National Cancer Institute; *USPSTF,* U.S. Preventive Services Task Force.

**Varying national guidelines for the initiation of colon cancer screening also warrant a complete discussion between patient and provider (Table 7.8).** A family history of polyps does not necessitate earlier onset of screening unless the polyps were advanced adenomas. If a single first-degree relative had colorectal cancer diagnosed after age 60, routine screening is recommended. Otherwise, screening should begin 10 years before the age at which the family member developed colorectal cancer.

Other screening tests, such as tests for hepatitis C and tuberculosis, should certainly be considered for women in high-risk groups, with comorbid medical conditions, or with certain family histories. The USPSTF also recommends offering one-time screening for hepatitis C in adults born between 1945 and 1965.

Endometrial cancer recommendations for early detection consist of advising women at menopause of their risk factors and the symptoms of endometrial cancer. Those symptoms include unexpected vaginal bleeding or spotting. Even in women known to be at increased risk of endometrial cancer, there is insufficient evidence to recommend screening.

Risk factors for endometrial cancer include the following:

- Unopposed estrogen treatment
- Tamoxifen therapy
- Late menopause
- Nulliparity
- Infertility or anovulation
- Obesity
- Hypertension
- Diabetes

Women with certain conditions, such as known hereditary nonpolyposis colorectal cancer, genetic mutation carriers, and strongly suspected carriers, should have an annual endometrial biopsy starting at age 35.

**TABLE 7.8** Colon Cancer Screening Guidelines

| | Initiate Screening, Age | End Regular Screening, Age |
|---|---|---|
| ACS, 2018 | 45 | 75 |
| USMSTF, 2017* | 50 | 75 |
| USPSTF, 2016† | 50 (45 if AA) | 75 |
| AAFP, 2016 | 50 | 75 |
| ACP, 2015 | 50 | 75 |
| NCCN, 2013 | 50 | 75 |

All organizations state that between ages 76 to 85 patients and their physicians, through shared decision making, may opt to continue screening.
All organizations recommend an absolute end to screening for patients older than 85.
*USMSTF is the U.S. Multi-society Task Force on Colorectal Cancer (consisting of the American College of Gastroenterology, the American Gastroenterological Association, and the American Society for Gastrointestinal Endoscopy). In 2018 they reviewed ACS recommendations and felt that evidence was limited to recommend screening beginning at age 45.
†A 2019 update is in progress evaluating beginning screening at age 45.
*AA,* African American; *AAFP,* American Academy of Family Physicians; *ACP,* American College of Physicians; *ACS,* American Cancer Society; *NCCN,* National Comprehensive Cancer Network; *USPSTF,* U.S. Preventive Services Task Force.

**The best source of updated recommendations for adult immunization schedules is the CDC's MMWR website (see Table 7.2).** All women should have a Tdap (tetanus, diphtheria, and pertussis) booster once in their adult lifetime and in each third trimester of pregnancy to facilitate some passive immunity to the fetus against *Bordetella pertussis*. Then, every 10 years, the regular Td (tetanus-diphtheria) booster is given. Influenza vaccination is recommended annually as well.

A highly efficacious HPV vaccine is advised for both men and women. In 2006 the Advisory Committee on Immunization Practices (ACIP) and then ACOG recommended vaccinating all girls and young women ages 9 to 26. The U.S. Food and Drug Administration (FDA) approved this in 2009. In 2011 ACIP recommended this vaccination for boys and young men as well. In 2014 the newest and most compressive vaccine, Gardasil 9, was approved for all people age 9 to 26. Finally, in 2018, the FDA approved Gardasil 9 for women and men through age 45; however, this has yet to be approved by ACIP. Ideally the vaccine should be administered before the onset of sexual activity to prevent cervical dysplasia and cancer and other diseases caused by low- and high-risk strains of HPV. See Chapter 29 for further details about cervical intraepithelial neoplasia.

For women in high-risk groups, MMR (measles-mumps-rubella) and hepatitis B vaccines should be given if indicated. The pneumococcal vaccine should be offered to women with chronic lung, liver, or cardiovascular disease; diabetes; asplenia; cochlear implants; and immunocompromising conditions. Herpes zoster vaccination (for shingles) is recommended for women age 50 and older. For women who are 65 and older, the pneumococcal vaccine should be given once.

In addition, women in all age groups should be offered appropriate immunizations and vaccinations when they travel to other countries. The hepatitis A vaccine is available and should be offered to women of all ages. In particular, the hepatitis A vaccine should be given to women who are traveling to areas with a high or intermediate endemicity of hepatitis A, use injection drugs, have chronic liver disease, receive clotting factor concentrates, or work with primates infected with hepatitis A.

Physicians should discuss risk behavior annually with their patients. In line with injury prevention, the patient should be reminded about the use of seat belts and helmets and other safety concerns mentioned earlier in this chapter. Fall precautions can be discussed with elderly patients.

Exposure of the skin to ultraviolet radiation and proper precautions to avoid overexposure should be discussed. Regular dental checkups should be encouraged. Adequate calcium and vitamin D intake for proper bone health and age-appropriate intake recommendations should be reviewed at the annual visit (Table 7.9).

## SPECIAL POPULATIONS

Data from the 2010 U.S. Census indicated there were an estimated 56 million noninstitutionalized people with a self-care disability in the United States. **Women with disabilities have some unique barriers to gynecologic care. Aside from communication obstacles and nonavailability of facilities with accessible examinations tables to make routine pelvic examinations easily performed, the patient may face ignorance or negative attitudes about a woman's life with disabilities.** Women with disabilities undergo screening for cervical and breast cancer less often than recommended. Contraception, sexuality issues, childbearing plans, and abuse issues may all have to be addressed.

Data from the 2006 to 2008 National Survey of Family Growth revealed that 1.1% and 3.5% of women identify as lesbian or bisexual, respectively. In addition, a small but substantial number of individuals identify as transgender. ACOG reflects that persons in these groups face barriers to health care, including discriminatory attitudes and treatment, confidentiality and disclosure concerns, limited health care access, and perhaps limited understanding of their risks. Physicians should not make assumptions about a patient's sexual orientation, gender identity, or type of sexual activity. Physicians sometimes conclude, incorrectly, that lesbian women do not need sexually transmitted infection or Pap screening because they are considered low risk. Fertility services should not be influenced by sexual orientation. ACOG has developed committee opinions with background information and recommendations (Committee Opinion no. 512 [ACOG, 2011] and Committee Opinion no. 525 [ACOG, 2012]).

**In summary, promoting good health is a continuing responsibility for both the physician and the patient.** It represents a challenge that includes education and observation on the physician's part and motivation on the patient's part. The U.S. Department of Health and Human Services has a division devoted to women's health titled the Office on Women's Health. Its website (www.womenshealth.gov) offers accurate patient information on screening recommendations for both healthy and at-risk women. Furthermore, the website lists symptoms of serious health conditions for heart attack and stroke, as well as for reproductive, breast, lung, digestive, bladder, skin, mental health, and muscle or joint problems. ACOG similarly has a comprehensive document for providing screening and prevention suggestions for women (www.acog.org/wellwoman).

**TABLE 7.9** Recommended Intakes of Calcium and Vitamin D

| Age (Years) | Intake Calcium (mg) | Intake Vitamin D (IU) |
|---|---|---|
| 14-18 | 1300 | 600 |
| 19-50 | 1000 | 600 |
| 51-70 | 1200 | 600 |
| 71+ | 1200 | 800 |
| Pregnancy and lactation | 1000 | 600 |

From Institute of Medicine, Food and Nutrition Board. *Dietary Reference Intakes for Calcium and Vitamin D.* Washington, DC: National Academy Press; 2010. Available at http://iom.nationalacademies.org/Reports/2010/Dietary-Reference-Intakes-for-Calcium-and-Vitamin-D/DRI-Values.aspx.

## REFERENCES

American College of Obstetricians and Gynecologists (ACOG). The utility of and indications for routine pelvic examination. ACOG Committee Opinion 754, 2018. https://www.acog.org/clinical/clinical-guidance/committee-opinion/articles/2018/10/the-utility-of-and-indications-for-routine-pelvic-examination.

American College of Obstetricians and Gynecologists (ACOG). Well-woman visit. ACOG Committee Opinion 755, 2018. https://www.acog.org/clinical/clinical-guidance/committee-opinion/articles/2018/10/well-woman-visit.

American College of Obstetricians and Gynecologists (ACOG). Breast cancer risk assessment and screening in average-risk women. ACOG Practice Bulletin 179, July 2017. https://www.acog.org/clinical/clinical-guidance/practice-bulletin/articles/2017/07/breast-cancer-risk-assessment-and-screening-in-average-risk-women.

Fontham EH, et al. Cervical Cancer Screening for Individuals at Average Risk: 2020 Guideline Update form the American Cancer Society. *Ca Cancer J Clin* 2020;70: 321-346

Moyer VA. Screening for HIV: U.S. Preventive Services Task Force Recommendation Statement. *Ann Intern Med.* 2013;159:51-60.

Saslow D, Solomon D, Lawson HW, et al. American Cancer Society, American Society for Colposcopy and Cervical Pathology, and American Society for Clinical Pathology screening guidelines for the prevention and early detection of cervical cancer. *CA Cancer J Clin.* 2012;62(3):147-172.

Senn CY, Eliasziw, M, Barata, P, Thurston WE, Newby-Clark, IR, Radtke HR, K Hobden KL. Efficacy of a Sexual Assault Resistance Program for University Women *N Engl J Med* 2015; 372:2326-2335 "http://www.nejm.org.offcampus.lib.washington.edu/toc/nejm/372/24/" June 11, 2015DOI: 10.1056/NEJMsa1411131

**Suggested readings for this chapter can be found on ExpertConsult.com.**

# 8 Interaction of Medical Diseases and Female Physiology

*Sarah K. Dotters-Katz, Fidel A. Valea*

## KEY POINTS

- Long-acting reversible contraception (LARC) methods are safe, effective, and have minimal risk of user error; thus they have become the recommended option for most women with complicated chronic illnesses.
- The severity of asthma symptoms increases around the time of menses.
- Many women with irritable bowel syndrome (IBS) and inflammatory bowel disease (IBD) have exacerbations of symptoms with menses.
- Women with chronic renal disease often experience menorrhagia and irregular menses, which often improves with transplant.
- Estrogen-containing contraceptives are not recommended in women with hypertension who are older than 35, use tobacco, have poorly controlled disease, or are on medications for hypertension.
- Progesterone stabilizes red cell membranes and significantly decreases the frequency of sickling crises.
- Withdrawal of progesterone (even in small amounts such as in the periovulatory period) leads to a significant decline in the seizure threshold and an increase in seizure frequency and severity.
- Women who have migraines with aura are more susceptible to stroke, and thus the use of estrogen-containing contraceptives (ECCs) in women with migraines with aura is contraindicated.
- Early referral of women with cancer to a reproductive endocrinologist with expertise in potential therapies to preserve fertility is important.

This chapter highlights the interactions with and influences of female physiology on major medical disease processes. The chapter also reviews how medical diseases affect female physiology. Many disease processes act directly; for example, renal failure commonly induces abnormal uterine bleeding. Other diseases act indirectly through their therapies, such as cancer chemotherapy, which may lead to ovarian failure. Multiple chapters in this text discuss important aspects of female physiology. This chapter serves as an addendum to those discussions. When considering specific drug interactions and doses, the clinician is encouraged to review current pharmacologic literature.

In general, **the impact of female physiology on medical disease is primarily via the effects of estrogen and to a lesser extent progesterone.** Other hormones, such as prolactin, oxytocin, and gonadotropins, play minor roles. Estrogen and progesterone affect almost all major organ systems in both tonic and cyclic modes. The effects of the female hormones are mediated directly through receptors (estrogen alpha, estrogen beta, progesterone) and indirectly through their effects on other organ systems, such as smooth muscle relaxation and changes in prostaglandin levels. The responses induced by estrogen and progesterone may be theorized, in a teleologic sense, as promoting successful reproduction. Pathology occurs when the normal hormonal effects overlap a disease process that is already present.

Medical diseases affect female physiology at all levels of the hypothalamic-pituitary-ovarian-genital axis, from anovulation to vaginal atrophy. Medical diseases also affect female physiology in a horizontal manner, throughout every stage of a woman's life. Thus medical diseases must be seen in both a vertical and a horizontal context (i.e., a three-dimensional manner). Because gynecologists commonly act as consultants to other health professionals, we are often asked to help with complications stemming from gynecologic issues. Though different clinicians direct the treatment of lupus, multiple sclerosis, or epilepsy, modulating the effects of female physiology on these disease processes is the role of the gynecologist.

## PULMONARY DISEASE

Asthma is more common in boys up until puberty. After puberty, the ratio reverses with women more at risk for asthma until menopause. **Asthma is one of several major diseases in which the severity of symptoms is increased around the time of menses** (Box 8.1). Premenstrual asthma is well described, affecting up to 40% of reproductive-age women who have asthma, with symptoms including increasing cough, wheezing, and shortness of breath. Up to 50% of hospitalizations for women with asthma in their 20s occur around the time of menses. Women with premenstrual asthma have been shown to have a measurable decline in respiratory function with the end of the menstrual cycle (Dratva, 2010). Data suggest that combination oral contraceptive pills (cOCPs) may blunt this effect and mildly decrease the severity of the asthma (Dratva, 2010). The variability of symptoms between cycles may be caused by the hormonal fluctuations from one cycle to the next.

Hormones can affect asthmatic symptoms through several mechanisms. One theory is that the increased symptomology is related to the estrogen- and progesterone-mediated increase in both serotonin and histamine release from granulocytes and mast cells (van den Berge, 2009). Estrogen also increases eosinophilic adhesion to the bronchial lining. In addition, progesterone induces degranulation of eosinophils. Interestingly, both estrogen and progesterone also have antiinflammatory properties, and it may be that the withdrawal of estrogen and progesterone at the end of the cycle contributes to a fluctuation in prostaglandin levels that leads to increased bronchial reactivity and premenstrual asthma.

Regarding the effects of asthma on female physiology, a few small series have noted an increased incidence of abnormal menstrual cycles in women with severe asthma (Real, 2007). Whether this is due to glucocorticoid medications or whether this is a direct effect from severe pulmonary disease on the hypothalamus is unclear. It should be noted that multiple studies have found that

**BOX 8.1** Major Diseases in Which Menstrual Hormonal Changes Affect Symptoms

Asthma
Atopic reactions
Epilepsy
Eating disorders
Irritable bowel syndrome
Menstrual migraines
Mental health disorders
Multiple sclerosis
Inflammatory bowel disease
Rheumatoid arthritis
Supraventricular tachycardia
Sickle cell disease
Type 1 diabetes

women with early menarche have twice the risk of asthma in early adulthood (Fida, 2012). Women who are taking inhaled glucocorticoids may be at increased risk for osteopenia and osteoporosis (Aljubran, 2014). Clinicians who care for women with asthma beyond their third decade should obtain vitamin D levels and council the women about adequate calcium intake. There are conflicting reports about the effect of menopause and hormone replacement therapy on asthma symptoms and severity; some have noted an improvement in symptoms, whereas others have noted a worsening (Tam, 2011; van den Berge, 2009). Increasing evidence exists to suggest that there may be a perimenopausal/menopausal phenotype of new-onset asthma characterized by neutrophilic airway inflammation and high frequency of severe exacerbations (Foschino Barbaro, 2010). Other data suggest that independent of asthma onset, asthma exacerbation after menopause tends to be more severe (Bialek-Gosk, 2018). Given these data, clinicians must be wary of any asthma in a perimenopausal or menopausal patient.

It is now common for women with cystic fibrosis (CF) to reach reproductive age. Tsang and colleagues, in a review of reproductive problems, noted that women with cystic fibrosis tend to have shorter stature, delayed puberty with delayed growth spurts, and delayed menarche (Tsang, 2010). The degree of delay is related to the severity of the disease. Additionally, because of the effects of estradiol on mucin production, periods of the menstrual cycle with high estradiol levels are associated with worse lung function (Tam, 2011). Girls with cystic fibrosis tend to be as sexually active as their peers; however, they tend to have less counseling regarding contraception than their peers. Estrogen-based contraceptives are acceptable for women with cystic fibrosis as long as they do not have pulmonary hypertension, active liver disease, or a history of thromboembolism (Tsang, 2010). Long-acting reversible contraception (LARC), including the progesterone intrauterine devices (IUDs) and progesterone implants, are also a safe, effective, and practical option for these young women. Issues of sexuality may be problematic for young women with severe cystic fibrosis because of poor body image secondary to chronic disease, infections, and gastrointestinal disturbances from pancreatic problems, as well as enlarged rib cages from chronic hyperventilation in some patients. Thus counseling on sexuality should occur in conjunction with contraceptive counseling.

There is an emerging body of evidence suggesting that fertility is affected in women with cystic fibrosis. Cervical mucus is thicker in women with cystic fibrosis, which may lead to altered fertility. **Oligomenorrhea, amenorrhea, and ovulatory dysfunction are increased in women with cystic fibrosis** proportionally to the severity of disease. Finally, alterations in uterine levels of bicarbonate, which affects sperm capacitation, also affect fertility in women with cystic fibrosis (Ahmad, 2013). Though a full discussion of the management of subfertility and infertility treatment options is beyond the scope of this chapter, intrauterine insemination, intracytoplasmic sperm injection, and in vitro fertilization have all been successfully performed in women with CF.

## Immune and Allergic Disease

The profound effect that female physiology has on immunity is best exemplified by the remarkably increased survival of women compared with men from infectious causes of disease. Estrogen and progesterone have multiple effects on the immune processes through numerous cellular sites. This is manifest in multiple disease processes (Box 8.2). In most women the effects are mild, but in women constitutionally or genetically predisposed to atopic reaction or autoimmune disease, the effects can be significant.

The overall effect may be grossly simplified in noting estrogen's effect on the B cell as an immune enhancer (Lang, 2004). In contrast, on T cells, estrogen tends to act as an inhibitor (Lang, 2004). Importantly, estrogen effects vary by the level and type of

**BOX 8.2** Effects of Estrogen and Progesterone on Cellular Processes of the Immune System

**B CELL**

Inhibited bone marrow B-cell lines with high concentrations of estrogen
Increased antibody production through inhibition of T-cell suppression
Enhanced interleukin-10 response

**T CELL**

Lower doses of estrogen are stimulatory, higher doses of estrogen are inhibitory, primarily through TNF
Stimulation of inhibitory T-cell pathways and T-cell cytokines
Low-level stimulation of interleukins

**MONOCYTES**

Increased monocyte apoptosis inhibiting differentiation
Inhibited dendritic cell differentiation (in vitro)
Inhibited migration of inflammatory cells with decreased migration at higher estrogen levels

**MAST CELLS AND GRANULOCYTES**

Estrogen increases serotonin and histamine release through estrogen alpha receptors
Progesterone promotes IgE production

**GENERAL INFLAMMATION**

Increased presence of estrogen beta receptors over estrogen alpha receptors with generalized inflammation
Increased sensitization of sensory neural tissue leading to increased neurogenic inflammation
Increased fibroblast activity and improved wound healing
Increased stimulation of the hypothalamus-pituitary-adrenal axis
Increased anaphylaxis* and allergic reactions

Data from Chen A, Rogan WJ. Isoflavones in soy infant formula: a review of evidence for endocrine and other activity in infants. *Annu Rev Nutr.* 2004;24:33-54; Lang JT, McCullough LD. Pathways to ischemic neuronal cell death: are sex differences relevant? *J Transl Med.* 2008;6:33; and Straub RH. The complex role of estrogens in inflammation. *Endocr Rev.* 2007;28(5):521-574.
*Includes drug induced and radiologic contrast media induced.
*IgE,* Immunoglobulin E; *TNF,* tumor necrosis factor.

estrogen. At lower levels, as in most of the menstrual cycle, estrogen stimulates immune responses. However, at high estrogen levels such as occur during pregnancy, estrogen generally inhibits immune cellular responses. The effects of estrogen on inflammation have important implications for wound healing. Women tend to heal more effectively than men because estrogen stimulates fibroblast activity and nerve growth. Estrogen's positive effect on reepithelialization lasts until several years after menopause (Straub, 2007). Interestingly, hormone replacement therapy improves wound healing (Peržel'ová, 2016).

B-cell–dominated autoimmune diseases have a higher incidence and severity in women (Straub, 2007). Estrogen enhances the hypersensitivity responses from both B-cell activity and granulocyte action in allergic responses (Chen, 2008). Women are more at risk for eczema, atopic irritations, hypersensitivity, and anaphylaxis from foods, medications, radiologic contrast media, and anesthesia compared with men (Chen, 2008). Granulocytes, eosinophils, mast cells, and basophils are all enhanced by estrogen (Chen, 2008). Estrogen also enhances serotonin and histamine release. In contrast, cellular-mediated immune mechanisms, primarily controlled through T cells, tend to be functionally inhibited by estrogen. At high, pregnancy levels of estrogen, there is functional inhibition of T-cell function, leading to improvement of T-cell–mediated autoimmune diseases such as rheumatoid arthritis or multiple sclerosis during pregnancy (Straub, 2007). During periods of estrogen withdrawal, late luteal phase, menstruation, postpartum, and early menopause, there are often clinical rebounds and an increase in disease flares with the release of T-cell suppression.

For the gynecologist asked to consult on women with autoimmune diseases, important strategies include completing screening for breast and cervical cancer routinely as one would for the general population; ensuring that any pregnancy is planned, not only to allow time for medication optimization, balancing disease stability with fetal risk, but also because the best pregnancy outcomes occur when autoimmune diseases are quiescent; and ensuring adequate and safe contraception for the reasons given earlier. **Estrogen-containing contraceptives (ECCs) (including the vaginal ring, the transdermal patch, and cOCPs) are acceptable for women with systemic lupus erythematosus (SLE) if they do not have antiphospholipid antibody syndrome (APAS) or a history of thrombosis** (Table 8.1) (CDC, 2010). Women with SLE are also at risk for menstrual irregularities; thus a hormonal contraceptive may also help with cyclic regulation (Tseng, 2011). However, LARC methods are also safe, have similar benefits as far as cyclic regulation, are more effective contraceptives, and are less susceptible to user error than all ECCs, but especially cOCPs. ECCs have not been shown to increase the severity of disease or the number of flares in premenopausal women with SLE (Sanchez-Guerrero, 2005).

Most autoimmune diseases do not flare around the time of menses. However, for those women with menstrual exacerbation, hormonal contraceptives may help decrease periodic variability. SLE does not seem to affect menstrual regularity or severity, nor does it appear to affect the timing of menopause. However, some antiinflammatory medications, including glucocorticoids and antineoplastic agents, affect not only the hypothalamic-pituitary-ovarian (HPO) axis but also the ovarian follicles, thus affecting both the menstrual cycle and menopausal timing (Table 8.2). Women with severe end-organ disease often develop downregulation of the HPO axis, also affecting the above (see Chapter 26). Hormone replacement therapy (HRT) is safe in women with mild disease and no history of APAS or thrombosis but has been shown to increase the number of mild, but not severe, flares in lupus patients (Andreoli, 2017; Sammaritano, 2012).

Multiple sclerosis (MS) is another autoimmune condition that merits discussion. Women are more commonly affected but usually have a less severe disease course than men (Ghezzi, 2008). Evidence is mixed regarding the effects of menstruation on disease flares. However, for women with cyclic disease flares, hormonal contraceptives are safe (Ghezzi, 2008). Women with severe multiple sclerosis have an increased risk of sexual dysfunction. Though data are limited, HRT may be useful for symptomatic postmenopausal women with MS without affecting disease activity.

**TABLE 8.1** Medical Disorders With Contraindicated Contraceptive Options

| Medical Disorder | Contraindicated Contraception | Rationale/Complication |
|---|---|---|
| Systemic lupus erythematosus with antiphospholipid antibodies or thrombosis | Estrogen-containing contraception* (ECC) | Increased venous thrombosis (VTE) risk |
| Crohn disease | Any oral contraception | Decreased absorption |
| | ECC† | Increased VTE risk |
| Severe dyslipidemia | ECC | Increased VTE risk |
| Hypertension with risk factors‡ | ECC | Increased VTE, stroke, and myocardial infarction risk |
| Renal transplant | ECC | Increased VTE risk<br>Increased metabolism |
| Thrombophilias | ECC | Increased VTE risk |
| Diabetes with risk factors§ | ECC | Increased VTE risk |
| Malabsorptive bariatric surgery | Any oral contraception | Decreased absorption |
| Migraine with aura | ECC | Increased VTE |
| Epilepsy on enzyme-inducing antiepileptic drugs | Progesterone-only oral contraception<br>Progesterone implant | Increased metabolism |

Modified from Centers for Disease Control and Prevention. U S. medical eligibility criteria for contraceptive use, 2010. *MMWR Recomm Rep.* 2010;59 (RR-4):1-86.

*Includes combined oral contraception, vaginal ring, and the transdermal patch.

†In cases of extensive or active disease, prior bowel resection, very active disease, corticosteroid use, or immobilization.

‡Risk factors include poor control, tobacco use, age older than 35, other chronic medical condition leading to vascular degradation, end organ damage, use of antihypertensives.

§Risk factors include end organ damage, vascular disease, hyperlipidemia, poorly controlled disease.

**TABLE 8.2** Antineoplastic and Chemotherapeutic Agents That May Produce Ovarian Failure

| Major Risk | Moderate Risk | Minimal Risk |
|---|---|---|
| Cyclophosphamide | Cisplatin | Methotrexate |
| Melphalan | Adriamycin | 5-Fluorouracil |
| Busulfan | Paclitaxel* | Vincristine |
| Chlorambucil | | Bleomycin |
| Procarbazine | | Actinomycin |
| Nitrogen mustard | | |

Modified from Sonmezer M, Oktay K. Fertility preservation in young women undergoing breast cancer therapy. *Oncologist.* 2006;11(5): 422-434.
*Unquantified risk at this time.

## GASTROINTESTINAL DISEASE

Estrogen and progesterone are critical in the modulation of the gastrointestinal tract. Estrogen plays a role in the secretory and absorptive function in gut epithelium, affects the gut's microbiome composition, and has receptors on enteric neurons, which regulate neurogenic reflexes (Mulak, 2014). Progesterone is known to affect the motility of the gut and the growth and metabolism of the bacteria in the gastrointestinal tract (Mulak, 2014). It is thus no surprise that many gastrointestinal disease processes affect women differently than they affect men.

Irritable bowel syndrome (IBS) is perhaps the best example of this effect. With a female-to-male prevalence as high as 5:1, up to half of women with IBS will have exacerbations of symptoms with menses. The rapid progesterone withdrawal at the end of the luteal phase and the increase in systemic prostaglandins both lead to exacerbations of symptoms, including bloating and abdominal pain (Mulak, 2014). cOCPs have been shown to decrease symptoms in women with IBS. For women in whom menstrual effects become debilitating, the use of gonadotropin-releasing hormone (GnRH) agonists or continuous cOCPs has been suggested. The incidence of IBS tends to decrease after menopause.

Celiac disease, like other autoimmune diseases, tends to preferentially affect women. Women are at twice the risk for developing celiac disease (Liu, 2014). Women with undiagnosed or poorly controlled celiac disease have later onset of menses, more irregular menstrual cycles, more secondary amenorrhea, and earlier age of menopause; these associations are not seen among women with treated disease (Casella, 2016). A meta-analyses regarding fertility and celiac disease suggested that women with unexplained infertility should be tested for celiac disease but that women with well-controlled disease do not have decreased fertility compared with women without celiac (Tersigni, 2014).

**Women with Crohn disease and ulcerative colitis tend to have symptomatic exacerbations around the time of menses—specifically, worsening nausea, constipation, and diarrhea.** Inflammatory bowel disease (IBD) has also been shown to have a negative effect on body image and sexuality (Moleski, 2011). Dyspareunia is also common, especially in those with Crohn disease. Women cite abdominal pain, fear of incontinence, and diarrhea as reasons for decreased levels of sexual activity (Moleski, 2011). Effective contraception is important for women with IBD because unplanned pregnancy in the setting of active disease is associated with worse maternal and fetal outcomes (Moleski, 2011). Though cOCPs are not associated with disease relapse, data suggest there is some risk of decreased absorption in women with Crohn disease and in women with increased intestinal transit secondary to previous bowel resection. For women with IBD who are at an increased risk for venous thromboembolism (VTE), including those with extensive or active disease, corticosteroid use, vitamin deficiencies, or immobilization, ECCs are not recommended (CDC, 2010). LARC methods are considered safe and effective in women with IBD, independent of disease severity, and thus often are preferred over oral contraceptive options and ECCs. It is also important to note that women with IBD are at increased risk for osteoporosis and osteopenia and should be screened accordingly.

Estrogen has been noted to have a protective effect on the development and progression of liver disease. Women with hepatitis C have a better response to therapy and a slower rate of disease progression than men (Rodríguez-Castro, 2014). Research also suggests estrogen plays a significant role in preventing carcinogenesis in the liver (Zhang, 2013). As such, hepatocellular carcinoma is less common in women. The literature also describes the use of hormone replacement in postmenopausal women to inhibit liver fibrosis (Zhang, 2013). In contrast, autoimmune-mediated liver diseases, such as primary biliary cirrhosis and autoimmune hepatitis, are more common in women. It is also important to note that for women with cirrhosis or severe liver disease, ECCs are contraindicated.

### Vascular and Hypertensive Diseases

In general, estrogens have a positive effect on the vascular system through improved lipid profiles. The presence of estrogen is associated with lower rates of atherogenic dyslipidemia, cardiovascular disease, and metabolic syndrome (Pellegrini, 2014). This effect is lost in postmenopausal women. However, women with dyslipidemias may have complications with estrogen because of its procoagulant effects, especially after the third or fourth decade. Women with dyslipidemia should avoid ECCs and HRT, although progesterone-only contraceptives, including LARC methods, are safe and effective for these women, independent of age.

In contrast, vascular and hypertensive diseases have important effects on women. Studies indicate that women with hypertension have much higher than expected levels of sexual dysfunction with impaired genital congestion and decreased arousal (Doumas, 2006). Data regarding the effects of antihypertensive medications on sexual function are mixed. Though beta-blockers are consistently associated with worsening sexual function, multiple studies have noted that adequate blood pressure control with medication actually leads to an improvement in sexual function (De Franciscis, 2013; Doumas, 2006; Fogari, 2004). Women with coronary artery disease and survivors of myocardial infarction have less sexual activity and increased sexual dysfunction (Basson, 2007). Thus it is helpful for gynecologists to inquire about sexual concerns in women with cardiovascular disorders.

Hormonally based contraceptives may be problematic in women who are taking antihypertensive medications or those with poorly controlled hypertension. **If there is no associated thrombosis, guidelines from the American College of Obstetricians and Gynecologists (ACOG) suggest that women may use ECCs as long as blood pressure is well controlled** (ACOG, 2006; WHO, 2015). A return office visit 2 or 3 months after initiation of any ECC to assess blood pressure and potential side effects is appropriate. Studies have shown a small increase in stroke and myocardial infarction in women on oral contraceptives with hypertension, but the absolute risk is quite small (ACOG, 2006; WHO, 2015). It should also be noted that women with a history of pregnancy-related hypertension who are currently normotensive are also at a slightly increased risk for myocardial infarction and VTE, though again, the absolute risk is small (ACOG, 2006; WHO, 2015). As long as a woman does not use tobacco or does not have other aspects of vascular disease besides mild hypertension, ECCs may be reasonable. However, LARC methods are preferable, especially after age 35.

Cardiac arrhythmias are also affected by gender, though the exact pathophysiologic reasons for this are unclear. Atrioventricular nodal reentrant tachycardia occurs twice as often in women as in men, though Wolff-Parkinson-White syndrome is more common in men (Curtis, 2012). Supraventricular tachycardias and ectopic ventricular beats occur more often and last longer in the luteal phase of the menstrual cycle (Curtis, 2012). The QT interval tends to be longer in women, increasing the risk for torsades de pointes. Though rates of atrial fibrillation are lower in women, women with atrial fibrillation are less likely to be anticoagulated and to undergo ablative procedures and are more likely to suffer a stroke (Curtis, 2012). Menopause does not appear to affect risk of developing atrial fibrillation (Guhl, 2017; Wong, 2017). Sudden cardiac death affects both genders equally.

### Renal Disease

Women with end-stage renal disease (ESRD) have high prolactin levels and gonadotropin-mediated disruption of the luteinizing hormone (LH) surge (Guglielmi, 2013). These hormonal alterations result in anovulatory cycles, amenorrhea, oligomenorrhea, menorrhagia, infertility, and decreased libido. The effects of chronic disease (see Chapter 26) on the HPO axis also contribute to an increased likelihood of anovulatory bleeding in this population. Many, though not all, menstrual irregularities improve with renal transplant. Though **many women with ESRD or on dialysis have irregular menstrual cycles and problems with infertility**, many are sexually active, and thus it is critical that contraception should be discussed with them. ECCs are contraindicated in this population, whereas progesterone-only methods, especially LARCS, are safe and effective (Wiles, 2018).

Women with ESRD have higher rates endometrial hyperplasia, likely related to anovulatory cycles. There is also an increased incidence of cervical dysplasia, thought to be due to increased susceptibility to human papillomavirus (HPV) infection. Mammography can be challenging in this population because of increased vessel calcifications. To avoid unnecessary procedures, the patient's history should be provided to the radiologist (Holley, 2007). CA-125 is also often falsely elevated in this population and should be interpreted with caution (Holley, 2007). Women with ERSD or who have undergone renal transplant have been shown to have a higher risk of surgical complications during gynecologic procedures (Heisler, 2010).

Up to 70% of women who are on hemodialysis, with chronic renal disease, and those who have had renal transplants have some degree of sexual dysfunction, including arousal disorders, decreased libido, and decreased genital blood flow, issues with lubrication, and orgasm problems. This may be related to lower levels of circulating estrogen. These women also go through menopause at an earlier age, 47 compared with 51 in women not undergoing dialysis, further exacerbating problems with sexual dysfunction (Guglielmi, 2013).

Peritoneal dialysis has many specific considerations in women. Fertility in this population is lower than in women receiving hemodialysis, likely related to a disruption in the ovum's path to the fallopian tube (Guglielmi, 2013). Additionally, these women may experience cyclic hemoperitoneum, usually related to retrograde menstruation (Guglielmi, 2013). The hemoperitoneum is often asymptomatic, though rarely it may cause obstruction to the dialysis catheter (Guglielmi, 2013). If the hemoperitoneum is recurrent or problematic, it may be treated with tubal ligation or hormonal suppression of ovulation (Guglielmi, 2013). Finally, women who undergo peritoneal dialysis may be at increased risk for uterine prolapse possibly related to changes in intraabdominal pressure associated with the dialysis.

## HEMATOLOGIC AND THROMBOTIC DISEASES

Estrogen affects hematologic diseases primarily through its prothrombotic effects. Progesterone decreases smooth muscle venous tone, which leads to increased clotting potential. Routine screening for thrombophilias in women without a history of thrombosis, before the use of ECCs or hormone replacement, is not indicated. **Women with a personal history of thrombosis related to estrogen should avoid estrogen-containing medications** (WHO, 2015). Women with known thrombophilias are great candidates for LARC methods but can also use progesterone-based oral contraceptives. Because supplemental estrogen is contraindicated in women with thrombophilias, these women may be more at risk for osteoporotic problems over time. These women should be regularly screened for a dietary history of calcium intake and for serum levels of vitamin D, with appropriate supplementation given.

Women with sickle cell disease (SCD) tend to go through menarche at a later age but do not have an increased rate of irregular cycles (Smith-Whitley, 2014). The menstrual cycle is often associated with increased pain crises. **Progesterone stabilizes red cell membranes and significantly decreases the frequency of sickling crises;** thus women with SCD may benefit from progesterone-containing contraceptives. Injectable medroxyprogesterone acetate has been used in women with frequent crises as an adjunct therapy with very good results (Smith-Whitley, 2014). The pain-mediating effects of progesterone-based IUDs and implants have not yet been well documented, though these are considered a safe contraceptive option for women with SCD. ECCs and HRT do not improve sickling but are not contraindicated (WHO, 2015).

Women who receive oral anticoagulants (OAs), either for treatment or prophylaxis, experience increased vaginal bleeding, menorrhagia, and metrorrhagia (Huq, 2011). Researchers reporting on a series of women noted that after starting the OA, the duration of bleeding increased, the percentage of women reporting heavy bleeding increased to almost 75%, and the number of women seeking medical treatment nearly doubled (Sjalander, 2007). Anovulatory cycles may be particularly troublesome for these women. A progesterone-based IUD or progesterone supplementation for the last 14 days of the cycle may be necessary to decrease heavy bleeding. **Estrogen-containing contraceptives are not recommended for women on anticoagulation** (CDC, 2010). Though the copper-containing IUD does not increase the risk of thrombosis, it is also generally not recommended given its association with increased menstrual bleeding (Huq, 2011). Women on OAs are also at an increased risk for ovulation-related bleeding and associated hemoperitoneum.

The most common inherited bleeding diathesis is von Willebrand disease. The association of von Willebrand disease and vaginal bleeding is discussed in Chapter 26. LARC methods are safe in these women. However, because estrogen increases von Willebrand factor, ECCs may be advantageous for women with von Willebrand disease and menorrhagia or ovarian cysts (Committee on Adolescent Health Care, 2013). Women with rare bleeding disorders fall into this category as well, and ECCs may be helpful for them. A consensus report discussed other therapies, including endometrial ablation or hysterectomy as potential options in women with bleeding disorders who do not desire fertility (James, 2009).

## Endocrine Disease

Women with type 2 diabetes or who are obese have increased rates of anovulation, infertility, and endometrial hyperplasia. **ECCs are acceptable in women with isolated diabetes (type 1 or 2) without end organ damage, as are progesterone-based contraceptives** (CDC, 2010). However, because many women with diabetes have coexisting vascular disease or hyperlipidemia, it is recommended that ECCs be limited to women who are nonsmokers and younger than 35 with no other significant pathologic condition. **LARC methods are safe, effective,**

**and recommended for women with any form diabetes, independent of severity.** In addition to the contraceptive effects, LARC methods also protect the endometrium in women who are anovulatory (ACOG, 2010).

Studies of sexuality in women with diabetes have noted increased sexual dysfunction, particularly for those with type 1 diabetes and those with long-standing disease. Sexual dysfunction is due to end organ disease, which leads to decreased genital blood flow, decreased lubrication, and orgasmic dysfunction. Young women with type 1 diabetes are also more likely to suffer from longer menstrual cycles and heavier menses compared with women without diabetes (Gaete, 2010). Though these issues are worse in women with a higher glycated hemoglobin (HbA1c), the problems persisted in women with well-controlled disease (Gaete, 2010). It should also be noted that insulin requirements and glycemic control vary with the hormonal fluctuations of the menstrual cycle, especially in the luteal phase and around menses. Discussion of this normal variation with younger women is important.

Obese women present an interesting conundrum regarding contraceptive options. Biologic plausibility for lower efficacy of many contraceptive options in obese women has long been stated. However, a 2016 review concluded that there did not appear to be an efficacy difference among obese and nonobese women taking cOCPs, though the review did recognize that data stratifying by body mass index (BMI) category was limited (Simmons, 2016). This same review also noted that the estrogen-containing patch (transdermal) has been found to be less efficacious in obese women, whereas the vaginal ring has not (Simmons, 2016). It should also be emphasized that given the increased risks of pregnancy-related complications in this population, some contraceptive effect is better than no contraception. The progestin-based IUD or progestin-based implant have the highest success rate, independent of weight, and should be considered a first-line treatment in the obese population (Robinson, 2013). Given the increased incidence of anovulation with obesity, the local effects of the progestin-based IUD are especially protective against endometrial hyperplasia as well (Robinson, 2013). Obese women also describe higher rates of sexual dysfunction than normal-weight women. However, this seems to improve with weight loss and improvement in body image (Kolotkin, 2012). This is true with both natural weight loss and bariatric surgery.

Obese women undergoing bariatric surgery should also be counseled about contraception and pregnancy planning. Malabsorptive procedures, particularly the Roux-en-Y procedure, have the potential to affect absorption of all oral contraception, including emergency contraception, and thus these methods should be discouraged in women who are undergoing or have undergone this sort of operations (Robinson, 2013). The efficacy of nonoral methods are not affected by bariatric surgery; thus the LARC methods are a good option for this population. After surgery, women may transition from being anovulatory to regular ovulation with weight loss and improved glucose control. It is recommended that women wait 12 to 18 months before attempting pregnancy after bariatric surgery, another reason that the LARC methods are a good option for these women (Mody, 2014).

Women with congenital adrenal hyperplasia (CAH) are usually treated with glucocorticoid replacement. These women are exposed to an androgenic environment throughout their lives; thus hormonally based contraceptives, including OCPs, are a good form of contraception. Though many of these women have difficulties with hirsutism, they should not be treated with spironolactone because it may affect mineralocorticoid regulation. Infertility secondary to chronically increased progesterone and androgen levels may occur, though this condition is correctable with steroid maintenance therapy (Reichman, 2014). Women with more severe phenotypes may need mineralocorticoid and progesterone suppression (Reichman, 2014). Women with CAH may also have problems with dyspareunia, vaginal stenosis, and lower sexual satisfaction (Nordenstrom, 2011). Sexual counseling for these women is helpful. Of note, thyroid disease is discussed in detail in Chapter 26.

## CENTRAL NERVOUS SYSTEM DISEASE

### Seizure Disorders

Estrogen and progesterone have significant effects on a woman's susceptibility to seizures. Estrogen is a proconvulsant, decreasing the seizure threshold. Estrogen increases neuronal excitability directly on nerve cells, as well as secondarily through inhibition of the GABA system. More potent, though, are the effects of progesterone, which acts primarily via its metabolite allopregnanolone, a neurosteroid. Allopregnanolone acts rapidly and directly on the GABA receptors to enhance their activity, producing potent neural inhibition throughout the central nervous system (CNS). **Withdrawal of progesterone (even in small amounts such as periovulatory) leads to a significant decline in seizure threshold and an increase in seizure frequency and severity.**

More than 1 million women in the United States have seizure disorders, and many have increased seizure activity related to changes in menstrual hormones. Catamenial epilepsy (from the Greek *katomenios*, meaning "monthly") has been defined as seizures that occur from 3 days before to 4 days after the onset of menses. Pure catamenial epilepsy affects 10% of all women with epilepsy (Crawford, 2009). However, nearly 80% of women have an increase in seizure activity related to menstrual cycles (Crawford, 2009). Progesterone-based contraceptives or a small amount of progesterone add-back during menses has been used to decrease seizure frequency. Continuous cOCPs with an every-3-month withdrawal may also be helpful. It is unclear if the progesterone-based IUD produces systemic progesterone levels high enough to affect the seizure threshold.

Though hormonal contraception is acceptable for women with seizure disorders, estrogen affects metabolism of some antiepileptic drugs (AEDs) (Table 8.3). Women who experience menstrual-related seizures should have serum levels of their anticonvulsant medications checked during menses. Some of these women will benefit from perimenstrual adjustments of their medications. In contrast, some antiepileptic drugs, referred to as *enzyme-inducing AEDs* (see Table 8.3), affect the metabolism of hormonal contraception. For women taking a medication from this family of AEDs, progesterone-only pills have decreased efficacy and are not recommended (Crawford, 2009). Similarly, progesterone implants are contraindicated in this population (Luef, 2009). Emergency contraception can be used in women with epilepsy, but those on enzyme-inducing AEDs may need a higher dose (Crawford, 2009).

Almost one-third of women with epilepsy exhibit some degree of sexual dysfunction, ranging from decreased interest to orgasmic dysfunction (Crawford, 2009). Thus providers caring for women with epilepsy should query patients regarding sexual

**TABLE 8.3** Interactions of Anticonvulsants (AEDs) and Oral Contraceptives

| Enzyme-Inducing AEDs | Non–Enzyme-Inducing AEDs |
|---|---|
| Barbiturates | Gabapentin |
| Carbamazepine | Lamotrigine |
| Phenytoin | Valproic acid |
| Topiramate | Ethosuximide |
| Vigabatrin | Levetiracetam |

Modified from the American College of Obstetrics and Gynecology (ACOG) Gynecologists' Committee on Practice (2019). ACOG Practice Bulletin No. 206: Use of hormonal contraception in women with coexisting medical conditions. *Obstet Gynecol* 133(2):e128–e150.

function and satisfaction. Epilepsy may predispose women to earlier menopause. **Seizures often increase in the perimenopausal transition, then decrease after menopause, especially in women who suffer from catamenial epilepsy** (Luef, 2009). HRT is associated with an increase in seizure frequency. Finally, women with epilepsy are at increased risk for osteoporosis related to the effects of AEDs on bone metabolism (Erel, 2011). Calcium and vitamin D supplements are recommended in this population, along with monitoring of bone mineral density (Crawford, 2009).

### Migraine Headaches

Women are three times more likely to have migraines than men. Fourteen percent of all women with migraines have pure menstrual migraines; 46% have exacerbation of severity and frequency of their migraines during menses. Approximately 17 million women are affected by this problem. A menstrual migraine is defined as a migraine headache, without aura, occurring within the last 2 days of the menstrual cycle and the first 3 days of menses and affecting two of every three cycles (Brandes, 2012). After menopause, the incidence of migraines decreases by two-thirds, and women and men have equal frequencies.

The cause of menstrual migraines is related to estrogen withdrawal. Migraines are primarily vascular headaches, and the withdrawal of the estrogen leads to a relative vascular instability (Mathew, 2013). Estrogen also affects the CNS serotonin receptors. The change in serotonin metabolism as estrogen is withdrawn affects the brainstem, which controls cerebral blood flow. Serotonin uptake is blocked by triptans, and triptans are noted to be extremely effective for both abortive treatment of menstrual migraines and short-term prophylaxis (prevention) (Mathew, 2013). **When menstrual migraines and menstruation-related migraines are diagnosed, therapeutic choices include modifying estrogen withdrawal with therapies such as the continuous OCPs, transdermal patches, or small amounts of estrogen add-back in the appropriate time window** (Brandes, 2012). Preventive therapies include tricyclic antidepressants, beta-blockers, and other medications (Brandes, 2012).

Women who have migraines with aura are more susceptible to stroke, and thus the use of estrogen-containing contraception in women with migraines with aura is contraindicated (WHO, 2015). However, progestin-only contraception and LARC methods are safe in this population.

## MENTAL HEALTH ISSUES

Changes in estrogen and progesterone levels have profound effects on psychiatric and psychological symptomology and on psychiatric diseases (Box 8.3). Estrogen and progesterone are neuromodulators; thus exacerbation of mental health conditions may occur with menstrual hormonal fluctuations. Premenstrual exacerbation has been shown to occur with anxiety disorder, panic disorder, obsessive-compulsive disorder, bipolar disease, eating disorders, and psychotic disorders (Pinkerton, 2010). Women without mental health disorders handle these fluctuations well, but women who have a predisposition to mental health disorders may be strongly affected by the hormonal fluctuations.

Premenstrual dysphoric disease (PMDD) affects up to 5% of women and is discussed in Chapter 37. Other mental health disorders are best managed by mental health providers. **However, the gynecologist may help provide hormonal stability. Continuous cOCPs can help improve depression that occurs around the time of menses** (Pinkerton, 2010). Sexual dysfunction may be a symptom of depression, but it can also be a side effect of antidepressant medications, including the serotonin reuptake inhibitors (SSRIs).

New-onset depression or worsening of known depression often occurs during the menopausal transition. Studies suggest this occurs in nearly 50% of women (Pinkerton, 2010). Screening for depression in this age group is important given the high incidence of disease. Treatment with antidepressant medications is the first-line therapy for moderate to severe depression in the menopausal transition and may help with hot flashes as well (Pinkerton, 2010). If there are only mild to moderate symptoms and the woman is an appropriate candidate, estrogen-containing HRT may be helpful (Pinkerton, 2010). Black cohosh and St. John's wort may also be beneficial in the treatment of perimenopausal depression, though they should be used with caution because safety data and production regulation are limited (Pinkerton, 2010).

**BOX 8.3** Emotional Symptoms Affected by Changes in Estrogen and Progesterone

- Anger
- Anxiety
- Appetite change
- Decreased self-esteem
- Depression
- Feelings of phobia
- Increased sense of fatigue
- Inhibited control of limbic system sensations
- Irritability
- Loss of pleasure
- Memory problems
- Mood lability
- Temperature fluctuations
- Vulnerability

Modified from Pinkerton JV, Guico-Pabia CJ, Taylor HS. Menstrual cycle-related exacerbation of disease. *Am J Obstet Gynecol.* 2010;202(3):221-231.

## CANCER

The gynecologist can play a valuable role in improving quality of life for women with cancer. Sexuality in cancer patients should be addressed from the beginning of cancer therapy. Issues of depression and sexual dysfunction are enhanced by ovarian failure, loss of hair, changes in body image, and changes in relationships (Lamb, 1995). Abnormal vaginal bleeding in the first few cycles of chemotherapy is frightening, and the role of the gynecologist is important at this phase of treatment.

Chemotherapy produces toxic effects on ovarian function that are related to dose, duration, and type of chemotherapy. Agents that are particularly toxic to the ovary are listed in Table 8.2. Of these, alkylating agents are the most toxic to the ovaries, but women who receive antineoplastic agents for control of severe autoimmune disease can also develop ovarian failure. Young women treated with oophorotoxic agents often become amenorrheic, but their menses and ovarian function may return after a few or several months (Sonmezer, 2006). They generally undergo menopause earlier. For older women, their chemotherapy-induced menopause is usually permanent. Radiation to the ovaries greater than or equal to 20 Gy may also produce ovarian failure, though oophoropexy to remove the ovaries from the field of radiation may mitigate this reaction (Mahajan, 2015).

In addition to the effects that chemotherapy has on the ovaries, the effects on the bone marrow, specifically thrombocytopenia, can lead to gynecologic issues. GnRH analogs have been shown to be effective in reducing episodes of severe vaginal bleeding associated with thrombocytopenia, without the potential risks associated with the estrogen-based options, especially

VTE (Bates, 2011). GnRH analogs may be used as prophylaxis for menorrhagia/menstrual suppression in women with expected thrombocytopenia for more than 30 days (Bates, 2011). Acute menorrhagia in women undergoing treatment for most cancers can be treated with tranexamic acid, relying on hormonal therapies as second-line agents (Bates, 2011).

Young women wishing to preserve ovarian function and fertility need consultation before treatments. Mature oocytes are the most susceptible to chemotherapy, whereas immature oocytes in prepubertal girls are somewhat resistant. Thus investigators have used GnRH antagonists to suppress follicular maturity and attempt to preserve ovarian function. The results are mixed, though a Cochrane review supports their usage (Chen, 2011). Other potential options to save oocyte function and preserve fertility include in vitro fertilization with freezing of embryos, harvesting/freezing of mature oocytes after ovarian stimulation, and ovarian cryopreservation, which is still in the investigational stage. The American Society of Clinical Oncology currently recommends discussion of both embryo and oocyte cryopreservation as methods of fertility preservation, and American Society of Reproductive Medicine notes these to be the first-line methods for fertility preservation (Loren, 2013; Martinez, 2017). The options should be reviewed in light of the patient's needs, fertility desires, and clinical situation. Early and urgent referral to a reproductive endocrinologist with expertise in potential therapies to preserve fertility is important (McLaren, 2012).

## SUMMARY

The interaction of female physiology and medical disease is complex. The gynecologist has several roles in the treatment of these women. **All providers who address women's health should regularly discuss issues of sexual function, particularly in the setting of coexisting chronic disease.** Additionally, the exacerbation of symptoms around the time of menses should be reviewed. Hormonal changes that increase the symptoms of women change over the course of a woman's reproductive life. Disease manifestation in a woman's 20s will not be the same as symptoms in her 40s or in her 60s. Many treatment options are available that can improve quality of life. Though gynecologists may not be the primary providers for nongynecologic diseases, they are best suited to act as consultants for adjunctive therapy, which may enhance the efficacy and treatment of medical disease.

### KEY REFERENCES

American College of Obstetricians and Gynecologists (ACOG). ACOG Practice Bulletin. No. 73: Use of hormonal contraception in women with coexisting medical conditions. *Obstet Gynecol.* 2006;107(6):1453-1472.

American College of Obstetricians and Gynecologists (ACOG). ACOG Practice Bulletin No. 110: Noncontraceptive uses of hormonal contraceptives. *Obstet Gynecol.* 2010;115(1):206-218.

Ahmad A, Ahmed A, Patrizio P. Cystic fibrosis and fertility. *Curr Opin Obstet Gynecol.* 2013;25(3):167-172.

Aljubran SA, Whelan GJ, Glaum MC, et al. Osteoporosis in the at-risk asthmatic. *Allergy.* 2014;69(11):1429-1439.

Basson R, Schultz WW. Sexual sequelae of general medical disorders. *Lancet.* 2007;369(9559):409-424.

Bates JS, Buie LW, Woodis CB. Management of menorrhagia associated with chemotherapy-induced thrombocytopenia in women with hematologic malignancy. *Pharmacotherapy.* 2011;31(11):1092-1110.

Bialek-Gosk K, Maskey-Warzechowska M, Krenke R, et al. Menopausal asthma-much ado about nothing? An observational study. *J Asthma.* 2018;55(11):1197-1204.

Brandes JL. Migraine in women. *Continuum (Minneap Minn).* 2012;18(4):835-852.

Centers for Disease Control and Prevention (CDC). U.S. Medical Eligibility Criteria for Contraceptive Use, 2010. *MMWR Recomm Rep.* 2010;59(RR-4):1-86.

Casella G, Orfanotti G, Giacomantonio L, et al. Celiac disease and obstetrical-gynecological contribution. *Gastroenterol Hepatol Bed Bench.* 2016;9(4):241-249.

Chen H, Li J, Cui T, et al. Adjuvant gonadotropin-releasing hormone analogues for the prevention of chemotherapy induced premature ovarian failure in premenopausal women. *Cochrane Database Syst Rev.* 2011;(11):CD008018.

Chen W, Mempel M, Schober W, et al. Gender difference, sex hormones, and immediate type hypersensitivity reactions. *Allergy.* 2008;63(11):1418-1427.

Committee on Adolescent Health Care, Committee on Gynecologic Practice. Committee Opinion No.580: von Willebrand disease in women. *Obstet Gynecol.* 2013;122(6):1368-1373.

Crawford PM. Managing epilepsy in women of childbearing age. *Drug Saf.* 2009;32(4):293-307.

Curtis AB, Narasimha D. Arrhythmias in women. *Clin Cardiol.* 2012;35(3):166-171.

De Franciscis P, Mainini G, Messalli EM, et al. Arterial hypertension and female sexual dysfunction in postmenopausal women. *Clin Exp Obstet Gynecol.* 2013;40(1):58-60.

Doumas M, Tsiodras S, Tsakiris A, et al. Female sexual dysfunction in essential hypertension: a common problem being uncovered. *J Hypertens.* 2006;24(12):2387-2392.

Dratva J. Use of oestrogen only hormone replacement therapy associated with increased risk of asthma onset in postmenopausal women. *Evid Based Med.* 2010;15(6):190-191.

Erel T, Guralp O. Epilepsy and menopause. *Arch Gynecol Obstet.* 2011;284(3):749-755.

Fida NG, Williams MA, Enquobahrie DA. Association of age at menarche and menstrual characteristics with adult onset asthma among reproductive age women. *Reprod Syst Sex Disord.* 2012;1(3):111.

Fogari R, Preti P, Zoppi A, et al. Effect of valsartan and atenolol on sexual behavior in hypertensive postmenopausal women. *Am J Hypertens.* 2004;17(1):77-81.

Foschino Barbaro MP, Costa VR, Resta O, et al. Menopausal asthma: a new biological phenotype? *Allergy.* 2010;65(10):1306-1312.

Gaete X, Vivanco M, Eyzaguirre FC, et al. Menstrual cycle irregularities and their relationship with HbA1c and insulin dose in adolescents with type 1 diabetes mellitus. *Fertil Steril.* 2010;94(5):1822-1826.

Ghezzi A, Zaffaroni M. Female-specific issues in multiple sclerosis. *Expert Rev Neurother.* 2008;8(6):969-977.

Guglielmi KE. Women and ESRD: modalities, survival, unique considerations. *Adv Chronic Kidney Dis.* 2013;20(5):411-418.

Guhl EN, Magnani JW. Atrial fibrillation and menopause: something else to worry about, or not? *Heart.* 2017;103(24):1930-1931.

Heisler CA, Casiano ER, Gebhart JB. Hysterectomy and perioperative morbidity in women who have undergone renal transplantation. *Am J Obstet Gynecol.* 2010;202(3):314.e311-314.

Holley JL. Screening, diagnosis, and treatment of cancer in long-term dialysis patients. *Clin J Am Soc Nephrol.* 2007;2(3):604-610.

Huq FY, Tvarkova K, Arafa A, et al. Menstrual problems and contraception in women of reproductive age receiving oral anticoagulation. *Contraception.* 2011;84(2):128-132.

James AH, Kouides PA, Abdul-Kadir R, et al. Von Willebrand disease and other bleeding disorders in women: consensus on diagnosis and management from an international expert panel. *Am J Obstet Gynecol.* 2009;201(1):12.e11-18.

Kolotkin RL, Zunker C, Østbye T. Sexual functioning and obesity: a review. *Obesity (Silver Spring).* 2012;20(12):2325-2333.

**Full references for this chapter can be found on ExpertConsult.com.**

# 9 Additional Considerations in Gynecologic Care

*Deborah S. Cowley, Anne Burke, Gretchen M. Lentz*

## KEY POINTS

- Depression, anxiety disorders, obsessive-compulsive disorder, and posttraumatic stress disorder are treatable with medications or psychotherapy.
- A history of manic or hypomanic symptoms increases the risk for a "switch" into mania with antidepressant treatment.
- Close follow-up, in 1 to 2 weeks, is recommended to monitor for increases in suicidal thoughts with antidepressants, especially in adolescents and young adults.
- Active suicidal thoughts and plans are a psychiatric emergency.
- Eating disorders are life-threatening conditions that are often unrecognized.
- Girls or women presenting with amenorrhea, menstrual dysfunction, low bone density, sexual dysfunction, infertility, anxiety, depression, or hyperemesis gravidarum should be screened for eating disorders.
- Women with anxiety disorders (especially panic disorder and posttraumatic stress disorder) are at increased risk for suicide and should be asked about suicidal thoughts or plans.
- Anxiety disorders respond well to reassurance, education, and treatment with psychotherapy and medications (especially SSRI antidepressants).
- Many substance use disorders, such as alcoholism, have a more rapidly progressive course in women than in men ("telescoping").
- More than seven drinks per week is considered heavy drinking for a woman.
- Motivational interviewing is a highly effective, brief intervention that increases engagement in substance abuse treatment and other behavior change.
- In cases of misuse of potentially habit-forming medications, a formal treatment agreement may be necessary.
- Understanding attachment styles can help providers to work effectively with "difficult" patients.
- Nonpharmacologic treatments for hypoactive sexual desire disorder include lifestyle changes for reducing stress and fatigue, recognizing and treating depression, increasing quality time with the partner, improving body image, and bringing novelty into the sexual repertoire.
- Environmental, staff, medical record, and physician-related measures can aid in engaging lesbian, bisexual, and transgender individuals in care and in ensuring high-quality health care.
- Lesbian, bisexual, and transgender individuals have an elevated rate of mental health problems, substance use disorders, and suicide attempts, especially during adolescence.
- Intimate partner violence crosses all ethnic, racial, educational, age, and socioeconomic lines and has a large burden of social, physical, mental, and public health implications.
- The physician has a responsibility to screen and acknowledge intimate partner violence and abuse, identify community resources for immediate referrals, assess safety, assist with reporting if necessary or desired, document appropriately using medicolegal tools, and provide ongoing clinical care.
- Gynecologists are often called on to provide or refer women for counseling related to grief; losses such as miscarriage, perinatal loss, and infertility; and end-of-life issues.
- Women suffering losses as a result of miscarriage, perinatal loss, unplanned pregnancy, or infertility benefit from support, counseling, and screening for depression and posttraumatic stress disorder.
- Complicated grief and grief accompanied by symptoms of depression benefit from antidepressant medication treatment in addition to psychotherapy.
- Women with terminal illness benefit from an engaged, genuine relationship with physicians and other health care providers, treatment of depression and anxiety states, psychological interventions and psychotherapy, and early integration of palliative care into treatment.

Gynecologists follow women across the life cycle, from puberty through old age. The gynecologist may be a woman's primary health care provider for much of this time. The gynecologist is thus in an important position to help a woman navigate normal developmental stages and challenges, to share in critical life events and to provide or obtain counseling for a woman as she works her way through emotional adjustments and problems.

Normal development includes challenges such as building an identity and self-esteem; dealing with sexuality and sexual development; forming meaningful relationships; pregnancy and motherhood; life roles and transitions; and losses, grief, and aging. In addition to these normal developmental transitions and challenges, a woman may have to deal with trauma related to difficult early childhood experiences, abuse, rape, or intimate partner violence. Psychiatric disorders such as depression, anxiety, posttraumatic stress disorder, and eating disorders are common in women, and conditions such as alcohol and drug use disorders often have a different presentation and course in women compared with men.

This chapter reviews common psychiatric disorders occurring in gynecologic patients, sexual function and disorders, and behavioral and psychosocial issues and traumas that may arise during a woman's lifetime, and it offers suggestions as to how the physician can aid the patient.

## DEPRESSION

**Major depression is common in women, with a lifetime prevalence of 20% to 25%.** Although boys and girls are equally likely to experience depression, major depression is about twice as common in women as in men, starting in adolescence. Worldwide, depression is one of the leading causes of functional impairment and disability. The diagnosis of major depression refers to persistent sadness or lack of interest or pleasure in usual activities, lasting for at least 2 weeks. It is accompanied by symptoms such as changes in eating habits, trouble sleeping, lack of energy and motivation, poor memory or concentration, and feelings of guilt, worthlessness, hopelessness, and despair. In severe cases, depression may lead to suicidal thoughts and actions. The diagnostic criteria for major depression are listed in Box 9.1. **The Patient Health Questionnaire (PHQ-9) (Table 9.1) is a useful screening tool for major depression**, can be filled out quickly by the woman in the waiting room or in the office before a visit, and helps in identifying depression, monitoring effects of treatment, and educating the woman about her own characteristic symptoms of depression. Scores of 5, 10, 15, and 20 are cutoff scores indicating mild, moderate, moderately severe, and severe depression, respectively.

**BOX 9.1** Diagnostic Criteria for Major Depressive Episode

Five or more of the following symptoms have been present during the same 2-week period and represent a change from previous functioning; at least one of the symptoms is either (1) depressed mood or (2) loss of interest or pleasure.

1. Depressed mood most of the day, nearly every day, as indicated by either subjective report (e.g., feels sad or empty) or observation made by others (e.g., appears tearful)
2. Markedly diminished interest or pleasure in all, or almost all, activities
3. Significant weight loss (when not dieting) or weight gain, or decrease or increase in appetite
4. Insomnia or hypersomnia
5. Psychomotor agitation or retardation observable by others
6. Fatigue or loss of energy
7. Feelings of worthlessness or excessive or inappropriate guilt
8. Diminished ability to think or concentrate, or indecisiveness
9. Recurrent thoughts of death (not just fear of dying), recurrent suicidal ideation, or a suicide attempt or specific suicide plan

Symptoms cause clinically significant distress or impairment.

Modified from American Psychiatric Association. *Diagnostic and Statistical Manual of Mental Disorders.* 5th ed. Washington, DC: American Psychiatric Association; 2013:160-161.

The cause of major depression is unclear. It may occur without a clear stress or precipitant, especially in women with a strong family history of depression who are genetically predisposed. A family history of depression, a prior depressive episode, and older age are all risk factors for depression. Rates of depression are higher in women who are socioeconomically disadvantaged. In addition, stressors such as loss of relationships and loved ones, divorce, role transitions, interpersonal conflicts, interpersonal violence, medical illness, or feelings of being trapped in a stressful situation without a way to escape or cope can precipitate depression. Depressive symptoms in a particular person may be uniquely determined by individual factors, such as family relationships while growing up and past experiences that are highly meaningful and evoke negative feelings and memories triggered by current situations or events.

The increased rate of depression in women starting at menarche has also been thought to result from hormonal factors. There are clear increases in risk for depressive symptoms premenstrually, with some women only experiencing mood symptoms at this time and others noting a worsening of underlying depression in the week or two before menses (for a discussion of premenstrual dysphoric disorder, see Chapter 35). The postpartum period is a high-risk time for depression and is the highest risk time in a woman's life for psychiatric hospitalization. There is also an increase in depressive symptoms at the time of menopause and the menopausal transition.

The differential diagnosis of major depression includes adjustment disorder, persistent depressive disorder (dysthymia), depression related to drugs and alcohol or secondary to a medical condition, and bipolar disorder. Adjustment disorder is a

**TABLE 9.1** Patient Health Questionnaire (PHQ-9)

| Over the past 2 weeks, how often have you been bothered by any of the following problems? | | | | |
|---|---|---|---|---|
| | **Not at All** | **Several Days** | **More than Half the Days** | **Nearly Every Day** |
| 1. Little interest or pleasure in doing things | 0 | 1 | 2 | 3 |
| 2. Feeling down, depressed, or hopeless | 0 | 1 | 2 | 3 |
| 3. Trouble falling or staying asleep, or sleeping too much | 0 | 1 | 2 | 3 |
| 4. Feeling tired or having little energy | 0 | 1 | 2 | 3 |
| 5. Poor appetite or overeating | 0 | 1 | 2 | 3 |
| 6. Feeling bad about yourself or that you are a failure or have let yourself or your family down | 0 | 1 | 2 | 3 |
| 7. Trouble concentrating on things, such as reading the newspaper or watching television | 0 | 1 | 2 | 3 |
| 8. Moving or speaking so slowly that other people could have noticed, or the opposite being so fidgety or restless that you have been moving around a lot more than usual | 0 | 1 | 2 | 3 |
| 9. Thoughts that you would be better off dead or of hurting yourself in some way | 0 | 1 | 2 | 3 |
| Total Score | ___ | + ___ | + ___ | + ___ |
| If you checked off any problems, how difficult have these problems made it for you to do your work, take care of things at home, or get along with other people? | | | | |
| ___ Not difficult at all ___ Somewhat difficult ___ Very difficult ___ Extremely difficult | | | | |

From Spitzer RL, Kroenke K, Williams JBW. For the Patient Health Questionnaire Primary Care Study Group. Validation and utility of a self-report version of PRIME-MD: the PHQ Primary Care Study. *JAMA.* 1999;282:1737-1744; Spitzer RL, Williams JBW, Kroenke K, et al. Validity and utility of the Patient Health Questionnaire in assessment of 3000 obstetrics-gynecologic patients. *Am J Obstet Gynecol.* 2000;183:759-769.

The PHQ was developed by Drs. Robert L. Spitzer, Janet B.W. Williams, Kurt Kroenke, and colleagues. PRIME-MD is a trademark of Pfizer Inc.

stress-related, short-term emotional or behavioral response to a stressful life circumstance. Depressive symptoms begin within 3 months of the onset of the stressor and resolve within 6 months once the stressful circumstance ends. The symptoms do not meet criteria for major depression. The physician can help a woman with an adjustment disorder by helping her to problem solve and cope with the situation she is in or by referring her for short-term therapy or counseling.

Persistent depressive disorder (previously called *dysthymic disorder*) is a chronic, low-grade depression, with symptoms present more than half the time for at least 2 years and no more than 2 months without depressive symptoms during that time. The best treatment is antidepressant medication and psychotherapy, but this condition is often harder to treat than major depression because of its chronicity. Depressive symptoms can also be caused by alcohol or drug use or by medical conditions, such as hypothyroidism, vitamin $B_{12}$ deficiency, anemia, or cancer (most classically pancreatic cancer). Women presenting with depression should be screened for medical disorders and asked about use of alcohol and drugs.

**Probably the greatest dilemma in deciding to prescribe antidepressants is the concern that if the woman has bipolar disorder, antidepressants can cause a "switch" into a manic episode.** Manic episodes are characterized by feelings of euphoria or irritability and increased energy or goal-directed activity, with symptoms such as decreased need for sleep, increased activity or agitation, talkativeness, racing thoughts, grandiose and unrealistic plans, and impulsive and risky behavior. If a woman has been hospitalized for mania or has had such symptoms for a week or more in the past, the diagnosis may be clear. However, people often do not recall their manic symptoms or have little insight into them, or they may have had briefer periods of a few days (hypomania) that still predispose them to mania with antidepressants. Screening questionnaires such as the Mood Disorder Questionnaire (MDQ) or clinician-administered Composite International Diagnostic Interview (CIDI) (STABLE Resource Toolkit; STABLE National Coordinating Council Resource Toolkit Workgroup, 2007, pp. 14-20) can be helpful in assessing the likelihood of a bipolar disorder. Difficulty determining whether or not a woman has bipolar disorder is an indication for psychiatric consultation because bipolar depression usually requires treatment with a mood stabilizer or atypical antipsychotic medication instead of, or combined with, an antidepressant.

Treatment of major depression can include antidepressant medication, psychotherapy, or both. **Because both antidepressant medication and psychotherapy are effective, the initial choice of treatment can be made according to the woman's preference,** although for more severe depression medication is indicated. Commonly prescribed antidepressant medications and dosages are listed in Table 9.2. A 2009 meta-analysis by Cipriani and colleagues suggested that the best combination of efficacy and tolerability is found with sertraline or escitalopram (Cipriani, 2009). **Because of their more benign side effect profiles, it is reasonable to start a selective serotonin reuptake inhibitor (SSRI) as the first antidepressant in most cases.** SSRI side effects include gastrointestinal symptoms (nausea, diarrhea, vomiting), which are minimized by taking the medication with a meal. Other common side effects include initial dizziness and headaches and sexual dysfunction, most commonly delayed orgasm or anorgasmia. Doses of the SSRI citalopram exceeding 40 mg daily are not recommended because of the risk of QT prolongation. SSRIs may also cause uncomfortable withdrawal symptoms if discontinued suddenly. Withdrawal symptoms can include gastrointestinal symptoms, headache, dizziness, and "electric shock" sensations. Fluoxetine, an SSRI with a long half-life, is not generally associated with withdrawal symptoms and women discontinuing other SSRIs can be switched to fluoxetine to minimize withdrawal. Fluoxetine also has the strongest evidence base for medication treatment of major depression in children and adolescents.

Serotonin and norepinephrine reuptake inhibitors (SNRIs) include venlafaxine and duloxetine. Venlafaxine is associated with a dose-related risk for gradual onset of hypertension, and blood pressure should be monitored carefully on this medication. SNRI side effects include gastrointestinal side effects, headaches, dizziness, anorgasmia, activation, and anxiety. Bupropion appears to exert its therapeutic effect by enhancing effects of dopamine and norepinephrine. It increases energy and can cause insomnia, increased anxiety, headaches, and gastrointestinal side effects. Bupropion also lowers the seizure threshold, especially at doses greater than 450 mg daily, and should not be used in women with a history of a seizure disorder or bulimia. Mirtazapine is an alpha$_2$-adrenergic, 5-HT2, and 5-HT3 receptor antagonist, which

**TABLE 9.2** *Commonly Prescribed Antidepressants*

| Antidepressant | Dose Range (mg/day) | Comments |
|---|---|---|
| **SEROTONIN REUPTAKE INHIBITORS (SSRIs)** | | |
| Citalopram | 20-40 | FDA warning of QT prolongation at doses >40 mg/day |
| Escitalopram | 10-20 | S-enantiomer of citalopram |
| Fluoxetine | 20-80 | Long half-life; unlikely to cause withdrawal symptoms with discontinuation or missed doses; best evidence base for use in children and adolescents |
| Paroxetine | 20-50 (25-62.5 controlled release) | High rate of withdrawal symptoms |
| Sertraline | 50-200 | |
| **SEROTONIN AND NOREPINEPHRINE REUPTAKE INHIBITORS (SNRIs)** | | |
| Duloxetine | 60-120 | May also be effective for neuropathic pain, urinary incontinence |
| Venlafaxine | 75-225 | Risk of elevated blood pressure |
| **OTHER** | | |
| Bupropion | 300-450 | Elevated risk of seizures, especially at doses >450 mg/day; contraindicated in patients with bulimia; may be effective for comorbid attention deficit disorder; activating; does not cause sexual dysfunction or weight gain; effective for smoking cessation |
| Mirtazapine | 15-45 | Sedating; causes weight gain |
| Trazodone | 25-100 (for insomnia) | Sedating; used as adjunctive treatment for insomnia |

*FDA,* Food and Drug Administration.

also has antihistaminic effects. Its common side effects include sedation and weight gain. Trazodone is a highly sedating serotonergic antidepressant that is used primarily at low doses (25 to 100 mg at bedtime) for insomnia. Tricyclic and monoamine oxidase (MAO) inhibitor antidepressants are infrequently prescribed because of side effects, in addition to dietary restrictions and the risk of hypertensive crisis with MAO inhibitors. **It is important to warn women that antidepressant medication can take up to 4 to 6 weeks to work and to schedule a follow-up visit** within that time to monitor treatment adherence, side effects, and therapeutic response. **The Food and Drug Administration (FDA) has required black box warnings regarding increases in suicidal ideation and behavior with antidepressants in children, adolescents, and young adults.** The mechanism for this is unclear but may be in part an increase in energy and motivation before improvement in mood. Women should be warned of this potential phenomenon and instructed to stop the medication and call the provider if this occurs. Overall, antidepressants reduce depression and risk for suicide, but this potentially serious side effect is another indication for close follow-up early in treatment. In particular, patients younger than 25 years should be seen 1 to 2 weeks after beginning antidepressant medication.

**Effective psychotherapies for depression include cognitive behavioral therapy (CBT) and interpersonal therapy (IPT). CBT addresses the negative thinking that is characteristic of depression, such as the belief that things are bad now, have always been bad, and will always be bad, or thoughts of worthlessness and guilt.** In addition, behavioral activation, or scheduling activities that provide a sense of accomplishment, mastery, or pleasure, is helpful in depression, and exercise has been shown to decrease depressive symptoms. **IPT addresses life changes and interpersonal challenges that contribute to depression.** These include grief, conflicts in interpersonal relationships including marital or intimate partner conflicts, and transitions in roles within work or the family. These therapies are usually weekly for an hour for 3 to 4 months. In cases of clear-cut couples issues, couples therapy may be indicated, especially after the woman has recovered from depression sufficiently to participate in such therapy. **Other nonmedication treatments for depression include morning light for seasonal or winter depression and electroconvulsive treatment (ECT) or repetitive transcranial magnetic stimulation (rTMS) for depression that does not respond to medication and psychotherapy.**

Both medication and psychotherapy are significantly more effective than placebo for treatment of major depression, with response rates varying between about 50% and 70%, depending on the patient population. Combined treatment with both psychotherapy and medication is more effective and is indicated for more severe depression.

**The goal of treatment for depression is complete remission, or resolution of all depressive symptoms, because even mild residual symptoms increase the risk of relapse.** Several measures can increase rates of remission (Cameron, 2014). First, close follow-up, with visits every 1 to 2 weeks at first and then every 2 to 4 weeks, will enhance adherence and response rates. One third of people prescribed an antidepressant discontinue the medication within 30 days. There is considerable stigma associated with taking psychotropic medication or having a psychiatric diagnosis, so addressing the woman's concerns that depression is a weakness or a character flaw can be helpful. Frequent visits also allow early identification of side effects that decrease adherence. Patient education about the lag in response to antidepressants and the need to take the medication every day for at least 6 to 12 months after symptomatic improvement is important. Tracking symptoms with a scale such as the PHQ-9 is helpful in monitoring progress and identifying residual symptoms. If there is little response in 2 to 4 weeks, a dose increase should be considered. A partial response at 8 weeks should prompt reassessment of the diagnosis; an attempt to ensure that the patient is taking the maximal tolerated dose of the antidepressant; and consideration of switching medications, adding an augmentation agent such as lithium, an atypical antipsychotic, or triiodothyronine (T3), or referral to a psychiatrist. Women who have had three or more episodes of major depression should be continued on maintenance antidepressant treatment.

Suicide is a feared and tragic outcome of depression and other mental health conditions. In the United States there were 47,173 suicide deaths in 2017; 6.1 per 100,000 women and 22.4 per 100,000 men died by suicide, and suicide was the 10th leading cause of death. Rates of suicide are highest among people aged 45 to 64 years compared with other age groups and in whites, and Native Americans compared with other ethnic groups. There are about 30 suicide attempts per every suicide death. Risk factors for suicide include depression or other mental health disorders; substance use disorders; a prior suicide attempt; a family history of psychiatric or substance use disorders; family violence, including physical or sexual abuse; access to means such as firearms in the house; and exposure to suicidal behavior by people such as family members, peers, or celebrities. **All depressed women should be asked about suicidal thoughts.** This should include asking about whether the woman feels hopeless or has had thoughts that life is not worth living or thoughts of ending her life, followed by more specific questions about whether she has made suicide plans and how far she has gone to carry these out. The Columbia Suicide Severity Rating Scale (Posner, 2011; scale available at http://cssrs.columbia.edu/wp-content/uploads/C-SSRS-Screener-with-Triage-Points-for-Primary-Care-2018-1.docx) provides a useful structured approach to asking about suicidal thoughts, with a screening form and triage recommendations tailored for primary care settings. **Active suicidal thoughts and plans are a psychiatric emergency.** The woman should not be left alone. The physician or staff should call 9-1-1 to have her taken to the nearest emergency room. Even in less acute cases, it is important to develop a safety plan with the patient, identifying family members, supportive people, and resources (e.g., crisis lines) she can call on, making a plan to remove firearms and other means of suicide from the home (means restriction), having someone else supervise the woman's medication, and seeking psychiatric or other mental health consultation as soon as possible.

## EATING DISORDERS

**Anorexia nervosa, bulimia nervosa, and binge eating disorder are the major eating disorders** and have a lifetime prevalence of 0.6%, 1%, and 3%, respectively (for a review of eating disorders, see Treasure, 2010). Eating disorders primarily affect younger people and have their peak onset between the ages of 10 and 19. These disorders are more common in women than in men. Many young women with eating disorders are secretive about their disorder, do not view it as a problem, and do not seek treatment for it. **Gynecologists may see such girls or women for related problems, such as amenorrhea, menstrual dysfunction, low bone density, sexual dysfunction, infertility, anxiety, depression, hyperemesis gravidarum, or other pregnancy complications. Because the woman may not volunteer information about disordered eating, it is important to have a high index of suspicion for eating disorders.** A simple five-question self-rating scale, the SCOFF questionnaire (Box 9.2), is highly sensitive and specific in detecting eating disorders in primary care settings and thus is a useful screening tool. The *Diagnostic and Statistical Manual*, Fifth Edition (DSM-5), diagnostic criteria for anorexia nervosa, bulimia nervosa, and binge eating disorder are listed in Box 9.3. Of note, the DSM-5 diagnosis of anorexia nervosa is also specified by current severity, with a body mass index (BMI) of 17 $kg/m^2$ being mild, 16 to 16.99 $kg/m^2$ moderate, 15 to 15.99 $kg/m^2$ severe, and less than 15 $kg/m^2$ extreme.

**BOX 9.2** SCOFF Screening Questionnaire for Eating Disorders

1. Do you make yourself sick because you feel uncomfortably full? ____ Yes ____ No
2. Do you worry you have lost control over how much you eat? ____ Yes ____ No
3. Have you recently lost more than one stone (14 pounds) in a 3-month period? ____ Yes ____ No
4. Do you believe yourself to be fat when others say you are too thin? ____ Yes ____ No
5. Would you say that food dominates your life? ____ Yes ____ No

Two or more "yes" answers indicate that the patient may have an eating disorder.

Modified from Morgan JF, Reid F, Lacey JH. The SCOFF questionnaire: assessment of a new screening tool for eating disorders. *BMJ.* 1999; 319:1467-1468.

Anorexia nervosa is characterized by a disturbed body image and fears of becoming fat or gaining weight, even though the person's body weight is less than expected. Weight loss is achieved by restricting food intake, overexercising, self-induced vomiting, or use of laxatives, emetics, and diuretics. Anorexia is most common in white teenage girls in industrialized Western societies. Societal pressures and standards of attractiveness for women, which emphasize thinness, have long been considered to increase the risk for anorexia nervosa, and a preoccupation with dieting is common in girls at menarche. Increasing evidence indicates, however, that there is clearly a significant genetic contribution to anorexia nervosa and other eating disorders, with heritability estimates of 50% to 80%. Other risk factors include a history of childhood sexual abuse and psychological traits of low self-esteem, perfectionism, and obsessive thinking.

**Medical signs and symptoms associated with anorexia nervosa include bradycardia, hypotension, hypothermia, leukopenia, hair loss, skin changes, and constipation.** Vomiting or laxative use may cause hypokalemia. Endocrine changes include

**BOX 9.3** Diagnostic Criteria for Eating Disorders

**ANOREXIA NERVOSA**

A. Restriction of energy intake relative to requirements, leading to a significantly low body weight in the context of age, sex, developmental trajectory, and physical health. *Significantly low weight* is defined as a weight that is less than minimally normal or, for children and adolescents, less than that minimally expected.
B. Intense fear of gaining weight or becoming fat, or persistent behavior that interferes with weight gain, even though at a significantly low weight.
C. Disturbance in the way in which one's body weight or shape is experienced, undue influence of body weight or shape on self-evaluation, or persistent lack of recognition of the seriousness of the current low body weight.

**Coding note:** The ICD-9-CM code for anorexia nervosa is **307.1,** which is assigned regardless of the subtype. The ICD-10-CM code depends on the subtype.

*Specify* whether:

**(F50.01) Restricting type:** During the last 3 months, the individual has not engaged in recurrent episodes of binge eating or purging behavior (i.e., self-induced vomiting or the misuse of laxatives, diuretics, or enemas). This subtype describes presentations in which weight loss is accomplished primarily through dieting, fasting, and/or excessive exercise.

**(F50.02) Binge-eating/purging type:** During the last 3 months, the individual has engaged in recurrent episodes of binge eating or purging behavior (i.e., self-induced vomiting or the misuse of laxatives, diuretics, or enemas).

*Specify* if:

**In partial remission:** After full criteria for anorexia nervosa were previously met, Criterion A (low body weight) has not been met for a sustained period, but either Criterion B (intense fear of gaining weight or becoming fat or behavior that interferes with weight gain) or Criterion C (disturbances in self-perception of weight and shape) is still met.

**In full remission:** After full criteria for anorexia nervosa were previously met, none of the criteria have been met for a sustained period of time.

D. *Specify* current severity:
The minimum level of severity is based, for adults, on current body mass index (BMI) or, for children and adolescents, on BMI percentile. The ranges are derived from World Health Organization categories for thinness in adults; for children and adolescents, corresponding BMI percentiles should be used. The level of severity may be increased to reflect clinical symptoms, the degree of functional disability, and the need for supervision.

**Mild:** BMI $\geq$ 17 kg/m$^2$
**Moderate:** BMI 16 to 16.99 kg/m$^2$
**Severe:** BMI 15 to 15.99 kg/m$^2$
**Extreme:** BMI $<$ 15 kg/m$^2$

**BULIMIA NERVOSA**

A. Recurrent episodes of binge eating. An episode of binge eating is characterized by both of the following:
   1. Eating, in a discrete period of time (e.g., within any 2-hour period), an amount of food that is definitely larger than most individuals would eat in a similar period of time under similar circumstances.
   2. A sense of lack of control over eating during the episode (e.g., a feeling that one cannot stop eating or control what or how much one is eating).
B. Recurrent, inappropriate compensatory behaviors in order to prevent weight gain, such as self-induced vomiting; misuse of laxatives, diuretics, or other medications; fasting; or excessive exercise.
C. The binge eating and inappropriate compensatory behaviors both occur, on average, at least once a week for 3 months.
D. Self-evaluation is unduly influenced by body shape and weight.
E. The disturbance does not occur exclusively during episodes of anorexia nervosa.

*Specify* if:

**In partial remission:** After full criteria for bulimia nervosa were previously met, some, but not all, of the criteria have been met for a sustained period of time.

**In full remission:** After full criteria for bulimia nervosa were previously met, none of the criteria have been met for a sustained period of time.

F. *Specify* current severity:
The minimum level of severity is based on the frequency of inappropriate compensatory behaviors. The level of severity may be increased to reflect other symptoms and the degree of functional disability.

**Mild:** An average of 1 to 3 episodes of inappropriate compensatory behaviors per week.
**Moderate:** An average of 4 to 7 episodes of inappropriate compensatory behaviors per week.
**Severe:** An average of 8 to 13 episodes of inappropriate compensatory behaviors per week.
**Extreme:** An average of 14 or more episodes of inappropriate compensatory behaviors per week.

**BOX 9.3** Diagnostic Criteria for Eating Disorders—cont'd

**BINGE-EATING DISORDER**

A. Recurrent episodes of binge eating. An episode of binge eating is characterized by both of the following:
   1. Eating, in a discrete period of time (e.g., within any 2-hour period), an amount of food that is definitely larger than what most people would eat in a similar period of time under similar circumstances.
   2. A sense of lack of control over eating during the episode (e.g., a feeling that one cannot stop eating or control what or how much one is eating).

B. The binge-eating episodes are associated with three (or more) of the following:
   1. Eating much more rapidly than normal.
   2. Eating until feeling uncomfortably full.
   3. Eating large amounts of food when not feeling physically hungry.
   4. Eating alone because of feeling embarrassed by how much one is eating.
   5. Feeling disgusted with oneself, depressed, or very guilty afterward.

C. Marked distress regarding binge eating is present.

D. Binge eating occurs, on average, at least once a week for 3 months.

E. The binge eating is not associated with the recurrent use of inappropriate compensatory behavior as in bulimia nervosa and does not occur exclusively during the course of bulimia nervosa or anorexia nervosa.

*Specify* if:

**In partial remission:** After full criteria for binge-eating disorder were previously met, binge eating occurs at an average frequency of less than one episode per week for a sustained period of time.

**In full remission:** After full criteria for binge-eating disorder were previously met, none of the criteria have been met for a sustained period of time.

*Specify* current severity:

The minimum level of severity is based on the frequency of episodes of binge eating. The level of severity may be increased to reflect other symptoms and the degree of functional disability.

**Mild:** 1 to 3 binge-eating episodes per week.

**Moderate:** 4 to 7 binge-eating episodes per week.

**Severe:** 8 to 13 binge-eating episodes per week.

**Extreme:** 14 or more binge-eating episodes per week.

From American Psychiatric Association. *Diagnostic and Statistical Manual of Mental Disorders.* 5th ed. Washington, DC: American Psychiatric Association; 2013: 338-339, 345, 350.

low estrogen and testosterone levels, amenorrhea, decreased libido, hypercortisolemia, and low bone density. Prolonged QT interval is a serious sequela of anorexia nervosa and has been associated with sudden death. The mortality rate of anorexia nervosa from all causes is 5% to 6% per decade of illness.

Psychiatric symptoms associated with anorexia nervosa include depression, anxiety, social difficulties, sleep disturbance, agitation, poor emotion regulation, rigidity, obsessional thinking, and compulsive behaviors. Interestingly, these symptoms occur in individuals without anorexia nervosa during starvation and resolve with weight gain and so are most likely caused, or at least exacerbated, by the illness.

Anorexia nervosa is difficult to treat (for a review, see Zipfel, 2015). Women do not usually seek help themselves but instead are brought to treatment by concerned family members. They fear gaining weight, do not see their illness as a problem, are often nonadherent with treatment, feel isolated and do not engage with treatment providers, and may have multiple relapses. About one third recover completely, but this may take a number of years. Early recognition and treatment improve outcome. Family members often become frustrated with the woman's multiple relapses, lack of insight, and apparent lack of cooperation with treatment and may need support themselves in dealing with her illness.

**The best treatment for anorexia nervosa involves referral to a multidisciplinary team, with medical, nutritional, psychological, and psychiatric expertise in this area.** The focus is on gradual refeeding to achieve weight gain and on outpatient treatment, with hospitalization only for acute, dangerous medical or psychiatric complications. In adolescents, family therapy focused on eating disorder behavior and weight gain or, in nonintact families, adolescent-centered individual psychotherapy is most effective (Lock, 2015). In adults, several different types of specialized psychotherapy show promise, including cognitive behavioral, psychodynamic, and supportive therapies adapted specifically for treatment of anorexia. In one randomized controlled trial (RCT), focal psychodynamic therapy seemed to help recovery most at 12 months, whereas enhanced CBT was more effective with speed of weight gain and improvement in eating disorder thinking (Zipfel, 2014). Few studies address relapse prevention, although a structured aftercare program after inpatient treatment reduces risk of relapse. **There is no clear evidence supporting treatment of anorexia with psychotropic medications.** Antidepressants do not promote weight gain or reduce eating disorder symptoms during acute treatment, and their efficacy for relapse prevention is unclear. The atypical antipsychotic olanzapine has been tried with the goal of addressing weight gain and distorted thinking about weight and body shape. A 16-week randomized placebo-controlled trial of 152 outpatients with anorexia nervosa (75 treated with olanzapine and 77 with placebo) showed greater weight gain with olanzapine but no significant differences in psychological symptoms such as obsessional thinking (Attia, 2019). In this study, olanzapine was prescribed at 2.5 mg daily for 2 weeks, 5 mg daily for 2 weeks, then 10 mg daily, as tolerated.

**Bulimia nervosa is characterized by binge eating, combined with inappropriate compensatory mechanisms to avoid weight gain, such as self-induced vomiting, misuse of laxatives or diuretics, or fasting or excessive exercise.** Binge eating and compensatory behaviors occur an average of once a week for 3 months (see Box 9.3 for full diagnostic criteria). Bulimia, like anorexia, is most common in young women, has a significant genetic component, may follow teasing or criticism about the woman's weight or shape, and is thought to involve disturbances in hunger-satiety pathways, the drive system and rewarding characteristics of food, or self-regulation. Comorbidity with mood and anxiety disorders, addictions, and suicidal thoughts and behaviors is common. All-cause mortality rates, including suicide rates, are elevated, with a mortality rate of 3.9% over 8 to 25 years of follow-up.

Women with bulimia nervosa and purging may develop hypokalemia, hyponatremia, hypochloremia, a metabolic alkalosis as a result of vomiting, or a metabolic acidosis with laxative abuse. Recurrent self-induced vomiting can result in loss of dental enamel, parotid gland enlargement, or calluses and scars on the dorsal aspect of the hand. Rare but serious complications include esophageal tears, gastric rupture, rectal prolapse, and cardiac arrhythmias.

**There is strong evidence for the efficacy of CBT for bulimia nervosa, although complete remission of binging and purging occurs in only 30% to 40%.** Other therapies for which there is some evidence of efficacy are IPT, dialectical behavior therapy (DBT) focusing on emotion regulation, and family therapy in adolescents. Antidepressants are superior to placebo in treatment of bulimia, with the agent of choice being fluoxetine 60 mg daily. Of note, the antidepressant bupropion is contraindicated in women with a history of bulimia because of an elevated risk of seizures, presumably because of electrolyte abnormalities. The outcome of bulimia is full recovery in 45%, significant improvement in 27%, and a chronic, protracted course in about 23%.

In binge eating disorder, the woman binge eats (as in bulimia nervosa) an average of once a week for at least 3 months, but she does not engage in compensatory behaviors such as purging, fasting, or excessive exercise. As a result, she may also develop obesity but does not develop the medical complications associated with purging or low weight. Treatment for binge eating disorder includes nutritional consultation, diet, physical activity, education, and specific psychotherapies. There is strong evidence for the efficacy of CBT in binge eating disorder and other psychotherapies, such as DBT and IPT, are also effective. Medication treatments include antidepressants such as SSRIs. Weight loss agents, topiramate, and stimulants may also be effective.

## OBESITY

Although obesity is not uniquely a gynecologic condition, obesity and overweight affect a substantial proportion of patients for whom gynecologists provide care. The prevalence of obesity continues to increase in the United States. The World Health Organization (WHO) definitions for BMI are shown in Table 9.3. Table 9.4 outlines classification by BMI. In 2016, 39.8% of U.S. adults were obese and 71.6% were overweight or obese. The prevalence of obesity is higher in adults aged 40 to 59, minority women, and low-income women and varies by geographic region. Non-Hispanic Black and Hispanic women have slightly higher prevalence of obesity than non-Hispanic white women, whereas non-Hispanic Asian women have the lowest prevalence. The WHO describes obesity as a global epidemic, contributing substantially to chronic disease and disability.

**Waist circumference is another parameter by which to measure obesity and when combined with BMI can be a predictor of obesity-related morbidity. Increased central adiposity is associated with increased risk of morbidity and mortality.** The waist circumference can be measured at the level of the anterior superior iliac spine, at the end of expiration. For women with a BMI of 25 to 34.9 kg/m² (overweight or class I obesity), a waist circumference of more than 35 inches (88 cm) is associated with heart disease and diabetes mellitus. Risks are increased even more for those with BMI of 35 kg/m² or greater (class II or III obesity).

**There is a strong relationship between mortality and increased BMI greater than 25 kg/m² (and less than 20 kg/m²)** (Fig. 9.1). Even in healthy people who have never smoked, at age 50 years there is still an elevated risk of death for persons whose BMIs are between 25 and 30 kg/m² (Adams, 2006). The risk of death increases 20% to 40% in the overweight group and by two to three times among obese persons. Severe obesity is a health hazard that carries a 12-fold increase in mortality.

Obesity often coexists with medical conditions such as hypertension, diabetes mellitus, dyslipidemias, arthritis, and obstructive sleep apnea (OSA). Obesity has been linked to increased operative morbidity and mortality, as well as obstetric and gynecologic conditions, including miscarriage, infertility, endometrial hyperplasia, and some types of cancer. High BMI has also been associated with increased vasomotor symptoms in menopause. One meta-analysis of increased BMI and cancer risk found a strong association between a five-point BMI increase and risk of endometrial cancer (relative risk [RR] 1.59, $P < .0001$), gallbladder cancer (RR 1.59, $P = .04$), esophageal adenocarcinoma (RR 1.51, $P < .0001$), and renal cancer (RR 1.34, $P < .0001$). A weaker positive association was found with postmenopausal breast, pancreatic, thyroid, and colon cancer plus leukemia, multiple myeloma, and non-Hodgkin lymphoma. The mechanisms of cancer's association with obesity

**TABLE 9.3** Body Mass Index Table

| BMI (kg/m²) | 19 | 20 | 21 | 22 | 23 | 24 | 25 | 26 | 27 | 28 | 29 | 30 | 31 | 32 | 33 | 34 | 35 |
|---|---|---|---|---|---|---|---|---|---|---|---|---|---|---|---|---|---|
| **Height (inches)** | | | | | | | | **Body Weight (lb)** | | | | | | | | | |
| 58 | 91 | 96 | 100 | 105 | 110 | 115 | 119 | 124 | 129 | 134 | 138 | 143 | 148 | 153 | 158 | 162 | 167 |
| 59 | 94 | 99 | 104 | 109 | 114 | 119 | 124 | 128 | 133 | 138 | 143 | 148 | 153 | 158 | 163 | 168 | 173 |
| 60 | 97 | 102 | 107 | 112 | 118 | 123 | 128 | 133 | 138 | 143 | 148 | 153 | 158 | 163 | 168 | 174 | 179 |
| 61 | 100 | 106 | 111 | 116 | 122 | 127 | 132 | 137 | 143 | 148 | 153 | 158 | 164 | 169 | 174 | 180 | 185 |
| 62 | 104 | 109 | 115 | 120 | 126 | 131 | 136 | 142 | 147 | 153 | 158 | 164 | 169 | 175 | 180 | 186 | 191 |
| 63 | 107 | 113 | 118 | 124 | 130 | 135 | 141 | 146 | 152 | 158 | 163 | 169 | 175 | 180 | 186 | 191 | 197 |
| 64 | 110 | 116 | 122 | 128 | 134 | 140 | 145 | 151 | 157 | 163 | 169 | 174 | 180 | 186 | 192 | 197 | 204 |
| 65 | 114 | 120 | 126 | 132 | 138 | 144 | 150 | 156 | 162 | 168 | 174 | 180 | 186 | 192 | 198 | 204 | 210 |
| 66 | 118 | 124 | 130 | 136 | 142 | 148 | 155 | 161 | 167 | 173 | 179 | 186 | 192 | 198 | 204 | 210 | 216 |
| 67 | 121 | 127 | 134 | 140 | 146 | 153 | 159 | 166 | 172 | 178 | 185 | 191 | 198 | 204 | 211 | 217 | 223 |
| 68 | 125 | 131 | 138 | 144 | 151 | 158 | 164 | 171 | 177 | 184 | 190 | 197 | 203 | 210 | 216 | 223 | 230 |
| 69 | 128 | 135 | 142 | 149 | 155 | 162 | 169 | 176 | 182 | 189 | 196 | 203 | 209 | 216 | 223 | 230 | 236 |
| 70 | 132 | 139 | 146 | 153 | 160 | 167 | 174 | 181 | 188 | 195 | 202 | 209 | 216 | 222 | 229 | 236 | 243 |
| 71 | 136 | 143 | 150 | 157 | 165 | 172 | 179 | 186 | 193 | 200 | 208 | 215 | 222 | 229 | 236 | 243 | 250 |
| 72 | 140 | 147 | 154 | 162 | 169 | 177 | 184 | 191 | 199 | 206 | 213 | 221 | 228 | 235 | 242 | 250 | 258 |
| 73 | 144 | 151 | 159 | 166 | 174 | 182 | 189 | 197 | 204 | 212 | 219 | 227 | 235 | 242 | 250 | 257 | 265 |
| 74 | 148 | 155 | 163 | 171 | 179 | 186 | 194 | 202 | 210 | 218 | 225 | 233 | 241 | 249 | 256 | 264 | 272 |
| 75 | 152 | 160 | 168 | 176 | 184 | 192 | 200 | 208 | 216 | 224 | 232 | 240 | 248 | 256 | 264 | 272 | 279 |
| 76 | 156 | 164 | 172 | 180 | 189 | 197 | 205 | 213 | 221 | 230 | 238 | 246 | 254 | 263 | 271 | 279 | 287 |

**TABLE 9.3** Body Mass Index Table—cont'd

| BMI (kg/m²) | 36 | 37 | 38 | 39 | 40 | 41 | 42 | 43 | 44 | 45 | 46 | 47 | 48 | 49 | 50 | 51 | 52 | 53 | 54 |
|---|---|---|---|---|---|---|---|---|---|---|---|---|---|---|---|---|---|---|---|
| **Height (inches)** | | | | | | | | | | **Body Weight (lb)** | | | | | | | | | |
| 58 | 172 | 177 | 181 | 186 | 191 | 196 | 201 | 205 | 210 | 215 | 220 | 224 | 229 | 234 | 239 | 244 | 248 | 253 | 258 |
| 59 | 178 | 183 | 188 | 193 | 198 | 203 | 208 | 212 | 217 | 222 | 227 | 232 | 237 | 242 | 247 | 252 | 257 | 262 | 267 |
| 60 | 184 | 189 | 194 | 199 | 204 | 209 | 215 | 220 | 225 | 230 | 235 | 240 | 245 | 250 | 255 | 261 | 266 | 271 | 276 |
| 61 | 190 | 195 | 201 | 206 | 211 | 217 | 222 | 227 | 232 | 238 | 243 | 248 | 254 | 259 | 264 | 269 | 275 | 280 | 285 |
| 62 | 196 | 202 | 207 | 213 | 218 | 224 | 229 | 235 | 240 | 246 | 251 | 256 | 262 | 267 | 273 | 278 | 284 | 289 | 295 |
| 63 | 203 | 208 | 214 | 220 | 225 | 231 | 237 | 242 | 248 | 254 | 259 | 265 | 270 | 278 | 282 | 287 | 293 | 299 | 304 |
| 64 | 209 | 215 | 221 | 227 | 232 | 238 | 244 | 250 | 256 | 262 | 267 | 273 | 279 | 285 | 291 | 296 | 302 | 308 | 314 |
| 65 | 216 | 222 | 228 | 234 | 240 | 246 | 252 | 258 | 264 | 270 | 276 | 282 | 288 | 294 | 300 | 306 | 312 | 318 | 324 |
| 66 | 223 | 229 | 235 | 241 | 247 | 253 | 260 | 266 | 272 | 278 | 284 | 291 | 297 | 303 | 309 | 315 | 322 | 328 | 334 |
| 67 | 230 | 236 | 242 | 249 | 255 | 261 | 268 | 274 | 280 | 287 | 293 | 299 | 306 | 312 | 319 | 325 | 331 | 338 | 344 |
| 68 | 236 | 243 | 249 | 256 | 262 | 269 | 276 | 282 | 289 | 295 | 302 | 308 | 315 | 322 | 328 | 335 | 341 | 348 | 354 |
| 69 | 243 | 250 | 257 | 263 | 270 | 277 | 284 | 291 | 297 | 304 | 311 | 318 | 324 | 331 | 338 | 345 | 351 | 358 | 365 |
| 70 | 250 | 257 | 264 | 271 | 278 | 285 | 292 | 299 | 306 | 313 | 320 | 327 | 334 | 341 | 348 | 355 | 362 | 369 | 376 |
| 71 | 257 | 265 | 272 | 279 | 286 | 293 | 301 | 308 | 315 | 322 | 329 | 338 | 343 | 351 | 358 | 365 | 372 | 379 | 386 |
| 72 | 265 | 272 | 279 | 287 | 294 | 302 | 309 | 316 | 324 | 331 | 338 | 346 | 353 | 361 | 368 | 375 | 383 | 390 | 397 |
| 73 | 272 | 280 | 288 | 295 | 302 | 310 | 318 | 325 | 333 | 340 | 348 | 355 | 363 | 371 | 378 | 386 | 393 | 401 | 408 |
| 74 | 280 | 287 | 293 | 303 | 311 | 319 | 326 | 334 | 342 | 350 | 358 | 365 | 373 | 381 | 389 | 396 | 404 | 412 | 420 |
| 75 | 287 | 295 | 303 | 311 | 319 | 327 | 335 | 343 | 351 | 359 | 367 | 375 | 383 | 391 | 399 | 407 | 415 | 423 | 431 |
| 76 | 295 | 304 | 312 | 320 | 328 | 336 | 344 | 353 | 361 | 369 | 377 | 385 | 394 | 402 | 410 | 418 | 426 | 435 | 443 |

From NHLBI Obesity Education Initiative. *Clinical Guidelines on the Identification, Evaluation, and Treatment of Overweight and Obesity in Adults.* NIH Publication No. 98-4083. Bethesda, MD: National Institutes of Health; 1998. Available at http://www.ncbi.nlm.nih.gov/books/NBK2003/pdf/Bookshelf_NBK2003.pdf.

**TABLE 9.4** Weight Classification by Body Mass Index (BMI)

| Weight | BMI* |
|---|---|
| Normal weight | 18.5-24.9 |
| Overweight | 25.0-29.9 |
| Obesity | >30 |
| Class I | 30.0-34.9 |
| Class II | 35.0-39.9 |
| Class III | >40 |

*BMI = weight in kilograms/height in square meters.

may be linked to hormone systems like insulin, insulin-like growth factor, sex steroids, adipokines, and other substances.

## Management of Obesity

**For overweight individuals or those with class I obesity, diet, exercise, and behavior modification are appropriate interventions. Those with class II or III obesity may benefit from medically supervised diet, exercise, and behavior modification or surgical management.** A systematic review of 12 trials found that intensive behavioral counseling, diet (reducing intake by ≥500 kcal/day), and exercise (≥150 minutes of walking/week) lead to clinically meaningful weight loss of 0.3 kg to 6.6 kg over 6 months (Wadden, 2014). Because sustained adherence to diet and exercise modifications can be difficult, surgical intervention (bariatric surgery) is likely to be the most effective approach for those with very high BMI.

## Diet

Organizations focused on weight management, such as Weight Watchers, may be successful for motivated individuals. Interventions that patients can manage themselves include tracking calorie intake, using smartphone apps for weight loss, avoiding food binges or eating at night, and practicing stress reduction or mindfulness-based training. A meta-analysis of 48 randomized trials of named diet programs reported that the largest weight loss was associated with low-carbohydrate diets and low-fat diets (Johnston, 2014), although differences in weight loss among these programs were minimal. It is more important to find a healthy diet that a person can adhere to long term. Because fat represents 9 Cal/g and protein and carbohydrate represent 4 Cal/g, a change in eating habits can allow an individual to eat more food while reducing unnecessary calories. Adherence to the U.S. Department of Agriculture (USDA) ChooseMyPlate dietary recommendations (https://www.choosemyplate.gov/), which emphasize fruits, vegetables, and grains over meat and dairy, is one way to make healthy diet changes that may facilitate weight loss. The use of portion-controlled servings has also been demonstrated to be effective for weight loss because people in general tend to underestimate how much they eat. Many diet programs prescribe or sell low-fat foods in an attempt to achieve a diet containing about 20% to 30% fat, though individuals may be able to achieve the same results through careful diet planning. Educating patients to change eating habits is important not only for losing weight but also for maintaining weight loss, which is more difficult. **Setting a realistic goal of 5% loss of body weight over 6 months is helpful.**

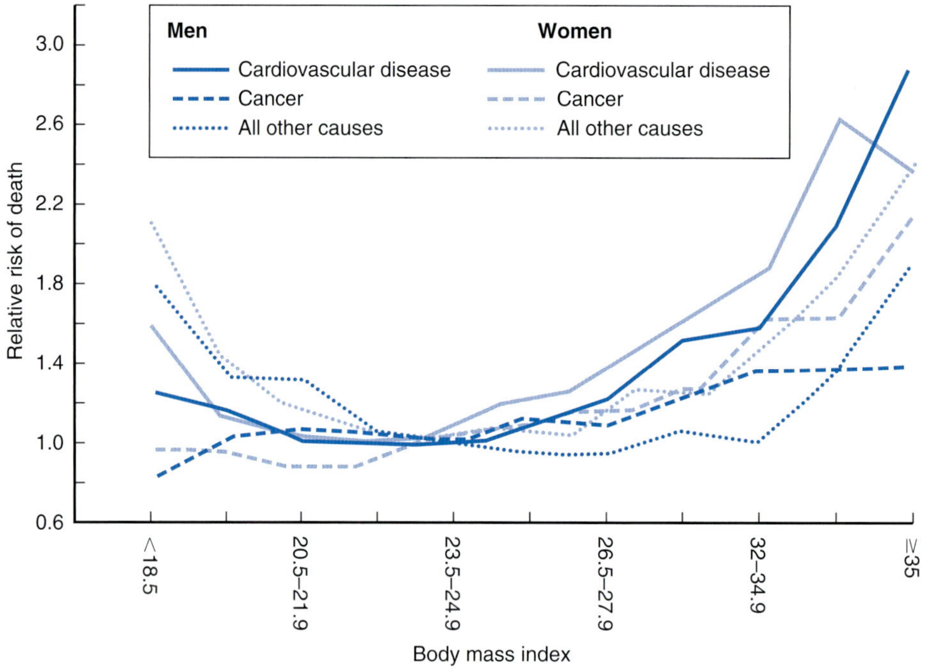


**Fig. 9.1** Relation between mortality and body mass index in men and women who have never smoked. (Data from Calle EE, Thun MJ, Petrelli JM, et al. Body-mass index and mortality in a prospective cohort of U.S. adults. *N Eng J Med.* 1999;341:1097-1105.)

Many individuals attempting weight loss have turned to fad diets such as juicing, detoxification, intermittent fasting, and paleo diets. Juicing and detoxification rely primarily on significant caloric restriction and are not sustainable (Cabo, 2019). Intermittent fasting and paleo diets are associated with short-term weight loss and may be more sustainable, but long-term data are lacking and long-term adherence may be problematic or impractical. Many of these diets may also be associated with adverse effects.

## Exercise

Exercise is a useful, and often necessary, addition to diet regimens. Several studies have demonstrated that although similar weight loss can be obtained by both diet alone and diet plus exercise programs, the latter will allow for a greater loss of fat stores while maintaining muscle mass. To maintain this advantage, exercise programs must be maintained. **Although exercise alone is not a good method for losing weight, it is beneficial for long-term weight management and overall health.** One study looked at amount of physical activity and weight gain in women and concluded that physical activity is inversely related to weight gain in women of normal weight but not in women who are overweight (Lee, 2010). Getting more active might be manageable for some women via their work commute. A U.K. study found that people who commuted to work by active methods (biking or walking) or public transport had significantly lower BMI and percentage of body fat than people who used private transportation (Flint, 2014). Presumably, using public transportation required more walking each day. Women in the United States may face challenges obtaining similar benefits because the built environment is often not conducive to exercise. Many areas lack accessible public transportation, and many individuals must commute long distances to work. Further, many in the United States live in neighborhoods where they do not feel safe walking or that lack sidewalks and other amenities that facilitate exercise.

Some attention has focused on what types of exercise may be most beneficial for weight loss. For example, several studies have focused on comparisons between moderate intensity training (MIT), such as distance running or cycling, and high-intensity training (HIT), which involves short bursts of high-intensity exercise. HIT seems to be associated with short-term weight loss and cardiovascular benefits but may not be feasible or safe for those with physical limitations or significant comorbidities, which may be concerns for many obese individuals. A systematic review reported small reductions in percentage of body fat with both HIT and MIT but noted that in the short term neither approach resulted in clinically meaningful reductions in body fat.

## Pharmacologic Interventions

**Pharmacologic therapy should be used as an adjunct to diet, exercise, and lifestyle modifications, rather than a solo approach.** FDA-approved formulations are associated with varying degrees of weight loss. Some medications are approved only for short-term (up to 12 weeks) use, whereas others can be used for a longer duration. Although surgical interventions generally result in greater levels of weight loss than do medications, many approved formulations have been associated with low to moderate weight loss in clinical studies. Medications may be a reasonable approach for those with BMI greater than 30 kg/m$^2$ or those with BMI 26 to 29.9 kg/m$^2$ and comorbidities. The initial choice of pharmacologic agent may depend on these and other factors.

Examples of pharmacologic weight loss therapy include orlistat, lorcaserin, phentermine-topiramate, and metformin, although there are several others as well.

- Orlistat inhibits dietary fat absorption and is considered first-line treatment because of its favorable safety profile. It is approved for up to 4 years of use. Most subjects can expect about 3% loss of initial weight, though side effects of fecal urgency, flatulence, and oily stools may occur.
- Lorcaserin is a serotonin 2c receptor agonist, which reduces appetite. It is an alternative for patients who cannot take orlistat. Over 1 year, about 50% of patients lost at least 3% of their body mass. Side effects include headache, dizziness, fatigue, nausea, and constipation.

TABLE 9.5 Guide to Selecting Treatment

| Body Mass Index Category | | | | | |
|---|---|---|---|---|---|
| **Treatment** | **25-26.9 kg/m²** | **27-29.9 kg/m²** | **30-34.9 kg/m²** | **35-39.9 kg/m²** | **>40 kg/m²** |
| Diet, physical activity, and behavior therapy | With comorbidities | With comorbidities | + | + | + |
| Pharmacotherapy | | With comorbidities | + | + | + |
| Surgery | | | With comorbidities | With comorbidities | With comorbidities |

From National Heart, Lung, and Blood Institute and North American Association for the Study of Obesity. *The Practical Guide: Identification, Evaluation, and Treatment of Overweight and Obesity in Adults.* Bethesda, MD: National Institutes of Health; 2000.
The + represents the use of indicated treatment regardless of comorbidities.

- Phentermine-topiramate is an acceptable option for postmenopausal women who do not have hypertension or cardiac disease. Up to 70% of individuals taking this medication will lose weight (Yanovski, 2014). Warnings include metabolic acidosis, increased heart rate, anxiety, insomnia, and increased creatinine levels. Both lorcaserin and phentermine-topiramate have warnings about memory, attention, and depression.
- Metformin is a reasonable initial therapy for individuals who require glycemic control in addition to weight loss.

There are other available medications as well; a comprehensive list is beyond the scope of this chapter. Long-term safety and efficacy data are limited for many weight loss medications. A guide to selecting treatment for obesity is given in Fig. 9.5.

## Bariatric Surgery

**Many bariatric surgery patients are women of reproductive age. Bariatric surgery is a proven intervention for weight loss and is associated with improvements in obesity-related medical comorbidities.** Eligible candidates for bariatric surgery include those with a BMI greater than 40 kg/m² or a BMI greater than 35 kg/m² with an obesity-associated comorbidity. Additional considerations include whether nonsurgical weight loss measures have failed, the woman is motivated and well informed, and there is acceptable surgical risk. The majority of postoperative obesity patients have resolution of or improvement in comorbid conditions such as diabetes, hypertension, dyslipidemia, and OSA (Puzziferri, 2014).

Types of bariatric surgery include malabsorptive procedures, restrictive procedures, and malabsorptive-restrictive procedures. Of the more common procedures, gastric banding is a restrictive procedure, and gastric bypass is both malabsorptive and restrictive. Surgeries can be performed via laparoscopic or open approaches. The chief benefit of bariatric surgery is weight loss, but improvements in comorbidities often occur. In an evaluation of 29 studies and 7971 patients, gastric bypass had better outcomes than gastric banding for long-term weight loss, type 2 diabetic control and remission, and improvements in hypertension and hyperlipidemia. Gastric bypass and sleeve gastrectomy were associated with weight loss exceeding 50% versus 31% in gastric band studies.

Surgical options can provide long-term weight loss but are not without complications. The 30-day mortality from bariatric surgical procedures ranges from 0.1% to 2%, depending on type of procedure and numerous patient factors. Short-term complications include thrombotic events, anastomotic leak, bleeding, and wound infection (all 2% or less), and long-term complications include thrombotic events, anastomotic or band complications, and nutritional deficiencies, particularly of iron and vitamin $B_{12}$. **Reproductive-aged patients are advised to avoid pregnancy for 12 to 24 months after surgery to allow stabilization of rate of weight loss and correct nutritional deficiencies.** Contraceptive counseling is an important role for the obstetrician-gynecologist in the postbariatric surgery period.

## Obesity in Adolescents

The percentage of young people who are overweight or obese has more than tripled since 1980. In the United States, 20.6% of adolescents aged 12 to 19 are obese, and the prevalence of obesity among adolescent girls is 21%. Standard adult BMI categories should not be applied to adolescents, whose BMI determination should incorporate growth chart data. For adolescents, *overweight* is defined as a BMI at or greater than the 85th percentile, *obesity* a BMI at or greater than the 95th percentile, and *severe obesity* a BMI greater than or equal to the 99th percentile for age.

Adolescents who are affected by obesity are at risk of developing impaired glucose tolerance, cardiovascular disease, nonalcoholic fatty liver disease, disordered breathing, and orthopedic problems. Consequences of these can continue and worsen into adulthood. Abnormal uterine bleeding and polycystic ovary syndrome (PCOS) are also more common among adolescents who are obese. Overweight and obesity during adolescence are also associated with psychosocial conditions, such as low self-esteem.

Diet, exercise, and behavioral modifications are the mainstay of treatment for children and adolescents who are overweight or obese. To be most successful, these interventions must be adopted by the entire family because children and adolescents are not in full control of their environments. A systematic review concluded that effective lifestyle interventions generally require a commitment of 28 hours or more to be effective. It further concluded that weight loss medications offer small benefit that is of unclear clinical significance. Orlistat is approved for use by adolescents and may result in weight loss, but gastrointestinal side effects may limit its use. Other weight loss medications may require further study before their use in adolescents can be recommended

Bariatric surgery may be appropriate for some obese adolescents who meet adult BMI criteria, and have attained at least Tanner IV stage of development or 95% of adult height based on bone age. For appropriately selected adolescent candidates, bariatric surgery can be an effective intervention to effect significant weight loss.

## Additional Considerations

**The Centers for Disease Control and Prevention (CDC) advised a multipronged approach to preventing obesity.** Recommendations include: (1) increasing consumption of fruits and vegetables; (2) regular physical activity, including for children; (3) increasing physical activity in overweight people to prevent the complications associated with obesity; and (4) breastfeeding, which is associated with a reduced risk of overweight children.

Population-based strategies and policies will likely be needed to have widespread impact.

The American College of Obstetricians and Gynecologists (ACOG) has issued guidance for the ethical care of patients with obesity. **Providers should be aware of their own implicit bias toward obese patients.** As with other aspects of care, obstetrician-gynecologists should incorporate principles of patient-centered counseling and open communication and focus on offering concrete strategies and goals to optimize overall health for individuals with obesity.

## ANXIETY DISORDERS, OBSESSIVE-COMPULSIVE DISORDER, AND POSTTRAUMATIC STRESS DISORDER

**Anxiety disorders are the most common psychiatric disorders in the general population. They usually have their onset in childhood, adolescence, or early adulthood and are more common in women than in men.** Anxiety is a normal, adaptive response to danger or threat and is associated with physical symptoms (e.g., increased heart rate, sweating, shaking) and cognitive symptoms (e.g., worry, fear). Increases in anxiety are common with life stressors, including medical appointments, diagnoses, and procedures. In addition, anxiety may result from a number of drugs (e.g., caffeine, cannabis, cocaine, methamphetamine, withdrawal of alcohol or opiates), medications (e.g., theophylline, steroids), or medical conditions (e.g., asthma, arrhythmias, temporal lobe epilepsy). Some people experience primary anxiety disorders, which involve excessive anxiety that interferes with daily functioning without apparent explanation or out of proportion to any stressor. Primary anxiety disorders include panic disorder, generalized anxiety disorder (GAD), social anxiety disorder, and specific phobias (for a review of primary anxiety disorders and their treatment, see Bandelow, 2017). Obsessive-compulsive disorder (OCD) and posttraumatic stress disorder (PTSD), although categorized separately from anxiety disorders in DSM-5, also involve significant anxiety and fear.

Panic disorder is characterized by sudden, intense attacks of fear. The symptom criteria for a panic attack are shown in Box 9.4. People with panic disorder have recurrent, unexpected panic attacks, with at least one of the attacks followed by a month or more of persistent concern about having additional attacks or worry about their consequences (e.g., losing control, having a heart attack, going crazy) or a maladaptive change in behavior because of panic attacks (e.g., avoiding certain situations for fear of having an attack). About one third of people in the general population have at least one panic attack during their lives, so that a woman presenting with a single panic attack can be reassured that this is very common. Panic attacks can be precipitated by frightening situations or heightened stress, in which case they are called *situational panic attacks.* People with only situational panic attacks are not diagnosed with panic disorder. Panic attacks without apparent precipitant are called *spontaneous.*

Panic disorder occurs in 1% to 2% of the population and is about twice as common in women than in men. Risk factors include a family history of panic disorder and significant life stress in the year before the development of symptoms. The disorder has a genetic component, with a heritability of about 30%. Complications include depression in about two thirds of people, and one third are depressed at the time of clinical presentation. Especially because panic attacks are unpredictable, they often lead to anticipatory anxiety (anxiety about having the next panic attack) and phobic avoidance, or avoidance of situations in which the person has had or would fear having a panic attack. These situations commonly include crowds, being in lines or in the middle of an audience, driving (especially in tunnels, over bridges, or in freeways), or other situations in which the woman would feel trapped, unable to get out, or publicly embarrassed. With time, the fear and avoidance surrounding panic attacks often become significantly more distressing and disabling than the attacks themselves and may lead to agoraphobia, or avoidance of multiple situations and activities. Panic disorder, like other anxiety disorders, is also associated with an increased rate of alcohol use as a form of self-medication. Finally, **panic and other anxiety disorders are associated with an increased risk for suicide attempts.** Thus even though a woman presents with anxiety and does not endorse depression, she should be asked about hopeless or suicidal thoughts.

**The treatment of panic disorder includes reassurance, education, general measures, medication, and psychotherapy. Fortunately, treatment response rates are high,** so it is possible to be optimistic that the woman has a highly treatable condition. She may fear that she is dying, has a life-threatening or serious medical illness, or that she is "going crazy," and she can be reassured that, although panic attacks are terrifying, none of these fears is true. Presenting a model of panic attacks as being the body's natural, healthy "alarm system" that is malfunctioning and being triggered for no reason is often helpful. As general measures, the woman should be counseled to avoid exacerbating factors, such as caffeine, alcohol, stimulants, or other illicit drugs, and to examine possible modifiable sources of increased life stress.

**BOX 9.4** Specifier With a Panic Attack

**Note:** Symptoms are presented for the purpose of identifying a panic attack; however, panic attack is not a mental disorder and cannot be coded. Panic attacks can occur in the context of any anxiety disorder as well as other mental disorders (e.g., depressive disorders, posttraumatic stress disorder, substance use disorders) and some medical conditions (e.g., cardiac, respiratory, vestibular, gastrointestinal). When the presence of a panic attack is identified, it should be noted with a specifier (e.g., "posttraumatic stress disorder with panic attacks"). For panic disorder, the presence of panic attack is contained within the criteria for the disorder and panic attack is not used with a specifier.

An abrupt surge of intense fear or discomfort that reaches a peak within minutes, and during which time four (or more) of the following symptoms occur:

**Note:** The abrupt surge can occur from a calm state or an anxious state.

1. Palpitations, pounding heart, or accelerated heart rate
2. Sweating
3. Trembling or shaking
4. Sensations of shortness of breath or smothering
5. Feeling of choking
6. Chest pain or discomfort
7. Nausea or abdominal distress
8. Feeling dizzy, unsteady, lightheaded, or faint
9. Chills or heat sensations
10. Paresthesias (numbness or tingling sensations)
11. Derealization (feelings of unreality) or depersonalization (being detached from oneself)
12. Fear of losing control or "going crazy"
13. Fear of dying

**Note:** Culture-specific symptoms (e.g., tinnitus, neck soreness, headache, uncontrollable screaming or crying) may be seen. Such symptoms should not count as one of the four required symptoms.

From American Psychiatric Association. *Diagnostic and Statistical Manual of Mental Disorders,* 5th ed. Washington, DC: American Psychiatric Association; 2013:214.

Panic disorder responds well to both medication and psychotherapy. In more severe cases or with significant comorbid phobic avoidance, a combination of both treatments is preferable. However, because both are effective, the approach to treatment can be determined by the woman's preference. **The first-line medication treatment for panic disorder is SSRIs.** There are two important differences in prescribing these medications for panic disorder versus for depression. First, **people with panic disorder are often very sensitive to medication side effects. Because panic attacks involve feeling out of control of physical sensations and one's own body, side effects can initially increase anxiety and panic.** Thus although ultimately doses need to be similar to antidepressant doses, it is wise to start treatment at a low dose (e.g., a daily dose of 12.5 mg sertraline, 5 mg citalopram), increasing the dose rapidly after a few days if the woman has no side effects. Second, **whereas antidepressants take 4 to 6 weeks or less to relieve depression, they can take up to 12 weeks to have their full effect on panic and anxiety**, with some effect expected by 6 weeks. It is important to educate the woman about this delayed and gradual onset of action. Many women present in distress and ask about something that will act more rapidly. In cases of severe disability resulting from panic attacks (e.g., inability to function, work, or go to school), it is reasonable to prescribe a benzodiazepine along with an SSRI, with the expectation that the SSRI will be the long-term treatment and the benzodiazepine will be tapered after at most 12 weeks. A benzodiazepine such as clonazepam, which has a longer half-life, requires only twice a day dosing and maintains more constant blood levels, is preferable to shorter-acting agents such as alprazolam. For women with a history of substance use disorders or who need to avoid the potential slowed reflexes, psychomotor impairment, and cognitive slowing associated with benzodiazepines, other alternative adjuncts to reduce anxiety and panic quickly could include hydroxyzine or gabapentin. **Buspirone has not been proven effective for panic disorder.** In those who do not tolerate SSRIs, most other antidepressants (e.g., venlafaxine, mirtazapine) are also effective for the long-term treatment of panic disorder, with the exception of bupropion, which can increase anxiety symptoms.

Psychotherapy is a highly effective treatment for panic disorder. **The best established therapy treatment is CBT, which focuses on addressing the catastrophic thoughts associated with panic attacks** (e.g., "I'm dying," "I'm going to crash my car and kill myself and other people"), learning coping and anxiety reduction strategies (e.g., relaxation, paced breathing to combat hyperventilation), and a gradual approach to feared situations to decrease disability. CBT for panic disorder is a weekly therapy for about 12 to 16 weeks, has significant improvement rates equal to or better than the 70% response rate with medication, yields long-term benefits after therapy is over, and increases the patient's sense of mastery and control, which is valuable in a disorder that makes people feel out of control. CBT can also help patients tolerate medication side effects and benzodiazepine withdrawal symptoms.

Overall, of the varied symptoms of panic disorder, panic attacks are the easiest to treat and quickest to resolve with both medication and therapy. Phobic avoidance and anticipatory anxiety usually linger for a longer time because of the unpredictability of panic attacks. People with panic disorder in most cases have a relapsing and remitting condition that requires long-term medication treatment (at least a year and often longer) and may recur in periods of increased stress.

**In contrast with the sudden attacks of fear in panic disorder, GAD is characterized by excessive anxiety and worry about a number of life situations** (e.g., work, school, family members) occurring more days than not for at least 6 months. The patient experiences her worries as excessive and difficult to control and as causing significant distress or trouble functioning. In addition, she has three or more of the following symptoms associated with her anxiety and worry: restlessness, insomnia, muscle tension, fatigue, trouble concentrating, or irritability. GAD usually begins early in life, is about twice as common in women than in men, has a genetic component, and has a lifetime prevalence of 5%. This is often a chronic disorder, with other lifetime psychiatric diagnoses (depression, other anxiety disorders, substance use disorders) superimposed in up to 90% of people. **The restlessness and trouble concentrating associated with GAD and anxiety in general may lead to a misdiagnosis of attention deficit disorder.**

The treatment of GAD often depends on the need to treat comorbid psychiatric conditions, which may have actually led the woman to seek medical help. **GAD itself responds to general measures such as avoiding caffeine, alcohol, and illicit drugs; medication; and psychotherapy. Antidepressants are effective for GAD, and the first-line long-term medication treatment is an SSRI. Buspirone 30 to 60 mg daily is effective for GAD and has few side effects.** Hydroxyzine and beta-blockers have been shown to be effective, as have benzodiazepines. However, given the chronic, often lifelong course of GAD, benzodiazepines are not recommended. Psychotherapy for GAD focuses on addressing and coping with worry ("What if" thoughts).

Social anxiety disorder (or social phobia) refers to anxiety in and avoidance of social situations, where the patient is or feels as though she is the center of attention and fears humiliation, embarrassment, or being judged negatively by other people (for diagnostic criteria, see Box 9.5). Symptoms of social anxiety disorder can include full-blown panic attacks, but these are provoked by social situations and are not spontaneous. In many cases, social anxiety disorder is restricted to specific situations, most often public speaking or other public performances. Some people have a more pervasive form of this disorder, in which fears and avoidance relate not just to public performance but to most social situations and interactions, such as meeting new people, parties, initiating and maintaining conversations, dating, group projects, speaking with authority figures, or asserting oneself.

Social anxiety disorder has lifetime and 12-month prevalences of 13% and 8%, respectively. Age of onset is usually early in life (mean 13 years), and women are more commonly affected than men. In Asian cultures, social anxiety often focuses on fears of giving offense to other people—for example, through making inappropriate eye contact, body odor, flatulence, or blushing. There is evidence for a genetic or familial risk for this condition. Women with social anxiety disorder may have associated poor self-esteem, difficulty asserting themselves, depression, or problematic alcohol use. Social anxiety disorder may be difficult to differentiate from shyness, although by definition social anxiety disorder involves marked distress or impairment in functioning.

Treatment of social anxiety disorder also includes medication and psychotherapy (Leichsenring, 2017). SSRIs are the first-line medication treatment and, as in other anxiety disorders, may take 8 to 12 weeks to have their full therapeutic effect. The SNRI venlafaxine is also effective. MAO inhibitors, though effective, bring with them dietary restrictions and risk of hypertensive crisis. Beta-blockers are helpful for performance anxiety but not for more generalized social anxiety disorder. Benzodiazepines are effective but should be used with caution because of the chronicity of this disorder, its comorbidity with alcohol use disorder, and risks of tolerance, dependence, withdrawal, sedation, psychomotor slowing, and cognitive effects with benzodiazepines. There is some evidence for efficacy of gabapentin or pregabalin. Women with social anxiety restricted to public speaking may benefit from practicing public speaking in a safe setting. CBT for social anxiety disorder is very effective. CBT includes individual treatment focusing on distorted thoughts about social situations (e.g., thoughts that the patient will make a fool of herself, has embarrassed herself, and that this will have catastrophic consequences) and on problem solving around and role-playing feared situations. Surprisingly, group CBT is also effective for social anxiety disorder.

**BOX 9.5** Diagnostic Criteria for Social Anxiety Disorder (Social Phobia)

A. Marked fear or anxiety about one or more social situations in which the individual is exposed to possible scrutiny by others. Examples include social interactions (e.g., having a conversation, meeting unfamiliar people), being observed (e.g., eating or drinking), and performing in front of others (e.g., giving a speech).
**Note**: In children, the anxiety must occur in peer settings and not just during interactions with adults.
B. The individual fears that he or she will act in a way or show anxiety symptoms that will be negatively evaluated (i.e., will be humiliating or embarrassing; will lead to rejection or offend others).
C. The social situations almost always provoke fear or anxiety.
**Note:** In children, the fear or anxiety may be expressed by crying, tantrums, freezing, clinging, shrinking, or failing to speak in social situations.
D. The social situations are avoided or endured with intense fear or anxiety.
E. The fear or anxiety is out of proportion to the actual threat posed by the social situation and to the sociocultural context.
F. The fear, anxiety, or avoidance is persistent, typically lasting for 6 months or more.
G. The fear, anxiety, or avoidance causes clinically significant distress or impairment in social, occupational, or other important areas of functioning
H. The fear, anxiety, or avoidance is not attributable to the physiologic effects of a substance (e.g., a drug of abuse, a medication) or another medical condition.
I. The fear, anxiety, or avoidance is not better explained by the symptoms of another mental disorder, such as panic disorder, body dysmorphic disorder, or autism spectrum disorder.
J. If another medical condition (e.g., Parkinson's disease, obesity, disfigurement from burns or injury) is present, the fear, anxiety, or avoidance is clearly unrelated or is excessive.

*Specify* if:
**Performance only:** If the fear is restricted to speaking or performing in public.

From American Psychiatric Association. *Diagnostic and Statistical Manual of Mental Disorders.* 5th ed. Washington, DC: American Psychiatric Association; 2013:202-203.

CBT and SSRIs yield response rates of 50% to 65% compared with a placebo response rate of 32%. Other psychotherapies, including mindfulness-based stress reduction, IPT, and psychodynamic therapy, appear promising but require further study.

Specific phobias occur in up to 20% of the general population and include fears of specific animals (e.g., snakes, spiders), phenomena (e.g., lightning), or situations (e.g., heights, flying in airplanes, driving, medical or dental procedures). People usually come to medical attention for specific phobias when these interfere with daily life or with their medical treatment. For example, people may develop specific phobias related to repeated medical events like chemotherapy treatments or to necessary aspects of their daily life, such as driving or traveling by plane. The best treatment for a specific phobia is desensitization, or gradually confronting the feared situation with the aid of an anxiety reducing strategy such as relaxation or imagery. In an acute situation, a benzodiazepine may help the woman to get through the particular event, but this will not reduce her future fear of the same situation.

**OCD is characterized by persistent, repetitive thoughts, ideas, or images that the patient finds irrational and intrusive (obsessions), and with repetitive behaviors or rituals (compulsions) designed to decrease the anxiety caused by obsessions.** Common obsessions include fears of contamination, dirt, germs, and illness; doubts (e.g., about having locked the door, turned off the oven, run over someone in one's car); needing to have things in order; and sexual or religious images or preoccupations. Compulsions include repetitive and excessive washing, cleaning, checking, putting things in order, or asking for reassurance. These obsessions and compulsions are distressing, time-consuming, or interfere with functioning. The full diagnostic criteria are shown in Box 9.6. Although most people with OCD realize that their obsessions and compulsions are irrational, some have poor or absent insight and think that their OCD-related beliefs may be true.

OCD has a lifetime prevalence of 2% to 3% and is more common in monozygotic than dizygotic twins and in first-degree relatives of affected individuals than in the general population. Rates are similar in men and women. However, men have an earlier peak age of onset than women (6 to 15 years old vs. 20 to 29 years old) and a higher comorbidity with Tourette's syndrome and tic disorders. In people with OCD, the incidence of Tourette's is 5% to 7% and of tics is 20% to 30%. Other conditions commonly associated with OCD, in both genders, include major depression, anxiety disorders, hypochondriacal concerns, and excessive use of alcohol and sedatives.

**Treatment of OCD includes both medications and psychotherapy** (Grant, 2014). The first-line treatment is serotonergic antidepressants, specifically SSRIs and clomipramine, which is a highly serotonergic tricyclic antidepressant. People with OCD may require higher doses of these medications than do depressed patients and take about 12 weeks for a full response. Response rates tend to be lower than in anxiety disorders and are generally 40% to 60%. It is uncommon for a patient with OCD to have complete resolution of symptoms, and this is usually a chronic, relapsing and remitting disorder requiring ongoing treatment. The specific psychotherapy treatment most helpful in OCD is exposure and response prevention. This treatment involves gradually increasing exposure to the feared situation, without performing the compulsive ritual (e.g., exposure to dirt without the ability to wash one's hands). Patients who agree to this treatment must tolerate significant anxiety, which, however, subsides with time after each exposure and diminishes over the course of treatment.

**PTSD refers to a characteristic set of responses to a traumatic situation that involves exposure to actual or threatened death, serious injury, or sexual violence, either to oneself or experienced by witnessing the trauma occurring to others,** learning that the trauma has happened to a close friend or family member, or working in a setting with repeated or extreme trauma exposure. The characteristic responses include symptoms of reexperiencing the event, avoidance of stimuli associated with the event, negative thoughts and mood associated with the trauma, and increased arousal. The full diagnostic criteria and lists of symptoms are given in Box 9.7. It is common for people to experience symptoms like this in the first month after a major trauma, in which case the diagnosis is acute stress disorder. After a month, when most people would have recovered, persistent symptoms are then diagnosed as PTSD.

PTSD has an estimated lifetime prevalence of 8% in adults in the United States. Rates of PTSD vary from one third to more than half of people exposed to specific traumas, such as combat, rape, or captivity. Risk factors for development of PTSD in people exposed to a specific trauma include female sex, younger age, severity and duration of the event, lack of social support, history of prior trauma, and history of preexisting psychiatric disorders. There is also evidence that people with greater autonomic arousal (higher heart rate and blood pressure) after the trauma are at increased risk. Although PTSD would appear to be a quintessentially environmentally determined disorder, the risk of development of PTSD after trauma appears to be heritable. PTSD is associated

**BOX 9.6** Diagnostic Criteria for Obsessive Compulsive Disorder

A. Presence of obsessions, compulsions, or both:

Obsessions are defined by (1) or (2):

1. Recurrent and persistent thoughts, urges, or images that are experienced, at some time during the disturbance, as intrusive and unwanted, and that in most individuals cause marked anxiety or distress.
2. The individual attempts to ignore or suppress such thoughts, urges, or images, or to neutralize them with some other thought or action (i.e., by performing a compulsion).

Compulsions are defined by (1) and (2):

1. Repetitive behaviors (e.g., hand washing, ordering, checking) or mental acts (e.g., praying, counting, repeating words silently) that the individual feels driven to perform in response to an obsession or according to rules that must be applied rigidly.
2. The behaviors or mental acts are aimed at preventing or reducing anxiety or distress, or preventing some dreaded event or situation; however, these behaviors or mental acts are not connected in a realistic way with what they are designed to neutralize or prevent, or are clearly excessive.

**Note:** Young children may not be able to articulate the aims of these behaviors or mental acts.

B. The obsessions or compulsions are time-consuming (e.g., take more than 1 hour per day), or cause clinically significant distress or impairment in social, occupational, or other important areas of functioning.

C. The obsessive-compulsive symptoms are not attributable to the physiologic effects of a substance (e.g., a drug of abuse, a medication) or another medical condition.

D. The disturbance is not better explained by the symptoms of another mental disorder (e.g., excessive worries, as in generalized anxiety disorder; preoccupation with appearance, as in body dysmorphic disorder; difficulty discarding or parting with possessions, as in hoarding disorder; hair pulling, as in trichotillomania [hair-pulling disorder]; skin picking, as in excoriation [skin-picking] disorder; stereotypies, as in stereotypic movement disorder; ritualized eating behavior, as in eating disorders; preoccupation with substances or gambling, as in substance-related and addictive disorders; preoccupation with having an illness, as in illness anxiety disorder; sexual urges or fantasies, as in paraphilic disorders; impulses, as in disruptive, impulse-control, and conduct disorders; guilty ruminations, as in major depressive disorder; thought insertion or delusional preoccupations, as in schizophrenia spectrum and other psychotic disorders; or repetitive patterns of behavior, as in autism spectrum disorder).

*Specify* if:

**With good or fair insight:** The individual recognizes that obsessive-compulsive disorder beliefs are definitely or probably not true or that they may or may not be true.

**With poor insight:** The individual thinks obsessive-compulsive disorder beliefs are probably true.

**With absent insight/delusional beliefs:** The individual is completely convinced that obsessive-compulsive disorder beliefs are true.

*Specify* if:

**Tic-related:** The individual has a current or past history of a tic disorder.

From American Psychiatric Association. *Diagnostic and Statistical Manual of Mental Disorders.* 5th ed. Washington, DC: American Psychiatric Association; 2013:237.

**BOX 9.7** Diagnostic Criteria for Posttraumatic Stress Disorder (PTSD)

**Note:** The following criteria apply to adults, adolescents, and children older than 6 years.

A. Exposure to actual or threatened death, serious injury, or sexual violence in one (or more) of the following ways:
1. Directly experiencing the traumatic event(s)
2. Witnessing, in person, the event(s) as it occurred to others
3. Learning that the traumatic event(s) occurred to a close family member or close friend. In cases of actual or threatened death of a family member or friend, the event(s) must have been violent or accidental
4. Experiencing repeated or extreme exposure to aversive details of the traumatic event(s) (e.g., first responders collecting human remains; police officers repeatedly exposed to details of child abuse).

**Note:** Criterion A4 does not apply to exposure through electronic media, television, movies, or pictures, unless this exposure is work related.

B. Presence of one (or more) of the following intrusion symptoms associated with the traumatic event(s), beginning after the traumatic event(s) occurred:
1. Recurrent, involuntary, and intrusive distressing memories of the traumatic event(s).

**Note:** In children older than 6 years, repetitive play may occur in which themes or aspects of the traumatic event(s) are expressed.

2. Recurrent distressing dreams in which the content and/or effect of the dream are related to the traumatic event(s).

**Note:** In children, there may be frightening dreams without recognizable content.

3. Dissociative reactions (e.g., flashbacks) in which the individual feels or acts as if the traumatic event(s) were recurring. (Such reactions may occur on a continuum, with the most extreme expression being a complete loss of awareness of present surroundings.)

**Note:** In children, trauma-specific reenactment may occur in play.

4. Intense or prolonged psychological distress at exposure to internal or external cues that symbolize or resemble an aspect of the traumatic event(s).
5. Marked physiologic reactions to internal or external cues that symbolize or resemble an aspect of the traumatic event(s).

C. Persistent avoidance of stimuli associated with the traumatic event(s), beginning after the traumatic event(s) occurred, as evidenced by one or both of the following:
1. Avoidance of or efforts to avoid distressing memories, thoughts, or feelings about or closely associated with the traumatic event(s).
2. Avoidance of or efforts to avoid external reminders (people, places, conversations, activities, objects, situations) that arouse distressing memories, thoughts, or feelings about or closely associated with the traumatic event(s).

D. Negative alterations in cognitions and mood associated with the traumatic event(s), beginning or worsening after the traumatic event(s) occurred, as evidence by two (or more) of the following:
1. Inability to remember an important aspect of the traumatic event(s) (typically due to dissociative amnesia and not to other factors such as head injury, alcohol, or drugs).

*Continued*

**BOX 9.7** Diagnostic Criteria for Posttraumatic Stress Disorder (PTSD)—cont'd

2. Persistent and exaggerated negative beliefs or expectations about oneself, others, or the world (e.g., "I am bad," "No one can be trusted," "The world is completely dangerous," "My whole nervous system is permanently ruined").
3. Persistent, distorted cognitions about the cause or consequences of the traumatic event(s) that lead the individual to blame himself/herself or others.
4. Persistent negative emotional state (e.g., fear, horror, anger, guilt, or shame).
5. Markedly diminished interest or participation in significant activities.
6. Feelings of detachment or estrangement from others.
7. Persistent inability to experience positive emotions (e.g., inability to experience happiness, satisfaction, or loving feelings).

E. Marked alterations in arousal and reactivity associated with the traumatic event(s), beginning or worsening after the traumatic event(s) occurred, as evidenced by two (or more) of the following:
1. Irritable behavior and angry outbursts (with little or no provocation) typically expressed as verbal or physical aggression toward people or objects.
2. Reckless or self-destructive behavior.
3. Hypervigilance.
4. Exaggerated startle response.
5. Problems with concentration.
6. Sleep disturbance (e.g., difficulty falling or staying asleep or restless sleep).

F. Duration of the disturbance (Criteria B, C, D, and E) is more than 1 month.

G. The disturbance causes clinically significant distress or impairment in social, occupational, or other important areas of functioning.

H. The disturbance is not attributable to the physiologic effects of a substance (e.g., medication, alcohol) or another medical condition.

*Specify* whether:

**With dissociative symptoms:** The individual's symptoms meet the criteria for posttraumatic stress disorder, and in addition, in response to the stressor, the individual experiences persistent or recurrent symptoms of either of the following:
1. **Depersonalization:** Persistent or recurrent experiences of feeling detached from, and as if one were an outside observer of, one's mental processes or body (e.g., feeling as though one were in a dream; feeling a sense of unreality of self or body or of time moving slowly).
2. **Derealization:** Persistent or recurrent experiences of unreality of surroundings (e.g., the world around the individual is experienced as unreal, dreamlike, distant, or distorted).

**Note:** To use this subtype, the dissociative symptoms must not be attributable to the physiologic effects of a substance (e.g., blackouts, behavior during alcohol intoxication) or another medical condition (e.g., complex partial seizures).

From American Psychiatric Association. *Diagnostic and Statistical Manual of Mental Disorders.* 5th ed. Washington, DC: American Psychiatric Association; 2013:271-272.

with depression, panic attacks and anxiety, substance abuse and dependence, suicidal thoughts and attempts, and, in severe cases, psychotic symptoms such as hallucinations or paranoia.

**Several types of individual and group psychotherapy are effective in the treatment of PTSD.** These therapies include coping with current life problems and triggers, exposure to and reexperiencing of the trauma through a trauma narrative with desensitization (e.g., prolonged exposure, eye movement desensitization, and reprocessing therapies), and examining any distorted thoughts about the trauma, such as guilt that the woman brought this on herself or could have done more to prevent or stop it (cognitive processing therapy). **It is important to recognize that many people are retraumatized and their symptoms worsened by retelling the story of the trauma, especially if this is not in the context of a structured, ongoing psychotherapeutic treatment.**

Medications are often used to address symptoms of PTSD. For example, SSRIs are effective in reducing depression, anxiety, and emotional numbing. Hypnotics may be helpful for insomnia. Prazosin, an alpha-adrenergic antagonist, may be helpful in reducing trauma-related nightmares and more general PTSD symptoms. Benzodiazepines should be used with caution, given the comorbidity with substance use disorders and reports of increased impulsivity in patients with PTSD given these medications. Acute management immediately after the trauma of a rape is discussed further later in the chapter.

## PSYCHOTROPIC MEDICATIONS AND ORAL CONTRACEPTIVES

The gynecologist often sees women who are taking psychotropic medications for one of the disorders described earlier or for other less common psychiatric disorders such as bipolar disorder or schizophrenia and may be called on to advise them about options for birth control. **There are several psychotropic medications that alter the metabolism and efficacy of oral contraceptives (OCs) or whose metabolism is in turn altered by OCs** (Oesterheld, 2008).

Induction of the hepatic cytochrome P450 3A4 enzyme can increase OC metabolism and cause contraceptive failure. Psychotropic medications that induce 3A4 and that have been associated with spotting, breakthrough bleeding, or unwanted pregnancy include the mood stabilizers carbamazepine (Tegretol) and oxcarbazepine (Trileptal), topiramate (Topamax; at doses >200 mg daily), and the wakefulness-enhancing agent modafinil (Provigil). St. John's wort, commonly used over the counter as an antidepressant, also induces 3A4 and can cause contraceptive failure. OC activity may be increased or prolonged by 3A4 inhibitors such as the antidepressants fluoxetine (Prozac) and possibly fluvoxamine (Luvox).

OCs are themselves moderate 1A2 and 2C19 inhibitors and mild 2B6 and 3A4 inhibitors. Thus OCs can increase levels and effects of amitriptyline (Elavil), bupropion (Wellbutrin), chlordiazepoxide (Librium), chlorpromazine (Thorazine), clozapine (Clozaril), diazepam (Valium), imipramine (Tofranil), and possibly olanzapine (Zyprexa). Drugs whose clearance is increased with OCs and therefore have lower blood levels include nicotine and the mood stabilizers lamotrigine (Lamictal) and valproic acid (Depakote). Lamotrigine levels have been found to be 84% higher in the week off ethinyl estradiol. Given the risk of Stevens-Johnson syndrome with fluctuating levels of lamotrigine and the likelihood of worsening mood symptoms with variations in blood levels of mood stabilizers such as lamotrigine and valproic acid, it is best to advise women taking these medications to use a continuous OC or another form of birth control.

## SUBSTANCE USE DISORDERS

Women have lower rates of alcohol and drug use and substance use disorders than men. However, substance use disorders are common in women and the rates are increasing. In the 2017 National Survey on Drug Use and Health, 13.7% of men and 8.8% of women 12 years or older reported past-month illicit drug use, 28.6% of men and 16.6% of women reported use of tobacco products, and 28.8% of men and 20.4% of women reported binge drinking. Rates of illicit drug use disorders in the past year were 3.6% in men and 2.0% in women, whereas 7.0% of men and 3.8% of women had past-year alcohol use disorder. Unlike other age groups, adolescents (ages 12 to 17) reported equal or higher rates of substance use problems in girls, with about 8% of each gender reporting past-month illicit drug use and 6.0% of girls and 4.6% of boys reporting past-month binge drinking. In 2015, 4.7% of pregnant women reported past-month illicit drug use (most often marijuana, followed by prescription opioids), 9.3% alcohol use, and 13.9% use of tobacco products. Alcohol, tobacco, and illicit drug use in women is of particular concern to gynecologists, not only because of the risks to the woman but also because of the risks to her children through teratogenic risks and effects on parenting abilities.

**Women consistently have been noted to have an accelerated progression of substance use disorders, with a shorter time between first use of a substance to onset of dependence and first treatment. This phenomenon is known as telescoping and is best established for alcohol, cannabis, cocaine, and prescription opiates** (McHugh, 2018). Women generally present for treatment with a more severe form of the disorder and more social, behavioral, and medical complications than men, despite a shorter period of heavy use. They are more likely than men to suffer psychosocial consequences, such as violence and victimization, and to have psychiatric comorbidity, especially depression, anxiety, eating disorders, and PTSD. **About 72% of women, as opposed to 57% of men, have coexisting psychiatric disorders, and in women these other disorders are more likely to have preceded, and to exacerbate, the substance use disorder.** Thus it is important to recognize and treat other mental health problems in women with alcohol and drug use disorders. Heavy drinking **in women increases general health risks, as it does in men, but also is associated with unplanned pregnancy, sexual assault, sexually** transmitted diseases, amenorrhea, anovulation, luteal phase dysfunction, and early menopause. The DSM-5 criteria for alcohol use disorder are shown in Box 9.8, and the DSM-5 includes similar criteria for other substances.

**Patients often do not report excessive alcohol or drug use or may not recognize their use as excessive.** As in primary care and mental health settings, patients seeing gynecologists are far less likely to be recognized as having a substance use disorder based on physician assessment and documentation. There are several screening tests that can help identify these disorders. Screening tests for alcohol use disorders are shown in Box 9.9. Although women with severe alcohol use disorders may have abnormalities in laboratory tests such as hepatic enzymes (alanine aminotransferase [ALT], aspartate aminotransferase [AST], gamma-glutamyl transferase [GGT]) or mean corpuscular volume (MCV), questionnaires provide a significantly more sensitive method of detecting problem drinking. The CAGE is a brief and widely used screening questionnaire. Although it is generally helpful in detecting heavy drinking, it is less sensitive in women and minorities. The T-ACE is a variation on the CAGE that replaces the "guilt" about drinking item with a question about tolerance. The T-ACE was developed specifically for use in

**BOX 9.8** Diagnostic Criteria for Alcohol Use Disorder

A problematic pattern of alcohol use leading to clinically significant impairment or distress, as manifested by at least two of the following, occurring within a 12-month period:

1. Alcohol is often taken in larger amounts or over a longer period than was intended.
2. There is a persistent desire or unsuccessful efforts to cut down or control alcohol use.
3. A great deal of time is spent in activities necessary to obtain alcohol, use alcohol, or recover from its effects.
4. Craving, or a strong desire or urge to use alcohol.
5. Recurrent alcohol use resulting in a failure to fulfill major role obligations at work, school, or home.
6. Continued alcohol use despite having persistent or recurrent social or interpersonal problems caused or exacerbated by the effects of alcohol.
7. Important social, occupational, or recreational activities are given up or reduced because of alcohol use.
8. Recurrent alcohol use in situations in which it is physically hazardous.
9. Alcohol use is continued despite knowledge of having a persistent or recurrent physical or psychological problem that is likely to have been caused or exacerbated by alcohol.
10. Tolerance, as defined by either of the following:
    a. A need for markedly increased amounts of alcohol to achieve intoxication or the desired effect
    b. A markedly diminished effect with continued use of the same amount of alcohol.
11. Withdrawal, as manifested by either of the following:
    a. The characteristic withdrawal syndrome for alcohol (refer to Criteria A and B of the criteria set for alcohol withdrawal, pp. 499-500).
    b. Alcohol (or a closely related substance, such as a benzodiazepine) is taken to relieve or avoid withdrawal symptoms.

*Specify* if:

**In early remission:** After full criteria for alcohol use disorder were previously met, none of the criteria for alcohol use disorder have been met for at least 3 months but for less than 12 months (with the exception that Criterion A4, "Craving, or a strong desire or urge to use alcohol," may be met).

**In sustained remission:** After full criteria for alcohol use disorder were previously met, none of the criteria for alcohol use disorder have been met at any time during a period of 12 months or longer (with the exception that Criterion A4, "Craving, or a strong desire or urge to use alcohol," may be met).

*Specify* if:

**In a controlled environment:** This additional specifier is used if the individual is in an environment where access to alcohol is restricted.

**Code based on current severity:** Presence of 2 to 3 symptoms.
**303.90 (F10.20) Moderate:** Presence of 4 to 5 symptoms.
**303.90 (F10.20) Severe:** Presence of 6 or more symptoms.

From American Psychiatric Association. *Diagnostic and Statistical Manual of Mental Disorders.* 5th ed. Washington, DC: American Psychiatric Association; 2013:490-491.

**BOX 9.9** Alcohol Use Disorder Screening Tests

**AUDIT**

The following questions pertain to your use of alcoholic beverages during the past year. A "drink" refers to a can or bottle of beer, a glass of wine, a wine cooler, or one cocktail or shot of hard liquor.

1. How often do you have a drink containing alcohol? (never, 0 points; monthly or less, 1 point; 2-4 times per month, 2 points; 2-3 times per week, 3 points; 4 or more times a week, 4 points)
2. How many drinks containing alcohol do you have on a typical day when you are drinking? (1-2 drinks, 0 points; 3-4 drinks, 1 point; 5-6 drinks, 2 points; 7-9 drinks, 3 points; 10 or more drinks, 4 points)
3. How often do you have 6 or more drinks on one occasion? (never, 0 points; less than once a month, 1 point; monthly, 2 points; weekly, 3 points; daily or almost daily, 4 points)
4. How often during the past year have you found that you were not able to stop drinking once you had started? (same scoring as question 3)
5. How often during the past year have you failed to do what was normally expected from you because of drinking? (same scoring as question 3)
6. How often during the past year have you needed a first drink in the morning to get yourself going after a heavy drinking session? (same scoring as question 3)
7. How often during the past year have you had a feeling of guilt or remorse after drinking? (same scoring as question 3)
8. How often during the past year have you been unable to remember what happened the night before because you were drinking? (same scoring as question 3)
9. Have you or someone else been injured as a result of your drinking? (no, 0 points; yes, but not in the past year, 2 points; yes, during the past year, 4 points)
10. Has a relative or friend, or a doctor, or other health care worker been concerned about your drinking or suggested you cut down? (same scoring as question 9)

Scoring: Add up points; score 0 to 40; score of 4 or above indicates possible alcohol abuse or dependence for women.

**CAGE**

C Have you ever felt you ought to cut down on your drinking?
A Have people annoyed you by criticizing your drinking?
G Have you felt bad or guilty about your drinking?
E Have you ever had a drink in the morning (eye opener) to steady your nerves or get rid of a hangover?

Scoring: 1 point for each "yes"; any yes response warrants further assessment.

**TWEAK**

T Tolerance: How many drinks can you hold (6 or more indicates tolerance) or how many drinks does it take before you begin to feel the first effects of the alcohol? (3 or more indicates tolerance)
W Worried: Have close friends or relatives worried or complained about your drinking in the past year?
E Eye opener: Do you sometimes take a drink in the morning when you first get up?
A Amnesia: Has a friend or family member ever told you about things you said or did while you were drinking that you could not remember?
K Kut down: Do you sometimes feel the need to cut down on your drinking?

Scoring: 2 points each for Tolerance or Worried; 1 point each for others; total

Possible = 7 points; 2 points or more warrants further assessment in women.

**T-ACE**

T Tolerance: How many drinks does it take to make you feel high? (3 or more indicates tolerance)
A Annoyed question from CAGE
C Cut down question from CAGE
E Eye opener question from CAGE

Scoring: 2 points for tolerance, 1 point each for "yes" on other items; 1 or more points warrants further assessment in women.

Modified from Bradley KA, Boyd-Wickizer J, Powell SH, Burman ML. Alcohol screening questionnaires in women: a critical review. *JAMA.* 1998;280:166-171.

pregnant women, given the high rate of guilt in women who consume any alcohol during pregnancy. Another effective screening test in detecting heavy alcohol use in groups of women of mixed ethnicity is the TWEAK. The AUDIT is a longer, 10-item screening test that has been well validated and includes self-reports of quantity and frequency of drinking. The first three items of the AUDIT (AUDIT-C) have a sensitivity of 0.60 to 0.73 and specificity of 0.91 to 0.96 for detection of alcohol use disorder in women, using a cutoff score of 3. The National Institute on Alcohol Abuse and Alcoholism (NIAAA) recommends a single-question screen, "How many times in the past year have you had 4 or more drinks in a day?" A response of one or more times is a positive screen. Similarly, the National Institute on Drug Abuse (NIDA) recommends a single question screen for drug use, "How many times in the past year have you used an illegal drug or used a prescription medication for nonmedical reasons?" A response of one or more times warrants further assessment. In general, women who score at or more than the cutoff score on any of these alcohol use screening tests, or who endorse any use of an illicit drug or tobacco, should be questioned further about the frequency, amount, and consequences of their use of alcohol and illicit drugs. The questions on the complete AUDIT questionnaire can be used to obtain further information about alcohol use, whereas the Drug Abuse Screening Test (DAST-10; Box 9.10) is helpful in further exploring the severity of illicit drug use. Each of these self-report questionnaires takes less than 5 minutes to administer. The gynecologist is often a woman's primary care provider and is in an ideal position to help the patient seek treatment for a substance use disorder. The patient may not realize that her use is problematic or dangerous. It can be useful to educate her about excessive levels of alcohol use, for example. For a woman, consuming eight or more drinks per week is considered heavy drinking, where a drink is a 12-ounce beer, 5-ounce glass of wine, or 1.5 ounces of 80-proof (40% alcohol) distilled spirits or liquor. Binge drinking is defined as drinking four or more drinks during a single occasion. Binge drinking and heavy drinking are associated with increased rates of accidents, injuries, risky sexual behaviors, and violence, including interpersonal violence and suicide. Heavy drinking over time has been linked to increases in mortality, cirrhosis, and breast cancer. Women also may benefit from education about adverse effects of alcohol, tobacco, and drugs to the fetus and newborn.

**Screening, Brief Intervention, and Referral to Treatment (SBIRT) is an evidence-based practice designed to identify and address problematic alcohol and drug use in any health care setting** and includes flowcharts, handouts, pocket guides, and

**BOX 9.10** Drug Abuse Screening Test (DAST-10)

1. Have you used drugs other than those required for medical reasons?
2. Do you use more than one drug at a time?
3. Are you always able to stop using drugs when you want to?
4. Have you had "blackouts" or "flashbacks" as a result of drug use?
5. Do you ever feel bad or guilty about your drug use?
6. Does your spouse (or parents) ever complain about your involvement with drugs?
7. Have you neglected your family because of your use of drugs?
8. Have you engaged in illegal activities in order to obtain drugs?
9. Have you ever experienced withdrawal symptoms (felt sick) when you stopped taking drugs?
10. Have you had medical problems as a result of your drug use (e.g. memory loss, hepatitis, convulsions, bleeding, etc.)?

Scoring: One point for each "yes" response, except question 3 ("no" = 1 point). Total score 0 = no problems reported; 1 to 2 = low level (monitor, reassess); 3 to 5 = moderate (investigate further); 6 to 8 = substantial; 9 to 10 = severe (scores of 6-10 warrant intensive assessment).

Modified from Skinner HA. The Drug Abuse Screening Test. *Addictive Behavior.* 1982;7:363-371.

brief educational and intervention materials (https://www.integration.samhsa.gov/clinical-practice/sbirt#why?). The brief intervention in SBIRT (https://www.integration.samhsa.gov/clinical-practice/sbirt/Brief-negotiated_interview_and_active_referral_to_treatment.pdf) includes a very specific, easy to use, succinct guide that takes the clinician through the process of asking about pros and cons of substance use, providing feedback about the patient's substance use and information about health risks, assessing readiness to change behavior, and negotiating next steps, including any referrals for treatment. Treatments include Alcoholics Anonymous, Women for Sobriety, Cocaine Anonymous, or Narcotics Anonymous; psychotherapy; medication-assisted treatment; and/or outpatient and inpatient substance abuse treatment centers. The Substance Abuse and Mental Health Services Administration (SAMHSA) provides a convenient list of drug and alcohol treatment programs by state and local area at http://www.samhsa.gov/find-help.

**The SBIRT brief intervention uses principles of motivational interviewing, an efficient and highly effective brief counseling technique that aims to accomplish behavior change by helping people explore and resolve ambivalence, because advice alone is often not sufficient to bring about behavior change, and patients vary in their stage of "readiness to change"** (Box 9.11). The goal of motivational interviewing is to move people through the stages of change listed in this box. Motivational interviewing was developed for substance use disorders but is also highly effective in promoting weight reduction, exercise, safe sex practices, and regular use of contraception.

**Motivational interviewing emphasizes reflective listening, rather than advice giving.** In the context of a trusting relationship, the physician expresses empathy and understanding of the patient's ambivalence and the obstacles to change, avoids arguments, points out discrepancies between the patient's behavior and her goals, helps problem solve ways to succeed in meeting goals, and supports the patient's own motivation and efforts to change. Training in motivational interviewing is readily available for clinicians desiring more detail than is provided in the SBIRT program. Motivational interviewing has been shown to be a highly effective intervention, and practicing this technique adds an average of only 3 minutes to a clinic visit. Resources and videos are listed in the 2009 ACOG Committee Opinion regarding motivational interviewing.

**BOX 9.11** Stages of Readiness for Change

- Precontemplation—The patient does not believe a problem exists. ("I won't get pregnant!")
- Contemplation—The patient recognizes a problem exists and is considering treatment or behavior change. ("Maybe I could get pregnant and there are things I could do to prevent this.")
- Action—The patient begins treatment or behavior change. ("I'll take that prescription for birth control pills.")
- Maintenance—The patient incorporates new behavior into daily life. ("I'm taking the pill every day.")
- Relapse—The patient returns to the undesired behavior. ("The pill makes me sick. I think I'll stop.")

Only about 10% of women needing treatment for a substance use disorder receive treatment. Furthermore, specific substances of abuse are associated with gender differences in patterns of use and treatment success (McHugh, 2018). Alcohol use in women is associated with the phenomenon of telescoping, or an accelerated course from onset of use to significant alcohol-related problems. Several biologic factors may contribute to this more rapid course, including the lower percentage of body water in women, lower levels of alcohol dehydrogenase in the gastric mucosa and thus decreased first pass metabolism, and slower rates of alcohol metabolism. Women also appear to have different motives for drinking, with a higher likelihood of drinking in response to stress, negative emotions, and underlying primary coexisting psychiatric disorders, and are more likely to seek care in mental health than in specialized substance use disorder treatment settings. Barriers to treatment include childcare responsibilities, financial resources, and greater stigma related to women's use of alcohol. Female patients may benefit from women-only treatment settings or groups addressing women's issues. Effective FDA-approved pharmacologic treatments for alcohol dependence in both genders include disulfiram, naltrexone, and acamprosate (Jonas, 2017). Naltrexone is contraindicated in patients with acute hepatitis or liver failure or who are on prescribed opioids because it can precipitate opiate withdrawal. Acamprosate is contraindicated in patients with renal impairment and may cause or worsen anxiety. Disulfiram can cause medically dangerous symptoms when combined with alcohol. Topiramate is not FDA approved but has been shown effective in the treatment of alcohol use disorder. Alcohol use during pregnancy is associated with fetal alcohol syndrome and fetal alcohol effects, and most women reduce their alcohol use once they know that they are pregnant.

Tobacco use is declining in both men and women, especially in adolescents, with only 4.9% of girls reporting past-month tobacco use in 2015, compared with 10.7% in 2007. However, in 2016, 9.1% of 12th grade girls reported electronic cigarette use. Although rates of nicotine use are higher in boys and men than in girls and women, women are at increased risk for heart attacks, chronic obstructive pulmonary disease, and lung cancer secondary to nicotine (Benowitz, 2010). Nicotine also is associated with early menopause and with spontaneous abortion, low birth weight, and preterm birth with in utero exposure. Only 3% of smokers are able to quit in any given year, and women appear to have more difficulty quitting than men. Women have more success quitting in the follicular versus the luteal phase of their cycle, but they are more likely to relapse because of weight gain associated with smoking cessation and have a high rate of relapse (about 65%) even if they have quit during pregnancy. Overall, outcomes of nicotine use disorder treatment are worse in women than in men. In randomized controlled trials of specific smoking cessation treatments, men respond better than women to nicotine replacement and women respond better to varenicline than to nicotine replacement or bupropion. However, bupropion may be particularly useful in women who have comorbid depression.

Marijuana use is increasing, with past-year use reported by 17.8% of men and 12.5% of women in 2017. Abuse is more common in men but has a more rapid progression in women. Marijuana use is associated with impaired memory, attention, and motivation; increases risk for the onset of panic attacks; may increase vulnerability to depression and psychotic disorders; and has been associated with preterm birth, low birth weight, and possible impairments in executive functioning with in utero exposure. Treatments include CBT, motivational interviewing, and contingency management.

Women may be more vulnerable than men to the reinforcing effects of stimulants, especially during the follicular phase when estrogen levels are high. The diagnosis of attention deficit disorder is increasingly being made in women, with a corresponding increase in therapeutic use of stimulants. In 2017, 7.0% of men and 6.7% of women reported past-year use of stimulants and 2.6% of men and 1.7% of women endorsed past-year stimulant misuse. Stimulant misuse is particularly common in 18 to 25 year olds and especially in college students (about 10%). Exposure to stimulants during pregnancy has been associated with higher rates of intrauterine growth restriction, low birth weight, preterm birth, and maternal hypertension. Attention-deficit/hyperactivity disorder (ADHD) has high rates of psychiatric comorbidity and can be confused with anxiety and mood disorders. It is important to recognize attention deficit disorder in women, but it is also important to avoid misdiagnosis and unnecessary treatment with stimulants. The diagnosis of ADHD requires that symptoms started in childhood (before the age of 12), and hyperactivity is less common in girls, who are more likely to present with inattention. In adults, assessing for childhood onset and ruling out other psychiatric conditions is crucial and may require psychiatric consultation. Treatments for attention deficit disorder include not only stimulants but also CBT, atomoxetine, and bupropion.

Use of heroin and other intravenous drugs is less common in women than in men, and women are more likely to inject drugs if their partner uses intravenous (IV) drugs and introduces them to injection. In contrast, overuse of prescription narcotics is more common in women than in men. Between 1999 and 2016, deaths from opiate overdose increased sevenfold in women versus fourfold in men. Studies of medication treatments for opiate use disorder, including studies of methadone and buprenorphine, show no gender differences in treatment outcome. Use of opiates, including methadone, during pregnancy is associated with neonatal abstinence syndrome, respiratory depression, preterm delivery, and fetal growth restriction.

## "DIFFICULT" PATIENTS AND CHALLENGING CLINICAL ENCOUNTERS

Every physician experiences clinical encounters that are challenging, and physicians describe about 15% of their patients as being "difficult" (for review, see Cowley, 2016). It is always possible for a physician to have a personality clash with an individual patient, but **"difficult" patients are a subset of patients who evoke negative feelings in many, if not most, physicians. These patients may be angry, argumentative, threatening, mistrustful, demanding, dissatisfied; may misuse habit-forming prescribed medications or appear to be "drug seeking"; may challenge the physician's approach and not comply with treatment recommendations; or may be difficult to engage in a productive treatment alliance.** In a classic 1978 paper, Groves described "hateful patients" as people who "kindle aversion, fear, despair, or even downright malice in their doctors." Feeling frustration, anxiety, or dislike in seeing patients significantly reduces a physician's satisfaction with providing medical care.

"Difficult" patients have also been described as "heartsink" patients, referring to the feeling that the provider has on seeing the patient's name on his or her schedule. This term emphasizes the physician's response to the patient, rather than attributing the difficulty of the interaction entirely to the patient. Indeed, there are physician characteristics that have been associated with describing patients as "difficult," including being younger (<40 years); working more than 55 hours per week; reporting higher stress; practicing in a medical subspecialty; having a higher number of patients with psychosocial problems or substance abuse; describing themselves as being anxious, perfectionistic, defensive, and/or "overly nice"; and having lower scores on psychosocial orientation to patient care.

A woman may not comply with treatment because of denial and fear of illness; cultural factors; having a different explanatory model of the symptoms, their cause, and their optimal treatment; or a misunderstanding of the diagnosis, treatment, or the physician's instructions and expectations. In these cases, education, reassurance where appropriate, use of a skilled interpreter, or gaining a better understanding of the woman's culture and view of her symptoms and illness may be very helpful. In some cases a formal cultural consultation may be needed. Although such situations may be challenging, their health care providers do not generally experience these women as being "difficult."

Groves grouped "hateful patients" into four different categories "dependent clingers," "entitled demanders," "manipulative help-rejecters," and "self-destructive deniers" and described their behavior patterns and ways in which the physician can intervene to work with them more effectively. In another paper, Strous and associates (2006) revisited Groves' original categories and suggested an overall framework for approaching these patients based on empathy and an understanding of the physician's own responses. Empathy refers to understanding another person's feelings, motives, and point of view. It is not synonymous with sympathy, because empathy does not involve pity. Understanding what a woman is experiencing and where the woman is coming from allows the physician to more calmly take a nonblaming, problem-solving approach. In addition, the physician can use his or her own responses to understand the woman better. For example, a woman who is feeling helpless and angry may, by complaining or demanding, evoke similar responses of helplessness or anger in her health care provider, allowing the provider insight into the woman's state of mind.

Groves' first group of "hateful patients," which he termed "dependent clingers," appears insatiable in their escalating demands for medical care and to represent a "bottomless pit." They require constant reassurance and inordinate amounts of time and attention, interfering with the rest of the physician's personal and professional life. These women may frequently and intrusively page, e-mail, call the physician at home or on the physician's cell phone, feeling unable to cope on their own. The physician cannot possibly fulfill all of the woman's demands, feels overwhelmed and angry, and tries to withdraw from caring for her. Groves suggested intervening as the woman's demands escalate and setting firm but reasonable limits (e.g., not giving out personal contact information, limiting visits or calls). The physician can empathically understand that the woman feels overwhelmed and unable to cope, but to preserve an effective treatment relationship the physician needs to be clear about what he or she realistically can and cannot do for the patient.

The second group, which Groves called "entitled demanders," displays a sense of entitlement, aggressively makes demands of the physician (e.g., for controlled substances, expensive diagnostic tests), and may make implicit or explicit threats, such as threats of litigation. This often leads the physician to feel angry and resist complying with the demands, even if some are reasonable. Groves recommended validating the patient's entitlement to good medical care but focusing on a shared therapeutic goal and the patient's role in working with the treatment team to accomplish that goal. Empathically recognizing the patient's fear of loss of control may allow the physician to respectfully point out destructive patterns of behavior and attempt to establish a more collaborative decision-making process.

"Manipulative help-rejecters" seek care but do not improve despite extensive workups and multiple attempts at treatment. Groves has suggested that these patients are afraid of losing the relationship with the physician if they improve. He recommended setting up a schedule of regular appointments that do not depend on having acute symptoms, much as one would do with a patient with chronic somatization and multiple physical symptoms of unclear etiology.

Finally, "self-destructive deniers" persist in self-destructive behavior such as drinking, smoking, risky sexual behavior, and use of drugs, despite obvious and significant medical problems that have resulted from this behavior. Groves conceptualized these people as having a form of chronic suicidal behavior and recommended ruling out depression, if needed with the help of a psychiatric consultation. In general, in cases in which the physician feels angry or overwhelmed and does not wish to treat the patient, consultation with colleagues, consultation with a psychiatrist, and having the woman see a psychiatrist, if she is willing to do so, can be very helpful in better understanding and managing the woman and the physician-patient relationship.

Women with the diagnosis of borderline personality disorder are often challenging for physicians to treat, given their chronic suicidal thoughts, self-harm behavior such as suicide attempts and cutting, intense and rapidly changing emotions, anger, and difficulty regulating and controlling their emotions rather than acting on them. Women with borderline personality disorder may also see one or more members of the treatment team as wonderful and other members of the team as being punitive or bad. This can lead to "splitting" within the treatment team, with team members having quite different views of and responses to the woman and resulting disagreements within the team about how to best manage the woman's care. It is important in these cases for the members of the team to have a unified approach, focusing on the best care of the woman and avoiding being overly punitive or gratifying. Psychiatric consultation can be very helpful, and there are well-validated, effective psychotherapies for people with this condition (for a review of borderline personality disorder, see Leichsenring, 2011).

Women who seek and misuse habit-forming prescription medications can also be experienced as "difficult" patients and may evoke feelings of anger, helplessness, and confusion in physicians. Such women may be quite skilled in presenting plausible reasons for their needing the medication, or they may present as "entitled demanders" and make actual or veiled threats. It is important to have clear limits regarding the circumstances under which the physician will or will not be willing to continue prescribing the medication and to convey these to the woman empathically and with her best interests in mind. It may be necessary to establish a formal treatment agreement with her, spelling out how the medication will be prescribed, in what amounts, and what will happen in the case of lost prescriptions or early refill requests. In an institutional setting, such as a hospital or clinic with multiple providers, it is important to include this treatment agreement in the medical record and make sure that it is consistent with institutional policies and values. Psychiatric consultation and addressing substance abuse or dependence issues directly may be necessary.

**An understanding of attachment styles can be useful in interacting with "difficult patients" and also in dealing with less extreme problems in delivering the best possible medical care.** Attachment theory was first elaborated by John Bowlby, a British psychiatrist, in the 1950s, and it posits that early interactions with caregivers in the first years of life influence an individual's later interpersonal relationships. These relationships include those with health care providers. When people become ill, often they "regress," become more vulnerable and childlike, and are less able to use more effective coping strategies. The position of being ill, with associated worries about loss of control, loss of health, needing to depend on others, and uncertainty about the future, amplifies any maladaptive patterns of attachment and interpersonal interactions stemming from relationships with early caregivers.

Most people have secure attachment styles and assume both that they themselves are deserving of care and that others can be trusted. There are three insecure attachment styles that affect relationships with medical providers and the quality of medical care: dismissing, preoccupied, and fearful attachment styles.

People with a dismissing attachment style have not been able to rely on early caregivers, have had to fend for themselves, and are compulsively self-reliant. They deny their own needs, tend to minimize symptoms or disability, have difficulty seeking and complying with medical care, and avoid seeking help or support. Women with this attachment style are hard to engage in regular care, especially for chronic illnesses, and may have worse health outcomes. Patients with diabetes with a dismissing attachment style have been shown to have significantly lower levels of exercise, foot care, and adherence to oral hypoglycemic medications. Such patients may either fall through the cracks in a busy practice or be frustrating for the physician who tries to engage them in more active treatment. Engaging such women requires respecting their need for autonomy and respect, being flexible about appointment frequency and duration, giving them control over their care where possible, and using tracking systems and appointment reminders to make sure that they are being followed appropriately.

A preoccupied attachment style is characterized by frequent care seeking. People with this attachment style have received inconsistent responses to their needs in the past and feel they must emphasize their symptoms and distress to evoke consistent care and support. Women with a preoccupied attachment style report more physical symptoms, despite comparable medical morbidity, and have high health care costs and utilization. Such women respond best to brief, frequent, regularly scheduled appointments and to a physician who is responsive but calm, consistent, and unflappable.

The main feature of a fearful attachment style is mistrust of oneself and others, usually based on a history of mistreatment or abuse in the past. The woman seeks help, but she mistrusts and may reject it. She seems anxious, demanding, and highly distressed on the one hand, but she misses appointments and is nonadherent on the other. A major challenge in treating these women is to be patient, accept them as they are, and not withdraw from care. It can be useful to provide care through a number of different clinic providers or a treatment team if possible, so that the woman can develop a relationship with the clinic rather than needing to trust a single person.

Understanding attachment styles and that women's interactions with the health care system reflect earlier formative relationships can be helpful in maintaining a nonpejorative stance toward the patient and in achieving the best health care outcome possible. In general, seeking an empathic understanding of the woman's point of view can allow the physician not to become caught up in negative feelings. Understanding the woman's fears and wishes does not mean that the physician needs to or should do what she wishes. However, it may help the physician to be able to set reasonable limits and expectations and pursue an approach that is in the woman's ultimate best interests, without feeling cruel, withholding, or intimidated. All physicians find some of their patients to be "difficult." Each physician can also increase his or her ability to manage these situations and reduce personal feelings of frustration, anger, or guilt, through consultation with colleagues, participating in a Balint group to discuss the psychological aspects of patient care, collaborating with other team members in discussing and making a plan for dealing with a patient, or consulting with a mental health specialist for or about the patient.

## SEXUAL FUNCTION AND DYSFUNCTION

Sexual satisfaction is one of the more important human experiences, yet it has been estimated that as many as 51% of women experience some sexual dissatisfaction. But self-reported distress about a woman's sex life was much less common, estimated to be 11% (Mitchell, 2013). Self-reported distress about the sexual problem is recommended to give a diagnosis of a sexual dysfunction.

**Although there is a strong physiologic basis for sexual function, it is impossible to separate sexual response from the many emotional, social, physical and other contributing factors that may influence a relationship.** Cultural or religious beliefs have influence on sexual function and dysfunction. For example, many African and some Asian and Middle Eastern countries practice female circumcision to varying degrees. The more extreme genital cutting or the trauma from the experience can result in reduced sexual activity, pain, and lowered frequency of orgasm.

In 1966 Masters and Johnson published their famous book *Human Sexual Response*, which was a discussion of observations made on the sexual cycles of 700 subjects. It is on this important work that our early understanding of the female sexual response was based. Masters and Johnson described four phases of the sexual response: excitement, plateau, orgasm, and resolution (Fig. 9.2).

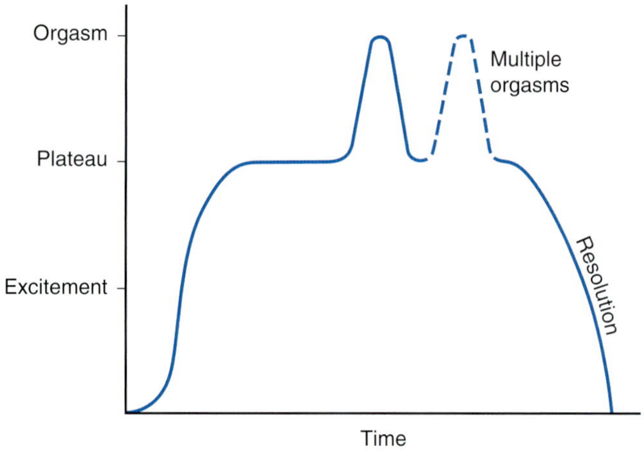


**Fig. 9.2** Sexual response cycle defined by Masters and Johnson. (From Masters WH, Johnson VE. *Human Sexual Response*. Boston: Little, Brown; 1966.)

The excitement phase may be initiated by a number of internal or external stimuli. Desire may be activated in the hypothalamus with dopaminergic activity. Physiologically this phase is associated with associated with an increase in sexual tension, which may manifest as the following:

Deep breathing
Increased heart rate and blood pressure
Warmth and erotic tension
Generalized vasocongestion
Skin flush
Breast engorgement and nipple erection
Engorgement of the labia and clitoris
Vaginal transudate

The clitoris generally swells and becomes erect because of increased genital blood flow and the neurotransmitter nitric oxide, causing it to be tightly applied to the clitoral hood. The dilation of the sinusoidal vascular spaces of the corporal tissue of the clitoris, vestibular bulbs, and spongiosal tissue lead to that engorgement. The vagina "sweats" a transudative lubricant, and the Bartholin glands may secrete small amounts of liquid. There is also a myotonic effect, which is most notable in nipple erection. Much of the response in the excitement phase is caused by stimulation of the parasympathetic fibers of the autonomic nervous system. Dynamic genital magnetic resonance imaging (MRI) studies enable the visualization of the physiologic arousal response that provides the direct observation of the time course and magnitude of this response, along with the variability that appears to occur in women with sexual arousal disorder. In some cases, anticholinergic drugs may interfere with a full response in this stage. A woman with diabetes with peripheral neuropathy may complain of poor arousal because of lack of sensation.

Next is the plateau stage, which is the culmination of the excitement phase and is associated with a marked degree of vasocongestion throughout the body. Breasts and their areolae are markedly engorged, as are the labia and the lower third of the vagina. The vasocongestion in the lower third of the vagina is such that it forms what has been called the *orgasmic platform*, causing a decrease in the diameter of the vagina by as much as 50% and thus allowing for greater friction against the penis. At this stage, the clitoris retracts tightly against the pubic symphysis, and the vagina lengthens, with dilation of the upper two thirds.

The next stage is orgasm, in which the sexual tension that has been built up in the entire body is released. Characteristics of orgasm are listed in Box 9.12. A myotonic response involves muscle systems of the entire body. There is contraction of the anal sphincter and the muscles surrounding the vagina. The uterus may also contract. Muscle contraction occurs 2 to 4 seconds after the woman begins to experience the orgasm and repeats at 0.8-second intervals. The actual number and intensity of contractions vary from woman to woman. Some women observed to have orgasmic contractions are not aware that they are having an orgasm. Masters and Johnson felt that prolonged stimulation during the excitement phase, during masturbation, or in conjunction with the use of a vibrator may lead to more pronounced orgasmic activity. Whereas the excitement phase is under the influence of the parasympathetic portion of the autonomic nervous system, orgasm seems to be related to the sympathetic portion. Brain changes with orgasm have been documented on functional MRI and positron emission tomography (PET), showing increased activation in the paraventricular nucleus of the hypothalamus, periaqueductal gray region of the midbrain, hippocampus, and cerebellum in women with spinal-cord injury. The release of endogenous opioids, serotonin, prolactin, and oxytocin also has been reported. Medication such as antihypertensive or antidepressant drugs, particularly SSRIs, may affect orgasmic response. A spinal cord injury may result in orgasmic disorder.

The resolution stage is last and represents a return of the woman's physiologic state to the preexcitement level. Although a

**BOX 9.12** Characteristics of Female Orgasm

Release of tension
Generalized myotonic contractions
Contractions of perivaginal muscles and anal sphincter
Uterine contractions

refractory period is typical of the sexual response cycle in a man, no such refractory periods have been identified in women. During the resolution phase, the woman generally experiences a feeling of personal satisfaction and well-being. Increased brain serotonergic activity and decreased dopamine release have been recorded.

**Alternative models of the human sexual response have been proposed that differ from the linear progression of Masters and Johnson's (1966) model and also incorporate women's motivations and reasons for engaging in sex. Basson (2006) proposed that the phases overlap and may even occur in a different order.** She proposed a more intimacy-based, circular model where arousal and desire are more interchangeable for women. In fact, in contrast to Masters and Johnson, desire may not always precede arousal. Women in established relationships may engage in sex, not because of sexual desire but because of a desire for intimacy with their partner (Fig. 9.3). Then endpoint might be more subjective and include satisfaction related to emotional closeness and affection rather than orgasm sometimes. That higher emotional intimacy in turn can lead to greater receptivity and entering the circular model at different points. There may be other stages of sexual response not accounted for in Masters and Johnson's work.

**A dual control model of sexual response offers a theoretical framework for sexual problems. There are inhibitory influences and excitatory influences that modulate sexual function.** Central neuroendocrine transmitters associated with excitatory signals are dopamine, norepinephrine, oxytocin and melanocortins, whereas inhibitory signals are associated with serotonin (5-HT), opioids, and endocannabinoids. High sexual excitation factors with low sexual inhibitions have been associated with out-of-control or high-risk sexual behaviors. Low sexual excitations with high sexual inhibition are associated with increased vulnerability for sexual dysfunctions. Neuroendocrine mechanisms and psychosocial aspects regulate that balance (Fig. 9.4). The strongest associations with both current and lifetime sexual problems were the inhibitory factors based on using the Sexual Excitation/Sexual Inhibition Inventory for Women, a 36-item self-report questionnaire. The two particular aspects related to sexual problems were "arousal contingency," meaning that everything has to be "just right" for sexual arousal to occur,

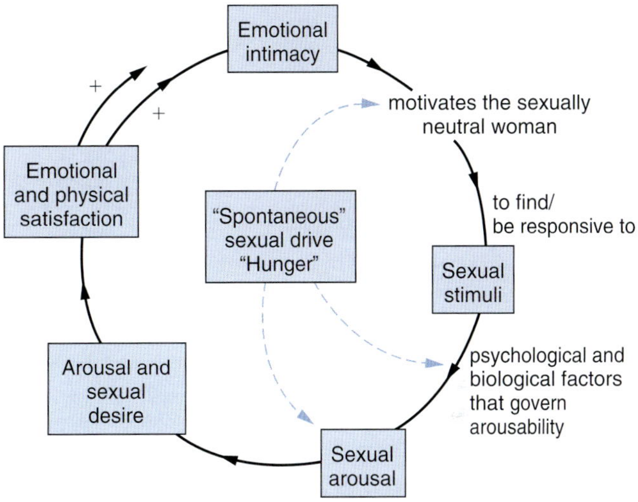


**Fig. 9.3** Blended intimacy-based and sexual drive–based cycles. (From Basson R. Female sexual response: the role of drugs in the management of sexual dysfunction. *Obstet Gynecol.* 2001;98:350-353.)

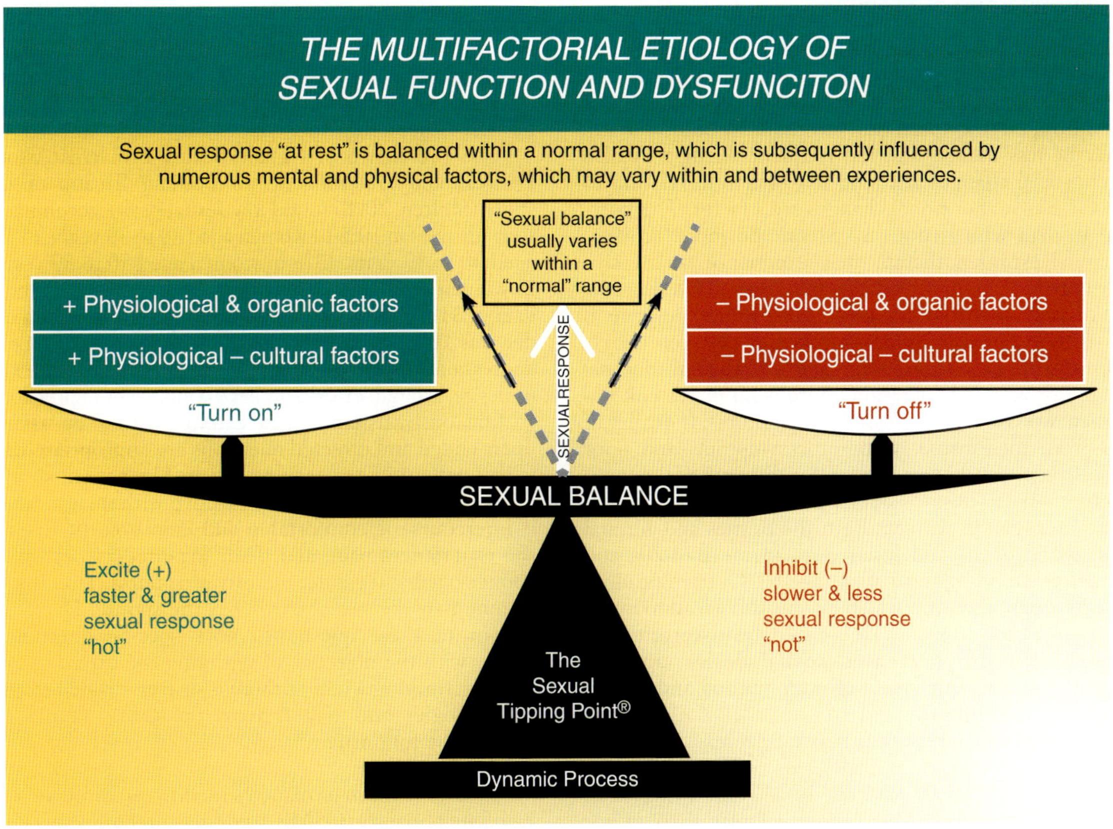


**Fig. 9.4** Dual control model or excitatory and inhibitory factors. (From Urologic Clinics of North America. Perelman, Michael A, PhD, Published May 1, 2011. Volume 38, Issue 2. Pages 125-139. Adapted from Perelman MA. The sexual tipping point: a mind/body model for sexual medicine. *J Sex Med.* 2009;6:630.)

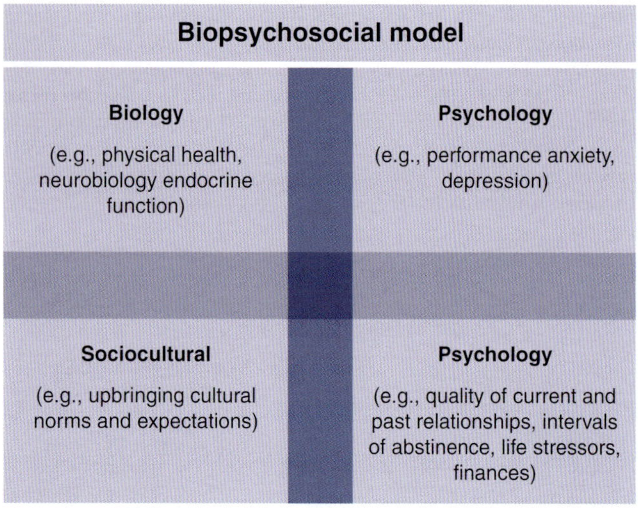


**Fig. 9.5** Biopsychosocial model of female sexual function. (From Thomas HN, Thurston RC. A biopsychosocial approach to women's sexual function and dysfunction at midlife: a narrative review. *Maturitas.* 2016(87):49-60.)

and "concerns about sexual function," relating to possible loss of arousal and worries about being a good lover or taking too long to reach orgasm.

All these models are helpful for conceptualizing varies aspects of female sexual function and dysfunction. Using a biopsychosocial framework helps appreciate the multidimensional aspects of sexual function (Fig. 9.5).

## Sexual Response and Menopause

**Many factors contribute to sexual changes as a woman enters menopause. Aging in general is associated with the slowing of sexual response and decreases in the intensity of response (Simon, 2018).** Specifically, arousal may be slower and orgasms may be less intense and less frequent. Aging may also lead to psychosocial changes affecting self-esteem in relation to desirability. Of course, hormonal changes are a factor. The postmenopausal woman who is not on systemic hormone replacement or vaginal estrogen therapy may experience progressive atrophy of vaginal epithelium, a change in vaginal pH, a decrease in quantity of vaginal secretions, and a decrease in the general circulation to the vagina and uterus. Although estrogen clearly plays a role in maintaining the integrity of the vaginal mucosal epithelium and promotes lubrication, there is no direct link between estrogen levels and sexual desire or symptoms. If quality of life is poor from menopausal vasomotor symptoms and poor sleep, then estrogen can improve overall well-being without directly affecting sexual desire complaints. Testosterone is the predominant androgen in women. Both the ovaries and adrenal gland produce androgens and levels peak in the mid-20s and decline thereafter. Levels plateau about age 60. Ovarian production ceases with oophorectomy, which may possibly lead to lower circulating levels of testosterone. **Decreased testosterone levels are associated with decreased sexual desire, arousal, sensation, and orgasm, but levels of endogenous androgens do not predict sexual function.**

A postmenopausal woman may experience other sexual problems relating to her partner, or if she is single, widowed, or divorced, to her lack of availability of male partners. In addition, her general health and the general health of her partner will play a role in her ability to respond sexually in a satisfactory manner. Pelvic organ prolapse, urinary incontinence and poor levator ani muscle function may contribute to poorer sexual function. Couples with marital or communication problems may find that menopause is an appropriate excuse to cease sexual activities. A concerned physician can help a couple sort out their needs and desire for sexual compatibility at this stage of life. Often, counseling aimed at dealing with problems of the relationship will alleviate sexual response difficulties.

Male partners of older women may suffer from medical conditions or be affected by medications, with a resultant decrease in arousal and difficulties in acquiring or maintaining an erection sufficient for intercourse. The physician should ask women about sexual function, and if male erectile dysfunction is evident, they should make suggestions for appropriate referral to physicians or other health care workers who may deal with male sexual dysfunction.

## Sexual Dysfunction

**Female sexual dysfunction is quite common, particularly the loss of desire for sex (ACOG, 2019).** Higher percentages of dysfunction are seen in couples presenting for couples therapy. Some women with loss of libido fear losing their partner. Both patient and physician wish for an easy solution, but the problem is often complex and not easily treated with drugs. Physicians caring for women should make a special effort to uncover sexual dysfunction because patients often do not bring up the problem unless asked. The DSM-V diagnoses for female sexual dysfunction include the following:

Sexual interest/arousal disorders (previously called hypoactive desire disorder which was separate from arousal disorders)
Orgasmic disorders
Genito-pelvic pain penetration disorders (previously dyspareunia, vaginismus)
Other specified and unspecified dysfunction
Substance/medication-induced dysfunction

To be classified as a dysfunction, the symptoms should lead to distress, which can mean frustration, grief, guilt, incompetence, loss, sadness, sorrow and worry. More than one condition may exist and there is often overlap such as lack of sexual interest, partner issues and genital pain.

The Prevalence of Female Sexual Problems Associated with Distress and Determinants of Seeking Treatment (PRESIDE) study (Shifren, 2008) found low sexual desire accompanied by personal distress in 10% of women aged 30 to 39 years, 11% in women aged 40 to 49 years, 13% in women aged 50 to 59 years, and 10% in women aged 60 to 69 years. A 2009 report with the PRESIDE data of 31,581 respondents found the prevalence of a desire disorder was 10%, but reduced to 6.3% for those without concurrent depression. Overall, 40% of those respondents with sexual disorder of desire, arousal, or orgasm have concurrent depression.

Obviously, assembling a careful history by asking general, open-ended and directed questions are appropriate when dealing with a patient in a gynecologic visit. The patient should be asked if she is sexually active; if she is active with men, women, or both; if intercourse is comfortable and enjoyable (if heterosexual); if she experiences pain; and if she experiences orgasm. Questions about sexual and gender identity are appropriate. It is best not to assume that the sexual partner is the spouse. Depending on the answer to these questions, more specific questioning should follow with the objective of outlining the extent of any problem and determining whether there is distress related to the problem.

Etiologies and risk factors for female sexual dysfunction include the following:

Medical issues such as diabetes mellitus, genitourinary syndrome of menopause (GSM), prior hysterectomy with or without oophorectomy, urinary incontinence, premature ovarian failure, neurologic illnesses, thyroid disease (both hyper- and hypo-), hyperprolactinemia

Psychological issues such as depression, anxiety, stress, sequelae of gynecologic or breast cancer and treatments, body image attitudes, negative sexual attitudes
Medications such as the following:
 Psychotropic (antidepressant such as SSRIs, SNRIs, tricyclic)
 Anticholinergic
 Antihypertensive (beta-blockers possibly)
 Histamine blockers
 Hormonal (GnRH agonists or other hormonal formulations)
 Antiepileptics
 Opioids
 Benzodiazepines
 Cancer treatments (especially breast and gynecologic cancer)
Traumatic issues such as history of sexual abuse, intimate partner violence, female genital mutilation, straddle injuries
Relationship discord
Substance abuse

Sexual response problems may be the result of a previous negative sexual experience or may be secondary to emotional or physical illness. Primary medical conditions causing female sexual dysfunction can be hormonal, anatomic, vascular, or neurologic. The problem may also be related to difficulties in the current relationship or to alcohol, marijuana, or drug abuse. Although an occasional alcoholic drink may decrease inhibitions and improve sexual response, in general, alcohol is a depressant and decreases a woman's ability to become sexually aroused and to become vaginally lubricated. Drugs with antihypertensive and anticholinergic activity, as well as those active at the alpha- and beta-adrenergic receptors, may decrease arousal or inhibit sexual interest. Narcotics, sedatives, and antidepressant drugs, such as SSRIs, may also depress sexual responsiveness. Finally, decreased arousal or ability to remain aroused may be due to distractions in the woman's life such as concerns for children, job, other stress or problems that may enter her consciousness during arousal.

## Sexual Interest/Arousal Disorders

**Hypoactive sexual desire disorder (low libido) is the most common sexual dysfunction and is reported by 5% to 14% of women surveyed.** While **the new DSM V category now puts sexual interest and arousal disorders in the same category** (as these are often coexistent), most research has separated these disorders, so the older terminology may be used. Hypoactive sexual desire disorder is defined as absent or decreased:

sexual interest,
sexual thoughts or fantasies,
initiation of sexual activity, or
responsiveness to a partner's attempts to initiate.

Studying functional MRI results has started to improve our understanding of etiology. Exposure to erotic material was associated with significant differences in both reports of subjective arousal and brain activation among women meeting criteria for hypoactive sexual desire disorder compared with normal control women (Fig. 9.6). There may be difference in attention level to one's own responses to sexual stimuli as well. This research also reinforced previous work suggesting there may be a weak relationship between measures of genital arousal and subjective arousal in women.

Because each individual has his or her own libidinal drive, it is not surprising that couples may have some incompatibility of needs. It is important, however, that these needs and desires be discussed openly and that reasons for lack of sexual desire that may involve experiences or problems inherent in the relationship be resolved. At times the problem may be a failure or inability to set aside appropriate time and effort for intimacy. The couple should be encouraged to give sexual activity a high priority within their relationship rather than leaving it last on the list of priorities. Couples should be encouraged to use arousal techniques that are appropriate for their relationship. Satisfactory foreplay of a mutually enjoyable nature should be encouraged. Adding novelty to the sexual experience may help the couple and this might be including new sexual positions, locations, time of day and new stimulation techniques. Broadening their definition of what their sexual experience might include can be helpful. Couples counseling and retreats might enhance their experience.

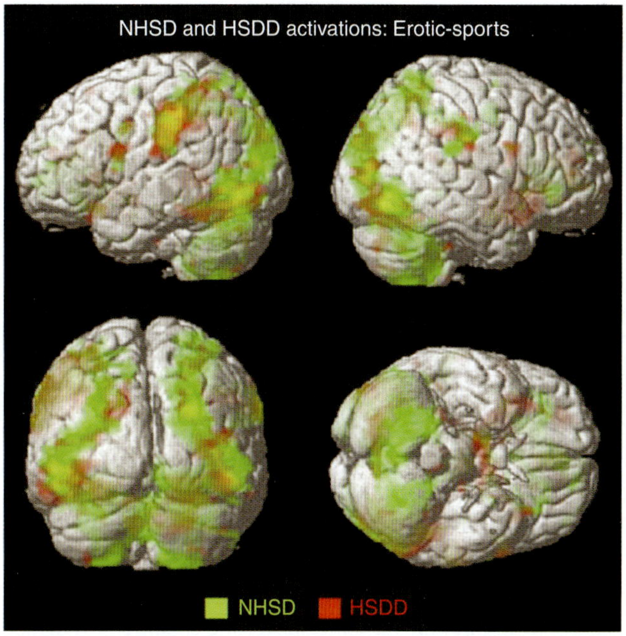


**Fig. 9.6** Functional magnetic resonance imaging of women with hypoactive sexual desire disorder compared with normal women. Surface rendering of NHSD (green) and HSDD (red) group average activations for the erotic-sports contrast, using a $P < .001$ threshold (uncorrected). Overlap of activation for the two groups appears as yellow. *NHSD,* no history of sexual dysfunction; *HSDD,* hypoactive sexual desire disorder. (From Arnow BA, Millheiser L, Garrett A, et al. Women with hypoactive sexual desire disorder compared with normal women: a functional magnetic resonance imaging study. *Neuroscience.* 2009;158(2):484-502. Copyright2009.)

Hormonal levels are often obtained in evaluating desire disorders. However, there is no evidence that low testosterone levels distinguish women with sexual desire disorder from others. A report on 1021 women who had androgen levels drawn from a random recruitment in Australia found neither total nor free testosterone nor dehydroepiandrosterone sulfate (DHEAS) levels discriminated between the women with and those without low sexual function. Testosterone testing in women is not recommended because the commonly available tests are not sensitive enough to detect the low concentrations in women, and the normal range in women has not been established.

There are two FDA-approved medication for hypoactive sexual desire disorder. Flibanserin is approved for premenopausal women, and daily use increased satisfying sexual events by about 1 per month. It is a centrally acting 5HT 1A agonist and a weak dopamine agonist. Alcohol must not be consumed. Side effects include drowsiness, hypotension, and syncope. In 2019 the FDA approved bremelanotide for use in premenopausal women. This activates melanocortin receptors, but the actual mechanism of action if unknown. In a randomized, double blind, placebo-controlled study, there was no change in the number of satisfying sexual events, but 25% of women had increases in sexual desire score and 35% had a decrease in the distress score. This is injected into the skin at least 45 minutes before anticipated sexual activity. It is contraindicated with hypertension, heart, kidney or liver disease.

Estrogen alone has not been shown to improve hypoactive sexual desire disorder. However, estrogen may improve sexual desire if hypoestrogenism is causing an overall lack of well-being from nighttime hot flashes and poor sleep or genital discomfort from atrophy. The risks of estrogen are discussed elsewhere. Androgen therapy is not at present FDA approved in women, but randomized controlled trials have noted some benefits in postmenopausal women with hypoactive sexual desire disorders and arousal disorders. Levels of endogenous androgens therapy that increase serum concentrations to the upper limit of normal have consistently been shown to improve female sexual desire and sexual activity. The transdermal testosterone patch has been evaluated with the higher-dose patch (300 μg) showing increases in desire over a 6-month study in selected populations of postmenopausal women. Improvements are modest. The group that has the most response to testosterone is women who have had surgical menopause.

A 2019 systematic review of 36 randomized controlled trials in 8480 participants also found testosterone significantly increased sexual function, including satisfactory sexual event frequency (about once per month), sexual desire, arousal, orgasm, well-being, and pleasure, in postmenopausal women (Islam, 2019). There was an increase in weight. There were no adverse changes in serum lipids when testosterone cream or a transdermal patch were used, but there were changes with oral routes. Again, the FDA has not approved the patch or any other testosterone preparation for women. Long-term safety and efficacy data are not available, and there are particular concerns about cardiovascular risk and breast cancer risks. Testosterone use in women remains controversial. Phosphodiesterase inhibitors have not been found to be effective (Davis, 2019). Bupropion has shown some effectiveness, even in women without depression, but further studies are needed. Trazadone is a serotonin 2a inhibitor and has some prosexual side effects of increased libido and orgasm. Again, few studies have been done.

**Because sex is a biopsychosocial experience, it is not surprising that no one treatment for low libido stands out. Studies narrowly focusing on orgasm, genital function, or frequency of intercourse without addressing satisfaction or quality of life may not get at the essence of the sexual experience.** At present, a sound approach to female sexual dysfunction is complex and needs to assess sexual education knowledge, a women's relationship with her partner, all forms of abuse including emotional abuse or traumatic experiences, body image issues, religious or cultural ideals, depression, concerns about sexually transmitted diseases, pain, other medical problems, and everyday fatigues and stresses. Exercise to improve blood flow to the pelvis and decrease fatigue, changing SSRI medication for depression if negative sexual side effects occur, and psychotherapy/sex therapy can all be beneficial. Improving overall health and body image attitudes with regular exercise, optimal diet, stress reduction (possibly with yoga and mindfulness-based training) may lead to a more satisfying sex life.

Sexual arousal disorder is characterized by a persistent inability to sense genital arousal. There may be difficulty attaining adequate lubrication and swelling response of sexual excitement. The prevalence of this disorder is uncertain but possibly 5% and often coexists with decreased sexual desire, chronic medical conditions (particularly vascular or neurologic injury) or vaginal atrophy. Sexual arousal disorders have received relatively little scientific inquiry. Masters and Johnson taught women sensate focus using masturbation training and working with the partners with apparently good results. Vaginal or systemic estrogen therapy improves arousal disorder by improving vaginal blood flow and lubrication in postmenopausal women. The FDA-approved EROS–CTD (Clitoral Therapy Device, UroMetrics, Inc., St. Paul, MN) is a cup that sits over the clitoris and a gentle vacuum is applied via a battery-powered device. The EROS-CTD has been reported to improve clitoral blood flow, engorgement, and genital sensation, which is effective in the ability to reach orgasm. Exercise may improve genital blood flow.

Although not classified in the DSM-5 criteria, persistent genital arousal has been increasingly reported. Although it is poorly understood, the unwanted genital arousal symptoms can be spontaneous, very unpleasant, and distracting. Tingling, throbbing, pulsating arousal can verge on pain in some women. The arousal is unrelieved by orgasm, and the feelings of arousal persist for hours or days. The prevalence is unknown, although cessation of antidepressants has been known to precipitate the persistent arousal. Others hypothesized the pudendal nerve or vascular changes as causes. Treatments are uncertain benefit but have ranged from cognitive therapy to using SSRIs to trials of neuromodulation.

## Genito-Pelvic Pain Penetration Disorders

Sexual pain is called genito-pelvic pain/penetration disorder in the DSM-5 criteria and includes the following:

Difficulty with vaginal penetration
Marked vulvovaginal or pelvic pain during penetration or attempts
Fear or anxiety about pain in anticipation of, during, or after penetration
Tightening or tensing of pelvic floor muscles during attempted penetration

A detailed history will include timing of pain, location of pain, diffuse or localized symptoms, length of problem and relation to injuries, hormonal changes, partner changes, urinary and gastrointestinal symptoms, and psychosocial factors. The examination includes the following:

Observation of vulvar skin rashes, adhesions, erythema, fissures, cracks, ulcers
Observation of perineal scarring or abnormality; sometimes putting the introitus on stretch will reveal a scar band
Introitus inspection of the urethra, hymen, vestibule
Vulvar vestibule Q-tip touching to appreciate hypersensitivity
Vaginal atrophy (pH), scarring, shortening, or stenosis
Anterior vaginal wall tenderness at the base of the bladder
Pelvic floor muscle tenderness, spasm, or trigger points
Bimanual examination of cervix, uterus, adnexa, uterosacral ligaments (nodules), posthysterectomy cuff

Common use of the terms *dyspareunia* and *vaginismus* persists; they have been used in prior research studies and so will be used here. Vaginismus is a condition in which the woman has difficulties allowing vaginal entry of a penis. It is thought to be secondary to involuntary contraction of vaginal introital and levator ani muscles. Recognizing the importance of pelvic floor muscle involvement has led to the use of terms such as *pelvic floor muscle hypertonus*, *levator ani syndrome*, and *levator ani muscle spasm*. Because of this spasm, penetration is either painful or impossible. With time, there can be fear of pain and phobic avoidance. Lamont's classic study has attempted to classify the degrees of vaginismus and, in a group of 80 patients, noted that 27 (34%) had first-degree vaginismus, defined as perineal and levator spasm relieved by reassurance during pelvic examination. Another 21 (26%) had second-degree vaginismus, defined as perineal spasm maintained throughout the pelvic examination. Another 18 (22.5%) demonstrated third-degree vaginismus, defined as levator spasm and elevation of the buttocks. A total of 10 (12.5%) had fourth-degree vaginismus, defined as levator and perineal spasm with withdrawal and retreat. Four of the 80 patients refused pelvic examination. These patients often complain not only of pain or fear of pain with coitus or pelvic examination but also of difficulty in inserting a tampon or vaginal medication. The condition may be primary, in which case the individual has never experienced successful coitus. This problem is generally based on either early sexual abuse or aversion to sexuality in general. There may be a lack of appropriate learning about sex secondary to cultural or familial teaching that sex is evil, painful, or undesirable. Vaginismus may also occur in patients who have been sexually active when an injury or vaginal infection has led to vaginal pain with attempted coitus. This has been seen in rape victims and in women who have had painful episiotomy repairs, severe yeast vaginitis, or vulvodynia. When the underlying cause for the vaginismus is understood, the matter may be discussed frankly with the patient and her partner to effect a relearning process that is conducive to relieving the symptoms.

Cognitive and behavioral therapy is encouraged, and then desensitization treatment can begin. Once desensitized to the fear and panic and by helping the woman feel in control, the actual vaginal spasm may be relieved by teaching the patient muscle relaxation and then self-dilation techniques, using fingers or dilators, in which she and her partner can participate. This is often greatly facilitated by having the woman working with a skilled pelvic floor physical therapist. There are little data from controlled trials.

When these strategies fail, botulinum neurotoxin type A injections have been studied in several trials with mixed results. Botulinum neurotoxin inhibits binding of intracellular acetylcholine vesicles to the cell membrane at the presynaptic level and decreases muscle spasm.

Dyspareunia is a sexual dysfunction in which genital pain occurs before, during, or after intercourse; it often has an organic basis. The prevalence is estimated to be 8% to 22% of women. The physician should obtain a careful history of when the dyspareunia occurs (e.g., on insertion of the penis, at the midvagina during thrusting, with deep penetration of the vault, with orgasm or after intercourse) because facts obtained by this history may point to organic causes, such as poor lubrication and vaginal atrophy, a painful bladder disorder, vulvodynia, poorly healed vaginal lacerations or episiotomy, and diseases such as pelvic inflammatory disease, pelvic congestion syndrome, or endometriosis. Box 9.13 lists some causes of dyspareunia.

**GSM with dyspareunia is thought to be due to vaginal atrophy.** Genitourinary syndrome of menopause (GSM) symptoms include vaginal dryness, vaginal and vulvar burning, dyspareunia, and dysuria due to hypoestrogenic effects on the genital tract. Low-dose vaginal estrogen, nonhormonal vaginal moisturizers, and vaginal lubricants are commonly recommended. Oral ospemifene is a selective estrogen receptor modulator that is approved for vulvovaginal atrophy and dyspareunia in postmenopausal women. This would be appropriate for women with hypoactive sexual desire disorder thought to be from pain from vaginal atrophy. Some data suggest this may also modestly improve sexual satisfaction with desire and arousal and orgasm. Vaginal dehydroepiandrosterone is an FDA-approved steroid for women with moderate to severe dyspareunia as a result of menopause. It is locally converted to estrogen and contraindicated in women with breast cancer. In a randomized trial it not only helped dyspareunia but also had some benefit for desire and orgasm. A side effect can be vaginal discharge. At present, no FDA-approved laser is available for gynecologic use.

Vulvodynia is chronic pain and burning in the vulva and affects up to 8.3% of women. Other symptoms might include stinging, irritation, or rawness in the vulva. The causes are largely unknown, but genetics, hormonal factors (maybe OCs), musculoskeletal factors (pelvic floor muscle hyperactivity, myofascial sources), inflammatory conditions, neurologic disorders, neuroproliferative conditions, environmental toxins, and structural abnormalities might be considered. Other pain syndromes can be reported, such as painful bladder syndrome, irritable bowel syndrome, endometriosis, and fibromyalgia. For women with localized provoked vulvar pain (vestibulodynia), researchers have found increased nerve endings and signs of inflammation in the vestibule. Avoiding soaps, detergents and scented products is recommended. A small study of extended-release gabapentin found improved sexual function. However, sexual function remained lower than in pain-free control participants. Topical gabapentin and topical lidocaine have been studied in small trials, with modest benefit. When no organic cause can be found for the dyspareunia, techniques similar to those used in evaluating and managing vaginismus are appropriate. Pelvic floor physical therapy may be beneficial for vaginismus, vulvodynia, and dyspareunia as well as sex therapy. With all the sexual pain disorders, it is not uncommon to treat the underlying organic cause with success and find the pain continues. It is often muscle tension problems from the pain-tension-pain cycle that remain (Fig. 9.7). Specific pathologic conditions should, of course, be treated. At times, changing coital position can relieve dyspareunia. Couples should be encouraged to experiment with female-dominant

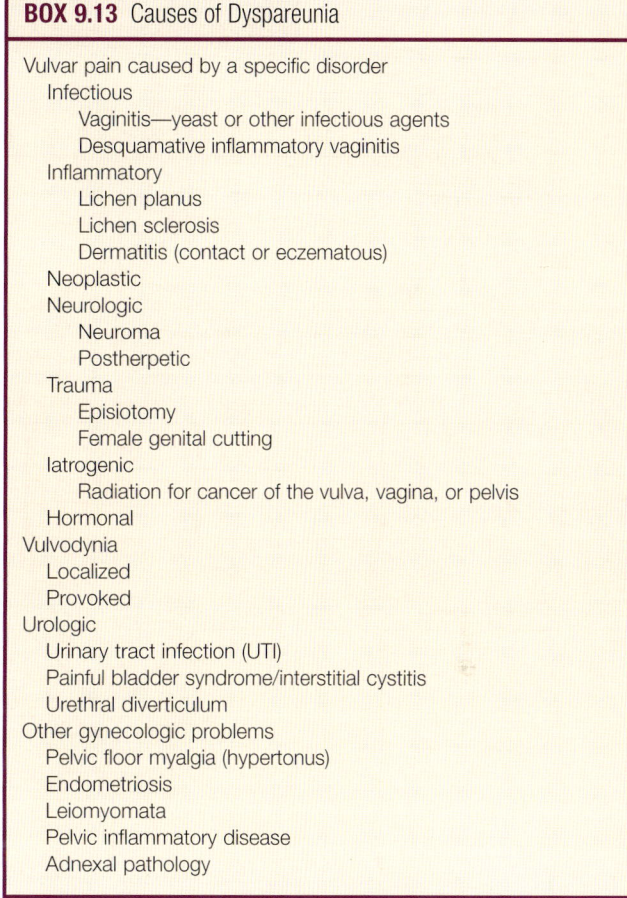

**BOX 9.13** Causes of Dyspareunia

- Vulvar pain caused by a specific disorder
  - Infectious
    - Vaginitis—yeast or other infectious agents
    - Desquamative inflammatory vaginitis
  - Inflammatory
    - Lichen planus
    - Lichen sclerosis
    - Dermatitis (contact or eczematous)
  - Neoplastic
  - Neurologic
    - Neuroma
    - Postherpetic
  - Trauma
    - Episiotomy
    - Female genital cutting
  - Iatrogenic
    - Radiation for cancer of the vulva, vagina, or pelvis
  - Hormonal
- Vulvodynia
  - Localized
  - Provoked
- Urologic
  - Urinary tract infection (UTI)
  - Painful bladder syndrome/interstitial cystitis
  - Urethral diverticulum
- Other gynecologic problems
  - Pelvic floor myalgia (hypertonus)
  - Endometriosis
  - Leiomyomata
  - Pelvic inflammatory disease
  - Adnexal pathology

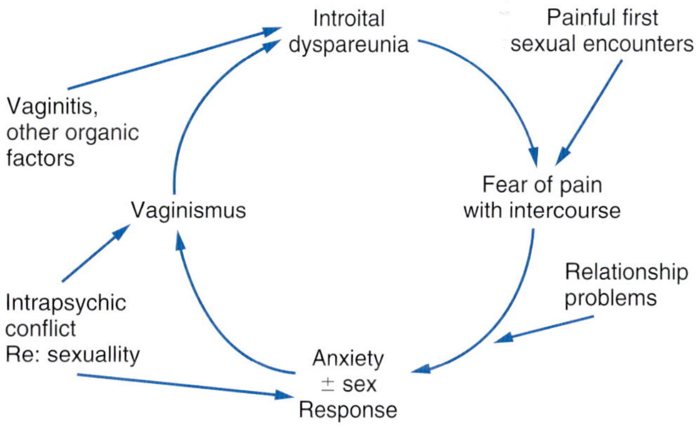


**Fig. 9.7** Dyspareunia and vaginismus cycle. (From Steege JF. Dyspareunia and vaginismus. *Clin Obstet Gynecol.* 1984;27:750-759.)

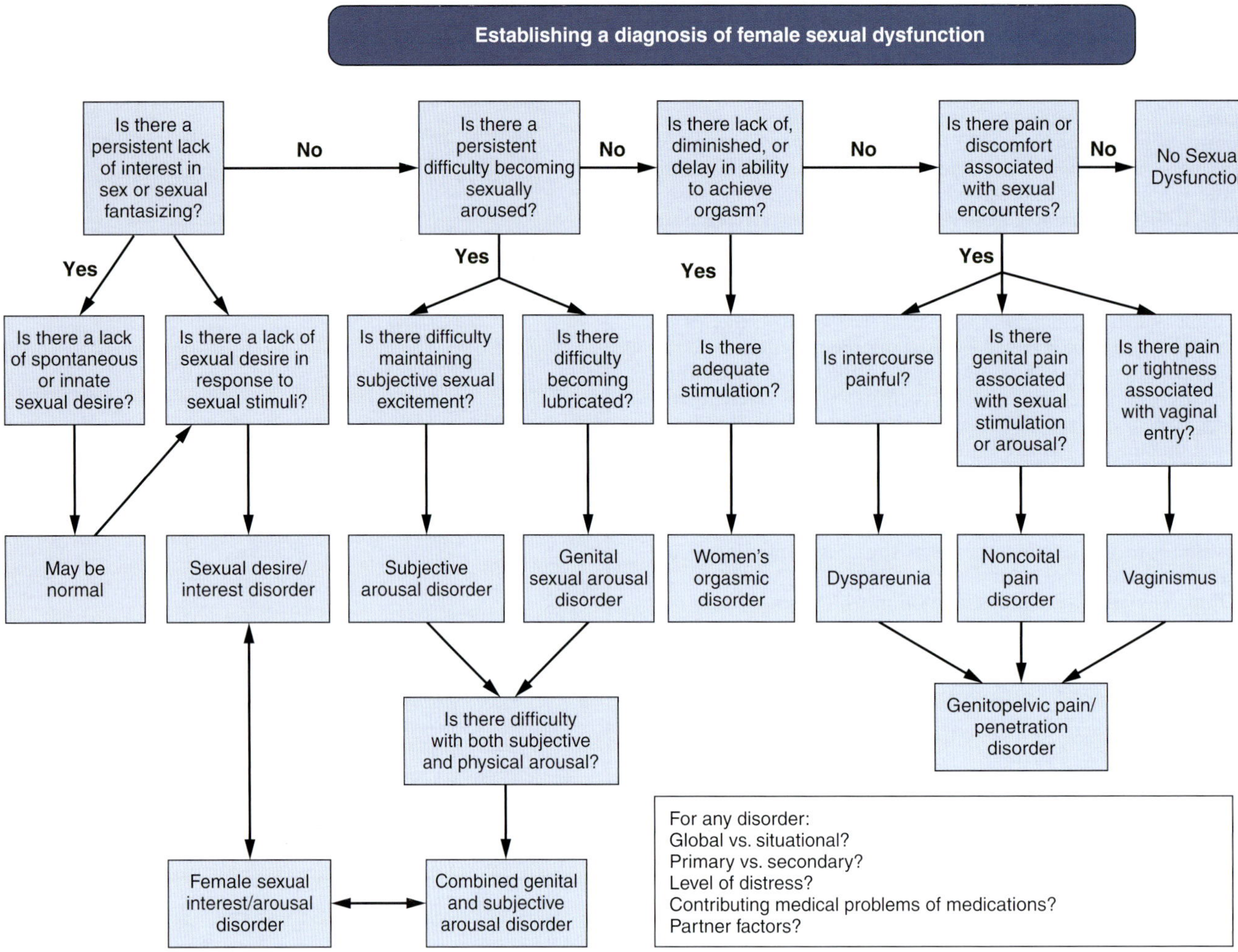


**Fig. 9.8** Arriving at the diagnosis of female sexual dysfunction. (From Erin Z. Latif M.D. and Michael P. Diamond M.D. Fertility and Sterility, 2013-10-01, Volume 100, Issue 4, Pages 898-904, Copyright 2013 American Society for Reproductive Medicine.)

and side-by-side positions to see if the pain can be prevented. Noncoital sexual expression can be encouraged. An algorithm for thinking about sexual dysfunction is shown in Fig. 9.8.

## Orgasmic Disorders

Orgasmic dysfunction is less common at 3% to 6% of women and is often situational. It is defined as persistent or recurrent delay in or absence of orgasm. As many as 10% to 15% of women have never experienced an orgasm through any form of sexual stimulation, and another 25% to 35% will have difficulty reaching an orgasm on any particular occasion. Many women may be orgasmic secondary to masturbation or oral sex but may not be orgasmic with penile intercourse. It is important to discern by history the extent of the patient's problem and to place it into proper perspective. If the patient is anorgasmic during intercourse but has experienced orgasms, communication with her partner may aid in bringing about an orgasm during intercourse by allowing her or her partner to stimulate her clitoral area with the intensity and timing necessary to bring about an orgasm. If the woman is anorgasmic, she may be given permission to learn masturbatory techniques and sensate focus exercises to become comfortable with her own body until she has an orgasm. Then these techniques may be applied to the coital situation, slowly increasing intimacy and trust, thereby developing the desired response during coitus. There may be psychological impacts interfering with the ability to attain orgasm, including body image, self-esteem, history of sexual abuse, or other negative beliefs. Couples should be encouraged to communicate their sexual needs so that appropriate stimulation is offered during the arousal period and during intercourse. For situational orgasmic disorder, the focus of dialogue should be the relationship. Developing this type of dialogue is often difficult but can be aided by counseling with a sensitive physician or sex therapist. Although treatment options are limited, CBT, sensate focus, Kegel exercises, enhancing partner communication, and direct clitoral stimulation have been beneficial.

Sexual response is a complex problem involving physiologic responses and psychosocial influences, which makes research studies hard to conduct. Although physicians and women may desire a pharmacologic solution, at present there is a paucity of good quality evidence. In fact, in the clinical trials of drug treatments for female sexual dysfunction, the placebo responses have been substantial. Whether attention to sexual function or changes in sexual behavior during a trial result in the marked placebo response, this definitely complicates the studies and needs to be considered in any treatment offered. Psychosexual counseling is often appropriate, as well as a comprehensive medical evaluation. There are many good books published on these topics. Treatments for sexual dysfunctions are summarized in Table 9.6.

**TABLE 9.6** *Treatments for Female Sexual Dysfunctions*

| Medication Category | Product Name | Formulation | Indication |
|---|---|---|---|
| **Pharmacologic Treatments** | | | |
| Local vaginal estrogens | Estradiol or CEE cream (Estrace, Premarin)<br>Estradiol vaginal tablet (Vagifem, Yuvafem)<br>Estradiol vaginal gel cap (Imvexxy)<br>Estradiol vaginal ring (Estring) | Cream<br>Vaginal tablet<br>Vaginal gel cap<br>Vaginal ring | Genitourinary syndrome of menopause |
| Selective estrogen receptor modulator | Ospemifene (Osphena) | Oral tablet | Genitourinary syndrome of menopause |
| DHEA | Prasterone (Intrarosa) | Vaginal suppository | Genitourinary syndrome of menopause |
| Testosterone (not FDA approved in women, approved in countries outside the United States) | Testosterone | Transdermal cream or gel | Hypoactive sexual desire disorder |
| Serotonin agonist/antagonist | Flibanserin (Addyi) | Oral tablet | Hypoactive sexual desire disorder |
| **Nonpharmacologic treatments** | | | |
| Lubricants | Multiple products | Water-based<br>Silicone-based<br>Hybrid (water- and silicone-based)<br>Oil-based | Used as needed for to reduce friction and enhance comfort with sexual activity |
| Moisturizers | Multiple products | NA | Used regularly for maintenance of vulvar/vaginal moisture |
| Sex therapy | NA | NA | Helpful for all FSD diagnoses |
| Pelvic floor physical therapy | NA | NA | For treatment of pelvic floor dysfunction |
| Mechanical devices | Vibrators<br>Clitoral vacuum device (Eros) | NA | Used to enhance vulvar, clitoral, and vaginal stimulation |
| Vaginal lasers (FDA cleared, but no specific indication for genitourinary syndrome of menopause) | Carbon dioxide fractional lasers<br>Erbium YAG lasers | NA | Genitourinary syndrome of menopause |

From Parish SJ, Hahn SR, Goldstein SW, et al. The International Society for the Study of Women's Sexual Health Process of Care for the Identification of Sexual Concerns and Problems in Women. *Mayo Clin Proc.* 2019;94(5):842-856. Copyright 2019 Mayo Foundation for Medical Education and Research.
*CEE,* Conjugated equine estrogen; *FDA,* Food and Drug Administration; *FSD,* female sexual dysfunction; *NA,* not applicable; *YAG,* yttrium-aluminum-garnet.

## LESBIAN, BISEXUAL, AND TRANSGENDER HEALTH CARE

Despite growing awareness of the health care issues and needs of lesbian, gay, bisexual, and transgender (LGBT) individuals, most physicians have received little or no training in this area. Reviews (e.g., Lapinski, 2018; Schulman, 2019) provide useful guidance for providing culturally competent, informed care. Terminology in this area is evolving, but in general the terms *lesbian*, *gay*, and *bisexual* refer to sexual orientation, whereas the term *transgender* refers to gender identity. In contrast to cisgender individuals, whose gender identity matches the gender assigned at birth, transgender individuals' gender identity differs from that assigned at birth. Other gender minority individuals may identify not as transgender but as genderfluid, bigender, or genderqueer. Polling data indicate that most 18 to 34 year olds see gender as being on a spectrum, 12% of millennials self-identify as transgender or gender nonconforming, and 56% of 13 to 20 year olds know someone who uses gender-neutral pronouns.

LGBT and gender minority people often experience chronic stress, including harassment and discrimination, a need for secrecy about one's sexual orientation or gender identity, and internalization of negative societal attitudes. LGBT populations have increased rates of victimization, adverse childhood events, bullying, interpersonal violence, unemployment, poverty, and health care disparities, and racial minority and disabled individuals are at particularly high risk.

**Multiple studies have now shown increased rates of depression, anxiety, substance use disorders, suicidal thoughts, and suicide attempts in LGBT individuals, especially adolescents.** The lifetime risk for suicide attempts is increased sixfold in bisexual and threefold in lesbian women, and 41% of transgender individuals report at least one suicide attempt (Grant, 2010). The risk for suicide attempts in LGBT youth has been reported to be four times that of heterosexual peers. A number of studies have now documented that lesbian women use mental health services at high rates, with 70% to 80% having been in therapy, primarily for depression and relationship problems. Family and community support and connectedness have been shown to increase resilience.

The DSM-5 includes a psychiatric diagnosis of gender dysphoria, defined as marked incongruence between one's experienced/expressed versus assigned gender, associated with clinically significant distress or impairment. This diagnosis, although providing a basis for reimbursement for desired medical and surgical interventions, has raised concerns about pathologization. In addition, historically the approach of mental health practitioners to LGBT individuals was to attempt to change their sexual orientation or gender identity through conversion therapy, which has been shown to be ineffective and harmful. **In the *International Classification of Diseases, Eleventh Revision* (ICD-11), gender incongruence has been moved from mental health disorders to sexual health conditions. A number of different measures have been recommended to provide an affirming health care**

**BOX 9.14** *Measures to Provide a Gender-Affirming Practice*

**PRACTICE ENVIRONMENT**

LGBT-relevant posters, brochures in waiting room
Gender-neutral restrooms

**INTAKE PROCESS**

Friendly staff with awareness of LGBT issues
Intake forms allowing a wide variety of gender identities
Asking about preferred pronouns

**CLINICAL CARE**

Open, respectful, nonjudgmental approach
Asking about and using preferred pronouns
Admitting incomplete knowledge and working to increase knowledge
Electronic health record allowing a wide range of gender identities and careful tracking of sexual orientation, natal gender, gender identity, organ inventory

**environment for LGBT patients and to enhance the likelihood of high-quality care (Box 9.14).** These include environmental, staff, medical record, and clinician factors.

Lesbians have a higher rate of cardiovascular risk factors, such as obesity and smoking. Smoking rates are especially high in lesbian adolescents. Lesbian and bisexual women are twice as likely to be obese as heterosexual women. Since the 1990s, lesbian women have become increasingly willing to disclose their sexual orientation to health care providers and to seek routine physical examinations. Nonetheless, their rates of routine physicals and Papanicolaou (Pap) smears are lower than national guidelines and lower than those of their heterosexual peers, and adolescents in particular have difficulty disclosing their sexual orientation to physicians. LGBT youth report that they think their health care provider should know their sexual orientation to provide the best possible care, but two thirds do not disclose this information. Lesbians prefer female and preferably lesbian health care providers and often use alternative health care providers such as nonphysicians, acupuncturists, and massage therapists. Lesbian women are 10 times less likely to be screened for cervical cancer than heterosexual women, even though their risk of developing the disease is comparable. This has been thought to be due to lack of concern and a belief that lesbian women were at low risk for cervical cancer. However, studies show human papillomavirus (HPV) screening and Pap smear frequency should be the same as the recommendations for heterosexual women. Sexually transmitted diseases also occur in lesbian women, particularly those who have had male partners.

Lesbians are increasingly having children through artificial insemination and adoption. Couples wishing to have children through donor insemination have concerns about coming out to their obstetrician, involving the nonpregnant partner, legal issues, family support, and parenting issues.

Transgender individuals are less likely to have health insurance, have poorer access to health care, and report discrimination and mistreatment in medical settings, with 28% reporting harassment, 19% being denied care, and 2% experiencing violence in a health care setting (Grant, 2010). Obstetrician-gynecologists may see such individuals at different stages of gender transition, including social (e.g., appearance, pronouns, preferred name, sexual behaviors), medical (e.g., use of hormones), or surgical. General principles of care include keeping an organ inventory for the patient and updating it annually (see Lapinski, 2018, for a sample organ inventory) to ensure appropriate preventive medical care and monitoring, and directing physical examinations and testing to the anatomy and hormonal interventions present, rather than to apparent gender. Patients may have specific questions or need counseling regarding effects of gender transition on fertility, fertility preservation, and changes in hormone treatment to allow pregnancy (e.g., a transgender man whose natal gender is female discontinuing testosterone treatment during pregnancy and breastfeeding).

In general, obstetrician-gynecologists need to be comfortable treating and advising LGBT and gender-minority individuals and couples, not just for pregnancy but also for general health issues or should refer them to an appropriate provider.

## RAPE, SEXUAL ASSAULT, AND INTIMATE PARTNER VIOLENCE

### Rape

**Rape, or the sexual assault of children, women, and men, is a common act. Sexual assault encompasses many acts, including rape, unwanted kissing or touching or genital touching. *Rape* is a legal term, redefined by the Federal Bureau of Investigation (FBI) in 2013 as any penetration, no matter how slight, of a body orifice (vagina or anus), with any body part or object, or oral penetration by a sex organ of another person, without the consent of the victim.** Sexual assault definitions and terms vary by state. Unfortunately, these are common problem all over the world. A 2014 worldwide systematic review found 7.2% of women had ever experienced nonpartner sexual violence. The rates were 8% to 13% in North America with higher rates in sub-Saharan Africa and lower in Asia. Another study found 19% of U.S. women reported they had experienced attempted or completed rape and nearly 80% had been first raped before the age of 25 years. In separating out by female age groups, 11% of high school adolescents reorted having been forced to have sex. The percentage increases the younger the adolescent is for involuntary first intercourse. Approximately 20% to 25% of women in college have been victims of actual or attempted sexual assault during college. Among women 18 years of age or older, 31.5% who were raped sustained physical injury and 36% of injured female victims received medical treatment. Of the rape victims who came to the emergency room, two thirds had general body trauma. Estimates suggest only 16% to 38% of rape victims report the rape to law enforcement. Victims are often reluctant to report sexual assault to the authorities because of embarrassment, fear of retribution, feelings of guilt, assumptions that little will be done, or simply lack of knowledge of their rights.

In the past, society has held many misconceptions about the rape victim, particularly female victims. These included the notion that the individual encouraged the rape by specific behavior or dress and that no person who did not wish to be raped could be raped. Furthermore, the feeling that rape was an indication of basic promiscuity was widely held. To some extent, many of these societal misconceptions are held today.

Sexual assault happens to people of all ages and races in all socioeconomic groups. The very young, the mentally and physically handicapped, and the very old are particularly susceptible. Recent studies found homeless women and women with mental illness are particularly vulnerable to sexual assaults compared with the general population. Although men can be victims of sexual violence, most victims are female. Sexual violence can be unwanted touching and rape, but it also includes nonphysical distressing acts of sexual harassment, threats, peeping, and taking nude photos without consent. The CDC reported in 2016 that lifetime estimates of rape or attempted rape of women range from 32.3% among multiracial women, 27.5% among American Indian/Alaska Native women, 21.2% among Black women,

20.5% among non-Hispanic white women, to 13.6% among Hispanic women. Furthermore, among sexual minorities, 46.1% and 13.1% of bisexual and lesbian women, respectively, have experienced rape at some point in their lives. Another vulnerable group appears to be women in the military. There are reports of high prevalence of military sexual trauma, sexual harassment, and assault during military service, which has prompted the Veterans Health Administration to enact several policies to address the detrimental health impacts of this experience.

Although the perpetrator may be a stranger, he or she is often an individual well known to the victim. In fact, for first rape experience in women, 30.4% of the time the perpetrator was known to be an intimate partner, 23.7% a family member, and 20% of the time an acquaintance.

Some situations have been defined as variants of sexual assault. These include marital rape, which involves forced coitus or related acts without consent but within the marital relationship, and "date rape." In the latter situation the woman may voluntarily participate in sexual play, but coitus is performed, often forcibly, without her consent. Date rape is often not reported because the victim may believe she contributed by partially participating. In fact, a 2014 U.S. Justice Department report said that up to 80% of sexual assaults in college settings are unreported.

Almost all states have statutes that criminalize coitus with women younger than certain specified ages. Such an act is referred to as *statutory rape.* Consent is irrelevant because the woman is defined by statute as being incapable of consenting.

During a rape, the victim loses control over his or her life for that period and often experiences anxiety and fear. When the attack is life threatening, shock with associated physical and psychological symptoms may occur. Burgess (1974) identified two phases of the rape-trauma syndrome. The immediate, or acute, phase lasts from hours to days and may be associated with a paralysis of the individual's usual coping mechanisms. Outwardly the victim may demonstrate manifestations ranging from complete loss of emotional control to a well-controlled behavior pattern. The actual reaction may depend on a number of factors, including the relationship of the victim to the attacker, whether force was used, and the length of time the victim was held against his or her will. Generally the victim appears disorganized and may complain of both physical and emotional symptoms. Physical complaints include specific injuries or general complaints of soreness, eating problems, headaches, and sleep disturbances. Behavior patterns may include fear, mood swings, irritability, guilt, anger, depression, and difficulties in concentrating. Often the victim will complain of flashbacks of the attack. Medical care is often sought during the acute period, and at this point it is the physician's responsibility to assess the specific medical problems and also to offer a program of emotional support and reassurance.

The second phase of the rape-trauma syndrome involves long-term adjustment and is designated the reorganization phase. During this time, flashbacks and nightmares may continue, but phobias may also develop. These may be directed against members of the offending sex, the sex act itself, or nonrelated circumstances, such as a newly developed fear of crowds or heights. During this period the victim may institute a number of important lifestyle changes, including job, residence, friends, and significant others. If major complications such as the contraction of a sexually transmitted infection (STI) or a pregnancy occur, resolution may be more difficult. The reorganization period may last from months to years and generally involves an attempt on the part of the victim to regain control over his or her life. During this time, medical care and counseling must be nonjudgmental, sensitive, and anticipatory. When the physician realizes that the patient is contemplating a major lifestyle change during this period, it is probably appropriate to point out to the patient why the change is being contemplated and the complicating effects it may have on the patient's overall well-being.

In some women, rape, like other trauma, can lead to ongoing, persistent PTSD, discussed earlier in this chapter, with disabling nightmares, flashbacks, hyperarousal, avoidance, depression, anxiety, poor sleep, and panic. Individuals with a history of trauma before the rape; greater severity, duration, and life-threatening nature of the assault; poor social support; and a history of depression or anxiety are more susceptible to developing PTSD. Among woman aged 40 to 60 years, 22% reported a history of sexual assault, and this group had significantly increased odds of depression, anxiety, and poor sleep (Thurstone, 2019). Approximately 15% to 20% of women ages 18 to 50 have chronic pelvic pain of more than a year's duration. An estimated 40% to 50% of those women have a history of physical or sexual abuse.

## Physician's Responsibility in Caring for a Rape Victim

Although any individual may become a rape victim, this discussion will be limited to the care of a woman, as is appropriate for a gynecology textbook (ACOG, 2019). **The physician's responsibility may be divided into three categories: medical, medicolegal, and supportive, as shown in Box 9.15.**

### Medical

The physician's medical responsibilities are to treat injuries and to perform appropriate tests for, to prevent, and to treat infections and pregnancies. It is important to obtain informed consent before examining the patient and collecting specimens. In addition to addressing legal requirements, it helps the victim to regain control over her body and her life. After acute injuries have been determined and stabilized, a careful history and physical examination should be performed. It is important to have a

**BOX 9.15** *Physician's* Responsibilities in Caring for a Rape Victim

**MEDICAL**

Treat injuries
Diagnose and treat STIs
Prevent pregnancy
Provide appropriate infectious disease prophylaxis

**MEDICOLEGAL**

Obtain informed consent and have chaperone.
Document history carefully
Examine patient thoroughly and specifically note injuries
Consider drawing and photographs of injuries
Obtain appropriate specimens for STI testing
Collect articles of clothing
Collect vaginal (rectal and pharyngeal) samples for sperm
Comb pubic hair for hair samples
Collect fingernail scrapings where appropriate
Collect saliva for secretion substance
Turn specimens over to forensic authorities and receive receipts for chart

**EMOTIONAL SUPPORT**

Discuss degree of injury, probability of infection, and possibility of pregnancy
Discuss the general course that can be predicted
Consult with a rape-trauma counselor
Arrange a follow-up visit for a medical and emotional evaluation in 1 to 4 weeks
Reassure as much as possible

*STI,* Sexually transmitted infection.

chaperone present while taking the history, performing the examination, and collecting the specimen, to reassure the victim and to provide support. The presence of such a third party probably reduces feelings of vulnerability on the part of the victim. She should be asked to state in her own words what happened; if she knew the attacker, and if not, to describe the attacker; and to describe the specific acts performed. A history of previous gynecologic conditions, particularly infections and pregnancy, use of contraception, and the date of last menstrual period, should be recorded. It is necessary to determine whether the patient may have a preexisting pregnancy or be at risk for pregnancy. It is also important to ascertain whether she has had a preexisting pelvic infection (Fig. 9.9).

Experience derived at the Sexual Assault Center in Seattle, Washington, demonstrated that between 12% and 40% of victims who are sexually assaulted have injuries. Most of these,

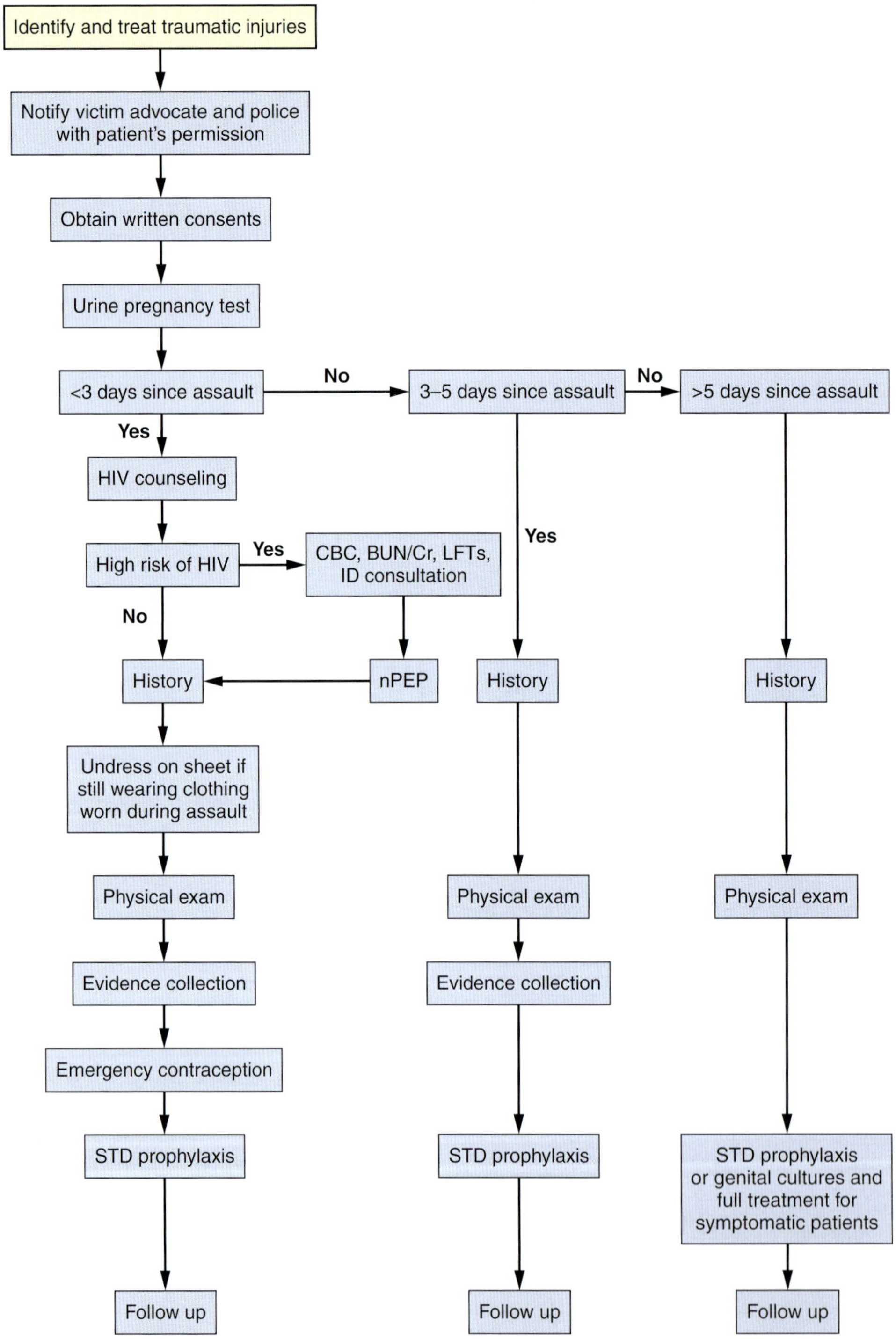


**Fig. 9.9** Sexual assault flowchart. *BUN,* Blood urea nitrogen; *CBC,* complete blood cell count; *Cr,* creatinine; *ID,* infectious disease; *LFT,* liver function test; *nPEP,* nonoccupational postexposure prophylaxis; *STD,* sexually transmitted disease. (From Fonge Y, Chisholm SL. Sexual assault. Emergency department management of patients after sexual assault. In Ferri F, ed. *Ferri's Clinical Advisor 2020.* St. Louis, MO: Elsevier; 2020.)

however, are minor and require simple reparative therapy. Only about 1% require hospitalization and major operative repair. Lack of genital injury does not rule out assault. Nonetheless, the victim will perceive the experience as having been life threatening because in many cases it may have been. Many injuries occur when the victim is restrained or physically coerced into the sexual act. Thus the physician should seek bruises, abrasions, or lacerations on the neck, back, buttocks, or extremities. Where a knife was used as a coercive tactic, small cuts may also be found. Erythema, lacerations, and edema of the vulva or rectum may occur because of manipulation of these areas with the hand or the penis. These are particularly common in children or virginal victims but may occur in any woman and should be looked for (Adams, 2018). Superficial or extensive lacerations of the hymen, posterior fourchette, or vagina may occur in virginal victims or in the elderly. Lacerations may also be noted in the area of the urethra, the rectum, and at times through the vaginal vault into the abdominal cavity. In addition, bite marks may be noted in any of these regions. Occasionally, foreign objects are inserted into the vagina, the urethra, or the rectum and may be found in situ.

***Summary of the Examination***

Go at the patient's pace and treat them with respect.

Have a chaperone and advocate for the woman.

Explain at regular intervals what you wish to do and why, remembering that consent is an ongoing process.

Have a good light source and use magnification as necessary.

Conduct a head to toe examination. Documentation of an injury should include:

- Abrasion
- Bruise
- Laceration
- Incision
- Bite marks
- Heat, chemical or electrical injury
- Size, shape, position, pattern
- Associated features (e.g., tenderness and swelling)

Consider the use of video colposcopy for the anogenital examination.

Record all negative and positive findings.

Most victims are concerned about possible infections transmission as a result of the rape. A review on the risk of infection in rape victims found it was difficult to separate new from existing infection but placed the prevalence of STIs as follows: *Neisseria gonorrhoeae* 0% to 26.3%, *Chlamydia trachomatis* 3.9% to 17%, *Treponema pallidum* 0% to 5.6%, *Trichomonas vaginalis* 0% to 19%, and HPV 0.6% to 2.3%. Few studies are available to predict the actual risk of acquiring an STI, but *C. trachomatis* may be the most commonly acquired infection incurred under these circumstances. Most victims fear acquiring HIV as a result of a sexual attack, but current risks are probably not high depending on the population involved and the sexual acts performed. Increased risk of HIV transmission occur with genital or rectal trauma leading to bleeding, multiple lacerations or deep wounds, and preexisting genital infection in the victim. In consensual sex, the risk for HIV transmission from vaginal intercourse is 0.1% to 0.2% and for receptive anal intercourse it is 0.5% to 3%.

Commercial "evidence kits" are available. State crime laboratory testing may include urine or serum for date rape drugs when amnesia or sedation is present. A speculum examination is not always necessary, but if bleeding is reported or noted on external vulvar examination, it is appropriate. It must be remembered that infection may not be limited to the vagina but may also include the pharynx or the rectum. Specific history to raise a suspicion of this possibility should be sought. Urine or nonculture nuclear amplification tests (NAATs) for *N. gonorrhoeae* and *C. trachomatis* are preferred according to the CDC 2015 guidelines. In addition,

**BOX 9.16** *Sexually Transmitted Diseases and Tests Available to Physicians Caring for a Rape-Trauma Victim*

NAATs for *Neisseria gonorrhoeae**
NAATs for *Chlamydia trachomatis**
NAATs from vaginal specimen for *Trichomonas vaginalis*
HIV—serology
Hepatitis B—screening serology
Syphilis—rapid plasma regain (RPR)
Point-of-care testing especially if vaginal discharge, malodor or itching
- *Trichomonas*—saline wet mount preparation and culture
- *Bacterial vaginosis*—pH, saline wet mount preparation
- *Candida*—potassium hydroxide wet mount preparation

Other considerations
- Herpes simplex—culture lesion or serology
- Cytomegalovirus—serology
- Condyloma virus—study lesion

*At sites of penetration or attempted penetration, urine or vaginal.
*NAAT,* Nucleic acid amplification test.

conventional cultures of the rectum and of the oral pharynx are indicated when the history suggests that this would be productive. A wet mount for *T. vaginalis* and bacterial vaginosis and a potassium hydroxide mount for *Candida albicans* are also useful (Box 9.16). Investigation for syphilis (rapid plasma regain [RPR]) is not routinely recommended at the Sexual Assault Center in Seattle, Washington, but may be done in follow-up. With rising syphilis rates nationwide, this may become routine.

Because the victim is also at risk for infection by the herpesvirus, hepatitis B virus, cytomegalovirus, HIV, condyloma acuminatum, and a variety of other STIs, the physician may wish to screen for those that seem appropriate at the time the victim is seen in the acute stage. Hepatitis B and HPV vaccination may be appropriate if the victim is not previously vaccinated and of appropriate age. Tetanus prophylaxis is appropriate in some cases as well. At follow-up visits the patient should again be investigated for signs and symptoms of the STIs, and appropriate repeat cultures, NAATs, and serologic studies should be obtained. Be aware that compliance with follow-up visits is poor. Prophylactic antibiotics are useful in acute rape management when the patient is concerned about contracting an STI or knows the assailant to be high risk. The CDC recommends the woman can be given a single dose of ceftriaxone 250 mg intramuscularly for gonorrhea prophylaxis plus single-dose azithromycin, 1 g PO, for chlamydia prophylaxis plus metronidazole 2 g PO in a single dose or tinidazole 2 g PO in a single dose for trichomoniasis. If the patient is pregnant, consider giving no medications, and follow-up screening should be done in 2 weeks. If prophylaxis is desired, these antibiotics are class B drugs in pregnancy (except doxycycline, which should not be given and is class D). This should prevent gonorrhea and chlamydia infection but will have no effect on herpes, condylomata, or many of the other problems mentioned. Postexposure HIV prophylaxis is available, and the CDC website has advice. It should be discussed with individuals initiating care less than 72 hours after assault and particularly if the victim has genital or rectal trauma. It is recommended if the assailant is known to have HIV or AIDS.

**Pregnancy**

The patient's menstrual history, birth control regimen, and pregnancy status should be assessed. If the patient is at risk for pregnancy at the time of the assault, an appropriate emergency contraception or "morning after" prophylaxis can be offered as long as the pregnancy test was negative and if given within 72 hours after unprotected intercourse (1.5 mg levonorgestrel). More alternatives are discussed in Chapter 13. In the experience of most sexual assault centers, the chance of pregnancy occurring is quite low. Some have estimated that approximately 5% of victims having a single, unprotected coitus will become pregnant. However, if the patient has been exposed at midcycle, the risk will be higher. The risk is higher in adolescents, who often are not on contraception and have higher fertility rates.

**TABLE 9.7** Survival Time of Sperm

| Source | Motile Sperm | Sperm | Acid Phosphatase |
|---|---|---|---|
| Vagina | Up to 8 hr | Up to 7-9 days | Variable (up to 48 hr) |
| Pharynx | 6 hr | Unknown | 100 IU* |
| Rectum | Undetermined | 20-24 hr | 100 IU* |
| Cervix | Up to 5 days | Up to 17 days | Similar to vagina |

From Anderson S. *Sexual Assault—Medical-Legal Aspects: An Unpublished Training Packet for Pediatric House Staff.* Seattle, WA: Harborview Medical Center; 1980.
*Minimum detectable.

## Medicolegal

To be meaningful, medicolegal material must be collected shortly after the assault takes place and definitely within 96 hours. The woman can be reassured that laws in all 50 states strictly limit use of past STIs or sexual history during a trial so as not to discredit her testimony. Commercially manufactured evidence kits are available and help with careful, thorough documentation and for preserving the chain of evidence for a legal case. Victims should be encouraged to come immediately to a center where they can be evaluated before bathing, urinating, defecating, washing out their mouths, changing clothes, or cleaning their fingernails. The U.S. Department of Justice, Office of Victims of Crime, supports Sexual Assault Nurse Evaluation (SANE) programs, which have models for acute care for sexual assault. Some institutions have Sexual Assault Response Teams (SARTs), so experts are available to do the appropriate psychological, medical, and legal evaluation. You should know the resources available in your community.

In general, evidence for coitus will be present in the vagina for as long as 48 hours after the attack, but in other orifices the evidence may last only up to 6 hours. Appropriate tests should document the patient's physical and emotional condition as judged by her history and physical examination and should include data that document the use of force, evidence for sexual contact, and materials that may help identify the offender. To document that force was used, the physician should carefully describe each injury noted and illustrate with either drawings or photographs. Detail is important, because injuries suffered by sexual assault victims have common patterns. Because *rape* and *sexual assault* are legal terms, they should not be stated as diagnoses; rather the physician should report findings as "consistent with use of force." Documentation of sexual contact must begin with a history of when the patient had intercourse before the attack. If sperm or semen is found in the vagina or cervix of a victim, it must not be confused with such substances deposited during the victim's prior consenting sexual acts. Sexual contact will be verified by analysis of secretions from the vagina or rectum by identifying motile sperm. Nonmotile sperm may be present as well if the attack occurred 12 to 20 hours previously. In some instances, motile sperm will be noted for as long as 2 to 3 days in the endocervix. Vaginal wet mount is no longer recommended for identifying sperm as it lacks reproducibility. Manufactured evidence kits are available.

It is difficult to ascertain whether ejaculation occurred in the mouth, because residual seminal fluid is rapidly destroyed by bacteria and salivary enzymes, making documentation of such an event difficult after more than a few hours have passed. Seminal fluid may be found staining the skin or the clothing several hours after the attack, and this should be looked for. Because acid phosphatase is an enzyme found in high concentrations in seminal fluid, substances removed for analysis should be tested for this enzyme. Table 9.7 demonstrates the survival time of sperm in the pharynx, rectum, and cervix.

In addition to documenting that intercourse has taken place, an attempt should be made to identify the perpetrator. In this regard, all clothing intimately associated with the area of assault should be collected, labeled, and submitted to legal authorities. In addition, smears of vaginal secretions or a Pap smear should be made to permanently document the presence of sperm. Vaginal secretions needed for DNA typing should be collected by wet or dry swab and refrigerated until a pathologist can process them. In the near future tests may also be available to identify prostate-specific antigen and seminal vesicle–specific antigen in vaginal secretions. Highly sensitive DNA fingerprinting is now readily available and is admissible in many jurisdictions. Pubic hair combings should be performed in an attempt to obtain pubic hair of the assailant. Saliva should be collected from the victim to ascertain whether she secretes an antigen that could differentiate her from substances obtained from the perpetrator. Finally, fingernail scrapings should be obtained for skin or blood if the victim scratched the perpetrator. Specific blood or DNA typing may be conducted to help identify the attacker. All materials collected should be labeled and turned over to the legal authority or pathologist, depending on the system used by the medical unit. A receipt should be obtained, and this should be documented in the patient's chart.

## Emotional Support for the Victim

After the physical needs of the patient have been met and after the physician has carefully documented the information concerning the sexual contact, he or she should discuss with the victim the degree of injury, probability of infection or pregnancy, general course that the victim might be expected to follow with respect to these, and how follow-up to aid prevention will be carried out. The physician must allow the victim to vent anxieties, fears and correct misconceptions. In doing this, the physician may call on other health personnel, such as individuals trained to help rape-trauma victims, to facilitate counseling and follow-up. The patient should not be released until specific follow-up plans are made and the patient understands what they are. A follow-up visit should be planned within 1 to 4 weeks to reevaluate the patient's medical, infectious disease, pregnancy, and psychological status. At this point, follow-up counseling should be encouraged. It is important at each visit to emphasize to the patient that she was a victim and holds no blame. At each step she must be allowed to vent her feelings and to discuss her current conceptions of the problem. It is important that the physician realize that some patients will appear to have excellent emotional control when seen immediately after a rape. This is an acute expression of the patient's defense mechanisms and should not be misinterpreted to indicate that the patient is coping with the circumstances. All the recommendations just listed should be followed *regardless* of the patient's apparent condition. Specific plans for follow-up are equally important in such an individual because it must be anticipated that she will follow the same postrape emotional process as anyone else. Finally, it is important to emphasize and reemphasize that at no time during the management or follow-up care of the rape victim should any comments be made by health care professionals suggesting that the patient was anything other than a victim. These women are sensitive to any accusations and insinuations and may even believe that they may have in some way been responsible for the rape. Their future well-being may be severely affected by creating such an impression.

## Female Circumcision

A form of sexual abuse only recently recognized in the Western world is female circumcision or genital cutting. It is a practice growing out of cultural and traditional beliefs dating back several thousand years. The WHO estimates that between 85 and 200 million women undergo these procedures each year. Although they are often performed in parts of Africa, the Middle East, and Southeast Asia, they are rarely performed in the United States or the rest of the Western world. About 168,000 women who have undergone such procedures currently live in the United States, and physicians may see the results of these procedures in patients who emigrate from countries where they are practiced.

The various forms of female genital mutilation include removal of the clitoral prepuce, excision of the clitoris, or removal of the clitoris and labia minora (Fig. 9.10). Occasionally the labia majora are also partially removed and the vagina partially sutured closed. The procedures are often performed between early childhood and age 14 and often without anesthesia under unsterile conditions by untrained practitioners. Therefore a variety of complications often occur, including infection, tetanus, shock, hemorrhage, and death. Long-term problems include chronic infection, scar formation, local abscesses, sterility, and incontinence. In addition, depression, anxiety, sexual dysfunction, dyspareunia, obstetric complications, and the psychosomatic conditions associated with sexual abuse may be seen. Physicians who care for women with this condition must develop an understanding of the cultural mores that lead to the performance of the procedure and the implications on these cultural beliefs that remedial surgery

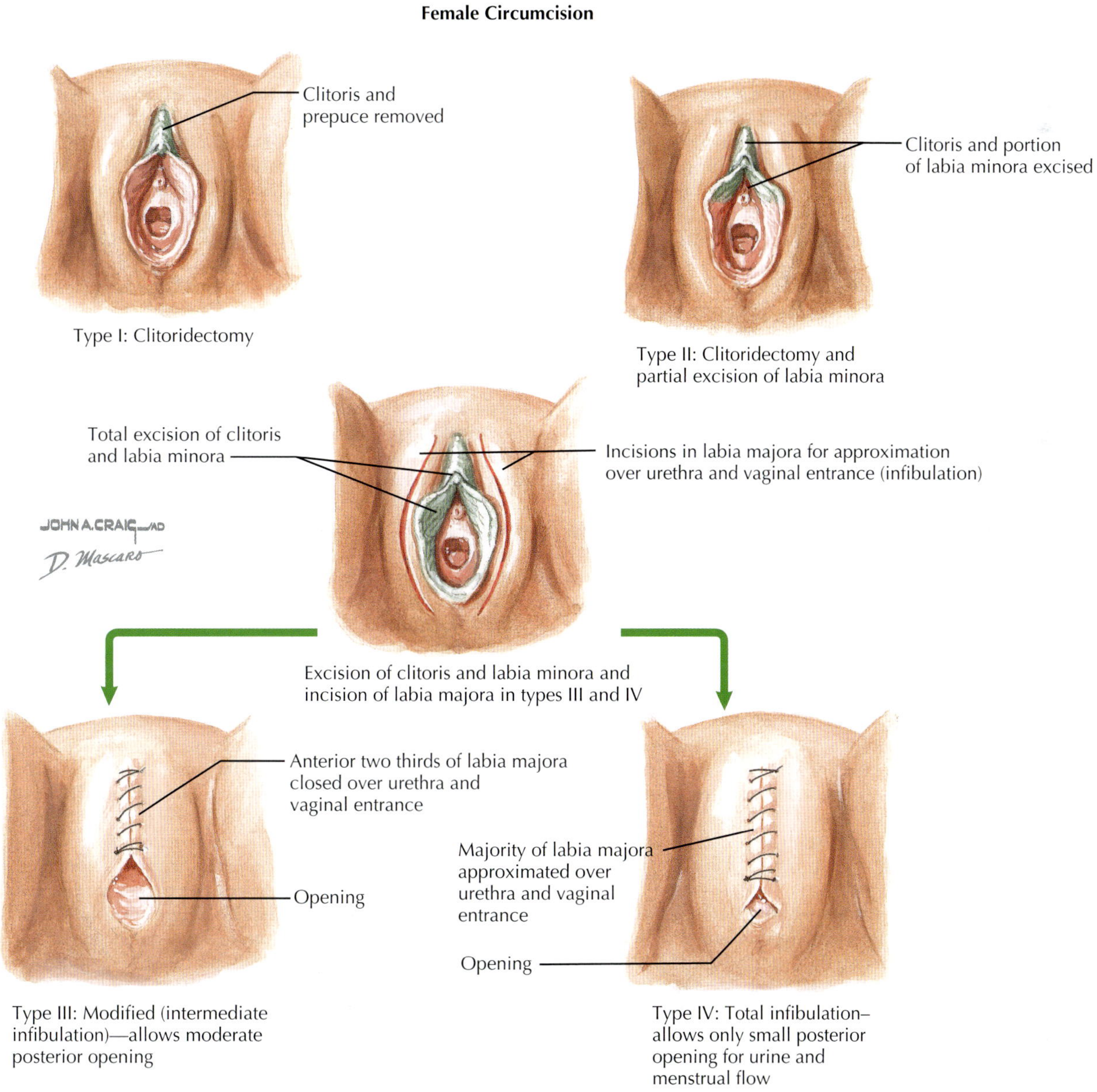


**Fig. 9.10** Female circumcision. (From Smith RP. *Netter's Obstetrics and Gynecology.* 3rd ed. Philadelphia, PA: Elsevier; 2018:188-190. 2018.)

may imply. Certainly the patient and her sexual partner should be involved in all decisions concerning intervention.

## Abuse

### Intimate Partner Violence

*Domestic violence*, *partner abuse*, *intimate partner violence*, *the battered woman*, and *spouse abuse* are terms that refer to violence occurring between partners in an ongoing relationship even if they are not married. A battered woman is defined as any woman older than age 16 with evidence of physical abuse on at least one occasion at the hands of an intimate male partner. The *battered wife syndrome* is defined as a symptom complex occurring as a result of violence in which a woman has at any time received deliberate, severe, or repeated (more than three times) physical abuse from her husband or significant male partner in which the minimal injury is bruising. ***Intimate partner violence*** **(IPV) is the CDC's preferred term because it allows for men or women to be the victim and intimate partners can be the same or opposite sex.** Actual or threatened physical, sexual, or psychological abuse by a current or former spouse (including common-law spouses), dating partner, boyfriend, or girlfriend is considered IPV. The American Medical Association (AMA) has treatment guidelines and **defines IPV as a "pattern of coercive behaviors that may include repeated battering and injury, psychological or emotional abuse, sexual assault, progressive societal isolation, economic deprivation, intimidation and stalking."** The actual physical abuse may vary from minimal activity, such as verbal abuse or threat of violence, to throwing an object, throwing an object at someone, pushing, slapping, kicking, hitting, beating, threatening with a weapon, or using a weapon. These acts may be spontaneous or intentionally planned. Most such violence is accompanied by mental abuse and intimidation. Partner abuse is often seen in conjunction with abuse of children and elderly persons in the same household. A 2008 study by Breiding and colleagues investigated risk factors for IPV in noninstitutionalized adults and found the victims to be female, of ethnic/racial minority, to have a lower income, to be less educated, and to be older. **There remain significant societal, cultural, and economic barriers for victims to seek help.**

It is difficult to ascertain the specific incidence of domestic violence, but it has been estimated that 4.5 million cases of IPV occur in the United States each year, and some authors have stated that at least 50% of family relationships are violent. In a 1984 U.S. Department of Justice study, 57% of 450,000 annual acts of family violence were committed by spouses or ex-spouses, and the wife was a victim in 93% of cases. In at least one fourth of these cases the violent acts had occurred at least three times in the previous 6 months. In 1990 statistics gathered by the FBI reported similar findings. A 2008 phone survey of noninstitutionalized adults provided some of the best IPV prevalence data to date. Nineteen percent of women reported threatened physical violence over their lifetime, 14.5% reported attempted physical violence, and 20.2% completed physical violence. The frequency of unwanted sex for an intimate partner was 10.2%. Within the previous 12 months, 1.4% of women reported completed physical or sexual violence.

**In addition, it has been estimated that between one third and one half of female homicide victims are murdered by their male partners,** whereas only 12% of male homicide victims are killed by their female partners. In 1992 the AMA published guidelines for the diagnosis and treatment of domestic violence. The association noted that 47% of husbands who beat their wives do so three or more times per year, that 14% of ever-married women reported being raped by their current or former husbands, and that rape is a significant or major form of abuse in 54% of violent marriages. The AMA guidelines also summarized various studies noting that battered women may account for 22% to 35% of women seeking care for any reason in emergency departments (the majority of whom are seen by medical or nontrauma services) and 19% to 30% of injured women seen in emergency departments. This was confirmed in a 2005 study in which 17% of women seeking care in an emergency department reported current abuse. **Nine percent to 14% of women seen in ambulatory care internal medicine clinics suffer IPV, and 26% to 28% of such women have been battered at some time.** The study states that 25% of women who attempt suicide, 25% who are receiving psychiatric services, and 23% of pregnant women seeking prenatal care have been victims of domestic violence. In addition, 45% to 59% of mothers of abused children have been abused, and 58% of women older than 30 who have been raped have been abused. In a gynecologic clinic in England, John and colleagues surveyed a cohort of 825 women. Twenty-one percent reported physical abuse, and of those, 48% also had forced sexual activity. A 2005 report confirmed the prevalence rates in health care facilities with 35% of obstetrics and gynecology patients reporting IPV and 13% of women seeking care reporting current abuse. Therefore it can be seen that domestic violence and battered women are common in our society today.

**The most common sites for injury are the head, neck, chest, abdomen, breast, and upper extremities.** Minor injuries such as scratches, bruises, sore muscles, and welts are common. The upper extremities may be fractured as the woman attempts to defend herself. Broken teeth, burns, laceration, head injury, and strangulation are also commonly observed. In a study from Yale, 84% of the injuries were severe enough to require medical treatment, and in 81% of the cases patients stated that the assailant had beaten them with the fists. In an English study of 100 women brought to a hostel for battered women, 44% suffered from lacerations and 59% stated that they had been kicked repeatedly. All women stated that they had been hit with a clenched fist. Fractures occurred in 32, and 9 of the women had been beaten and taken to the hostel unconscious. A 2006 study also found significant injury among victims; of 519,031 cases, 41% of assaults caused observable injuries and 28% required medical treatment.

Murder and suicide are common components of the domestic violence problem. In a large study from Denver, Walker reported that three quarters of the battered patients felt that the batterer would kill them during the relationship, and almost half felt that they might kill the batterer. Of these victims, 11% stated that they had actually tried to kill the batterer, and 87% believed that they themselves would be the ones to die if someone were killed. This is not an exaggeration because IPV resulted in 1544 deaths in 2004. One third of these women stated that they seriously considered committing suicide. Walker noted that victims and their attackers often are depressed and may move rapidly between suicidal and homicidal intent.

**There is a strong relationship between spouse battering and child abuse.** In Walker's study, 53% of men who abused their partners were noted also to abuse their children. Another one third had threatened to abuse their children. Interestingly, in the same relationship, 28% of the wives who themselves were abused stated that they had abused their children while living in the violent household, and an additional 6% thought that they might abuse their children at the time they were evaluated.

**Physical abuse in pregnancy is common and may be referred to as *prenatal child abuse*.** The incidence is somewhere between 1% and 20%, depending on the study population. In one study, 81 of 742 (10.9%) patients visiting a prenatal clinic stated that they had been victims of abuse at some time in the past, and 29 of these women stated that the abuse had continued into the pregnancy. Violence may increase postpartum. One fifth of these women noted an increase in abuse during pregnancy, and one third noted a decrease. In a study of a group of Medicaid-eligible postpartum women, a constellation of factors associated with violence during pregnancy was noted. Of the patients in this study, 7% suffered battering, and significant correlates including anxiety, depression, housing problems, inadequate prenatal care, and drug and alcohol abuse were identified. The women in the study who were battered during pregnancy suffered a more severe constellation of symptoms than did those who were battered only before pregnancy. In the case of pregnant patients, most studies note that battering is often directed to the breasts and abdomen.

It is important that physicians increase their ability to recognize the signs of intimate partner violence. A study classic study by Hilberman and Monson (1977) demonstrated that 25% of women treated for injuries in an emergency room were victims of wife battering. The physicians who were treating these patients made the correct diagnosis originally in only 3% of cases. Viken has listed a profile of the characteristics of the abused wife. These include a history of having been beaten as a child, raised in a single parent home, married as a teenager, and pregnant before marriage. Such women frequently visit clinics and emergency rooms with a variety of somatic complaints, including headaches, insomnia, choking sensation, hyperventilation, gastrointestinal symptoms, and chest, pelvic, and back pain. Noncompliance with the advice of physicians with respect to these complaints is common (Box 9.17).

In visits to the physician's office or emergency room, the patient often appears shy, frightened, embarrassed, evasive, anxious, or passive and often cries. The batterer may accompany the patient on such visits and stay close at hand to monitor what she says to the physician. Thus the woman may be hesitant to provide information about how she was injured, and the explanation given may not fit the injuries observed. Alcohol or other drug abuse is common in such individuals.

**Physicians should become comfortable with asking the patient whether she has been physically abused. Every pregnant woman should be screened for IPV.** Introductory questions such as "Has anyone hurt you or tried to injure you?" "Has an intimate partner ever threatened you with physical violence?" and "Have you ever been physically abused either recently or in the past?" are appropriate. The physician should follow up on any positive answers in a nonjudgmental manner in an attempt to learn what is happening. Physical examinations should be complete with particular attention to bruises, lacerations, burns, improbable injury, and other signs of injury. If the patient is wearing sunglasses, she should be asked to remove them so that the physician can determine whether there are eye injuries. If the patient is pregnant, bruises seen on the breasts or abdomen should always be discussed. Physicians should carefully note evidence for abuse in the patient's record.

**BOX 9.17** Somatic Complaints in Abused Women

Headaches
Insomnia
Choking sensation
Hyperventilation
Chest, back, or pelvic pain

**OTHER SIGNS AND SYMPTOMS**

Shyness
Fright
Embarrassment
Evasiveness
Jumpiness
Passivity
Frequent crying
Often accompanied by male partner
Drug or alcohol abuse (often overdose)
Injuries

From American College of Obstetricians and Gynecologists. The battered woman. *ACOG Technical Bull.* 1989;124.

Battering acts tend to run in cycles consisting of three phases. The first phase is tension building, in which tension between the couple gradually escalates, manifested by discrete acts that cause family friction. Name-calling, intimidating remarks, meanness, and mild physical abuse such as pushing are common. The batterer often expresses dissatisfaction and hostility in a somewhat chronic form. The victim may attempt to placate the batterer in hopes of pleasing him or calming him. She may actually believe at this point that she has the power to avoid aggravating the situation. She may not respond to his hostile actions and may even be successful from time to time in apparently reducing tensions. This, of course, will reinforce her belief that she can control the situation. As the tension phase builds, the batterer's anger is less controlled, and the victim may withdraw, fearing that she will inadvertently set off explosive behavior. Often this withdrawal is the signal for the batterer to become more aggressive. Anything may spark the hostile act, and the acute battering then takes place. This is the cycle's second phase and is represented by an uncontrollable discharge of tension that has built up through the first phase. The attack may take the form of both verbal and physical abuse, and the victim is often left injured. In self-defense the victim may actually injure or kill the batterer. In approximately two thirds of cases reported by Walker, alcohol abuse was involved. However, the alcohol use may have been the excuse rather than the reason for the battering. After the abuse has taken place, the third phase generally follows. In this situation, the batterer apologizes, asks forgiveness, and frequently shows kindness and remorse, showering the victim with gifts and promises. This gives the victim hope that the relationship can be saved and that the violence will not recur. Batterers are often charming and manipulative, offering the victim justification for forgiveness. The cycles, however, do repeat themselves, with the first phase increasing in length and intensity, the battering becoming more severe, and the third phase tending to decrease in both duration and intensity. The batterer learns that he can control the victim without obtaining much forgiveness. The victim becomes more demoralized and loses her ability to leave the situation even if she has the means and opportunity to do so.

Batterers, too, tend to have a specific profile in most cases. They are men who refuse to take responsibility for their behavior, blaming their victims for their violent acts. They often have strong controlling personalities and do not tolerate autonomy in their partners. They have rigid expectations of marriage and sexual behavior and consider their wives or partners as chattel. They wish to be cared for in their most basic needs, frequently make unrealistic demands on their wives, and show low tolerance for stress. Depression and suicide attempts are often a part of their behavior pattern, but in general they are aggressive and assaultive in most of their behavior, generally using violence to solve their problems. On the other hand, they are often charming and manipulative, especially in their relationships outside the marriage. They often exhibit low self-esteem, feelings of inadequacy, and a sense of helplessness, all of which are generally made worse by the prospects of losing their wives. It is typical behavior for male batterers to exhibit contempt for women in their usual activities. Therapy is usually ineffective and seems to work only when the man can be made to give up violence as his primary means of solving problems.

Once the physician discovers that a woman is living in an abusive relationship, it is important to acknowledge to the patient the seriousness of the situation. To do otherwise is to give the impression that the physician approves or at least accepts the violent condition. It is important to attend to the patient's injuries and to assess the patient's emotional status from the standpoint of a psychiatric condition such as a suicidal ideation, depression, anxiety, or signs of abuse of drugs, alcohol, or other medications. The physician should also attempt to estimate the woman's ability to assess her own situation and her readiness to take appropriate action. If problems involving mental illness are present, a referral to an appropriate mental health worker who is sensitive to the issues of domestic violence should be made. Physicians should know the community resources available for handling family violence. The police department, crisis hotline, rape relief centers, domestic violence programs, and legal aid services for abused women can offer help in the acute situation. Hospital emergency rooms and shelters for battered women and children are also excellent resources. Health care workers in these organizations or private practitioners who specialize in the care of battered women, their spouses, and their children can offer counseling and follow-up care. Such individuals may be social workers, psychologists, psychiatrists, or other mental health workers trained specifically for this purpose. The physician's job is to recognize the problem and either offer counseling or get counseling for the patient so that she understands her rights and alternatives and learns to protect herself and her children from future harm. The victim of abuse likely will not wish to leave her home because of economic concerns and a fear that the batterer may continue to pursue her. Although she may have the batterer arrested and served with restraining orders, she may be convinced that she and her children cannot be protected from the batterer. She may also believe that there is a possibility of reconciliation and of change in behavior on the part of the batterer. It is therefore reasonable to discuss an exit plan with the victim to be used should the violence recur. This exit plan should include the following:

1. Have a change of clothes packed for both her and her children including toilet articles, necessary medications, and an extra set of keys to the house and car. These can be placed in a suitcase and left with a friend or family member.
2. Keep some cash, a checkbook, and a savings account book with the friend or family member.
3. Other identification papers, such as birth certificates, social security cards, voter registration cards, utility bills, and driver's license, should be kept available because children will need to be enrolled in school and the woman may have to seek financial assistance.
4. Have something special, such as a toy or book, for each child.
5. Have financial records available, such as mortgage papers, rent receipts, and an automobile title.
6. Determine a plan on exactly where to go regardless of the time of day or night. This may be to a friend or relative's house or to a shelter for battered women and children.
7. Ask neighbors to call police if violence begins.
8. Remove weapons.
9. Teach children to call 9-1-1.

Rehearsing an exit plan, as one would conduct a fire drill, makes it possible for the battered woman to respond even under the stress of the battering. **Long-term aid and referral of the patient, her children, and the batterer to the appropriate resources is an important aspect of the care of such patients.** The ACOG has prepared a patient education brochure that physicians can keep in their offices and give to individuals who suffer from this problem. Making the brochures available in the office waiting room may encourage women with these needs to get help.

**These women often suffer from severe psychiatric problems, such as anxiety, depression, PTSD, and other pathologic conditions that may require psychotherapy.** Women who are both physically and sexually assaulted have significantly higher levels of PTSD compared with women who are physically abused only. However, women who suffer any abuse, including emotional abuse without physical or sexual abuse, have a higher rate of mental health problems, including postpartum depression. Group counseling or individual counseling may also help them to rebuild their lives as single individuals or single parents. It is often necessary to help them develop a skill that will enable them to be employable. Counseling programs take these things into consideration. Children of victims who may be victims as well also require counseling to avoid behavior patterns that will lead to aggressive behavior in their later lives.

IPV is a common problem that affects the family unit in particular and society in general. It can occur in all segments of society and reflects the violence that is a part of life today and the behavior of many (USPSTF, 2018 recommends screening reproductive age women). Physicians should learn to detect its presence in their patients and offer ways the victim can seek help. The help may include counseling for the victim, batterer, and children or constructing a plan for the woman to exit the relationship and rebuild her life in safety. There are many possible barriers for physicians screening for IPV and acting on their suspicions (Box 9.18). Ferguson's 2010 address about IPV gave multiple recommendations regarding clinical practice, education and training, and research needs in this area in hopes of "ending this blight against women."

If the male batterer has not undergone anger management therapy, family counseling or intervention can be extremely dangerous, as it often raises issues that exacerbate the violence and increase the risk of serious harm to the woman and her children. Therefore this should not be advised until such time as the male batterer has addressed and eliminated his violent behavior. In general, success in such attempts with respect to the male partner is usually minimal.

Although all states have requirements for reporting child abuse, not all states require the reporting of domestic violence. However, many states have aggressive programs for intervening in domestic violence cases, and physicians should become aware of the programs in effect in their area. The patient should always be encouraged to leave a violent situation and may need community resources to help with economic and social adjustment, as well as protection for herself and her children from the violent partner. ACOG's website has a page on resources for violence against women and lists each state's coalitions for sexual assault

**BOX 9.18** Possible Barriers to Physician Screening for Intimate Partner Violence (IPV)

- Belief that "someone else will take care of it"
- Forgetfulness
- Not a physician's responsibility/role
- IPV "should be private"
- "Cannot offer much"
- Lack of scientific evidence that screening improves outcomes
- Cynicism: "nothing will happen"
- Legal entanglement
- Worry about offending/angering patients
- Screening will take too much time
- Insufficient training
- Uncertainty about training requirements
- Uncertainly about legal implications if screen is positive
- Uncomfortable discussing issues of IPV
- "Do not need to ask; the patient will volunteer the information"
- Beliefs about victims of spouse abuse
- Fear of retaliation against patient
- Frustration over lack of patient disclosure
- Not scientific, "sexy"

From Ferguson JE 2nd. Why doesn't SOMEBODY do something? *Am J Obstet Gynecol.* 2010;202(6):635-643.

and domestic violence (https://www.acog.org/womens-health/faqs/intimate-partner-violence).

### The Elderly

The Select Committee on Aging, in investigating domestic violence against the elderly, held hearings before the Subcommittee of Human Services of the House of Representatives in 1980. The committee noted that approximately 500,000 to 2.5 million cases involving abuse of the elderly occur per year in the United States. **The committee documented that abuse of the elderly may be as large a nationwide problem as child abuse.** Usually the abused person is a woman older than age 75, often with a physical impairment. She is generally white, widowed, and living with relatives. The abuser is generally an adult child living within the family but may also be a spouse. Counseling issues involve the entire family but particularly the individual causing the abuse. Physicians who care for older patients should be alert for signs and symptoms of this type of domestic abuse; when it is found, community resources should be activated. All 50 states have passed legislation protecting the elderly from domestic violence and neglect. Forty-two states have mandatory reporting laws.

## GRIEF AND LOSS

The term *grief* is usually used to refer to the emotional, behavioral, and functional response to the death of a loved one. However, many people experience symptoms of grief in response to losses other than death, such as losing a marriage, a job, one's health, or hope of having children, as in infertility. **Gynecologists are likely to see women at times of uncomplicated grief, complicated grief, or grief-related major depression.** Recognizing when a grief reaction is following an expectable course, as opposed to being complicated or involving major depression, is important in ensuring that the woman receives needed treatment.

**Uncomplicated or "normal" grief has been postulated to follow defined stages, including initial numbness or shock, then sadness and depression, reorganization, and recovery.** However, the literature suggests that grief experiences vary significantly among different cultures, people, and individual losses, often with intermingling of different "stages" of grief at the same time. Grief is now thought to be a process with a wide spectrum of individual responses and a variable course, including not only painful feelings but also positive emotions and memories.

Shear (2015) has reviewed the nature of uncomplicated grief, complicated grief, and grief-related depression. **Acute grief occurs early after the loss, is intensely painful, and includes sadness, longing, preoccupation with thoughts of the deceased or of the loss, disturbed sleep and appetite, trouble concentrating, and separation from and lack of interest in other people and usual activities.** Bereavement may include benign hallucinations, such as hearing the voice, seeing, or sensing the presence of the deceased. Such experiences are normal and not of clinical concern. The loss of a loved one is associated with heightened risks of health problems such as myocardial infarction and Takotsubo (stress) cardiomyopathy, as well as depression, anxiety, and substance use disorders. Within a few months, acute grief gives way to integrated grief, a state in which the deceased or what has been lost is thought of often with sadness, but the woman is not preoccupied and can once more participate in pleasurable and meaningful activities and relationships. Triggers, including birthdays, anniversaries, or situations that remind her of the loss, may precipitate waves of grief, which gradually become less intense and less frequent over time. Uncomplicated grief does not require formal treatment but instead gradually lessens with the support of family, friends, and community such as church and clergy; reassurance; information about the expected course of grief; and sometimes the help of support groups.

**Complicated grief, or prolonged grief disorder, occurs in about 10% to 20% of people who lose a romantic partner and is more common than this with the death of a child.** It is more likely when the death is sudden or violent (e.g., homicide, suicide, or an accident). Symptoms include intense pain and longing, difficulty accepting the loss, anger, intrusive thoughts and ruminations, guilt, feelings of estrangement from other people, and suicidal thoughts. Risk factors include a history of mood and anxiety disorders, multiple losses, adverse life events, and other stressors reducing the woman's ability to cope. Complicated grief requires treatment to avoid becoming chronic and unremitting. Treatment should include psychotherapy specific for complicated grief or, if this is not available, therapy focusing on adapting to loss, restoring functioning, and returning to meaningful activities and goals. Antidepressant medication (citalopram) has been shown to be superior to placebo in treating depressive symptoms associated with complicated grief (Shear, 2016).

Acute grief may also be associated with symptoms that meet the criteria for major depression; 40% to 50% of bereaved people meet criteria at 1 month, about 20% to 25% at 2 months, and about 16% at 1 year. Bereavement-related depression is similar in clinical characteristics, course, and treatment response to major depression occurring after a range of other stressors or without any identifiable trigger. Women with a history of depression, or moderate to severe depressive symptoms as part of grief, should be treated aggressively, even in the first month or two after the loss, with antidepressant medication and psychotherapy, whereas those with milder depression can be monitored or referred for psychotherapy alone.

**Obstetricians and gynecologists may need to counsel patients experiencing grief related to several areas of reproduction, including spontaneous abortion, stillbirth, and infertility** (Bhat, 2016). About 15% to 20% of recognized pregnancies end in miscarriage. After a miscarriage, a woman may experience sadness, guilt, self-blame, anger, PTSD symptoms, and anxiety about future pregnancies. **Nongestational are also affected, although members of a couple may grieve in different ways.** A miscarriage most commonly represents the loss not of an established relationship but of hopes and expectations for the future, including pregnancy and parenthood. Despite this difference in the nature of the loss, the feelings of grief after miscarriage resemble those that may arise after losing a loved one, and the course of recovery is similar to that of other types of grief. However, grief after early pregnancy loss often is not acknowledged or supported, exacerbating feelings of isolation. Acute symptoms of grief usually lessen significantly within about 6 months may subside sooner if the patient becomes pregnant again, but have also been reported to last for up to 2 years.

A routine follow-up appointment to discuss with the woman or couple the cause of the miscarriage and implications for future pregnancies has been shown to lower anxiety symptoms and is recommended at 6 weeks after a miscarriage (Bhat, 2016) because a woman's response to miscarriage at 6 weeks predicts her response at 1 year. Several studies have examined specific psychological interventions after miscarriage. For example, Swanson and associates (2009) studied 341 couples, randomly allocated to four different interventions at 1, 5, and 11 weeks after the miscarriage. Interventions were couples-focused counseling by a nurse in the couple's home for three sessions, a set of three video and workbook modules, a combination of one nurse counseling session with the three-video and workbook modules, and no intervention. All interventions used previously established models, Swanson's Caring Theory and the Meaning of Miscarriage Model, took a supportive approach, and focused on discussing the miscarriage, losses and gains resulting from the miscarriage, sharing the loss and rejoining public life, "getting through it," and trying again. The most effective intervention overall, for both depression and grief, was the three sessions of counseling by the nurse. In the absence of this resource, the obstetrician-gynecologist can help the patient and couple by normalizing feelings of depression and grief, giving the expectation that these will resolve, but also monitoring carefully for more severe or persistent symptoms of depression, PTSD, or suicidal thoughts indicating a need for referral for mental health treatment.

Stillbirth occurs in about 0.5% of pregnancies. Stillbirth is associated with grief; increased rates of depression, anxiety, and PTSD symptoms; feelings of guilt; and a higher rate of complicated grief than other kinds of losses. Women with poor social support, preexisting mental health problems, recurrent perinatal losses, and no living children are at higher risk for more intense and prolonged complicated grief. PTSD is reported in about 20% of women during the next pregnancy. Partners also experience similar symptoms of grief after a stillbirth and experience anxiety and PTSD with the next pregnancy. Loss of a baby may cause relationship strain or breakup, especially if the intensity or timing of grief differs significantly between the two parents. In addition, siblings may, depending on their age, be confused about what has happened, feel that they are to blame, or feel loss. Parents preoccupied by their own grief may have difficulty recognizing or helping their other children with these feelings.

Recommendations for clinicians include giving the woman and her partner clear information about what is going wrong and what is being done, involving the parents in decision making as much as possible, ensuring that the woman has access to postpartum medical care (e.g., suppression of lactation, contraception, help with gynecologic and sexual problems), and holding a meeting 1 to 2 months later to review what is known about the cause of the baby's death and to answer questions regarding future pregnancies. Couples are commonly advised, at the time of the loss, to create memories of the child, including holding the dead baby, giving the baby a name, taking photographs, and having a funeral. Many parents may want this and find it very important. However, holding the dead baby is especially controversial and in different studies has been associated with both better and poorer psychological outcomes. Couples may benefit from support groups, and those women or their partners who experience more severe or persistent depression, complicated grief, anxiety, PTSD, or suicidal thoughts should be referred for mental health treatment with psychotherapy and medication as indicated.

A special counseling challenge involves the care of a woman with an unplanned pregnancy. Such individuals often suffer conflicting feelings, which may include shame and guilt, a genuine desire to have a child, fear of social and family consequences, and fear for their own future and physical well-being. In addition, they may suffer from guilt about the termination of pregnancy if abortion is considered. Although many such women have good social support (e.g., family, significant others, friends, and religious counselors), others will rely on the physician for advice and direction. The physician can discuss all possible options with the woman, including having and raising the child, offering the child for adoption, or terminating the pregnancy. Issues involving the role of the baby's father, the effect of any decision on the future life of the woman, and the risks of procedures should be considered. The woman should be aided in reaching the most appropriate decision for her circumstances and supported in carrying out her decision. When necessary, appropriate referrals to social agencies (e.g., adoption, abortion counseling, or welfare services) should be made. The woman may experience depression, anxiety, or grief in this situation, even when making what she thinks is the best decision possible.

The inability to have a child, or infertility, affects about 1 in 10 couples and can precipitate feelings of isolation, inadequacy, poor self-esteem, guilt, anger, loss of control over one's life, depression, difficulty being around pregnant women or couples with young children, changes in one's identity and sense of meaning, and relationship strain. Infertility treatment involves significant cost, medical treatments and procedures, and psychological stress. Among women presenting for infertility treatment, 40% meet criteria for a psychiatric disorder, including 23% with an anxiety disorder and 17% to 19.5% with major depression (Bhat, 2016). Failed infertility treatment engenders further stress and depression. Psychological distress has been reported to be the primary reason for dropout from infertility treatment, and pretreatment depression is predictive of dropout after one in vitro fertilization (IVF) cycle. There is some evidence that higher levels of psychological stress are associated with lower success rates of infertility treatment. Only about 50% of couples have a child as a result of infertility treatment, and those not succeeding commonly experience a grief reaction. The SCREENIVF (Verhaak, 2010) is a screening tool for pretreatment anxiety and depression, helplessness about and low acceptance of fertility problems, and lack of social support for use at the beginning of infertility treatment, in conjunction with access to mental health evaluation and treatment as needed (Bhat, 2016).

Many infertile couples gain information and support from the Internet, although using this as one's sole source of support has been linked with higher levels of psychological distress. Women and their partners may benefit from support groups or individual or group psychotherapy. Interventions proved effective in reducing distress, and in some studies in improving conception rates, include CBT, ongoing counseling and education throughout the infertility treatment process, relaxation, stress management, coping skills, and group support. CBT and fluoxetine have been shown to reduce both distress and depressive symptoms in mildly to moderately depressed infertile women (Faramarzi, 2013). Women with severe depression, grief, or suicidal thoughts should be referred for evaluation and antidepressant or other psychotropic medication treatment.

## DEATH AND DYING

Gynecologists, especially gynecologic oncologists, care for women who are dying. **There are several challenges for physicians caring for dying patients. First, physicians have been shown to be optimistic and inaccurate in their prognoses for terminally ill patients and to overestimate their ability to combat disease. This makes it difficult to know when to shift the conversation with a patient from a focus on cure or fighting the disease to a focus on palliative care.** Making this transition may be difficult for the physician, who does not wish to give up hope prematurely. On the other hand, most patients are very concerned about issues of quality of life in confronting dying and hope for a process in which they can retain dignity, feel like themselves as much as possible, have adequate time and opportunity to put their "house in order," and have maximal possible comfort and pain relief. It is important for physicians to help women by discussing with them issues of "do not resuscitate" (DNR) orders, treatment of pain, referral to hospice, and other end-of-life issues. In fact, introducing palliative care discussions earlier in treatment appears to be helpful. For example, in a study of 151 patients with metastatic non-small-cell lung cancer, patients randomly allocated to early palliative care integrated with oncologic care had a better quality of life and mood, less aggressive care at the end of life, and longer survival (Temel, 2011).

Psychological issues for dying patients are highly variable, depending on the person's stage of life, sense of the meaning of her life and of the illness, coping style, relationships and family support, spiritual beliefs, and economic circumstances. Feelings of grief, sadness, despair, fear, anxiety, and loneliness are present at some stage for nearly all dying patients, but some are able to achieve a high degree of equanimity and acceptance.

Developmentally, young adults with terminal illness commonly struggle with anger about the unfairness of the illness, grief and loss about life experiences they will not have, and issues related to being dependent on their parents for care. Parents of young children are concerned about the impact of their illness and death on their children, losing the opportunity to see their children grow up, and how to maintain a normal life and routine for their children and family in the face of their illness. For women in later stages of life, feelings about death depend on the degree of satisfaction and meaning that they feel with their life and what they have done, the kinds and quality of attachments they have, whether they feel robbed of retirement and later life, and whether they have lost their spouse or intimate partner already.

Block (2006) provided a comprehensive overview of psychological issues faced by dying patients and ways to explore with them issues related to the meaning of the illness, meaning of their life and achievements, spirituality, relationship issues, other life stressors, maintaining a sense of self, and fears and hopes that the patient has. Terminally ill patients benefit from the treatment of depression or anxiety states to improve the quality of the remainder of their lives. Dying patients also benefit from psychological interventions, including listening, the opportunity to share feelings and the chance to reflect on past experiences and future hopes. Specific therapies for patients with advanced cancer include general counseling; CBT, especially for symptoms of anxiety and depression; meaning-centered therapy focusing on meaning, legacy, and courage; dignity, life review, and narrative therapy; compassion and self-compassion; communication skills training to help with communication with health care providers; and music and writing (Teo, 2019). The gynecologist can help a dying woman by maintaining an engaged, genuine relationship with the woman as an individual throughout the dying process, helping the woman and family to anticipate and address practical issues such as enrolling in hospice and other palliative care services, and maximizing comfort and pain control.

## KEY REFERENCES


ACOG Committee on Health Care for Underserved Women. ACOG Committee Opinion No. 423: Motivational interviewing: a tool for behavior change. *Obstet Gynecol.* 2009;113(1):243-246.

ACOG Committee Opinion No. 777: Sexual Assault. *Obstet Gynecol.* 2019;133(4):e296-e302.

ACOG Practice Bulletin #213, Female Sexual Dysfunction. *Obstet Gynecol.* 2019;134(1):e1-e18.

Adams JA, Farst KJ, Kellogg ND. Interpretation of medical findings in suspected child sexual abuse: an update for 2018. *J Pediatr Adolesc Gynecol.* 2018;31(3):225-231.

Adams KF, Schatzkin A, Harris TB, et al. Overweight, obesity, and mortality in a large prospective cohort of persons 50 to 71 years old. *N Engl J Med.* 2006;355:763-778.

Attia E, Steinglass JE, Walsh BT, et al. Olanzapine versus placebo in adult outpatients with anorexia nervosa: a randomized clinical trial. *Am J Psychiatry.* 2019;176(6):449-456.

Bandelow B, Michaelis S, Wedekind D. Treatment of anxiety disorders. *Dialogues Clin Neurosci.* 2017;19:93-107.

Basson R. Sexual desire and arousal disorders in women. *N Engl J Med.* 2006;354:1497-1506.

Benowitz NL. Nicotine addiction. *N Engl J Med.* 2010;362:2295-2303.

Bhat A, Byatt N. Infertility and perinatal loss: when the bough breaks. *Curr Psychiatry Rep.* 2016;18:31.

Block SD. Psychological issues in end-of-life care. *J Palliat Med.* 2006;9:751-766.

Bradley KA, Boyd-Wickizer J, Powell SH, Burman ML. Alcohol screening questionnaires in women: a critical review. *JAMA.* 1998;280(2):166-171.

Breiding MJ, Black MC, Ryan GW. Prevalence and risk factors of intimate partner violence in eighteen US states/territories. *Am J Prev Med.* 2008;34:112-118.

Burgess AW, Holmstrom LL. Rape trauma syndrome. *Am J Psychiatry.* 1974;131(9):981-986.

Cameron C, Habert J, Anand L, Furtado M. Optimizing the management of depression: primary care experience. *Psychiatry Res.* 2014;220(S1):545-557.

Cipriani A, Furukawa TA, Salanti G, et al. Comparative efficacy and acceptability of 12 new-generation antidepressants: a multiple-treatments meta-analysis. *Lancet.* 2009;373:746-758.

Cowley DS. Challenging patient encounters. Clinical Updates in Women's Health Care monograph series. *Am Coll Obstet Gynecol.* 2016;15(5).

Davis SR, Baber R, Panay N, et al. Global consensus position statement on the use of testosterone therapy for women. *J Sex Med.* 2019;16(9): 1331-1337.

Faramarzi M, Pasha H, Esmailzadeh S, et al. The effect of cognitive behavioral therapy and pharmacotherapy on infertility stress: a randomized controlled trial. *Int J Fertil Steril.* 2013;7(3):199-206.

Ferguson II JE. Why doesn't SOMEBODY do something? *Am J Obstet Gynecol.* 2010;202(6):635-643.

Flint E, Cummins S, Sacker A. Associations between active commuting, body fat, and body mass index: population based, cross sectional study in the United Kingdom. *BMJ.* 2014;349:g4887.

Grant JE. Clinical practice: obsessive-compulsive disorder. *N Engl J Med.* 2014;371(7):646-653.

Grant JM, Mottet LA, Tanis J. *National Transgender Discrimination Survey Report on Health and Health Care;* 2010. Available at https://cancer-network.org/wp-content/uploads/2017/02/National_Transgender_Discrimination_Survey_Report_on_health_and_health_care.pdf. Accessed June 26, 2019.

Groves JE. Taking care of the hateful patient. *N Engl J Med.* 1978;298: 883-887.

Hilberman E, Monson K. Sixty battered women. *Victimology.* 1977;2:460.

Johnston BD, Kanters S, Bandayrel K, et al. Comparison of weight loss among named diet programs in overweight and obese adults: a meta-analysis. *JAMA.* 2014;312(9):923-933.

Islam RM, Bell RJ, Green S, Page MJ, Davis SR. Safety and efficacy of testosterone for women: a systematic review and meta-analysis of randomised controlled trial data. *Lancet Diabetes Endocrinol.* 2019;7(10): 754-766.

Jonas DE, Garbutt JC. Screening and counseling for unhealthy alcohol use in primary care settings. *Med Clin North Am.* 2017;101:823-837.


**Full references and Suggested readings for this chapter can be found on ExpertConsult.com.**

# 10 Endoscopy in Minimally Invasive Gynecologic Surgery

*Licia Raymond, Gretchen M. Lentz*

## KEY POINTS

- Technological developments in hysteroscopy and laparoscopy favor a smaller footprint to facilitate ambulatory procedures, with a trend toward smaller-caliber endoscopes and instruments and creative specimen removal with attention to safety.
- Indications for hysteroscopy include removal of endometrial polyps or submucous myomas, retained intrauterine devices or Essure coils, the diagnosis and treatment of intrauterine adhesions, and resection of a uterine septum or cesarean niche. Hysteroscopy can serve as a diagnostic examination in the setting of recurrent pregnancy loss, infertility, myomectomy planning, and persistent abnormal uterine bleeding with inability to rule out endometrial pathologic conditions by ultrasound/blind biopsy.
- Indications for gynecologic laparoscopy include hysterectomy, myomectomy, treatment of endometriosis, removal of ectopic pregnancy, removal of adnexal pathologic tissue, evaluation of pelvic pain with treatment of any pathologic condition amenable to conservative surgery in a person interested in future childbearing, risk-reducing adnexal surgery, sterilization, appendectomy, drainage of pelvic/intraabdominal abscess, release of pelvic/intraabdominal adhesions, repair of cesarean section niche and congenital anomalies, and oncologic surgical staging.
- An appropriately placed paracervical block with local anesthetic to affect the hypogastric nerves in close proximity to the uterosacral ligaments is more effective than topical or intracervical anesthesia for hysteroscopy. A longer-acting paracervical block can be included for postoperative pain management with hysterectomy or myomectomy and in endometriosis surgery as part of an enhanced recovery after surgery protocol. Local instillation of anesthetic at the laparoscopic port sites at the beginning or conclusion of surgery is also beneficial to the patient.
- Vaginoscopic technique, minimizing speculum usage, avoidance of a tenaculum, use of a small-caliber hysteroscope, and short operating time correlate with patient comfort during hysteroscopy. Mechanical morcellation is increasingly being used to remove intrauterine pathologic tissue, and operative times are shorter compared with resectoscopic procedures. Interestingly, the use of either energy modality for even a simple polyp removal has become more commonplace, potentially increasing cost in the office environment.
- Saline is the standard as a hysteroscopic distention medium, with an allowable fluid deficit of up to 2.5 L. Electrolyte disturbance and complications of fluid overload can occur at less than that deficit level, so be diligent about hysteroscopic fluid management.
- Complications of hysteroscopy include uterine perforation with risk of injury to the surrounding vascular and visceral structures, pelvic infection, bleeding, and overabsorption of the distending media.
- Complications specific to laparoscopy include trocar entry injuries to blood vessels or internal organs, port site hernias, hypercapnia from absorption of carbon dioxide, and ventilatory compromise from the compressive effects of the pneumoperitoneum and/or steep Trendelenburg position.
- The primary laparoscopic trocar placement can cause up to 50% of vascular and bowel injuries in gynecologic laparoscopy. It is important for the laparoscopic surgeon to strategically plan for the where and the how of initial trocar placement and be familiar with the three entry techniques.
- Laparoscopic surgery is usually multiport, with a trend to small-diameter instruments. Single-site surgery has a learning curve and can be done through an umbilical or vaginal approach; the robotic platform has both single-site and multiport options. Any surgery, of course, can be a hybrid of different approaches. Examples of this include hand-assist surgery and laparoscopic-assisted vaginal surgery.
- Thermal or mechanical bowel or urinary tract injuries can occur in laparoscopic surgery and might not be recognized intraoperatively. Sequelae from a delay in diagnosis can have serious consequences; diligent teamwork is required for optimal postoperative care. Cystoscopy can provide reassurance about bladder integrity and ureteral patency but not necessarily show a thermal injury.
- As a risk-reducing measure to prevent future malignant transformation to ovarian carcinoma, bilateral salpingectomy should be offered to all women desiring sterilization and to all women undergoing hysterectomy. If the ovaries are preserved, care should be taken to remove the entire fimbria because this is the site of greatest risk for malignant transformation, and to avoid disruption of the ovarian blood supply from the infundibulopelvic ligament.
- Safe specimen removal in laparoscopic surgery requires mindfulness and careful preoperative review with the patient regarding options. Specimen extraction using nonpower morcellation is often done from within a bag from a vaginal approach; alternatives include extension of an abdominal port, usually midline at a suprapubic incision or the umbilicus.
- Simulation training in endoscopic surgery improves surgical skills and can results in improved "muscle memory" with regard to the handling of laparoscopic and hysteroscopic equipment, dissection techniques, suturing, and knot tying.

**Accompanying video for this chapter is available on ExpertConsult.com.**

## INTRODUCTION

Endoscopic procedures such as laparoscopy and hysteroscopy are performed with a telescope and a light source, which when linked to a camera and video monitor provide for visualization and documentation of internal structures. ***Laparoscopy* refers to viewing the peritoneal cavity, including the pelvis, and *hysteroscopy* refers to the uterine cavity. Endoscopy is an integral component of minimally invasive gynecologic surgery, providing an important mode of access for the diagnosis and operative management of many gynecologic conditions.**

The traditional hysteroscopic access to the uterine cavity and abdominal multiport laparoscopic approach to the peritoneal cavity are the backbone of a growing array of access modalities, instrumentation, and operative procedures in gynecologic surgery. These include the diagnosis and management of the following:

- Benign and malignant neoplasms
- Acquired and congenital anomalies
- Endometriosis
- Pelvic infection and adhesive disease
- Infertility and pregnancy complications
- Pelvic pain
- Abnormal bleeding
- Removal of adnexal structures
- Pelvic prolapse
- Myomectomy
- Hysterectomy

**Gynecologists also perform cystoscopy during laparoscopic and urogynecologic procedures to evaluate the bladder and visualize the ureteral orifices, to examine for intraoperative injury and inadvertent needle or mesh placement, and to assess for invasive pathologic conditions such as deep infiltrative endometriosis, mesh erosion, or metastatic gynecologic cancer affecting the urinary tract.** Retroperitoneal placement of an endoscope allows for extraperitoneal lymph node dissection in oncologic surgery. Robotic assistance facilitates complex laparoscopic surgery such as oncologic staging and surgery in patients who are morbidly obese. **With Vnotes (vaginal natural orifice transluminal endoscopic surgery), the surgeon uses the vagina as an access point for the endoscope, building on techniques used in single-site transumbilical laparoscopic surgery and using the vagina as a portal to the abdominal cavity instead of the umbilicus.**

**Endoscopy is a cornerstone of minimally invasive gynecologic surgery (MIGS)** and has advanced dramatically since the pioneering work of Raoul Palmer and Kurt Semm in the 1960s and 1970s (Palmer, 1974; Semm, 1979). The emergence of educationally focused endoscopic organizations across the globe, enhanced collaboration between surgical specialties, practice focus on MIGS, and the establishment of MIGS fellowship programs and advanced training programs have positively affected the depth, breadth, and quality of research and technical advances in gynecologic endoscopy. The integration of MIGS into the fields of benign gynecology, gynecologic oncology, and urogynecology has served to move minimally invasive surgery into the mainstream as a standard of care for the majority of gynecologic surgical procedures. This chapter is an evidence-based overview of gynecologic endoscopy, intended to encourage skilled, cost-effective, appropriate endoscopic care, with an aim to optimize gynecologic outcomes.

## PREOPERATIVE DECISION MAKING

Contemporary hysteroscopy and laparoscopic procedures are less often preoperatively placed in "diagnostic" or "operative" categories and more typically done as "see and treat" interventions, in part because of what can be accomplished during the preoperative workup and in part because of the expanded smorgasbord of what can be accomplished with the hysteroscope and laparoscope. The patient who presents with abnormal uterine bleeding, pelvic pain, a pelvic mass, or signs of a pelvic infection will have a thorough history and physical examination (H&P), appropriate laboratory studies, and almost universally some type of imaging study to inform the clinical decision-making process before surgery. An attentive, thorough H&P is paramount in the preoperative workup. This will guide decision making regarding which laboratory tests to order, be it a pregnancy test, blood count, thyroid study, chemistries, chlamydia and gonorrhea, or tumor markers. It will help determine which imaging tests are needed. The optimal preoperative evaluation incorporates a patient-centered approach to decision making. Careful attention to preoperative discovery helps guide the appropriate surgical intervention because operative findings can then be anticipated and the patient's preferences are understood.

### Preoperative Imaging: Ultrasound

**Surgical readiness is facilitated by preoperative imaging, which almost universally involves a sonographic study.** Gynecologic ultrasound is a cost-effective, noninvasive, and accessible imaging technique that can help elucidate the nature and extent of pelvic disease (Benacerraf, 2015). Ultrasound is easily integrated into the process of gynecologic investigation and preoperative planning; for example, a transabdominal "visceral slide-test" can yield information about the likelihood of adhesive disease at the site of planned trocar placement, decreasing procedure-related complications and increasing patient safety (Yildirim, 2019). The observer-dependent nuances of an ultrasound examination in real time can be informative for the gynecologic surgeon, assessing the presence and nature of uterine or adnexal pathologic changes, elucidating the likelihood of infiltrative endometriosis or pelvic adhesions, and helping to clarify what surgical options are reasonable or contraindicated. When ultrasound is performed as a point-of-care study, the patient becomes an integral part of the ongoing discussion of findings, and this enhances the process of shared decision making.

Minimally invasive surgical options for definitive diagnosis with the twin goal of symptom relief can be offered to the patient, guided by ultrasound findings and concomitant physical examination. Uterine fibroids might be visualized within the myometrium by ultrasound in a perimenopausal woman with heavy and painful menses, or the clinician might surmise that adenomyosis has infiltrated throughout the myometrium by the diffuse inhomogenous echotexture and thickened uterine wall apparent on transvaginal ultrasound. A classic ovarian endometrioma or an ovarian dermoid cyst might be visualized sonographically in the setting of a palpable pelvic mass. Should the ultrasound appearance of the adnexa be suspicious for an ovarian malignancy, prompt referral to a gynecologic oncologist can be arranged.

In the setting of abnormal bleeding, a thin endometrial lining of normal contour in a postmenopausal patient or in the early follicular phase of a premenopausal patient by ultrasound essentially rules out intracavitary pathologic conditions (Wheeler, 2017). It is acceptable then to forego a potentially painful endometrial biopsy in such a patient and concentrate on causative factors for the abnormal bleeding other than endometrial pathologic conditions in the initial workup. An endometrial polyp or submucosal fibroid can be identified by a properly timed ultrasound as a mass within the uterine cavity and is often missed by an endometrial biopsy (Rotenberg, 2015). With ultrasound as first-line triage in the setting of abnormal uterine bleeding or infertility, when an endometrial mass is visualized, it is not unreasonable for hysteroscopy to be the next step, as the only invasive intervention for diagnosis and treatment of what is likely an endometrial polyp or myoma.

### Additional Imaging Options

Adjuncts to the standard gray-scale ultrasound evaluation include Doppler flow to evaluate lesion vascularity in the uterus or adnexa, informing the gynecologist about the likelihood of an endometrial polyp versus intracavitary fibroid versus a mere blood clot and providing information indicating the likelihood of a benign versus malignant process in the adnexa. **Sonohysterography involves placing a small catheter to instill either saline or gel into the uterine cavity under ultrasound guidance and can help rule out the presence of an endometrial mass in the setting of a relatively thickened endometrial appearance when no discrete mass is seen by standard ultrasound.** If no mass is apparent, an endometrial biopsy could suffice for endometrial diagnosis and hysteroscopy deferred. **Sonohysterography has been shown to be comparable to hysteroscopy in delineating the presence of**

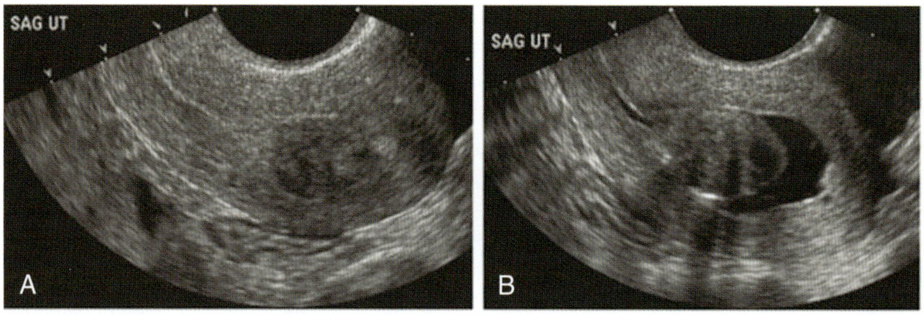


**Fig. 10.1 (A)** Ultrasound image of a uterine fibroid. **(B)** Saline-infusion sonogram of the same patient, outlining the submucous fibroid. (From Khan Z, Stewart EA. Benign uterine diseases. In: Strauss J, Barbieri R. *Yen & Jaffe's Reproductive Endocrinology*. 8th ed. Philadelphia: Elsevier; 2019:643-661.e15. Images courtesy Dr. Mary Frates, Department of Radiology, Brigham and Women's Hospital and Harvard Medical School, Boston, Massachusetts.)

**intrauterine pathologic conditions such as polyp or submucosal fibroid formation** (Fig. 10.1), retained products of conception, a cesarean section scar defect, or uterine septum (Van Dongen, 2007). Three-dimensional (3-D) ultrasound is an excellent tool to ascertain the presence of uterine anomalies or an intrauterine device (IUD) location and can be used in lieu of magnetic resonance imaging (MRI) to delineate fibroids before a complex laparoscopic myomectomy; 3-D ultrasound with gel instillation has been referred to as "virtual hysteroscopy" and can be helpful as an adjunct to ultrasound for preoperative planning before a more complicated hysteroscopic myomectomy.

**Preoperative MRI imaging is helpful in selective patients to assess a fibroid uterus for signs of adenomyosis or sarcoma or map fibroids before a laparoscopic or hysteroscopic myomectomy procedure**. Computed tomography (CT) is less helpful in the pelvis for elucidating gynecologic pathologic conditions but can be informative with delineation of the urinary tract and gastrointestinal systems and in investigating pelvic abscess formation. Fluorescence studies are increasingly helpful intraoperatively in delineation of disease. In addition, intraoperative transabdominal or laparoscopic ultrasound can provide crucial information to guide surgical interventions.

## HYSTEROSCOPY

**Hysteroscopy is the direct visualization of the endometrial cavity and its contents via the cervix using an endoscope and a light source**. Technological developments with a trend toward smaller-caliber hysteroscopes have enabled more office-based procedures and facilitated operating room procedures with intravenous (IV) sedation rather than general anesthesia.

### Indications for Hysteroscopy

**Endometrial polyps are a common cause of abnormal uterine bleeding, found in up to 35% of patients with postmenopausal bleeding** (Bakour, 2012) and not infrequently in women on tamoxifen. These usually benign endometrial growths can cause abnormal bleeding and subfertility in premenopausal woman. **Submucosal fibroids within the endometrial cavity can cause profoundly heavy uterine bleeding and anemia in premenopausal women and can contribute to infertility and pregnancy loss, as well as IUD expulsion. Because both endometrial polyps (Fig. 10.2) and submucosal fibroids are often missed by a blind endometrial biopsy, ultrasound is an evidence-based initial step in the investigation of abnormal uterine bleeding in both reproductive-age and postmenopausal patients, with hysteroscopic evaluation the gold standard for diagnosis and treatment of these intracavitary lesions.** Indications for hysteroscopy include

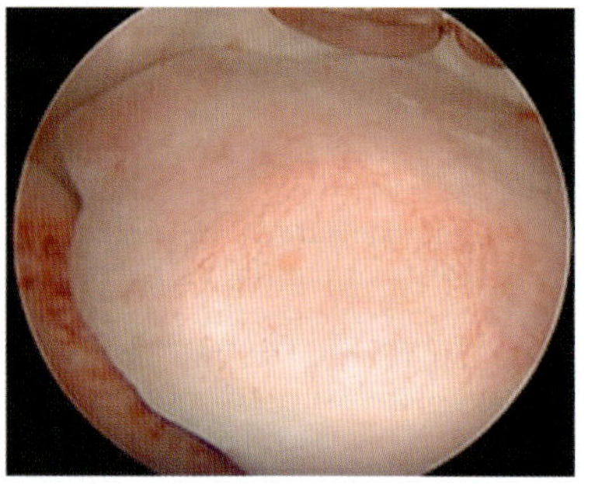

**Fig. 10.2** Hysteroscopic view of intrauterine polyp

diagnosis and treatment in patients with abnormal bleeding and the finding of an endometrial mass on ultrasound or sonohysterography. In patients with nondiagnostic imaging, endometrial biopsy can be performed in lieu of or at the time of hysteroscopy to rule out endometrial carcinoma or precancerous endometrial pathologic conditions.

Intrauterine adhesions are usually caused by prior uterine instrumentation and can present with amenorrhea and infertility as a condition called Asherman syndrome (Asherman, 1948). This agglutination is best diagnosed by hysteroscopy and can be treated with scissors or instrumental dissection under hysteroscopic visualization. Another indication for hysteroscopy is the management of a retained or impacted intrauterine device, which can be removed under direct visualization with a hysteroscopic 5-French grasper. Uterine anomalies such as septal defects (Fig. 10.3) can be confirmed hysteroscopically and resected with a small 5-French bipolar tip or hysteroscopic scissors; other energy sources can also be used, with care taken not to damage the endometrium. Retained products of conception remote from delivery or after a pregnancy loss might be amenable to cold-loop resection or mechanical morcellation under hysteroscopic guidance (Fig. 10.4). A cesarean scar defect can be evaluated hysteroscopically concomitant with laparoscopic surgical correction or, if the patient is not interested in a future pregnancy and abnormal bleeding is a problem, treated with hysteroscopic resection under ultrasound guidance (Fig. 10.5).

Hysteroscopic sterilization is anticipated to again be an option in the future; its global use from 2002 to 2018 is now historical because there is no longer a device on the market for blockage of the proximal aspect of the fallopian tubes by hysteroscopic means. Hysteroscopy can be used to remove Essure implants when a significant component of a retained sterilization device is present in the uterine cavity; familiarity with the implant is necessary to ensure the entire coil set is extracted.

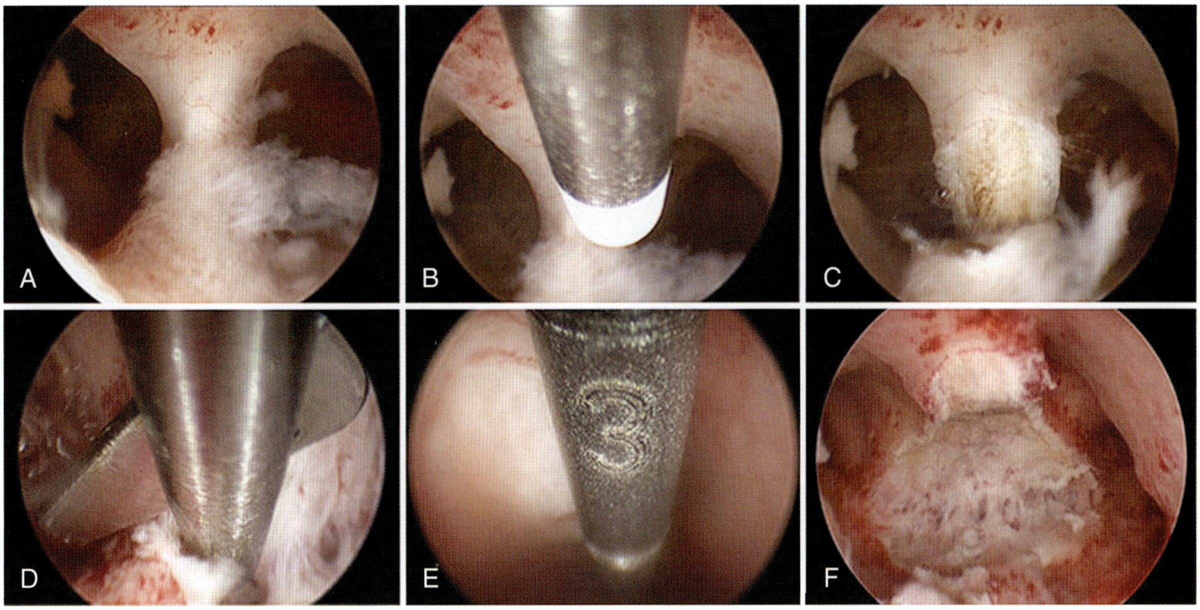


**Fig. 10.3** Uterine septum resection. Hysteroscopic metroplasty with miniaturized instruments on a U2a uterus (i.e., a partial septate uterus). The first 2.5 cm of the septum are resected using a 5F bipolar electrode (Karl Storz) **(A–C)** followed by the last 0.5 cm, which are incised using **(D)** blunt scissors **(D)** because care is taken to avoid cutting intraseptal blood vessels. **(E)** The use of an intrauterine millimetric palpator (KARL STORZ, Germany) introduced via the working channel of the hysteroscope allows checking the actual depth of metroplasty, which may be combined with ultrasound measurements (3 cm of sectioned septum). **(F)** The final view of the uterine cavity. (From Di Spiezio Sardo A, Zizolfi B, Bettocchi S, et al. Accuracy of hysteroscopic metroplasty with the combination of presurgical 3-dimensional ultrasonography and a novel graduated intrauterine palpator: a randomized controlled trial. *J Minim Invasive Gynecol.* 2016;23(4):557-566.)

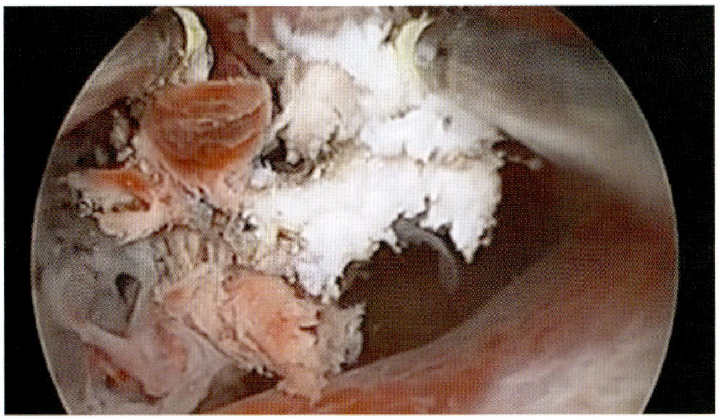

**Fig. 10.4** Hysteroscopic removal of retained products of conception. (From Alosnso L, Nieto L, Carugno J. Hysteroscopic removal of retained products of conception implanted over a focal area of adenomyosis: a case report. *J Minim Invasive Gynecol.* 2018;25(3):382-383.)

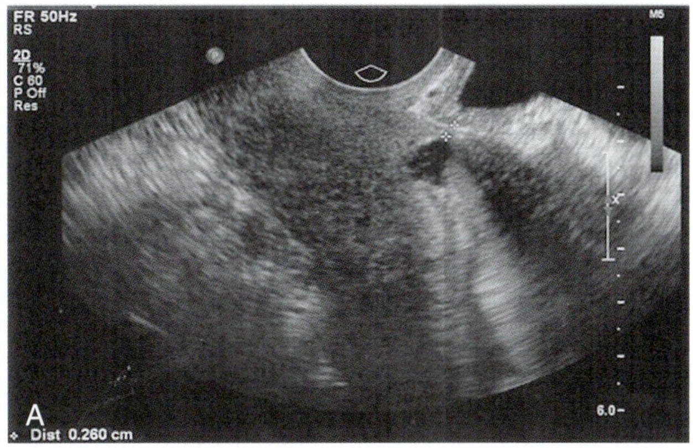


**Fig. 10.5** Ultrasound of an isthmocele. (From Cohen SB, Mashiach R, Baron A, et al. Feasibility and efficacy of repeated hysteroscopic cesarean niche resection. *Eur J Obstet Gynecol Reprod Biol.* 2017;217:12-17.)

**BOX 10.1** Indications for Hysteroscopy

- Endometrial diagnosis (abnormal uterine bleeding, recurrent pregnancy loss)
- Endocervical and endometrial polypectomy
- Hysteroscopic myomectomy
- Lysis of intrauterine adhesions
- Uterine septum repair
- Assessment and possible resection of cesarean scar defect
- Removal of foreign body, such as retained intrauterine device or intracavitary Essure implant
- Removal of retained products of conception
- Recurrent pregnancy loss

Indications for hysteroscopy are listed in Box 10.1. Relative contraindications for hysteroscopy include pregnancy and genital tract infections, including active herpes.

## Hysteroscopic Equipment

A hysteroscope can be rigid (Fig. 10.6) or flexible, and the tip diameter can range in size from approximately 3 to 9 mm. The wider the tip of the hysteroscope, the greater the potential for patient discomfort and cervical trauma because progressive cervical dilation will likely be required for the larger hysteroscope to be advanced through the endocervical canal and into the endometrial cavity. The tip of a rigid hysteroscope can be 0 degrees or angled, depending on the operator's preference; 12- to 30-degree lenses are

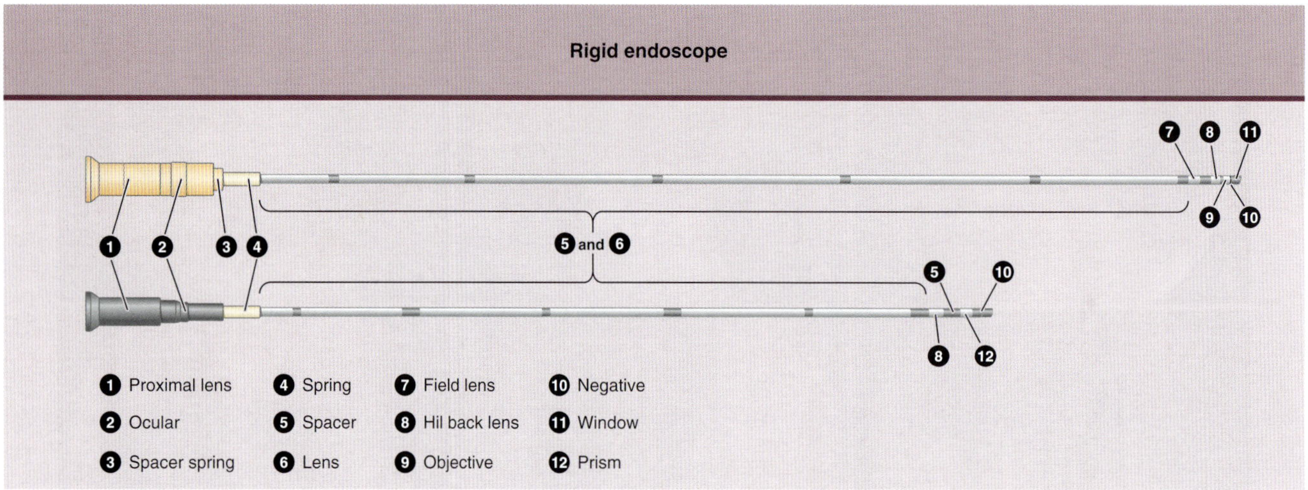


**Fig. 10.6** Anatomy of a rigid endoscope. (From Beiber EJ, Sanfilippo JS, Horowitz IR. *Clinical Gynecology.* Philadelphia: Elsevier, 2006.)

most often used. A light source is required, and a camera with attached video monitor is usually included. The reimbursement profile for hysteroscopy has shifted to significantly favor office-based procedures, supporting the capital investment in equipment. One obstacle to office-based hysteroscopy can be the reprocessing of instruments, but this challenge is not insurmountable. A case-by-case expenditure is an alternative with disposable setups and hysteroscopes, although these are not as versatile as most reusable systems. Future trends in instrumentation will likely include reposable, hybrid systems with LED and Bluetooth mechanisms.

## Fluid Management

**Hysteroscopy requires a mechanism for intrauterine distention to facilitate visualization.** Most hysteroscopes have a mechanism for continuous flow of input and output fluid to optimize visualization within the uterine cavity. Isotonic solutions are considered the safest option, as opposed to electrolyte-free hypotonic solutions, which carry a higher risk of potentially life-threatening hyponatremia in association with excess fluid absorption. Saline has become the distention medium of choice for both office and operating room hysteroscopy.

**Saline is an isotonic electrolyte solution that can be used with bipolar electrosurgical energy, laser energy, and mechanical interventions. Hypotonic electrolyte-free fluids are compatible with monopolar electrosurgical platforms and can also be used with mechanical instruments or laser.** Carbon dioxide gas has had a role as a distention medium in diagnostic hysteroscopy but has the potential for gas embolism and is not conducive to operative interventions because visualization can be limited.

The continuous inflow of the distention solution to optimize visualization can have implications on patient hemodynamics. Fluid overload and the resultant altered physiology can cause life-threatening hyponatremia, cerebral edema, and congestive heart failure; therefore a team awareness of fluid balance with hysteroscopy is crucial. The lower safety profile of hypotonic fluids relative to isotonic solutions such as physiologic saline is due to the greater risk of hyponatremia and fluid overload per quantity absorbed. **Because of well-documented complications that can arise from excessive hysteroscopic fluid absorption with any medium, an important safety measure with any hysteroscopic procedure includes judicious measurement of the fluid deficit, the difference between fluid in and fluid out.**

Guidelines mandate discontinuation of a hysteroscopic procedure before a fluid deficit of 1 L with a hypotonic solution such as glycine or mannitol. Guidelines allow for a fluid deficit of 2.5 L with isotonic fluids such as saline (AAGL, 2013). Fluid management systems are available to provide a more precise measurement of fluid input and output and to heighten safety when high fluid volumes are anticipated. Certain fluid management systems allow for adjustment of flow pressures to optimize visualization. For more simple office-based procedures, fluid overload can be avoided by limiting from the onset the amount of fluid to be infused to an amount under the deficit guidelines.

## Hysteroscopic Instruments

Hysteroscopes have an operative port through which graspers, scissors, tenacula, or bipolar tips can be placed (Fig. 10.7). These working instruments are usually 5 French in diameter, fit easily into a standard 5-mm hysteroscope, and can release, incise, grasp, or biopsy endometrial pathologic tissue under direct visualization. The polyp, small leiomyoma, or biopsy specimen can often then be extracted along with the hysteroscope. Endometrial polyp forceps and specialized myoma forceps can be used to gently grasp and remove any endometrial pathologic tissue inadvertently released within the uterine cavity, and ultrasound guidance can be used to assist with this process if desired. This simple technique works well with endometrial polyps and can also be used with fragments of myomas from resectoscopic surgery. These small 5-French instruments can also be used through an operative port to remove a retained IUD or Essure coil and to treat intrauterine adhesions or an intrauterine septum.

Specialized hysteroscopes are available that can incorporate an energy-based modality for operative intervention under direct visualization. These options for intracavitary treatment include the electrosurgical resectoscope (Fig. 10.8) and the mechanical morcellator (Fig. 10.9), and they are especially helpful with fibroid removal and also with larger polyps. Advanced technology has resulted in ever smaller prototypes of these hysteroscopes, essentially the equivalent of a 5-mm office hysteroscope, and so these procedures as well are being moved into the office setting. For challenging cases, however, such as those requiring significant dilation of a stenotic cervix or for which a large-bore hysteroscope is needed, IV sedation in the operating room setting might be imperative.

# Office-Based Hysteroscopy and Minimal Impact Technique

The office or clinic is a cost-effective venue for many hysteroscopic procedures, efficient for the gynecologist, and convenient

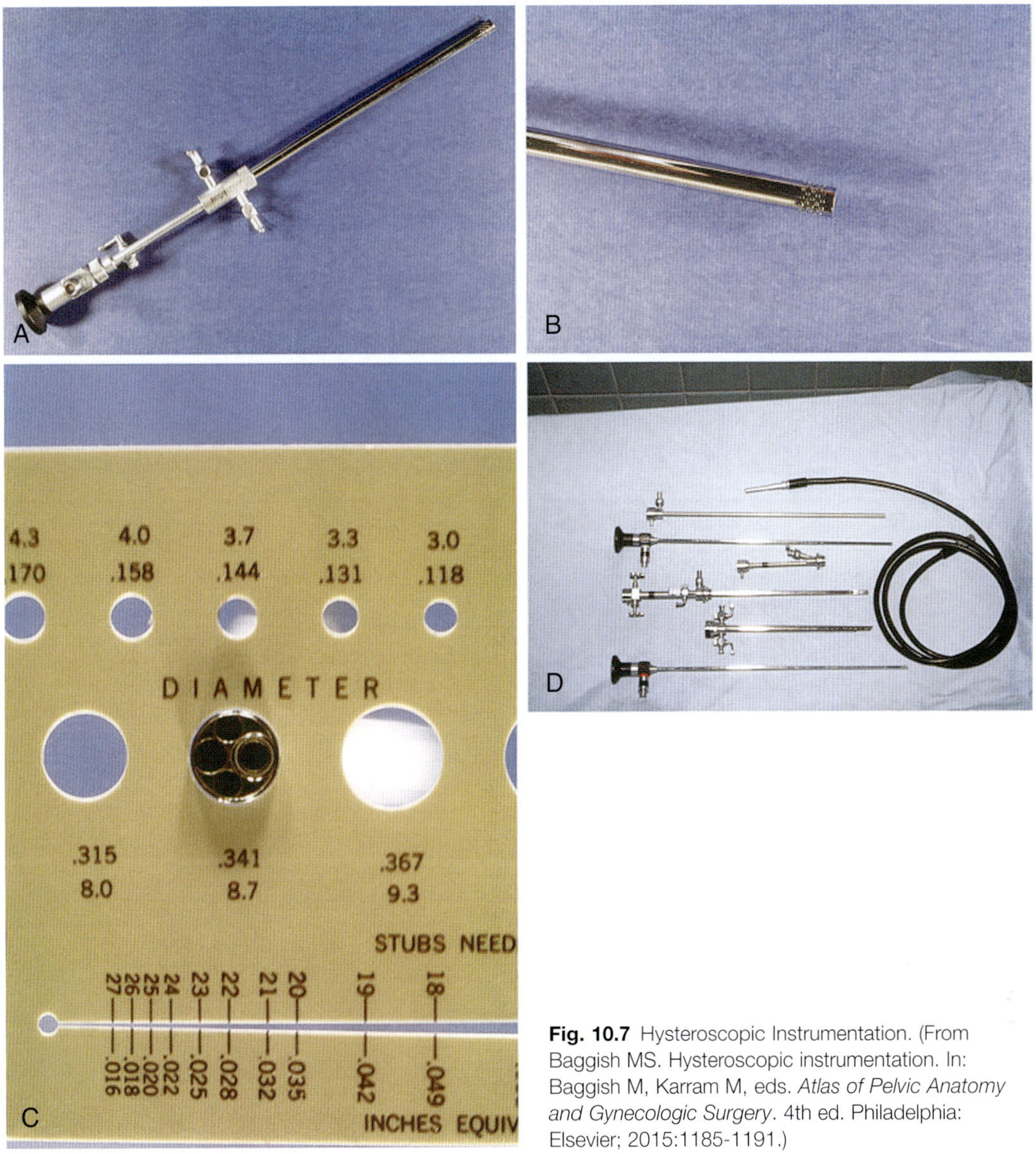


**Fig. 10.7** Hysteroscopic Instrumentation. (From Baggish MS. Hysteroscopic instrumentation. In: Baggish M, Karram M, eds. *Atlas of Pelvic Anatomy and Gynecologic Surgery*. 4th ed. Philadelphia: Elsevier; 2015:1185-1191.)

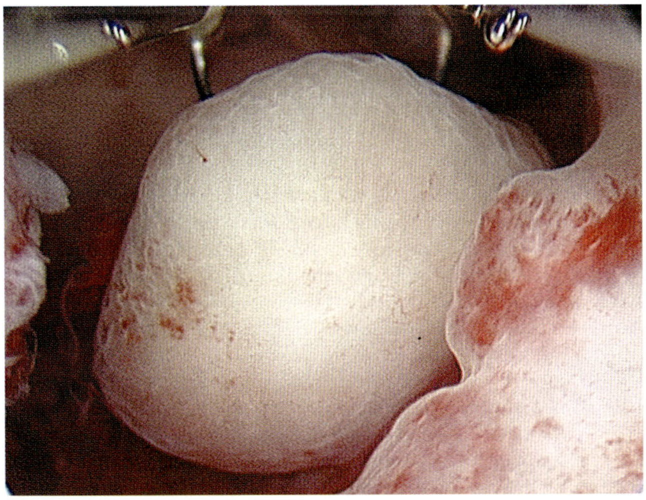

**Fig. 10.8** A uterine polyp with the hysteroscopic resection tool behind the polyp. (From Goldberg JM, Falcone T. *Atlas of Endoscopic Techniques in Gynecology.* London: WB Saunders; 2000:187.)

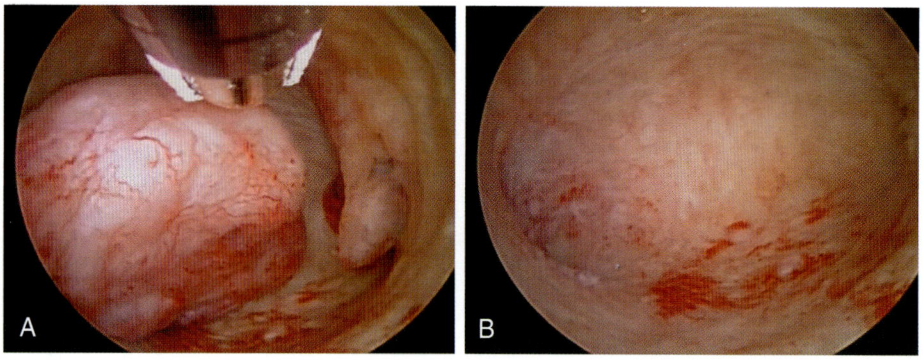


**Fig. 10.9** Intrauterine polyp before **(A)** and after **(B)** hysteroscopic morcellation. (Courtesy Dr. Howard Topel and Smith & Nephew.)

**BOX 10.2 Equipment for Office Hysteroscopy**

Hysteroscope of choice, with attendant light source and monitor
Saline solution, inflow/outflow tubing
Under-buttocks drape and blue pads
Accounting system for fluid management
Open-sided speculum, as thin as possible to reduce patient discomfort
Ring forceps with sterile gauze or cotton balls
Chlorhexidine 4% (off label) or povidone-iodine scrub
Paracervical block equipment
- 22-gauge spinal needle
- Control syringe
- Anesthetic solution

Tenaculum
Microdilators and standard cervical dilators on standby
Hysteroscopic grasping forceps preloaded into the scope
Scissors and tenaculum on standby
Endometrial polyp forceps
Energy devices, as deemed appropriate
Emergency kit for vagal response, Foley catheter for bleeding

**BOX 10.3 Optimizing Office Hysteroscopy**

Administer preprocedure analgesic, such as ibuprofen.
Ensure the patient is in a nonfasting state.
Use a small-diameter hysteroscope.
Know the uterine axis.
Use the vaginoscopic "no-touch" technique.
Paracervical block can be performed with a longer-acting agent such as chloroprocaine.
Minimize speculum use.
Use chlorhexidine as a cleansing solution.
Avoid tenaculum if possible; use anesthetic at the site if needed.
Minimize cervical dilation. Use the scope to advance under vision.
Dilate the distal cervix if stenosis is encountered. Place the scope into the cervical opening and attempt to use the scope to advance through the endocervix under vision with fluid running to decrease the risk of perforation.

for the patient (Box 10.2). A meta-analysis comparing office hysteroscopy with operating room hysteroscopy showed no significant difference in adverse events or treatment success (Bennett, 2019). Office hysteroscopy was substantially less expensive in all randomized trials compared with the operating room counterpart. There was greater reported postoperative pain associated with the office venue, however, and the authors' conclusion was that a shift to an office venue should be "thoughtfully considered." Effective strategies can be employed to enhance patient comfort (Box 10.3).

Preoperative nonsteroidal medication has been shown to decrease postoperative discomfort after office hysteroscopy, and can be taken by the patient in advance of the appointment. Ingestion of a light meal is encouraged because it might also ward off any tendency to a vasovagal reaction and can help decrease any NSAID-associated gastrointestinal upset. Engagement with the patient is helpful, and this can include live observation of the procedure on the video monitor, as well as conversation, humor, and music.

## Smaller-Caliber Hysteroscopes

There has been a trend toward smaller-diameter hysteroscopes with improved optics to facilitate the performance of high-quality operative procedures in the office setting, often without the need for a speculum, cervical dilation, anesthesia, or sedation. A thinner scope is ideal for an office-based procedure because the smaller the hysteroscope caliber, the more likely the scope can be placed into the cervical os and advanced into the endometrial cavity under direct vision, without having to dilate the endocervical canal or use anterior countertraction on the cervix. This direct entry approach, limiting the use of a tenaculum and instrumental cervical dilation and minimizing speculum use, is associated with less patient discomfort. This can facilitate a more simple, safe, convenient office-based procedure allowing for completion of the intended task without need for sedation and in certain cases without need for a local anesthetic.

## Paracervical Block

A paracervical block can be administered to lessen discomfort associated with passage of instruments through the cervix and with the operative procedure in general. A well-placed, high-volume paracervical instillation of anesthetic can be helpful even when performing hysteroscopy under IV sedation in the operating room because it can facilitate avoidance of general anesthesia. Diffusion of a large volume of anesthetic to the hypogastric nerves lateral to the uterosacral ligaments is accomplished by a very superficial paracervical injection at five and seven o'clock, just barely into the vaginal epithelium, creating a large "wheal" with at least 10 mL at each site, for a total of at least 20 mL of anesthetic. This more medial, superficial instillation will lessen the risk of an intravascular injection into a descending branch of the uterine artery and is the same paracervical block that can be used in the operating room with longer-acting bupivacaine as an adjunct for postoperative pain control in laparoscopic hysterectomy and myomectomy procedures. Intravascular administration can cause a transient anesthesia reaction. A small-bore 22G spinal needle is recommended, and a control syringe is optimal for safety. One should pause to let the anesthetic take effect before proceeding with instrumentation. Additional anesthetic can be applied superficially at the anterior cervix if a tenaculum is to be used.

### Vaginoscopy

There is considerable positive experience with "vaginoscopy," by which the hysteroscope introduced into the vagina and through the cervix without use of a speculum or paracervical block. One randomized trial comparing vaginoscopy with a standard hysteroscopic approach showed vaginoscopy to be faster and less painful, with the conclusion it should be the technique of choice for outpatient hysteroscopy (Smith, 2019). There appears to be no increased risk for infection in a study of nearly 43,000 office hysteroscopies; antibiotic prophylaxis is not routinely prescribed (Florio, 2019).

An alternative to vaginoscopy is to use an open-sided speculum to place any necessary paracervical block, then set the hysteroscope tip into the cervical os and remove the speculum. The hysteroscope can then be advanced under vision without the interference of the rigid speculum. Removal of the speculum is also often appreciated by the patient. Should a tenaculum be required, local anesthetic can first be superficially instilled into the anterior cervix.

### Cervical Stenosis and Risk of Uterine Perforation

**Should cervical stenosis be encountered, the insertion of the hysteroscope will be more challenging, requiring anterior traction and use of graduated cervical dilators.** Minicervical dilators can be used for this purpose. When cervical dilation is required, it is possible to only dilate the outer aspect of the cervical canal, place the hysteroscope into the cervical opening and under flow with direct vision, then advance the rest of the way into the cavity. **Advancing the hysteroscope under direct vision might decrease the risk of uterine perforation, a complication that occurs more commonly in the setting of cervical stenosis.**

Uterine perforation is usually not clinically consequential but could conceivably be of serious consequence if the perforation is lateral into the uterine vasculature or involves the active use of an energy device, in which case damage can occur to adjacent structures such as bowel, bladder, or blood vessels. There is conflicting evidence about the use of preoperative misoprostol as a cervical ripening agent before gynecologic transcervical procedures to reduce the risk of difficult insertion and associated cervical trauma and uterine perforation. The effect of preoperative administration of misoprostol as a cervical ripening agent before hysteroscopy is uncertain, and evidence does not support its routine use for operative hysteroscopy (Selk, 2011).

## Hysteroscopic Procedures

### Hysteroscopic Polypectomy

**Endometrial polyps can be isolated or multiple and are best resected from the uterine wall under hysteroscopic visualization.** The simplest, most cost-effective method is with use of a reusable 5-French hysteroscopic forceps focused at the attachment site. Specimen removal from the endometrial cavity is often accomplished by maintaining a grasp on the polyp while withdrawing the hysteroscope. If this is not successful, extraction of the resected lesion does not necessarily require hysteroscopic visualization and can be accomplished with careful use of handheld endometrial polyp forceps. Reinsertion of the hysteroscope can confirm all pathologic tissue has been removed. An endometrial biopsy specimen can then be obtained as a global endometrial screen if desired.

Mechanical morcellation and resectoscopic techniques intended for submucosal fibroid removal are increasingly used for hysteroscopic polypectomy, despite the fact that polyp removal can usually be accomplished without energy. Endometrial polyps can be resected using electrosurgical energy with a bipolar (or monopolar) resectoscope. Care should be taken not to thermally damage the endometrial base in women planning future pregnancies. The electromechanical morcellator can remove endometrial polyps, and newer reusable systems are now available that could benefit cost effectiveness.

### Hysteroscopic Myomectomy

The removal of submucosal fibroids is indicated for heavy bleeding and to improve fertility. **Hysteroscopic myomectomy is performed on type 0 to 2 submucosal fibroids (Fig. 10.10), using either a bipolar resectoscope to shave the myoma in fragments or a mechanical morcellator that chops the fibroid into pieces and then aspirates the fragments into a collection container.** Use of a monopolar resectoscope is a less commonly used option for resectoscopic treatment of intracavitary fibroids, with use of a nonelectrolyte solution and lower threshold for fluid deficit. The achievement of complete fibroid resection is dependent on the size and location of the fibroid, the degree of intramural extension, and the extent of fluid loss, which is often the limiting factor in completing of tumor removal of larger, more imbedded fibroids.

The mechanical morcellator has a shorter learning curve and studies show it to be consistently faster than the resectoscope, likely because of the specimen collection mechanism, but it has limitations in removal of the imbedded myometrial components of type 1 and type 2 fibroids compared with resectoscopic surgery. Morcellators tend to be disposable and can be more costly per item compared with the resectoscope; reusable models are becoming available.

### Endometrial Ablation

**Endometrial ablation is a procedure intended to destroy the endometrium and thereby treat heavy menstrual bleeding in women who have completed childbearing and for whom medical management has failed, as an alternative to hysterectomy.** First-generation endometrial ablation is performed under direct hysteroscopic vision with a resectoscope or rollerball, and second-generation techniques use a global device that destroys the endometrium after blind placement of an energy device into the endometrial cavity. Similar rates of amenorrhea and patient satisfaction have been reported, but ablation by resectoscopic technique or rollerball is associated with longer operative times, more frequent use of general anesthesia, and higher rates of irrigation fluid overload and cervical laceration compared with nonresectoscope modes. Pregnancy after an endometrial ablation is contraindicated because implantation is more likely to occur in the myometrium, resulting in the potential for adverse pregnancy outcomes.

Endometrial ablation is less often performed, in great part because of the efficacy of the levonorgestrel intrauterine device in controlling quality of menses (Silva-Filho, 2013) and also because of concerns about the long-term ability to assess the endometrium after ablation and screen for uterine cancer. Approximately 10% to 15% of women end up having a hysterectomy after an ablation. Endometrial ablation has been supplanted by the levonorgestrel IUD, which provides comparable reductions in menstrual blood loss and contraception, in addition to endometrial protection from hyperplasia and carcinoma. In patients with abnormal

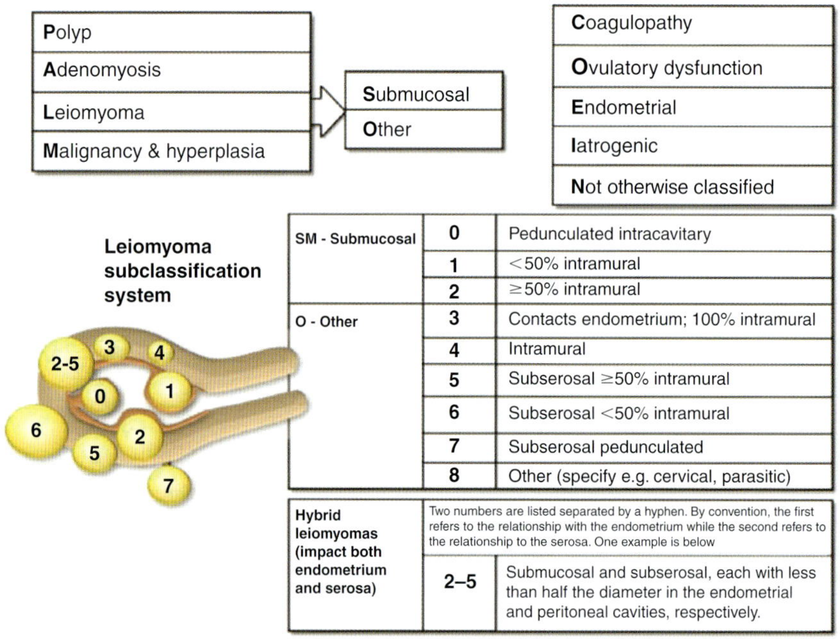
Polyp
Adenomyosis
Leiomyoma
Malignancy & hyperplasia
Submucosal
Other
Coagulopathy
Ovulatory dysfunction
Endometrial
Iatrogenic
Not otherwise classified
Leiomyoma subclassification system
SM - Submucosal
0 Pedunculated intracavitary
1 <50% intramural
2 ≥50% intramural
O - Other
3 Contacts endometrium; 100% intramural
4 Intramural
5 Subserosal ≥50% intramural
6 Subserosal <50% intramural
7 Subserosal pedunculated
8 Other (specify e.g. cervical, parasitic)
Hybrid leiomyomas (impact both endometrium and serosa)
Two numbers are listed separated by a hyphen. By convention, the first refers to the relationship with the endometrium while the second refers to the relationship to the serosa. One example is below
2–5 Submucosal and subserosal, each with less than half the diameter in the endometrial and peritoneal cavities, respectively.
2-5
3
4
0
1
6
5
2
7

**Fig. 10.10** International Federation of Gynecology and Obstetrics (FIGO) classification of uterine fibroids (Munro). (Malcolm G. Munro MD, FACOG, FRCS(c). *Best Practice & Research: Clinical Obstetrics & Gynaecology*, 2017-04-01, Volume 40, Pages 3-22, Copyright © 2016.)

**BOX 10.4** Long-Term Complications of Endometrial Ablation

- Postablation syndrome, with associated pelvic pain
- Potential for high-risk pregnancy
- Trapped hematometra within a scarred endometrium, retrograde bleeding
- Endometrial scarring compromising future endometrial evaluation
- Endometrial scarring obscuring signs and symptoms of endometrial cancer

uterine bleeding after endometrial ablation, evaluation of the endometrial cavity can be hindered because of scarring, and this can result in a return to the operating room for definitive hysterectomy. A Cochrane review determined that hysterectomy is superior to ablation in terms of long-term satisfaction, and that any cost benefit to ablation fades over time because of the need for reoperation (Fergusson, 2013). Long-term complications of endometrial ablation are listed in Box 10.4.

## Complications of Hysteroscopic Surgery

**Hysteroscopy has a low risk of adverse events, with an increased occurrence in the setting of more complex procedures such as myomectomy, septum excision, and use of energy devices** (Munro, 2015) **(Table 10.1).**

Most uterine perforations occur on entry, are midline, and are clinically inconsequential. A lateral perforation, however, might cause vascular trauma and bleeding; an anterior perforation could injure the bladder; and a posterior perforation might perforate the rectum. Uterine perforation with an energy device deployed may have dire consequences, hence the dictum to only trigger energy when coming toward and not away from yourself. In difficult cases ultrasound guidance can be useful. Suspect uterine perforation if the operative view suddenly disappears, the fluid deficit suddenly increases, or the hysteroscope suddenly inserts farther than the fundus. Thermal injury to surrounding organs may occur with deep resections or perforations with the electrocautery instrument. If perforation is suspected during operative hysteroscopy, an intraperitoneal evaluation may be necessary. Unrecognized uterine perforation might result in postoperative

**TABLE 10.1** Short-Term Complications of Hysteroscopy

| Complication | Rate (%) |
|---|---|
| **Overall Complication Rate** | |
| Diagnostic hysteroscopy | 0.95 |
| Operative hysteroscopy | 2-3 |
| Hysteroscopic myomectomy | 1-5 |
| **Uterine Perforation** | |
| Operative hysteroscopy | 1 |
| Endometrial ablation—resectoscope | 2-2+ |
| Endometrial ablation—nonresectoscope | 1 |
| Fluid overload | 0.06-2 |
| Bleeding | 0.03-3 |
| Pelvic infection | 0.01 |
| Death—fluid overload or septicemia | 0.01 |
| Embolism; gas, air | * |
| Cervical laceration | * |
| Creation of false cervical passage | * |
| Failure to complete the procedure | * |
| Electrocautery injury | * |
| Urinary tract or bowel injury | * |
| Pulmonary and cerebral edema | * |
| Dissemination of cervical or endometrial cancer | * |

*Rare complication or exact rate of complication unknown.

abdominal or pelvic pain beyond what would normally be expected, abdominal distention, heavy vaginal bleeding, hypotension, nausea or vomiting, or hematuria. Bowel injury, particularly thermal injuries, may present with delayed onset of symptoms.

Although not common, if intrauterine bleeding is excessive during hysteroscopy, electrocautery coagulation at the bleeding point may be sufficient. An inflatable 30-mL Foley balloon can be inserted via the cervix, inflated, and left for 12 to 24 hours to tamponade the uterine cavity, facilitating hemostasis. A systemic hemostatic agent such as tranexamic acid may also be given. A suture can be applied to a bleeding cervical laceration.

The risk of infection after hysteroscopy is quite low, and although prophylactic antibiotics are not routinely administered, antibiotics might be prudent should there be any concerns about infection or in patients with a history of pelvic inflammatory disease. Patients should be appropriately screened for sexually transmitted infections before instrumentation.

A patient might have a vasovagal reflex from cervical dilation and instrumentation of the uterine cavity that can result in syncope. This reflex can be diminished by ensuring the patient is well hydrated and can be prevented by encouraging patients to eat before they come in for an office procedure. If a tenaculum is to be placed, local anesthesia should be instilled first. A paracervical block can also be helpful in alleviating patient discomfort.

Finally, the spectra of hyponatremia and electrolyte disturbance with fluid overload resulting in congestive heart failure and pulmonary or cerebral edema are serious complications that the gynecologist and surgical team must work diligently to prevent, being mindful of fluid dynamics and patient status at all times.

## GYNECOLOGIC LAPAROSCOPY

**Laparoscopy is a keystone of modern abdominal surgery, involving the insertion of thin instruments through small incisions to perform an intraabdominal operation and a distention pneumoperitoneum for visualization within the abdomen and pelvis.** The first published case report of a laparoscopic surgery was 1910 in Sweden, describing an intraperitoneal opportunity for visual diagnosis using a cystoscope (Jacobaeus, 1910). Since the 1990s, laparoscopy has become the standard of care for abdominal access in a majority of surgical cases. This is because **laparoscopic surgery benefits the patient in many ways compared with "open" laparotomic surgery with a larger incision: less postoperative pain and faster recovery, less risk of surgical site infection, blood loss, and thromboembolism, fewer purported postoperative adhe**sions. These advantages are particularly important for obese patients, who have a relatively greater risk of wound infection, thromboembolic events, and other complications from laparotomy compared with laparoscopy. Laparoscopic optics are enhanced by magnification, and visualization in the pelvis can in certain situations be improved compared with open surgery. In fact, the visual magnification and anatomic detail evident in contemporary gynecologic laparoscopy has sparked an appreciation for the safety benefits of retroperitoneal dissection and nuanced surgical dissection with nerve-sparing intention.

In 1936, Bösch of Switzerland published on laparoscopic sterilization as an operative intervention, and by the 1970s laparoscopic tubal ligation was the method of choice for female sterilization. Kurt Semm (1927-2003) was a German gynecologist who pioneered numerous endoscopic surgeries in the 1960s until his retirement in 1995. He is considered the father of modern laparoscopy, reporting on instrument development and technical advances enabling laparoscopic interventions from 1973 onward. His skills as a toolmaker contributed to the development of numerous surgical instruments: an electronic $CO_2$ insufflator, uterine manipulators, coagulation and cutting instruments, and knot-tying devices. He performed the first laparoscopic appendectomy in 1980 and truly had to have his head examined: At the insistence of coworkers at the University of Kiel, he was forced to undergo a brain scan to prove there was no brain damage instigating his passion for endoscopic surgery.

Although gynecologists were at the forefront of laparoscopic exploration in the latter part of the 20th century and the field of gynecologic oncology has shifted to mainstream endoscopic surgery into the surgical armamentarium for gynecologic cancer care, benign gynecologists in the early 21st century have been slower to incorporate advanced laparoscopy and have underperformed in the conversion of open cases to laparoscopic procedures. Gynecologists operate in the pelvis, which is easily accessed through the familiar transverse lower abdominal Pfannenstiel incision performed for most cesarean sections. This may explain why laparoscopy has been more slowly adopted for major benign gynecologic procedures compared with our general surgery counterparts, who had great incentive to replace a morbid and painful right upper quadrant incision with laparoscopic cholecystectomy. It has been postulated that training programs in obstetrics and gynecology do not provide adequate caseloads in MIGS, and it may be that gynecologic surgeons with busy obstetric practices who are less familiar with advanced laparoscopic surgery follow the adage *First, do no harm,* and adhere to the open surgical principles they know well and trust.

The development of a laparoscopic surgeon requires commitment to requisite training, continuing ongoing education, and a sufficient case load to become and stay proficient. It has been demonstrated that a practice focus on minimally invasive surgery with targeted education, training opportunities, and surgical tracking can result in optimization of the percentage of cases performed in a minimally invasive manner (Abel, 2019; Loring, 2015).

### Indications for Laparoscopy

It is not uncommon for the obstetrician/gynecologist (OB/GYN) generalist to be called on to perform an emergency surgery for adnexal torsion or an ectopic pregnancy or to schedule an ovarian cystectomy for a dermoid excision or a bilateral salpingectomy for permanent sterilization. Each of these procedures requires surgical skill, familiarity with the requisite anatomy, and competent decision making and can be accomplished laparoscopically by a proficient gynecologic surgeon with all the advantages to the patient associated with laparoscopic surgery. **Patients found to have a gynecologic condition amenable to laparoscopic intervention are potential candidates for any one of a number of minimally invasive procedures:**

- Treatment of endometriosis and pelvic adhesive disease
- Removal of pathologic adnexal structures
- Sterilization
- Treatment of ectopic pregnancy or pelvic infection
- Staging of gynecologic malignancy with nerve-sparing pelvic dissection
- Correction of prolapse with sacrocolpopexy or uterosacral suspension
- Laparoscopic hysterectomy or myomectomy.

**Careful consideration needs to be exercised in the following situations:**

- Intestinal obstruction
- Hemoperitoneum with hemodynamic instability
- Severe cardiovascular or pulmonary disease
- Tuberculous peritonitis

### Preparation for Laparoscopic Surgery

The major hazards of laparoscopy are the general anesthesia, which is almost uniformly required, and the placement of laparoscopic trocars. In addition, complication rates increase with the complexity of surgery. Collaboration with the anesthesia provider, the surgical team, and the nursing staff both in advance of and during laparoscopic surgery is important. Establish a good working relationship with specialists who might be called on to give advice or participate in patient care before, during, and after surgery: hospitalists, gastroenterologists, urologists, general and colorectal surgeons, and oncologists.

### Enhanced Recovery After Surgery

The goal of enhanced recovery after surgery (ERAS) pathways is to decrease the physiologic stress of surgery and thereby augment a safer and speedier recovery process. Components include the following (ACOG, 2018):

- Preoperative education
- Focus on nutrition
- Maintenance of normothermia
- Use of nonopioid analgesics and adjunctive regional anesthetics
- Early postoperative feeding and mobilization
- Minimization of catheter usage
- Optimization of thromboprophylaxis
- Antimicrobial therapy
- Fluid balance

### Surgical Site Infection

Smaller incisions, use of a chlorhexidine-based solution for surgical site preparation, and clipping instead of shaving excess hair are local measures that the available evidence shows can be prevent surgical site infections (SSIs). Guidelines exist for judicious and appropriate use of prophylactic antibiotics for many gynecologic procedures. Careful attention to surgical technique is important.

### Operating Room Setup

No surgery is simple, yet every surgery can be simply prepared for. **Surgical readiness is key and starts with surgical team communication on what might be anticipated so that appropriate equipment is accessible.** The patient will be in dorsal lithotomy position, on a gel pad or other device to prevent sliding while in Trendelenburg. The patient's arms are carefully tucked and padded to prevent nerve injury, with hands supinated (thumbs up). Lower positioning with the buttocks at the caudal edge of the table fold also helps to prevent cephalad slide during the procedure. The legs are positioned comfortably in stirrups, semiflexed, and supported for the duration of the case. The distal lower extremities can be raised to achieve hip flexion during portions of the case when vaginal access is required (i.e., for placement of a paracervical block or a uterine manipulator and for vaginal specimen removal). An indwelling Foley catheter can be placed for the duration of a laparoscopic procedure or, alternatively, the bladder can be drained in and out at the start of a shorter surgical case. Backfilling a Foley catheter with saline or carbon dioxide can help delineate the bladder margins during a difficult dissection.

**The exposure and tension provided by appropriate use of a uterine manipulator is invaluable for many laparoscopic surgeries, increasing surgical access to the cul-de-sacs and sidewalls and protecting the ureters during parametrial dissection and the hysterectomy colpotomy.** Tubal patency can also be assessed with instillation of dilute methylene blue solution into the uterine manipulator.

Improved 5-mm laparoscope optics are adequate for most laparoscopic procedures. This smaller scope allows for port hopping, the risk of hernia formation is reduced, and sutures are not necessary for closure. Some surgeons prefer a 10-mm laparoscope. Use of an angled 30-degree scope tip can optimize visualization. Graspers should be ergonomically friendly, and a simple accessible locking mechanism can be helpful. Atraumatic graspers are predominantly used. A laparoscopic blunt probe is helpful with surgical dissection of the retroperitoneum and dense adhesions of endometriosis. A suction irrigator is important, in the event of unanticipated bleeding and also to irrigate at the conclusion of a case because blood is adhesiogenic and clearing the surgical field might be helpful in adhesion prevention. The tip edges of the suction irrigator are relatively sharp and can cause trauma; care should be taken when using this instrument for blunt dissection.

**It is important for the surgeon to be familiar with the energy modality to be used in a case, whether it be electrosurgical, ultrasonic, or laser. An energy device ideally performs both a coagulation and a cutting mechanism.** Options include a disposable bipolar vessel-sealing device, an ultrasonic dissector, laser, or simply combining the use of reusable bipolar forceps and monopolar scissors. Most energy instruments are compatible with 5-mm ports. Care must be taken with deployment of energy and dissection of surgical planes that inadvertent thermal injury to visceral structures is avoided. It is imperative to be mindful of instrument tip location at all times.

Needle holders, a laparoscopic tenaculum, specimen bags, and accessory trocars should be available. A suture or fixation device can be used to optimize exposure, and a rectal probe might be used to delineate the rectum in cases of rectovaginal endometriosis. Hemostatic agents and laparoscopic clip appliers can be useful for problematic bleeding requiring intervention beyond pressure, coagulation, or suturing. The endoscopic ligature loop provides cost-effective ligation of the appendix through a port size as little as 3 mm; laparoscopic staplers are a more costly alternative and require a 10-mm port size but may be preferable with a more complicated appendectomy.

Cystoscopic equipment might be needed to evaluate the ureteral orifices, confirm ureteral patency and bladder integrity; alternatively the laparoscope can be used as a cystoscope at the conclusion of an operative procedure (O'Hanlan, 2007).

## Laparoscopic Port Placement

### Initial Entry

**More than 50% of all complications in laparoscopic surgery are related to the initial trocar insertion, with potentially life-threatening associated vascular and bowel injuries.** Techniques and instrumentation have evolved to mitigate against such serious injury, including use of bladeless (Fig. 10.11) rather than bladed trocars. **The umbilicus is the thinnest site of the abdominal wall, and is the preferred site for the initial laparoscopic entry in most cases. An alternative entry site is Palmer point in the left upper quadrant, which is particularly helpful in the setting of suspected periumbilical adhesions, the presence of a larger abdominal mass, or umbilical mesh (Fig. 10.12).**

The location of the great vessels in relation to the umbilicus is in part dependent on body habitus, with the umbilicus more caudad in

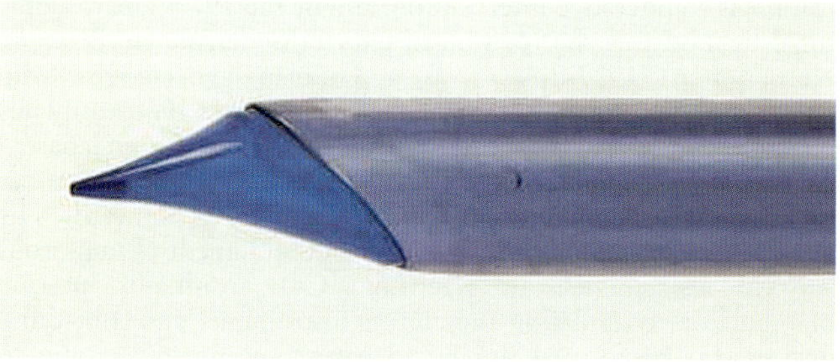

**Fig. 10.11** Blunt tip trocar

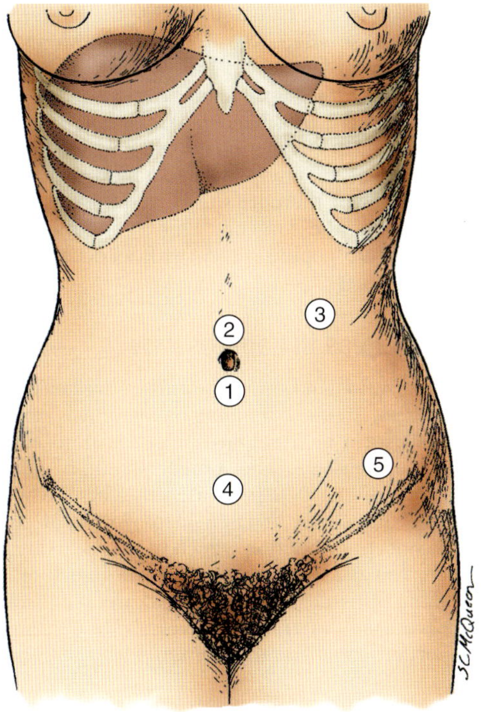


**Fig. 10.12** Usual sites for insertion of insufflating needle in laparoscopy: *(1)* infraumbilical fold, *(2)* supraumbilical fold, *(3)* left costal margin, *(4)* midway between umbilicus and pubis, and *(5)* left McBurney's point. (From Corson SL. Operating room preparation and basic techniques. In: Phillips JM, ed. *Laparoscopy.* Baltimore: Williams & Wilkins; 1977.)

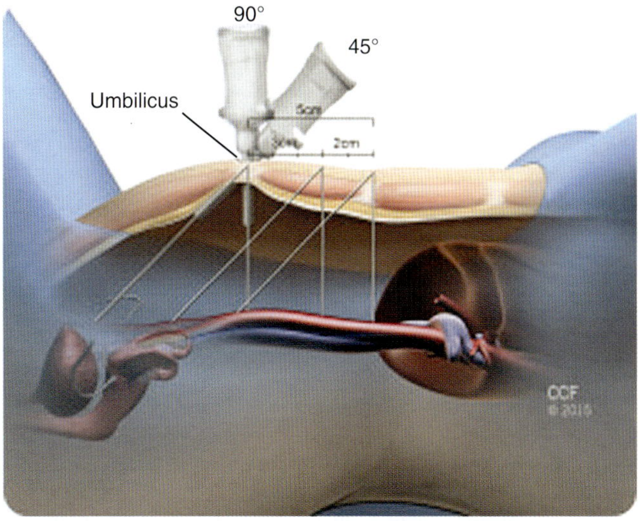


**Fig. 10.13** Intraumbilical primary trocar insertion for laparoscopic access: the relationship between points of entry and retroperitoneal vital vasculature by imaging. (Distances to retroperitoneal vasculature. Relationship of laparoscopic access points, angles of entry, and distances to retroperitoneal vasculature. *Stanhiser. Supraumbilical laparoscopic entry and distances to retroperitoneal vasculature. Am J Obstet Gynecol 2015.*)

relation to the vessels in the setting of obesity as opposed to directly above the vessels in thinner patients. **During laparoscopic entry the patient should be flat and not in an inadvertent Trendelenburg position and legs should be down minimizing hip flexion, otherwise the aorta and vena cava will be relocated more directly under the umbilicus and more at risk for injury (Fig. 10.13).** It is important to verbally check in with the anesthesiologist before making the initial incision and confirm the operating table is indeed flat. To decrease the risk of visceral injury the bladder should be empty, and in the setting of a planned left upper quadrant entry the stomach should be deflated with an orogastric tube.

As the optics with smaller-caliber laparoscopes have improved, 5-mm access ports can be used for most surgeries, allowing for "port-hopping" with the 5-mm laparoscope from different vantage points. The first trocar is inserted in an open or closed fashion. The open or Hasson technique consists of layer-by-layer dissection through the skin, subcutaneous tissue, fascia, and then peritoneum, with visual placement of a blunt specialized trocar to which fascial sutures are affixed to aide in closure (Hasson, 1974). This technique is favored by general surgeons and many gynecologic oncologists.

The two closed-entry techniques are (1) Verres needle (Fig. 10.14) insertion, then carbon dioxide insufflation, then trocar insertion; and (2) direct trocar insertion without first instilling carbon dioxide. One advantage of direct trocar insertion compared with first insufflating with the Verres needle is that entry into the abdominal cavity is achieved more quickly. Intraabdominal $CO_2$ pressure as measured with the Verres needle is the most accurate assessment of intraperitoneal placement and should be less than 10 mm. A higher $CO_2$ pressure is usually indicative of inadvertent preperitoneal placement of the Verres needle or a submental needle location, neither of which has clinical import other than the need to redo the Verres needle

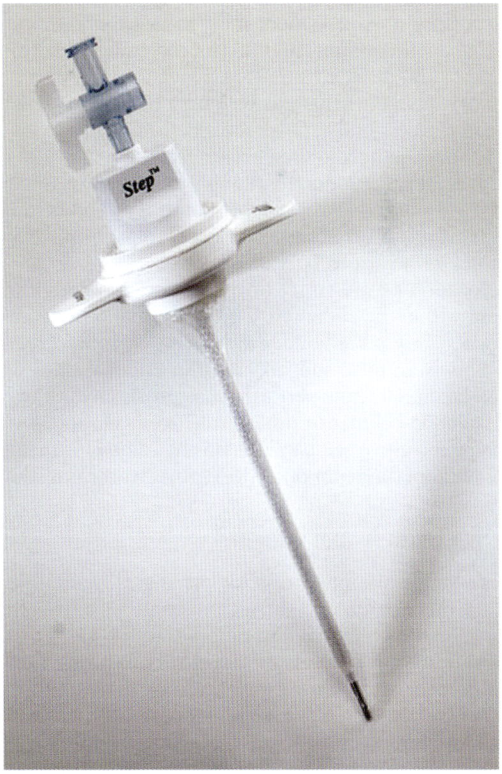


**Fig 10.14** Example of Veress needle.

insertion. The surgeon must be mindful of the risk of visceral or vascular injury. The stopcock of the Verres needle should be open, so that if a vascular injury occurs, blood will be promptly seen.

During the initial insertion process at the umbilicus one must be careful to maintain a midline trajectory to avoid off-side injury to the more lateral but ever-present iliac vessels. The abdominal wall should be sufficiently elevated to protect against injury to the aorta, vena cava, and other intraabdominal or retroperitoneal structures. Towel clips can help maximize elevation of the abdominal wall to increase safety during entry.

With either the Verres needle technique or direct entry, having the laparoscope within an optical trocar to guide the insertion process can be invaluable. A Cochrane review found that no single technique or instrument prevents the occurrence of vascular or visceral injury associated with laparoscopic entry. What is most important to successful laparoscopic entry is surgeon expertise and familiarity with the nuances of a particular entrance method. It is recommended that the choice of entry technique be based on surgeon preference, experience, and comfort level (Ahmad, 2019).

### Accessory Port Placement

**Accessory ports are placed under laparoscopic visualization from the entry port site and so are less fraught with risk.** Radially dilating or bladeless trocars are generally safer than bladed trocars. The smaller the incision, the lower the risk of future hernia formation. Any port site can be enlarged, if need be, for specimen removal or larger caliber equipment; this would preferentially be a midline port to avoid lateral nerve entrapment with wound closure. A general rule is a port site with a diameter greater than 11 mm will have fascial closure to prevent a postoperative port site hernia, though hernias have occurred even in 5-mm port sites. Microsized 2- to 3-mm percutaneous instruments are available, some in reposable fashion such that the equivalent of a larger instrument can be added to the tip of the device from within the abdomen.

The surgeon should operate with both hands, and decisions about accessory port placement must reflect this requirement. A diamond-shaped configuration allows for equal opportunity for both right- and left-sided surgeons. Once a surgeon masters use of the suprapubic port this can be a very useful constellation for laparoscopic access and exposure, dissection, suturing, and tissue removal. Some gynecologists prefer ipsilateral port placement because it is more ergonomic, though it is less versatile and less cosmetic. All surgeons should be mindful of body mechanics when operating; shorter surgeons need to "step up" for better ergonomics with various port placements.

The location of the target operative site also determines port placement within the abdomen. The vagina can be an access point for a trocar, easily placed under direct vision in the posterior cul-de-sac. This is an ideal spot to insert an endobag into which an ovary can be placed while performing a cystectomy in the pelvis. A vaginal balloon occluder or other malleable occlusion device such as a sponge in a glove can be placed in the vagina for maintenance of the pneumoperitoneum once the vaginal trocar is removed.

### Single-Site Surgery and Vnotes

There are single-site platforms for placing all operative instruments and the laparoscope through a single port, usually 2.5 to 3 cm in diameter. Operative dissection, traction, resection, suturing, and specimen removal can be performed through this single incision, which is traditionally located at the umbilicus. The learning curve for single-site laparoscopy is steeper than multiport laparoscopy, mainly because of issues with triangulation. The robotic platform allows for greater ease with orientation. Instruments with flexible tips are useful. The vagina can also be an access point for single-site surgery, and this is the basis of Vnotes. An accessory abdominal port can always be placed to assist with a single-site surgery, as a hybrid procedure.

## HAND-ASSISTED LAPAROSCOPY

Another example of hybrid surgery is hand-assisted laparoscopy, in which an access port large enough to accommodate the surgeon's hand is used. Challenging cases with severe adhesive disease, a large mass effect, or innumerous fibroids requiring removal might benefit from the placement of a hand in the pelvis and continuation of the laparoscopic procedure. This can be achieved by placement of a hand port. The platform has a gel covering through which the operator's hand can be placed without losing either pneumoperitoneum or laparoscopic visualization. The length of the port site corresponds in centimeters to the glove size of the surgeon. This is one of many hybrid approaches to laparoscopic surgery, with a focus on minimally invasive surgical access.

## Surgical Principles in Laparoscopy

Adequate visualization and surgical exposure are key components of optimal surgery. An understanding of anatomy is paramount so that tissue planes can be developed in avascular spaces to delineate structures and disease. The surgeon should be familiar with the nuances of any energy device used in a case, whether it be electrosurgical, ultrasonic, or laser. Deployment of energy also includes the concept of traction, which when occurring either on or off camera can cause unsuspected tissue injury or bleeding. Gentle handling of tissue (Fig. 10.15) and careful dissection technique with avoidance of trauma to vessels, bowel, and urinary tract is important, as is communication with the surgical team throughout the case.

## Anesthesia

General anesthesia with endotracheal intubation is preferred for gynecologic laparoscopic surgery because it facilitates both the pneumoperitoneum and Trendelenburg position by relaxing the abdominal wall and providing ventilation. This enhances visualization and exposure of pelvic structures. The surgeon should be aware of the physiologic effects of the carbon dioxide pneumoperitoneum and attempt to maintain as low an intraabdominal pressure as necessary. Similarly, the degree of Trendelenburg should be only that necessary to achieve adequate exposure and can vary from case to case. Communication between the anesthesiologist and laparoscopic surgeon before, during, and immediately after an operative procedure is extremely important.

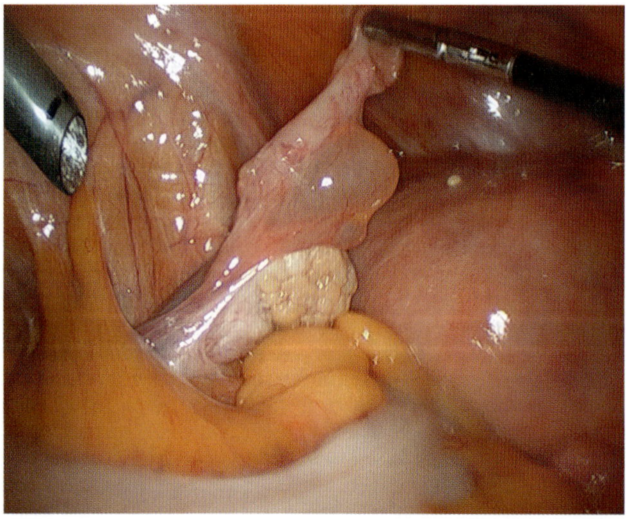

**Fig 10.15** Laparoscopic view of left pelvis viewing left lower quadrant port and right atraumatic grasper holding left fallopian tube with paratubal cyst and normal ovary. (Courtesy Dr. Seine Chiang, University of Washington.)

## Laparoscopic Procedures

### Laparoscopic Hysterectomy

Vaginal hysterectomy is the preferred method for benign hysterectomy when feasible (ACOG, 2017). **Laparoscopic hysterectomy is the preferred alternative to open surgery for patients in whom vaginal hysterectomy is not appropriate, such as when adnexal pathologic tissue is present, endometriosis needs to be evaluated and treated, or an enlarged and distorted fibroid uterus (Fig. 10.16) extends toward the pelvic sidewall.**

The most common indication for hysterectomy of any type is symptomatic fibroids. These usually benign myometrial tumors occur in up to 70% of women and can cause pain, abnormal bleeding, anemia, and pressure symptoms, significantly affecting quality of life in those patients who choose removal of the uterus as a definitive surgery. Endometriosis is the second most common indication for hysterectomy in the United States, and advanced surgical skills are usually required for optimal results. Other indications for hysterectomy include gynecologic cancer, pelvic infection, definitive management of chronic uterine pain or abnormal uterine bleeding. The incidence of benign hysterectomy is decreasing because the expense has risen exponentially and there is more concentrated focus on medical management of pelvic pain and abnormal bleeding.

Use of a uterine manipulator to optimize surgical access to operative sites and to protect the ureters is helpful during laparoscopic hysterectomy. A long-acting, appropriately placed paracervical block can be helpful in postoperative pain management. If the patient chooses a total laparoscopic hysterectomy with the cervix removed, the largest incision then is the colpotomy site at the top of the vagina, through which the specimen can be removed. Specimen extraction of larger uteri requiring morcellation for removal in laparoscopic surgery is discussed later in this chapter. Precursors for ovarian cancer can arise in the fallopian tubes, and so it is recommended that laparoscopic hysterectomy for benign conditions with intended ovarian preservation be accompanied by bilateral salpingectomy to reduce the risk of future ovarian cancer.

### Laparoscopic Myomectomy

Uterine fibroids are the most common pelvic tumor in women and, when symptomatic, can be managed with hormonal manipulation and menstrual suppression, uterine artery embolization, radiofrequency ablation, MRI-guided focused ultrasound, hysterectomy, or fibroid removal (myomectomy). Myomectomy is the preferred nonmedical treatment in women intending to preserve future childbearing potential and can be accomplished laparoscopically in a majority of cases. Medical treatments such as gonadotropin-releasing hormone agonists or antagonists, selective progesterone receptor modulators, or progesterone antagonists can be used preoperatively if surgical status might benefit from correction of anemia or shrinkage of the mass effect.

Placement of a uterine manipulator allows for variable access to the uterus and attachment of a dye-filled syringe can confirm tubal patency and help identify the endometrial cavity. A long-acting paracervical block can decrease postoperative cramping and facilitate same-day discharge. Dilute vasopressin injected just under the serosal surface where any uterine incision will be made can contribute to a seemingly bloodless surgery. Temporary ligation of the uterine artery at its origin in the pelvic sidewall can be performed to reduce intraoperative blood loss. Tourniquet application is an option. Port placement and the trajectory of the uterine incision are determined by both the anatomy and the operator's preference for suturing. Optimally the hysterotomy incision to the level of the pseudocapsule is made with minimal thermal damage. Traction with a laparoscopic tenaculum can be helpful while atraumatically dissecting the fibroid from healthy myometrium. Hysterotomy closure is performed in layers as indicated. Often, barbed suture is used because it reapproximates the tissue in a balanced manner without undue tension. The final layer can be sutured as a hidden subcuticular closure, at which the barbed suture excels. Alternatively, a whipped suture line or baseball in-and-out suture can be placed as the final layer of closure. Specimen removal can be accomplished either abdominally or vaginally in a contained or open fashion, depending on the patient and operator preference.

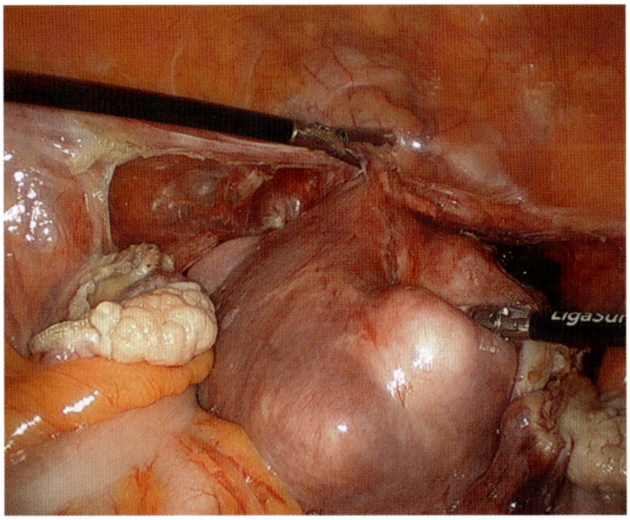

Fig. 10.16 The beginning of a laparoscopic hysterectomy for uterine fibroids showing the creation of the bladder flap with the left grasper elevating the bladder peritoneum and a bipolar/cutting device in the right hand. (Courtesy Dr. Seine Chiang, University of Washington.)

### Treatment of Endometriosis

Endometriosis is an inflammatory disease process manifested by pain, infertility, bowel and bladder dysfunction, and a multitude of other heterogenous presentations. It is a condition in which lesions microscopically resembling the glands and stroma of endometrial tissue are located in aberrant foci outside of the endometrial lining. The most common form of endometriosis is superficial peritoneal disease, which is often located in close proximity to the hypogastric nerve complex in the vicinity of the uterosacral ligaments. More deeply infiltrative forms of endometriosis in the pelvis can cause dense pelvic adhesive disease and obliteration of the posterior cul-de-sac, invade bowel or bladder, destroy fallopian tubes, and essentially replace the ovaries with endometrioma formation. There is not necessarily a linear correlation between the severity of disease and the degree of pain symptoms. Nodular fixation or prominence with tenderness of the uterosacral ligaments on pelvic examination can raise suspicion for endometriosis. An adnexal mass might be palpated and ultrasound then demonstrate the typical appearance of an ovarian endometrioma; however, there is no valid noninvasive diagnostic test for endometriosis, and laparoscopy remains the gold standard for the diagnosis of this benign but potentially debilitating condition. This is especially problematic for the subset of patients with significant, chronic pain but no objective findings outside of the operating room, in whom there can be a significant delay in diagnosis.

**Conservative surgery for endometriosis is usually performed laparoscopically, with attention to restoration of normal anatomy, releasing adhesions, and excising or ablating any pathologic findings. Appendectomy may be required** (Fig 10.17). Advanced laparoscopic skills are often required. As with hysterectomy and myomectomy, a uterine manipulator is essential for adequate

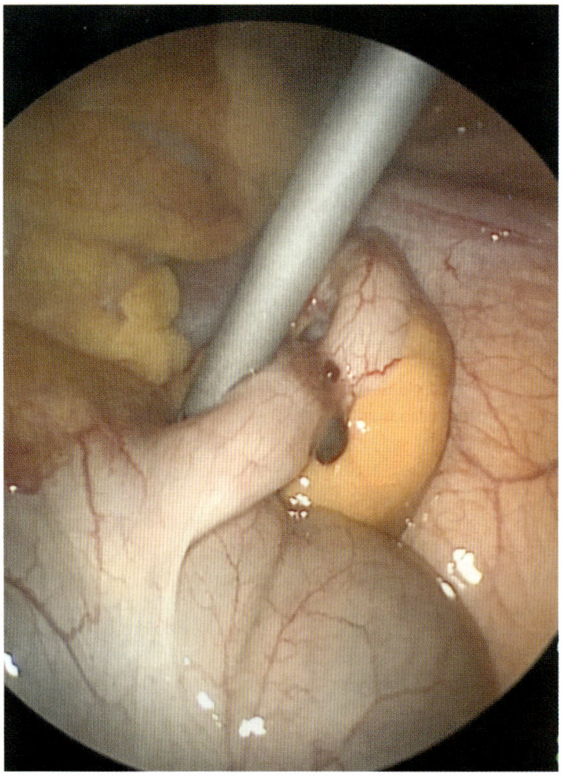

**Fig. 10.17** Endometriosis on the appendix. (Courtesy Dr. Licia Raymond, University of Washington.)

inspection and optimal treatment and can also provide a conduit with which to assess tubal patency. Surgical care is usually combined with medical treatments and complementary approaches to pain and/or fertility management, as indicated. Future interventions will likely block angiogenesis and ameliorate neuroinflammation.

### Surgical Management of Ectopic Pregnancy

An ectopic pregnancy is an extrauterine pregnancy and is most often located in the fallopian tube. Early ectopic pregnancies are often amenable to medical management without having to resort to surgery. In ideal circumstances this condition is diagnosed before any symptoms occur and before the pregnancy is large enough to be visualized by ultrasound, by a process of elimination demonstrating that a nonviable pregnancy is not located within the uterus. **Laparoscopy is the treatment of choice when surgery is needed or medical management fails and can include removal of the affected fallopian tube (salpingectomy) or removal of the ectopic pregnancy from an incision in a retained fallopian tube (salpingostomy) or merely extracting the ectopic from the distal aspect of the fallopian tube in cases of a tubal abortion**. Indications for ectopic surgery include failed medical management, inability to comply with the medical management protocol or a contraindication to methotrexate, impending or ongoing rupture, hemodynamic instability, and patient preference.

Ectopic pregnancies can also occur in the abdominal cavity, on the ovary, within the cervix, in the interstitial segment of tube within the uterus, in the upper lateral horn of a bicornuate uterus, and within a cesarean section scar. Heterotopic pregnancies, in which an ectopic pregnancy coexists with an intrauterine pregnancy, occur more commonly in the setting of assisted reproduction. These variants are associated with a greater risk of life-threatening rupture, in part because of anatomic considerations. Combined medical and surgical intervention may be required.

## ADNEXAL PATHOLOGY

**Laparoscopy is ideal for the diagnosis and management of tubal and ovarian masses, with adnexal preservation an option in the setting of a fertility-sparing procedure**. Appropriate preoperative workup is indicated to avoid operating on functional cysts. Torsed adnexal structures can usually be unwound to preserve adnexal function. Careful dissection with attention to minimizing thermal damage to the preserved tube and ovarian tissue is important when excising pathology, to preserve ovarian reserve and future reproductive potential. At the conclusion of an ovarian cystectomy, transient pressure on the retained ovary usually suffices for hemostasis; this can be applied while irrigating and surveying the abdomen. Cautery or hemostatic agents are rarely needed.

**Atraumatic dissection is requisite to minimize the risk of specimen rupture in the setting of ovarian cystectomy of a potential malignancy**. Peritoneal washings can be obtained for cytologic testing and contained specimen removal performed using an appropriately sized endoscopic bag. The ovary can be placed into the specimen bag during dissection, to minimize content spillage in case of cyst rupture.

When releasing dense adhesions of adnexal structures to the lateral pelvic sidewall, ureterolysis can be helpful to protect the ureter. Making a window in the broad ligament to isolate the infundibulopelvic ligament before ligation of the ovarian vessels when performing an oophorectomy ensures no harm comes to the ureter at the pelvic brim. It is important for the laparoscopist to be familiar with the retroperitoneal space, and this maneuver enhances skill development in retroperitoneal dissection.

### Risk-Reducing Adnexal Surgery

Removal of the ovaries and fallopian tubes is a means by which to prevent future adnexal cancer and is the most effective strategy for reducing the incidence of ovarian cancer and mortality in high-risk women with hereditary mutations such as *BRCA1* and *BRCA2*. The preoperative workup should include a recent pelvic ultrasound and CA-125 level. Risk-reducing laparoscopic bilateral salpingo-oophorectomy includes a careful survey of peritoneal and serosal surfaces and biopsies as appropriate. Pelvic washings are obtained for cytologic testing, and care must be taken to remove the entire fallopian tube. The ovarian vessels are ligated at the pelvic brim, at least 2 cm proximal to the ovary. Special pathologic sectioning of the specimen is required because of the increased potential for occult malignancy.

Adnexal removal at the time of hysterectomy in women with average risk is a strategy to reduce the risk of future adnexal disease, and counseling should take into consideration a patient's age and willingness to use replacement estrogen. Prophylactic bilateral salpingectomy with the removal of the fallopian tubes alone more than halves the risk for ovarian cancer and is recommended when feasible in women who have completed childbearing and are undergoing laparoscopic surgery, including hysterectomy (Falconer, 2015).

## STERILIZATION

Sterilization is intended as a permanent procedure. Laparoscopic options include mechanical ligation of the fallopian tubes, electrosurgical desiccation of the fallopian tubes, and removal of the fallopian tubes. The latter procedure provides the greatest protection against future ovarian cancer and the highest efficacy and is recommended whenever feasible. Care must be taken to remove all of the fimbria and to not affect the ovarian blood supply.

## PELVIC INFLAMMATORY DISEASE

Pelvic inflammatory disease (PID) can be related to an ascending infection from a sexually transmitted pathogen such as chlamydia or gonorrhea, from gynecologic instrumentation or surgery, from IUD placement or a pregnancy-related condition, or from a nongynecologic source such as appendicitis or diverticulitis. Pelvic inflammatory disease is multimicrobial and can result in tuboovarian abscess formation. Broad-spectrum antibiotics are often effective treatment; however, surgical intervention might be needed in the setting of inadequate response to medical management. Laparoscopic drainage of pelvic abscesses, with concomitant washout with saline irrigation and lysis of adhesions, can serve as a minimally invasive and efficacious approach to abscess-related PID.

## ONCOLOGY

Laparoscopy plays an important role in gynecologic oncology and is especially beneficial for patients who are overweight, with an associated decrease in perioperative morbidity. It is increasingly being used in endometrial cancer staging, with randomized clinical trials showing equivalent oncologic safety and benefits in terms of perioperative outcomes (Walker, 2012). There was a trend favoring laparoscopic radical hysterectomy for cervical cancer, which reversed in 2018 when available evidence suggested compromised long-term oncologic outcomes. Laparoscopic staging is performed in cases of ovarian cancer, and a Cochrane review has determined that laparoscopy can be helpful in determining which cases of advanced ovarian cancer should first undergo neoadjuvant chemotherapy versus primary surgical debulking (Van de Vrie, 2019).

## PELVIC PROLAPSE

Abdominal sacral colpopexy by laparotomy is considered the gold standard for vaginal vault prolapse, and laparoscopic techniques have been developed to similarly suspend the vaginal apex to the anterior longitudinal ligament of the sacrum, with apparent equivalence in surgical outcomes. Favorable outcomes support the use of laparoscopic sacral hysteropexy for women interested in uterine preservation. Laparoscopic uterosacral ligament colpopexy is an option for apical support at the time of hysterectomy.

## COMPLICATIONS OF LAPAROSCOPY

Complications of laparoscopy are listed in Box 10.5.

## SPECIMEN REMOVAL

Inherent in surgical treatment of disease is the potential need to remove pathologic tissue, and the small access ports of endoscopic surgery can pose a challenge in this regard. Hysteroscopic removal of lesions and tissue fragments from the uterine cavity are removed with suction devices or careful use of specifically designed forceps. Specimen removal with laparoscopic surgery is often efficiently accomplished with use of endoscopic bags placed through a laparoscopic abdominal port or a vaginal port; this is particular true of adnexal cysts because once the fluid is expelled from within the exteriorized bag, what little tissue is left in the bag is easily retrieved in a "contained" fashion.

Removal of solid, larger masses can represent a challenge, especially if there is concern that damaging the integrity of the mass with open morcellation within the abdominal cavity might cause an adverse outcome in the setting of tissue dispersion of an undiagnosed malignancy. Of particular concern is the possibility that a rare leiomyosarcoma could be mistaken for a benign leiomyoma. In years past, electromechanical morcellation without containment was commonly used to dismantle fibroids and hysterectomy specimens for removal through a laparoscopic port, particularly during laparoscopic myomectomy procedures and supracervical hysterectomies. This resulted in case reports of the inadvertent dissemination of benign and unsuspected malignant tissue within the abdomen and pelvis. Recognition of the potential adverse effect of this practice led to the U.S. Food and Drug Administration (FDA) to issue a warning in 2014 against the use of laparoscopic power morcellators. As a result of that and subsequent FDA warnings, the use of power morcellation and uncontained morcellation has plummeted, as has the incidence of supracervical hysterectomy (AAGL, 2018).

Preoperative counseling in the setting of presumed benign disease should include a discussion of the potential for an undiagnosed malignancy and address the matter of safe specimen removal. Techniques for contained removal of larger specimens have been developed, and the patient may express a preference for the site of extraction, be it the umbilicus, a suprapubic site, or the vagina. With a total laparoscopic hysterectomy, the colpotomy site is the largest operative incision and is an obvious site for specimen extraction, contained or otherwise. Use of a ringed wound retractor within a containment bag can facilitate access for hand morcellation of an enlarged uterus, whether extraction takes place from the vagina or an enlarged umbilical incision or suprapubic site (Fig. 10.18). An FDA-approved containment system is available for use with an electronic morcellator, which is intended for abdominal use only.

### Laparoscopy in Pregnancy

Laparoscopic surgery can be safely performed on a pregnant patient in any trimester, with fewer wound complications, less risk of thromboembolism, less uterine manipulation, better visualization, and faster recovery compared with open surgery. Appendicitis and biliary concerns are the most common indications for abdominal surgery during pregnancy (Fig. 10.19). Early surgical management of both cholecystitis and suspected appendicitis is encouraged for pregnant patients because a delay in aggressive management can lead to increased morbidity and

**BOX 10.5** Laparoscopic Complications

- Lacerations of major blood vessels: aorta, vena cava, iliac, obturator, epigastric
- Trocar or Veress needle injury
- Intestinal injury
- Urinary tract injury
- Thermal injury—immediate or delayed
- Positional injury and/or nerve compression
- Adverse consequences of pneumoperitoneum, such as hypercapnia, reduced cardiac output, ventilatory compromise, gas embolism, pneumothorax, cardiac arrhythmias
- Incisional hernia

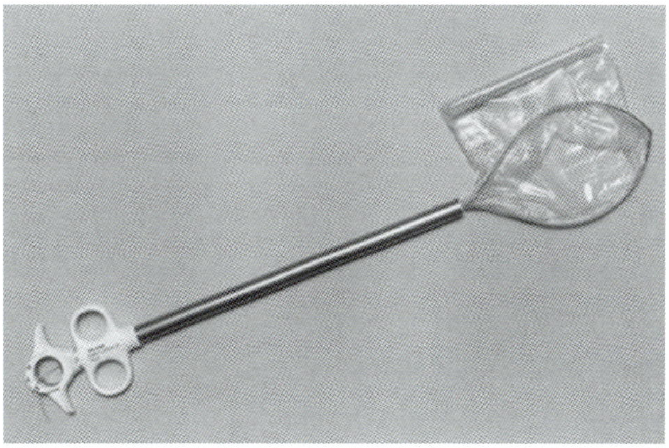

**Fig. 10.18** Specimen extraction bag.

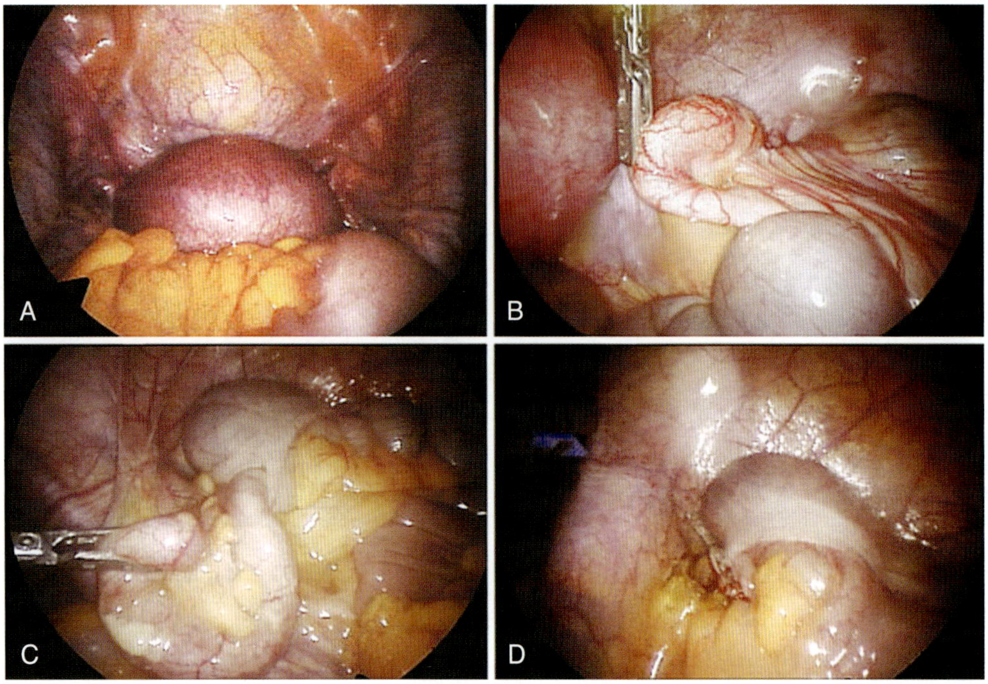


**Fig. 10.19** Laparoscopy for appendectomy in pregnancy. (Seon Hye Park, Moon Il Park, Joong Sub Choi, Jung Hun Lee, Hyung Ook Kim and Hungdai Kim. *European Journal of Obstetrics & Gynecology and Reproductive Biology*, 2010-01-01, Volume 148, Issue 1, Pages 44-48, Copyright © 2009 Elsevier Ireland Ltd.)

fetal loss. Additional indications for laparoscopic surgery in pregnancy include adnexal torsion, a symptomatic or suspicious adnexal mass, trauma, and intrauterine access for fetoscopic surgeries. To reduce compression of the vena cava and any subsequent adverse effect on cardiac output and placental blood flow, patients in more advanced stages of pregnancy are positioned in supine or lithotomy with a leftward tilt. The intraabdominal pressure is ideally maintained at less than 12 mm Hg because $CO_2$ insufflation of the abdomen to pressures greater than 15 mm may adversely affect maternal ventilatory status, cardiac output, and placental perfusion.

In the second and third trimesters of pregnancy, initial abdominal entry has an increased risk of inadvertently injuring the enlarged uterus. To decrease this risk, an open entry technique and entry in the left upper quadrant at the Palmer point should be considered. Secondary trocars are inserted under direct visualization, with the index finger placed near the trocar tip to control entry into the abdomen and avoid injury. A sponge stick in the vagina may be used to gently tilt the uterus, avoiding use of a standard uterine manipulator.

The American College of Chest Physicians (ACCP) guidelines recommend thromboprophylaxis for all pregnant patients undergoing surgery. Mechanical compression devices are reasonable for shorter laparoscopic procedures. The addition of low-molecular-weight heparin is suggested for procedures lasting longer than 45 minutes. Early ambulation should be encouraged postoperatively. Prophylactic tocolytics are not routinely administered but can be provided to treat any increase in uterine activity. If the fetus is of a viable gestational age, fetal heart rate monitoring should be performed before and after the surgical procedure.

## Robotics in Laparoscopy

Robotic technology inserts computer assistance into a remote surgical field and was initially developed for military application. The robotic platform for laparoscopic assistance was FDA approved for use in gynecologic surgery in 2005, and for some surgeons it is a preferred method by which to perform certain advanced laparoscopic procedures. The surgeon's console is remote from the patient and has both finger-controlled handles and foot pedals. A surgical cart with robotic arms is at the bedside, as is a surgical scrub technician and often an additional surgical assistant. A second surgeon's console can be used by a trainee. The surgeon sits outside the sterile surgical field at the console and has control of all docked laparoscopic equipment, including the 3-D camera. This places camera control and most of the surgical field exposure entirely in the purview of the operating surgeon and takes it out of the hands of the assistant, who is at the bedside providing instrument and needle exchanges, suction, and traction. With robotic surgery the docked instruments add an element of abdominal wall elevation, which can aid in exposure, especially helpful with patients who are morbidly obese. Articulated needle holders, graspers, and energy devices enhance the surgeon's ability to dissect and suture. Uterine manipulation and specimen removal take place at the bedside.

Robotic technology in its current state has a relatively cumbersome footprint and adds cost to the operating room environment. Robotics adoption has outpaced high-level evidence supporting its use in gynecologic surgery; despite innumerable scientific articles being published on surgical robotics, it is difficult to separate evidence from the power of marketing. In its current state, robotic assistance in gynecologic surgery does not appear to significantly add to the surgical armamentarium of an advanced laparoscopic surgeon with an experienced surgical team; however, the integrated system of robotic surgical simulation for training, the ability of the surgeon to completely control operating field exposure, and the articulated instrumentation simplifying suturing and enhancing surgical dissection have resulted in an increasing number of gynecologists adopting robotics into practice.

Although the evidence suggests that for laparoscopic surgeries performed by an expert gynecologist the current robotic platform holds no advantage over conventional laparoscopic surgery, it appears that for certain complex procedures such as oncologic surgery, surgery in the obese, multiple myomectomy, challenging hysterectomy, and sacrocolpopexy, and for certain surgeons who otherwise would perform an open procedure, there is a role for robotic-assisted laparoscopy. Advances in artificial intelligence and sensor technology will reshape the role of robotic assistance in minimally invasive surgery, providing multiple platforms for bedside automation of tasks such as vaginal cuff suturing, for delineation of anatomy and pathology by augmented reality with image overlay, and for optimization of surgical strategy. This focus on smart technology with a smaller footprint could conceivably revolutionize minimally invasive surgery in the future.

## HOW WE LEARN: THE ROLE OF ENDOSCOPIC SIMULATION

**Surgical simulation plays a vital role in skill acquisition both for trainees and for established gynecologic surgeons learning new techniques, and endoscopic simulation is being increasingly integrated into surgical skill development.** The time invested in learning the principles of good surgical technique and acquiring skills has been shown to improve surgical prowess (Lichtman, 2018). Muscle memory is developed by repetition of simulated endoscopic tasks, and both speed and accuracy can be improved with accumulated hours of practice.

As of 2020, the American Board of Obstetrics and Gynecology requires candidates to have certification in fundamentals of laparoscopic surgery (FLS), which includes an assessment of simulation skills and a written examination. The five required hands-on tasks demonstrate eye-hand coordination and the ability to work with two hands in an ambidextrous, efficient fashion. Both time and accuracy are evaluated in the testing scenarios.

The American College of Obstetricians and Gynecologists (ACOG) endeavors to provide a standardized curriculum for surgical skill training through its Simulations Working Group and, together with the Council on Resident Education in Obstetrics and Gynecology (CREOG) Surgical Skills Task Force, has designed a curriculum that includes endoscopic modules. Video recordings of operative techniques and procedures are increasingly used in gynecologic education, both to demonstrate surgical techniques and to review surgical performance. Live surgery is thereby optimized, enhancing excellence in gynecologic care.

## GYNECOLOGIC SURGERY: THE TRIPLE AIM

In 2008, the Institutes for Healthcare Improvement identified the Triple Aim as a 3-D approach to improving health care outcomes (Box 10.6). Endoscopic surgery certainly supports one primary goal of the Institute for Healthcare Improvement's Triple Aim: enhancing the patient experience. Improvements in technology, techniques, and pain management have led to more outpatient and office-based procedures, as well as more complex and complicated endoscopic endeavors. Technological advances will likely come to support computer assistance and 3-D visualization for conventional laparoscopy, safer dissection algorithms, automated suturing, smaller port size with more versatile equipment, and better tissue extraction methods.

The American Board of Obstetrics and Gynecology now designates a practice focus in minimally invasive gynecology. Fellowships in MIGS provide postresidency training and have improved the caliber of gynecologic surgery and research in the United States. As of 2020, graduating residents in obstetrics and gynecology in the United States must attain certification in fundamentals of laparoscopic surgery, and a certification examination dedicated to the field of gynecology called Essentials in Minimally Invasive Gynecology (EMIG) is being suggested as a specialty-specific assessment tool.

Operative cases traditionally completed by open techniques will more often in experienced hands be performed via an endoscopic approach, with attendant shorter hospital stays and recovery time but also potentially with longer operative times and case-specific costs. Enhanced, ongoing surgical training is paramount for those gynecologists who choose to provide surgical services, and adequate surgical volume is important. Video documentation has provided a modern avenue for endoscopic surgical education and assessment. Simulation training in endoscopy is being increasingly integrated into surgical skill development to facilitate proper surgical technique and safe instrumentation. The complexity of medical, technological, and procedural advances in gynecologic care has engendered a cost shift and training burden on our health care systems, challenging our very definition of the obstetrician-gynecologist, and there is strong evidence to support postresidency surgical tracking, with exceptions for practitioners in rural and underserved areas. Thoughtful engagement, transparency, and nonbiased scrutiny will help us strike a balance with the other two primary goals of the Triple Aim: improving population health and controlling health care costs.

**BOX 10.6** The Triple Aim: Improving Health Care

Improve the patient experience of health care.
Improve the health of the population.
Reduce the per capita cost of health care.

## REFERENCES


AAGL Practice Report: Practice guidelines for the management of hysteroscopic distending media. *J Minim Invasive Gynecol.* 2013;20(2):137–148.

AAGL Tissue Extraction Task Force. Morcellation during uterine tissue extraction: an update. *J Minim Invasive Gynecol.* 2018;25(4):543–550.

Abel MK, Kho K, Walter A, Zaritsky E. Measuring quality in minimally invasive gynecologic surgery: what, how, and why? *J Minim Invasive Gynecol.* 2019;26(2):321–326.

Ahmad G, Baker J, Finnerty J, et al. Laparoscopic entry techniques. *Cochrane Database Syst Rev.* 2019;1:CD006583.

American College of Obstetricians and Gynecologists. Choosing the route of hysterectomy for benign disease. Committee Opinion # 701. *Obstet Gynecol.* 2017;129(6):e155.

American College of Obstetricians and Gynecologists. Preoperative pathways: Enhanced Recovery after Surgery (ERAS). Committee Opinion #750. *Obstet Gynecol.* 2018;132:e120–e130.

Asherman JG. Amenorrhoea traumatic (atretica). *J Obstet Gynaecol Br Emp.* 1948:55(1):23–30.

Bakour SH, Timmermans A, Mol BW, et al. Management of women with postmenopausal bleeding: evidence-based review. *Obstet Gynaecol.* 2012;14(4):243–249.

Benacerraf BR, Abuhamad AZ, Bromley B, et al. Consider ultrasound first for imaging the female pelvis. *Am J Obstet Gynecol.* 2015;212(4):450–455.

Bennett A, Lepage C, Thavorn K, et al. Effectiveness of outpatient versus operating room hysteroscopy for the diagnosis and treatment of uterine conditions: a systematic review and meta-analysis. *J Obstet Gynaecol Can.* 2019;41(7):930–941.

Falconer H, Yin L, Grönberg H, Altman D. Ovarian cancer risk after salpingectomy: a nationwide population-based study. *J Natl Cancer Inst.* 2015;107(2):dju410.

Fergusson RJ, Lethaby A, Sheppard S, Farquhar C. Endometrial resection and ablation versus hysterectomy for heavy menstrual bleeding. *Cochrane Database Syst Rev.* 2013;29:CD000329.

Florio P, Nappi L, Mannini L, et al. Prevalence of infections after in-office hysteroscopy in premenopausal and postmenopausal women. *J Minim Invasive Gynecol.* 2019;26(4):733–739.

Hasson HM. Open laparoscopy: a report of 150 cases. *J Reprod Med.* 1974;12:234–238.

Jacobaeus HC. Concerning the possibility of applying cystoscopy in the examination of serous cavities. *Münch Med Wochenschr.* 1910;57:2090–2092.

Lichtman AS, Parker W, Goff B, et al. A randomized multicenter study assessing the educational impact of a computerized interactive hysterectomy trainer on gynecology residents. *J Minim Invasive Gynecol.* 2018;25(6):1035–1043.
Loring M, Morris SN, Isaacson KB. Minimally invasive specialists and rates of laparoscopic hysterectomy. *JSLS.* 2015;19(1):e2014.00221.
Munro M, Christianson L. Complications of hysteroscopic and uterine resectoscopic surgery. *Clin Obstet Gynecol.* 2015;58(4):765–797.
O'Hanlan KA. Cystoscopy with a 5mm laparoscope and a suction irrigator. *J Minim Invasive Gynecol.* 2007;14(2):260–263.
Palmer R. Safety in laparoscopy. *J Reprod Med.* 1974;13(1):1–5.
Rotenberg O, Renz M, Reimers L, et al. Simultaneous endometrial aspiration and sonohysterography for the evaluation of endometrial pathology in women aged 50 years and older. *Obstet Gynecol.* 2015;125(2):414–423.
Selk A, Kroft J. Misoprostol in operative hysteroscopy. A systemic review and meta-analysis. *Obstet Gynecol.* 2011;118(4):941–949.
Semm K. New methods of pelviscopy (gynecologic laparoscopy) for myomectomy, ovariectomy, tubectomy, and adnectomy. *Endoscopy.* 1979;11(2):85–93.
Silva-Filho AL, Pereira Fde A, de Souza SS, et al. Five-year follow-up of levonorgestrel-releasing intrauterine system versus thermal balloon ablation for the treatment of heavy menstrual bleeding: a randomized controlled trial. *Contraception.* 2013;87:409–415.
Smith PP, Kolhe S, O'Connor S, Clark TJ. Vaginoscopy against standard treatment: a randomized controlled trial. *BJOG.* 2019;126(7):891–899.
Van de Vrie R, Rutten MJ, Asseler JD, et al. Laparoscopy for diagnosing resectability of disease in women with advanced ovarian cancer. *Cochrane Database Syst Rev.* 2019;3:CD009786.
Van Dongen H, de Kroon CD, Jacobi CE, et al. Diagnostic hysteroscopy in abnormal uterine bleeding: a systematic review and meta-analysis. *BJOG.* 2007;114(6):664–675.
Walker JL, Piedmont MR, Spirtos NM, et al. Recurrence and survival after random assignment to laparoscopy versus laparotomy for comprehensive surgical staging of uterine cancer: Gynecology Oncology Group Study LAP2. *J Clin Oncol.* 2012;30:695–700.
Wheeler KC, Goldstein SR. Transvaginal ultrasound for the diagnosis of abnormal uterine bleeding. *Clin Obstet Gynecol.* 2017;60(1):11–17.
Yildirim I, Yildirim D, Yesiralioglu S, et al. The visceral slide test for the prediction of abdominal wall adhesions: a prospective cohort study. *East J Med.* 2019;24(1):91–95.

**Suggested readings for this chapter can be found on ExpertConsult.com.**

PART III General Gynecology

# 11 Congenital Abnormalities of the Female Reproductive Tract

## Anomalies of the Vagina, Cervix, Uterus, and Adnexa

*Beth W. Rackow, Roger A. Lobo, Gretchen M. Lentz*

### KEY POINTS

- Gender identification in a newborn infant has emotional and psychological implications and should be performed as accurately as possible. However, in the setting of ambiguous genitalia, gender assignment should not be considered without definitive testing and multidisciplinary participation.
- Congenital adrenal hyperplasia is an autosomal recessive condition, most commonly the result of an inborn error of metabolism involving the enzyme 21-hydroxylase. Homozygous individuals account for 1 of every 490 to 67,000 births, averaging 1 in 14,000, and are at risk of moderate to severe manifestations. Approximately 1 in 20 to 1 in 250 individuals are heterozygotes (carriers), and they can have a more mild presentation. Differences in incidence depend on the ethnic background of the population tested.
- Vaginal agenesis is most often associated with Mayer-Rokitansky-Küster-Hauser syndrome, also known as müllerian agenesis. Up to 50% of these women have urologic abnormalities, and approximately one in eight have skeletal abnormalities as well.
- Approximately 15% of women with a history of first-trimester recurrent miscarriage and 25% of those with a second-trimester miscarriage may have a uterine anomaly.
- The uterine septum is the only uterine anomaly that can be easily corrected with a surgical procedure. In women with poor reproductive outcomes, surgery can normalize their chances of miscarriage and live birth.

Congenital abnormalities of the female reproductive tract are common and can affect the external genitalia and müllerian structures. These abnormalities can be caused by **genetic errors or by teratogenic events during embryonic development**. Minor abnormalities may be of little consequence, but major abnormalities may lead to severe impairment of menstrual and reproductive functions and can be associated with anomalies of the urinary tract. This chapter reviews a number of such abnormalities and discusses diagnosis and treatment. Anomalies can present at varying times in a woman's life—at birth, before puberty, with the onset of menses, and during a pregnancy with adverse pregnancy outcomes—but **many women with congenital anomalies of the reproductive tract are asymptomatic**. Based on large studies, **the incidence of müllerian anomalies is considered to be 1% to 3%** (Nahum, 1998), and the prevalence of uterine anomalies is suggested to be 5% to 8% (Chan, 2011). Because of the profound psychological effects such abnormalities can have, the gynecologist must approach the problems of genital and müllerian anomalies with sensitivity and an understanding of the effects on the woman and her family. Most tertiary centers have a diverse multidisciplinary team available for the evaluation, treatment, and support of the patient with a serious disorder of sexual development.

## AMBIGUOUS GENITALIA

After delivery, the obstetrician is often the provider who identifies the gender of the neonate. Thereafter, a more detailed assessment of the neonate's genital anatomy is necessary. The physician should systematically observe the newborn's perineum, beginning with the mons pubis. The clitoris should be examined for any obvious enlargement, the opening of the urethra should be identified, and the labia should be gently separated to see if the introitus can be visualized. If it is possible to separate the labia, the hymen might be observed. Generally the hymen is perforate, revealing the entrance to the vagina. At times the labia are joined by filmy adhesions, which usually separate during childhood but can be treated with the application of estrogen cream when medically indicated. Posteriorly the labia fuse in the midline at the posterior fourchette of the perineum. Posterior to the perineal body the rectum can be visualized, and it should be tested to be sure that it is perforate. Meconium staining around the rectum is evidence of perforation. If there is doubt, the rectum may be penetrated with a moistened cotton-tipped swab. Palpation of the inguinal area and labia for any masses is also important.

In newborns with ambiguous genitalia, a range of abnormalities involving the clitoris, urethra, labia, and introitus can be identified, and immediate evaluation is necessary. **The current diagnostic terminology for individuals with abnormal external genitalia and associated issues is *disorder of sexual development (DSD)*,** and these disorders can be related to in utero androgen exposure (too much or too little) that has affected development of the external genitalia. Women (individuals with XX karyotypes) with masculinized or virilized external genitalia are identified as 46,XX DSD, and men (with 46,XY karyotypes)

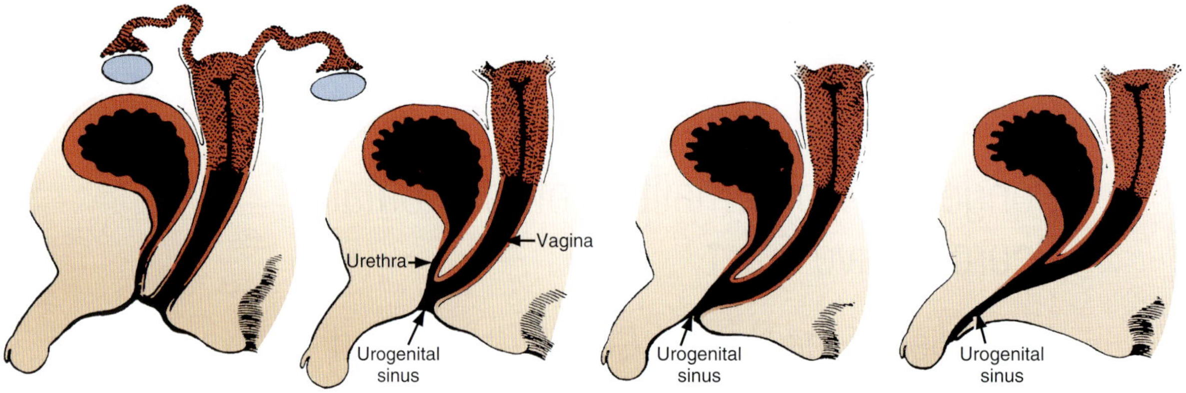


**Fig. 11.1** Examples of 46,XX disorders of sexual development induced by prenatal exposure to androgens. Exposure after 12th fetal week leads only to clitoral hypertrophy *(left)*. Exposure at progressively earlier stages of differentiation *(from left to right)* leads to retention of the urogenital sinus and labioscrotal fusion. If exposure occurs sufficiently early, the labia fuse to form a penile urethra. (From Grumbach MM, Hughes IA, Conte FA. Disorders of sex differentiation. In Larsen RP, Kronenberg HM, Melmed S, Polonsky KS, eds. *Williams Textbook of Endocrinology.* 10th ed. Philadelphia: WB Saunders; 2003:916.)

**with undervirilized external genitalia are identified as 46,XY DSD** (Lee, 2006). For women, the timing of antenatal (embryonic) exposure to androgen influences the degree of masculinization (Fig. 11.1) (Grumbach, 2003). The vaginal plate separates from the urogenital sinus at about 12 weeks of fetal development. **Androgen exposure before 12 weeks can result in labioscrotal fusion and retention of the urogenital sinus,** which creates a single tract that the urethra and vagina empty into before reaching the perineum. **Androgen exposure after 12 weeks primarily presents with clitoral hypertrophy** (Low, 2003).

The finding of ambiguous genitalia occurs in a wide spectrum of possibilities, from labioscrotal fusion and an enlarged clitoris with a penile urethra to a urogenital sinus to clitoromegaly and a normal introitus. With labial fusion, the physician should palpate the groins and labial folds for evidence of gonads. Gonads palpable in the inguinal canal, labioinguinal region, or labioscrotal folds are usually testes, and this finding is typically seen in a male with ambiguous genitalia rather than a virilized woman. Conversely, an infant with ambiguous genitalia but without palpable testes in the scrotum is more likely to be a virilized woman, most often the result of congenital adrenal hyperplasia. A rectal examination may allow palpation of a cervix and uterus, thus helping with gender assignment. If a bifid clitoris and labial fusion are noted, this anomaly is usually associated with extrophy of the bladder. As with any congenital anomaly, the neonate should be thoroughly evaluated for other congenital anomalies.

**The initial evaluation of ambiguous genitalia involves checking a karyotype, performing a transabdominal pelvic ultrasound to assess pelvic anatomy, and obtaining blood for serum electrolytes and steroid hormone levels.** In a female neonate an ultrasound can easily identify a uterus because the estrogenized tissue is easy to visualize. If further evaluation of neonatal pelvic anatomy is necessary, cystoscopy and vaginoscopy can be performed with a pediatric cystoscope to assess the pelvic structures, including the location of the urethra and vagina and the presence of a cervix. Possible causes of 46,XX DSD include congenital adrenal hyperplasia, other genetic mutations that affect the steroid pathway, maternal ingestion of androgens, and maternal production of excess androgens (Box 11.1) (Grumbach, 2003).

It is important to systematically evaluate the newborn's genitalia to make the appropriate gender assignment when possible. In the past, gender was assigned primarily on the principle of "phallic adequacy," meaning neonates with an ambiguous phallus were assigned female gender. In contrast, **the current approach is to initiate a thorough evaluation of the neonate and to defer gender assignment until the clinical picture is clear.** Most tertiary centers use a multidisciplinary team for the evaluation and management of an individual with DSD, including specialists in medical genetics, pediatric urology, pediatric endocrinology, gynecology, and psychiatry (Allen, 2009).

**BOX 11.1** Classification of 46,XX DSD

**I. ANDROGEN-INDUCED**

**A. Fetal Source**

1. Congenital adrenal hyperplasia
   a. Virilism only, defective adrenal 21-hydroxylation (CYP21)
   b. Virilism with salt-losing syndrome, defective adrenal 21-hydroxylation (CYP21)
   c. Virilism with hypertension, defective adrenal 11β-hydroxylation (CYP11B1)
   d. Virilism with adrenal insufficiency, deficient 3β-HSD 2 (HSD3B 2)
2. P450 aromatase (CYP19) deficiency
3. Glucocorticoid receptor gene mutation

**B. Maternal Source**

1. Iatrogenic
   a. Testosterone and related steroids
   b. Certain synthetic oral progestogens and, rarely, diethylstilbestrol
2. Virilizing ovarian or adrenal tumor
3. Virilizing luteoma of pregnancy
4. Congenital virilizing adrenal hyperplasia in mother*

**C. Undetermined Source**

1. Virilizing luteoma of pregnancy

**II. NON–ANDROGEN-INDUCED DISTURBANCES IN DIFFERENTIATION OF UROGENITAL STRUCTURES**

From Grumbach MM, Hughes IA, Conte FA. Disorders of sex differentiation. In: Larsen RP, Kronenberg HM, Melmed S, Polonsky KS, eds. *Williams Textbook of Endocrinology.* 10th ed. Philadelphia: Saunders; 2003.

*In pregnant patient whose disease is poorly controlled or who is noncompliant, especially during the first trimester.

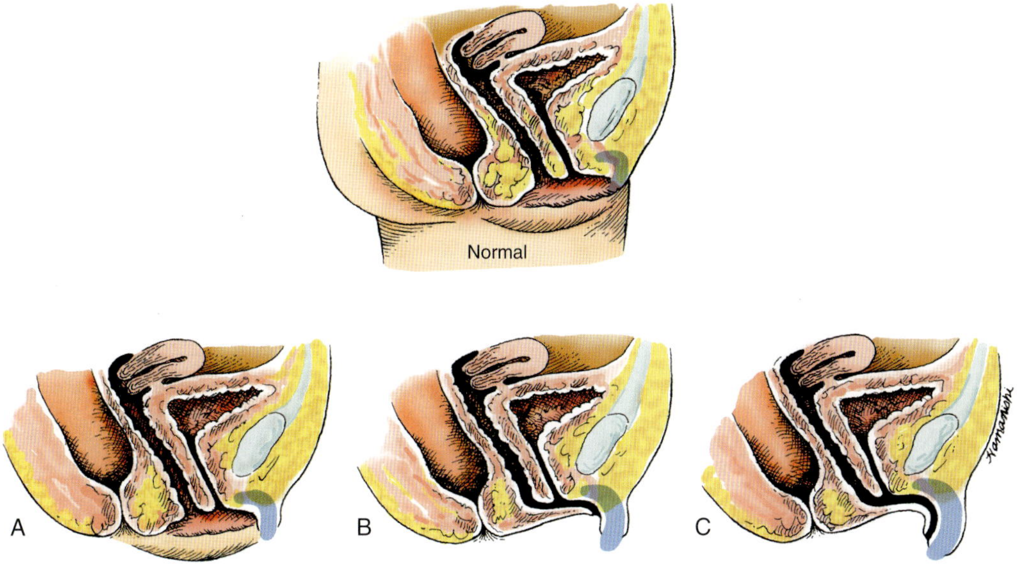


**Fig. 11.2** Sagittal views of genital deformities seen in female infants who are masculinized. **A,** Minimal masculinization with slight enlargement of the clitoris. **B,** Labial fusion and more marked enlargement of the clitoris. **C,** Complete labial fusion, enlargement of the clitoris, and formation of a partial penile urethra. (Modified from Verkauf BS, Jones HW Jr. Masculinization of the female genitalia in congenital adrenal hyperplasia: relationship to the salt losing variety of the disease. *South Med J.* 1970;63:634-638.)

## Perineal and Hymenal Anomalies

### Clitoral Anomalies

In an adult woman the clitoris is generally 1 to 1.5 cm long and 0.5 cm wide in the nonerect state. The glans is partially covered by a hood of skin, and the urethra opens near the base of the clitoris. Abnormalities of the clitoris are unusual, although it may be enlarged as a result of androgen stimulation. In such circumstances the shaft of the clitoris may be quite enlarged and partial development of a penile urethra may have occurred (Fig. 11.2) (Verkauf, 1970). Extreme cases of androgen stimulation are generally associated with fusion of the labia. These findings occur in infants with congenital adrenal hyperplasia and in those with in utero exposure to exogenous or endogenous androgens (Fig. 11.3) (Black, 2003). Similar in appearance to infants with congenital adrenal hyperplasia, men with partial androgen insensitivity syndrome have underdeveloped male external genitalia and a small phallus that appears as clitoral hypertrophy (Fig. 11.4) (Black, 2003).

A bifid clitoris (Fig. 11.5) is usually seen in association with extrophy of the bladder, which occurs rarely (1 per 30,000 births) and has a male predominance (3:1). However, when it occurs in women, it is often associated with a bifid clitoris. **Approximately half of female patients with bladder extrophy may have associated reproductive tract anomalies** such as vaginal anomalies and müllerian duct fusion disorders. In such cases an anterior rotation and a shortening of the vagina with labial fusion are quite common.

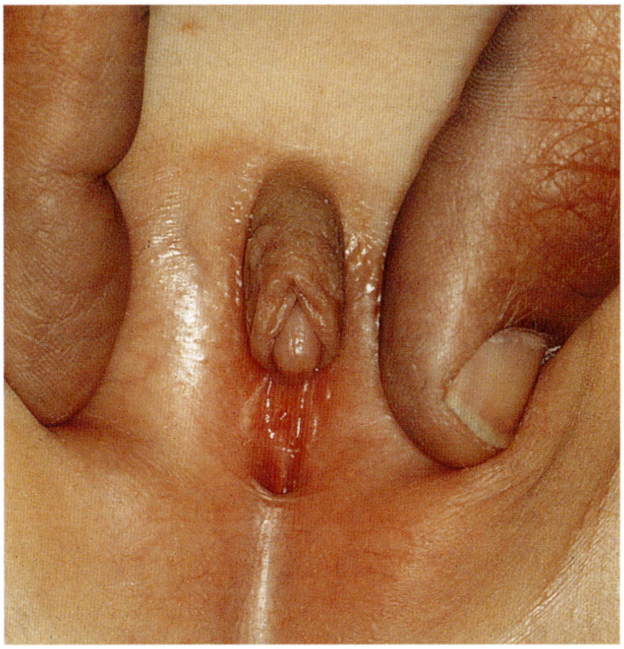

**Fig. 11.3** Clitoromegaly with posterior labial fusion in a child with congenital adrenal hyperplasia. (From McKay M. Vulvar manifestations of skin disorders. In: Black M, McKay M, Braude P, et al, eds. *Obstetric and Gynecologic Dermatology.* 2nd ed. Edinburgh: Mosby; 2003:120.)

### Labial Fusion

Labial fusion may occur without clitoromegaly. The resultant ambiguous genitalia implies a form of DSD. The diagnoses 46,XX DSD and 46,XY DSD apply to individuals with a pure XX or XY karyotype but with the external genitalia of the opposite sex of the karyotype or ambiguous genitalia. **The term *hermaphrodite* was derived from** the child of the Greek gods Hermes and Aphrodite, Hermaphroditus, who was part female and part male. It is no longer used. True hermaphroditism is now called ***ovotesticular DSD*; a person with this condition has both ovarian (including follicular elements) and testicular tissue, either in the same or opposite gonads.** Ovotesticular DSD is extremely rare in North and South America but more common (though still very rare) in Africa.

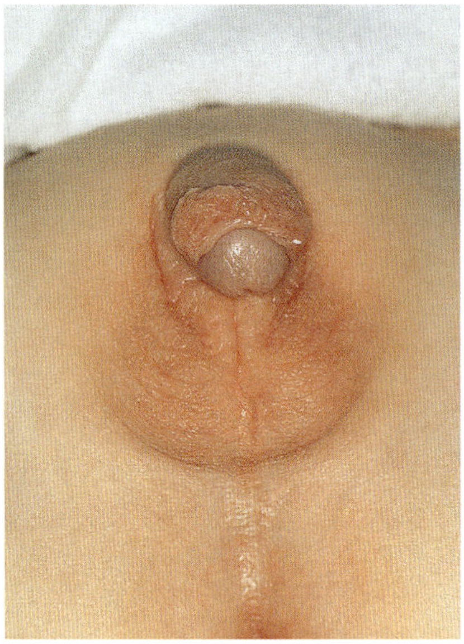

**Fig. 11.4** Ambiguous genitalia in a 46,XY child with partial androgen insensitivity. (From McKay M. Vulvar manifestations of skin disorders. In: Black M, McKay M, Braude P, et al, eds. *Obstetric and Gynecologic Dermatology.* 2nd ed. Edinburgh: Mosby; 2003:121.)

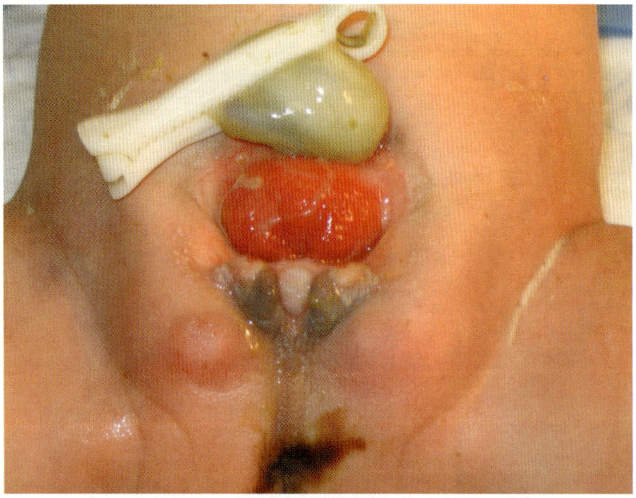

**Fig. 11.5** An example of a bifid clitoris in an infant with extrophy of the bladder. (Courtesy Richard Grady, MD.)

**Ovotestes are present in individuals with ovaries that usually have both an SRY antigen and testicular tissue present.** The degree to which müllerian and wolffian development occurs depends on the amounts of testicular tissue present in the ovotestes and the proximity to the developing duct system. When considerable amounts of testicular tissue are present within the organ, there is a tendency for descent toward the labial/scrotal area. Thus palpation of the gonad in the inguinal canal or within the labial scrotal area is fairly common. Ovulation and menstruation may occur if the müllerian system is appropriately developed. In a similar fashion, spermatogenesis may occur as well. **When testicular tissue is present, there is an increased risk for malignant degeneration, and these gonads should be removed after puberty.** Germ cell tumors, such as gonadoblastomas and

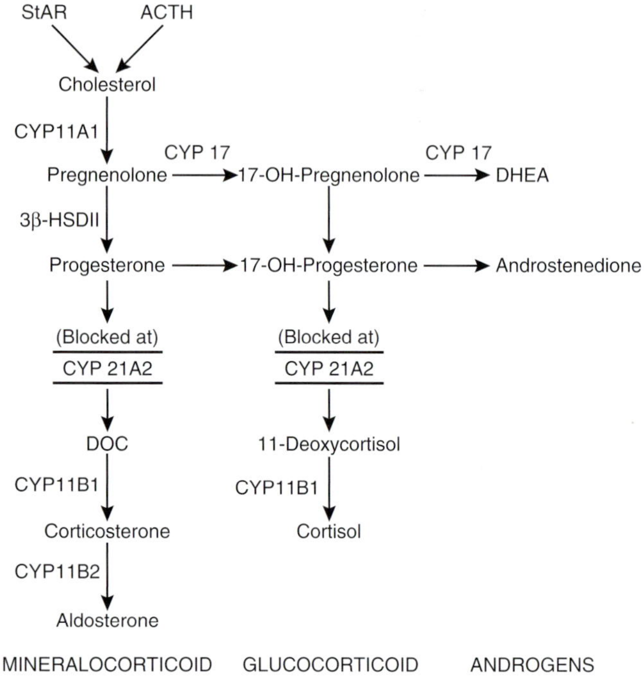


**Fig. 11.6** Steroid pathway in congenital adrenal hyperplasia with absence of 21-hydroxylase. *ACTH,* Adrenocorticotropic hormone; *3β-HSDII,* 3β-hydroxysteroid dehydrogenase; *DHEA,* dehydroepiandrosterone; *DOC,* deoxycorticosterone; *StAR,* Steroid acute regulatory protein. (From Grumbach MM, Hughes IA, Conte FA. Disorders of sex differentiation. In: Larsen RP, Kronenberg HM, Melmed S, Polonsky KS, eds. *Williams Textbook of Endocrinology.* 10th ed. Philadelphia: WB Saunders; 2003:533.)

dysgerminomas, have been reported in the ovarian portion of ovotestes.

## Congenital Adrenal Hyperplasia

Although labial fusion may result from exposure to exogenous androgens or be associated with defects of the anterior abdominal wall, by far the most common cause is congenital adrenal hyperplasia. **The most common form of congenital adrenal hyperplasia results from an inborn error of metabolism involving deficiency of the 21-hydroxylase enzyme** (Fig. 11.6). This condition is transmitted as an autosomal recessive gene coded on chromosome 6, and both severe and mild gene mutations have been identified. With the severe mutation, because of the absence of the 21-hydroxylase enzyme, the major biosynthetic pathway to cortisol is blocked; instead, 17-OH-progesterone is produced and then converted to the androgen androstenedione. The fetal hypothalamic-pituitary axis senses inadequate levels of cortisol and secretes excess adrenocorticotropic hormone (ACTH), which leads to increasing levels of androstenedione from the female adrenal gland and subsequent masculinization of the external genitalia. Homozygous individuals occur with an incidence as high as 1 per 490, depending on the geographic location and population studied. Screening programs have noted the incidence to be approximately 1 in 14,500 births (Pang, 1988). Depending on the population, carriers of the gene (heterozygotes) are present in a frequency ranging from 1 per 20 to 1 per 250. Two other less common enzyme defects, also transmittable as autosomal recessive traits, may produce similar abnormal findings: the **11-hydroxylase deficiency and the 3b-hydroxysteroid dehydrogenase deficiency**. These two enzyme defects and 21-hydroxylase deficiency may cause ambiguous genitalia with masculinized women.

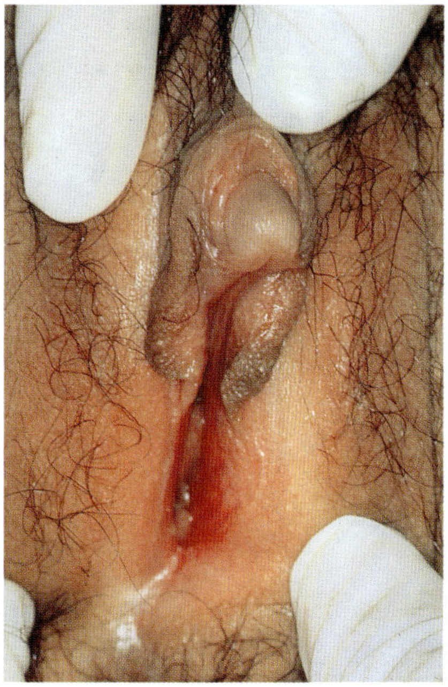

**Fig. 11.7** An 11-year-old girl with clitoromegaly and thick genital hair who presented with facial hair and was found to have 21-hydroxylase deficiency. (From McKay M. Vulvar manifestations of skin disorders. In: Black M, McKay M, Braude P, et al, eds. *Obstetric and Gynecologic Dermatology.* 2nd ed. Edinburgh: Mosby; 2003:120.)

Congenital adrenal hyperplasia (CAH) may be demonstrated at birth by the presence of ambiguous genitalia in 46,XX individuals or may present later in childhood. The majority of newborns (75%) who are **homozygous for a CAH mutation are at risk for the development of a life-threatening neonatal adrenal crisis as a result of sodium loss because of lack of aldosterone production.** In individuals with a milder disease presentation, delayed diagnosis may result in accelerated bone maturation because of high levels of androgens being aromatized to estradiol, thus leading to premature closure of the epiphyseal plates and short stature. The development of premature secondary sexual characteristics in men and further virilization in women may also occur (Fig. 11.7) (Black, 2003). Most U.S. states have mandatory neonatal 17-OH progesterone testing to screen for CAH.

**Treatment of congenital adrenal hyperplasia involves cortisol replacement.** This suppresses ACTH output, decreasing the stimulation of the cortisol-producing pathways of the adrenal cortex and subsequently decreasing androgen production. For women known to be at risk, those diagnosed with CAH, and those who have had children with CAH, antenatal therapy may be offered, but this remains controversial. After a positive pregnancy test, daily administration of dexamethasone suppresses the fetal adrenal glands until the fetal gender can be verified with prenatal diagnosis. Although this intervention remains an option, it should not be carried out routinely and **is still considered experimental by the major societies** (e.g., the Endocrine and Pediatric Endocrine Societies). Many female infants exposed to high levels of androgens in utero may need corrective surgery. Children who have had initial corrective surgeries may need follow-up vaginoplasty as teenagers because of vaginal stenosis. Furthermore, because of the profound gender identity issues related to ambiguous genitalia in women with CAH, and also for women with other DSDs, **ongoing psychological support and counseling are important**. When available, multidisciplinary team support is recommended for the gynecologic, urologic, endocrinologic, and psychological care of these individuals.

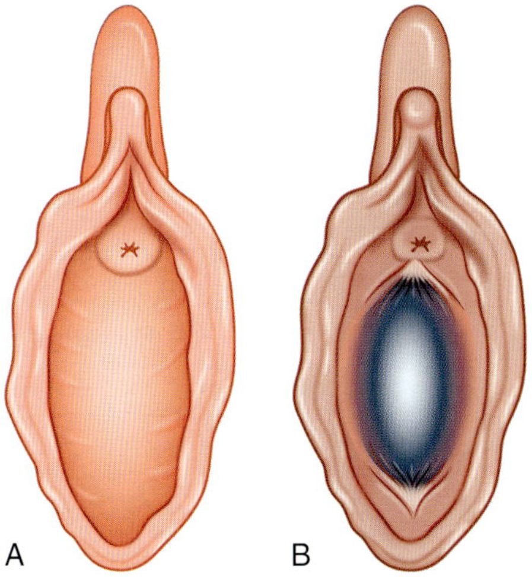


**Fig. 11.8** Diagrammatic depiction of an imperforate hymen (**A**) and a bulging hymen (**B**) caused by hematocolpos. (Modified from Dietrich JE, Miller DM, Quint EH. Obstructive reproductive track anomalies. *J Pediatr Adoles Gyn.* 2014;27(6):396-402.)

## Hymenal Anomalies

The hymen represents the junction of the sinovaginal bulbs with the urogenital sinus and is composed of endoderm from the urogenital sinus epithelium. The hymen is initially a solid membrane of tissue, and the central cells of the membrane typically dissolve during late fetal development to establish a connection between the lumen of the vaginal canal and the vestibule. If this perforation does not take place, the hymen is imperforate (Dietrich, 2014) (Fig. 11.8). The incidence of an imperforate hymen is thought to be approximately 1 in 1000 live-born female infants (Usta, 1993). Occasionally, a hydrocolpos or mucocolpos may occur in neonates or infants when fluid or vaginal secretions build up behind an imperforate hymen. Although this fluid collection may spontaneously resolve, if it forms a mass that obstructs the urinary tract, then the hymen must be incised to release the obstructing fluid.

Menarche typically occurs within 2 to 3 years from the start of thelarche (breast development), and young women with an imperforate hymen may experience cyclic cramping but no menstrual flow. **An imperforate hymen is commonly diagnosed after puberty in the setting of primary amenorrhea, hematocolpos, and possibly hematometra, which can cause pelvic pain, urinary retention, and difficulty with bowel movements.** In more advanced cases, because of retrograde menstruation, the menstrual blood may distend the fallopian tubes and form endometrial implants in the peritoneal cavity. Surprisingly, some women have minimal symptoms with this condition.

The diagnosis can be determined by history and physical examination; a bulging membrane with a bluish hue is appreciated at the introitus, and a vaginal mass is palpable on rectal examination. Surgical intervention is necessary to relieve the obstruction of the reproductive tract. Under anesthesia, a cruciate incision is made into the hymen extending from 10 to 4 o'clock and 2 to 8 o'clock. Once the imperforate hymen has been carefully incised and the hematocolpos drained, the excess hymenal tissue is trimmed and hemostasis is achieved with interrupted fine absorbable sutures. The tissue often heals quickly and well, leaving a patent hymen.

**Several variations of partial hymenal perforation exist: microperforate, cribriform and septate hymen, and incomplete perforate hymen** (Fig. 11.9) (Moore, 2003). Women with partial hymenal perforation commonly present with difficulty

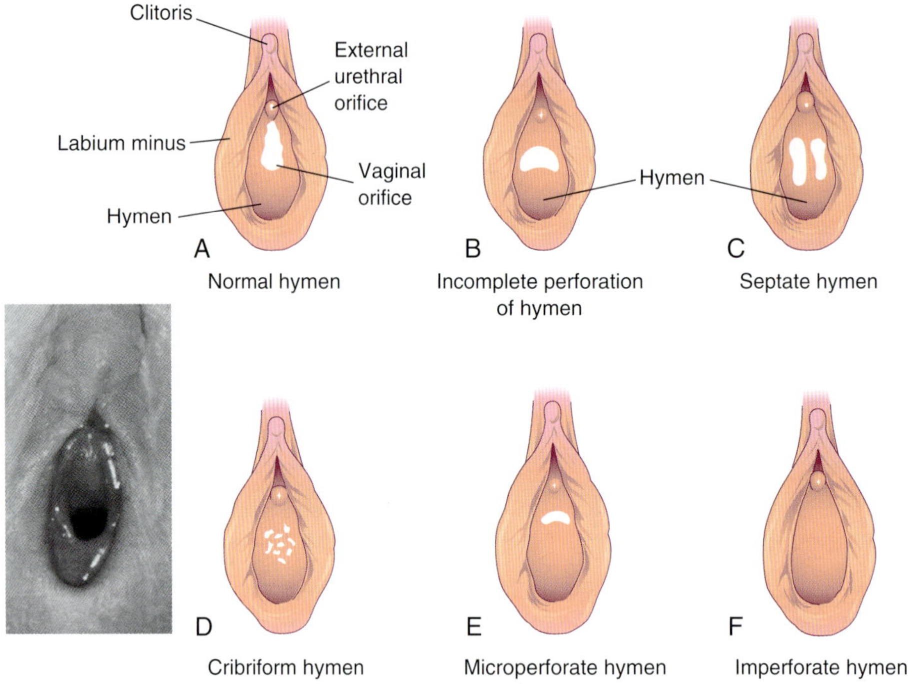


**Fig. 11.9** Congenital anomalies of the hymen. Panels **A** through **F** show different types of hymen abnormalities. The photograph shows a normal hymen as in **A**. (From Moore KL, Persaud TVN. *The Developing Human.* 7th ed. Philadelphia: WB Saunders; 2003:322.)

inserting a tampon or difficulty with sexual activity. Occasionally a young woman is able to insert a tampon past the hymen anomaly, but once the tampon expands with blood, it cannot be removed because of the partial hymenal obstruction. Surgical correction may be necessary to remove the excess hymenal tissue and restore normal hymenal anatomy.

## MÜLLERIAN ANOMALIES

Müllerian anomalies, otherwise known as ***congenital anomalies of the female reproductive tract,*** occur as a result of defects in development of the müllerian ducts, which are the embryologic origin of the fallopian tubes, uterus, cervix, and a portion of the vagina. Before reviewing these disorders, it is important to understand the development of the female reproductive tract.

### Embryology

**Although genetic sex is determined when sperm fertilizes the oocyte, male or female phenotype is not defined until after the sixth week of development.** Between the third and fifth weeks of embryologic development, both the wolffian (mesonephric) and müllerian (paramesonephric) ducts are present. The müllerian ducts form from clefts between the mesonephros and the developing gonad. The paired wolffian ducts connect the embryologic kidney (mesonephros) to the cloaca between 5 and 10 weeks of gestation; development of the functional kidney (metanephros) is stimulated by an outgrowth of the wolffian duct known as the ureteric bud. **The fate of these various embryonic elements is closely entwined; an insult to or abnormal development of one embryonic element usually affects the others.**

The subsequent steps of müllerian duct development are elongation, fusion, canalization, and septal resorption. The müllerian ducts elongate caudally and eventually fuse in the midline as they descend into the pelvis, reaching the urogenital sinus at an elevation known as the *müllerian tubercle.* At this point the ducts are two solid tubes of tissue that are fused medially; this occurs by 10 weeks' gestation. Next, central absorption of the cells occurs, leading to two hollow tubes of tissue that remain fused medially. Last, the midline septum between the two tubes of tissue undergoes resorption; this process commonly occurs in a caudal to cephalad direction, leading to a midline unified structure. The inferior portion of the müllerian ducts becomes the upper vagina, followed by the cervix and uterus, and the cephalad unfused portion of the ducts develops into the fallopian tubes. **This process is completed by week 20 of embryologic development.** Although this is the common theory of müllerian duct development, based on the variety of anomalies that arise from this process, many variations can occur.

The vagina develops from both müllerian duct tissue and the urogenital sinus. Once the müllerian ducts reach the urogenital sinus at approximately 10 weeks' gestation, cells proliferate from the upper portion of the urogenital sinus to form solid aggregates known as the *sinovaginal bulbs.* These cell masses develop into a cord, the vaginal plate, which extends from the müllerian ducts to the urogenital sinus. This plate canalizes, starting at the hymen, which is where the sinovaginal bulb attaches to the urogenital sinus, and proceeding cranially to the developing cervix, which by this time has already canalized. The process is completed by 20 weeks' gestation.

As previously mentioned, abnormalities in any or multiple parts of müllerian and urogenital sinus development can occur and lead to a constellation of structural defects of the female reproductive tract. Anomalies in müllerian duct elongation, fusion, canalization, and septal resorption have been identified, as have anomalies in vaginal plate resorption. Common müllerian anomalies are discussed in the next few sections.

### Anomalies of Müllerian Duct Development

Müllerian anomalies are commonly classified into **three categories of disordered duct development: agenesis and hypoplasia,**

**lateral fusion defects, and vertical fusion defects.** Reproductive tract abnormalities caused by in utero exposure to diethylstilbestrol (DES), a synthetic estrogen that has not been used for several decades, constitute a fourth group of anomalies. Agenesis and hypoplasia can occur for a portion of or an entire müllerian duct or for both ducts, affecting one or multiple müllerian-derived structures. Lateral fusion defects are the most common category of müllerian defects and originate from failure of migration of one or both ducts, midline fusion of the ducts, or absorption of the midline septum between the ducts. A range of anomalies can occur, including symmetric or asymmetric and nonobstructed or obstructed müllerian structures. Vertical fusion defects occur as a result of disordered fusion of the müllerian ducts with the urogenital sinus or abnormal vaginal canalization, and they may present with menstrual flow obstruction. The next sections discuss specific abnormalities of müllerian duct development.

## Vaginal Agenesis

Vaginal agenesis, also called *müllerian agenesis* or *müllerian aplasia*, occurs as a result of failure of müllerian duct development or marked aberrations in the typical steps of müllerian development. This condition is also known as the ***Mayer-Rokitansky-Küster-Hauser (MRKH) syndrome***, named after the four physicians who discovered the syndrome (Fig. 11.10) (Baramki, 1984). **Vaginal agenesis is characterized by a congenital abnormality of the vagina, ranging from an absent vagina to a shortened one, and variable development of the uterus; 7% to 10% of women with vaginal agenesis have rudimentary uterine tissue present** (Fedele, 2007). The syndrome occurs in **approximately 1 in 5000 women**. These individuals have normal pubertal development, normal ovarian function, and a 46,XX karyotype, and they commonly present with primary amenorrhea at age 15 to 16 years. The cause of this disorder is currently unknown, but research into possible genetic disorders leading to MRKH syndrome is ongoing.

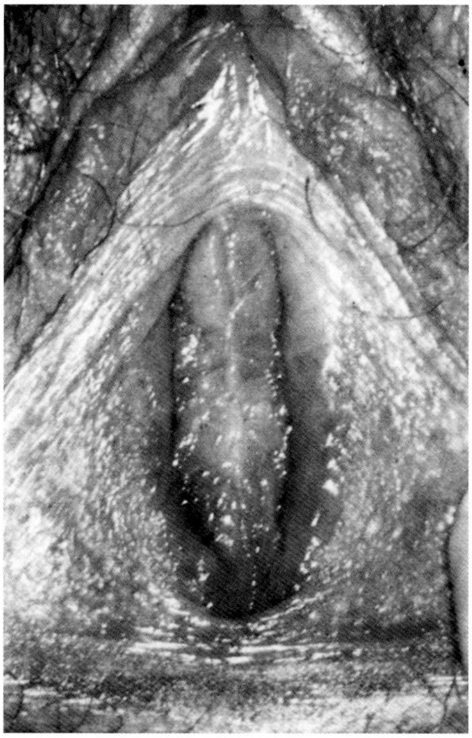

Fig. 11.10 External genitalia of a female patient with congenital absence of the vagina. (From Baramki TA. Treatment of congenital anomalies in girls and women. *J Reprod Med.* 1984;29(6):376-384.)

Complete vaginal agenesis is discovered in 75% of women with MRKH syndrome and approximately 25% have a short vaginal pouch. **Some women may have rudimentary uterine horns and can have myomas or adenomyosis in the rudimentary myometrium. If the uterine horns contain some endometrium with an epithelial lining, called functional rudimentary horns, menstruation into a blocked system can occur, which can lead to monthly cramping, pelvic pain, and endometriosis from retrograde menstruation.** A study by Fedele and colleagues noted that 92 of 106 women with müllerian agenesis had small müllerian remnants (Fedele, 2007). In women with müllerian agenesis, the ovaries are normal and the fallopian tubes are usually present.

Other congenital anomalies are associated with the diagnosis of müllerian agenesis. Because of the concomitant development of the müllerian and urinary tracts, **up to 50% of women with müllerian agenesis have concurrent urinary tract anomalies.** Phelan and coworkers reported that of 72 patients with vaginal agenesis, 25% had urologic abnormalities noted on intravenous pyelography (Phelan, 1953). A later study by Baramki demonstrated that 40% of 92 patients with müllerian agenesis had urologic abnormalities (Baramki, 1984). These anomalies can include renal agenesis, pelvic kidney, multicystic dysplastic kidney, and ureteral duplication. **One study described a 12% incidence of skeletal anomalies**, usually involving congenital fusion or absence of vertebrae in these patients. **Other anomalies associated with müllerian agenesis include cardiac defects and hearing loss**. Hence, women with müllerian agenesis require dedicated imaging of the urinary tract and other evaluation as indicated.

Girls with müllerian agenesis present with normal pubertal development and primary amenorrhea. Physical examination demonstrates the absence of a vaginal opening or the presence of a short vaginal pouch, and there is an inability to palpate a uterus on rectal examination. When evaluating a female patient with primary amenorrhea and a distal vaginal obstruction, the differential diagnosis includes vaginal agenesis, transverse vaginal septum, imperforate hymen, and androgen insensitivity syndrome. With müllerian agenesis, measurement of reproductive hormones reveals normal levels, and the karyotype is 46,XX. Although ultrasound examination may verify the presence of normal ovaries and the absence of a uterus, magnetic resonance imaging (MRI) offers detailed evaluation of the soft tissues of the pelvis and can confirm the diagnosis of müllerian agenesis; it can also assess if any rudimentary uterine tissue is present. Surgical evaluation by laparoscopy is not necessary unless the evaluation of pelvic pain and possible removal of functional rudimentary horns is necessary. The ovaries of these patients are normal and should not be removed.

### Androgen Insensitivity

Although androgen insensitivity syndrome is not a müllerian anomaly, it presents in a similar manner to vaginal agenesis and therefore is reviewed in this chapter. Androgen insensitivity occurs in individuals with a 46,XY karyotype who have certain genetic abnormalities that cause **defective androgen receptors**. The syndrome formerly was termed *testicular feminization syndrome*. Because the developing fetus cannot sense any testosterone, **the external genitalia are feminized** and a short vaginal pouch can develop from the urogenital sinus. Because of the testicular production of antimüllerian hormone, the müllerian ducts are resorbed and the wolffian duct–derived tissue persists. **Because of the lack of functional androgen receptors, the testes remain undescended.** These individuals undergo normal pubertal development, and the testes make increasing amounts of testosterone, which is aromatized to estrogen; however, without functional androgen receptors, there is no testosterone action (e.g., male muscle mass and hair production). **These phenotypic women commonly present with**

**primary amenorrhea, and they tend to be tall and have sparse to no pubic hair. After an estrogen-induced growth spurt, the undescended testes should be removed to prevent the development of a gonadoblastoma.**

**Treatment of Vaginal Agenesis**

Once the diagnosis of vaginal agenesis is determined, this information should be shared with the patient and her support system during a face-to-face conversation. This diagnosis has significant emotional, physical, sexual, and reproductive consequences for the patient, and psychological counseling should be encouraged to help her cope with the diagnosis and its implications. **The treatment of vaginal agenesis involves creation of a neovagina for future sexual function.** Additionally, the patient should be aware that achieving motherhood is possible using her own eggs and a gestational carrier, through adoption, or possibly through the developing field of uterine transplantation.

Both nonoperative and operative methods are available to achieve creation of a neovagina. The purpose of a vagina is sexual function, although some patients may wish to pursue this intervention before they are ready to become sexually active. **The first-line treatment to create a neovagina is a nonoperative option involving the use of vaginal dilators, which is more than 90% successful in female patients with vaginal agenesis** (ACOG, 2018). This is a time-consuming process that requires the daily use of dilators for 15 to 20 minutes, and it can take 3 to 6 months or longer to create a functional vagina. Each set of dilators has several sizes that increase in width and length, and the dilator is pressed at the vaginal dimple to stretch the skin. Lidocaine jelly can be applied to the vagina before each session to reduce discomfort. Appropriate instruction should be provided before initiating dilation and intermittently throughout the process to make sure that proper technique is being used. Once the neovagina is created, maintenance dilation must be performed several times per week unless the patient is sexually active. These women must be counseled that they should still use condoms to protect against sexually transmitted infections.

**Multiple options are available for operative reconstruction of the vagina.** The goal of the operation is to develop the potential space between the bladder and the rectum and insert into this space a new tissue that will develop into a vagina. **Common tissues used include a split-thickness skin graft, buccal mucosa, peritoneum, bowel (sigmoid or small bowel), and synthetic tissue grafts** (ACOG, 2018). After the vaginal space is opened and the new tissue is inserted, the patient must wear a mold for a number of months to maintain the vaginal shape as the surgical site heals. Thereafter, if she is not having intercourse regularly, she must use vaginal dilators several times per week to maintain the neovagina. Other surgical procedures to create a neovagina exist, but that discussion is beyond the scope of this chapter.

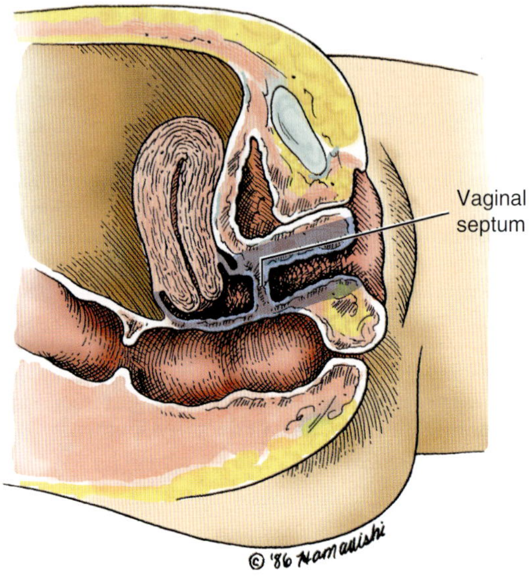


**Fig. 11.11** Diagram of transverse vaginal septum.

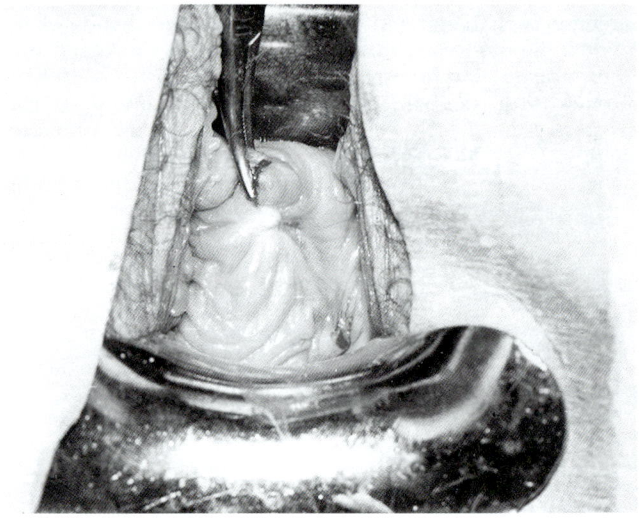

**Fig. 11.12** Patient with complete transverse vaginal septum.

## Transverse Vaginal Septum

A transverse vaginal septum occurs as a result of partial canalization of the vaginal plate, leaving a band of tissue across the vagina (Fig. 11.11). **This septum may be partial (perforate) or complete, and it most commonly lies at the junction between the upper third and lower two-thirds of the vagina** (Fig. 11.12). Transverse vaginal septae occur less often in the midvagina and lower vagina, and the general incidence is approximately 1 per 75,000 women. Partial transverse vaginal septa have been reported in DES-exposed women. **This diagnosis is rarely made in prepubertal girls unless there is development of a mucocolpos or mucometrium behind the septum, which can cause an unexplained abdominal mass to form.** At the time of menarche, the presence of a complete septum leads to hematocolpos and hematometra, similar to that seen with an imperforate hymen, except that because the obstruction is higher in the vagina and the septum is made of thicker tissue than the hymen, there is no bulging tissue at the introitus. With this anomaly, the female patient presents with primary amenorrhea and reports cyclic cramping and worsening pelvic pain. In contrast, the female patient with an incomplete (perforate) transverse septum usually menstruates but can develop hematocolpos over time, along with foul-smelling vaginal discharge, or she might report normal menstrual function but the inability to insert a tampon or have intercourse. The transverse vaginal septum is often less than 1 cm thick; however, some septa can be more than 2 cm thick. With a thin transverse vaginal septum, the septal tissue is excised and the proximal and distal vaginal tissue are sutured together to create a normal vagina. A similar procedure is performed for a perforate transverse vaginal septum. The procedure to correct a thick vaginal septum is more difficult; once the septum is excised, a tissue graft may be needed to bridge the distance between the proximal and distal vaginal tissue edges. With all these vaginal reconstructive procedures, the female patient may need to wear a stent or use dilators to prevent scarring and narrowing at the surgical site. Longitudinal septa of the vagina are discussed later in this chapter along with duplication of the uterus and cervix.

## Vaginal Adenosis

In the woman who was exposed to DES in utero, the junction between the müllerian ducts and the sinovaginal bulb may not be sharply demonstrated. If müllerian elements invade the sinovaginal bulb, remnants may remain as areas of adenosis in the adult vagina. Vaginal adenosis is generally palpated submucosally, although it may be observable at the surface.

## Abnormalities of the Cervix

Cervical anomalies can occur along with uterine and vaginal anomalies or can occur in isolation. **Cervical duplication occurs when the müllerian ducts have incomplete or no fusion; it can result in two separate and distinct cervices or two cervices that are fused at the midline.** Additionally, a septate cervix can occur when the midline septum within the cervix does not resorb. These anomalies do not typically obstruct menstrual flow. In contrast, **cervical agenesis and hypoplasia occur as a result of incomplete or absent duct development and often present with obstructed menstrual flow** with associated cyclic or chronic pain and hematometra. These rare anomalies require ultrasound or MRI examination to clarify the anatomic disorder. Several management options are available, including long-term menstrual suppression with hormones, cervical reconstruction, and hysterectomy. In addition, other cervical anomalies, such as hoods, collars, and adenosis, are possible in women with in utero DES exposure.

## Abnormalities of the Uterus

Abnormalities of the uterus can occur as a result of agenesis or hypoplasia of one or both müllerian ducts, or lateral fusion defects can result from disordered duct fusion and septal resorption. There are several classification systems for müllerian anomalies; in 1988, the American Fertility Society (Fig. 11.13) provided a straightforward classification system of uterine anomalies based on embryologic origin (American Fertility Society, 1988). A comparison of the American Fertility Society (now American Society for Reproductive Medicine [ASRM]) system with that of the European Society of Human Reproduction and Embryology (ESHRE) found that the latter would lead to overdiagnosis of certain conditions that were not true anomalies (Ludwin, 2014). An updated publication by Ludwin compared the prevalence of the diagnosis of a septate uterus using three different classifications (Fig. 11.14). **This study reconfirmed that there is an overdiagnosis of a septum using ESHRE/European Society of Gynecological Endoscopy criteria and that, using ASRM criteria, a septum was not associated with infertility but with miscarriage** (Ludwin, 2019).

Hypoplasia/*agenesis* (category I) and *unicornuate* (category II) denote anomalies with developmental failure of one or both müllerian ducts; *didelphys* (category III) and *bicornuate* (category IV) describe anomalies involving a varying degree of failure of midline fusion; *septate* (category V) and *arcuate*

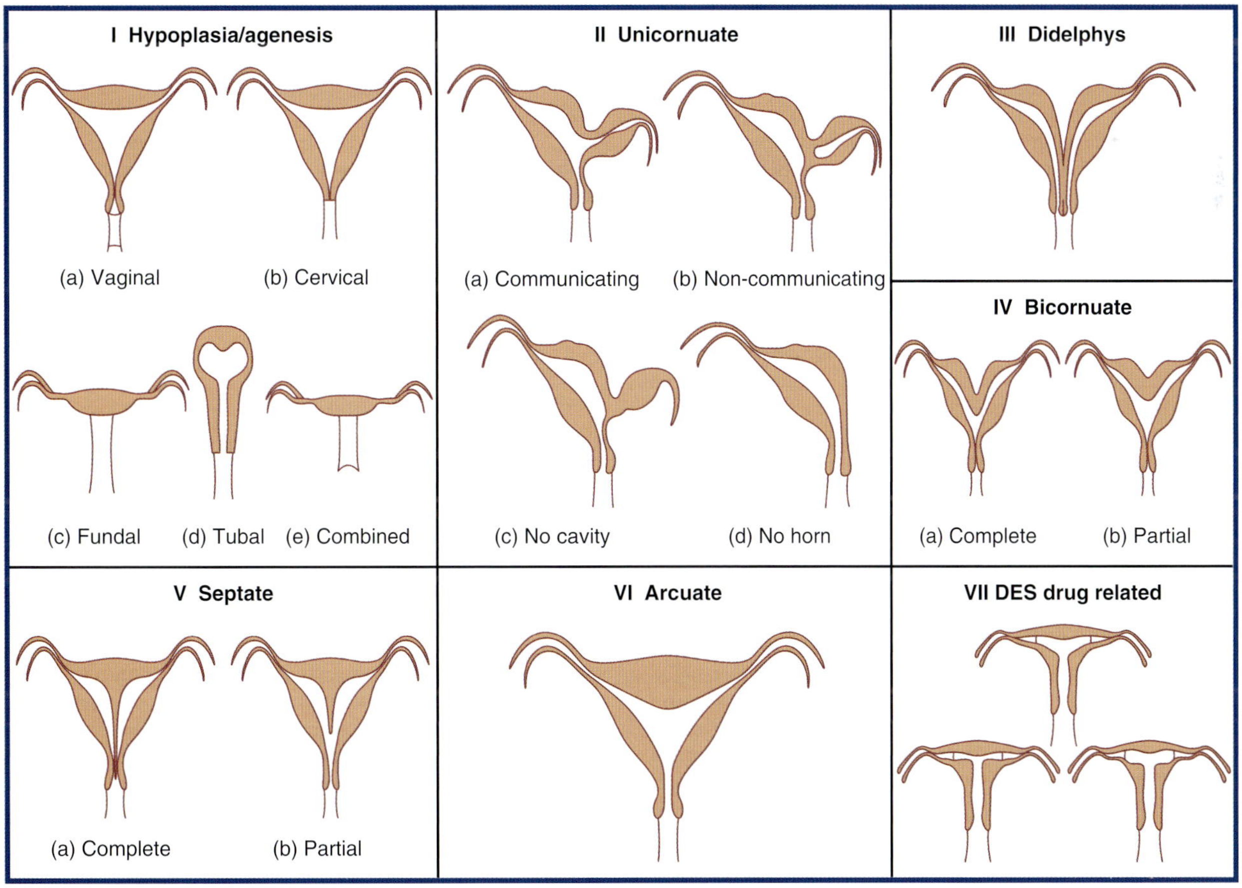


**Fig. 11.13** American Fertility Society classification. *DES,* Diethylstilbestrol. (From The American Fertility Society classification of adnexal adhesions, distal tubal occlusion, tubal occlusion secondary to tubal ligation, tubal pregnancies, müllerian anomalies and intrauterine adhesions. *Fertil Steril.* 1988;49(6):944-955.)

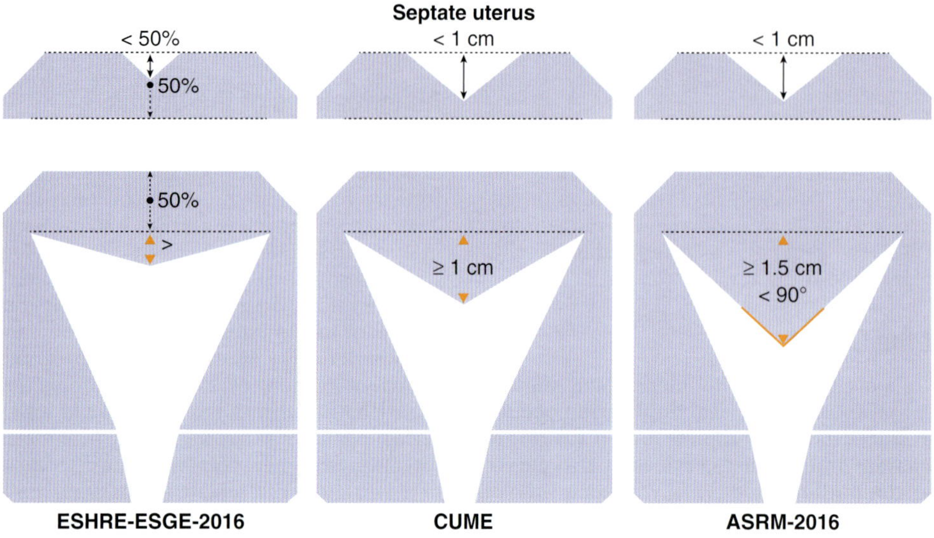


**Fig. 11.14** Comparisons of the diagnosis of a septate uterus according to the classifications of three different societies: European Society of Human Reproduction and Embryology (ESHRE) and the European Society of Gynecological Endoscopy (ESGE) 2016, American Society for Reproductive Medicine (ASRM) 2016, and the Congenital Uterine Malformation by Experts (CUME) 2018. (From Ludwin A, Ludwin I, Coelho Neto MA, et al. Septate uterus by updated ESHRE/ESGE, ASRM and CUME definitions: association with infertility, previous miscarriage, and warnings for women and healthcare systems, and associated cost analysis. *Ultrasound Obstet Gynecol.* 2019.)

(category VI) identify anomalies with some degree of failure of resorption of the midline septum. With this classification system, associated anomalies of the vagina, cervix, fallopian tubes, and urinary system must be documented separately. **It should also be recognized that numerous anomalies exist that are exceptions to the standard theory of müllerian duct development.**

Often constellations of müllerian abnormalities occur together. A didelphys uterus is commonly seen with a duplicated vagina, and this presents similar to a longitudinal vaginal septum. In some cases the vaginal septum obstructs one side of the duplicated system, causing a female patient to present with worsening pain during menstruation as a result of hematocolpos and hematometra on the obstructed side. A bicornuate uterus can present with a single cervix or a duplicated cervix, and a longitudinal vaginal septum can also be present. A septate uterus can present with a single, septate, or duplicated cervix and may also occur with a longitudinal vaginal septum. A unicornuate uterus may occur in isolation or be associated with a contralateral rudimentary uterine horn that may contain functional endometrial tissue. Another classification by Toaff (Toaff, 1984) depicts some of these variations (Fig. 11.15).

Urinary tract anomalies such as renal agenesis or pelvic kidney are common in women with uterus didelphys with an obstructing longitudinal vaginal septum causing an obstructed vagina and uterus and in those with a unicornuate uterus with a rudimentary horn ipsilateral to the anomalous or obstructed side. **Hence, in female patients with a müllerian anomaly, and especially in those with a unilateral obstruction, imaging of the urinary tract is important to look for concomitant anomalies** (Oppelt, 2007).

## Imaging

**MRI is the gold standard for the diagnosis of uterine abnormalities. However, three-dimensional (3D) ultrasound (US) is also beneficial and is considered to be equivalent in most circumstances** (Benacerraf, 2015; Bermejo, 2010; Grimbizis, 2016). Fig. 11.16 compares MRI and 3D US images of some abnormalities using the American Fertility Society classification. Imaging with a hysterosalpingogram, which can show two upper uterine cavities (Fig. 11.17), cannot differentiate between a bicornuate and septate uterus. Conventional two-dimensional (2D) US is also not able to make this distinction because it cannot visualize the coronal plane, which is necessary to assess the external contour of the uterus; this is accomplished either by 3D US or MRI (Troiano, 2004). Although 2D US is an appropriate first imaging technique for a low-risk female patient, but a woman who is at higher risk for a uterine anomaly should be assessed with 3D US (Grimbizis, 2016).

## Symptoms and Signs

It is important to recognize several gynecologic and obstetric signs and symptoms that may indicate a müllerian anomaly and to also remember that many girls and women with congenital uterine anomalies are asymptomatic. Uterine agenesis presents with primary amenorrhea. Primary amenorrhea and worsening pelvic pain may identify a complete obstruction of the reproductive tract at the level of the vagina, cervix, or uterus. Women with a unilateral obstructive anomaly may report cyclic or noncyclic pelvic pain and dysmenorrhea, and these symptoms can begin several months after menarche or into adulthood. Obstructive uterine anomalies are associated with hematometra, retrograde menstruation, and endometriosis. Endometriosis is a common finding in women with obstructive and nonobstructive müllerian anomalies. Abnormal bleeding can also occur with uterine anomalies and has been associated with septate uteri. Furthermore, vaginal anomalies may occur in conjunction with uterine anomalies, and abnormal bleeding may be due to a partial or microperforate vaginal obstruction or a longitudinal vaginal septum. A longitudinal vaginal septum, which is associated with septate, didelphys, and bicornuate uteri, may be a woman's first presentation with a uterine anomaly; associated symptoms include difficulty with tampon insertion, bleeding around one tampon

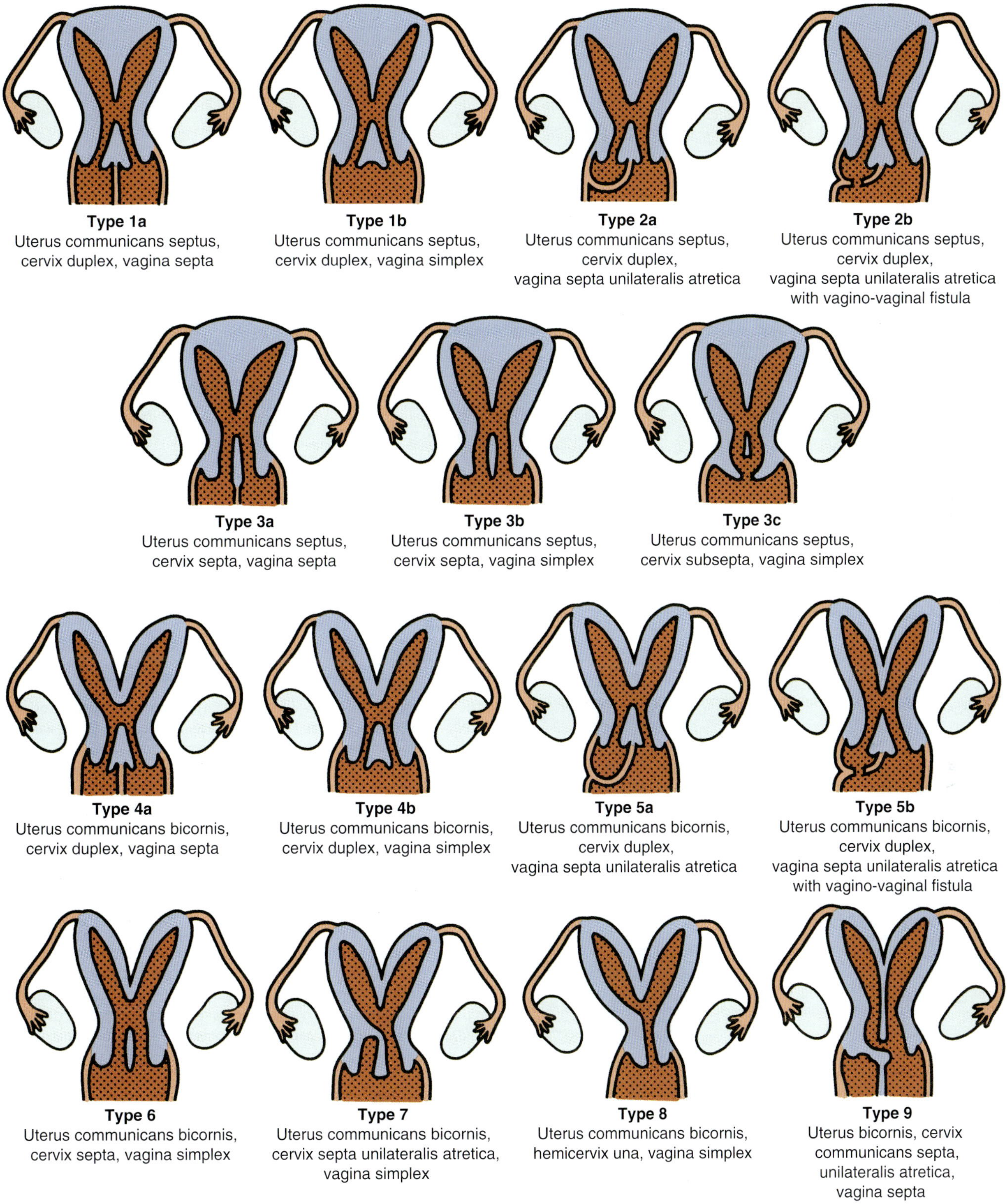


**Fig. 11.15** Morphologic classification of communicating uteri. All have an isthmic communication except type 9, which has a low cervical communication. (From Toaff ME, Lev-Toaff AS, Toaff R. Communicating uteri: review and classification with introduction of two previously unreported types. *Fertil Steril.* 1984;41(5):661-679. Copyright 1984, with permission from The American Society for Reproductive Medicine.)

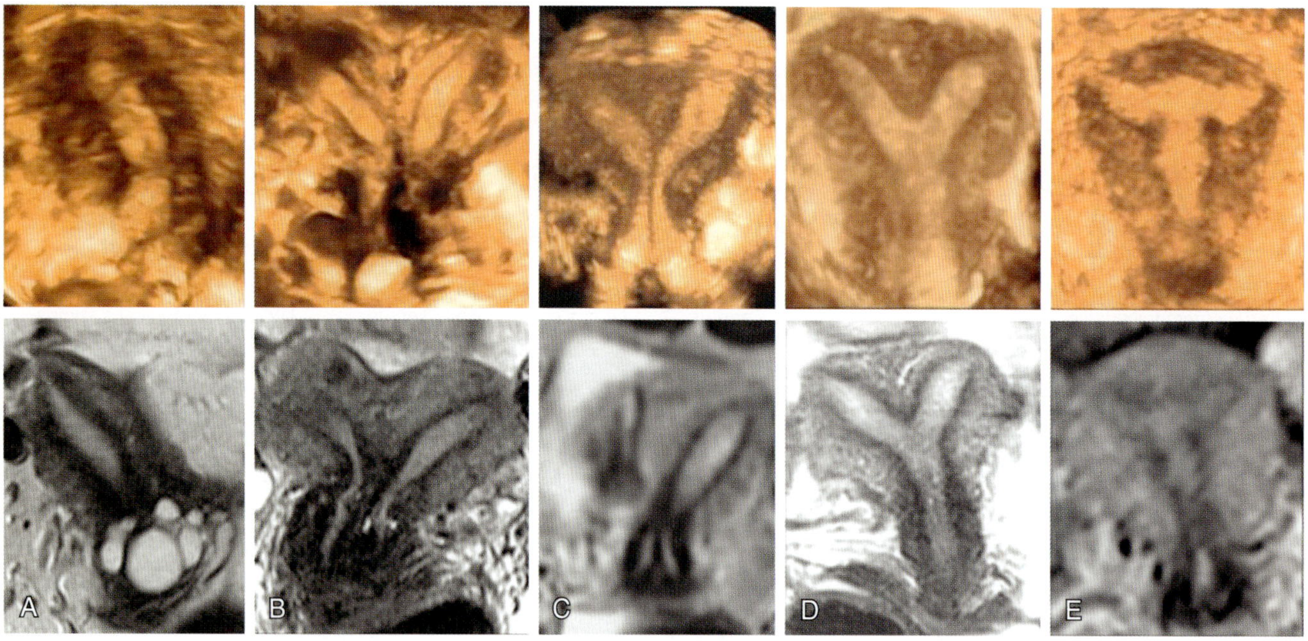


**Fig. 11.16** Comparison of müllerian anomalies as viewed by three-dimensional (3D) ultrasound and magnetic resonance imaging (MRI). The comparisons of 3D ultrasound *(top row)* and MRI *(bottom row)* are very similar. **A,** unicornuate uterus; **B,** bicornuate bicollis uterus; **C,** complete septate uterus with two cervices; **D,** partial septate uterus; **E,** uterus with diethylstilbestrol-related malformation. (From Bermejo C, Martinez Ten P, Cantarero R, et al. Three-dimensional ultrasound in the diagnosis of müllerian duct anomalies and concordance with magnetic resonance imaging. *Ultrasound Obstet Gynecol.* 2010;35(5):593-601.)

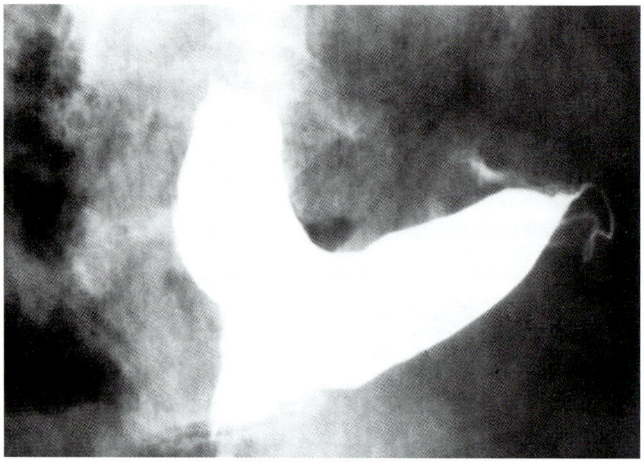

**Fig. 11.17** Hysterosalpingogram (HSG) of a bicornuate uterus seen in a woman with repetitive abortions; a partial uterine septum would look similar on HSG. When an anomaly is appreciated on HSG, further testing is indicated to assess the myometrial contour of the uterus, which helps to make the correct diagnosis.

(two are required), and dyspareunia. Hence, if a vaginal anomaly is identified, uterine imaging is warranted.

Congenital uterine anomalies are associated with a higher rate of poor obstetric outcomes, including recurrent pregnancy loss (RPL), first- and second-trimester pregnancy loss, intrauterine growth restriction, preterm labor and delivery, placental abruption, malpresentation, and intrauterine fetal demise. **Among women with RPL, the incidence of uterine anomalies is highly variable and ranges from 6% to 38%, but based on meta-analyses it is likely closer to 12% to 16% and is as high as 25% in women with second-trimester pregnancy loss** (Chan, 2011; Saravelos, 2008). In one study the odds ratio for preterm birth less than 34 weeks in women with a uterine anomaly was 7.4 (Hua, 2011). However, many studies have reported that in women with uterine anomalies, despite the high risk of miscarriage and midtrimester pregnancy loss, the chance of a live birth is greater than 50% (Grimbizis, 2001). Uterine dysfunction is thought to occur as a result of diminished cavity size, impaired ability to distend, abnormal myometrial and cervical function, inadequate vascularity, or abnormal endometrial development. Because of higher rates of fetal malpresentation, an increased rate of cesarean delivery can occur in women with uterine anomalies. **Additional obstetric complications, such as cervical incompetence, pregnancy-induced hypertension (caused by renal anomalies), and antepartum and postpartum bleeding, are also associated with uterine anomalies.** IN addition, pregnancy may occur in an obstructed or rudimentary uterine horn or in the fallopian tube associated with a rudimentary horn. **Uterine horn pregnancies are surgical emergencies because of an 89% rate of rupture and the related maternal morbidity and mortality** (Jaysinghe, 2005).

## Diagnosis

Diagnosis of a uterine anomaly may be indicated by an individual's history, suggested by physical examination, and confirmed with pelvic imaging. Depending on the population studied and the quality of the imaging, either the arcuate uterus or the septate uterus is the most common uterine anomaly. Several imaging modalities are possible, as discussed previously. In general, MRI is best able to assess more complex müllerian anomalies that may involve the uterus, cervix, and vagina, and simultaneous assessment of the urinary tract is possible.

Additionally, 3D US has been shown to achieve at least equivalent assessment of uterine anomalies (Grimbizis, 2016). Because of the availability of high-quality, reliable imaging, **it is rarely necessary to perform surgery to diagnose a uterine anomaly.** It must be emphasized that with müllerian anomalies, the evaluation of the urinary tract is commonly indicated to identify any concomitant abnormalities.

### Management

Surgical intervention is indicated for women with obstructive anomalies and associated pelvic pain and endometriosis and may be indicated for women with poor obstetric outcomes such as RPL, second-trimester loss, or preterm delivery. The goals of surgery include restoration of pelvic anatomy, preservation of fertility, and treatment of pelvic pain and endometriosis. Before attempting surgery for women with uterine anomalies and RPL or preterm delivery, it is important to rule out extrauterine causes of these obstetric issues. Of the uterine anomalies, the septate uterus is most amenable to surgical correction; **hysteroscopic metroplasty is a minimally invasive procedure that incises the uterine septum and unifies the uterine cavity**. In contrast, **the unicornuate uterus is never considered operable**, but excision of a functional rudimentary uterine horn and the attached fallopian tube is recommended to prevent a horn or tubal gestation and to treat hematometra and pelvic pain. The bicornuate and didelphys uteri are considered operable only in select, rare circumstances; abdominal or laparoscopic metroplasty can be performed to unify a bicornuate or didelphys uterus, but it is only performed in rare patients with poor obstetric outcomes. Furthermore, when indicated, a cervical cerclage can be used to attempt to improve pregnancy outcomes in women with uterine anomalies and a history of poor reproductive outcomes.

**Hysteroscopic metroplasty** to correct a partial or complete septate uterus can improve reproductive outcomes and is indicated in women with poor obstetric outcomes, including RPL or second-trimester pregnancy loss (ASRM, 2016; Homer, 2000). During the procedure, the septum is visualized and incised with a cutting device such as scissors, an electrode, or a laser, and the cavity achieves a normal contour. **After the hysteroscopic procedure, the risk of pregnancy loss or other adverse perinatal outcomes decreases dramatically;** live birth rates improve from 50% to approximately 80%, and miscarriage rates decrease from 45% to approximately 15% (Grimbizis, 2001; Homer, 2000). Because of its safety, simplicity, and excellent postoperative results, the hysteroscopic approach is preferred for surgical treatment of a uterine septum; laparoscopy can be used to assess the fundal contour and guide the extent of septum resection but is not mandatory. The surgical treatment of uterine septa in asymptomatic women is controversial, but after careful counseling, some women elect to undergo surgery because of concerns regarding the obstetric risks associated with a uterine septum (ASRM, 2016).

## Ovarian Abnormalities

### Accessory Ovary and Supernumerary Ovary

In 1959, Wharton defined *accessory ovary* and *supernumerary ovary*. The former term is used when excess ovarian tissue is noted near a normally placed ovary and is connected to it. Supernumerary ovary occurs when a third ovary is separated from the normally situated ovaries; such ovaries may be found in the omentum or retroperitoneally. Wharton estimated that the occurrence of either accessory ovary or supernumerary ovary is rare, finding approximately one case of accessory ovary per 93,000 patients and one case of supernumerary ovary in 29,000 autopsies. In Wharton's review, 3 of 4 patients with supernumerary ovary and 5 of 19 patients with accessory ovary had additional congenital defects, most often abnormalities of the genitourinary tract (Wharton, 1959).

#### REFERENCES


Allen L. Disorder of sexual development. *Obstet Gynecol Clin North Am.* 2009;36(1):25-45.

American College of Obstetrics and Gynecology (ACOG). ACOG Committee Opinion 728. Mullerian agenesis: diagnosis, management and treatment. *Obstet Gynecol.* 2018;131:e35-e42.

Baramki TA. The treatment of congenital anomalies in girls and women. *J Reprod Med.* 1984;29:376-384.

Benacerraf BR, Abuhamad AZ, Bromley B, et al. Consider ultrasound first for imaging the female pelvis. *Am J Obstet Gynecol.* 2015;212(4):450-455.

Bermejo C, Martinez Ten P, Cantarero R, et al. Three-dimensional ultrasound in the diagnosis of Müllerian duct anomalies and concordance with magnetic resonance imaging. *Ultrasound Obstet Gynecol.* 2010;35:593-601.

Black M, McKay M, Braude P, et al. *Obstetric and Gynecologic Dermatology.* 2nd ed. Edinburgh: Mosby; 2003:121.

Chan YY, Jayaprakasan K, Zamora J, et al. The prevalence of congenital uterine anomalies in unselected and high-risk populations: a systematic review. *Hum Reprod Update.* 2011;17:761-771.

Dietrich JE, Millar DM, Quint EH. Obstructive reproductive tract anomalies. *Pediatr Adolesc Gynecol.* 2014b;27:396-402.

Fedele L, Bianchi S, Frontino G, et al. Laparoscopic findings and pelvic anatomy in Mayer-Rokitansky-Kuster-Hauser syndrome. *Obstet Gynecol.* 2007;109:1111-1115.

Grimbizis GF, Camus M, Tarlatzis BC, et al. Clinical implications of uterine malformations and hysteroscopic treatment results. *Hum Reprod Update.* 2001;7:161-174.

Grimbizis GF, DiSpezio Sardo A, Saravelos SH, et al. The Thessaloniki ESHRE/ESGE consensus on diagnosis of female genital anomalies. *Hum Reprod.* 2016;31:2-7.

Grumbach MM, Hughes IA, Conte FA. Disorders of sex differentiation. In: Larsen RP, Kronenberg HM, Melmed S, Polonsky KS, eds. *Williams Textbook of Endocrinology.* 10th ed. Philadelphia: WB Saunders; 2003.

Homer HA, Li TJ, Cooke ID. The septate uterus: a review of management and reproductive outcome. *Fertil Steril.* 2000;73:1-14.

Jaysinghe Y, Rane A, Stalewski H, et al. The presentation and early diagnosis of the rudimentary uterine horn. *Obstet Gynecol.* 2005;105:1456-1467.

Lee PA, Houk CP, Ahmed SF, et al. Consensus statement on management of intersex disorders. International Consensus Conference on Intersex. *Pediatrics.* 2006;118(2):e488-e500.

Low Y, Hutson JM. Murdoch Children's Research Institute Sex Study Group: rules for clinical diagnosis in babies with ambiguous genitalia. *J Paediatr Child Health.* 2003;39:406-413.

Ludwin A, Ludwin I, Pitynski K, et al. Are the ESHRE/ESGE criteria of female genital anomalies for diagnosis of septate uterus appropriate? *Hum Reprod.* 2014;29(4):867-868.

Ludwin A, Ludwin I, CoelholNeto MA, et al. Septate uterus by updated ESHRE/ESGE, ASRM and CUME definitions: association with infertility, previous miscarriage, and warnings for women and healthcare systems, and associated cost analysis. *Ultrasound Obstet Gynecol.* 2019;54(6):800–814.

Moore KL, Persaud TVN. *The Developing Human Clinically Oriented Embryology.* 7th ed. Philadelphia: WB Saunders; 2003.

Nahum GG. Uterine anomalies—how common are they, and what is their distribution among subtypes. *J Reprod Med.* 1998;43:877-887.

Oppelt P, von Have M, Paulsen M, et al. Female genital malformations and their associated abnormalities. *Fertil Steril.* 2007;87:335-342.

Pang SY, Wallace MA, Hofman L, et al. Worldwide experience in newborn screening for classical congenital adrenal hyperplasia due to 21-hydroxylase deficiency. *Pediatrics.* 1988;81:866-874.

Phelan JT, Counseller VS, Greene LF. Deformities of the urinary tract with congenital absence of the vagina. *Surg Gynecol Obstet.* 1953;97:1.

Practice Committee of the American Society of Reproductive Medicine (ASRM). Uterine septum: a guideline. *Fertil Steril.* 2016;106:530-540.

Saravelos SH, Cocksedge KA, Li TC. Prevalence and diagnosis of congenital uterine anomalies in women with reproductive failure: a critical appraisal. *Hum Reprod Update.* 2008;14:415-429.
The American Fertility Society classifications of adnexal adhesions, distal tubal occlusion, tubal occlusion secondary to tubal ligation, tubal pregnancies, müllerian anomalies and intrauterine adhesions. *Fertil Steril.* 1988;49:944-955.
Toaff ME, Lev-Toaff AS, Toaff R. Communicating uteri: review and classification with introduction of two previously unrecorded types. *Fertil Steril.* 1984;41:661-679.
Troiano RN, McCarthy SM. Müllerian duct abnormalities: imaging and clinical issues. *Radiology.* 2004;233:19-34.
Usta IM, Awwad JT, Usta JA, et al. Imperforate hymen: report of an unusual familial occurrence. *Obstet Gynecol.* 1993;82:655-656.
Verkauf BS, Jones Jr HW. Masculinization of the female genitalia in congenital adrenal hyperplasia: relationship to the salt losing variety of the disease. *South Med J.* 1970;63:634-638.
Wharton LR. Two cases of supernumerary ovary and one of accessory ovary within an analysis of previously reported cases. *Am J Obstet Gynecol.* 1959;78:1101-1119.

**Suggested readings for this chapter can be found on ExpertConsult.com.**

# 12 Pediatric and Adolescent Gynecology

## Gynecologic Examination, Infections, Trauma, Pelvic Mass, Precocious Puberty

*Eduardo Lara-Torre, Fidel A. Valea*

### KEY POINTS

- It is important to give the child a sense that she will be in control of the examination process. Emphasize that the most important part of the examination is just "looking" and that there will be conversation during the entire process.
- Many gynecologic conditions in children can be diagnosed by inspection alone.
- The vaginal epithelium of the prepubertal child appears redder and thinner than the vaginal epithelium of a woman in her reproductive years.
- The prepubertal vagina is also narrower, thinner, and lacks the ability to distend like that of the vagina of a reproductively mature woman.
- The vagina of a child is 4 to 5 cm long and has a neutral pH.
- During the physical examination, including rectal examination, of the prepubertal child, no pelvic masses except the cervix should be palpable. The normal prepubertal uterus and ovaries are nonpalpable. The relative size ratio of cervix to uterus is 2:1 in a child.
- Many adolescent girls do not want other observers, such as mothers, in the examining room.
- It is estimated that 80% to 90% of outpatient visits of children to gynecologists involve the classic symptoms of vulvovaginitis: introital irritation and discharge.
- Positive identification of gonorrhea or chlamydia in a child with premenarcheal vulvovaginitis is considered diagnostic of sexual abuse. However, many infants are infected with *Chlamydia trachomatis* during birth and remain infected for up to 2 to 3 years in the absence of specific antibiotic therapy.
- The major factor in childhood vulvovaginitis is poor perineal hygiene.
- A vaginal discharge that is both bloody and foul-smelling strongly suggests the presence of a foreign body.
- In the period surrounding the time of puberty, children often develop a physiologic discharge secondary to the increase in circulating estrogen levels.
- The foundation of treating childhood vulvovaginitis is the improvement of local perineal hygiene.
- The majority of cases of persistent or recurrent nonspecific vulvovaginitis respond to improved hygiene and treatment of irritation resulting from trauma or irritating substances.
- The classic symptom of pinworms *(Enterobius vermicularis)* is nocturnal vulvar and perianal itching, the treatment for which is the anthelmintic agent mebendazole.
- The most common vaginal foreign body in preadolescent girls is a wad of toilet tissue.
- Persistent vaginal bleeding is an extremely rare symptom in a preadolescent girl. However, it is important to do a thorough workup because of the serious sequelae of some of the causes of vaginal bleeding.
- Labial adhesions do not require treatment unless they are symptomatic or voiding is compromised. If necessary, small amounts of daily topical estrogen to the labia may be used for treatment.
- The usual cause of genital trauma during childhood is an accidental fall. Most such traumas involve straddle injuries.
- Accidental genital trauma often produces extreme pain and overwhelming anxiety for the child and her parents. Because of compassion and empathy, the gynecologist may underestimate the extent of the anatomic injuries.
- Small follicular cysts in preadolescent girls are usually self-limiting.
- Ultrasound should be used as the initial diagnostic imaging technique for the evaluation of the pelvis in children and adolescents.
- Ovarian tumors constitute approximately 1% of all neoplasms in premenarcheal children. In preadolescent girls, both benign and malignant ovarian tumors are usually unilateral. Routine biopsy of the normal-appearing contralateral ovary should be avoided.
- Approximately 75% to 85% of ovarian neoplasms necessitating surgery are benign, with cystic teratomas being the most common.
- The most common malignancy in preadolescent girls is a germ cell tumor.
- Even though ovarian neoplasms are rare in children, this diagnosis must be considered in a young girl with abdominal pain and a palpable mass.
- The surgical therapy of an ovarian neoplasm in a child should have two goals: the appropriate surgical removal of the neoplasm and the preservation of future fertility.
- Ovarian torsion should be managed conservatively with untwisting and preservation of the adnexa, regardless of the appearance.
- Presence or absence of Doppler flow in the ovary on ultrasound is not diagnostic of ovarian torsion, and the decision to pursue surgical intervention should be based on the level of clinical suspicion.

Gynecologic diseases are uncommon in children, especially compared with the incidence and prevalence of diseases in women of reproductive age. This chapter considers gynecologic diseases of children from infancy through adolescence. Congenital anomalies, precocious development, and amenorrhea are covered in more detail in other chapters.

The **evaluation of children's gynecologic problems** involves considerations of physiology, psychology, and developmental issues that **are different from those of adult gynecology**. The evaluation of young girls is age dependent. For example, the physical presence of the mother often may facilitate examining a 4-year-old girl but may inhibit the cooperation of a 14-year-old adolescent. Thus the office visit and the gynecologic physical examination are performed differently in a prepubertal child compared with an adolescent girl or a mature reproductive-age woman.

## GYNECOLOGIC VISIT AND EXAMINATION OF A CHILD

### General Approach

Considerable effort should be devoted to gaining the child's confidence and establishing rapport. Young girls **should feel that they are participating in their examination**, not that they are being coerced or forced to have a gynecologic exam. If the interaction is poor during the first visit, the negative experience will detract from future physician-patient interactions (Lara-Torre, 2008).

The pediatric gynecologic visit may be unique to both the child and the parent. Most pediatric visits are preventive in nature, but the **pediatric gynecologic visit is usually problem oriented**. This may create considerable and understandable anxiety in the child and parent. **The majority of** children's gynecologic **problems are treated by medical**, rather than surgical, **means**.

The **most common** gynecologic **condition** of children **is vulvovaginitis**. Other commonly seen diagnoses at a pediatric gynecology visit include labial adhesions, vulvar lesions, suspicion of sexual abuse, and genital trauma. Many if not most of these conditions may eventually require an examination to determine the cause of the problem. An organized stepwise approach in a nonthreatening environment is more likely to result in a successful evaluation of the genitalia.

**A successful gynecologic examination** of a child **demands** that the physician employ an exam pace that conveys both **gentleness and patience** with the time spent, without seeming to be hurried or rushed. One excellent technique is for the physician to sit, not stand, during the initial encounter. This conveys an unhurried approach. The ambiance of the examining room may decrease the anxiety of the child if familiar and friendly objects such as children's posters are present. Interruptions should be avoided. **Speculums and instruments** that might frighten a child or parent **should be within drawers** or cabinets and out of sight during the evaluation. If a child is scheduled to be seen in the middle of a busy clinic, the staff needs to be alerted that the pace and general routine will be different during her visit.

### Performance of the Gynecologic Exam in a Child

The components of a complete pediatric examination include a history, inspection with visualization of the external genitalia and noninvasive visualization of the vagina and cervix, and, if necessary, a rectal examination (Jacobs, 2014).

Obtaining a history from a child is not an easy process. Children are not skilled historians and will often ramble, introducing many unrelated facts. **Much of the history must be obtained from the parents**. However, young children can help define their exact symptoms on direct questioning.

In addition, while obtaining a history, an opportunity exists to **educate the child on vocabulary to describe the genital area**. One way to describe genital area and breasts is to call them "**private areas**" and define this as meaning areas that are covered by a bathing suit. The examination also allows a period of opportunity to counsel children, in an age-appropriate manner, about potential sexual abuse.

After the history has been obtained, the parents and the child should be **reassured that the examination will not hurt**. It is important to give the child a sense that she will be in control of the examination process. A helpful technique is to place the child's hand on top of the physician's hand as the abdominal examination is being performed and to give her some choices, such as having a doll, an electronic tablet, or a toy with her. This will give the child a sense of control and divert the child's attention if she is ticklish or is squirming. Emphasize that **the most important part of the examination is just "looking"** and there will be conversation during the entire process. To successfully examine a child, one needs the cooperation of the patient, the parent, and a medical assistant.

A child's reaction will depend on her age, emotional maturity, and previous experience with health care providers. **She should be allowed to visualize and handle any instruments** that will be used. Many young children's primary contact with providers involves immunizations; children should be assured that this visit does not involve any "shots." It is also helpful to assure the adult accompanying the child that speculums are not part of the examination.

**Occasionally it is best to defer the genital examination until a second visit.** This is a difficult decision and is based on the extent of the child's anxiety in relation to the severity of the clinical symptoms. Physicians may elect to treat the primary symptoms of vulvovaginitis for 2 to 3 weeks, realizing that on rare occasions they could be missing something more serious. It is recommended that **the examination start with the nongenital areas**, such as listening to the heart and lungs; an abdominal examination and inspection of the skin should be performed. This allows one to establish a rapport and mimics the traditional visits the child has with the pediatrician. A child **should never be restrained for a gynecologic examination**. Often reassurance and sometimes delay until another day are the best approaches. In rare circumstances, it may be necessary to use continuous intravenous conscious sedation or general anesthesia to complete an essential examination. The most important technique to ensure cooperation is to involve the child as a partner. Ideally children should feel they are part of the examination rather than having an exam "done to them."

Draping for the gynecologic examination may produce more anxiety than it relieves and is unnecessary in the preadolescent child. A handheld mirror may help in some instances when discussing specifics of genital anatomy. It is critical to have all tools, culture tubes, and equipment within easy reach during a pediatric genital examination. Children often cannot hold still for long intervals while instruments are being located.

The first aspect of the pelvic examination is evaluation of the external genitalia (Fig. 12.1). An infant may be examined on her mother's lap. Pads should be placed in the mother's lap because examination often is associated with urination. Young children may be examined in the frog leg position, and children as young as 2 to 3 years of age may be examined in the lithotomy position with use of stirrups, although this is generally used for girls aged 4 to 5 years and older.

Once the child is positioned, the vulvar area and introitus should be inspected. **Many gynecologic conditions in children may be diagnosed by inspection**. The introitus will gape open with **gentle pressure downward and outward** on the lower thigh or undeveloped thigh or labia majora area (**traction**) (Fig. 12.2). Asking the child to pretend to blow out candles on a birthday cake

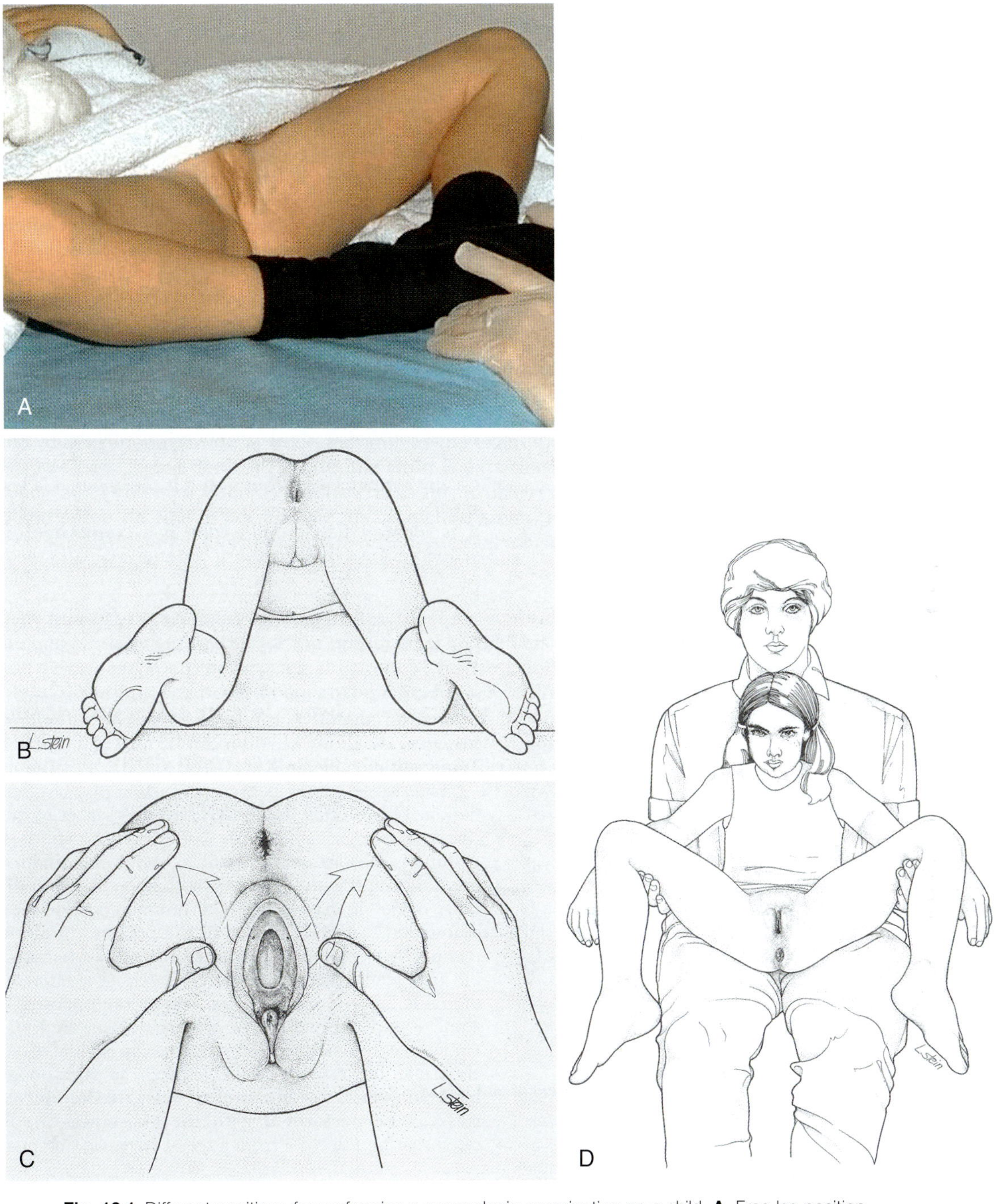


**Fig. 12.1** Different positions for performing a gynecologic examination on a child. **A,** Frog leg position. **B,** Knee-chest position. **C,** Prone position. **D,** Sitting on mom's lap. (**A,** from John J. McCann, M.D., F.A.A.P., David L. Kerns, M.D., F.A.A.P. Examination technique, frog leg position. Union, MO: Evidentia Learning; 2016. Available at www.childabuseatlas.com; **B** and **C** and **D,** from Finkel MA, Giardino AP, eds. *Medical Examination of Child Sexual Abuse: A Practical Guide.* 2nd ed. Thousand Oaks, CA: Sage, 2002:46-64.)

may facilitate the process. Visualization of the introitus is better achieved using the previously described traction and the Valsalva maneuver than separation because it gives a deeper view of the structures and partial visualization of the vagina.

The second phase of the examination involves **evaluation of the vagina**. This can be accomplished without the insertion of any instruments. One method is to **use the knee-chest position** (see Fig. 12.1, *B*). The child lies prone and places her buttocks in the air with legs wide apart. The vagina will then fill with air, aiding the evaluation. The child is told to have her abdomen sag into the table. An assistant pulls upward and outward on the labia majora on one side while the examiner does the same with the nondominant hand on the contralateral labia. Then an otoscope or **ophthalmoscope is used as a magnifying instrument and light source but *is not* inserted into the vagina.**

While the light from the otoscope or ophthalmoscope is shone into the vagina, the examiner can evaluate the vaginal walls and visualize the cervix as a transverse ridge, or flat button, that is redder than the vagina. This technique is generally successful in cooperative children unless there is a very high crescent-shaped hymen,

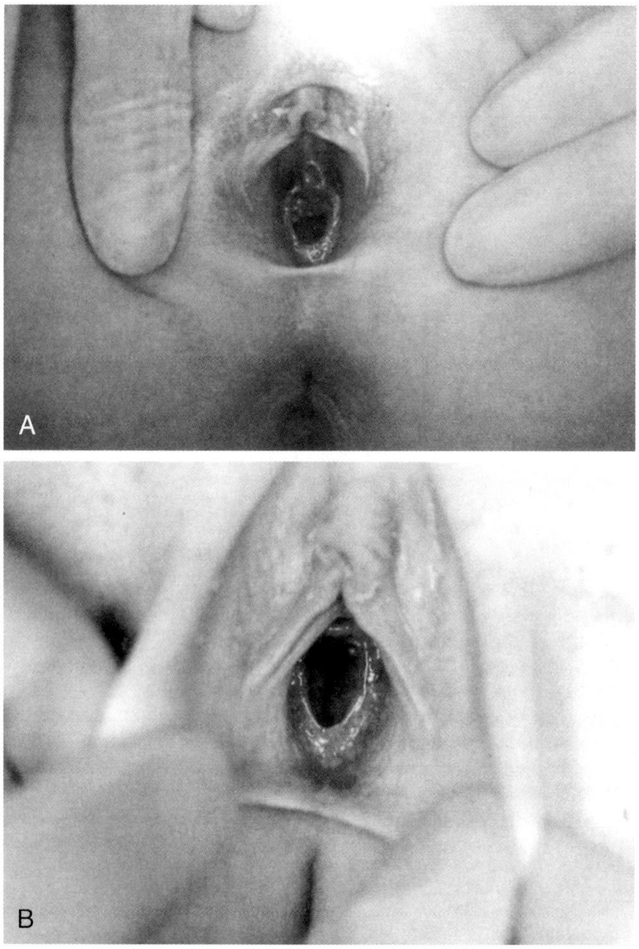

**Fig. 12.2** Examination of the vulva, hymen, and anterior vagina by gentle lateral retraction (**A**) and gentle gripping of the labia and pulling anteriorly (**B**). (From Emans SJ. Office evaluation of the child and adolescent. In: Emans SJ, Laufer MR, Goldstein DP, eds. *Pediatric and Adolescent Gynecology.* 4th ed. Philadelphia: Lippincott-Raven; 1998.)

in which case it is too difficult to shine the light into the small aperture of the vaginal introitus. A foreign object and the cervix may be visualized using this technique. After inspection of the vagina and cervix, vaginal secretions may be obtained for microscopic examination and culture (the technique is described later).

## Normal Findings: Hymen and Vagina of a Prepubertal Child

**The hymen of a prepubertal child exhibits a diverse range of normal variations and configurations** (Fig. 12.3). Hymens are often crescent shaped but may be annular or ringlike. They may have septums, microperforations, or fingerlike extensions or be completely imperforate. There are no reported cases of congenital absence of the hymen. A mounding of hymeneal tissue is often called a *bump*. Bumps are usually a normal variant and are often attached to longitudinal ridges within the vagina. Hymens in newborns are estrogenized, resulting in a thick, pink, elastic redundancy. Older unestrogenized girls have thin, nonelastic hymens with significant signs of vascularity. Not every variant of hymen is normal, and **transections between 3 and 9 o'clock should raise a suspicion for abuse** because these are likely acquired rather than congenital (discussed further in Chapter 9).

The vaginal epithelium of the prepubertal child appears redder and thinner than the vagina of a woman in her reproductive years. **The vagina is 4 to 6 cm long**, and the secretions in a prepubertal child **have a neutral or slightly alkaline pH**. Recurrent vulvovaginitis, persistent bleeding, suspicion of a foreign body or neoplasm, and congenital anomalies may be indications to perform a vaginoscopy and examine the inside of the vagina.

**Vaginoscopy in a prepubertal child most often requires sedation** with a brief inhalation or intravenous anesthetic, but in select circumstances it can also be performed in the office with older, cooperative children. The introduction of any instrument into the vagina of a young child takes skillful patience. The prepubertal vagina is narrower, thinner, and lacks the distensibility of the vagina of a woman in her reproductive years. There are many narrow-diameter endoscopes that will suffice, including the Kelly air cystoscope, contact hysteroscopes, pediatric cystoscopes, small-diameter laparoscopes, plastic vaginoscopes, handheld disposable hysteroscopes (e.g., Endosee Handheld Hysteroscopy System, CooperSurgical Inc., Trumbull, CT), and special smaller, narrower speculums designed by Huffman and Pederson. **The ideal pediatric endoscope is a cystoscope or hysteroscope because the accessory channel** facilitates the retrieval of foreign bodies while at the same time allowing a vaginal lavage to be performed. A nasal speculum or otoscope can also be used, but they are usually too short for older girls and thus are less than optimal. Local anesthesia of the vestibule may be obtained with 2% topical viscous lidocaine (Xylocaine) or longer-acting products such as lidocaine/prilocaine cream. **A complete vaginal evaluation should never be performed under duress or by force;** to avoid this, sedation can be used when performing this examination on children.

The last step in the pelvic examination may be a rectal examination. This is often the most distressing aspect of the examination and may be omitted, depending on the child's symptoms. Common **reasons to perform a rectal examination include genital tract bleeding, pelvic pain, and suspicion of a foreign body or pelvic mass.** The child should be warned that the rectal examination will feel similar to the pressure of a bowel movement. The normal prepubertal uterus and ovaries are nonpalpable on rectal examination. The relative size ratio of cervix to uterus is 2:1 in a child, in contrast to the opposite ratio in an adult. Except for the cervix, any mass discovered on rectal examination in a prepubertal examination should be considered abnormal. In this age of reliable access to ultrasonography, **the internal genital examination to evaluate the uterus and ovaries can be performed with the assistance of sonography**, often sparing the child from a rectal or pelvic examination.

## The Office Visit and Examination of the Adolescent Girl

***Adolescence*** is the period of life during which an individual physically matures and **begins to transition psychologically from a child into an adult**. This period of transition involves important physical and emotional changes. Before puberty, the girl's reproductive organs are in a resting, dormant state. Puberty produces dramatic alterations in the external and internal female genitalia, as well as the adolescent's hormonal milieu. Because the pubertal changes are often a cause of concern for adolescent girls and their parents, the gynecologist must offer the adolescent patient an empathetic, kind, knowledgeable, and gentle approach. These interactions between the physician and the adolescent girl allow the physician an opportunity to gain the patient's trust and educate the pubertal teenager about pelvic anatomy and reproduction.

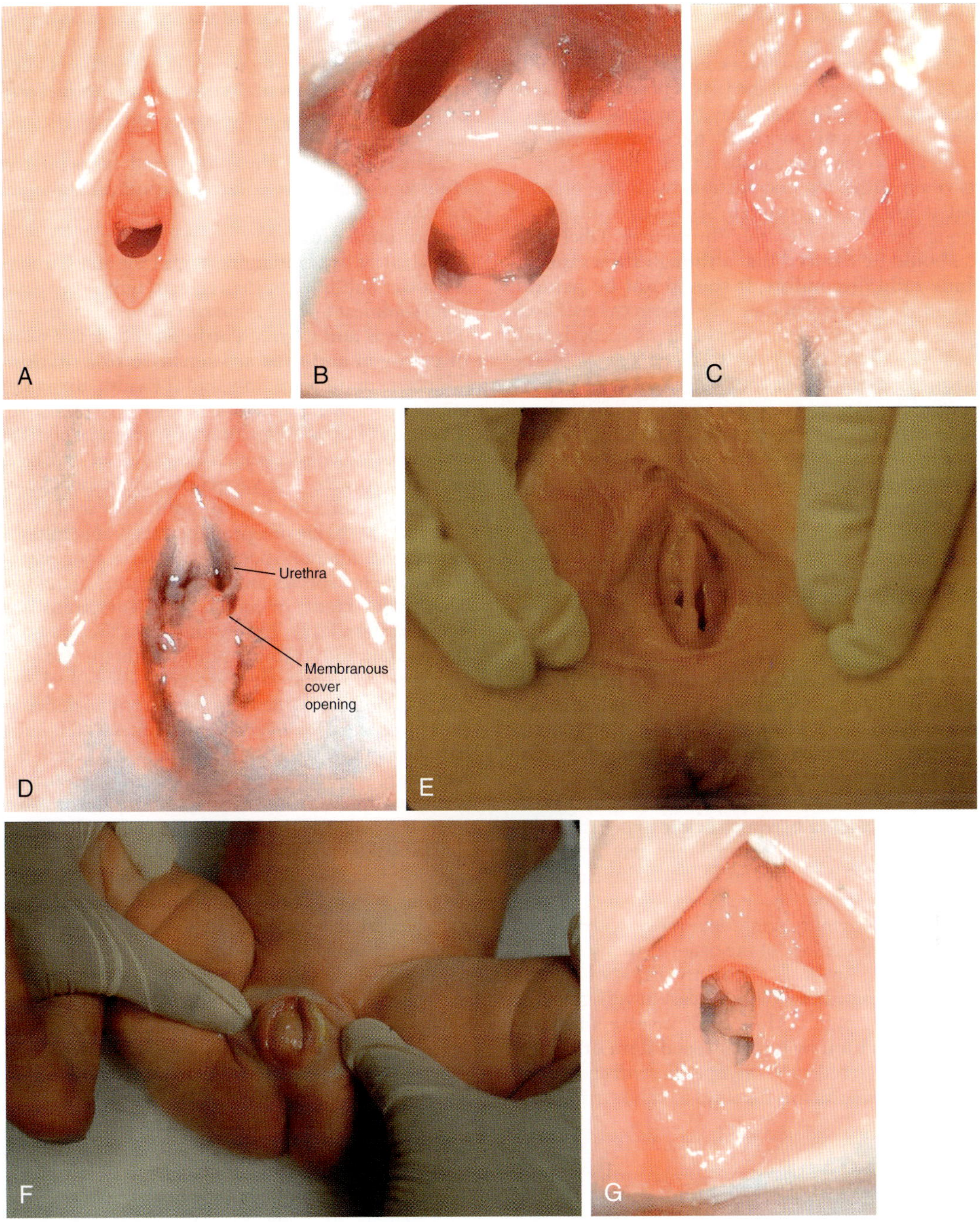


**Fig. 12.3** Types of hymens. **A,** Crescentic. **B,** Annular. **C,** Redundant. **D,** Microperforate. **E,** Septated. **F,** Imperforate. **G,** Hymeneal tags. (**A** through **F,** from Perlman SE, Nakajima ST, Hertweck SP. *Clinical Protocols in Pediatric and Adolescent Gynecology.* London: Parthenon Publishing Group; 2004; **G,** from John J. McCann, M.D., F.A.A.P., David L. Kerns, M.D., F.A.A.P. Hymenal tag, a congenital variation. Union, MO: Evidentia Learning; 2016. Available at www.childabuseatlas.com.)

The critical factors surrounding the pelvic examination of an adolescent girl are different from those of examinations of children 2 to 8 years old. Many adolescent girls do not want their mother, guardian, or other observers in the examining room, and **in many adolescent gynecology visits, a full pelvic examination is unnecessary** (Lara-Torre, 2008). Common indications for a pelvic examination in an adolescent are listed in Box 12.1.

Each adolescent is at a different stage of development, and the approach to the **examination may require variations that fit her developmental stage.** A patient in early adolescence (aged 12

**BOX 12.1** Common Indications for Pelvic Examination in the Adolescent

- Delayed puberty
- Pelvic pain
- Suspicion of intraabdominal disease
- Dysfunctional uterine bleeding
- Undiagnosed vaginal discharge
- Inability to insert tampons

to 14 years) may behave similarly and need similar support as those in the prepubertal stages. They may ask for their mothers to be there, be fearful of the examination concept, and need more than one visit to achieve the goals of the visit. Those in middle or late adolescence (aged 15 to 19 years) may be more accepting of the idea of an examination and more likely to cooperate with the proper counseling and in the appropriate setting.

Adolescents often come for examinations with the preconceived idea that it will be very painful. Slang terminology for speculums among teens includes the threatening label "the clamp." **Teens should be assured that although the examination may include mild discomfort, it should not be painful.** Providers can counsel patients that they will inform them of each step in the process and then ask the teen if she is ready before performing each step. This places the teen in control of the tempo and allows her to anticipate the next element of the examination. Allowing the patient to see and touch the instruments also may assist in demystifying the examination and allow it to flow more smoothly. In this setting **it may be helpful to use the "extinction phenomenon,"** in which the examiner provides pressure on the perineum lateral to the introitus before insertion of the speculum.

## Problems in Prepubertal Children

### Vulvovaginitis

***Vulvovaginitis* is the most common gynecologic problem in prepubertal girls.** It is estimated that 80% to 90% of outpatient visits of children to gynecologists involve the classic symptoms of vulvovaginitis: introital irritation (discomfort/pruritus) or discharge (Table 12.1) (Farrington, 1997).

The prepubertal vagina is neutral or slightly alkaline. **With puberty**, the prepubertal **vagina becomes acidic** under the influence of bacilli dependent on a glycogenated estrogen-dependent vagina. Breast budding is a reliable sign that the vaginal pH is shifting to an acidic environment.

The severity of vulvovaginitis symptoms varies widely from child to child. The pathophysiology of the majority of instances of vulvovaginitis in children involves a primary irritation of the vulva, which may be accompanied by secondary involvement of the lower one-third of the vagina. **Most cases involve an irritation of the vulvar epithelium by normal rectal flora or chemical irritants.** This is referred to as ***nonspecific vulvovaginitis.*** There often are predisposing factors that lead to vulvar irritations,

**TABLE 12.1** Clinical Features of Children Presenting With Vulvovaginitis

| Features | Number | Percentage |
|---|---|---|
| **Symptoms** | | |
| Itch | 81 | 40 |
| Soreness | 108 | 54 |
| Bleeding | 37 | 19 |
| Discharge | 104 | 52 |
| **Signs** | | |
| Genital redness | 167 | 84 |
| Visible discharge | 66 | 33 |
| Perianal soiling | 35 | 18 |
| Specific skin lesion | 28 | 14 |
| None | 5 | 2-4 |

From Pierce AM, Hart CA. Vulvovaginitis: causes and management. *Arch Dis Child.* 1992;67(4):509-512.

such as the use of perfumed soaps or the pressure from tight seams of jeans or tights, which create denudation, allowing the rectal flora to easily infect the irritated epithelium. **Cultures from the vagina indicate normal rectal flora or *Escherichia coli.*** In a primary care setting, nonspecific vulvovaginitis accounts for the majority of vulvovaginitis cases.

There are both physiologic and behavioral reasons why a child is susceptible to vulvar infection. Physiologically the child's vulva and vagina are exposed to bacterial contamination from the rectum more often than are the adult's. Because the child lacks the labial fat pads and pubic hair of the adult, when a child squats, the lower one-third of the vagina is unprotected and open. There is no significant geographic barrier between the vagina and anus. The **vulvar and vaginal epithelium lack the protective effects of estrogen and thus are sensitive to irritation or infection.** The labia minora are thin, and the vulvar skin is red because the abundant capillary network is easily visualized in the thin skin. The vaginal epithelium of a prepubertal child has a neutral or slightly alkaline pH, which provides an excellent medium for bacterial growth. The vagina of a child lacks glycogen, lactobacilli, and a sufficient level of antibodies to help resist infection. The normal vagina of a prepubertal child is colonized by an average of nine different species of bacteria: four aerobic and facultative anaerobic species and five obligatory anaerobic species.

**A major factor** in childhood vulvovaginitis **is poor perineal hygiene** (Box 12.2). This results from the anatomic proximity of the rectum and vagina coupled with the fact that, after toilet training, most youngsters are unsupervised when they defecate. Many youngsters wipe their anus from posterior to anterior and thus inoculate the vulvar skin with intestinal flora. A minor vulvar irritation may result in a scratch-itch cycle, with the possibility of secondary seeding because children wash their hands infrequently. Children's clothing is often tight fitting and nonabsorbent, which keeps the vulvar skin irritated, warm, moist, and at risk for vulvovaginitis.

In some cases, nonspecific vulvovaginitis may be caused by carrying viral infections from coughing into the hands directly to the abraded vulvar epithelium. Similarly, a child with an upper respiratory tract infection may autoinoculate her vulva, especially with specific organisms (see Box 12.2). Vulvovaginitis in children may also be caused by a variety specific **pathogens such as group A or group B b-hemolytic streptococci, *Haemophilus influenzae*, and *Shigella boydii*;** *Neisseria gonorrhoeae*, *Trichomonas vaginalis*, and *Chlamydia trachomatis* may also be responsible in cases associated with abuse but are significantly less common.

**Pinworms are another cause of vulvovaginitis in prepubertal children.** Approximately 20% of female children infected with pinworms *(Enterobius vermicularis)* develop vulvovaginitis. The classic symptom of pinworms is nocturnal vulvar and perianal itching. At night the milk-white, pin-sized adult worms migrate from the rectum to the skin of the vulva to deposit eggs. They may be discovered by means of a flashlight or by dabbing of the vulvar skin with clear cellophane adhesive tape, ideally before the child has arisen in the morning. The tape is subsequently examined under the microscope.

Despite widespread belief, mycotic **(yeast) vaginal infections are *not* common in prepubertal children** because the alkaline pH of the vagina does not support fungal growth. Mycotic vaginal infections may be seen in immunosuppressed prepubertal girls such as those with human immunodeficiency syndrome (HIV) or diabetes or on chronic steroid therapy. It can also present as a chronic colonization (diaper rash) in patients using diapers. Other specific causes of vulvovaginitis may include systemic diseases and chickenpox and herpes simplex infection.

There is nothing specific about the symptoms or signs of childhood vulvovaginitis. Often the first awareness comes when the mother notices staining of the child's underwear or the child complains of itching or burning. The quantity of discharge can

**BOX 12.2** Etiologic Factors of Premenarcheal Vulvovaginitis

**NONSPECIFIC**

1. Poor perineal hygiene
2. Intestinal parasitic invasion with pruritus
3. Foreign bodies
4. Urinary tract infections with irritation

**SPECIFIC**

**Bacterial**

1. Group A β-hemolytic streptococci
2. *Streptococcus pneumoniae*
3. *Haemophilus influenzae/parainfluenzae*
4. *Staphylococcus aureus*
5. *Neisseria meningitides*
6. *Escherichia coli*
7. *Shigella flexneri/sonnei*
8. Other enterics
9. *Neisseria gonorrhoeae*
10. *Chlamydia trachomatis*

**Protozoal**

1. *Trichomonas*

**Mycotic**

1. *Candida albicans*
2. Other

**HELMINTHIASIS**

1. *Enterobius vermicularis*

**Viral/Bacterial Systemic Illness**

1. Chickenpox
2. Measles
3. Pityriasis rosea
4. Mononucleosis
5. Scarlet fever
6. Kawasaki disease

**Other Viral Illnesses**

1. Molluscum contagiosum in genital area
2. Condylomata acuminate
3. Herpes simplex type 2

**Physical/Chemical Agents**

1. Sandboxes
2. Trauma
3. Bubble baths
4. Other

**Allergic/Skin Conditions**

1. Seborrhea
2. Lichen sclerosus
3. Psoriasis
4. Eczema
5. Contact dermatitis

**Tumors**

**Other**

1. Prolapsed urethra
2. Ectopic ureter

From Blythe MJ, Thompson L. Premenarchal vulvovaginitis. *Indiana Med.* 1993;86(3):236-239.

vary greatly, from minimal to copious. The color ranges from white or gray to yellow or green. **A discharge that is both bloody and purulent is likely not from vulvovaginitis but from a foreign body** (see Vaginoscopy for Prepubertal Bleeding without Signs of Puberty later in this chapter), although patients infected with some pathogens, particularly ***Shigella boydii,*** often present with a **bloody or blood-tinged discharge.** The signs of vulvovaginitis are variable and not diagnostic, but they include vulvar erythema, edema, and excoriation.

The **differential diagnosis** of persistent or recurrent vulvovaginitis not responsive to treatment should include considerations of a **foreign body, primary vulvar skin disease (allergic or contact dermatitis), ectopic ureter, and child abuse.** If the predominant symptom is pruritus, then pinworms or an irritant/nonspecific vulvitis is the most likely diagnosis.

The vulvar skin of children may also be affected by systemic skin diseases, including lichen sclerosus, seborrheic dermatitis, psoriasis, and atopic dermatitis. The classic **perianal figure eight or hourglass rash is indicative of lichens sclerosus** with white patches and in some cases local trauma. An ectopic ureter emptying into the vagina may only intermittently release a small amount of urine; thus this rare congenital anomaly should be considered in the differential diagnosis in young children.

## Treatment of Vulvovaginitis

**The foundation of treating childhood vulvovaginitis is the improvement of local perineal hygiene.** Both parent and child should be instructed that the vulvar skin should be kept clean, dry, and cool and irritants should be avoided. The child should be instructed to void with her knees spread wide apart (even while facing the toilet to improve urine draining) and taught to wipe from front to back after defecation. Loose-fitting cotton undergarments should be worn. Chemicals that may be allergens or irritants, such as bubble bath, must be discontinued, and harsh soaps and chemicals should be avoided. Instructing patients to use nonmedicated, nonscented wipes rather than toilet paper may prevent the self-inoculation of the vagina with small pieces of toilet paper, which can initiate a chronic discharge.

Most episodes of childhood vulvovaginitis are cured solely by improved local hygiene. The majority of symptoms improve with hygienic changes and sitz baths (warm water, no soaps or chemicals). Using this approach for a 2-week period should resolve most symptoms in patients with nonspecific vulvovaginitis. When **this intervention fails**, there should be greater suspicion of bacterial colonization; in this case a reasonable approach is the **use of broad-spectrum oral antibiotics such as amoxicillin or trimethoprim/sulfamethoxazole given for 10 to 14 days.** Without continuation of the hygiene measures, however, broad-spectrum antibiotics will only offer temporary relief and the problem is likely to recur (Bercaw-Pratt, 2014).

If patients are going to be treated with antibiotics, one should attempt to **collect a sample** of the vulvovaginal discharge for culture **before** initiation of the **antibiotics.** In noncooperative children, treatment should not be withheld if a specimen cannot be collected and empiric treatment may be started., many techniques have been described for attempting to collect a specimen, including the use of a very slim urethral Dacron swab moistened with nonbacteriostatic saline (used for collection of male urethral cultures). Pokorny has described another method for collecting fluid from a child's vagina **using a catheter within a catheter** (Pokorny, 1987). This easily assembled adaptation uses a No. 12 red rubber bladder catheter for the outer catheter and the hub end of an intravenous butterfly catheter for the inner catheter (Fig. 12.4). The outer catheter serves as an insulator, and the inner catheter is used to instill a small amount of saline and aspirate into the vaginal fluid. The results of the vaginal culture may demonstrate a single organism that is a respiratory, intestinal, or sexually transmitted disease pathogen. The presence of sexually transmitted organisms in a child is usually a strong indication that sexual abuse may have taken place, and appropriate referral and follow-up is necessary (see Chapter 9).

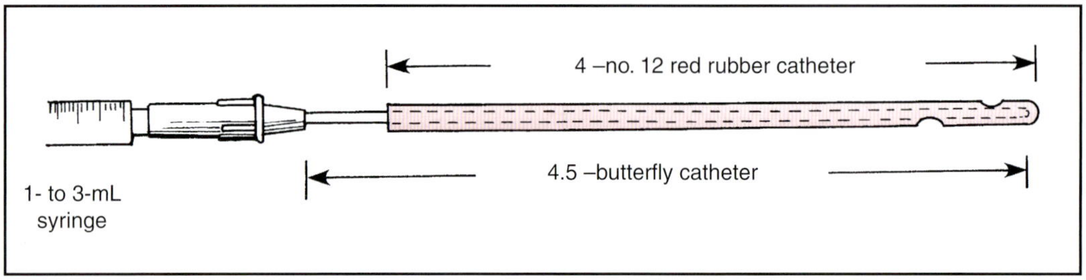


**Fig. 12.4** Assembled catheter within a catheter, as used to obtain samples of vaginal secretions from prepubertal patients. (Modified from Pokorny SF, Stormer J. Atraumatic removal of secretions from the prepubertal vagina. *Am J Obstet Gynecol.* 1987;156(3):581-582.)

## Other Prepubertal Gynecologic Problems

### Labial Adhesions

***Labial adhesions*** literally means the labia minora have adhered or agglutinated together at the midline. Another term sometimes used to describe this condition **is *adhesive vulvitis***. Denuded epithelium of adjacent labia minora agglutinates and fuses the two labia together, creating a flat appearance of the vulvar surface. A telltale somewhat translucent vertical midline line is visible on physical examination at the site of agglutination. This narrow vertical line is pathognomonic for labial adhesions (Fig. 12.5). Labial adhesions are often partial, only involving the upper or lower aspects of the labia. Small adhesions are common in preschool children, and perhaps **as many as 20% will have** some degree of **labial adhesions on routine examination** (Bacon, 2015).

Inexperienced examiners may confuse labial adhesions for an imperforate hymen or vaginal agenesis. Although the physical examination findings are significantly different, all these conditions may occlude the visualization of the vaginal introitus. In the patient with an imperforate hymen, the labia minora normally appear like an upside-down V and no hymeneal fringe is visible at the introitus. In vaginal agenesis the hymeneal fringe is typically normal but the vaginal canal ends blindly behind the hymeneal fringe.

Labial adhesions are **most common** in girls **between 2 and 6 years** of age, with up to 90% of cases occurring before age 6. Estrogen reaches a nadir during this time, predisposing the non-estrogenized labia to denudation.

There is considerable variation in the length of agglutination of the two labia minora. In the most advanced cases there is fusion over both the urethral and the vaginal orifices. **It is extremely rare for this fusion to be complete**, and most children urinate through openings at the top of the adhesions, even when the urethra cannot be visualized (pinpoint opening). However, the partially fused labia may form a pouch in which urine is caught and later dribbled, presenting as incontinence. Associated urinary infections have also been reported and may be the presenting symptom leading to the diagnosis. Most patients will be asymptomatic or present with intermittent dysuria.

The recommended **treatment in asymptomatic patients is observation** (Bacon, 2015). Most of the time treatment requests are driven by the parental concern of a closed vagina and their interpretation that this may lead to an inability to have children in the future or engage in intercourse. Although they do not explicitly say this, on further questioning, many parents disclose this kind of concern. With appropriate counseling and reassurance of the benign and common nature of this condition, as well as the likely resolution during puberty, most parents are reassured and follow advice. The majority of patients will fall into this category and can be reassured and followed over time to **spontaneous resolution when they produce their own endogenous estrogen.** If spontaneous separation does not occur at puberty and manual separation is required, the presence of better estrogenized skin decreases the **chances of recurrence**, which in children can range **from 25% to 65%**.

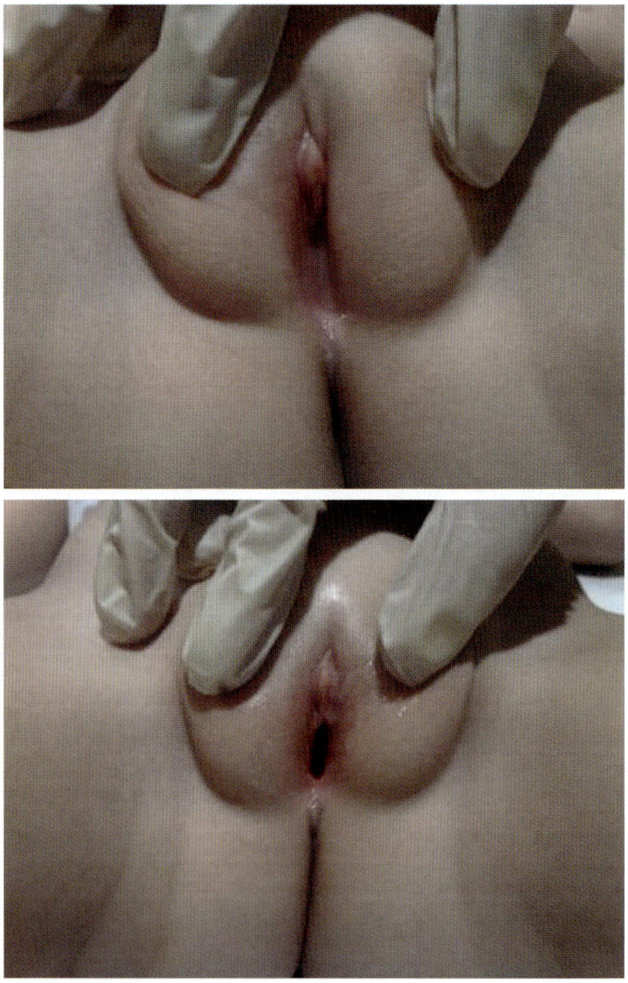

**Fig. 12.5** Labial adhesions before and after treatment. (From Acker A, Jamieson MA. Use of intranasal midazolam for manual separation of labial adhesions in the office. *J Pediatr Adolesc Gynecol.* 2013;26(3): 196-198.)

Some children present with symptoms, which may include voiding difficulties, dysuria, frequent urinary infections, urine dribbling after voiding, recurrent vulvovaginitis, discomfort from the labia pulling at the line of adhesions, and, in rare cases, bleeding from the line of adhesion pulling apart.

**Do not attempt to separate the adhesions in the office** by pulling briskly on the labia minora. It is very painful, and the raw edges are likely to adhere again because the child will be reticent to allow application of medication after being subjected to this degree of pain. Even with local anesthesia, such as lidocaine ointments or creams, the potential pain and traumatic experience for the child should deter providers from this intervention except in the well-motivated, mature child.

The **most common treatment** of this condition is **topical estrogen cream** applied to the labia two times per day at the site of fusion. This usually results in spontaneous separation, typically in approximately 2 to 8 weeks. In cases in which resolution takes longer than several weeks, the clinician can reexamine the patient. If increased pigmentation is noted lateral to the midline of agglutination, the caregiver should be reinstructed to apply the cream to the line because the lateral pigmentation indicates the estrogen is being applied lateral to the actual adhesion. The action of estrogen and the application over the adhesion line itself make the treatment more effective. Care should be taken to **not administer topical estrogen for more than 6 to 8 weeks** because prolonged use has been associated with breast budding and, less commonly, vaginal bleeding from the peripheral effects of the absorption of estrogen. Failure of separation within the normal time frame should trigger an alternative treatment.

**When estrogen** therapy **fails** and symptoms persist, the use of **midpotency topical steroids, such as betamethasone**, twice a day for 6 to 8 weeks has also shown adequate results and can be considered as a first- or second-line treatment.

Once the condition has been resolved, **recurrence can often be prevented by applying a bland ointment** (such as zinc oxide cream or petroleum jelly) to the raw epithelial edges for at least 1 month or even longer. As previously mentioned, recurrences are common.

McCann and colleagues reported the association between injuries of the posterior fourchette and labial adhesions in sexually abused children (McCann, 1988). Labial agglutination alone is so common that immediate suspicion of child abuse based solely on this finding in 2- to 6-year- olds is unwarranted. However, the combination of labial adhesions and scarring of the posterior fourchette, especially in children with new-onset labial adhesions after age 6, should prompt the clinician to consider sexual abuse in the differential diagnosis.

## Physiologic Discharge of Puberty

In the **early stages of puberty**, children often **develop a physiologic vaginal discharge** typically described as having a gray-white coloration, although it may appear slightly yellow; it is not purulent. The physiologic discharge represents desquamation of the vaginal epithelium. The estrogenic environment allows acid-producing bacilli to become part of the normal vaginal ecosystem, and the acids the bacilli produce cause desquamation of the prepubertal vaginal epithelium. When the physiologic discharge is examined with the microscope, sheets of vaginal epithelial cells are identified.

Clinically there are usually very few symptoms associated with this discharge. Occasionally the thickness of the discharge causes the vulva to be "pasted" to undergarments and causes some symptoms of irritation and erythema. Usually the only **treatment** necessary **is reassurance** of both mother and child that this is a normal physiologic process that will subside with time. Symptomatic children may be treated with sitz baths and frequent changing of underwear.

## Urethral Prolapse

**Prolapse of the urethral mucosa** is not a rare event in children. The most common **presentation is** not urinary symptoms but **prepubertal bleeding**. Often a sharp increase in abdominal pressure, such as coughing, precedes the urethral prolapse. On examination the distal aspect of urethral mucosa may be prolapsed along the entire 360 degrees of the urethra (Fig. 12.6). This forms a red donutlike structure. The prolapse may be partial or incomplete, presenting as a ridge of erythematous tissue. It is critical to distinguish this from grapelike masses of sarcoma botryoides that originate from the vagina. Occasionally the prolapse becomes necrotic and blue-black in color.

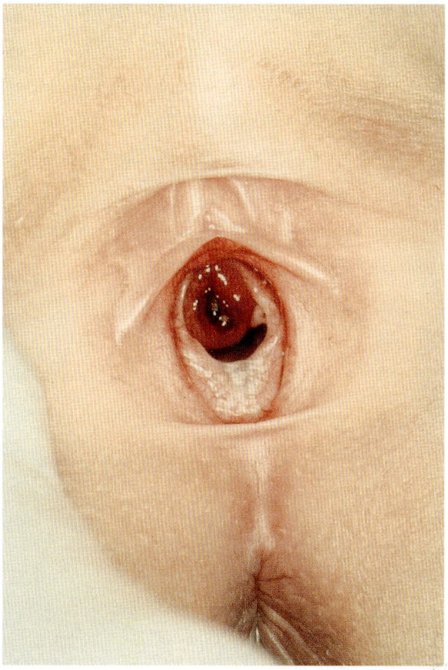

**Fig. 12.6** Prepubertal urethral prolapse with high, crescent-shaped hymen.

The most common treatment is conservative and nonoperative. **Topical estrogen has been found to be effective** in the management of this condition in many case reports and series. Although no randomized controlled trials exist, the short duration of treatment and demonstrated benefits in these series support treatment to prevent necrosis. Surgery is seldom necessary, except in rare cases where necrosis is obviously present.

## Lichen Sclerosus

***Lichen sclerosus*** (LS), or lichen sclerosus atrophicus, is a skin dystrophy most commonly seen in postmenopausal women and prepubertal children. The cause is unclear, although there is some evidence that it may be **associated with autoimmune phenomena**. This has not been confirmed by prospective studies. Histologically there is thinning of the vulvar epithelium with loss of the rete pegs. The **most common symptoms are pruritus** and vulvar discomfort. Other presentations may include prepubertal bleeding from trauma, constipation, and dysuria (Bercaw-Pratt, 2014).

The appearance of LS varies, but lesions are always limited by the labia majora. If lesions go beyond the labia majora, the condition is unlikely to be LS. **The lesion** often appears in an **hourglass or figure eight formation** involving the genital and perianal area (Fig. 12.7). The skin may be lichenified with a **hypopigmented** parchmentlike appearance. Parents may note that the genital area appears **whitened.** Pruritus is a typical presenting symptom. Secondary changes may occur subsequent to the patient excoriating the area. When this occurs, there are often

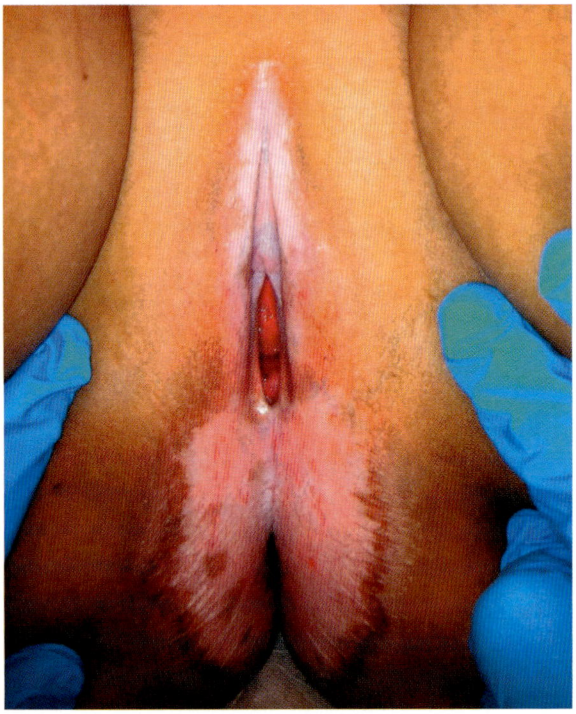

**Fig. 12.7** Typical appearance of lichen sclerosus in a 9-year-old with a 1-year history of vulvar pruritus. (From Bercaw-Pratt JL, Boardman LA, Simms-Cendan JS. North American Society for Pediatric and Adolescent Gynecology. Clinical recommendation: pediatric lichen sclerosus. *J Pediatr Adolesc Gynecol.* 2014;27(2):111-116.)

signs of trauma and breaks in the integument, which in turn can become colonized with skin bacteria and create a superimposed bacterial dermatitis.

Given the abnormal appearance of LS with secondary changes, clinicians unfamiliar with this skin dystrophy often arrive at the misdiagnosis of sexual abuse. However, clinicians experienced in pediatric or postmenopausal gynecology usually have no difficulty arriving at the correct diagnosis. Given the classic appearance **in children** and the lack of association with cancer at this age, **a biopsy is not necessary or indicated before treatment**. In cases in which the diagnosis is unclear or the disease is recalcitrant to therapy, a small punch biopsy may confirm the diagnosis. Performing a biopsy in prepubertal children is often difficult. Many children will not tolerate a local injection, and holding down children to perform a biopsy is clearly not acceptable. Sedation anesthesia is preferable in this situation. Rarely, children will tolerate a biopsy using local anesthesia.

The **treatment** of LS in children should always start with **avoiding irritation or trauma** to the genital epithelium. Children should be encouraged to avoid straddle activities such as bicycle or tricycle riding when symptomatic. Patients should clean the labia by soaking in sitz baths. Parents sometimes may assume lack of cleanliness is contributing to the disorder and scrub the area with soap, which may actually exacerbate the disease. Tightly fitting clothing such as jeans or tights may also abrade and irritate the vulva.

The North American Society of Pediatric and Adolescent Gynecology (NASPAG) recommends the use of **high-potency steroids such as clobetasol** as the initial step in treatment of this condition. **Tapering** the steroid level should be considered as soon as a response is seen or **within 4 to 6 weeks**. The tapering can be achieved by following the initial treatment with a 2- to 3-week of midpotency steroid such as betamethasone and conclude with 1% hydrocortisone for another 2 weeks (Fig. 12.8). The use of **ointments is preferred over creams** given there is less irritation compared with creams and the petroleum base of ointments appear to help it stay in place longer. The parents should apply the drug sparingly but consistently, avoiding application to nonaffected areas to prevent systemic effects of the drug such as adrenal suppression.

Recurrences, or **"flares,"** of the condition **are common** and continue for a significant time in most patients. In the past it was believed that LS **improves with puberty**; however, though improvement and resolution occur sometimes, many patients continue to have symptoms or physical findings. **Second-line** treatment, including immune modulators such as **tacrolimus 0.1% ointment** twice daily for up to 3 months, may have moderate success.

## Prepubertal Bleeding Without Secondary Signs of Puberty

**Female puberty** in the is the process of biologic change and physical development after which sexual **reproduction becomes possible**. This is a time of accelerated linear skeletal growth and development of secondary sexual characteristics, such as breast development and the appearance of axillary and pubic hair. The usual **sequence** of the physiologic events of puberty begins with a somatic change: an **increase in growth velocity** followed by either **breast development** (thelarche) or the appearance of **pubic hair** (adrenarche), followed by the period of maximal growth velocity (approximately 9 cm/year), and, last, **menarche**. The onset of thelarche typically precedes adrenarche in white girls. In contrast, African American girls often have adrenarche before thelarche (up to 15% of girls) (Appelbaum, 2012).

The cross-sectional Pediatric Research in Office Settings (PROS) study of more than 1700 American girls provided contemporary data on pubertal timing (Herman-Giddens, 1997). In this study approximately one-third of the African American girls had thelarche or adrenarche at age 7 and almost 50% by age 8. Approximately 15% of white girls had initiated puberty by age 8 and almost 40% by age 9. Mean ages for thelarche and adrenarche were 8.9 and 8.8 for African American girls and 10 and 10.5 years for white girls, respectively. The mean age of menarche was almost 12.2 years for the African American girls compared with 12.8 years in the white girls. It should be noted that these ages of pubertal onset were significantly earlier, and the sequences somewhat different, than previous, much older, classic descriptions of British children published by Marshall and Tanner (Marshall, 1969).

Recommendations from the PROS have included a new guideline regarding the definition of precocious development. They propose that **precocious puberty** should be defined as **thelarche or adrenarche before age 6 in African American girls or 7 in white girls**. These recommendations are controversial because some serious pathologic causes (e.g., endocrine or central nervous system [CNS] conditions) could be overlooked if these guidelines were strictly upheld. Certainly, in girls younger than 8 with CNS or behavioral issues, a pathologic cause of development should be entertained. A common clinical problem that is sometimes mistaken for precocious puberty is prepubertal bleeding in children without any other signs of puberty such as breast development (Box 12.3).

### Vaginal Bleeding

The normal sequence of puberty is that thelarche precedes menarche. In children with **prepubertal bleeding without breast budding, there is almost never an endocrinologic** cause, with the **exception** being a rare presentation of **McCune-Albright**

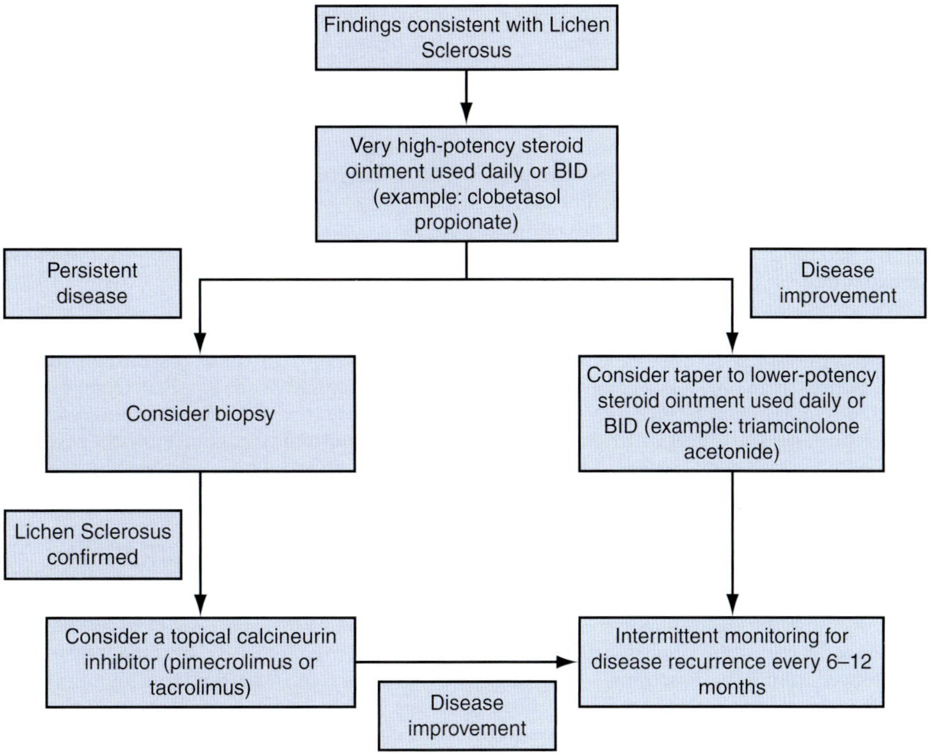


**Fig. 12.8** Algorithm for treatment of lichen sclerosus in children. *BID,* Twice daily. (From Bercaw-Pratt JL, Boardman LA, Simms-Cendan JS, North American Society for Pediatric and Adolescent Gynecology. Clinical recommendation: pediatric lichen sclerosus. *J Pediatr Adolesc Gynecol.* 2014;27(2):111-116.)

**BOX 12.3** Differential Diagnosis of Prepubertal Bleeding Without Any Breast Development

Foreign object
Genital trauma
Sexual abuse
Lichen sclerosus
Infectious vaginitis (especially from *Shigella*)
Urethral prolapse
Breakdown of labial adhesions
Friable genital warts or vulvar lesions
Vaginal tumor
Rare presentation of McCune-Albright syndrome (typically have breast development)
Isolated menarche (controversial)
Dermatologic conditions with secondary excoriation
Nongenital bleeding; mistaken as genital: rectal and urinary

syndrome (polyostotic fibrous dysplasia) or the uncommon presentation of isolated premature menarche.

The **differential diagnosis** of vaginal bleeding without pubertal development includes **foreign body, vulvar excoriation, lichen sclerosus, shigella vaginitis, separation of labial adhesions, trauma** (abuse and accidental), **urethral prolapse, and friable genital warts** (see Box 12.2). **Rare** causes include malignant tumors (**sarcoma botryoides** and endodermal sinus tumors of the vagina) and an unusual presentation of McCune-Albright syndrome. Lists of the differential diagnoses of prepubertal bleeding often also include accidental estrogen exposure (e.g., from ingestion of a mother's birth control pills or prolonged used of estrogen topical therapy). However, in reality such exposure would rarely provide enough endometrial stimulation to produce withdrawal bleeding without breast budding. Neonates may develop a white mucoid vaginal discharge or a small amount of vaginal spotting because of the withdrawal of maternal estrogens. The discharge and vaginal spotting are self-limited.

It should be remembered that although the differential diagnosis of prepubertal bleeding includes sexual abuse, most sexually abused children do not have prepubertal bleeding. In some settings, such as emergency departments, it is more likely that cases of prepubertal bleeding are due to sexual abuse compared with patients seen in primary pediatric offices or tertiary referral practices.

## Foreign Bodies

Symptoms secondary to a vaginal **foreign body** are responsible for approximately **4% of pediatric gynecologic** outpatient **visits.** The majority of foreign bodies are found in girls **aged 3 to 9 years.** The history is usually not helpful because an adult has not witnessed, nor does the child remember, putting a foreign object into the vagina. Many types of foreign bodies have been discovered; however, the most common are small wads of toilet paper. Other common foreign objects include small, hard objects such as hairpins, parts of a toy, and tips of plastic markers; crayons; and sand or gravel. Some of these objects are not radiopaque. When small swabs are used to perform vaginal cultures, the examiner may note an odd sensation of touching something other than vaginal mucosa. Objects such as coins and plastic toys are often easily visible on vaginal examination, especially in the knee-chest position. **Children** may **insert foreign bodies** because the genital area is **pruritic**, or it may occur when naturally curious children are **exploring their bodies.**

The **classic symptom is a foul, bloody vaginal discharge**. However, the discharge is often purulent and without blood. The natural history probably reflects the object initially causing irritation, creating a purulent discharge; then, as the object imbeds itself into the vaginal epithelium, bleeding and spotting may occur. There is often a lag between insertion of the object and the vaginal bleeding. Over time the foreign body **may become** partially "buried" or **embedded** within the vaginal wall. These embedded objects are often difficult to remove without discomfort, and **removal may require sedation**.

The presence of **unexplained vaginal bleeding is an indication for a vaginoscopy**. Especially in children younger than 6 years without of signs of an endocrinopathy (breast budding, estrogenization of the hymen), this should be done expeditiously to rule out malignant vaginal tumors. If an object is seen on examination, in a cooperative child the clinician may be able to either grasp the object with a forceps or flush out the object by irrigation. The catheter technique described previously may be used. **The use of a pediatric feeding tube** with room temperature or warmed saline **can also be used to flush the vagina**. With either technique, care should be taken to minimize contact with the hymen because it is a sensitive area at this age and the sensation can be enough for the child to stop cooperating with the procedure. In many instances this is not possible because the child cannot cooperate or because a solid object is embedded into the vaginal wall. In these cases the object can be removed during vaginoscopy.

Children who insert foreign objects often have recurrences. This may be secondary to persistent pain or pruritus in the genital area that was not addressed at the initial encounter, and the child uses the object (solid or toilet paper) to rub or scratch the genital area. If the foreign object is toilet paper, then having the child use wipes instead of toilet paper may reduce recurrences.

### *Shigella* Vaginitis

Approximately half of all cases of ***Shigella* vaginitis present with prepubertal bleeding**. Generally there are no concurrent gastrointestinal symptoms. Cultures for *Shigella* should be strongly considered in any child with no obvious cause for prepubertal bleeding. Rarely, vaginitis caused by other organisms can also present with prepubertal bleeding.

### Rare Causes: Vaginal Tumors and McCune-Albright Syndrome

**McCune-Albright** syndrome **is a rare somatic mutation that occurs in neural crest cells** during embryogenesis. Because the mutation does not occur in the germline, it is **not inherited**. The mutation **affects G protein receptors** and has a variable expression, depending on how many early cells are affected (an example of mosaicism). **The *GNAS1* gene** is the affected area. Patients with the syndrome may manifest the **classic triad of café-au-lait spots, abnormal bone lesions, and precocious puberty**. Most McCune-Albright patients present with prepubertal bleeding along with thelarche. Rarely a child may present with bleeding and no breast budding. Examination of the child with prepubertal bleeding should include examination of the skin for café-au-lait spots, and the historical intake should include queries about frequent bone fractures. In cases of unexplained prepubertal bleeding, the possibility of McCune-Albright should be considered, and serial breast examinations may reveal breast budding.

### Sarcoma Botryoides and Endodermal Sinus Tumors of the Vagina

**Almost all cases** of **sarcoma botryoides** of the vagina in prepubertal children **occur before age 6** (although cases in children up to age 8 have been reported), and **endodermal sinus tumors occur before age 2**. Although these tumors are extremely rare causes of prepubertal bleeding, they must be considered in every young child. Both are aggressive malignancies, and prompt diagnosis is critical. In young children with no evident cause of prepubertal bleeding, a vaginoscopy should be done to rule out these malignancies.

### Vaginoscopy for Prepubertal Bleeding Without Signs of Puberty

Many times, no clear cause of prepubertal bleeding is determined at vaginoscopy. In these cases there likely was a small foreign object that has been expelled from the vagina or has disintegrated. Even though many vaginoscopies are negative, it is especially important for clinicians to perform them promptly in young prepubertal girls with bleeding to exclude rare but aggressive vaginal malignancies.

## ACCIDENTAL GENITAL TRAUMA

The usual cause of accidental genital trauma during childhood is a fall. Seventy-five percent of cases of accidental trauma to the vulva and vagina involve straddle injuries. However, sexual abuse is obviously an important consideration in the differential diagnosis (Bond, 1995). Sexual abuse in a child is discussed later in this chapter.

### Vulvar Trauma: Lacerations and Straddle Injury

One of the **most common causes of genital trauma** in a child is a **straddle injury**. This problem occurs when a child stands, or hovers, with her legs apart over a hard object and then falls with the perineum hitting against the object. Common straddle injuries in children occur on playground climbing structures, such as a monkey bar, or fence rails and around the edges of pools. A straddle injury generally **results in unilateral and superficial injury** and **rarely involves the hymen**. In two separate series involving more than 130 children with straddle injuries, only three had hymeneal transection (Dowd, 1994).

In cases of **hymeneal transection** with a history of straddle injury, **sexual abuse should be strongly considered**. In the rare cases in which the hymen is transected as a result of accidental trauma, there is usually a history of a penetrating injury such as falling onto a stick horse or broom. **If hymeneal transection** has occurred, the examiner must confirm that the object has not penetrated into the vaginal wall, which could result in a dangerous hematoma, perforation into the cul-de-sac, or perforation of the abdominal cavity with potential visceral damage. **A vaginoscopy or laparoscopy (or both) is generally required** to rule out these possibilities. Perforations into the abdomen may not result in significant vaginal bleeding.

In children presenting with trauma and genital **bleeding, the examiner must first ascertain the site and extent of injury** and amount of bleeding. Viscous lidocaine or a longer-acting topical agent such as lidocaine/prilocaine cream can be applied and allowed appropriate time to provide anesthesia. Then the area can be gently washed by irrigating the labial area with sterile warmed water. Typical lacerations may involve denudation around the urethra or labia. The posterior fourchette is less commonly involved. In children with vulvar trauma, considerations should be given to providing a booster injection of tetanus toxoid if the last immunization was more than 5 years before the trauma.

**Superficial lacerations** (equivalent to first-degree obstetric lacerations) **generally do not require repair**, in contrast to deeper lacerations. Often, superficial lacerations can be adequately treated by applying oxidized cellulose or a similar product to stop the bleeding. Slightly deeper lacerations can be repaired with small adhesive wound closure strips (e.g., Steri-Strips). In some deeper lacerations, one well-placed suture will stop substantial bleeding. This scenario is typical of lacerations on the inferior aspect of the labia minora. Placement of the suture may be aided by injection of lidocaine in cooperative children or by conscious sedation in the emergency department.

**General anesthesia is usually required for diagnosis and treatment of extensive or deep lacerations** or in children who are unable to tolerate repair in the office or emergency department. In patients in whom the extent of the laceration cannot be fully visualized, an examination under anesthesia should be performed to prevent missing deeper lacerations than what is visualized in the emergency room. While anesthetized, the laceration should be irrigated and debrided, the vessels ligated, and the injuries repaired. Occasionally it is necessary to perform laparoscopy or an exploratory laparotomy for a suspected retroperitoneal hematoma or intraabdominal injury. Appropriate consultation with urology or pediatric surgery specialists is recommended when the extent of the laceration is beyond the vulvovaginal areas.

### Vulvar Hematomas

If the vulva strikes a blunt object, a hematoma usually results. The lack of the mature reproductive woman's fat pad in the vulvar area predisposes a young child to bleeding from trauma. If the object is sharp, such as a fence post or skating blade, the injury may be a laceration with the potential for penetration of the perineum and injury to internal pelvic organs. Other common causes of vulvar and vaginal trauma include sexual abuse, automobile and bicycle accidents, kicks sustained in a fight, and self-inflicted wounds (Fig. 12.9).

The size of vulvar and vaginal hematomas varies widely. Initially there is bleeding into the loose connective tissue. When the pressure from the expanding hematoma exceeds the venous pressure, **in most cases the hematoma will stop growing**. In the majority of cases, **surgical exploration should be avoided.** It is rare to find a specific vessel to ligate except in cases in which the hematoma is quickly expanding over 1 to 2 minutes of observation, which likely represents a rare arterial laceration. The extent of the hematoma should be determined by both visualization and palpation. **The treatment of nonexpanding vulvar hematomas is observation** by serial examinations and the use of an ice pack or cool sitz bath and pain medications. Patients may have difficulty voiding secondary to a urethral injury, urinary obstruction, or urinary injury or because they are anxious to void onto abraded vulvar surfaces.

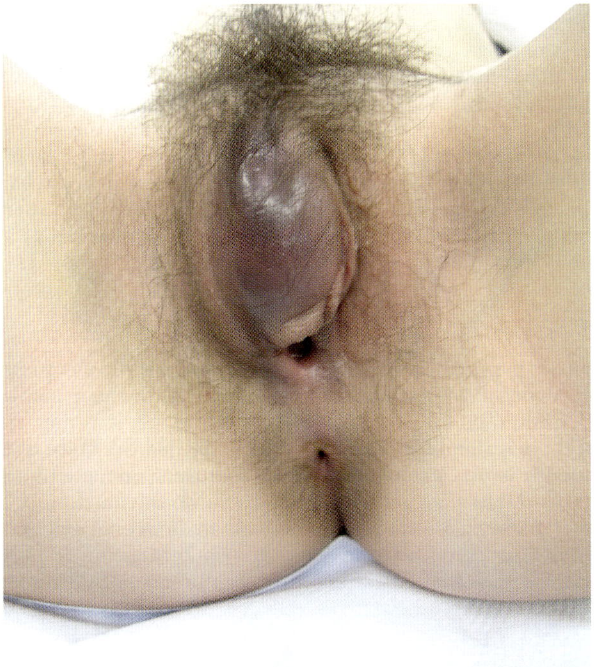

**Fig. 12.9** Vulvar hematoma in an adolescent girl as a result of a straddle injury. (From Mok-Lin EY, Laufer MR: Management of vulvar hematomas: use of a Word catheter. *J Pediatr Adolesc Gynecol.* 2009;22(5):e156-e158.)

## Sexual Abuse

Sexual abuse in reproductive women is covered in Chapter 9. This chapter contains information specifically related to sexual abuse in the prepubertal child. For a detailed and complete description of evaluation and treatment of the potentially sexually abused child, practitioners should refer to the American Academy of Pediatrics guidelines, initially published in 2009 and reaffirmed in 2013 (Kellogg, 2009), as well as the Sexually Transmitted Diseases Treatment Guidelines from the Centers for Disease Control and Prevention (CDC, 2015). These documents also contain a detailed table that describes the implications of commonly encountered sexually transmitted or sexually associated infections in the diagnosis and reporting of sexual abuse in children (Jenny, 2013).

### Scope of the Problem

Unfortunately, the sexual abuse of children is extremely common in the United States. Estimates indicate that approximately **20% of girls are involved in some type of sexual activity** during childhood. Globally this number is even higher, with approximately one-fourth of all girls victimized sexually during childhood. Although abduction cases with subsequent sexual abuse by a person unknown to the family attract national media coverage, this scenario is rare. **Most perpetrators are male acquaintances known and trusted by the families.** Fathers are responsible approximately 21% of the time and other male relatives 19% of the time. It is often not appreciated that mothers are involved 4% to 8% of the time. Babysitting is a common modus operandi for abusers to gain access to children.

### History in Sexual Abuse

There are two situations in which health care providers need to garner information regarding potential sexual abuse. One is the child or family who presents with potential sexual abuse as the chief complaint. The other situation is when the child is seen for another complaint, such as a purulent discharge, but the provider considers the possibility of sexual abuse based on historical information or physical examination.

Telephone calls regarding potential sexual abuse are a challenge for practitioners. **Urgent evaluation is necessary if the abuse has occurred within 72 hours (for forensic evidence)**, if the child is currently in a danger of repeated abuse or self-harm, or for obvious injuries such as lacerations that require treatment. If none of these criteria are encountered, the child and her family can be evaluated on a nonurgent basis. This is important because specially trained personnel should become involved as soon as possible in these situations (**pediatric forensic nurse examiners**). In many settings these children can be referred to a sexual abuse team on a nonemergency basis. In settings where teams are not available, it is critical that practitioners are aware of other community resources. If at all possible, it is usually better if the child and family are interviewed separately by a qualified mental health provider (such as a social worker or psychologist) who is experienced in evaluating sexual abuse. Guidelines have been published on appropriate methods of interviewing children who may be victims of sexual abuse. Often state departments of children's services or the social work department of the community hospital can refer providers to appropriate mental health providers.

Unless there are compelling medical reasons not to do so, this **interview should be performed before a genital examination.** There are several reasons for this recommendation. First, latency-age children may not be able to separate the examination from touching involved in abuse, making the history more difficult to obtain. Second, in the majority of abused children the examination is completely normal. It is important that families not rely on an examination to decide whether to seek counseling or intervention that would keep their child safe. Although providers should ask relevant questions, the more complete interview by an experienced mental health provider minimizes repetitive questioning of the child. The interview may also allow rapport to be created between the mental health professional doing the interview and the family so that the relationship can transition to therapy if indicated.

Practitioners may also consider sexual abuse based on historical complaints or physical examination findings. In this situation it is critical for the provider to query the guardian or parent in a nonthreatening manner. The approach should be "We are all on the same team and we all want to ensure the safety of your child." **Queries directed to the child should be open ended and nonjudgmental. Leading questions should be avoided.**

## Legal Issues in Reporting Possible Sexual Abuse

Providers must be aware of their state's laws and how to file a report alleging sexual abuse. **Every state requires that suspected and known child abuse be reported.** The word *suspected*, however, deserves definition. *Isolated* complaints that may be associated with sexual abuse (e.g., nightmares or genital bleeding) often do not require a report. Clinicians may suspect sexual abuse based on a variety of historical complaints and physical examination findings. Consideration of other causes of these complaints and findings is also critical. For example, in children who present with genital bleeding, the differential diagnosis may also include urethral prolapse, foreign bodies, lichen sclerosus, vaginal tumors, and nonabusive trauma.

**If** a provider is **unsure** whether a report is required, he or she should **discuss the situation with local child protective services** or a social worker. These professionals can help providers avoid filing vague and unnecessary reports, which clog the services of overburdened state agencies. They can also aid in filing reports in borderline cases that justify exploration to ensure the safety of children. In addition, discussion with agencies may help protect providers from prosecution for failure to report. It is important to document discussions in patient charts. Guidelines have been developed by the American Academy of Pediatrics regarding appropriate filing of abuse reports (Kellogg, 2009). **Providers should not be hesitant to file because of fear of liability** for an alleged false report. Although suits have been filed against physicians, states generally ensure immunity. It should, however, be noted that there have been successful malpractice actions against providers who have failed to diagnose or report sexual abuse.

## Physical Examination and Evaluation for Sexually Transmitted Infections

The examination of a potentially sexually abused child should include a general examination, with attention directed at evaluating the skin for bruising, lacerations, or trauma. Parents or concerned adults should be counseled that the results of a genital examination in children who have been abused are usually normal. **Physical evidence is present in less than 5% of children.** The genital examination should be carried out as described earlier in this chapter. In addition, a thorough physical examination looking for signs of physical abuse must be documented in the chart (Christian, 2000).

**In situations in which abuse has occurred within 72 hours, careful collection of forensic evidence is important.** Collection of all clothing and undergarments is critical because approximately two-thirds of forensic evidence is obtained from linens and clothing. Motile sperm will be present in the prepubertal vagina for approximately 8 hours and nonmotile sperm for approximately 24 hours. Because prepubertal children do not have cervical mucous, sperm do not remain in the cervical canal for the longer durations seen in reproductive-age women. Rape kits also often include testing for a protein specific to the prostate. Vaginal specimens may be obtained by using small swabs within the vagina, similar to the method described for obtaining vaginal cultures.

Given that only approximately **5% of abused children acquire a sexually transmitted infection** (STI), providers must decide when STI testing is indicated. Both gonorrhea and chlamydia cause a vaginitis, not a cervicitis, in prepubertal children, so a vaginal culture should be done. In the United States a **vaginal *culture* for gonorrhea and chlamydia, not DNA testing, should be performed** as recommended by the Centers for Disease Control and Prevention (CDC, 2015). There are several issues with the nucleic acid amplification tests that are commonly used in reproductive-age women. Because nonculture methods are not labeled for use in children, positive testing may not be admissible in court. The prevalence of gonorrhea and chlamydia in children is usually lower than in appropriately screened adolescents and adults; therefore the actual positive predictive values of a positive test are lower.

Testing in prepubertal children is also influenced by the typical incubation intervals of STIs. If a child was abused in an isolated incident, an STI may not be found on testing immediately after the abuse. However, a purulent discharge would prompt testing and be a red flag for possible ongoing abuse rather than an isolated incident.

When a child presents in a nonacute setting, the provider must decide whether to perform testing for STIs. It is rare for a child to have gonorrhea or chlamydia without a vaginal discharge (Bell, 1992). Standards of care regarding this issue may differ in various locations, and consultation with the local sexual assault team is warranted.

## Hymen in the Evaluation of Sexual Abuse

There is a general misunderstanding regarding the significance of hymeneal changes. The transverse diameter of the hymen was previously used as a marker of abuse. However, it is now clear that there is significant variation in children and **the state of the hymen it is not a reliable marker of abuse**. Complete transections of the hymen, and clefts that extend to the junction of the hymen between 3 o'clock and 9 o'clock, are not congenital, but if present they could be from abuse or a child inserting an object. Controversies exist regarding the significance of incomplete transections (Fig. 12.10).

## Genital Warts

**Human papillomavirus (HPV)**, the causative agent of genital warts, **may be transmitted to children** from the maternal genital tract **at delivery or by sexual or nonsexual transmission** after birth. The incubation interval from transmission to the presence of visible genital warts has not been defined in children;

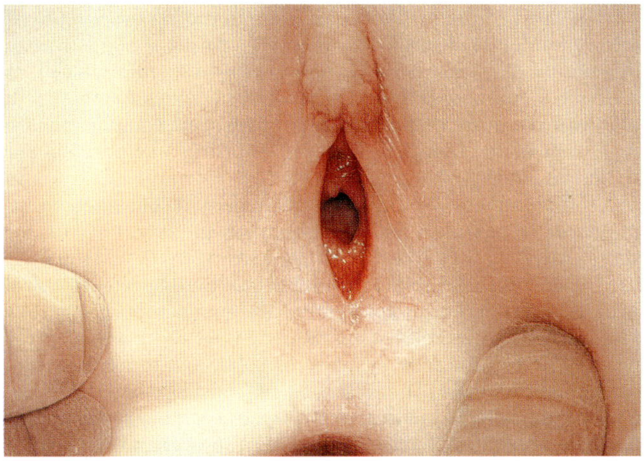

**Fig. 12.10** Hymenal bump alongside an incomplete transection of the hymen at approximately 7 to 8 o'clock.

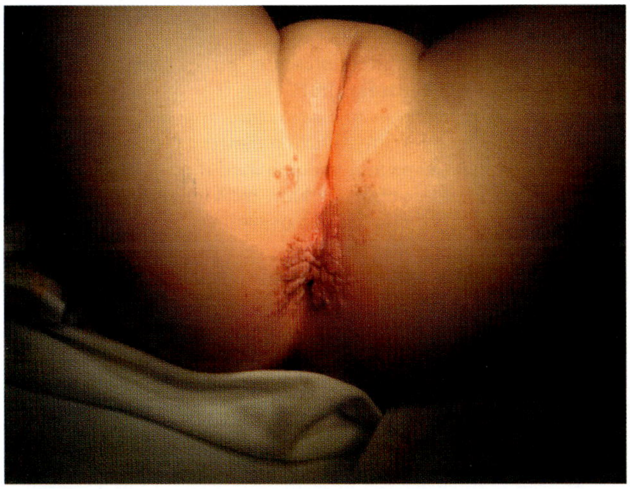

**Fig. 12.11** A 3-year-old with genital warts. (From Leclair E, Black A, Fleming N. Imiquimod 5% cream treatment for rapidly progressive genital condyloma in a 3-year-old girl. *J Pediatr Adolesc Gynecol.* 2012;25(6):e119-e121.)

however, it appears likely that **most warts appearing before age 3 years are from maternal-child transmission** (Fig. 12.11). If the child is aged 3 years or older, serious consideration should be given to the possibility of sexual transmission. However, genital warts "discovered" in a 4-year-old may have been present for some time before being noticed. This is particularly a problem in the perianal area, which may not be examined carefully even in children undergoing a cursory genital examination as part of well-child annual care (Handley, 1993).

Approximately **half of lesions will regress over 5 years. Expectant management is reasonable**, but parents may prefer treatment. Treatment in children is difficult. Caustic treatments such as trichloroacetic acid are painful even if children are pretreated with local anesthesia. **Topical imiquimod cream** is labeled for use in children 12 years and older and can cause significant vulvar irritation but **has been used successfully** in younger children; however, if the child accidentally carries imiquimod cream to the cornea, it could cause damage to the eye. Laser and/or ultrasonic treatment is an option for significant wart tissue but must be performed under anesthesia and can be associated with significant postoperative pain.

## The Ovary and Adnexa in Pediatric and Adolescent Gynecology: Cysts, Tumors, and Torsion

**Most ovarian masses** in this age group **are functional ovarian cysts, and** if a tumor is present, it most often is a **benign teratoma** (dermoid). However, **malignancies** can occur and **are** most often of **germ cell origin**, but they can **also** be **sex cord–stromal** in origin such as a granulosa cell tumor (Amies, 2016; Lara-Torre, 2002).

Physiologic and functional cysts of the ovaries arise from gonadotropin stimulation of the follicles. They may present in the fetus, newborn, or infant; at puberty; and in adolescence. The appropriate management may depend on the age and on the appearance of the cyst on ultrasound. Cysts of follicular development will be clear without significant solid components and almost always are less than 7 to 10 cm in size in reproductive-age adolescents. Management of adolescent functional cysts is essentially the same as the management in reproductive-age women. **Cysts in neonates can generally be observed** until resolution. Neonates and children can be observed **for any signs of torsion.** If they have exceptionally large cysts their caregivers should be advised to seek immediate medical attention. Torsion can certainly occur and is not rare. Many neonatal cysts are initially identified on antenatal ultrasound. There are few studies, all with small numbers, regarding the natural history of antenatal or neonatal ovarian cysts. Cysts during the preschool and early grade school years are unusual, reflecting that gonadotrophins are low.

Corpus luteum cysts are often more complex than other follicular cysts. Management is similar to that in mature reproductive-age women, and observation is warranted unless signs of malignancy are present. Consideration should be given to dermoids and the possibility of germ cell tumors if a mass has both solid and cystic components. In rare cases of intersex, such as mixed gonadal dysgenesis, suspicion of malignancy should be high. Pediatric ovarian cysts **can be a rare presentation of hypothyroidism.**

### Prenatal Ovarian Cysts

Obstetric ultrasound of a female fetus often demonstrates a **simple ovarian cyst (up to 80% of fetuses).** Before a diagnosis of an ovarian cyst is made, it is critical to exclude urinary or gastrointestinal anomalies. Fetal malignancy is rare.

There is controversy regarding the management of large antenatal cysts. Antenatal aspiration for the large antenatal cyst (4 cm or more) has been proposed by some to avoid potential antenatal torsion. The obvious disadvantage is the risk involved in antenatal surgery and the fact that resolution is a typical clinical course. Size and appearance enter heavily into management decisions; for example, if the cyst seems to be wandering around the abdomen on repetitive ultrasounds, it may be of greater risk of torsion. Also, large cysts (probably greater than 9 cm) may require the mother to give birth by cesarean section.

The natural histories of both antenatal and neonatal cysts are difficult to define. Data generated from a few small series may be misleading because the outcome may be dependent on size, mobility, and how the cyst first presented. The presence of what appears to be torsion may not result in the loss of an ovary. The relative rarity of the congenital absence of one ovary makes it likely that untwisting occurs. The incidence of congenital unilateral ovarian agenesis is quite low; it is perhaps as rare as 1 in approximately 10,000 female fetuses. **Ovarian malignancy is extremely rare in this age** group and is not a consideration in the therapeutic approach. For these reasons observation is reasonable in these cases (Bryant, 2004).

## Neonatal Ovarian Cysts

Simple cystic ovarian masses in newborns and neonates are common and can be followed expectantly. Parents should be given ovarian torsion warnings, and if the infant presents with acute vomiting or abdominal pain, she should be immediately evaluated for ovarian torsion. **Repeat serial ultrasonography should be performed every 4 to 6 weeks until the cyst resolves.** Almost all will resolve if they do not undergo torsion. **Malignancy is not a consideration in newborns** when deciding on therapy. Aspiration is an option for large cysts.

## Ovarian Cysts in Children and Adolescents

The **management** of cystic ovarian structures in children and adolescents should also be **expectant unless they are extremely large (>10 cm)**, in which case the possibility of functional cysts becomes less likely. Many times, physiologic and functional cysts are discovered on an abdominal ultrasound performed for complaints such as abdominal pain. Often the presence of a cyst is incidental and unrelated to the complaint. However, **in patients with pain, the possibility of ovarian torsion should be entertained.** Pain from ovarian cysts generally stems from three sources: (1) expansion of the ovarian cortex (which is typical during the growth phase of follicles and lasts less than 72 hours), (2) peritoneal bleeding from rupture (particularly common in bleeding disorders and patients on anticoagulation), and (3) ovarian torsion. These causes of pain do not typically present as chronic pelvic or abdominal pain. **Recurrent functional ovarian cysts may be prevented** by the use of anovulatory agents, such as **combined oral contraceptives**, in adolescents, but these agents **do not assist in the resolution of cysts that are** actively **present**.

## Ovarian Tumors in Children and Adolescents

A variety of tumors, both benign and malignant, can be seen in the childhood and adolescent years. One should always **consider** the possibility of a **malignancy**, particularly in patients **with solid ovarian masses or cystic and solid components on ultrasound**. A malignant diagnosis should also be considered in patients with presumed functional ovarian cysts that do not resolve during serial monitoring.

Germ cell tumors are the most common gynecologic neoplasm in this age group, and fortunately, most are benign ovarian teratomas. The **most common malignant** germ cell tumor is a **dysgerminoma**, followed by endodermal sinus tumors and immature teratomas. These tumors are covered in detail in Chapter 33, but several issues are especially pertinent to children and adolescents.

Bilateral tumors are seen in 10% to 15% of dysgerminomas, but this condition is rare in all of the other germ cell tumors of the ovary except for immature teratomas. **Sex cord tumors**, such as granulosa and thecal cell tumors, can also be seen in this age group and **often produce steroids** (estrogen and testosterone respectively). Rare tumors such as **gonadoblastoma**, a germ cell and sex cord tumor, are **seen in patients with intersex disorders** such as mixed gonadal dysgenesis.

**Recurrent abdominal pain is** a common complaint of school-age children and is often a **presenting symptom** in patients **with ovarian neoplasms**. A young child may not be able to differentiate lower abdominal pain from pelvic pain because of the small size of the preadolescent female pelvis, making the ovaries essentially abdominal organs. One can understand why increasing abdominal girth is a common finding associated with ovarian enlargement.

The most common clinical manifestation of an ovarian tumor is lower abdominal pain or the presence of a mass. Some ovarian tumors in children produce only vague discomfort, such as abdominal fullness or bloating. However, **adnexal masses in children are more often associated** with acute complications—such as **torsion, hemorrhage, and rupture**—than are similar tumors in adults.

Ovarian tumors constitute approximately 1% of all neoplasms in premenarcheal children. Ultrasound, magnetic resonance imaging (MRI), or abdominal computed tomography (CT) may be used in the evaluation of a suspected pelvic mass or abdominal pain of uncertain origin in children. Abdominal ultrasonography may be used to establish that the origin of the mass is in the pelvis, whether the mass is cystic or solid, and the presence of ascites (Anthony, 2012) and should be considered as the initial imaging modality. **Calcifications** in an ovarian mass may appear toothlike, indicating a likely diagnosis of an ovarian **teratoma**.

As part of the preoperative workup, the child may be screened for elevated serum levels of **tumor markers** such as **alpha-fetoprotein, both alpha and beta human chorionic gonadotropin (HCG), inhibin (A and B), lactate dehydrogenase, estradiol, and testosterone**; even tumor markers that are associated with other neoplasms can be detected in girls. HCG may be positive for either the alpha or beta subunit, so a pregnancy test that only tests for the beta subunit is inadequate.

Ovarian tumors in preadolescent girls, both benign and malignant, are **usually unilateral**. Thus it is imperative to be as conservative as possible in managing the opposite ovary to protect potential future fertility. During surgery the opposite ovary should be carefully inspected and palpated if possible. It is generally unnecessary and potentially harmful to perform a biopsy on a normal-appearing contralateral ovary in a preadolescent girl. This is especially true in patients with dermoids. Careful inspection of the contralateral ovary in patients with a dysgerminoma or an immature teratoma—malignancies in which bilateral tumors are not as rare—is also appropriate, reserving biopsy only for when an abnormality is detected by clinical inspection. In the past it was common practice to perform a wedge biopsy of the contralateral ovary, but that practice was not evidence based and was abandoned because it clearly increased the possibility of scarring and infertility.

Children with suspected ovarian cancer should be referred to specialists who are up to date on the most current data from research groups such as the Pediatric Oncology Group and the Gynecologic Oncology Group, now part of NRG Oncology (Cushing, 1999). Providers should be skilled in providing their patients proper staging procedures, including lymph node assessment, and evidence-based adjuvant therapy as indicated by standard national guidelines such as the guidelines of the National Comprehensive Cancer Network (NCCN) (Morgan, 2013). The role of adjuvant therapy should be individualized for each patient. The use of tumor markers to help differentiate patients with benign teratoma from malignancies is helpful in triaging appropriate referrals. However, regardless of what the makers show, referral is prudent.

Approximately **75% to 85% of ovarian neoplasms that necessitate surgery in premenarcheal girls are benign** and approximately 15% to 25% are malignant neoplasms. The risk is less in young children. In a review of ovarian masses in children, Brown and coworkers reported that the risk of malignancy was only 3% up to age 8 (Brown, 1993).

In summary, even though ovarian neoplasms are rare in children, this diagnosis should be considered in a young girl with abdominal pain and a palpable mass. The surgical therapy should have **two goals**: first and most important, the appropriate surgical procedure, including selective evaluation of lymph nodes and **appropriate staging procedures**; second, the **preservation of future fertility**, because hysterectomy is usually not necessary, even in rare cases of bilateral childhood or adolescent ovarian malignancy. The uterus should be retained to keep the patient's options for future fertility intact. Even in the absence of ovaries, fertility may be possible with artificial reproductive technology and the use of donor eggs.

## Ovarian Torsion

Ovarian torsion is covered in more detail in Chapter 18. Issues unique to children and adolescents are covered in this discussion. Torsion in prepubertal girls may be secondary to a pelvic mass or caused by mechanical factors that occur in the peripubertal interval. In early puberty the ovaries drop from their prepubertal position at the pelvic brim into the pelvis. This drop occurs under the influence of gonadotropins that surge at puberty. Some young women may have longer supportive ligaments, predisposing them to twisting. Approximately **two-thirds of the time**, ovarian **torsion occurs on the right side**, increasing the likelihood of the process being confused with appendicitis. The sigmoid colon in the left lower quadrant helps prevent the left ovary from twisting.

Although both appendicitis and torsion can present with acute pain and rebound, the gradual progression of appendicitis is quite different from the acute severe pain of torsion. Nausea and emesis often ensue immediately with torsion as a result of the severity of the pain. Appendicitis tends to present with anorexia, which gradually worsens. The young girl with an **acute onset of pain and simultaneous emesis** likely has **ovarian torsion** rather than appendicitis.

Approximately one-third of ovarian torsion cases in children and adolescents are not associated with a predisposing ovarian mass such as a dermoid, large functional cyst, or malignancy. Nevertheless, even in children without an ovarian mass, after torsion the ovary will become swollen and enlarged as the lymphatic flow is blocked. In children and adolescents **the differentiation between torsion and appendicitis is a common dilemma**. Radiologic evaluation to rule out appendicitis may reveal a pelvic mass. Unfortunately, **the presence of vascular flow in the ovary does not rule out torsion**. In fact, many cases of surgically proven torsion had normal vascular flow on ultrasound evaluation. Once a torsion is identified at the time of surgery, it is important to consider the patient's future fertility. There are numerous reports in the literature demonstrating the benefit of **untwisting the gonad, regardless of its appearance**, because most will regain function after the edema resolves. Risk of **embolus** from a thrombosed ovarian vein **has not been reported** in the literature. In institutions where pediatric surgeons manage these patients, consultation and **co-management with gynecology** will likely **result in better outcomes and fewer adnexectomies.**

## REFERENCES


American College of Obstetricians and Gynecologists (ACOG). *Guidelines for Women's Health Care.* 4th ed. Washington, DC: ACOG; 2014.

Amies Oelschlager AE, Gow KW, Morse CB, et al. Management of large ovarian neoplasms in pediatric and adolescent females. J Pediatr Adolesc Gynecol. 2016;29:88-94.

Anthony EY, Caserta MP, Singh J, et al. Adnexal masses in female pediatric patients. *Am J Roentgenol.* 2012;198(5):W426-W431.

Appelbaum H, Malhotra S. A comprehensive approach to the spectrum of abnormal pubertal development. *Adolesc Med.* 2012;23(1):1-14.

Bacon JL, Romano ME, Quint EH. Clinical recommendation: pediatric labial adhesions. *J Pediatr Adolesc Gynecol.* 2015;28(5):405-409.

Bell TA, Stamm WE, Wang S, et al. Chronic Chlamydia trachomatis infections in infants. *JAMA.* 1992;267(3):400-402.

Bercaw-Pratt JL, Boardman LA, Simms-Cendan JS. North American Society for Pediatric and Adolescent Gynecology (NASPAG): Clinical recommendation: pediatric lichen sclerosus. *J Pediatr Adolesc Gynecol.* 2014;27(2):111-116.

Bond GR, Dowd MD, Landsman I, et al. Unintentional perineal injury in prepubescent girls: a multicenter, prospective report of 56 girls. *Pediatrics.* 1995;95(5):628-631.

Brown MF, Hebra A, McGeehin K, et al. Ovarian masses in children: a review of 91 cases of malignant and benign masses. *J Pediatr Surg.* 1993;28:930–933

Bryant AR, Laufer MR. Fetal ovarian cysts. *J Reprod Med.* 2004;49(5): 329-337.

Centers for Disease Control and Prevention (CDC). Sexually transmitted diseases treatment guidelines, 2015. *MMWR Recomm Rep.* 2015; 64(RR-12):1-140.

Christian CW, Lavelle JM, Dejong AR, et al. Forensic evidence findings in prepubertal victims of sexual assault. *Pediatrics.* 2000;106(1 Pt 1): 100-104.

Cushing B, Giller R, Ablin A, et al. Surgical resection alone is effective treatment for ovarian immature teratoma in children and adolescents: a report of the Pediatric Oncology Group and the Children's Cancer Group. *Am J Obstet Gynecol.* 1999;181(2):353-358.

Dowd MD, Fitzmaurice L, Knapp J, et al. The interpretation of urogenital findings in children with straddle injuries. *J Pediatr Surg.* 1994; 29(1):7-10.

Farrington PF. Pediatric vulvo-vaginitis. *Clin Obstet Gynecol.* 1997; 40(1):135-140.

Handley J, Dinsmore W, Maw R, et al. Anogenital warts in prepubertal children: sexual abuse or not? *Int J STD AIDS.* 1993;4(5):271-279.

Herman-Giddens ME, Slora EJ, Wasserman RC, et al. Secondary sexual characteristics and menses in young girls seen in office practice: a study from the Pediatric Research in Office Settings network. *Pediatrics.* 1997;99(4):505-512.

Jacobs AM, Alderman E. Gynecologic examination of the pre-pubertal girl. *Pediatr Rev.* 2014;35:97-105.

Jenny C, Crawford-Jakubiak JE. Committee on Child Abuse and Neglect, American Academy of Pediatrics: The evaluation of children in the primary care setting when sexual abuse is suspected. *Pediatrics.* 2013;132(2):e558-e567.

Kellogg ND. Committee on Child Abuse and Neglect, American Academy of Pediatrics: clinical report—the evaluation of sexual behaviors. *Pediatrics.* 2009;124(3):992-998.

Lara-Torre E. Ovarian neoplasias in children. *J Pediatr Adolesc Gynecol.* 2002;15(1):47-52.

Lara-Torre E. The physical examination in pediatric and adolescent patients. *Clin Obstet Gynecol.* 2008;51:205-213.

Marshall WA, Tanner JM. Variations in pattern of pubertal changes in girls. *Arch Dis Child.* 1969;44(235):291-303.

McCann J, Voris J, Simon M. Labial adhesions and posterior fourchette injuries in childhood sexual abuse. *Am J Dis Child.* 1988;142(6): 659-663.

Morgan Jr RJ, Alvarez RD, Armstrong DK, et al. Ovarian cancer, version 2.2013. *J Natl Compr Canc Netw.* 2013;11(10):1199-1209.

Pokorny SF, Stormer J. Atraumatic removal of secretions from the prepubertal vagina. *Am J Obstet Gynecol.* 1987;156(3):581-582.


**Suggested readings for this chapter can be found on ExpertConsult.com.**

# 13 Contraception and Abortion

Katherine Rivlin, Anne R. Davis

KEY POINTS

- Approximately 45% of all pregnancies in the United States are unintended, and among women who experience unintended pregnancy, more than half are not using contraception. By age 45, at least half of U.S. women will experience an unintended pregnancy, and one in four will have had an abortion.
- Failure rates in the first year of contraceptive use are highest for coitus-related methods (e.g., withdrawal, periodic abstinence, condoms, barrier methods) followed by combined contraceptives (pill, patch, ring) and the progestin injection. Intrauterine devices (IUDs), implants, and sterilization have typical use failure rates of less than 1%, similar to that of sterilization.
- Combined hormonal contraceptives increase a woman's risk of venous thromboembolism (VTE) about threefold to approximately 1 in 1000 per year. Women with risk factors for VTE or cardiovascular disease (e.g., obesity, age older than 35, smoking, a personal or family history of clotting disorder) should use effective birth control methods without estrogen.
- The most effective method of emergency contraception is the copper IUD, followed by a single dose of oral ulipristal acetate. An oral dose of levonorgestrel is somewhat less effective but available over the counter.
- First- and second-trimester medical and surgical abortions are common and safe. Overall, abortions have a lower complication risk than carrying a pregnancy to term. Access to legal and safe abortion is a cornerstone of maternal health.

## CONTRACEPTION OVERVIEW

**Contraception is nearly a universal health care need among those who can become pregnant.** About 99% of women aged 15 to 44 who have ever had sexual intercourse report use of at least one contraceptive method at some point (Daniels, 2013). In the United States, 70% of the 64 million women aged 15 to 44 are at risk of unintended pregnancy; they are sexually active, not infertile, and not trying for pregnancy. Of those at risk, about 10% do not use contraception. **About 45% of pregnancies in the United States are unintended, and among women who experience unintended pregnancy, more than half are not using contraception** (Mosher, 2010).

Tubal sterilization (18.6%), the oral contraceptive pill (12.6%), long-acting reversible contraceptive (LARC) methods (10.3%), and condoms (8.7%) comprise the most commonly used methods (Table 13.1) (Daniels, 2018). Distinct advantages and disadvantages characterize contraceptive methods. Clinicians should be able to explain the unique features of each method, must identify medical contraindications to a given method and offer safe and effective alternatives, and should keep the risks of pregnancy in mind when discussing methods. **For healthy women, and especially for medically challenging patients, pregnancy risks generally exceed risks related to contraception.**

## CONTRACEPTIVE COUNSELING

Health care outcomes improve when provider counseling incorporates patient preferences. In contraception counseling, communication between the patient and provider can affect initiation and continuation of birth control. Most women value personal autonomy when making decisions about contraception more than they do in other areas of medicine (Dehlendorf, 2010).

**Shared decision making (SDM) provides a useful counseling tool.** Using this model, the clinician contributes medical expertise, and the patient contributes her values and preferences. Priorities vary; therefore counseling should be tailored to each individual woman. SDM works particularly well in contraception counseling because most methods of birth control are safe for most women. **A shared decision-making approach correlates with improved patient satisfaction compared with decisions driven solely by the provider or the patient** (Dehlendorf, 2017).

### Medical Eligibility Criteria for Contraceptive Use

Most women initiating contraception are healthy, and in general the risks of pregnancy outweigh the risks of most contraceptive methods. However, there are certain medical conditions that may contraindicate using a particular method. The health care provider must be aware of these specific contraindications to ensure that a given method is both acceptable to the patient *and* safe.

The **World Health Organization** (WHO) publishes detailed guidelines listing the medical eligibility criteria for the use of individual contraceptive methods. These regularly updated guidelines can be downloaded from the WHO website (www.who.int/reproductivehealth) (WHO, 2015). The **Centers for Disease Control and Prevention (CDC)** also publishes regularly updated medical eligibility criteria tailored to U.S. practice; CDC guidelines are available for download along with a companion app (www.cdc.gov/reproductivehealth) (Curtis, 2016).

## CONTRACEPTIVE EFFECTIVENESS

All contraceptive methods have a typical use effectiveness (pregnancy rate given actual, real-life conditions including occasional inconsistent or incorrect use) and perfect use effectiveness (pregnancy rate given correct and consistent use with every act of intercourse). Pregnancy rates can vary widely between typical and perfect use depending on the method (Table 13.2). In general, coitus-related methods and more user-dependent methods are less effective than "forgettable methods" such as LARC. **Combining any method with a condom decreases the risk of sexually transmitted infection acquisition.**

This chapter presents contraceptive methods according to efficacy, with the methods that most effectively prevent

**TABLE 13.1** Percentage Distribution of Women Aged 15 to 44, by Current Contraceptive Status: United States, 2015-2017

| Characteristic | % |
|---|---|
| Using contraception | 64.9 |
| Female sterilization | 18.6 |
| Male sterilization | 5.9 |
| Pill | 12.6 |
| Male condom | 8.7 |
| Long-acting reversible contraceptives | 10.3 |
| Depo-Provera, contraceptive ring, or patch | 3.2 |
| All other contraceptive methods | 5.6 |
| Not using contraception | 35.1 |
| Never had sexual intercourse or did not have sex in the past 3 months | 17.0 |
| Pregnant, postpartum, or seeking pregnancy | 7.5 |
| Nonuser who had sexual intercourse in the past 3 months | 7.9 |
| All other nonusers | 2.7 |

Data from Daniels K, Abma J. Current contraceptive status among women aged 15-49: United States, 2015-2017. *NCHS Data Brief.* 2018;(327). Available at https://www.cdc.gov/nchs/data/databriefs/db327-h.pdf.

pregnancy presented first followed by the less effective methods. This framework of contraceptive effectiveness follows the communication tool offered by the WHO (Fig. 13.1) but is not a one-size-fits-all formula for counseling. For example, one study found lack of side effects and affordability were key to acceptability, in addition to efficacy (Lessard, 2012). Identifying preferences is key because a patient may feel misunderstood or reluctant to seek health care if her provider emphasizes effectiveness when she places greater value on another feature such as bleeding patterns.

## Initiating Contraception

Once selected, method initiation can usually begin immediately if desired. In the case of regular menstrual cycles, all methods can be initiated in days 1 through 5 of the menstrual cycle with expected immediate contraceptive protection. Outside of these cycle days, **providers can also recommend initiation when reasonably sure, based on history and urine pregnancy testing, that a woman is not pregnant** (CDC, 2013). This is **the quick start method.** Quick start helps to avoid pregnancies that occur while waiting for menses to begin. After quick starting, the copper intrauterine device (IUD) is immediately effective. For other methods, providers should recommend a backup method such as abstinence or a barrier contraceptive for 1 week while awaiting contraceptive protection. When a health care provider is not reasonably certain about pregnancy, the benefits of initiating methods such as the birth control pill, implant, or injectable likely outweigh the risks. For intrauterine devices, the patient and provider should use SDM to explore the benefits of the device against the risks of an unlikely but possible pregnancy. After a quick start, initiators should be encouraged to repeat a pregnancy test if menses does not return or if pregnancy symptoms emerge. Occasionally pregnancy may occur after initiating a method using quick start. Contraceptive hormones are not teratogenic, and it is safe to continue pregnancies after a quick start or in other instances of contraceptive failure if desired.

## Permanent Contraception: Sterilization

Fallopian tube and vas deferens occlusion (sterilization) offer safe and highly effective contraception. In contrast to reversible or temporary methods, sterilization is permanent.

The decision to undergo sterilization should be made solely by the individual in consultation with a provider. The history of sterilization in the United States raises ethical concerns that must be considered, even today. Thousands of forced sterilization procedures occurred in the United States, disproportionately to poor women and women of color, whereas other women were denied sterilization because of provider beliefs (ACOG, 2017). **Prospective studies document that up to 20% of women younger than age 30 report regret after sterilization** (Hillis, 1999). If women wish to conceive after tubal sterilization, in vitro fertilization is likely necessary and is performed more often than tubal reconstructive surgery in these patients. Age should not be a barrier, however; younger women who are well informed and desire permanent sterilization can be offered the procedure. Providers offering sterilization should understand federal and local rules related to waiting periods, age, and disability status.

### Vasectomy

**Vasectomy is a safe and highly effective** outpatient procedure that takes about 20 minutes. More than 300,000 vasectomies are performed annually in the United States. After identifying and cutting the vas deferens, the ends of the vas are closed by ligation or fulguration and then replaced in the scrotal sac. This procedure prohibits sperm from passing into the ejaculate. **After about 13 to 20 ejaculations, the ejaculate becomes sperm free but otherwise unchanged.**

Vasectomy offers important advantages over tubal sterilization. The procedure is relatively low cost (it is the most cost-effective method) and can be performed in an office setting using local anesthesia. No entry into the peritoneal cavity occurs, and efficacy is easily verified when a semen sample confirms the absence of sperm. Until that time, another method of birth control must be used. In the United States, reversal requests range from 5% to 7% among men who have had a vasectomy. Vas reanastomosis, a difficult and meticulous procedure, offers a success rate of approximately 50% (ASRM, 2004).

### Tubal Sterilization

Tubal sterilization prevents fertilization by cutting, occluding, or removing the fallopian tubes. Methods in the United States include laparoscopy anytime outside of pregnancy and postpartum sterilization concurrent with cesarean delivery or immediately after a vaginal delivery. About half of sterilization procedures occur in the postpartum period (Chan, 2010).

Tubal sterilization is highly effective, with failure rates similar to LARC methods. The Collaborative Review of Sterilization (CREST), a prospective study of more than 10,000 women who underwent transabdominal sterilization that included 14 years of follow-up, provided information related to many aspects of tubal sterilization. Findings included a 5-year cumulative failure probability of 13 per 1000 procedures, with failures sometimes occurring years later. Younger women had a higher risk of failure. Postpartum partial salpingectomy carried the lowest 10-year cumulative risk of failure (7.5 per 1000 procedures); the rate with bipolar fulguration was higher (Peterson, 1996).

The CREST study occurred before the widespread adoption of Filshie clips, transcervical sterilization, and salpingectomy techniques. Some data show a 10-year cumulative failure rate of **2 to 3 per 1000 procedures for the Filshie clip** (Shaw, 1999). Data are less clear for transcervical sterilization; Gariepy calculated a first-year failure rate of 57 in 1000 (Gariepy, 2014).

**TABLE 13.2** Percentage of U.S. Women Experiencing an Unintended Pregnancy During the First Year of Typical Use and the First Year of Perfect Use of Contraception and the Percentage Continuing Use at the End of the First Year

| Method | % of Women Experiencing an Unintended Pregnancy Within the First Year of Use | | % of Women Continuing Use at 1 Year‡ |
|---|---|---|---|
| | Typical Use* | Perfect Use† | |
| No method§ | 85 | 85 | |
| Spermicides‖ | 21 | 16 | 42 |
| Female condom¶ | 21 | 5 | 41 |
| Withdrawal | 20 | 4 | 46 |
| Diaphragm** | 17 | 16 | 57 |
| Sponge | 17 | 12 | 36 |
| Parous women | 27 | 20 | |
| Nulliparous women | 14 | 9 | |
| Fertility awareness–based methods†† | 15 | | 47 |
| Ovulation method† | 23 | 3 | |
| TwoDay method† | 14 | 4 | |
| Standard Days method† | 12 | 5 | |
| Natural Cycles†† | 8 | 1 | |
| Symptothermal method†† | 2 | 0.4 | |
| Male condom¶ | 13 | 2 | 43 |
| Combined and progestin-only pills | 7 | 0.3 | 67 |
| Evra patch | 7 | 0.3 | 67 |
| NuvaRing | 7 | 0.3 | 67 |
| Depo-Provera | 4 | 0.2 | 56 |
| Intrauterine contraceptives | | | |
| ParaGard (copper T) | 0.8 | 0.6 | 78 |
| Skyla (13.5 mg LNG) | 0.4 | 0.3 | |
| Kyleena (19.5 mg LNG) | 0.2 | 0.2 | |
| Liletta (52 mg LNG) | 0.1 | 0.1 | |
| Mirena (52 mg LNG) | 0.1 | 0.1 | 80 |
| Nexplanon | 0.1 | 0.1 | 89 |
| Tubal occlusion | 0.5 | 0.5 | 100 |
| Vasectomy | 0.15 | 0.1 | 100 |

From Trussell J, Aiken ARA. Contraceptive efficacy. In: Hatcher RA, Nelson AL, Trussell J, et al, eds. *Contraceptive Technology.* 21st ed. New York: Ayer Company Publishers; 2018.

*Among *typical* couples who initiate use of a method (not necessarily for the first time), the percentage who experience an accidental pregnancy during the first year if they do not stop use for any reason other than pregnancy. Estimates of the probability of pregnancy during the first year of typical use for fertility awareness–based methods, withdrawal, the male condom, the pill, and Depo-Provera are taken from the 2006-2010 National Survey of Family Growth (NSFG) corrected for underreporting of abortion.

†Among couples who initiate use of a method (not necessarily for the first time) and who use it *perfectly* (both consistently and correctly), the percentage who experience an accidental pregnancy during the first year if they do not stop use for any other reason. See the text for the derivation of the estimate for each method.

‡Among couples attempting to avoid pregnancy, the percentage who continue to use a method for 1 year.

§This estimate represents the percentage who would become pregnant within 1 year among women now relying on reversible methods of contraception if they abandoned contraception altogether.

‖150 mg gel, 100 mg gel, 100 mg suppository, 100 mg film.

¶Without spermicides.

**With spermicidal cream or jelly.

††About 80% of segments of Fertility Awareness Based Methods (FABM) use in the 2006-2010 National Survey of Family Growth (NSFG) were reported as calendar rhythm. Specific FABM methods are too uncommonly used in the U.S. to permit calculation of typical use failure rates for each using NSFG data; rates provided for individual methods are derived from clinical studies. The Ovulation and TwoDay methods are based on evaluation of cervical mucus. The Standard Days method avoids intercourse on cycle days 8 through 19. Natural Cycles is a fertility app that requires user input of basal body temperature (BBT) recordings and dates of menstruation and optional luteinizing hormone (LH) urinary test results. The Symptothermal method is a double-check method based on evaluation of cervical mucus to determine the first fertile day and evaluation of cervical mucus and temperature to determine the last fertile day.

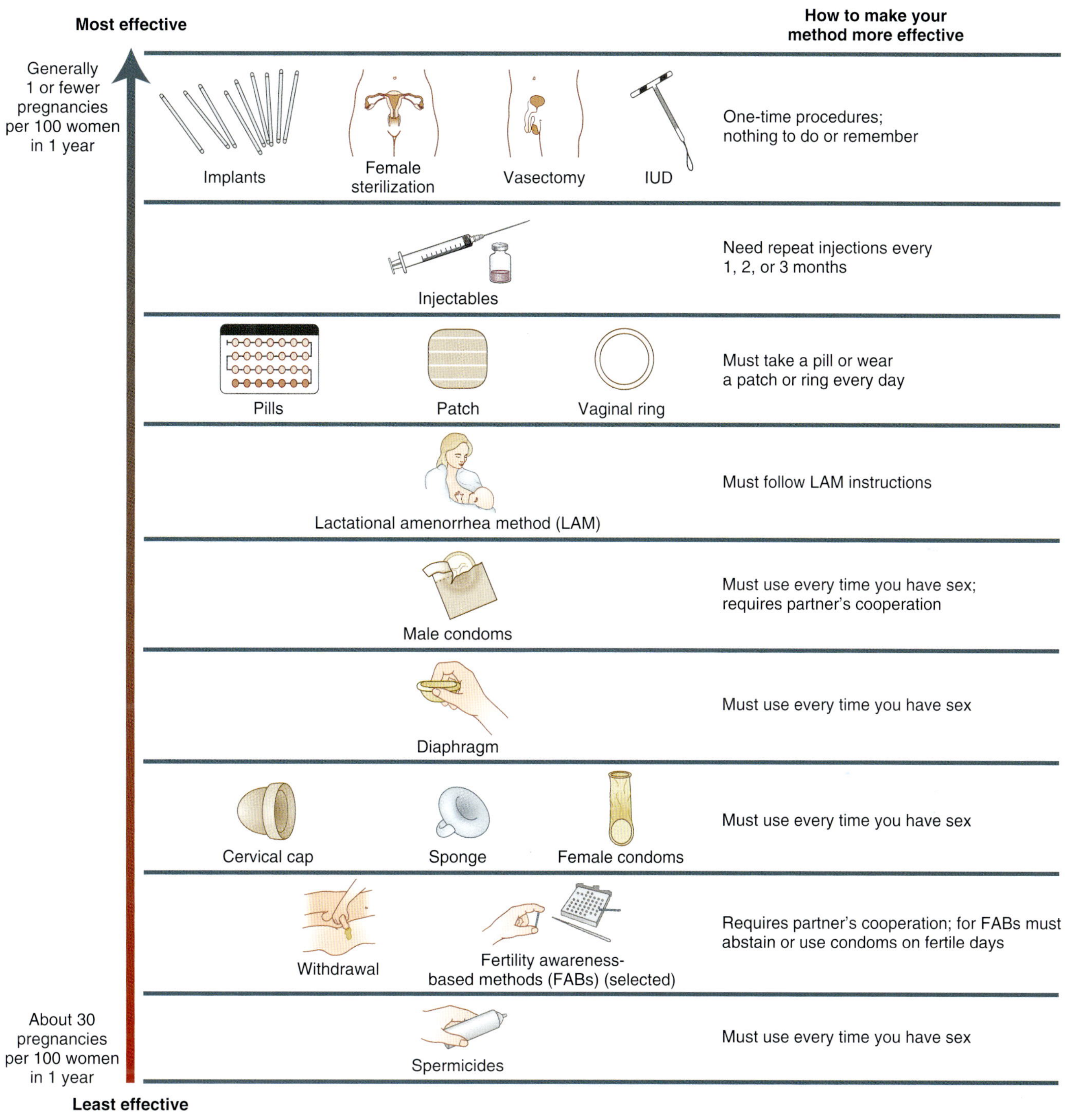
Most effective
How to make your method more effective
Generally 1 or fewer pregnancies per 100 women in 1 year
Implants
Female sterilization
Vasectomy
IUD
One-time procedures; nothing to do or remember
Injectables
Need repeat injections every 1, 2, or 3 months
Pills
Patch
Vaginal ring
Must take a pill or wear a patch or ring every day
Lactational amenorrhea method (LAM)
Must follow LAM instructions
Male condoms
Must use every time you have sex; requires partner's cooperation
Diaphragm
Must use every time you have sex
Cervical cap
Sponge
Female condoms
Must use every time you have sex
Withdrawal
Fertility awareness-based methods (FABs) (selected)
Requires partner's cooperation; for FABs must abstain or use condoms on fertile days
About 30 pregnancies per 100 women in 1 year
Spermicides
Must use every time you have sex
Least effective

**Fig. 13.1** The World Health Organization's tiered approach contraception counseling tool comparing typical effectiveness of contraceptive methods. *IUD,* Intrauterine device. (Redrawn from Association of Reproductive Health Professionals. You Decide Tool Kit: Contraceptive Efficacy Tools. Adapted from World Health Organization. *Comparing Typical Effectiveness of Contraceptive Methods.* Geneva, Switzerland: WHO; 2006.)

Clinicians lack sufficient information on expected failure rates for salpingectomy; however, the low failure rate of partial salpingectomy may serve as a proxy. **If pregnancy occurs after tubal sterilization, location should be ascertained immediately because these pregnancies are often ectopic.**

### Surgical Approach

Tubal occlusion can occur during cesarean section, immediately postpartum through an infraumbilical minilaparotomy while the uterus is still enlarged and the tubes can be easily identified, or, as is commonly used outside the United States, during an interval minilaparotomy. Ligation and resection of a portion or the entirety of both fallopian tubes using a technique such as bilateral salpingectomy or the modified Pomeroy method is common (Fig. 13.2). These methods typically involve general or regional anesthesia. Laparoscopic sterilization methods include salpingectomy, bipolar cautery, the Filshie clip, and the Silastic band (Falope ring).

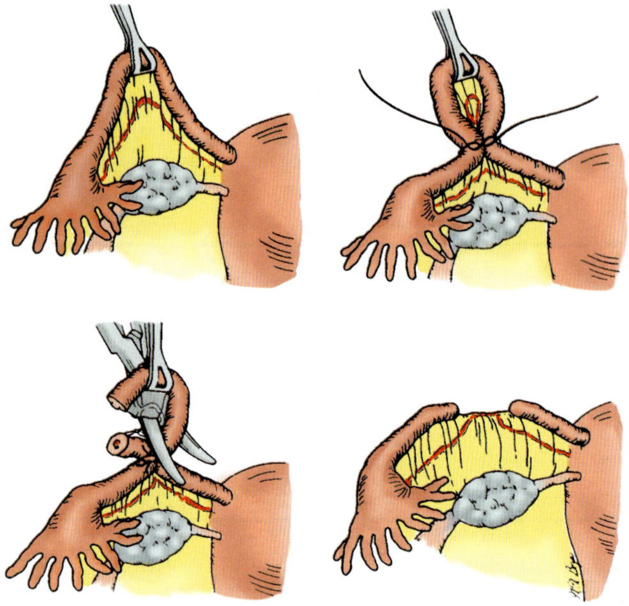

**Fig. 13.2** Modified Pomeroy technique of female sterilization. (From Sciarra JJ. Surgical procedures for tubal sterilization. In: Sciarra JJ, Zatuchni GI, Daly MJ. *Gynecology and Obstetrics.* Vol. 6. Philadelphia: Harper & Row; 1984.)

No hysteroscopic sterilization methods are available in the United States. The Essure device, which involved hysteroscopic placement of microinserts in the fallopian tubes with eventual tubal tissue ingrowth and occlusion, was **voluntarily withdrawn by the manufacturer in 2018** because of a decrease in sales after an increase in patient reports of adverse events (Bayer, 2018). **Women with Essure devices in place can continue using it safely.** For patients experiencing complications, management options include removal via laparoscopic salpingotomy, salpingectomy or cornuectomy, hysteroscopic removal, and hysterectomy if clinically indicated (ACOG, 2019).

### Cancer Prevention

Tubal sterilization with occlusion methods reduces the risk of ovarian cancer. Strong data suggest that many serous, endometrioid, and clear cell carcinomas begin in the fallopian tube rather than the ovary. Opportunistic salpingectomy, or the removal of both fallopian tubes in their entirety for the purposes of ovarian cancer risk reduction, appears to be a safe method of permanent sterilization with risks comparable to occlusion methods of tubal ligation. The risks and benefits of both techniques should be discussed with patients who desire permanent sterilization (ACOG, 2019).

## Long-Acting Reversible (LARC) Methods

The intrauterine device and implant (LARC methods) are highly effective and provide an option of years-long use without further clinician visits or medication refills. Unlike sterilization, **LARC methods are immediately reversible with a rapid return to fertility**. Very few medical contraindications to LARC exist. Although upfront costs can be high, these methods do not incur maintenance costs. LARC users typically report high continuation rates and user satisfaction. **The American Congress of Obstetricians and Gynecologists (ACOG) recommends that it is safe to offer nulliparous women and adolescents LARC methods**. (ACOG, 2018).

Practitioners should be mindful that women can face biased or even coercive contraceptive counseling practices and feel pressured to choose long-acting methods like LARC based on the priorities of the clinician rather than the patient (Higgins, 2016). This becomes particularly important for low-income women and women of color, who more often report lower quality family planning health care interactions than their higher-income and white counterparts. In some studies, providers were more likely to recommend IUDs to black and Hispanic women of low socioeconomic status (Dehlendorf, 2010). Conflict and coercion can arise when a patient requests LARC removal and a clinician expresses reluctance or delays or even refuses to perform a removal. Patient requests for LARC removal should be honored, regardless of clinicians' wishes.

The LARC methods available in the United States include the Paragard T380A copper intrauterine device, several levonorgestrel intrauterine systems (LNG-IUSs), and a single-rod etonogestrel subdermal implant (Nexplanon). No LARC methods contain estrogenic components. In the United States, LARC use increased among contraceptive users from 2% in 2002 to 8.5% in 2009 and 11.6% in 2012 (Kavanaugh, 2015).

## Intrauterine Devices

The IUD is the most commonly used reversible method of contraception worldwide and offers a safe and highly effective method with similar failure rates for typical and perfect use. **First-year failure rates with the copper T380A IUD and the LNG-releasing IUD (LNG-IUD) are less than 1%,** with the annual incidence of accidental pregnancy decreasing steadily thereafter. After 12 years, the cumulative pregnancy rate of the copper T380A IUD reaches 1.7%. At 5 years of use, the pregnancy rate for the LNG-IUD is about 1.1%. These pregnancy rates are comparable to those after surgical sterilization. Contraindications to IUD insertion include pregnancy, pelvic inflammatory disease, endometritis, uterine or cervical malignancy, and a müllerian anomaly or myomas that significantly distort the uterine cavity. For additional information on medical contraindications, please see the CDC Medical Eligibility Criteria (MEC) (Curtis, 2016).

The copper T380A IUD (Paragard) (Fig. 13.3, *A*) is the only copper-bearing IUD currently marketed in the United States, although other copper IUDs are undergoing U.S. clinical trials. Because of the constant dissolution of copper (in amounts less than that ingested in the normal diet), copper IUDs require periodic replacement. **The copper T380A is currently approved for use in the United States for 10 years and maintains its effectiveness for at least 12 years.**

A progestin reservoir in the vertical arm of a T-shaped IUD also provides long-term effectiveness. Two LNG-IUD types, **Mirena and Liletta** (see Fig. 13.3, *B*), contain a total of 52 mg of levonorgestrel, which is released at a rate of about **20 μg** of LNG daily into the endometrial cavity. These LNG-IUDs maintain a high level of effectiveness **for 5 years; data suggest high effectiveness continues for 7 years** (McNicholas, 2015), and both are undergoing clinical trials for further extended use. **Progestin-releasing IUDs reduce menstrual blood loss and treat heavy menstrual bleeding and related iron deficiency anemia**.

In addition, **a 13.5-μg LNG-releasing IUD device with a slightly smaller body than the Liletta and the Mirena is approved for up to 3 years of use (Skyla), and another device with 19.5 mg LNG was approved for 5 years of use (Kyleena).** For the purposes of this chapter, we refer to the with 20-μg releasing LNG IUD devices when discussing the LNG-IUD.

### Mechanisms of Action

All IUDs induce a local and sterile inflammatory response within the endometrium that incapacitates sperm thereby preventing

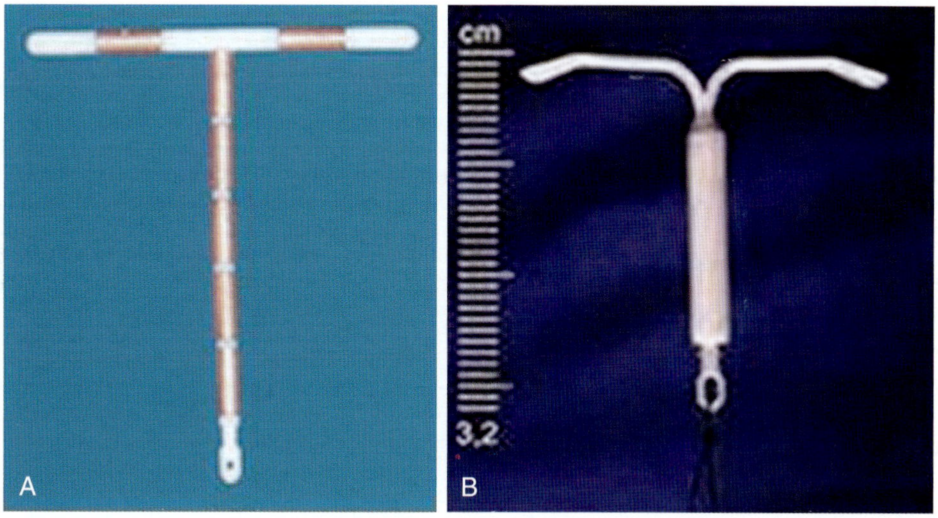


**Fig. 13.3 A,** Copper T intrauterine device. **B,** The levonorgestrel intrauterine system (LNG-IUS) Mirena. (**A,** From Yu J, Li H, Li J, et al. Comparative study on contraceptive efficacy and clinical performance of the copper/low-density polyethylene nanocomposite IUD and the copper T220C IUD. *Contraception.* 2008; 78(4):319-323; **B,** From Searle ES. The intrauterine device and the intrauterine system. *Best Pract Res Clin Obstet Gynaecol.* 2014;28(6):807-824.)

fertilization of the ovum. This sterile inflammatory response was the only mechanism of inert historical IUDs. **Modern IUDs contain either copper or progestin that augments local effects and improves efficacy. No IUD causes abortion; all contraceptive effects are preimplantation.**

Copper markedly increases the extent of the inflammatory reaction with accumulation throughout the uterine lumen, the cervix, and probably the fallopian tubes. In addition, **copper impedes sperm transport and viability in the cervical mucus.** Because of these changes, very few, if any, sperm reach the oviducts, and the ovum usually does not become fertilized. The very small numbers of fertilizations that do occur underlie the failure rate of these devices. The **primary effect of the progestin in the LNG-IUD is to thicken cervical mucus.** Thickened mucous impedes sperm mobility and access to the upper genital tract. Additionally, **the LNG-IUD decreases tubal motility and produces a thin, inactive endometrium.** The low levels of circulating steroid sometimes inhibit ovulation. Systemic LNG levels are lower in IUD users than users of LNG-containing implants or oral pills.

## Adverse Effects

### Pain

Most insertions are straightforward and accomplished on the first attempt. Women who are nulliparous and/or experience dysmenorrhea report more pain during insertion than parous women and those without menstrual pain (Maguire, 2012). Cervical preparation with misoprostol does not increase the success of insertion and increases pain. Ibuprofen or naproxen administered before insertion does not reduce insertion pain but is helpful for cramping during the hours afterward. Multiple trials show that topical anesthesia does not affect insertion pain, although a paracervical block may decrease it, particularly in nulliparous women. Clinicians should receive training in correct insertion technique as detailed in the product labeling

### Uterine Bleeding

Most women who discontinue use of the copper IUD do so for heavy or prolonged menses or intermenstrual bleeding related to increased local prostaglandin release in response to the IUD. **On average, copper IUD users experience about 1 additional day of bleeding per cycle. Heavy bleeding decreases with time and rarely leads to anemia. In contrast, LNG-IUD users experience a reduction in menstrual bleeding as early as 3 months after insertion that persists for the duration of use.** After 24 months, **50% of users report amenorrhea and 25% oligomenorrhea**; providers should discuss the possibility of eventual amenorrhea with patients before insertion because some may find this unacceptable.

### Uterine Perforation

Uterine perforation is a rare (**1 in 1000 insertions**) but potentially serious complication. Perforation is usually fundal and **occurs at the time of insertion.** IUDs correctly inserted entirely within the endometrial cavity do not migrate through the uterine muscle into the peritoneal cavity. With experienced providers, the risk of perforation is less. Straightening the uterine axis with a tenaculum and measuring the cavity with a uterine sound before IUD insertion reduces perforation risk. **Perforation risk is slightly higher in women currently breastfeeding.**

The clinician should rule out perforation if the user cannot feel the IUD strings and did not observe that the device was expelled. To assess missing strings, the provider can use ultrasound to locate the device. **If the device is not located with ultrasonography, a radiograph visualizing the abdomen and pelvis should be performed**; all IUDs will be visible on a plain radiograph. IUDs outside the uterus usually can be removed by means of laparoscopy. In a study of 61,448 women with at least a year of follow-up, no IUD perforations led to serious clinical complications beyond the need for laparoscopic retrieval (Heinemann, 2015).

The widespread use of transvaginal ultrasound has led to the discovery that IUDs can sit in the uterine cavity below the fundus. **In asymptomatic individuals, the device should be left in place if entirely within the uterine cavity.** However, if the stem of the device is visible at the external cervical os or any part of the IUD is visualized below the internal os on ultrasound, the IUD should be removed.

### Complications Related to Pregnancy

A pregnancy with an IUD in place is rare. **Among the few IUD users who do become pregnant, an ectopic location is more likely than among pregnant women without an IUD.** Therefore in the case of a positive pregnancy test, a pelvic ultrasound must be performed to locate the pregnancy. If intrauterine, the device should be removed. **Pregnancies that occur with an IUD in place have a higher incidence of spontaneous abortion or infection.** After IUD removal, the complication rate becomes similar to that of a pregnancy without an IUD. In the case of an undesired pregnancy, a vacuum aspiration can be performed to remove both the pregnancy and the device.

### Infection

**The risk of infection after IUD insertion is small and decreases with time.** The placement process, not the device itself or its threads, creates a transient risk of infection, as does any transcervical procedure. In a meta-analysis of randomized controlled trials (RCTs), routine use of prophylactic antibiotics preceding IUD insertion did not change the risk of pelvic infection (Grimes, 1999). An IUD may be placed without results from cervical screening for infection; however, if a provider has clinical suspicion of infectious endocervicitis, testing for gonorrhea and chlamydia should be performed and the IUD insertion delayed. **Providers caring for women undergoing routine insertion or care with an IUD in place should follow standard sexually transmitted infection (STI) screening guidelines.**

Positive gonorrhea or chlamydia screening tests that occur with an IUD in place can be successfully treated without removing the IUD. For patient with symptoms of pelvic inflammatory disease (PID) and an IUD, an antibiotic regimen for PID approved by the CDC should be used with close clinical follow-up. If the infection does not improve within 48 to 72 hours of treatment or if there is evidence of tubo-ovarian abscess, the device should be removed and an alternative method initiated (Hauk, 2015).

Routine cytologic testing can identify *Actinomyces* organisms during cervical screening with IUDs in place. If the woman is asymptomatic, no treatment is indicated. In the rare event of pelvic infection, treatment includes IUD removal and an appropriate course of antibiotics (usually penicillin).

## Overall Safety

Several long-term studies indicate IUD use is associated with a reduction in risk of developing cervical and endometrial cancer. Data are promising for the use of the LNG-IUS as a fertility-sparing treatment of early stage endometrial cancer. To date, few studies have evaluated whether hormonal IUD use changes the risk of breast cancer; however, it is an active research question.

## Subdermal Implants

Subdermal implants, which consist of one or more thin flexible rods containing a progestin hormone rank, among the most effective methods of contraception, with an effectiveness equal or superior to that of sterilization and IUDs. In the United States one implant is available, **Nexplanon, which contains 68 mg of etonogestrel (ENG).** Nexplanon is approved **for 3 years of use**; however, preliminary studies indicate continued effectiveness for 5 years (McNicholas, 2015). The **implant inhibits ovulation and thickens cervical mucus.** After removal, serum etonogestrel levels decline to undetectable within a week. Ninety percent of users ovulate within 1 month after removal.

In clinical trials, continuation rates are high at 50% to 80% until 2 years. **Bleeding irregularities are the most common reason for discontinuation, accounting for about 60% of early removals.** As with other progestin-only methods, nearly all women experience changes in their regular bleeding pattern. Women may experience amenorrhea or infrequent, frequent, or prolonged bleeding. Unlike depo-medroxyprogesterone acetate (DMPA) or the LNG-IUS, the bleeding patterns of individual women will be unpredictable.

**U.S. providers must complete a Food and Drug Administration (FDA)–mandated training program before providing Nexplanon implants.** After skin infiltration with local anesthesia, the implant is inserted superficially into the subdermal tissue of the nondominant upper arm posterior to the groove between the bicep and triceps. The insertion site is closed with adhesive without the need for suture (Fig. 13.4), and the procedure usually takes less than a minute to complete. From the subdermal space, the steroid diffuses into the circulation at a constant rate. At the end of use, the implant must be removed. The removal site is infiltrated with local anesthetic and the implant removed through a 2- to 3-mm incision then closed with adhesive (see Fig. 13.4). Correct, superficial insertion enhances the ease of removal; improperly placed deep implants are more difficult to remove. If nonpalpable, an implant can be identified using imaging of the upper arm. Rare cases (1 per 100,000 insertions) of distant migration of the implant to the pulmonary artery have been reported (Reed, 2019).

### Hormonal Contraceptives Methods Mechanisms of Action

Systemically absorbed hormonal contraceptives primarily prevent pregnancy by suppressing gonadotropins. The progestin component suppresses the luteinizing hormone (LH) surge, which inhibits ovulation. Methods that contain estrogen prevent a rise in follicle-stimulating hormone (FSH), which inhibits follicular development through a synergistic effect with the progestin. Estrogen also stabilizes the endometrium, which prevents unscheduled bleeding. In addition, secondary contraceptive effects of progestins include thickening cervical mucus, which makes it less permeable to sperm; thinning the endometrium, which makes it less suitable for implantation; and impairing tubal motility, which interferes with gamete transport.

### Drug Interactions

When taken together with other drugs metabolized through the same hepatic cytochrome P450 pathway, hormonal contraceptive

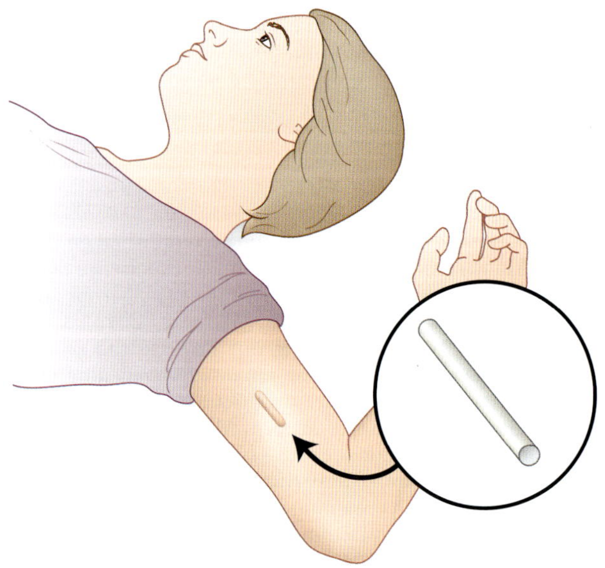

**Fig. 13.4** Insertion of a contraceptive implant. (Modified from and used with permission of Mayo Foundation for Medical Education and Research. All rights reserved.)

levels may be affected, which may affect efficacy. Clinicians should be aware that, among others, certain anticonvulsants (phenytoin, carbamazepine, oxcarbazepine), antibiotics (rifampin), and antiretrovirals (efavirenz, nevirapine) may decrease the efficacy of some hormonal contraceptives. Levels of lamotrigine used for seizures and mental health conditions will decrease with coadministration of estrogen-containing contraceptives. Specific prescribing and interactions guidelines are available through the CDC MEC.

#### Hormonal Method Side Effects

Some hormonal contraception users report various negative physical and psychological side effects such as headache, weight gain, mood disorders, breast changes, bloating, and sexual problems. Such effects may lead to method discontinuation. Clinicians should be attentive to an individual's symptoms and concerns, offer reassurance, and be willing to change to a different contraceptive on request. In discussing these experiences, providers and patients should also recall that negative physical feelings and symptoms are very common among women of reproductive age who do not use hormonal contraception. Research from placebo-controlled studies provides insight and suggests some users can overestimate how much their method contributes. In a 6-month double-blind RCT of 507 women, those administered oral contraceptive pills or placebo reported types and numbers of side effects that were indistinguishable and a similar percentage of women discontinued over the course of the study (Redmond, 1999). **The widespread belief in such side effects may contribute to a disinclination to continue or even to start oral contraceptives.**

### Noncontraceptive Health Benefits of Hormonal Contraceptives

In addition to preventing pregnancy, hormonal contraceptives may provide additional health benefits to patients. **Studies consistently demonstrate a strong protective effect between progestin-containing contraceptives and endometrial cancer**. Compared with nonusers, women who use oral contraceptives (OCs) for at least 1 year have a decreased risk of developing endometrial cancer between ages 40 and 55. This protective effect is related to duration of use, increasing **from a 20% reduction in risk with 1 year of use to a 40% reduction with 2 years of use to about a 60% reduction with 4 years of use**. This protective effect **persists for at least 15 years** after stopping use of the OCs.

In addition, OCs **reduce the risk of ovarian cancer by about 20% for every 5 years of use.** For woman using OCs for 15 years or more, the risk is almost halved and even 1 year of use may provide a protective effect (Grimbizis, 2010). Using OCs **also reduces the risk of ovarian cancer in women with *BRCA1* and *BRCA2* mutations and in those with a family history of ovarian cancer** (Moorman, 2013)

Beyond cancer reduction, some of the immediate benefits of hormonal contraceptive use include improvement of heavy menstrual bleeding dysmenorrhea and endometriosis. The antiestrogenic action of the progestins suppresses proliferation of the endometrial glands, thereby **reducing blood loss** and intrauterine prostaglandins at the time of endometrial shedding. The decreased blood loss makes iron deficiency anemia less likely in OC users than nonusers. **Endometriosis improves during use of hormonal methods** because progestins suppress endometrial proliferation, and hormonal methods that inhibit ovulation can also reduce ovulatory disorders such as Mittelschmerz and premenstrual syndrome.

**Estrogen-containing methods of birth control such as OCs, the patch, or the ring may improve acne.** The effect of a method on acne relates to three properties: the androgenicity of the progestin component, the reduction of free androgens as a result of an estrogen-driven increase in serum hormone-binding globulin, and the activity of 5α-reductase, the enzyme that converts testosterone to dihydrotestosterone. In double-blind, placebo-controlled studies, low-dose OCs had a greater reduction of acne with no difference in adverse events compared with placebo pills (Redmond, 1997).

Hormonal contraceptives may be ideal treatments for gynecologic conditions such as polycystic ovary syndrome (PCOS) and pelvic pain. In the setting of PCOS, estrogen-containing methods reduce circulating androgens by suppressing gonadotropins and inducing the production of sex hormone–binding globulin. All progestin-containing methods protect the endometrium from an arrested proliferative phase that is common in PCOS and the concurrent increased risk of endometrial hyperplasia.

## Injectable Suspensions

**DMPA (Depo-Provera) is the only injectable contraceptive available in the United States.** Worldwide, other short-term injectables composed of progestin alone or a combination of progestins and estrogens are also available.

Medroxyprogesterone acetate (MPA) is a long-acting derivative of progesterone formulated as an injectable crystalline suspension. **When used consistently, the failure rate at 1 year is 0.2%.** Typical use **failure rates are around 6%**, related to delayed injections. These effectiveness rates apply to women of all body weights.

The intramuscular formulation contains **150 mg DMPA, given every 13 weeks** deep into the gluteal or deltoid muscle with slow release into the systemic circulation. Repeat injections can be given up to 2 weeks late without requiring additional contraceptive protection (Curtis, 2016). The **subcutaneous formulation contains 104 mg of MPA and is injected also every 13 weeks** into the subcutaneous tissue of the anterior thigh or abdominal wall. Self-administration of subcutaneous DMPA is feasible; women who self-administered after teaching had similar MPA levels and continuation rates compared with women receiving clinic administration (Beasley, 2014).

### Return of Fertility

Return to fertility may be delayed because of the lag time in clearing DMPA from the circulation. The median delay to conception is 9 to 10 months after the last injection, with a wide range in resumption of ovulation, from 15 to 49 weeks from the last injection. Women who wish to become pregnant after discontinuing DMPA may experience a delay in the resumption of fertility. After this initial delay, fecundity is similar to that found after discontinuing a barrier contraceptive (Fig. 13.5). Use of DMPA delays but does not prevent return of fertility.

### Clinical Side Effects

#### Bleeding Patterns

A major side effect of DMPA is a change in the menstrual cycle. In the first 3 months after the first injection, about 30% of women experience amenorrhea and another 30% to 40% experience light irregular bleeding and spotting. As the duration of use extends, the incidence of bleeding steadily declines. By 1 year more than half of women experience amenorrhea and at 2 years that rises to about 70% (Fig. 13.6). After discontinuation, half of women resume a regular cyclic menstrual pattern within 6 months and about three fourths have regular menses within 1 year.

#### Weight Changes

About **one-fourth of women using DMPA gain weight, usually in the first 6 months of use**. Several longitudinal studies

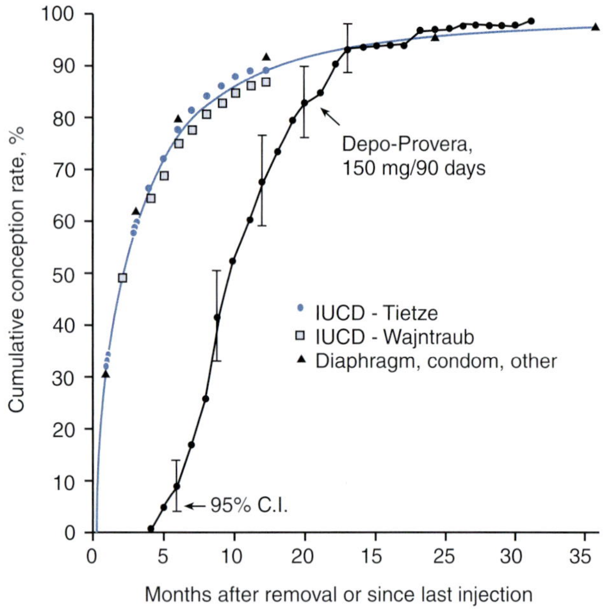


**Fig. 13.5** Cumulative conception rates of women who discontinued a contraceptive method to become pregnant. *IUCD,* Intrauterine contraceptive device. (From Schwallie PC, Assenzo JR. The effect of depo-medroxyprogesterone acetate on pituitary and ovarian function, and the return of fertility following its discontinuation: a review. *Contraception.* 1974;10(2):181-202.)

indicate that DMPA users gain between 1.5 (2.2 pounds) and 4 kg (8.8 pounds) in their first year of use and continue to gain weight thereafter. The mechanism of weight gain in women using DMPA is poorly understood, and some suggest that the injection be used with caution in patients who are already overweight or obese.

**Bone Density**

Because DMPA suppresses production of estradiol, bone resorption is increased and associated with a modest decrease in bone mineral density (BMD). Longer-term studies indicate that bone density changes reverse after DMPA discontinuation. Given that changes are temporary, measurement of BMD during DMPA use is unnecessary and medical therapy should not be offered in DMPA users with low BMD. Even in women younger than 18 and older than 45, age groups at higher risk of fracture, the WHO has endorsed the use of DMPA in conjunction with an adequate explanation of risks and benefits. DMPA can be used as a long-term birth control method, and there is no time limit or restriction prohibiting extended use (Cromer, 2006).

**DMPA Health Benefits**

In addition to those noncontraceptive benefits that apply to all hormonal methods, DMPA can be used for women with hormonally sensitive (catamenial) epilepsy to suppress estrogen fluctuations and avoid progestin withdrawal that triggers seizures in spontaneously cycling women. In some studies, DMPA seems to have beneficial effects on sickle cell pain crises.

## Oral Contraceptives

Effective and easy to use, OCs became the most widely used reversible contraceptive method within a few years of their introduction to the United States in 1960. The high-dose original pill formulations caused side effects such as nausea, breast tenderness, and weight gain that often led to discontinuation. Since that time, other formulations with steadily decreasing dosages of both the estrogen and progestin components have become available. **Reductions in the dose of the contraceptive steroid ethinyl estradiol (EE) has coincided with a lower incidence of severe adverse cardiovascular effects and side effects without increasing the failure rate.** Today, the most widely used OCs combine EE with one of several synthetic progestins.

### Pharmacology and formulations

The three major types of OC formulations include daily progestin-only pills (POPs), also known as minipills, fixed-dose (monophasic) combination pills, and multiphasic combination pills. The combination formulations are the most widely used and incorporate several different types of progestins. **The modifications in chemical structure of different synthetic progestins affect their biologic activity.** One should consider biologic activity, not just the amount of steroid present, to characterize the

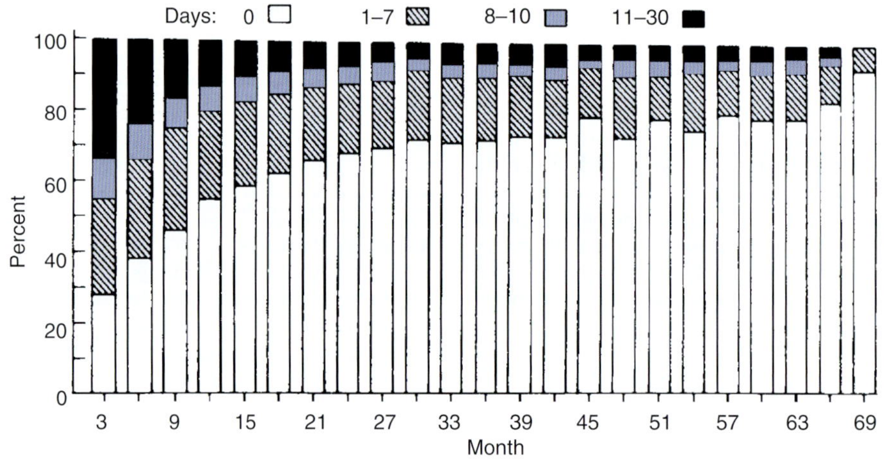


**Fig. 13.6** Percentage of patients with bleeding or spotting on days 0, 1 to 7, 8 to 10, or 11 to 30 per 30-day cycle while receiving injectable depo-medroxyprogesterone acetate (DMPA), 150 mg every 3 months. (From Schwallie PC, Assenzo JR. Contraceptive use: efficacy study utilizing medroxyprogesterone acetate administered as an intramuscular injection once every 90 days. *Fertil Steril.* 1973;24:331-339, from The American Society for Reproductive Medicine.)

pharmacologic activity of the progestin. Monophasic products contain tablets with the same dose combination of an estrogen and progestin each day. In multiphasic formulations, pills containing several different dose combinations come in the same pack. A different tablet color corresponds to each dose combination. Depending on the number of dose combinations, formulations may be further classified as biphasic, triphasic or quadriphasic.

**In the United States most OC regimens are packaged in a 28-day (4-week) cycle.** Many combination OC formulations provide active pills for 21 days (3 weeks) followed by a 7-day hormone-free interval (HFI). Most OCs are packaged with inactive spacer (placebo) pills during the HFI. Some formulations provide an iron or folate supplement in the spacer pills. Uterine bleeding occurs secondary to hormone withdrawal during the HFI, typically 1 to 3 days after taking the last active pill. Some formulations provide active tablets for 24 days, reducing the HFI to only 4 days, and these may be more effective than 21-day active pill formulations.

Other dosing strategies include extended and continuous cycles. Extended cycle regimens contain 84 days of active pills followed by a 7-day HFI that results in scheduled withdrawal bleeding only four times a year. Another product provides a continuous daily regimen with 28 active pills to eliminate scheduled withdrawal bleeds. Some providers recommend extended use of generic, less expensive monophasic OCs, instructing patients to discard the placebo pills and begin a new cycle pack after 21 days for a similar effect. This strategy assumes access to early refills.

## Effectiveness

OCs have a 1% failure rate with perfect use and an 8% failure rate with typical use. In a cohort study of U.S. women, 24-day OC regimens containing a progestin with a long half-life had higher contraceptive effectiveness compared with 21-day regimens (Dinger, 2011). No other difference in clinical effectiveness has been demonstrated among the various combination formulations available in the United States.

Clinicians should ensure easy access to refills. Accidental pregnancies occurring during OC use probably reflect delayed initiation of a new pill pack or missing more than one or two tablets. The pill-free interval must not extend beyond 7 days; to maintain ovulatory suppression the most important pill to take on time is the first one of each cycle. When a woman misses two or more pills in a pack, she should take emergency contraception and use backup for a week.

#### Physiology

The balance between estrogen and progestin influences the bleeding profile of a combination OC. Estrogen induces endometrial proliferation. Progestins oppose the mitotic action of estrogen, leading to a thinner and stable decidualized endometrium. Even though women taking combined OCs are exposed to both hormones at the same time rather than sequentially as in a spontaneous menstrual cycle, they typically undergo some endometrial proliferation. ***Withdrawal bleeding* refers to bleeding OCs users experience during the hormone-free interval. *Breakthrough bleeding* refers to unscheduled bleeding occurring during days with active pill use.**

Breakthrough bleeding and absence of withdrawal bleeding (amenorrhea) can occur as a result of relatively insufficient estrogen to support the endometrium. If pregnancy is ruled out, neither of these bleeding changes are inherently worrisome. If desired, clinicians can increase the amount of estrogen in the pill formulation or change the progestin to offset those effects. **Randomized studies comparing cyclic to extended and continuous dosing regimens document a decrease in the total scheduled bleeding days but an increase in breakthrough bleeding and spotting with extended or continuous use of hormonal contraceptives.** Bleeding patterns typically improve over time, with rates of unscheduled bleeding highest in early cycles. Women who experience prolonged breakthrough bleeding during continuous OC use might benefit from discontinuing the active pills for 3 days to allow for a short period of withdrawal bleeding and then restarting. Greater gaps could result in ovulation and unintended pregnancy.

#### Metabolic Effects

Weight gain represents a common experience of women using hormonal contraception. Weight gain is common in the U.S. population, and the extent to which hormonal methods cause additional weight gain appears limited. Many OC users do not gain weight; one 2013 study assessed weight after OC initiation in women with obesity and normal weight, weighing participants before and after 3 months of OCP use. Neither group experienced a substantial change in weight (Mayeda, 2014).

### Return to Fertility

After discontinuation of low-dose OCs, the suppressive effect on the hypothalamic-pituitary-ovarian axis disappears quickly. After the initial recovery, completely normal endocrine function occurs. There is little, if any, effect of duration of OC use on the time to subsequent conception. There is no risk of congenital malformations or other adverse outcomes in pregnancies among women who conceive while taking OCs or shortly thereafter.

### Neoplastic Risks and Benefits

For a discussion of neoplastic risks and benefits, see Noncontraceptive Benefits of Hormonal Contraceptives earlier in this chapter.

### Breast Cancer

Breast cancer is hormonally mediated; therefore, women using hormonal methods of contraception may be concerned about the risk. The absolute risk of breast cancer is low given the young age of most OC users. However, **studies indicate that current OC use may be associated with a 20% to 25% increased risk of early breast cancer.** Some evidence indicates that those breast cancers diagnosed during OC use are more likely to be localized. The increased risk is transient; the lifetime risk of developing breast cancer in women who have used OC is comparable to those who have never used OCs even in women with a high risk of developing breast cancer, including women with an immediate family history of breast cancer and those with *BRCA1* and *BRCA2* mutations (Milne, 2005).

#### Cervical Cancer

The epidemiologic data regarding the risk of invasive cervical cancer and cervical intraepithelial neoplasia with OC use are conflicting. **Confounding factors could account for contrasting results in different studies. Studies indicate that the risk of both invasive and in situ cervical cancer increases with increasing duration of OC use.** These risks persist after adjusting for human papillomavirus (HPV) infection, squamous cell or adenocarcinoma, number of sexual partners, cervical cytology screening, smoking, and use of barrier contraceptives (Appleby, 2007; Smith, 2003).

**There is no evidence that OC use alters the incidence or rate of the progression of cervical dysplasia to invasive cancer.** Women with treated cervical dysplasia can use OCs, as can those with newly diagnosed dysplasia awaiting evaluation. More data are needed to assess the impact of OC use on cervical dysplasia and cancer in HPV-vaccinated women.

### Liver Adenoma and Colorectal Cancer

The development of a benign hepatocellular adenoma is an extremely rare occurrence. An increased risk of this tumor was reported in early OC studies of prolonged use of high-dose formulations but seems to be far lower for women taking lower OC doses. Women with active liver disease should not use hormonal contraception because the liver is a major site for the metabolism of synthetic steroids.

A meta-analysis of published studies of the relationship between OCs and colorectal cancer showed that OC ever use was associated with a 15% to 20% reduction in the risk of colorectal cancer (Fernandez, 2001).

### Coagulation Parameters

Epidemiologic studies consistently demonstrate that the risk of both venous and arterial thrombosis increases among users of combined OCs compared with nonpregnant nonusers. However, although combined OCs (COCs) increase the risk of venous thromboembolism (VTE), they offer significant protection against pregnancy, a condition associated with a substantially higher risk of thrombosis—roughly twofold higher—than that observed with OCs.

The increased risk is related to the estrogen component of the pill and is dose dependent (Gerstmann, 1991). A woman's baseline risk of VTE increases by three times if she uses an estrogen-containing OC. If a woman already has an increased baseline risk, such as having a personal history of VTE or being a carrier of a prothrombotic gene, she should not take an estrogen-containing contraceptive. Screening for coagulation disorders should only be considered before starting an OC if the woman has a family history of thrombotic events. Although progestins alone do not affect coagulation parameters, whether newer progestins increase the coagulation risk of OC use remains controversial. It has been suggested that COCs with the newer progestins increase the risk over that of the older, early-generation products.

Obesity is a modest risk factor for VTE (Fig. 13.7), and obesity with a body mass index [BMI] greater than 40 can be considered a relative contraindication to use of a combined hormonal method, especially in older OC users. Use of COCs by women older than age 35 who also smoke tobacco or electronic cigarettes is contraindicated because of the risk of myocardial infarction.

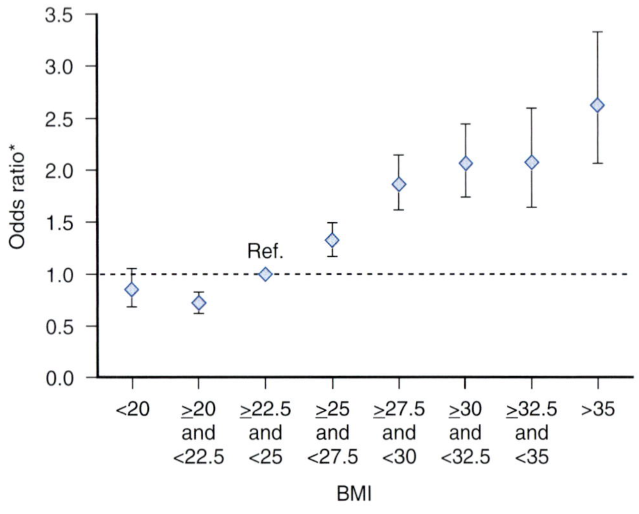


| | | | | | | | | |
|---|---|---|---|---|---|---|---|---|
| $n_p$ | 160 | 416 | 817 | 925 | 704 | 402 | 190 | 220 |
| $n_c$ | 256 | 865 | 1236 | 1102 | 626 | 311 | 154 | 133 |

*Adjusted for age and sex.

**Fig. 13.7** Relative risk (with 95% confidence intervals) of deep vein thrombosis by categories of body mass (BMI), adjusted for age and sex. (From Pomp ER, le Cessie S, Rosendaal FR, Doggen CJ. Risk of venous thrombosis: obesity and its joint effect with oral contraceptive use and prothrombotic mutations. *Br J Haematol.* 2007;139:289-296.)

## Contraindications to Oral Contraceptive Use

OCs can be prescribed safely for the majority of women of reproductive age because these women are young and generally healthy. There are, however, certain absolute contraindications, including a history of vascular disease (thromboembolism, thrombophlebitis, atherosclerosis, myocardial infarction, and stroke) and systemic disease that may affect the vascular system (active lupus erythematosus with vascular involvement and diabetes with retinopathy or nephropathy). Cigarette smoking by OC users older than age 35, migraine with true aura, and uncontrolled hypertension are also contraindications. Women with active liver disease should not take OCs. Women who have recovered from liver disease, such as viral hepatitis, and whose liver function tests have returned to normal can safely take OCs.

Relative contraindications to OC use include heavy cigarette smoking younger than age 35 and undiagnosed causes of amenorrhea or genital bleeding. Women younger than 35 who have migraine headache without with aura can use COC, and if headache occurs only during the hormone-free interval, continuous dosing can help control the symptoms. Women with diabetes without cardiovascular progression can take low-dose OC formulations because these agents do not affect glucose tolerance or accelerate diabetes mellitus.

## Progestin-Only Pills

The available POP formulation consists of tablets containing a low dose of progestin, without estrogen, taken every day without a steroid-free interval. **Because the dose of progestin in POPs is less than the ovulation inhibition dose, other progestogenic effects such as cervical mucous thickening become the primary mechanism of action.** Clinicians should counsel their patients using POPs to take pills consistently at the same time of day to ensure that progestin concentrations do not fall to less than the effective level. **Newer POPs entering the U.S. market contain progestins that inhibit ovulation consistently.** Because women using POPs may still ovulate, endogenous estradiol and progesterone produced by the ovary will affect endometrial bleeding patterns, resulting in regular menses, irregular bleeding, spotting, or amenorrhea, depending on an individual woman's response.

# Contraceptive Patch

The contraceptive skin patch (Fig. 13.8) contains 75 μg ethinyl estradiol and 6 mg norelgestromin (Xulane). The patch is applied to the skin each week for 3 consecutive weeks followed by a patch-free week to allow scheduled withdrawal bleeding. The patch may be applied to the buttocks, upper outer arm, lower abdomen, or upper torso, excluding the breasts. After skin application, both steroids appear in the circulation rapidly and reach a plateau within 48 hours. The primary mechanism of action, effectiveness, and metabolic and clinical effects are similar to COCs. Results from early clinical trials suggest that patch efficacy may be slightly lower in women with body weight more than 90 kg; however, even in the heaviest women the patch was 90% effective. Newer patch results show similar effectiveness across body weights.

# Contraceptive Vaginal Ring

Steroids pass easily through the vaginal epithelium directly into the circulation. A flexible **ring-shaped device containing 2.7 mg of ethinyl estradiol and 11.7 mg of etonogestrel** (Fig. 13.9), the contraceptive ring (NuvaRing), is placed in the

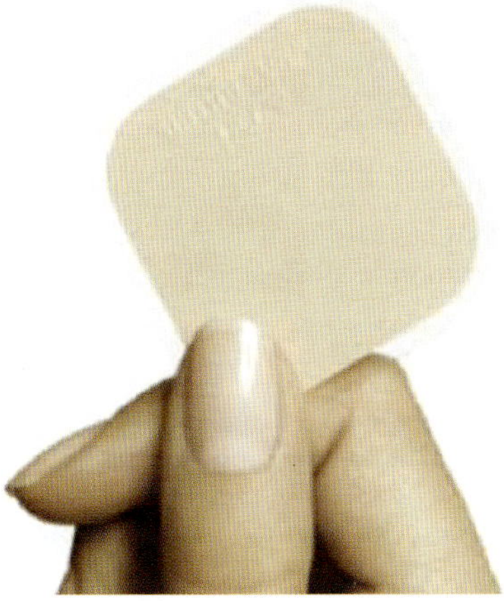

**Fig. 13.8** The contraceptive skin patch releasing ethinyl estradiol and norelgestromin.

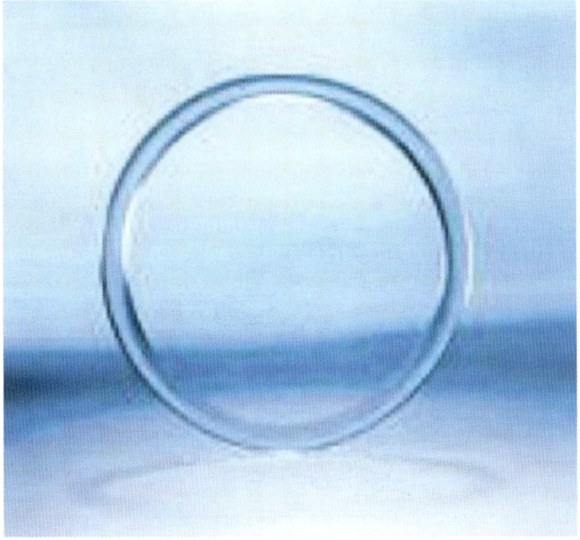

**Fig. 13.9** The contraceptive vaginal ring releasing ethinyl estradiol and etonogestrel.

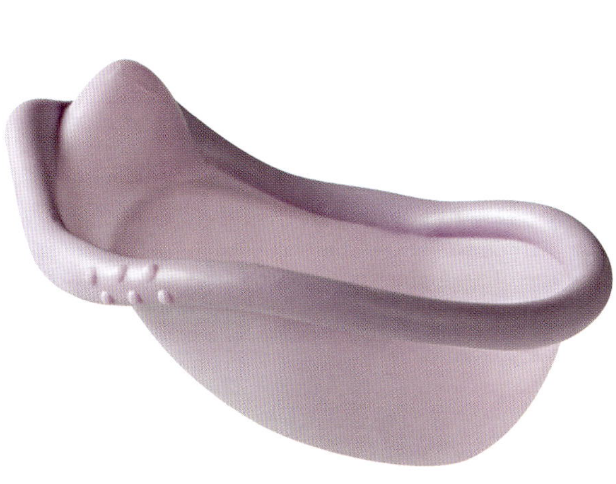

**Fig. 13.10** The Caya diaphragm. (Courtesy Kessel Medintim GmbH, www.medintim.de.)

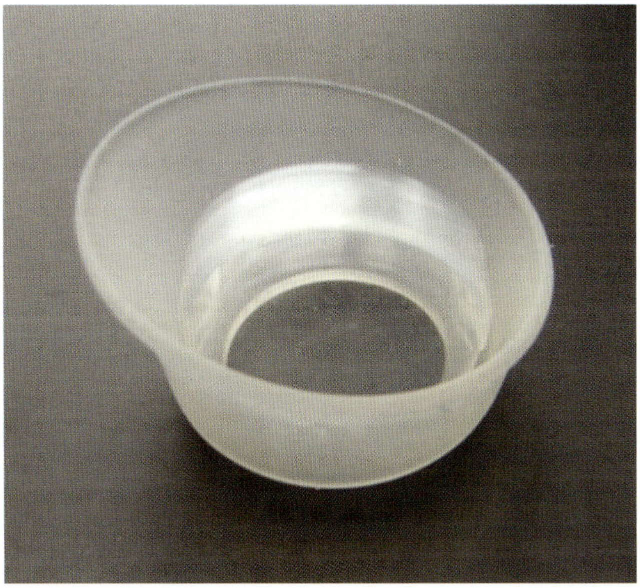

**Fig. 13.11** The female barrier method FemCap.

vagina for 21 days and then removed for up to 7 days to allow withdrawal bleeding. After this ring-free interval the woman inserts a new ring. Ring expulsion is uncommon, and both users and their partners typically report high acceptability. Mechanisms of actions, efficacy, and side effects are similar to those of COCs. Continuous use has been studied, and results are similar to those observed with continuous COCs.

Clinical trials showed no difference in ring efficacy for women in the heaviest weight category (>166 lb [75 kg]) (Westhoff, 2005), but few overweight or obese women were enrolled in those trials. A pharmacokinetic study showed therapeutic progestogen and ethinyl estradiol levels adequate to inhibit ovulation without increases in follicular activity in both women with obesity and those with normal weight (Dragoman, 2013).

## Barrier Methods

### Diaphragm and Cervical Cap

When Margaret Sanger introduced the vaginal diaphragm to the United States in 1916, it became the most widely used female-controlled reversible contraceptive method for 4 decades before the introduction of COCs. The diaphragm is a thin, dome-shaped membrane of latex rubber or silicone with a flexible rim. The device is collapsed for insertion and then expands within the vagina to create a mechanical barrier and spermicide reservoir between the vagina and the cervix. Traditionally, health care providers fitted diaphragms to find the largest comfortable size, though no data have assessed whether a "good fit" correlates with improved effectiveness. **The FDA-approved Caya, a single-size diaphragm that does not require fitting by a practitioner, is intended for use over the counter** (Fig. 13.10).

A cervical cap is a cup-shaped silicone or rubber device that fits around the cervix fitted by a clinician. **The only cap currently on the U.S. market is the FemCap.** This product, made of soft, durable, hypoallergenic silicone rubber, is designed to contact the vaginal walls as the dome of the device sits over the cervix (Fig. 13.11).

**The diaphragm and cervical cap are used with a spermicide and left in place for at least 6 hours after the last coital act.** If repeated intercourse takes place, additional spermicide should be used vaginally. **The failure rate during the first year of use for the diaphragm or cervical cap ranges from 13% to**

**17% among all users and may be as low as 4% to 8%** with perfect use. The diaphragm and cervical cap may also reduce the risk of cervical dysplasia and cancer.

### Male and Female Condoms

The latex and polyurethane male condoms are the only contraceptive method with FDA-approved labeling that supports both **prevention of pregnancy and the transmission of STIs.** Clinicians should review proper condom use with both men and women and encourage their use for STI protection. The male condom should be applied to the erect penis before any contact with the vagina or vulva. The tip should extend beyond the end of the penis by about half an inch to collect the ejaculate. After ejaculation, the penis must be removed from the vagina while still somewhat erect and the base of the condom grasped to ensure the condom is removed without spillage of the ejaculate. Water-based lubrication may reduce condom breakage. The typical-use failure rate for the male condom is around 15% (Hatcher, 2011).

The female condom consists of a soft, loose-fitting polyurethane sheath with two flexible rings. One ring lies at the closed end of the sheath and serves as an insertion mechanism and internal anchor for the condom inside the vagina. The outer ring forms the external edge of the device and remains outside the vagina after insertion, thus providing protection to the introitus and the base of the penis during intercourse (Fig. 13.12). The female condom is prelubricated and intended for single use. Like male condoms, the device is available over the counter, does not require fitting, and protects against sexually transmitted infections. It can be inserted before the onset of sexual activity and left in place after ejaculation has occurred. The typical use failure rate at 1 year is estimated to be 21% (Hatcher, 2011).

## Lactational Amenorrhea Method

Because prolactin inhibits gonadotropin pulsatility, breastfeeding women typically remain amenorrheic for a variable length of time after giving birth. Higher frequency and longer duration of breastfeeding contribute to menstrual suppression, and night nursing is highly correlated with anovulation and amenorrhea.

The criteria for successful use of the lactational amenorrhea method (LAM) are continuous amenorrhea and exclusive breastfeeding (no formula or food supplements) for up to 6 months after delivery. Night nursing is highly protective. LAM failure rate in the first 6 months postpartum is less than 2%.

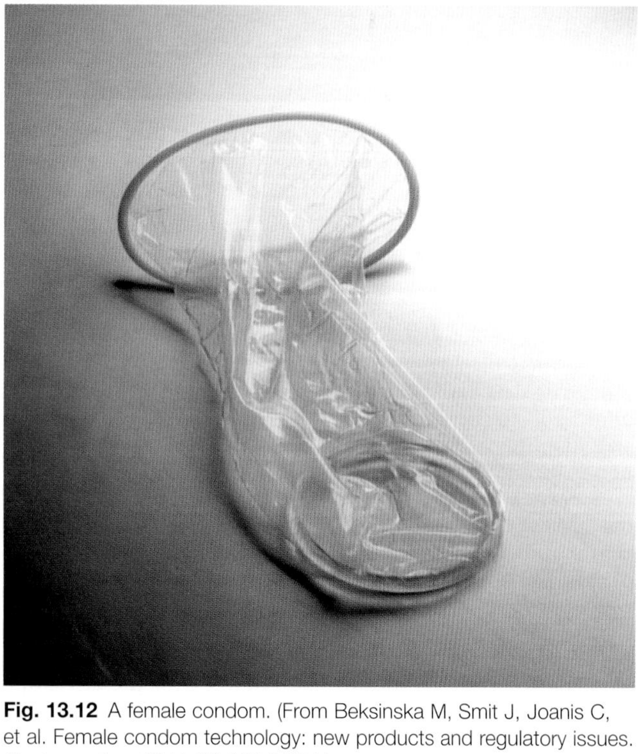

**Fig. 13.12** A female condom. (From Beksinska M, Smit J, Joanis C, et al. Female condom technology: new products and regulatory issues. *Contraception.* 2011;83(4):316-321.)

## Fertility Awareness

Many couples use abstinence from sexual intercourse or a barrier method during the "fertile window" of the menstrual cycle (the 5 days preceding ovulation or the day of ovulation) to prevent pregnancy. Several techniques are used to estimate the timing of ovulation.

**The oldest of these is the calendar rhythm method.** With this method, the period of abstinence is determined by calculating the length of the individual woman's previous menstrual cycle and using three assumptions: (1) The human ovum can be fertilized for only about 24 hours after ovulation, (2) sperm can fertilize for 3 to 5 days after coitus, and (3) ovulation usually occurs 12 to 16 days before the onset of menses. The woman therefore establishes her fertile period by subtracting 18 days from the length of her previous shortest cycle and 11 days from her previous longest cycle and abstains from coitus during this time. This method assumes a normal and predictable menstrual cycle.

Other fertility awareness methods rely on cyclic physiologic changes. Increasing levels of progesterone occurring after ovulation cause a detectible rise in **daily basal body temperature (BBT).** Using the BBT method, the woman must abstain from intercourse from the cessation of menses until the third consecutive day of elevated basal temperature, or when she is postovulatory. The cervical mucus method requires that the woman recognize and interpret the presence and consistency of cervical mucus. Increasing estradiol levels increase the production of cervical mucus. Intercourse can occur after menses ends until the first day that copious, slippery mucus is observed to be present and again 4 days after the last day when the characteristic mucus was present.

The calendar, temperature, and cervical mucus methods can be used separately or in combination with one another—the symptothermal method. Overall typical failure rates are around 24%. Women with irregular cycles, those who are older than 35, and those who are immediately postpartum should not use fertility awareness methods that rely on regular cycles and predictable ovulation. Women using these methods should also have control over when intercourse occurs.

## Birth Control Method Apps

Most U.S. women of reproductive age have smartphones, and there are more than 165,000 easy-to-access apps related to women's health and pregnancy. Though widely available and often free, these apps are not monitored by regulatory agencies. Some people may use these apps to track fertility to avoid pregnancy. **In a systematic evaluation of the accuracy and functionality of more than 1000 fertility tracking apps, only 20 were both free and medically accurate** (Moglia, 2016). Similarly, most apps were unable to predict the true "fertile window" when data from seven real cycles were sent to almost 100 fertility-tracking apps (Duane, 2016). Although such apps may empower women to monitor their menstrual cycles more closely, they should be used with caution because most are inaccurate and may even contain misleading information. Patients should also be cautioned about uncertain privacy protections for their personal information.

### Coitus-Related Methods

#### Spermicides

Spermicides consist of an active agent and a carrier. The active agent is a surfactant that immobilizes or kills sperm on contact by destroying the sperm cell membrane. The carriers include gels, foams, creams, tablets, films, and suppositories. Spermicides must be placed into the vagina before each coital act, often in combination with a barrier contraceptive to increase effectiveness. The contraceptive sponge, a cylindric piece of soft polyurethane impregnated with 1 mg of **nonoxynol-9 spermicide**, must be inserted into the vagina before intercourse and is effective for 24 hours. **The failure rate ranges from 15% to 25%.**

#### Coitus Interruptus (Withdrawal)

Removal of the penis from the vagina before ejaculation to prevent pregnancy is an ancient male-controlled method of contraception without contraindications, devices, or cost. Withdrawal can fail because of sperm present in some preejaculate, the fluid produced by the penis during sexual excitement and before ejaculation. More commonly, the method fails if withdrawal is not performed in a timely fashion. Correct and consistent use with every act of intercourse should be stressed, not only during suspected fertile times. A major drawback of the method is the lack of any protection against sexually transmitted infections. **Failure rates range from 4% with perfect use to 22% with typical use.**

## EMERGENCY CONTRACEPTION

Emergency contraception (EC) allows women to reduce the risk of pregnancy after unprotected intercourse. Though commonly described as the morning-after pill, **EC can actually be used up to 120 hours after intercourse**, depending on the method. The effectiveness of EC is greater the closer it is taken to the time of intercourse. Developed in the 1970s, the Yuzpe method involves the ingestion of various forms and doses of combined OCs after unprotected intercourse. If the dose of OCs is high enough, ovulation may be inhibited. This method has been used infrequently in the United States since the 1990s because other EC methods have greater effectiveness.

The most well-known and commonly used EC is a 1.5-mg levonorgestrel single-dose pill taken orally within 72 hours of unprotected sex. This method of EC is available over the counter and works by delaying or inhibiting ovulation. Because this effect is preovulatory, its effectiveness depends on the cycle day it is taken. If taken after ovulation has occurred, this method is no longer effective.

Another orally available EC is a 30-mg single dose of the selective progesterone receptor modulator ulipristal acetate (UPA, ella). Ovulation is delayed for 5 days in women who take ulipristal acetate. Women can take it closer to the time of ovulation than other methods and still successfully delay ovulation, even after the LH surge has occurred. Thus UPA is approved for use up to 120 hours from the time of unprotected intercourse and is more effective at preventing pregnancy than the levonorgestrel-only method (Glasier, 2010). Levonorgestrel pills are less effective as EC in women with obesity, but UPA effectiveness is maintained in these women (Praditpan, 2017).

The copper IUD is the most effective form of EC. Insertion up to 5 days after unprotected intercourse is 99% effective at preventing pregnancy. When appropriate, another benefit is the potential fulfillment of a woman's long-term contraceptive needs. Studies evaluating the LNG-IUD placement for use as EC are under way, but there is insufficient evidence to recommend its use for this purpose at this time.

## OTHER CONTRACEPTIVE CONCERNS

### Postpartum

On average, resumption of ovulation with return to fertility occurs 45 days postpartum in women who are not breastfeeding. Antenatal care visits provide an ideal time to review plans and contraceptive methods. In addition to usual medical considerations, the postpartum time requires special attention to the risk of thrombosis and the impact on breastfeeding. **The risk of venous thromboembolism (VTE) remains elevated for 6 weeks postpartum.** Combined hormonal methods (COCs, the patch, and the ring) further increase VTE risk and should not be initiated until 6 weeks postpartum. **Progestin-only methods, such as POPs, implants, and the LNG-IUD, do not increase the risk of VTE and can be safely initiated immediately**. Obstetricians can place IUDs after placental delivery at the time of cesarean or vaginal birth. This timing provides immediate contraception without the need for further visits, examinations, or procedures. However, IUD expulsion rates immediately after delivery exceed rates for interval placement. Expulsion rates vary by device and delivery type; rates are highest for LNG-IUD placement after vaginal birth (up to 25%) and about 10% for copper IUDs or LNG-IUDs placed at the time of cesarean delivery, compared with rates of about 5% for either device placed 6 weeks after delivery (Whitaker, 2018).

## BREASTFEEDING

Women who breastfeed exclusively—that is, with minimal or no nonmilk supplements—can expect contraceptive protection as a result of ovulatory suppression and resulting lactational amenorrhea for 6 months postpartum. Such exclusive breastfeeding practices remain uncommon in the United States. Providers should address contraceptive options with all women, regardless of breastfeeding intentions. Choosing the right birth control method while breastfeeding can be challenging for women who have concerns related to the impact of hormonal methods. Because withdrawal from progesterone after delivery initiates lactogenesis, use of a hormonal method of birth control while breastfeeding could theoretically affect milk production. Women and clinicians can be generally reassured; although data are limited, the LNG-IUD, the progestin-only implant, and progestin-only pills appear to have little to no impact on breastfeeding or infant growth and development (Curtis, 2016). The DMPA injection similarly appears to have little effect; however, evidence from animal studies have led the WHO to recommend delaying DMPA until 6 weeks postpartum in breastfeeding women. Clinical trials are ongoing to better answer this question.

Little high-quality research has addressed the impact of combined hormonal methods, and theoretically the effects of estrogens could reduce milk supply. Studies examining the impact of estrogen-containing contraception (pills, patch, vaginal ring) on breastfeeding have similarly inconsistent results. Some show no affect, whereas others show a reduction in breastfeeding duration and breast milk volume. These effects are no longer present once breastfeeding has been established or after 6 weeks postpartum (Bahamondes, 2013). In addition, in the first 6 weeks postpartum, estrogen-containing methods should be avoided because of the increased VTE risk. Therefore the CDC recommends a delay in estrogen-containing methods until 6 weeks postpartum in both breastfeeding and nonbreastfeeding women. In contrast, the WHO advises a delay in estrogen-containing methods until 6 months postpartum in breastfeeding women, particularly in low-resource settings, given the importance of breastfeeding on infant health. A provider may use contraceptive shared decision making in these situations, weighing the theoretical concerns of

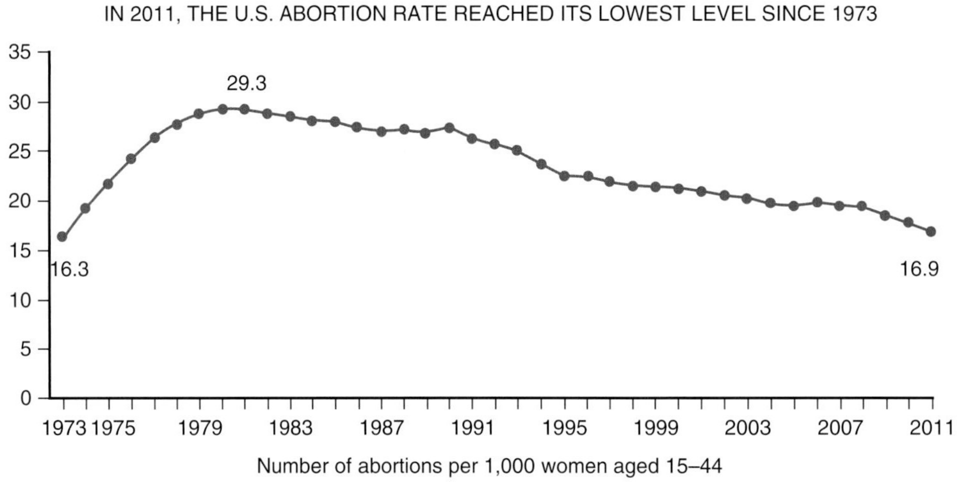


**Fig. 13.13** Trends in abortion. The U.S. abortion rate reached a historic low in 2017. (From Guttmacher Institute. Induced Abortion in the United States. 2019. Available at https://www.guttmacher.org/fact-sheet/induced-abortion-united-states.) Accessed on September 18, 2019

a given method on breastfeeding against the methods contraceptive and noncontraceptive benefits

## INDUCED ABORTION

**Access to safe, legal abortion services forms a cornerstone of maternal health care.** Unfortunately, illegal abortion continues and comprises a leading cause of preventable maternal death in many countries. Induced abortion is common in the United States and worldwide. **By age 45, about half of all U.S. women experience unintended pregnancy; 1 in 20 of all US women will have an abortion by age 20, 1 in 5 by age 30, and 1 in 4 by age 45.** (Jones, 2017). Impressive gains in contraceptive safety, access, and use have contributed to decreasing abortion rates in the U.S. since a peak in the 1980s (Fig. 13.13). In 2017 about 862,320 abortions were performed, representing a rate of 13.5 per 1000 women, the lowest rate ever observed in the United States (Jones, 2019). Despite decreases, however, U.S. abortion rates remain higher than other Western countries.

Ninety percent of abortions occur within the first 12 weeks of pregnancy; fewer than 1% occur after 20 weeks. The most common reasons for abortion include poverty and lack of resources to raise a child, responsibility for other dependents, problems with a partner, young age, and being in school. About 60% of women who have an abortion already have children (Jerman, 2016; Jones, 2018). Some women seek abortion for medical reasons related to their health, pregnancy complications, or a fetal condition. **Abortion often follows contraception failure; half of women report using a contraceptive method such as condoms or pills in the month they became pregnant** (Jones, 2018).

Access to abortion services is sparse or absent in many parts of the United States, especially in rural areas. In 2017, 89% of U.S. counties lacked a clinic to provide abortion care (Jones, 2019). Since the landmark *Roe v. Wade* decision that legalized abortion across the country in 1973, many states have steadily enacted laws restricting access. These state laws, which number in the hundreds, mandate waiting periods before an abortion, gestational age limits, restrictions on use of public or private insurance, and parental consent requirements, among others. Abortion care is more restricted than at any time since legalization in 1973, though a few states have increased access. Some clinics and providers who work in abortion care in the United States have experienced harassment and even overt violence.

## METHODS OF ABORTION

### Aspiration

**Curettage by vacuum aspiration** is the predominant abortion technique in the first trimester. Early pregnancy aspiration can be completed with a flexible or rigid plastic cannula connected to a syringe. This technique, called **manual vacuum aspiration (MVA)**, accomplishes uterine evacuation **up to a gestational age of 10 weeks**. Dilation of the cervix is usually required before aspiration. After 10 weeks, an **electric vacuum aspiration (EVA) system** can offer more efficient evacuation with continuous suction. In early gestations, randomized trials shown similar patient satisfaction with MVA and EVA.

After any vacuum aspiration, good practice includes careful tissue inspection to check for complete removal of the gestational sac, placenta, and fetal tissues (visible on inspection after about 9 weeks). If products of conception cannot be visualized, a sonogram can identify retained tissue. In the case of very early pregnancy, it can be difficult to identify a gestational sac. Serial human chorionic gonadotropin (HCG) evaluation or a repeat ultrasound in 1 week can ensure that pregnancy termination is complete. The MVA technique provides a low-cost and highly efficient technique to manage miscarriage in an office setting, including incomplete or missed abortion.

### Dilation and Evacuation

**Dilation and evacuation (D&E) is the standard surgical technique used for abortion after about 14 weeks.** Among midtrimester abortions performed in the United States, about 95% are D&Es. Alternatives to D&E include medical induction abortion and hysterotomy, a surgical procedure with much greater morbidity.

Because a greater volume of fetal tissue is present than in the first trimester, preoperative cervical dilation is needed to allow for safe, appropriate instrumentation. **Cervical preparation with osmotic dilators can be achieved after several hours or by placement the day prior.** The most commonly used dilators are small tents of dried and sterilized seaweed, ***Laminaria japonica.*** By gently opening the cervix over several hours, the osmotic dilators reduce the risk of uterine perforation and cervical injury. **Another strategy for cervical preparation is**

**the administration of misoprostol, a prostaglandin and E1 analog, typically given in a dosage of 400 or 600 mg vaginally or buccally a few hours before vacuum aspiration or D&E.** Misoprostol softens the cervix to facilitate mechanical dilation. Mifepristone can be used in some cases to augment dilation protocols before D&E. Surgeons use a combination of suction and uterine forceps to remove fetal and decidual tissue. In some cases, intraoperative ultrasound guidance may assist the surgeon during D&E. Inspection to identify expected fetal tissues and the placenta confirms a complete procedure.

## Medication Abortion

### First-Trimester Medication Abortion

In September 2000 the U.S. FDA approved the combination of mifepristone and misoprostol as a safe and effective alternative to surgical abortion. These medications are used by a growing proportion of women undergoing early abortions. In 2017 medication abortion accounted for 39% of all nonhospital abortions and for about 60% of abortions before 10 weeks' gestation (Jones, 2019).

Mifepristone (Mifeprex), also known as RU-486, is a competitive inhibitor of the endometrial progesterone receptor. Mifepristone combined with the administration of the prostaglandin misoprostol 24 to 72 hours later results in a complete abortion more than 95% of the time. Either drug is much less effective when administered alone as a single dose. The most commonly used evidence-based regimen combines 200 mg oral mifepristone with 800 μg buccal or vaginal misoprostol. If mifepristone is not available, repeat doses of misoprostol provide another approach.

Those undergoing a medication abortion pass the products of conception at home after misoprostol administration and can follow up to confirm a complete abortion using repeat ultrasound or HCG testing. Most providers recommend nonsteroidal antiinflammatory drugs (NSAIDs) for uterine cramping during the process. Side effects can include nausea, vomiting, and chills, and bleeding lasts from 7 to 14 days. On rare occasions, prolonged or heavy bleeding can lead to the need for emergency curettage or even blood transfusion. Women who choose a medication approach report high satisfaction with this method.

### Induction Abortion after the First Trimester

Nonsurgical midtrimester induction abortion is usually performed with the administration of misoprostol. When available, adding mifepristone the day before misoprostol is preferred because mifepristone substantially shortens the induction-to-delivery interval. Professional organizations recommend 200 mg mifepristone followed by 800 μg misoprostol administered vaginally 24 to 48 hours later, then 400 μg misoprostol administered vaginally or sublingually every 3 hours up to 5 doses. If mifepristone is not available, guidelines recommend a vaginal loading dose of 600 to 800 μg misoprostol followed by 400 μg misoprostol vaginally or sublingually every 3 hours up to 5 doses (ACOG, 2013). This regimen appears to be safe in women with a prior cesarean delivery because uterine rupture is very rare. Some advantages of a medical induction of labor over D&E include the avoidance of surgery and the chance to view or hold the fetus if desired. If no provider skilled in D&E is available, labor induction may be the only safe option. Access to adequate pain control throughout the process is a key consideration. Disadvantages include a required inpatient hospitalization, increased costs compared with outpatient D&E, an unknown and possibly prolonged induction interval (can exceed 24 hours), and a higher risk of retained placenta necessitating D&C in about 15% of cases.

### Approaches to Pain Control

For surgical abortion, providers should discuss available options to weigh associated risks and benefits. Options can range from local to general anesthesia. For early-term office-based procedures, many women do well with a paracervical block, usually using lidocaine, and an NSAID; some providers add anxiolytics. If available, moderate or deep sedation can also be offered. Some degree of sedation is usually required for procedures in the midtrimester. Administering sedation requires attention to maintaining safe respiration.

### Complications

Modern, legal abortion in the United States is very safe (National Academies of Science, 2018). **Serious complications are rare, and the overall mortality is less than 1 per 100,000 procedures**. The U.S. maternal mortality rate, by comparison, was 17.2 per 100,000 births from 2011 to 2015 (Petersen, 2019). Two important determinants of complications are the gestational age and method of abortion chosen. Beyond 10 weeks, abortion complication rates increase progressively with gestational age. Therefore access to abortion maintains safety and barriers to care increase the risk of complications.

Serious complications after first trimester aspiration abortion, such as hospital admission, surgery, or blood transfusion, occur very rarely, in less than 1% of cases (National Academies of Science, 2018). The most common complications include infection, retained products of conception, hemorrhage, and the need for a repeat procedure (up to 5% may experience one of these complications); perforation is less common. The routine use of preoperative antibiotic prophylaxis is recommended to reduce the risk of infection. The risk of complications increases somewhat for D&E procedures, with an overall rate of up to 4% and a serious complication rate of about 1% (National Academies of Science, 2018). Existing research indicates abortion does not increase a women's risk of infertility, abnormal placentation, breast cancer, depression, or anxiety (National Academies of Science, 2018).

### REFERENCES


American College of Obstetricians and Gynecologists (ACOG). Committee on Practice Bulletins-Gynecology; ACOG Practice Bulletin no. 208: Benefits and risks of sterilization. *Obstet Gynecol.* 2019; 133(3):592-594.

American College of Obstetricians and Gynecologists (ACOG). Committee Opinion No. 735: Adolescents and Long-Acting Reversible Contraception: Implants and Intrauterine Devices. *Obstet Gynecol.* 2018;131(5):e130-e139.

American College of Obstetricians and Gynecologists (ACOG). Committee on Gynecologic Practice; Long-Acting Reversible Contraception Working Group: ACOG Committee Opinion no. 642: Increasing access to contraceptive implants and intrauterine devices to reduce unintended pregnancy. *Obstet Gynecol.* 2015;126(4):e44-e48.

ACOG Practice Bulletin 135: second trimester abortion. *Obstet Gynecol.* 2013;121(6):1394-1406.

Centers for Disease Control and Prevention (CDC). U.S. selected practice recommendations for contraceptive use, 2013. *MMWR.* 2013;62(5):5-7.

Curtis KM, Jatlaoui TC, Tepper NK, et al. U.S. selected practice recommendations for contraceptive use, 2016. *MMWR Recomm Rep.* 2016; 65(RR-4):1-66.

Daniels K, Abma J. Current contraceptive status among women aged 15-49: United States, 2015-2017. *NCHS Data Brief.* 2018;(327).

Daniels K, Mosher WD, Jones J. Contraceptive methods women have ever used: United States, 1982-2010. *Natl Health Stat Report.* 2013;(62):1-15.

Dehlendorf C, Grumbach K, Schmittdiel JA, Steinauer J. Shared decision making in contraceptive counseling. *Contraception.* 2017;95(5):452-455.

Dehlendorf C, Ruskin R, Grumbach K, et al. Recommendations for intrauterine contraception: a randomized trial of the effects of patients'race/ethnicity and socioeconomic status. *Am J Obstet Gynecol.* 2010;203:319.e1-319.e8.

Dinger J, Minh T, Buttmann N, Bardenheuer K. Effectiveness of oral contraceptive pills in a large U.S. cohort comparing progestogen and regimen. *Obstet Gynecol.* 2011;117(1):33-40.

Gerstman BB, Piper JM, Tomita DK, Ferguson WJ, Stadel BV, Lundin FE. Oral contraceptive estrogen dose and the risk of deep venous thromboembolic disease. *Am J Epidemiol.* 1991;133(1):32-37.

Glasier A, Cameron S, Fine P, et al. Ulipristal acetate versus levonorgestrel for emergency contraception: a randomised non-inferiority trial and meta-analysis. *Lancet.* 2010;375(9714):555-562.

Grimbizis G, Tarlatzis B. The use of hormonal contraception and its protective role against endometrial and ovarian cancer. *Best Pract Res Clin Obstet Gynaecol.* 2010;24(1):29-38.

Grimes D, Schulz K. Prophylactic antibiotics for intrauterine device insertion: a metaanalysis of the randomized controlled trials. *Contraception.* 1999;60(2):57-63.

Hatcher R, Trussell J, Nelson AL, et al., eds. *Contraceptive Technology.* 20th rev. ed. New York: Ardent Media; 2011.

Hauk L. CDC Releases 2015 Guidelines on the Treatment of Sexually Transmitted Disease. *Am Fam Physician.* 2016;93(2):144-154.

Higgins JA, Kramer RD, Ryder KM. Provider Bias in Long-Acting Reversible Contraception (LARC) promotion and removal: perceptions of young women. *Am J Public Health.* 2016;106(11):1932-1937.

Hillis S, Marchbanks P, Tylor L, Peterson H. Poststerilization regret: findings from the United States Collaborative Review of Sterilization. *Obstet Gynecol.* 1999;93(6):889-895.

Jones RK, Witwer E, Jerman J, *Abortion Incidence and Service Availability the United States, 2017.* New York: Guttmacher Institute; 2019. Available at https://www.guttmacher.org/report/abortion-incidence-service-availability-us-2017.

Kavanaugh ML, Jerman J, Finer LB. Changes in use of long-acting reversible contraception methods among U.S. women, 2009-2012. *Obstet Gynecol.* 2015;126:917-927.

Lessard LN, Karasek D, Ma S, et al. Contraceptive features preferred by women at high risk of unintended pregnancy. *Perspect Sex Reprod Health.* 2012;44:194-200.

Mayeda ER, Torgal AH, Westhoff CL. Weight and body composition changes during oral contraceptive use in obese and normal weight women. *J Womens Health (Larchmt).* 2014;23(1):38-43.

McNicholas C, Maddipati R, Zhao Q, Swor E, Peipert JF. Use of the etonogestrel implant and levonorgestrel intrauterine device beyond the U.S. Food and Drug Administration-approved duration. *Obstet Gynecol.* 2015;125(3):599-604.

Milne RL, Knight JA, John EM, et al. Oral contraceptive us and risk of early-onset breast cancer in carriers and noncarriers of BRCA1 and BRCA2 mutations. *Cancer Epidemiol Biomarkers Prev.* 2005;13:350.

Mosher WD, Jones J. Use of contraception in the United States: 1982-2008. *Vital Health Stat 23.* 2010;(29):1-44.

National Academies of Sciences, Engineering, and Medicine. *The Safety and Quality of Abortion Care in the United States.* Washington, DC: National Academies Press; 2018.

Petersen EE, Davis NL, Goodman D, et al. Vital Signs: Pregnancy-Related Deaths, United States, 2011-2015, and Strategies for Prevention, 13 States, 2013-2017. *MMWR Morb Mortal Wkly Rep.* 2019;68:423-429.

Peterson HB, Xia Z, Hughes JM, Wilcox LS, Tylor LR, Trussell J. The risk of pregnancy after tubal sterilization: findings from the U.S. Collaborative Review of Sterilization. *Am J Obstet Gynecol.* 1996;174(4):1161-1168.

Redmond G, Godwin AJ, Olson W, Lippman JS. Use of placebo controls in an oral contraceptive trial: methodological issues and adverse event incidence. *Contraception.* 1999;60(2):81-85.

Whitaker A, Chen B. Society of Family Planning Guidelines: postplacental insertion of intrauterine devices. *Contraception.* 2018;97:2-13.

World Health Organization (WHO). *Medical Eligibility Criteria for Contraceptive Use.* 5th ed. Geneva, Switzerland: WHO, 2015. Available at: https://www.who.int/reproductivehealth/publications/family_planning/MEC-5/en/. Accessed October 23, 2020.

**Suggested readings for this chapter can be found on ExpertConsult.com.**

# 14 Menopause and Care of the Mature Woman

## Endocrinology, Consequences of Estrogen Deficiency, Effects of Hormone Therapy, and Other Treatment Options

*Roger A. Lobo*

### KEY POINTS

- The average age of menopause in the United States is 51.3 years; it is younger in certain ethnic groups, and is genetically predetermined and is not related to the number of ovulations, race, socioeconomic conditions, education, height, weight, age at menarche, or age at last pregnancy.
- Because most diseases in women occur after menopause, the onset of menopause heralds an important opportunity to institute prevention strategies for prolonging and improving the quality of life for women.
- Vasomotor symptoms or hot flushes may persist for 10 or more years, with bothersome flushes occurring for about 7 years. Estrogen is the best therapy for the hot flush; other effective therapies are progestogens, selective serotonin reuptake inhibitors (SSRIs), gabapentin, clonidine, some phytoestrogens, acupuncture, and stellate ganglion blockade.
- Dual-energy x-ray absorptiometry (DEXA) is the most accurate method to measure bone density. A country-specific algorithm (FRAX) using DEXA has been developed to calculate the 10-year risk of fracture. In addition to estrogen (with and without progestogen), alendronate, risedronate, ibandronate, zoledronic acid, raloxifene, calcitonin, denosumab, romosozumab and teriparatide will reduce postmenopausal bone loss, and some agents will stimulate bone formation as well.
- The primary indication for estrogen therapy is symptoms of menopause (hot flushes as well as quality-of-life issues); bone health may also be an indication in some women. In younger postmenopausal women who are receiving hormonal therapy for symptoms, the benefits outweigh risks. There are consistent data for a reduction in all-cause mortality of 20% to 30% in younger women who initiate estrogen therapy at the onset of menopause. These findings suggest a potential role of estrogen as a prevention therapy after menopause

**Menopause** is defined by the last menstrual period. Because cessation of menses is variable and many of the symptoms thought to be related to menopause may occur before cessation of menses, there is seldom a precise timing of this event. Other terms used are ***perimenopause,*** which refers to a variable time beginning a few years before and continuing after the event of menopause, and ***climacteric,*** which merely refers to the time after the cessation of reproductive function. Although the terms *menopausal* and *postmenopausal* are used interchangeably, the former term is less correct because *menopausal* should only relate to the time around the cessation of menses.

As life expectancy increases beyond the eighth decade worldwide, particularly in developed countries, an increasing proportion of the female population is postmenopausal. **With the average age of menopause being 51 years, more than a third of a woman's life is now spent after menopause.** Here, symptoms and signs of estrogen deficiency merge with issues encountered with natural aging. As the world population increases and a larger proportion of this population is made up of individuals older than 50, medical care specifically directed at postmenopausal women becomes an important aspect of modem medicine. **Indeed an opportunity exists at the onset of menopause for providers to address the long-term needs of women after menopause and to have an impact on longevity and quality of life** (Lobo, 2016). In the United States, the number of women entering menopause is projected to have doubled in the 30 years between 1990 and 2020, and the total number of postmenopausal women is expected to be in range of 60 million (Table 14.1).

Age of menopause, which is a genetically programmed event, is subject to some variability. **The age of menopause in Western countries (between 51 and 52 years)** is thought to correlate with general health status; socioeconomic status is associated with an earlier age of menopause. Higher parity, on the other hand, has been found to be associated with a later menopause. Smoking has consistently been found to be associated with menopause onset taking place 1 to 2 years earlier. Hysterectomy has also been cited as resulting in an earlier menopause, presumably because of a diminution in the blood supply to the ovary; however, the data have not been consistent. Although body mass has been thought to be related to age of menopause (with greater body mass index [BMI] associated with later menopause), the data have not been consistent. However, physical or athletic activity has not been found to influence the age of menopause. There also appear to be ethnic differences in the onset of menopause. In the United States black and Hispanic women have been found to have menopause approximately 2 years earlier than white women. Although parity is generally greater around the world than in the United States, the age of menopause appears to be somewhat earlier outside the United States. Malay women have menopause at approximately age 45, Thai women at age 49.5, and Filipina women between ages 47 and 48. Menopause has also been reported to occur at an average age of 46.2 years in women from India (Ajuja, 2016). Women in countries at higher altitude (Himalayas or Andes) have been shown to have menopause 1 to 1.5 years earlier. Because the average age of menopause in the United States is 51 to 53 years, menopause before age 40 is considered premature and before age 45 is considered early. Conversely, by age 58, 97% of women will have gone through menopause. **The primary determinate of age of menopause is genetic.** Based on family studies, de Bruin and colleagues (de Bruin, 2001) showed that heritability for age of menopause averaged 0.87, suggesting that

**TABLE 14.1** U.S. Population Entering the Postmenopausal Years, Ages 55 through 64

| Year | Population (in Millions) |
|---|---|
| 1990 | 10.8 |
| 2000 | 12.1 |
| 2010 | 17.1 |
| 2020 | 19.3 |

Modified from U.S. Bureau of the Census. *Current Population Reports: Projections of the Population of the United States 1977 to 2050.* Washington, DC: U.S. Government Printing Office; 1993.

genetics explains up to 87% of the variance in menopausal age. The maternal contribution is around 50%.

Other than specific gene mutations that have been shown to cause **premature ovarian failure or insufficiency** (explained later in this chapter), no specific genes have been implicated to account for this genetic influence. However, several genes are likely to be involved in determining the age of menopause; they include genes regulating immune function and DNA repair (Stolk, 2012) and may also include genes coding telomerase activity, which affects aging in general.

## PREMATURE OVARIAN INSUFFICIENCY

Premature ovarian failure (POF) or premature ovarian insufficiency (POI), which is a newer term, is defined as **hypergonadotropic ovarian failure occurring before age 40. POI occurs in 5% to 10% of women who are evaluated for amenorrhea**; thus the incidence varies according to the prevalence of amenorrhea in various populations. Estimates of the overall prevalence of POI in the general population range between 0.3% and 0.9% of women. Throughout life, there is an ongoing rate of atresia of oocytes. Because this process is accelerated with various forms of gonadal dysgenesis because of defective X chromosomes, one possible cause of POI is an increased rate of atresia that has yet to be explained. A decreased germ cell endowment or an increased rate of germ cell destruction can also explain POI. Nevertheless, about 1000 (of the original 2 million) primarily follicles may remain. Although most of these oocytes are likely to be functionally deficient, **spontaneous pregnancies occur occasionally in young women in the first few years after the diagnosis of POI.** There are several possible causes of POI (Box 14.1).

Defects in the X chromosome may result in various types of gonadal dysgenesis with varied times of expression of ovarian failure. Even patients with classical gonadal dysgenesis (e.g., 45,XO) may undergo a normal puberty, and occasionally a pregnancy may ensue as a result of genetic mosaicism. **Very small defects in the X chromosome may be sufficient to cause POI**. Familial forms of POI may be related to either autosomal dominant or sex-linked modes of inheritance. Mutations in the gene encoding the follicle-stimulating hormone (FSH) receptor (e.g., mutation in exon 7 in the gene on chromosome 2p) have been described, but these are extremely rare outside of the Finnish population, in whom these mutations were originally described. An expansion of a trinucleotide repeat sequence in the first exon on the *FMR1* gene (Xq 27.3) leads to fragile X syndrome, a major cause of developmental disabilities in men.

The permutation in fragile X syndrome has been shown to be associated with POI. Type 1 blepharophimosis/ptosis/epicanthus inversus (BPES) syndrome, an autosomal dominant disorder caused by mutations in the forkhead transcription factor FOXL2, includes POI. Triple X syndrome has also been associated with POI. It has been suggested that functional mutations of antimüllerian hormone (AMH) may also be associated with POI.

Dystrophic myotonia has also been linked to POI, although the mechanism underlying this relationship is unclear. Under the category of enzymatic defects, galactosemia is a major cause of POI that is related to the toxic buildup of galactose in women who are unable to metabolize the sugar. Even in women with fairly well-controlled galactose-free diets, POI tends to occur. Another enzymatic defect linked to POI is 17α-hydroxylase deficiency. This rare condition manifests differently from the other causes discussed here because the defect in the production of sex steroids leads to sexual infantilism and hypertension.

The degree to which **autoimmunity may be responsible for POI** is unclear, but it has been suggested to be associated in 17.5% of cases. Virtually all autoimmune disorders have been found to be associated with POI, including autoimmune polyendocrinopathies such as autoimmune polyendocrinopathy/candidiasis/ectodermal dystrophy (APECED), which is caused by mutations in the autoimmune *(AIRE)* gene on band 21 q22. The presence of the thymus gland appears to be required for normal ovarian function because POI has been associated with hypoplasia of the thymus. In patients who have undergone ovarian biopsy as part of their evaluation, lymphocytic infiltration surrounding follicles has been described, as well as resumption of menses after immunosuppression. Immunoassays using antibodies directed at ovarian antigens have been developed and have demonstrated positive findings in some patients with POI, although the relevance of these findings remains unsettled. Ovarian autoantibodies could also conceivably be a secondary phenomenon to a primary cell-mediated form of immunity. Specific enzymes such as 3β-hydroxysteroid dehydrogenase (3βHSD) may also be the target of ovarian autoimmunity. Approximately 2% to 4% of women with autoimmunity for POI will have antiadrenal antibodies as well (Chen, 1996). This can be screened for by an assay for 21-hydroxlase antibodies. Adrenal function, more practically, can be assessed by measuring dehydroepiandrosterone sulfate (DHEA-S) levels, which are higher in younger women than in menopausal women, unless the adrenal gland is affected. It may also be helpful to assess ovarian volume and follicular presence by vaginal ultrasound in these women as well. The ovaries in younger women with POI are more normal in size and have follicles present compared with the smaller atrophic ovary in menopause.

From a practical standpoint, **screening for the common autoimmune disorders is appropriate in women found to have POI.** Not practical to measure, however, are abnormalities in the structure of gonadotropins, in their receptors, or in receptor binding, which could be associated with POI; these measurements are difficult. Although abnormal urinary forms of gonadotropins have been reported in women with POI, these data have not been replicated. Abnormalities of FSH receptor binding, as mediated by a serum inhibitor, have been described. A genetic defect that may lead to alterations in FSH receptor structure was mentioned previously.

**BOX 14.1** Possible Causes of Premature Ovarian Failure

- Genetic
- Enzymatic
- Immune
- Gonadotropin defects
- Ovarian insults
- Idiopathic

Under the category of ovarian insults, POI may be induced by ionizing radiation, chemotherapy, or overly aggressive ovarian surgery. Although not well documented, viral infections have been suggested to play a role, particularly mumps. **A dose of 400 to 500 rads is known to cause ovarian failure 50% of the time**, and older women are more vulnerable to experiencing permanent failure. A dose of approximately 800 rads is associated with failure in all women. Ovarian failure (transient or permanent) may be induced by chemotherapeutic agents, although younger women receiving this insult have a better prognosis. **Alkalizing agents**, particularly cyclophosphamide, appear to be most toxic. By exclusion, the majority of women are considered to have idiopathic POI because no demonstrable cause can be pinpointed. Among these women, small mutations in genes lying on the X chromosome or yet to be identified autosomal genes may be the cause.

## Management of Premature Ovarian Insufficiency

Evaluation of POI in women younger than 30 should include screening for autoimmune disorders and a karyotype; detailed recommendations for screening of such women are available (Rebar, 2000). In addition, vaginal ultrasound may be useful for assessing the size of the ovaries and the degree of follicular development, which, if present, may signify an immunologic defect. **Women with POI caused by immunologic defects should be screened carefully for thyroid, adrenal, and other autoimmune disorders.**

Treatment of all cases usually consists of **estrogen replacement.** Although in menopausal therapy clinicians have steered away from the term *replacement* therapy, in this specific instance of POI, estrogen treatment is truly *replacement* therapy. If fertility is a concern, the most efficacious treatment is oocyte donation. Various attempts at ovarian stimulation are usually unsuccessful; sporadic pregnancies that may occur (~5%) are just as likely to occur spontaneously as with any intervention, and often while on physiologic estradiol ($E_2$) replacement. In this setting it has been our preference not to use oral contraceptive pills for replacement in women wishing to conceive. In a long-term follow-up of a large number of women diagnosed with POI, within a year spontaneous ovarian function was observed in 24% of the women and over time **the rate of spontaneous pregnancies was 4.4%** (Bidet, 2011).

Estrogen replacement in these young women with POI is extremely important and is not analogous to hormone therapy (HT) after menopause because these young women are at substantial long-term risk for osteoporosis and cardiovascular disease (CVD). Coronary heart disease and death are specifically increased in approximately 70% of women with POI, but not stroke. Another review emphasized the increased risks in several organ systems, including brain, cardiovascular, and bone, and early mortality with untreated premature or early menopause (Faubion, 2015). A more extreme example of this phenomenon is with premature oophorectomy, with which the risk of CVD is many-fold increased (Fig. 14.1) (Atsma, 2006). Women with POI should be offered estrogen replacement, with some form of progestogen in women with a uterus, at least up to the natural age of menopause.

# MENOPAUSAL TRANSITION (PERIMENOPAUSE)

A workshop was convened in 2001 to build consensus on describing various stages of the menopausal transition. A follow-up conference, the **Study of Reproductive Aging Workshop (STRAW+10)**, had more streamlined bleeding criteria for the

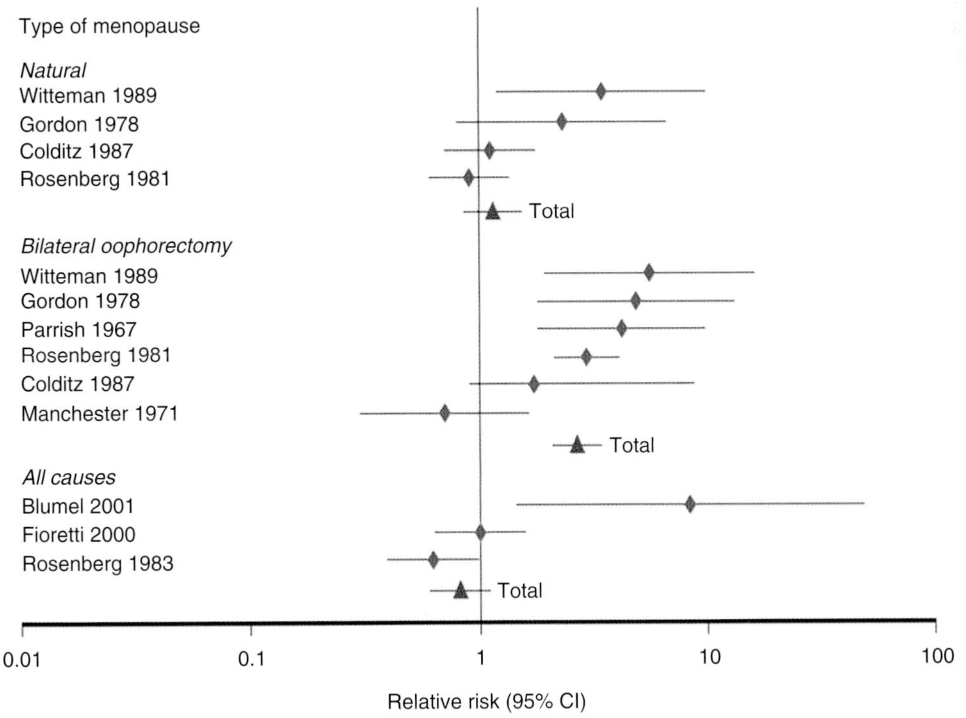


**Fig. 14.1** Effect of type of "early" menopause on cardiovascular disease. Data taken from a meta-analysis. *CI,* Confidence interval. (From Atsma F, Bartelink ML, Grobbee DE, et al. Postmenopausal status and early menopause as independent risk factors for cardiovascular disease: a meta-analysis. *Menopause.* 2006;13(2):265-279.)

Menarche (at stage −5) FMP (0) (between stages −1 and +1a)

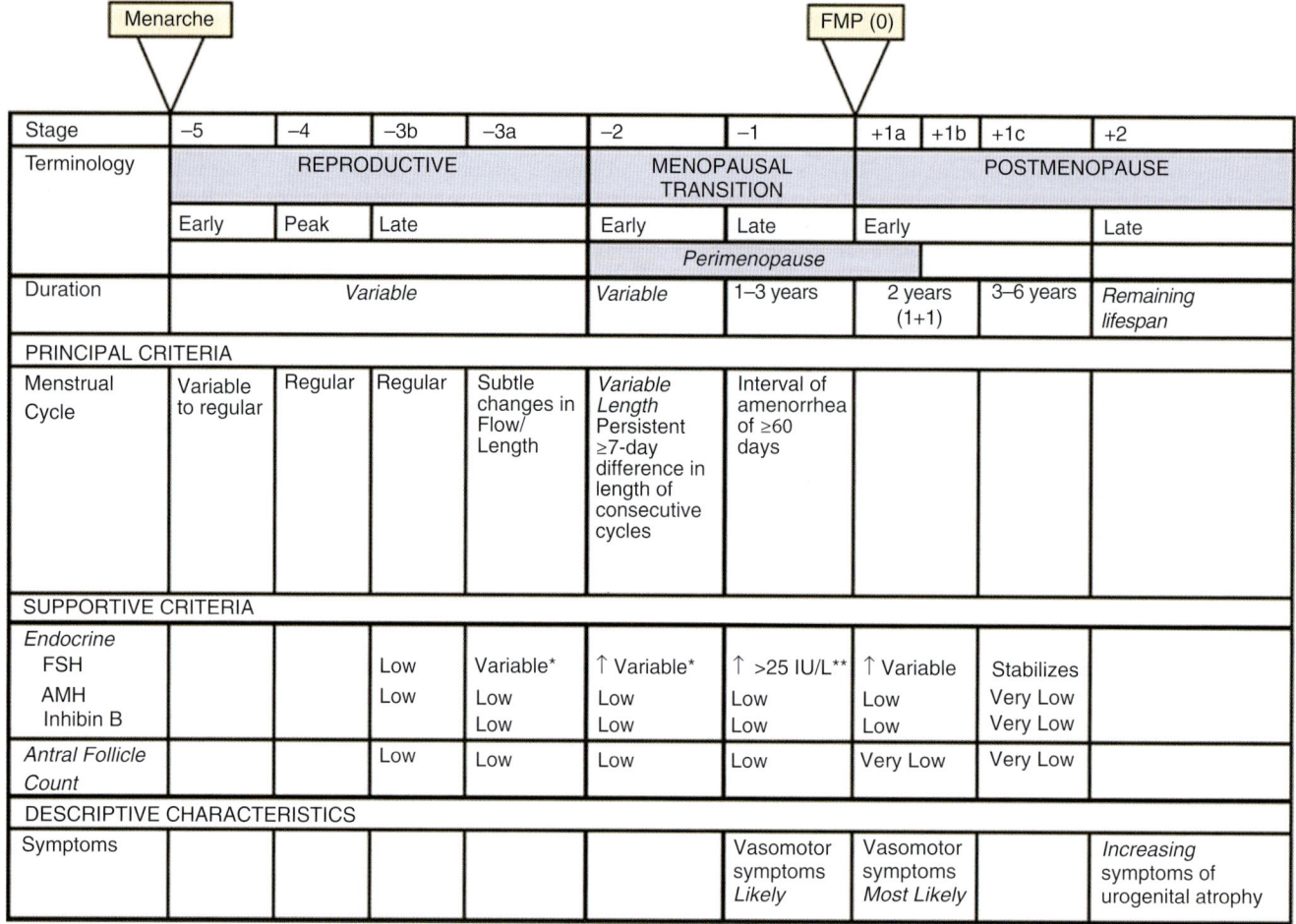

| Stage | −5 | −4 | −3b | −3a | −2 | −1 | +1a | +1b | +1c | +2 |
|---|---|---|---|---|---|---|---|---|---|---|
| Terminology | REPRODUCTIVE | | | | MENOPAUSAL TRANSITION | | POSTMENOPAUSE | | | |
| | Early | Peak | Late | | Early | Late | Early | | | Late |
| | | | | | *Perimenopause* | | | | | |
| Duration | *Variable* | | | | *Variable* | 1–3 years | 2 years (1+1) | | 3–6 years | *Remaining lifespan* |
| PRINCIPAL CRITERIA | | | | | | | | | | |
| Menstrual Cycle | Variable to regular | Regular | Regular | Subtle changes in Flow/ Length | *Variable Length* Persistent ≥7-day difference in length of consecutive cycles | Interval of amenorrhea of ≥60 days | | | | |
| SUPPORTIVE CRITERIA | | | | | | | | | | |
| *Endocrine* FSH | | | Low | Variable* | ↑ Variable* | ↑ >25 IU/L** | ↑ Variable | | Stabilizes | |
| AMH | | | Low | Low | Low | Low | Low | | Very Low | |
| Inhibin B | | | | Low | Low | Low | Low | | Very Low | |
| *Antral Follicle Count* | | | Low | Low | Low | Low | Very Low | | Very Low | |
| DESCRIPTIVE CHARACTERISTICS | | | | | | | | | | |
| Symptoms | | | | | | Vasomotor symptoms *Likely* | Vasomotor symptoms *Most Likely* | | | *Increasing* symptoms of urogenital atrophy |

**Fig. 14.2** The Stages of Reproductive Aging Workshop + 10 staging system for reproductive aging in women. *AMH,* Antimüllerian hormone; *FMP,* Final menstrual period; *FSH,* follicle-stimulating hormone. (From Harlow SD, Gass M, Hall JE, et al. Executive summary of the stages of reproductive aging workshop + 10: addressing the unfinished agenda of staging reproductive aging. *J Clin Endocrinol Metab.* 2012;97(4):1159-1168.)

various stages and expanded the stages including the use of biochemical markers such as inhibin B and AMH, in addition to FSH (Harlow, 2012) (Fig. 14.2). This scheme is important from a descriptive standpoint for the physiology behind the normal menopausal transition and is useful for characterization of women in various stages in research studies. **The earliest sign of impending menopause during the menopause transition is a change in menstrual length.**

The ovary changes markedly from birth to the onset of menopause (Fig. 14.3). The greatest number of primordial follicles is present in utero at 20 weeks' gestation, and the follicles undergo a regular rate of atresia until around the age of 37. After this time, the decline in primordial follicles appears to become more rapid between age 38 and menopause (Fig. 14.4), when no more than 1000 follicles remain. These remaining follicles are primarily atretic in nature.

These changes are reflected in circulating levels of AMH, which decline rapidly with ovarian aging. **When levels of serum AMH become undetectable, menopause is likely to occur in 4 to 5 years.**

## Ovarian Changes During Perimenopause

Although perimenopausal changes are generally thought to be endocrine in nature and result in menstrual changes, a marked diminution of reproductive capacity precedes this period by several years. This decline may be referred to as *gametogenic ovarian failure* and is reflected by decreased AMH, inhibin B levels, and antral follicle counts and a rising FSH. The concept of dissociation in ovarian function is appropriate. These changes may occur with normal menstrual function and no obvious endocrine deficiency; however, they may occur in some women as early as age 35 (10 or more years before endocrine deficiency ensues). Although subtle changes in endocrine and menstrual function can occur for up to 3 years before menopause, it has been shown that **the major reduction in ovarian estrogen production does not occur until approximately a year before menopause** (Fig. 14.5) (Randolph, 2011). There is also a slow decline in androgen status (i.e., androstenedione and testosterone), which cannot be adequately detected at the time of perimenopause. **The decline in androgen is largely a phenomenon of aging.** Products of the granulosa cell are most important for the feedback control of FSH. As the functional capacity of the follicular units decreases, the secretion of substances that suppress FSH also decreases. A marker of this is inhibin B, in which levels are lower in the early follicular phase in women in their late 30s (Fig. 14.6). Inhibin B is seldom measured clinically; rather AMH (which also reflects granulosa cell function) is most often assessed, as noted previously. Indeed, FSH levels are higher throughout the cycle in older ovulatory women than in younger

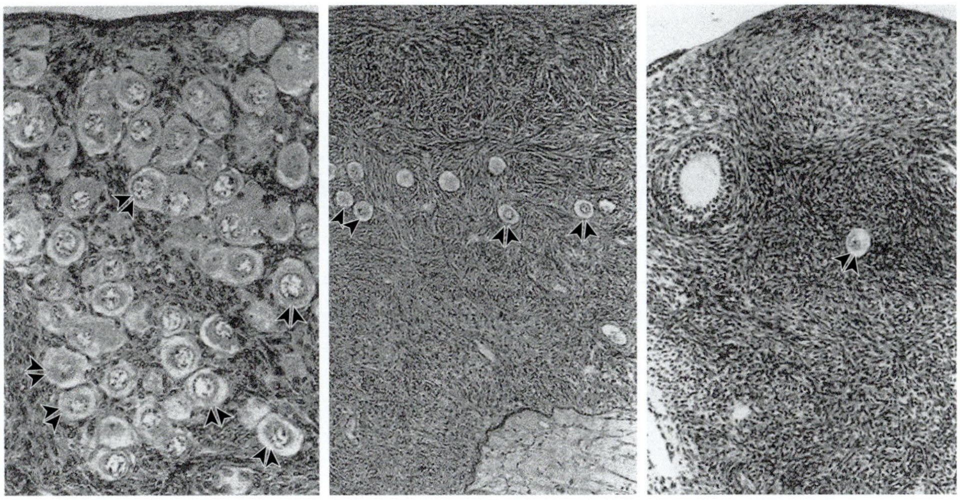


**Fig. 14.3** Photomicrographs of the cortex of human ovaries from birth to age 50 years. Small nongrowing primordial follicles *(arrowheads)* have a single layer of squamous granulosa cells. (Modified from Erickson GF. An analysis of follicle development and ovum maturation. *Semin Reprod Endocrinol.* 1986;3:233.)

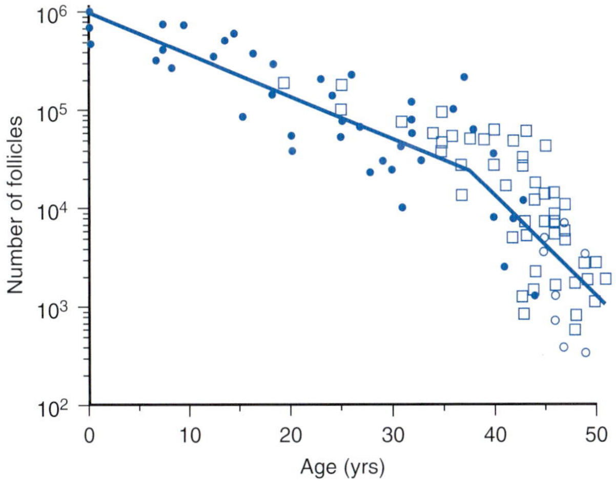


**Fig. 14.4** The age-related decrease in the total number of primordial follicles (PFs) within both human ovaries from birth to menopause. As a result of recruitment (initiation of PF growth), the number of PFs decreases progressively from about 1 million at birth to 25,000 at 37 years. At 37 years, the rate of recruitment increases sharply, and the number of PFs declines to 1000 at menopause (about age 51 years). (Modified from Faddy MJ, Gosden RJ, Gougeon A, et al. Accelerated disappearance of ovarian follicles in mid-life: implications for forecasting menopause. *Hum Reprod.* 1992;7:1342.)

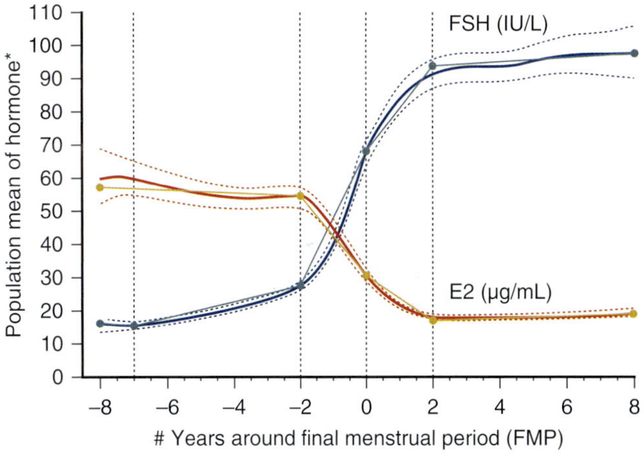


**Fig. 14.5** Adjusted population means (95% confidence interval) for segmented mean profiles for follicle-stimulating hormone (FSH) and estradiol ($E_2$) across the final menstrual period in the Study of Women's Health Across the Nation (N = 1215). (From Randolph JF Jr, Zheng H, Sowers MR, et al. Change in follicle-stimulating hormone and estradiol across the menopausal transition: effect of age at the final menstrual period. *J Clin Endocrinol Metab.* 2011;96(3):746-754.)

women (Fig. 14.7). The functional capacity of the ovary is also diminished as women enter into perimenopause. With gonadotropin stimulation, although $E_2$ levels are not very different between younger and older women, total inhibin production by granulosa cells is decreased in women older than 35. From a clinical perspective, subtle increases in FSH on day 3 of the cycle, or increases in the clomiphene challenge test, correlate with decreased ovarian responses to stimulation and decreased fecundability. AMH serves as the most practical marker of reproductive aging. Levels decrease throughout life, being undetectable at menopause, and show less variability during the menstrual cycle compared with other markers such as FSH. However, values are lower by up to 20% in women on oral contraceptives, and this should be taken into account when assessing levels in younger women. When values reach an undetectable range (<0.05 ng/mL), menopause has been found to occur within 5 years, as stated previously (Fig. 14.8).

Although there is a general decline in oocyte number with age, an accelerated atresia occurs around age 37 or 38 (see Fig. 14.4). The reason for this acceleration is not clear, but one possible theory relates to activin secretion. Because granulosa cell–derived activin is important for stimulating FSH receptor expression, the rise in FSH levels could result in more activin production, which in turn enhances FSH action. A profile of elevated activin with lower inhibin B has been found in older

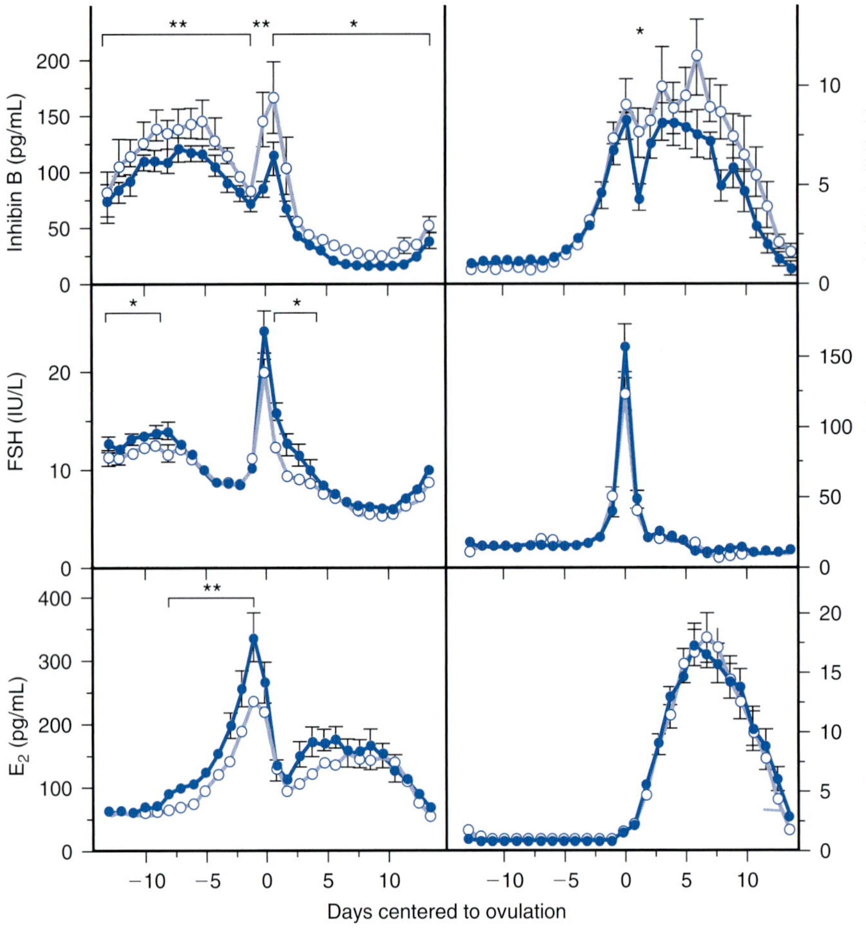


**Fig. 14.6** An inhibin B, follicle-stimulating hormone (FSH), estradiol ($E_2$), inhibin A, and progesterone ($P_4$) levels in cycling women 20 to 34 years old (^) and 35 to 46 years old (•). Hormone levels are depicted as centered to the day of ovulation (* $P < .04$; ** $P < .02$) when comparing the two age groups. (From Welt CK, McNicholl DJ, Taylor AE, et al. Female reproductive aging is marked by decreased secretion of dimeric inhibin. *J Clin Endocrinol Metab.* 1999;84(1):105.)

women (Fig. 14.9). This autocrine action of activin, involving enhanced FSH action, might be expected to lead to accelerated growth and differentiation of granulosa cells. Furthermore, activin has been shown to increase the size of the pool of preantral follicles in the rat. At the same time, these follicles become more atretic. Clinical treatment of perimenopausal women should address three general areas of concern: (1) irregular bleeding; (2) symptoms of early menopause, such as **hot flushes**; and (3) the inability to conceive. Treatment of irregular bleeding is complicated by the fluctuating hormonal status. Estrogen levels may be higher than normal in the early follicular phase and progesterone secretion may be normal or slightly decreased, although not all cycles are ovulatory. For these reasons, short-term use of an oral contraceptive (usually 20 $\mu$g ethinyl estradiol) may be an option for otherwise healthy women who do not smoke to help them cope with irregular bleeding. Early symptoms of menopause, particularly vasomotor changes, may occur as the result of fluctuating hormonal levels. In this setting an oral contraceptive may be an option if symptoms warrant therapy. Alternatively, lower doses of estrogen used alone may be another option.

## Hormonal Changes With Established Menopause

Fig. 14.10 depicts the typical hormonal levels of postmenopausal women compared with those of ovulatory women in the early follicular phase. The most significant findings are the marked reductions in $E_2$ and estrone ($E_1$). **Serum E2 is reduced to a greater extent than E1**. Serum $E_1$, on the other hand, is produced primarily by peripheral aromatization from androgens, which decline principally as a function of age. Levels of $E_2$ average 15 pg/mL and range from 10 to 25 pg/mL but are closer to 10 pg/mL or less in women who have undergone oophorectomy. More sensitive assays for $E_2$ using mass spectroscopy give lower levels of $E_2$ with average levels around 3 to 5 pg/mL. Serum $E_1$ values average 30 pg/mL but may be higher in women with obesity because aromatization increases as a function of the mass of adipose tissue. Estrone sulfate ($E_1$ S) is an estrogen conjugate that serves as a stable circulating reservoir of estrogen, and levels of $E_1$ S are the highest among estrogens in postmenopausal women. In premenopausal women, values are usually more than 1000 pg/mL; in postmenopausal women, levels average 350 pg/mL. Apart from elevations in FSH and luteinizing hormone (LH), other pituitary hormones are not affected. The rise in FSH, beginning in stage −2 as early as age 38 (see Fig. 14.2), fluctuates considerably until approximately 4 years after menopause (stage +1c), when values are consistently greater than 20 mIU/mL. Specifically, growth hormone (GH), thyroid-stimulating hormone (TSH), and adrenocorticotropic hormone (ACTH) levels are normal. Serum prolactin levels may be slightly decreased because prolactin levels are influenced by estrogen status. Both the

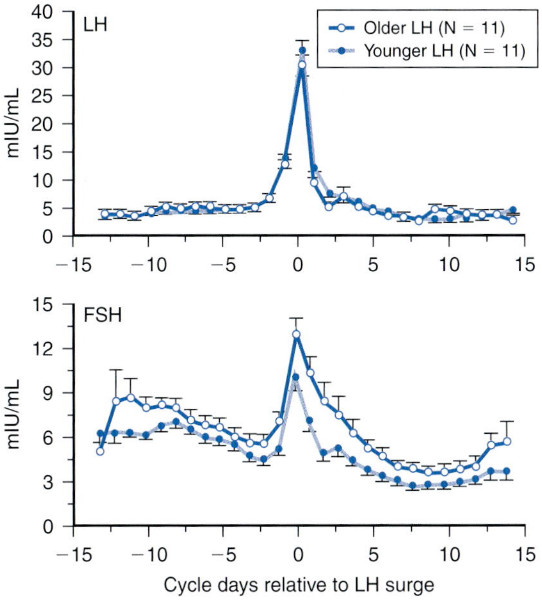


**Fig. 14.7** The daily serum follicle-stimulating hormone (FSH) and luteinizing hormone (LH) levels throughout the menstrual cycle of 11 women in each group (mean ± standard error). The gonadotropin secretion pattern in normal women of advanced reproductive age in relation to the monotropic FSH rise. (Modified from Klein NA, Battaglia DE, Clifton DK, et al. The gonadotropin secretion pattern in normal women of advanced reproductive age in relation to the monotropic FSH rise. *J Soc Gynecol Investig.* 1996;3:27.)

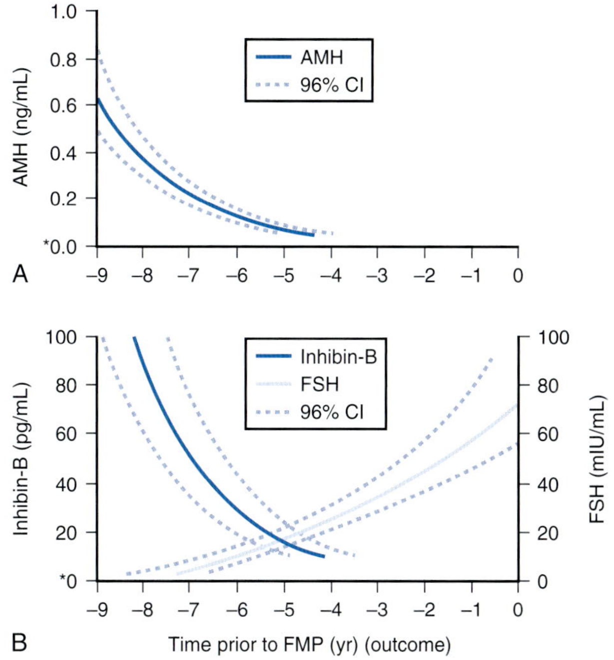


**Fig. 14.8** **A,** Antimüllerian hormone (AMH) decreases to undetectable levels (0.05 ng/mL) 5 years before the final menstrual period. **B,** Inhibin B (10 pg/mL) does so 4 years before the last menstrual period. *CI,* Confidence interval; *FMP,* Final menstrual period; *FSH,* follicle-stimulating hormone. (From Sowers MR. Eyvazzadeth AD, McConnell D, et al. Antimüllerian hormone and inhibin in the definition of ovarian aging and the menopause transition. *J Clin Endocrinol Metab.* 2008;93(9):L34768-L34783.)

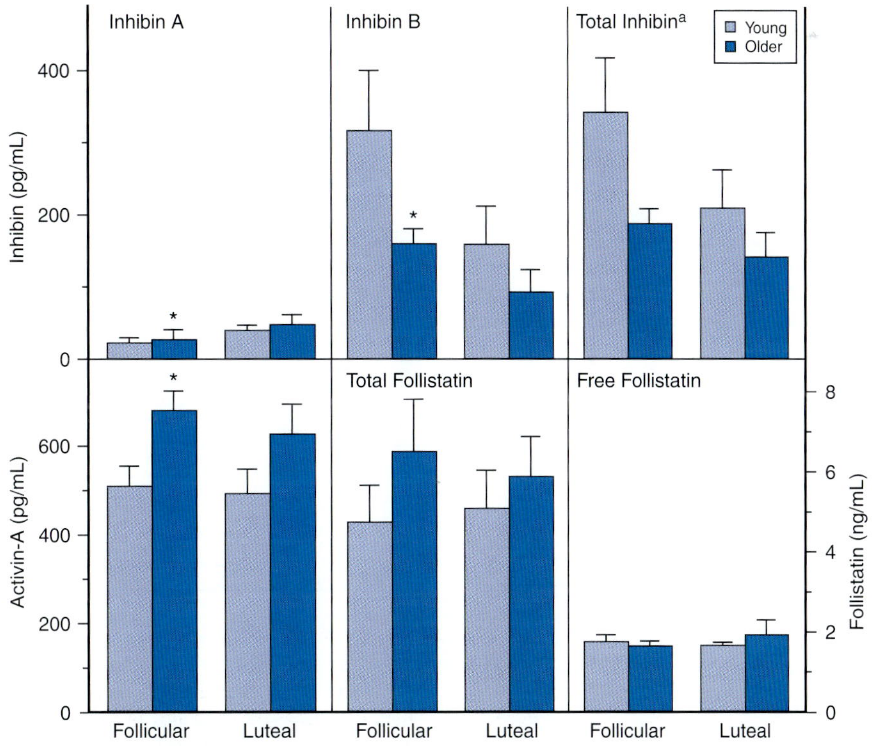


**Fig. 14.9** Mean concentrations of gonadal proteins from the same subjects. Total inhibin is a derived number from the sum of inhibin A and inhibin B. *Group differences; $P < .05$. Net increase in stimulatory input resulting from a decrease in inhibin B and an increase in activin A may contribute in part to the rise in follicular phase follicle-stimulating hormone in aging cyclic women. (Modified from Reame NE, Wyman TL, Phillips DJ, et al. Net increase in stimulatory input resulting from a decrease in inhibin B and an increase in activin A may contribute in part to the rise in follicular phase follicle-stimulating hormone of aging cyclic women. *J Clin Endocrinol Metab.* 1998;83:3302.)

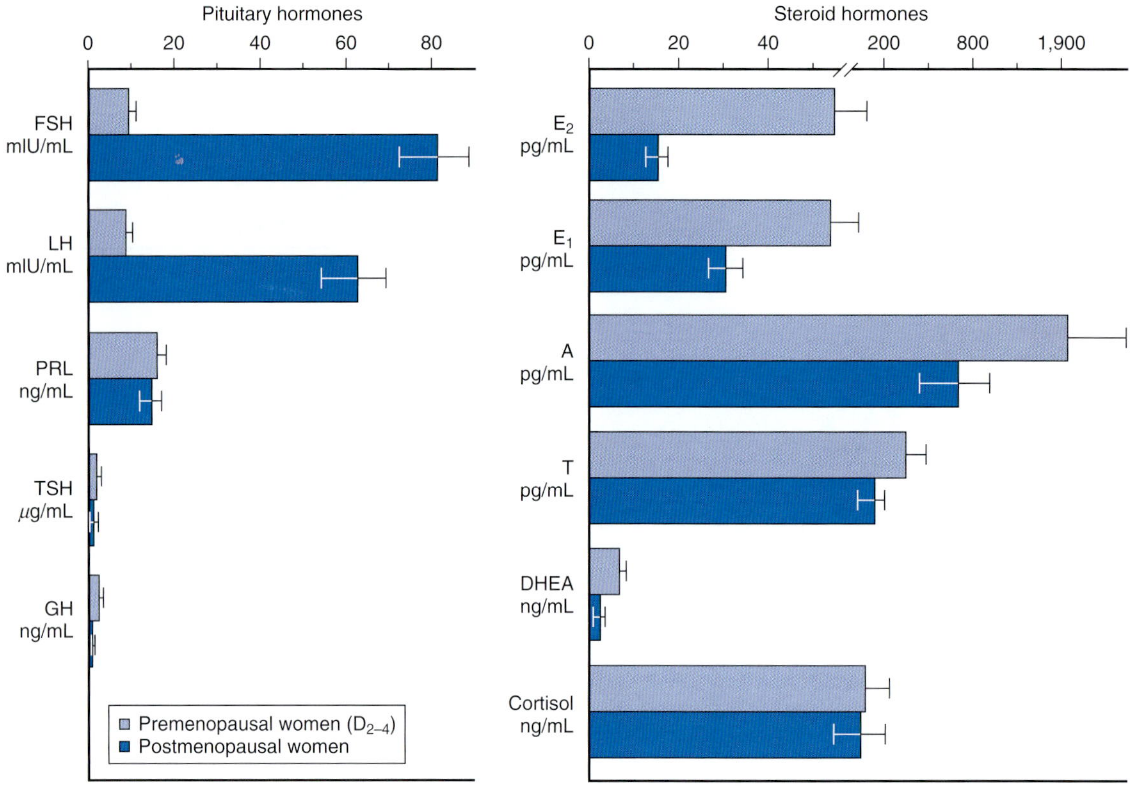


**Fig. 14.10** Circulating levels of pituitary and steroid hormones in postmenopausal women compared with levels in premenopausal women studied during the first week (days 2 to 4 [$D_{2-4}$] of the menstrual cycle. *A,* Androstenedione; *DHEA,* dehydroepiandrosterone; *$E_1$,* estrogen; *$E_2$,* estradiol; *FSH,* follicle-stimulating hormone; *GH,* growth hormone; *LH,* luteinizing hormone; *PRL,* prolactin; *T,* testosterone; *TSH,* thyroid-stimulating hormone. (Modified from Yen SSC. The biology of menopause. *J Reprod Med.* 1977;18:287.)

postmenopausal ovary and the adrenal gland continue to produce androgen. The ovary continues to produce androstenedione and testosterone but not $E_2$, and this production has been shown to be at least partially dependent on LH. Androstenedione and testosterone levels are lower in women who have experienced bilateral oophorectomy, with values averaging 0.8 ng/mL and 0.1 ng/mL, respectively. The adrenal gland also continues to produce androstenedione, DHEA, and DHEA-S; primarily as a function of aging, these values decrease somewhat (adrenopause), although cortisol secretion remains unaffected. Most "ovarian" testosterone production may actually arise from the adrenal gland by way of precursors (Couzinet, 2001). Most likely, the adrenal gland supplies precursor substrates (DHEA and androstenedione) for ovarian testosterone production. More recent measurements of 11-oxygenated androgens, which are mainly adrenal derived, will be important to investigate, but there are few data on this at present. Although DHEA-S levels decrease with age (approximately 2% per year), data have suggested that levels transiently rise in perimenopause before the continuous decline thereafter (Fig. 14.11). This interesting finding from the Study of Women Across the Nation (SWAN) also suggested that DHEA-S levels are highest in Chinese women and lowest in African American women.

Testosterone levels also decline as a function of age, which is best demonstrated by the reduction in 24-hour means levels (Fig. 14.12). Because of the role of the adrenal gland in determining levels of testosterone after menopause, adrenalectomy or dexamethasone treatment results in undetectable levels of serum testosterone. Compared with total testosterone, the measurement

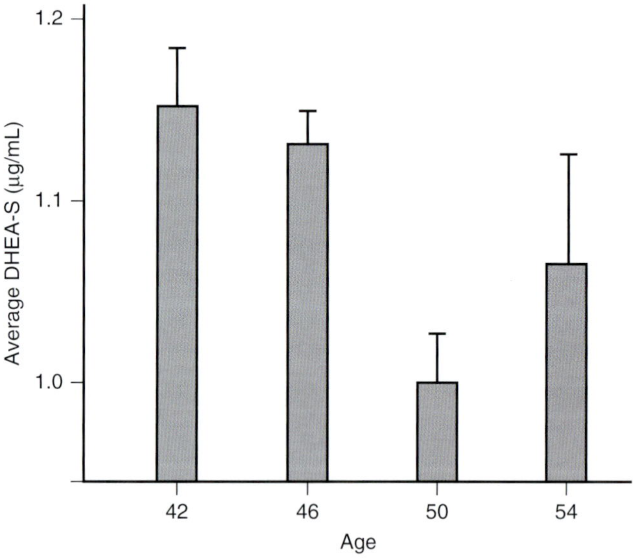


**Fig. 14.11** Mean (± standard error) circulating dehydroepiandrosterone sulfate (DHEA-S) at each year of age of the entire study population before and after adjustment for age, current smoking, menopausal status, log body mass index (BMI), ethnicity, site, and the interaction between ethnicity and log BMI. (Modified from Lasley BL, Santoro N, Randolf JF, et al. The relationship of circulating dehydroepiandrosterone, testosterone, and estradiol to stages of the menopausal transition and ethnicity. *J Clin Endocrinol Metab.* 2002;87:3760-3767.)

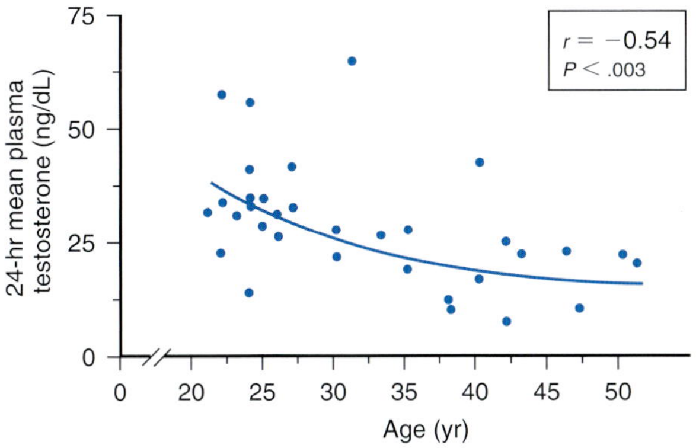


**Fig. 14.12** The 24-hour mean plasma total testosterone (T) level compared with age in normal women. The regression equation was T (nmol/L) = 37.8 × age (years) − 1.12($r = -0.54$; $P < .003$). (Modified from Zumoff B, Strain GW, Miller LK, et al. Twenty-four hour mean plasma testosterone concentration declines with age in normal premenopausal women. *J Clin Endocrinol Metab.* 1995;80:1429.)

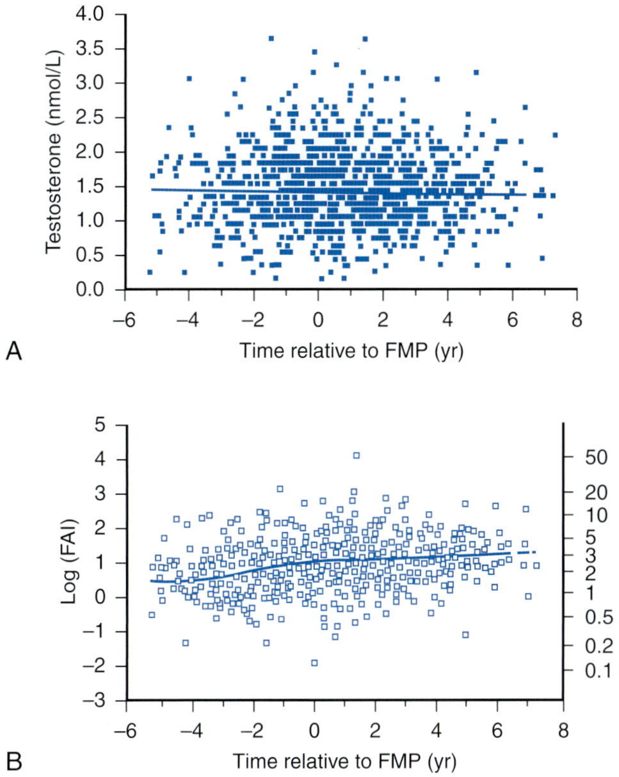


**Fig. 14.13 A,** Linear regression model: observed testosterone (T) and fitted levels of mean T across the menopausal transition. **B,** Double logistic model: observed free androgen index (FAI) and fitted levels of mean FAI across the menopausal transition. The left and right axes show FAI levels on the log and antilog scales, respectively. The horizontal axis represents time (years) with respect to first menstrual period (FMP); negative (positive) numbers indicate time before (after) FMP. (From Burger HG, Dudley EC, Cui J, et al. A prospective longitudinal study of serum testosterone, dehydroepiandrosterone sulfate, and sex hormone-binding globulin levels through the menopause transition. *J Clin Endocrinol Metab.* 2000;85:2832.)

of bioavailable, or "free," testosterone is more useful in postmenopausal women. After menopause, sex hormone–binding globulin (SHBG) levels decrease, resulting in relatively higher levels of bioavailable testosterone or a higher free androgen index (Fig. 14.13). In women receiving oral estrogen, bioavailable testosterone levels are extremely low because SHBG levels are increased. How this relates to the decision to consider androgen therapy in postmenopausal women is discussed later in this chapter.

Elevated gonadotropin (FSH/LH) levels arise from reduced secretion of $E_2$ and inhibin, as described earlier. Although some aging effects of the brain are likely to exist, there is abundant human evidence that menopause in women is an ovarian-induced event.

## EFFECTS OF MENOPAUSE ON VARIOUS ORGAN SYSTEMS

### Central Nervous System

The brain is an active site for estrogen action and estrogen formation. Estrogen activity in the brain is mediated via estrogen receptor (ER) $\alpha$ and ER$\beta$. Whether or not a novel membrane receptor (non-ER $\alpha$ /ER $\beta$) exists is still being debated. However, both genomic and nongenomic mechanisms of estrogen action clearly exist in the brain. Fig. 14.14 illustrates the predominance of ER $\beta$ in the cortex (frontal and parietal) and the cerebellum, based on work in rats. Although 17$\beta$ $E_2$ is a specific ligand for both receptors, certain synthetic estrogens (e.g., diethylstilbestrol) have greater affinity for ER$\alpha$, whereas phytoestrogens have a greater affinity for ER$\beta$.

Estrogen has multiple actions on the brain, as reviewed by Henderson (Box 14.2); thus some important functions linked to estrogen contribute to well-being in general and, more specifically, to cognition and mood. The hallmark feature of declining estrogen status in the brain is the hot flush, which is more generically referred to as a *vasomotor episode. Hot flash* usually refers to the acute sensation of heat, and the flush or vasomotor episode includes changes in the early perception of this event and other skin changes (including diaphoresis).

Hot flushes usually occur for 2 years after the onset of estrogen deficiency but can persist for 10 or more years. **Prospective data suggest that the average time for persistence of bothersome hot flushes is 7.4 years** (Avis, 2015), and up to 42% of women aged 60 to 65 years have bothersome symptoms. In 10% to 15% of women, these symptoms are severe and disabling. In the United States the incidence of these episodes varies in different ethnic groups. Symptoms are greatest in Hispanic and black women, intermediate in white women, and lowest among Asian women (Fig. 14.15). The severity and persistence of hot flushes for 10 or more years may cause a series of "irregular" symptoms, such as irritability, which may affect quality of life (Oldervave, 1993) (Fig. 14.16). The fall in estrogen levels precipitate the vasomotor symptoms. It has been found that some women who experience hot flushes have a thermoregulatory disruption with a much narrower temperature range between sweating and shivering. Freedman has shown that the difference in temperature at which shivering occurs and when sweating occurs, termed the *thermoneutral zone*, is wide in asymptomatic women (Freedman, 2007). This zone is substantially more narrowed in symptomatic women, explaining their vulnerability to vasomotor symptoms (Fig. 14.17). Although these data have validity, our current **understanding of hot flush generation relates to the thermoregulatory region of the brain (**Fig. 14.18**),** which is innervated by afferent neurokinin-kisspeptin-dynorphin neurons. **With menopause these neurons swell and activate the thermoregulatory centers, triggering flush activity. This can be attenuated by estrogen, and more specifically by the use of NK3 receptor antagonists, which provide a therapeutic**

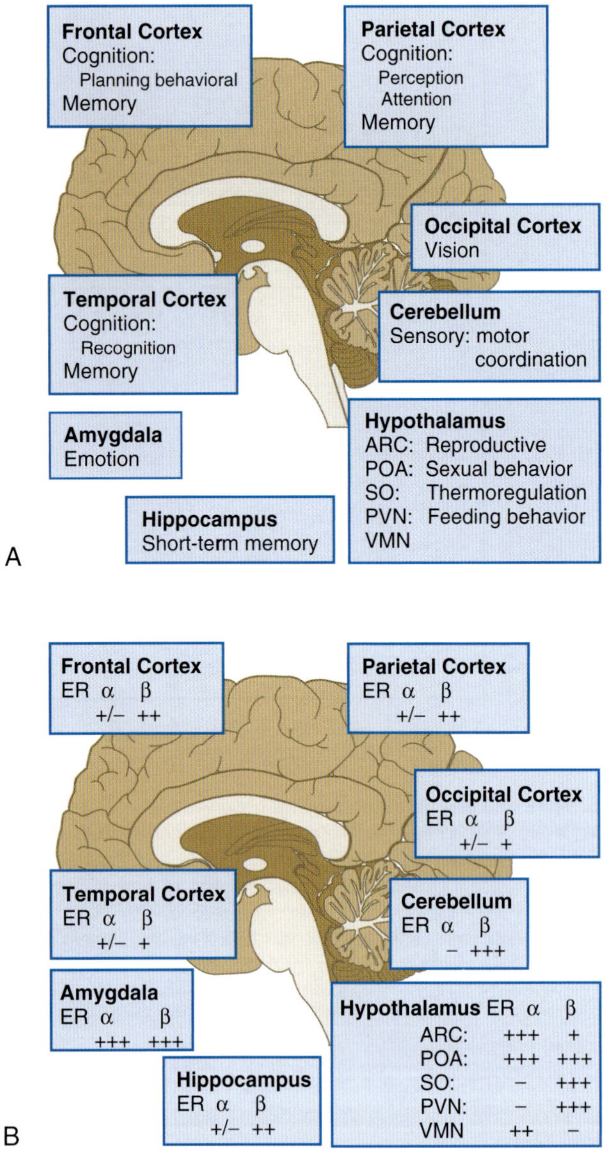


**Fig. 14.14** **A,** Each region of the brain has an important role in specific brain functions. Optimal brain activity is maintained by means of the integration of different areas by neural tracts. **B,** Distribution of ERα and ERβ messenger RNA in the rat brain. *ARC,* Arcuate nucleus; *ER,* estrogen receptor; *POA,* preoptic area; *PVN,* paraventricular nucleus; *SO,* supraoptic nucleus; *VMN,* ventromedial nucleus. (**B,** Adapted from Cela V, Naftolin F. Clinical effects of sex steroids on the brain. From Lobo RA, ed. *The Treatment of the Post-menopausal Woman: Basic and Clinical Aspects.* 2nd ed. Philadelphia: Lippincott Williams & Wilkins; 1999:247-262.)

**opportunity for nonhormonal treatment of hot flushes (Prague, 2017).**

The flush has been well characterized physiologically. It results in heat dissipation, as witnessed by an increase in peripheral temperature (fingers, toes); a decrease in skin resistance, associated with diaphoresis; and a reduction in core body temperature (Fig. 14.19). **There are hormonal correlates of flush activity, such as an increase in serum LH and in plasma levels of proopiomelanocortin peptides (ACTH, β-endorphin) at the time of the flush,** but these occurrences are thought to be epiphenomena that result as a consequence of the flush and are not related to its cause. One of the primary complaints of women with hot flushes is **sleep disruption.** They may awaken several times during the night and require a change of bedding and clothes because of diaphoresis. Nocturnal sleep disruption in postmenopausal women with hot flushes has been well documented by electroencephalographic (EEG) recordings. Sleep efficiency is lower, and the latency to rapid eye movement (REM) sleep is longer in women with hot flushes compared with asymptomatic women. This disturbed sleep often leads to fatigue and irritability during the day, and sleep may be disrupted even if the woman is not conscious of being awakened from sleep. In this setting, EEG monitoring has indicated sleep disruption occurs in concert with physiologic measures of vasomotor episodes. The frequency of awakenings and hot flushes is reduced appreciably with estrogen treatment (Fig. 14.20).

In postmenopausal women, estrogen has been found to improve depressed mood regardless of whether or not this is a specific complaint (critics of some of this work point out that mood is affected by the symptomology and by sleep deprivation). Blinded studies carried out in asymptomatic women have also shown benefit. In an estrogen-deficient state such as occurs after menopause, a higher incidence of depression (clinical or subclinical) is often manifest. However, menopause per se does not cause depression, and although estrogen does generally improve depressive moods, it should not be used for psychiatric disorders. Nevertheless, very high pharmacologic doses of estrogen have been used to treat certain types of psychiatric depression.

**BOX 14.2** Effects of Estrogen on Brain Function

**ORGANIZATIONAL ACTIONS**

Effects on neuronal number, morphology, and connections occurring during critical stages of development

**NEUROTROPHIC ACTIONS**

Neuronal differentiation
Neurite extension
Synapse formation
Interactions with neurotrophins

**NEUROPROTECTIVE ACTIONS**

Protection against apoptosis
Antioxidant properties
Antiinflammatory properties
Augmentation of cerebral blood flow
Enhancement of glucose transport into the brain
Blunting of corticosteroid response to behavioral stress
Interactions with neurotrophins

**NEUROTRANSMITTERS AFFECTED**

Acetylcholine
Noradrenaline
Serotonin
Dopamine
Glutamate
Gamma-aminobutyric acid
Neuropeptides

**EFFECTS ON GLIAL CELLS**

**PROTEINS INVOLVED IN ALZHEIMER DISEASE EFFECTED**

Amyloid precursor protein
Tau protein
Apolipoprotein E

Modified from Henderson VW. Estrogen, cognition, and a woman's risk of Alzheimer's disease. *Am J Med.* 1997;103(Suppl 3A):11.

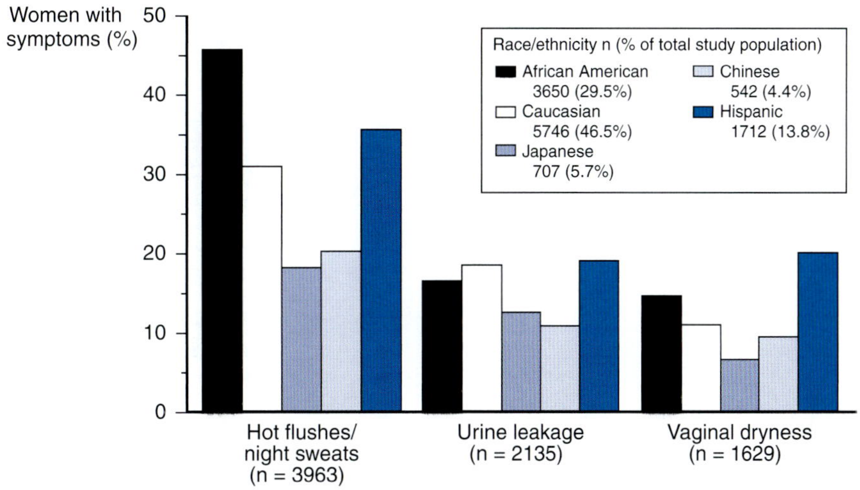


**Fig. 14.15** The Study of Women's Health Across the Nation (SWAN). Symptom severity. (Modified from Gold EB, Sternfeld B, Kelsey JL, et al. Relation of demographic and lifestyle factors to symptoms in a multi-racial/ethnic population of women 40 to 55 years of age. *Am J Epidemiol.* 2000;152:463.)

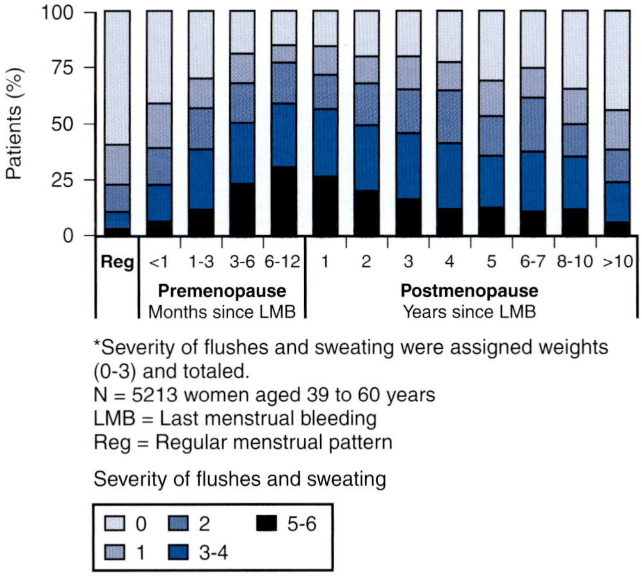


**Fig. 14.16** Impact of menopause on well-being. (Modified from Oldenhave A, Jaszmann LJ, Haspels AA, et al. Impact of climacteric on well-being: a study based on 5213 women 39 to 60 years old. *Am J Obstet Gynecol.* 1993;168:772.)

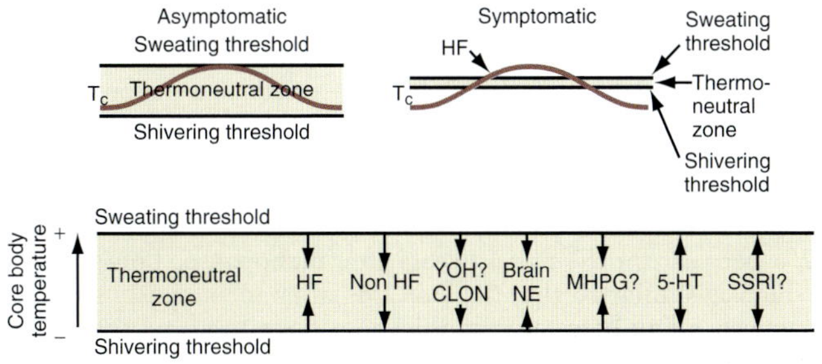


**Fig. 14.17** Narrowing of the thermoregulatory zone in symptomatic women. *5-HT,* 5-Hydroxytryptamine; *HF,* Hot flush; *SSRI,* selective serotonin reuptake inhibitor. (Data from Freedman RR. Menopausal hot flashes. In: Lobo RA, ed. *Treatment of the Postmenopausal Woman.* 4th ed. New York: Academic Press; 2007:187-198.)

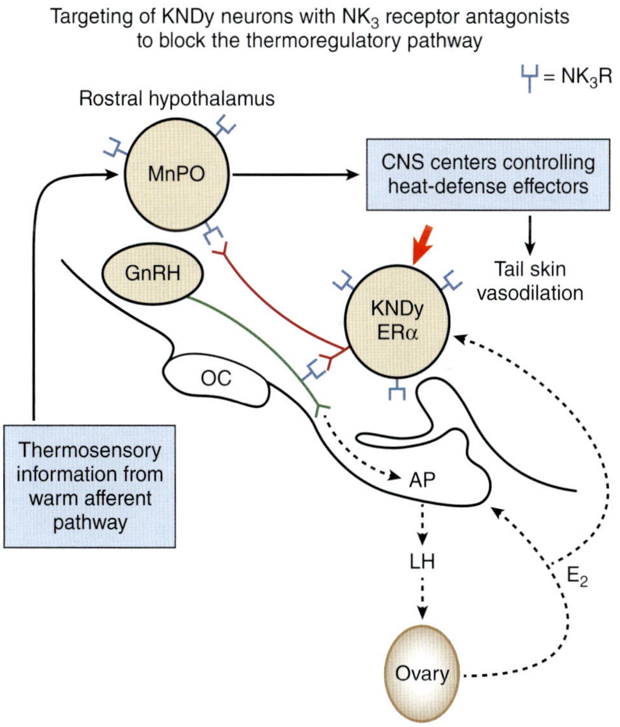


**Fig. 14.18** Targeting the KNDy neuron with neurokinin 3 (NK3) receptor antagonists to block the thermoregulatory pathway, which has neuronal connections from the mid hypothalamus to the rostral hypothalamus where thermoregulatory control occurs (rat model). *CNS,* central nervous system; *$E_2$,* estradiol; *ER,* estrogen receptor; *GnRH,* gonadotropin-releasing hormone; *KNDy,* kisspeptin/neurokinin B/dynorphin; *LH,* luteinizing hormone. Modified from Mittelman-Smith MA, Williams H, Krajewski-Hall SJ, et al. Role for kisspeptin/neurokinin B/dynorphin (KNDy) neurons in cutaneous vasodilatation and the estrogen modulation of body temperature. *Proc Natl Acad Sci U S A.* 2012;109(48):19846-19851.

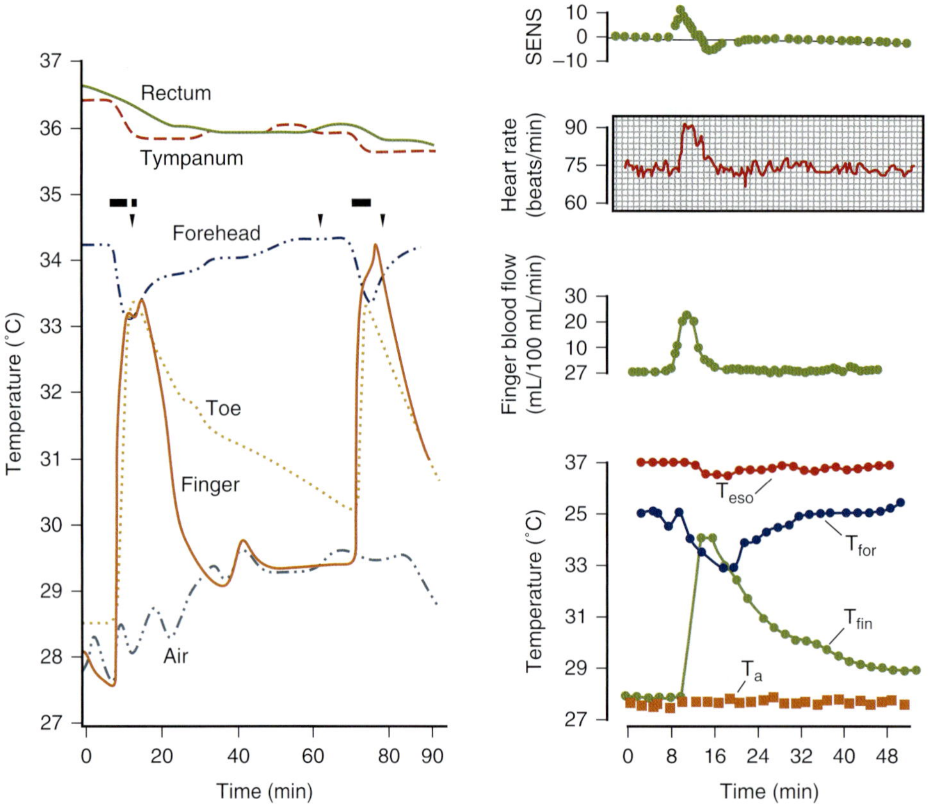


**Fig. 14.19** Temperature responses to two spontaneous flashes and evoked flash. *Down arrow* indicates finger stab for blood sample. *Black bars* indicate time of flush. *SENS,* sensation; $T_{fin}$, temperature at various places on the body. (Data from Molnar GW: Body temperature during menopausal hot flushes. *J Appl Physiol.* 1975;38(3):499-303.)

Progestogens as a class generally attenuate the beneficial effects of estrogen on mood, although this effect is highly variable.

Cognitive decline in postmenopausal women is related to aging and to estrogen deficiency. The literature is somewhat mixed about whether there are benefits of estrogen in terms of cognition. **Studies have suggested that in natural menopause, there is an early decline in cognitive function at the onset of menopause, but this spontaneously improves over time,** (Greendale, 2009). **Verbal memory appears to be enhanced with estrogen** and has been found to correlate with acute changes in brain imaging, signifying brain activation. Dementia increases as women age, and the most common form of dementia is Alzheimer disease (AD). Box 14.2 lists several neurotropic and neuroprotective factors related to how estrogen deficiency may be expected to result in the loss of protection against the development of AD. In addition, estrogen has a positive role in enhancing neurotransmitter function, which is deficient in women with AD. This function of estrogen has particular importance and relevance for the cholinergic system, which is affected in AD. **Estrogen use after menopause appears to decrease the likelihood of developing or delaying the onset of AD according to several observational studies and meta-analyses.** However, once a woman is affected by AD, estrogen is unlikely to provide any benefit. Data from the Women's Health Initiative (WHI), however, suggested a lack of benefit of estrogen or estrogen/progestogen, or even a worsening of cognition, in women initiating hormonal therapy after age 65. This suggests that **timing of initiation of HT is critical**, and this has also been supported by basic science studies, which have found that early exposure to estrogen decreased the possibility of brain damage from free radicals and also promoted maintenance of neuronal and synaptic activity. However, prospective trials in younger women still have not been able to confirm the older observational data, suggesting a cognitive benefit of estrogen. Therefore this area remains somewhat inconclusive. In summary, **although early treatment with estrogen in younger women at the onset of menopause *may* be beneficial for cognition as it is with certain types of mood (although not proved yet), later treatment (e.g., after age 65) has no benefit and may even be detrimental, depending on the regimen of hormones used.**

## Collagen and Other Tissues

**Estrogen has a positive effect on collagen**, which is an important component of bone and skin and serves as a major support tissue for the structures of the pelvis and urinary system. Both estrogen and androgen receptors have been identified in skin fibroblasts. **Nearly 30% of skin collagen is lost within the first 5 years after menopause**, and collagen decreases approximately 2% per year for the first 10 years after menopause. This statistic, which is similar to that of bone loss after menopause, strongly suggests a link between skin thickness, bone loss, and the risk of **osteoporosis.** Although the literature is not entirely consistent, **estrogen therapy generally improves collagen content after menopause and improves skin thickness substantially** after about 2 years of treatment (Dunn, 1997). There is a possible bimodal effect with high doses of estrogen causing a reduction in skin thickness. The supportive effect of estrogen on collagen has

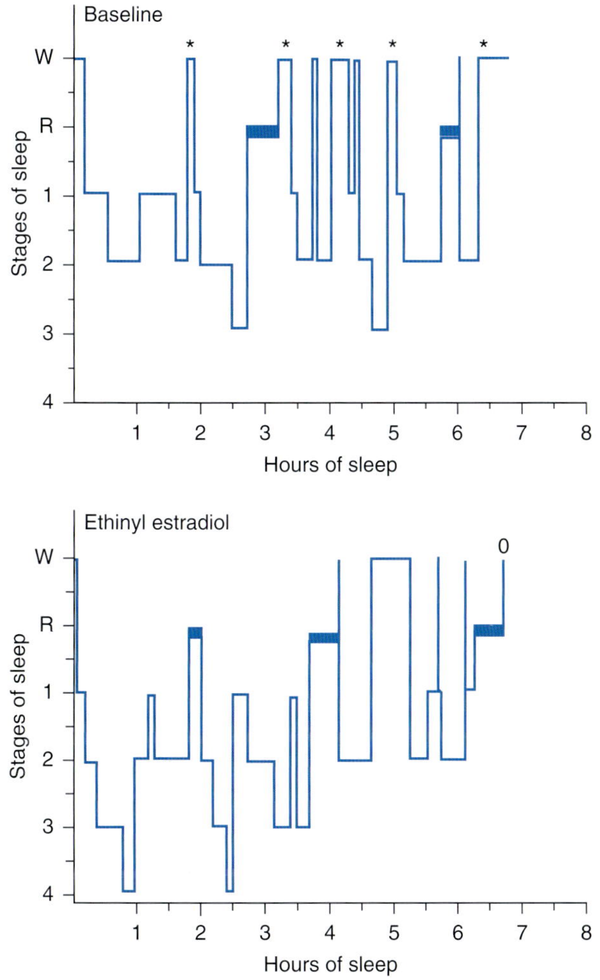


**Fig. 14.20** Sleep grams measured in a symptomatic patient before and after a 30-day administration of ethinyl estradiol, 50 μg four times daily. (Modified from Erlik Y, Tataryn IV, Meldrum DR, et al. Association of waking episodes with menopausal hot flushes. *JAMA.* 1981; 245:1741.)

important implications for bone homeostasis and for the pelvis after menopause. Here, reductions in collagen support and atrophy of the vaginal and urethral mucosa have been implicated in a variety of symptoms, including prolapse and urinary symptoms (Falconer, 1996). Vaginal estrogen has also been shown to reduce recurrent urinary tract infections. Symptoms of urinary incontinence and irritative bladder symptoms occur in 20% to 40% of perimenopausal and postmenopausal women. Uterine prolapse and other gynecologic symptoms related to poor collagen support, as well as urinary complaints, may improve with estrogen therapy. Although estrogen generally improves symptoms, urodynamic changes have not been shown to be altered. Estrogen has also been shown to decrease the incidence of recurrence of urinary tract infections. Restoration of bladder control in older women with estrogen has been shown to decrease the need for admission to nursing homes in Sweden. Estrogen may also have an important role in normal wound healing. In this setting, estrogen enhances the effects of growth factors such as transforming growth factor-β (TGF-β) (Ashcroft, 1997).

Although still not completely settled, it appears that oral estrogen does not improve stress urinary incontinence in postmenopausal women and may even cause such symptoms in previously asymptomatic older women. Estrogen may, however, improve urge and other irritative urinary symptoms.

**TABLE 14.2** Genitourinary Syndrome of Menopause (GSM): Symptoms and Signs

| Symptoms | Signs |
|---|---|
| Genital dryness | Decreased moisture |
| Decreased lubrication with sexual activity | Decreased elasticity |
| Discomfort or pain with sexual activity | Labia minora resorption |
| Postcoital bleeding | Pallor/erythema |
| Decreased arousal, orgasm, desire | Loss of vaginal rugae |
| Irritation/burning/itching of vulva or vagina Dysuria | Tissue fragility/fissures/petechiae |
| Urinary frequency/urgency | Urethral eversion or prolapse<br>Loss of hymenal remnants<br>Prominence of urethral meatus<br>Introital retraction<br>Recurrent urinary tract infections |
| Supportive findings: pH > 5, increased parabasal cells on maturation index, and decreased superficial cells on wet mount or maturation index. | |

Modified from Portman DJ, Gass MLS. Genitourinary syndrome of menopause: new terminology for vulvovaginal atrophy from the International Society for the Study of Women's Sexual Health and The North American Menopause Society. *Menopause.* 2014;21:1063-1068.

## Genitourinary Syndrome of Menopause

*Genitourinary syndrome of menopause (GSM)* is now the accepted terminology and replaces terms such as atrophic vaginitis or vulvovaginal atrophy. The definition encompasses subjective and objective findings of the vulva, vagina, and lower urinary tract. The constellation of established symptoms and signs may be found in Table 14.2 (Portman, 2014).

Vulvovaginal complaints are often associated with estrogen deficiency. During perimenopause, symptoms of dryness and atrophic changes occur in 21% and 15% of women, respectively. However, these findings increase with time, and by 4 years these incidences are 47% and 55%, respectively. With this change, an increase in sexual complaints also occurs, with an incidence of dyspareunia of 41% in sexually active 60-year-old women. Estrogen deficiency results in a thin, paler vaginal mucosa. The moisture content is low, the pH increases (usually >5), and the mucosa may exhibit inflammation and small petechiae.

With estrogen treatment, particularly when used locally, vaginal cytologic changes have been documented, transforming from a cellular pattern of predominantly parabasal cells to one with an increased number of superficial cells. Along with these changes, the vaginal pH decreases, the vaginal blood flow increases, and the electropotential difference across the vaginal mucosa increases to that found in premenopausal women. Vaginal DHEA (0.25% to 1.0%) has been used with some suggested efficacy; the mechanism is presumed to be the local conversion of DHEA into estrogen, with possibly some other modulating effects as well (Heo, 2019).

Ospemifene 60 mg, a selective estrogen receptor agonist (SERM), has been approved as an oral treatment for vulvovaginal atrophy. This SERM has particular properties of acting as an agonist in the vagina and as an antagonist in other tissues such as the breast.

The approach to urinary symptoms will be addressed in different chapters.

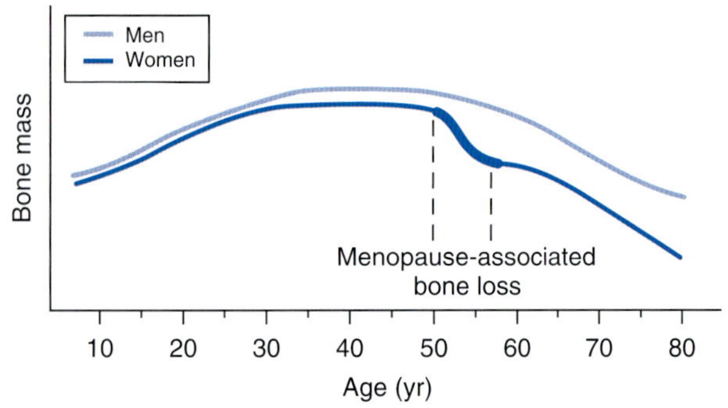


**Fig. 14.21** Bone mass by age and sex. (Modified from Finkelstein JS: Osteoporosis. In: Goldman L, Bennet JC, eds. *Cecil Textbook of Medicine.* 21st ed. Philadelphia: Saunders; 1999:1366-1373; and Riggs BL, Melton LJ III. Involutional osteoporosis. *N Engl J Med.* 1986;314:1676.)

## Bone Health

**Estrogen deficiency has been well established as a cause of bone loss.** This loss can be noted for the first time when menstrual cycles become irregular in perimenopause from 1.5 years before menopause to 1.5 years after menopause, and spine bone mineral density (BMD) has been shown to decrease by 2.5% per year, compared with a premenopausal loss rate of 0.13% per year. Loss of **trabecular bone** (spine) is greater with estrogen deficiency than is loss of **cortical bone**.

Postmenopausal bone loss leading to osteoporosis is a substantial health care problem. In Caucasian women, 35% of all postmenopausal women have been estimated to have osteoporosis based on BMD. Furthermore, the lifetime fracture risk for these women is 40%. The morbidity and economic burden of osteoporosis is well documented. Interestingly, some data suggest that up to 19% of Caucasian men also have osteoporosis. Bone mass is substantially affected by sex steroids through classic mechanisms to be described later in this chapter. Attainment of peak bone mass in the late second decade (Fig. 14.21) is key to ensuring that the subsequent loss of bone mass with aging and estrogen deficiency does not lead to early osteoporosis. $E_2$ together with GH and insulin-like growth factor-1 act to double bone mass at the time of puberty, beginning the process of attaining peak bone mass. Postpubertal estrogen deficiency (amenorrhea from various causes) substantially jeopardizes peak bone mass. Adequate nutrition and calcium intake are also key determinants. Although estrogen is of predominant importance for bone mass in both women and men, testosterone is important in stimulating periosteal apposition; as a result, cortical bone in men is larger and thicker.

However, even in men estrogen appears to be important for bone health in that in male individuals with aromatase deficiency (inability to convert androgen to estrogen) osteoporosis ensues (Carani, 1997).

Estrogen receptors are present in osteoblasts, osteoclasts, and osteocytes. Both ER$\alpha$ and ER$\beta$ are present in cortical bone, whereas ER$\beta$ predominates in cancellous or trabecular bone (Bord, 2001). However, the more important actions of $E_2$ are believed to be mediated via ER$\alpha$. Estrogens suppress bone turnover and maintain a certain rate of bone formation. Bone is remodeled in functional units, called *bone multicenter units* (BMUs), where resorption and formation should be in balance. Multiple sites of bone go through this turnover process over time. Estrogen decreases osteoclasts by increasing apoptosis, thus reducing their life span. The effect on the osteoblast is less consistent, but $E_2$ antagonizes glucocorticoid-induced osteoblast apoptosis. Estrogen deficiency increases the activities of remodeling units, prolongs resorption, and shortens the phase of bone formation. It also increases osteoclast recruitment in BMUs, and thus resorption outstrips formation. The molecular mechanisms of estrogen action on bone involve the inhibition of production of proinflammatory cytokines, which increase with a decrease in estrogen at menopause, leading to increased bone resorption (Pacifici, 1996). These cytokines include interleukin-1, interleukin-6, tumor necrosis factor-$\alpha$, colony-stimulating factor-1, macrophage colony-stimulating factor, and prostaglandin $E_2$, all of which may contribute to increased resorption. $E_2$ also upregulates TGF-$\beta$ in bone, which inhibits bone resorption. Receptor activation of nuclear factor kappa B (NF$\kappa$B) ligand (RANKL) is responsible for osteoclast differentiation and action. A scheme for how all these factors interact has been proposed (Fig. 14.22) (Riggs, 2000). In women, Riggs has suggested that bone loss occurs in two phases. With estrogen levels declining at the onset of menopause, an accelerated phase of bone loss, which is predominantly of cancellous bone, occurs. Approximately 20% to 30% of cancellous bone and 5% to 10% of cortical bone can be lost in a span of 4 to 8 years. Thereafter, a slower phase of loss (1% to 2% per year) ensues, during which more cortical bone is lost. This phase is thought to be induced primarily by secondary hyperparathyroidism. The first phase is also accentuated by the decreased influence of stretching or mechanical factors, which generally promotes bone homeostasis, as a result of estrogen deficiency. Genetic influences on bone mass are more important for the attainment of peak bone mass (heritable component, 50% to 70%) than for bone loss. Polymorphisms of the vitamin D receptor gene, TGF-$\beta$ gene, and the Spl binding site in the collagen type 1 Al gene have all been implicated as being important for bone mass (Nguyen, 2000).

Bone mass can be detected by a variety of radiographic methods (Table 14.3). Dual-energy x-ray absorptiometry (DEXA) scans have become the standard of care for detection of **osteopenia** and osteoporosis. By convention, the **T score** is used to reflect the number of standard deviations of bone loss from the peak bone mass of a young adult. Osteopenia is defined by a T score of –1 to –2.5 standard deviations; osteoporosis is defined as greater than 2.5 standard deviations.

Various biochemical assays are also available to assess bone resorption and formation in both blood and urine (Table 14.4). At present, serum markers appear to be most useful for assessing changes, with antiresorptive therapy having less variability compared with the urinary assessments. Although these biochemical measurements cannot reliably predict bone mass, they may be useful as markers of the effectiveness of treatment. For example, an increased resorption marker may decrease within months into the normal range with an antiresorptive therapy, whereas it takes 1 to 2 years to see a change in BMD with DEXA.

Fracture risk is determined not only by bone mass but by many factors, the most important of which is bone strength. This in turn is determined by bone mass and by bone turnover, for which biochemical assessments may be helpful. **A research method employs a high-resolution quantitative computed tomography of bone, which is intended to provide a "virtual" bone biopsy.** This may be available in the future. **The World Health Organization (WHO) has made available an algorithm to predict the 10-year fracture risk of men and women living around the world. This model, called *FRAX,* can be assessed at www.shef.ac.uk/FRAX and is calculated based on individual patient history data and the results from DEXA.** Although there are other assessment tools as well, FRAX is perhaps the most used, but it requires a DEXA measurement. The FRAX tool is used as a rationale for pharmacologic therapy. For example, with osteopenia, if the FRAX score shows a **10-year risk of hip fracture of more than 3% or a 10-year risk of any other osteoporotic fracture of more than 20%, treatment should be initiated.**

In terms of the use of DEXA, U.S. Preventative Task Force guidelines suggest screening with DEXA at age 65 or older in

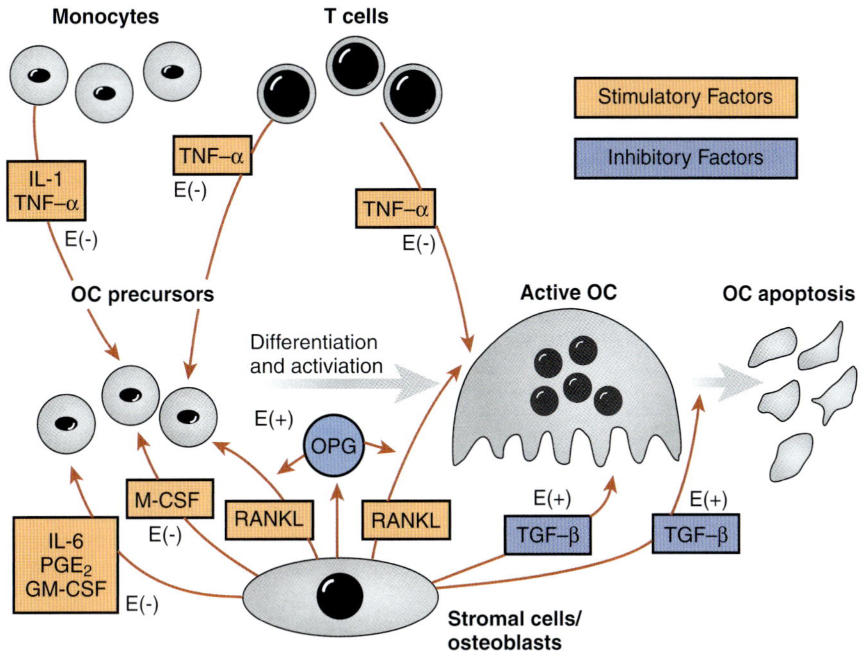


**Fig. 14.22** Model for mediation of effects of estrogen *(E)* on osteoclast formation and function by cytokines in bone marrow microenvironment. Stimulatory factors are shown in orange and inhibitory factors are shown in blue. Positive (+) or negative (−) effects of E on these regulatory factors are shown in red. The model assumes that regulation is accomplished by multiple cytokines working together in concert. *GM-CSF,* Granulocyte-macrophage colony-stimulating factor; *IL,* interleukin; *M-CSF,* macrophage colony-stimulating factor; *OC,* osteoclast; *OPG,* osteoprotegerin; *PGE*$_2$, prostaglandin E$_2$; *RANKL,* receptor activation of B ligand; *TGF-β,* transforming growth factor beta; *TNF-α,* tumor necrosis factor alpha. (Modified from Riggs BL. The mechanisms of estrogen regulation of bone resorption. *J Clin Invest.* 2000;106:1203.)

**TABLE 14.3** Techniques for the Detection of Bone Mass

| | | Precision in | Examination and Analysis | Estimated |
|---|---|---|---|---|
| | | Effective | | |
| **Technique** | **Anatomic Site of Interest** | **Vivo (%)** | **Time (min)** | **Dose** |
| Equivalent (uSv) | | | | |
| Conventional radiographs | Spine, hip<br>2000 | NA | <5 | 2000 |
| Radiogrammetry | Hand | 1-3 | 5-10 | <1 |
| Radiographic absorptiometry | Hand | 1-2 | 5-10 | <1 |
| Single x-ray absorptiometry | Forearm, heel | 1-2 | 5-10 | <1 |
| Dual x-ray absorptiometry | Spine, hip, forearm, total body | 1-3 | 5-20 | 1-10 |
| Quantitative computed tomography | Spine, forearm, hip | 2-4 | 10-15 | 50-100 |
| Quantitative ultrasound | Heel, hand, lower leg | 1-3 | 5-10 | None |

Modified from van Kuijk C, Genant HK. Detection of osteopenia. In: Lobo RA, ed. *Treatment of the Postmenopausal Woman: Basic and Clinical Aspects.* 2nd ed. Philadelphia: Lippincott Williams & Wilkins; 1999:287-292.
*NA,* Not applicable.

all women and in younger women with traditional risk factors for fracture (U.S. Preventive Services Task Force, 2018). These traditional risk factors include advanced age, previous fracture, glucocorticoid therapy, parental history of hip fracture, low body mass, cigarette smoking, excessive alcohol use, rheumatoid arthritis and secondary osteoporosis as a result of factors such as hypogonadism/POI, malabsorption, and liver disease.

Many agents are now available for preventing osteoporosis. Guidelines for initiating treatment are history of a fracture, osteoporosis as determined on DEXA, or osteopenia with FRAX scores, as noted earlier. It is important to make a distinction about using various agents for the *prevention* of osteoporosis (e.g., in a woman who has risk factors and is osteopenic: T score greater than −2.5) as opposed to using drugs to *treat* established osteoporosis (T scores greater than −2.5).

**TABLE 14.4** Bone Turnover Markers

| Marker | Specimen |
|---|---|
| **Bone Resorption Markers** | |
| Cross-linked N-telopeptide of type I collagen (NTX) | Urine, serum |
| Cross-linked C-telopeptide of type I collagen (CTX) | Urine (αα and ββ forms), serum (ββ form) |
| MMP-generated telopeptide of type I collagen (ICTP or CTX-MMP) | Serum |
| Deoxypyridinoline, free and peptide bound (fDPD, DPD) | Urine, serum |
| Pyridinoline, free and peptide bound (fPYD, PYD) | Urine serum |
| Hydroxyproline (OHP) | Urine |
| Glycosyl hydroxylysine (GylHyl) | Urine, serum |
| Helical peptide (HelP) | Urine |
| Tartrate resistant acid phosphatase | Serum, plasma |
| 5b Isoform specific for osteoclasts (TRACP 5b) | |
| Cathepsin K (Cath K) | Urine, serum |
| Osteocalcin fragments (uOC) | Urine |
| Bone Formation Markers | |
| Osteocalcin (OC) | Serum |
| Procollagen type I C-terminal propeptide (PICP) | Serum |
| Procollagen type I N-terminal propeptide (PINP) | Serum |
| Bone-specific alkaline phosphatase (bone ALP) | Serum |

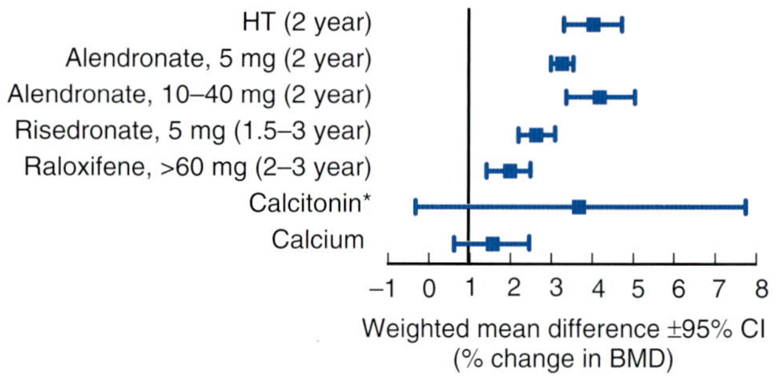


**Fig. 14.23** Meta-analysis of osteoporosis therapies: total hip bone mineral density (BMD). *CI,* Confidence interval; *HT,* Hormone therapy. (From Cranney A, Guyatt G, Griffith L, et al. Meta-analyses of therapies for postmenopausal osteoporosis. IX: summary of meta-analyses of therapies for postmenopausal osteoporosis. *Endocr Rev.* 2002;23:570; data from Cranney A, Tugwell P, Wells G, et al. Meta-analyses of therapies for postmenopausal osteoporosis. I. Systematic reviews of randomized trials in osteoporosis: introduction and methodology. *Endocrine Rev.* 2002;23:496.)

The use of estrogen depends on whether there are other indications for estrogen treatment and whether there are any possible contraindications. Estrogen has been shown to reduce the risk of osteoporosis and to reduce osteoporotic fractures. A dose equivalent of 0.625 mg of conjugated equine estrogens (CEEs) was once thought to be necessary for the prevention of osteoporosis, but we now know that lower doses (0.3 mg of CEE or its equivalent) in combination with progestogens, or even with adequate calcium alone, can prevent bone loss, although there are no long-term fracture data with lower-dose therapy. Whether the addition of progestogens by stimulating bone formation increases bone mass beyond that produced by estrogen alone is unclear. The androgenic activity of certain progestogens such as norethindrone acetate (NET) also has been suggested to play a role by stimulating bone formation. Fig. 14.23 provides data on changes in BMD at the hip using various agents (Cranney, 2002). Companion figures from the same review (not shown) provide data on vertebral and other nonvertebral fractures. Although these data from an earlier meta-analysis have been updated, the graphic comparisons are basically unchanged. A more recent network meta-analysis suggests that for prevention of hip fracture, compared with placebo, only the following agents have efficacy: romosozumab, an anabolic agent (relative risk [RR], 0.44); alendronate (RR, 0.61); zoledronate (RR, 0.60); risedronate (RR, 0.73); denosumab (RR, 0.56), estrogen/progestogen (RR, 0.72); and calcium with vitamin D (RR, 0.81) (Barrionuevo, 2019).

**SERMs** such as **raloxifene**, droloxifene, and tamoxifen all have been shown to decrease bone resorption. Raloxifene has been shown to decrease vertebral fractures in a large prospective trial (Ettinger, 1999). All of these agents are used for *prevention.* In younger women, one complicating factor is that agents such as raloxifene may induce hot flushes; however, they do afford some protection for breast cancer risk because they act as estrogen antagonists at the level of the breast. SERMs such as raloxifene act as a low-dose estrogen and can prevent vertebral fractures but not hip fractures. **Tibolone** (structurally related to 19-nor progestins) has also been shown to be an effective treatment for the prevention of osteoporosis. Tibolone (not marketed in the United States) has SERM-like properties, but it is not specifically a SERM because it has mixed estrogenic, antiestrogenic, androgenic, and progestogenic properties as a result of its metabolites. The drug does not seem to cause uterine or breast cell proliferation and also is beneficial for vasomotor symptoms. It prevents osteoporosis and has been shown to be beneficial in treatment of osteoporosis as well at a dose of 2.5 mg daily.

**Bisphosphonates** have been shown to have a significant effect on the *prevention and treatment* of osteoporosis, using similar doses for both indications. With this class of agents (etidronate, alendronate, risedronate, ibandronate, and zoledronic acid), incorporation of the bisphosphonate with hydroxyapatite in bone increases bone mass. The skeletal half-life of bisphosphonates in bone can be as long as 10 years, and their effects on the skeleton are sustained for a few years after discontinuation, which does not occur with other agents. These agents reduce both spine and hip fractures (see Fig. 14.23). Most data have been derived with **alendronate**, which, at a dosage of 5 mg daily (35 mg weekly), prevents bone loss; at 10 mg daily (70 mg weekly), alendronate is an effective treatment for osteoporosis, with evidence available that this treatment reduces vertebral and hip fractures (Cummings, 1998). Similar data are available for **risedronate** (35 mg weekly). **Ibandronate** has been approved as a once-a-month treatment (150 mg), and some data to date support the reduction in vertebral fractures. It can also be injected (3 mg) every 3 months. **Zoledronic acid 5 mg is available as an intravenous infusion** (over 15 minutes) once a year for the treatment of osteoporosis and every 2 years for prevention. **This class of medications has the property of causing esophageal irritation, and care must be taken in administering the oral doses in an upright position with a full glass of water.**

Some concern has been raised about bisphosphonates and osteonecrosis of the jaw, fractures of long bones such as the femur with long-term use, and atrial fibrillation. Jaw problems only occur with high doses when poor dentition is present. Femur fractures with long-term use are extremely rare, and atrial fibrillation, although statistically increased with bisphosphonate use, is also rare. Nevertheless, we do not have long-term data (>10 years), and these drugs should not be used for more than 10 years and not with another antiresorptive agent. Their use in younger postmenopausal women (<60 years) should be limited unless there is significant osteoporosis present.

**RANKL** secreted by osteoblasts causes bone resorption (see Fig. 14.22). **Denosumab** is a monoclonal antibody that binds up RANKL, thus preventing bone resorption. It is an effective treatment for osteoporosis, and although it can also be used for prevention, it is largely viewed as a secondary agent, particularly for women intolerant to other treatments. Denosumab 60 mg is administered subcutaneously every 6 months, and it is effective both at the vertebrae and at the hip, with an efficacy that is similar to or greater than that of the bisphosphonates. Unlike the bisphosphonates, however, the effects wear off immediately after discontinuation of treatment. Although denosumab does not carry the small risks of jaw osteonecrosis and long bone fractures, as an immune therapy, long-term effects of immune modulation are not known.

Calcitonin (50 IU subcutaneous injections daily or 200 IU intranasally) has been shown to inhibit bone resorption, and vertebral fractures have been shown to decrease with calcitonin therapy. Long-term effects, however, have not been established, and this is not a first-line therapy today.

Fluoride has been used for women with osteoporosis because it increases bone density. A lower dose (50 $\mu g$ daily) of slow-release sodium fluoride does not seem to cause adverse effects (gastritis) and has efficacy in preventing vertebral fractures.

**Intermittent parathyroid hormone (PTH) (teriparatide, abaloparatide)** is effective at increasing bone mass in women with significant osteoporosis. In a randomized trial lasting 3 years, average bone density increased in the hip and spine, with fewer fractures observed. This is a second-tier therapy reserved for severe cases of osteoporosis. Teriparatide at 20 $\mu g$ needs to be injected subcutaneously on a daily basis for no longer than 18 months (Murad, 2012).

**Romosozumab,** mentioned earlier, an anabolic agent that is a **monoclonal antibody against sclerostin, is** now approved for the treatment of severe osteoporosis. Sclerostin is a product of osteocytes and inhibits bone formation; thus **romosozumab, as an antibody, increases bone formation and reduces fractures.** Like teriparatide, it is a second-line therapy in patients with an intolerance to other drugs and for severe osteoporosis. Romosozumab 210 mg injected subcutaneously once monthly performed as well as or better than teriparatide in head to head clinical trials.

Adjunctive measures for prevention of osteoporosis are calcium, vitamin D, and exercise.

It should be noted that with all the drug therapies noted here, women should not be deficient in calcium or vitamin D, and supplements are usually required.

Calcium with vitamin D, used together, has been shown to increase bone only in older individuals and was found to be better than placebo for preventing hip fractures in the meta-analysis reviewed earlier. However, this will not be sufficient to prevent bone loss in younger women at the onset of menopause, and these modalities alone are not thought to be effective for the treatment of osteoporosis. A woman's total intake of elemental calcium should be 1500 mg daily if no agents are being used to inhibit resorption, and 400 to 800 IU of vitamin D should also be ingested. Caution should be exercised in prescribing excessive calcium, particularly in older individuals, because this has been linked to coronary events. Exercise has been shown to be beneficial for building muscle and bone mass and for reducing falls.

There has been a realization that many women in the United States are **vitamin D deficient**, particularly those in the northern parts of the country because of less sunlight exposure. Vitamin D may also be important as an antimitotic agent that may prevent certain types of cancer. Although there is some controversy about what a normal vitamin D level should be, a blood level of 25-hydroxyvitamin D (25[OH]D) less than 30 ng/mL usually warrants supplemental treatment with 25(OH)D.

Although it is clear that women with established osteoporosis (fractures or a T score of −2.5 or greater) should receive an antiresorptive agent (usually a bisphosphonate), there is more controversy regarding initiating preventive strategies in patients with T scores in the osteopenia range (–1.0 to −2.5) unless there are significant risk factors, as noted earlier. Many women, however, may sustain fractures when in this range of T scores. Age and risk factors largely help determine the need to treat those with osteopenia. In this setting, depending on the age of the woman, her family history, and whether she has vasomotor symptoms, she may be offered HT, a SERM, or a bisphosphonate. **The FRAX algorithm should be used as a guide to therapy.**

## DEGENERATIVE ARTHRITIS

Degeneration of intervertebral discs is a process that occurs rapidly after menopause. This is consistent with changes in collagen, as noted previously. There is evidence that this is benefited by estrogen after menopause.

Osteoarthritis is a source of significant distress. **Estrogen is powerful inhibitor of damage to chondrocytes**. The WHI study found that estrogen alone (but not combination hormone therapy) significantly decreased osteoarthritis. A 2018 Korean health assessment study showed that knee osteoarthritis was reduced by 30% in users of HT (Jung, 2018). However, much more work is needed in this area.

## CARDIOVASCULAR EFFECTS

Women have a very low incidence of CVD before menopause, but after menopause the risk increases significantly. Data from the Framingham study have shown that the incidence is three times lower in women before menopause than in men (3.1 per 1000 per year in women ages 45 to 49). The incidence is approximately equal in men and women aged 75 to 79 (53 and 50.4 per 1000 per year, respectively). This trend also pertains to gender differences in mortality resulting from CVD. **Coronary artery disease is the leading cause of death in women, and the lifetime risk of death is 31% in postmenopausal women versus a 3% risk of dying of breast cancer.**

Although CVD becomes more prevalent only in the later years after a natural menopause, premature cessation of ovarian function (before the average age of menopause) constitutes a significant risk. Premature menopause, occurring before age 35, has been shown to increase the risk of myocardial infarction two- to threefold, and oophorectomy before age 35 increases the risk sevenfold (Lobo, 2007).

When the possible reasons for the increase in CVD are examined, the most prevalent finding is an accelerated rise in total cholesterol in postmenopausal women. The changes of weight, blood pressure, and blood glucose with aging, although important, are not thought to be as important as the rate of rise in total cholesterol, which is substantially different in women after menopause versus men. This increase in total cholesterol is explained by increases in levels of low-density lipoprotein cholesterol (LDL-C). The oxidation of LDL-C is also enhanced, as are levels of very-low-density lipoproteins and lipoprotein (a). High-density lipoprotein cholesterol (HDL-C) levels trend downward with time, but these changes are small and inconsistent relative to the increases in LDL-C.

Coagulation balance is not substantially altered as a counterbalance of changes occurs. Some procoagulation factors increase (factor VII, fibrinogen), but so do counterbalancing factors such as antithrombin III, plasminogen, protein C, and protein S. Blood flow in all vascular beds decreases after menopause; prostacyclin production decreases, endothelin levels increase, and vasomotor responses to acetylcholine are constrictive, reflecting reduced nitric oxide synthetase activity. Most of these latter changes primarily are due to the fairly rapid reduction in estrogen levels, in that with estrogen all these parameters (generally) improve, and coronary arterial responses to acetylcholine are dilatory, with a commensurate increase in blood flow.

Circulating plasma nitrites and nitrates have also been shown to increase with estrogen, and angiotensin-converting enzyme levels tend to decrease. Estrogen and progesterone receptors have been found in vascular tissues, including coronary arteries (predominantly ERβ). In addition, some membrane effects are mediated by estrogen.

Overall, the direct vascular effects of estrogen are considered to be as important, or more important, than the changes in lipid and lipoproteins after menopause. Although replacing estrogen has been thought to be beneficial for the mechanisms previously cited, these beneficial arterial effects may only be seen in younger (stage +1[a-c]) postmenopausal women (Fig. 14.24) (Mendelsohn, 2005). Women with significant atherosclerosis or risk factors such as those studied in secondary prevention trials, who have established atherosclerosis and prior coronary disease, do not respond well to this treatment because of coronary plaque burden (see Fig. 14.24), which prevents estrogen action. Some of this lack of effect may be accounted for by increased methylation of the promoter region of ERα, which occurs with atherosclerosis and aging. Another mechanism is the significant conversion of cholesterol to 27-OH cholesterol, which also impedes estrogen's production of nitric oxide (Fig. 14.25).

In normal, nonobese postmenopausal women, carbohydrate tolerance also decreases as a result of an increase in insulin resistance. This, too, may be partially reversed by estrogen, although the data are mixed, and high doses of estrogen with or without progestogen cause a deterioration in insulin sensitivity. Biophysical and neurohormonal responses to stress (stress reactivity) are exaggerated in postmenopausal women compared with premenopausal women, and this heightened reactivity is blunted by estrogen. Whether these changes influence cardiovascular risk with estrogen deficiency is not known, but clearly estrogen treatment returns many parameters into the range of premenopausal women in early postmenopausal women. Several trials including data from both hormonal trials of the WHI have shown a reduction in the development of diabetes with HT (Bonds, 2006; Lobo, 2014).

These consistently strong basic science and clinical data for the protective effects of estrogen on the cardiovascular system together with strong **epidemiologic evidence for a protective effect of estrogen** (Fig. 14.26) led to the belief that estrogen should be prescribed to prevent CVD in women. Clinical trial data, however, have refuted this notion in women with established disease, as noted previously. **Results from several randomized trials in women have failed to show a protective effect in women with established coronary disease.** Furthermore, **a trend toward increased cardiovascular events (early harm) has been observed in this setting** in some women within the first 1 to 2 years. The WHI trial, which compared CEE/medroxyprogesterone acetate (MPA) with placebo, came to similar conclusions. Though considered to be a primary prevention trial, it studied participants in a large range of ages (mean age 63). These women did not have vasomotor symptoms and

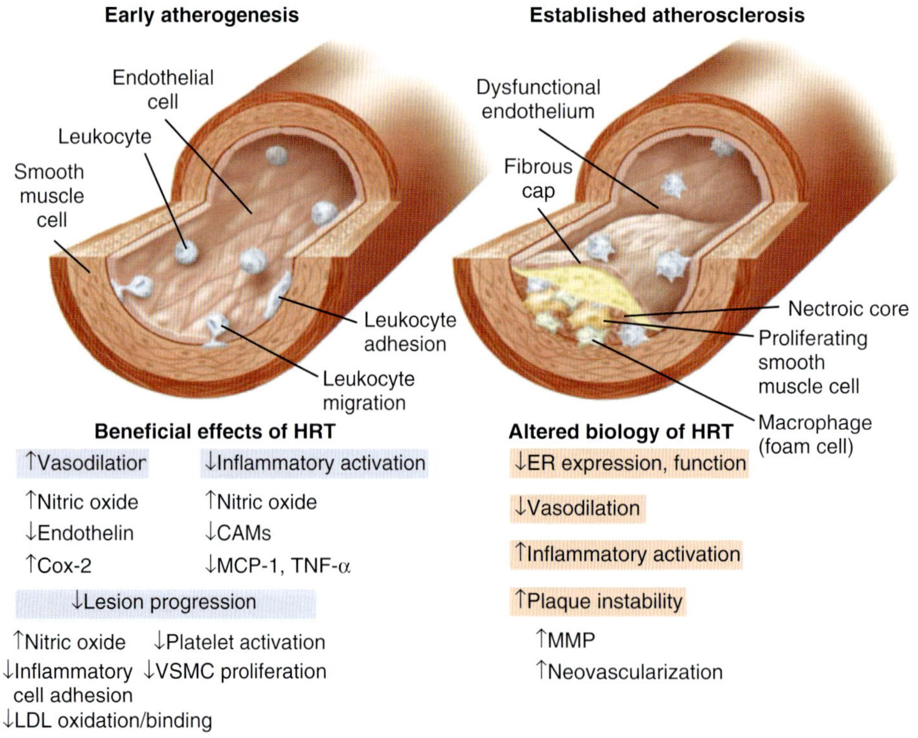


**Fig. 14.24** Mechanisms of benefit of hormonal therapy with estrogen in early menopause (relatively clean coronary vessels) and the lack of effect in older women and those with significant atherosclerotic plaque burden. *CAM,* Cellular adhesion molecule; *Cox-2,* cyclooxygenase 2; *ER,* estrogen receptor; *HRT,* hormone replacement therapy; *LDL,* low-density lipoprotein; *MCP-1,* Macrophage chemoattractant protein -1; *MMP,* matrix metalloproteinase; *TNF-α,* tumor necrosis factor alpha; VSMC, vascular smooth muscle cell. (From Mendelsohn ME, Karas RH. Molecular and cellular basis of cardiovascular gender differences. *Science* 2005;308(5728): 1583-1587.)

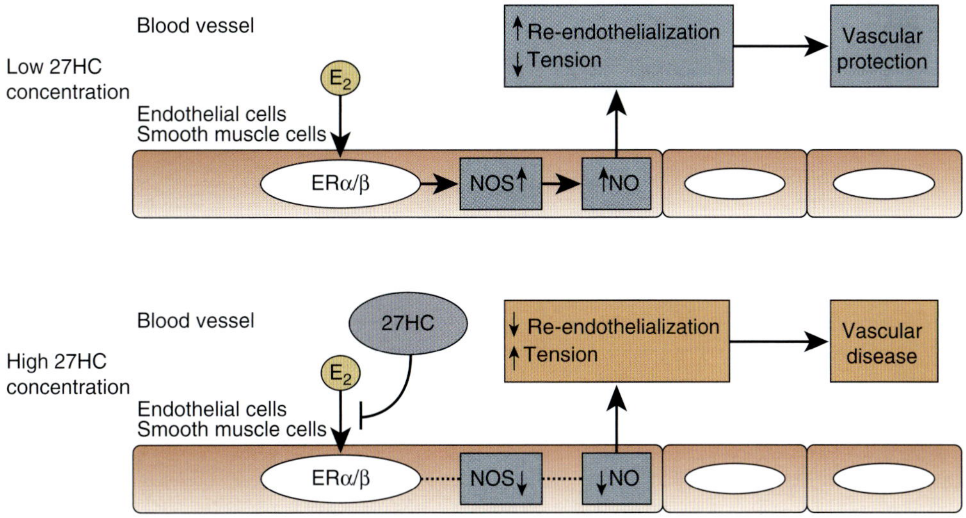


**Fig. 14.25** Hypothesis of how elevated (27-hyroxycholesterol, 27HC) can influence the effect of estradiol ($E_2$). *ER,* Estrogen receptor, *NO,* nitric oxide, *NOS,* nitric oxide synthetase. (From Umetani M, Domoto H, Gormley AK, et al. 27-Hydroxycholesterol is an endogenous SERM that inhibits the cardiovascular effects of estrogen. *Nat Med.* 2007;13(10):1185-1192.)

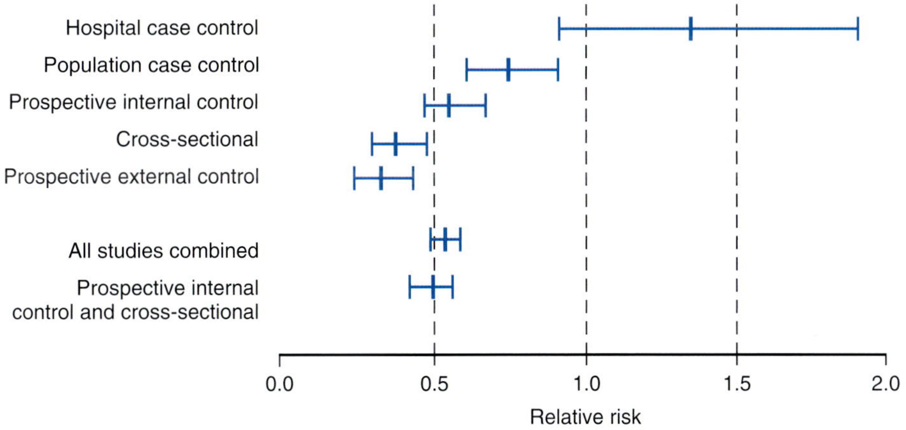


**Fig. 14.26** Estrogen replacement therapy and coronary heart disease. Relationship between relative risk and study type. (Modified from Stampfer MJ, Colditz GA. Estrogen replacement therapy and coronary heart disease: a quantitative assessment of the epidemiologic evidence. *Prev Med.* 1991;20:47.)

had more risk factors than the healthy women studied in observational cohorts, as shown in Fig. 14.26.

The protective effect of estrogen demonstrated in the observational trials such as the Nurse's Health Study (NHS) (see Fig. 14.26) occurred predominantly in young, healthy, symptomatic women. Table 14.5 compares the demographics of the participants of the WHI and the NHS. Trials carried out in a monkey model have shown a 50% to 70% protective effect against coronary atherosclerosis when estrogen is begun at the time of oophorectomy, with or without an atherogenic diet; delaying the initiation of hormonal therapy for even 2 years (in the monkey) prevents this protective effect (Fig. 14.27). This has been called the *timing hypothesis*, in which early intervention shows benefit and late intervention with hormonal therapy is possibly harmful for the cardiovascular (CV) system. This has been shown in clinical trial data (see later) and also pertains to the beneficial effects of estrogen on glucose tolerance and insulin sensitivity.

The perception of coronary harm and other risks in older women receiving combined CEE/MPA in WHI led to widespread confusion and concern about HT in general and led to most women stopping HT and not starting it even when there were significant symptoms. As will be discussed later, **more recent data now have confirmed that HT is safe for young, healthy women, and it is particularly indicated in women**

**TABLE 14.5** Demographics of Women in WHI and NHS

| | WHI | NHS |
|---|---|---|
| Mean age or age range at enrollment (years) | 63 | 30-55 |
| Smokers (past and current) | 49.9% | 55% |
| Body mass index (BMI: mean) | 28.5 kg/m$^2$ | 25.1 kg/m$^2$ |
| Aspirin users | 19.1% | 43.9% |
| Menopausal symptoms | Rare | Common |

*NHS,* Nurse's Health Study; *WHI,* Women's Health Initiative.

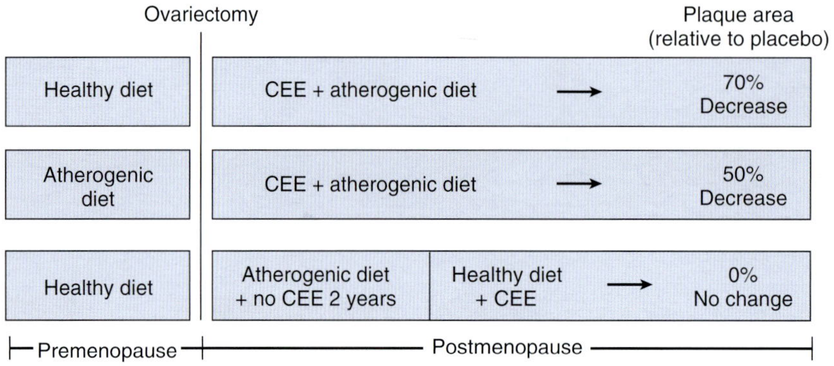


**Fig. 14.27** Importance of timing of intervention on the effect of estrogens on atherogenesis in nonhuman primates. *CEE*, Conjugated equine estrogen. (Modified from Clarkson TB, Anthony MS, Jerome CP. Lack of effect of raloxifene on coronary artery atherosclerosis of postmenopausal monkeys. *J Clin Endocrinol Metab*. 1998;83:721; data from Adams MR, Register TC, Golden DL, et al. Medroxyprogesterone acetate antagonizes inhibitory effects of conjugated equine estrogens on coronary artery atherosclerosis. *Arterioscler Thromb Vasc Biol*. 1997;17:217; Clarkson TB, Anthony MS, Morgan TM. Inhibition of postmenopausal atherosclerosis progression: a comparison of the effects of conjugated equine estrogens and soy phytoestrogens. *J Clin Endocrinol Metab*. 2001a;86:41; and Williams JK, Anthony MS, Honore EK, et al. Regression of atherosclerosis in female monkeys. *Arterioscler Thromb Vasc Biol*. 1995;15:827.)

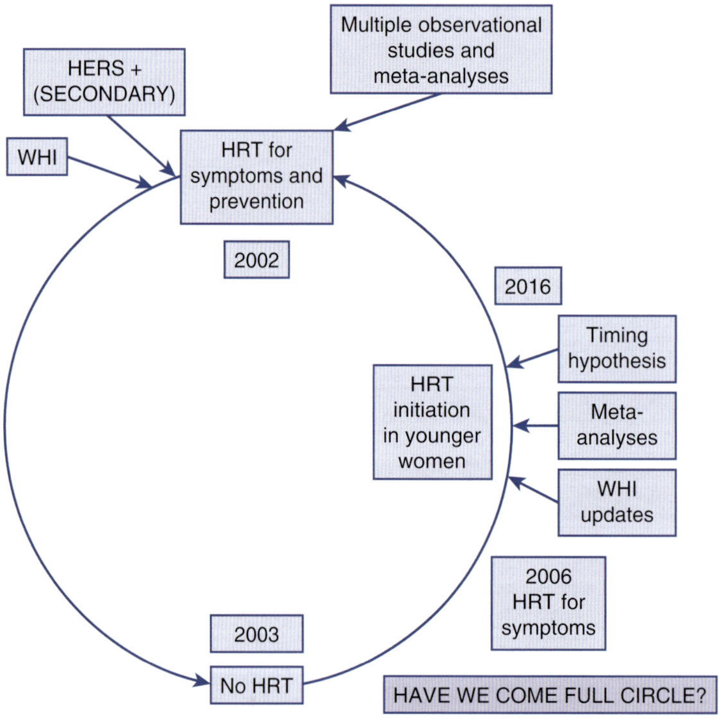


**Fig. 14.28** Diagrammatic depiction asking whether we have come full circle in the prescribing of hormone replacement therapy (HRT). HRT use before 2002, based on strong epidemiologic data and meta-analyses, was for symptom control and prevention. HRT use essentially stopped soon thereafter. Some limited use for symptoms began again around 2006. The suggestion in the figure is that the use should be coming around full circle based on new data as depicted by the arrows. *HERS*, Heart Estrogen/progestin Replacement Study; *WHI*, Women's Health Initiative. (From Lobo RA, Pickar JH, Stevenson JC, Mack WJ, Hodis HN. Back to the future: Hormone replacement therapy as part of a prevention strategy for women at the onset of menopause Atherosclerosis 2016;254:282-290.)

**with symptoms**. It appears we have come full circle as many of the original concepts of cardioprotection and reduction in all-cause mortality with estrogen have been once again confirmed from the randomized trials, when one examines the effects in younger women close to menopause (Lobo, 2016) (Fig. 14.28). However, what we have learned from the WHI is that although younger women benefit, older women do not (the timing hypothesis) and may endure harm, as several secondary prevention trials (in women with established coronary disease) have shown. No clear explanation exists for what may cause the observed "early harm," but these effects were not observed in those women receiving statins concurrently. This finding suggests that HT (in the doses used) may lead to plaque destabilization and thrombosis in some women with established (although possibly silent) coronary disease. The molecular mechanisms for this effect may be due to estrogen upregulating matrix metalloproteinase-9 and inhibiting its natural inhibitor within the mural area of the plaque; the resultant disruption of the gelatinous covering then leads to thrombosis. The antiinflammatory effects of statins inhibit this process. Additional lessons learned from WHI and more recent data are findings that **estrogen** is what is protective, and **progestogens**, depending on the type and dose, are likely to attenuate or eliminate any protective effect and also may be implicated in the risk of breast cancer.

## What Are the Current Data on the Effects of Estrogen and Estrogen/Progestogen on the Cardiovascular System?

Data from WHI first reported that the younger women, aged 50 to 59, receiving CEE alone had a significantly reduced coronary score. In 2007 the WHI reported that women aged 50 to 59 receiving CEE and CEE/MPA (combined analysis) had a significant 30% reduction in all-cause mortality (Rossouw, 2007). Subsequently pooled analyses of prospective studies, including data from the WHI, showed a statistical benefit in the reduction of coronary disease with estrogen in women less than 10 years from menopause or younger than age 60 years. A Bayesian meta-analysis (looking at retrospective and prospective studies) showed consistent data for a reduction in all-cause mortality of about 30% in younger women receiving hormonal treatment (Salpeter, 2009) (Fig. 14.29).

As discussed previously, the 13-year follow-up data from the WHI, including the intervention and follow-up phases of the trial, showed a significant benefit in younger women receiving CEE alone (Manson, 2013) (Fig. 14.30). The data with CEE/MPA were in the same direction for mortality but were less robust. These data have been updated for 18 years of follow-up, but the data have not changed in any substantial way. The most recent follow-up data regarding estrogen alone in younger women, at this writing, suggests an additional benefit for women who had experienced a bilateral salpingo-oophorectomy (Manson, 2019). Mortality at the 18-year follow-up was substantially and significantly lower in users of estrogen.

Several prospective trials in younger women deserve some discussion. A prospective trial in Denmark of 1000 recently postmenopausal women who received $E_2$ alone or $E_2$ and norethindrone (in women with a uterus) or no treatment for up to 10 years, with follow-up for up to 16 years, showed significant coronary benefit (Schierbeck, 2012). Cardiovascular death, myocardial infarction, and hospitalizations for congestive heart failure were significantly reduced in users of HT (Fig. 14.31). ELITE tested the "timing" hypothesis by treating women who were within 6 years of menopause and another group of women who were more than 10 years past menopause. Oral $E_2$ 1 mg or placebo was used in both groups, with vaginal progesterone for endometrial protection. The primary endpoint was carotid intima media thickness, which was significant reduced in recently menopausal women but not in the older women, confirming the hypothesis (Hodis, 2014) (Fig. 14.32).

A Cochrane analysis reviewed cardiovascular (CV) and overall mortality with HT and found no change in mortality when all ages and both primary and secondary prevention trials were combined (Boardman, 2015). **However, in women less than 10 years from menopause the data were consistent with findings noted previously, with significant protective effects of 30% in all-cause mortality and 40% to 50% protection from CV mortality.** However, a significant increase was noted in venous thromboembolism (VTE), which is well known to occur with oral therapy (as also occurs with oral contraceptives) but does not affect mortality. Stroke was not affected in this younger population. The complications of VTE and potentially of ischemic stroke are discussed later.

The two risk areas for CVD, even in younger women, at least potentially, are VTE and ischemic stroke. **It is now accepted that there is a two- to threefold increase in venous thrombosis risk with oral hormonal therapy.** However, the prevalence of this risk is low, particularly in young, healthy women. This two- to threefold risk is similar to that with the use of oral contraceptives. For pulmonary embolism risk, in women aged 50 to 60 years, the background risk is approximately 10 to 20 events per 100,000 woman-years. Thus with HT the twofold increase may result in 40 events per 100,000 woman-years, which is less than the rate in normal pregnancy (approximately 60/100,000 women). This risk is related to age, weight, dose, and route of administration of estrogen. It has also been suggested that some progestogens increase this risk further, although this has not been established. Most events (deep vein thrombosis or pulmonary emboli) occur early (within the first year) and decrease thereafter, suggesting an aberrant thrombophilic interaction with oral estrogen. The risk has been found not to be increased with transdermal estrogen (Canonico, 2008) (Fig. 14.33), which warrants consideration of the use of transdermal therapy in more high-risk women (e.g., those with obesity or hypertension).

Stroke (ischemic, not hemorrhagic) was found to be increased in the WHI trials (both HT and estrogen therapy [ET]). There was an approximately 30% increase over the 5 to 6 years of the trial, but this outcome was confined primarily to older women in the trial. These data are similar to data from the NHS trial where even younger women had a very small but statistically increased risk of ischemic stroke with standard doses of oral estrogen. The increase in younger women is extremely small and may not be statistically significant. In the 13-year follow-up data from the WHI (Manson, 2013) and in the Cochrane review (Boardman, 2015), stroke was not significantly increased in the younger age groups. Thus although a rare event, ischemic stroke risk may be increased in women taking standard doses of oral estrogen (women using CEE at 0.625 mg or more) but not with lower doses (e.g., CEE 0.3 mg). Similarly, transdermal therapy has not been associated with an increased risk. These and other data point to a thrombotic risk with oral estrogen (in susceptible women). The mechanism of ischemic stroke risk in younger women is not likely to be due to atherosclerosis, as it is in coronary disease in older women, but is due to acute thrombosis (Lobo, 2011) (Fig. 14.34). The thrombosis risk in younger women, much like the risk of venous thrombosis, likely is due to an aberrant interaction of estrogen with thrombotic factors, at times because of an underlying thrombophilia.

In summary, there should be no concern regarding increased cardiovascular risk for young, healthy women at the onset of menopause who are contemplating HT for treatment of symptoms. In this setting there is no evidence of increased risk, and indeed these women may be found to benefit from a cardiovascular standpoint.

## CANCER RISKS IN POSTMENOPAUSAL WOMEN

Just as CVD is a concern for women after menopause, the risk of cancer also increases with time after menopause, but this is a function of aging and not a consequence of menopause per se. ***Prevention*** requires healthy lifestyle measures and screening for early detection, which will be emphasized again later in the chapter.

Although breast cancer is generally believed to be the leading cause of death in postmenopausal women, in fact it is lung cancer. Indeed, mortality from breast cancer tends to decrease after menopause, on an age-specific basis, but cardiovascular mortality increases, and these lines transect around the time of menopause (Fig. 14.35). The gynecologist should be well

**Study year**

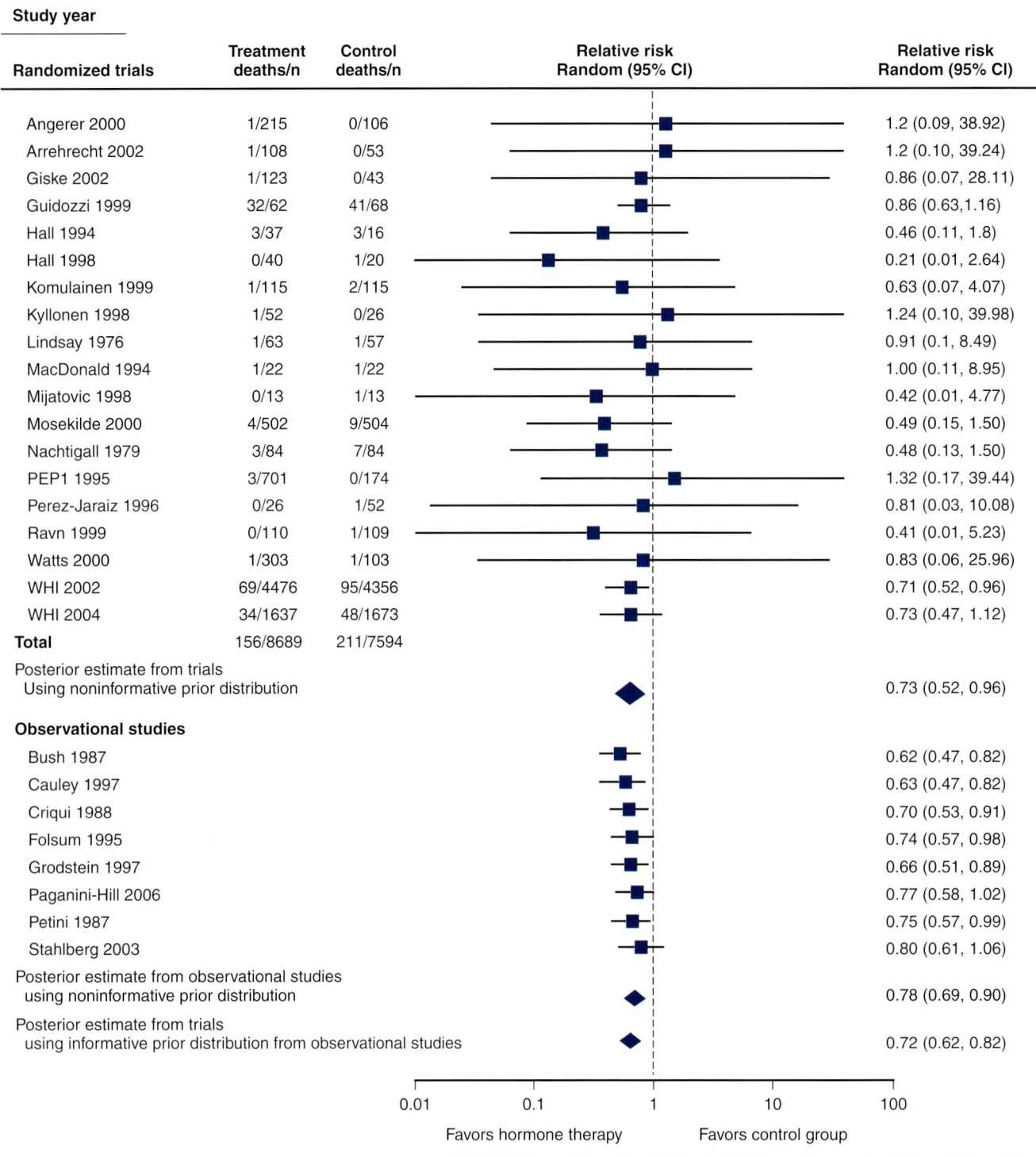

| Randomized trials | Treatment deaths/n | Control deaths/n | Relative risk Random (95% CI) |
|---|---|---|---|
| Angerer 2000 | 1/215 | 0/106 | 1.2 (0.09, 38.92) |
| Arrehrecht 2002 | 1/108 | 0/53 | 1.2 (0.10, 39.24) |
| Giske 2002 | 1/123 | 0/43 | 0.86 (0.07, 28.11) |
| Guidozzi 1999 | 32/62 | 41/68 | 0.86 (0.63,1.16) |
| Hall 1994 | 3/37 | 3/16 | 0.46 (0.11, 1.8) |
| Hall 1998 | 0/40 | 1/20 | 0.21 (0.01, 2.64) |
| Komulainen 1999 | 1/115 | 2/115 | 0.63 (0.07, 4.07) |
| Kyllonen 1998 | 1/52 | 0/26 | 1.24 (0.10, 39.98) |
| Lindsay 1976 | 1/63 | 1/57 | 0.91 (0.1, 8.49) |
| MacDonald 1994 | 1/22 | 1/22 | 1.00 (0.11, 8.95) |
| Mijatovic 1998 | 0/13 | 1/13 | 0.42 (0.01, 4.77) |
| Mosekilde 2000 | 4/502 | 9/504 | 0.49 (0.15, 1.50) |
| Nachtigall 1979 | 3/84 | 7/84 | 0.48 (0.13, 1.50) |
| PEP1 1995 | 3/701 | 0/174 | 1.32 (0.17, 39.44) |
| Perez-Jaraiz 1996 | 0/26 | 1/52 | 0.81 (0.03, 10.08) |
| Ravn 1999 | 0/110 | 1/109 | 0.41 (0.01, 5.23) |
| Watts 2000 | 1/303 | 1/103 | 0.83 (0.06, 25.96) |
| WHI 2002 | 69/4476 | 95/4356 | 0.71 (0.52, 0.96) |
| WHI 2004 | 34/1637 | 48/1673 | 0.73 (0.47, 1.12) |
| **Total** | 156/8689 | 211/7594 | |
| Posterior estimate from trials Using noninformative prior distribution | | | 0.73 (0.52, 0.96) |
| **Observational studies** | | | |
| Bush 1987 | | | 0.62 (0.47, 0.82) |
| Cauley 1997 | | | 0.63 (0.47, 0.82) |
| Criqui 1988 | | | 0.70 (0.53, 0.91) |
| Folsum 1995 | | | 0.74 (0.57, 0.98) |
| Grodstein 1997 | | | 0.66 (0.51, 0.89) |
| Paganini-Hill 2006 | | | 0.77 (0.58, 1.02) |
| Petini 1987 | | | 0.75 (0.57, 0.99) |
| Stahlberg 2003 | | | 0.80 (0.61, 1.06) |
| Posterior estimate from observational studies using noninformative prior distribution | | | 0.78 (0.69, 0.90) |
| Posterior estimate from trials using informative prior distribution from observational studies | | | 0.72 (0.62, 0.82) |

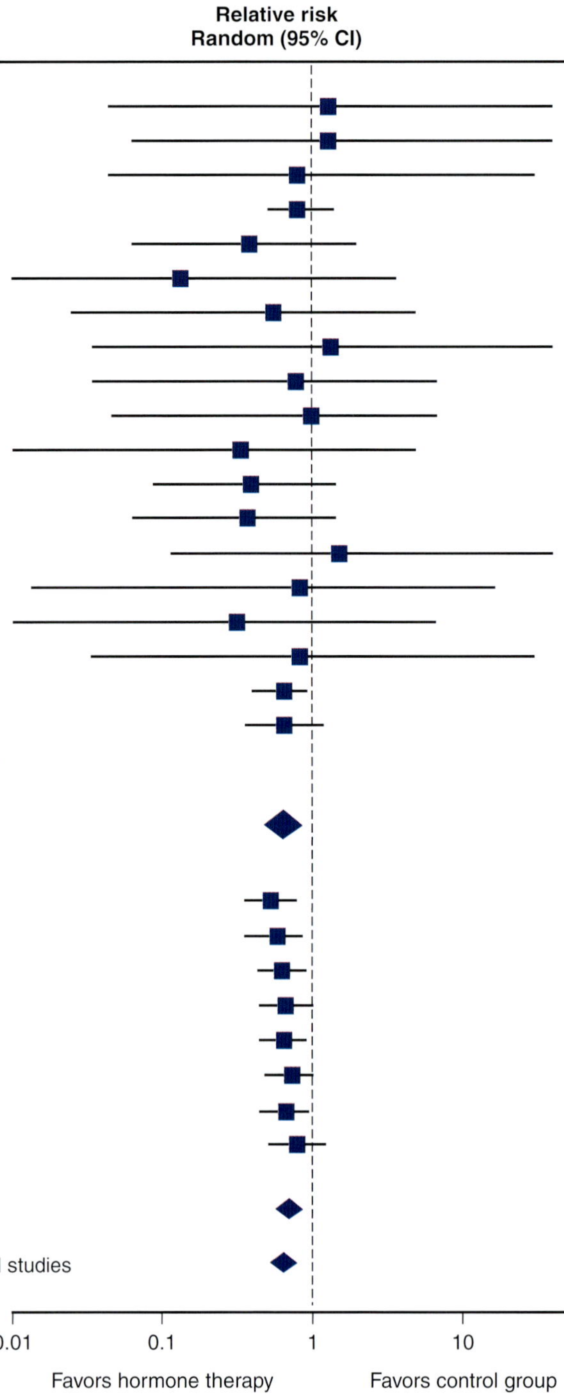


**Fig. 14.29** Bayesian meta-analysis of reduction in mortality with hormone therapy in younger women. *CI,* Confidence interval; CI, confidence interval; *PEP1,* Postmenopausal Estrogen/Progestin Interventions study; *WHI,* Women's Health Initiative. (Modified from Salpeter SR, Cheng J, Thabane L, et al. Bayesian meta-analysis of hormone therapy and mortality in younger postmenopausal women. *Am J Med.* 2009;122(11): 1016-1022.)

versed in the epidemiology of and preventive strategies for breast, lung, cervical, endometrial, ovarian, and colorectal cancer. Further discussions of these cancers may be found in Part IV (Gynecologic Oncology) of this text. What follows is a discussion of the potential effects of HT on endometrial, breast, ovarian, and colorectal cancer.

**Endometrial cancer** is a common cancer in postmenopausal women and is increased in women using **unopposed estrogen therapy**. Although a woman's risk for endometrial cancer with unopposed estrogen use is two- to eightfold higher than that for the general population, precursor lesions (primarily endometrial hyperplasia) signal the presence of an abnormality in most

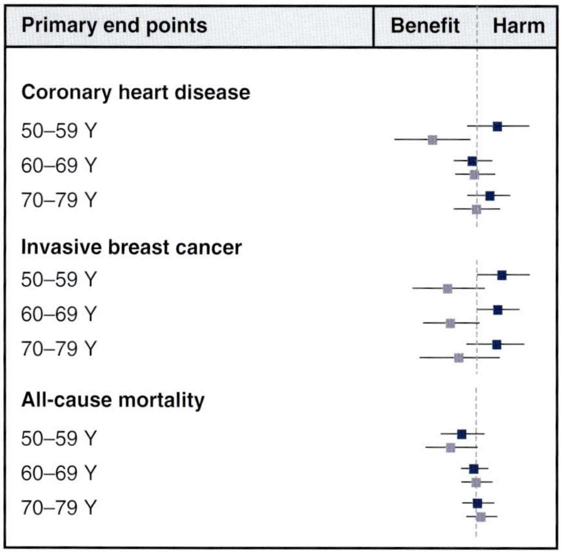


**Fig. 14.30** Cumulative 13-year follow-up data, intervention and follow-up phases with conjugated equine estrogen (CEE) and CEE/medroxyprogesterone acetate (MPA) arms of the Women's Health Initiative in different age groups *(CEE, light blue; CEE/MPA, dark blue)*. (Modified from Manson JE, Chlebowski RT, Stefanick ML, et al: Menopausal hormone therapy and health outcomes during the intervention and extended poststopping phases of the Women's Health Initiative randomized trials. *JAMA* 310(13):1353-1368, 2013.)

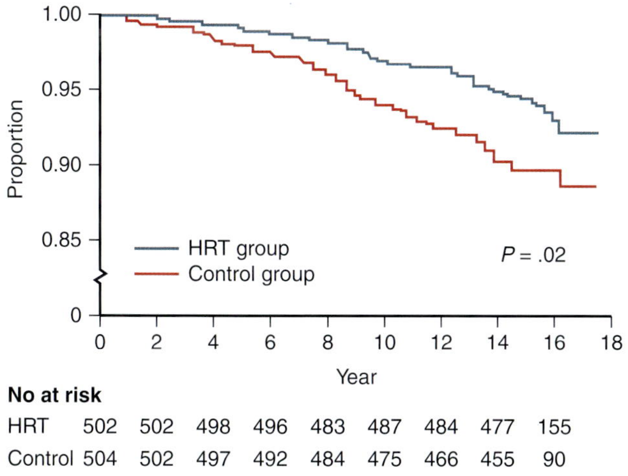


**Fig. 14.31** Sixteen-year follow-up of women randomly allocated to hormone therapy (HT) showing a reduction in death, heart failure, and myocardial infarction (MI). (Modified from Schierbeck IL, Renmark L, Tofteng CL, et al. Effect of hormone replacement therapy on cardiovascular events in recently postmenopausal women: randomized trial. *BMJ.* 2012;345:e6409.)

patients, and the cancer is usually well differentiated and hormonally responsive, as are hyperplasias.

One study showed that the risk of endometrial hyperplasia was 20% after 1 year of using 0.625 mg of oral CEE. In another study, the 3-year postmenopausal Estrogen/Progestin Interventions Trial, this risk of hyperplasia was approximately 40% at the end of 3 years. No cancers were reported in either of these two studies, and the addition of a progestogen essentially eliminated the hyperplasia risk. Use of CEE alone at 0.3 mg/day for 2 to 3 years results in a hyperplasia risk of 5% to 10%. With the same

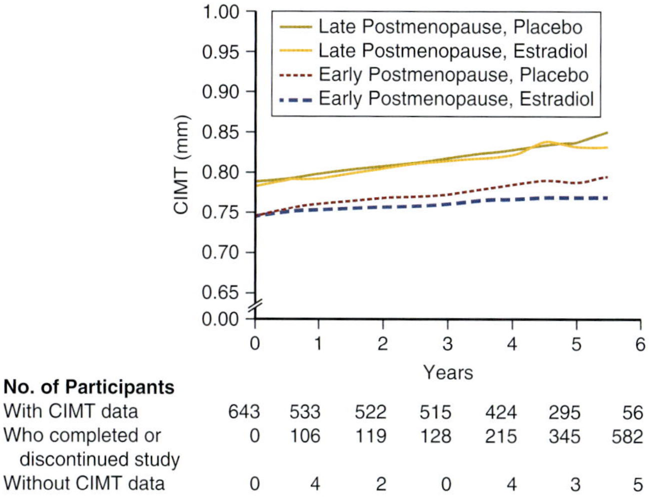


**Fig. 14.32** Carotid intima media thickness (CIMT) changes in younger and older postmenopausal women treated with estradiol versus placebo (the ELITE trial). Younger women, but not older women, with *early* initiation of estradiol had significant attenuation of CIMT. (From Hodis HN, Mack WJ, Henderson VW, et al. Vascular effects of early versus late postmenopausal treatment with estradiol. *N Engl J Med.* 2016;374:1221-1231.)

dose of esterified estrogens (which are less potent), no hyperplasia was found after 2 years.

**The risk for endometrial cancer in women taking estrogen and progestogen is similar to that of women in the general population** because combination therapy merely eliminates the excess risk attributed to estrogen; a few studies, however, have suggested a lower risk of endometrial cancer with **continuous combined hormone treatment.** It is important to remember that some endometrial cancers occurring in postmenopausal women are not hormonally related; thus some women may develop a **serous** type of cancer (poorly differentiated) while on HT, making continuous surveillance important. It could be argued that these serous cancers, which are usually receptor negative, may have arisen independently of HT use.

Although the risk for endometrial cancer is increased substantially in estrogen users, the risk of death from this type of endometrial cancer does not increase proportionately. Endometrial cancers associated with estrogen use are thought to be less aggressive than spontaneously occurring cancers, in part because tumors in women taking estrogen are more likely to be discovered and treated at an earlier stage, thus improving survival rates.

## Risk of Breast Cancer With Estrogen Use

Several studies and meta-analyses have shown a borderline or small statistical increase in the risk of breast cancer (RR, 1.2 to 1.4) after approximately 5 years of estrogen use. This risk is related to the dose of estrogen and to duration of use. Data have pointed to the addition of progestogen as a major contributor to this increased risk of breast cancer. A 2019 meta-analysis did not reach different conclusions, but several important papers were missing from this analysis. (Collaborative Group, 2019). There is some biologic plausibility to this notion in that progesterone in the normal luteal phase increases breast mitotic activity and HT increases mammographic tissue density relative to ET alone. Several small case-control studies found no increase with ET alone, but the same studies showed a statistically significant increase with progestogen use (in the range of a 1.3 or 1.4 RR). In the WHI trial, the increase

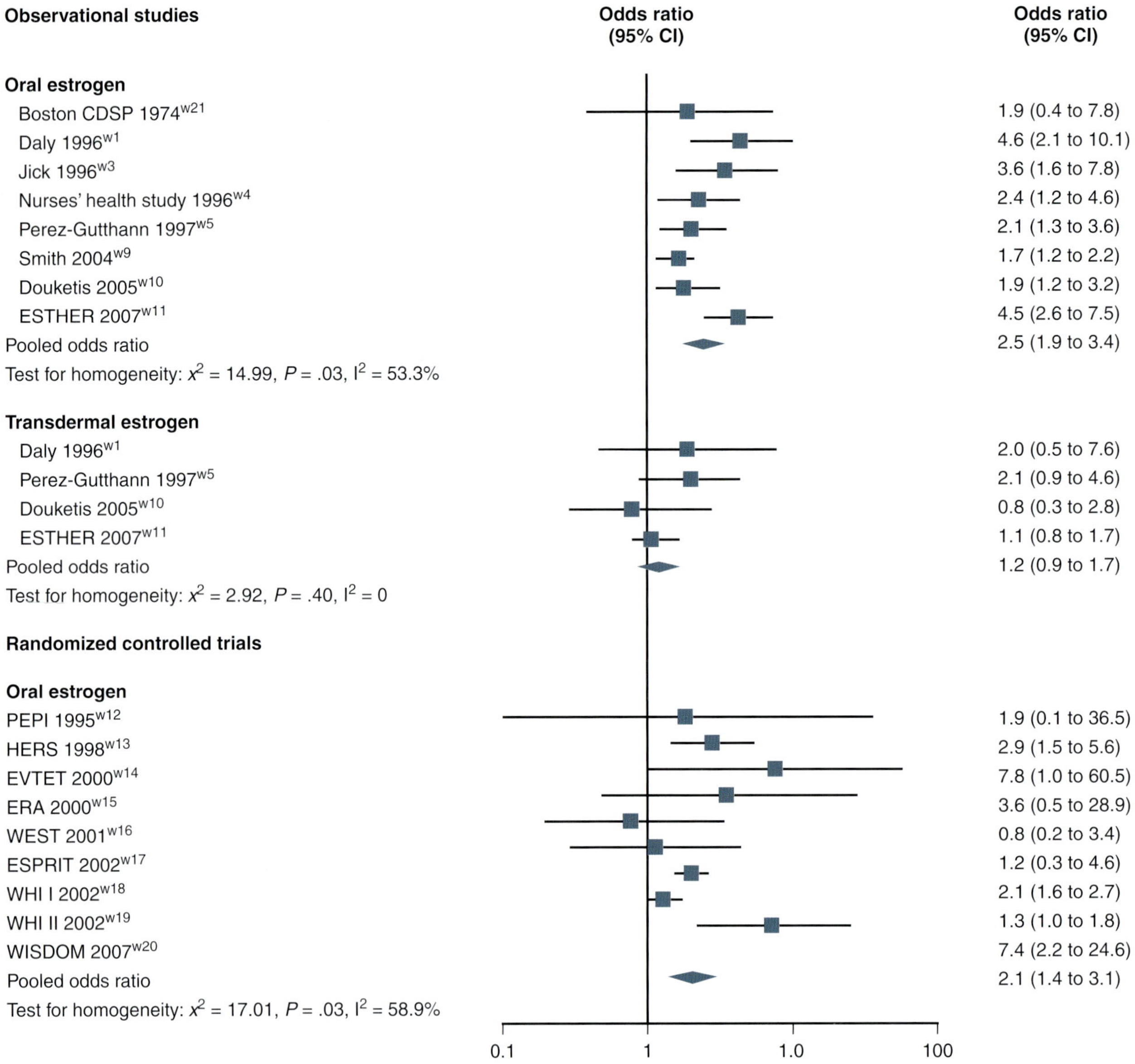


**Fig. 14.33** Meta-analysis of various studies showing no increased risk of thrombosis with transdermal therapy. *CI,* Confidence interval; *w,* week. (Modified from Canonico M, Plu-Bureau G, Lowe GD, et al. Hormone replacement therapy and risk of venous thromboembolism in postmenopausal women: systematic review and meta-analysis. *BMJ.* 2008;336(7655):1227-1231.)

in breast cancer risk was of borderline significance with CEE/MPA (hazard ratio [HR], 1.24 [1.01 to 1.54]). A reanalysis by Anderson and coworkers found that when correcting for variables known to affect breast cancer risk, the average risk was no longer statistically significant: 1.20 (0.94 to 1.53) (Anderson, 2006). It is important to note that the total duration of therapy is very important for the risk with estrogen/progestogen therapy. In the WHI trial the significant increase over 5 years was only found in prior users of HT, suggesting a longer cumulative effect. *There was no statistical increase over 5 years with CEE/MPA in women in the WHI trial who had not used HT in the past* (Anderson, 2006). A large collaborative case-control study also has shown that continuous combined estrogen-progestogen therapy is associated with increased breast cancer risk over time.

The effect of estrogen/progestogen therapy and breast cancer risk is thought to be one of promotion, rather than carcinogenesis per se. Occult breast tumors are extremely common in breast tissue and take up to 10 years of slow growth to be clinically detectable. It has been suggested that certain doses of estrogen, and particularly estrogen/progestogen therapy, stimulate the growth of these occult receptor positive tumors, which shortens the time to clinical detection, thus allowing them to be recognized as a consequence of HT. Using the modeling of growth kinetics by Santen and applying these numbers to findings in the WHI lends credence to this notion (Santen, 2012).

In the estrogen-only arm of the WHI, after 6½ years there was a borderline significant ***decrease*** **in breast cancer risk** (HR, 0.77 [0.59 to 1.01]). In a more complete analysis of these findings, Stefanick and associates found the risk to be significantly decreased for ductal cancer (0.71 [0.52 to 0.99]), and **in a sensitivity analysis among adherent women, the decrease was statistically significant (0.67 [0.47 to 0.9])** (Stefanick, 2006) (Fig. 14.36). Thus although it is unclear why there should be a decrease in breast cancer risk, we may conclude that standard-dose ET

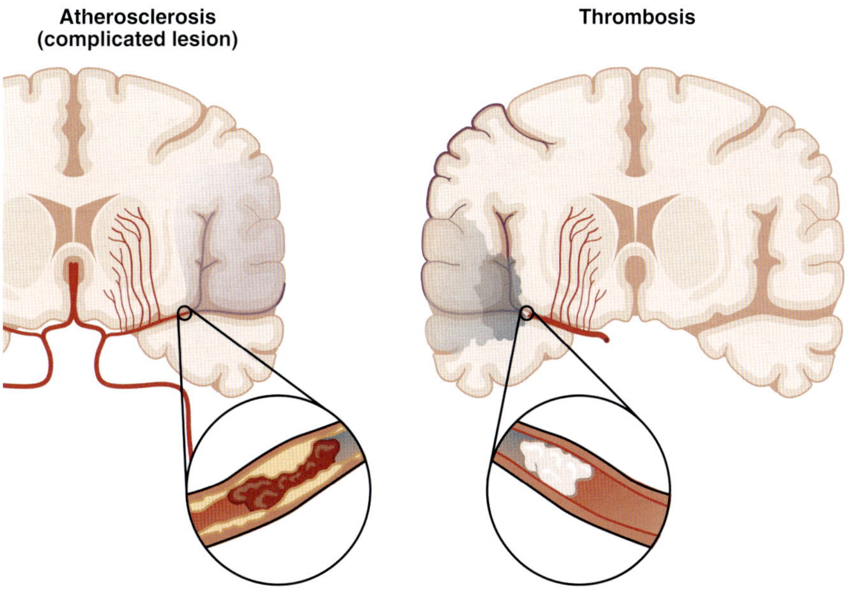


**Fig. 14.34** Mechanisms of ischemic stroke risk with estrogen in older women as a result of atherosclerosis with complicated lesions *(left)* and as a result of thrombosis in younger women *(right)*.

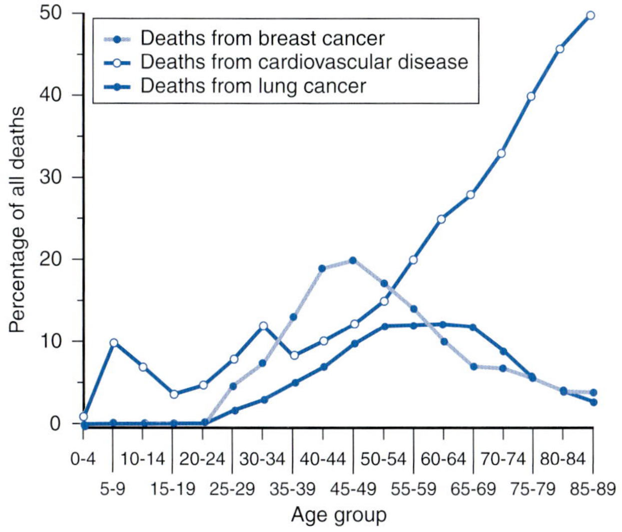


**Fig. 14.35** Risks of breast cancer and lung cancer versus cardiovascular disease in various age categories. (Modified from Phillips KA, Glendon G, Knight JA. Putting the risk of breast cancer in perspective. *N Engl J Med.* 1999;340:141. Copyright 1999 Massachusetts Medical Society.)

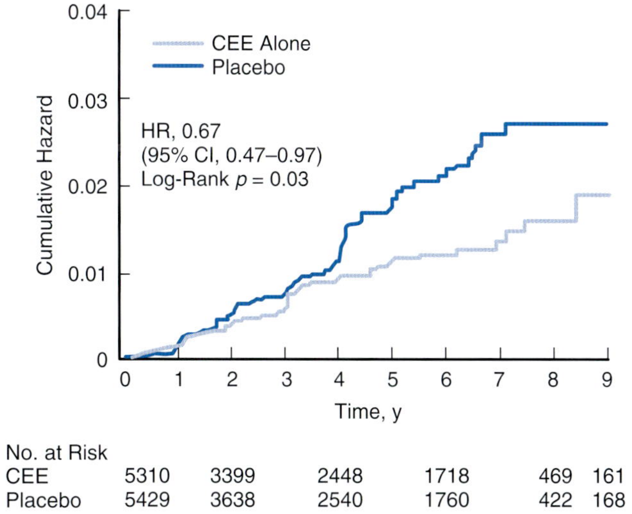


**Fig. 14.36** Cumulative hazard for invasive breast cancer: sensitivity analysis. *CEE,* Conjugated equine estrogen; *CI,* confidence interval; *HR,* hazard ratio. (From Stefanick ML, Anderson GL, Margolis KL, et al. Effects of conjugated equine estrogens on breast cancer and mammography screening in postmenopausal women with hysterectomy. *JAMA.* 2006;295:1647.)

(0.625 mg CEE) is not associated with a risk of breast cancer except for very long-term users. In an analysis from the NHS, Chen and colleagues found that this risk only increases significantly after 20 years (Table 14.6). This risk is predominantly seen in lean women because women who are overweight or obese already have an increased risk of breast cancer, which is not further increased. A theory proposed by Jordan has suggested that the decrease in risk is confined to women who did not receive hormones immediately after menopause, but some time later. **The theory suggests that this lag allowed the occult breast cancers to undergo apoptosis when later exposed to estrogen, thus decreasing the risk of breast cancer.**

The promotional effect of hormones and breast cancer is thought to be enhanced by the use of progestogens. Some observational data from France have shown that use of natural progesterone may not enhance the risk as has been noted with synthetic progestins (Fournier, 2008).

Putting these risks into perspective is important for patient counseling. The background risk for breast cancer in a woman between the ages of 50 and 60 is 2.8 per 100 women. According to data from the WHI, the overall relative risk for women taking CEE/MPA for 5 years was approximately 1.24. Note that this applies to women who had also used hormones in the past, as noted earlier. **This 24% increase translates into an overall risk of 3.47 per 100 women, less than 1% greater than the background risk.** This risk is expected to be even lower with different regimens, including lower-dose therapy, and potentially with different progestogens, such as natural progesterone, which

**TABLE 14.6** Risk of Invasive Breast Cancer by Duration of ET Use among All Postmenopausal Women Who Had Undergone Hysterectomy and Those with ER+/PR+ Cancer Only*

| | All Postmenopausal Women | | | | | | | |
|---|---|---|---|---|---|---|---|---|
| | Who Had Undergone Hysterectomy | | | | ER+/PR+ Cancers Only | | | |
| **ET Use and Duration (Years)** | All | | Screened Cohort† | | All | | Screened Cohort† | |
| | Cases | Risk | Cases | Risk | Cases | Risk | Cases | Risk |
| Never | 226 | 1.00 | 104 | 1.00 | 87 | 1.00 | 48 | 1.00 |
| Current | | | | | | | | |
| <5 | 99 | 0.96 (0.75-1.22) | 59 | 1.06 (0.76-1.47) | 38 | 1.00 (0.67-1.49) | 26 | 1.04 (0.64-1.70) |
| 5-9.9 | 145 | 0.90 (0.73-1.12) | 95 | 0.91 (0.68-1.21) | 70 | 1.19 (0.86-1.66) | 50 | 1.08 (0.72-1.62) |
| 10-14.9 | 190 | 1.06 (0.87-1.30) | 141 | 1.11 (0.85-1.44) | 85 | 1.27 (0.93-1.73) | 77 | 1.29 (0.89-1.86) |
| 15-19.9 | 129 | 1.18 (0.95-1.48) | 95 | 1.19 (0.89-1.58) | 61 | 1.48 (1.05-2.07) | 58 | 1.50 (1.02-2.21) |
| ≥20 | 145 | 1.42 (1.13-1.77) | 127 | 1.58 (1.20-2.07) | 69 | 1.73 (1.24-2.43) | 74 | 1.83 (1.25-2.68) |
| *P* for trend for current use | | <.001 | | <.001 | | <.001 | | <.001 |

From Chen WY, Manson JE, Hankinson SE, et al. Unopposed estrogen therapy and the risk of invasive breast cancer. *Arch Intern Med.* 2006;166:1027.
*All cases are reported as number of cases; risks are reported as multivariate relative risk (95% CI), controlled for age (continuous), age at menopause (continuous), age at menarche (continuous), BMI (quintiles), history of benign breast disease (yes or no), family history of breast cancer in first-degree relative (yes or no), average daily alcohol consumption (0, 0.5-5, 5-10, 10-20, or ≥20 g/day), parity/age at first birth (nulliparous; 1-2 children and age at first birth ≤22 years; 1-2 children and age at first birth 23-25 years; 1-2 children and age at first birth 25 years; ≥3 children and age at first birth ≤22 years; ≥3 children and age at first birth 23-25 years; ≥3 children and age at first birth >25 years).
†Screened cohort defined as those women starting in 1988 who reported either a screening mammogram or clinical breast examination in the previous 2 years. All cases before 1988 are excluded.
*BMI*, Body mass index; *CI*, confidence interval; *ER+/PR+*, positive for both estrogen and progesterone receptors; *ET*, unopposed estrogen therapy.

has been shown in observational studies not to increase the risk. A relative risk of 1.24 for breast cancer is less than that for obesity alone (3.3) or for being a flight attendant (1.87) because of the increase in cosmic radiation. Furthermore, for estrogen alone there is probably no increased risk at moderate to low doses for up to 20 years of exposure, as noted by Chen and colleagues. **The risk of breast cancer is much higher with certain endogenous risk factors such as obesity and increased breast density than it is with any type of HT** (Fig. 14.37).

With some exceptions in the literature, **most reports have shown that the mortality rate in users of ET/HT is improved compared with those women not receiving hormones** who are diagnosed with breast cancer. Fig. 14.38 depicts the 10-year follow-up data from WHI with women receiving CEE alone; both breast cancer mortality and total mortality were reduced in users of estrogen (Anderson, 2012). It should be appreciated that women receiving HT are likely to have (and should have) closer surveillance (examinations and mammography); accordingly, most tumors, if they occur, will be detected at an early stage.

Family history and genetic mutations (e.g., *BRCA1* and *BRCA2*) substantially increase the risk of a woman developing breast cancer. However, the literature suggests that the use of HT does not increase this risk further. Nevertheless, for many women it is unacceptable to consider a potentially promotional effect of using HT, and they may opt for risk reduction strategies such as the use of tamoxifen or other SERMs.

If there is a concern regarding hormones and breast cancer, it is with larger doses, a longer duration, and specifically the use of a progestogen. Accordingly, for longer-term therapy, if warranted (>5 years), lower doses of estrogen should be used, and progestogen exposure should be minimized.

## Ovarian Cancer

Several studies have suggested an increased risk of ovarian cancer with long-duration use of estrogen or estrogen/progestogen therapy. However, the data are inconsistent, and the purported risk is less than a twofold relative risk. Prospective randomized trials such as the WHI have found no statistical increase in risk. A 2015 meta-analysis suggested a modest risk of 30% to 40% (Collaborative Group, 2019). In this analysis it is unclear if adequate attention was paid to confounders, and there was no association with length of exposure regarding risk, which does not make sense physiologically. Further, estrogen and estrogen/progestogens both carried some risk, whereas use of oral contraceptives are known to decrease ovarian cancer risk. According to this meta-analysis, **the risk was calculated to be approximately 1 extra case of ovarian cancer per 1000 women over 5 years, which suggests if this association is real, it is extremely rare.**

## Colorectal Cancer

The third most common cancer in women, colorectal cancer, is often preventable by the detection and treatment of polyps. Women older than 50 should have a colorectal evaluation by some means (detection of occult blood, sigmoidoscopy, or a colonoscopy). **Data have been fairly consistent in identifying a reduction in risk with the use of hormones**. Several meta-analyses have shown an approximate **33% decrease in risk**, as did the observational data from the NHS and the prospective randomized trial data of the CEE/MPA arm of the WHI. It is unclear why in the ET arm of WHI a decrease was not observed. No definitive mechanism for this protective effect has been found, although several theories have been advanced (e.g., changes in the composition of bile acids, antiinflammatory effects).

## Other Cancers

More attention is being paid to lung cancer, in part because it is the leading cause of cancer mortality in women. The data on HT, however, have not been consistent and are without convincing evidence of any increased risk of lung cancer with HT use.

# DISEASE PREVENTION AFTER MENOPAUSE

**Because all major diseases, including CVD, obesity, metabolic diseases (particularly diabetes), cancer, and AD, as well**

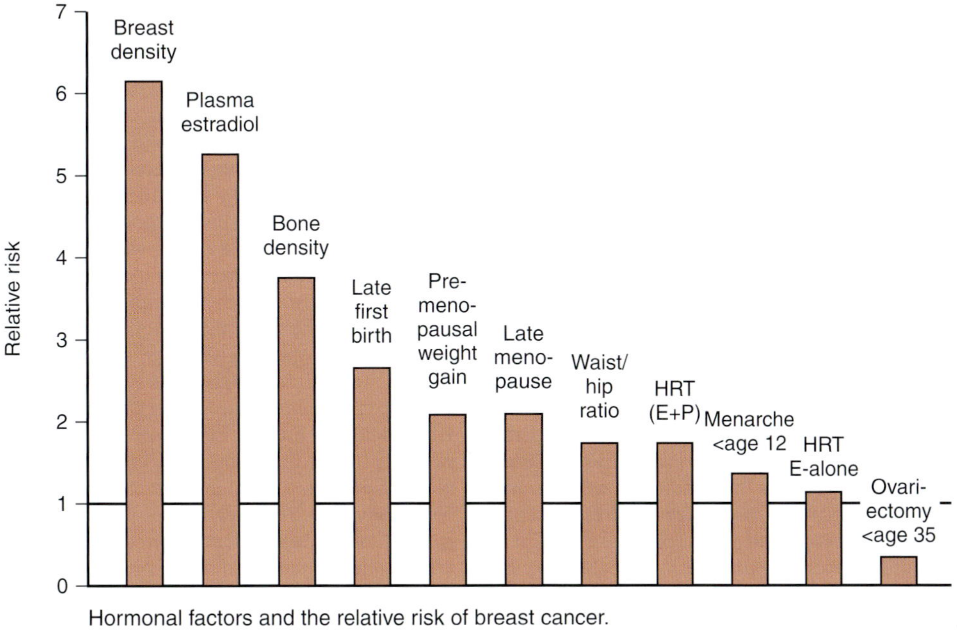


**Fig. 14.37** Risks of breast cancer with various exposures and endogenous traits, particularly increased breast density. *E,* Estrogen; *HRT,* hormone replacement therapy; *P,* progestogen. (Modified from Gompel A, Santen RJ: Hormone therapy and breast cancer risk 10 years after the WHI. *Climacteric.* 2012;15(3):241-249.)

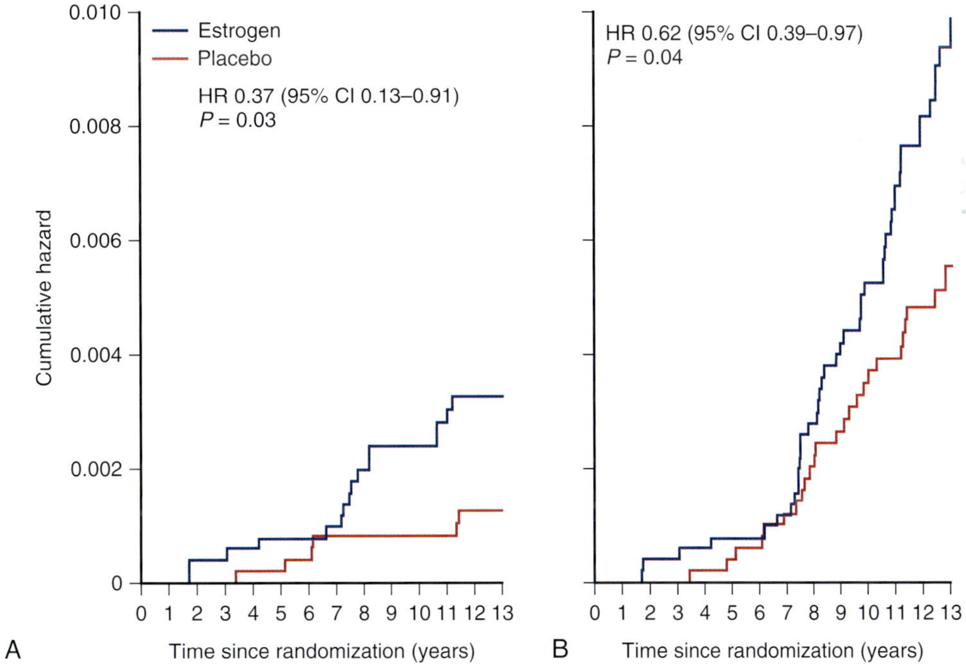


**Fig. 14.38** In women with breast cancer, women taking estradiol ($E_2$) had significantly reduced mortality; breast cancer (**A**) and total (**B**). *CI,* confidence interval; *HR,* hazard ratio. (Modified from Anderson GL, Chlebowski RT, Aragaki AK, et al. Conjugated equine oestrogen and breast cancer incidence and mortality in postmenopausal women with hysterectomy: extended follow-up of the Women's Health Initiative randomized placebo-controlled trial. *Lancet Oncol.* 2012;13(5):476-486.)

**as cognitive decline increase after menopause, menopause itself heralds an important opportunity to screen for and prevent many of these problems** (Lobo, 2014).

Details of this approach may be found in the review cited, but in essence it stresses the introduction of screening procedures for these disorders and then beginning prevention strategies such as prescribing diet and exercise regimens and the consideration of HT. Primary strategies for the prevention of CVD in men, such as statins and aspirin, have not been shown to be of benefit in women (Lobo, 2014). Thus apart from lifestyle measures, there are no good prevention strategies for women, with the possible exception of HT. As discussed previously, in a young healthy population of women close to menopause, estrogen-based therapy has been shown to significantly decrease coronary disease and mortality, with minimal to rare risks of adverse outcomes. As Fig. 14.28 shows, the use of HT was considered for prevention until the time of the various secondary prevention trials (such as the Heart and Estrogen/Progestin Replacement Study [HERS]) and then the WHI, and this concept is now being reconsidered, although it remains controversial. Table 14.7 lists a compilation of several studies and meta-analyses that are **remarkably consistent in showing a reduction in mortality in younger women receiving estrogen after menopause, which strengthens the argument for considering the use of estrogen for prevention.**

Because "early harm" was reported in **older women** taking standard doses of CEE/MPA in secondary prevention trials and in the WHI, it has been suggested (by some) that women have a cardiovascular risk assessment before initiating HT. **The American Heart Association (www.heart.org) offers an easy-to-use rapid risk assessment calculator, which defines women at low risk if they have a less than 7.5% chance of sustaining a myocardial infarction in 10 years.** Although some investigators have questioned the validity of this approach, risk assessment is not an unreasonable course in general, along the lines of stressing the need for *prevention* after menopause. Because most of the CV-related risks of HT relate to oral therapy, "higher"-risk women may benefit more by being placed on transdermal estrogen.

In summary, apart from the need to screen carefully for all diseases at the onset of menopause and stressing healthy lifestyle measures, the decision to initiate HT should be straightforward in symptomatic women who will benefit more in terms of absolute numbers of women affected by treatment (see Fig. 14.39). Fig. 14.39, generated from newer data and data from the WHI in the 50- to 59-year-old age group, shows the absolute benefits and risks associated with the use of estrogen, strongly emphasizing benefits. However, when these absolute numbers are compared with the benefit of the reduction in hot flushes in women receiving estrogen, the latter appears to be the predominant effect (Fig. 14.40). The decision to use HT at the onset of menopause probably applies for women who are at greater risk for osteoporosis as well, based on family history and their physical characteristics. Otherwise, it is not unreasonable to consider HT in otherwise healthy women with adequate counseling and discussion of the risks and benefits. This should be an individual decision. For some women, the fear of breast cancer, particularly in those with some family history of the disease, will overshadow any potential benefits, and this view has to be respected. Women who decide to initiate HT should be made aware that this need not be a long commitment, and therapy should be reassessed annually based on needs and symptoms.

Finally, the data to date regarding protection are strongest for the use of estrogen; certain progestogens may eliminate or attenuate the benefit, and some progestogens increase the promotional risk of breast cancer. Philosophically, therefore, HT should be about using the lowest amount of a progestogen necessary to prevent endometrial disease.

**TABLE 14.7** Consistency in the Reduction in All-Cause Mortality in Younger Women Receiving Estrogen at the Onset of Menopause

| Study | Point Estimate (Relative Risk) |
|---|---|
| Observational meta-analysis | 0.78 (0.69-0.90)* |
| Randomized trials meta-analysis | 0.73 (0.52-0.96)* |
| Bayesian | 0.72 (0.62-0.82)* |
| WHI combined groups | 0.70 (0.62-0.82)† |
| WHI 13-year cumulative CEE | 0.78 (0.59-1.03)‡ |
| WHI 13-year cumulative CEE/MPA | 0.88 (0.70-1.1)‡ |
| Cochrane meta-analysis | 0.70 (0.52-0.95)§ |
| Finnish registry data (pre-WHI) | 0.57 (0.48-0.66)‖ |
| Finnish registry data (post-WHI) | 0.46 (0.32-0.64)‖ |

*Salpeter SR, Cheng J, Thabane L, et al. Bayesian meta-analysis of hormone therapy and mortality in younger postmenopausal women. *Am J Med.* 2009;122(11):1016-1022.

†Rossouw JE, Prentice RL, Manson JE, et al. Postmenopausal hormone therapy and cardiovascular disease by age and years since menopause. *JAMA.* 2007;297(13):1465-1477.

‡ Manson JE, Chlebowski RT, Stefanick ML, et al. Menopausal hormone therapy and health outcomes during the intervention and extended poststopping phases of the Women's Health Initiative randomized trials. *JAMA.* 2013;310:1353-1368.

§ Boardman HMP, Hartley L, Main C, et al. Hormone therapy for preventing cardiovascular disease in post-menopausal women (review). *Cochrane Database Syst Rev.* 3:CD002229, 2015.

‖Tuomikoski P, Lyytinen H, Korhonen P, et al. Coronary heart disease mortality and hormone therapy before and after the Women's Health Initiative. *Obstet Gynecol.* 2014;124: 947-953. (Coronary mortality including all women but with similar point estimates as in women <60 years.)

*CEE,* Conjugated equine estrogen; *MPA,* medroxyprogesterone acetate; WHI, Women's Health Initiative.

## Hormone Regimens

The various hormonal preparations and osteoporosis drugs that are available for treatment are listed in Box 14.3. A more complete list may be found in the Consumer section of the North American Menopause Society website at www.menopause.org. For the clinician and patient, as noted earlier, the decision to start estrogen therapy need not involve a long-term commitment. For short-term treatment of symptoms, estrogen should be used at a low dose that can control hot flushes or can be administered via the vaginal route for symptoms of dryness or dyspareunia. There are no definitive data on what doses are necessary for CV protection, but whereas low doses of estrogen may be sufficient to prevent bone loss (discussed earlier), the doses necessary to afford CV protection may need to be higher, although there are no definitive data. Therefore lower doses are still recommended, which are sufficient for symptom control.

Oral estrogen results in higher levels of $E_1$ than $E_2$; this is true for oral micronized $E_2$ as well as oral $E_1$ products. CEE is a mixture of at least 10 conjugated estrogens derived from equine pregnant urine. $E_1$ S is the major component, but the biologic activities of equilin, 17$\alpha$-dihydroequilin, and several other B-ring unsaturated estrogens, including $\delta$5 dehydroestrone, have been documented. Table 14.8 compares the standard doses of the most commonly prescribed oral estrogens and the levels of $E_1$ and $E_2$ achieved. Much of the following clinical information may be found in systematic reviews.

Synthetic estrogens, given orally, are more potent than natural $E_2$. Ethinyl estradiol is used in oral contraceptives, with a dose of 5 $\mu$g being equivalent to the standard ET doses used (0.625 mg CEE or 1 mg micronized $E_2$). Standard ET doses are five or six times less than the amount of estrogen used in oral contraceptives. Although there are incomplete data available to compare the equivalencies of CEE and micronized $E_2$ (because of different end organ effects and the mixture of estrogens in CEE, which are difficult to measure), 0.625 mg CEE is probably equivalent to 1.5 mg of micronized $E_2$. Oral estrogens have a potent hepatic first-pass effect that results in the loss of approximately 30% of their activity with a single passage after oral administration. However, this results in stimulation of hepatic proteins and enzymes. Some of these changes are not particularly beneficial (e.g., an increase in procoagulation factors and an increase in C-reactive protein),

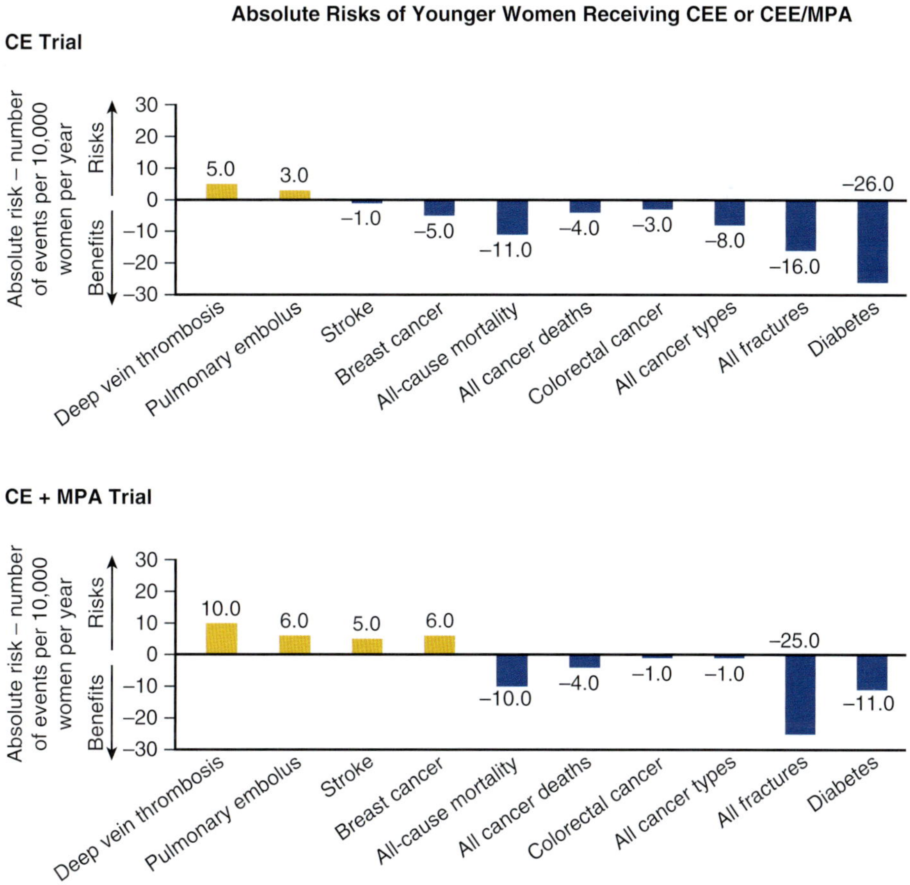


**Fig. 14.39** Absolute risks in younger women receiving estrogen or estrogen/progestogen. *CEE,* Conjugated equine estrogen; *MPA,* medroxyprogesterone acetate. (Data from Women's Health Initiative; modified from Lobo RA, Pickar JH, Stevenson JC, Mack WJ, Hodis HN. Back to the future: hormone replacement therapy as part of a prevention strategy for women at the onset of menopause. *Atherosclerosis.* 2016;254:282-290.)

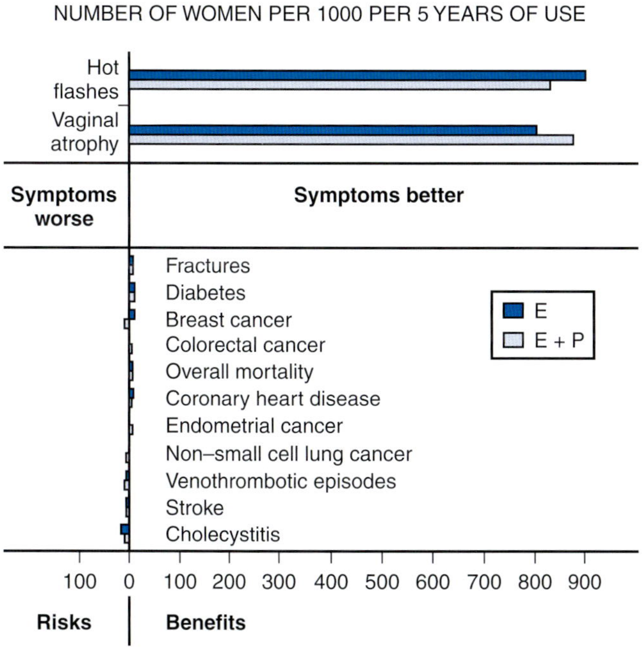


**Fig. 14.40** Putting risks and benefits in perspective for the 50- to 59-year-old. (Modified from Santen R. Endocrine Society position paper. *J Clin Endocrinol Metab.* 2010;95[7 Suppl 1]:s1-s66.)

whereas other changes are beneficial (an increase in HDL-C and a decrease in fibrinogen and plasminogen activator inhibitor-1).

$E_2$ can be administered in patches, gels, lotions, sprays, and subcutaneously. These routes of administration are not subject to major hepatic effects as with oral therapy. Accordingly, there is no increase in C-reactive protein and minimal if any change in coagulation factors, but there is also only a minimal increase in HDL-C. Patches are available in doses from 0.014 mg to 0.1 mg, available for administration once or twice weekly. An ultra-low dose patch (0.014 mg/day) has been marketed for osteoporosis prevention in older women and not for treating hot flushes. Matrix patches are preferable to the older alcohol-based preparations because there is less skin reaction and estrogen delivery is more reliable. Whereas levels of $E_2$ with oral therapy may vary widely among women and within the day (peaks and valleys), levels with transdermal therapy are more constant within each woman, yet values achieved may vary from woman to woman based on absorption and metabolic characteristics. With the 0.05-mg patch, $E_2$ levels should be in the 40 to 50 pg/mL range, but a woman can have a value as high as 200 pg/mL or a level that is less than 20 pg/mL. This issue of interpatient variability is based on skin absorption, metabolism, and body distribution. Accordingly, regardless of symptomatic control, it is valuable to assess at least once what the $E_2$ level is in a woman using a patch. This becomes more critical for women in whom the clinician wishes to keep the levels low, because of concerns of thrombosis, for example, or that sufficient $E_2$ is being delivered if the patch is being used for the prevention of osteopenia or osteoporosis.

**BOX 14.3** Hormonal and Osteoporosis Treatments: Available and Approved for Use in Postmenopausal Women

**ESTROGENS**

**Oral**

CEE, 0.3, 0.45, 0.625, 0.9, 1.25, and 2.5 mg
Piperazine estrone sulfate, equivalent of 0.625, 1.25, and 2.5 mg
Esterified, 0.3, 0.625, 0.9, 1.25, and 2.5 mg
Micronized estradiol, 0.5, 1, and 2 mg

**Transdermal**

Estradiol patches, 0.014, 0.025, 0.0375, 0.05, 0.75, and 0.10 mg/day
Estradiol gels, 0.25 to 1.5 mg/day various brands
Estradiol spray, 1.53 mg/day

**Vaginal**

Cream, CEE (0.0625%), estradiol (0.01%)
Estradiol ring, 2 mg: release for atrophy 7.5 μg/day for 3 months
Estradiol acetate ring for vasomotor symptoms: 50 to 100 μg/day for 3 months
Estradiol hemihydrate (tablet) 10 μg: 1 tablet per day for 2 weeks, then twice/week
Estradiol soft gel inset, 4 μg and 10 μg: daily use for 2 weeks, then twice/week

**Parenteral**

Intramuscular injections should be avoided

**PROGESTINS**

**Oral**

Medroxyprogesterone acetate, 2.5, 5, and 10 mg
Norethindrone acetate, 5 mg
Micronized progesterone, 100 and 200 mg

**Vaginal**

Micronized progesterone, 100 mg
Progesterone gel, 4% and 8%

**COMBINATIONS**

**Oral**

CEE + MPA (0.625 mg) + MPA (2.5 or 5 mg)
CEE + MPA (0.3 mg + MPA, 1.5 mg)
Micronized estradiol (1 mg) + norethindrone, acetate (0.5 mg); or 0.5 mg with 0.1 norethindrone acetate
Micronized estradiol (1 mg) + 0.5 mg drospirenone; or 0.5 mg estradiol and 0.25 mg drospirenone
Ethinyl estradiol (5 μg), norethindrone acetate (1 mg or 2.5 μg), and 0.5 mg norethindrone acetate
CEE + bazedoxifene (SERM), 0.45 + 20 mg/day
Micronized estradiol (1 mg) + micronized progesterone (100 mg) in single tablet

**Transdermal**

Patch, 0.05 mg estradiol with 140 μg or 250 μg norethindrone acetate
Patch, 0.045 mg estradiol with levonorgestrel 0.015 mg

**ANDROGENS**

**Oral**

Esterified estrogen and methyl testosterone (0.625/1.25 mg and 1.25/2.5 mg)

**Transdermal**

Patch, 150 μg/300 μg, approved outside the United States

**OTHER NONHORMONAL PRODUCTS**

Ospemifene (SERM), 60 mg/day for vulvovaginal atrophy
Paroxetine (SSRI), 7.5 mg/day for vasomotor symptoms

**MEDICATIONS FOR OSTEOPOROSIS**

**Bisphosphonates**

Alendronate, 5 and 10 mg daily; 35 and 70 mg weekly
Risedronate, 5 mg; 35 mg weekly
Ibandronate, 150 mg monthly and 3l mg IV every 3 months
Zoledronic acid 5 mg once yearly
Etidronate, 200 mg (intermittent)

**Selective Estrogen Receptor Modulators (SERMs)**

Raloxifene, 60 mg

**Others for Osteoporosis**

Tibolone, 2.5 mg (not approved in the United States)
Denosumab, 60 mg subcutaneously every 6 months
Human parathyroid hormone 1-34; 20 μg subcutaneously daily
Romosozumab 105 mg × 2 (prefilled syringes) subcutaneously once/month

*CEE,* Conjugated equine estrogens; *IV,* intravenously; *MPA,* medroxyprogesterone acetate.

**TABLE 14.8** Mean Serum Estradiol ($E_2$) and Estrone ($E_1$)

| | Level (pg/mL) | Level (pg/mL) |
|---|---|---|
| Estrogen dose (mg) | $E_2$ | $E_1$ |
| CEE (0.3)* | 18 | 76 |
| CEE (0.625) | 39 | 153 |
| CEE (1.25) | 60 | 220 |
| Micronized $E_2$ (1) | 35 | 190 |
| Micronized $E_2$ (2) | 63 | 300 |
| $E_1$ sulfate (0.625) | 34 | 125 |
| $E_1$ sulfate (1.25) | 42 | 220 |

*Conjugated equine estrogen (CEE) contains biologically active estrogens other than $E_2$ and $E_1$.

Note also that many commercial assays for $E_2$ are not reliable and do not accurately reflect $E_2$ status, although sensitive assays using mass spectroscopy have been incorporated into clinical assays.

In women with GSU, vaginal therapy is most appropriate. Cream formulations of $E_2$ or CEE are available, as well as tablets, inserts, and an estrogen ring. With creams, systemic absorption occurs but with levels that are one-fourth that achieved after similar doses administered orally. Absorption decreases as the mucosa becomes more estrogenized. For CEE, only 0.5 g (0.3 mg) or less is necessary; for micronized $E_2$, doses as low as 0.25 mg are sufficient. Other products (tablets, inserts and rings) are available that have been designed to limit systemic absorption. A Silastic ring is available that delivers $E_2$ to the vagina for 3 months with only minimal systemic absorption. A vaginal preparation of DHEA (prasterone 6.5 mg vaginal inserts) has also been approved for use to treat dyspareunia. DHEA as a prehormone relies on local (vaginal) conversion to other androgens and estrogen, which may exert a beneficial local effect. Prasterone has been found to be equivalent in efficacies to other hormonal preparations (Heo, 2019).

Estrogen may be administered continuously (daily) or for 21 to 26 days each month. **If the woman has a uterus, a progestogen should be added to the regimen.** For women who are totally intolerant of progestogens (regardless of the dose and route of administration) and take unopposed estrogen, even at lower doses, periodic endometrial sampling is necessary. In this setting, endometrial thickness by ultrasound may be a guide.

## Dealing With Side Effects

Apart from the thrombotic risks of larger doses of oral estrogen (discussed previously), there may be an "idiosyncratic" blood pressure response to oral estrogen. This has been described primarily with the use of CEE and occurs about 5% of the time. Estrogen typically causes no change in blood pressure and often can lower blood pressure, even in women with hypertension. A hypertensive response is often dealt with by changing the dose, preparation, or route of administration. The important clinical point is that blood pressure should be checked after initiation of therapy.

Other somatic effects of estrogen include potential breast tenderness, fluid retention, and bloating (more common with progestogens). All these symptoms are easily dealt with by changing the dose or preparation and potentially by changing the route of administration as well. There should be a great deal of flexibility in the prescribing of estrogen because there is no ideal product for all women.

## Use of a Progestogen

There are many ways to administer progestogens. The most commonly used oral progestins are medroxyprogesterone acetate (MPA) in doses of 2.5 and 5 to 10 mg, norethindrone (NET) in doses of 0.3 to 1 mg, and micronized progesterone in doses of 100 to 300 mg. Equivalent doses to prevent hyperplasia when administered for at least 10 days in a woman receiving ET (equivalent to 0.625 mg CEE) are as follows: MPA, 5 mg; NET, 0.35 mg; and micronized progesterone, 200 mg. Larger doses of estrogen may require larger doses and particularly more prolonged regimens of a progestogen. In the sequential administration of progestogens, the number of days (length of exposure) is more important than the dose. Thus, if a woman is receiving oral ET continuously, a regimen of at least 10 to 12 days' exposure is preferable to a 7-day regimen.

When progestogens are administered sequentially (10 to 14 days each month), withdrawal bleeding occurs in about 80% of women. Continuous administration of both estrogen and progestogen (continuous combined therapy) was developed to achieve amenorrhea. In the first 3 to 6 months, breakthrough bleeding and spotting are common. In some women on this regimen, amenorrhea is never completely achieved. The most common combinations in the United States are single tablets containing 0.45 or 0.625 mg CEE with 1.5 and 2.5 mg MPA, respectively, and 5 $\mu g$ of $E_2$ with 1 mg NET and 1 mg micronized $E_2$ with 0.5 mg NET. The Food and Drug Administration (FDA) has approved a single capsule containing $E_2$ 1 mg with natural progesterone 100 mg for daily dosing. Transdermal patches $E_2$ and NET or $E_2$ and levonorgestrel are also available.

Progesterone administered vaginally (in low doses) avoids systemic effects and results in high concentrations of progesterone in the uterus. This can be accomplished with capsules, suppositories, or a 4% gel. Intrauterine delivery of progestogens is ideal for targeting the uterus and minimizing systemic effects. However, the only marketed product, the Mirena intrauterine system, delivers too high a dose of levonorgestrel (52 mg in the system) for lower doses of estrogen therapy; a 13.5-mg system (Skylar) has been made available. Progestogens, particularly when taken orally, may lead to problems of continuance or compliance because of adverse effects, including mood alterations and bleeding. This requires flexibility in prescribing habits. Most short-term clinical trials have demonstrated an attenuating effect of progestogens on cardiovascular endpoints that are improved with estrogen; these effects include lipoprotein changes (an attenuation of the rise in HDL-C) and arterial and metabolic effects, and potentially a further increase in thrombotic risk. The cardiovascular effects found in the WHI with CEE alone and CEE with MPA, which showed a more favorable effect without MPA, also suggest some detrimental effects of added progestogen. However, two different populations of women were studied in the two WHI trials, which limits any direct comparison. The most inert progestogens, such as micronized progesterone, or vaginal delivery of progesterone should have the fewest attenuating effects. As noted earlier, it is most likely that progestogen exposure is what increases the risk of breast cancer with HT. Natural micronized progesterone was found not to increase the risk of breast cancer in several French observational studies (Fournier, 2008). Progestogens should not be used in women who have had a hysterectomy.

## Androgen Therapy

In a subtle way, some women are relatively androgen deficient or insufficient. Clinicians have proposed adding androgen to ET or HT for complaints or problems relating to libido and energy that are not relieved by adequate estrogen. Although well-controlled trials using parenteral testosterone have shown benefit in younger oophorectomized women, there have been few data showing a benefit to using more physiologic therapy. Data using a testosterone patch or pellet (with near physiologic levels) have indicated improvement in several scales of well-being and sexual function (Simon, 2005). A 2019 systematic review and meta-analysis showed that testosterone is both safe and efficacious when used to treat low sexual desire in women (Islam, 2019). Although testosterone is typically administered nonorally, an oral preparation (esterified estrogens 0.625 mg with 1.25 mg of methyl testosterone) was shown to improve sexual motivation and enjoyment in women with hypoactive sexual desire who were unresponsive to estrogen alone. The latter findings correlated with an increase in circulating unbound testosterone levels. **At present, androgen therapy should be individualized and considered for those women who have symptoms that are not adequately relieved with traditional hormonal therapies.** Measuring testosterone before therapy is not helpful in making this determination, but it is essential to monitor testosterone levels during therapy because the normal range of testosterone is narrow in women and there is a tendency to get higher levels, which can lead to adverse effects, particularly masculinizing symptoms such as acne and hirsutism. Administration of DHEA at 25 to 50 mg/day may also be an option for raising endogenous testosterone, but data have not shown it to be beneficial for symptoms such as hypoactive sexual desire.

Another SERM-like compound that is used worldwide but is not approved in the United States is tibolone. This progestogen-like compound exhibits estrogenic, antiestrogenic, and androgenic effects by virtue of its structure and metabolites. At 2.5 mg, tibolone suppresses hot flushes, prevents osteoporosis, and has a positive effect on mood and sexual function. There is also limited (or no) uterine stimulation. However, there is suppression of HDL-C, but at the same time a decrease in triglycerides. In monkeys no deleterious effect of tibolone on coronary arteries was identified.

## "Bioidentical" Hormone Therapy

It has become popular to have compounding pharmacies dispense a mixture of "bioidentical" hormones in a cream or suspension for topical administration. These preparations usually contain one or more estrogens, progesterone, testosterone, and often other precursors such as pregnenolone. **As an unregulated industry, without approval by the FDA, there is inadequate**

**quality control for these products, with batch-to-batch variation and the inclusion of some steroid hormones that may not be necessary.** Claims that these compounded products are safer than pharmaceutical grade hormones is completely unsubstantiated. Nevertheless, use of these preparations has dramatically increased since the reports from the WHI, with the perception that they are safer. Ironically, during this time, as use of traditional hormone products has decreased, an increased incidence of endometrial cancer has been witnessed (Constantine, 2019). Also, "titrating" preparations to salivary hormone levels is not accurate and has never been validated. Indeed micronized $E_2$, orally or as a transdermal product, and micronized progesterone are bioidentical products approved by the FDA and should be first-line therapies. Several major societies have come out with strong statements against the use of compounded bioidentical preparations, and there is a combined statement from the American Society for Reproductive Medicine (ASRM) and the American College of Obstetricians and Gynecologists (ACOG) (Practice Committee, 2012).

### Tissue Selective Estrogen Complex Concept

The tissue selective estrogen complex (TSEC) concept is a newer therapy for menopause that pairs together an estrogen and a SERM, which when complexed together have specific and different tissue properties than either one would exert independently. A specific SERM, bazedoxifene (BZA)—which has agonistic effects (acting like an estrogen) on bone, antagonistic effects on the uterus and breast, and minimal effects on the central nervous system (CNS)—when paired with CEE maintains the effects of CEE on reducing hot flushes, yet prevents endometrial hyperplasia. Accordingly, a progestogen is not needed, and this continuous regimen results in a low rate of vaginal bleeding. It is beneficial for osteoporosis protection and at least theoretically should be safer for the breast as well (Kagan, 2012). It is available as a combination product of CEE 0.45 mg and 20 mg of BZA.

## ALTERNATIVE THERAPIES FOR MENOPAUSE

There are several nonhormonal alternatives for symptoms of menopause, which are listed in Box 14.4, although none of these is as effective as estrogen. Nevertheless, for women who cannot or choose not to take a hormonal preparation, some of these are viable substitutes. Because there is a fairly significant placebo effect in the reduction in hot flushes (up to 40% reduction), at least in the short term, randomized trials against placebo are necessary to establish efficacy.

Not listed here, because this list includes nonhormonal preparations, rather than estrogen or estrogen/progestogen regimens, there is an established efficacy of using progestogens alone. MPA 10 to 20 mg, and NET 5 to 10 mg (as well as other progestogen regimens) used alone have shown some benefit in women with hot flushes, but this is less beneficial than the use of estrogen and has more side effects, particularly with more long-term therapy (>3 months). Also, if a woman cannot or will not take estrogen, it is unlikely that she would take a progestogen alone. Therefore this is often an impractical choice for dealing with symptoms.

**BOX 14.4** Nonhormonal Therapies for Vasomotor Symptoms

Antidepressants (SSRIs/SNRIs)
Gabapentin
Clonidine
Isoflavones, red clover, black cohosh
Cognitive behavior therapy
Acupuncture
Stellate ganglion block

*SNRI*, selective norepinephrine reuptake inhibitor; *SSRI*, selective serotonin reuptake inhibitor.

### Antidepressants (Selective Serotonin Reuptake Inhibitors/Serotonin Norepinephrine Reuptake Inhibitors)

Several well-controlled clinical studies have demonstrated efficacies of several antidepressant drugs for hot flushes that were initially used in women with breast cancer. These include fluoxetine (20 mg), venlafaxine (75 mg), paroxetine (12.5 mg, 25 mg), and escitalopram (10 mg, 20 mg). Apart from some side effects, such as nausea, dry mouth, and sexual dysfunction, all these agents are superior to placebo in reducing hot flushes. However, only one product, paroxetine, is approved by the FDA, at a lower dose of 7.5 mg. This has a moderate effect, and in breast cancer patients it may interfere with tamoxifen therapy.

### Gabapentin

Gabapentin has been shown to be superior to placebo in doses ranging from 300 to 900 mg. Side effects include somnolence, dizziness, fatigue, and ataxia, which are dose related. If doses are titrated up to 2400 mg (a very large dose), the efficacy has been shown to be similar to that of CEE at 0.625 mg (Reddy, 2006).

### Antihypertensives

Clonidine has been the most studied antihypertensive, but methyldopa also has efficacy over placebo in reducing hot flushes. Typically a 0.1-mg patch is used daily. There is an obvious hypotensive response, and the efficacy is not very large, precluding its routine use unless the patient is also hypertensive.

### Phytoestrogens

It has been suggested that 30% to 60% of women with symptoms at menopause seek "natural" therapies, and the majority are botanicals such as phytoestrogens. The Dietary Supplement Health and Education Act of 1994 classifies most botanical medicines as food supplements and removes them from regulatory oversight and scrutiny by the FDA. Adulteration, contamination, and poor quality control in their harvesting, manufacture, and formulation yield products of questionable efficacy and safety.

The FDA has determined that more than 25% of Chinese patent medicines are adulterated with hidden pharmaceutical drugs. These kinds of deficiencies make it difficult for consumers and practitioners to employ botanicals with confidence and security. Furthermore, clinical trial data obtained using one brand of herbal product cannot necessarily be extrapolated to other brands using the same plant.

Phytoestrogens are a class of plant-derived estrogen-like compounds conjugated to glycoside moieties. Phytoestrogens are not biologically active in their native forms unless taken orally. After oral ingestion, colonic bacteria cleave the glycosides, producing active compounds that are subject to the enterohepatic circulation. These compounds can produce estrogen-agonistic effects in some tissues, whereas in other tissues they produce antagonistic effects.

Few randomized trials have examined the efficacy of phytoestrogens. For large daily doses (60 mg isoflavone), there appears to be some limited efficacy in relieving hot flushes, although the literature on this issue is mixed. In placebo-controlled trials, red clover and black cohosh have been found to have similar effects as placebo (Fig. 14.41) (Geller, 2009).

With doses of 30 to 40 mg of soy isoflavone, cholesterol levels may be reduced, but this is not a consistent finding. Phytoestrogens do not appear to have much of an effect on bone loss or on vaginal atrophy.

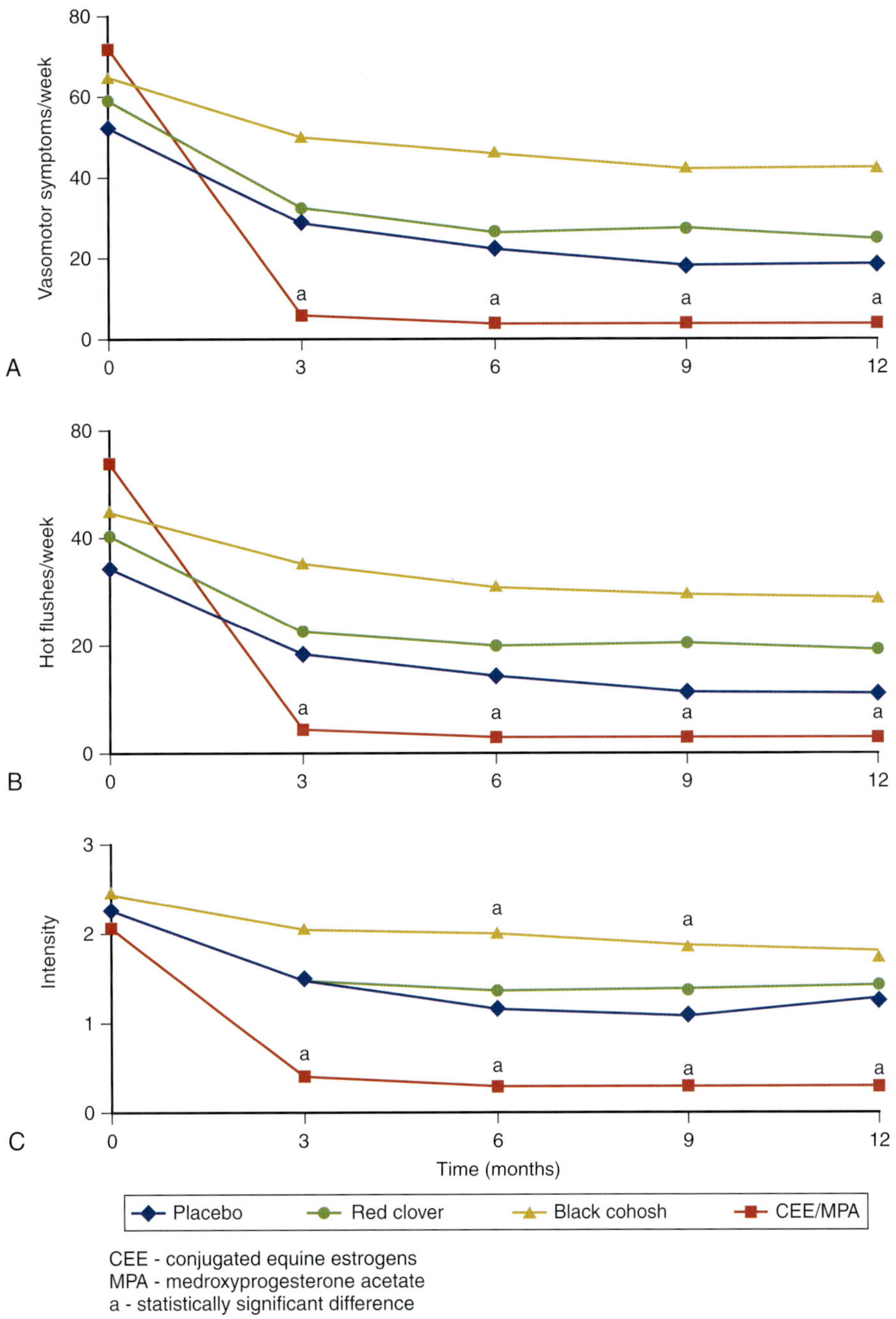


**Fig. 14.41** **A,** Number of vasomotor symptoms per week. **B,** Number of hot flushes per week. **C,** Intensity of the hot flushes. Black cohosh and red clover are not different from placebo. *E*, Estrogen; *P*, progestogen. (Modified from Geller SE, Shulman LP, van Breemen RB, et al. Safety and efficacy of black cohosh and red clover for the management of vasomotor symptoms: a randomized controlled trial. *Menopause.* 2009;16(6): 1156-1166.)

## Cognitive Behavioral Therapy

"Talk therapy," which teaches coping skills that may change one's cognitive appraisal of the symptoms, may be beneficial (van Driel et al., 2019). It is not clear if this treatment is sustained over time.

## Acupuncture

Acupuncture has been used in several trials to assess the treatment of hot flushes and other menopausal symptoms. A meta-analysis confirmed that acupuncture may be effective in alleviating the frequency and severity of hot flushes (Chiu, 2015).

## Stellate Ganglion Blockade

Although somewhat invasive, needle injection of the stellate ganglion has been shown to be effective in some women, such as those being treated for breast cancer. In one study, image-guided stellate ganglion blockade with 5 mL of 0.5% bupivacaine was shown to be beneficial compared with sham injection with saline for vasomotor symptoms (Walega, 2014).

## KEY REFERENCES


Anderson GL, Chlebowski RT, Rossouw JE. Prior hormone therapy and breast cancer risk in the Women's Health Initiative randomized trial of estrogen and progestin. *Maturitas.* 2006;55:107-115.

Ashcroft GS, Dodsworth J, van Boxtel E, et al. Estrogen accelerates cutaneous wound healing associated with an increase in TGF-beta 1 levels. *Nat Med.* 1997;3:1209-1215.

Atsma F, Bartelink ML, Grobbee DE, et al. Postmenopausal status and early menopause as independent risk factors for cardiovascular disease: a meta-analysis. *Menopause.* 2006;13(2):265-279.

Avis NE, Crawford Sl, Greendale G, et al. Duration of menopausal vasomotor Symptoms. *JAMA Intern Med.* 2015;175(4):531-539.

Barrionuevo P, Kapoor E, Asi N, et al. Efficacy of pharmacological therapies for the prevention of fractures in postmenopausal women: a network meta-analysis. *J Clin Endocrinol Metab.* 2019;104:1623-1630.

Bidet M, Bachelot A, Bissauge E, et al. Resumption of ovarian function and pregnancies in 358 patients with premature ovarian failure. *JCEM.* 2011;96:38964-38972.

Boardman HMP, Hartley L, Main C, et al. Hormone therapy for preventing cardiovascular disease in post-menopausal women (review). *Cochrane Database Syst Rev.* 2015;3:CD002229.

Bonds DE, Lasser N, Qi L, et al. The effect of conjugated equine oestrogen on diabetes incidence: the Women's Health Initiative randomized trial. *Diabetologia.* 2006;49(3):459-468.

Canonico M, Plu-Bureau G, Lowe GD, et al. Hormone replacement therapy and risk of venous thromboembolism in postmenopausal women: systematic review and meta-analysis. *BMJ.* 2008;336(7655):1227-1231.

Carani C, Quin K, Simoni M, et al. Effect of testosterone and estradiol in a man with aromatase deficiency. *N Engl J Med.* 1997;337:91-95.

Chen S, Sawicka J, Betterle C, et al. Autoantibodies to steroidogenic enzymes in autoimmune polyglandular syndrome, Addison's disease, and premature ovarian failure. *J Clin Endocrinol Metab.* 1996;81(5):1871-1876.

Chiu H-Y, Shyu, Y-K, Chang Pi-Chen et al. Effects of acupuncture on menopause-related symptoms in breast cancer survivors: a meta-analysis of randomized controlled trials. *Cancer Nurs.* 2016;39(3):228-237.

Chu MC, Cosper P, Orio F, et al. Insulin resistance in postmenopausal women with metabolic syndrome and the measurements of adiponectin, leptin, resistin, and ghrelin. *Am J Obstet Gynecol.* 2006;194(1):100-104.

Collaborative Group on Hormonal Factors in Breast Cancer. Type and timing of menopausal hormone therapy and breast cancer risk: individual participant meta-analysis of the worldwide epidemiological evidence. *Lancet.* 2019;394(10204):1159-1168.

Collins JA, Allen I, Donner A, Adams O. Oestrogen use and survival in endometrial cancer. *Lancet.* 1980;2:961-963.

Cooper AR, Baker VL, Sterling EW, et al. The time is now for a new approach to primary ovarian insufficiency. *Fertil Steril.* 2011;95(6):1890-1897.

Constantine GD, Kessler G, Graham S, et al. Increased incidence of endometrial cancer following the Women's Health Initiative: an assessment of risk factors. *J Womens Health.* 2019;28(2):237-243.

Couzinet B, Meduri G, Lecce MG, et al. The postmenopausal ovary is not a major androgen-producing gland. *J Clin Endocrinol Metab.* 2001;86:5060-5066.

Cummings SR, Black DM, Thompson DE, et al. Effect of alendronate on risk of fracture in women with low bone density but without vertebral fractures: results from the fracture intervention trial. *JAMA.* 1998;280:2077-2082.

Dawson-Hughes B, Looker AC, Tosteson AN, et al. The potential impact of new National Osteoporosis Foundation guidance on treatment patterns. *Osteoporos Int.* 2010;21(1):41-52.


**Full references and Suggested readings for this chapter can be found on ExpertConsult.com.**

# 15 Breast Diseases

## Detection, Management, and Surveillance of Breast Disease

*Samith Sandadi, David T. Rock, James W. Orr Jr., Fidel A. Valea*

### KEY POINTS

- The breast consists of approximately 20% glandular tissue and 80% fat and connective tissue; increasing proportions of fibroglandular to fatty tissues are the mark of denser breasts. Breast density is associated with increased risks of malignancy.
- Lymph drainage of the breast usually flows toward the most adjacent group of nodes. This concept represents the basis for sentinel node mapping in breast cancer. In most instances, breast cancer spreads in an orderly fashion within the axillary lymph node basin based on the anatomic relationship between the primary tumor and its associated regional (sentinel) nodes.
- The breast undergoes normal maturational changes throughout a woman's lifetime. The normal maturation involves a gradual increase in fibrous tissue around the lobules; with time the glandular elements are completely replaced by fibrous tissue.
- The incidence of benign breast disorders begins to rise during the second decade of life and peaks in the fourth and fifth decades. In malignant diseases the incidence continues to increase after menopause.
- Fibroadenomas are the most common benign breast neoplasm and are most often present in adolescents and women in their 20s.
- Approximately 35% of fibroadenomas will disappear, and 10% will become smaller after many years.
- More than two-thirds of women will experience breast pain at some time during their reproductive years, most commonly in the perimenopausal years. Approximately 90% of conditions that cause breast pain are benign.
- Cyclic bilateral breast pain is the classic symptom of fibrocystic breast change. The signs of fibrocystic changes include increased engorgement and density of the breasts, excessive nodularity, rapid change and fluctuation in the size of cystic areas, increased tenderness, and, occasionally, spontaneous nipple discharge.
- The majority of nipple discharge complaints have a benign cause; however, 55% present with a coexisting mass, of which 19% are malignant. An underlying malignancy is more likely when the discharge is spontaneous (vs. induced with nipple pressure), arises from a single duct, is blood stained, and is unilateral and persistent (occurring more than twice weekly).
- Intraductal papilloma and fibrocystic changes are the two most common causes of spontaneous nonmilky nipple discharge.
- Lactational mastitis commonly occurs in the first pregnancy during the first 6 weeks of breastfeeding. Continued breastfeeding or manual pumping of the affected breast is recommended to decrease engorgement.
- One out of eight women (12.5%) in the United States will develop carcinoma of the breast over the course of her lifetime.
- Approximately 50% of newly diagnosed breast cancers are attributable to known risk, whereas 10% are associated with a positive family history.
- Approximately 5% to 10% of breast cancers have a familial or genetic link. A genetic predisposition to develop breast carcinoma has been recognized in some families. In these families, breast cancer tends to occur at a younger age, and there is a higher prevalence of bilateral disease.
- Mutations in the *BRCA* family of genes have been identified that confer a lifetime risk of breast cancer that approaches 85%. *BRCA1* and *BRCA2* genes are involved in the majority of inheritable cases of breast cancer. These genes function as tumor suppressor genes, and several mutations have been described on each of these genes.
- Once a woman has developed carcinoma of one breast, her risk is approximately 1% per year of developing cancer in the other breast.
- Both tamoxifen and raloxifene significantly decrease the relative risk of developing breast carcinoma. Aromatase inhibitors are a reasonable alternative to SERMs for postmenopausal women.
- Screening mammography is the primary imaging technique for breast cancer detection. The sensitivity of mammography ranges from 80% to 90% and decreases in women with dense breasts.
- The incidence of carcinoma in biopsy specimens corresponds directly with the patient's age. Approximately 20% of breast biopsy results in women age 50 are positive, and this figure increases to 33% in women age 70 or older.
- Breast cancer is usually asymptomatic before the development of advanced disease. Breast pain is experienced by only 10% of women with early breast carcinoma. The classic sign of a breast carcinoma is a solitary, solid, three-dimensional, dominant breast mass. The borders of the mass are usually indistinct.
- Microscopic metastatic disease occurs early via both hematogenous and lymphatic routes. For example, 30% to 40% of women without gross adenopathy in the axilla will have positive nodes discovered during histologic examination. With the additional assessment tools of immunohistochemical staining for the presence of cytokeratin and serial sectioning of axillary nodes, 10% to 30% of patients considered to have negative nodes by standard histologic analysis are found to be node positive.
- The initial size of the breast carcinoma is the single best predictor of the likelihood of positive axillary nodes. The presence and number of axillary node metastases are the best predictors of survival.
- Carcinomas make up the majority of breast malignancies and originate in the epithelium of the collecting ducts (ductal) or the terminal lobular ducts (lobular). Invasive ductal carcinoma is the most common, constituting approximately 70% to 80% of malignancies.
- A multidisciplinary team approach is necessary in the treatment of breast cancer. Determination of local or systemic treatment is based on several prognostic and predictive factors, including tumor histologic characteristics, tumor hormone receptor status (estrogen/progesterone), tumor HER2 status, multigene testing, axillary lymph node status, evaluation of metastatic disease, patient age, comorbidities, and menopausal status.
- The primary therapy for the majority of women with stages I and II breast cancer is conservative surgery, which preserves the breast, followed by radiation therapy.
- Gynecologists should actively address the psychosexual problems that breast cancer causes in women early in the evaluation of the disease and for several years.

The gynecologist's role in managing breast problems is broad because they often serve as a woman's primary health care advocate. Historically, gynecologists have played a leadership role in the modern development of women's breast cancer care. In 1913 they were instrumental in the organization of the American Cancer Society (initially known as the American Society for the Control of Cancer), and in 1976 they assumed a major role in the organization of the American Society of Breast Disease. Strategically, gynecologists, commonly acting as primary health care advocates, continue to maintain a vital and advantageous role in the diagnosis and management of benign, premalignant, and malignant breast disease. In fact, the prevalence and significant psychological and psychosocial effect of breast disease necessitate that a comprehensive plan for the diagnosis and management of breast disease becomes a critical component of high-quality women's health care. This chapter intends to present a clinically oriented approach to improve the understanding of breast anatomy, the important diagnostic and therapeutic aspects of benign breast disease, and the epidemiology, detection, and management of breast cancer.

In the United States 7.8% of office visits by women (>51 million/year) related to breast disease. Breast pain is a common and chronic symptom in women, with a prevalence of 52% in the general population, and adversely affects the quality of life in more than 40% of women (Kushwaha, 2018). Additionally, breast cancer accounts for 30% of all new cancer diagnoses in women, is the second most common cause of cancer- related death in women, and is the leading cause of premature mortality from cancer in U.S. women (as measured by total years of life lost).

The role of the gynecologist in the management of breast disease has been addressed in a number of published clinical opinions and practice bulletins from the American College of Obstetrics and Gynecology. The role of the gynecologist, with shared decision making, includes the following:

- Compiling a comprehensive personal and family history in an effort to identify risk factors and institute care accordingly
- Performing clinical breast examinations when deemed appropriate in average risk individuals and in those at high risk or with breast symptoms.
- Promoting breast self-awareness and offering instructions for breast self-evaluation as indicated or desired
- Distinguishing between benign and malignant disease and offering successful therapy for benign disease.
- Discussing the risks and benefits of screening mammography and encouraging compliance with guidelines
- Performing diagnostic procedures or referral to those who specialize in breast disease when clinically indicated (i.e., when a palpable mass has been detected)

Despite the fact that 50% of cases of breast cancer in women 50 years and older and 71% of cases of breast cancer in women younger than 50 years are detected by women themselves (ACOG Practice Bulletin Number 179, 2015), most guidelines have questioned the benefit of breast self-examination. Thus the term *breast self-awareness* has been coined to imply the potential benefit of women being aware of their breasts and looking for abnormalities or changes, without mention of frequency or proper technique. Additionally, these guidelines indicate that there is insufficient evidence to assess the additional benefit of clinical breast examination (CBE) beyond screening mammography in women aged 40 years or older (Siu, 2016). However, the American College of Obstetrics and Gynecology and the National Comprehensive Cancer Network suggest that CBE be offered or performed at 1- to 3-year intervals in patients aged 25 to 39 years and annually after 40 (ACOG Practice Bulletin 179, 2015).

## ANATOMY/EMBRYOLOGY

Breast (mammary gland) development begins from the integument along the epithelial mammary ridges during the sixth gestational week in utero. Ducts and acini are derived from ectoderm, whereas supporting tissue arises from mesenchyme. Embryologic development requires a series of orderly events regulated by systemic and local hormones and growth factors. Before puberty, male and female mammary glands are identical. Ductal tissue and secretory lobule development occurs under the influence of the hormonal changes that occur during puberty (see Chapter 38 ). Actual milk production is initiated by hormonal changes that occur during and after pregnancy.

The breasts are large, structurally dynamic, modified apocrine/sweat glands located on the superficial fascia anterior to the deep pectoralis major fascia of the chest wall. Posteriorly the retromammary space, a loose connective tissue plane, allows free movement over the chest wall (i.e., the breast is not firmly attached to the deep fascia). Breast tissue is suspended from the clavicle and deep clavipectoral fascia by the **suspensory ligaments of Cooper** that weave through the breast tissue and attach to the dermis of the skin (Fig. 15.1). These fibrous septa maintain the natural shape of the breast. Clinically, malignant involvement (particularly locally advanced disease) of these ligaments often produces skin retraction.

Breast size and shape depend on genetic, racial, and dietary factors as well as age, parity, and menopausal status. The "average" adult breast during reproductive years weighs approximately 250 g. Typically a superolateral projection of glandular tissue (the axillary tail of Spence) pierces the deep fascia and extends toward the axilla. Glandular tissue comprises approximately 20% of the mature breast, with the remainder composed of adipose and connective tissue. The major determinant of breast size is adipose tissue volume. The periphery of the breast is predominantly adipose, and glandular tissue comprises a higher proportion of the central breast (Fig. 15.2). Typically, glandular tissue regresses and is replaced by adipose tissue after menopause.

*Breast density* refers to the proportion of fibrous or glandular tissue to adipose tissue. Breast density is only determined mammographically, because dense breasts are not clinically characterized

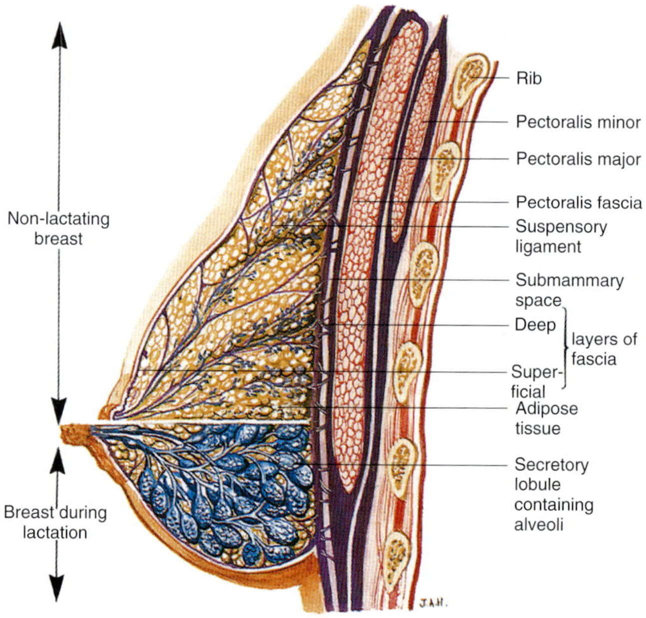


**Fig. 15.1** Lactating breast. (From Shah P, ed. Breast. In: Standring S, ed. *Gray's Anatomy*. London: Churchill Livingstone; 2005:969.)

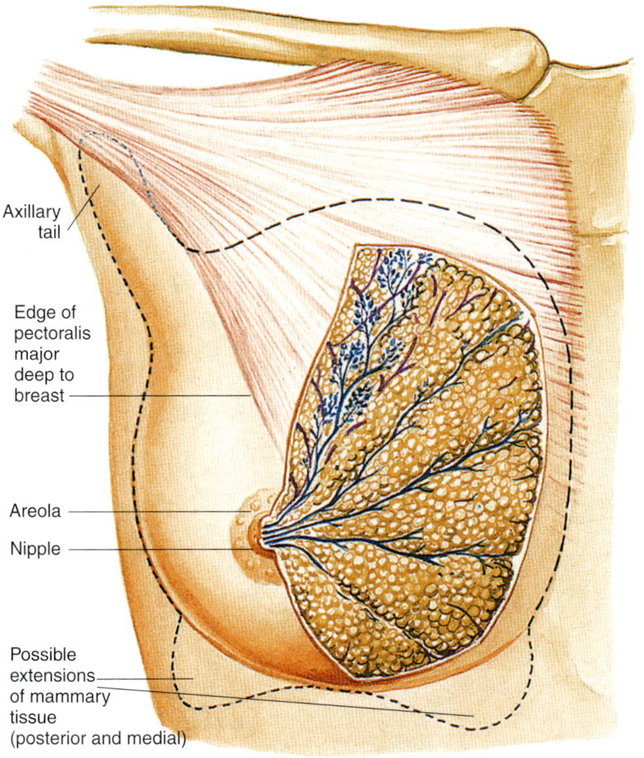


**Fig. 15.2** The structures of the breast. (From Shah P, ed. Breast. In: Standring S, ed. *Gray's Anatomy.* London: Churchill Livingstone; 2005:969.)

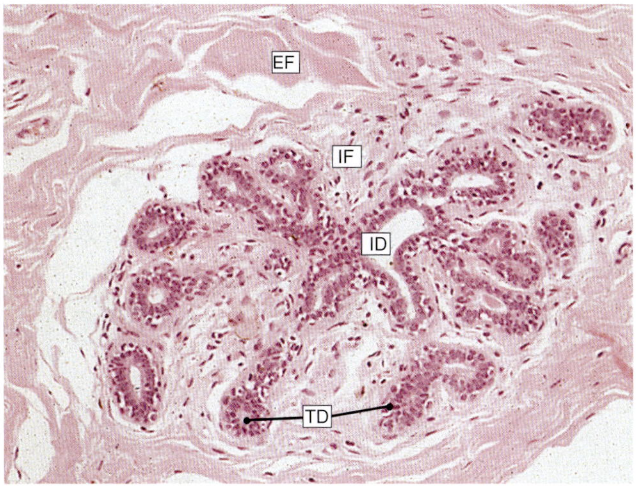


**Fig. 15.3** Histologic photograph of a mammary lobule. Note the ductal tissue surrounded by fibrous tissue. Terminal ductules *(TD)* surround the central ductule *(ID). EF,* Extralobular fibrocollagenous tissue. (From Stevens A, Lowe J. *Human Histology.* 3rd ed. Philadelphia: Mosby; 2005:390.)

by a certain size or shape, and they may or may not be palpably firm. The percentage of breast density on a mammogram correlates with breast cancer risk. Importantly, when comparing the lowest density category with highest, the relative risk is increased more than fivefold.

A breast is composed of 10 to 20 variably sized, triangular-shaped **lobes** distributed radially from the nipple. Each lobe contains its own duct system draining the 10 to 100 lobules with alveoli (acini). These functional lobules include epithelial (ductal) and stromal components and are affected by hormonal changes (estrogen, progesterone, and prolactin) resulting in development, maturation, and differentiation (Fig. 15.3). The organization of the ductal system is stimulated at puberty. Secretory cells drain into alveoli, which drain into "terminal" ducts that coalesce into larger collecting ducts and join with ducts from other lobules to end in lactiferous ducts, terminating at the excretory ducts of the nipple.

Approximately 5 to 20 **areolar (Montgomery) glands** produce an oily secretion functioning to keep the nipple supple and protected, which is particularly important during breastfeeding. They also produce a volatile compound that has been implicated in stimulating infants' appetite through olfactory pathways (Doucet, 2009). These generally sensitive glands are located in the areola and nipple. Infection, blockage, or irritation can result in significant clinical symptoms or problems.

The principal blood supply of the breast is derived from the perforating branches of the internal mammary arteries that originate from the internal thoracic artery. Additional sources include the lateral thoracic and thoracoacromial arteries, which originate from the axillary artery, and the posterior third, fourth, and fifth intercostal arteries, which are branches of the thoracic aorta. The inferior and central portions of the breast are less vascular.

Breast lymphatics converge in the subareolar plexus of **Sappy**. Approximately 75% of the lymphatics, particularly from the outer quadrants, drain to the 30 to 60 ipsilateral axillary regional nodes. The axillary nodes are classified by three anatomic levels defined by their relationship to the pectoralis minor muscle. Level I nodes are located lateral to the lateral border of the pectoralis minor muscle. Level II nodes are located posterior to the pectoralis minor muscle. Level III nodes include the infraclavicular nodes medial to the pectoralis minor muscle. The remaining lymphatics drain to the internal mammary or parasternal nodes, which have direct drainage to the mediastinum, the medial quadrants of the opposite breast, or the inferior phrenic nodes. The latter is important because it provides a route for metastatic disease to the liver, ovaries, and peritoneum (Fig. 15.4). Lymphatic fluid usually flows toward the most adjacent group of nodes, forming the foundation for using sentinel node mapping to evaluate for nodal spread in breast cancer. In most instances, breast cancer spreads in an orderly fashion within the axillary lymph node basin based on the anatomic relationship between the primary tumor and its associated regional (sentinel) nodes. However, lymphatic metastases from one specific area of the breast may be found in any or all of the groups of regional nodes.

Breast ductal epithelium is extremely sensitive to cyclic hormonal changes. Parenchymal proliferation of the ducts is seen during the follicular phase, and there is dilation of the ductal system and differentiation of the alveolar cells into secretory cells during the luteal phase. Alveolar elements respond to both estrogen and progesterone. The stroma and myoepithelial cells also respond to estrogen and progesterone. Women often experience cyclic breast fullness and tenderness likely related to the 25 to 30 mL average volume fluctuation of the premenstrual breasts. Additionally, premenstrual breast symptoms are produced by an increase in blood flow, leading to vascular engorgement, and water retention. A parallel enlargement of the ductal lumen and an increase in ductal and acinar cellular secretory activity also occur. Menstruation brings a regression of cellular activity in the alveoli, and the ducts become smaller. These changes are clinically reflected by the cyclic changes noted on breast examination.

The breast undergoes normal maturational changes. In addition to the pubertal and pregnancy-induced changes in the lactiferous duct lobule, the fibrous and adipose components also evolve. Normal maturation involves a gradual increase in fibrous tissue around the lobules, and with time the glandular elements are completely replaced by fibrous tissue. Women in their 20s and 30s have a

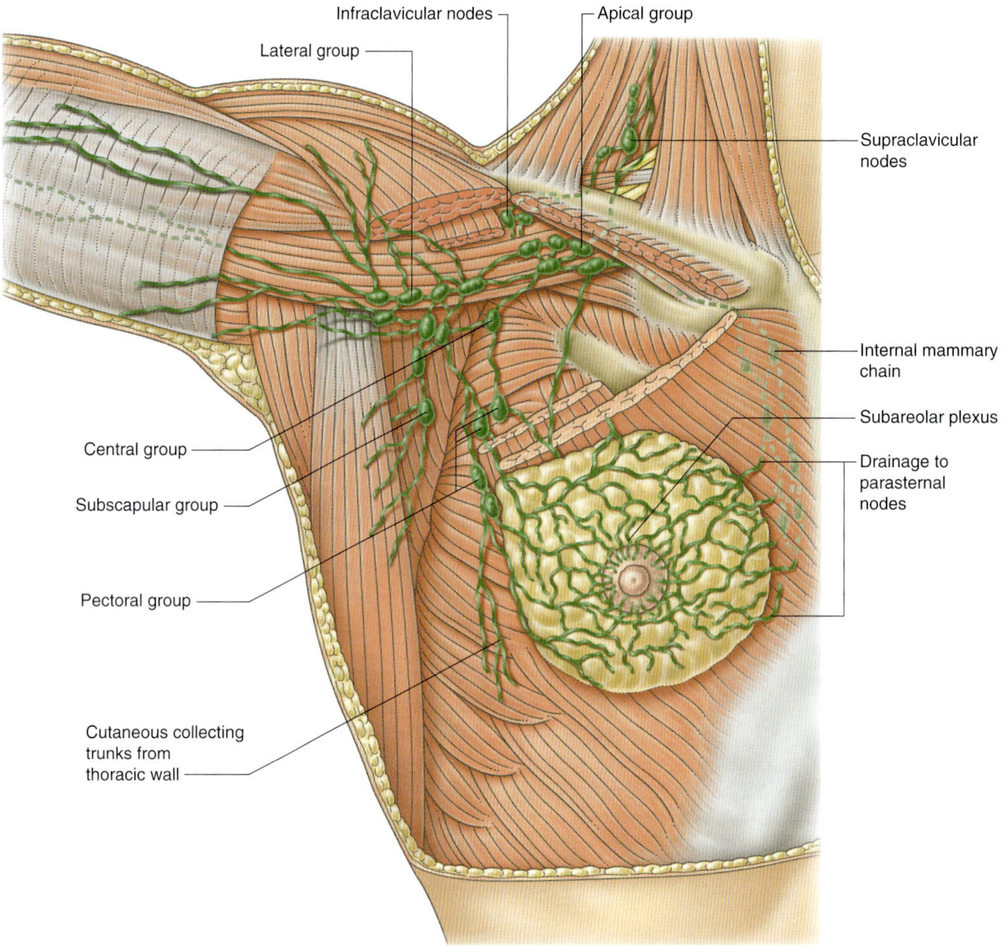


**Fig. 15.4** Lymph vessels of the breast and axillary lymph nodes. (From Shah P, ed. Breast. In: Standring S, ed. *Gray's Anatomy*. London: Churchill Livingstone; 2005:971.)

gradual increase in nodularity as the lobular tissue increases with repetitive cyclic hormonal stimulation. Compared with the prepregnancy or postpregnancy state and lactation, breasts may decrease in size and shape. Thus breast examination often yields different findings in the 20-year-old and the 40-year-old, as well as in women experiencing perimenopause and postmenopause. These changes underscore the value of breast self-awareness because each woman should personally know those changes in her breast at different times in her cycle and life (Fig. 15.5).

## CONGENITAL DEVELOPMENTAL BREAST ABNORMALITIES

### Nipple

Accessory nipples may occur along the breast or milk lines running from the axilla to the groin. **Polythelia** (supernumerary or accessory nipples) occurs in less than 1% (white European descent) to 2.5% (Jewish population) of women. They most commonly present in the inframammary region (90%), may be unilateral or bilateral, and occur in equal frequency in men and women. Development may be partial or complete, and the condition is both sporadic and familial. Obstructive or duplicative urologic anomalies may be present as well, and an increased risk of renal cancer has been reported. When present, accessory nipples have the same risk for disease as normal nipples. Treatment is generally restricted to managing irritation or improving cosmesis when necessary.

Congenital nipple inversion occurs in 2% of women, typically in those with a family history of the same condition. The cause is related to shortening and tethering of breast ducts or the development of fibrous bands during intrauterine life. Although nipple inversion may increase mechanical problems with breastfeeding, surgical correction often leads to loss of sensation and inability to breastfeed.

Athelia, complete unilateral or bilateral absence of nipple and areola, can be familial (autosomal dominant) and is associated with amastia (absent nipple, areola, and breast tissue) or other rare syndromes (e.g., Poland syndrome). Associated ectodermal abnormalities (such as absence of the pectoral muscles) should be excluded. Treatment includes nipple and areola reconstruction commonly using tissue flaps and tattooing.

### Breast Tissue

Aplasia is diagnosed when the nipple and areola are present but glandular tissue is absent. Amastia, complete absence of both breast tissue and the nipple-areola complex, occurs with regression or failure to develop the mammary ridge. It is often associated with other ectodermal defects, including cleft palate.

**Polymastia**, accessory breast tissue or supernumerary breasts, occurs in approximately 1% to 2% of the general population, with a female preponderance. Accessory breast tissue most commonly presents in the axilla, and multiple site occurrence is not uncommon (~33%). The initial diagnosis is often at puberty or during pregnancy, when the accessory breast tissue development

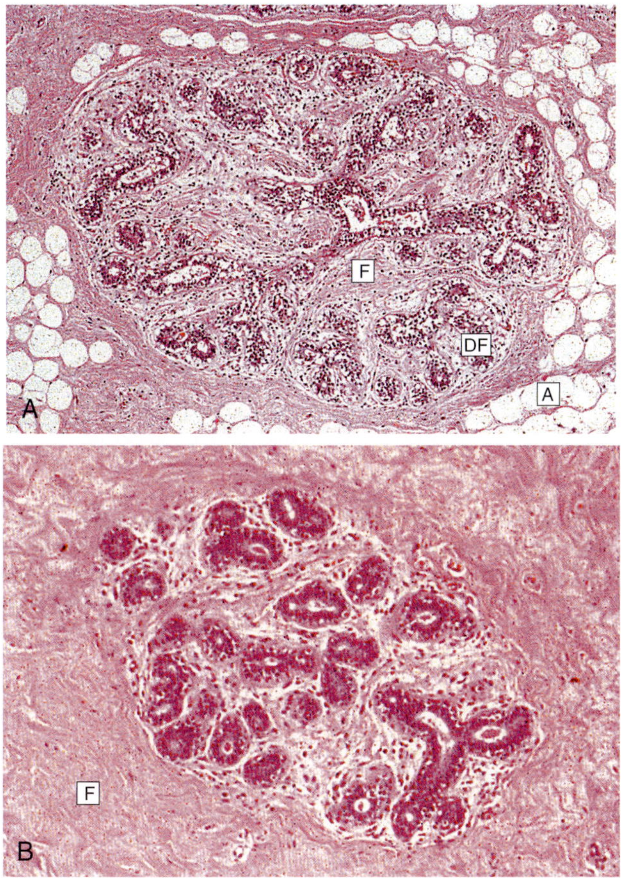


**Fig. 15.5 A,** Micrograph showing normal breast tissue from a 23-year-old woman. At the center is a breast lobule in which the system of terminal ducts and ductules is embedded in loose intralobular fibrocollagenous stroma *(F)*. There is a narrow surrounding zone of dense extralobular fibrocollagenous support tissue *(DF)*, outside of which is the soft adipose tissue *(A)* that forms the bulk of the breast. **B,** Micrograph showing normal breast tissue from a 43-year-old woman. As women age, the amount of fibrocollagenous tissue *(F)* in the breast increases, replacing some of the adipose tissue. The mammary lobules become enclosed in dense collagen. (From Stevens A, Lowe J. *Human Histology.* 3rd ed. Philadelphia: Mosby; 2005:393.)

and stimulation parallel that of normal breast tissue. Supernumerary breast tissue, be it rudimentary or fully developed, is customarily asymptomatic; however, it can cause discomfort and may be considered cosmetically unacceptable. Importantly, supernumerary breast tissue is subject to normal changes and is susceptible to the entire disease spectrum that occurs in the normal breast. Conservative management is encouraged because surgery can be associated with unattractive scars, restriction of movement, pain, and other complications. Liposuction may useful to decrease the fatty element of accessory breasts.

Asymmetric breast development, common in adolescence and in maturity, represents a benign, normal variation unless an associated palpable abnormality is present. In the extreme a breast can be hypoplastic or absent (aplasia), which can occur in isolation or in association with a defect in (one or both) pectoral muscles. Significant asymmetry can be deeply disturbing and may affect a teenager's self-image. Full breast development usually occurs by age 18 to 21 years, and if deemed necessary, corrective augmentative or reduction surgery should be timed accordingly.

**Breast hypertrophy** may be related to excessive development of glandular tissue during puberty, weight gain, or naturally occurring fat deposition of breast tissue associated with aging. It may be asymmetric and is separated into pubertal (virginal hypertrophy), gestational (gravid macromastia), and adult types. Medical treatment is typically not successful, and reduction mammoplasty is not indicated until a significant volume of breast tissue requires removal to relieve associated symptoms such as headache, neck or back pain, upper extremity paresthesia, brassiere strap grooving, or intertrigo. The best surgical outcome can be expected when the planned procedure occurs after 6 to 12 months of breast size stabilization.

Tubular breasts or tuberous breast deformity is associated with a constriction in the lower pole of the breast. This unilateral or bilateral congenital breast abnormality occurs in both sexes. During puberty, breast development is stymied and the breasts fail to develop normally and fully. The transverse breast diameter is narrowed and the base constricted related to glandular hypoplasia with a deficiency in the circumferential skin envelope of the breast base. The breast appears to herniate into an oversized and protuberant areola. The exact cause of this condition is as yet unclear; however, a genetic link to a disorder of collagen deposition is suspected. Corrective procedures can be divided into operations that involve augmentation, mastopexy, combined augmentation/mastopexy, lipomodeling, and tissue expansion followed by augmentation (Winocour, 2013).

## Benign Breast Disorders

Benign breast disorders (BBDs) and their wide range of symptoms represent the majority (~90%) of breast-related complaints and abnormalities evaluated in an obstetrician/gynecologist's office. This heterogeneous group of lesions or abnormalities may be incidental or may be detected clinically or radiographically.

BBDs are often misdiagnosed and misunderstood secondary to their varied spectrum at presentation and associated anxiety concerning the possibility and fear of malignancy. Understanding the causes and management of BBD is essential to provide proper clinical management and to psychologically allay patients' and families' fears. Various terminology has been used to describe BBD. Most emphasize clinical signs, symptoms, or histologic findings. BBDs can be classified as follows:

1. Aberrations of normal development and involution (ANDI)
2. Pathologic classification
3. Clinical classification
4. Classification based on the risk for malignancy

The **ANDI classification** incorporates symptoms, signs, histology, physiology, pathogenesis, and degree of breast abnormality, classified in relation to the normal processes of reproductive life and involution through a spectrum of breast conditions that range from "normal" to "disorder" to "disease" (Hughes, 1991). Thus ANDI classification suggests that BBDs are a result of minor aberrations in the normal development process, hormonal response, and involution of the breast (see Table 15.1).

Commonly, BBDs are subdivided histologically by their potential future cancer risk (ACOG Practice Bulletin 164, 2016):

- Nonproliferative disorders: no increased risk
- Proliferative disorders without atypia: mild to moderate increase in risk
- Atypical hyperplasia: substantial increase in risk (relative risk 3 to 5×) (Table 15.2)

Finally, a clinical classification is often used in which abnormalities can be subgrouped as follows:

- Physiologic swelling and tenderness
- Nodularity
- Breast pain (not usually associated with malignancy)
- Palpable breast lumps
- Nipple discharge including galactorrhea
- Breast infection and inflammation—typically associated with lactation

**TABLE 15.1** ANDI Classification of Benign Breast Disorders

| | Normal | Disorder | Disease |
|---|---|---|---|
| Early reproductive years (age 15-25) | Lobular development<br>Stromal development<br>Nipple eversion | Fibroadenoma<br>Adolescent hypertrophy<br>Nipple inversion | Giant fibroadenoma<br>Gigantomastia<br>Subareolar abscess |
| Later reproductive years (age 25-40) | Cyclical changes of menstruation<br>Epithelial hyperplasia of pregnancy | Cyclical mastalgia<br>Nodularity<br>Bloody nipple discharge | Incapacitating mastalgia |
| Involution (age 35-55) | Lobular involution<br>Duct involution<br>Dilation<br>Sclerosis<br>Epithelial turnover | Macrocysts<br>Sclerosing lesions<br>Duct ectasia<br>Nipple retraction<br>Epithelial hyperplasia | Periductal mastitis<br>Epithelial hyperplasia with atypia |

*ANDI*, Aberrations of normal development and involution.

**TABLE 15.2** Breast Lesions and Breast Cancer Risk

| Lesion Type | Lesion Subtype* | Aggregate Relative Risk of Future Breast Cancer (95% CI) |
|---|---|---|
| Nonproliferative | Simple cysts<br>Mild hyperplasia (usual type)<br>Papillary apocrine change | 1.17 (0.94-1.47)† |
| Proliferative without atypia | Fibroadenoma<br>Giant fibroadenoma<br>Intraductal papilloma<br>Moderate/florid hyperplasia (usual type)<br>Sclerosing adenosis<br>Radial scar | 1.76 (1.58-1.95)† |
| Atypical hyperplasia | Atypical ductal hyperplasia<br>Atypical lobular hyperplasia | 3.93 (3.24-4.76)† |
| Lobular carcinoma in situ | | 6.9-11‡ |

*Dupont WD, Page DL. Risk factors for breast cancer in women with proliferative breast disease. N Engl J Med 1985;312:146–51.
†Dyrstad SW, Yan Y, Fowler AM, Colditz GA. Breast cancer risk associated with benign breast disease: systematic review and meta-analysis. Breast Cancer Res Treat 2015;149:569–75.
‡Confidence interval not reported.
Data from Morrow M, Schnitt SJ, Norton L Current management of lesions associated with an increased risk of breast cancer. Nat Rev Clin Oncol 2015;12:227–38.

Most commonly BBD involves pain, discharge, or a mass. Infection or mastitis is less common. These symptoms and subsequent physical findings may result in denial, anxiety, and fear as patients worry that the symptoms represent cancer. The increase in size, density, and nodularity during the second half of the menstrual cycle is often associated with increased sensitivity or breast pain. Importantly, cancer-related breast pain is generally a late symptom and is a lone presenting symptom in less than 6% of women with malignant disease. Nipple discharge is also a less common sign of cancer. The correlation of a mass with malignancy is dependent on the patient's age. The incidence of BBD begins to rise during the second decade of life and peaks in the fourth and fifth decades, as opposed to malignant diseases, whose incidence continues to increase after menopause.

Simple breast cysts, occurring in 35% of reproductive aged women, represent the most common nonproliferative breast lesion (ACOG Practice Bulletin 164, 2016). Radiologically simple breast cysts (without septa or mural thickening) are almost always benign and can be managed expectantly. Aspiration is typically reserved to alleviate symptoms. Mild hyperplasia and simple papillary apocrine change are relatively rare benign nonproliferative lesions.

**Fibroadenomas**, composed of fibrous and epithelial elements, are the most common benign solid breast neoplasms (15% to 20%) and are often noticed accidentally while bathing. They most often occur in adolescents and young women (peak incidence at age 20 to 24) and are related to an aberration in normal lobular development. They demonstrate hormonal dependence, lactate during pregnancy, and involute to be replaced by hyaline connective tissue during perimenopause. Fibroadenomas represent 12% of breast masses after menopause. Clinically they usually present as solitary, slow-growing, painless, freely mobile, firm, solid breast masses. The average size is 2.5 cm, and they usually remain fairly constant in size. Giant fibroadenoma, larger than 5 cm, are rare. Hyperplastic lobules histologically resembling fibroadenomas are present in virtually all breasts. All the cellular elements of fibroadenomas are normal on conventional and electron microscopy, and the epithelium and myoepithelium maintain a normal relationship.

On clinical examination it may be difficult to distinguish a fibroadenoma from a cyst. In fact, diagnosis based solely on CBE is correct 66% of the time. Importantly, imaged complex cysts and any cysts with solid areas should be biopsied or excised. Ultrasound is the initial noninvasive study to differentiate a solid versus a cystic mass because mammography is rarely indicated in a woman younger than 35 with fibroadenomas. Core needle biopsy is indicated when the cause of a palpable mass cannot be established. Surgical evaluation is appropriate for any mass (at any age) that exhibits a rapid increase in size. Fibroadenomas can be followed clinically. Surgical excision of fibroadenomas should be considered if they are symptomatic or to relieve anxiety related to the palpable mass. They have a "rubbery" consistency, are usually well circumscribed, and are easily delineated from surrounding breast tissue in approximately 95% of cases (Fig. 15.6). Nonoperative management can be considered for small, asymptomatic fibroadenomas in women younger than 35 if clinical examination, imaging evaluation (either mammogram or ultrasound), and biopsy (usually core needle) results are 100% concordant. Approximately 35% of fibroadenomas will disappear, and approximately 10% shrink when followed. Conservative management requires continued surveillance at 6-month intervals for at least 2 years. Despite the option of conservative management, many women prefer to have the fibroadenoma excised. Excision should be performed through a cosmetically placed inframammary, axillary, or

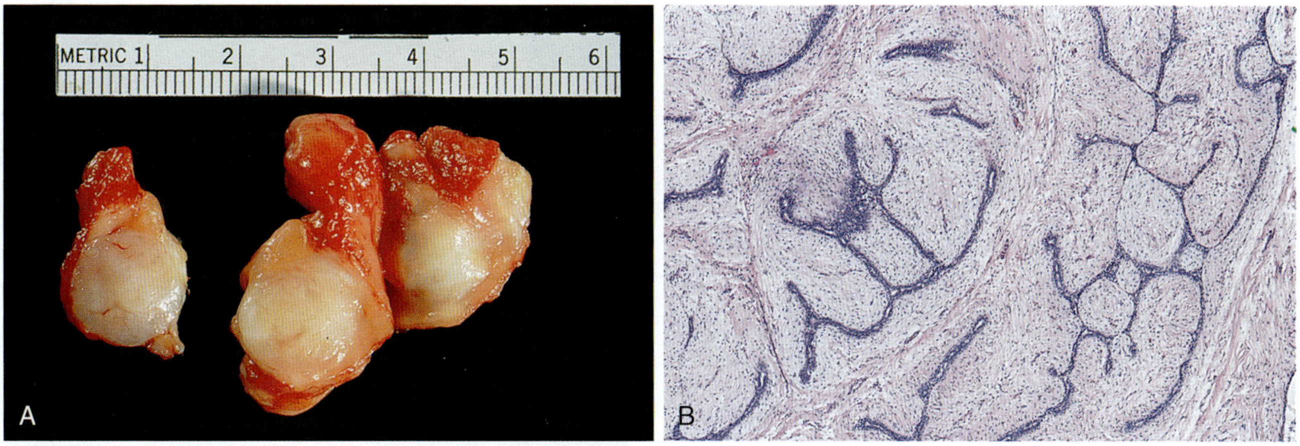


**Fig. 15.6 A,** Fibroadenoma with a characteristic tan, well-circumscribed nodule. **B,** Histologic section of fibroadenoma with epithelial cells surrounded by loose mesenchymal fibrous tissue. (From Voet RL. *Color Atlas of Obstetric and Gynecologic Pathology.* St. Louis: Mosby-Wolfe; 1997:204.)

circumareolar incision. Fibroadenomas are a proliferative disorder, and particularly when accompanied by complex cysts larger than 3 mm in diameter, sclerosing adenosis, epithelial calcification, or papillary changes, are associated with an increased risk of breast cancer; the later development of invasive breast cancer risk also is increased (approximately twofold). Women with fibroadenomas should be made aware of this risk and encouraged to maintain continued close surveillance. The postoperative risk of recurrent fibroadenoma is approximately 20%. Studies support the successful use of ultrasound-guided high-intensity focused ultrasound or cryoablation as an alternative treatment to surgery (Peek, 2018).

**Phyllodes tumors**, previously termed *Cystosarcoma phyllodes*, represent the opposite end of the spectrum of fibroepithelial tumors. Phyllodes tumors are rare, representing only 2.5% of fibroepithelial tumors and less than 1% of breast malignancies. The typical age of onset is 15 to 20 years later than fibroadenomas (fourth and fifth decades of life). They are almost exclusively seen in women and may be benign, borderline, or malignant. Differentiating benign from malignant phyllodes can be difficult and involves assessment of the size, histologic stroma/epithelium ratio, border of the lesion, stromal cellularity, number of stromal mitoses, and presence or absence of necrosis. All three generally present as a breast mass, often grow rapidly, and are typically larger at diagnosis than a fibroadenoma or ductal carcinoma. Histologically, stromal elements dominate and will invade the ducts in a leafy projection; hence the name *phyllodes*, or "leaf" (Fig. 15.7). Even the most experienced pathologists may have difficulty distinguishing among fibroadenoma, benign phyllodes tumors, and malignant cystosarcoma phyllodes. Phyllodes tumors' mammographic appearance as a rounded density with smooth borders is similar to that of fibroadenomas. Mammography and ultrasonography are therefore unreliable in differentiating among fibroadenomas, benign phyllodes tumors, and malignant phyllodes tumors.

These tumors can be locally aggressive and require wide local excision with 1-cm margins. Unlike fibroadenomas, phyllodes tumors should not be shelled out because this surgical technique will result in an unacceptably high recurrence rate. Unfortunately, the pathologic appearance of a phyllodes tumor does not always predict the neoplasm's clinical behavior; however, risk of local recurrence of the tumor is associated with microscopic margin involvement. Malignant tumors metastasize hematogenously, and the risk of metastases is 25%; local recurrence is common (>20%), even with benign and borderline tumors.

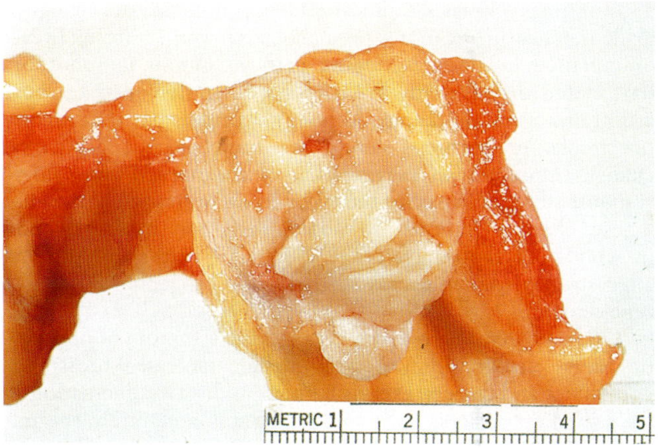


**Fig. 15.7** Phyllodes tumor with leaflike projections within the fleshy mass. (From Voet RL. *Color Atlas of Obstetric and Gynecologic Pathology.* St. Louis: Mosby-Wolfe; 1997:205.)

## Fibrocystic Change

Many breast symptoms stem from **fibrocystic changes**, previously designated fibrocystic *disease*, which is a common and natural maturation of breast tissue over time. The functional unit of the breast (the lobule), the alterations associated with the interaction among hormones, and the epithelial and stromal components of the lobule are responsible for many cases of BBDs. Initial or immature lobules, primarily developing in the early reproductive years (ages 15 to 25 years), are typically replaced during pregnancy and subsequently by mature lobules. Lobular changes manifest most commonly during the menstrual cycle. Late cycle peak mitosis, followed by apoptosis, provides a milieu for stromal or ductal tissues to transform from a normal to an abnormal state. Over time these deviations produce marked differences in the structure and appearance of the breast tissue, which is histologically described as *fibrosis* or *adenosis* and is often observed in women with no clinical complaint or finding.

Involutional breast changes, clinically apparent before age 35 years, affect stromal and epithelial components of the lobules. Early stromal involution can result in the formation of microcysts from the remaining epithelial acini. Microcyst formation is common and is often present in healthy breasts. Ductule obstruction facilitates progression of microcysts to macrocysts. Loose, hormonally receptive connective tissue in the stroma is replaced by denser connective tissue, and epithelial involution results in gradual disappearance of the ductal elements. Epithelial involution is dependent on the continuing presence of surrounding specialized stroma. Thus cyclical and involutional changes are concurrently present for more than 30 years, and the involutional changes will be extensive, with few ductal and lobular structures spared by the time menopause occurs.

Fibrocystic change, is the most common of all benign breast conditions. Clinicians use the nonspecific term *fibrocystic change* to describe the clinical, mammographic, and histologic findings associated with multiple irregularities in contour and texture typically associated with cyclical breast pain. Fibrocystic change presents as a spectrum of changes throughout a woman's reproductive age, with significant patient variation. *Fibrocystic change* has an extensive list of synonyms and terminology that includes more than 35 different names and terms. The 10th revision of the *International Statistical Classification of Diseases and Related Health Problems* (ICD-10) calls this *diffuse cystic mastopathy*.

The true frequency of fibrocystic change is unknown; however, autopsy evidence of histologic fibrocystic change is noted in 53% of normal breasts. Clinical evidence of fibrocystic change is evident in nearly one in two premenopausal women during breast examination; however, depending on the definition, some authors have noted that as many as 90% of women demonstrate some aspect of fibrocystic change. Although no consistent abnormality of circulating hormone levels has been proved, fibrocystic changes represent an exaggeration of the normal physiologic response of breast tissue to the cyclic levels or ovarian hormones. These changes, unusual in adolescence, are most common in women of reproductive age (20 to 50 years) and unusual after menopause unless associated with exogenous hormone replacement.

Cyclic bilateral breast pain is the classic symptom of fibrocystic breast change. Clinical signs include increased breast engorgement and density, excessive breast nodularity, fluctuation in the size of cystic areas, increased tenderness, and, rarely, spontaneous nipple discharge. Signs and symptoms are typically more prevalent during the premenstrual state.

Associated mastalgia is bilateral, often difficult to localize, and most common in the upper, outer breast quadrants. Pain may radiate to the shoulders and upper arms. Severe localized pain occurs when a simple cyst rapidly expands. The pathophysiology that produces these symptoms and signs includes cyst formation, epithelial and fibrous proliferation, and varying degrees of fluid retention. The differential diagnosis of breast pain includes referred pain from a dorsal radiculitis or inflammation of the costochondral junction (Tietze syndrome). The latter two conditions have symptoms that are not cyclic and are unrelated to the menstrual cycle.

The physical findings of excessive nodularity as a result of fibrocystic changes have been described as similar to palpating the surface of multiple peas. There may be multiple areas of seemingly ill-defined thickening or areas of palpable lumpiness that seem more two dimensional than the three-dimensional mass usually associated with a carcinoma (Fig. 15.8). Larger cysts may be ballotable, analogous to a water-filled balloon.

There are three general clinical stages of fibrocystic change, with each stage having characteristic histologic findings. Clinically these stages are variable and overlap, but they are described to assist in the understanding of the natural history. The first stage, mazoplasia (mastoplasia), is associated with intense stromal proliferation and occurs in the early reproductive years (20s). Breast pain is noted primarily in the upper, outer breast quadrants, with most tenderness in the axillary tail.

The second clinical stage, adenosis, is characterized by marked proliferation and hyperplasia of ducts, ductules, and alveolar cells

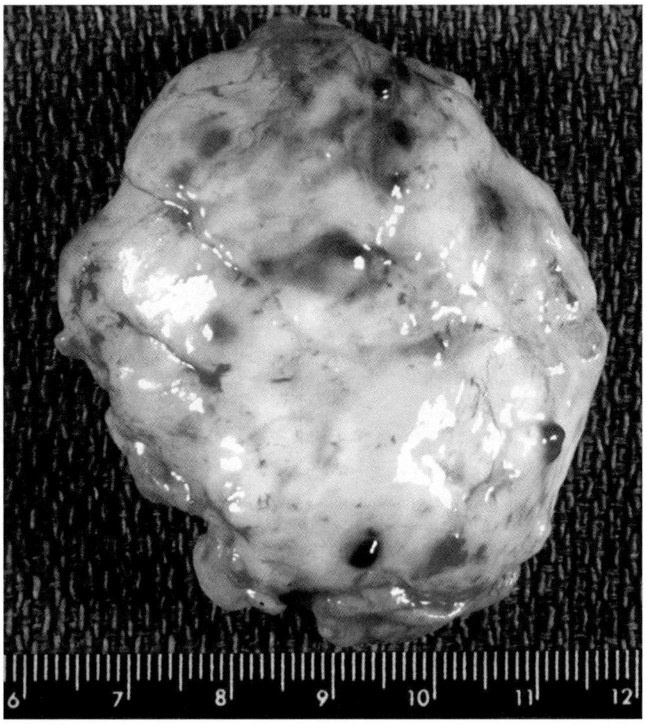


**Fig. 15.8** Breast biopsy specimen from a 38-year-old woman demonstrating the characteristic gross appearance of fibrocystic changes. Note the multiple cysts interspersed between the dense fibrous connective tissue. (Courtesy Fidel A. Valea, MD.)

and typically occurs in women in their 30s. Premenstrual breast pain and tenderness is less severe. Multiple small breast nodules varying from 2 to 10 mm in diameter are present.

The cystic phase is the last stage and typically occurs another decade later, in women in their 40s. Typically there is no breast pain unless a cyst increases rapidly in size, with associated sudden pain, point tenderness, and a lump. Cysts are tender to palpation and vary from microscopic to 5 cm in diameter. Although breast cysts may occur at any age, they are generally simple and may be managed with aspiration alone. Complex cysts have internal septations, debris, or solid components and may require core needle biopsy if stability cannot be documented. The fluid aspirated from a large cyst is typically straw colored, dark brown, or green, depending on the chronicity of the cyst.

Women with a clinical diagnosis of fibrocystic change have a wide variety of histopathologic findings. The histologic aspect of fibrocystic change is characterized by proliferation and hyperplasia of the lobular, ductal, and acinar epithelium (Fig. 15.9). Usually the proliferation of fibrous tissue occurs and accompanies epithelial hyperplasia. Many histologic variants of fibrocystic change have been described, including cysts (from microscopic to large, blue, domed cysts), adenosis (florid and sclerosing), fibrosis (periductal and stromal), duct ectasia, apocrine metaplasia, intraductal epithelial hyperplasia, and papillomatosis. Ductal epithelial hyperplasia with atypia and apocrine metaplasia with atypia are the most prominent histologic findings directly associated with the subsequent development of breast carcinoma. If either of these two conditions is discovered on breast biopsy, the chance of future breast carcinoma is increased fivefold.

Clinical management of fibrocystic change is age dependent and includes appropriate use of breast imaging. Initial evaluation should exclude malignancy, particularly in the presence of a mass or with a concerning or uncertain examination. Thereafter, successful symptom control may involve a number of medical options.

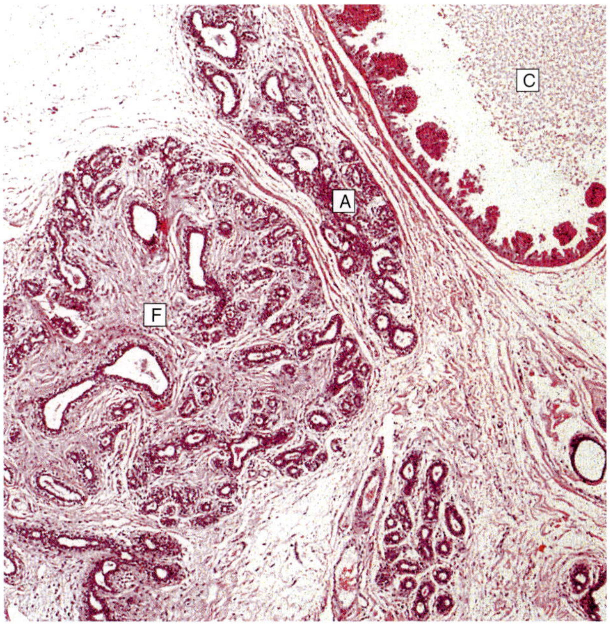


**Fig. 15.9** Fibrocystic changes from histologic section. Note fibrosis *(F)*, adenomatous changes with increased ductal tissue *(A)*, and cysts *(C)*. (From Stevens A, Lowe J. *Human Histology.* 3rd ed. Philadelphia: Mosby; 2005:392.)

Initial therapy for fibrocystic change involves mechanical support using a firm support or sports bra. Dietary changes to reduce methylxanthines or caffeine exposure have been helpful in relieving symptoms for some women. Although confirmatory medical studies evaluating the benefit of these dietary changes are lacking, there seems to be little harm to trying this inexpensive option for 3 to 6 months. The only dietary substance that seems to correlate with fibrocystic symptoms is dietary fat, particularly saturated fat. Studies have demonstrated a dose-related effect between increased saturated fat and fibrocystic breast symptoms. Incorporating a low-fat, nutrient-dense diet makes sense, and limiting intake of saturated fat intake should be considered as a simple therapeutic tool for the management of women with symptomatic, refractory fibrocystic changes. Additionally, some advocate limiting or eliminating alcohol consumption to lessen estrogen levels. Diuretics are sometimes prescribed during the premenstrual phase and may lessen symptoms of breast discomfort and engorgement.

Oral contraceptives or supplemental progestins administered during the secretory phase of the cycle have also been used to treat fibrocystic changes. Oral contraceptives are reported to decrease the incidence of fibrocystic changes by 30% (Schindler, 2013). Unfortunately, 40% of women will have recurrent symptoms after discontinuation.

Danazol, dosed at 100, 200, and 400 mg daily for 4 to 6 months, suppresses gonadotropins and effectively relieves symptoms and decreases breast nodularity in ~90% of patients. Unfortunately, virilizing side effects such as hirsutism, acne, and voice changes often limit its use. Danazol therapy for 6 months or more should be tapered to eliminate side effects. The beneficial effects of danazol persist for several months after discontinuation.

Oral tamoxifen, 20 mg daily, is superior to placebo in randomized, double-blind trials, and pain relief is reported to be sustained in 72% of women for more than 1 year after discontinuation. Tamoxifen administration restricted to the luteal phase of the menstrual cycle abolishes pain in 85% of women; however, adverse side effects are common (21%). After treatment, 25% of women suffer recurrent pain within 1 year. Tamoxifen 10 mg daily can be prescribed during the luteal phase of the menstrual cycle and results in similar improvements in symptoms but with a marked reduction in adverse effects.

The selective estrogen receptor modulator (SERM) centchroman (Ormeloxifene; 30 mg twice weekly), a weak estrogen receptor (ER) agonist and a strong ER antagonist, demonstrated significant efficacy in the management of breast pain and fibrocystic nodularity. On rare occasions, gonadotropin-releasing hormone (GnRH) agonists may benefit women with severe fibrocystic change.

## Mastalgia (Breast Pain)

More than two-thirds of women will experience breast pain at some time during their reproductive years, most commonly in the perimenopausal years. Eleven percent experience moderate to severe cyclic breast pain and 58% experience mild discomfort. Breast pain commonly interferes with usual sexual activity in 48% and with physical (37%), social (12%), and school (8%) activity in others. Approximately 90% of conditions that cause breast pain are benign. Breast pain is typically divided into cyclic pain, related to the menstrual cycle, and noncyclic pain. Cyclic pain is diffuse and bilateral and most commonly associated with fibrocystic changes. Noncyclic breast pain is commonly localized and related to a cyst. Noncyclic breast pain should be evaluated, particularly in older women, because there is a small association with malignancy. Mammography and additional imaging can be valuable. The differential diagnosis includes a cyst, chest wall pain, radicular pain, costochondritis, mastitis, pregnancy-related pain, prolactinomas, and medication exposure (Box 15.1). Laboratory evaluation should include human chorionic gonadotropin (HCG) and prolactin levels in premenopausal women. Breast cysts occur in as many as 7% of women during their lifetime and may be therapeutically aspirated if they are simple. A negative postaspiration breast examination is reassuring. Recurring simple cysts can be followed with ultrasound, typically withholding repeat aspiration for symptomatic cysts. For a more complex cyst, a more detailed workup is usually necessary. Patients with complex cysts should have a tissue diagnosis performed with a core needle biopsy if the cysts are symptomatic or show progressive changes on serial sonography. Pain as a presenting symptom of malignancy is uncommon in general and is extremely rare in the absence of mass or skin changes. Breast pain treatment is directed at the cause; however, nonsteroidal antiinflammatories are often useful when pain is idiopathic.

**BOX 15.1** Medications Associated with Mastalgia

Antihypertensives
Atenolol and other beta-blockers
Hydrochlorothiazide
Methyldopa
Minoxidil
Spironolactone
Antidepressants and antipsychotic agents
Amitriptyline and other tricyclic antidepressants
Chlorpromazine/promethazine
Fluoxetine
Haloperidol
Hormonal agents
Estrogens
Progestins
Androgens
Ginseng
Clomiphene citrate
Digoxin
Chlorpropamide

## Mastitis and Inflammatory Disease

Breast infection is often subdivided into lactational, nonlactational, and postoperative. Although decreasing in overall incidence, mastitis, an infection of the ductal systems or smaller sebaceous glands, is most commonly related to *Staphylococcus aureus*. Empiric treatment with an agent that covers gram-positive organisms is appropriate. If there is poor response to the initial course of antibiotics, cultures for methicillin-resistant *S. aureus* (MRSA) should be performed and an agent such as a doxycycline or sulfamethoxazole/trimethoprim is indicated; however, these two agents are contraindicated if a woman is pregnant or lactating.

**Lactational mastitis** commonly occurs in the first pregnancy during the first 6 weeks of breastfeeding. Curiously, mastitis in pregnancy usually responds to first-line antibiotics such as a cephalosporin, even in the presence of MRSA; however, infection may progress to a breast abscess in 5% to 11% of patients. Continued breastfeeding or manual pumping of the affected breast is recommended to decrease engorgement.

**Nonpuerperal mastitis** is often associated with breast cysts and cyst rupture. Ultrasonography assists in excluding an abscess. Obviously, one should always consider and exclude the presence of malignant breast disease, particularly inflammatory cancer. Additional testing for diabetes and human immunodeficiency virus (HIV) may be indicated, particularly if yeast is the offending organism. Syphilis, tuberculosis, atypical bacterial, and fungal infections may rarely cause nonpuerperal mastitis. In patients with recurrent mastitis, consider choosing an antibiotic to cover MRSA, such as clindamycin, sulfamethoxazole/trimethoprim, doxycycline, or vancomycin. Nipple piercing, particularly in smokers, is associated with mastitis and a 20-fold increase in subareolar abscess formation. As with any infection, the clinician should strongly consider removal of the foreign body. The American College of Obstetricians and Gynecologists (ACOG) recommends counseling women who are planning to get piercings to have prepiercing hepatitis B and tetanus vaccinations.

Idiopathic granulomatous mastitis (IGM), also called **idiopathic granulomatous lobular mastitis (IGLM)**, is a rare cause of breast inflammation and may affect any age group. This disease may present with a mass, abscess, inflammation, or granuloma formation. The granulomas are often found within the lobules and on biopsy are noted to be sterile. Mammography may be equivocal or may be suspicious for malignancy. Steroid treatment has been reported to be effective in small series with equivocal results. The disease is usually self-limited, resolving within months. Skin scarring and residual small abscesses may remain, often necessitating surgical treatment. Chronic inflammatory diseases, such as lupus, sarcoidosis, and Wegner granulomatosis, are rare causes of noninfectious mastitis, and evaluation for these diseases should be performed if antibiotics are not effective. Importantly, any breast inflammation not responsive to adequate antibiotic treatment warrants a tissue diagnosis. Core needle biopsy is often performed when there is a lack of response to antibiotics. The diagnosis is commonly made when the biopsy specimen indicates sterile granulomas after excluding other causes of granulomatous mastitis such as tuberculosis.

## Nipple Discharge

Nipple discharge is responsible for 7% of physician visits involving breast complaints. The majority have a benign cause; however, 55% present with a coexisting mass, of which 19% are malignant. An underlying malignancy is more likely when the discharge is spontaneous (vs. induced with nipple pressure), arises from a single duct, is blood stained, and is unilateral and persistent (occurring more than twice weekly). Age is important because an underlying malignancy is present in 3% of women younger than 40, 10% of women between 40 and 60, and 32% of women older than 60 when nipple discharge is the *only* presenting symptom.

**Intraductal papilloma** and fibrocystic changes are the two most common causes of spontaneous nonmilky discharge. Galactorrhea is likely when breast discharge is bilateral, copious, milky pale in color, and occurs from multiple ducts. Importantly, numerous medications and conditions can affect the hypothalamic-pituitary axis and lead to prolactin secretion and galactorrhea. As many as 65% of premenopausal women may have a normal benign physiologic discharge with gentle squeezing of the nipple. Evaluation includes physical examination, mammography, and sonography. The patient's history may not differentiate spontaneous discharge from elicited discharge because a woman may continually attempt to express the discharge, which causes more fluid to leak.

Evaluation and diagnosis include clinically separating the discharges into those that are spontaneous and those that only are expressed by pinching or squeezing the nipple (Fig. 15.10). Nipple discharges range in color from milky to green, brown, purple, and bloody. Hemoccult testing for detection of blood in the discharge is neither sensitive nor specific. Malignancy should be excluded in any woman with a bloody discharge or any discharge associated with a mass or if the discharge originates from only one or two adjacent ducts.

Assessment of *pathologic* nipple discharge involves a careful breast examination to identify the presence or absence of a breast mass. Firm areola pressure can assist in identifying the site of any dilated duct (pressure over a dilated duct will produce the discharge); this finding helps to define where an incision should be made for any subsequent surgery. The nipple is squeezed with firm, gentle digital pressure, and if fluid is expressed, the site and character of the discharge are recorded. Although bloodstained breast discharge is more likely to be associated with malignancy, fewer than 20% of patients who have a bloodstained discharge or who have a discharge containing moderate or large amounts of blood will have an underlying malignancy. Importantly, the absence of blood in nipple discharge does not exclude an underlying malignancy. Cytologic examination of nipple discharge can be helpful but has a poor sensitivity (<50%).

Management of a suspicious discharge begins with a physical examination and mammography, ultrasound, or magnetic resonance imaging (MRI). Any mass associated with discharge requires appropriate biopsy. A number of techniques have been evaluated to determine the cause and avoid unnecessary extirpative surgery. Ductoscopy (using a microendoscope passed into the offending duct) allows direct visualization. Ductal lavage involves duct canalization, and collection of fluid for cytologic evaluation. This technique increases cell yield by 100 times that of simple discharge cytologic examination but can be uncomfortable for the patient. Ductography (imaging of the ductal system by infecting contrast into the symptomatic duct), also called a **galactogram**, has 60% sensitivity for detecting malignancy. This study can identify intraductal filling defects or cutoff lesions, which have a high positive predictive value for the presence of either a papilloma or a carcinoma. The procedure can be technically challenging and cause significant patient discomfort. Surgical excision of the duct and its associated lobular unit is both diagnostic and therapeutic. With the patient anesthetized, a 4-0 lacrimal probe is passed through the duct. A periareolar flap is then created, and the retroareolar duct with the probe can be identified and excised individually.

## Intraductal Papilloma

Intraductal papillomas are broad-based or pedunculated polypoid epithelial lesions that may obstruct and distend the involved duct. They are most commonly diagnosed in perimenopausal women. Classically their clinical presentation includes an intermittent but spontaneous discharge from one nipple involving one or two ducts. The associated discharge can be watery, serous, or bloody,

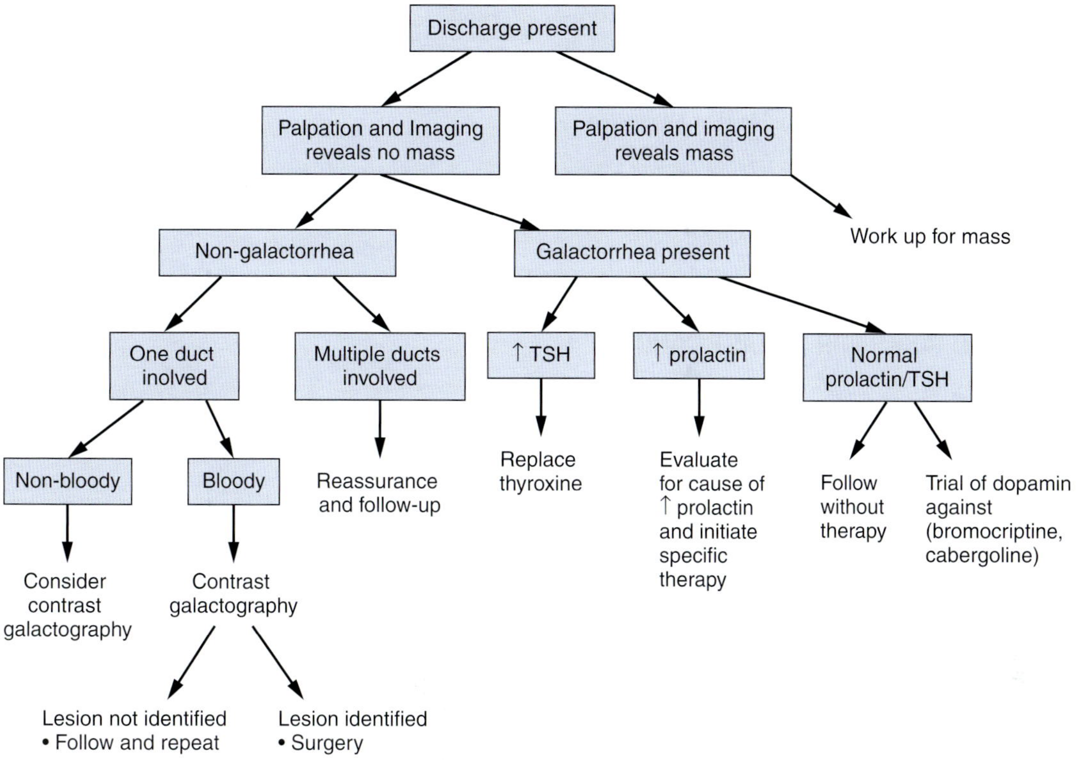


**Fig. 15.10** Algorithm for Evaluation of Nipple Discharge. (From Santen RJ. Benign breast disease in women. [Updated May 25, 2018.] In: Feingold KR, Anawalt B, Boyce A, et al., eds. *Endotext.* South Dartmouth, MA: MDText.com, Inc.; 2000.)

and of variable volume. Approximately 75% of intraductal papillomas are located beneath the areola, are small and soft, and are often difficult to palpate, typically measuring 1 to 3 mm in diameter. During examination of the breast it is important to circumferentially put radial pressure on different areas of the areola. This technique helps to identify whether the discharge emanates from a single duct or multiple openings. When the discharge comes from a single duct, the differential diagnosis includes both intraductal papilloma and carcinoma.

Treatment of intraductal papilloma involves excisional biopsy of the involved duct and a small amount of surrounding tissue. Although these tumors tend to regress in postmenopausal women, excision should be considered to rule out malignancy. Careful surveillance at 3- to 4-month intervals is necessary if the papilloma is not surgically excised. Women with a solitary papilloma have a twofold increase in subsequent development of breast carcinoma.

## Fat Necrosis

**Fat necrosis**, a benign nonsuppurative inflammatory process of adipose tissue, is a condition with a wide variety of presentations on mammography, ultrasound, and MRI. The incidence of fat necrosis of the breast is estimated to be 0.6%, representing 2.75% of all breast lesions. Fat necrosis is found in 0.8% of breast tumors and 1% in breast reduction mammoplasty cases, and the average age of patients is 50 years. Fat necrosis is most commonly the result of trauma to the breast, although it can be associated with radiotherapy, anticoagulation (warfarin), infection, or breast procedures, including breast aspiration or biopsy, lumpectomy, reduction mammoplasty, implant removal, and breast reconstruction. Other rare causes for fat necrosis include polyarteritis nodosa, Weber-Christian disease, and granulomatous angiopanniculitis.

Patients commonly present with a firm, tender, indurated, ill-defined mass that may have coexisting ecchymosis, erythema, inflammation, pain, skin retraction or thickening, nipple retraction, and occasionally lymphadenopathy. As many as 70% present as an occult lesion without a history of trauma. The area of fat necrosis may liquefy and become cystic, forming an oil cyst with a characteristic calcified rim. Mammography may demonstrate coarse calcifications, focal asymmetries, or microcalcifications. Treatment of fat necrosis is excisional biopsy. There is no relationship between fat necrosis and the development of subsequent breast carcinoma.

# BREAST CARCINOMA

Globally, breast carcinoma is the most common malignancy of women, and in the United States it is the second most common cause of all cancer deaths in women. Approximately 12.35% of women (1 in 8 women) will develop carcinoma of the breast at some point during their lifetime. In 2020, approximately 276,480 women in the United States were diagnosed with invasive breast cancer, with 42,170 women dying from the disease (Siegel, 2020). The importance of early detection and diagnosis of breast carcinoma cannot be overemphasized. An increase in public awareness combined with improvements in mammography and newer imaging techniques have facilitated earlier detection of breast carcinoma. Earlier detection, combined with improvements in therapy, has resulted in improved survival rates. With the advent of chemoprevention in high-risk women, there is an opportunity to alter the natural course of the disease.

**Breast carcinoma** generally presents in one of two ways: either with clinical symptoms or found on screening evaluation. In the United States most breast cancer is diagnosed as a result of an abnormal screening test. Screening includes examination by a health provider (referred to as *clinical breast examination*) and imaging. The ideal time to initiate screening, along with determination of intervals, is individualized for each woman based on her risk factors. A thorough understanding of the epidemiology of breast cancer is warranted when calculating the risk of developing breast cancer. Several models are available that help assess a patient's risk. If no risk factors are noted, she is said to be at average or normal risk, corresponding to the 12% (or 1 in 8) risk for a woman of developing breast malignancy during her lifetime. Because a woman's risk may change as her family history evolves or new findings develop on imaging, risk assessment should be ongoing.

## EPIDEMIOLOGY AND RISKS FOR BREAST CANCER

Breast cancer continues to be the most commonly diagnosed cancer in women worldwide. It is caused by a progressive accumulation of mutations in the cell's DNA. Epidemiologic studies help identify factors that through either exposure or inheritance place a woman at risk for a greater chance of cellular change. Approximately 50% of newly diagnosed breast cancers are attributable to known risk, whereas 10% are associated with simply a positive family history. The degree of risk is important to know in order to advise women and establish plans for screening or interventions.

Most epidemiologic literature when reporting breast cancer risks describes the risk from any given factor as a relative risk. Relative risk is the risk of subjects in an exposed group compared with subjects in a nonexposed group. In contrast, clinical and genetic studies usually report results as a woman's lifetime risk: the risk of developing or dying from a disease over the course of one's lifetime. The distinction can be confusing for patients and families. For example, a *BRCA* mutation may increase the relative risk 10-fold and the lifetime risk up to 85%. Clinicians must be aware of the difference when reviewing the literature and subsequently when counseling patients and their families.

The risk factors for breast cancer may be divided into several categories (Table 15.3): demographic, estrogen exposure, lifestyle, personal breast characteristics, familial and inherited genetic mutations, and radiation exposure (Clemons, 2001; Labuy-Secretan, 2016). Risk is generally grouped as minor and major. Minor risk factors increase a woman's lifetime risk from 12% to approximately 15%. Importantly, epidemiologic studies have also noted factors that decrease a woman's risk (Table 15.4).

**TABLE 15.3** Risk Factors for Breast Cancer

| Risk Factor | Qualification | Relative Risk |
|---|---|---|
| Age | ≤49 y<br>50-59 y<br>Age 60-69 y<br>≥70 y | 2.0<br>2.3<br>3.5<br>6.7 |
| Geographic | Common in Western countries | |
| Age at menarche | >14 y (low risk) vs. <12 y | 1.5 |
| Age at first full-term pregnancy | <20 y (low risk) vs. >30 y | 1.9-3.5 |
| Late menopause | <45 y (low risk) vs. >55 y (high risk) | 2.0 |
| Hormone replacement therapy | No use vs. current | 1.2 |
| Contraceptive pill use | None vs. past or current use | 1.07-1.2 |
| Alcohol use | None vs. 2-5 drinks/day | 1.4 |
| Postmenopausal weight gain | Women with a higher BMI | 1.1 per 5 BMI units |
| Bone density | Lowest vs. highest quartile | 2.7-3.5 |
| Nightshift work | Exposed to nightshift work | 1.48 |
| Smoking | History of smoking | 1.10* |
| Benign breast disease | None vs. positive biopsy result | 1.7 |
| Breast density (as measured by mammography) | 0% vs. ≥75% | 1.8-6.0 |
| Hyperplasia with atypia | None vs. positive biopsy result | 3.7 |
| Multiple relatives, not first degree, with breast cancer | | |
| One first-degree relative with breast cancer (mother or sister) | None vs. yes | 2.6 |
| Two or more first-degree relatives | Increased risk if the cancers are premenopausal | |
| Deleterious *BRCA1/BRCA2* genes | Negative vs. positive | 2.0-7.0 |
| Mantle radiation for treatment of malignancy | Very high risk, which increases with age | |

*Summary relative risk.

## DEMOGRAPHIC ASSOCIATIONS

Age continues to remain the strongest risk factor for developing breast cancer. The risk of breast carcinoma increases directly with the patient's age (Table 15.5). Data from the Surveillance, Epidemiology, and End Results (SEER) database report the probability of a woman developing breast cancer from birth to age 49 as 2% (1 in 49 women) compared with 7% (1 in 14 women) at age 70 or older (Siegel, 2020).

The incidence of breast cancer varies based on geographic region. The highest rates are found in North America, Australia/New Zealand, and Western and Northern Europe. Women in Eastern Europe, South Africa, Japan, and the Caribbean form a middle group in terms of incidence. The lowest incidences are found in Asia and sub-Saharan Africa.

In the United States white women have the highest rate of breast cancer; however, black women have higher breast cancer mortality. Data from 2005 to 2009 the rate of newly diagnosed breast cancer was 122 per 100,000 white women and 117 per 100,000 black women. Black women more commonly presented with regional or advanced disease (45% vs. 35%) and had a 41% higher breast cancer–specific mortality rate (32 vs. 22 deaths per 100,000 women) (Centers for Disease Control and Prevention [CDC], 2012). This difference may be due to several factors, including both socioeconomic aspects and the histologic variety of tumors.

## ESTROGEN-RELATED EXPOSURE RISKS

Breast cancer risk is increased with high endogenous estrogen levels in both premenopausal and postmenopausal women. This effect is especially noted in hormone receptor–positive breast cancer. Various studies have shown that both prolonged exposure to and higher concentrations of estrogen are associated with a higher risk of breast cancer. Breast cancer is rare in prepubertal girls. Women who have breast cancer and undergo oophorectomy have a lower recurrence rate. Interestingly, the rate

**TABLE 15.4** Factors Associated with a Decreased Risk for Breast Cancer

| Demographic | Qualification | Relative Risk |
|---|---|---|
| Born and living outside Western countries | | |
| Late menarche | After age 14 | |
| Oophorectomy | Yes vs. no | 0.3 |
| Lactation | >16 mo vs. none | 0.73 |
| Parity | ≥5 vs. 0 | 0.73 |
| Postmenopausal body mass (kg/m$^2$) | <22.9 vs. >30.7 | 0.63 |
| Physical activity | Yes vs. no | 0.70 |
| Vitamin D | Low levels associated with risk | |
| Intake of vitamin D | Associated with decreased risk | |
| Olive oil and omega-3 fatty acids | | |
| Low-fat diet | Results suggestive but not yet conclusive | |
| Aspirin | >1×/wk for ≥16 mo vs. no use | 0.79 |

**TABLE 15.5** A Woman's Risk of Having Developed Breast Cancer

| Age | Risk |
|---|---|
| 25 | 1 in 19,608 |
| 30 | 1 in 2525 |
| 35 | 1 in 622 |
| 40 | 1 in 217 |
| 45 | 1 in 93 |
| 50 | 1 in 50 |
| 55 | 1 in 33 |
| 60 | 1 in 24 |
| 65 | 1 in 17 |
| 70 | 1 in 14 |
| 75 | 1 in 11 |
| 80 | 1 in 10 |
| 85 | 1 in 9 |
| Ever | 1 in 8 |

Data from National Cancer Institute. Painter K. Factoring in cost of mammograms. *USA Today.* December 5, 1996, p 11D.

of recurrence in oophorectomized women is decreased, even in women with hormone receptor–negative cancers.

Reproductive factors must also be considered in determining the risk of developing breast cancer. Nulliparous women are at an increased risk of breast cancer compared with parous women, but the protective effect of pregnancy is not noted until 10 years after delivery. It is unclear whether an association exists between either multiparity or nulliparity and breast cancer. The age at which a woman delivers her first child is an important risk factor. Age at first pregnancy was analyzed in the Nurses' Health Study. Compared with nulliparous women at or near menopause, women who delivered their first child at age 20, 25, or 35 years had a cumulative incidence of breast cancer (up to age 70) that was 20% lower, 10% lower, and 5% higher, respectively (Colditz, 2000). Early age at menarche is associated with a higher risk of breast cancer. Women with menarche at or after age 15 years of age were less likely to develop ER-positive breast cancer compared with those with menarche before the age of 13 years. Additionally, a 16% decreased risk of ER-negative breast cancer was noted in women with menarche at or after age 15 years.

Breastfeeding decreases the risk of breast cancer. A pooled analysis of data from 47 studies involving 50,302 women with breast cancer and 96,973 women without the disease found a direct correlation between the length of time of lactation and decreasing risk for breast malignancy (Collaborative Group on Hormonal Factors in Breast Cancer, 2002). Women who breastfed longer were more protected against breast cancer. The relative risk of breast cancer decreased by 4.3% per 12 months of breastfeeding. This decrease did not vary significantly by parity, ethnicity, age of menarche and menopause, and geographic factors. Newcomb and colleagues reported that after adjusting for parity, age at first delivery, and other confounding factors, lactation was associated with a slight reduction in the risk of breast cancer among premenopausal women compared with those who had never lactated (relative risk [RR], 0.78; confidence interval [CI], 0.6 to 0.91) (Newcomb, 1994). Overall, breastfeeding decreases the risk of breast cancer in a dose-response relationship.

Hormone replacement—specifically the use of combined estrogen and progesterone—is an established risk factor for breast cancer. Data from the Women's Health Initiative (WHI) showed that compared with the placebo group, combined hormone replacement increases the risk of breast cancer by 24%. Of note, estrogen-only use in women with a history of a hysterectomy did not increase the risk of breast cancer (Chlebowski, 2003). The decision to use hormone replacement therapy in patients with and without other risk factors should be individualized and the risks and benefits discussed so that the woman may make an informed decision. Unlike combination hormonal replacement (estrogen and progesterone), oral contraceptives and other forms of estrogen-related contraception do not increase the risk of breast cancer. Multiple studies have noted that the oral contraceptives used since the 1980s do not pose an increased risk compared with the extremely high levels of estrogen used in oral contraceptives in the 1960s and 1970s. There is no association between abortion and breast cancer incidence.

## LIFESTYLE AND DIETARY RISK FACTORS

The relationship between dietary habits and the risk of breast cancer is not clear. A direct association between dietary fat and the risk of breast cancer has not been clearly established, and various studies have failed to show a significant association between the highest and the lowest category of consumed dietary fat and an increased risk of breast cancer. In the WHI study of postmenopausal women, the dietary arm of the study evaluated 48,835 healthy postmenopausal women who tried to reduce fat intake (Prentice, 2006). There was a minimal effect on decreasing malignancy in the breast (RR, 0.91; CI, 0.83 to 1.01) after a mean follow-up of 8.1 years. Although no direct association between dietary fat intake and breast cancer risk has been established, there may be a modest effect when comparing extremes of fat intake. In the AARP Diet and Health Study, women in the highest quintile of fat intake had rates of invasive breast cancer 11% to 22% higher than those of women in the lowest quintile (Thiébaut, 2007). Although obesity is associated with a general increase in morbidity and mortality, the risk of breast cancer related to body mass index (BMI) is linked to the menopausal status of women (Lauby-Secretan, 2016). Obese women are at a higher risk for developing breast cancer during their postmenopausal years, with increased amounts of peripheral conversion of androstenedione to estrone. In premenopausal women, an increased BMI is associated with a lower risk of breast cancer.

Studies also have found a significant association with decreased levels of vitamin D and decreased calcium and increased risks of breast cancer and increased morbidity once breast cancer is diagnosed. An increase in plasma 25-hydroxyvitamin D (25[OH]D) levels between 27 and 35 ng/mL was associated with a decrease in breast cancer risk in postmenopausal women (Bauer, 2013). No association between 25(OH)D levels and breast cancer risk has been noted in premenopausal women. Antioxidant supplementation (vitamin A, E, or C, or beta-carotene) has not been shown to be protective for breast cancer. Data regarding the effect of nonsteroidal antiinflammatory drugs (NSAIDs) on breast cancer risk are varied. Several small studies and a nested study from the WHI noted aspirin to decrease risk for breast cancer, breast cancer recurrence, and breast cancer mortality; however, data from the Nurses' Health Study showed no association between use of aspirin, NSAIDs, or acetaminophen and the incidence of breast cancer (Zhang, 2012).

Alcohol consumption has been associated with increased risk for multiple cancers, including breast cancer. Older studies reported a 40% to 50% increase in the relative risk of developing breast cancer related to alcohol consumption. The alcohol effect was primarily in ER-positive tumors. Breast cancer risk is higher in women consuming both low and high levels of alcohol compared with no consumption. Longnecker showed that the risk of breast cancer was strongly related to the amount of alcohol consumed and that even light drinking was associated with a 10% increase in relative risk (Longnecker, 1994). A 2013 meta-analysis of 110 epidemiologic studies reported a 5% increase (RR, 1.05%) in female breast cancer with light alcohol intake (Bagnardi, 2013).

Phytoestrogens are naturally occurring plant substances with a chemical structure similar to 17-beta estradiol. They consist mainly of isoflavones (found in high concentrations in soybeans and other legumes) and lignans (found in a variety of fruits, vegetables, and cereal products). There is low-quality evidence that soy-rich diets in Western women prevent breast cancer. A 2008 meta-analysis of eight studies evaluated the effect of soy food intake and breast cancer risk (Wu, 2008). A higher intake of isoflavones (≥20 mg per day) was associated with a 29% reduction in breast cancer risk in Asian women, but no association with soy intake was noted among Western women. Of note, the highest level of soy intake in Western women was only about 0.8 mg daily, which may not have been an adequate amount to detect an effect.

Various miscellaneous environmental exposures have been studied for possible associations with the development of breast cancer. In a 2005 meta-analysis of 13 studies, Megdal and associates found that altered day/night exposure, shift work, and increased light exposures were associated with an increased risk of breast cancer (RR, 1.48; CI, 1.36 to 1.61). Suppression of nocturnal melatonin production by the pineal gland secondary to nocturnal light exposure may contribute to the increased risk of developing breast cancer. Magnetic radiation, power lines, computer terminals, and electric blanket exposure do not increase the risk of breast cancer. Breast implants have not been shown to increase the risk for breast cancer.

## BREAST HISTORY AND BREAST CHARACTERISTICS

Women with a personal history of breast cancer or ductal carcinoma in situ are at an increased risk of developing invasive breast cancer in the contralateral breast. Analysis of SEER data showed the incidence of invasive contralateral breast cancer in women with a history of primary breast cancer was 4% during a 7.5-year follow-up period (Nichols, 2011). The risk of a contralateral breast cancer depends on the age at the time of the index breast cancer diagnosis in conjunction with the hormone receptor status

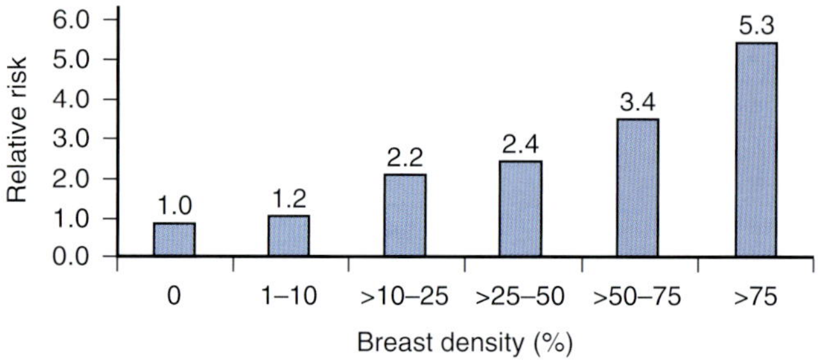


**Fig. 15.11** Risks of breast cancer with increasing breast density. (Modified from Santen RJ, Mansel R. Benign breast disorders. *N Engl J Med.* 2005;353(3):275-285.)

of the primary tumor. The presence of ductal carcinoma in situ did not modify the rate of contralateral breast cancer.

Boyd and coworkers reported that women with dense breasts, as defined by more fibrous tissue, have a relative risk of 4.7 (CI, 2 to 6.2) for breast cancer (Fig. 15.11) (Boyd, 2007). This finding has been verified in other studies, and the increased risk is not due to a more difficult or later diagnosis but to the biologic characteristics of the breast itself. Women with dense breasts noted on mammograms (dense tissue involving at least 75% of the breast) have a risk of breast cancer four to five times greater compared with women with less dense tissue. Both usual and atypical hyperplasia increases the risk of breast cancer. There is a mild increase in risk when biopsy results have shown hyperplasia; however, hyperplasia with atypia increases the risk by 4 to 6 orders of magnitude. The cumulative incidence of breast cancer among women with atypical hyperplasia approaches 30% at 25 years of follow-up.

## INHERITED AND FAMILIAL RISKS

Most cases of breast cancer are sporadic in nature and not an inherited cancer. About 5% to 10% of all breast cancers are caused by an inherited gene mutation. There are at least four specific breast cancer syndromes, each associated with a specific mutation. Each of these syndromes is autosomal dominant and involves mutations in the proteins that repair DNA. The most common are the mutations in the breast cancer susceptibility genes, *BRCA1* and *BRCA2*. Less common are Li-Fraumeni syndrome, associated with *P53* gene mutations, and Cowden syndrome, associated with *PTEN* gene mutations (Table 15.6).

Women with genetic syndromes tend to develop breast cancer at earlier ages and tend to have more aggressive tumors with a higher prevalence of bilateral disease. **Hereditary breast and ovarian cancer (HBOC) syndrome** is the most common cause of hereditary breast and ovarian cancers. This syndrome is associated with *BRCA1* and *BRCA2* mutations and is responsible for approximately 5% of breast cancer cases in the United States. Although the incidence of *BRCA* mutation is 1:250 in the United States, because of the founder effect the prevalence of *BRCA1* and *BRCA2* mutations is variable among ethnic groups and geographic areas. It is highest among people of Ashkenazi Jewish heritage, in whom approximately 2% of the population carries a deleterious *BRCA1* or *BRACA2*.

The *BRCA* genes code for very large tumor suppressor proteins. Germline mutations in *BRCA* genes result in mutation carriers losing one of their wild-type alleles. These mutation carriers have only one functional allele of these genes in their cells. Tumors in carriers tend to demonstrate loss of the other wild-type allele through other somatic mutations or loss of heterozygosity. This genomic instability of women with *BRCA* mutations causes them to be more susceptible to further mutations of DNA, which subsequently leads to malignant transformation of breast and ovarian epithelial cells.

**TABLE 15.6** Major Inherited Gene Mutation Syndromes Associated with Breast Cancer

| Syndrome | Gene | Incidence | Lifetime Breast Cancer Risk | Associated Cancer Risks |
|---|---|---|---|---|
| *BRCA1* | *BRCA1* | 1/500-1/1000 | 85% | Ovary and pancreas |
| *BRCA2* | *BRCA2* | Unclear | 85% | Ovary and pancreas |
| Cowden | *PTEN* | 1/100,000-1/200,000 | 50% | Thyroid and endometrium |
| Li-Fraumeni | *TP53* | 1/20,000 | 90% | Sarcoma, brain, and leukemia |

Other syndromes, including Peutz-Jeghers syndrome, ataxia telangiectasia, *CHEK2* gene mutation, and Fanconi syndrome, have much smaller lifetime risks with poorer penetrance.

*BRCA1* has 1863 amino acids, with several different functions, and was mapped at 17q21. In combination with several other genes including *BARD1*, *BRCA2*, *CHK1*, and *RAD51*, *BRAC* is involved in repair of double-strand DNA breaks and control of cell cycle checkpoints. Women with a *BRCA1* mutation have a risk of breast cancer of approximately 55% to 70% to age 70 and an average lifetime risk of ovarian cancer approaching 40%. The *BRCA2* gene was mapped to chromosome 13q12 and the DNA sequence determined by Schutte and coworkers in 1995. Women with a *BRCA2* gene mutation have a 45% to 70% risk of breast cancer to age 70 and a 15% to 20% lifetime risk of ovarian cancer. The risk of a contralateral breast cancer in women with a deleterious *BRCA1* or *BRCA2* mutation has been estimated to range from 10% to 65%. The contralateral breast cancer risk also depends on the age of first breast cancer presentation, with the risk being higher when the age of diagnosis is younger than 40 compared with older than 50 years. *BRCA2* mutations are also associated with male breast cancers, conferring a 5% to 10% risk for a man who has inherited the mutation. Because male breast cancer is so rare, any man with breast cancer should be tested for a *BRCA* mutation.

Data also suggest a potential role of *BRCA1* and *BRCA2* mutations in sporadic breast and ovarian cancers, in particular triple-negative breast cancers (i.e., breast cancers that lack expression of the estrogen receptor, progesterone receptor, and human epidermal growth factor receptor 2 [HER2]), some of which exhibit hypermethylation of *BRCA1*, *BRCA2*, or other downstream genes, leading to abnormal gene expression. The genomic instability of *BRCA1*- and *BRCA2*-deficient cells in hereditary and triple-negative breast cancer provides an opportunity for therapeutic development, especially drugs that target DNA repair pathways. This includes platinum-type drugs that generate double-stranded DNA breaks or poly (adenosine diphosphate–ribose) polymerase (PARP) inhibitors, which are involved in the repair of DNA single-strand breaks.

Women with a family history of breast cancer have an increased risk of developing breast cancer. Approximately 15% of breast cancers are related to familial risk. Women in such families have a combination of low penetrance polygenic inheritance contributing to their personal risk. The risk for breast cancer is significantly affected by the number of female first-degree relatives with and without cancer. The risk increases for a woman the more relatives she has with breast cancer. Additionally, the age at diagnosis of the affected first-degree relative is another factor that influences the risk for breast cancer. The risk is threefold higher if the first-degree relative was diagnosed before age 30. Models that will predict a woman's breast cancer risk are discussed later.

## RADIATION EXPOSURE

Exposure to therapeutic ionizing radiation is a recognized risk factor for the development of breast cancer. The risk of developing breast carcinoma is consistent with a linear dose-response relationship. This was first recognized in Japanese women who survived the atomic bombs dropped during World War II, with a high incidence of women exposed as teenagers developing breast carcinoma in their 30s. Other historical examples of ionizing radiation–induced breast cancer include women with a history of radiation treatments for postpartum mastitis, irradiation of the thymus in infancy, or multiple fluoroscopic examinations during treatment for tuberculosis. Currently, women at highest risk from radiation exposure are those who were treated with radiation for childhood malignancies, in particular Hodgkin lymphoma. Those with prepubertal exposure represent the most vulnerable age group; however, increased risk is evident in women exposed as late as age 45 years. It is important to differentiate therapeutic ionizing radiation from radiation exposure as a result of diagnostic imaging. One 64-slice chest computed tomography (CT) adds less than 1% to a woman's lifetime risk of breast cancer.

## RISK ASSESSMENT AND PREVENTION

Stratification of a woman's risk of developing breast cancer is paramount. This should be an ongoing and dynamic process because her risk increases with age and with changes in both personal and family history. The chance of developing a malignancy can be calculated based on her risk profile. This profile will influence the recommendations for both her screening and for preventive measures such as chemoprevention.

The risk factors that influence a woman's chances of developing a malignancy are multifactorial. With the exception of certain genetic mutations, a single risk factor is not sufficient by itself to stratify a woman into a risk group. Consequently, individualized counseling is the most effective approach to evaluating risk. Risk factors can be stratified into (1) major factors that increase relative risk greater than two times normal and (2) minor factors (see Table 15.3). A women's personal risk of developing breast cancer is divided into three levels: average, moderate, and high. Additionally, within the latter group a very high-risk group is identified for purposes of prophylactic options (Table 15.7). Women of average risk have a personal risk of about 12% of developing breast cancer, the risk of the general population. In the moderate risk group, women have personal risks from 12% to 15% of developing breast malignancy during their lifetime and have one or more minor risk factors. These women do not need any changes in screening recommendations compared with those for the general population. Women at high risk include those who have greater than a 15% personal risk of developing breast cancer, usually from a major risk factor. In the very high-risk category, women have a personal risk greater than 25%, which includes women with a *BRCA* mutation and those who have had mantle radiation. They are often referred to breast specialists for ongoing evaluation.

Several models have been empirically developed to estimate a woman's risk of breast cancer. The most widely available and accepted tool is the Breast Cancer Risk Assessment Tool (BCRAT) developed by Dr. Mitchell Gail, which is commonly known as the **Gail model**. The original model was based on data acquired from the Breast Cancer Detection and Demonstration Project to

TABLE 15.7 Risk Levels for the Development of Breast Cancer

| Level | Lifetime Risk for Breast Cancer | Recommendations for Screening |
|---|---|---|
| Average | 12% | Yearly exams and mammograms beginning at age 40 |
| Moderate | 12%-15% | Yearly exams and mammography beginning at age 40 |
| High | 15%-20% | Yearly exams and mammography beginning at age 40; offer chemoprevention |
| Very high risk | >20% | Exams every 6 months; mammography alternating with MRI should be started on an individualized basis depending on the risk factor (e.g., for women with mantle radiation, imaging should begin at age 30 or 8 years after radiation is finished); offer chemoprevention |

*MRI,* Magnetic resonance imaging.

calculate the risk of a women developing breast cancer over the next 5 years until age 90. The model was developed in white women, taking into account age, race, age of menarche, number of births, number of first-degree relatives with breast cancer, and number of breast biopsy results that have shown atypia. This model has been updated to estimate the risk for African American women using data from the Contraceptive and Reproductive Experiences Study and for Asian American and Pacific Islander women using data from the Asian American Breast Cancer Study (Gail, 2007; Matsuno, 2011). The BCRAT was designed for women who have never had a diagnosis of breast cancer, ductal carcinoma in situ (DCIS), or lobular carcinoma in situ (LCIS) and who do not have a strong family history suggesting an inherited gene mutation. It is not applicable to women with more than two first-degree relatives with breast cancer and does not consider more distant relatives, the age at which relatives developed breast cancer, or a family history of ovarian cancer. It is not useful for women with a strong family history of breast cancer on the paternal side. Most important, it does not estimate the risk of carrying a deleterious *BRCA1* or *BRCA2* gene.

The **Clauss model**, developed by Elizabeth Clauss in 1994, uses data from the Cancer and Steroid Hormone Study. This model uses first- and second-degree relatives, both maternal and paternal, to calculate risk but does not use risk factors beyond family history and also is not as robust in woman who are not white. The Clauss model provides the lifetime risks for a woman over any given decade of her life.

Computerized risk prediction models have been developed to assess not only the risk of breast cancer but also the risk of carrying a deleterious *BRCA1* or *BRCA2* genes, and include the BRCAPRO model (incorporates six predictive models for inherited or familial breast cancer), the International Breast Cancer Intervention Study or Tyrer-Cuzick model (incorporates both genetic and nongenetic risk factors to determine the risk of developing breast cancer and estimates of *BRCA1/2* mutation probabilities), and the BOADICEA model (developed to determine breast and ovarian cancer susceptibility because of genetic mutations).

All cancers are a result of mutations in certain genes. Mutations may be sporadic or inherited from a parent. Hereditary cancers develop secondary to mutations associated with an increased risk for certain cancer. These high-penetrance phenotypes are passed on to offspring from the mother and/or father. They are characterized by an early age of onset and have an autosomal dominant inheritance. Genetic counseling is an integral component in the management of hereditary cancers. Many patients who undergo genetic testing do not receive adequate counseling. In one series of 5080 patients surveyed, only 43.5% received formal genetic counseling (Katz, 2018). An initial risk evaluation should be completed in an effort to determine whether a formal assessment is warranted. When evaluating a woman's breast cancer risk, an important role of the clinician is to determine which women should be evaluated for the inherited cancer syndromes. Several risk factors can raise suspicion for an inherited mutation. If a woman has a 5% to 10% probability (based on probability models) of having a *BRCA* mutation, she should be referred to a genetic counselor for a comprehensive assessment and workup of the family history. Reasons for referral to a genetic counselor for hereditary cancer risk evaluation include female patients with breast cancer diagnosed at a young age (≤45 years), a triple-negative receptor tumor, two or more synchronous primary breast cancers, male patients with breast cancer, and invasive ovarian/fallopian tube/primary peritoneal cancer. Additional criteria include women with first-degree (sister, mother, or daughter) relatives with a history of breast cancer, a confirmed mutation in another family member, and women of Ashkenazi Jewish heritage, especially those with a family history of ovarian or breast cancer. Pre- and postgenetic counseling is essential and includes discussing the issues and implications of the results, legal and insurance aspects, noninformative results, and choices for chemoprevention or surgical prophylaxis. Women with negative or noninformative *BRCA* results may still need high-risk screening because their risks may be greater than that of the general population.

Multigene testing has been possible because of next-generation sequencing. This form of testing allows the detection of pathogenic or likely pathogenic variants not detected in single-gene testing. Comprehensive risk panels include a large number of genes associated with several cancer types. The aim of this testing is to identify pathogenic or likely pathogenic variants that are clinically actionable The National Comprehensive Cancer Network (NCCN) provides guidelines for the management of patients with known genetic mutations (Table 15.8). Depending on the specific genetic mutation, management options may range from close observation and imaging to consideration for a risk-reducing mastectomy. Testing should only be conducted when pre- and posttest counseling is available. Multigene testing increases the possibility of detecting a **variant of uncertain significance (VUS)**, which contributes to the complexity of genetic counseling. In a cross-sectional study involving next-generation sequencing of 2158 individuals with breast cancer, 33% to 40% were found to have a VUS (Tung, 2015).

The benefits of screening have been emphasized by major health societies and professional organizations (Table 15.9). The U.S. Preventive Services Task Force (USPSTF) recommendations updated the screening guidelines for breast cancer in 2016. The task force's recommendations were designed for women age 40 and older who do not show any signs or symptoms of breast cancer, who have no personal history of breast cancer, and who do not have a known genetic mutation or a history of chest radiation at a young age. The updated recommendations are as follows: (1) Routine screening of average-risk women should begin at age 50, (2) routine screening should end at age 74, (3) women should get screening mammograms every 2 years, and (4) teaching breast self-examination is not recommended. These recommendations were based on evidence that shows the value of mammography increases with age, with women aged 50 to 74

**TABLE 15.8** Known Genetic Mutations in Breast Cancer and their Management

| Genetic Mutation | Breast Cancer Risk | Management |
|---|---|---|
| *ATM* | Increased by 15–40% | Annual mammography starting at age 40 with consideration for breast tomosynthesis/MRI |
| *BARD1* | Limited evidence for increased risk but stronger for triple negative breast Ca. | Annual mammography starting at age 40 with consideration for breast tomosynthesis/MRI |
| *BRCA1*<br>*BRCA2* | Both carry increased absolute risk greater than 60% | Breast awareness starting at age 18<br>Clinical breast exam, every 6–12 months starting at age 25 years.<br>Breast screening:<br>Age 25–29 years: annual breast MRI screening with contrast or mammogram with consideration of tomosynthesis, only if MRI is unavailable or individualized based on family history if a breast cancer diagnosis before age 30 is present.<br>Age 30–75 years: annual mammogram with consideration of tomosynthesis and breast MRI screening with contrast.<br>Age >75 years: management should be individualized<br>Consider risk-reducing mastectomy |
| *BRIP1* | Potential increase in risk | Management based on family history |
| *CDH1* | Increased absolute risk 41–60% | Annual mammogram with consideration of tomosynthesis or breast MRI with contrast starting at age 30 |
| *CHECK2* | Increased absolute risk 15–40% | Annual mammography starting at age 40 with consideration for breast tomosynthesis/MRI |
| *MSH2*<br>*MLH1*<br>*MSH6*<br>*PMS2*<br>*EPCAM* | Limited evidence of increased risk, absolute risk is <15% | Management based on family history |
| *NBN* | Increased risk of breast cancer with variant 657del5 | Management based on family history |
| *NF1* | Increased absolute risk 15–40% | Annual mammography starting at age 30 with consideration for breast tomosynthesis/MRI |
| *PALB2* | Increased absolute risk 41–60% | Annual mammography starting at age 30 with consideration for breast tomosynthesis/MRI<br>Consider risk-reducing mastectomy |
| *PTEN* | Increased absolute risk 40–60% | Breast awareness starting at age 18<br>Clinical breast exam, every 6–12 months starting at age 25 years (or 5–10 years before earliest known breast cancer in the family)<br>Breast screening:<br>Age 25–29 years: annual breast MRI screening with contrast or mammogram with consideration of tomosynthesis, only if MRI is unavailable or individualized based on family history if a breast cancer diagnosis before age 30 is present.<br>Age 30–75 years: annual mammogram with consideration of tomosynthesis and breast MRI screening with contrast.<br>Age >75 years: management should be individualized<br>Consider risk-reducing mastectomy |
| *RAD51C* | Increased absolute risk 15–40% | Management based on family history |
| *RAD51D* | Increased absolute risk 15–40% | Management based on family history |
| *STK11* | Increased absolute risk 40–60% | Annual mammography alternating with Breast MRI every 6 months starting at age 30 and clinical breast exam every 6 months |
| *TP53* | Increased absolute risk >60% | Breast awareness starting at age 18<br>Clinical breast exam, every 6–12 months starting at age 20 years.<br>Breast screening:<br>Age 20–29 years: annual breast MRI screening with contrast or mammogram with consideration of tomosynthesis, only if MRI is unavailable or individualized based on family history if a breast cancer diagnosis before age 30 is present.<br>Age 30–75 years: annual mammogram with consideration of tomosynthesis and breast MRI screening with contrast.<br>Age >75 years: management should be individualized<br>Consider risk-reducing mastectomy |

benefiting the most. In this age group screening is most beneficial and has the least amount of harm when performed every 2 years.

ACOG recommends that women of average risk be offered screening mammography beginning at age 40. Women at average risk should have screening mammography every 1 to 2 years. After age 55, biennial screening mammography is a reasonable option and should continue until at least age 75 years (ACOG Practice Bulletin 179, 2015).

The American Cancer Society (ACS) screening guidelines for women with an average risk of breast cancer were revised in

TABLE 15.9 Professional Society Recommendations for Screening Mammography

| Organization | Age to Initiate Mammography | Age to Conclude Mammography | Interval between Screenings |
|---|---|---|---|
| American Academy of Family Physicians | Routinely at ≥50 y<br>Screening before age 50 should be individualized | Screening recommended to age 74 y<br>Evidence insufficient for age ≥75 y | Not stated for age 40-49 y<br>2 y for age 50-74 y |
| American Cancer Society | Routinely at ≥45 y<br>Offered for age 40-45 y | While in good health and is expected to live ≥10 y | 1 y for age 45-54 y<br>2 y for age ≥55 y (with option of 1 y) |
| American College of Obstetricians and Gynecologists | Offer staring at age 40<br>Recommend by no later than age 50 if not already initiated | Age 75 | 1 or 2 y |
| American College of Physicians | Routinely at ≥50 y<br>40 y based on benefits, harms, preferences, and risk profile | When life expectancy is ≤10 y | 2 y |
| American College of Radiology | 40 y | No upper age limit | 1 y for all ages |
| American Society of Breast Surgeons | 40 y | When life expectancy is <10 y | 1 y for all ages |
| National Comprehensive Cancer Network | 40 y | When severe comorbidities limit life expectancy to ≤10 y | 1 y for all ages |
| U.S. Preventive Services Task Force, 2017 | Routinely at ≥50 y<br>Screening before age 50 should be individualized | Screening recommended to age 74 y<br>Evidence insufficient for age ≥75 y | 2 y for age 50-74 y |

2015. The updated recommendations are as follows: (1) Regular screening mammography should start at age 45 years; (2) annual screening should be offered to women aged 45 to 54 years, (3) women 55 years and older should undergo biennial screening or have the opportunity to continue screening annually, (4) women between the ages of 40 and 44 years should have the opportunity to begin annual screening, and (5) screening mammography should be continued as long as a woman's overall health is good and she has a life expectancy of 10 years or longer (Oeffinger, 2015).

No data exist regarding the ideal age at which to begin CBEs. In the asymptomatic, low-risk patient it is unclear at what age to begin CBEs. The occurrence of breast cancer is rare before age 20 years and uncommon before age 30 years. ACOG guidelines recommend that CBE be offered every 1 to 3 years for women 25 to 39 years old and annually for women 40 years and older. The NCCN recommends that CBE be performed every 1 to 3 years in women aged 20 to 39 years and annually for women 40 years and older. Per the USPSTF guidelines, insufficient evidence exists to assess the additional benefits and harms of CBE beyond screening mammography in women 40 years or older. The ACS does not recommend CBE for breast cancer screening among average-risk women at any age.

## CHEMOPROPHYLAXIS AND CHEMOTHERAPEUTIC RISK REDUCTION

Breast cancer risk reduction should be considered throughout a woman's life. For women who are high risk, endocrine therapy should be discussed to reduce the risk of invasive or in situ breast cancers. The American Society of Clinical Oncology (ASCO) and the USPSTF both provide recommendations regarding the use of endocrine therapy. Selection criteria in identifying women who would benefit from endocrine therapy include age older than 60 years, age older than 35 years with a history of lobular carcinoma in situ, ductal carcinoma in situ or atypical proliferative lesion of the breast (atypical ductal or lobular hyperplasia), women 35 to 59 years with a Gail model risk of breast cancer 1.66% or more over 5 years, and women with known *BRCA1* or *BRCA2* mutations who do not undergo prophylactic mastectomy.

Tamoxifen and raloxifene, both **selective estrogen receptor modulators**, are proven options that can decrease the risk of breast cancer in high-risk women (Table 15.10). Tamoxifen blocks the effects of endogenous estrogens in both the normal breast and the one with breast cancer. In the National Surgical Adjuvant Breast and Bowel Project (NSABP) B-14 trial, tamoxifen users had a significant decrease in the incidence of contralateral breast cancers compared with placebo. As a result, the Breast Cancer Prevention Trial (BCPT) was designed to assess whether tamoxifen would decrease the incidence of breast cancer in a high-risk population as determined by the Gail model for breast cancer risk assessment (Fisher, 1998). The trial enrolled 13,388 women in a double-blind, randomized, placebo-controlled trial to evaluate the effects of tamoxifen on risk reduction. The trial was closed prematurely because of a large discordance between the two groups. Tamoxifen significantly reduced the incidence of breast cancer in this population of patients by 49% compared with controls ($P < .00001$). It did not reduce the incidence of ER-negative cancers. A 2013 meta-analysis by the USPSTF analyzed data from four trials comparing tamoxifen to placebo (Nelson, 2013). The results showed a reduction in the risk of invasive breast cancer (RR, 0.70; 95% CI, 0.59 to 0.82), primarily noted in ER-positive breast cancer. A significant reduction in the incidence of nonvertebral fractures was also seen (RR, 0.66; 95% CI, 0.45 to 0.98). Additionally, the long-term follow-up results from the International Breast Cancer Intervention Study I (IBIS-1) showed a long-term reduction in the risk of hormone receptor–positive breast cancer (Cuzick, 2015). In this study of more than 7000 women, tamoxifen compared with placebo reduced the risk of invasive breast cancer between years 0 and 10 (hazard ratio [HR], 0.72; 95% CI, 0.59 to 0.88) and after 10 years (HR, 0.69; 95% CI, 0.53 to 0.91). This risk reduction was observed in hormone receptor–positive breast cancer (HR, 0.66; 95% CI, 0.54 to 0.81). Although treatment with tamoxifen compared with placebo is associated with an increased incidence in thromboembolic events and an increased incidence of endometrial cancer, the overall incidence of adverse events is small.

**TABLE 15.10** Breast Cancer Chemoprevention

| Results | Tamoxifen vs. Placebo* | Raloxifene vs. Placebo* | Raloxifene vs. Tamoxifen* |
|---|---|---|---|
| **BENEFITS** | | | |
| Invasive breast cancer | 0.70 (0.59-0.82) | 0.44 (0.27-0.71) | 1.02 (0.82-1.28) |
| Estrogen receptor–positive invasive breast cancer | 0.58 (0.42-0.79) | 0.33 (0.18-0.61) | 0.93 (0.72-1.24) |
| Estrogen receptor–negative invasive breast cancer | 1.19 (0.92-1.55) | 1.25 (0.67-2.31) | 1.15 (0.75-1.77) |
| Noninvasive breast cancer | 0.85 (0.54-1.35) | 1.47 (0.75-2.91) | 1.40 (0.98-2.00) |
| All-cause mortality | 1.07 (0.90-1.27) | 0.91 (0.81-1.02) | 0.94 (0.71-1.26) |
| Vertebral fracture | 0.75 (0.48-1.15) | 0.61 (0.54-0.69) | 0.98 (0.65-1.46) |
| Nonvertebral fracture | 0.66 (0.45-0.98) | 0.97 (0.87-1.09) | Insufficient data |
| **HARMS** | | | |
| Thromboembolic events | 1.93 (1.41-2.64) | 1.60 (1.15-2.23) | 0.70 (0.54-0.91) |
| Coronary events | 1.00 (0.79-1.27) | 0.95 (0.84-1.06) | 1.10 (0.85-1.43) |
| Stroke | 1.36 (0.89-2.08) | 0.96 (0.67-1.38) | 0.96 (0.64-1.43) |
| Endometrial cancer | 2.13 (1.36-3.32) | 1.14 (0.65-1.98) | 0.62 (0.35-1.08) |
| Cataracts | 1.25 (0.93-1.67) | 0.93 (0.84-1.04) | 0.79 (0.68-0.92) |

Modified from Nattinger AB. In the clinic. Breast cancer screening and prevention. *Ann Intern Med.* 2010;152(7):ITC41.

*All values are risk ratio (95% confidence interval). Four trials compared tamoxifen with placebo, two trials compared raloxifene with placebo, and one trial compared raloxifene with tamoxifen.

Raloxifene was approved by the Food and Drug Administration (FDA) for breast cancer risk reduction after the results of the Study of Tamoxifen and Raloxifene (STAR) trial (Vogel, 2006). A reduced incidence of thromboembolic events and endometrial cancer was noted in the raloxifene group compared with tamoxifen. In an 81-month median follow-up analysis, long-term raloxifene retained 76% of the effectiveness of tamoxifen in preventing invasive disease and grew closer over time to tamoxifen in preventing noninvasive disease. Less toxicity in regard to the development of endometrial cancer, uterine hyperplasia, and thromboembolic events was observed in the raloxifene group.

**Aromatase inhibitors (AIs)** are a reasonable alternative to SERMs for postmenopausal women. In the International Breast Cancer Intervention Study (IBIS-II), postmenopausal women at high risk of breast cancer were randomly allocated to treatment with anastrozole or placebo for 5 years (Cuzick, 2014). After a median follow-up of 5 years, a 50% reduction in the number of invasive breast cancer was noted with anastrozole compared with the placebo group (HR, 0.47; 95% CI, 0.32 to 0.68) along with a similar decrease in the incidence of DCIS. However, musculoskeletal side effects, vaginal dryness, and vasomotor symptoms were significantly greater in the anastrozole group.

Women with *BRCA1* mutations have significantly less benefit from tamoxifen. This is because almost all *BRCA1*-associated tumors are hormone receptor negative, unlike *BRCA2* carriers, who should be offered chemoprevention. Though these medications are effective, many women do not want to take them because of the side effects related to premature or perimenopausal symptoms. These women should be offered additional medications to control the side effects.

Surgical prophylaxis is another option for the woman who wants to reduce risk. In a retrospective cohort of 639 patients, Hartmann was able to demonstrate a 90% breast cancer risk reduction for the patient with a high risk of breast cancer after prophylactic bilateral mastectomy. In a follow-up study, Hartmann was able to demonstrate a similar risk reduction in a population of women with *BRCA* gene mutations (Hartmann, 2001). Although prophylactic bilateral mastectomy provides the greatest risk reduction, it is usually reserved for the very high-risk patient because of the associated physiologic and complicated psychological consequences. Although most women who have undergone prophylactic bilateral mastectomy do not regret having undergone the procedure, approximately 5% to 20% report dissatisfaction.

## DETECTION AND DIAGNOSIS

In the United States and countries with established screening programs, most breast cancers are diagnosed as a result of an abnormal mammogram. However, a significant number are also noted during patient or clinician breast examination, and up to 15% of women are diagnosed with breast cancer not detected on mammography. Breast cancer is usually asymptomatic prior to the development of locally advanced disease. Approximately 10% of women with early breast carcinoma experience breast pain that is associated; however, focal mastalgia is usually associated with a benign condition. The classic sign of a breast carcinoma is a solitary, solid, immovable, dominant breast mass with irregular borders. About 75% of breast cancers present as a palpable breast mass. Axillary adenopathy is a potential sign of more advanced locoregional disease. Nipple discharge is an even less common symptom of breast cancer. Findings suggestive of inflammatory breast cancer include erythema, skin thickening, and skin edema causing the appearance of an orange peel (peau d'orange). With increased screening, many cancers and in situ lesions are found before any symptoms are experienced.

Screening uses tests in asymptomatic women at periodic intervals to discover breast malignancies. There is more scientific evidence regarding screening for breast cancer than for any other cancer. The kinetics of growth in breast carcinoma is the basis for the recommendations for screening and detection. The average breast mass doubles in volume every 100 days, and the diameter doubles every 300 days. A breast carcinoma grows for 6 to 8 years before reaching a diameter of 1 cm, after which it doubles in less than another year. The mean diameter of a breast mass discovered by women who perform BSE at monthly intervals is 2 cm.

Three potential screening modalities include **BSE, CBE, and imaging with mammography**. BSE has the major advantages of no cost to the patient and convenience. However, studies have failed to show a beneficial effect of regular BSE in rates of breast cancer diagnosis, mortality, or tumor stage or size. BSE is associated with higher rates of breast biopsy for benign disease. As a result, BSE is not recommended as a screening tool. CBE and mammography are complementary procedures, and therefore the effectiveness of CBE in screening by itself is difficult to assess. As part of the screening process, the sensitivity of CBE was estimated to be 54% and specificity 94% (Barton, 1999). Various imaging modalities are available for identifying lesions that are suspicious for breast cancer. Mammography continues to be the primary choice in screening for breast cancer. It is important to note that a negative mammogram does not rule out breast carcinoma. Ultrasound is used as an adjunct to mammography for diagnostic follow-up of an abnormality seen on screening mammography. Additional imaging techniques include MRI and tomosynthesis. Current data do not support the use of MRI in screening women at average risk for breast cancer. Its use is limited to screening in high-risk patients. Newer tests, such as tomography, are under evaluation.

In summary, present protocols for screening of breast carcinoma are not ideal and continue to evolve. Nevertheless, screening tests result in a reduction in the mortality rate from breast cancer of approximately 25% to 30%.

## Self-Examination of the Breasts

Few randomized trials regarding breast self-examination exist. A 2003 Cochrane systematic review included two large population studies from China and Russia. Twice as many biopsies with benign results were performed in the screening group compared with the control group (RR, 1.89; 95% CI, 1.79 to 2.00) (Gemignani, 2011). Several other studies did not show an advantage of breast self-examination in the rates of breast cancer diagnosis, breast cancer death, or tumor stage or size. Although this procedure has long been advocated, breast self-examination in itself does not decrease breast cancer mortality. However, research has shown that routine breast self-examination does play a role in detecting breast cancer compared with finding a breast lump by chance or simply knowing what is normal for each woman. For this reason, some societies continue to recommend some form of self-breast examination. ACOG recommends breast self-awareness, which for some patients includes performing a BSE and reporting changes to their physician. The ACS recommends educating women about the benefits and limitations of BSE and to report any changes. BSE is an option for women starting in their 20s. The USPSTF, however, recommends against teaching breast self-examination.

Women who choose to perform a BSE should do so when their breasts are least likely to be tender or swollen. In premenopausal women, a few days immediately after a menstrual period are the best time to detect changes in normal lumps or texture of the breasts. Postmenopausal women or women who have had a hysterectomy can perform BSE on the same calendar days each month if they choose. Breast changes that women should be aware of include development of a lump or mass, swelling of the breast, nipple abnormalities or discharge, and skin irritation or dimpling. The examination is best done in both supine and upright positions using the finger pads of the three middle fingers. Three different levels of pressure (light, medium, and firm) are used to examine the breast. Women should be consistent in their technique used. One of the easier techniques to follow is to palpate the breasts in a clockwise fashion beginning at the nipple and gradually circumscribing larger circles; however, some advocate the vertical pattern (up and down pattern) as the most effective for examining the entire breast without missing any breast tissue.

## Clinical Breast Examination

Several studies have investigated the use of physical examination in addition to mammography; however, for ethical reasons no randomized trial comparing physical examination without mammography has been conducted. In a meta-analysis investigating the effectiveness of CBE, Barton and colleagues included all controlled trials and case-control studies in which CBE was at least part of the screening process (Barton, 1999). CBE alone detected between 3% and 45% of breast cancers that were missed during mammography screening. The authors estimated CBE sensitivity at 54% and specificity at 94%. Factors associated with greater accuracy included longer duration of examination and a higher number of specific techniques used during the examination.

Considerable variability exists among physicians' ability to detect breast lumps. Fletcher and coworkers tested the physical examination techniques of 80 different physicians using simulated breasts (Fletcher, 1985). Detection rates ranged from 17% to 83%. The ability to detect the mass was directly related to the size of the mass; 87% of 1-cm, 33% of 0.5-cm, and 14% of 0.3-cm masses were discovered. Physicians with higher discovery rates spent more time performing the examination.

Differing guidelines exist in the medical literature regarding the use of CBE in breast cancer screening protocols. However, it must be noted that no group recommends CBE alone. The ACS does not recommend CBE for breast cancer screening at any age among average-risk women. ACOG recommends CBE for everyone every 3 years from age 20 to 39 and annually thereafter. The USPSTF recommendations state that current evidence is insufficient to assess the additional benefits and harms of CBE beyond screening mammography in women 40 years or older.

Several palpation techniques exist for the CBE, and limited comparative data on the efficacy of these techniques are available. A complete breast examination involves inspecting and palpating the breasts with the patient in the sitting and the supine position. Initially in the sitting position with the patient's arms at her sides, the clinician observes the contour, symmetry, and vascular pattern of the breasts and the skin for irritation, retraction, or edema. The patient is next asked to raise her arms over her head and any tethering of breast tissue to the chest wall should be noted. Examination of the axilla and supraclavicular nodes is best performed with the patient sitting upright. The breast examination is then performed in the supine position with both the woman's arms at her side and raised above her head. The examination includes palpation of all quadrants of the breast, axilla, supraclavicular areas, and adjacent chest wall. Palpation should use the pads of the first three fingers placed together, exerting firm but gentle pressure. It is important to examine both nipples for retraction or skin irritation. The areola should be compressed to identify any discharge. The normal breast has a small depression directly below the nipple. The skin of the breast is again carefully inspected for unusual vascular patterns, edema, erythema, or retraction (Fig. 15.12).

## Mammography

The goal of screening mammography is the detection of cancer before it is clinically palpable and less likely to have progressed to the regional nodes or distant metastases. Mammography may identify cancer up to 4 years before it comes clinically evident. The 5-year survival rate for women whose breast cancer is believed to be localized to the breast with negative axillary nodes is approximately 99% versus 84% with regionalized disease (when axillary nodes are involved). In contrast to screening mammography, diagnostic mammography is performed when women have complaints such as breast pain, a palpable lump (or mass), nipple

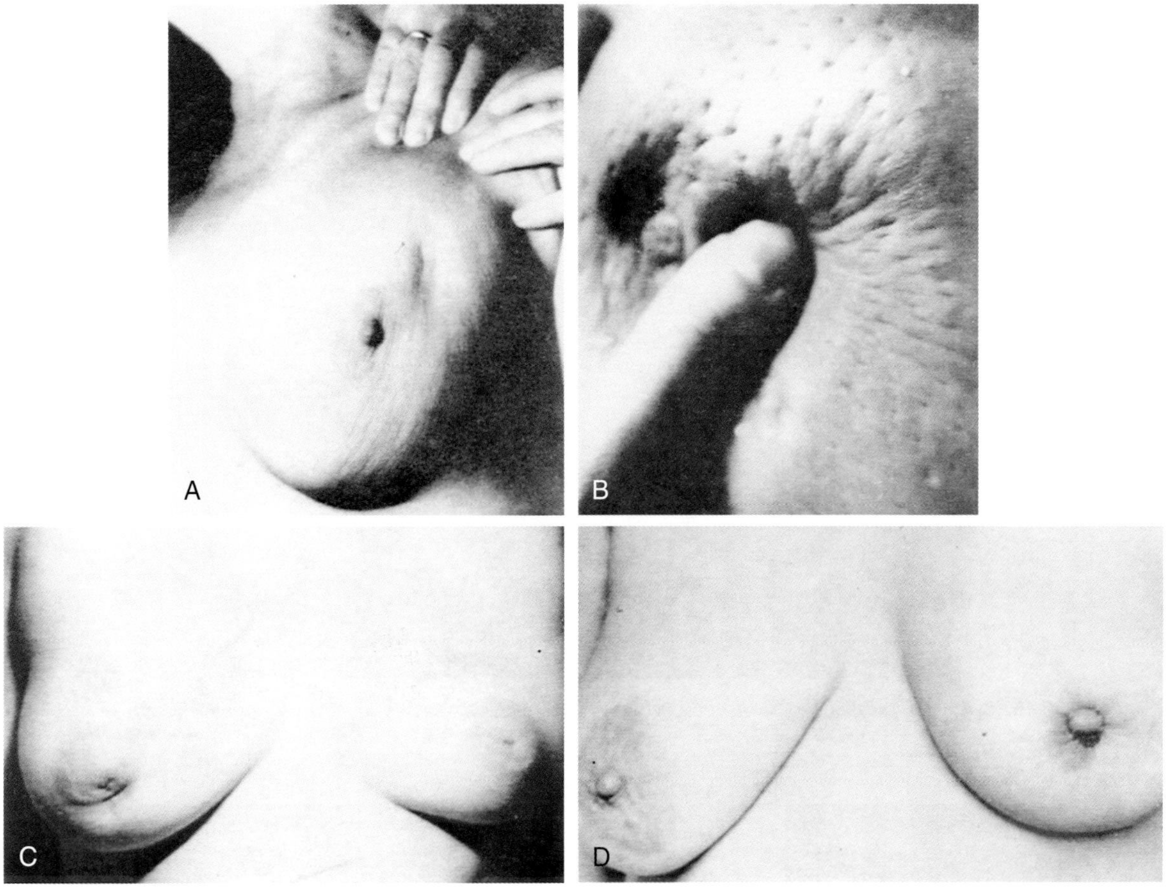


**Fig. 15.12** Signs of breast carcinoma. **A,** Retraction found during physical examination. **B,** Peau d'orange from underlying carcinoma. **C,** Retraction of right nipple. **D,** Retraction of left nipple from carcinoma. (From Degrell I. *Atlas of Diseases of the Mammary Gland.* Basel, Switzerland: S Karger; 1976:20.)

discharge, or abnormality on a screening study or to follow women who have been treated for breast cancer.

Screening mammography is the primary imaging technique for breast cancer detection and the only breast imaging method found to reduce breast cancer–related mortality. Mammography uses x-ray photons and can identify fine calcifications or small asymmetric densities associated with breast neoplasms months to years before the carcinoma enlarges to a size that may be palpated on physical examination. Nine randomized controlled trials using mammography with or without a CBE have been conducted. Systematic reviews of the trials differentiating mammogram screening with no screening indicate a protective effect among women ages 40 to 69. A 2012 meta-analysis of randomized trials showed a 20% relative risk reduction for breast cancer mortality in women who underwent screening compared with controls (Independent UK Panel on Breast Cancer Screening, 2012). However, critics suggest that breast cancer screening now may be less effective as the majority of these trials were initiated before 1990 and do not reflect modern therapy or modern imaging.

The sensitivity of mammography ranges from 80% to 90% in the detection of breast cancer and decreases in women with dense breasts. Density is not a function of the size or firmness of the breast but refers to the ratio of glandular tissue to fatty elements. It is also a significant risk factor for the development of breast cancer. In cases where a woman is noted by plain-film mammography to have dense breasts, she should be referred for digital mammography preferably with tomosynthesis, or if she has dense breasts and she is in a known high-risk group, with greater than 20% risk of the development of breast cancer, she should be offered an MRI.

Mammographic views can be generalized into two groups: standard views and supplementary views. The mediolateral oblique (MLO) view and the craniocaudal (CC) view (Fig. 15.13) are the two standard projections performed on routine screening. The MLO view is the most important projection as it depicts the greatest amount of breast tissue and is the only view that includes all of the upper outer quadrant and axillary tail. The amount of visible pectoral muscle in the MLO view determines the amount of breast tissue included in the image. This is an important factor in reducing the number of false negatives and increasing the sensitivity of mammography. Additionally, it is important to visualize the upper outer quadrant in the MLO view because most pathologic breast changes develop in this area. An optimal CC view depicts the external lateral portion of the breast, the retromammary fat tissue (Chassaignac bag), the pectoral muscle on the posterior edge, and the nipple.

Abnormalities noted on mammography include calcifications, masses, asymmetry, and architectural distortion. The most specific mammographic feature of malignancy is a focal mass with spiculated margins (Fig. 15.14). The positive predictive value of a mass with a spiculated margin is 81% and with irregular shape it is 73%. Clustered microcalcifications (Fig. 15.15) are noted in approximately 60% of cancers detected mammographically. Microcalcifications range from 0.1 to 1 mm in diameter, and the presence of five or more calcifications within a volume of 1 $cm^3$ is termed a **cluster**. Subsequent breast biopsies will find 25% of

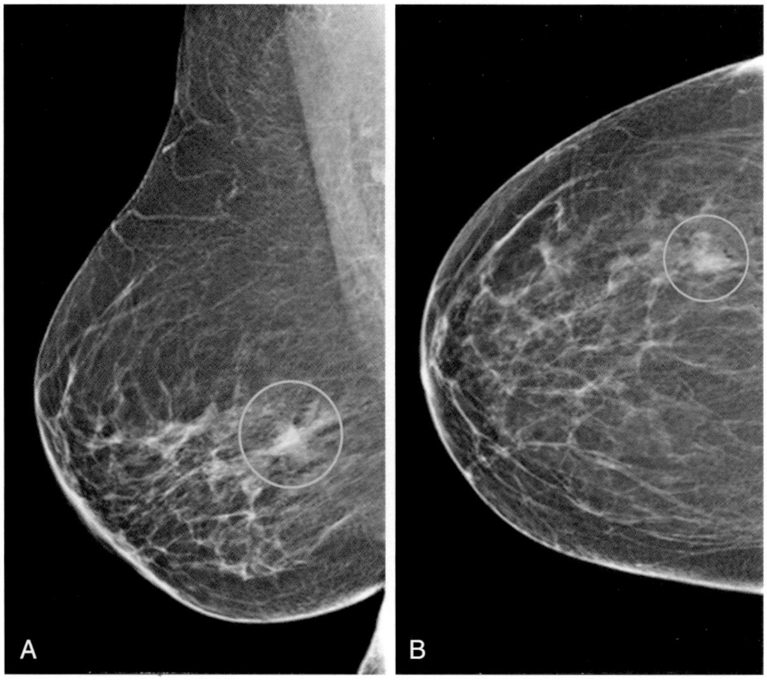


**Fig. 15.13** **A,** Right breast, mediolateral oblique view. **B,** Right breast, craniocaudal view. (Courtesy Laura Isley, MD.)

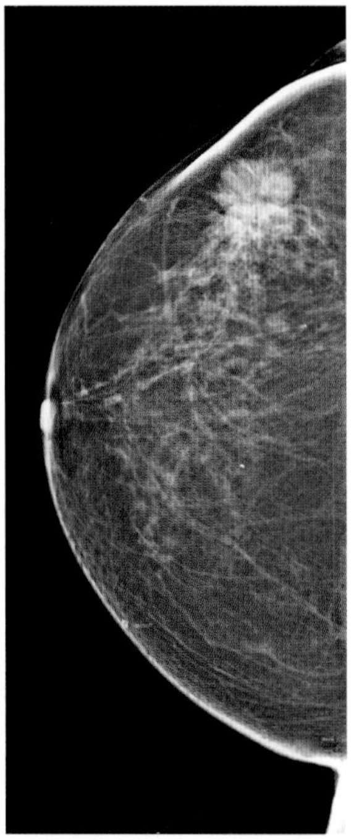

**Fig. 15.14** Spiculated breast mass. (Courtesy Laura Isley, MD.)

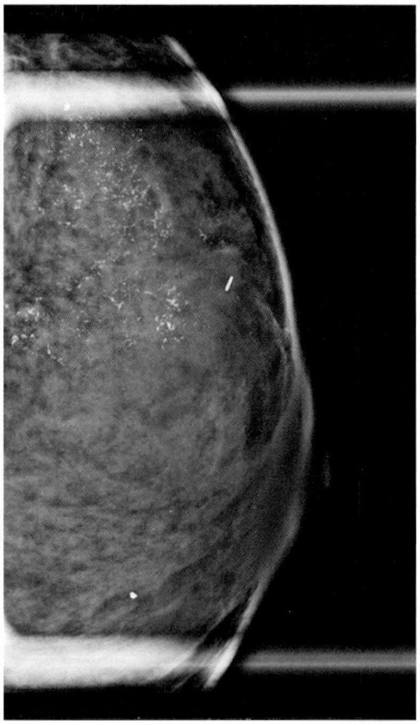

**Fig. 15.15** Breast microcalcifications. (Courtesy Laura Isley, MD.)

clusters associated with cancer and 75% with benign disease. Clustered microcalcifications can be associated with intraductal calcifications in areas of necrotic tumor or calcifications within mucin-secreting tumors. Linear branching microcalcifications have a higher predictive value for malignancy than do granular microcalcifications, particularly for high-grade DCIS. Breast cancers, including DCIS, are more often diagnosed with the granular type of calcifications.

Mammographic findings are summarized employing the American College of Radiology **Breast Imaging Reporting and Data System (BI-RADS)** (Fig. 15.16). This reporting system was devised to standardize mammographic terminology, reduce confusing interpretations, and facilitate the monitoring of outcomes. There are six assessment categories, each associated with a specific risk of cancer. Category 0 is an incomplete assessment and therefore requires additional evaluation, which may include

| BI-RAD class | Description | Probability of malignancy | Follow-up |
|---|---|---|---|
| 0 | Needs additional | N/A | Additional imaging evaluation +/– prior imaging for comparison |
| 1 | Negative | 0 | Routine mammography screening |
| 2 | Benign | 0 | Routine mammography screening |
| 3 | Probably Benign | < 2% | Short interval followup or continued surveillance mammography |
| 4 | Suspicious | >2 % but < 95% | Biopsy/Tissue diagnosis |
| 4A | Low suspicion | >2 % but ≤10% | |
| 4B | Moderate suspicion | >10 % but ≤50% | |
| 4C | High suspicion | >50 % but < 95% | |
| 5 | Highly Suspicious | ≥ 95% | Biopsy/Tissue diagnosis |
| 6 | Known/Proven Malignancy | N/A | Surgery when appropriate |
| BI-RADS Breast Imaging Reporting and Data Systems | | | |

**Fig. 15.16** BI-RAD (Breast Imaging Reporting and Data Systems) classification of mammographic lesions. (From Pazdur R, Coia LR, Hoskins WJ, Wagman LD, eds. *Cancer Management: A Multidisciplinary Approach.* 4th ed. Melville, NY: Cligott Publishing Group; 2006:143.)

further imaging. Categories 1 and 2 are nonmalignant. Category 3 represents a lesion that is felt to be benign but requires interval follow-up imaging to confirm stability. Categories 4 and 5 are lesions felt to be suspicious enough to warrant biopsy. Category 6 represents malignancy that has been proved. The BI-RADS final assessment is provided to standardize the reporting of mammographic findings and provide recommendations for further management.

## Digital Mammography

**Digital mammography** is the technique by which the radiographic image is obtained with digital detectors and recorded electronically in a digital format. The image is further processed and displayed as a gray-scale image that can be displayed in multiple formats. Digital mammography has several advantages compared with conventional film screen mammography. Image acquisition, display, and storage are much faster. Image manipulation through adjustments in contrast, brightness, and magnification of selected regions enables radiologists to obtain superior views. This technology makes it possible to subtract various layers of computerized imagery to examine suspicious areas and improve the ability to detect and diagnose breast carcinoma. Greater contrast resolution allows better screening of women with dense breasts and breast implants. With the ability to manipulate and postprocess the images, subtle abnormalities are increasingly detected. Images can be stored easily for future reference and can be sent electronically to be read at multiple viewing stations, thereby allowing double reading when necessary. The main disadvantages of digital mammography include the cost of the equipment and the reduced spatial resolution compared with film.

Digital mammography has been compared with film screen mammography in various studies with little difference reported in cancer detection rates. In the Digital Mammographic Imaging Screening Trial (DMIST), 49,528 asymptomatic women underwent both film and digital mammography (Pisano, 2008). Although there was no significant difference in overall diagnostic accuracy, digital mammography was more accurate for premenopausal and perimenopausal women. Furthermore, it was superior for women with dense breasts. Approximately 25,000 women aged 45 to 69 years were randomized to either digital or film screen mammography in the Oslo II Study (Skaane, 2007). The breast cancer detection rate at 2 years was significantly higher in the full field digital mammography group compared with film screen mammography (0.59% and 0.38%, respectively). In the United States the majority of imaging centers use digital mammography. It may provide a small screening advantage in women younger than 50 years old. However, it must be noted that film mammography is an acceptable screening method for all women.

## Magnetic Resonance Imaging

**MRI** is another imaging modality used to detect breast cancer. It does not use ionizing radiation. Malignant tumors with increased tumor angiogenesis are differentiated from benign tumors based on the rapid uptake and release of contrast (Fig. 15.17). Lesions are classified as mass or nonmass. The reported sensitivity of MRI ranges from 71% to 100%. The lower specificity, less than 65%, is secondary to the overlap in the enhancement pattern of benign and malignant lesions. Although the specificity of MRI is lower than that for mammography, the sensitivity is higher, and it is especially useful in women with dense fibroglandular breasts and implants.

Screening recommendations are that women with a 20% or higher lifetime risk of breast cancer should be scheduled for annual MRI and mammogram screening, usually alternating every 6 months. In women of average risk, breast MRI has poor specificity. Additional potential uses or indications for MRI are to improve imaging of structures close to the chest wall, to improve

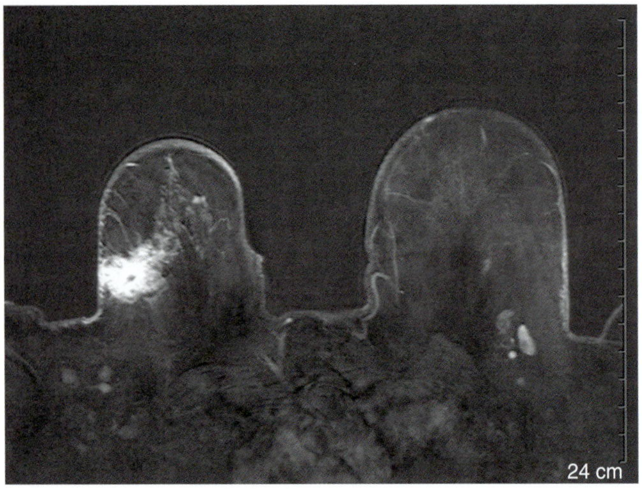


**Fig. 15.17** Breast magnetic resonance image showing mass. (Courtesy Laura Isley, MD.)

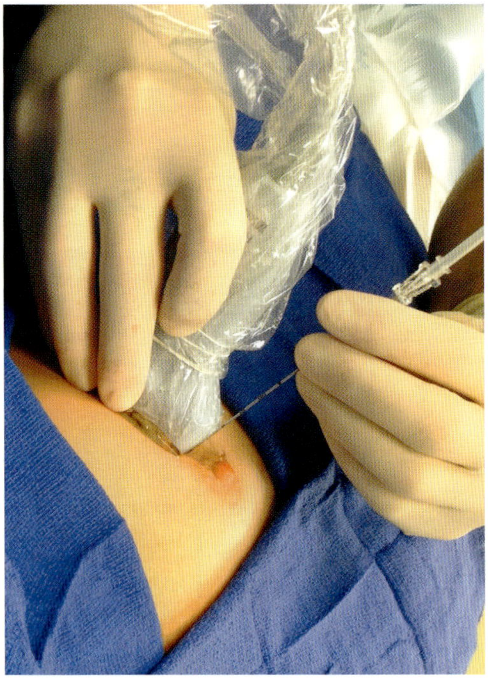

**Fig. 15.18** Intraoperative ultrasound-guided wire bracketing of a nonpalpable breast lesion for excision. (Courtesy David T. Rock, MD.)

imaging of women with breast implants, to detect occult primary tumors, and to evaluate for silicone implant integrity. MRI is useful in the documentation of response to neoadjuvant chemotherapy and diagnosis of recurrence and for screening of high-risk patients. MRI may be useful in the identification of multifocal, multicentric, or contralateral disease.

Several limitations of breast MRI exist. It cannot identify microcalcifications, and there is loss of image quality with respiratory movements. Breast MRI with gadolinium is not performed during pregnancy. MRI is contraindicated in patients with a history of gadolinium allergy, diminished renal function, and cardiac pacemakers, defibrillators, or other implanted devices whose operation may be disturbed by the MRI magnet.

## Ultrasound

**Ultrasound** has an established role in conjunction with mammography for evaluating abnormalities and is often used in the diagnostic follow-up of an abnormal screening mammogram. It should not be used by itself as a screening tool in average risk women. No randomized trials exist comparing combination ultrasound and mammography versus mammography alone for screening in average-risk women. However, women with dense breasts may benefit from the addition of ultrasound to screening mammography. Ultrasound screening increased the detection of otherwise occult cancers by 37% in a study involving 3626 women age 42 to 67 with dense breasts and no visible abnormalities on mammography. In women with dense breasts as their only risk factor, the American College of Radiology recognizes that ultrasound as an addition to screening mammography may be useful for incremental cancer detection.

Ultrasonography of the breast is a highly operator- and reader-dependent test with a great deal of variation among different centers. Ultrasound uses sound waves to image tissues and is particularly effective in differentiating cystic from solid masses. The accuracy rate of ultrasound to diagnose a cystic mass is 96% to 100%, which exceeds the combined accuracy of mammography and physical examination. It can be used in examining the axilla and determining lymph node status.

Ultrasound is often used to guide needle aspiration or direct core needle biopsy. It has also been used to localize tumors intraoperatively without a guidewire with excellent success rates (Fig. 15.18). In pregnant women or women younger than 30 years old with focal breast symptoms or findings, ultrasound is the first line of imaging. Although MRI is superior at detecting silicone implant ruptures, ultrasound is usually more readily available and can be used in cases where MRI is contraindicated. In summary, ultrasound should not be used as a sole imaging technique for breast disease. Because of its lack of sensitivity and specificity for early breast carcinoma, it should not be used in an attempt to detect subclinical disease in the general population at this time.

## Computed Tomography

CT is not routinely used for breast cancer screening or diagnosis. Because of higher radiation doses and longer study times, CT has limited value compared with mammography. The thickness of cross-sectional slices with CT misses the majority of areas of microcalcification. It is useful for contrast-enhancing lesions, for lesions close to the chest wall, and for studying the most medial and lateral aspects of the breast. It is sometimes used for preoperative wire location of a mass that is difficult to localize by mammography. However, the increased expense and radiation exposure virtually eliminate CT scans from screening programs.

## Tomosynthesis

Breast tomosynthesis, commonly referred to as **three-dimensional (3D) mammography**, is a modification of digital mammography. The 3D image is created by taking multiple low-dose images per view along an arc over the breast. The compressed breast remains stationary while the x-ray tube rotates approximately 1 degree for each image in a 15- to 50-degree arc. The 11 to 49 acquired images are projected as cross-sectional "slices" of the breast, with each slice typically 1-mm thick. Thin slice reconstruction with tomosynthesis allows true lesions to be distinguished from spurious lesions caused by overlapping structures identified on routine mammography. Breast tomosynthesis has been approved in the United States for breast cancer screening when used in combination with mammography. Friedewald and colleagues compared screening by digital mammography with digital mammography plus tomosynthesis (Friedewald, 2014). In this large retrospective study with data collected from 13 sites, the addition of tomosynthesis to digital mammography resulted in an overall decrease in recall rate of 16 per 1000 screens (95% CI, 18 to 14; $P < .001$) and more invasive cancers detected (4.2 cancers vs. 5.4 cancers per 1000 studies; $P < .001$). The detection rate for ductal carcinoma in situ was similar in both groups.

Disadvantages of tomosynthesis include increased radiation exposure and reading time. The radiation exposure is approximately double the usual radiation dose associated with mammography and can be even greater in patients with dense or thick breasts. Facilities with newer techniques that have a lower radiation dose are expensive and not widely available.

## Breast Tissue Sampling

The evaluation of a breast mass includes a clinical examination, imaging, and tissue sampling. This triple test has been advocated as a reliable alternative to excisional biopsy. If the physical examination, imaging findings, and cytologic evaluation of the mass all confirm the same benign process, the patient can be followed to monitor the mass. However, if any of these assessments indicate cancer, a biopsy should be performed. The false-negative rate of triple test diagnosis approaches that of surgical biopsy, and the false-positive rate is comparable with that for frozen section.

Common indications for tissue biopsy include bloody discharge from the nipple, a persistent 3D mass, or suspicious mammography. Additionally, nipple retraction or elevation and skin changes, such as erythema, induration, or edema, are also indications for breast biopsy. Imaging should precede biopsy because the inflammation and bleeding that can occur secondary to the biopsy may significantly impair needed visualization of the breast with imaging. The choice of initial biopsy methods is dependent on the lesion characteristics, including whether it is palpable, and location. The least invasive technique that is likely to produce a diagnostic specimen should be used.

## Fine-Needle Aspiration

**Fine-needle aspiration (FNA)** is the least invasive first-line sampling technique, followed by core needle biopsy. FNA is a simple, office-based procedure. It is appropriate for new, well-circumscribed, usually tender masses that are thought to be simple (not complex) cysts. If the lesion is not palpable, ultrasound guidance may be used to localize the lesion. It is also valuable in the evaluation of ipsilateral axillary lymph nodes.

The skin over the breast is the most sensitive area, but the breast tissue itself has few pain fibers. Some providers choose to inject a small amount of local anesthetic (1 mL of 1% lidocaine). Care must be taken to avoid the development of a hematoma, which may obscure the mass and decrease the accuracy of the FNA. A small (18- to 21-gauge) needle is used when performing an FNA. The breast mass is secured with one hand, and the other hand introduces the needle attached to a 10- or 20-mL syringe into the mass. If the mass is found to be a cyst, the procedure can be converted to a cyst aspiration. The color of the fluid obtained via aspiration varies from clear to grossly bloody. Samples should be sent to a cytopathologist for evaluation. However, if the aspirated fluid is clear, it is not necessary to submit it for cytologic evaluation, and the patient should be reevaluated in 1 to 2 months. If the cyst recurs, imaging should be performed to confirm its benign nature and reaspiration performed under ultrasound guidance. Less than 20% of cysts recur after a single aspiration, and fewer than 10% recur after two aspirations. A biopsy should be performed on cysts that recur within 2 weeks or that necessitate more than one repeat aspiration. In cases of a solid mass, a fixed specimen is obtained and submitted for cytopathologic evaluation. Several passes are made through the mass with continuous suction from the syringe. Moving the needle within a single tract will give a satisfactory cellular yield in the majority of cases.

Complications of needle aspiration are rare and include hematoma formation and infection. The theoretic risk of spreading cancer along the needle track has not been substantiated. Finally, it is difficult to determine the difference between carcinoma in situ and invasive cancer from the cytologic specimen obtained from FNA.

## Core Needle Biopsy and Excisional Biopsy

**Core needle biopsy** retrieves more tissue than FNA, permitting the differentiation between invasive versus in situ cancer. A more definitive histologic assessment, including tumor grade angiolymphatic invasion and hormone receptor status, can be made. In addition, core needle biopsy usually provides adequate tissue for genomic analysis or cancer profiling. Vacuum-assisted directional biopsy can be used to acquire a greater volume of tissue. Excisional biopsy should be reserved for certain situations when a diagnosis is not established using the diagnostic triad.

Core needle biopsy is usually performed using a larger needle (9 to 14 gauge) than FNA. After administration of local anesthetic, a small skin incision is made and the core biopsy needle is inserted. Three to five cores of solid tissue are collected for pathologic evaluation. A biopsy clip must be placed at the time of the biopsy for future localization of the lesion. Core needle biopsy may be performed with ultrasound, mammographic, or MRI guidance. Mammographic or stereotactic guidance is primarily used for biopsy of calcifications. The breast is imaged at 30-degree angles with two-dimensional mammography, and the lesion is localized using computer-assisted positioning and targeting devices.

Nonpalpable breast lesions discovered by breast imaging techniques, including screening mammography, require preoperative localization by the radiologist. Under mammographic, ultrasound, or MRI guidance, a wire is placed percutaneously so that the tip of the wire is fixed in the lesion. Image-guided techniques play a vital role in preoperative staging of breast cancer patients and in the planning of definitive surgery.

## Classification

Carcinomas make up the majority of breast malignancies and originate in the epithelium of the collecting ducts (ductal) or the terminal lobular ducts (lobular). Sarcomas are rare, constituting less than 1% of primary breast cancers, and arise from stromal or connective tissue. Tumor grade is based on tubule formation, nuclear pleomorphism, and mitotic counts using the Nottingham score to determine low, intermediate, or high grade. Higher grade is associated with a poorer long-term prognosis.

Initially, breast carcinoma may be divided into invasive and in situ lesions (Table 15.11). Invasive ductal carcinoma accounts for the majority, approximately 80%, of invasive carcinomas. Invasive lobular carcinomas constitute approximately 10% to 15% of cases. Other subtypes include mucinous, tubular, medullary, micropapillary, and papillary. Both in situ and invasive carcinomas are often found in the same quadrant of the breast. Additionally, multifocal carcinomas are not uncommon, and bilateral breast carcinomas occur in 1% to 2% of newly diagnosed cases.

# DUCTAL CARCINOMA IN SITU

**DCIS** is a noninvasive lesion in which the cellular abnormalities are limited by the basement membrane of the breast ducts. The risk of DCIS increases with age, and it accounts for approximately

**TABLE 15.11** Simplified Classification of Breast Carcinoma Based on Histology

| Type of Carcinoma | Percentage of All Cases Diagnosed |
|---|---|
| Ductal carcinoma | |
| In situ | 5 |
| Infiltrating | 70 |
| Infiltrating with uniform histologic appearance | 10 |
| Medullary, colloid, comedo, tubular, papillary | |
| Lobular carcinoma | |
| In situ | 3 |
| Infiltrating | 9 |
| Inflammatory carcinoma | 2 |
| Paget disease | 1 |

20% of newly diagnosed breast cancers. It is most commonly discovered in perimenopausal and postmenopausal women, and mammography has significantly increased the detection of this lesion. DCIS, evidenced by clustered microcalcifications, is not usually detectable by palpation. Diagnosis is confirmed with a core needle biopsy, usually using stereotactic guidance.

The histologic diagnosis of ductal carcinoma in situ includes a heterogeneous group of tumors with varying malignant potential. Classification is based on architectural pattern (comedo, micropapillary, cribriform, or solid), tumor grade (high, intermediate, or low), and evidence of necrosis. Identification of microinvasion, a minute focus of stromal invasion, is crucial because treatment recommendations may change.

The goal of treatment is to prevent the development of invasive cancer. Treatment approaches include surgery, radiation therapy, and adjuvant endocrine therapy. Mastectomy is curative for more than 98% of DCIS patients. Breast-conserving surgery (lumpectomy, partial mastectomy) followed by radiation therapy has shown equivalent survival compared with mastectomy. Chemoprevention with either a SERM or aromatase inhibitor is recommended for women with ER-positive DCIS who have undergone breast conservation therapy to reduce the risk of developing additional invasive or noninvasive breast cancers.

## LOBULAR CARCINOMA IN SITU

**Lobular carcinoma in situ (LCIS)** is a noninvasive lesion arising from the lobules and terminal ducts of the breast. Historically, LCIS is found with an invasive carcinoma in approximately 5% of malignant breast specimens. Although it does not have the same malignant potential as DCIS, women with LCIS are at an increased risk of developing breast cancer. Approximately 80% to 90% of cases occur in premenopausal women.

LCIS has a greater tendency to be bilateral and multifocal. The latent period for development of malignancy is longer than with DCIS. Approximately one fifth of women diagnosed with LCIS develop invasive breast carcinoma over a 20- to 25-year follow-up period. To rule out an invasive component, NCCN guidelines recommend reexcision in cases where LCIS is diagnosed by core needle biopsy. LCIS is not managed as a precursor lesion. In cases in which LCIS is diagnosed on an excisional biopsy, obtaining histologically negative margins is not mandatory because LCIS is often multicentric. Breast cancer chemoprevention with a SERM or an aromatase inhibitor may be indicated for women diagnosed with LCIS.

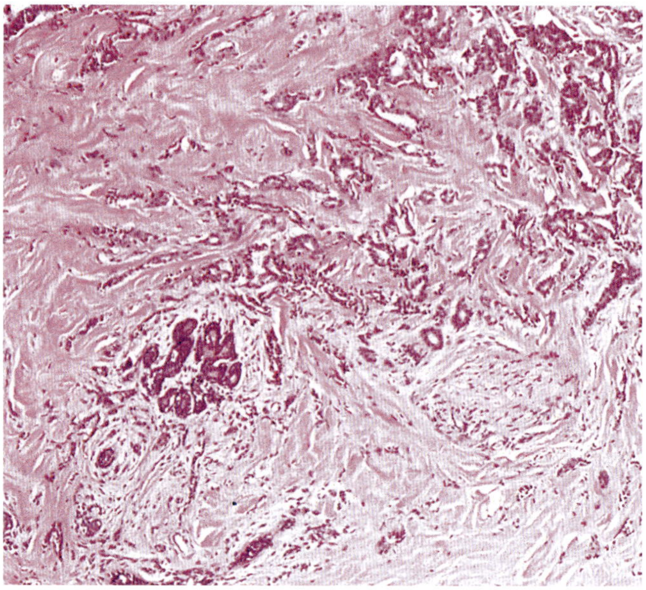

**Fig. 15.19** Invasive ductal carcinoma of the breast. Malignant cells are invading the fibrous tissue. (From Stevens A, Lowe J. *Human Histology.* 3rd ed. Philadelphia: Mosby; 2005:392.)

## INFILTRATING OR INVASIVE DUCTAL CARCINOMA

Infiltrating or **invasive ductal carcinoma** is the most common breast malignancy, comprising approximately 70% to 80% of breast malignancies. Histologically, nonuniform malignant epithelial cells of varying sizes and shapes infiltrate the surrounding tissue (Fig. 15.19). Cytologic features range from bland to highly malignant, and tumors are graded based on architectural and cytologic characteristics. Typically, infiltrating ductal carcinomas are firm and gray-white. The degree of fibrous response as a result of the invading malignant cells is responsible for the firm palpable mass, radiologic density, and texture during biopsy.

## INFILTRATING LOBULAR CARCINOMA

**Infiltrating lobular carcinomas** constitute approximately 10% to 15% of invasive lesions and are the second most common type of invasive breast cancer. These lesions are characterized by the uniformity of the small, round neoplastic cells that infiltrate the stroma and adipose tissue in a single-file fashion (Fig. 15.20). This neoplasia tends to have a multicentric origin in the same breast and tends to involve both breasts more often than infiltrating ductal carcinoma. Infiltrating lobular carcinomas are more commonly ER positive. Unlike infiltrating ductal carcinomas, the excised breast tissue often has a normal consistency and no mass lesion is grossly evident. Histologic subdivisions of infiltrating lobular carcinoma include small cell, round cell, and signet cell carcinomas.

## INFLAMMATORY BREAST CANCER

**Inflammatory breast cancer** is rare and accounts for approximately 1% to 5% of breast cancers. This type is recognized clinically as a rapidly growing malignant carcinoma with highly angiogenic and angioinvasive characteristics. Because of its aggressive features, most inflammatory breast cancers are diagnosed as either stage III or IV, and most are invasive ductal carcinomas. Infiltration of malignant cells into the dermal lymphatics of the skin produces a clinical picture that appears like a skin infection (Fig. 15.21). The breast is firm, warm, and enlarged with thickened, erythematous, peau d'orange skin

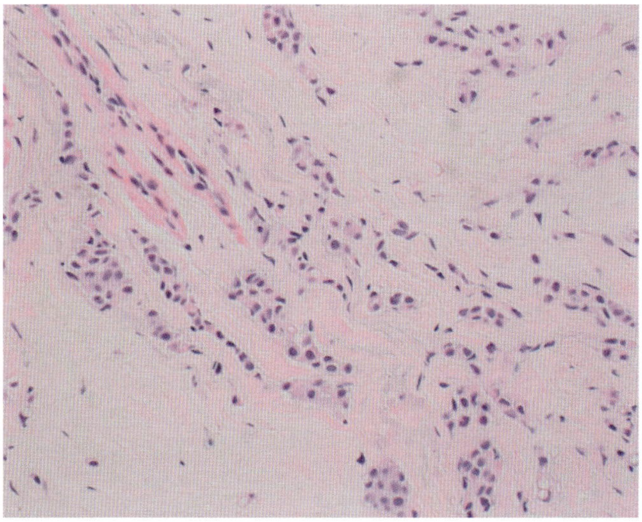

**Fig. 15.20** Infiltrating lobular carcinoma of the breast. Neoplastic cells infiltrating the stroma and adipose tissue in a single-file fashion. (Courtesy Panagiotis J. Tsakalakis, MD.)

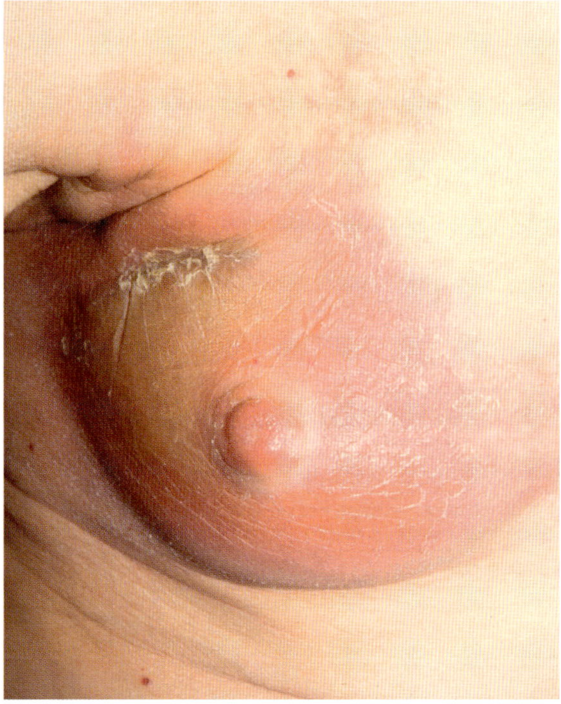

**Fig. 15.21** Inflammatory breast carcinoma—cellulitic-appearing plaque. (From Marks J, Miller J. *Lookingbill and Marks' Principles of Dermatology.* 4th ed. Philadelphia: Saunders; 2006.)

changes. Histologically, dermal lymphatic invasion by malignant cells is noted.

## PAGET DISEASE

**Paget disease** of the breast is rare, constituting 1% to 3% of new breast carcinomas (Fig. 15.22). This lesion has an innocent appearance and looks like eczema or dermatitis of the nipple. The clinical picture of a scaly, raw, or ulcerated lesion of the nipple and areola is usually the result of an infiltrating ductal carcinoma that invades the epidermis. The majority of patients (97%) with

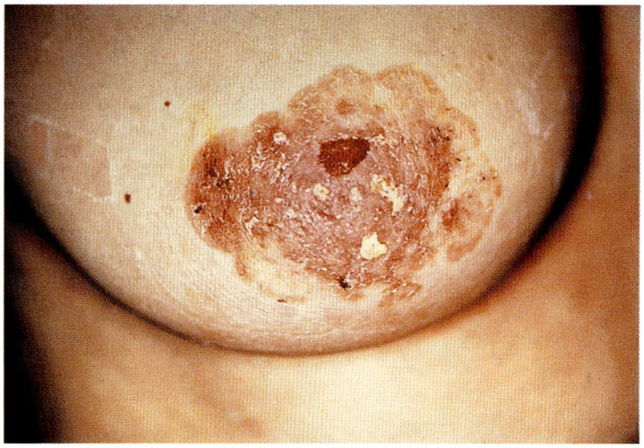

**Fig. 15.22** Paget disease of the breast. Note the erythematous plaques around the nipple. (From Callen JP. Dermatologic signs of systemic disease. In: Bolognia JL, Jorizzo JL, Rapini RP, eds. *Dermatology.* Edinburgh: Mosby; 2003:714.)

Paget disease also have an underlying cancer, either DCIS or invasive cancer, somewhere else in the breast. Punch biopsy or a full-thickness wedge biopsy of the nipple is used for diagnosis. Intraepithelial adenocarcinoma cells (Paget cells) are noted on histologic examination, presenting either singly or in small groups within the epidermis of the nipple.

## GENOMIC PROFILING

Historically, the treatment of breast cancer was based on tumor histologic characteristics, axillary node status, tumor size, receptor patterns, and grade of differentiation. In addition to simplified histologic classification, a classification based on gene expression or profiling, including the presence of hormone receptors, has evolved. Identification of tumor receptor status is critical because endocrine therapy is used both for adjuvant therapy and in the management of advanced disease. The **genomic analysis** of tumors has led to the molecular subtyping of breast cancers. In the early 2000s, Perou and coworkers classified breast tumors into four different molecular subtypes: luminal, basal, HER2, and normal (Perou, 2000). Subsequently, the luminal group was further differentiated into luminal-A and luminal-B subgroups. Basal-like tumors include triple-negative tumors, tumors that are estrogen, progesterone, and HER2 negative by immunohistochemistry. A more aggressive subtype of triple-negative tumors, claudin-low tumors, has also been described. These divisions are detailed in Table 15.12.

The lactiferous ducts have two layers: the inner layer closest to the lumen and the outer layer next to the basement membrane with more myoepithelial elements. Cancers that appear to have expression of genes similar to luminal cells are usually hormonally estrogen sensitive. Luminal-A tumors make up approximately 40% of all breast cancers. These tumors generally have the best prognosis and are low grade, estrogen and progesterone receptor positive, and HER2 (Neu) negative. These are more commonly found in older women.

Luminal-B tumors account for approximately 20% of all breast cancers and have a more aggressive behavior compared with the luminal-A subtype. These tumors have overexpression of HER2 (Neu) and have a higher expression of the proliferation-related genes. Often they are estrogen and progesterone as well as *P53* gene mutation positive (these are acquired *p53* mutations as opposed to inherited mutations).

The third subtype, HER2 enriched, constitutes 10% to 15% of breast cancers. It is characterized by a high expression of both

**TABLE 15.12** Classification of Breast Carcinoma Based on Gene Profiling and Hormone Receptor

| Expression Type | Grade | Characteristic Behavior | Hormone Receptor Status* |
|---|---|---|---|
| Luminal A | Usually low grade | Good prognosis | E and P+ |
| Luminal B | All grades | Mixed prognosis | E and P+, Her2 (Neu)+ |
| Her2 (Neu) | Higher grades | Poor prognosis | E and P–, Her2 (Neu)+ |
| Basal | Usually grade 3 | Poor prognosis | Triple negative |
| Normal breast† | Usually low grade | Good prognosis | Triple negative |

**E*, Estrogen receptor; *P*, progesterone receptor.
†Normal breast does not express gene profiling of basal elements and myoepithelial gene expression.

HER2 and proliferation gene clusters. These tumors are usually estrogen and progesterone negative, high grade, have a high rate of *P53* mutations, and have a poor prognosis.

The basal subtype makes up 15% to 20% of breast cancers. It is similar to basal-type duct cells in terms of expression of more myoepithelial gene profiling. These triple-negative tumors are usually high grade and exhibit a low expression of the luminal and *HER2* gene clusters. *BRCA1* tumors are up to 95% basal type.

A fifth type of breast cancer, claudin-low tumors, constitutes approximately 10% of breast cancers. Claudin-low tumors are also triple-receptor negative (estrogen, progesterone, and HER2 [Neu]). They have a high proliferation capability and are more aggressive than other subtypes.

## MANAGEMENT

A multidisciplinary team approach is necessary in the treatment of breast cancer. Local disease is treated with surgery, radiation therapy, or both. Systemic treatment includes chemotherapy, endocrine therapy, biologic therapy, or a combination of these regimens. Determination of local or systemic treatment is based on several prognostic and predictive factors, including tumor histologic characteristics, tumor hormone receptor status (estrogen/progesterone), tumor HER2 status, multigene testing, axillary lymph node status, evaluation of metastatic disease, patient age, comorbidities, and menopausal status.

The primary algorithm of treatment is primarily determined by the tumor stage. The tumor-node-metastasis (TNM) system is a widely recognized staging system based on both clinical and pathologic criteria (Table 15.13). The goal of treatment for stage 0, pure noninvasive carcinomas (LCIS, DCIS), is preventing the development of invasive disease or diagnosing the development of an invasive component when still confined to the breast. In cases of invasive disease, treatment is based on the stage-appropriate guideline for invasive carcinoma. The major objectives of treating breast carcinoma are control of local disease, treatment or prevention of distant metastases, and improved quality of life for women treated for the disease. With multiple therapeutic options in both local and systemic therapy for breast carcinoma, women have an active role in deciding their own treatment regimen. There are several methods for controlling local disease. Breast conservation with lumpectomy or quadrantectomy is a common choice for the control of local disease.

**TABLE 15.13** TNM Staging of Breast Cancer

| | | | |
|---|---|---|---|
| **PRIMARY TUMOR (T)** | | | |
| TX | Primary tumor cannot be assessed | | |
| T0 | No evidence of primary tumor | | |
| Tis* | Carcinoma in situ; intraductal carcinoma, lobular carcinoma in situ, or Paget disease of the nipple with no tumor | | |
| T1 | Tumor is ≤2 cm in greater dimension | | |
| T1a | Tumor is ≤0.5 cm in greatest dimension | | |
| T1b | Tumor is >0.5 cm but not more than 1 cm in greatest dimension | | |
| T1c | Tumor is more than 1 cm but not more than 2 cm in greatest dimension | | |
| T2 | Tumor is >2 cm but not more than 5 cm in greatest dimension | | |
| T3 | Tumor is >5 cm in greatest dimension | | |
| T4 | Tumor of any size with direct extension to chest wall or skin | | |
| T4a | Extension to chest wall | | |
| T4b | Edema (including peau d'orange) or ulceration of the skin of the breast or satellite skin nodules confined to the same breast | | |
| T4c | Both T4a and T4b above | | |
| T4d | Inflammatory carcinoma | | |
| **REGIONAL LYMPH NODE INVOLVEMENT (N) (CLINICAL)** | | | |
| NX | Regional lymph nodes cannot be assessed (e.g., previously removed) | | |
| N0 | No regional lymph node metastasis | | |
| N1 | Metastasis to movable ipsilateral axillary lymph node(s) | | |
| N2 | Metastasis to ipsilateral axillary lymph node(s) fixed to one another or the other structures | | |
| N3 | Metastasis to ipsilateral mammary lymph node(s) | | |
| **DISTANT METASTASIS (M)** | | | |
| MX | Presence of distant metastasis cannot be assessed | | |
| M0 | No distant metastasis | | |
| M1 | Distant metastasis (includes metastasis to ipsilateral supraclavicular lymph node[s]) | | |
| **STAGE GROUPING** | | | |
| Stage 0 | Tis | N0 | M0 |
| Stage I | T1 | N0 | M0 |
| Stage IIa | T0<br>T1<br>T2 | N1<br>N1*<br>N0 | M0<br>M0<br>M0 |
| Stage IIb | T2<br>T3 | N1<br>N0 | M0<br>M0 |
| Stage IIIa | T0<br>T1<br>T2<br>T3 | N2<br>N2<br>N2<br>N1, N2 | M0<br>M0<br>M0<br>M0 |
| Stage IIIb | T4<br>Any T | Any N<br>N3 | M0<br>M0 |
| Stage IV | Any T | Any N | M1 |

From Eberlein TJ. Current management of carcinoma of the breast. *Ann Surg.* 1994;220(2):121-136.
Paget disease associated with a tumor is classified according to the size of the tumor. Chest wall includes ribs, intercostal muscles, and serratus anterior muscle but not pectoral muscle.
*The prognosis of patients with pN1a is similar to that of patients with pN0.

Sentinel node biopsy has become standard practice in the treatment of early-stage breast cancer. Chemotherapy is used not only for patients with proven metastatic disease but also for women at high risk for developing distant or recurrent disease. An emphasis on conservative surgery plus radiation therapy to control multifocal cancer in the same breast and on reconstructive surgery after mastectomy has improved the quality of life for women with breast carcinoma.

## Surgical Therapy

The decision concerning appropriate therapy and the extent of the surgical operation to treat breast carcinoma should be made by the patient in consultation with the surgeon, radiation oncologist, and medical oncologist who will treat her. The size of the tumor, the initial extent of disease, the virulence of the neoplasm, and the presence of estrogen, progesterone, or HER2 receptors are key medical factors in the decision. The initial size of the breast carcinoma is the single best predictor of the likelihood of positive axillary nodes. The presence and number of axillary node metastasis are the best predictors of survival. Traditionally the evaluation for localized invasive disease includes bilateral diagnostic mammography, possible subsequent ultrasonography, tumor hormone receptor status, HER2 receptor status, and pathology review. MRI for the evaluation and determination of the extent of disease has been controversial. Supporters cite high sensitivity in evaluating the extent of disease, especially for invasive cancer and in dense breasts, as well as the identification of second cancers. Arguments against MRI use include a high percentage of false-positive findings resulting in additional diagnostic workup or more extensive surgery than necessary.

Locoregional treatment of clinical stage I, IIA, IIB, or T3N1MO (a subset of stage IIIA) invasive breast cancer includes lumpectomy (or total mastectomy ± reconstruction) with surgical axillary staging. Intensive discussions concerning breast reconstruction or external prostheses are important to help the patient contemplate the effects of surgery on body image. Morris and coworkers have studied the psychological and social adjustments to mastectomy in 160 women, who were followed at intervals of 3, 12, and 24 months after surgery (Morris, 1977). One in four women was still having problems with depression and associated marital and sexual problems 2 years after the initial therapy. Until the 1980s, radical mastectomy was the standard operation for carcinoma of the breast. Radical mastectomy was designed to control local disease by an extensive en bloc removal of the breast and underlying pectoralis major and pectoralis minor muscles and complete axillary dissection. It is a cosmetically disfiguring operation, leaving a major deformity of the chest wall. With an increased understanding that cancer of the breast is often a systemic disease and that prognosis is similar with conservative surgery, the therapeutic emphasis has changed to less radical surgery and increased use of radiotherapy and chemotherapy (Table 15.14).

**TABLE 15.14** Ten-Year Disease-Free Survival Rates of Women with Breast Cancer

| | Conservation Surgery and Radiation | Radical or Modified Radical Mastectomy Alone |
|---|---|---|
| Minimal breast cancer | 92% | 95% |
| Stage I | 78% | 80% |
| Stage II | 73% | 65% |

From Montague ED. Conservation surgery and radiation therapy in the treatment of operable breast cancer. *Cancer.* 1984;53(3 Suppl):700-704.

Often patients are not cured even with extensive local therapy. Thus protocols were established for more conservative approaches to treat local disease. The modified radical mastectomy removes the breast and only the fascia over the pectoralis major muscle. The pectoralis minor muscle may be removed to facilitate the axillary dissection. Simple mastectomy includes removal of the breast without underlying muscle tissue. A nipple-areola–sparing mastectomy can be considered in select patients undergoing a therapeutic mastectomy followed by immediate reconstruction. Candidates include women with small to moderate breast size with minimal ptosis and tumors smaller than 2 cm with a tumor to nipple–areolar complex distance larger than 2 cm. Contraindications to this procedure include inflammatory breast cancer, clinical involvement of the nipple–areolar complex, nipple retraction, Paget disease, and bloody nipple discharge. For patients having a mastectomy for prophylactic indications, a skin-sparing or nipple-sparing mastectomy is an option with good cosmetic results.

Breast-conserving therapy (**lumpectomy**, axillary **sentinel lymph node** biopsy followed by whole breast irradiation) has been shown to be equivalent to mastectomy and axillary lymph node dissection in the primary treatment of women with stages I and II breast cancer. In a 20-year follow-up comparing total mastectomy, lumpectomy, and lumpectomy plus irradiation, no differences were noted in overall survival, disease-free survival, or distant disease-free survival (Table 15.15). Resection of a wider area of the breast than lumpectomy is referred to as a quadrantectomy. In cases of positive margins, surgical reexcision is recommended. Mastectomy may be necessary in cases of positive margins after further surgical reexcision. Contraindications to lumpectomy include the need for radiation therapy during pregnancy, extensive disease not amenable to resection by a local excision with a single incision resulting in satisfactory cosmetic outcome, and diffuse suspicious or malignant-appearing microcalcifications. Relative contraindications include tumor size greater than 5 cm, history of previous radiation therapy to the breast or chest wall, and active connective tissue disease such as scleroderma or lupus that is adversely affected by radiation therapy. When planning for breast conservation surgery, tumors may be localized preoperatively with wire or needle localization using ultrasound or mammography. MRI has also been used to bracket lesions. In addition, some surgeons have employed the SAVI SCOUT surgical guidance system (Cianna Medical, Aliso Viejo, CA) for localization. This system uses a nonradioactive

**TABLE 15.15** Twenty-Year Follow-up Comparing Total Mastectomy, Lumpectomy, and Lumpectomy Plus Irradiation

| | Total Mastectomy | Lumpectomy Alone | Lumpectomy and Irradiation |
|---|---|---|---|
| Overall survival | 47% ± 2% | 46% ± 2% | 46% ± 2% |
| Cumulative incidence of a recurrence in ipsilateral breast | N/A | 39.2% | 14.3% |
| Disease free survival | 36% ± 2% | 35% ± 2% | 35% ± 2% |
| Distant disease free survival | 49% ± 2% | 45% ± 2% | 46% ± 2% |

From Fisher B, Anderson S, Bryant J, et al. Twenty-year follow-up of a randomized trial comparing total mastectomy, lumpectomy, and lumpectomy plus irradiation for the treatment of invasive breast cancer. *N Engl J Med.* 2002;347(16):1233-1241.
*N/A*, Not applicable.

infrared-activated electromagnetic wave reflector, about the size of a grain of rice, which is placed under guidance to localize the area of question. Using a nonradioactive hand wand, it can locate the lesion and facilitate the excision of nonpalpable breast lesions. An advantage of this system is that the reflector may be inserted up to 30 days before surgery.

Surgical axillary staging is recommended for stages I, IIA, IIB, and IIIA breast cancer. Sentinel lymph node mapping and resection is recommended in the surgical staging of the clinically negative axilla for stages I, IIA, IIB, and IIIA breast cancer. Sentinel node biopsy has decreased the need for complete axillary lymphadenectomy. Compared with standard axillary lymphadenectomy, sentinel lymph node (SLN) biopsy results in less arm and shoulder pain, lymphedema, and sensory loss. By injecting with radioactive colloid tracers and dyes, the surgeon can identify the first set of regional lymph nodes that receive lymphatic drainage from the tumor. These are termed *sentinel lymph nodes.* Subsequently these nodes can be removed and the axillary dissection can be deleted if they are negative. In a large multi-institutional trial, Krag and colleagues were able to identify the sentinel nodes in 93% of the cases. The accuracy of sentinel node mapping for predicting the status of axillary nodes in this series was 97%. The positive predictive value was 100%, and the negative predictive value was 96% (Krag, 1998). In the American College of Surgeons Oncology Group (ACOSOG) Z0011 study, women 18 years or older with T1/T2 tumors, fewer than three positive SLNs, and who were undergoing breast-conserving surgery followed by whole breast radiation were randomly allocated to SLN resection alone versus axillary lymph node (ALN) dissection. No difference was noted in local recurrence, disease-free survival, or overall survival. Locoregional recurrences at a follow-up of 6.3 years occurred in 4.1% of the ALN group and 2.8% of the SLN group ($P = .11$). Median overall survival was 92% in both groups. No further axillary surgery is recommended in patients with a T1 or T2 tumor with less than three positive SLNs who did not receive neoadjuvant therapy and were treated with lumpectomy and whole breast radiation (Giuliano, 2010). Axillary lymph nodes are classified into three levels based on their relationship to the pectoralis minor muscle. Level 1 nodes are inferior and lateral to the pectoralis minor muscle; level II nodes are posterior to the pectoralis minor and below the axillary vein; and level III nodes are medial to the pectoralis minor and against the chest wall. Level I or II axillary dissection is recommended in patients with clinically positive nodes at the time of diagnosis confirmed by FNA or core biopsy and in cases where sentinel nodes are not identified. The boundaries of an axillary lymphadenectomy are the axillary vein superiorly, the serratus anterior muscle medially, and the latissimus dorsi muscle laterally (Fig. 15.23). The long thoracic and thoracodorsal nerves must be identified because injury to the long thoracic nerve may result in a protruding or "winged" scapula deformity. The thoracodorsal nerve innervates the latissimus dorsi muscle, and injury may result in mild weakness of internal rotation and shoulder adduction.

Breast reconstruction must be considered for any woman undergoing mastectomy for breast cancer. Although reconstruction is an optional procedure that does not influence the probability of disease recurrence or death, it is associated with an improvement in the patient's quality of life. Consultation with a reconstructive plastic surgeon should be offered. Various factors influence the type of reconstruction including patient preference, smoking history, body habitus, comorbidities, and radiation therapy plans. Obesity and smoking increase the risk of wound-healing complications and flap failure.

Postmastectomy reconstruction with implants can be performed by immediate placement of a permanent subpectoral implant or by placement of a subpectoral tissue expander implant. The pectoral muscle is stretched with gradual expansion of the expander implant by the addition of saline. Implants may contain silicone gel, saline, or a combination of both. Reconstruction techniques with autologous tissue include abdominal flaps: a **transverse rectus abdominis (TRAM) flap** and the **deep inferior epigastric perforator (DIEP) flap**, a gluteus maximus myocutaneous flap, and a latissimus dorsi flap reconstruction. Another option is only offered in a few centers. Called the **transverse upper gracilis (TUG)** flap, it does not use skin or muscle from the abdominal wall or buttocks but instead uses skin, fat,

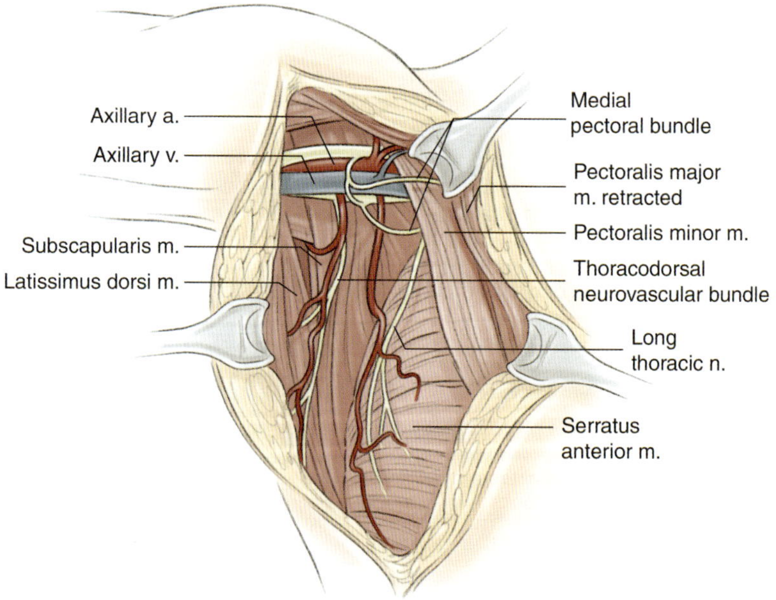


**Fig. 15.23** Anatomy of the axilla. The boundaries of an axillary lymphadenectomy are the axillary vein superiorly, the serratus anterior muscle medially, and the latissimus dorsi muscle laterally. (From Keurer HM. *Kuerer's Breast Surgical Oncology.* New York: McGraw Hill; 2010.)

and muscle from the upper inner thigh (ACS, 2015) (Fig. 15.24). In patients undergoing postmastectomy radiation, placement of a tissue expander at the initial procedure followed by implant placement after completion of radiation therapy is preferred. If autologous tissue is used, reconstruction should be delayed until at least 6 months after completion of radiation therapy.

## Radiation Therapy

The majority of women treated with breast-conserving surgery are candidates for breast radiation therapy. After breast-conserving surgery, external beam whole breast irradiation is usually administered. In the 2011 meta-analysis by the Early Breast Cancer Trialists' Collaborative Group (EBCTCG) of 10,801 women in 17 trials, whole breast irradiation resulted in a significant reduction in the 10-year risk of any first recurrence compared with breast-conserving surgery alone (19.3 vs. 35%; RR, 0.52; 95% CI, 0.48 to 0.56). Additionally, a significant reduction in the 15-year risk of breast cancer death (21.4% vs. 25.2%; RR, 0.82; 95% CI, 0.75 to 0.90) was noted in the whole breast irradiation group (EBCTCG, 2011a). A radiation therapy boost to the tumor bed is offered to women at higher risk of recurrence (positive lymph nodes,

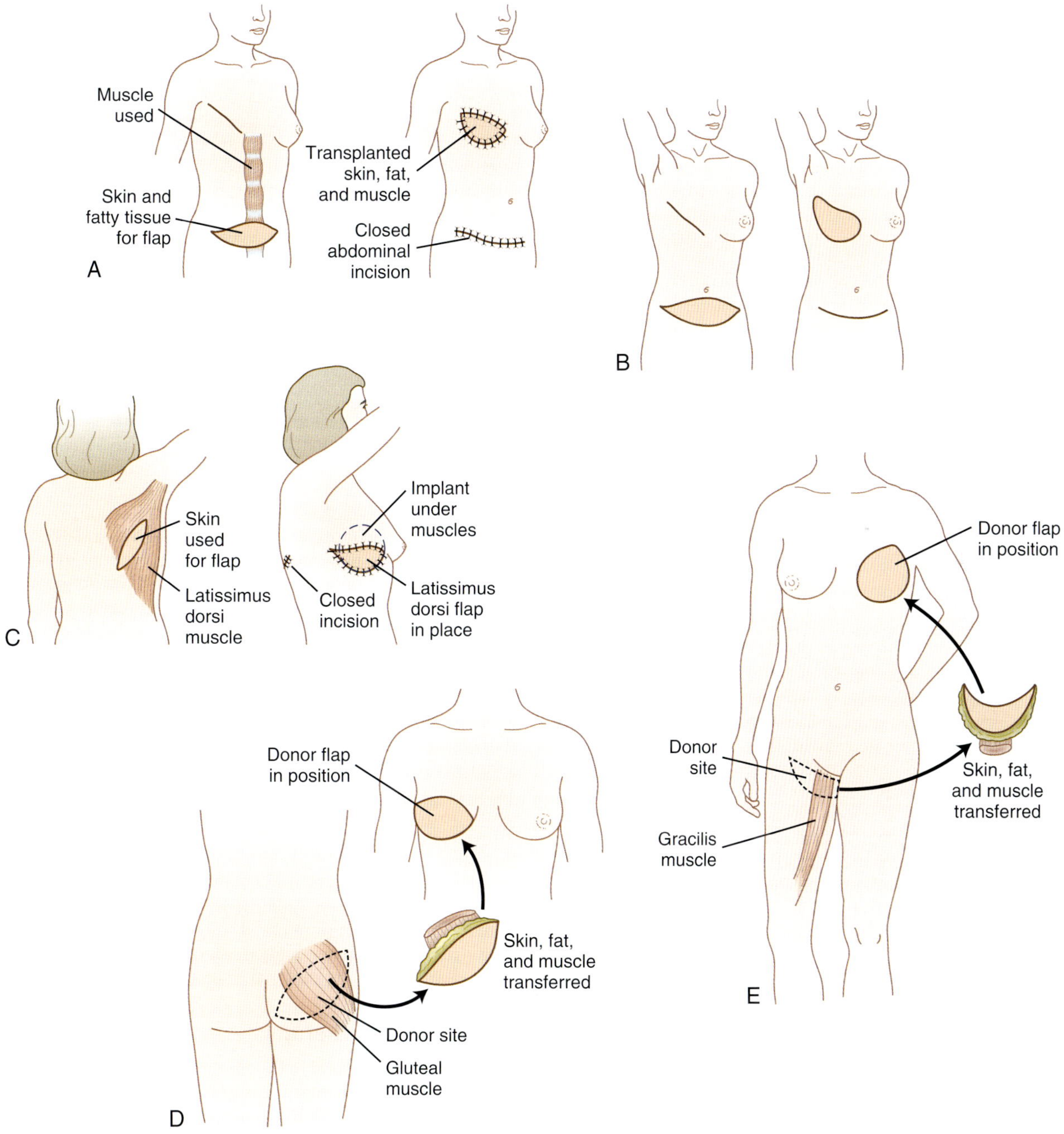


**Fig. 15.24 A,** Pedicle transverse rectus abdominis (TRAM) flap incisions through which the flap of muscle, fat, and skin are tunneled under the skin to fill the defect in the breast. **B,** Incisions used for the deep inferior epigastric perforator (DIEP) flap. **C,** Latissimus dorsi flap. **D,** Gluteal-free flap. **E,** Transverse upper gracilis (TUG) flap. (Modified from American Cancer Society (ACS). *Breast Reconstruction After Mastectomy;* 2015. Available at http://www.cancer.org/acs/groups/cid/documents/webcontent/002992-pdf.pdf.)

lymphovascular invasion, young age, or high-grade disease after lumpectomy). In women 70 years or older with node-negative, stage 1, ER-positive breast cancer, postoperative radiation therapy may be omitted if they receive postoperative endocrine therapy because the risk of an in-breast recurrence is low.

Women with positive axillary lymph nodes after mastectomy and axillary lymphadenectomy are also candidates for breast radiation therapy. Randomized trials have shown both a disease-free and overall survival advantage of chest wall and regional node irradiation in these women. NCCN guidelines recommend irradiation after mastectomy in women with four or more positive axillary lymph nodes and strong consideration of radiation in women with one to three positive axillary lymph nodes (NCCN, 2020). Chest wall irradiation is also recommended in women with negative nodes but with a primary tumor greater than 5 cm or positive surgical margins.

## Medical Therapy

Along with earlier detection, advancements in systemic adjuvant therapy have resulted in a decrease in the breast cancer mortality rate. Clinicopathologic factors including stage, tumor grade, and vascular space invasion are used to calculate the risk of disease recurrence. The two major factors in predicting the likelihood of systemic disease in breast carcinoma are the diameter of the primary tumor and the number of positive axillary nodes. Women whose initial tumor is less than 1 cm in diameter and who have negative axillary nodes have excellent chances for disease-free survival. The 10-year relapse rate is less than 10%.

## Hormonal Therapy

The presence and concentration of receptors should be obtained at the initial diagnostic biopsy or surgery. Women with hormone receptor–positive breast cancer are candidates for **endocrine therapy**. Receptor status may change after radiotherapy or chemotherapy. Estrogen receptors are of two types, ER-alpha and ER-beta. Most laboratories test only for the ER-alpha receptors, and its biology is better understood. ER-beta receptors' role in malignancy is still under investigation. As tumors mutate and metastasize, the expression of estrogen receptors decreases. Hormonal therapies become less effective in controlling disease. Progesterone receptor positivity is a sign of better differentiation and a greater response to hormonal therapy. Progesterone receptors are often lost as tumors metastasize as well. In general, luminal-A receptor–positive tumors are usually better differentiated and exhibit a less aggressive clinical behavior, including a lower risk of recurrence and lower capacity to proliferate. When estrogen receptors are positive, approximately 60% of breast cancers will respond to hormonal therapy; an 80% response rate is noted when both estrogen and progesterone receptors are present. If estrogen receptors are negative, less than 10% of tumors respond to hormonal manipulation.

Hormonal therapy is usually accomplished by drugs that change endocrine function by blocking receptor sites or blocking synthesis of hormones. Hormonal therapy is effective in producing a response in advanced metastatic carcinoma for approximately 1 year. Metastatic disease in soft tissue and bone is the most sensitive to hormonal manipulation. Tamoxifen, a selective estrogen receptor modulator, is a commonly prescribed hormonal agent for breast carcinoma. The 2011 EBCTCG meta-analysis compared tamoxifen treatment for 5 years with no endocrine treatment (EBCTCG, 2011b). Analysis showed a significant reduction in the risk of breast cancer recurrence at 15 years (RR, 0.61; 95% CI, 0.57 to 0.65) and a significant reduction in the risk of breast cancer mortality at 15 years (RR 0.70; 95% CI, 0.64 to 0.75). Treatment with tamoxifen was associated with an increased risk of thromboembolic disease, strokes, and intrauterine polyps as well as endometrial hyperplasia and carcinoma. The overall incidence of uterine cancer was low and confined to women older than 55 years. Most tamoxifen-related endometrial cancers were stage I, grade 1, and were successfully treated with surgery alone.

Tamoxifen has the greatest effect in postmenopausal women. As one would expect, tamoxifen is of greater benefit in women with tumors that have estrogen receptors than in tumors that are negative for estrogen receptors. There is no significant improvement in survival rates in patients with ER-negative tumors. However, even in receptor-negative patients, 5 years of tamoxifen use will decrease the risk of a second primary or contralateral breast cancer by as much as 45%. Trials of tamoxifen in the adjuvant treatment setting for breast cancer showed that 10 years of tamoxifen improved outcomes compared with 5 years. In the worldwide Adjuvant Tamoxifen: Longer Against Shorter (ATLAS) trial, approximately 13,000 women were randomly allocated to continue tamoxifen to 10 years or stop at 5 years (Davies, 2013). Among women with ER-positive disease, continuation of tamoxifen reduced the risk of breast cancer recurrence, reduced breast cancer mortality, and reduced overall mortality. The reductions in adverse breast cancer outcomes appeared to be less extreme before than after year 10 with halved breast cancer mortality during the second decade after diagnosis. Extended tamoxifen use had no effect on breast cancer outcome in the cohort of women with ER-negative disease and an intermediate effect among women with unknown ER status. Based on these results and those of other major trials, ASCO updated their practice guidelines on the optimal duration of treatment of adjuvant endocrine therapy, particularly adjuvant tamoxifen (Burstein, 2014). Pre- or perimenopausal women who have received 5 years of adjuvant tamoxifen should be offered tamoxifen for 10 years. Postmenopausal women who have received 5 years of adjuvant tamoxifen should be offered the choice of continuing tamoxifen or changing to an aromatase inhibitor for 10 years' total adjuvant endocrine therapy.

Aromatase inhibitors (AIs) (anastrozole, letrozole, and exemestane) block the peripheral conversion of adrenal androgens to estrone. They are ineffective in women with intact ovarian function, including those who experienced chemotherapy-induced amenorrhea, because AIs may cause an inadvertent rise in gonadotropins from the ovary, limiting their effectiveness. Cessation of ovarian function can be definitively attained by oophorectomy or pelvic radiation. Ovarian suppression can also be accomplished with pharmacologic interventions that inhibit ovarian production of estrogen, such as the gonadotropin-releasing hormone (GnRH) agonists. In premenopausal women with ER-positive breast cancer, combined results of the Suppression of Ovarian Function Trial (SOFT) and Tamoxifen and Exemestane Trial (TEXT) indicated that ovarian suppression plus an AI compared with ovarian suppression plus tamoxifen in premenopausal women with ER-positive breast cancer results in better disease-free survival but not overall survival (Pagani, 2014). Compared with tamoxifen, AIs have been shown to improve outcomes for postmenopausal women with hormone receptor–positive breast cancer. In a meta-analysis of approximately 32,000 postmenopausal women with ER-positive breast cancer, AIs compared with tamoxifen were noted to reduce recurrence rates by approximately 30%, have a higher risk of osteoporosis/fractures, and have a lower risk of endometrial cancer (EBCTCG, 2015).

## HER2-Directed Therapy

The determination of HER2 tumor status is recommended for newly diagnosed invasive breast cancers and for recurrences of breast cancer. The **HER2/neu gene**, *ERBB2*, is an epithelial growth factor determinant (human epidermal receptor), and amplification or overexpression HER2 oncogene is found in 18% to 20% of women with breast cancer. When overexpressed on tumor cells, the HER2/neu gene is a poor prognostic sign and a marker for aggressive disease. Breast tumors are classified as HER2 positive if the tumor has either an immunohistochemical (IHC) stain of 3+ (defined as uniform membrane staining for HER2 in 10% or more of tumor cells), a HER2/chromosome enumeration probe 17 (CEP17) fluorescent in situ hybridization (FISH) amplification ratio of 2 or greater, or a HER2/CEP17 ratio less than 2 with an average HER2 copy number greater than 6 signals/cell.

HER2-targeted therapy is recommended in patients with *ERBB2*-positive tumors. **Trastuzumab** is a humanized monoclonal antibody directed against the extracellular domain of the *ERBB2* receptor. Several trials have shown significant improvement in outcome and were stopped early because of the improved outcomes compared with placebo. The drug affects multiple steps in the cell cycle and importantly sensitizes cells to other chemotherapy agents. It also increases antibody-dependent, cell-mediated cytotoxicity. Trastuzumab given for 1 year in conjunction with chemotherapy in patients with HER2-positive tumors improved disease-free and overall survival (Moja, 2012). Treatment with trastuzumab is associated with a higher risk of cardiotoxicity including congestive heart failure and a decrease in left ventricular ejection fraction. Caution must be used when patients are also receiving anthracycline-based chemotherapy, and patients should undergo routine cardiac monitoring. Pertuzumab, a monoclonal antibody that binds to HER2 and prevents dimerization of HER2 with other HER receptors, may be used in conjunction with chemotherapy and trastuzumab regimens to overcome trastuzumab resistance because of HER2:HER3 heterodimer formation. The addition of pertuzumab does not appear to increase toxicity.

### Chemotherapy

Chemotherapy is used in the treatment of breast cancer in both the adjuvant and neoadjuvant settings and is recommended for the treatment of most triple-negative breast cancers, HER2-positive breast cancers, and high-risk luminal tumors. The benefit of chemotherapy is more pronounced in ER-negative tumors.

The decision to use adjuvant chemotherapy is based on several variables including the surrogate intrinsic phenotype determined by ER/PR, HER2, and Ki-67 assessment with the selective help of first-generation genomic testing. The two most commonly used molecular prognostic profiles are the **Oncotype DX** *test* and the **MammaPrint assay**. The Oncotype DX Breast Cancer Assay measures the expression of 16 cancer genes and 5 reference genes to produce a recurrence score (RS) from 0 to 100. It is used to estimate both the risk of recurrence of early-stage breast cancer and the benefit from adjuvant chemotherapy. This assay is indicated in women with negative nodes or one to three positive nodes and ER-positive breast cancer. The MammaPrint test analyzes 70 genes (Amsterdam 70 gene prognostic profile) and calculates either a high-risk or low-risk recurrence score for early-stage breast cancer. This clinically validated prognostic profile can be used in patients with breast cancers that are either hormone receptor positive or negative and node negative or with one to three positive nodes and in patients with HER2-positive disease.

Combination therapy of cytotoxic drugs is vastly superior to single-agent regimens. Anthracycline-containing combinations are more effective than regimens that do not contain anthracyclines. Paclitaxel therapy has excellent activity in breast cancer. The addition of four to five cycles of paclitaxel to four to six cycles of the doxorubicin (Adriamycin) and cyclophosphamide regimen improved disease-free and overall survival rates in patients with node-positive breast cancer. Overall, chemotherapy regimens based on anthracyclines and taxanes reduce breast cancer mortality by about one-third.

In the neoadjuvant setting, chemotherapy has the potential to change unresectable tumors to resectable ones and decrease the extent of surgery necessary to achieve adequate resection. Neoadjuvant chemotherapy may be considered for patients who desire breast-conserving surgery but initially are not candidates because of tumor size. Neoadjuvant therapy is commonly used in patients with inflammatory breast cancer and may confer a survival benefit in this population of patients. The chemotherapy regimens used in the neoadjuvant setting are the same as those used in the adjuvant setting. Endocrine- and HER2-targeted therapy may also be used in the preoperative setting. HER2-positive breast cancer and triple-negative breast cancer are the most chemosensitive and are excellent subtypes for neoadjuvant chemotherapy. These patients have the highest pathologic complete response rate. In HER2-positive breast cancer, neoadjuvant therapy should include trastuzumab and pertuzumab with a taxane.

## BREAST CANCER DURING PREGNANCY

Breast cancer is not commonly diagnosed during pregnancy. Less than 5% of breast cancers diagnosed before the age of 50 are during pregnancy or in the postpartum period. However, most breast cancers diagnosed during pregnancy are poorly differentiated, ER/PR negative and ALN positive and have a large primary tumor size. Diagnosis of cancer during pregnancy is often delayed by 2 months or longer. Similar to nonpregnant women, in pregnant or postpartum women a breast mass is usually the presenting sign. A mass that persists for more than 2 weeks should be evaluated. Mammography is not contraindicated in pregnancy, although abdominal shielding is recommended. Breast ultrasonography can also be used to better define a mass and guide biopsy. A clinically suspicious mass should be biopsied either by FNA or core needle biopsy. Staging studies should be tailored in an effort to minimize fetal exposure to radiation.

Treatment options during pregnancy are not very different from the nonpregnant state and include mastectomy, breast-conserving therapy, and systemic therapy, but not radiation therapy. Although radical mastectomy is the most common surgery, breast-conserving therapy is an option if radiation therapy can be delayed to the postpartum period. According to the NCCN guidelines, SLN biopsy may be safely performed during pregnancy with a radiolabeled sulfur colloid. The use of blue dye is contraindicated in pregnancy. Systemic chemotherapy should be avoided in the first trimester and not be given after week 35 of pregnancy or within 3 weeks of delivery to avoid transient neonatal myelosuppression and other complications. The risk of fetal malformation during the second and third trimesters is approximately 1.3%. Most data regarding chemotherapy in pregnancy are with anthracycline and alkylating chemotherapy. Fewer data exist regarding taxanes. NCCN guidelines recommend weekly administration of paclitaxel after the first trimester if indicated. Trastuzumab is not recommended for use during pregnancy and should be delayed to the postpartum period. Endocrine therapy is also contraindicated during pregnancy.

Various studies have shown no significant difference in outcomes between women diagnosed with breast cancer during pregnancy and nonpregnant women. In a meta-analysis of 30 studies including 37,100 controls and 3628 cases of pregnancy-associated breast cancer, a higher risk of death was noted in women diagnosed in the postpartum period (HR, 184; 95% CI, 1.28 to 2.65) rather than during pregnancy (HR, 1.29; 95% CI, 0.72 to 2.24) (Azim, 2012). Termination of pregnancy does not appear to improve survival.

## SURVEILLANCE

As of 2019, there were approximately 16.9 million cancer survivors in the United States (Miller, 2019). The number of cancer survivors has increased in part because of aging and growth of the population and also because of advancements in early detection and treatment. Breast cancer patients account for almost 44% of female cancer survivors, and close surveillance after treatment is paramount. Although most breast cancer recurrences occur in the first 5 years after treatment, recurrence may be diagnosed decades after treatment. Ongoing age-appropriate screening and preventive care for other conditions not related to breast cancer should continue as recommended for the general populations.

The NCCN guidelines are not stratified according to stage at time of diagnosis or treatment. Interval history and physical examination are recommended every 4 to 6 months for 5 years and annually thereafter, with mammography every 12 months. Women on tamoxifen are recommended to have an annual gynecologic examination every 12 months if the uterus is present. Regular bone mineral density determination is recommended for women on an aromatase inhibitor. Adherence to adjuvant endocrine therapy and maintaining an ideal body weight are also recommended. Other routine laboratory tests and imaging are not recommended for routine surveillance. The use of estrogen, progesterone, or SERMs in the treatment of osteoporosis or osteopenia is discouraged, although it may be considered in select cases. In general, bisphosphonates are preferred for bone mineral density health. Similar to the NCCN guidelines, ASCO recommendations for the follow-up and management of breast cancer include regular history, physical examination, and mammography. The ASCO guidelines recommend a history and physical examination every 3 to 6 months for the first 3 years, every 6 to 12 months for years 4 and 5, and annually thereafter. Additional testing is recommended only if symptoms arise. For women who have undergone breast-conserving surgery, a posttreatment mammogram should be obtained 12 months after the initial mammogram and at least 6 months after completion of radiation therapy. Thereafter, annual mammography is recommended. Women should have regular gynecologic follow-up, and those who received tamoxifen should report any vaginal bleeding because they are at an increased risk of developing endometrial cancer.

Treatment of breast cancer with chemotherapy or hormonal therapy may cause menopausal symptoms. Women often report that sexual activity is less enjoyable and more painful, and women who have undergone mastectomy report problems with body image and interest in sex. Depression is associated with sexual dysfunction in breast cancer survivors. Physicians must regularly inquire about sexual functioning, and women with complaints of dyspareunia or other sexual disorders should be offered a referral to a sexual health expert. Women who report dyspareunia or difficulty reaching orgasm may benefit from vaginal dilators, vaginal lubricants and moisturizers, or counseling. The risks and benefits of local or vaginal estrogen therapy should be discussed and individualized based on patient symptoms and tumor characteristics. The use of vaginal estrogens in this setting is aimed at improving the patient's quality of life and should not be underestimated.

## KEY REFERENCES


American Cancer Society (ACS). *Breast Reconstruction After Mastectomy;* 2015. Available at http://www.cancer.org/acs/groups/cid/documents/webcontent/002992-pdf.pdf.

American College of Obstetricians and Gynecologists (ACOG). Practice Bulletin No. 164. Diagnosis and management of benign breast disorders. *Obstet Gynecol.* 2016;127:e141-e156. (Reaffirmed in 2018.)

American College of Obstetricians and Gynecologists (ACOG). Practice Bulletin No. 179. Breast cancer risk assessment and screening in average-risk women. *Obstet Gynecol.* 2017;130:e1-e16. (Reaffirmed in 2019.)

Azim Jr HA, Santoro L, Russell-Edu W, et al. Prognosis of pregnancy-associated breast cancer: a meta-analysis of 30 studies. *Cancer Treat Rev.* 2012;38(7):834-842.

Bagnardi V, Rota M, Botteri E, et al. Light alcohol drinking and cancer: a meta-analysis. *Ann Oncol.* 2013;24(2):301-308.

Barton MB, Harris R, Fletcher SW. The rational clinical examination. Does this patient have breast cancer? The screening clinical breast examination: should it be done? How? *JAMA.* 1999;282(13):1270-1280.

Bauer SR, Hankinson SE, Bertone-Johnson ER, et al. Plasma vitamin D levels, menopause, and risk of breast cancer: dose-response meta-an alysis of prospective studies. *Medicine (Baltimore).* 2013;92(3):123-131.

Boyd NF, Guo H, Martin LJ, et al. Mammographic density and the risk and detection of breast cancer. *N Engl J Med.* 2007;356(3):227-236.

Burstein HJ, Temin S, Anderson H, et al. Adjuvant endocrine therapy for women with hormone receptor-positive breast cancer: American society of clinical oncology clinical practice guideline focused update. *J Clin Oncol.* 2014;32(21):2255-2269.

Centers for Disease Control and Prevention (CDC). Vital signs: racial disparities in breast cancer severity-United States, 2005-2009. *MMWR Morb Mortal Wkly Rep.* 2012;61(45):922-926.

Chlebowski RT, Hendrix SL, Langer RD, et al. Influence of estrogen plus progestin on breast cancer and mammography in healthy postmenopausal women: the Women's Health Initiative Randomized Trial. *JAMA.* 2003;289(24):3243-3253.

Clemons M, Goss P. Estrogen and the risk of breast cancer. *N Engl J Med.* 2001;344:276.

Colditz GA, Rosner B. Cumulative risk of breast cancer to age 70 years according to risk factor status: data from the Nurses' Health Study. *Am J Epidemiol.* 2000;152(10):950-964.

Collaborative Group on Hormonal Factors in Breast Cancer. Breast cancer and breastfeeding: collaborative reanalysis of individual data from 47 epidemiological studies in 30 countries, including 50302 women with breast cancer and 96973 women without the disease. *Lancet.* 2002;360(9328):187-195.

Cuzick J, Sestak I, Cawthorn S, et al. Tamoxifen for prevention of breast cancer: extended long-term follow-up of the IBIS-I breast cancer prevention trial. *Lancet Oncol.* 2015;16(1):67-75.

Cuzick J, Sestak I, Forbes JF, et al. Anastrozole for prevention of breast cancer in high-risk postmenopausal women (IBIS-II): an international, double-blind, randomised placebo-controlled trial. *Lancet.* 2014;383(9922):1041-1048.

Davies C, Pan H, Godwin J, et al. Long-term effects of continuing adjuvant tamoxifen to 10 years versus stopping at 5 years after diagnosis of oestrogen receptor-positive breast cancer: ATLAS, a randomised trial. *Lancet.* 2013;381(9869):805-816.

Doucet S, Soussignan R, Sagot P, et al. The secretion of areolar (Montgomery's) glands from lactating women elicits selective, unconditional responses in neonates. *PLoS One.* 2009;4(10):e7579.

Early Breast Cancer Trialists' Collaborative Group (EBCTCG), Darby S, McGale P, et al. Effect of radiotherapy after breast-conserving surgery on 10-year recurrence and 15-year breast cancer death: meta-analysis of individual patient data for 10,801 women in 17 randomised trials. *Lancet.* 2011a;378(9804):1707-1716.

Early Breast Cancer Trialists' Collaborative Group (EBCTCG), Davies C, Godwin J, et al. Relevance of breast cancer hormone receptors and other factors to the efficacy of adjuvant tamoxifen: patient-level meta-analysis of randomised trials. *Lancet.* 2011b;378(9793):771-784.

Early Breast Cancer Trialists' Collaborative Group (EBCTCG);, Dowsett M, Forbes JF, et al. Aromatase inhibitors versus tamoxifen in early breast cancer: patient-level meta-analysis of the randomised trials. *Lancet.* 2015;386(10001):1341-1352.

Fisher B, Costantino JP, Wickerham DL, et al. Tamoxifen for prevention of breast cancer: report of the National Surgical Adjuvant Breast and Bowel Project P-1 Study. *J Natl Cancer Inst.* 1998;90(18):1371-1388.

Fletcher SW, O'Malley MS, Bunce LA. Physicians' abilities to detect lumps in silicone breast models. *JAMA.* 1985;253(15):2224-2228.

Friedewald SM, Rafferty EA, Rose SL, et al. Breast cancer screening using tomosynthesis in combination with digital mammography. *JAMA.* 2014;311(24):2499-2507.

Gail MH, Costantino JP, Pee D, et al. Projecting individualized absolute invasive breast cancer risk in African American women. *J Natl Cancer Inst.* 2007;99(23):1782-1792.

Gemignani ML. Breast cancer screening: why, when, and how many? *Clin Obstet Gynecol.* 2011;54(1):125-132.

Giuliano AE, McCall L, Beitsch P, et al. Locoregional recurrence after sentinel lymph node dissection with or without axillary dissection in patients with sentinel lymph node metastases: the American College of Surgeons Oncology Group Z0011 randomized trial. *Ann Surg.* 2010; 252(3):426-432; discussion 432-433.

Gram IT, Park SY, Kolonel LN, et al. Smoking and risk of breast cancer in a racially/ethnically diverse population of mainly women who do not drink alcohol: The MEC Study. *Am J Epidemiol.* 2015;182:917.

Hartmann LC, Sellers TA, Schaid DJ, et al. Efficacy of bilateral prophylactic mastectomy in BRCA1 and BRCA2 gene mutation carriers. *J Natl Cancer Inst.* 2001;93(21):1633-1637.

Hughes LE. Classification of benign breast disorders. The ANDI classification based on physiological processes within the normal breast. *Br Med Bull.* 1991;47(2):251-257.


**Full references and Suggested readings for this chapter can be found on ExpertConsult.com.**

# 16 Early and Recurrent Pregnancy Loss

## Etiology, Diagnosis, Treatment

Jenna Turocy, Zev Williams

### KEY POINTS

- Pregnancy loss affects approximately 10% to 30% of all clinically recognized pregnancies, with nearly 80% occurring in the first trimester. The majority of pregnancy losses are sporadic and result from genetic causes that are greatly influenced by maternal age.
- Fewer than 5% of women will experience two consecutive pregnancy losses and only 1% experience three or more. Women with two prior losses and no live births experience a loss rate of 25%, which increases to 45% with three consecutive losses.
- Evaluation of recurrent pregnancy loss should proceed after two consecutive clinical pregnancy losses and may include screening for genetic factors and antiphospholipid syndrome, assessment of uterine anatomy, and testing for hormonal and metabolic factors.
- Treatment of recurrent pregnancy loss should be guided by underlying cause. Women with unexplained recurrent pregnancy loss should be offered psychological support and counseling and reassurance. More than 50% of patients with unexplained recurrent pregnancy loss achieve live birth with no intervention.
- Cases in which women are diagnosed with early pregnancy loss can be managed surgically, with medication or expectantly. Studies have noted no difference in subsequent pregnancy rates, and the management choice is typically based on patient preference.

Pregnancy loss is by far the most common complication of pregnancy, affecting more than 20% of clinically recognized pregnancies, and is often physically and emotionally distressing. The terms *spontaneous abortion*, *miscarriage*, and *pregnancy loss* are used interchangeably in the literature (ACOG, 2018). Though used colloquially, for the purposes of this chapter, the term *miscarriage* will not be used because it imputes a failure on the part of the woman to properly carry the pregnancy. ***Early pregnancy loss*** is defined as a nonviable intrauterine pregnancy with either an empty gestational sac *(anembryonic gestation, blighted ovum)* or with a gestational sac containing an embryo or fetus without fetal heart activity within the first 12 6/7 weeks of gestation. Although the terms *embryo* and *fetus* are used synonymously, ***embryo* is the correct term before 10 weeks' gestation.** *Biochemical* or *chemical pregnancy loss* refers to a loss that occurs after a positive beta-human chorionic gonadotropin (β-HCG) and before detection on ultrasound. **After 20 weeks' gestation, pregnancy loss is called an *intrauterine fetal demise*** if no delivery or *preterm birth* or *stillbirth* if delivery occurred (Kutteh, 2007).

In the past the terms ***threatened abortion*, *inevitable abortion*, and *missed abortion*** were used in reference to the appearance of the patient on presentation. *Threatened abortion* refers to patients with vaginal bleeding in the setting of a viable intrauterine pregnancy with a closed cervical os; *inevitable abortion* refers to patients with an open cervical os. The term *missed abortion* describes patients diagnosed with a loss of pregnancy without the passage of products of conception (POCs). These vague terms are no longer widely used because they often lead to confusion and do not affect the management options for pregnancy loss.

**Recurrent pregnancy loss (RPL)** traditionally has been defined as three or more consecutive, clinically recognized losses (Rai, 2006). More recent definitions have recommended including two or more clinically recognized losses (ASRM, 2012). The term *habitual abortion* has now been almost completely replaced by *RPL*. In addition, **RPL may be further stratified into *primary* or *secondary*.** *Primary RPL* refers to pregnancy loss in women who have never carried to viability. In contrast, *secondary RPL* refers to pregnancy loss in a woman who has had a previous live birth. *Nonconsecutive pregnancy loss* describes women who have had multiple spontaneous pregnancy losses interspersed with normal pregnancies.

This chapter discusses the epidemiology, etiology, diagnosis, and management of pregnancy loss before 20 weeks' gestation. Because pregnancy loss may occur spontaneously or as a result of a recurring cause, spontaneous early pregnancy loss and RPL are discussed throughout the chapter.

## EPIDEMIOLOGY

### Spontaneous Early Pregnancy Loss

**Pregnancy loss is common, affecting 10% to 30% of clinically recognized pregnancies** (Kutteh, 2007). Extremes of age increase the risk of pregnancy loss; loss is more common in women younger than 18 years and older than 35 years and rises both with increasing parity and number of prior losses (Fig. 16.1). The loss rate is believed to approach 80% in women age 45 and older (ASRM, 2012).

Nearly 80% of all pregnancy losses occur in the first trimester, and the incidence declines with advancing gestational age (Harlap, 1980) (Fig. 16.2). The loss rate when a gestational sac is visualized by ultrasound is 11.5%; it falls to 6% to 8% if embryonic cardiac activity is observed at 6 weeks and falls to 2% to 3% if cardiac activity persists at 8 to 12 weeks. Compared with their younger counterparts, women older than age 34 experience a loss rate twice as high, even after visualization of a fetal heartbeat (Achiron, 1991). Women with bleeding in the first trimester and

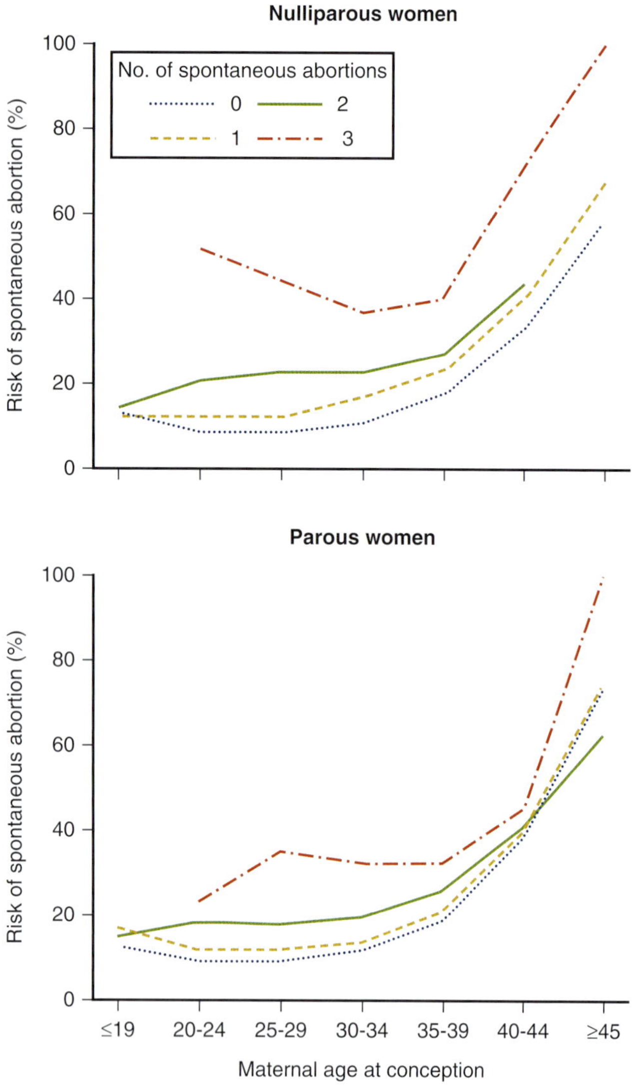


**Fig. 16.1** Risk of spontaneous abortion in nulliparous and parous women according to maternal age at conception and number of spontaneous abortions in preceding 10 years. (From Nybo Andersen AM, Wohlfahrt J, Christens P, et al. Maternal age and fetal loss: population based register linkage study. *BMJ.* 2000;320(7251):1708-1712.)

confirmed presence of fetal cardiac activity have a 15% risk of suffering a pregnancy loss (Hasan, 2009).

Evaluation of the medical literature should take into account that the majority of patients with a prior pregnancy loss will eventually have a successful pregnancy; a study of more than 53,000 parous women reported that 43% experienced one or more prior first trimester pregnancy losses (Cohain, 2017). Remembering that 90% of pregnancy losses are not recurrent, watchful waiting may prove the best, albeit emotionally the hardest thing to do.

## Recurrent Pregnancy Loss

Although sporadic pregnancy loss is common, fewer than 5% of women will experience two consecutive pregnancy losses, and only 1% experience three or more (ASRM, 2012). Women with two prior losses and no live births experience a loss rate of 25%, which increases to 45% with three consecutive losses (Knudsen, 1991) (Table 16.1).

Historically, RPL has been defined as three or more consecutive pregnancy losses. The American Society of Reproductive Medicine (ASRM) defines RPL as two or more failed clinical pregnancies, documented by ultrasonography or histopathologic examination, that are not necessarily consecutive (ASRM, 2012). For epidemiologic studies, however, ASRM recommends that ideally three or more losses be used as the threshold for RPL. The European Society of Human Reproduction Embryology (ESHRE) released a consensus statement in 2014 proposing that *RPL* describes repeated pregnancy loss, including nonvisualized pregnancy losses, but did not recommend a number of losses required to be defined as recurrent loss (Kolte, 2015). The rationale to include nonvisualized pregnancies (biochemical pregnancy losses and/or pregnancies of unknown location) in the definition of RPL comes from a retrospective cohort study of 587 women who had three or more consecutive pregnancy losses before 12 weeks of gestation (Kolte, 2014). Nonvisualized pregnancy losses had the same negative impact on future live birth as clinical pregnancy losses.

It is important to emphasize to **patients with RPL that their overall prognosis is good, with more than 80% of women with RPL younger than 30 years and 60% to 70% of women with RPL ages 31 to 40 achieving a successful pregnancy within 5 years of their first visit to a physician** (Lund, 2012).

## RECURRENT PREGNANCY LOSS EVALUATION

For a pregnancy to successfully progress to term, a remarkable number of biological processes and events must occur properly both in the embryo/fetus and mother; failure or deficiencies in any of these can result in a pregnancy loss. Thus the evaluation and management of a woman or couple with RPL is based on careful and systematic evaluation for those factors that can contribute to the loss, followed by targeted correction of any deficiencies. Most clinicians begin the diagnostic evaluation for RPL after two failed clinical pregnancies because one early pregnancy loss is relatively common. If a pregnancy loss occurs in the second trimester, the cause is more likely to recur. **Thus a diagnostic evaluation should be considered after a woman has had only one second-trimester loss.**

The evaluation for women with RPL starts with a history and physical examination, including pertinent questions regarding previous uterine instrumentation, menstrual regularity, exposure to environmental toxins, history of venous or arterial thrombosis, and family history of pregnancy losses or birth defects and open-ended questions that explore the patient's ideas about causation. The history should include a description of the gestational age of all previous pregnancies because RPL typically occurs at a similar gestational age in consecutive pregnancies and the most common causes of RPL vary by trimester. For example, pregnancy losses related to chromosomal or endocrine defects tend to occur earlier in gestation compared with losses caused by anatomic or immunologic abnormalities. Physical examination should include a general physical assessment with attention to signs of endocrinopathy (e.g., galactorrhea) and uterine abnormalities (e.g., uterine septum, fibroids).

The patient's history should be used to guide laboratory evaluation. Any history suggestive of thyroid disease may prompt studies for thyroid-stimulating hormone (TSH) level and the presence of antithyroid antibodies. Other studies may include laboratory testing for prolactin, hemoglobin A1C, and

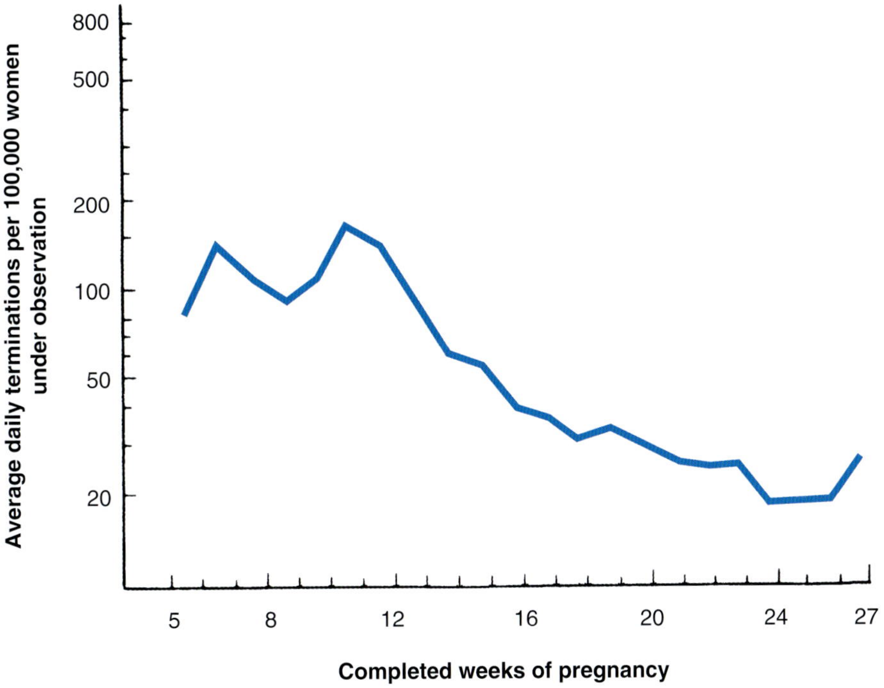


**Fig. 16.2** Pregnancy loss by week of pregnancy. (From Harlap S, Shiono PH, Ramcharan S. A life table of spontaneous abortions and the effects of age, parity, and other variables. In: Porter IH, Hook EB, eds. *Human Embryonic and Fetal Death.* New York: Academic Press; 1980.)

**TABLE 16.1** Risk of Subsequent Pregnancy Ending in a Pregnancy Loss*

| Number of Previous Pregnancy Losses | Number of Pregnancies Studied | Pregnancy Loss Risk (%) |
|---|---|---|
| 0 | 18,164 | 10.7 (10.3-11.2) |
| 1 | 21,054 | 15.9 (15.4-16.4) |
| 2 | 2,231 | 25.1 (23.4-27.0) |
| 3 | 353 | 45.0 (39.8-50.4) |
| 4 | 94 | 54.3 (43.7-64.4) |
| Overall | 19,737 | 11.3 (10.9-11.8) |

From Knudsen UB, Hansen V, Juul S, et al. Prognosis of a new pregnancy following previous spontaneous abortions. *Eur J Obstet Gynecol Reprod Biol.* 1991;39:31.

*The table is calculated from a 6.6% sample of the study pregnancies. Figures in parentheses: 95% confidence limits; $\chi^2$ (trend) = 728; *df* = 1: $P < .001$.

antiphospholipid antibodies. Anatomic causes of RPL can be diagnosed using a three-dimensional ultrasound or sonohysterography. POC cytogenetic testing should also be offered if available. If no other cause is identified, a parental karyotype should be performed to determine whether a balanced structural chromosomal abnormality exists. More controversial testing includes testing for ovarian reserve, inherited thrombophilias, autoantibodies, HLA typing, luteal phase progesterone, and sperm DNA fragmentation; routine cervical cultures; screening for diabetes; and endometrial biopsy. Table 16.2 **lists the accepted basic diagnostic workup for RPL. A thorough evaluation, including genetic analysis, will reveal a cause of recurrent loss in approximately 90% of couples who seek treatment** (Popescu, 2018).

## ETIOLOGY

Pregnancy loss may be caused by fetal and/or maternal factors. Fetal causes may be related to chromosomal, genetic, or structural abnormalities. Maternal factors include medical conditions such as endocrinopathies and certain thrombophilias, environmental exposures, and structural issues of the uterus. These categories can overlap; for example, maternal diabetes with poor glycemic control may cause a lethal heart defect in the fetus.

## CHROMOSOMAL

Chromosomal abnormalities are the most common cause of early pregnancy loss, accounting for approximately 50% to 60% of all

**TABLE 16.2** Summary of the Recommendations for Investigations and Treatments of Couples With Recurrent Pregnancy Loss From the American Society of Reproductive Medicine (ASRM) and European Society of Human Reproduction and Embryology (ESHRE)

| Investigation | American Society for Reproductive Medicine (ASRM) Recommendations | European Society of Human Reproduction and Embryology (ESHRE) Recommendations | Potential Treatment | Reference |
|---|---|---|---|---|
| Genetic analysis of pregnancy tissue | Recommend | Not routinely recommended; may be performed for explanatory purposes | Guide further investigation | Stephenson, 2002 |
| Parental karyotype | Recommend | Not routinely recommended; could be carried out after individual assessment of risk | Genetic counseling and information on preimplantation genetic testing | Franssen, 2005<br>Stephenson, 2006<br>Hassold, 2007 |
| Uterine anatomy<br>• Transvaginal 3D ultrasound<br>• Sonohysterography<br>• Hysterosalpingogram<br>• Pelvic MRI<br>• Hysteroscopy | Recommend | Recommend | Surgery for selective uterine abnormalities | Grimbizis, 2001<br>Grimbizis, 2016 |
| Thyroid screening<br>• TSH<br>• Thyroid peroxidase antibodies | Recommend | Recommend | Levothyroxine for hypothyroidism | Abalovich, 2007<br>Vissenberg, 2015<br>Maraka, 2016 |
| Prolactin screening | Recommend | Not routinely recommended; only if clinical symptoms of hyperprolactinemia (oligo/amenorrhea) | Bromocriptine for hyperprolactinemia | Hirahara, 1998<br>Li, 2013 |
| Insulin resistance<br>• Hemoglobin A1C<br>• Glucose tolerance test | Recommend | Not recommended | Lifestyle and pharmacologic therapy for glycemic control | Wang, 2011<br>Morley, 2017 |
| Antiphospholipid antibodies<br>• Lupus anticoagulant<br>• Anticardiolipin antibodies IgG and IgM<br>• β2 Glycoprotein | Recommend after 3 unexplained losses before tenth week of gestation | Recommend after two pregnancy losses | Low-dose aspirin and a prophylactic dose heparin | Miyakis, 2006<br>Van den Boogaard, 2013 |
| Hereditary thrombophilia<br>• Factor V Leiden<br>• Prothrombin gene mutations<br>• Protein C or protein S<br>• Antithrombin deficiencies | Not recommended; only if personal history of thromboembolism or first-degree relative with high-risk thrombophilia | Not recommended; only with additional risk factors for thrombophilia | Anticoagulation | De Jong, 2011<br>Bates, 2016 |

Testing not routinely recommended: ovarian reserve, luteal phase insufficiency, alloimmune factors (anti-HY antibodies, natural killer cell testing, anti-HLA antibodies), infectious causes, sperm DNA fragmentation

From Practice Committee of the American Society for Reproductive Medicine. Evaluation and treatment of recurrent pregnancy loss: a committee opinion. *Fertil Steril.* 2012; 98(5):1103-1111; and Atik RB, Christiansen OB, Elson J, et al. ESHRE guideline: recurrent pregnancy loss. *Human Reproduction Open.* 2018;2:1-12.

*3D,* Three dimensional; *HLA,* human leukocyte antigen; *Ig,* immunoglobulin; *MRI,* magnetic resonance imaging; *TSH,* thyroid-stimulating hormone.

pregnancy losses (ACOG, 2018). Pregnancy loss in the first trimester is more likely to be due to cytogenetic defects compared with losses in the second trimester (Romero, 2015).

Chromosomal abnormalities can be classified into those caused by an abnormal number of chromosomes and those caused by abnormal chromosome structure. Most chromosomal abnormalities are numeric abnormalities resulting from errors during gametogenesis (chromosomal nondisjunction during meiosis), fertilization (triploidy as a result of digyny or diandry), or division of the fertilized ovum (tetraploidy or mosaicism). In a study using chromosomal microarray analysis, cytogenetic abnormalities were found in 59% of the 2389 post–pregnancy loss POC samples: aneuploidy accounted for 85%, triploidy for 10%, and structural anomalies or tetraploidy for the remaining 4% (Levy, 2014). Unlike karyotyping, which requires live cells to culture, **chromosomal microarray analysis (CMA) using**

**single-nucleotide polymorphism (SNP)–based arrays can be performed on DNA extracted from formalin-fixed and paraffin-embedded (FFPE) tissues.** A retrospective study of more than 7000 POC samples successfully analyzed 92% of fresh tissue samples and 86% of FFPE samples using CMA (Sahoo, 2017). **Clinically significant abnormalities were identified in 53.7%** of specimens (3975 of 7396), 94% of which were considered causative of pregnancy loss.

Aneuploidy is usually caused by errors in the first meiotic division of the oocyte, although some trisomies are due to errors in paternal meiotic division. Aneuploidies occur with increasing frequency as maternal age increases, though the rate is not linear, and the rate of increasing frequency of numeric anomalies increases with advanced maternal age (Hassold, 2001; Franasiak 2014) (Fig. 16.3). Trisomies represent the largest class of aneuploidies, with trisomy 16 being the most common autosomal trisomy followed by trisomy 22. While monosomy for autosomes is infrequent, monosomy X has been observed in 11.2% of chromosomally abnormal pregnancy losses (Sahoo, 2017). However, nearly 1 in 300 monosomy X gestations will survive to viability (Hassold, 2007). **Monosomy X is unique in being paternally derived in approximately 75% of cases** (Uematsu, 2002).

Most chromosomal abnormalities in the embryo arise de novo. Rarely the abnormality is inherited from a parent who may have a balanced chromosomal translocation. Couples with RPL should undergo peripheral karyotyping to detect any balanced structural chromosomal abnormalities. **Of couples with RPL, 3% to 5% have a major chromosomal rearrangement** (vs. 0.7% of the general population) (Hassold, 2007). About 50% of these rearrangements are balanced translocations, 25% are Robertsonian translocations, and another 12% are female sex chromosome mosaicism. The remainder of major chromosomal rearrangements are either inversions or other types of sporadic abnormalities. **Balanced translocations are more common in women and more likely to result in a pregnancy loss if the translocation is of maternal origin.** Genetic counseling is recommended when a structural genetic factor is identified. The likelihood of subsequent live birth depends on the chromosome(s) involved and the type of rearrangement. **Large studies have shown spontaneous live birth rates of up to 71% in carriers of a structural rearrangement** (Stephenson, 2006). Preimplantation genetic testing (PGT), amniocentesis, and chorionic villus sampling are options to detect inherited genetic abnormalities in offspring.

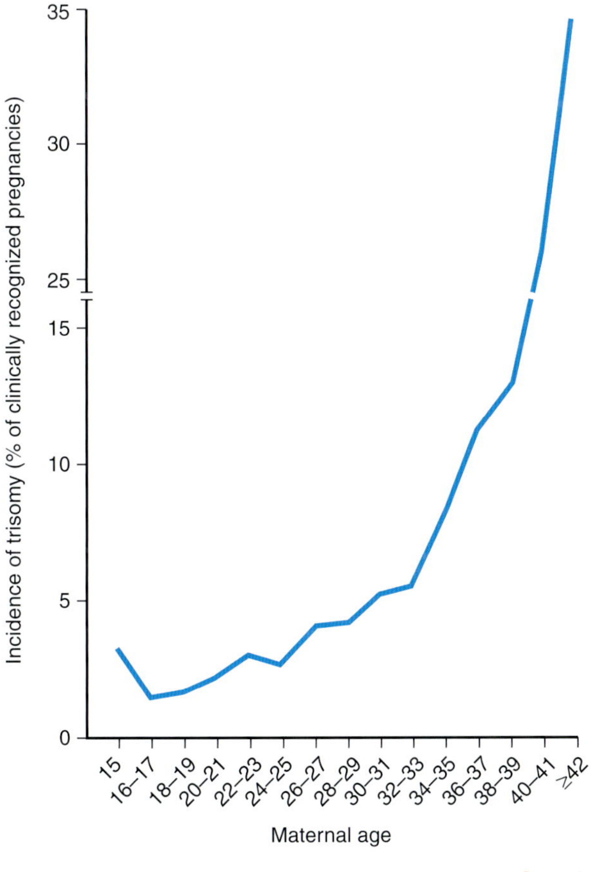


**Fig. 16.3** Maternal age and trisomy Incidence of trisomy relative to maternal age among all clinically recognized pregnancies. (From Hassold T, Hunt P. To err (meiotically) is human: the genesis of human aneuploidy. *Nat Rev Genet.* 2001;2(4):280-291.)

In contrast to sporadic pregnancy losses, most RPLs are not caused by chromosomal abnormalities. Stephenson and colleagues analyzed 420 karyotypes of aborted pregnancy samples from 285 couples with RPL and found that 54% of recurrent losses had normal cytogenetic evaluations (Stephenson, 2002) (Table 16.3). In women younger than 36, recurrent loss primarily was due to causes other than chromosomal abnormalities. The American College of Obstetricians and Gynecologists (ACOG) and ASRM recommend chromosomal evaluation of POC samples as part of the clinical evaluation of couples with RPL (ACOG, 2013; ASRM, 2012). *Rescue karyotyping* refers to the cytogenetic evaluation of archived POCs that have been formalin fixed and paraffin embedded and may be useful in cases where tissue has been collected but not cytogenetically tested (Kudesia, 2014). **By identifying the women whose pregnancy loss is due to a gross chromosomal abnormality, cytogenetic testing can prevent patients from undergoing costly and unnecessary evaluations**, whereas a negative result warrants further evaluation of a variety of anatomic, endocrinologic, hematologic, and immunologic disorders.

## UTERINE ANOMALIES

Uterine abnormalities, either congenital or acquired, may not provide the optimal environment for the developing embryo and thus may result in the loss of a genetically normal embryo.

### Anomalies of Uterine Development

Women with uterine anomalies have higher rates of first and second-trimester pregnancy losses compared with women with a normal uterus. **Uterine anomalies are present in approximately 12.6% of patients (range, 1.8% to 37.6%) with RPL compared with 4.3% of the general population (range, 2.7% to 16.7%)** (Grimbizis, 2001). The wide range reflects the differences in diagnostic and imaging techniques used. Several imaging modalities may be used to evaluate the uterus, including hysterosalpingogram, transvaginal ultrasonography, and sonohysterography. Magnetic resonance imaging (MRI) and three-dimensional transvaginal ultrasonography may help better characterize the anomaly.

The septate uterus is the most common uterine anomaly in the general population and is also associated with poorest reproductive outcomes. Composed of fibromuscular tissue, the septum has a decreased blood supply, which may lead to poor

**TABLE 16.3** Frequency of Cytogenetic Diagnoses in 420 Pregnancy Losses from 285 Couples With Recurrent Pregnancy Loss

| Diagnosis | Number of Pregnancy Losses | Frequency (%) |
|---|---|---|
| Euploid, female* | 120 | 29 |
| Euploid, male† | 105 | 25 |
| Trisomy 1 | 0 | 0 |
| Trisomy 2 | 4 | 0.95 |
| Trisomy 3 | 0 | 0 |
| Trisomy 4 | 1 | 0.24 |
| Trisomy 5 | 1 | 0.24 |
| Trisomy 6 | 3 | 0.7 |
| Trisomy 7 | 3 | 0.7 |
| Trisomy 8 | 4 | 0.95 |
| Trisomy 9 | 4 | 0.95 |
| Trisomy 10 | 1 | 0.24 |
| Trisomy 11 | 1 | 0.24 |
| Trisomy 12 | 1 | 0.24 |
| Trisomy 13 | 11 | 2.6 |
| Trisomy 14 | 11 | 2.6 |
| Trisomy 15 | 22 | 5.2 |
| Trisomy 16 | 19 | 4.5 |
| Trisomy 17 | 2 | 0.48 |
| Trisomy 18 | 4 | 0.95 |
| Trisomy 19 | 0 | 0 |
| Trisomy 20 | 2 | 0.48 |
| Trisomy 21 | 11 | 2.6 |
| Trisomy 22 | 16 | 3.8 |
| Double trisomy | 9 | 2.1 |
| Sex trisomy (47,XXY) | 1 | 0.24 |
| Monosomy X (45,X) | 18 | 4.3 |
| Monosomy X and trisomy 21 | 1 | 0.24 |
| Triploidy | 27 | 6.4 |
| Tetraploidy | 10 | 2.4 |
| Unbalanced translocations | 8 | 1.9 |
| Total | 420 | 100 |

From Stephenson MD, Awartani KA, Robinson WP. Cytogenetic analysis of miscarriages from couples with recurrent miscarriage: a case control study. *Hum Reprod.* 2002;17:446-451.
*Consisting of 118 cases of 46,XX and two cases of balanced translocations.
†Consisting of 105 cases of 46,XY.

implantation, resulting in early pregnancy loss. Later in gestation, the septum may compromise available space for growth, leading to pregnancy loss, malpresentation, or preterm term birth. Other congenital anomalies associated with pregnancy loss include unicornuate, didelphys, and bicornuate uteruses (ASRM, 2012).

Hysteroscopic septum incision, or metroplasty, is the treatment of choice for women with a septate uterus and a history of pregnancy loss. **A large meta-analysis found that hysteroscopic resection of the uterine septum increased live birth rates from 6.1% before surgery to 83.2%** after metroplasty. However, many of the retrospective studies included in this meta-analysis used patients as their own controls, which limits the interpretation of these results. The benefits of hysteroscopic metroplasty have not yet been assessed by a prospective randomized trial. In cases of bicornuate uterus, metroplasty may be performed transabdominally or laparoscopically but has not been shown to increase the live birth rate. Thus **metroplasty is not recommended for women with bicornuate uterus**. Uterine reconstruction is not feasible for the unicornuate uterus.

## Acquired Uterine Defects

### Fibroids

Fibroids are common benign uterine tumors that are present in more than one-third of women of reproductive age (Baird, 2003). The size and location of the fibroid is an important factor in determining the risk posed. Submucosal fibroids protrude into and distort the endometrial cavity and can increase the risk of pregnancy loss, possibly as a result of abnormal vascularization, impaired uterine contractility, and rapid distention of the uterus early in pregnancy. An association between pregnancy loss and intramural and subserosal myomas is less clear. Subserosal fibroids with greater than 50% of their mass outside the myometrium are unlikely to cause adverse pregnancy outcomes. The role of intramural fibroids in pregnancy is controversial (Klatsky, 2008; Pritts, 2009).

A meta-analysis of 23 studies (including 1 randomized trial) found the spontaneous pregnancy loss rate to be higher in women with submucosal or intramural fibroids with an intracavitary component (Pritts, 2009). Studies of women with fibroids that did not distort the uterine cavity have also shown an increased risk of pregnancy loss; however, these studies may have included women with fibroids with intracavitary distortion that was missed on imaging studies such as a hysterosalpingogram or an ultrasound.

Myomectomy is recommended for women with RPL and a fibroid that is submucosal or intramural with an intracavitary portion. Studies have shown a decrease in pregnancy loss rate after a myomectomy. In a large review published in 1981, Buttram and Reiter reported that among 1941 women, an abdominal myomectomy reduced the rate of pregnancy loss from 41% to 19% (Buttram, 1981). A smaller 2004 study by Marchionni and colleagues showed that pregnancy loss rates decreased from 69% to 25% after a myomectomy (Marchionni, 2004). Hysteroscopic myomectomy is the procedure of choice for submucosal myomas. With advances in laparoscopic suturing, most myomectomies for intramural fibroids may be performed laparoscopically. An abdominal myomectomy may be performed when there are multiple intramural fibroids or when the uterus is significantly enlarged.

### Endometrial Polyps

Endometrial polyps are a relatively common acquired anomaly, with an incidence of 7.8% to 34.9% (Lieng, 2009; Sillo-Seidl, 1971). Observational studies have reported improved spontaneous pregnancy rates after hysteroscopic polypectomy (Spiewankiewicz 2003; Varasteh, 1999), possibly because of changes in endometrial receptivity (Rackow, 2011). A 2019 systematic review showed that hysteroscopic resection of endometrial polyps was associated with an increased rate of clinical pregnancy in patients who underwent intrauterine insemination (IUI) (Zhang, 2019). However, clinical pregnancy and miscarriage rates were not improved in patients undergoing in vitro fertilization (IVF) cycles. **Thus the effect of hysteroscopic polypectomy on pregnancy outcomes remains unclear**. Although there are no adequate studies showing a benefit for polypectomy in RPL, given the underlying premise of restoring anatomy to normal and the low risk associated with polypectomy, **removal of polyps may be considered in women with RPL** (Jaslow, 2014).

## Intrauterine Adhesions (Asherman Syndrome)

Intrauterine adhesions (IUAs), or synechiae, are scar tissue within the uterine cavity and are referred to as Asherman syndrome when associated with symptoms such as amenorrhea, infertility, or pregnancy loss. Pregnancy loss is thought to be a result of insufficient endometrium to support fetoplacental growth.

Adhesions are commonly caused by previous intrauterine surgery (Table 16.4). Any intrauterine surgery may traumatize the basalis layer of the endometrium, which then heals by forming granulation tissue. Granulation tissue on opposing walls of the uterus can fuse, forming filmy adhesions composed of endometrial tissue and dense adhesions consisting entirely of connective tissue. These adhesions may result in partial or complete obliteration of the uterine cavity.

Postpartum complications such as hemorrhage or retained placenta are major risk factors for adhesion formation. A greater number of intrauterine surgical procedures increases the risk of IUA formation. **In a meta-analysis of 10 prospective studies, the risk of IUA development was 2.1-fold higher for two or more curettage procedures compared with one curettage procedure** (Hooker, 2014). Adhesions can also form in a nongravid uterus as a result of procedures that injure the endometrium such as a myomectomy. In a study by Taskin and coworkers, hysteroscopic resection of multiple submucosal leiomyomas had the highest risk of IUA formation compared with other hysteroscopic procedures (Taskin, 2000).

**TABLE 16.4** Reported Incidence of Intrauterine Adhesion After Various Conditions and Procedures

| Condition | Procedure | Incidence | Reference |
|---|---|---|---|
| **Gravid** | | | |
| SAB | Suction D&C | 15%<br>19% | Gilman, 2016<br>Hooker, 2014 |
| First trimester TOP | Suction D&C | 21% | Hooker, 2016 |
| Retained POC | Hysteroscopic resection | 6%<br>13%<br>19% | Smorgick, 2014<br>Hooker, 2016a<br>Barel, 2015 |
| | Suction D&C | 30% | Hooker, 2016b |
| **Gynecologic** | | | |
| Septum | Hysteroscopic septum resection (bipolar) | 24% | Yu, 2016 |
| Fibroids | Hysteroscopic myomectomy (bipolar) | 8% | Touboul, 2009 |
| | Abdominal myomectomy | 22% | Bhandari, 2016 |

*D&C*, Dilation and curettage; *POC*, product of conception; *SAB*, spontaneous abortion; *TOP*, termination of pregnancy.

Suspected IUAs may be seen in imaging studies such as ultrasound, saline infusion sonogram (Fig. 16.4), and hysterosalpingogram (Fig. 16.5). On hysterosalpingogram, the defects are typically irregular, with sharp contours and homogeneous opacity that persist in multiple views. The diagnosis is best confirmed and treated by hysteroscopy (Makris, 2007).

**The recommended treatment for symptomatic IUA is hysteroscopic lysis of the adhesions**. The goal of surgery is to restore the size and shape of the uterine cavity. Unfortunately, **adhesion recurrence rates have been reported to be**

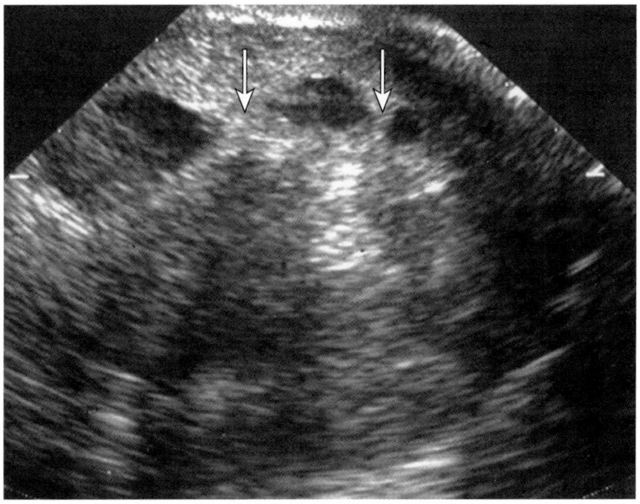

**Fig. 16.4** Sonohysterography of intrauterine adhesions *(arrows)*. (From Goldberg JM, Falcone T. *Atlas of Endoscopic Techniques in Gynecology*. London: WB Saunders; 2000:27.)

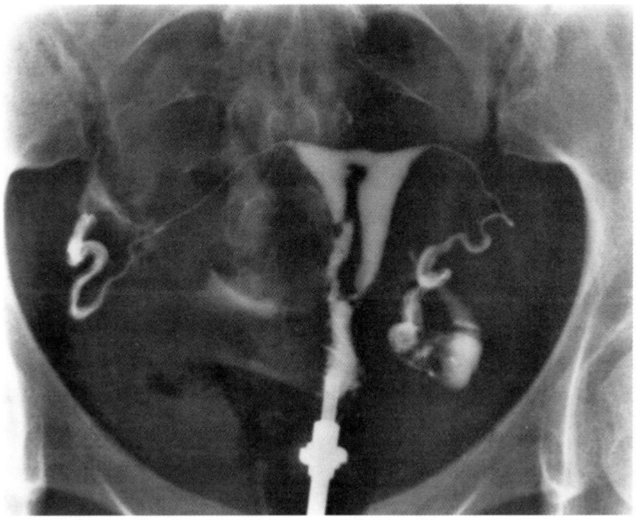

**Fig. 16.5** Endometrial adhesions. The patient was a 23-year-old gravida 5, para 0, spontaneous abortus 4, ectopic 1, with previous left linear salpingostomy, being evaluated for recurrent pregnancy loss. Irregular, linear filling defect represents adhesions between anterior and posterior walls of the endometrial cavity, extending from the internal os to a level near the fundus. (From Richmond JA. Hysterosalpingography. In: Mishell DR Jr, Davajan V, eds. *Infertility, Contraception, and Reproductive Endocrinology*. 3rd ed. Oradell, NJ: Medical Economics Books; 1991.)

**as high as 30% to 66% after surgical lysis** (Hanstede, 2015). The prevention of adhesion recurrence is challenging, and no single method has shown superiority (Salazar, 2017). Suggested postlysis management approaches include placement of a mechanical barrier such as a pediatric balloon in the intrauterine cavity, postoperative treatment with estrogen and timed progestin therapy, and a repeat hysteroscopy (Johary, 2014). In a meta-analysis of trials comparing multiple types of antiadhesion therapies with placebo or no intervention, treatment did not affect the subsequent live birth rate (odds ratio [OR], 0.99; 95% confidence interval [CI], 0.46 to 2.13; 3 studies, 150 women), although antiadhesion therapy was associated with fewer recurrent IUAs at the time of a second-look hysteroscopy (OR, 0.36; 95% CI, 0.20 to 0.64; 7 studies, 528 women) (Bosteels, 2015). **In women with severe IUAs, we suggest repeating an office hysteroscopy after the initial surgery.** At that point, any new adhesions will be filmy and can be gently taken down. This process can then be repeated until the cavity has fully healed from surgery.

Gel barriers and regenerated cellulose adhesions barriers (Interceed) have also been investigated to reduce the recurrence of adhesions. Although studies have suggested that gel barriers (hyaluronic acid gel and polyethylene oxide-sodium carboxymethylcellulose) have a role in preventing IUA reformation (Acunzo, 2003; Guida, 2004), a meta-analysis reported no definitive conclusion could be made because of the heterogeneity of study designs and lack of reproducibility of the study results (Healy, 2016). Because the optimal approach to the prevention of IUAs is not yet known, the discussed treatment options are reasonable alternatives.

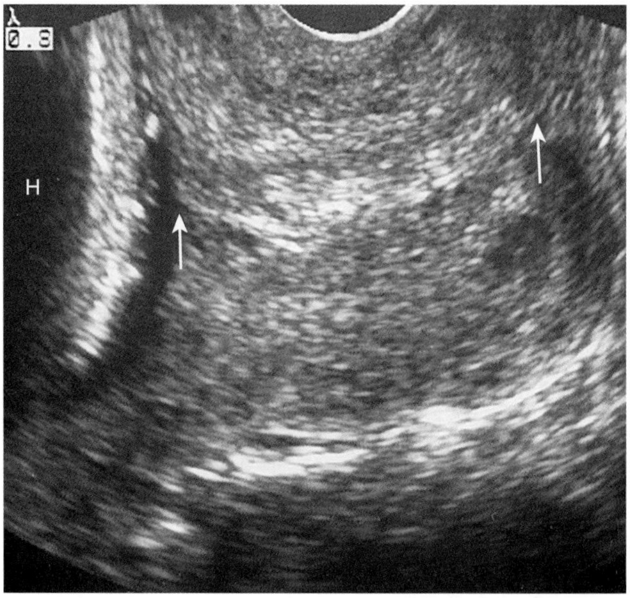


**Fig. 16.6** Transvaginal ultrasound of a normal-appearing cervix. *Large arrow* to small area denotes canal from external os to internal os, respectively. *H,* Fetal head. (From Fong KW, Farine D. Cervical incompetence and preterm labor. In: Rumack CM, Wilson SR, Charboneau JW, eds. *Diagnostic Ultrasound.* 2nd ed. St. Louis: Mosby; 1998.)

### Cervical Incompetence (Cervical Insufficiency)

Cervical incompetence is characterized by an asymptomatic dilation of the internal cervical os, leading to dilation of the cervical canal during the second trimester (Figs. 16.6 and 16.7). Cervical abnormalities, either congenital or as a result of trauma, are risk factors for structural cervical weakness.

Cervical trauma may result from treatment of cervical intraepithelial neoplasia such as conization or loop electrosurgical excision procedures, rapid mechanical dilation before a gynecologic procedure, and obstetric lacerations. Congenital abnormalities that have been associated with cervical weakness include uterine anomalies, genetic disorders affecting collagen (e.g., Ehlers-Danlos syndrome), and in utero diethylstilbestrol exposure. **Cervical insufficiency may be a cause of recurrent second-trimester loss but is not typically associated with early pregnancy loss.**

## ENDOCRINE FACTORS

## Luteal Phase Deficiency

Progesterone is required for implantation and maintenance of pregnancy; therefore **disorders related to impaired progesterone are likely to affect pregnancy success.** For the first 7 weeks of gestation, progesterone is produced by the corpus luteum and maintains the endometrium.

After the corpus luteum regresses, progesterone is synthesized by the trophoblast and maintains the decidual tissue. If progesterone secretion from the corpus luteum is low or if the endometrium has inadequate response to normal circulating levels of progesterone, endometrial development may be unable to support the implanted blastocyst, leading to pregnancy loss.

There is no consensus on the best method of diagnosis or treatment for luteal phase deficiency (ASRM, 2015a). The diagnosis of luteal insufficiency historically was made by performing a histologic examination of the endometrium; however, histologic dating of the endometrium has proven unreliable and not reproducible (Murray, 2004). Similarly, the measurement of progesterone levels in the luteal phase is not considered a reliable diagnostic test. **There is no standard progesterone value that defines normal luteal function because the corpus luteum varies from cycle to cycle in a normal fertile woman.** In a 2015 committee opinion, the ASRM concluded "there is no reproducible, pathophysiologically relevant, and clinically practical standard to diagnose luteal phase deficiency and distinguish fertile from infertile women" ( 2015). **Therefore we do not recommend performing luteal phase testing.**

Abnormal luteal phase progesterone production may also occur as a result of medical conditions such as elevated prolactin or abnormal thyroid function and treatment of the underlying condition is recommended.

## Thyroid Disease

**Risk of pregnancy loss is increased in women with poorly controlled thyroid disease, including hypo- and hyperthyroidism.** Studies have also shown that subclinical hypothyroidism (SCH), defined as TSH greater than 4 mIU/L, is associated with pregnancy loss and treatment with levothyroxine improves pregnancy rates and decreases the rate of pregnancy loss. **A meta-analysis of 18 cohort studies by Maraka and colleagues reported that SCH doubles the risk of pregnancy loss compared with euthyroid women** (Maraka, 2016). The normal reference range for TSH changes in pregnancy. **The upper limit of normal in most laboratories is 4 mIU/L for nonpregnant women and 2.5 mIU/L during the first trimester of pregnancy.** The use of the first trimester pregnancy thresholds to diagnose and treat subclinical hypothyroidism in women attempting pregnancy remains

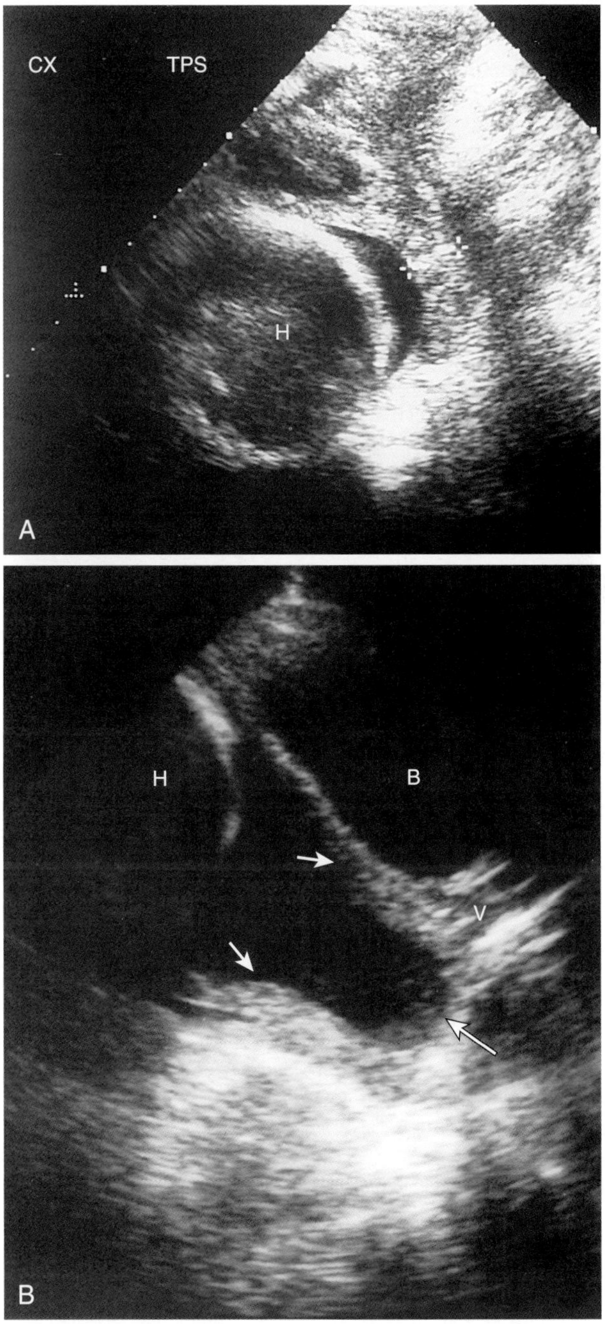


**Fig. 16.7 A,** Cervical shortening, the cervix was measured as 15 mm. Cursors are on the cervix. **B,** Advanced funneling or herniation of the membranes into the canal. This view was seen on transabdominal scan (*small arrows,* internal os; *large arrow,* external os). *B,* Maternal bladder; *CX,* cervix; *H,* fetal head; *TPS,* transperineal scan; *V,* vagina. (From Fong KW, Farine D. Cervical incompetence and preterm labor. In: Rumack CM, Wilson SR, Charboneau JW, eds. *Diagnostic Ultrasound.* 2nd ed. St. Louis: Mosby; 1998.)

controversial. According to the ASRM, if TSH levels before pregnancy are between 2.5 and 4 mIU/L, management options include either monitoring levels and treating when TSH is 4 mIU/L or greater or treating with levothyroxine to maintain TSH at 2.5 mIU/L or less (ASRM, 2015b). The Endocrine Society recommends that patients with RPL be treated to keep a TSH level between 1 and 2.5 mIU/L. **Once pregnant, women being treated for hypothyroidism often require an increase in thyroxine during pregnancy, beginning as early as the fifth week of pregnancy.**

Studies regarding treating euthyroid patients with positive thyroid antibodies are conflicting. A large randomized controlled trial of 952 euthyroid women with positive antithyroid antibodies showed no benefit when treated with levothyroxine (Dhillon-Smith, 2019). Routine screening for antithyroid antibodies in women with RPL is not currently recommended but may be considered if repeated TSH values are 2.5 mIU/L or more or when other risk factors for thyroid disease are present.

## Hyperprolactinemia

Hyperprolactinemia has been associated with pregnancy loss. Elevated levels of prolactin can alter the hypothalamic-pituitary axis, resulting in impaired folliculogenesis, decreased oocyte maturation, and a short luteal phase. **Normalization of prolactin levels with a dopamine agonist improves pregnancy outcomes in women with RPL.** In a randomized controlled trial, 64 hyperprolactinemic women with RPL were randomly assigned bromocriptine therapy or no bromocriptine; treatment resulted in an 85.7% live-born rate compared with 52.4% in the untreated group (Hirahara, 1998). Prolactin levels in early pregnancy were significantly greater in women who miscarried.

## Diabetes Mellitus, Insulin Resistance, and Polycystic Ovary Syndrome

Women with poorly controlled diabetes mellitus are at significantly increased risk for pregnancy loss. High hemoglobin A1C values early in pregnancy (particularly values above 8%) have been linked to increase frequencies of pregnancy loss and congenital malformations (Greene, 1989). The increased risk may be due to hyperglycemia, maternal vascular disease and possibly immunologic factors. Conversely, women with well controlled diabetes are no more likely than women without diabetes to suffer pregnancy loss (Milas, 1988).

**Insulin resistance, as seen in women with polycystic ovary syndrome (PCOS), may also be a factor in pregnancy loss.** The pregnancy loss rate in women with PCOS may be as high as 20% to 40% (Glueck, 2002; Rai, 2000). The sex hormone abnormalities in women with PCOS may cause premature or delayed ovulation and poor endometrial receptivity. **Insulin, at levels found in patients with insulin resistance, has been shown to be directly toxic to primary trophoblast cells from first trimester placentas, and this toxic effect is prevented by the addition of metformin** (Vega, 2019). High testosterone and androstenedione concentrations and insulin resistance may also adversely affect the endometrium. Observational studies suggest that metformin reduces the risk of pregnancy loss in women with PCOS. However, **a Cochrane review in 2017 concluded that metformin treatment has no effect on the risk of pregnancy loss in the entire PCOS population** (Morley, 2017). **Treatment with metformin for prevention of pregnancy loss is not routinely recommended for patients with PCOS.**

# IMMUNOLOGIC FACTORS

**Both autoimmune and alloimmune mechanisms have been implicated as causes of pregnancy loss.** Autoimmunity involves an immune response directed against an antigen normally present within the body; autoimmune diseases such as systemic lupus erythematous and antiphospholipid syndrome have been linked to RPL. Alloimmune disorders involve an abnormal maternal immune response to fetal or placental antigens.

## Alloimmune Disorders

The physiologic mechanism by which foreign fetal tissue is protected from the mother's immunologic system is poorly understood (Williams, 2012). Since the 1960s, investigators have hypothesized that pregnancy loss, and recurrent loss in particular, may be associated with abnormalities in this maternal alloimmune response. Allogenic factors may cause pregnancy loss by a mechanism similar to a graft rejection in transplant recipients. To date, however, immunologic treatments have not shown to be effective.

Prevention of an immune rejection of the fetus requires local immunologic adaptions within the mother. It is thought that in normal pregnancy the maternal immune response system recognizes the paternally derived antigens on the embryonic tissues and produces several alloantibodies that protect against the cytotoxic maternal immune response. The placenta and fetal membranes are directly exposed to maternal blood and tissues. Thus unique features of these cells that compose this interface must have the ability to protect the genetically distinct fetal tissue to inhabit the maternal host. Multiple strategies to avoid maternal immune cells and antibody-mediated cell destruction have been proposed, including altered human leukocyte antigen (HLA) expression, synthesis of immune regulatory molecules, and expression of high levels of complement regulatory proteins that protect the extraembryonic tissues from maternal antipaternal cytotoxic antibodies.

**It has also been suggested that women with RPL may lack essential components that provide immunologic protection to the embryos, such as an altered expression of complement regulatory proteins.** Other theories include cytokine dysregulation, a higher proportion of natural killer cells, and the formation of antipaternal lymphocytic antibodies. The degree of shared major histocompatibility locus antigens between a couple with RPL has also been investigated. **Studies have produced inconsistent data that have not been reproduced in more than one laboratory** (ASRM, 2012).

**Proposed immunomodulatory treatments for RPL have not been proven effective.** A **Cochrane review of 20 randomized trials concluded that immunotherapies such as paternal cell immunization, third-party donor leukocytes, trophoblast membranes, and intravenous immunoglobulin do not improve the live birth rate compared with placebo treatment** (Wong, 2014). Glucocorticoids have several antiinflammatory effects, including suppression of natural killer cell activity. The live birth rate was similar in a trial of 202 women with RPL and a variety of autoantibodies (antinuclear, anti-DNA, antilymphocyte, anticardiolipin, lupus anticoagulant) who were randomly assigned to receive either prednisone (0.5 to 0.8 mg/kg body weight per day) and aspirin (100 mg/day) or placebo (Laskin, 1997). **Glucocorticoids are not recommended for the treatment of RPL** because of uncertain efficacy and known increases in complications such as preterm premature rupture of membranes, gestational diabetes, and maternal hypertension.

**A randomized trial using weight-based dosing of granulocyte colony-stimulating factor (G-CSF) in women with unexplained RPL did show a benefit, with a higher live birth rate (82.8% vs. 48.5%, *P* = .0061; OR, 5.1; 95% CI, 1.5 to 18.4)** (Scarpellini, 2009). **A subsequent randomized trial using fixed and higher dosing of G-CSF did not show benefit, but overdosing of patients may have resulted in paradoxical responses (Eapen, 2019).**

## Antiphospholipid Syndrome

Antiphospholipid syndrome (APLS), an autoimmune disorder associated with RPL, may be present in 5% to 15% of patients with RPL (Reindollar, 2000). APLS may occur as a primary condition or in the setting of an underlying disease such as systemic lupus erythematous (SLE). Phospholipids are present throughout the body and found in almost all vasculature, particularly placental vasculature. Antiphospholipid antibodies react with proteins on the endothelium and induce platelet activation and thrombosis. Additionally, the antiphospholipid antibodies have a deleterious effect on the developing trophoblast. Abnormal endovascular trophoblastic invasion may explain early pregnancy losses and the development of uteroplacental vascular insufficiency later during pregnancy in women with APLS.

**The diagnostic criteria for APLS are outlined in** Box 16.1; **diagnosis requires at least one clinical and one laboratory feature.** The authors of the international consensus statement list several clinical events that should trigger testing for APLS (Miyakis, 2006), including thromboembolic events (arterial or venous) and pregnancy loss. The group concluded that **testing for APLS is indicated in the setting of three or more unexplained pregnancy losses before the tenth week of gestation when maternal anatomic or hormonal abnormalities and paternal and maternal chromosomal causes have been excluded.** Most pregnancy losses in women with RPL occur before 10 weeks' gestation; however, a greater proportion of losses related to APLS occur after 10 weeks' gestation. **Thus a single unexplained loss of a morphologically normal fetus at or beyond 10 weeks' gestation also warrants testing for APLS. Preterm birth at less than 34 weeks and associated with preeclampsia with severe features or placental insufficiency (intrauterine growth restriction) are also indications**

**BOX 16.1** International Consensus Definition for the Diagnosis of Antiphospholipid Syndrome

Diagnosis requires one of the following clinical criteria and one of the laboratory criteria:

**CLINICAL CRITERIA**

1. Vascular thrombosis
2. Pregnancy morbidity
   (a) One or more unexplained deaths of a morphologically normal fetus at or beyond the tenth week of gestation, or
   (b) One or more premature births of a morphologically normal neonate before the thirty-fourth week of gestation because of eclampsia, severe preeclampsia, or features consistent with placental insufficiency, or
   (c) Three or more unexplained consecutive spontaneous losses before the tenth week of pregnancy

**LABORATORY CRITERIA**

1. Lupus anticoagulant present on two or more occasions at least 12 weeks apart
2. Anticardiolipin antibody of IgG or IgM isotype in medium to high titer (i.e., greater than 40 GPL or MPL, or greater than the 99th percentile) on two or more occasions, at least 12 weeks apart
3. Anti-β2 glycoprotein-1 antibody of IgG or IgM isotype in 99th percentile titer on two or more occasions, at least 12 weeks apart

Data from Committee on Practice Bulletins—Obstetrics, American College of Obstetricians and Gynecologists. Practice Bulletin No. 132: antiphospholipid syndrome. *Obstet Gynecol.* 2012;120(6):1514-1521.

*Ig,* Immunoglobulin; *GPL,* IgG phospholipid units; *MPL,* IgM phospholipid units.

**for APLS testing.** Other clinical criteria include venous, arterial, and small vessel thrombosis. **Testing for antiphospholipid antibodies should be performed in women with a prior unexplained venous thromboembolism or a new venous thromboembolism during pregnancy.** Superficial venous thrombosis does not satisfy the criteria for thrombosis for APLS.

The three antiphospholipid antibodies included in the diagnosis of APLS are (1) lupus anticoagulant (LAC), (2) anticardiolipin (ACL), and (3) anti-β2 glycoprotein. **Positive test results should be performed twice because low-positive to midpositive levels can be due to viral illness and revert to normal.**

Lupus anticoagulant was first described in a woman with lupus; it binds with phospholipids and increases clotting time, inhibiting coagulation in vitro. However, in vivo lupus anticoagulant is a strong procoagulant. Detection of the lupus anticoagulant is generally based on delayed clotting in phospholipid-dependent coagulation tests (activated partial thromboplastin time, kaolin clotting time, or dilute Russell's viper venom time). Notably, the Venereal Disease Research Laboratory (VDRL) test for syphilis uses a phospholipid assay. Therefore **the presence of lupus anticoagulant may induce a false-positive VDRL result. Anticardiolipin antibody titers are considered positive if titers of immunoglobulin G (IgG) or IgM are in the 99th percentile; in 3% to 5% of general population, low levels may be observed that are of uncertain significance.** A high titer of **antibodies to anti-β2 glycoprotein** is also considered sufficient to establish the diagnosis. Assays for other antiphospholipid antibodies are not standardized, and routine screening is not warranted.

**Treatments used for APLS have included antiplatelet agents (aspirin [ASA]), anticoagulants (heparin, low molecular weight heparin [LMWH]), and immunosuppressive therapy (prednisone, intravenous immunoglobins).** We suggest that treatment for women with APLS and a history of stillbirth or recurrent fetal loss **should include low-dose ASA (81 mg/day) and a prophylactic dose of LMWH. Treatment should be initiated with a positive pregnancy test.** Unfractionated heparin and low-dose ASA are reasonable alternatives. A 2005 **Cochrane review found that the combination of ASA and heparin reduced pregnancy loss in women with antiphospholipid antibodies by 54% compared with ASA alone** (Empson, 2005). For women with laboratory criteria for APLS and a history of preeclampsia or placental insufficiency, low-dose ASA therapy alone beginning at the end of the first trimester and continuing through delivery may be sufficient. Prophylactic-dose LMWH may be added when placental examination shows extensive decidual inflammation, vasculopathy, and thrombosis (Viall, 2015). **Pregnant women with the incidental finding of persistent positive antiphospholipid antibody tests without any of the clinical criteria for APLS may treated with low-dose ASA** (Tincani, 2003). Women with a history of arterial or venous thrombosis and laboratory criteria for APLS are at high risk of recurrent thrombosis. The American College of Chest Physicians Evidence-Based Clinical Practice Guidelines recommends therapeutic dosing of LMWH for anticoagulation during pregnancy with resumption of warfarin postpartum (Bates, 2012).

**Other therapies, including prednisone and intravenous immunoglobulin, have not been proven to show any benefit, and their use is therefore not recommended.** Multiple large randomized trials that evaluated the use of heparin or ASA in women with unexplained RPL not meeting the diagnosis of APLS have not shown a benefit.

### Celiac Disease

Celiac disease is a systemic autoimmune disease caused by an allergy to gluten. Typically patients present with gastrointestinal symptoms related to intestinal malabsorption. Celiac disease has been associated with RPL in some but not all studies (Kumar, 2011; Greco, 2004). **It is hypothesized that antigliadin antibodies are toxic to trophoblasts.** Suppression of the antibodies through dietary control appears to improve pregnancy rates. A study of women with RPL and celiac disease by Tursi and coworkers noted improved pregnancy outcomes when women were placed on gluten-free diets (Tursi, 2008). **Any woman with a personal or family history of celiac disease or gluten intolerance should be tested for antigliadin and antiendomysial antibodies.** The prevalence of celiac disease in first-degree relatives of patients with celiac disease is 10%. Women with gastrointestinal symptoms may also try a gluten-free diet to determine whether symptoms improve with diet changes.

## INHERITED THROMBOPHILIA

Pregnancy is a state of hypercoagulability, which is further increased in various thrombophilias. Thrombogenic properties are increased as a self-protective physiologic adaption to prevent hemorrhage during implantation, placentation, and the third stage of labor. Inherited thrombophilia is a genetic tendency to venous thrombosis. **If the mother has an inherent thrombotic tendency such as thrombophilia, this thrombogenic microenvironment in the placenta can intensify, leading to multiple small infarctions at the uteroplacental interface.** Thrombosis of the spiral arteries and intervillous space on the maternal side of the placenta can impair adequate placental perfusion. This abnormal, enhanced thrombotic environment may lead to adverse pregnancy outcomes such as pregnancy loss, abruption, intrauterine growth restriction (IUGR), and preeclampsia. A relationship to early pregnancy loss is less clear.

The potential for thrombosis of the microvasculature of the placenta has been used to explain the association between thrombophilia and RPL. However, the literature is contradictory on the association between maternal inherited thrombophilia and RPL in the first trimester. A growing body of evidence suggests that treatment with anticoagulants does not improve these outcomes.

**The association between thrombophilia and pregnancy loss appears to be stronger for second-trimester and later losses compared with early pregnancy losses.** The European Prospective Cohort on Thrombophilia (EPCOT) showed the overall risk of pregnancy loss was increased, with an OR of 1.35, in women with thrombophilia (Preston, 1996). However, the OR was only statistically significant for stillbirth (defined as fetal loss after 28 weeks' gestation) compared with pregnancy loss (defined as fetal loss before 28 weeks' gestation). In a case-control trial of 3496 women with unexplained pregnancy loss and matched controls, an association was seen between factor V Leiden and prothrombin gene mutation and pregnancy loss after 10 weeks (Lissalde-Lavigne, 2005). No association found with less than 10 weeks' gestation. Although there are clear differences in the definition of losses between the studies, both show a stronger association between thrombophilia and late, rather than early, pregnancy losses. This finding is logical given that placental development has not taken place very early in pregnancy. Consequently, **thrombosis of placental vasculature in women with thrombophilia is less likely to explain early pregnancy loss.**

Other prospective studies have not shown an association between thrombophilia and pregnancy loss. The Eunice Kennedy Shriver National Institute of Child Health and Human Development's Maternal-Fetal Medicine Units Network prospectively studied 134 pregnant women who were **heterozygous for factor V Leiden and found no increase in the incidence of fetal loss** (Dizon-Towson, 2005). **A secondary analysis was conducted for maternal carriers of prothrombin G20210A mutation and again no increased risk was noted** (Silver, 2010).

**BOX 16.2** Thrombophilias Associated with Pregnancy loss

Antiphospholipid antibodies—anticardiolipin, lupus anticoagulant, and anti-β2 glycoprotein
Antithrombin III deficiency
Elevated factor VIII levels
Factor V Leiden mutation
MTHFR mutations*
Plasminogen activator inhibitor-1 deficiency
Protein C deficiency
Protein S deficiency
Prothrombin G20210A mutation
Thrombocytosis (thrombocythemia—platelet counts >750,000)

*Methylenetetrahydrofolate reductase mutations. (Mild hyperhomocysteinemia is technically not a thrombophilia, though it may be associated with thrombosis. Many laboratories include testing for the mutations in thrombophilia panels.)

The prevalence of thrombophilia, both acquired and inherited, is up to 15% of the general population; thus it is difficult to conclude if the presence of thrombophilia is the definitive cause of a specific adverse pregnancy event. Factor V Leiden mutation and the prothrombin gene mutation account for 50% to 60% of cases of an inherited hypercoagulable state in Caucasian populations. Deficiencies in protein S, protein C, and antithrombin (AT) account for most of the remaining cases (Box 16.2). These disorders appear to be responsible for or at least contribute to at least half of venous thromboembolisms during pregnancy. Mild hyperhomocysteinemia is sometimes considered a thrombophilia, but data suggest that it is a weak risk factor. **There is insufficient evidence to recommend screening for MTHFR polymorphisms or to measure fasting homocysteine levels as part of the evaluation of thrombophilia as a cause for venous thromboembolism.**

**Routine screening of women with RPL for inherited thrombophilia is not recommended** (ACOG, 2013; ASRM, 2012; Atik, 2018). If a patient has a personal history of venous thromboembolism in the setting of a nonrecurrent risk factor (such as surgery) or a first-degree relative with a known or suspected high-risk thrombophilia, screening patients for inherited thrombophilia (superficially factor V Leiden, prothrombin gene mutations, protein C, protein S, and AT deficiencies) may be clinically justified. Treatment of this inherited thrombophilia involves subcutaneous heparin or LMWH regimens. Without a personal or family history of thromboembolism, there is insufficient evidence that antepartum prophylaxis with unfractionated heparin or LMWH prevents recurrence of pregnancy loss.

## INFECTIONS

**Acute maternal infections may result in pregnancy loss as a result of fetal or placental infection.** An estimated 15% of early spontaneous pregnancy loss is associated with infection. Untreated syphilis leads to 21% increased risk of fetal loss and still birth (Gomez, 2013). Pregnant women infected with listeria monocytogenes are at risk for central nervous system infection and bacteremia, which may lead to fetal death. Viral infections such as cytomegalovirus, varicella, and rubella have been associated with both first- and second-trimester losses. The incidence of fetal loss in women infected with parvovirus B19 is estimated to be 8%, and risk of loss is 5.6 times higher with infection in the first trimester compared with the second trimester (Xiong, 2019). Women with a cytomegalovirus (CMV) infection are 2.5 times more likely to experience pregnancy loss compared with those not infected (Rasti, 2016).

There is no convincing data that infections cause RPL. Given the lack of evidence linking any infectious agent to RPL, routine screening for infectious organisms and the use of antibiotics empirically is not recommended for couples with RPL.

## ENVIRONMENTAL FACTORS

### Personal Habits (Smoking, Alcohol, Caffeine, Nonsteroidal Antiinflammatory Drugs)

### Smoking

**Smoking tobacco increases the risk of pregnancy loss in a dose-dependent manner.** In a large retrospective study of 47,146 women, an increased risk of pregnancy loss was seen in women who smoked as few as 10 cigarettes per day (Armstrong, 1992). A meta-analysis of 112 articles confirmed the risk of pregnancy loss was increased with the amount smoked (1% increase in relative risk per cigarette smoked per day) (Pineles, 2014). The mechanism responsible is unknown but may relate to the vasoconstrictive and antimetabolic effects of tobacco smoke. **Cigarette smoke contains several toxic agents such as nicotine, carbon monoxide, and mutagens, which may be harmful to the developing embryo.** Nicotine's vasoconstrictive effect can reduce the blood flow to the placenta. Smoking cessation should be recommended for all who wish to conceive.

### Alcohol

Observational studies have generally, but not consistently, found that moderate to high alcohol consumption increases the risk of pregnancy loss (Table 16.5). Windham and colleagues reported there was an increased risk of pregnancy loss in women who consumed more than three drinks per week during the first 12 weeks of pregnancy (Windham, 1997). After studying 24,679 singleton pregnancies, Kesmodel and colleagues found more than a threefold increased risk of first-trimester pregnancy loss for women who drank on average more than five drinks per week (Kesmodel, 2002). Interpretation of studies examining alcohol use in pregnancy is complicated by the many confounding factors and underreporting of actual alcohol consumption. **We recommend women who are pregnant or trying to conceive avoid alcohol consumption because alcohol is a known teratogen and a safe level of alcohol intake has not been established for any stage of pregnancy.**

### Caffeine

Caffeine is a stimulant found in tea, coffee, soft drinks, chocolate, and some over-the-counter medications. Coffee is one of the most common sources of high caffeine intake. **During pregnancy, caffeine clearance from the mother's blood slows down significantly**. Results from observational studies suggest that excess intake of caffeine may be an independent risk factor for pregnancy loss. However, other systematic reviews failed to show an association between caffeine intake and pregnancy loss, with the possible exception of intake of very high levels (e.g., 1000 mg, or 10 cups of coffee, over 8 to 10 hours) (Brent, 2011). Studies are limited by potential recall bias, confounding factors, and difficulty of quantifying caffeine consumption accurately (e.g., different cup sizes, coffee brands, and brewing methods). **Given the limited data, we recommend pregnant women and women trying to conceive limit daily caffeine intake to less than 300 mg/day (equivalent to 3 cups of coffee)** (Cnattingius, 2000).

TABLE 16.5 Frequency (%) of Alcohol Consumption Among Women Experiencing Early Pregnancy Losses (Cases) and Women Delivering at 28 Weeks' Gestation or Later (Controls)

| Frequency of Alcohol Consumption during Pregnancy | Percentage Distribution | | | |
|---|---|---|---|---|
| | Cases | Controls | Adjusted Odds Ratio | 95% Confidence Interval |
| Never | 42.6 | 43.7 | 1.00 | 0.59-0.99 |
| Twice a month and less | 28.9 | 38.0 | 0.77 | 0.71-1.52 |
| Daily | 4.5 | 1.4 | 3.00 | 1.39-6.49 |
| Total | 648 | | | 645 |

From Kline J, Stein Z, Susser M, et al. Environmental influences on early reproductive loss in a current New York City study. In: Porter IH, Hook EB, eds. *Human Embryonic and Fetal Death.* New York: Academic Press; 1980.

## Nonsteroidal Antiinflammatory Drugs

Several observational studies have suggested that nonsteroidal antiinflammatory drugs (NSAIDs) use may increase the risk of pregnancy loss; however, other studies have not detected an increased risk. A cohort study of 1097 women showed an increase risk of pregnancy loss in women who used NSAIDs during early pregnancy compared with unexposed controls and with women who used acetaminophen (Li, 2018). The effect was dose dependent, with NSAID use for more than 14 days leading to a higher risk of pregnancy loss compared with NSAID use of 14 days or less. After adjusting for multiple confounders, including maternal age, previous pregnancy loss, caffeine intake, and smoking, **the effect remained, but only for women who used NSAIDs around conception (adjusted hazard ratio [HR], 1.9; 95% CI, 1.3 to 2.7). These findings are consistent with the hypothesis that inhibition of prostaglandin production by NSAIDs impairs embryo implantation.**

These findings are contradictory to a large cohort study by Daniel and colleagues that linked data from medication dispensing records to information on obstetric outcomes for 65,457 pregnancies, including 6508 pregnant women with spontaneous pregnancy losses and 4495 pregnant women exposed to NSAIDs (Daniel, 2014). Daniel and colleagues found no significant increase in the risk of pregnancy loss after NSAID exposure after controlling for numerous factors, including maternal age, diabetes, hypothyroidism, obesity, hypercoagulation or inflammatory conditions, RPL, IVF, and tobacco use.

Although data are conflicting, **it is reasonable to advise that women trying to conceive avoid the use of NSAIDS to minimize the risk of pregnancy loss, particularly when alternatives such as acetaminophen are available.**

## Extremes of Maternal Weight

Body mass index (BMI) less than 18.5 or more than 25 kg/m$^2$ has been associated with an increased risk of infertility and pregnancy loss. A case-control study with more than 1600 patients with obesity (BMI $\geq$ 30 kg/m$^2$) compared with age-matched controls (BMI 19 to 24.9 kg/m$^2$) found an increased risk of early pregnancy loss (OR, 1.2; 95% CI, 1.01 to 1.46) and RPL (OR, 3.5; 95% CI, 1.03 to 12.01) (Lashen, 2004). An observational cohort study of 372 women with early RPL found that women with obesity have an increased frequency of euploid pregnancy losses (Boots, 2014). The pathophysiology of the association between obesity and pregnancy loss is unclear. A proposed mechanism includes leptin resistance and its detrimental effect on endometrial receptivity. **We encourage women who desire pregnancy to maintain a normal BMI.**

## Stress

The evidence linking stress to pregnancy loss is weak and conflicting. Severe stress is a well-documented cause of pregnancy loss in animal models. Chronic stress can lead to increased cortisol levels, decreased immunity, and an increased susceptibility to infections, all of which increase the risk of pregnancy loss (Frazier, 2018; Nepomnaschy 2006; Sastra 2013; Wainstock, 2013). **Given the multifactorial causes of stress, it is difficult to determine causation. Thus data linking psychological stress to sporadic pregnancy loss and RPL remain inconclusive.**

## Other Factors

Numerous therapeutic medications are considered teratogenic in pregnancy (e.g., isotretinoin) and may increase the risk of early pregnancy loss. Diethylstilbestrol (DES) was prescribed to women throughout the 1950s and mid-1960s and led to uterine malformations (e.g., T-shaped uterus). Women exposed to DES during their fetal life have a significantly greater incidence of spontaneous pregnancy loss than controls. Because DES was withdrawn from the U.S. market in 1971, it not a current cause of pregnancy loss, except in women at the end of their childbearing years. Exposure to toxins, pollutants, and other environmental factors may increase the risk of pregnancy loss by causing cell death or interfering with growth of normal tissue and cell differentiation. Ionizing radiation, excessive lead and mercury exposure, temperature extremes, and air pollution have all been linked to early pregnancy loss.

# MALE FACTORS

Despite being responsible for half of the genetic contribution to the embryo, little is known about how male factors contributes to pregnancy loss. **Researchers have speculated that various male factors such as abnormal sperm morphology, sperm DNA fragmentation, and advanced parental age are associated with pregnancy loss.** *Sperm DNA fragmentation* refers to sperm with DNA damage. Theoretically, the higher the percentage of damaged DNA in sperm, the worse the sperm will function and the higher the risk of pregnancy loss. In an analysis of 2969 couples, Robinson and colleagues demonstrated that **sperm DNA fragmentation is associated with sporadic pregnancy loss, with a relative risk of 2.16 (95% CI, 1.54 to 3.03)** (Robinson, 2012). Similarly, McQueen and colleagues performed an analysis on 579 men with RPL and found that male partners of women with a history of RPL have a significantly higher rate of sperm DNA fragmentation compared with the partners of fertile control women (mean difference 11.91; 95% CI, 4.97 to 18.86) (McQueen, 2019).

Higher percentages of DNA fragmentation have been seen in men of advanced paternal age and may result from correctable environmental factors such as exogenous heat, toxic exposures, varicoceles, and increased reactive oxygen species in semen. Oxidative stress can lead to DNA damage and may be exacerbated by smoking, obesity, and excessive exercise. The effects of lifestyle, occupational exposure, and semen quality were examined in a study by Ruixue and colleagues using semen analyses and detailed questionnaires from 68 couples with RPL and 63 randomly selected healthy controls (Ruixue, 2013). Semen from men in the RPL group had significantly reduced total progressive motility, increased abnormal morphology, and a higher mean percentage of DNA-damaged sperm compared with those of controls. Furthermore, the risk of RPL was significantly increased when smoking, drinking, and occupational exposure to environmental factors were superimposed (OR, 11.965; 95% CI, 1.49 to 95.62). **In couples with RPL, male factors such as sperm quality, occupational exposure, and lifestyle (smoking, alcohol consumption, exercise pattern, and body weight) should be assessed in addition to female factors**.

## UNEXPLAINED RECURRENT PREGNANCY LOSS

Even if no cause is identified, patients with RPL should be encouraged that the chance of live birth is good, with more than 50% of patients with unexplained RPL achieving live birth with no intervention (Scott, 1994). This rate must be considered when evaluating therapies for unexplained RPL. Many clinicians offer progesterone supplementation in early pregnancy to women with unexplained RPL, despite conflicting evidence. In a randomized, placebo-controlled trial of more than 800 women with unexplained RPL, vaginal progesterone did not change the pregnancy loss or live birth rate, with approximately two-thirds of women in each group delivering a live infant (progesterone and placebo birth rates: 66% vs. 63%, relative rate 1.04; 95% CI, 0.94 to 1.15) (Coomarasamy, 2015). Thus use of vaginal progesterone once a pregnancy has been established has not been shown to improve outcomes.

It is not known if intramuscular progesterone or other progestin therapies provide a benefit. Investigators have hypothesized that the therapeutic effect of progesterone may be related to immune modulation and that earlier initiation of progesterone, such as during the luteal phase, may improve outcome. As an example, in a small study of women with RPL and abnormal endometrial development as defined by elevated levels of nCyclinE expression, luteal phase treatment with micronized progesterone improved the 10-week pregnancy rate (Stephenson, 2017). No live birth rates were reported.

Studies evaluating the value of IVF and PGT for aneuploidy (PGT-A) in women with unexplained RPL have yielded mixed results. Researchers have argued that the percentage of aneuploidy losses in women with unexplained RPL may be underestimated given that conventional karyotyping using tissue culture is not definitive and studies on POCs are not often performed in very early losses. Garrisi and associates published a controlled clinical trial comparing the rate of pregnancy loss after IVF/PGT-A in patients with unexplained pregnancy loss to their own expected loss rate (Garrisi, 2009). For patients 35 years or older, the expected loss rate was 34% but the observed loss rate was 13.6% after IVF/PGT-A. These authors concluded that PGT-A improves pregnancy outcome in women with unexplained RPL, particularly those older than 35 years. This is in contrast to a retrospective cohort study of 300 women with RPL in which the pregnancy, live birth, and pregnancy loss rates were similar for women who underwent IVF/PGT-A and women who elected expectant management (Murugappan, 2016). The medical risks and financial burden of IVF/PGT-A should also be justified before recommending routine use of this intervention.

Pregnancy loss has a significant emotional impact on the affected couple. Couples who suffer from RPL are at risk for heightened anger, depression, anxiety, and feelings of grief and guilt. Many studies have demonstrated that these women benefit from extensive counseling and emotional support throughout early gestation. In a study by Stray-Pedersen and colleagues, a cohort of 158 couples with 3 or more consecutive unexplained pregnancy losses were divided into two groups, one receiving routine obstetric care during the pregnancy and the other receiving additional tender loving care (TLC) (Stray-Pedersen, 1984). TLC was defined as psychological support with weekly medical and ultrasonographic examinations and instructions to avoid heavy work, travel, and sexual activity. The difference in live births was significant: 36% in the control group and 85% in the TLC group. Results, however, should be interpreted with caution because the groups were not randomly allocated and only patients who lived within a reasonable distance to the hospital were offered TLC. Clifford and associates also reported that women with unexplained RPL given psychological support early in pregnancy had a 74% viable birth rate without other therapy (Clifford, 1997). Although data linking the cause of RPL to psychological factors is inconclusive, it is advisable to offer patients with RPL support and counseling.

## PREGNANCY LOSS DIAGNOSTIC EVALUATION

### Clinical Presentation

Early pregnancy loss may occur in the presence or absence of symptoms and with or without the passage of tissue. Vaginal bleeding may be described as light or heavy, intermittent or constant, and with or without feelings of pain. Abdominal pain is often described as a cramping sensation and can vary from mild to severe. Pain often worsens with the passage of pregnancy tissue. Women may note a reduction in pregnancy symptoms such as decreased breast tenderness, nausea, or vomiting. Alternatively, some women are asymptomatic and pregnancy loss is diagnosed on routine ultrasound.

Bleeding in the first trimester of pregnancy is common and occurs in 20% to 30% of all pregnancies; most will not result in pregnancy loss (Everett, 1997; Strobino, 1989). One prospective study of more than 4000 pregnant women reported pregnancy loss in 12% of women with first-trimester vaginal bleeding (Hasan, 2010). Bleeding may result from implantation of the pregnancy, discrete cervical or vaginal lesions, ectopic pregnancy, or disruption of blood vessels in the decidua. A speculum examination should be performed to assess the source and quantity of bleeding. A visibly dilated cervical os or pregnancy tissue present at the os is concerning for an ongoing or inevitable pregnancy loss.

Although bleeding may be heavy with the passage of pregnancy tissue, almost all women remain hemodynamically stable; rarely a woman may become hemodynamically unstable and necessitate transfusion and immediate surgical evacuation. Women with hemorrhage typically present with heavy vaginal bleeding combined with orthostatic vital signs, anemia, and tachycardia. Occasionally, young pregnant women may experience massive hemorrhage without demonstrating tachycardia or hypotension. Care should be taken to avoid unnecessary delay in the management of such patients.

### Laboratory Evaluation

A "discriminatory zone" of β-hCG levels has been used to predict when an intrauterine gestational sac should be visible on imaging. **A β-hCG of 1500 IU has traditionally been accepted as the level at which transvaginal ultrasound should reveal an intrauterine gestational sac in a viable pregnancy.** However, this level remains controversial (Barnhart, 2012). An analysis of 651 pregnancies reported **discriminatory β-hCG levels at which structures would be predicted to be seen 99% of the time were 3510 mIU/mL for the gestational sac, 17,716 mIU/mL for the yolk sac, and 47,685 mIU units/mL for the fetal pole** (Connolly, 2013). Levels peak around 100,000 IU at 10 weeks, with the steepest rate of increase observed in the first 6 weeks, followed by a slower rise and eventual fall after the peak.

Caution should be used when trying to interpret a single β-hCG level. In a normally developing pregnancy, the level of β-hCG should rise in a predictable fashion. Two studies that included more than 1000 women with early pregnancies found viable pregnancies had a minimal increase in β-hCG of 35% over 48 hours (Morse, 2012; Seeber, 2006). The rate of increase may be less predictable at low levels. Three serial β-hCGs are typically needed to establish a trend. A decreasing or plateaued β-hCG concentration is most consistent with a failed pregnancy (nonviable intrauterine pregnancy or involuting ectopic pregnancy). A low serum progesterone level may also be predictive of pregnancy loss. Progesterone levels less than 12 ng/mL are also concerning (Lek, 2017) but should not be used for diagnosis of pregnancy loss because of high variability.

## Imaging

Transvaginal ultrasound is generally performed in all pregnant women with signs or symptoms suggestive of pregnancy loss to confirm either an intrauterine gestation or pregnancy demise. The first sonographic finding of a pregnancy is the gestational sac, which should be seen by 4.5 to 5 weeks' gestation (Table 16.6; Fig. 16.8). It appears as a small, fluid-filled saclike structure eccentrically located within the endometrium. This structure and its echogenic rim represent the chorionic cavity, implanting chorionic villi, and associated decidual tissue. Caution should be used when making the presumptive diagnosis of a gestational sac in the absence of a definitive embryo or yolk sac because the intrauterine fluid collection may represent a pseudogestational sac related to an ectopic pregnancy. The yolk sac is the first anatomic structure to appear within the gestational sac, at the beginning of the fifth week of gestation. The embryonic disc (i.e., the thickened region along the outermost margin of the yolk sac) should be visualized by approximately 5 to 6 weeks' gestational age. **A mean gestational sac diameter 8 mm or larger in diameter with no yolk sac or a distorted or large yolk sac 7 mm or larger is considered abnormal. A nonviable pregnancy may be diagnosed if neither the yolk sac nor the embryonic pole is visible by the time the mean diameter of the gestational sac is 25 mm** (Doubilet, 2013).

**TABLE 16.6** Ultrasound Findings in Early Pregnancy

| Ultrasound Findings | Gestational Age from LMP (days) | Approximate HCG (IU) | Approximate Risk of Pregnancy Loss* |
|---|---|---|---|
| Gestational sac | 23-29 | 1500 | <12% |
| Yolk sac | 32-45 | 5000 | <9%[†] |
| Embryonic disc | 35-45 | | <8% |
| Fetal cardiac activity | >42 with CRL × 5 mm | 13,000-15,000 | <8% |
| Embryo 2 cm with heart rate | 56 | | <2% |

*If no vaginal bleeding.
[†]If the gestational sac is 10 mm.
*CRL*, Crown-rump length; *HCG*, human chorionic gonadotropin; *LMP*, last menstrual period.

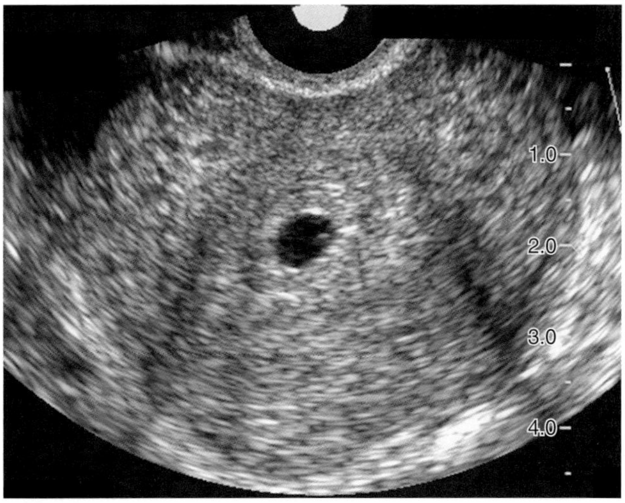


**Fig. 16.8** Endovaginal ultrasound 6 days after a gestational sac, with mildly increased decidual reaction surrounding the echolucent sac. *UT*, Uterus. (From Lyons EA, Levi CS, Dashefsky SM. The first trimester. In: Rumack CM, Wilson SR, Charboneau JW, eds. *Diagnostic Ultrasound.* 2nd ed. St. Louis: Mosby; 1998.)

Fetal cardiac activity can first be seen at 5.5 to 6 weeks' gestation. Initially the fetal heart rate should be in the 80 to 110 beats per minute (bpm) range and can often increase to 180 to 220 bpm, but by 12 weeks the fetal heart rate should return to 110 to 160 bpm. **A slow fetal heart rate (<100 bpm at 5 to 7 weeks' gestation) has been associated with early pregnancy loss** (Doubilet, 1999).

Bleeding in the first trimester may be due to disruption of decidual vessels at the maternal-fetal interface and can appear as a **subchorionic hematoma** on an ultrasound. Small subchorionic hematomas are common in the first trimester; **the risk of pregnancy loss increases if the subchorionic hematoma is greater than 25% of the volume of the gestational sac** (Pearlstone, 1993). **In a meta-analysis of seven comparative studies, women with a subchorionic hematoma were twice as likely to experience pregnancy loss compared with women without (18% vs. 9%; OR, 2.18; 95% CI, 1.29 to 3.68)** (Tuuli, 2011). Location of the hematoma also appears to affect outcome, with worse outcomes reported for retroplacental versus marginal hematomas.

## PREGNANCY LOSS DIAGNOSIS

Diagnosis of pregnancy loss should be made after a thorough medical history and a physical examination combined with an ultrasound and β-hCG values. Once an intrauterine pregnancy is identified on ultrasound, pregnancy loss is diagnosed if a subsequent ultrasound shows no intrauterine pregnancy or there is a loss of previously seen cardiac activity.

The diagnosis of pregnancy loss may also be made on the initial transvaginal ultrasound based on strict criteria. Early studies of the transvaginal ultrasound for determination of fetal viability used **a crown-rump length (CRL) of 5 mm without cardiac activity or an empty intrauterine gestational sac with a mean sac diameter (MSD) of 16 mm** to diagnose a pregnancy loss. However, more recent data have prompted the Society of

Radiologists in Ultrasound Multispecialty Panel on Early First Trimester Diagnosis of Miscarriage and Exclusion of a Viable Intrauterine Pregnancy to recommend more conservative guidelines (Doubilet, 2013). **These newer criteria require a CRL of 7 mm or more with no heartbeat or an MSD of 25 mm or more with no embryo to diagnose an early pregnancy loss.** The aim of these criteria is to facilitate achievement of 100% specificity with a zero false-positive rate in the diagnosis of a nonviable pregnancy. The guidelines also give findings suggestive, but not diagnostic, of pregnancy loss (Box 16.3).

When caring for women experiencing possible early pregnancy loss, providers should consider other clinical factors when interpreting the Society of Radiologists in Ultrasound guidelines. These factors include the woman's desire to continue the pregnancy; her willingness to postpone intervention to achieve 100% certainty of pregnancy loss; the potential consequences of waiting for intervention, including unwanted spontaneous passage pregnancy tissue; the need for an unscheduled visit or procedure; and the patient's anxiety (ACOG, 2018). **The patient should be included in the diagnostic process, and guidelines should be individualized to the patient's circumstances.**

## BLEEDING IN EARLY PREGNANCY

Pregnant women who present with vaginal bleeding but do not meet the diagnostic criteria for pregnancy loss may be managed expectantly. Patients should be asked to call their doctor if they experience additional vaginal bleeding, pelvic cramping, or passage of tissue from the vagina. A pelvic ultrasound may be repeated weekly until a viable pregnancy is confirmed or excluded.

Avoidance of excessive physical activity or exercise and intercourse is typically advised, but this has not been shown to improve outcomes. Bed rest should not be recommended. Other interventions such as muscle relaxants or vitamin supplementation have not been found to be beneficial.

The benefit of supplemental progestin treatment for prevention of pregnancy loss in women with vaginal bleeding is not clear, in part because of differing types of progestins, varying routes of administration, and differing outcomes assessed. A Cochrane review of seven randomized trials that involved women with bleeding in early pregnancy who were administered progesterone agents showed a significantly lower risk of pregnancy losses among women who received progesterone compared with those who received placebo or no treatment (OR, 0.64; 95% CI, 0.47 to 0.87; 7 trials; 696 women) (Wahabi, 2018). Of note, the trials included were small; the largest trial had a sample size of 191. In a 2019 randomized controlled trial, 4153 women with vaginal bleeding in early pregnancy were randomly assigned to receive either 400 mg of vaginal progesterone or placebo twice daily until 16 weeks' gestation. Pregnancy loss and live birth rates were similar between the two groups (pregnancy loss rate 20% vs. 22%, relative rate 0.91; 95% CI, 0.81 to 1.01; live birth rate 75% vs. 72%, relative rate 1.03; 95% CI, 1.00 to 1.07) (Coomarasamy, 2019). In women with three or more consecutive pregnancy losses, progestin administration may be of some potential benefit. According to ACOG, "for threatened early pregnancy loss, the use of progestins is controversial, and conclusive evidence supporting their use is lacking" (ACOG, 2018).

**BOX 16.3** Society of Radiologists in Ultrasound Guidelines for Transvaginal Ultrasonographic Diagnosis of Early Pregnancy Loss*

**FINDINGS DIAGNOSTIC OF EARLY PREGNANCY LOSS†**

Crown-rump length of 7 mm or greater and no heartbeat
Mean sac diameter of 25 mm or greater and no embryo
Absence of embryo with heartbeat 2 weeks or more after a scan that showed a gestational sac without a yolk sac
Absence of embryo with heartbeat 11 days or more after a scan that showed a gestational sac with a yolk sac

**FINDINGS SUGGESTIVE, BUT NOT DIAGNOSTIC, OF EARLY PREGNANCY LOSS‡**

Crown-rump length of less than 7 mm and no heartbeat
Mean sac diameter of 16 to 24 mm and no embryo
Absence of embryo with heartbeat 7 to 13 days after an ultrasound scan that showed a gestational sac without a yolk sac
Absence of embryo for 6 weeks or longer after last menstrual period
Empty amnion (amnion seen adjacent to yolk sac, with no visible embryo)
Enlarged yolk sac (>7 mm)

Small gestational sac in relation to the size of the embryo (<5 mm difference between mean sac diameter and crown-rump length)

Data from Committee on Practice Bulletins—Obstetrics, American College of Obstetricians and Gynecologists. Practice Bulletin No. 150: early pregnancy loss. *Obstet Gynecol.* 2015;125(5):1258–1267.

*Criteria are from the Society of Radiologists in Ultrasound Multispecialty Consensus Conference on Early First Trimester Diagnosis of Miscarriage and Exclusion of a Viable Intrauterine Pregnancy, October 2012.

†These are the radiologic criteria only and do not replace clinical judgment.

‡When there are findings suspicious for early pregnancy loss, follow-up ultrasonography at 7 to 10 days to assess the pregnancy for viability is generally appropriate.

## MANAGEMENT OF EARLY PREGNANCY LOSS

Once a nonviable pregnancy has been diagnosed, a thorough discussion with the patient and her partner or support person should ensue. Her feelings surrounding the pregnancy, as well as cultural preferences and past experience, may influence her decision regarding intervention. Provided there is no evidence of infection, expectant management, medical therapy, and surgical evacuation of the uterus are all viable, effective options. For women who prefer to avoid surgery and anesthesia, expectant or medical management may be chosen. Women who choose these options should be counseled; about 10% to 20% will require surgical intervention for complete evacuation. Overall, serious complications after early pregnancy loss treatments are rare and comparable across treatment types. **The choice of method is typically based on patient preference.**

### Expectant Management

Expectant management is an option for patients with stable vital signs and no signs of infection. The majority of tissue will pass after the first 2 weeks of diagnosis of pregnancy, and an interval of 3 to 4 weeks between diagnosis and expulsion is not unusual. Luise and colleagues expectantly followed 686 patients with suspected first-trimester pregnancy loss for up to 4 weeks (Luise, 2002). Successful spontaneous abortion occurred in 81% of all expectantly managed patients, 91% of those with incomplete pregnancy loss, 76% of those with missed abortion, and 66% of those with anembryonic pregnancies. Complications such as infection and excessive pain or bleeding occurred in 1% of expectantly managed patients.

**If expulsion has not occurred after 4 weeks, surgical evacuation is recommended.** Retention of the deceased embryo in the uterus beyond 5 weeks after the demise is associated with consumptive coagulability and hypofibrinogenemia.

## Medical Management

Women with a nonviable pregnancy up to 12 weeks and 6 days may be candidates for outpatient medical management provided there are no signs of infection, hemorrhage, severe anemia, or bleeding disorders. Women may prefer medical management to expectant management to expedite the process and potentially increase the likelihood of expulsion. In most cases, collection of POCs for cytogenetic analysis may be possible after medical management, though success rates in collection of tissue for cytogenetic testing are lower than with surgical management (Kucheroy, 2018).

Medical management most often includes misoprostol, a prostaglandin E1 analog. Misoprostol is administered either orally or vaginally, with the vaginal route preferred to maintain steady serum levels and to avoid gastrointestinal side effects. Results of a large randomized controlled trial showed success rates of 71% after a single dose and 84% after a second dose of 800 μg misoprostol per vagina (Zhang, 2005).

Mifepristone, a progesterone receptor antagonist, may be used as a pretreatment followed by misoprostol. A randomized trial of 300 women with a diagnosed pregnancy loss between 5 and 12 weeks' gestation reported that mifepristone pretreatment followed by misoprostol therapy resulted in higher rates of complete expulsion (84% vs. 67%) and lower rates of surgical uterine aspiration (9% vs. 24%) compared with misoprostol alone (Schreiber, 2018). Women with an absent gestational sac and/or open cervical os were excluded from the study because of the known high efficacy of misoprostol alone in this group (approximately 90%). This trial contrasts with earlier studies that reported mifepristone pretreatment did not improve outcomes (Gronlund, 2002; Stockheim, 2006). The earlier studies used higher doses of mifepristone (600 vs. 200 mg) and lower doses of misoprostol (400 vs. 800 μg), which may have contributed to the discrepant findings. The availability of mifepristone is limited by the U.S. Food and Drug Administration. ACOG recommends 800 μg vaginal misoprostol with a repeat dose as needed and the consideration of mifepristone (200 mg orally) when available (ACOG, 2018).

## Surgical Management

Surgical treatment is preferable for women who desire a shorter time to complete treatment and wish to avoid the experience of pain and bleeding that accompanies the passage of the POCs. POCs may also be sent for cytogenetic evaluation to determine the karyotype and potential cause of the pregnancy loss. Surgical evacuation of the uterus should also be performed in patients who present with hemorrhage, hemodynamic instability or signs of infection.

The procedure is typically performed under intravenous conscious sedation with or without a paracervical block. At 10 weeks' gestation or less, manual uterine evacuation and electric vacuum aspiration have similar rates of successful evacuation and patient acceptability (Goldberg, 2004; Wen, 2008). **The use of suction curettage is superior to the use of sharp curettage alone,** and the routine use of sharp curettage along with suction curettage in the first trimester does not provide any additional benefit as long as the provider is confident the uterus is empty. Hysteroscopic removal of pregnancy tissue may be preferable in complicated cases, such as in women with a known uterine septum. Prophylactic antibiotics are given to decrease the risk of infection. Experts have recommended **administration of a single 200-mg dose of doxycycline 1 hour before surgical management.** Potential surgical complications, although rare, include uterine perforation, cervical trauma, intrauterine adhesion formation, and anesthesia-related complications.

Surgical evacuation is associated with a lower risk of unplanned hospital admissions and a need for subsequent treatment compared with expectant and medical management. This was illustrated in the MIST trial, in which 1200 women diagnosed with pregnancy loss at less than 13 weeks' gestation were randomly assigned to expectant, medication (mifepristone and misoprostol), or surgical management (Trinder, 2006). **Significantly more unplanned admissions and unplanned surgical curettage occurred after expectant and medical management than after surgical management.** No differences were found in the incidence of infection; blood transfusions occurred in 2% of women in the expectant management group, 1% in the medication group, and no patients in the surgery group. In a follow-up study, future reproductive outcomes were assessed; live birth rates 5 years after the initial pregnancy loss were similar in the three management groups (Smith, 2009). **Women can be reassured that long-term subsequent pregnancy rates are not affected by their choice of pregnancy loss management.**

## Alloimmunization Prevention

If a woman is Rh(D) negative and unsensitized, Rh(D) immune globulin should be considered. Although the risk of alloimmunization is low in first-trimester pregnancy loss, ACOG **recommends women receive Rh(D) immune globin immediately after surgical management or within 72 hours of the diagnosis of early pregnancy loss with planned medical or expectant management in the first trimester** (ACOG, 2018). Women who undergo surgical evacuation are at higher risk of alloimmunization resulting from the procedure. Women with clinically significant vaginal bleeding without pregnancy loss are also at risk for alloimmunization because bleeding is often attributed to marginal separation of the placenta, which could result in maternofetal bleeding (Von Stein, 1992). **A 50-μg** dose is effective through the twelfth week of gestation because of the small volume of red blood cells in the fetoplacental circulation (mean red cell volume at 8 and 12 weeks is 0.33 mL and 1.5 mL, respectively); however, **it is reasonable to use the more readily available 300-μg dose if the 50-μg dose is unavailable.**

## Septic Abortion

***Septic abortion*** **refers to a pregnancy loss accompanied by an intrauterine infection.** Although uncommon, septic abortion can be life threatening, with a fatality rate of 0.4 to 0.6 per 100,000 first-trimester pregnancy losses. Elevated temperature, leukocytosis, lower abdominal pain, cervical motion tenderness, and a purulent vaginal discharge are all signs of septic abortion. Infection can spread from the endometrium through the myometrium and eventually affect the parametrium and peritoneum. **The cause is most often polymicrobial,** with *Escherichia coli* and other aerobic gram-negative rods involved. Group B streptococci, anaerobic streptococci, *Bacteroides*, and *Clostridium perfringens* may also be implicated. Shock can occur from the release of endotoxins.

Patients presenting with signs and symptoms of septic abortion should be stabilized with fluids and blood products as needed. Blood and cervical cultures should be obtained, followed by the administration of broad-spectrum intravenous antibiotics. Choice of antibiotics is typically the same as for pelvic inflammatory disease. Evacuation of the uterus should be performed with extra care given the increased risk of perforation in an infected gravid uterus. Hysterectomy may be warranted for patients who fail to respond to uterine evacuation and antibiotics, develop pelvic abscess, or are found to have clostridial necrotizing myonecrosis (gas gangrene).

## Management of Second-Trimester Pregnancy Loss

Both surgical and medical methods can be used in the management of second-trimester pregnancy losses. When comparing management options, providers should consider safety, effectiveness, logistics, and patient preference. Dilation and evacuation (D&E) is safe and effective but requires clinicians proficient in a midtrimester D&E. Compared with a first-trimester procedure, a D&E in the second trimester has a higher risk of complications, including uterine perforation, hemorrhage, and infection. Cervical preparation with osmotic dilators or prostaglandin analogs may be used to decrease the risk of cervical trauma. Medical management is often performed in the hospital setting and includes the use of one or more of the following: prostaglandin analogs, mifepristone, osmotic cervical dilators, Foley catheters, and oxytocin. Misoprostol, either alone or in combination with other agents, is recommended because of its high efficacy, low cost, and ease of use (ACOG, 2013). Oxytocin is not commonly used in the second trimester because of the inefficient response of the uterus during this gestational period. Surgical evacuation may be needed for retained POCs after medical management. Medical management or intact D&E may be preferable when autopsy is desired.

## Follow-up Care

Women diagnosed with pregnancy loss should be scheduled for follow-up appointments, and passage of the pregnancy should be confirmed. After surgical evacuation, POCs should be sent for histopathologic examination. Placental villi may be visualized, confirming intrauterine pregnancy. For women who pass the POCs spontaneously or with medication, pelvic ultrasound may be performed to document the absence and presumed passage of a previously seen gestational sac. Endometrial thickness may be measured; however, there is no defined criteria for an empty uterus. **Serum** β-hCG values may be followed and typically return to normal within 2 to 6 weeks after a completed loss. If the β-hCG level does not return to undetectable, women should be evaluated for retained POCs, an undiagnosed ectopic pregnancy, or a gestational trophoblastic disease. Menses typically resumes within 6 weeks. Rarely IUAs may occur after surgical evacuation of the uterus, and in its severe form, menses may not resume.

**Some patients may benefit from grief counseling**. Grieving and depression are common after pregnancy loss. Women may complain of fatigue, anorexia, sleeplessness, and somatic symptoms such as headache and back pain. If symptoms of depression are apparent, then counseling and therapy with antidepressants should be pursued. Open-ended questions are the best way to assess a patient's mood and status. Many women experience guilt after pregnancy loss, believing that the loss was caused by an action that they performed. In fact, one study found that 80% of women had guilt associated with a particular act or habit that was perceived as causing the pregnancy loss (Bardos, 2015). Most commonly believed causes of pregnancy loss were stress (76%), lifting a heavy object (64%), prior IUD use (28%), and prior oral contractive use (22%). It is important to dispel these beliefs to reassure patients their actions or habits did not cause the loss.

Potential causes of the pregnancy loss and future pregnancy planning should also be discussed at the follow-up visit. **There is no compelling evidence showing that delaying conception after an early pregnancy loss decreases subsequent pregnancy loss risk.** In an observational study of nearly 1100 women with a history of pregnancy loss, women who tried to conceive within 0 to 3 months of a loss were more likely to conceive and achieve live birth (53% vs. 36%) compared with women who waited more than 3 months to attempt conception (Schliep, 2016). If another pregnancy is not desired, hormonal-based contraception may be initiated immediately after completion of the early pregnancy loss if appropriate.

Testing for RPL may be performed after two first-trimester pregnancy losses. Given the heightened anxiety, couples with RPL often request "any possible cure." The clinician is all too commonly requested "to try anything." Thus couples with RPL are all too often offered treatment not supported by data. When treating patients with RPL, practitioners should provide empathy and understanding while guiding families through this difficult time using the best evidence available.

### Acknowledgment

The authors would like to acknowledge the contributions of Sanaz Keyhan, Lisa Muasher, and Suheil J. Muasher for their work on the previous edition of this chapter; some of their work has been retained here.

### KEY REFERENCES

Abalovich M, Mitelberg L, Allami C, Gutierrez S, Alcaraz G, Otero P, et al. Subclinical hypothyroidism and thyroid autoimmunity in women with infertility. *Gynecol Endocrinol.* 2007;23(5):279-283.

Achiron R, Tadmor O, Mashiach S. Heart rate as a predictor of first-trimester spontaneous abortion after ultrasound-proven viability. *Obstet Gynecol.* 1991;78(3 Pt 1):330-334.

Acunzo G, Guida M, Pellicano M, et al. Effectiveness of auto-cross-linked hyaluronic acid gel in the prevention of intrauterine adhesions after hysteroscopic adhesiolysis: a prospective, randomized, controlled study. *Hum Reprod.* 2003;18:1918-1921.

American College of Obstetricians and Gynecologists Women's Health Care Physicians (ACOG). ACOG Committee on Genetics. Committee Opinion No 581: the use of chromosomal microarray analysis in prenatal diagnosis. *Obstet Gyncol.* 2013;122:1374-1377.

American College of Obstetricians and Gynecologists Women's Health Care Physicians (ACOG). ACOG Practice Bulletin No. 135: second-trimester abortion. *Obstet Gynecol.* 2013;121(6):1394-1406.

American College of Obstetricians and Gynecologists Women's Health Care Physicians (ACOG). ACOG Practice Bulletin No. 138: inherited thrombophilias in pregnancy. *Obstet Gynecol.* 2013;122(3):706-717.

American College of Obstetricians and Gynecologists Women's Health Care Physicians (ACOG). ACOG Practice Bulletin No. 200: early pregnancy loss. *Obstet Gynecol.* 2018;132(5)e197-e207.

Armstrong BG, McDonald AD, Sloan M. Cigarette, alcohol, and coffee consumption and spontaneous abortion. *Am J Public Health.* 1992;82(1): 85-87.

Atik RB, Christiansen OB, Elson J, et al. ESHRE guideline: recurrent pregnancy loss. *Hum Reprod Open.* 2018;2:1-12.

Baird DD, Dunson DB, Hill MC, et al. High cumulative incidence of uterine leiomyoma in black and white women: ultrasound evidence. *Am J Obstet Gynecol.* 2003;188:100.

Bardos J, Hercz D, Friedenthal J, et al. A national survey on public perceptions of miscarriage. *Obstet Gynecol.* 2015;125:1313.

Barel O, Krakov A, Pansky M, et al. Intrauterine adhesions after hysteroscopic treatment for retained products of conception: what are the risk factors? *Fertil Steril.* 2015;103:775-779.

Barnhart KT. Early pregnancy failure: beware of the pitfalls of modern management. *Fertil Steril.* 2012;98(5):1061-1065.

Bates SM, Greer IA, Middeldorp S, et al. VTE, thrombophilia, antithrombotic therapy, and pregnancy: Antithrombotic Therapy and Prevention of Thrombosis, 9th ed: American College of Chest Physicians Evidence-Based Clinical Practice Guidelines. *Chest.* 2012;141:e691S.

Bates SM, Middeldorp S, Rodger M, James AH, Greer I. Guidance for the treatment and prevention of obstetric-associated venous thromboembolism. *J Thromb Thrombolysis.* 2016;41(1):92-128.

Bhandari S, Ganguly I, Agarwal P, et al. Effect of myomectomy on endometrial cavity: a prospective study of 51 cases. *J Hum Reprod Sci.* 2016; 9:107-111.

Boots CE, Stephenson MD. Does obesity increase the risk of miscarriage in spontaneous conception: a systematic review. *Semin Reprod Med.* 2011;29(6):507-513.
Boots CE, Bernardi LA, Stephenson MD. Frequency of euploid miscarriage is increased in obese women with recurrent early pregnancy loss. *Fertil Steril.* 2014;102(2):455-459.
Bosteels J, Weyers S, Kasius J, et al. Anti-adhesion therapy following operative hysteroscopy for treatment of female subfertility. *Cochrane Database Syst Rev.* 2015;(11):CD011110.
Brent RL, Christian MS, Diener RM. Evaluation of the reproductive and developmental risks of caffeine. *Birth Defects Res B Dev Reprod Toxicol.* 2011;92:152.
Buttram VC Jr, Reiter RC. Uterine leiomyomata: etiology, symptomatology, and management. *Fertil Steril.* 1981;36:433-445.
Choi BC, Polgar K, Xiao L, Hill JA. Progesterone inhibits in-vitro embryotoxic Th1 cytokine production to trophoblast in women with recurrent pregnancy loss. *Hum Reprod.* 2000;15(Suppl 1):46.
Clifford K, Rai R, Regan L. Future pregnancy outcome in unexplained recurrent first trimester miscarriage. *Hum Reprod.* 1997;12(2):387-389.
Cnattingius S, Signorello LB, Annerén G, et al. Caffeine intake and the risk of first-trimester spontaneous abortion. *N Engl J Med.* 2000; 343(25):1839-1845.
Cohain JS, Buxbaum RE, Mankuta D. Spontaneous first trimester miscarriage rates per woman among parous women with 1 or more pregnancies of 24 weeks or more. *BMC Pregnancy Childbirth.* 2017;17:437.
Connolly A, Ryan DH, Stuebe AM, Wolfe HM. Reevaluation of discriminatory and threshold levels for serum β-hCG in early pregnancy. *Obstet Gynecol.* 2013;121:65.
Coomarasamy A, Williams H, Truchanowicz E, et al. A randomized trial of progesterone in women with recurrent miscarriages. *N Engl J Med.* 2015;373:2141.
Coomarasamy A, Devall AJ, Cheed V, et al. A randomized trial of progesterone in women with bleeding in early pregnancy. *N Engl J Med.* 2019;380:1815.
Dalton VK, Harris L, Weisman CS, et al. Patient preferences, satisfaction, and resource use in office evacuation of early pregnancy failure. *Obstet Gynecol.* 2006;108:103.
Daniel S, Koren G, Lunenfeld E, et al. Fetal exposure to nonsteroidal anti-inflammatory drugs and spontaneous abortions. *CMAJ.* 2014;186: E177.

**Full References for this chapter can be found on ExpertConsult.com.**

# 17 Ectopic Pregnancy

## Etiology, Pathology, Diagnosis, Management, Fertility Prognosis

*Hye-Chun Hur, Roger A. Lobo*

KEY POINTS

- The rate of ectopic pregnancy in the United States has remained fairly constant since the early 2000s and is approximately 6.6 in 1000 pregnancies in women aged 15 to 24.
- Risks of ectopic pregnancy include age, smoking, pelvic inflammatory disease, infertility, and prior tubal surgery. After tubal sterilization, the risk of ectopic pregnancy if a pregnancy occurs is about 30%, reaching 50% if the sterilization technique was tubal desiccation.
- Human chorionic gonadotropin (HCG) trends can help diagnose ectopic pregnancies. About 85% of women with an ectopic pregnancy have serum HCG levels lower than in normal pregnancy. In early pregnancy the normal HCG doubling time is 1.4 to 3 days, with 85% of pregnancies demonstrating a 66% HCG increase every 48 hours. An HCG rise less than 53% in 48 hours is 99% sensitive for an abnormal pregnancy.
- Ectopic pregnancies can be managed surgically with salpingectomy or salpingostomy. Randomized trial data suggest there is no difference in overall subsequent pregnancy outcomes between women who are treated by salpingostomy versus salpingectomy.
- Asymptomatic persistent ectopic pregnancy can be treated expectantly or with methotrexate (MTX). The success of MTX depends on the size and age of the gestation and the initial HCG level. After the methotrexate injection, the HCG level should fall at least 15% between days 4 and 7 and at least 15% weekly thereafter.

**Ectopic pregnancy** occurs when the fertilized ovum/developing blastocyst implants at a site outside the endometrial cavity. It was probably first described in the year 963 by Albucasis, an Arab writer. In 1876, before the initiation of surgical therapy, the mortality rate from ectopic pregnancy was estimated to be 60%. The first successful operative treatment of ectopic pregnancy was performed in 1883 by Lawson Tait in England. In 1887, he reported that he had performed salpingectomy on four women with ectopic pregnancy and that they all survived.

## EPIDEMIOLOGY

**The incidence of ectopic pregnancy has been estimated to be between 1% to 2% of all pregnancies.** Although the incidence of ectopic pregnancy increased sixfold between 1970 and 1992, it has remained stable since then. In the United States in 1989, the annual ectopic pregnancy rate per 10,000 women aged 15 to 44 was 15.5, similar to that in Finland but higher than the rate in France. The last national data reported by the Centers for Disease Control and Prevention (CDC) showed that **the overall incidence of ectopic pregnancy had plateaued to approximately 20 in 1000 pregnancies** in the early 1990s. The current incidence of ectopic pregnancy is difficult to estimate from available hospitalization and insurance records because the number of ectopic pregnancy cases requiring inpatient hospital treatment has decreased. The incidence varies among different countries, with rates as high as 1 in 28 and 1 in 40 pregnancies reported in Jamaica and Vietnam, respectively. The risk of ectopic pregnancy associated with assisted reproductive technology is increased compared with the general population, with rates from 0.8% to 8.6%. **Data from the National Assisted Reproductive Technology Surveillance System from 2001 to 2011 showed that the rate of ectopic pregnancy declined from 2% to 1.6%** out of 553,577 pregnancies in the United States (Perkins, 2015).

There has been an increasing trend toward treating ectopic pregnancy conservatively (without resorting to salpingectomy) and on an ambulatory basis without overnight hospitalization. With earlier detection of ectopic pregnancy, a steadily increasing percentage of women with this problem are now being treated before tubal rupture occurs, by outpatient laparoscopic procedures or by medical treatment with methotrexate. An analysis of both hospital discharge data and an ambulatory medical care survey revealed that the estimated number of hospitalizations for ectopic pregnancy in the United States declined from nearly 90,000 in 1989 to about 45,000 in 1994. However, in 1992, about half of all women with ectopic pregnancy in the United States were treated as outpatients, and the estimated number of total ectopic pregnancies in this year was 108,000, for a rate of 19.7 per 1000 reported pregnancies. Thus in the United States in 1992, about 2 of every 100 women who were known to conceive had an ectopic gestation. The increased incidence of ectopic pregnancy is thought to be due to two factors: (1) the increased incidence of salpingitis, caused by increased infection with *Chlamydia trachomatis* or other sexually transmitted pathogens; and (2) improved diagnostic techniques, which enable the diagnosis of unruptured ectopic pregnancy with more precision and earlier in gestation, before asymptomatic resolution of the pregnancy occurs.

**The rate of ectopic pregnancy increases with increasing age.** However, because of the lower pregnancy rate in older women, overall only about 11% of ectopic pregnancies in the United States occur in women aged 35 to 44, whereas more than half, 58%, occur in women aged 25 to 34 years. Most ectopic pregnancies occur in multigravid women. Only 10% to 15% of ectopic pregnancies occur in nulligravid women, whereas more than half occur in women who have been pregnant three or more times. In the United States, the rates of ectopic pregnancy are similar in each section of the country, but the rates are higher for nonwhite women compared with white women. About 3% of all reported pregnancies in nonwhite women aged 35 to 44 in the United States are ectopic.

## MORTALITY

Even with the increased use of surgery and blood transfusions and earlier diagnosis, **ectopic pregnancy remains a major cause of maternal death in the United States today.** From the last CDC report, **6% of pregnancy-related mortality during the period of 1991 to 1999 was due to ectopic pregnancies.** In the United States, 876 deaths were attributed to ectopic pregnancy between 1980 and 2007. Ectopic pregnancy is the most common cause of maternal death in the first half of pregnancy. The ectopic pregnancy–to–mortality ratio has declined by 57% from the period 1980 to 1984 to 2003 to 2007, from 1.15 to 0.5 (Creanga, 2011). The mortality ratio was 6.8 times higher for African American women than for white women and 3.5 times higher for women older than 35 years compared with women younger than 25 years. Of the 76 deaths among women hospitalized with ectopic pregnancy between 1998 and 2007, 70% of the ectopic pregnancies were located in the fallopian tubes. Unmarried women of all races have a 1.7 times greater chance of dying of ectopic pregnancy than married women. **Overall the risk of death from ectopic pregnancy is about 10 times greater than the risk of childbirth and more than 50 times greater than the risk of legal abortion.**

The major cause of mortality from ectopic pregnancy is blood loss. Most cases of mortality (70%) result from gestations in the tube, and the other 30% are interstitial cornual or abdominal gestations. Because the overall incidence of ectopic pregnancy occurring in these latter locations is slightly less than 4%, interstitial and abdominal ectopic pregnancies have about a five times greater risk of being fatal. About three-fourths of the women with fatal ectopic pregnancies initially developed symptoms and died in the first 12 weeks of gestation. Of the remaining one-fourth who developed symptoms and died after the first-trimester, 70% had interstitial or abdominal pregnancies. Patient delay in consulting a physician after development of symptoms accounted for one-third of the deaths, whereas treatment delay resulting from misdiagnosis contributed to the half the deaths.

## ETIOLOGY

### Factors Contributing to the Risk

**The major factor contributing to the risk of ectopic pregnancy is *salpingitis*.** Salpingitis results from infectious causes such as pelvic inflammatory disease (PID) or inflammatory causes such as endometriosis. Its morphologic sequelae account for about half of the initial episodes of ectopic pregnancy. However, **in about 40% of cases the cause cannot be determined** and is presumed to be a physiologic disorder resulting from the delay of passage of the embryo into the uterine cavity. Ovulation from the contralateral ovary has been implicated as a cause of the delay of blastocyst transport, and it has been suggested that contralateral ovulation occurs in about one-third of tubal pregnancies, although this has not been confirmed.

Another possibility in the etiology of ectopic pregnancy is a hormonal imbalance; an elevated circulating level of either estrogen or progesterone can alter normal tubal contractility. An **increased rate of ectopic pregnancies has been reported in women who conceive with physiologically and pharmacologically elevated levels of progestogens.** The latter condition can be produced locally with a progestogen-releasing intrauterine device (IUD) and systemically with progestin-only oral contraceptives. Iatrogenic, physiologically increased levels of estrogen and progesterone occur after ovulation induction and the use of assisted reproductive technology (ART) with either **clomiphene citrate or human menopausal gonadotropins, and an increased rate of ectopic pregnancies has been reported in women conceiving after each of these treatment modalities.**

Another possible cause is an abnormality of embryonic development. Although aneuploidy has been found to be prevalent in ectopic pregnancies, it may not be higher than the normal rate of aneuploidy and is unlikely to be a cause of ectopic pregnancies. Inherited genetic abnormalities most probably are not a cause of ectopic pregnancy either. Also, there is no increased incidence of ectopic pregnancy among first-degree relatives.

Several epidemiologic studies have indicated that **cigarette smoking is associated with about a twofold increased risk of ectopic pregnancy,** even when the data were controlled for the presence of other risk factors. The risk of ectopic pregnancy was directly related to the number of cigarettes smoked per day, with a fourfold increased risk noted among women who smoked 30 or more cigarettes per day. Known risk factors for ectopic pregnancy, presented as odds ratios and attributable risk, are depicted in Table 17.1 (Bouyer, 2003).

The major causes of ectopic pregnancy are discussed in more detail next.

**TABLE 17.1** Odds Ratios for Ectopic Pregnancy (Compared With Women With Recent Successful Pregnancies) and the Attributable Risks Associated With Different Risk Factors

| | Odds Ratio | Attributable Risk* |
|---|---|---|
| Probable salpingitis | 2 | |
| Confirmed salpingitis | 3.5 | |
| History of tubal surgery | 3.5 | 0.18† |
| Smoking | | 0.35 |
| Ex-smoker | 1.5 | |
| 1-9 cigarettes per day | 2 | |
| 10-19 cigarettes per day | 3 | |
| ≥20 cigarettes per day | 4 | |
| Age (years) | | 0.14 |
| 30-39 | 1.5 | |
| ≥40 | 3 | |
| Spontaneous abortion | 3 | 0.07 |
| Elective abortion | 2 | 0.03 |
| IUD history | 1.5 | 0.05 |
| Previous infertility | 2.5 | 0.18 |

From Fernandez H, Gervaise A. Ectopic pregnancies after infertility treatment: modern diagnosis and therapeutic strategy. *Hum Reprod Update.* 2004;10(6):503-513.

Odds ratios for ectopic pregnancy (compared with deliveries) and attributable risks of the principal risk factors.

*IUD, Intrauterine device.*

*From Auvergne registry data (Bouyer J, Coste J, Shojaei T, et al. Risk factors for ectopic pregnancy: a comprehensive analysis based on a large case-control, population-based study in France. *Am J Epidemiol.* 2003;157:185).

†Risk attributable to history of genital infection and tubal surgery together is 0.33.

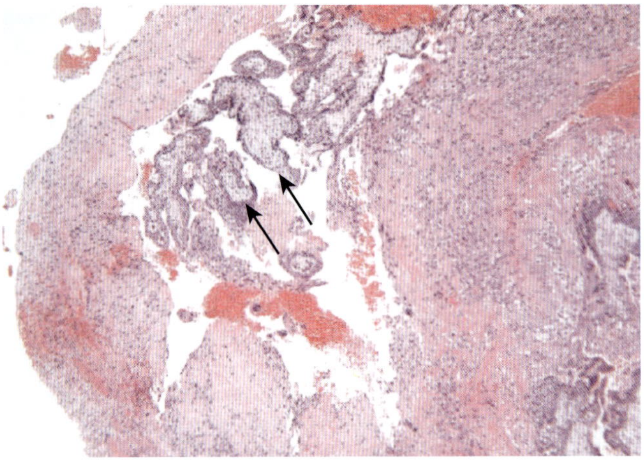

**Fig. 17.1** Histologic results of ectopic pregnancy. Note the trophoblastic tissue *(arrows)* in the fallopian tube lumen. (Modified from www.imagingpathways.health.wa.gov.au.)

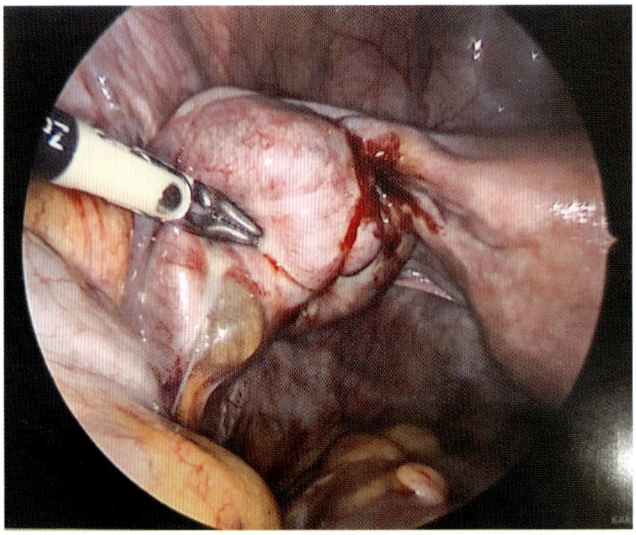

**Fig. 17.2** Left ovarian endometrioma behind clubbed left tube with hydrosalpinx and adjacent bowel adhesions.

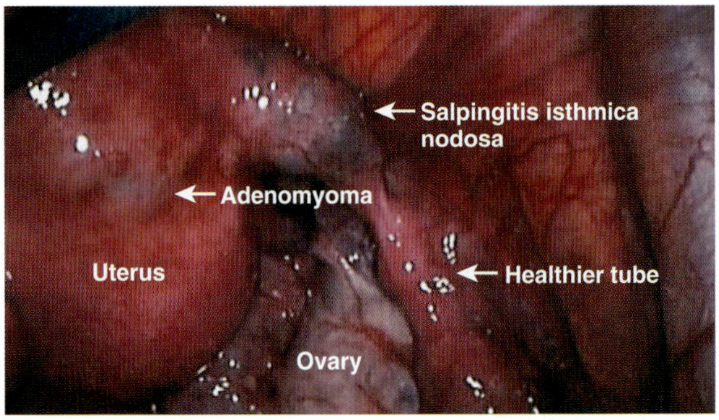


**Fig. 17.3** Laparoscopic view of salpingitis isthmica nodosa in the isthmic tube and cornual regions of the uterus. Note the normal distal tube. (From www.dan martinmd.com.)

## Tubal Pathology Leading to Ectopic Risk

Disruption of normal tubal anatomy from infection, surgery, congenital anomalies, or inflammatory disease such as endometriosis is a major cause of ectopic pregnancy. The agglutination of the plicae (folds) of the endosalpinx produced by salpingitis can allow passage of sperm but prevent the normal transport of the larger morula. The morula can be trapped in blind pockets formed by adhesions of the endosalpinx. In their 20-year longitudinal study, Weström and colleagues found that nearly half (45.3%) of the women with ectopic pregnancy had a clinical history or histologic findings of a prior episode of acute salpingitis (Weström, 1981). This is in agreement with the 40% incidence of prior salpingitis found on histologic examination by several groups of investigators in women with ectopic pregnancy (Fig. 17.1).

Weström and colleagues prospectively followed 900 women aged 15 to 34 years who had laparoscopically confirmed acute salpingitis and found that the subsequent ectopic pregnancy rate was 68.8 per 1000 conceptions, yielding **a sixfold increase in the risk of ectopic pregnancy**. The risk of ectopic pregnancy after acute salpingitis increased both with the number of episodes of infection and with the increasing age of the women at the time of infection. The odds ratios for ectopic pregnancy after two and after three or more episodes of chlamydial infection were 2.1 and 4.5, respectively. Data also suggest that a history of chlamydial infection results in the production of PROKR2 protein, which creates a microenvironment that predisposes to tubal implantation.

### Endometriosis

Inflammation and adhesions of the fallopian tubes as a result of conditions such as endometriosis are risk factors for ectopic pregnancy. Fig. 17.2 portrays an example of endometriosis resulting in a left ovarian endometrioma, tubal inflammation, and adhesions, with subsequent clubbed tube and hydrosalpinx. Compared with women without endometriosis, women with endometriosis had two times the risk for ectopic pregnancy (relative risk, 1.9; 95% confidence interval [CI], 1.8 to 2.1) (Hjordt Hansen, 2014).

### Salpingitis Isthmica Nodosa

Salpingitis isthmica nodosa (SIN) is defined as the microscopic presence of tubal epithelium within the myosalpinx or beneath the tubal serosa (Fig. 17.3). In two histopathologic studies of tubes removed from women with ectopic pregnancy, it was found that about half contained lesions of SIN compared with 5% in a control group. With serial sectioning, it has been determined that **SIN is actually a diverticulum or intrauterine extension of the tubal lumen**. Associated histologic evidence of chronic salpingitis was seen in only 6% of the tubes, suggesting that **SIN was not necessarily the result of infection**. The **tubal pregnancy** has been found to have usually implanted in a portion of the tube distal to the SIN, indicating that **mechanical entrapment of the morula is not the mechanism whereby SIN causes tubal gestation.** It is possible that SIN itself or the associated tubal anomalies may be responsible for dysfunction of the tubal transport mechanism without anatomic obstruction.

It is likely that adhesions between the tubal serosa and bowel or peritoneum may interfere with normal tubal motility and cause ectopic pregnancy because, as reported, 17% to 27% of women with ectopic pregnancy have had previous abdominal surgical procedures not involving the oviduct. On the other hand, neither endometriosis nor congenital anomalies of the tube have been associated with an increased incidence of ectopic pregnancy.

### Tubal Surgery

An operative procedure on the tube itself is a cause of ectopic pregnancy whether the tube is morphologically normal, as occurs with sterilization procedures, or abnormal, as occurs with post salpingitis reconstructive surgery. **The incidence of ectopic pregnancy occurring after salpingoplasty or salpingostomy procedures to treat distal tubal disease ranges from 15% to 25%,** probably because the damage to the endosalpinx remains. The rate of ectopic pregnancy after reversal of sterilization procedures is lower, about 4%, because the tubes have not been damaged by infection. The rate of ectopic pregnancy after sterilization is discussed later in this chapter.

### History of Ectopic Pregnancy

Women who have had a prior ectopic pregnancy, even if treated medically or by unilateral salpingectomy, are at increased risk for having a subsequent ectopic pregnancy. **The odds of a recurrent ectopic pregnancy among women with history of ectopic pregnancy compared with other pregnant women is almost threefold greater (adjusted odds ratio [AOR], 2.72; 95% CI 1.66 to 2.8)** (Li, 2015). Of women who conceive after having one ectopic pregnancy, about **25% of subsequent pregnancies are ectopic.** The **rates of recurrent ectopic pregnancy after single-dose methotrexate treatment, salpingectomy, and linear salpingostomy are 8%, 9.8%, and 15.4%,** respectively, among women who conceive (Yao, 1997).

### Diethylstilbestrol Exposure

Although it is less commonly encountered today, the incidence of ectopic gestation is significantly greater (four to five times) in women who have been exposed to diethylstilbestrol (DES) in utero and has been reported at the rate of 4% to 5%. This is likely because of abnormal tubal morphology and impaired function of the fimbriae. In women exposed to DES whose hysterosalpingograms demonstrated abnormalities in the uterine cavity, the ectopic pregnancy rate was as high as 13%.

## Contraception Failure

## Tubal Sterilization

For several decades, sterilization has been the most popular method of contraception used by couples in the United States. Since the development of laparoscopic surgery, female tubal sterilization is performed about twice as often as vasectomy. In an analysis of the long-term risk of pregnancy after tubal sterilization reported by Peterson and coworkers, **it was found that within 10 years after the procedure, the cumulative life table probability of pregnancy was 1.85%.** The 10-year failure rate after bipolar electrosurgical sterilization of the tubes was 2.48%, which rose to 5.43% if the sterilization procedure was performed when the woman was younger than 28 years. These investigators reported that for all 143 pregnancies occurring after tubal sterilization, 43 (30.1%) were ectopic pregnancies (Peterson, 1997).

Several investigators have reported that if pregnancy occurred after tubal sterilization with electrosurgical devices (monopolar or bipolar instruments), the ectopic pregnancy rate was as high as 50%. It has been hypothesized that fistulas may develop, allowing sperm to pass into the distal segment of the oviduct and fertilize the egg (Fig. 17.4) (Corson, 1986). Such fistulas can be demonstrated radiographically in about 11% of women after laparoscopic electrosurgical sterilization. Peterson and colleagues reported that within 10 years after the sterilization procedure, women sterilized with bipolar devices had twice as many ectopic pregnancies compared with those sterilized with metal clips or silicone bands. The overall ectopic pregnancy rate after bipolar sterilization was 1.7%.

Because about one-third of pregnancies that occur after all tubal sterilizations are ectopic, women should be counseled that if they do not experience the expected menses at any time after tubal sterilization before menopause, a test to detect human chorionic gonadotropin (HCG) should be performed rapidly, and if they are pregnant, a diagnostic evaluation to exclude the presence of ectopic pregnancy is necessary. In women who have an ectopic pregnancy after sterilization with the use of electrosurgery, because the site of the fistula usually cannot be determined clinically, salpingectomies should be carried out.

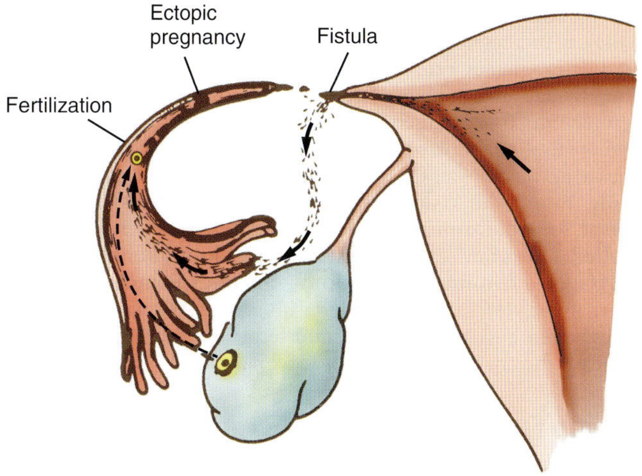


**Fig. 17.4** Mechanism of ectopic pregnancy after sterilization. (From Corson SL, Batzer FR. Ectopic pregnancy: a review of the etiologic factors. *J Reprod Med.* 1986;31:78.)

More often tubal sterilizations are now completed with bilateral salpingectomies. Compared with bipolar electrosurgical sterilization, in which a portion of the tube is desiccated, bilateral salpingectomies offer complete removal of the fallopian tube. This offers several advantages, including reduced risk of post-tubal fistula formation, diminished risk of tubal stump ectopic pregnancy, decreased risk of poststerilization hydrosalpinx. and opportunistic salpingectomies, which decrease one's lifetime risk of ovarian cancer (Clark, 2018).

## Intrauterine Device

In general, individuals using contraception have a lower incidence of ectopic pregnancy compared with those not using contraception because the likelihood of conceiving is lower. Among contraceptive failures, women using diaphragms or combination oral contraceptives do not have an increased risk of ectopic pregnancy, whereas contraceptive failures with the IUD lead to an increased risk of ectopic pregnancy. **Among IUD contraceptive failures, the risk of ectopic pregnancy is approximately 6% for the copper IUD versus 50% for the levonorgestrel IUD (Backman, 2004).** This is because the progestogen-releasing IUD inhibits tubal contractions, resulting in a higher ectopic rate than the copper IUD. Women who use this method of contraception have about twice the risk of ectopic pregnancy (7.5 per 1000 woman-years) if they conceive compared with women who use no method of contraception (3.5 per 1000 woman-years). Women using IUDs who elect to have their pregnancies terminated should have a histologic examination of the tissue removed from the uterine cavity to be certain the pregnancy was intrauterine.

## Hormonal Alterations

## Ovarian Stimulation

As occurs with exogenous progesterone administration, if increased levels of exogenous or endogenous estrogens are present shortly after the time of ovulation, the incidence of ectopic pregnancy is increased. Several investigators have reported that the ectopic pregnancy rate is about 1.5% for conceptions that occur after ovulation has been induced with clomiphene citrate. The ectopic rate in pregnancies occurring after ovulation with human menopausal gonadotropins (HMGs) has been reported to range between 3% and 4%. Fernandez and colleagues, in a case-control study, found the **risk of ectopic pregnancy was increased about fourfold among ovulatory women treated with controlled ovarian hyperstimulation—clomiphene citrate, HMG, or a combination of both—for unexplained infertility** (Fernandez, 1991). These reports indicate that increased levels of estrogen and progesterone interfere with tubal motility and increase the chance of an ectopic pregnancy.

## In Vitro Fertilization

Ectopics occur more often after in vitro fertilization and embryo transfer. The reason for this increased incidence likely is due to one or more of several factors: increased sex steroid hormone levels, the presence of proximal tubal disease (although the ratio is similar in women with normal tubes), and flushing an embryo directly into the tube. Data from the National ART Surveillance System identified that **1.7% of more than 550,000 pregnancies were ectopic** between the period of 2001 and 2011. The ectopic pregnancy rate was also noted to be associated with multiple embryo transfer. **The rate of ectopic pregnancy was 1.6% when one embryo was transferred compared with 1.7%, 2.2%, and 2.5% when two, three, or four or more embryos were transferred,** respectively (Perkins, 2015).

# SITES OF ECTOPIC PREGNANCY

Most ectopic pregnancies occur in the tube. In Breen's series and more recent series (Bouyer, 2002; Breen, 1970), 97.7% of the ectopic pregnancies were tubal, 1.4% were abdominal, and less than 1% were ovarian or cervical (Fig. 17.5). **The majority of tubal pregnancies, 70% to 81%, were located in the ampullary portion of the tube**, being about equally divided between the distal and middle third of the tube. About 12% of tubal gestations occur in the isthmus and 5% to 11% in the fimbrial region. Although Breen considered pregnancies located in the cornual area of the uterus to be uterine in origin, they are in fact pregnancies implanted in the interstitial portion of the tube. **About 2% of all ectopic pregnancies are interstitial, and these are often associated with severe morbidity** because they become symptomatic later in the gestation, are difficult to diagnose, and often produce massive hemorrhage when they rupture (Fig. 17.6) (Bolaji, 2010). A true **cornual pregnancy** is one located in the rudimentary horn of a bicornuate uterus, which is quite rare. In a review of 240 true cornual pregnancies reported by O'Leary and O'Leary, about 90% of them ruptured with massive hemorrhage (O'Leary, 1963).

**About 1 in 200 ectopic pregnancies are true ovarian pregnancies.** The four criteria that fulfill the diagnosis of ovarian pregnancy originally described by Spiegelburg are as follows:

1. The tube and fimbria must be intact and separate from the ovary.
2. The gestational sac must occupy the normal position of the ovary.
3. The sac must be connected to the uterus by the ovarian ligament.
4. Ovarian tissue should be demonstrable in the walls of the sac.

Many women with ovarian pregnancies are believed to have a ruptured corpus luteum cyst, and the correct diagnosis was made during the surgical procedure only 28% of the time. The hemorrhagic mass (ovarian ectopic) should be located adjacent to the corpus luteum, never within it. Ovarian pregnancy is also associated with profuse hemorrhage, with 81% of reported to have a **hemoperitoneum** greater than 500 mL. Nevertheless, most can be successfully treated by ovarian resection and not oophorectomy.

**Most abdominal pregnancies occur secondary to tubal abortion with secondary implantation in the peritoneal cavity** (Fig. 17.7). On rare occasions a primary abdominal pregnancy may occur, and all of the following three criteria originally set forth by Studdiford must be present:

1. The tubes and ovaries must be normal, with no evidence of recent or past injury.
2. There must be no evidence of a uteroplacental fistula.

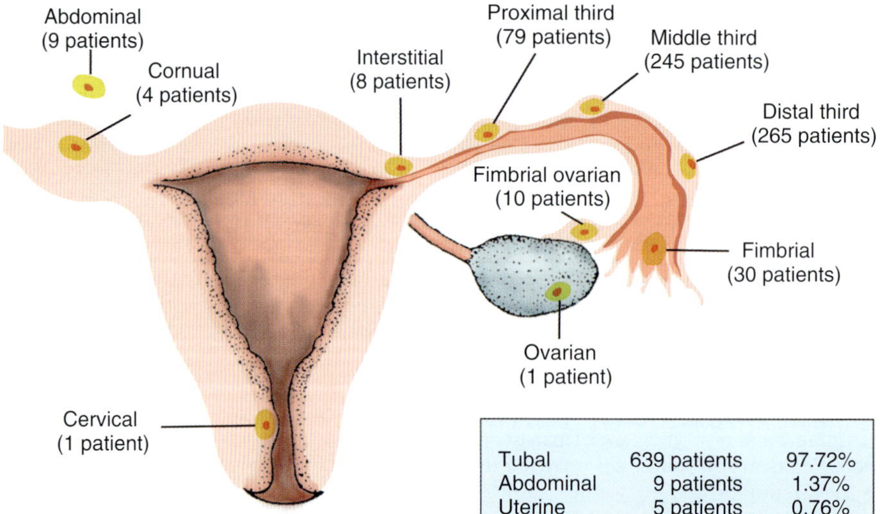


| | | |
|---|---|---|
| Tubal | 639 patients | 97.72% |
| Abdominal | 9 patients | 1.37% |
| Uterine | 5 patients | 0.76% |
| Ovarian | 1 patient | 0.15% |
| Total | 654 patients | 100.00% |

**Fig. 17.5** Anatomic sites of ectopic pregnancy. (From Breen JL. A 21 year survey of 654 ectopic pregnancies. *Am J Obstet Gynecol.* 1970;106:1004.)

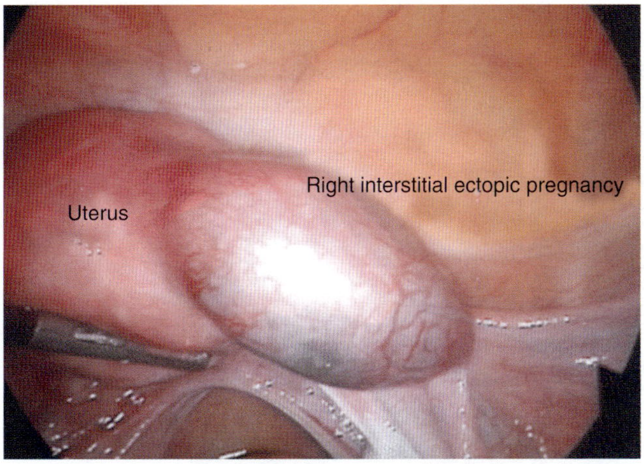


**Fig. 17.6** Right interstitial pregnancy at laparoscopy. (Modified from Bolaji I, Gupta S. Medical management of interstitial pregnancy with high beta selective human chorionic gonadotropin. *Ultrasound.* 2010;18(2):60-67.)

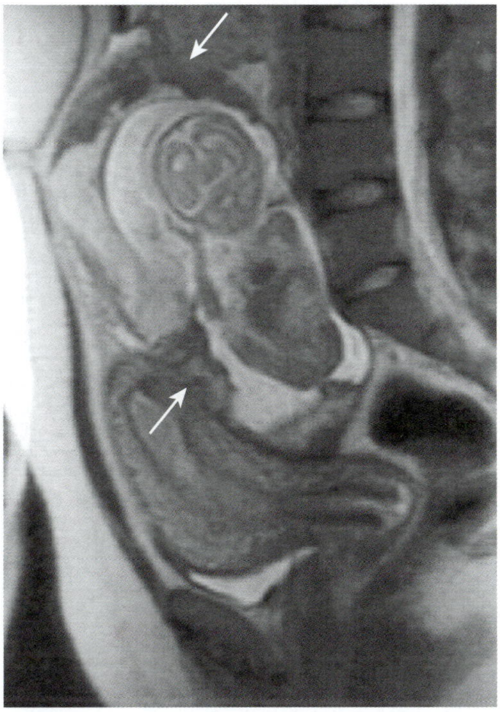

**Fig. 17.7** Magnetic resonance image of abdominal pregnancy showing placental infarction. Note the distance of the pregnancy from the uterus. (From https://www.researchgate.net/figure/MRI-of-advanced-intraligamentar-abdominal-pregnancy-Holzhacker-et-al-2008_fig4_221918569.)

3. The pregnancy must be related only to the peritoneal surface, and it must be early enough in gestation to eliminate the possibility of secondary implantation after primary tubal nidation (Studdiford, 1942).

An unusual type of primary abdominal pregnancy occurs when implantation is in the spleen or liver, producing massive intraperitoneal hemorrhage.

The prognosis for fetal survival in abdominal pregnancy is poor (11%) and is difficult to diagnose. Once the diagnosis is established, a laparotomy with removal of the fetus should be performed immediately to prevent a possible fatal hemorrhage. An adjunctive option is to administer methotrexate. On occasion, when the placenta is tightly adherent to bowel and blood vessels, it should be left in the abdominal cavity. In such instances the placental tissue usually resorbs. Retained placenta in the abdomen can lead to symptoms of abdominal pain and intermittent fever that may last for many months, as well as possible partial bowel obstruction and abscess formation. Therefore, if it is surgically feasible, removal of the entire placenta is the ideal goal. Furthermore, partial removal of the placenta may result in massive hemorrhage. Therefore, given all of these risks, it is important to carefully consider the best surgical approach because the decision making is challenging and critical.

The four pathologic criteria for the diagnosis of **cervical pregnancy** as reported by Rubin and colleagues are as follows (Fig. 17.8):

1. Cervical glands must be present opposite the placental attachment;
2. The attachment of the placenta to the cervix must be intimate;
3. The placenta must be below the entrance of the uterine vessels or below the peritoneal reflection of the anteroposterior surface of the uterus; and
4. Fetal elements must not be present in the corpus uteri.

The usual characteristic clinical findings of cervical pregnancy are uterine bleeding after amenorrhea without cramping pain, a softened cervix that is disproportionately enlarged, complete confinement and firm attachment of the products of conception to the endocervix, and a closed internal os.

**Most cervical pregnancies are associated with previous cervical or uterine surgery, such as curettage or cesarean delivery**. The differential diagnosis is difficult and includes incomplete abortion, placenta previa, carcinoma of the cervix, and a degenerating leiomyoma. Although cervical ectopic pregnancies previously have been associated with a high mortality because of massive hemorrhage, now, with better methods of diagnosis and treatment, death is rare. In the past, more than half of women with a cervical pregnancy required a hysterectomy for treatment, and this was nearly always necessary if the pregnancy had advanced beyond 18 weeks. There have been several case reports in which a cervical pregnancy was successfully treated by systemic methotrexate. Other case reports have shown that after angiographic uterine artery embolization, evacuation of the pregnancy can be easily performed transcervically with minimal blood loss. Transvaginal ultrasound–guided injections of potassium chloride directly into the gestational sac have successfully terminated pregnancies, as has the local injection of methotrexate, with or without uterine artery embolization.

**Cesarean scar ectopic pregnancy** is a rare but potentially serious complication of early pregnancy. In this type of ectopic pregnancy, the gestational sac is located in the previous cesarean scar and is surrounded by myometrium and connective tissue (Fig. 17.9). **It occurs in about 1 in 2000 pregnancies and 6% of ectopic pregnancies** among women with previous cesarean deliveries (Rotas, 2006). In a large series of 268 cesarean scar ectopic pregnancies, Sadeghi and colleagues reported four cases of uterine rupture, including one case of fetomaternal death at 38 weeks' gestation (Sadeghi, 2010). The incidence does not appear to correlate with the number of cesarean deliveries. It is believed that the mechanism for implantation is related to the migration of the embryo through a small defect in the previous incision site or a microscopic fistula within the scar. Adenomyosis, in vitro fertilization, previous dilation and curettage, and manual removal of the placenta are also reported as risk factors.

Another uncommon form of ectopic gestation is combined intrauterine and extrauterine (heterotopic) pregnancy (94% tubal and 6% ovarian). Heterotopic pregnancy is traditionally considered a rare occurrence, with an incidence between 1 in 16,000 or

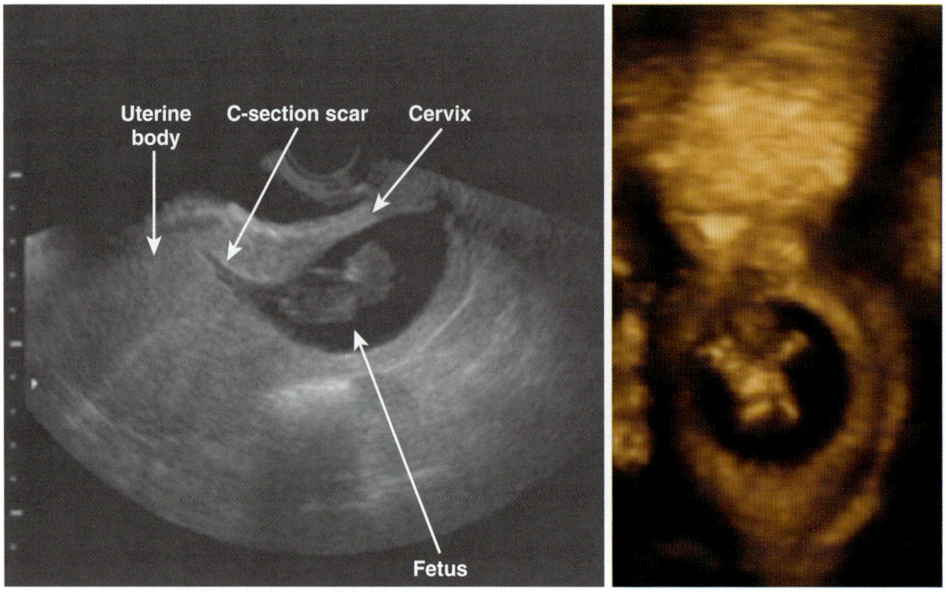


**Fig. 17.8** Cervical pregnancy as viewed by two-dimensional ultrasound *(left panel)*. Note the normal endometrium to the left of the gestational sac and the larger fetal pole. The right panel shows the same cervical ectopic on three-dimensional ultrasound. Note the ballooned-out cervix and narrowed uterine isthmus/lower segment above it. *C-section,* Cesarean section.

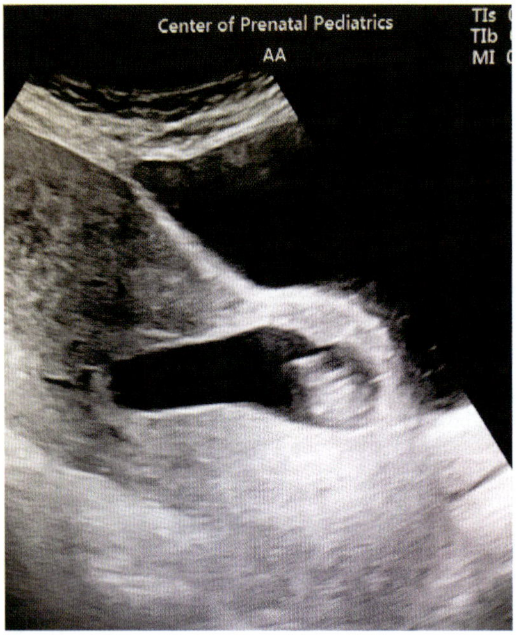


**Fig. 17.9** Ultrasound image of cesarean scar ectopic pregnancy.

1 in 30,000 pregnancies. With the increase of use of ovulation-inducing agents and ART, the overall incidence of heterotopic pregnancy has risen to approximately 1 in 3900 pregnancies. In a series of all registered ART pregnancies in the United States from 1999 to 2002, **the incidence of heterotopic pregnancy was 1.5 per 1000 ART pregnancies**. The incidence has been reported to be higher when tubal damage was present or when four or more embryos were transferred.

A **chronic ectopic pregnancy** occurs when the intraperitoneal hemorrhage associated with tubal abortion or rupture is relatively minor and ceases spontaneously, but the ectopic gestation neither resolves completely nor implants and continues to develop as an abdominal pregnancy. The trophoblast continues to secrete HCG in small amounts, with the circulating levels less than 1000 mIU/mL in 50% of cases and less than 100 mIU/mL in 20% of cases. In one series, about 6% of all surgically treated ectopic pregnancies in one institution were classified as chronic. The most common (72%) gross pathologic finding was dense adhesions produced by the inflammatory response to the trophoblast. These adhesions attach omentum and bowel to the site of the ectopic pregnancy. In one-third of the cases, a collection of clotted blood or old hematoma was present. It has been reported that because of the extensive disease, it was necessary to perform a hysterectomy in 25% of cases, and for chronic ovarian ectopic pregnancies, an oophorectomy was necessary in 60% of patients.

## HISTOPATHOLOGY

When the morula implants in the tube, it does not grow mainly in the tubal lumen as has been assumed for many years. A review of the pathology of tubal gestation found that after implanting on the mucosa of the endosalpinx, the trophoblast invaded the lamina propria and then the muscularis of the tube and grew mainly between the lumen of the tube and its peritoneal covering. Growth occurred both parallel to the long axis of the tube and circumferentially around it. As the trophoblast invades vessels, retroperitoneal tubal hemorrhage occurs that is mainly extraluminal but may extrude from the fimbriated end and create a hemoperitoneum before tubal rupture (Fig. 17.10) (Budowick, 1980).

The stretching of the peritoneum covered by this hemorrhage results in episodic pain before the final perforation into the peritoneal cavity. Rupture occurs when the serosa is maximally stretched, producing necrosis secondary to an inadequate blood supply.

Hemoperitoneum is nearly always found in advanced **ruptured ectopic pregnancy** other than that which is cervical in origin. Usually there is a combination of clotted and unclotted blood in the peritoneal cavity. The unclotted blood does not clot on removal from the peritoneal cavity because it originates from lysis of blood that has previously coagulated, similar to what occurs during menstrual bleeding. The hematocrit value of this nonclotting blood is nearly always greater than 15%, such a finding being reported in 98% of specimens obtained by **culdocentesis** in a series of ectopic pregnancies. Historically, at the time

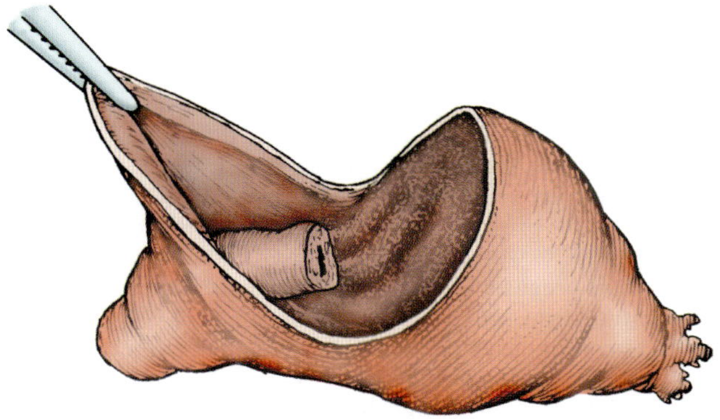

**Fig. 17.10** Artist's rendition of a dissected ampullary ectopic pregnancy showing space between the tube and the peritoneum, revealed when blood clots and placenta were removed. Toward the fimbriated end, no dissection was performed, and the external appearance is that of a dilated tube. (From Budowick M, Johnson TRB, Genadry R, et al. The histopathology of the developing tubal ectopic pregnancy. *Fertil Steril.* 1980;34:169. Courtesy The American Fertility Society.)

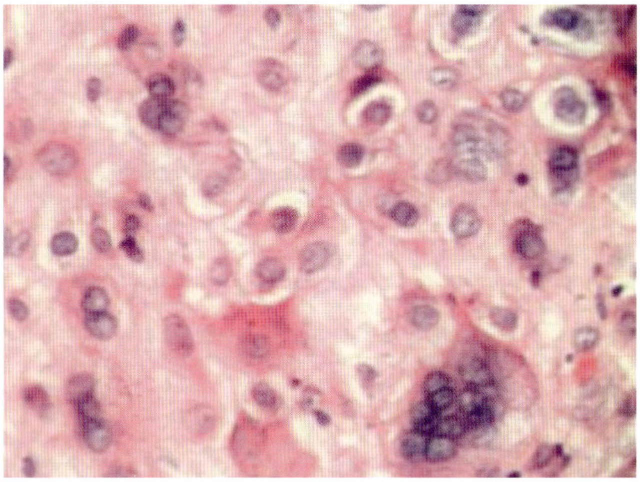

**Fig. 17.11** Histologic view of an Arias-Stella reaction. Note the enlarged secretory endometrial cells, which are hypertrophied, hyperchromatic, and pleomorphic. (From https://www.researchgate.net/figure/MRI-of-advanced-intraligamentar-abdominal-pregnancy-Holzhacker-et-al-2008_fig4_221918569.)

of laparotomy for a ruptured ectopic pregnancy, about half of the women have less than 500 mL of hemoperitoneum, one-fourth between 500 and 1000 mL, and one-fifth more than 1000 mL.

**When the tube is removed and examined histologically, inflammatory cells are nearly always seen**. These include plasma cells, lymphocytes, and histiocytes. The presence of chorionic villi, which are often degenerated or hyalinized, and nucleated red cells establish the diagnosis of ectopic pregnancy. Decidual reaction in the tube is uncommon.

Because of limited space or inadequate nourishment, **the trophoblastic tissue of most ectopic pregnancies does not grow as rapidly as that of pregnancies within the uterine cavity**. As a result, HCG production does not increase as rapidly as in a normal pregnancy, and although steroid production of the corpus luteum is initiated, elevated progesterone levels cannot be maintained. Thus initially the endometrium becomes decidualized because of continued progesterone production by the corpus luteum. **Sometimes the secretory cells of the endometrial glands become hypertrophied with hyperchromatism, pleomorphism, and increased mitotic activity, as originally described by Arias-Stella** (Fig. 17.11). The **Arias-Stella reaction** can be confused with neoplasia, but it is not unique for ectopic pregnancy because it can occur with an intrauterine pregnancy (IUP) and after ovarian stimulation with clomiphene citrate. In a histologic study of the endometrium in 84 women with ectopic pregnancies, 40% of cases had secretory endometrium, with the remainder being about equally divided among the findings of proliferative endometrium, decidual reaction, and Arias-Stella reaction. When progesterone levels fall as a result of insufficient HCG, endometrial integrity is no longer maintained and it breaks down, producing uterine bleeding. Sometimes nearly all the decidua is passed through the cervix in an intact way, producing a **decidual cast** that may be clinically confused with a spontaneous abortion (Fig. 17.12).

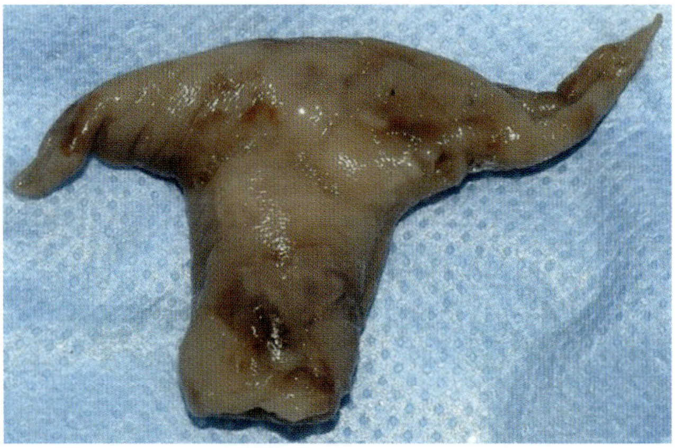

**Fig. 17.12** Decidual cast. (From https://www.researchgate.net/figure/MRI-of-advanced-intraligamentar-abdominal-pregnancy-Holzhacker-et-al-2008_fig4_221918569.)

## SYMPTOMS

Among women with risk factors for ectopic pregnancy, with the use of early hormonal testing and vaginal sonography, it is now often possible to establish the diagnosis of ectopic pregnancy before symptoms develop. However, symptoms often develop when intraperitoneal bleeding occurs from extrusion of blood through the fimbriated end of the tube in cases of tubal pregnancies or from disruption of overlying tubal, ovarian, or myometrial tissue from rupture of the gestational sac.

The most common symptoms of ectopic pregnancy are abdominal pain, absence of menses, and irregular vaginal bleeding. Abdominal pain is nearly a universal symptom of intraperitoneal bleeding, but its characteristics are similar with different causes of bleeding. Before rupture occurs, the pain may be characterized as only a vague soreness or be colicky in nature. Its location may be generalized, unilateral, or bilateral. Shoulder pain occurs in about one-fourth of women with ruptured ectopic pregnancy as a result of diaphragmatic irritation from the hemoperitoneum. During rupture of the tube, the pain usually becomes intense. Syncope occurs in about one-third of women with tubal rupture. Other symptoms that occur after tubal rupture include dizziness and an urge to defecate.

The majority of women with ectopic pregnancy fail to have menses at the expected time but have one or more episodes of irregular vaginal bleeding when the decidual endometrial tissue is sloughed. The interval of amenorrhea is usually 6 weeks or more. The bleeding is usually characterized as spotting but may simulate menstrual bleeding. It is rarely as heavy as that which occurs in spontaneous abortion. About 5% to 10% of women with an advanced ectopic pregnancy will note passage of a decidual cast, as noted previously (see Fig. 17.12).

## SIGNS

The most common presenting sign in a woman with symptomatic ectopic pregnancy is abdominal tenderness, which, together with adnexal tenderness elicited at the time of the bimanual pelvic examination, is present in nearly all women with an advanced or ruptured ectopic pregnancy. It is possible to palpate an adnexal mass in half of the women, and about one-third have some degree of uterine enlargement that is nearly always smaller than a normal 8-week intrauterine gestation except when an interstitial gestation is present. Tachycardia and hypotension can occur after rupture if blood loss is profuse, but temperature elevation is an uncommon finding, present in only about 5% to 10% of women with tubal rupture, and is rarely greater than 38° C.

### Differential Diagnosis of Symptomatic Ectopic Pregnancy

The diagnosis is usually obvious for women with the classic symptoms of ruptured ectopic pregnancy: a history of irregular bleeding followed by sudden onset of pain and syncope accompanied by signs of peritoneal irritation. However, before rupture the symptoms and signs are nonspecific and may also occur with other gynecologic disorders. Entities often confused with ectopic pregnancy include salpingitis, threatened or incomplete abortion, ruptured corpus luteum, appendicitis, dysfunctional uterine bleeding, adnexal torsion, degenerative uterine leiomyoma, and endometriosis.

In the past, studies have found that women with an ectopic pregnancy were seen multiple times before a correct diagnosis was made. Because of the possibility of a fatal outcome from undiagnosed ruptured ectopic pregnancy, it is essential that the diagnosis of ectopic pregnancy be considered in any woman of childbearing age with abdominal pain and irregular uterine bleeding even if she has had a previous tubal sterilization procedure or is using an effective method of reversible contraception.

Ectopic pregnancy should be suspected in any woman who develops the symptoms listed earlier, particularly if she has previously had a pelvic operation, especially tubal surgery, either a tubal reconstructive procedure or a sterilization procedure. Other risk factors include one or more episodes of salpingitis, a previous ectopic gestation, current use of a progesterone-releasing IUD, use of a progestin-only oral contraceptive, use of pharmacologic methods of ovulation induction, and a history of infertility. In any woman with the symptoms of ectopic gestation, the diagnosis is facilitated by a quantitative assay for HCG and pelvic ultrasonography and can be established and treated by laparoscopy or laparotomy. Culdocentesis and measurement of serum progesterone levels have also been used for diagnostic assistance. Before the development of pelvic vaginal ultrasound, the finding of nonclotting blood at the time of culdocentesis, especially if the hematocrit was more than 15%, was of great assistance in establishing the diagnosis of ruptured ectopic pregnancy. **With the use of high-resolution pelvic ultrasound, the presence of intraperitoneal fluid can be easily visualized and culdocentesis is no longer routinely done.**

### Procedures Used for the Diagnostic Evaluation of the Asymptomatic or Mildly Symptomatic Woman With Suspected Ectopic Pregnancy

#### Human Chorionic Gonadotropin

About 85% of women with ectopic pregnancy have serum HCG levels lower than those seen in normal pregnancy at a similar gestational age. However, **a single quantitative HCG assay cannot be used to diagnose ectopic pregnancy** because the actual dates of ovulation and conception are often not known. Even if the date of ovulation is known, 2.5% of women with normal gestations will have HCG levels lower than the normal 95% confidence limits. Furthermore, low HCG levels are also found in women with various stages of spontaneous abortion, conditions that must be considered in the differential diagnosis. Intact HCG and free β-HCG levels were measured in a large group of women in early pregnancy who presented with symptoms of ectopic pregnancy. Although mean levels of intact HCG and free β-HCG were significantly lower in the group of women with ectopic pregnancy and those who aborted than in those with viable intrauterine pregnancies, the individual HCG levels among the three conditions overlapped too much to devise a cutoff level for diagnostic purposes (Ledger, 1994).

Fig. 17.13, as constructed by Barnhart, shows the expected changes (increases) in HCG levels in women with an intrauterine pregnancy and in spontaneous abortion. **Ninety-nine percent of normal intrauterine pregnancies have an increase of at least 53% in 2 days, which is less than the rise that was previously accepted (approximately 66%).** This rate of increase should be similar in single or multiple gestations (Barnhart, 2009). **In women with an ectopic pregnancy, the rate of rise in HCG can mimic an intrauterine pregnancy 21% of the time and can mimic a spontaneous abortion 8% of the time.** Note the overlap in this increase or decrease in HCG levels as depicted in Fig. 17.13.

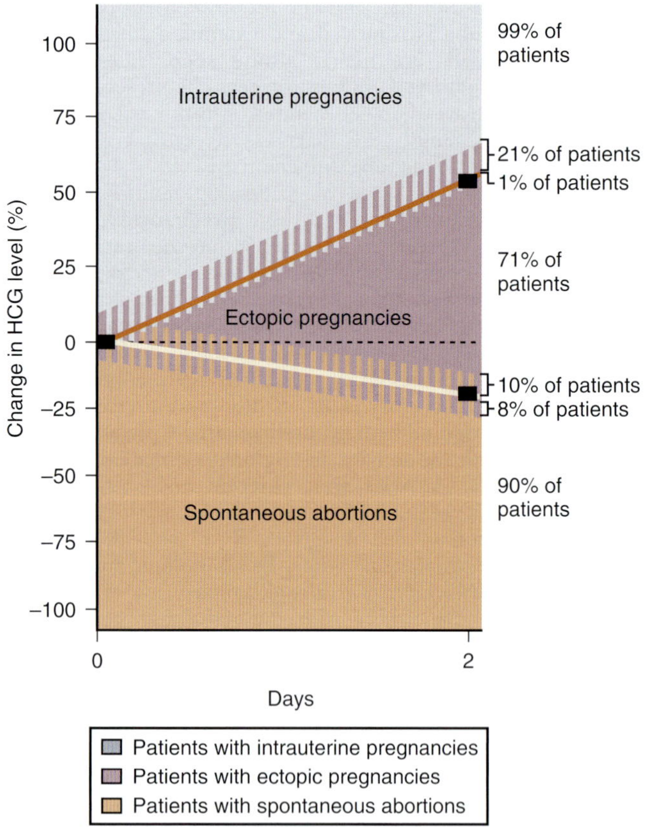


**Fig. 17.13** Change in the human chorionic gonadotropin (HCG) level in intrauterine pregnancy, ectopic pregnancy, and spontaneous abortion. An increase or decrease in the serial HCG level in a woman with an ectopic pregnancy is outside the range expected for that of a woman with a growing intrauterine pregnancy or a spontaneous abortion 71% of the time. However, the increase in the HCG level in a woman with an ectopic pregnancy can mimic that of a growing intrauterine pregnancy 21% of the time, and the decrease in the HCG level can mimic that of a spontaneous abortion 8% of the time. (Modified from Barnhart K. Ectopic pregnancy. *N Engl J Med.* 2009;361(4):384.)

Today the key to the diagnosis of ectopic pregnancy is transvaginal ultrasound (TVUS). The concept of a "discriminatory zone" has been advanced and is defined as the serum HCG level above which **a gestational sac should be visualized by TVUS if an IUP is present. In most institutions, a serum HCG level of 1500 to 2000 mIU/mL is used. Setting the discriminatory zone at 2000 mIU/mL instead of 1500 mIU/mL may minimize the risk of intervening when an intrauterine pregnancy is viable** but may increase the risk of delaying the diagnosis of an ectopic pregnancy. When an IUP is not seen on TVUS at the set discriminatory zone, an abnormal pregnancy is diagnosed and an ectopic pregnancy needs to be ruled out. It has been suggested further that as reliable as using the discriminatory zone is, the length of gestational sac is at least as important when accurate dating is available (as occurs with luteinizing hormone [LH] surge monitoring, etc.). Clearly by 5.5 weeks from the last menstrual period (LMP) (in a woman with normal ovulatory cycle length) an intrauterine sac should be visible in a normal intrauterine pregnancy. **Important ultrasound findings include visualization of a yolk sac at 5.5 weeks, a fetal pole by 6 weeks, and cardiac activity at 6.5 weeks. An abnormal pregnancy is likely if there is absence of a fetal pole with a gestational sac of 2 cm and if no cardiac activity is noted with a crown-rump length of more than 0.5 cm.**

Thus serial measurements of HCG are of great assistance in the early diagnosis of unruptured ectopic pregnancy. However, a differentiation between ectopic pregnancies and impending spontaneous abortion cannot be made with this technique because the rate of increase of HCG in women with an ectopic pregnancy is often similar to that found in women with an impending intrauterine abortion. An algorithm for possible treatment is presented here.

## Progesterone

Serum progesterone values are lower in an ectopic pregnancy, with levels in normal intrauterine pregnancies at 10 ng/mL or greater. An abnormal IUP will also have low values. However, a rising progesterone level is helpful in determining that there is a normal IUP (Fig. 17.14) (McCord, 1996). The clearance of progesterone from the circulation in a failed pregnancy or ectopic is also faster than that of HCG. Therefore progesterone levels have been used as a diagnostic aide for ectopic pregnancy. Nevertheless, it is not commonly used today in practice.

## Ultrasonography

Development of the transvaginal transducer probes with 7-MHz scanning frequency has enabled more precise imaging of the pelvic organs in early pregnancy than is possible with transabdominal ultrasonography. With these probes it is usually possible to identify an intrauterine gestational sac when the HCG level reaches 1500 mIU/mL and virtually always when the HCG level exceeds 2500 mIU/mL (First International Reference Preparation [First IRP], now called the *Third International Standard*), about 5 to 6 weeks after the last menses. Kadar and colleagues reported that in both singleton and multiple gestations a gestational sac should always be seen sonographically beyond 24 days after conception, 38 days' gestational age (Kadar, 1981). Because a heterotopic (combined extrauterine and intrauterine) pregnancy is a rare event, the finding of an intrauterine gestational sac should nearly always exclude the presence of an ectopic pregnancy. When a gestational sac is not present and the HCG level is in the discriminatory zone, a pathologic pregnancy, either an ectopic or a nonviable intrauterine gestation, is most likely present and should be suspected. Usually an adnexal mass or a gestational saclike structure can be identified in the tube when an ectopic pregnancy is present that produces levels of HCG greater than 2500 mIU/mL.

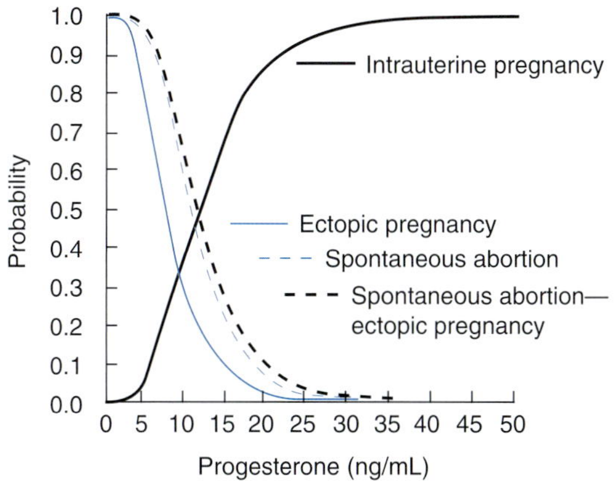


**Fig. 17.14** Predicted pregnancy outcome versus progesterone concentrations. The probability of ectopic pregnancy and spontaneous abortion decreases with rising progesterone levels, forming a negative-sloping, sigmoid-shaped curve, a mirror image of the intrauterine pregnancy curve, with its slope decreasing sharply at approximately 5 ng/mL (15.9 nmol/L) and increasing sharply at approximately 17 ng/mL (54.1 nmol/L). (From McCord ML, Arheart KL, Muram D, et al. Single serum progesterone as a screen for ectopic pregnancy: exchanging specificity and sensitivity to obtain optimal test performance. *Fertil Steril.* 1996;66:513. Copyright 1996, The American Society for Reproductive Medicine.)

Thus diagnostic criteria for the ultrasonographic diagnosis of ectopic pregnancy with the use of a vaginal probe include the detection of a complex or cystic adnexal mass (often called an echogenic "bagel" sign) or visualization of an embryo fetal pole in the adnexa (Fig. 17.15). This is in the absence of an intrauterine gestational sac when the gestational age is known to be more than 38 days or if the HCG level is more than a certain threshold, usually between 1500 and 2500 mIU/mL.

About two-thirds of women presenting with symptoms of ectopic pregnancy have HCG levels greater than 2500 mIU/mL, and when this occurs, the diagnosis of ectopic pregnancy can usually be made by ultrasound. For the other one-third with lower HCG levels, unless a gestational sac is evident on ultrasonography, other diagnostic techniques, such as measurement of a serum

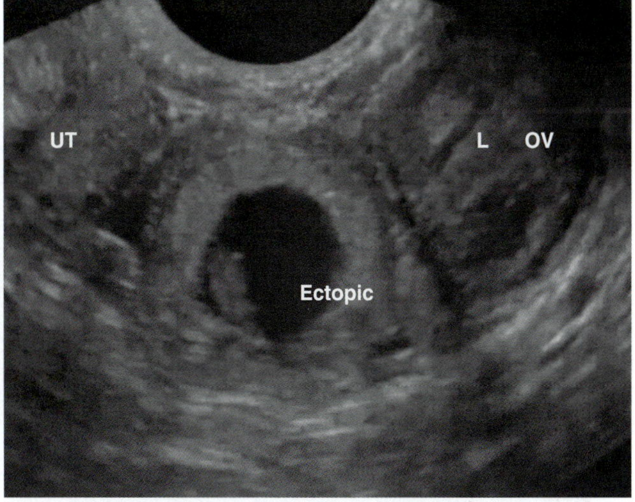


**Fig. 17.15** Ultrasound showing a left tubal ectopic. Note the bagel appearance of gestational sac, which here has a fetal pole. *L OV,* Left ovary; *U,* uterus. (Modified from embryology.med.unsw.edu.au.)

progesterone level and serial HCG determination, should be performed. Repeat ultrasonographic examinations at 3- to 5-day intervals are often helpful in establishing a correct diagnosis.

Several investigators have shown that the use of endovaginal color Doppler flow imaging allows the diagnosis of ectopic pregnancy with greater sensitivity and specificity compared with ordinary endovaginal sonography. With endovaginal color flow imaging of the pelvic structures in the presence of an ectopic pregnancy, **about a 20% difference in the degree of tubal blood flow between the adnexa has been found compared with less than an 8% difference with intrauterine gestations.** Use of **endovaginal color flow compared with routine transvaginal sonography increased the sensitivity of the diagnosis of ectopic pregnancy from 71% to 95%, with a specificity of 96% to 100% in** various studies (Fig. 17.16).

## Dilation and Curettage

When serum HCG levels are more than 1500 mIU/mL, the gestational age exceeds 38 days, or the serum progesterone level is less than 5 ng/mL and no intrauterine gestational sac is seen with vaginal ultrasonography**, a curettage of the endometrial cavity (by dilation and curettage [D&C]) with histologic examination of the removed tissue, by frozen section if desired, can be undertaken** to determine whether any gestational tissue is present. This is a pragmatic approach reserved for those women who do not desire a pregnancy. Note that it has been shown that an endometrial biopsy (e.g., Pipelle) is inadequate in this scenario. Spandorfer and coworkers reported that frozen section was 93% accurate in identifying chorionic villi. If no chorionic villi are visualized in the removed tissue, serial HCGs can be followed. A presumptive diagnosis of ectopic pregnancy can be made with rising serum HCGs and treatment undertaken. An analysis by Ailawadi suggested that performing a D&C in this setting results in fewer complications and is at least as cost effective as the empiric use of methotrexate (Ailawadi, 2005). **When chorionic villi are detected and an IUP is evacuated, the serum HCG should drop by at least 15% the day after curettage.**

## Diagnostic Evaluation of Women With Suspected Ectopic Pregnancy

Several authors have developed flow sheets to aid the clinician in establishing the diagnosis of an asymptomatic or mildly symptomatic ectopic pregnancy. They involve the use of vaginal probe

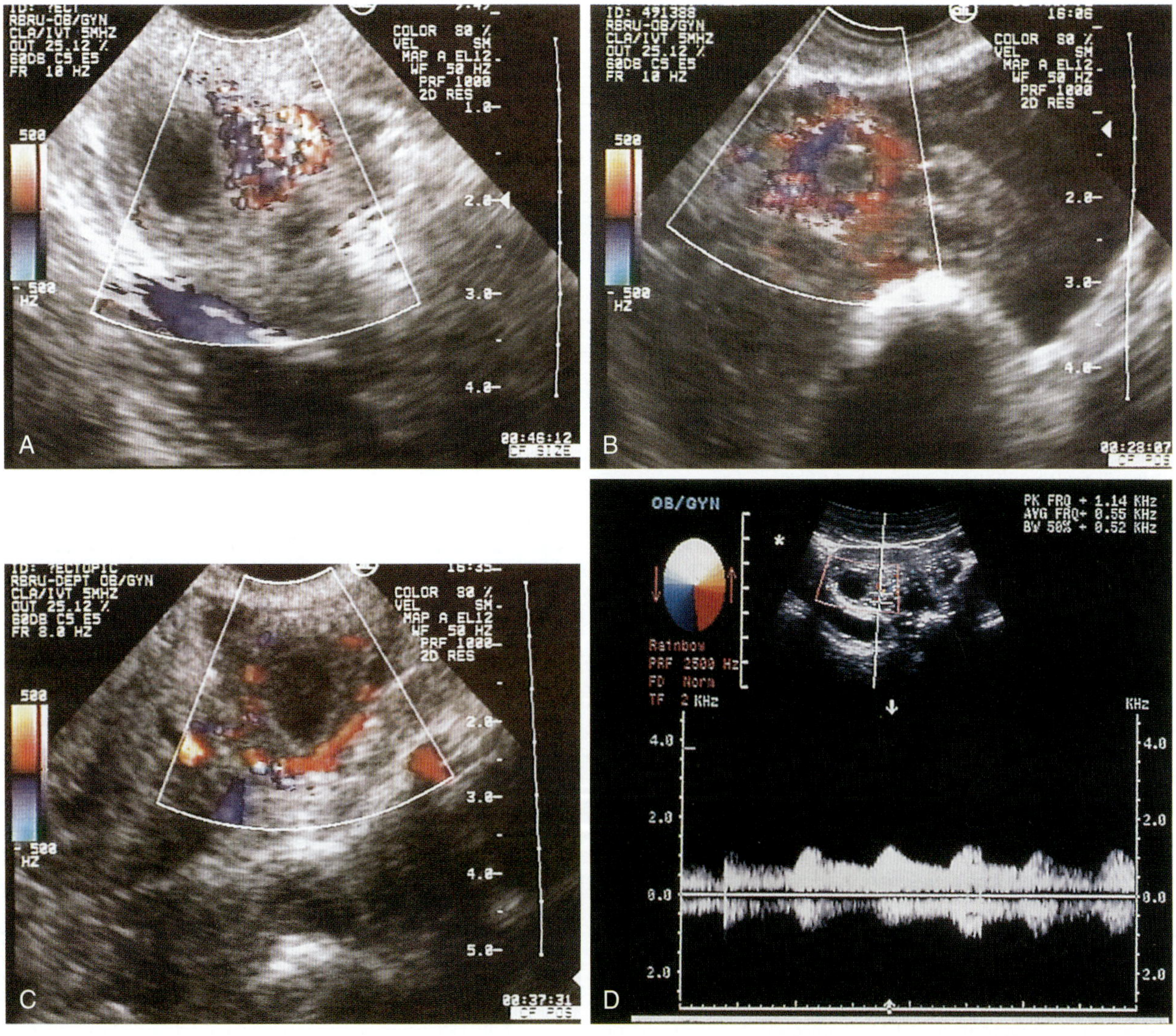


**Fig. 17.16** Ectopic pregnancy showing enhanced blood flow using color Doppler. **A-C,** Examples of color "lighting up" ectopic pregnancies on ultrasound, which can be quantified **(D).**

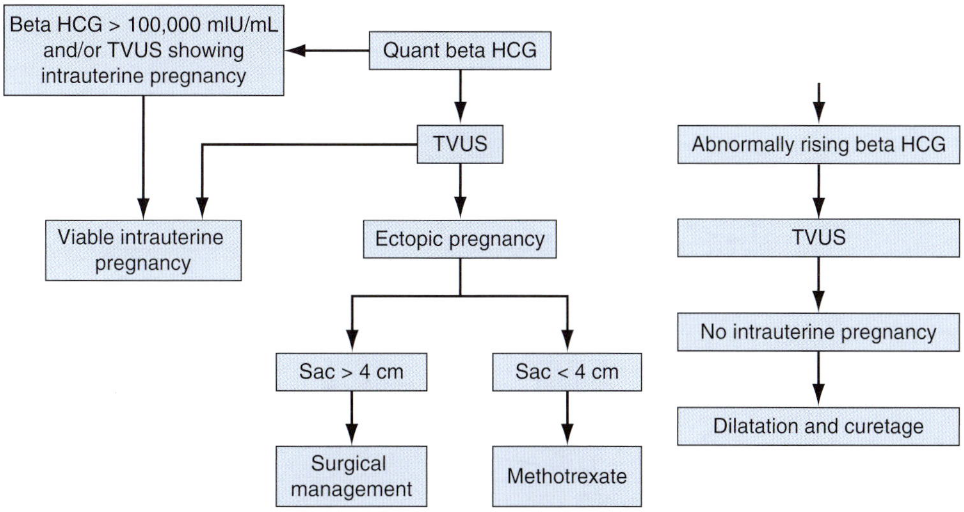


**Fig. 17.17** Possible algorithm for use of methotrexate versus surgery for ectopic pregnancy. *HCG,* Human chorionic gonadotropin; *Quant,* quantitative; *TVUS,* transvaginal ultrasound.

pelvic ultrasonography, measurements of serial quantitative HCG and single serum progesterone levels, and uterine curettage. One suggested algorithm is presented in Fig. 17.17. Note that because of clinical variability, this is merely a guide to management.

These diagnostic aids are of particular use when following an asymptomatic woman with risk factors for ectopic pregnancy, beginning shortly after conception. Performing a quantitative HCG assay twice weekly, calculating the rate of increase (measuring serum progesterone levels at 4, 5, and 6 weeks' gestational age), and performing serial ultrasonography beginning 3 weeks after ovulation will help establish the diagnosis of ectopic pregnancy before tubal rupture. The combination of these two techniques is particularly applicable for stable women treated in institutions with adequate facilities for ultrasound and rapid serial quantitative β-HCG assays. If a woman with or without risk factors for ectopic pregnancy develops mild symptoms consistent with an ectopic gestation and is hemodynamically stable, vaginal sonography, measurement of serial HCG levels, and possibly serum progesterone level, as well as uterine curettage if indicated, will aid in establishing the diagnosis. **The use of a quantitative serum HCG assay and transvaginal sonography enables the diagnosis of ectopic gestation in hemodynamically stable women to be made with a sensitivity of 97% to 100% and a specificity of 95% to 99%** (Fig. 17.18) (Gracia, 2001).

Both suggested algorithms include the use of D&C. Although, as stated previously, this approach has been deemed to be cost effective, some women, particularly those who have been attempting pregnancy, are reluctant to have this treatment. In this setting it is reasonable to continue serial HCG and ultrasound monitoring. Unless HCG falls, it will be clear that with time, treatment of a nonviable pregnancy is needed, which could be with either a D&C or the use of methotrexate.

In an in vitro fertilization setting, if HCG criteria suggest an abnormal pregnancy of unknown location, a suction cannula can be used in an outpatient setting to aid in the diagnosis. Using this approach to rule out an ectopic pregnancy resulted in avoiding the use of methotrexate in more than two-thirds of patients (Brady, 2014).

If a woman develops symptoms of a ruptured ectopic pregnancy that are of sufficient hemodynamic severity to require emergency care, a sensitive qualitative pregnancy test and vaginal sonography are usually all the diagnostic aids necessary to establish the diagnosis. If vaginal sonography is not immediately available on an emergent basis, culdocentesis may be performed. If HCG is present and peritoneal fluid is seen sonographically, it is most likely that an ectopic pregnancy is present, and laparoscopy should be performed.

## MANAGEMENT

### Surgical Treatment

#### Tubal Pregnancy

Laparoscopy is the procedure of choice for ruptured ectopic pregnancy as well as for cases when medical therapy (methotrexate) is contraindicated or refused. Laparoscopy is also useful at times when an accurate diagnosis cannot be made. Older studies have suggested that there is a false-positive and false-negative rate of approximately 2% with the use of laparoscopy for ectopic pregnancies (i.e., either not being able to see the ectopic or confusing findings with hemorrhagic corpus luteal cysts, hematosalpinx, and other findings).

Conservative treatment (i.e., preserving the tube and not performing a salpingectomy) for an unruptured ectopic pregnancy has been considered to be the method of choice for women who desire future fertility. A prospective randomized trial suggested similar long-term pregnancies rates for salpingostomy versus salpingectomy and a somewhat increased rate of retained trophoblastic tissue after salpingostomy (Mol, 2014). However, in a large review by Yao and Tulandi of women with an ectopic pregnancy attempting to conceive after salpingostomy, 60% had an IUP and 15% an ectopic pregnancy. After salpingectomy, 38% had an IUP and 10% an ectopic pregnancy (Yao, 1997).

The conservative surgical techniques used include salpingotomy (in which the tubal incision is closed primarily but is unnecessary and has worse subsequent pregnancy rates [discussed later]), salpingostomy (in which the tubal incision is allowed to close by secondary intention), fimbrial evacuation, and partial salpingectomy, also called ***segmental resection*** of the portion of

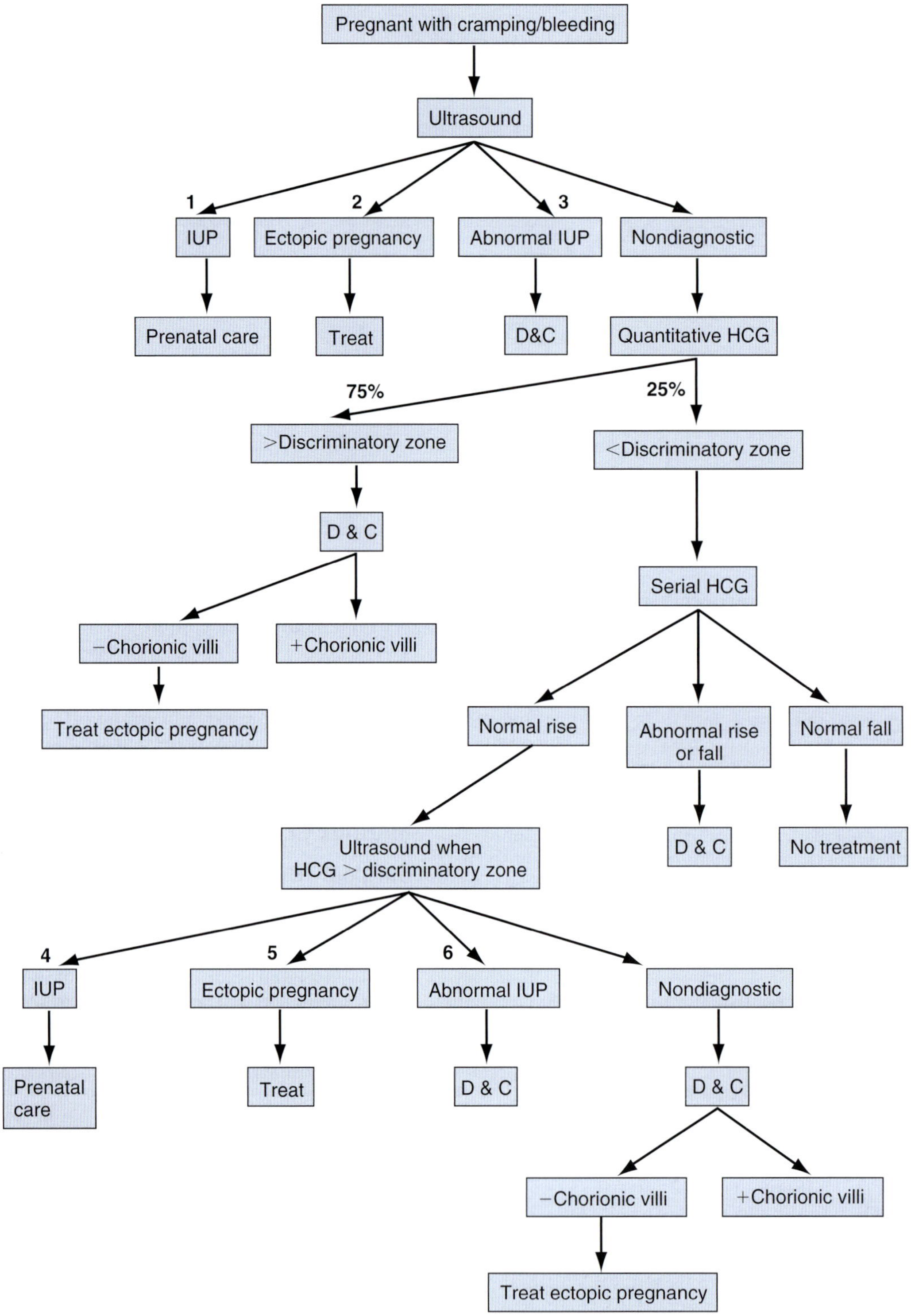


**Fig. 17.18** Sample schematic. Numbers refer to probabilities. *D&C,* Dilation and curettage; *HCG,* human chorionic gonadotropin; *IUP,* intrauterine pregnancy. (From Gracia C, Barnhart KT. Diagnosing ectopic pregnancy. *Obstet Gynecol.* 2001;97:465.)

the tube containing the ectopic pregnancy. Fimbrial evacuation usually traumatizes the endosalpinx and is associated with a high rate of recurrent ectopic pregnancy (24%), about twice as high as the rate after salpingectomy. In addition, this procedure may not remove the entire tubal gestation, and another procedure may be required a few days later.

The best results with conservative management occur after salpingostomy (Fig. 17.19) (Leach, 1989). Tulandi and Guralnick reported that the 2-year cumulative rates of IUP after salpingotomy and salpingostomy were similar, about 45%, but the 1-year rates were twice as great when salpingostomy was performed (45% versus 21%), indicating that there is a more rapid return of normal

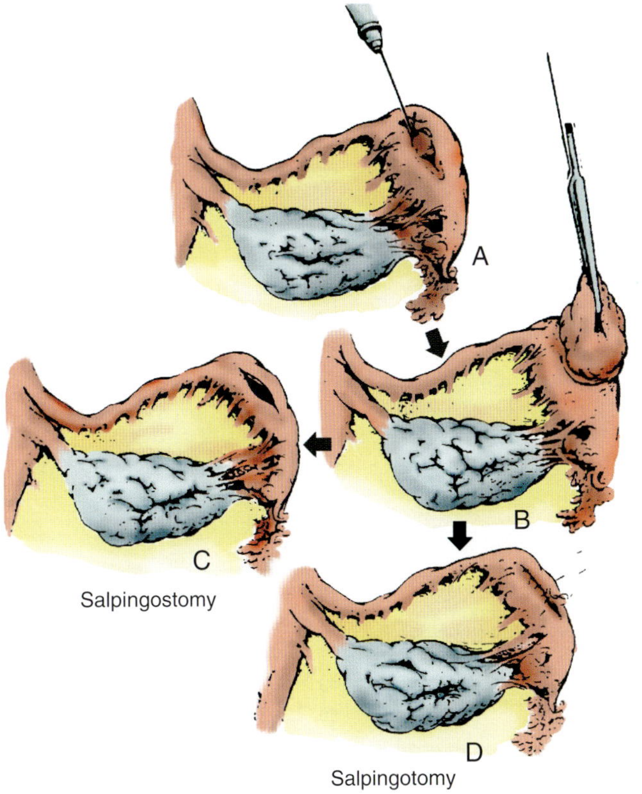


**Fig. 17.19** **A,** Incision is made into the antimesenteric border of the fallopian tube. **B,** Ectopic pregnancy is gently removed from within the fallopian tube. **C,** Salpingostomy site is allowed to heal by secondary intention. **D,** Salpingotomy is completed by primary closure. (From Leach RE, Ory SJ. Modern management of ectopic pregnancy. *J Reprod Med.* 1989;34:325.)

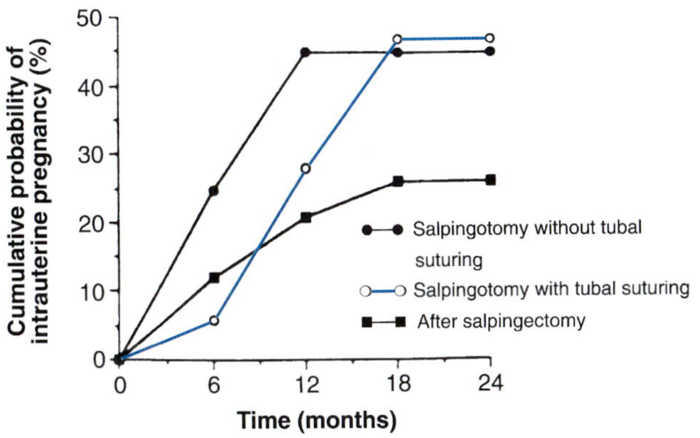


**Fig. 17.20** Cumulative probability of intrauterine pregnancy after conservative surgical treatment of tubal ectopic pregnancy by salpingotomy without tubal suturing, salpingotomy with tubal suturing, and after salpingectomy. (From Tulandi T, Guralnick M. Treatment of tubal ectopic pregnancy by salpingotomy with or without tubal suturing and salpingectomy. *Fertil Steril.* 1991;55:53. Copyright 1991, The American Society for Reproductive Medicine.)

tubal function when the incision heals by secondary intention than when it is sutured (Fig. 17.20) (Tulandi, 1991).

The techniques described here can be used to treat the majority of unruptured tubal pregnancies, although this long-held belief has been challenged with the randomized trial referred to earlier (Mol, 2014).

If a woman who is nulliparous has an unruptured ectopic pregnancy and strongly desires a conservative approach, salpingostomy should seriously be considered. The findings of the randomized trial showing equal future pregnancy rates even if salpingectomy is carried out (Mol, 2014) (Fig. 17.21) should also be weighed in the decision making.

## Interstitial Pregnancy

An interstitial pregnancy in the cornual area of the uterus can be treated laparoscopically; but it may require laparotomy with resection. A deep cornual resection is not deemed necessary and does not decrease the risk of recurrent ectopic pregnancy. It has been proposed that a laparoscopic cornuotomy using a temporary tourniquet suture and diluted vasopressin injection can be effective for these cases (Fig. 17.22). Choi and colleagues described eight cases of patients who underwent this technique. They described a low estimated blood loss (50 ± 22 mL) without major complications such as hemorrhage, and no postoperative adjuvant therapy was required. They concluded that this procedure is safe and effective in interstitial pregnancy with the advantage of preserving reproductive function compared with cornual resection (Choi, 2009).

Subsequent intrauterine pregnancies after previous cornual ectopic pregnancy should be delivered by cesarean section.

## Ovarian Pregnancy

Rare ovarian pregnancies can be treated by laparoscopic surgical excision. Many times this occurs when the expected surgery is for a ruptured tubal ectopic pregnancy or hemorrhagic corpus luteum. The surgical treatment alternatives include an ovarian wedge resection or unilateral salpingo-oophorectomy, the latter of which should be avoided and does not improve the subsequent pregnancy rate or lower the risk of recurrence.

## Abdominal Pregnancy

Abdominal pregnancy is a rare situation. From an analysis of 11 abdominal pregnancy–related deaths and an estimated 5221 abdominal pregnancies in the United States, it has been estimated that there were 10.9 abdominal pregnancies per 100,000 live births and 9.2 per 1000 ectopic pregnancies. **The mortality rate was 5.1 per 1000 cases.** In a literature review Hymel found 31 cases of late abdominal pregnancies (more than 20 weeks' gestation) from 1965 to 2012 (Hymel, 2015). The most common sites of placental implantation were in the uterus or adnexa (47.8%), bowel (30%), and the potential spaces surrounding the uterus (8.7%). Five cases of intraabdominal abscess were identified in the 14 patients in whom the placenta had been left in situ. Maternal outcomes were documented in 26 cases, with 7 deaths; 27 fetal outcomes were documented in 22 cases, with 3 fetal deaths (13.6%). Treatment is always surgical, and interventional radiology and endovascular surgery must be considered for assistance.

## Cervical Pregnancy

Surgical treatment of cervical ectopic pregnancies consists of evacuation with D&C or vacuum aspiration. This often occurs after methotrexate treatment, which facilitates a decrease in the size and vascularity of the pregnancy. What must be considered is the risk of hemorrhage, which can be avoided by a prophylactic suture ligation of the cervical branches of the uterine artery, with absorbable sutures, at 3 and 9 o'clock under transabdominal ultrasound guidance and a running-lock absorbable suture around the entire edge of the cervix.

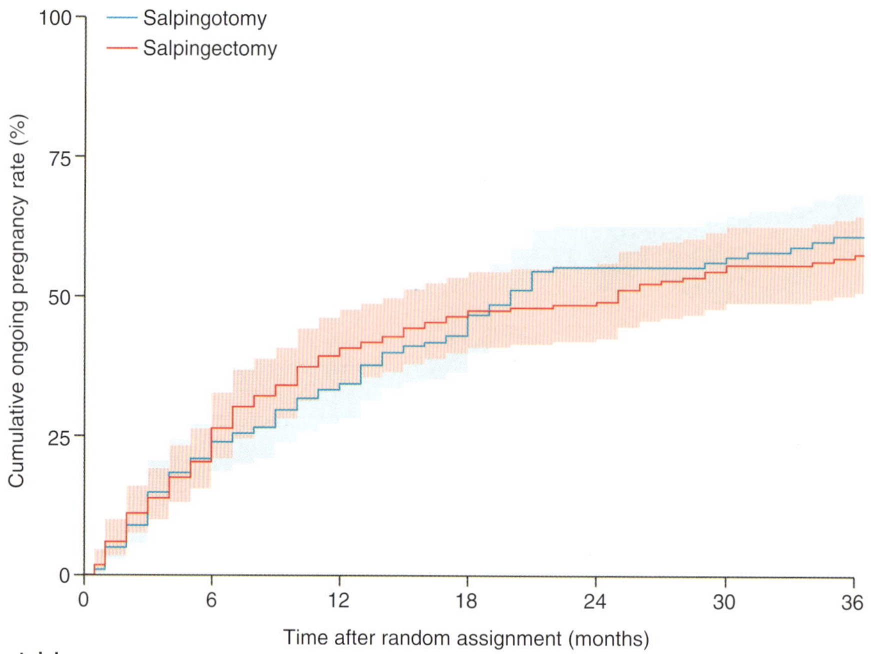

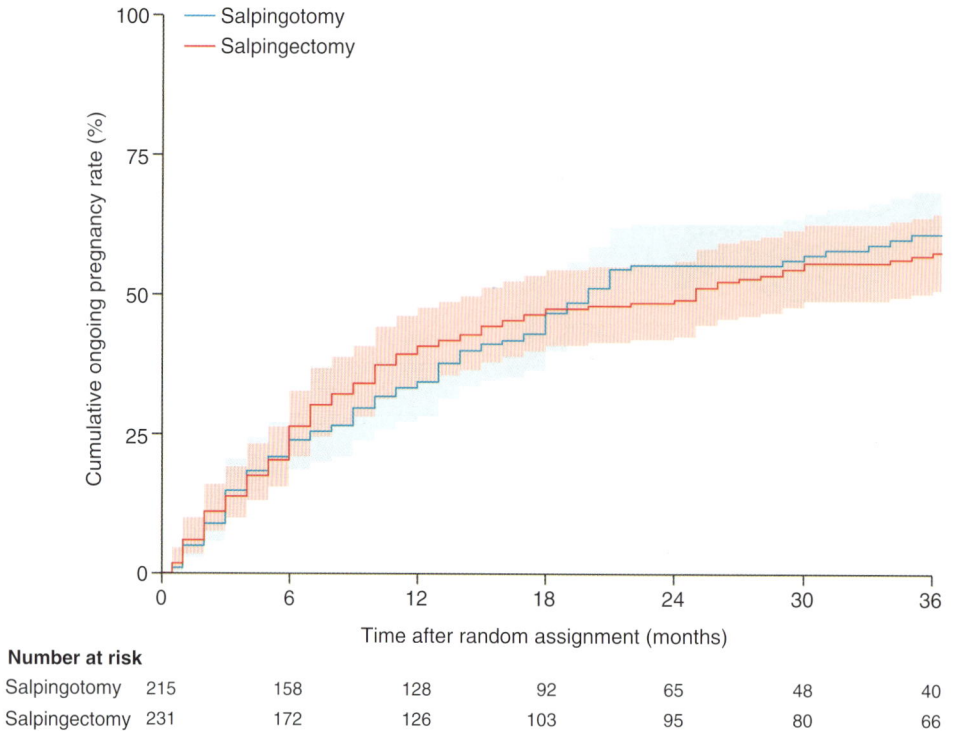

**Fig. 17.21** Kaplan-Meier curves for time to ongoing pregnancy by natural conception. Shaded areas show 95% confidence interval (CI). Median time to ongoing pregnancy by natural conception after salpingotomy was 20 months (95% CI, 17 to 23) and after salpingectomy was 26 months (95% CI, 15 to 37); cumulative rate of ongoing pregnancy by natural conception after 36 months was 60 × 7% after salpingotomy and 56 × 2% after salpingectomy. log rank *P* = .678; $\chi^2$ = 0.172 (1 *df*). (From Mol F, van Mello NM, Strandell A, et al. Salpingostomy versus salpingectomy in women with tubal pregnancy [ESEP study]: an open-label, multicentre, randomised controlled trial. *Lancet.* 2014;383(9927):1483-1489.)

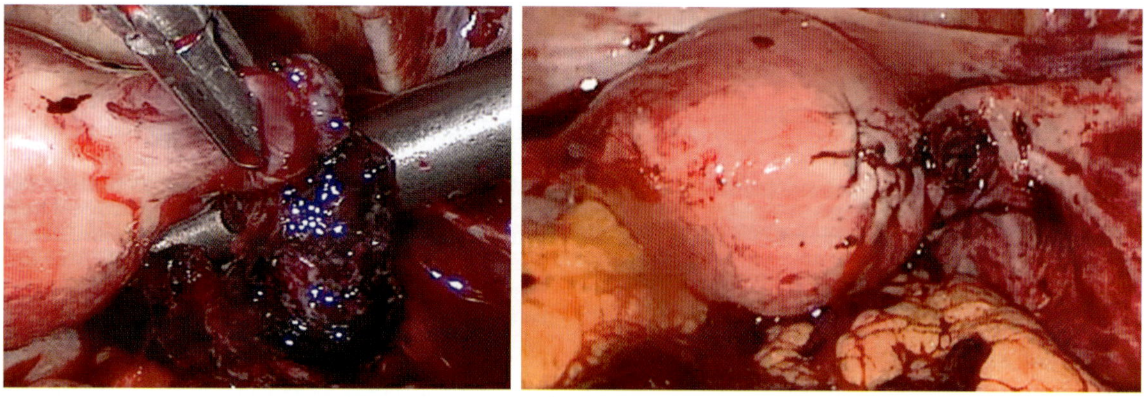

**Fig. 17.22** Laparoscopic surgery for interstitial pregnancy in the cornual area of the uterus. The ectopic is evacuated after a linear incision is made and the defect is sutured as shown. (Courtesy Columbia University MIS Program.)

## Cesarean Scar Pregnancy

Surgical treatment of cesarean scar pregnancies also consists of evacuation with D&C or vacuum aspiration under transabdominal ultrasound and/or laparoscopic guidance. To prevent hemorrhage, temporary laparoscopic bilateral artery occlusion with silicone tubing has been described. Hysteroscopy coupled with curettage followed by uterine artery embolization is also an alternative surgical approach for these cases (Qian, 2015). **Another surgical option includes laparoscopic excision of the cesarean scar pregnancy with vasopressin injection and/or preoperative uterine artery embolization.**

## Persistent Ectopic Pregnancy

With increasing use of conservative surgical treatment instead of salpingectomy for the treatment of ectopic pregnancy, persistent ectopic pregnancy (PEP) is becoming more common. The overall mean incidence of PEP after linear salpingostomy is about 5%, being higher when the procedure is performed laparoscopically and lower when performed by laparotomy. After fimbrial expression or tubal abortion, the incidence of persistence ranges from 12% to 15%.

PEP is uncommon when the preoperative HCG level is less than 3000 mIU/mL. When preoperative HCG levels are greater than 3000 mIU/mL, the incidence of PEP has been reported to

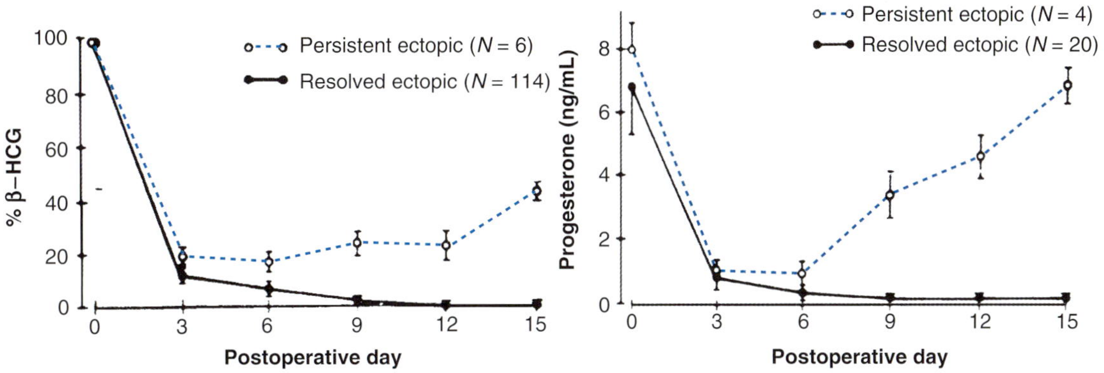


**Fig. 17.23** **A,** Serum β-human chorionic gonadotropin (β-HCG) patterns in persistent and resolved ectopic gestations after conservative surgery. **B,** Serum progesterone patterns in persistent and resolved ectopic gestations after conservative surgery. (From Vermesh M, Silva PD, Rosen GF, et al: Persistent tubal ectopic gestation: patterns of circulating beta-human chorionic gonadotropin and progesterone, and management options. *Fertil Steril.* 1988;50:584. Copyright 1988, The American Society for Reproductive Medicine.)

range from about 22% to 42%. If the HCG level is more than 1000 mIU/mL 7 days after surgery or is more than 15% of the original level at this time, PEP is nearly always present. If the day 7 HCG level is less than 1000 mIU/mL or less than 15% of the initial value, PEP is unlikely. Vermesh and associates measured both HCG and progesterone levels preoperatively and every 3 days after conservative tubal surgery for an unruptured ectopic gestation in a group of 114 women (Vermesh 1988). Of this group, six (5.3%) had PEP, all of whom had an initial sharp drop in HCG levels to 25% of the pretreatment levels 6 days after surgery, similar to the remainder of the group who did not have PEP. After 6 days, titers of the former group plateaued or rose slightly (Fig. 17.23, *A*).

Based on these data, PEP is presumed to be present if a day 9 serum HCG level is more than 10% of the initial level or a day 9 serum progesterone level is more than than 1.5 ng/mL (Fig. 17.23, *B*). It is now recommended that after linear salpingostomy either HCG or progesterone levels be measured initially on day 6 postoperatively and at 3-day intervals thereafter. Increasing levels of either of these hormones beyond day 6 or a day 6 level of HCG more than 1000 mIU/mL or more than 15% of the original value are all indicators of PEP. Because tubal rupture is likely to occur with PEP, it is best to treat the entity before this emergency situation occurs.

Methods used to treat PEP include salpingectomy, salpingostomy, methotrexate, and expectant management. Expectant management is usually reserved for the asymptomatic woman whose HCG titers plateau but do not rise. Surgical management should be used for women who develop symptoms of persistent lower abdominal pain. The remaining women with PEP are best treated with methotrexate. A single dose of 50 mg/m$^2$ of methotrexate is usually sufficient to resolve PEP. Graczykowski and Mishell performed a randomized trial in which a single dose of methotrexate or placebo was given within 24 hours after salpingostomy. The use of methotrexate reduced the risk of developing PEP by nearly 90%. The prophylactic use of a single dose of methotrexate may be considered in women with larger ectopic pregnancies or higher initial levels of HCG or when the surgery was difficult.

## Medical Treatment

For stable patients, methotrexate (MTX) has become established as a reasonable primary treatment for ectopic pregnancy and is comparable with surgical therapy in observational studies. For medical and surgical therapy, rates of tubal pregnancy (62% to 90%) and recurrence rates (8% to 15%) are comparable.

MTX should be used in asymptomatic women who qualify for such treatment (see Fig. 17.17) and who have no contraindications (Table 17.2) (Practice Committee ASRM, 2008). Before treatment, several tests should be obtained, including a complete blood cell count (CBC), liver function test, blood urea nitrogen (BUN) test, and tests of creatinine, blood type, and Rh.

**TABLE 17.2** Contraindications to Medical Management of Ectopic Pregnancy With Systemic Methotrexate

| Contraindication | ACOG | ASRM |
|---|---|---|
| Absolute contraindications | Breastfeeding; laboratory evidence of immunodeficiency; preexisting blood dyscrasias (bone marrow hypoplasia, leukopenia, thrombocytopenia, or clinically significant anemia); known sensitivity to methotrexate; active pulmonary disease; peptic ulcer disease; hepatic, renal, or hematologic dysfunction; alcoholism; alcoholic or other chronic liver disease | Breastfeeding: evidence of immunodeficiency; moderate to severe anemia, leukopenia, or thrombocytopenia; sensitivity to methotrexate; active pulmonary or peptic ulcer disease; clinically important hepatic or renal dysfunction; intrauterine pregnancy |
| Relative contraindications | Ectopic mass >3.5 cm; embryonic cardiac motion | Ectopic mass >4 cm detected by transvaginal ultrasonography; embryonic cardiac activity detected by transvaginal ultrasonography; patient declines blood transfusion; patient is not able to participate in follow-up; high initial HCG level (>5000 mIU/mL) |
| Choice of regimen based on HCG level | Multidose regimen of methotrexate may be appropriate if presenting HCG value >5000 mIU/mL | Single-dose regimen of methotrexate better in patients with a low initial HCG level |

Data from American Society for Reproductive Medicine. The Practice Committee: medical treatment of ectopic pregnancy. *Fertil Steril.* 2008;90:S206.

*ACOG,* American College of Obstetricians and Gynecologists; *ASRM,* American Society for Reproductive Medicine; *HCG,* human chorionic gonadotropin.

There are two main protocols for MTX: multidose and single-dose regimens (Tables 17.3 and 17.4) (Practice Committee ASRM, 2008). There is also an intermediate two-dose regimen, which will be discussed later. The multidose regimen is more successful but involves more dosing and therefore potentially has more side effects; however, it also includes the use of leucovorin (folinic acid), an antagonist to MTX, to reduce the risk of side effects. As shown in Table 17.3, the multidose regimen can be stopped if there is an appropriate decrease in HCG with treatment. The complications of MTX are listed in Box 17.1. **In all regimens, the reduction in HCG is key to success, but complete resolution of HCG usually takes 2 to 3 weeks, and it can linger for up to 8 weeks after treatment.**

**TABLE 17.3** Multiple-Dose MTX Treatment Protocol

| Treatment Day | Laboratory Evaluation | Intervention |
|---|---|---|
| Pretreatment | HCG, CBC with differential, liver function tests, creatinine, blood type and antibody screen | Rule out spontaneous Ab Rhogam if Rh negative |
| 1 | HCG | MTX 1.0 mg/kg IM |
| 2 | | LEU 0.1 mg/kg IM |
| 3 | HCG | MTX 1.0 mg/kg IM if <15% decline on days 1-3 |
| | | If >15%, stop treatment and start surveillance |
| 4 | | LEU 0.1 mg/kg IM |
| 5 | HCG | MTX 1.0 mg/kg IM if <15% decline on days 3-5 |
| | | If >15%, stop treatment and start surveillance |
| 6 | | LEU 0.1 mg/kg IM |
| 7 | HCG | MTX 1.0 mg/kg IM if <15% decline on days 5-7 |
| | | If >15%, stop treatment and start surveillance |
| 8 | | LEU 0.1 mg/kg IM |

From The Practice Committee of the American Society for Reproductive Medicine. Medical treatment of ectopic pregnancy. *Fertil Steril.* 2008;90(5 Suppl):S206-S212.
Surveillance every 7 days (until HCG < 35 mIU/mL). Screening laboratory studies should be repeated 1 week after the last dose of MTX.
*CBC,* Complete blood cell count; *HCG,* human chorionic gonadotropin; *IM,* intramuscularly; *LEU,* leucovorin; *MTX,* methotrexate.

**TABLE 17.4** Single-Dose MTX Treatment Protocol

| Treatment Day | Laboratory Evaluation | Intervention |
|---|---|---|
| Pretreatment | HCG, CBC with differential, liver function tests, creatinine, blood type, and antibody screen | Rule out spontaneous Ab Rhogam if Rh negative |
| 1 | HCG | MTX 50 mg/m$^2$ IM |
| 4 | HCG | |
| 7 | HCG | MTX 50 mg/m$^2$ IM if $\beta$-HCG decreased <15% between day 4 and day 7 |

From The Practice Committee of the American Society for Reproductive Medicine: Medical treatment of ectopic pregnancy. *Fertil Steril* 90(5 Suppl):S206-S212, 2008.
Surveillance every 7 days (until HCG < 5 mIU/mL).
*HCG,* Human chorionic gonadotropin; *IM,* intramuscularly; *MTX,* methotrexate.

**BOX 17.1** Treatment and Side Effects Associated With MTX

**TREATMENT EFFECTS**

Increase in abdominal girth
Increase in HCG during initial therapy
Vaginal bleeding or spotting
Abdominal pain

**DRUG SIDE EFFECTS**

Gastric distress, nausea, and vomiting
Stomatitis
Dizziness
Severe neutropenia (rare)
Reversible alopecia (rare)
Pneumonitis (rare)

From The Practice Committee of the American Society for Reproductive Medicine. Medical treatment of ectopic pregnancy. *Fertil Steril.* 2008; 90(5 Suppl):S206-S212.
*HCG,* Human chorionic gonadotropin; *MTX,* methotrexate.

**BOX 17.2** Predictors of MTX Treatment Failure

Adnexal fetal cardiac activity
Size and volume of the gestational mass (>4 cm)
High initial HCG concentration (>5000 mIU/mL)
Presence of free peritoneal blood
Rapidly increasing HCG concentrations (>50%/48 hours) before MTX
Continued rapid rise in HCG concentrations during MTX

From The Practice Committee of the American Society for Reproductive Medicine. Medical treatment of ectopic pregnancy. *Fertil Steril.* 2008; 90(5 Suppl):S206-S212.
*HCG,* Human chorionic gonadotropin; *MTX,* methotrexate.

Meta-analyses have confirmed **the overall success of MTX to be 78% to 96%.** The single-dose regimen has been reported to have a success of 88.1%, and the multidose regimen was significantly more successful at 89% to 96%. It is clear that there is a high failure rate with the single-dose regimen, and this is clearly related to the viability of the ectopic, based on its size and the level of HCG (Box 17.2). **A yolk sac in the adnexa accompanied by a level of HCG greater than 5000 mIU/mL affords a poorer prognosis after MTX single-dose therapy.** Mol and associates performed a systematic review and meta-analysis comparing laparoscopic salpingostomy and methotrexate. They concluded that the clinical treatment is more cost effective with less hospitalization, faster recovery, and no significant difference in subsequent spontaneous conception rates or recurrent ectopic pregnancies (Mol, 2008).

Fig. 17.24 provides the correlation of failure rates with high levels of HCG (Practice Committee ASRM, 2008). Box 17.2 lists the predictions of failed responses. A two-dose regimen has been proposed as well, which is intermediate between the single high-dose and multidose regimens. In the two-dose regimen, which

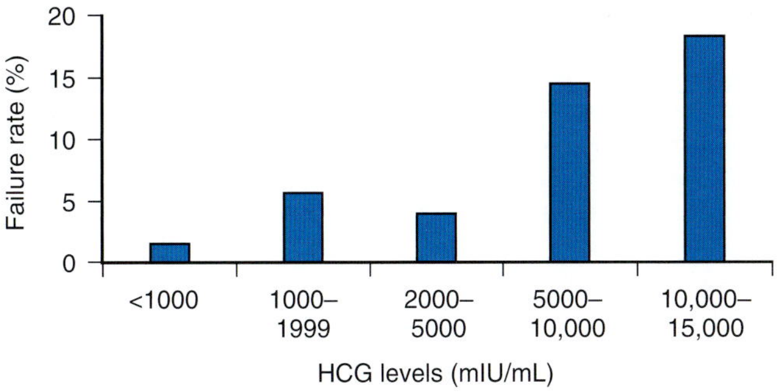


**Fig. 17.24** Single-dose methotrexate (MTX) treatment failure based on human chorionic gonadotropin (HCG) level. (From The Practice Committee of the American Society for Reproductive Medicine. Medical treatment of ectopic pregnancy. *Fertil Steril.* 2008;90(5 Suppl): S206-S212.)

may be considered for patients who have HCG levels greater than 5000 mIU/mL, MTX (50 mg/m$^2$) is administered on days 1 and 4 without leucovorin.

About 85% of patients treated with methotrexate have a transient rise in HCG level between 1 and 4 days after treatment. **Between 4 and 7 days after methotrexate is administered, the HCG levels should fall at least 15%.** If this amount of decrease does not occur or there is less than a 15% decrease in HCG levels in each subsequent week, **an additional dose of methotrexate should be given for a maximum of three doses.** If after three doses of methotrexate HCG levels do not decline by 15% weekly, a surgical procedure should be performed. Serum progesterone levels fall more rapidly than HCG levels after methotrexate, and a progesterone level of less than 1.5 ng/mL has been found to be an excellent predictor of resolution of the ectopic pregnancy. Between 3 and 7 days after initiating therapy, severe pelvic pain lasting up to 12 hours commonly occurs. This symptom, probably caused by tubal abortion, must be differentiated from the symptoms of tubal rupture. Serial monitoring of vital signs and measurement of hematocrit levels are helpful. If the woman remains hemodynamically stable and the pain disappears, a tubal abortion has probably taken place and no further therapy is necessary.

To avoid the toxicity of systemic methotrexate administration, a smaller dose of the drug has been administered directly into the tube with either laparoscopic or ultrasound visualization. In a summary of 11 series involving 295 women treated with tubal injection of methotrexate, 83% had successful resolution of the ectopic pregnancy; subsequent tubal patency rates were 88% and fertility rates were 82%.

Because of the lower success rate and need for direct needle placement with local injection, most clinicians now use systemic methotrexate administration. There have also been several reports of direct intratubal injection of other substances, including potassium chloride, hypertonic glucose, and prostaglandins, but use of these agents is generally less successful than the use of methotrexate.

Methotrexate plays an important role in the treatment of nontubal ectopic pregnancies. It can be administrated intramuscularly or intraamniotically and may be used in combination with other therapies, such as intraamniotic administration of potassium chloride, vaginal mifepristone, or uterine artery embolization. For nontubal ectopic pregnancies, such as cervical or interstitial or in a cesarean scar, if methotrexate alone is not effective, additional treatments such as curettage, hysteroscopy, or even hysterectomy can be considered.

Some new drugs are being studied for the clinical management of the ectopic pregnancies, with drugs such as selective progesterone receptor modulators (i.e., mifepristone) and epidermal growth factor receptor inhibitors combined with methotrexate. Further studies are required to confirm the efficacy of these medications.

## Expectant Management

Although **expectant management is not advised,** it is useful to know some ectopic pregnancies may resolve spontaneously without treatment, with an overall success rate of 69% reported for expectant management. The lower the initial HCG level, the greater the success with spontaneous resolution.

Trio and coworkers, using multivariate analysis, reported that an initial HCG titer of less than 1000 mIU/mL and a decrease in HCG levels between the initial serum sample and one obtained a few days later were each independent predictors of successful spontaneous resolution, whereas sonographic visualization of an ectopic gestational sac was not an independent predictor of failure. In their series of 49 women managed expectantly, 88% of those with an initial HCG level of less than 1000 mIU/mL had successful resolution.

Korhonen and associates measured serial HCG levels among 118 women with ectopic pregnancies undergoing expectant management. This group comprised one fourth of all the ectopic pregnancies diagnosed at their institution during a 3-year period. Among those with spontaneous resolution, HCG levels declined to undetectable levels within 4 to 67 days, with a mean of 20 days. When comparing those who did and did not require surgery, a distinct difference in the rate of decline of HCG levels was not observed until 7 days after the initial examination (Fig. 17.25) (Korhonen, 1994). **If HCG levels did not diminish by more than two-thirds of the initial level within 7 days, two-thirds of this group needed surgical treatment for rising HCG levels, clinical symptoms, or sonographic findings of intraperitoneal bleeding.** It is important to note that serial sonography of tubal pregnancies being managed expectantly can demonstrate an increase in size and vascularity as they resolve. Although insight

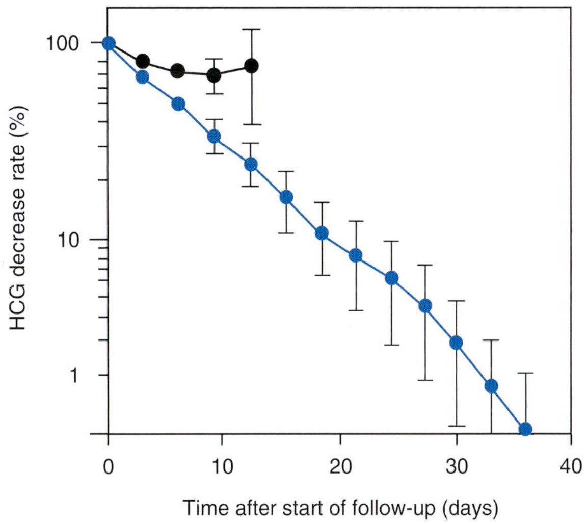


**Fig. 17.25** Mean value and 95% confidence limits for ratio of serum human chorionic gonadotropin (HCG) concentrations to starting value during expectant management in patients with a spontaneous resolution *(blue circles)* and in those later treated by laparoscopy *(black circles).* The two groups diverged at 7 days. (From Korhonen J, Stenman UH, Ylöstalo P. Serum human chorionic gonadotropin dynamics during spontaneous resolution of ectopic pregnancy. *Fertil Steril.* 1994;61: 632. Copyright 1994, The American Society for Reproductive Medicine.)

regarding expectant management of ectopic pregnancies is important, if an unruptured ectopic pregnancy is diagnosed by β-HCG and ultrasound, methotrexate or laparoscopy would be the preferred treatment course over expectant management.

### Women With a History of Infertility

In women with a history of infertility, **methotrexate therapy is preferred unless a hydrosalpinx is present on the affected tube with the ectopic pregnancy**, in which case salpingectomy should be preferred. The Cochrane database has shown that methotrexate therapy is equivalent to laparoscopic surgery; it has also been deemed more cost effective.

## PROGNOSIS FOR SUBSEQUENT FERTILITY

If a woman wishes to conceive after having an ectopic pregnancy, three possibilities exist: She may remain infertile, she may conceive and have an intrauterine gestation (with a viable birth or spontaneous abortion), or she may conceive and have an ectopic gestation. **Overall, the subsequent conception rate in women after all ectopic pregnancies is about 60%, with the other 40% remaining infertile.**

Among those who conceive after the initial ectopic pregnancy, about one-third result in another ectopic pregnancy and one-sixth are spontaneous abortions. Therefore only about half the pregnancies are viable, with only one-third of all women with an ectopic pregnancy have a subsequent live birth. However, these overall figures are modified by several factors, particularly age, parity, history of infertility, evidence of contralateral tubal disease, whether the ectopic pregnancy is ruptured or intact, and use of an IUD at the time of the ectopic gestation.

**The subsequent fertility rate is significantly higher in parous women younger than age 30.** Women with high parity (more than three births) who develop an ectopic pregnancy have a relatively high rate, about 80%, of subsequent conception. If the ectopic pregnancy occurs in a woman's first pregnancy, her overall subsequent conception rate is only about 35%, being lower with a history of infertility and higher with no such history. The subsequent conception rate is also lower in women who have a history of salpingitis and among those with visual changes in the contralateral tube suggesting prior salpingitis. Alternatively, several studies suggest that women with IUD-related ectopic pregnancies have normal rates of subsequent fertility and no increased risk of a subsequent ectopic pregnancy.

In addition, future fertility is significantly higher in women who have an unruptured tubal pregnancy than in those with tubal rupture, so early diagnosis is desirable. Only 65% of women with a ruptured ectopic pregnancy subsequently conceive, whereas the conception rate in women with an unruptured tubal pregnancy is approximately 82%. In two large groups of women with unruptured ectopic pregnancy treated by conservative surgery, a high incidence of subsequent fertility (80% to 86%) and a low incidence of subsequent ectopic pregnancy (11% to 22%) have been reported. The IUP rates were 64% to 70%. In both series the IUP rates were highest (82% to 86%) in women with no history of infertility or gross evidence of prior salpingitis. The IUP rates were significantly lower (41% to 56%) in women with infertility. It has been shown that in women with evidence of prior tubal infection or a history of infertility, subsequent IUP rates were higher when they were treated with salpingostomy (73% to 76%) than when treated with salpingectomy (43% to 44%).

Although most studies in the literature indicate that the overall subsequent ectopic pregnancy rate is similar among women treated by salpingostomy or salpingectomy, the data suggest that conservative surgery with salpingostomy is most beneficial for women with evidence of contralateral tubal damage or a history of infertility. When assessing salpingostomy outcomes by mode of incision, the women treated by laparoscopy conceived sooner than those treated by laparotomy, and there were more ectopic pregnancies in the laparotomy group. Overall, when comparing the laparoscopy and laparotomy groups, 68% versus 71% had an IUP, and 5% versus 19% had an ectopic pregnancy, respectively.

Among women with an unruptured ectopic pregnancy, the following are independent factors that decrease the rate of subsequent fertility and increase the risk of subsequent ectopic pregnancy: a history of infertility (particularly resulting from tubal disease), previous salpingitis, a prior ectopic pregnancy, or the presence of only one tube (Fig. 17.26). Therefore, **if more than one of these factors are present, salpingectomy should be considered over salpingostomy because 80% of recurrent ectopic pregnancies occur in the same tube as the initial ectopic pregnancy**.

The rate of repeat ectopic pregnancy after a single ectopic pregnancy ranges from 8% to 27%, with a mean of about 20%. Because the overall pregnancy rate is in the 60% to 80% range, about 1 in 3 to 4 conceptions after an ectopic pregnancy is a repeat ectopic pregnancy.

**Women with an ectopic pregnancy who become pregnant again should be monitored by ultrasound early in pregnancy.**

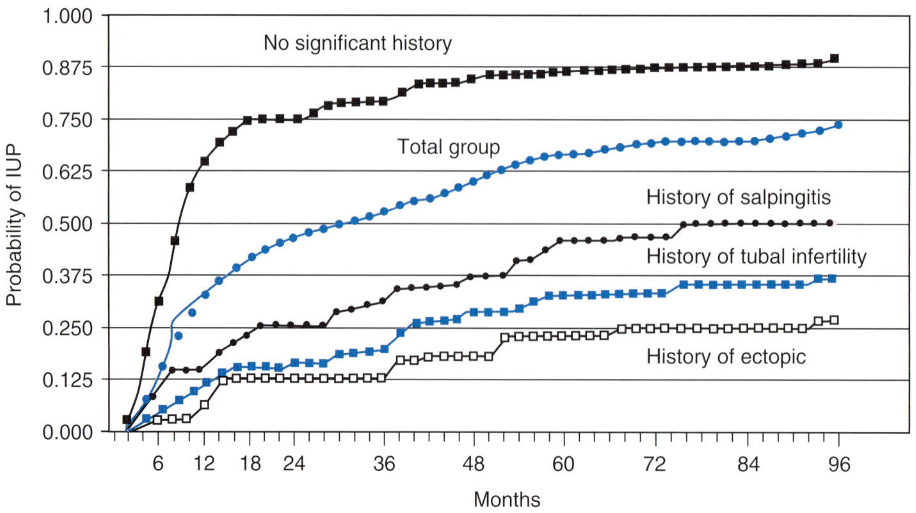


**Fig. 17.26** Cumulative pregnancy rate according to the patient's history. *IUP,* Intrauterine pregnancy.

Only about 1 in 3 nulliparous women who have had an ectopic pregnancy ever conceives again (35%), and about one-third of these conceptions are an ectopic pregnancy, for an overall rate of 13%. Risk factors for a repeat ectopic pregnancy were ectopic pregnancy as the first pregnancy, age younger than 25, evidence of tubal infection, and history of infertility (see Table 17.1). With two ectopic pregnancies, the subsequent fertility rate decreases even further. Of women who have had two consecutive ectopic pregnancies treated by salpingostomy, about half will subsequently conceive, but the majority of these will be a repeat ectopic pregnancy. There have been several reports on salpingostomy or salpingotomy in women with an unruptured tubal pregnancy in the only remaining tube. In the great majority of the subjects, the other tube had been removed because of another ectopic gestation. Of 90 women so treated in six different centers, the conception rate was 81%, with an IUP rate of 57%. About one-fourth of the women who conceived had a subsequent ectopic pregnancy, which is similar to the rate among all ectopic pregnancies. Thus conservative surgery or medical therapy may be considered when an unruptured ectopic pregnancy occurs in the only remaining tube.

Lund Karhus and colleagues performed a study of long-term reproductive outcomes in women whose first pregnancy was an ectopic. They concluded that **compared with women with a first miscarriage, women with a first ectopic pregnancy had a relative risk of a term pregnancy of 0.55; miscarriages, 0.46; and induced abortions, 0.72; and a 4.7-fold increased risk of further ectopic pregnancy** (Lund Karhus, 2013).

## REFERENCES


Ailawadi M, Lorch SA, Barnhart KT. Cost-effectiveness of presumptively medical treating women at risk for ectopic pregnancy compared with first performing a dilatation and curettage. *Fertil Steril.* 2005;83(2):376.

Barnhart K. Ectopic pregnancy. *N Engl J Med.* 2009;361(4):379-387.

Bolaji I, Gupta S. Medical management of interstitial pregnancy with high beta selective human chorionic gonadotropin. *Ultrasound.* 2010;18(2):60-67.

Bouyer J, Coste J, Fernandez, et al. Sites of ectopic pregnancy: a 10 year population-based study of 1800 cases. *Hum Reprod.* 2002;17:3224.

Bouyer J, Coste J, Shojaei T, et al. Risk factors for ectopic pregnancy: a comprehensive analysis based on a large case-control, population-based study in France. *Am J Epidemiol.* 2003;157:185.

Brady P, Imudia AN, Awonuga AO, et al. Pregnancies of unknown location after in vitro fertilization: minimally invasive management with Karman cannula aspiration. *Fertil Steril.* 2014;101(2):420-426.

Breen JL. A 21-year survey of 654 ectopic pregnancies. *Am J Obstet Gynecol.* 1970;106:1004.

Budowick M, Johnson TR, Genadry R, et al. The histopathology of the developing tubal ectopic pregnancy. *Fertil Steril.* 1980;34:169.

Choi YS, Eun DS, Choi J, et al. Laparoscopic cornuotomy using a temporary tourniquet suture and diluted vasopressin injection in interstitial pregnancy. *Fertil Steril.* 2009;91(15):1933-1937.

Corson SL, Batzer FR. Ectopic pregnancy: a review of the etiologic factors. *J Reprod Med.* 1986;31:78.

Creanga AA, Shapiro-Mendoza CK, Bish CL, et al. Trends in ectopic pregnancy mortality in the United States 1980-2007. *Obstet Gynecol.* 2011;117(4):837.

Fernandez H, Coste J, Job-Spira N. Controlled ovarian hyperstimulation as a risk factor for ectopic pregnancy. *Obstet Gynecol.* 1991;78:656.

Gracia C, Barnhart KT. Diagnosing ectopic pregnancy. *Obstet Gynecol.* 2001;97:465.

Hjordt Hansen MV, Dalsgaard T, Hartwell D, et al. Reproductive prognosis in endometriosis. A national cohort study. *Acta Obstet Gynecol Scand.* 2014;93(5):483-489.

Hymel JA, Hughes DS, Gehlot A, et al. Late abdominal pregnancies (≥20 weeks gestation): a review from 1965 to 2012. *Gynecol Obstet Invest.* 2015;80(4):253-258.

Kadar N, Caldwell BV, Romero R. A method of screening for ectopic pregnancy and its indications. *Obstet Gynecol.* 1981;58:162.

Korhonen J, Stenman UH, Ylostalo P. Serum human chorionic gonadotropin dynamics during spontaneous resolution of ectopic pregnancy. *Fertil Steril.* 1994;61:632.

Leach RE, Ory SJ. Modern management of ectopic pregnancy. *J Reprod Med.* 1989;34:325.

Ledger WL, Sweeting VM, Chatterjee S. Rapid diagnosis of early ectopic pregnancy in an emergency gynaecology service—are measurements of progesterone, intact and free beta human chorionic gonadotrophin helpful? *Hum Reprod.* 1994;9:157.

Lund Karhus L, Egerup P, Wessel Skovlund C, et al. Long-term reproductive outcomes in women whose first pregnancy is ectopic: a national controlled follow-up study. *Hum Reprod.* 2013;28(1):241-246.

McCord ML, Arheart KL, Muram D, et al. Single serum progesterone as a screen for ectopic pregnancy: exchanging specificity and sensitivity to obtain optimal test performance. *Fertil Steril.* 1996;66:513.

Mol F, Mol BW, Ankum WM, et al. Current evidence on surgery, systemic methotrexate and expectant management in the treatment of tubal ectopic pregnancy: a systematic review and meta-analysis. *Hum Reprod Update.* 2008;14:309-319.

Mol F, van Mello NM, Strandell A, et al. Salpingotomy versus salpingectomy in women with tubal pregnancy (ESEP study): an open-label, multicenter, randomized controlled trial. *Lancet.* 2014;383(9927):1483-1489.

O'Leary JL, O'Leary JA. Rudimentary horn pregnancy. *Obstet Gynecol.* 1963;22:371.

Perkins KM, Boulet SL, Kissin DM, et al. Risk of ectopic pregnancy associated with assisted reproductive technology in the United States 2001-2011. *Obstet Gynecol.* 2015;125(1):70.

Peterson HB. The risk of ectopic pregnancy after tubal sterilization. U.S. Collaborative Review of Sterilization Working Group. *N Engl J Med.* 1997;336:762.

Practice Committee of American Society for Reproductive Medicine. Medical treatment of ectopic pregnancy. *Fertil Steril.* 2008;90(3):S206-S212.

Qian ZD, Huang LL, Zhu XM. Curettage or operative hysteroscopy in the treatment of cesarean scar pregnancy. *Arch Gynecol Obstet.* 2015;292(5):1055-1061.

Rotas MA, Haberman S, Levgur M. Cesarean scar ectopic pregnancies: etiology, diagnosis, and management. *Obstet Gynecol.* 2006;107:1373.

Sadeghi H, Rutherford T, Rackow BW, et al: Cesarean scar ectopic pregnancy: case series and review of the literature. *Am J Perinatol.* 2010;27(2):111-120.


**Suggested readings for this chapter can be found on ExpertConsult.com.**

# 18 Benign Gynecologic Lesions

## Vulva, Vagina, Cervix, Uterus, Oviduct, Ovary, Ultrasound Imaging of Pelvic Structures

*Mary Segars Dolan, Cherie C. Hill, Fidel A. Valea*

### KEY POINTS

- The most common large cyst of the vulva is a cystic dilation of an obstructed Bartholin duct, with a lifetime risk estimated to be 2%. These cysts occur most often during the third decade. Inflamed cysts may be treated with oral antibiotics or incision and drainage.
- The vulva contains 1% of the skin surface of the body, but 5% to 10% of all malignant melanomas in women arise from this region. Melanoma is the second most common malignancy arising in the vulva and accounts for 2% to 3% of all of the melanomas occurring in women.
- Ideally all vulvar nevi should be excised and examined histologically. Special emphasis should be directed toward the flat junctional nevus and the dysplastic nevus because they have the greatest potential for malignant transformation. The dysplastic nevus is characterized by being more than 5 mm in diameter, with irregular borders and patches of variegated pigment.
- The management of nonobstetric vulvar hematomas is usually conservative unless the hematoma is greater than 10 cm in diameter or rapidly increasing.
- In adult women, 50% of cases of chronic vulvovaginal pruritus are due to allergic and irritant contact dermatitis. The most common causes of vulvar contact dermatitis are cosmetic and local therapeutic agents. Initial treatment of severe lesions is removal of all irritants or potential allergens and application of topical steroids until the skin returns to normal.
- Women usually develop psoriasis during their teenage years, with approximately 3% of adult women being affected. Approximately 20% of these have involvement of the vulvar skin. The margins of psoriasis are better defined than the common skin conditions in the differential diagnosis, including candidiasis, seborrheic dermatitis, and eczema.
- Psoriasis does not involve the vagina, only the vulva.
- Lichen sclerosus does not involve the vagina, whereas lichen planus may involve the vagina.
- Vulvar pain (vulvodynia) is one of the most common gynecologic problems, reported by up to 16% of women in the general population; 30% of women will have spontaneous relief of their symptoms without any treatment.
- Classically the symptoms associated with the urethral diverticulum are extremely chronic in nature and do not resolve with multiple courses of oral antibiotic therapy.
- Cervical stenosis may occur after loop electrocautery excision procedures (LEEPs). The volume of tissue removed and repeated excisional procedures have been reported to increase the risk for cervical stenosis.
- Endocervical polyps are smooth, soft, red, fragile masses found most commonly in multiparous women in their 40s and 50s. After the endocervical polyp is removed, endometrial sampling should be performed to diagnose a coexisting endometrial hyperplasia or carcinoma.
- Endometrial polyps are noted in approximately 10% of women when the uterus is examined at autopsy. Approximately one in four women with abnormal bleeding will have an endometrial polyp.
- Leiomyomas are the most common benign neoplasms of the uterus. The lifetime prevalence of leiomyomas is greater than 80% among African American women and approaches 70% among white women.
- Cytogenetically, leiomyomas are chromosomally normal and arise from a single cell (they are clonal). All the cells are derived from one progenitor myocyte.
- Abnormal bleeding is experienced by a third of women with myomas, the most common pattern being intermenstrual spotting. Women with myomas and abnormal bleeding should be thoroughly evaluated for concurrent causes of bleeding.
- Adenomyosis is often asymptomatic. If multiple serial sections of the uterus are obtained, the incidence may exceed 60% in women aged 40 to 50 years.
- Adenomyosis rarely causes uterine enlargement greater than a size that corresponds to 14 weeks' gestation unless there is concomitant uterine pathologic change.
- The initial management of a suspected follicular cyst is conservative observation. The majority of follicular cysts disappear spontaneously by either reabsorption of the cyst fluid or silent rupture within 4 to 8 weeks of the initial diagnosis.
- The practice of aspirating cysts laparoscopically should be limited to cysts that are completely simple and associated with normal CA-125 levels. The intraoperative spillage of malignant cystic tumors should be avoided if possible, although the true risk that spillage poses is unknown.
- The differential diagnosis of a woman with acute pain and a suspected ruptured corpus luteum cyst includes ectopic pregnancy, a ruptured endometrioma, and adnexal torsion.
- The treatment of unruptured corpus luteum cysts is conservative. However, if the cyst persists or intraperitoneal bleeding occurs, necessitating operation, the treatment is cystectomy.
- Drainage or fenestration is effective for follicular cysts and poorly effective for cystadenomas. They will tend to recur. When cysts are drained, it is essential to remember that the cytologic examination of cyst fluid has poor predictive value and poor sensitivity in differentiating benign from malignant cysts.
- Theca lutein cysts arise from either prolonged or excessive stimulation of the ovaries by endogenous or exogenous gonadotropins or increased ovarian sensitivity to gonadotropins. The condition of ovarian enlargement secondary to the development of multiple luteinized follicular cysts is termed *hyperreactio luteinalis*. Approximately 50% of molar pregnancies and 10% of choriocarcinomas have associated bilateral theca lutein cysts.

*Continued*

KEY POINTS—cont'd

- Benign ovarian teratomas vary from a few millimeters to 25 cm, may be single or multiple, and are bilateral 10% to 15% of the time. Dermoids are believed to arise during fetal life from a single germ cell. They are 46,XX in karyotype.
- Operative treatment of benign cystic teratomas is via cystectomy with preservation of as much normal ovarian tissue as possible.
- Fifty percent of patients with an ovarian fibroma will have ascites if the tumor is greater than 6 cm. The incidence of associated ascites is directly proportional to the size of the tumor.
- Transitional cell tumors (Brenner tumors) are small, smooth, solid, fibroepithelial tumors of the ovary. They usually occur in women between the ages of 40 and 60 and are predominantly unilateral.
- Adnexal torsion occurs most commonly in the reproductive years, with the average age of patients being in the mid-20s. Pregnancy predisposes to adnexal torsion.
- Ovarian tumors are discovered in 50% to 60% of women with adnexal torsion.
- Abnormal color Doppler flow is highly predictive of torsion of the ovary. However, approximately 50% of women with surgically confirmed adnexal torsion will have a normal Doppler flow study.
- Conservative surgery, either through the laparoscope or via laparotomy, entails gentle untwisting of the pedicle, possibly cystectomy, and stabilization of the ovary with sutures. Detorsion and fixation of the ovary is a safe procedure that reduces the risk of recurrence.
- The risk of pulmonary embolus with adnexal torsion is approximately 0.2%. The risk is similar regardless of whether the condition is managed by conservative surgery with untwisting or adnexal removal without untwisting.

## INTRODUCTION

This chapter reviews benign gynecologic lesions; however, the symptoms and differential diagnoses of these lesions have definite similarity with those of malignant disease. As in many areas of medicine, gynecologic problems do not fall into definitive categories, and those that include malignant disease often overlap with those that include benign disease. When the diagnosis from the history, physical examination, and laboratory tests is clear, management is usually self-evident. When a specific diagnosis is unclear, tissue biopsy may be appropriate. Thus the clinical approach to patient complaints or findings must be broad and not so focused as to prematurely exclude dangerous pathologic conditions within the differential diagnosis.

The discussions in this chapter are arranged anatomically, beginning with the vulva and subsequently covering the vagina, cervix, uterus, oviducts, and ovaries. This chapter does not attempt to be encyclopedic; rather, lesions have been selected based on their clinical importance and prevalence. Therefore extremely rare lesions have been omitted. Because several nonneoplastic abnormalities and lesions present in ways similar to those of benign tumors, this chapter also discusses entities that are not specifically abnormal growths. Clinical problems such as torsion of the ovary, lacerations of the vagina, and hematomas of the vulva are examples of common conditions included in this chapter. Gynecologic infections and associated changes are discussed in Chapter 23.

The successful clinician uses both deductive and inductive reasoning in making a diagnosis. To master both these techniques, one must be adept at history taking and physical examination and be able to form a complete list of possible causes that may be related to the patient's complaint. An understanding of the problems discussed in this chapter will be helpful in that endeavor.

## VULVA

### Urethral Caruncle and Urethral Prolapse

Urethral caruncle and urethral prolapse are conditions that primarily affect postmenopausal women and premenarchal girls. They are thought to occur as a result of decreased estrogen. A urethral caruncle is a small, fleshy mass that occurs at the posterior portion of the urethral meatus. The tissue of the caruncle is soft, smooth, friable, and bright red and initially appears as an eversion of the urethra (Fig. 18.1). Urethral caruncles are generally small, single, and sessile, but they may be pedunculated and grow to be 1 to 2 cm in diameter. Urethral caruncles are believed to arise from an ectropion of the posterior urethral wall associated with retraction and atrophy of the postmenopausal vagina. The growth of the caruncle is secondary to chronic irritation or infection.

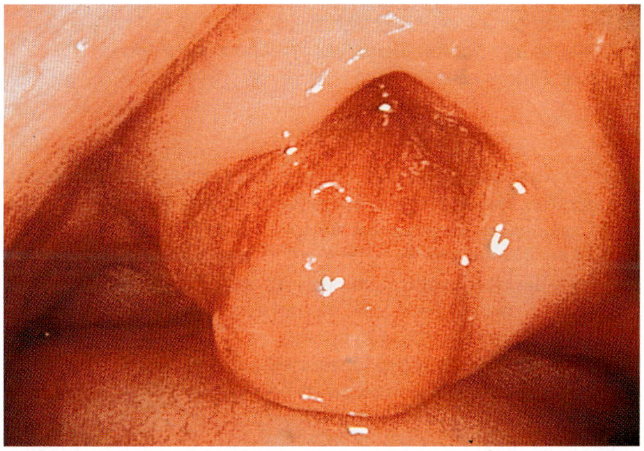

**Fig. 18.1** Photo of urethral caruncle at the base of the meatus. (From Cundiff GW, Bent AE. *Endoscopic Diagnosis of the Female Lower Urinary Tract.* London: WB Saunders; 1999.)

Histologically the caruncle is composed of transitional and stratified squamous epithelium with a loose connective tissue, and often the submucosal layer contains relatively large dilated veins. Caruncles are often subdivided by their histologic appearance into papillomatous, granulomatous, and angiomatous varieties.

They are often secondarily infected, producing ulceration and bleeding. The symptoms associated with urethral caruncles are variable. Many women are asymptomatic, whereas others experience dysuria, frequency, and urgency. Sometimes the caruncle produces point tenderness after contact with undergarments or during intercourse. Ulcerative lesions usually produce spotting on contact more commonly than hematuria. The diagnosis of a urethral caruncle is established by biopsy under local anesthesia because it can appear similar to a neoplasm.

Initial therapy is oral or topical estrogen and avoidance of irritation. If the caruncle does not regress or is symptomatic, it

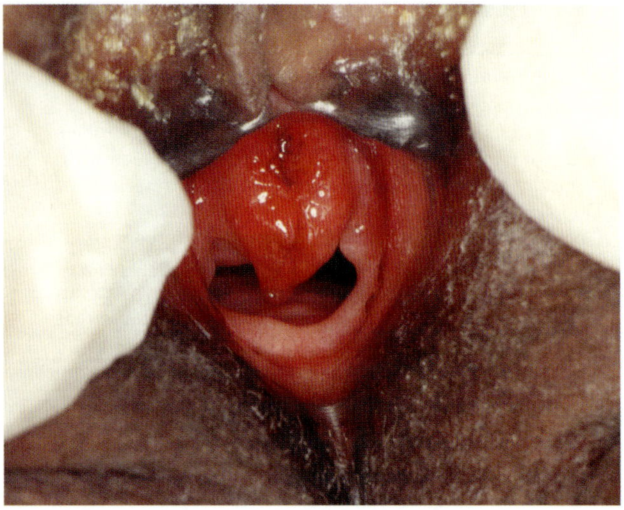

Fig. 18.2 Urethral prolapse found incidentally in a 5-year-old girl on a colposcopic examination for suspected abuse with an edematous red collar of tissue surrounding the urethral meatus. (From Hudson MJ, Swenson AD, Kaplan R, et al. Medical conditions with genital/anal findings that can be confused with sexual abuse. In: Jenny C, ed. *Child Abuse and Neglect: Diagnosis, Treatment and Evidence.* St. Louis: Elsevier; 2011.)

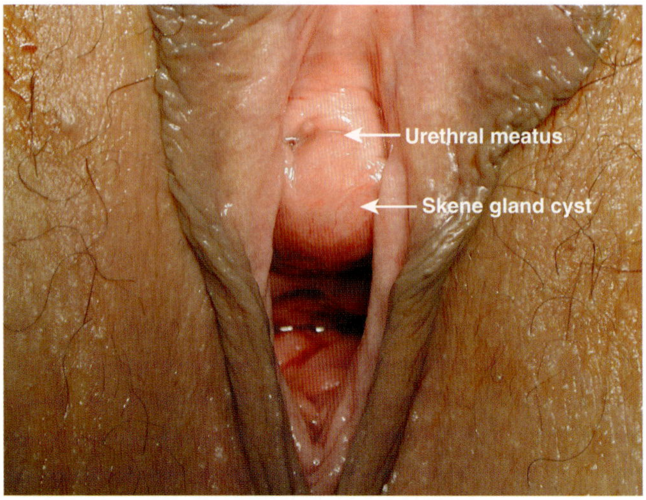


Fig. 18.3 Skene gland cyst. (From Shah SR, Nitti VW. Benign vaginal wall masses and paraurethral lesions. In: Nitti VW, ed. *Vaginal Surgery for the Urologist.* Philadelphia: Elsevier; 2012.)

may be destroyed by cryosurgery, laser therapy, fulguration, or operative excision. After operative destruction, a Foley catheter is usually left in place for 48 to 72 hours to prevent urinary retention. Follow-up is necessary to ensure that the patient does not develop urethral stenosis. It is not uncommon for the caruncle to recur. Small, asymptomatic urethral caruncles do not need treatment.

Urethral prolapse is predominantly a disease of the premenarcheal girl, although it can occur in postmenopausal women (Fig. 18.2). Patients may have dysuria; however, most are asymptomatic. The annular rosette of friable, edematous, prolapsed mucosa does not have the bright red color of a caruncle and is easily distinguished from a caruncle because it is circumferential (Tunitsky, 2012). It may be ulcerated with necrosis or grossly edematous. Therapy for a prolapsed urethra is hot sitz baths and antibiotics to reduce inflammation and infection. Topical estrogen cream is sometimes an effective treatment. In rare cases it may be necessary to excise the redundant mucosa.

The differential diagnosis of urethral caruncles includes primary carcinoma of the urethra and prolapse of the urethral mucosa. Malignant lesions are usually hard and irregular in shape and typically are within the urethra itself (Tunitsky, 2012). Urethral carcinoma is primarily a disease in elderly women. The symptoms of a urethral carcinoma include bleeding, urinary frequency, and dysuria. The majority of urethral carcinomas are of squamous cell origin. Most of these rare carcinomas arise from the distal urethra.

The differential diagnosis of a periurethral mass also includes urethral diverticulum, leiomyoma, vaginal wall inclusion cyst, Skene gland cyst or abscess, and, less commonly, Gartner duct cyst and ectopic ureterocele (Tunitsky, 2012). These are discussed later in this chapter in the Vagina section.

## Cysts

The most common large cyst of the vulva is a cystic dilation of an obstructed Bartholin duct. Bartholin glands open into the vulvar vestibule at about the 5 and 7 o'clock position, distal to the hymenal ring. Bartholin duct cysts and abscesses are fairly common, with a lifetime risk estimated to be 2% (Edwards, 2011). They occur most often during the third decade. Noninflamed cysts contain sterile, clear, mucinous fluid. They do not require treatment unless large enough to cause discomfort. Inflamed cysts may be treated with oral antibiotics or incision and drainage. Lesions in the Bartholin gland can occur as carcinomas, a rare tumor that accounts for 2% to 7% of vulvar carcinomas.

Occasionally the ducts of mucous glands of the vestibule become occluded. The resulting small cysts (usually 0.5 to 2 cm) may be clear, yellow, or blue. Similar small mucous cysts occur in the periurethral region. Wolffian duct cysts or mesonephric cysts are rare, but when they do occur, they are found near the clitoris and lateral to the hymeneal ring. These cysts have thin walls and contain clear serous fluid.

Skene duct cysts are rare, usually small, located on the anterior wall of the vagina along the distal urethra, and may present with symptoms of discomfort or be found on routine examination. These cysts arise secondary to infection and scarring of the small ducts (Fig. 18.3). The differential diagnosis includes urethral diverticula; however, clinically, physical compression of the cyst, unlike compression of a urethral diverticula, should not produce fluid from the urethral meatus. Imaging studies such as magnetic resonance imaging (MRI) and ultrasound may also assist in establishing the diagnosis. Asymptomatic cysts in premenopausal women may be managed conservatively. Treatment is excision with careful dissection to avoid urethral injury.

The most common small vulvar cysts are epidermal (or epidermoid) cysts, which are firm, smooth-surfaced, white, yellow, slightly pink, or skin-colored papules or nodules averaging 0.5 to 2 cm in size (Edwards, 2011). They are most commonly located on the hair-bearing areas. One or several lesions may be present, usually nontender and slow growing. They are firm to shotty in consistency, and their contents are usually under pressure. When noninflamed, they are asymptomatic and no treatment is necessary. If confirmation is needed, incision reveals white, caseous material, like thick cheese. Vulvar epidermal cysts do not have sebaceous cells or sebaceous material identified on microscopic examination but have keratin produced by keratinocytes in the lining of the cyst wall (Edwards, 2011). With rupture or leakage of a cyst, inflammation can occur, necessitating treatment with heat applied locally and possibly incision and drainage. Cysts that become recurrently infected or produce pain should be excised when the acute inflammation has subsided. The typical epidermoid cyst

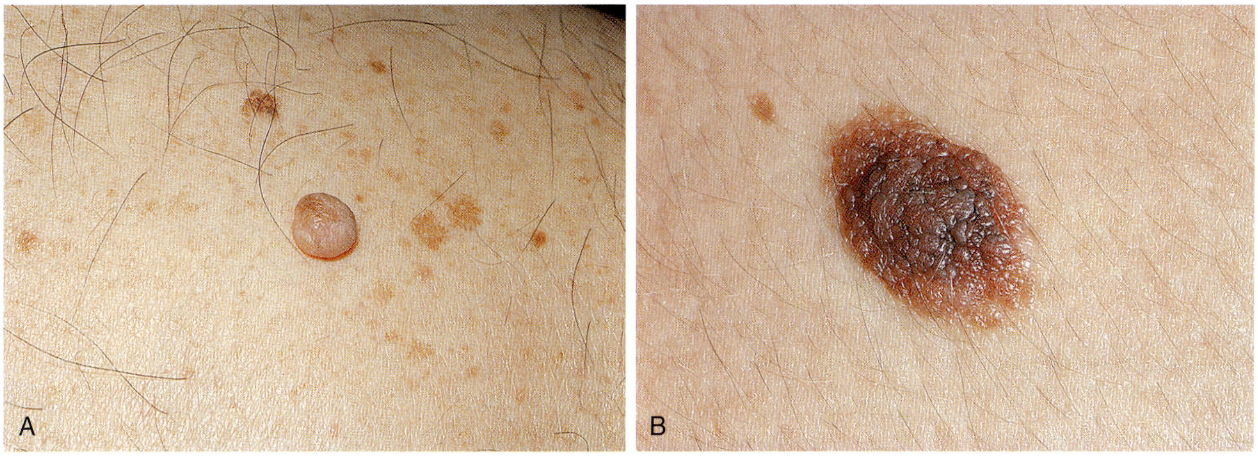


**Fig. 18.4** Vulvar nevi. **A,** Dome-shaped intradermal nevus. **B,** Compound nevus with irregular pigmentation. (From Fisher BK, Margesson LJ. *Genital Skin Disorders: Diagnosis and Treatment.* St. Louis: Mosby; 1998.)

develops from embryonic remnants of an anatomically malformed pilosebaceous unit.

An "inclusion cyst" may arise when bits of epithelium are implanted in the skin during surgery or trauma sufficient to break the skin surface. These may be seen at the site of an episiotomy or obstetric laceration. Large epidermal cysts may be confused with fibromas, lipomas, and hidradenomas.

## Nevus

A nevus, commonly referred to as a *mole*, is a localized nest or cluster of melanocytes. These undifferentiated cells arise from the embryonic neural crest and are present from birth. Many nevi are not recognized until they become pigmented at the time of puberty. Vulvar nevi are one of the most common benign neoplasms in women. As with nevi in other parts of the body, they exhibit a wide range in depth of color, from blue to dark brown to black, and some may be amelanotic. The diameter of most common nevi ranges from a 3 to 10 mm. Grossly a benign nevus may be flat, elevated, or pedunculated. The borders are sharp, the color even, and the shape is symmetric. Dysplastic nevi are commonly 6 to 20 mm with one or more atypical features such as speckling of color, diffuse margination, additional red, white, or blue hues, and asymmetry. Other pigmented lesions in the differential diagnosis include hemangiomas, endometriosis, malignant melanoma, vulvar intraepithelial neoplasia, and seborrheic keratosis.

Vulvar nevi are generally asymptomatic. Most women do not closely inspect their vulvar skin; however, during examination, the use of a mirror held by the patient may facilitate teaching self-vulvar exam. Histologically the lesions are subdivided into three major groups: junctional (a symmetric macule), compound, and intradermal nevi (both papules) (Fig. 18.4).

Melanoma is the second most common malignancy arising in the vulva and accounts for 2% to 3% of all of the melanomas occurring in women, even though the vulva contains approximately 1% of the skin surface area of the body. The incidence of vulvar melanoma is stable or slightly decreasing. It is more common in older, white women, with a mean age at diagnosis of 68 years (Sugiyama, 2007). It is estimated that 50% of malignant melanomas arise from a preexisting nevus. Family history of melanoma is one of the strongest risk factors for the disease.

Ideally, all vulvar nevi should be excised and examined histologically. Special emphasis should be directed toward the flat junctional nevus and the dysplastic nevus because they have the greatest potential for malignant transformation (Fig. 18.5). The lifetime risk of a woman developing melanoma from a congenital

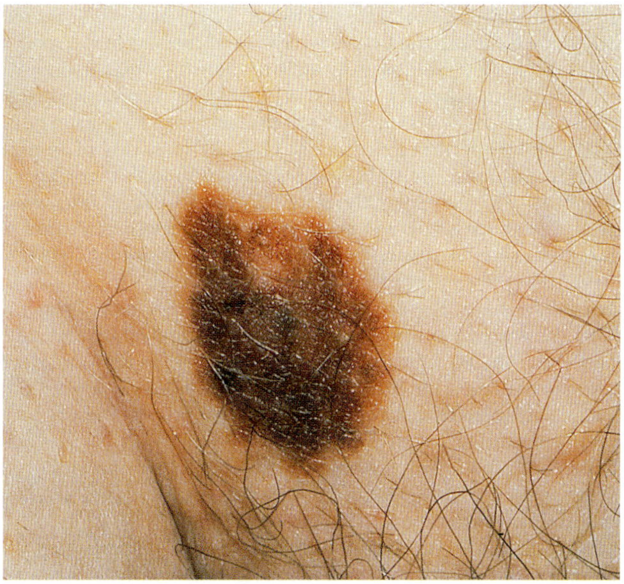

**Fig. 18.5** Suprapubic dysplastic nevus with an irregular shape, reddish hue to the edges, and indistinct margins. (From Fisher BK, Margesson LJ. *Genital Skin Disorders: Diagnosis and Treatment.* St. Louis: Mosby; 1998.)

junctional nevus that measures greater than 2 cm in diameter is estimated to be approximately 10%. The lifetime risk of a melanoma forming in women with dysplastic nevi is 15 times that of the general population.

Removal may be accomplished with local anesthesia or coincidentally with obstetric delivery or gynecologic surgery. Proper excisional biopsy should be three-dimensional and adequate in width and depth. Approximately 5 to 10 mm of normal skin surrounding the nevus should be included, and the biopsy specimen should include the underlying dermis as well.

Some patients are reluctant to have a "normal" appearing nevus removed. Nevi that are raised or contain hair rarely undergo malignant change. However, if they are often irritated or bleed spontaneously, they should be removed. Recent changes in growth or color, ulceration, bleeding, pain, or the development of satellite lesions mandate biopsy. The characteristic clinical features of an early malignant melanoma may be remembered by thinking *ABCD: asymmetry, border* irregularity, *color* variegation, and a *diameter* usually greater than 6 mm.

## Hemangioma

Hemangiomas are rare malformations of blood vessels rather than true neoplasms. Vulvar hemangiomas often are discovered initially during childhood. They are usually single, 1 to 2 cm in diameter, flat, and soft, and they range in color from brown to red or purple. Histologically the multiple channels of hemangiomas are predominantly thin-walled capillaries arranged randomly and separated by thin connective tissue septa. These tumors change in size with compression and are not encapsulated. Most hemangiomas are asymptomatic; occasionally they may become ulcerated and bleed.

There are at least five different types of vulvar hemangiomas. The strawberry and cavernous hemangiomas are congenital defects discovered in young children. The strawberry hemangioma is usually bright red to dark red, is elevated, and rarely increases in size after age 2. Approximately 60% of vulvar hemangiomas discovered during the first years of life spontaneously regress in size by the time the child goes to school. Cavernous hemangiomas are usually purple and vary in size, with the larger lesions extending deeply into the subcutaneous tissue. These hemangiomas initially appear during the first few months of life and may increase in size until age 2. Similar to strawberry hemangiomas, spontaneous resolution generally occurs before age 6. Senile or cherry angiomas are common small lesions that arise on the labia majora, usually in postmenopausal women. They are most often less than 3 mm in diameter, multiple, and red-brown to dark blue. Angiokeratomas are approximately twice the size of cherry angiomas, are purple or dark red, and occur in women between the ages of 30 and 50. They are noted for their rapid growth and tendency to bleed during strenuous exercise. In the differential diagnosis of an angiokeratoma is Kaposi sarcoma and angiosarcoma. Pyogenic granulomas are an overgrowth of inflamed granulation tissue that grow under the hormonal influence of pregnancy, with similarities to lesions in the oral cavity. Pyogenic granulomas are usually small, slightly pedunculated nodules approximately 1 cm in diameter, appearing "pinched in" at the base. They may be mistaken clinically for malignant melanomas, basal cell carcinomas, vulvar condylomas, or nevi. Treatment of pyogenic granulomas involves wide and deep excision to prevent recurrence.

The diagnosis is usually established by gross inspection of the vascular lesion. Asymptomatic hemangiomas and hemangiomas in children rarely require therapy. In adults, initial treatment of large symptomatic hemangiomas that are bleeding or infected may require subtotal resection. When the differential diagnosis is questionable, excisional biopsy should be performed. A hemangioma that is associated with troublesome bleeding may be destroyed by cryosurgery, sclerotherapy, or with the use of lasers. Cryosurgical treatment usually involves a single freeze/thaw cycle repeated three times at monthly intervals. Obviously, if the histologic diagnosis is questionable, any bleeding vulvar mass should be treated by excisional biopsy so that the definitive pathologic diagnosis can be established. Surgical removal of a large, cavernous hemangioma may be technically difficult. Lymphangiomas of the vulva do exist but are extremely rare.

Another rare malformation is the vulvar venous malformation. These lesions may become symptomatic at any age and are relatively prone to thrombosis. Venous malformations are different from vulvar varicosities, which are exacerbated with pregnancy and tend to regress postpartum. There are reports of the successful use of sclerotherapy for the treatment of the malformations.

## Fibroma

Fibromas are the most common benign solid tumors of the vulva. They are more common than lipomas, the other common benign tumors of mesenchymal origin. Fibromas occur in all age groups and most commonly are found in the labia majora (Fig. 18.6). However, they actually arise from deeper connective tissue. Thus they should be considered as dermatofibromas. They grow slowly and vary from a few centimeters to one gigantic vulvar fibroma reported to weigh more than 250 pounds. Most are between 1 and 10 cm in diameter. The smaller fibromas are discovered as subcutaneous nodules. As they increase in size and weight, they become pedunculated. Smaller fibromas are firm; however, larger tumors often become cystic after undergoing myxomatous degeneration. Sometimes the vulvar skin over a fibroma is compromised by pressure and ulcerates.

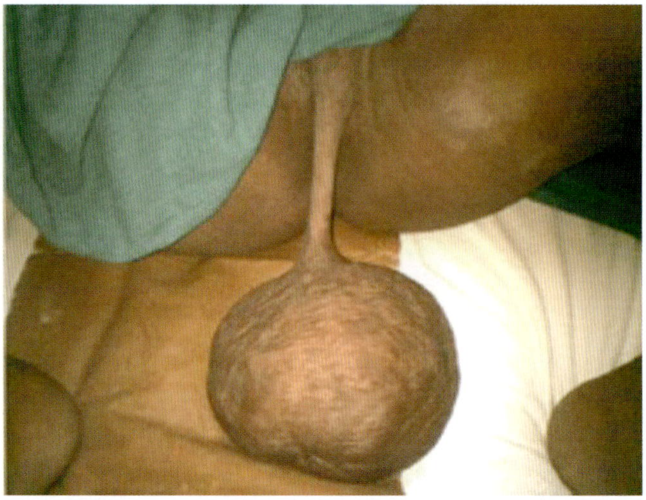

**Fig. 18.6** Clinical photograph of a patient showing a pedunculated fibroma from the labia majora. (From Najam R, Chowdhury HH, Awasthi S. A large fibroma polyp of labia majora—a case report. *J Clin Case Rep.* 2013;3:297.)

Fibromas have a smooth surface and a distinct contour. On cut surface the tissue is gray-white. Fat or muscle cells microscopically may be associated with the interlacing fibroblasts. Fibromas have a low-grade potential for becoming malignant. Smaller fibromas are asymptomatic; larger ones may produce chronic pressure symptoms or acute pain when they degenerate. Treatment is operative removal if the fibromas are symptomatic or continue to grow. Occasionally they are removed for cosmetic reasons.

## Lipoma

Lipomas are the second most common type of benign vulvar mesenchymal tumor. A common hamartoma of fat, lipomas of the vulva are similar to lipomas of other parts of the body. In the vulva, they are most commonly located periclitorally or within the labia majora (Edwards, 2011). When discovered they are softer and usually larger than fibromas (Fig. 18.7). The majority of lipomas in the vulvar region are smaller than 3 cm. The largest vulvar lipoma reported in the literature weighed 44 pounds. They are slow growing, and their malignant potential is extremely low.

When a lipoma is cut, the substance is soft, yellow, and lobulated. Histologically, lipomas are usually more homogeneous than fibromas. Prominent areas of connective tissue occasionally are associated with the mature adipose cells of a true lipoma. Unless extremely large, lipomas do not produce symptoms. Computed tomography and MRI may be used to evaluate tumor extensions and anatomic connections with surrounding structures. MRI has been reported to facilitate the differentiation of vulvar lipomas from vulvar liposarcomas (Jayi, 2014). Excision is

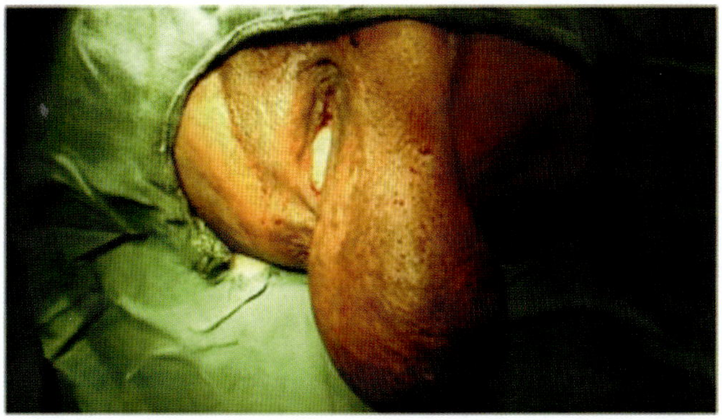

**Fig. 18.7** Vulvar lipoma arising from the left labia majora. (From Hasija S, Khoiwal S, Bilwal B. Vulvar lipoma—a rare case report. *Am J Med Case Rep.* 2015;3(12):413-414.)

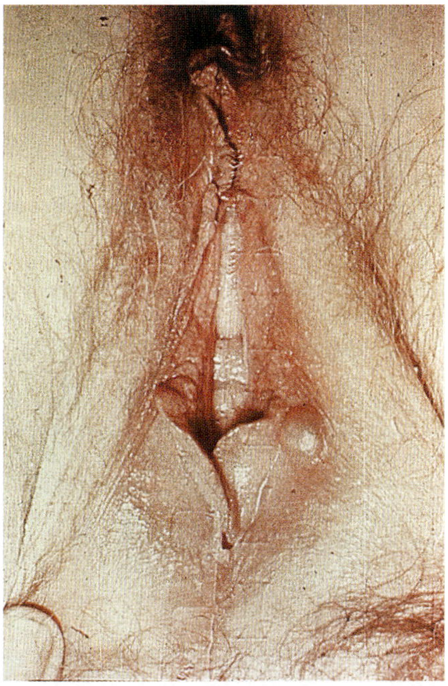

**Fig. 18.8** Hidradenoma. (From Shea CH, Stevens A, Dalziel KL, et al. The vulva: cysts, neoplasms, and related lesions. In: Robboy SJ, Anderson MC, Russell P, eds. *Pathology of the Female Reproductive Tract.* Edinburgh: Churchill Livingstone; 2002.)

usually performed to establish the diagnosis, although smaller tumors may be followed conservatively.

## Hidradenoma (Mammary-Like Gland Adenoma)

The hidradenoma is a rare, small, benign vulvar tumor thought to be derived from mammary-like glands located in the anogenital area of women (Fig. 18.8). In a review of 46 cases, the tumors occurred only in postpubertal women aged 30 to 90 (Scurry, 2009). Clinically, hidradenoma are small, smooth-surfaced, medium soft to firm nodules found most commonly on the labia majora or labia minora. They appear cystic and are usually asymptomatic; however, some patients report itching, bleeding, and mild pain. Hidradenomas may be cystic or solid, and approximately 50% are less than 1 cm in diameter. These tumors have well-defined capsules and arise deep in the dermis. Histologically, because of its hyperplastic, adenomatous pattern, a hidradenoma may be mistaken at first glance for an adenocarcinoma. On close inspection,

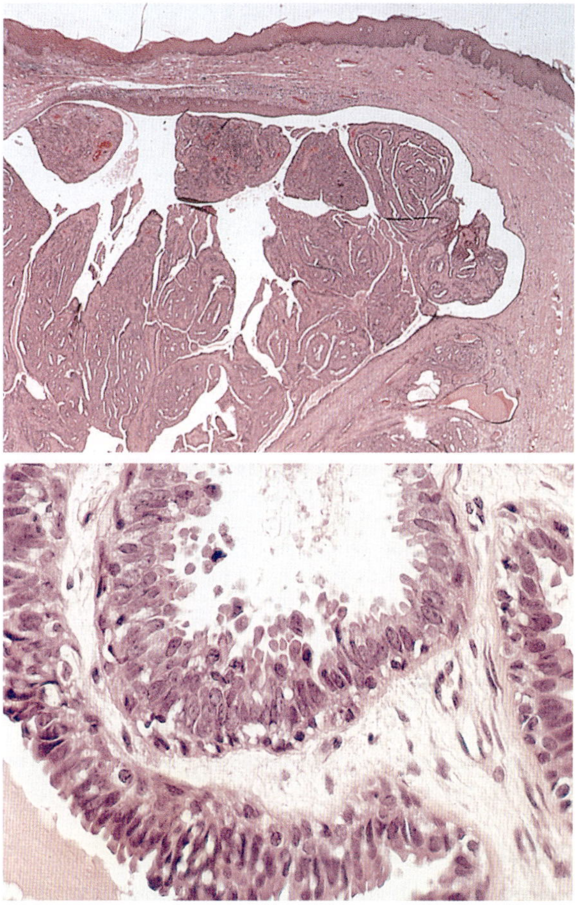

**Fig. 18.9** Histologic views: low- and high-power micrographs of hidradenoma. (From Clement PB, Young RH. *Atlas of Gynecologic Surgical Pathology.* Philadelphia: WB Saunders; 2000.)

however, although there is glandular hyperplasia with numerous tubular ducts, there is a paucity of mitotic figures and a lack of significant cellular and nuclear pleomorphism (Fig. 18.9). Excisional biopsy is the treatment of choice.

## Syringoma

The syringoma is a benign skin adnexal neoplasm thought to be of eccrine origin. It is common on the face and eyelids but unusual on the vulva. In the vulvar area these small, asymptomatic papules (usually less than 5 mm in diameter) are located on the labia majora. The papules are skin colored or yellow and may coalesce to form cords of firm tissue. They may be hormonally active because pregnancy may aggravate associated pruritus and progesterone receptors have been detected in this neoplasm (Heller, 2012). This tumor is usually treated by excisional biopsy, cryosurgery, or laser therapy. The most common differential diagnosis is Fox-Fordyce disease, a condition of multiple retention cysts of apocrine glands accompanied by inflammation of the skin. The latter disease often produces intense pruritus, whereas syringoma is generally asymptomatic. Fox-Fordyce disease improves with pregnancy and oral contraceptive use and remits after menopause. It is treated with topical steroids, topical tretinoin cream, and oral isotretinoin.

## Endometriosis

Endometriosis of the vulva is uncommon. Only 1 in 500 women with endometriosis present with vulvar lesions. The firm, small nodule or nodules may be cystic or solid and vary from a few millimeters to several centimeters in diameter. The subcutaneous lesions are blue, red, or purple, depending on their size, activity, and closeness to the surface of the skin. The gross and microscopic pathologic picture of vulvar endometriosis is similar to endometriosis of the pelvis (see Chapter 19). Vulvar adenosis may appear similar to endometriosis. The former condition occurs after laser therapy of condylomata acuminata.

Endometriosis of the vulva is usually found at the site of an old, healed obstetric laceration, an episiotomy site, an area of operative removal of a Bartholin duct cyst, or along the canal of Nuck. The pathophysiology of vulvar endometriosis development may be secondary to metaplasia, retrograde lymphatic spread, or potential implantation of endometrial tissue during operation. In one series, 15 cases of vulvar endometriosis were believed to be associated with prophylactic postpartum curettage performed in 2028 deliveries, since there was not a single case in 13,800 deliveries without curettage. In general, symptoms do not appear for many months after implantation.

The most common symptoms of endometriosis of the vulva are pain and introital dyspareunia. The classic history is cyclic discomfort and an enlargement of the mass associated with menstrual periods. Treatment of vulvar endometriosis is by wide excision or laser vaporization depending on the size of the mass. Recurrences are common after inadequate operative removal of the entire involved area, and as a result most would also recommend medical therapy with continuous oral contraceptives, progestins, or gonadotropin-releasing hormone (GnRH) agonists.

## Granular Cell Myoblastoma

Granular cell myoblastoma is a rare, slow-growing, solid vulvar tumor originating from neural sheath (Schwann) cells and is sometimes called a *schwannoma*. These tumors are found in connective tissues throughout the body, most commonly in the tongue, and occur in any age group. Approximately 7% of solitary granular cell myoblastomas are found in the subcutaneous tissue of the vulva. Twenty percent of multiple granular cell myoblastomas are located in the vulva. The tumors are usually located in the labia majora but occasionally involve the clitoris.

These tumors are subcutaneous nodules, usually 1 to 5 cm in diameter. They are benign but characteristically infiltrate the surrounding local tissue. The tumors are slow growing, but as they grow, they may cause ulcerations in the skin. The overlying skin often has hyperplastic changes that may look similar to invasive squamous cell carcinoma. Grossly these tumors are not encapsulated, and the cut surface of the tumor is yellow. Histologically, there are irregularly arranged bundles of large, round cells with indistinct borders and pink-staining cytoplasm. Initially the cell of origin was believed to be striated muscle; however, electron microscopic studies have demonstrated that this tumor is from cells of the neural sheath.

The tumor nodules are painless. Treatment involves wide excision to remove the filamentous projections into the surrounding tissue. If the initial excisional biopsy is not sufficiently aggressive, these benign tumors tend to recur. Recurrence occurs in approximately one in five of these vulvar tumors. The appropriate therapy is a second operation with wider margins, as these tumors are not radiosensitive.

## Von Recklinghausen Disease

The vulva is sometimes involved with the benign neural sheath tumors of von Recklinghausen disease (generalized neurofibromatosis and café-au-lait spots). The vulvar lesions of this disease are fleshy, brownish red, polypoid tumors. Approximately 18% of women with von Recklinghausen disease have vulvar involvement. Excision is the treatment of choice for symptomatic tumors.

## Other Abnormal Tissues Presenting as Vulvar Masses

The differential diagnosis of vulvar masses includes a large array of rare lesions and aberrant tissues, including leiomyomas, squamous papillomas, sebaceous adenomas, dermoids, accessory breast tissue and müllerian or wolffian duct remnants, epidermal inclusion cysts, sebaceous cysts, mucous cysts, and skin diseases such as seborrheic keratosis, condylomata acuminata, and molluscum contagiosum. Some of these diseases are discussed in this chapter, others in Chapter 23.

## Hematomas

Hematomas of the vulva are usually secondary to blunt trauma such as a straddle injury from a fall, an automobile accident, or a physical assault. Traumatic injuries producing vulvar hematomas have been reported secondary to a wide range of recreational activities, including bicycle, motorcycle, and go-cart riding; sledding; water skiing; cross-country skiing; and amusement park rides (Fig. 18.10). Spontaneous hematomas are rare and usually occur from rupture of a varicose vein during pregnancy or the postpartum period.

The management of nonobstetric vulvar hematomas is usually conservative unless the hematoma is greater than 10 cm in diameter or is rapidly expanding. The bleeding that produces a vulvar hematoma is usually venous in origin. Therefore it may be controlled by direct pressure. Compression and application of an ice pack to the area are appropriate therapy. If the hematoma continues to expand, operative therapy is indicated in an attempt to identify and ligate the damaged vessel. Often identification of the "key responsible vein" is a futile operative procedure. However, obvious bleeding vessels are ligated, and a pack is placed to promote hemostasis. During the operation, careful inspection and, if needed, endoscopy are performed to rule out injury to the urinary bladder and rectosigmoid.

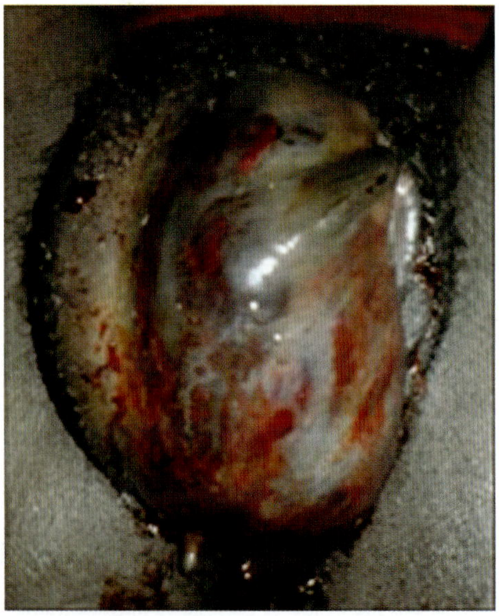

**Fig. 18.10** Traumatic hematoma of the left vulva. (From Taingson MC, Adze JA, Bature SB, Durosinlorun AM, Caleb M, Amina A. Haematoma of the labia minora following consensual sexual intercourse. *Sahel Med J.* 2018;21:52-54.)

The majority of small hematomas regress with time; however, a "chronic expanding hematoma" may become particularly problematic. The most familiar clinical example of this type of problem is the chronic subdural hematoma, but a similar situation may accompany vulvar hematomas. The underlying pathophysiology is repetitive episodes of bleeding from capillaries in the granulation tissue of the hematoma, which result in a chronic, slowly expanding vulvar mass. Treatment of a chronic expanding hematoma is drainage and debridement.

## DERMATOLOGIC DISEASES

The skin of the vulva is similar to the skin over any surface of the body and is therefore susceptible to any generalized skin disease or involvement by systemic disease. The most common skin diseases involving the vulva include contact dermatitis, neurodermatitis, psoriasis, seborrheic dermatitis, cutaneous candidiasis, and lichen planus. The majority of vulvar skin problems are red, scalelike rashes, and the woman's primary complaint is of pruritus. The diagnosis and treatment of these lesions are often obscured or modified by the environment of the vulva. The combination of moisture and heat of the intertriginous areas may produce irritation, maceration, and a wet, weeping surface. Patients will commonly apply ointments and lotions, which may produce secondary irritation. Therefore it is important that the gynecologist examine the skin of the entire body because the patient may have more classic lesions of the dermatologic disease in another location. The skin of the vulva is susceptible to acute infections produced by *Streptococcus* or *Staphylococcus*, such as folliculitis, furunculitis, impetigo, and a chronic infection, hidradenitis suppurativa.

The nonspecific symptom complex of vulvar pruritus and burning is presented next as an introduction to the discussion of dermatologic diseases of the vulva.

### Pruritus

Pruritus is the single most common gynecologic problem; it is a symptom of intense itching with an associated desire to scratch and rub the affected area. Not uncommonly, secondary vulvar pain develops in association or subsequent to pruritus. In some women pruritus becomes an almost unrelenting symptom, with the development of repetitive "itch-scratch" cycles. The itch-scratch cycle is a complex of itching leading to scratching, producing excoriation and then healing. The healing skin itches, leading to further scratching. Pruritus is a nonspecific symptom. The differential diagnosis includes a wide range of vulvar diseases, including skin infections, sexually transmitted diseases, specific dermatosis, vulvar dystrophies, lichen sclerosus, premalignant and malignant disease; contact dermatitis; neurodermatitis; atrophy; diabetes; drug allergies; vitamin deficiencies; pediculosis, scabies; psychological causes; and systemic diseases such as leukemia and uremia.

The management of pruritus involves establishing a diagnosis, treating the offending cause, and improving local hygiene. For successful treatment the itch-scratch cycle must be interrupted before the condition becomes chronic, resulting in lichenification of the skin (lichen simplex chronicus). Lichenification clinically is recognized by palpably thickened skin, exaggerated skin markings, and lichen-type scale. The resulting dry, scaly skin often cracks, forms fissures, and becomes secondarily infected, thus complicating the treatment (see Chapter 30).

### Contact Dermatitis

The vulvar skin, especially the intertriginous areas, is a common site of contact dermatitis. The vulvar skin is more reactive to exposure by irritants than other skin areas such as the extremities. Contact dermatitis is usually caused by one of two basic pathophysiologic processes: a primary irritant (nonimmunologic) or a definite allergic (immunologic) origin. A large proportion of adult patients with chronic vulvovaginal pruritis are symptomatic because of contact dermatitis. Substances that are irritants produce immediate symptoms such as a stinging and burning sensation when applied to the vulvar skin. The symptoms and signs secondary to an irritant disappear within 12 hours of discontinuing the offending substance. In contrast, allergic contact dermatitis requires 36 to 48 hours to manifest its symptoms and signs.

Allergic contact dermatitis is a cell-mediated delayed-type (type IV) hypersensitivity reaction. There is development of antigen-specific T cells that may return to the skin at the next contact with the allergen. Often the signs of allergic contact dermatitis persist for several days despite removal of the allergen. Rarely, some women will be allergic to latex or semen. These elicit type 1, immunoglobulin E (IgE)–mediated, immediate reactions. Angioedema and urticarial plaques and papules arise within minutes of contact, and anaphylaxis may result.

Excessive cleansing of the vulvar skin and urinary or fecal incontinence may precipitate an irritant dermatitis. The majority of chemicals that produce hypersensitivity of the vulvar skin are cosmetic or therapeutic agents, including vaginal contraceptives, lubricants, sprays, perfumes, douches, fabric dyes, fabric softeners, synthetic fibers, bleaches, soaps, chlorine, dyes in toilet tissues, and local anesthetic creams (Fig. 18.11). External chemicals that trigger the disease process must be avoided. Some of the most severe cases of contact dermatitis involve lesions of the vulvar skin secondary to poison ivy or poison oak. Women with a history of atopy or eczema are more at risk for contact dermatitis and tend to be more sensitive to skin irritations.

Acute contact dermatitis results in a red, edematous, inflamed skin. The skin may become weeping and eczematoid. The most severe skin reactions form vesicles and at any stage may become secondarily infected. The common symptoms of contact dermatitis

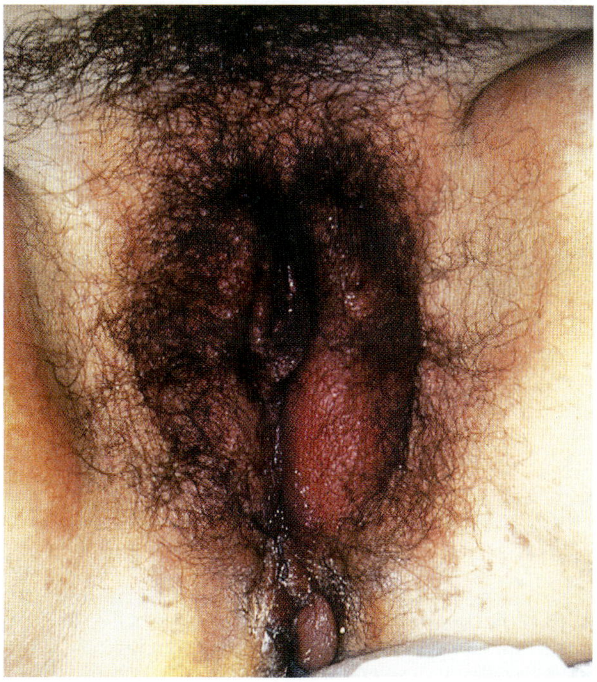

**Fig. 18.11** Acute contact dermatitis to chlorhexidine. Edema and erythema are present in areas where the antiseptic chlorhexidine solution was applied. (From Stevens A, Dalziel KL. Vulvar dermatoses. In: Robboy SJ, Anderson MC, Russell P, eds. *Pathology of the Female Reproductive Tract.* Edinburgh: Churchill Livingstone; 2002.)

include superficial vulvar tenderness, burning, and pruritus. Chronic untreated contact dermatitis can evolve into a syndrome of lichenification, with the skin developing a leathery appearance and texture, known as *lichen simplex chronicus* (Fig. 18.12).

The foundation of treatment of contact dermatitis is withdrawal of the offending substance. Sometimes the distribution of the vulvar erythema helps to delineate the irritant. For example, localized erythema of the introitus often results from vaginal medication, whereas generalized erythema of the vulva is secondary to an allergen in clothing. It is possible to use a vulvar chemical innocuously for many months or years before the topical vulvar "allergy" develops.

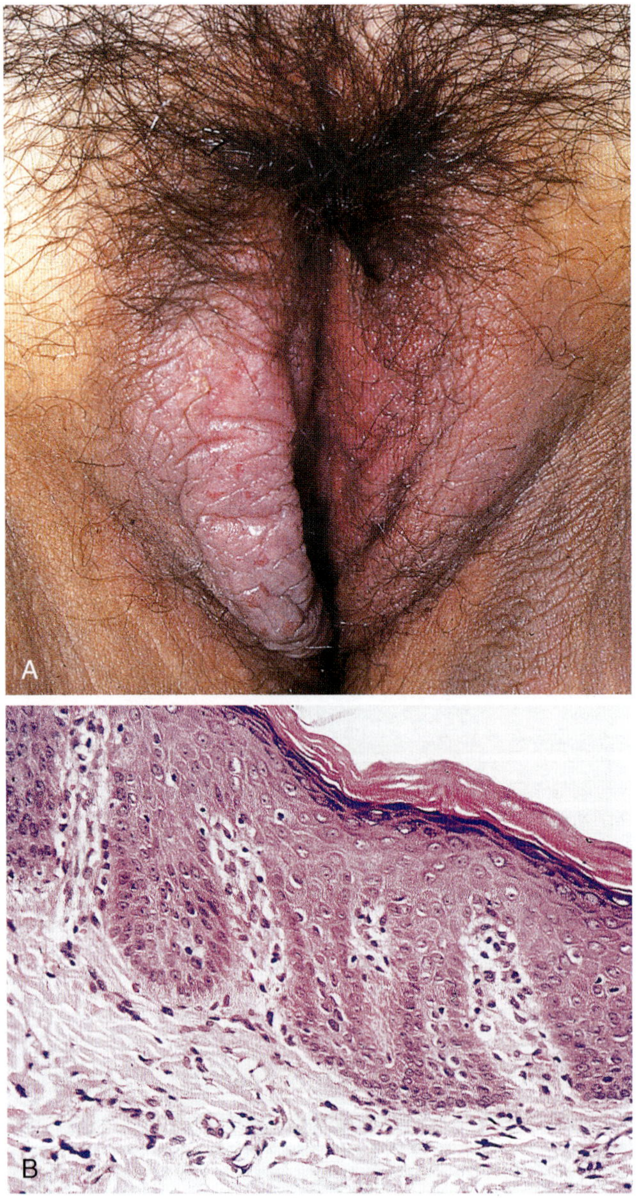


**Fig. 18.12 A,** Lichen simplex chronicus manifesting of the right labium majus. There is thickening and accentuation of skin markings, with surface excoriation caused by recent scratching. **B,** Lichen simplex chronicus. The epidermis shows thickening of rete ridges, thickening of the granular layer, and overlying hyperkeratosis. (From Stevens A, Dalziel KL. Vulvar dermatoses. In Robboy SJ, Anderson MC, Russell P, eds. *Pathology of the Female Reproductive Tract.* Edinburgh: Churchill Livingstone; 2002.)

Once the offending substances and all potential allergens have been eliminated, topical steroids can be applied to the vulva until the skin returns to normal. The vulvar skin should be kept clean and dry. Use of a barrier product such as zinc oxide ointment or vitamin A and D ointment may be needed to keep urine and feces away from the skin in patients with incontinence. The pain and burning can be treated with tepid water bath soaks several times a day for the first few days. Use of a lubricating agent such as petroleum jelly or Eucerin cream will reduce the pruritus by rehydrating the skin and should be applied after the soaks. Cotton undergarments that allow the vulvar skin to aerate should be worn, and constrictive, occlusive, or tight-fitting clothing such as pantyhose should be avoided. Use of a nonmedicated cornstarch baby powder may facilitate vulvar dryness. Hydrocortisone (0.5% to 1%) and fluorinated corticosteroids (Valisone, 0.1%, or Synalar, 0.01%) as lotions or creams may be rubbed into the skin two to three times a day for a few days to control symptoms. Synthetic systemic corticosteroids (prednisone, starting with 50 mg/day for 7 to 10 days in a decreasing dose) are sometimes necessary for treatment of poison ivy and poison oak or severe reactions. Antipruritic medications, such as antihistamines, are not of great therapeutic benefit except as soporific agents. Women often experience pruritus after steroid therapy for vulvar dermatitis. This is not necessarily a recurrence but rather represents a type of withdrawal reaction. This rebound pruritus is seen most commonly with prolonged and higher doses of steroids. After examination, the optimal treatment is a step-down to a short course of a low-potency topical steroid such as 1% hydrocortisone. Topical steroids should be continued for a month or more after clinical improvement because microscopic evidence of inflammation remains for a considerable period (Edwards, 2011).

## Psoriasis

Psoriasis is a common, generalized skin disease of unknown origin. Generally, women develop psoriasis during their teenage years, with approximately 3% of adult women affected. Approximately 20% of these cases involve vulvar skin. Similar to candidiasis, psoriasis may be the first clinical manifestation of human immunodeficiency virus (HIV) infection. Psoriasis is chronic and relapsing, with an extremely variable and unpredictable course marked by spontaneous remissions and exacerbations. Twenty-five percent of women have a family history of the disease. Genetic susceptibility to develop psoriasis is believed to be multifactorial. Common areas of involvement are the scalp and fingernails. When psoriasis involves the vulvar skin, it produces both anxiety and embarrassment.

Vulvar psoriasis usually affects intertriginous areas and is manifested by red to red-yellow papules. These papules tend to enlarge, becoming well-circumscribed, dull-red plaques (Fig. 18.13). Though the presence of classic silver scales and bleeding on gentle scraping of the plaques may help establish the diagnosis, the scales are less common in the vulva than on other areas of the body.

With psoriasis on the vulvar region, the number of scales is extremely variable and often they are absent. Under the influence of the moisture and heat of the vulva, vulvar psoriasis may resemble candidiasis. Importantly for the diagnosis, psoriasis does not involve the vagina. Sometimes dermatologists treat refractory cases of psoriasis with oral retinoids. The margins of psoriasis are more well defined than the common skin conditions in the differential diagnosis, including candidiasis, seborrheic dermatitis, and eczema. Initial treatment for mild disease is 1% hydrocortisone cream. If the patient has pain secondary to chronic fissures or more moderate disease, a 4-week course of a fluorinated corticosteroid cream should be given. If this treatment is not successful, a dermatologist should be consulted. Several newer antipsoriatic treatments may benefit this condition, especially when it becomes moderate to severe, including vitamin D analogs, topical retinoids,

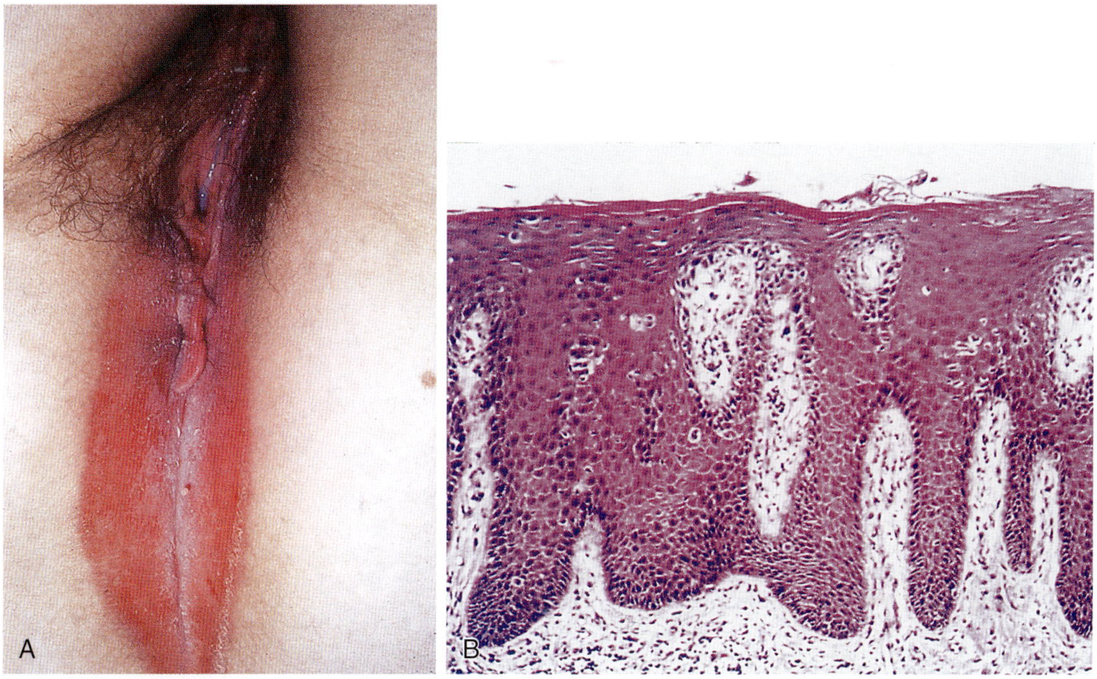


**Fig. 18.13 A,** Psoriasis of perineum and vulva. Flexural psoriasis often lacks the typical parakeratotic scale of psoriasis on other body sites. Painful erosion of the natal cleft is common. **B,** Psoriasis. There is psoriasiform hyperplasia of rete ridges with papillary dermal edema and telangiectasia. The parakeratotic scale on the skin surface is not prominent in vulvar psoriasis. (From Stevens A, Dalziel KL. Vulvar dermatoses. In: Robboy SJ, Anderson MC, Russell P, eds. *Pathology of the Female Reproductive Tract.* Edinburgh: Churchill Livingstone; 2002.)

calcineurin inhibitors, salicylic acid, coal tar cyclosporine, and drugs that alter the immune system (biologics). Systemic steroids often produce a rebound flare-up of the disease.

## Seborrheic Dermatitis

Seborrheic dermatitis is a common chronic skin disease of unknown origin that classically affects the face, scalp, sternum, and the area behind the ears. Rarely, the mons pubis and vulvar areas may be involved. Vulvar lesions are pale to yellow-red, erythematous, and edematous, and they are covered by a fine, nonadherent scale that is usually oily. Excessive sweating and emotional tension precipitate attacks. Although the cause is unknown, an abnormal reaction in the skin to a commensal yeast, *Pityrosporum ovale,* has been implicated in the pathogenesis. Treatment with topical and oral antifungal agents causes improvement; however, they are not as effective as topical steroids (Edwards, 2011). Approximately 2% to 4% of women have some form of the disease. The pruritus associated with seborrheic dermatitis varies from mild to severe. Treatment is similar to that for contact dermatitis, with hydrocortisone cream being the most effective medication. The differential diagnosis of seborrheic dermatitis includes psoriasis, cutaneous candidiasis, and contact dermatitis. Often it is difficult to differentiate between the cutaneous manifestations of psoriasis and seborrheic dermatitis. Clinically and pragmatically the exact diagnosis is only of academic interest because the treatment is similar.

## Lichen Planus

Lichen planus is an uncommon vulvovaginal dermatosis. Women complain of soreness, burning, itching, and dyspareunia. The disease presents most commonly as a hypertrophic, coalesced plaque similar to lichen sclerosis. Lichen sclerosis, though, does not involve the vagina, whereas lichen planus can. Three types of vulvar lichen planus have been described: erosive, classical, and hypertrophic. Erosive lichen planus is the most common and is characterized by erosions around the introitus, clitoris, and labia majora and minora (Fig. 18.14). A lacy white edge is commonly seen. Vaginal involvement is common, and patients may also present with contact bleeding, erythema, and scarring with synechiae. Many patients may also report mouth pain and have gingival lesions that appear erosive and desquamative. The classical type presents with small purple, polygonal papules, with sometimes a reticulate lace pattern. Hyperkeratotic lichen planus presents as single or multiple white, hyperkeratotic papules and plaques. Lichen planus is an inflammatory condition with unknown cause; however, evidence suggests it to be an autoimmune disease of cellular immunity (Edwards, 2011). The autoimmune phenomenon can be triggered by certain drugs, including beta-blockers, angiotensin-converting enzyme (ACE) inhibitors, and other medications. It may also arise spontaneously. The correct diagnosis is confirmed by a small punch biopsy of the vagina or vulva. Histologic findings (Fig. 18.15) include degeneration of the basal layers, a lymphocytic infiltrate of the dermis, and epidermal acanthosis.

This chronic disease tends to have spontaneous remissions and exacerbations that last for weeks to months. Treatment of local lesions is by use of a potent topical steroid ointment such as clobetasol applied twice daily. Steroid suppositories may be inserted intravaginally at night. If the patient is intensely symptomatic, oral steroids may be necessary. In postmenopausal women, topical or systemic estrogen replacement can also be crucial to avoid additional mucosal thinning. Other treatments for resistant cases include methotrexate, oral retinoids, oral griseofulvin, dapsone, azathioprine, cyclophosphamide, and topical cyclosporine. Surgery may be necessary to separate vaginal adhesions or uncover a buried clitoris. Postoperatively the use of vaginal dilators can prevent scar re-formation. Women with this condition should be monitored at periodic intervals because of an associated increased risk of developing vulvar squamous cell carcinoma.

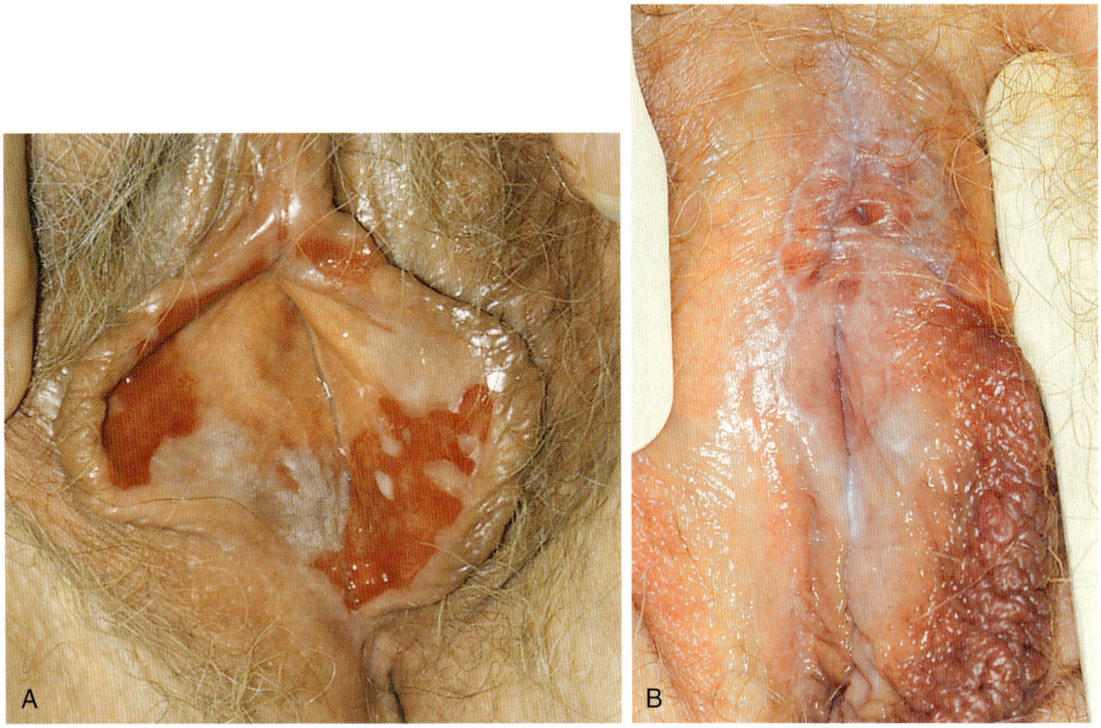

Fig. 18.14 Lichen planus. **A,** Eroded ulcers in the vulva. **B,** Lacy reticulated pattern of lichen planus with periclitoral scarring in a 71-year-old woman who has had oral lichen planus for 10 to 15 years, cutaneous lichen planus of arms and legs for 18 months, and bouts of erosive vaginal lichen planus with scarring and partial vaginal stenosis. (From Fisher BK, Margesson LJ. *Genital Skin Disorders: Diagnosis and Treatment.* St. Louis: Mosby; 1998.)

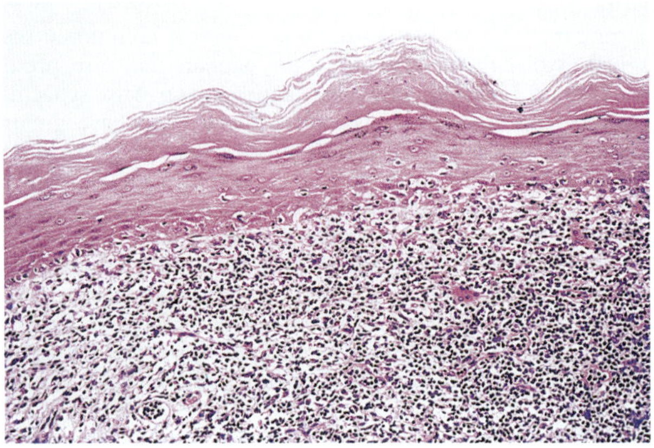

**Fig. 18.15** Lichen planus, histologic view. Note hyperkeratosis with extensive basal layer destruction and a dense lichenoid infiltrate at the dermoepidermal junction. (From Stevens A, Dalziel KL. Vulvar dermatoses. In: Robboy SJ, Anderson MC, Russell P, eds. *Pathology of the Female Reproductive Tract.* Edinburgh: Churchill Livingstone; 2002.)

## Behçet Disease

Behçet disease is a rare disorder initially described as a triad of oral aphthous ulcers, genital aphthous ulcers, and uveitis. It is now known to be a multisystem disease with potential development of problems in many organ systems: skin, joints, cardiovascular, central nervous system, and gastrointestinal tract. The prevalence is high in the Mediterranean region, Middle East, and Japan. Turkey has the highest prevalence, with a rate of 100 to 400 in 100,000 individuals (Edwards, 2011). The diagnosis is made after exclusion of herpetic lesions and other ulcerative diseases. The symptoms respond to topical anesthetics. Severe disease may require antineoplastic therapy including methotrexate, steroids, or other medications.

## Hidradenitis Suppurativa

Hidradenitis suppurativa is a chronic, unrelenting, refractory infection of skin and subcutaneous tissue that contains apocrine glands. The apocrine glands are found mainly in the axilla and the anogenital region. The disease is rare before puberty; 98% of cases are found in reproductive-age women, and most all disease regresses after menopause. As the infection progresses over time, deep scars and pits are formed (Fig. 18.16). The patient undergoes great emotional distress as this condition is both painful and is associated with a foul-smelling discharge. Theories of the cause of this condition favor an inflammation beginning in the hair follicles (Fig. 18.17). Thus the term sometimes used synonymously is *acne inversa.* The lesions involve the mons pubis, the genitocrural folds, and the buttocks. The differential diagnosis of hidradenitis suppurativa includes simple folliculitis, Crohn disease of the vulva, pilonidal cysts, and granulomatous sexually transmitted diseases. The differentiation from Crohn disease is usually made by history with an absence of gastrointestinal (GI) involvement. The early phase of the disease involves infection of the follicular epithelium, at first appearing as a boil. This is followed by erythema, involvement of multiple follicles, and chronic infections that burrow and form cysts that break open and track through subcutaneous tissue, creating odiferous and painful sinuses and fistula in the vulva. The chronic scarring, fibrosis, and hyperpigmentation with foul-smelling discharge and soiling of underclothes lead to a socially debilitating condition. The diagnosis should be confirmed by biopsy.

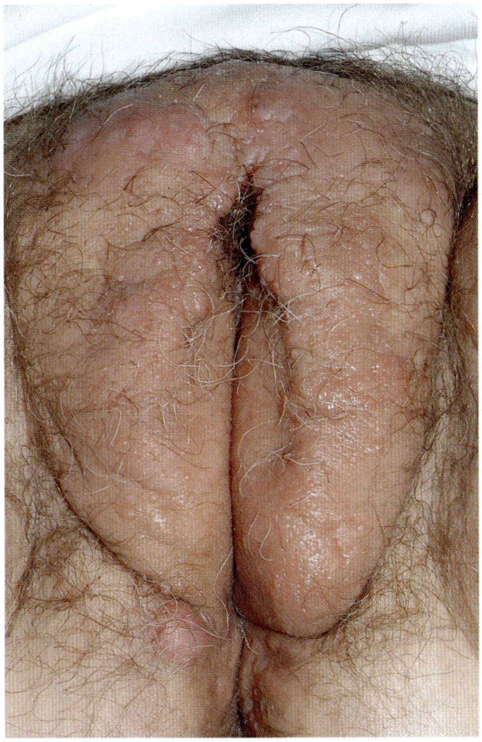

**Fig. 18.16** Hidradenitis suppurativa: multiple vulvar abscesses with edema of the mons pubis and labia majora. Notice the "pitting" and "scars" from chronic infection. (From Amankwah Y, Haefner H. Vulvar edema. *Dermatol Clin.* 2010;28(4):765-777.)

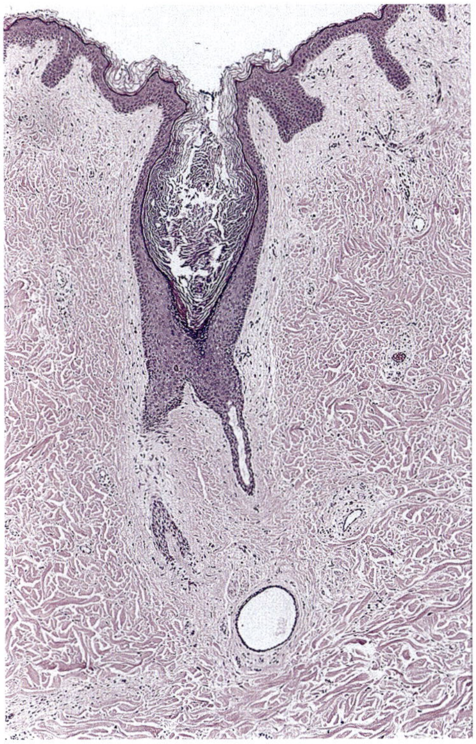

**Fig. 18.17** Hydradenitis suppurativa. Biopsy with follicular plugging and connection to dilated apocrine duct. (From Kelly P. Folliculitis and the follicular occlusion tetrad. In Bolognia JL, Jorizzo JL, Rapini RP, eds. *Dermatology.* Edinburgh: Mosby; 2003.)

Early on in the disease process there are small furuncles and folliculitis, for which topical and oral clindamycin is usually effective in the short term, usually requiring a 3-month course of antibiotics. Unfortunately, relapse is common; if treatment with long-term antibiotic therapy and topical steroids is unsuccessful, other medical therapies have included antiandrogens, isotretinoin, and cyclosporine. The treatment of refractory cases is aggressive, wide operative excision of the infected skin.

## Edema

Edema of the vulva may be a symptom of either local or generalized disease. Two of the most common causes of edema of the vulva are secondary reactions to inflammation or to lymphatic blockage. Vulvar edema is often recognized before edema in other areas of the female body is noted. The loose connective tissue of the vulva and its dependent position predispose to early development of pitting edema. Systemic causes of vulvar edema include circulatory and renal failure, ascites, and cirrhosis. Vulvar edema also may occur after intraperitoneal fluid is instilled to prevent adhesions or for dialysis. Local causes of vulvar edema include allergy, neurodermatitis, inflammation, trauma, and lymphatic obstruction caused by carcinoma or infection. Infectious diseases that are associated with vulvar edema include necrotizing fasciitis, tuberculosis, syphilis, filariasis, and lymphogranuloma venereum.

### Vulvar Pain Syndromes: Vulvar Vestibulitis, Vestibulodynia, and Dysesthetic Vulvodynia

Vulvar pain (vulvodynia) is one of the most common gynecologic problems, reported by up to 16% of women in the general population (Stockdale, 2014). Vulvodynia is a pain disorder that occurs without visible findings, infection, inflammation, neoplasia, or a neurologic disorder. The disease has a wide spectrum of symptomology and response to treatment; therefore causation is most likely multifactorial. The diagnosis is made after excluding other treatable causes. A complete history identifying the onset of pain, other associated symptoms, duration of pain, medical and sexual history, treatments tried, allergies, and triggers for pain should be taken. A physical examination with a cotton swab to identify specific areas of pain should be documented. Large population-based studies have noted that symptoms wax and wane, with many women having spontaneous remission (up to 10% of the time).

The terms *vulvar pain syndrome*, *vulvodynia*, and *vulvar vestibulitis* are often used interchangeably. Vulvar vestibulitis is somewhat of a misnomer because it is not inflammation. Vulvar pain syndrome is further subdivided into two categories: vestibulodynia and dysesthetic vulvodynia. The two conditions have a significant amount of overlap, although with different causes and clinical courses. In general, vestibulodynia is found in younger women, most commonly white, with onset shortly after puberty through the mid-20s. Dysesthetic vulvodynia is most common in peri- and postmenopausal women who have rarely if ever had previous vulvar pain.

The differential diagnosis of vulvar pain includes neurologic diseases, herpes simplex infection, chronic infections, abuse, pain syndromes, neoplasia, contact dermatitis, and psychogenic causes. Chronic pain is considered to be part of the vulvodynia spectrum once the diagnoses of infection, invasive disease, and inflammation have been excluded. Severe chronic pain can be socially debilitating, and these patients have a wide spectrum of associated affective symptomology as well. Women with vulvodynia have greater psychological distress than women who have other vulvar problems. Importantly, these psychological concerns must be addressed as part of the therapeutic management.

Vestibulodynia involves the symptom of allodynia, which is hyperesthesia, a pain that is related to nonpainful stimuli. The

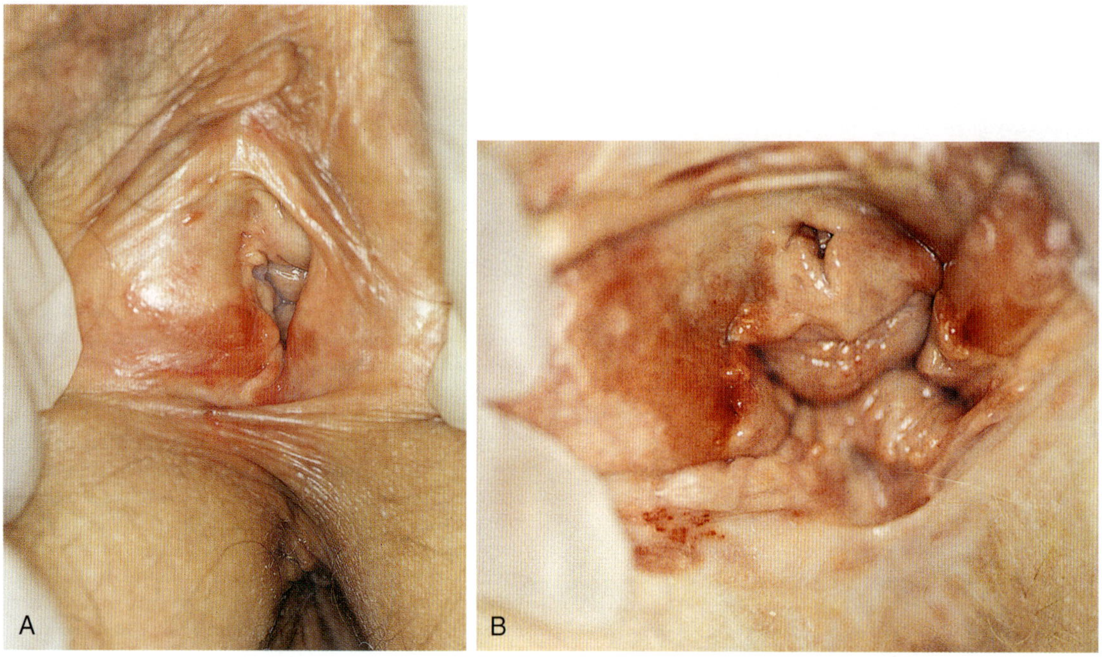


**Fig. 18.18** Vulvar vestibulitis. **A,** Redness localized to the right Bartholin duct opening and, below it, vulvar vestibulitis. **B,** Discrete localized periglandular erythema in vulvar vestibulitis in a 60-year-old woman. (From Fisher BK, Margesson LJ. *Genital Skin Disorders: Diagnosis and Treatment.* St. Louis: Mosby; 1998.)

pain is not present without stimulation. The diagnostic maneuver to establish the presence of allodynia is to lightly touch the vulvar vestibule with a cotton-tipped applicator. The vulvar areas most likely to be affected are from the 4 to 8 o'clock positions along the vulvar-vaginal borders. Erythema is not always present, but when present, it is confined to the vulvar vestibule (Fig. 18.18). Additionally, patients with vestibulodynia experience intolerance to pressure in the vulvar region. This pain is neurogenic in origin. The intolerance to pressure may be caused by tampon use, sexual activity, or tight clothing, and the pain is described as raw and burning. It is not a spontaneous pain; it is invoked. However, it is severe in nature. Some authors have suggested that symptoms be present for at least 6 months before establishing the diagnosis. The symptoms may appear around the time of first intercourse, or within the next 5 to 15 years.

Studies of women with vulvar vestibulodynia have found no increased incidence of sexual abuse compared with controls. However, many women are found to have erotophobia. Some even noted an increased nerve density and normal estrogen receptors compared with controls. In contrast, other investigators have noted an increase in alpha-estrogen receptors. Theories regarding the cause cite potential immunologic and infectious factors, though no theory has been proved to date. Oral contraceptive use in younger women and hormone replacement in older women have no association with vestibulodynia.

Vulvar dysesthesia, or vulvodynia, is a nonlocalized pain that is constant (not provoked by touch), mimicking a neuralgia. Allodynia is rarely noted, and erythema is also much less common than in vulvar vestibulodynia. Women with vulvodynia are more often perimenopausal or postmenopausal. Dyspareunia is currently present but has usually not been present before the development of dysesthesia. Similar to women with vulvar vestibulodynia, there is not an increased history of sexual abuse compared with controls. Women with dysesthesia also have an increased incidence of chronic interstitial cystitis. In general, both groups of women have an increased incidence of atopy. In some, a history of inflammation from topical agents may be elicited. These agents have usually either been self-prescribed or prescribed by a professional to treat initially what seems to be infection. Patients are often depressed and anxious, but this is thought to be a secondary reaction to the chronic pain. An outline for evaluating these patients is presented in Box 18.1. Before the diagnosis, one should exclude infection by atypical *Candida* (which may not be obvious on inspection and should be diagnosed by culture) and by group B *Streptococcus.* Some would recommend that before extensive treatment a punch biopsy should be obtained to rule out dermatitis presenting atypically, including lichen sclerosis.

The therapeutic approach for these two conditions emphasizes a sensitivity to the debilitating social aspects of the problem. Similar to other chronic pain syndromes, tricyclic antidepressants or gabapentin have been found to be successful in several series. Doses of gabapentin range from 300 to 3600 mg, usually given with increasing doses every week. Most authors start at 300 mg daily, increase to 300 mg twice daily, then three times a day, then 600 mg three times per day to 900 three times per day,

**BOX 18.1** Evaluation of Patients With Vulvar Pain

- Examination of vulva for abnormal redness, erosions, crusting, ulceration, hypopigmentation
- Cotton swab test to identify areas of pain on pressure (e.g., vestibule)
- Sensory neurologic examination for allodynia and symmetric sensation
- Examination for vaginal redness, erosions, pallor, dryness
- Biopsy of specific skin findings for evaluation by dermatopathologist
- Microscopic evaluation of vaginal secretions for yeast, pH, increased white blood cells
- Culture for *Candida* (exclusive of *C. albicans*) and bacteria (especially group B *Streptococcus*)
- Evaluation for depression and impact on quality of life
- Classification of vulvar vestibulitis syndrome or dysesthetic vulvodynia

and so on; the average effective dose is approximately 1800 mg daily. Approximately 66% to 75% of women have a response to treatment with gabapentin. When the medication is discontinued, it should be tapered.

Biofeedback and behavior modification therapy have also produced relief. Topical 5% lidocaine ointment has been described as a local treatment option with limited success.

In the past, women with refractory vulvar vestibulitis have been treated with surgical removal of the vulvar vestibule and reapproximation of tissue. The surgery is difficult, with a significant complication rate, but results are generally good. In one series of 126 women with vulvar vestibulitis, the complication rate was 39%; 89% of women felt that the surgery improved their condition enough to recommend it to other women (Traas, 2006). Importantly, 30% of women have spontaneous relief of their symptoms without any treatment. Reports have indicated that multilevel nerve block given simultaneously for refractory cases has produced some response. Botulinum neurotoxin is also effective in some women, particularly those with concurrent vaginismus and levator ani spasm. Series of treatments and combinations of treatments are often used.

For women with vestibulodynia unresponsive to other therapies, surgery is usually recommended. Vestibulectomy and modified vestibulectomy (partial or limited from 3 to 9 o'clock) have resulted in resolution in 60% to 90% of patients compared with 40% to 80% for nonsurgical interventions (Stockdale, 2014). Surgery has been noted to be most effective in younger women. Some advocate for partial vestibulectomy because most pain and painful skin occur in the lower half of the vestibule. Complications from vestibulectomy include occlusion of the Bartholin gland, leading to development of cysts. This problem requires surgical "unroofing" of the duct.

## VAGINA

### Urethral Diverticulum

A urethral diverticulum is a permanent, epithelialized, saclike projection that arises from the posterior urethra. Most are thought to be acquired and occur in women between ages 30 and 60 years (Lee, 2005). It often presents as a mass on the anterior vaginal wall, and urethral diverticula represent approximately 84% of periurethral masses (Table 18.1). It is a common problem, being discovered in approximately 1% to 3% of women. Most urogynecologists have noted a decline in the prevalence of this condition since the early 1990s. The majority of cases are initially diagnosed in reproductive-age women, with the peak incidence in the fourth decade of life. The symptoms of a urethral diverticulum are nonspecific and are identical to the symptoms of a lower urinary tract infection. To diagnose this elusive condition, one should suspect urethral diverticulum in any woman with chronic or recurrent lower urinary tract symptoms. The urologic aspects of this condition are discussed in Chapter 21. Histologically the diverticulum is lined by epithelium; however, there is a lack of muscle in the saclike pocket.

Urethral diverticula may be congenital or acquired. Few urethral diverticula are present in children; therefore it is assumed that most diverticula are not congenital. The anatomy of the urethra has been described as a tree with many stunted branches that represent the periurethral ducts and glands. It is assumed that the majority of urethral diverticula result from repetitive or chronic infections of the periurethral glands. The suburethral infection may cause obstruction of the ducts and glands, with subsequent production of cystic enlargement and retention cysts. These cysts may rupture into the urethral lumen and produce a suburethral diverticulum. Persistent inflammation and stasis can lead to stone formation (10%). Malignancy has been reported in 6% to 9% of cases, mostly adenocarcinoma (Foley, 2011). Urethral diverticula are small, from 3 mm to 3 cm in diameter. The majority of urethral diverticula open into the midportion of the urethra (Table 18.2). Occasionally, multiple suburethral diverticula occur in the same woman.

Classically the symptoms associated with the urethral diverticulum are extremely chronic in nature and have not resolved with multiple courses of oral antibiotic therapy. The most common symptoms associated with urethral diverticula are urinary urgency and frequency and dysuria, which is the presenting symptom in about 90% of cases. Approximately 15% of women with urethral diverticula experience hematuria. Other authors have stressed the three *D*s associated with a diverticulum: *dysuria*, *dyspareunia*, and *dribbling* of the urine. Although for years, postvoiding dribbling has been termed a classic symptom of urethral diverticulum, it is reported by fewer than 10% of women with this condition. In Lee's series a palpable, tender mass was discovered in 56 of 108 patients (Lee, 2005). It is interesting that in most large series, approximately 20% of the women are asymptomatic. A classic sign of a suburethral diverticulum is the expression of purulent material from the urethra after compressing the suburethral area during a pelvic examination. Although the sign of producing a discharge by manual expression is specific, its sensitivity is poor.

The foundation of diagnosing urethral diverticulum is the physician's awareness of the possibility of this defect occurring in women with chronic symptoms of lower urinary tract infection. Historically the two most common methods of diagnosing urethral diverticulum have been the voiding cystourethrography and cystourethroscopy. Approximately 70% of urethral diverticula will be filled by contrast material on a postvoiding radiograph with a lateral view. Cystourethroscopy will demonstrate the

**TABLE 18.1** Final Diagnosis of Periurethral Mass and Frequency

| Diagnosis | N (%) | 95% Confidence Interval (%) |
|---|---|---|
| Urethral diverticulum | 66 (84) | 73,91 |
| Diverticulum with malignancy | 4 (6) | 2,14.8 |
| Vaginal cyst | 6 (7) | 3,15 |
| Leiomyoma | 4 (5) | 1,12 |
| Vaginal squamous cell carcinoma | 2 (2.5) | 0.03,8.8 |
| Ectopic ureter | 2 (2.5) | 0.03,8.8 |
| Granuloma | 1 (1) | 0.03,6.8 |

From Blaivas JG, Flisser AJ, Bleustein CB, Panagopoulos G. Periurethral masses: diagnosis in a large series of women. *Obstet Gynecol.* 2004;103(5 Pt 1):842-847.

**TABLE 18.2** Location of the Ostium in 108 Female Patients With Diverticulum of the Urethra

| Site | Number of Patients |
|---|---|
| Distal (external) third of the urethra | 11 |
| Middle third of the urethra | 55 |
| Proximal (inner) third of the urethra (including vesical neck) | 18 |
| Multiple sites | 18 |
| Unknown | 6 |

From Lee RA. Diverticulum of the urethra: clinical presentation, diagnosis, and management. *Clin Obstet Gynecol.* 1984;27:490-498.

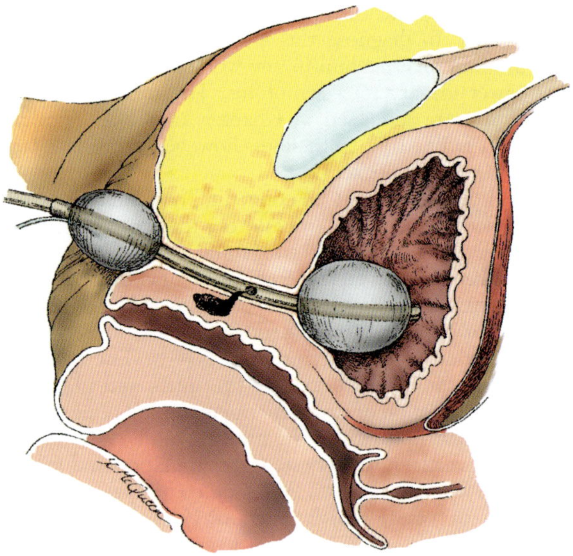

**Fig. 18.19** Double-balloon catheter in use for positive-pressure urethrography.

urethral opening of the urethral diverticulum in approximately 6 of 10 cases. Other diagnostic tests used to identify urethral diverticula include urethral pressure profile recordings, transvaginal ultrasound, computed tomography (CT) scans, MRI, and positive-pressure urethrography. For diagnosis of urethral diverticulum, MRI sensitivity is 100% because the resolution is excellent (Tunitsky, 2012). Ultrasonography, done translabially (or introitally), may assist in the assessment of the mass as cystic or solid. Positive-pressure urethrography is done with a special double-balloon urethral catheter (Davis catheter) (Fig. 18.19). Classically the recordings of the pressure profile of the urethra demonstrate a biphasic curve in a woman with a urethral diverticulum. If a woman has a urethral diverticulum and urinary incontinence, performing a stress urethral pressure profile will help differentiate the cause. The differential diagnosis includes Gartner duct cyst, an ectopic ureter that empties into the urethra, and Skene glands cysts.

Several different operations can correct urethral diverticula. Excisional surgery should be scheduled when the diverticulum is not acutely infected. Operative techniques can be divided into transurethral and transvaginal approaches, with most gynecologists preferring the transvaginal approach as described by Lee (Lee, 2005). The majority of diverticula enter into the posterior aspect of the urethra. Diverticula of the distal one-third may be treated by simple marsupialization. After operations, approximately 80% of patients obtain complete relief from symptoms. Some diverticula have multiple openings into the urethra. Complete excision of this network of fistulous connections is important. The recurrence rate varies between 10% and 20%, and many failures are due to incomplete surgical resection. The most serious consequences of surgical repair of urethral diverticula are urinary incontinence and urethrovaginal fistula. Postoperative incontinence usually follows operative repairs of large diverticula that are near the bladder neck. This incontinence may be secondary to damage to the urethral sphincter. The incidence of each of these complications is approximately 1% to 2%.

## Inclusion Cysts

Inclusion cysts are the most common cystic structures of the vagina. In a series of 64 women with cystic masses of the vagina, 34 had inclusion cysts (Deppisch, 1975). The cysts are usually discovered in the posterior or lateral walls of the lower third of the vagina. Inclusion cysts vary from 1 mm to 3 cm in diameter. Similar to inclusion cysts of the vulva, inclusion cysts of the vagina are more common in parous women. Inclusion cysts usually result from birth trauma or gynecologic surgery. Often they are discovered in the site of a previous episiotomy or at the apex of the vagina after hysterectomy.

Histologically, inclusion cysts are lined by stratified squamous epithelium. These cysts contain a thick, pale yellow substance that is oily and formed by degenerating epithelial cells. Often these cysts are erroneously called sebaceous cysts in the misbelief that the central material is sebaceous. Similar to vulvar inclusion cysts, the cause is either a small tag of vaginal epithelium buried beneath the surface after a gynecologic or obstetric procedure or a misplaced island of embryonic remnant that was destined to form epithelium.

The majority of inclusion cysts are asymptomatic. If the cyst produces dyspareunia or pain, the treatment is excisional biopsy.

## Dysontogenetic Cysts

Dysontogenetic cysts of the vagina are thin-walled, soft cysts of embryonic origin. Whether the cysts arise from the mesonephros (Gartner duct cyst), the paramesonephricum (müllerian cyst), or the urogenital sinus (vestibular cyst) is predominantly of academic rather than clinical importance. The cysts may be differentiated histologically by the epithelial lining (Fig. 18.20). Most mesonephric cysts have cuboidal, nonciliated epithelium. Most perimesonephric cysts have columnar, endocervical-like epithelium. Occasionally pressure produced by the cystic fluid produces flattening of the epithelium, which makes histologic diagnosis less reliable. Although most commonly single, dysontogenetic cysts may be multiple. Usually the cysts are 1 to 5 cm in diameter

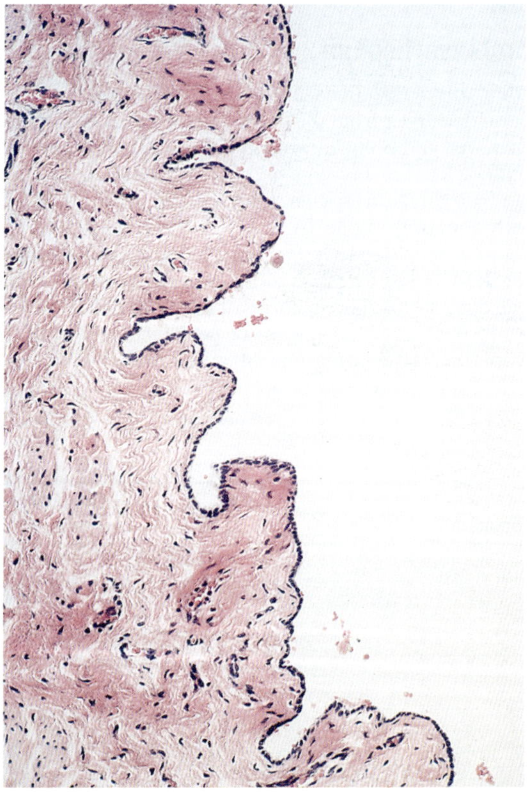

**Fig. 18.20** Histologic examination of a Gartner duct cyst from the lateral vaginal wall. The cyst is lined by nonciliated cells. (From Clement PB, Young RH. *Atlas of Gynecologic Surgical Pathology.* Philadelphia: WB Saunders; 2000.)

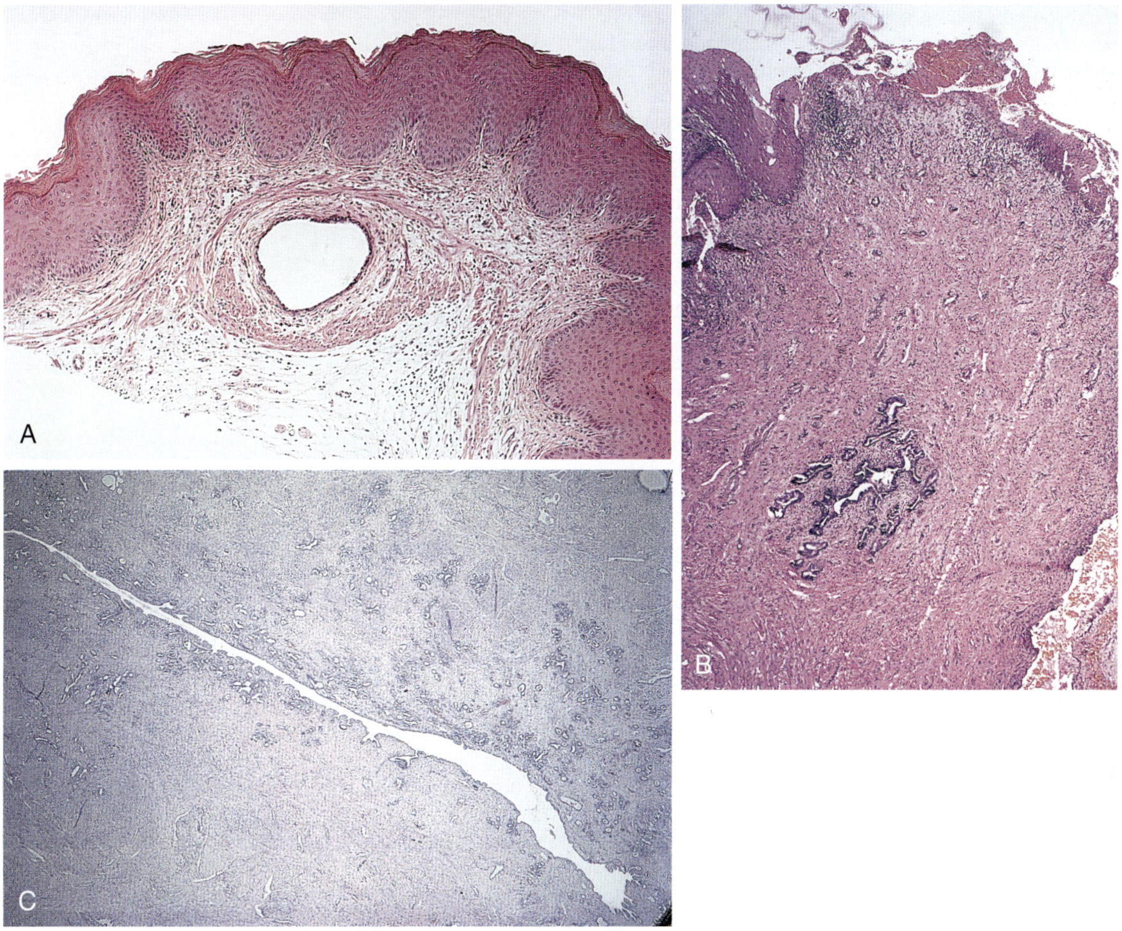


**Fig. 18.21 A,** Normal mesonephric duct. On cross section it is a single duct in the submucosa surrounded by clusters of smooth muscle bands. **B,** Mesonephric duct. The mother duct, located deep in the wall of the vagina, is surrounded by smaller arborized offshoots. **C,** Elongated mesonephric duct. (From Robboy SJ, Anderson MC, Russell P, et al. The vagina. In: Robboy SJ, Anderson MC, Russell P, eds. *Pathology of the Female Reproductive Tract.* Edinburgh: Churchill Livingstone; 2002.)

and are discovered in the upper half of the vagina (Fig. 18.21). Sometimes multiple small cysts may present like a string of large, soft beads. A large cyst presenting at the introitus may be mistaken for a cystocele, anterior enterocele, or obstructed aberrant ureter. Approximately 1 in 200 women develop these cysts.

Embryonic cysts of the vagina, especially those discovered on the anterior lateral wall, are usually Gartner duct cysts. In the embryo the distal portion of the mesonephric duct runs parallel with the vagina. It is assumed that a segment of this embryonic structure fails to regress, and the obstructed vestigial remnant becomes cystic. These cysts are most commonly found in the lower one-third of the vagina.

Most of these benign cysts are asymptomatic, sausage-shaped tumors that are discovered only incidentally during pelvic examination. Small asymptomatic Gartner duct cysts may be followed conservatively. In a series of 25 women undergoing operations for symptomatic dysontogenetic cysts, a wide range of symptoms were reported, including dyspareunia, vaginal pain, urinary symptoms, and a palpable mass. Sometimes large cysts interfere with the use of tampons. MRI can be useful in delineating the course and anatomic arrangement of vaginal cysts (Wai, 2004).

Operative excision is indicated for chronic symptoms. Rarely, one of these cysts becomes infected, and if operated on during the acute phase, marsupialization of the cyst is preferred. Excision of the vaginal cyst may be a much more formidable operation than anticipated. The cystic structure may extend up into the broad ligament and anatomically be in proximity to the distal course of the ureter.

Rare tumors of the vagina include fibromas, angiomyxomas, and hemangiomas. All are usually found by the patient and require surgical excision.

## Tampon Problems

The vaginal tampon has achieved immense popularity and ubiquitous use. It is not surprising that there are rare associated risks with tampon usage: vaginal ulcers, the "forgotten" tampon, and toxic shock syndrome. The latter, related to toxins elaborated by *Staphylococcus aureus*, is discussed in Chapter 23.

Wearing tampons for a few days has been associated with microscopic epithelial changes. The majority of women develop epithelial dehydration and epithelial layering, and some will develop microscopic ulcers. These minor changes take between 48 hours and 7 days to heal. Using colposcopy to evaluate the vaginal epithelium after tampon use, Friedrich found serial changes of epithelial drying, peeling, layering, and ultimately microulceration in 15% of women wearing tampons only during the time of normal menstruation. No clinical symptoms were associated with these microscopic changes. Theoretically these microulcerations are a potential portal of entry for HIV.

Large macroscopic ulcers of the vaginal fornix have been described in women using vaginal tampons for prolonged times for persistent vaginal discharge or spotting. The ulcers have a base of clean granulation tissue with smooth, rolled edges. One can even find tampon fibers in the biopsy specimens of these ulcers. The pathophysiology of the ulcer is believed to be secondary to drying and pressure necrosis induced by the tampon. Obviously, many of these young women use tampons for the identical symptoms that are associated with a vaginal ulcer—that is, spotting and vaginal discharge. Often the intermenstrual spotting is believed to be breakthrough bleeding from oral contraceptives, and the possibility of a vaginal ulcer from chronic tampon usage is overlooked.

Vaginal ulcers are not uncommon secondary to several types of foreign objects, including diaphragms, pessaries, and medicated silicon rings. Management is conservative because the ulcers heal spontaneously when the foreign object is removed. Any persistent ulcer should be biopsied to establish the cause.

A woman with a "lost" or "forgotten" tampon presents with a classic foul vaginal discharge and occasionally spotting. The tampon is usually found high in the vagina. The odor from a forgotten tampon is overwhelming. The tampon is removed using a "double glove technique" where two gloves are donned on the removal hand and, on grasping the tampon, the outer glove is pulled over the tampon and tied as the tampon is removed. The woman should be treated with an antibiotic vaginal cream or gel (such as metronidazole or clindamycin) for the next 5 to 7 days.

## Local Trauma

The most common cause of trauma to the lower genital tract of adult women is coitus. Approximately 80% of vaginal lacerations occur secondary to sexual intercourse. Other causes of vaginal trauma are straddle injuries, penetration injuries by foreign objects, sexual assault, vaginismus, and water-skiing accidents. The management of vulvar and vaginal trauma in children is discussed in Chapter 12.

The predisposing factors believed to be related to coital injury include virginity, the state of the postpartum and postmenopausal vaginal epithelium, pregnancy, intercourse after a prolonged period of abstinence, hysterectomy, and inebriation. In one series of 19 injuries from normal coitus, 12 of the women were between the ages of 16 and 25 and 5 were older than 45 (Smith, 1983). The most common injury is a transverse tear of the posterior fornix. Similar linear lacerations often occur in the right or left vaginal fornices. The location of the coital injury is believed to be related to the poor support of the upper vagina, which is supported only by a thin layer of connective tissue. The most prominent symptom of a coital vaginal laceration is profuse or prolonged vaginal bleeding. Many women experienced sharp pain during intercourse, and 25% noted persistent abdominal pain. The most troublesome but extremely rare complication of vaginal laceration is vaginal evisceration. Coital injury to the vagina should be considered in any woman with profuse or prolonged abnormal vaginal bleeding. Sensitive but thorough history regarding abuse is always appropriate.

Management of coital lacerations involves prompt suturing under adequate anesthesia. Secondary injury to the urinary and gastrointestinal tracts should be ruled out.

# CERVIX

## Endocervical and Cervical Polyps

Endocervical and cervical polyps are the most common benign neoplastic growths of the cervix, reported in 4% of gynecologic patients. Endocervical polyps are most common in multiparous women in their 40s and 50s. Cervical polyps usually present as a single polyp, but multiple polyps do occur occasionally. The majority are smooth, soft, reddish purple to cherry red, and fragile. They readily bleed when touched. Endocervical polyps may be single or multiple and are a few millimeters to 4 cm in diameter. The stalk of the polyp is of variable length and width (Fig. 18.22). Polyps may arise from either the endocervical canal (endocervical polyp) or ectocervix (cervical polyp). Endocervical polyps are more common than are cervical polyps. Often the terms *endocervical* and *cervical* polyps are used to describe the same abnormality. Polyps whose base is in the endocervix usually have a narrow, long pedicle and occur during the reproductive years, whereas polyps that arise from the ectocervix have a short, broad base and usually occur in postmenopausal women.

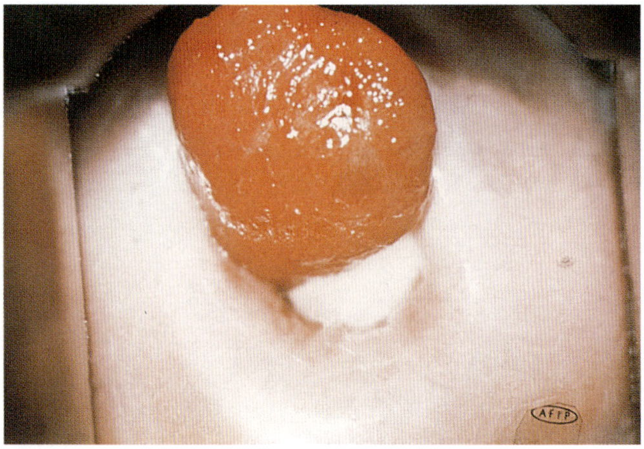

**Fig. 18.22** Cervical polyp. A large polyp protrudes from the external cervical os. The surface is red and rough, covered by endocervical epithelium. (From Anderson MC, Robboy SJ, Russell P, et al. The cervix—benign and non-neoplastic conditions. In: Robboy SJ, Anderson MC, Russell P, eds. *Pathology of the Female Reproductive Tract.* Edinburgh: Churchill Livingstone; 2002.)

The hypothesis of the origin of endocervical polyps is that they are usually secondary to inflammation or abnormal focal responsiveness to hormonal stimulation. Focal hyperplasia and localized proliferation are the response of the cervix to local inflammation. The color of the polyp depends in part on its origin, with most endocervical polyps being cherry red and most cervical polyps grayish white.

The classic symptom of an endocervical polyp is intermenstrual bleeding, especially after contact such as coitus or a pelvic examination. Sometimes an associated leukorrhea emanates from the infected cervix. Many endocervical polyps are asymptomatic and recognized for the first time during a routine speculum examination. Often the polyp seen on inspection is difficult to palpate because of its soft consistency.

Histologically the surface epithelium of the polyp is columnar or squamous epithelium, depending on the site of origin and the degree of squamous metaplasia (Fig. 18.23). The stalk is composed of an edematous, inflamed, loose, and richly vascular connective tissue. Six different histologic subtypes have been described: adenomatous, cystic, fibrous, vascular, inflammatory, and fibromyomatous. Greater than 80% are of the adenomatous type. During pregnancy, focal areas of decidual changes may develop in the stroma. Often there is ulceration of the stalk's most dependent portion, which explains the symptom of contact bleeding. Malignant degeneration of an endocervical polyp is extremely rare; the reported incidence is less than 1 in 200. Considerations in the differential diagnosis include endometrial polyps, small prolapsed myomas, retained products of conception, squamous papilloma, sarcoma, and cervical malignancy. Microglandular endocervical hyperplasia sometimes presents as a

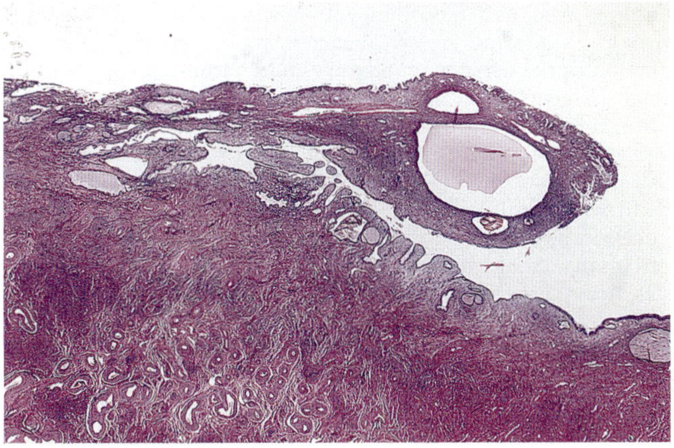

**Fig. 18.23** Cervical polyp. The stroma is fibromuscular and the base contains thick-walled blood vessels. Endocervical crypts, some dilated, are present within the polyp. (From Anderson MC, Robboy SJ, Russell P, et al. The cervix—benign and non-neoplastic conditions. In: Robboy SJ, Anderson MC, Russell P, eds. *Pathology of the Female Reproductive Tract.* Edinburgh: Churchill Livingstone; 2002.)

1- to 2-cm polyp. This is an exaggerated histologic response, usually to oral contraceptives.

Most endocervical polyps may be managed in the office by grasping the base of the polyp with an appropriately sized clamp. The polyp is avulsed with a twisting motion and sent to the pathology laboratory for microscopic evaluation. The polyp is usually friable. If the base is broad or bleeding ensues, the base may be treated with chemical cautery, electrocautery, or cryocautery. After the polyp is removed, the endometrium should be evaluated in women older than 40 who have presented with abnormal bleeding, to rule out coexisting pathologic changes because a significant endometrial pathologic condition is found in approximately 5% of asymptomatic women with endocervical polyps.

## Nabothian Cysts

Nabothian cysts are retention cysts of endocervical columnar cells occurring where a tunnel or cleft has been covered by squamous metaplasia. These cysts are so common that they are considered a normal feature of the adult cervix. Many women have multiple cysts. Grossly these cysts may be translucent or opaque whitish or yellow in color, and they vary from microscopic to macroscopic size, with the majority between 3 mm and 3 cm in diameter. Rarely, a woman with several large nabothian cysts may develop gross enlargement of the cervix. These mucous retention cysts are produced by the spontaneous healing process of the cervix. The area of the transformation zone of the cervix is in an almost constant process of repair, and squamous metaplasia and inflammation may block the cleft of a gland orifice. The endocervical columnar cells continue to secrete, and thus a mucous retention cyst is formed. Nabothian cysts are asymptomatic, and no treatment is necessary.

## Lacerations

Cervical lacerations may occur during obstetric deliveries. Obstetric lacerations vary from minor superficial tears to extensive full-thickness lacerations at 3 and 9 o'clock, respectively, which may extend into the broad ligament. Lacerations may occur in nonpregnant women with mechanical dilation of the cervix. The atrophic cervix of the postmenopausal woman increases the risk of cervical laceration when the cervix is mechanically dilated for dilation and curettage (D&C) or hysteroscopy.

Acute cervical lacerations bleed and should be sutured. Cervical lacerations that are not repaired may give the external os of the cervix a fish-mouthed appearance; however, they are usually asymptomatic. The use of laminaria tents to slowly soften and dilate the cervix before mechanical instrumentation of the endometrial cavity has reduced the magnitude of iatrogenic cervical lacerations. Furthermore, the practice of routine inspection of the cervix after every second- or third-trimester delivery has enabled physicians to discover and repair extensive cervical lacerations. Extensive cervical lacerations, especially those involving the endocervical stroma, may lead to incompetence of the cervix during a subsequent pregnancy.

## Cervical Myomas

Cervical myomas are smooth, firm masses that are similar to myomas of the fundus (Figs. 18.24 and 18.25). A cervical myoma is usually a solitary growth in contrast to uterine myomas, which, in general, are multiple. Depending on the series, 3% to 8% of myomas are categorized as cervical myomas. Because of the relative paucity of smooth muscle fibers in the cervical stroma, the majority of myomas that appear to be cervical actually arise from the isthmus of the uterus.

Most cervical myomas are small and asymptomatic. When symptoms do occur, they are dependent on the direction in which the enlarging myoma expands. The expanding myoma produces symptoms secondary to mechanical pressure on adjacent organs. Cervical myomas may produce dysuria, urgency, urethral or ureteral obstruction, dyspareunia, or obstruction of the cervix. Occasionally a cervical myoma may become pedunculated and protrude through the external os of the cervix. These prolapsed myomas are often ulcerated and infected. A very large cervical myoma may produce distortion of the cervical canal and upper vagina. Rarely a cervical myoma causes dystocia during childbirth.

The diagnosis of a cervical myoma is by inspection and palpation. Grossly and histologically, cervical myomas are identical to and indistinguishable from myomas of the corpus of the uterus. Occasionally the histologic picture of cervical myomas will demonstrate many hyalinized, thick-walled blood vessels that are postulated to be the source of the neoplastic smooth muscle tumor. This latter subtype of cervical myoma is termed a *vascular*

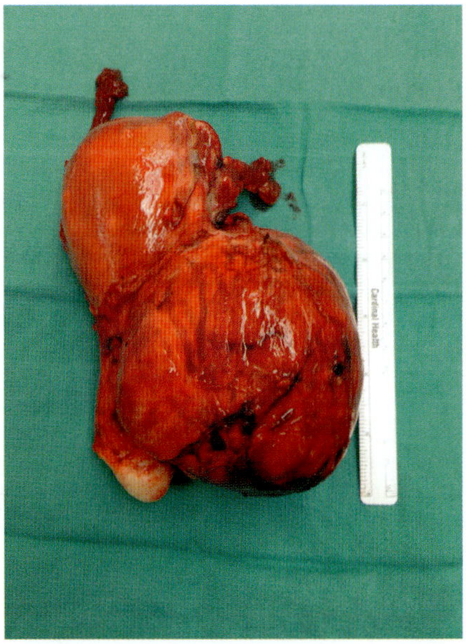

**Fig. 18.24** Large fibroid originating from the lateral wall of the cervix and growing into the broad ligament. (Courtesy Fidel A. Valea, MD.)

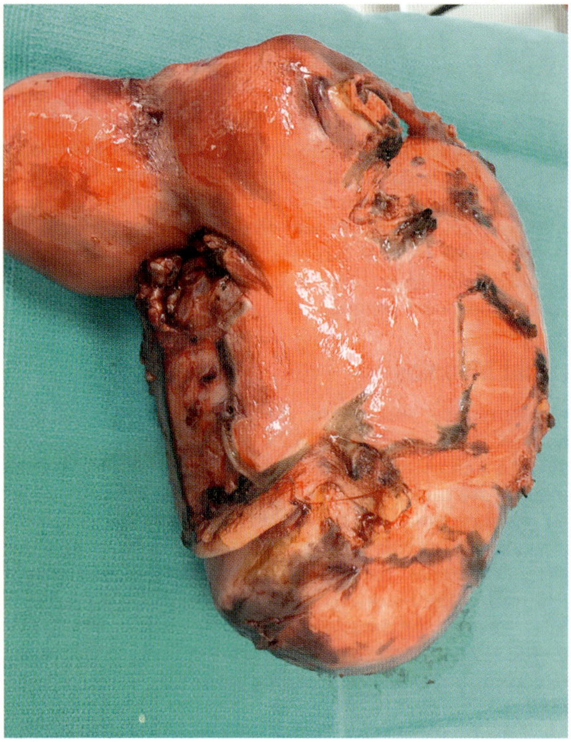

**Fig. 18.25** Posterior view of the uterus with a large fibroid that is prolapsing through a very dilated cervix and completely distorts the anatomy of the lower uterine segment. (Courtesy Fidel A. Valea, MD.)

*leiomyoma.* Management is similar to that of uterine myomas in that asymptomatic, small myomas may be observed for rate of growth. The occurrence and persistence of symptoms from a cervical myoma are an indication for medical therapy with GnRH agonists or myomectomy or hysterectomy, depending on the patient's age and future reproductive plans. Because of both a complex blood supply and involvement with the distal course of the ureter, treatment of cervical myomas that grow laterally may become a challenge if myomectomy is the operation of choice. Cervical myomas may be treated by radiologic catheter embolization. Prolapsed uterine myomas are discussed later in this chapter.

### Cervical Stenosis

Cervical stenosis most often occurs in the region of the internal os and may be divided into congenital or acquired types. The causes of acquired cervical stenosis are operative, radiation induced, infectious, neoplastic, or atrophic changes. Loop electrocautery excision procedure (LEEP), cone biopsy, and cautery of the cervix (either electrocautery or cryocoagulation) are the operations most commonly associated with cervical stenosis, which often depends on the volume of tissue removed. The symptoms of cervical stenosis depend on whether the patient is premenopausal or postmenopausal and whether the obstruction is complete or partial. Common symptoms in premenopausal women include dysmenorrhea, pelvic pain, abnormal bleeding, amenorrhea, and infertility. The infertility is usually associated with endometriosis, which is commonly found in reproductive-age women with cervical stenosis. Postmenopausal women are usually asymptomatic for a long time. Slowly they develop a hematometra (blood), hydrometra (clear fluid), or pyometra (exudate).

The diagnosis is established by inability to introduce a 1- to 2-mm dilator into the uterine cavity. If the obstruction is complete, a soft, slightly tender, enlarged uterus is appreciated as a midline mass, and ultrasound examination demonstrating fluid within the uterine cavity. Management of cervical stenosis is dilation of the cervix with dilators under ultrasound guidance. If stenosis recurs, monthly laminaria tents may be used. Similarly, office follow-up and sounding of the cervix of women who have had a cone biopsy or cautery of the cervix is important to establish patency of the endocervical canal. Postmenopausal women with pyometra usually do not need antibiotics. After the acute infection has subsided, endometrial carcinoma and endocervical carcinoma should be ruled out by appropriate diagnostic biopsies. After cervical dilation, it is often useful to leave a T tube or latex nasopharyngeal airway as a stent in the cervical canal for a few days to maintain patency.

## UTERUS

### Ultrasound

Ultrasound, primarily endovaginal, is the most common and most efficient imaging technique for pelvic structures. For endovaginal ultrasound, transducers are configured on vaginal probes and placed in a sterile sheath, usually a glove or condom, before an examination. During the examination the woman is in a dorsal lithotomy position and has an empty bladder. Because the transducer is closer to the pelvic organs than when a transabdominal approach is employed, endovaginal resolution is usually superior. However, if the pelvic structures to be studied have expanded and extend into the patient's abdomen, the organs are difficult to visualize with an endovaginal probe. Most ultrasound machines are equipped with both types of transducers.

For transabdominal gynecologic examinations, a sector scanner is preferable. It provides greater resolution of the pelvis and an easier examination than the linear array. During abdominal pelvic ultrasound examination, it is helpful for the patient to have a full bladder. This serves as an acoustic window for the high-frequency sound waves. Ultrasound is more than 90% accurate in recognizing the presence of a pelvic mass, but it does not establish a tissue diagnosis.

Ultrasonography employs an acoustic pulse echo technique. The transducer of the ultrasound machine is made up of piezoelectric crystals that vibrate and emit acoustic pulses. Acoustic echoes return from the tissues being scanned and cause the crystals to vibrate again and release an electric charge. A computer within the ultrasound machine then integrates the electric charges to form the image. Present equipment provides resolution of less than 0.2 mm.

Doppler ultrasound techniques assess the frequency of returning echoes to determine the velocity of moving structures. Measurement of diastolic and systolic velocities provides indirect indices of vascular resistance. Muscular arteries have high resistance. Newly developed vessels, such as those arising in malignancies, have little vascular wall musculature and thus have low resistance. Three-dimensional ultrasound is a computer technique in which multiple two-dimensional images are compiled to render either a surface- or volume-based image that appears to occupy space, as opposed to being flat. Three-dimensional ultrasound has of yet not been shown to have a specific diagnostic advantage in gynecology compared with other modalities.

A disadvantage of ultrasound is its poor penetration of bone and air; thus the pubic symphysis and air-filled intestines and rectum often inhibit visualization. Advantages of ultrasound include the real-time nature of the image, the absence of radiation, the ability to perform the procedure in the office before, during, or immediately after a pelvic examination, and the ability to describe the findings to the patient while she is watching. One of the most reassuring aspects of sonography is the absence of adverse clinical effects from the energy levels used in diagnostic studies.

Sonographic evaluation of endometrial pathologic changes involves measurement of the endometrial thickness or stripe. The normal endometrial thickness is 4 mm or less in a postmenopausal woman not taking hormones. The thickness varies in premenopausal women at different times of the menstrual cycle and in women taking hormone replacement (Fig. 18.26), making endometrial thickness measurements less reliable in that setting. The endometrial thickness is measured in the longitudinal plane, from outer margin to outer margin, at the widest part of the endometrium. Ultrasound is not a screening tool in asymptomatic women. However, several studies of postmenopausal women with vaginal bleeding have documented that malignancy is extremely rare in women with an endometrial thickness of 4 mm or less. Systematic reviews have noted that ultrasound may be reliably used to predict 96% to 99% of endometrial cancers in women with postmenopausal bleeding. The flip side of the coin is that 1% to 4% of malignancies will be missed using a cutoff of less than 4 mm (Tabor, 2002). In addition, papillary-serous adenocarcinomas of the endometrium do not always develop the same endometrial stripe thickness as endometrioid cancer. Two caveats for using ultrasound in screening of postmenopausal bleeding are (1) ultrasound does not provide a diagnosis—a tissue specimen is necessary for a diagnosis; and (2) all women with bleeding, no matter the endometrial thickness, should have a tissue biopsy. If an endometrial biopsy obtains inadequate tissue and the endometrial thickness is 5 mm or greater, a repeat biopsy, hysteroscopically directed biopsy, or curettage should be performed.

Sonohysterography is an easily accomplished and validated technique for evaluating the endometrial cavity. The technique involves instilling saline into the uterine cavity. Sonohysterography is an alternative to office hysteroscopy. In this procedure a thin balloon-tipped catheter or intrauterine insemination catheter is inserted through the cervical os, and 5 to 30 mL of warmed saline is slowly injected into the uterine cavity. Meta-analyses of sonohysterography have found the procedure to be successful in obtaining information in 95% of women, with minimal complications. Contraindications are active cervical or uterine infection. Some clinicians will have patients take a dose of ibuprofen before the procedure. Preferably, sonohysterography is performed in the proliferative phase of the cycle when the endometrial lining is at its lowest level. Sonohysterography has also been helpful in the evaluation of polyps, filling defects, submucous myomas, and uterine septae (Fig. 18.27). Importantly, sonohysterography, as with all types of ultrasound, does not make a tissue diagnosis.

Sonography is the method of choice to locate a "missing" intrauterine device (IUD). It will help in diagnosing perforation of the uterus or unrecognized expulsion of the device. Endovaginal ultrasound transducers equipped with needle guides are often used for oocyte aspiration as part of *in vitro* fertilization.

In summary, ultrasound has become an extremely valuable adjunct to the bimanual examination. In many patients, particularly those with obesity, it is superior to perform bimanual examination alone. An endovaginal ultrasound of an early pregnancy has become a mainstay in the evaluation of the pregnant woman with first-trimester vaginal bleeding.

## Endometrial Polyps

Endometrial polyps are localized overgrowths of endometrial glands and stroma that project beyond the surface of the endometrium. They are soft, pliable, and may be single or multiple. Most polyps arise from the fundus of the uterus. *Polypoid hyperplasia* is a benign condition in which numerous small polyps are discovered throughout the endometrial cavity. Endometrial polyps vary from a few millimeters to several centimeters in diameter, and it is possible for a single large polyp to fill the endometrial cavity. Endometrial polyps may have a broad base (sessile) or be attached by a slender pedicle (pedunculated). They occur in all age groups but have a peak incidence between the ages of 40 and 49. The prevalence of endometrial polyps in reproductive-age women is 20% to 25%, and they are noted in approximately 10% of women when the uterus is examined at autopsy. The cause of endometrial polyps is unknown. Because polyps are often associated with endometrial hyperplasia, unopposed estrogen has been implicated as a possible cause.

The majority of endometrial polyps are asymptomatic. Those that are symptomatic are associated with a wide range of abnormal bleeding patterns. No single abnormal bleeding pattern is diagnostic for polyps; however, menorrhagia, premenstrual and postmenstrual staining, and scanty postmenstrual spotting are the most common. Occasionally a pedunculated endometrial polyp with a long pedicle may protrude from the external cervical os. Sometimes large endometrial polyps may contribute to infertility.

Polyps are succulent and velvety, with a large central vascular core. The color is usually gray or tan but may occasionally be red or brown. Histologically, an endometrial polyp has three components: endometrial glands, endometrial stroma, and central vascular channels (Fig. 18.28; see Fig. 18.27). Epithelium must be identified on three sides, like a peninsula. Approximately two out of three polyps consist of an immature endometrium that does not respond to cyclic changes in circulating progesterone. This immature endometrium differs from surrounding endometrium and often appears as a "Swiss cheese" cystic hyperplasia during all phases of the menstrual cycle (Fig. 18.29). The other one-third of endometrial polyps consist of functional endometria that will undergo cyclic histologic changes. The tip of a prolapsed polyp often undergoes squamous metaplasia, infection, or ulceration. The clinician cannot distinguish whether the abnormal bleeding originates from the polyp or is secondary to the commonly coexisting endometrial hyperplasia. Approximately one in four reproductive-age women with abnormal bleeding will have endometrial polyps discovered in her uterine cavity.

Malignancy in an endometrial polyp is related to patient's age and is most often of a low stage and grade. In one series of 67 women from the United Kingdom with endometrial polyps, 86% were benign, 13% hyperplastic, and 3% malignant. Another series of 61 women with polyps found 88% were benign and 5% were malignant. In a review and meta-analysis of the oncogenic potential of reported endometrial polyps, the prevalence of premalignant or malignant polyps was 5.42% in postmenopausal women compared with 1.7% in reproductive-age women. Furthermore, the prevalence of endometrial neoplasia within polyps in women with symptomatic bleeding was 4.15% compared with 2.16% for those without bleeding. Among symptomatic postmenopausal women with endometrial polyps, 4.47% had a malignant polyp compared with 1.51% in asymptomatic postmenopausal women (Lee, 2010). The question of an association of endometrial polyps with endometrial carcinoma is still debated. A population-based, case-control study from Sweden estimated that the increased risk of subsequent endometrial carcinoma in women with endometrial polyps is only twofold. It is interesting that benign polyps have been found in approximately 20% of uteri removed for endometrial carcinoma.

Unusual polyps have been described in association with chronic administration of the nonsteroidal antiestrogen tamoxifen. The endometrial abnormalities associated with chronic tamoxifen therapy include polyps, 20% to 35%; endometrial hyperplasia, 2% to 4%; and endometrial carcinoma, 1% to 2%; and often with multiple irregular sonolucencies suggesting the presence of cysts.

Most endometrial polyps are asymptomatic, and the diagnosis is not usually established until the uterus is opened after hysterectomy for other reasons. Endometrial polyps may be discovered by vaginal ultrasound, with or without hydrosonography, hysteroscopy, or hysterosalpingography, during the diagnostic workup of a woman with a refractory case of abnormal uterine bleeding or

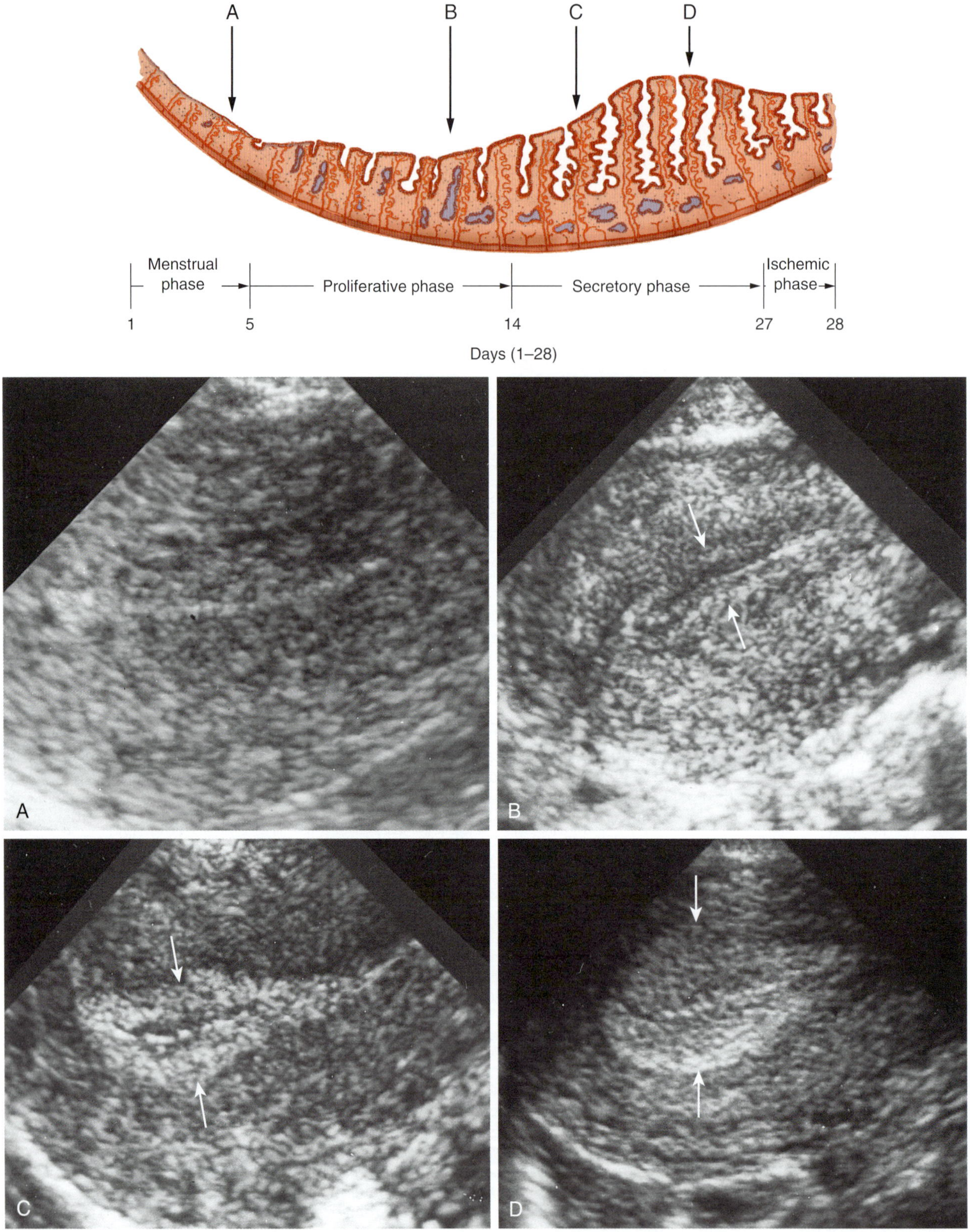


**Fig. 18.26** Variation in endometrium during menstrual cycle. **A,** Early proliferative phase. **B,** Late proliferative phase. **C,** Periovulatory phase. **D,** Late secretory phase. Note increase in endometrial thickness throughout the menstrual cycle. Also note multilayered appearance in the late proliferative phase. (From Fleischer AC, Kepple DM. Benign conditions of the uterus, cervix, and endometrium. In: Nyberg DA, Hill LM, Bohm-Velez M, et al, eds. *Transvaginal Ultrasound.* St. Louis: Mosby–Year Book; 1992.)

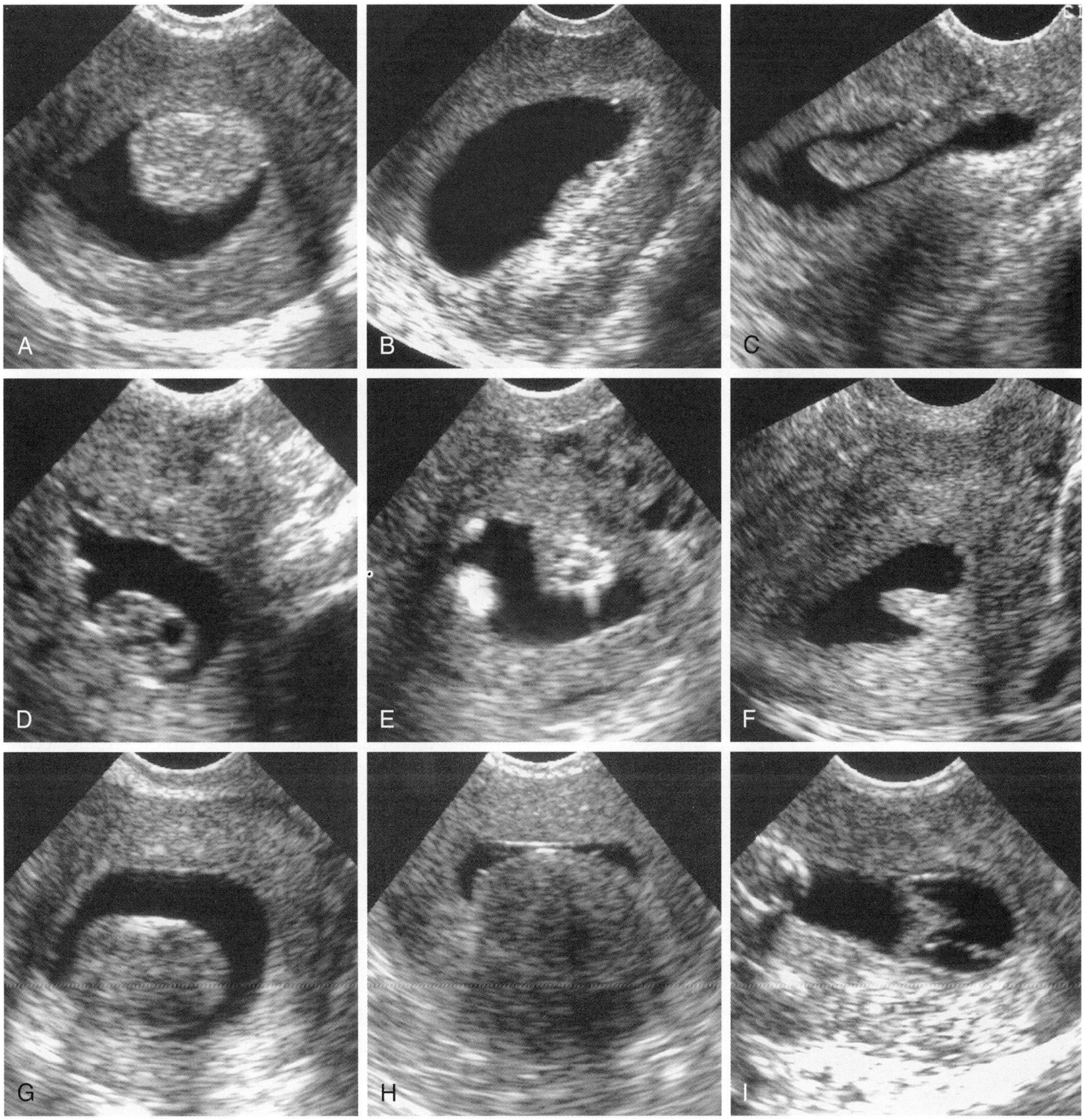


**Fig. 18.27** Sonohysterograms. **A,** Well-defined, round echogenic polyp. **B,** Carpet of small polyps. **C,** Polyp on a stalk. **D,** Polyp with cystic areas. **E,** Small polyp. **F,** Small polyp. **G,** Hypoechoic submucosal fibroid. **H,** Hypoechoic attenuating submucosal fibroid. **I,** Endometrial adhesions. Note bridging bands of tissue within fluid-filled endometrial canal. (From Salem S. The uterus and adnexa. In Rumack CM, Wilson SR, Charboneau JW, eds. *Diagnostic Ultrasound.* 2nd ed. St. Louis: Mosby; 1998:538.)

pelvic mass. Endometrial polyps are often confused with endocervical polyps (Fig. 18.30). A well-defined, uniformly hyperechoic mass that is less than 2 cm in diameter, identified by vaginal ultrasound within the endometrial cavity, is usually a benign endometrial polyp (see Fig. 18.27, *A-C*). Most endometrial polyps usually resolve after a few years, although new polyps can form.

The optimal management of endometrial polyps is removal by hysteroscopy with D&C. Because of the common association of endometrial polyps and other endometrial pathologic conditions, it is important to examine histologically both the polyp and the associated endometrial lining. Polyps, because of their mobility, often tend to elude the curette. Postcurettage hysteroscopic studies have demonstrated that routine use of a long, narrow polyp forceps at the time of curettage at best results in discovery and removal of only approximately one in four endometrial polyps. The differential diagnosis of endometrial polyps includes submucous leiomyomas, adenomyomas, retained products of conception, endometrial hyperplasia, carcinoma, and uterine sarcomas.

## Hematometra

A hematometra is a uterus distended with blood and is secondary to gynatresia, which is partial or complete obstruction of any portion of the lower genital tract. Obstruction of the isthmus of the uterus, cervix, or vagina may be congenital or acquired. The two most common congenital causes of hematometra are an imperforate hymen and a transverse vaginal septum. Among the leading

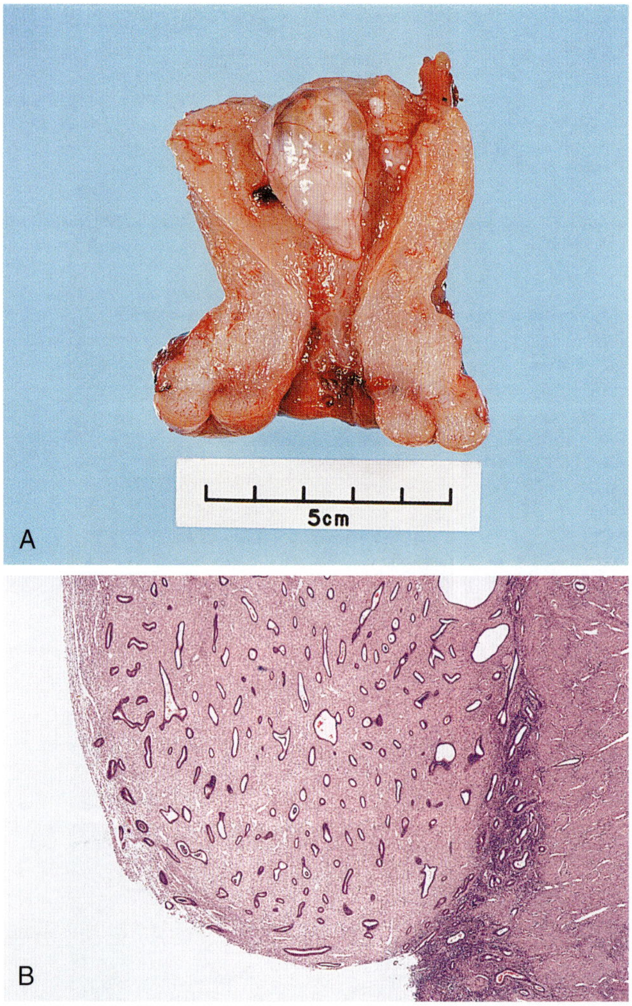


**Fig. 18.28** Endometrial polyp. **A,** Note cystic glands in the polyp. **B,** The fibrous stroma of the polyp contrasts with the cellular stroma of the adjacent endometrium. (From Anderson MC, Robboy SJ, Russell P, et al. Endometritis, metaplasias, polyps, and miscellaneous changes. In: Robboy SJ, Anderson MC, Russell P, eds. *Pathology of the Female Reproductive Tract.* Edinburgh: Churchill Livingstone; 2002.)

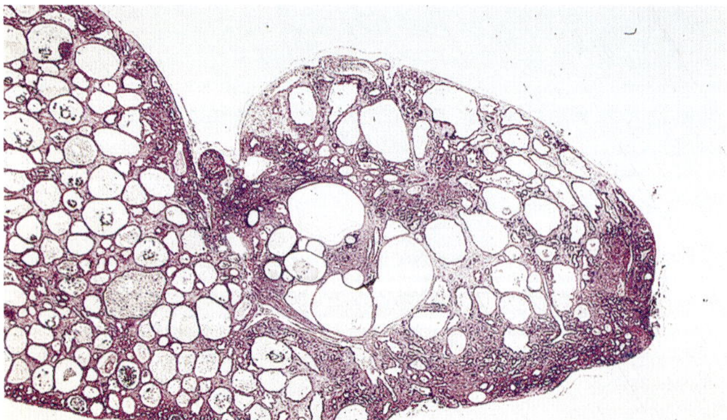

**Fig. 18.29** Endometrial polyp showing multiple cystic glands with flattened epithelial lining. (From Anderson MC, Robboy SJ, Russell P, et al. Endometritis, metaplasias, polyps and miscellaneous changes. In: Robboy SJ, Anderson MC, Russell P, eds. *Pathology of the Female Reproductive Tract.* Edinburgh: Churchill Livingstone; 2002.)

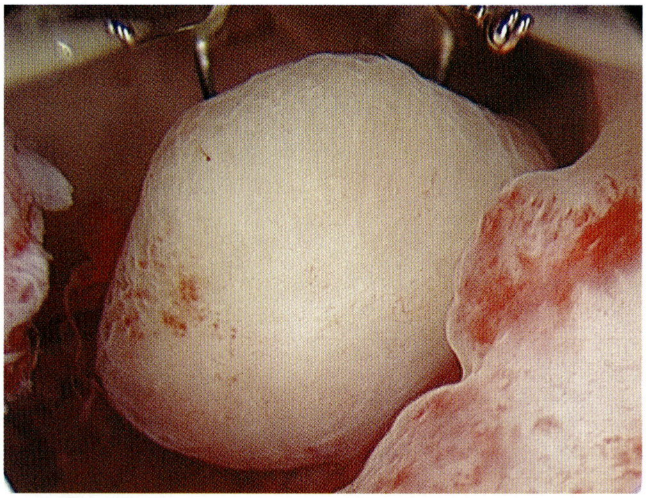

**Fig. 18.30** Endocervical polyp was seen at hysteroscopy. (From Goldberg JM, Falcone T. *Atlas of Endoscopic Techniques in Gynecology.* London: WB Saunders; 2000.)

causes of acquired lower tract stenosis are senile atrophy of the endocervical canal and endometrium, scarring of the isthmus by synechiae, cervical stenosis associated with surgery, radiation therapy, cryocautery or electrocautery, endometrial ablation, and malignant disease of the endocervical canal.

The symptoms of hematometra depend on the age of the patient, her menstrual history and the rapidity of the accumulation of blood in the uterine cavity, and the possibility of secondary infection producing pyometra. Thus common symptoms of hematometra include primary or secondary amenorrhea and possibly cyclic lower abdominal pain. During the early teenage years, the combination of primary amenorrhea and cyclic, episodic cramping lower abdominal pains suggests the possibility of a developing hematometra. Occasionally the obstruction is incomplete, and there is associated spotting of dark brown blood. Hematometra in postmenopausal women may be entirely asymptomatic. On pelvic examination a mildly tender, globular uterus is usually palpated. Ultrasound may be used to confirm the diagnosis.

The diagnosis of hematometra is generally suspected by the history of amenorrhea and cyclic abdominal pain. The diagnosis is usually confirmed by vaginal ultrasound or probing the cervix with a narrow metal dilator, with release of dark brownish black blood from the endocervical canal. Sometimes the blood retained inside the uterus becomes secondarily infected and has a foul odor.

Management of hematometra depends on operative relief of the lower tract obstruction. Treatment of congenital obstruction is discussed in Chapter 11. Appropriate biopsy specimens of the endocervical canal and endometrium should be obtained to rule out malignancy when the cause of hematometra is not obvious. If the uterus is significantly enlarged or if there is any suspicion that the retained fluid is infected, drainage should be accomplished first. Biopsy should be postponed for approximately 2 weeks to diminish the chances of infection or uterine perforation. Hematometra after operations or cryocautery usually resolves with cervical dilation. Rarely, a hematometra may form after a first-trimester abortion. This is treated by repeat suction aspiration of the products of conception that are blocking the internal os.

## Leiomyomas

Leiomyomas, also called *myomas*, are benign tumors of muscle cell origin. These tumors are often referred to by their popular names, *fibroids* or *fibromyomas*, but such terms are semantic misnomers if one is referring to the cell of origin. Most leiomyomas contain varying amounts of fibrous tissue, which is believed to be secondary to degeneration of some of the smooth muscle cells.

Leiomyomas are the most common benign neoplasms of the uterus. The lifetime prevalence of leiomyomas is greater than 80% among African American women and approaches 70% among white women (Baird, 2003). In general, a third of myomas will become symptomatic, causing abnormal and excessive uterine bleeding, pelvic pain, pelvic pressure, bowel and bladder dysfunction, infertility, recurrent miscarriage, and abdominal protrusion. Leiomyomas are a tremendous public health burden and the most common indication for hysterectomy in the United States. Approximately 42 per 1000 women are hospitalized annually because of fibroids, but African American women have higher rates of hospitalization, myomectomies, and hysterectomies compared with white women (relative risk [RR] of 3.5, 6.8, and 2.4, respectively) (Wechter, 2011). In black women, vitamin D deficiency has been linked with increased fibroid risk (Baird, 2013). Why some women develop myomas and others do not is unknown. Therefore effective treatment is limited by the poor understanding of their pathogenesis.

Risk factors associated with the development of myomata include increasing age, early menarche, low parity, tamoxifen use, obesity, and in some studies a high-fat diet. Smoking has been found to be associated with a decreased incidence of myomata, believed to be due to relative estrogen deficiency. African American women have the highest incidence, whereas Hispanic and Asian women have similar rates to white women. There appears to be a familial tendency to develop myoma. Studies of twins have noted that when identical and fraternal twins are compared, a significant proportion of myoma tend to have an inherited basis. Rare genetic conditions such as hereditary leiomyomatosis and renal cell cancer (Launoned, 2001) and Alport syndrome (Uliana, 2011) feature development of myomas. The growth of myomas is dependent on gonadal steroids, and there are increased numbers of steroid receptors in myomas compared with normal myometrium. They have a limited malignant potential with less than 1% transformation into malignancy. Cytogenetically, most fibroids are chromosomally normal and arise from a single cell (are clonal). Although fibroids are clonal in nature, heterogeneity exists and they may vary greatly in size, location, and appearance within the same uterus. There is accumulating evidence that suggests hypoxia is implicated in early cellular events that lead to the myometrial smooth muscle cell to transform into leiomyoma (Tal, 2014). Angiogenesis and vascularization are factors that control the growth of tumors. Tal and Segars reviewed the molecular regulation of the growth factors involved in angiogenesis of fibroids and described the potential implications for future therapy (Tal, 2014).

Although leiomyomas arise throughout the body in any structure containing smooth muscle, in the pelvis the majority are found in the corpus of the uterus. Occasionally, leiomyomas may be found in the fallopian tube or the round ligament, and approximately 5% of uterine myomas originate from the cervix. Rarely, myomas will arise in the retroperitoneum and produce symptoms secondary to "mass effects" on adjacent organs.

Myomas may be single but most often are multiple. They vary greatly in size from microscopic to multinodular uterine tumors that may weigh more than 50 pounds and literally fill the patient's abdomen (Fig. 18.31). Initially most myomas develop from the myometrium, beginning as intramural myomas. As they grow, they remain attached to the myometrium with a pedicle of varying width and thickness. Small myomas are round, firm, solid tumors. With continued growth, the myometrium at the edge of the tumor is compressed and forms a pseudocapsule. Although myomas do not have a true capsule, this pseudocapsule is a valuable surgical plane during a myomectomy.

Myomas are classed into subgroups by their relative anatomic relationship and position to the layers of the uterus (Fig. 18.32).

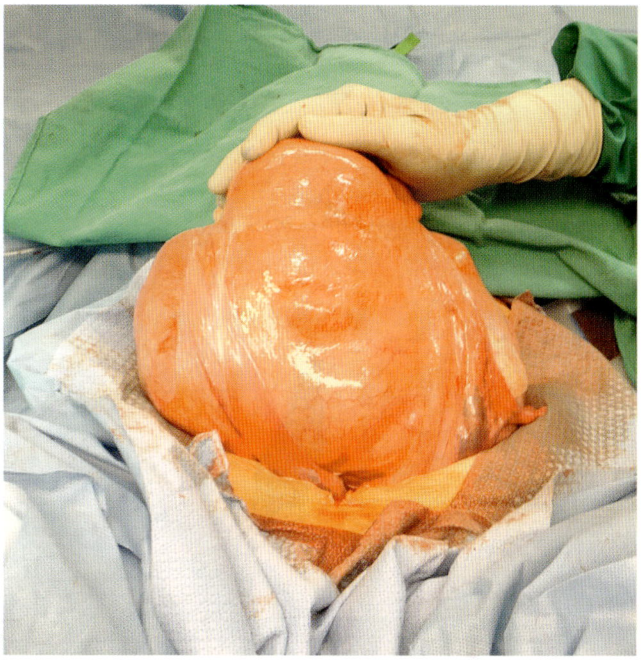

**Fig. 18.31** Image of large fibroid uterus before hysterectomy. (Courtesy Fidel A. Valea, MD.)

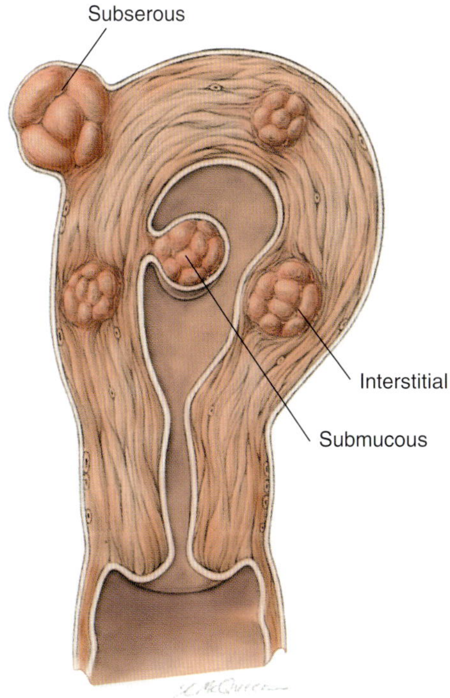


**Fig. 18.32** Drawing of cut surface of uterus showing characteristic whorl-like appearance and varying locations of leiomyomas. (From Novak ER, Woodruff JD, eds. *Novak's Gynecologic and Obstetric Pathology.* 6th ed. Philadelphia: WB Saunders; 1967:215.)

The three most common types of myomas are intramural, subserous, and submucous, with special nomenclature for broad ligament and parasitic myomas (Fig. 18.33). Continued growth in one direction determines which myomas will be located just below the endometrium (submucosal) and which will be found just beneath the serosa (subserosal) (Fig. 18.34). Although only 5% to 10% of

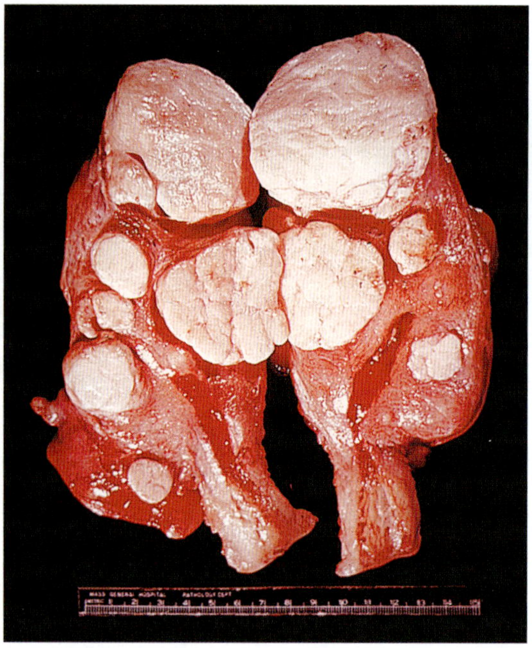

**Fig. 18.33** Multiple leiomyomas. These are predominantly intramural. The bulging cut surfaces are clearly shown. (From Anderson MC, Robboy SJ, Russell P. Uterine smooth muscle tumors. In: Robboy SJ, Anderson MC, Russell P, eds. *Pathology of the Female Reproductive Tract.* Edinburgh: Churchill Livingstone; 2002.)

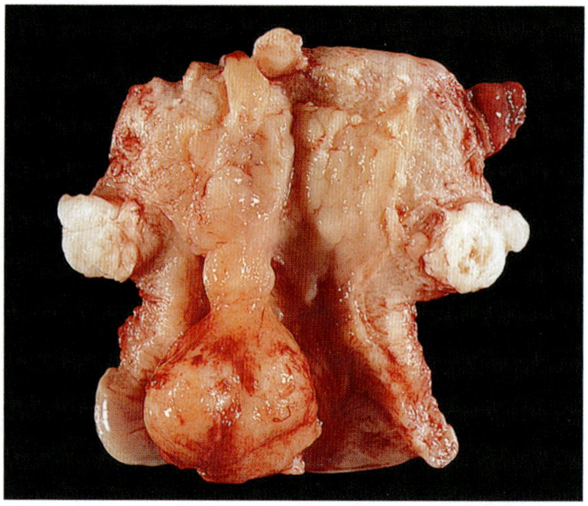

**Fig. 18.35** Uterus with multiple myomata. Note the large central submucosal myoma. (From Voet RL. *Color Atlas of Obstetric and Gynecologic Pathology.* St. Louis: Mosby-Wolfe; 1997.)

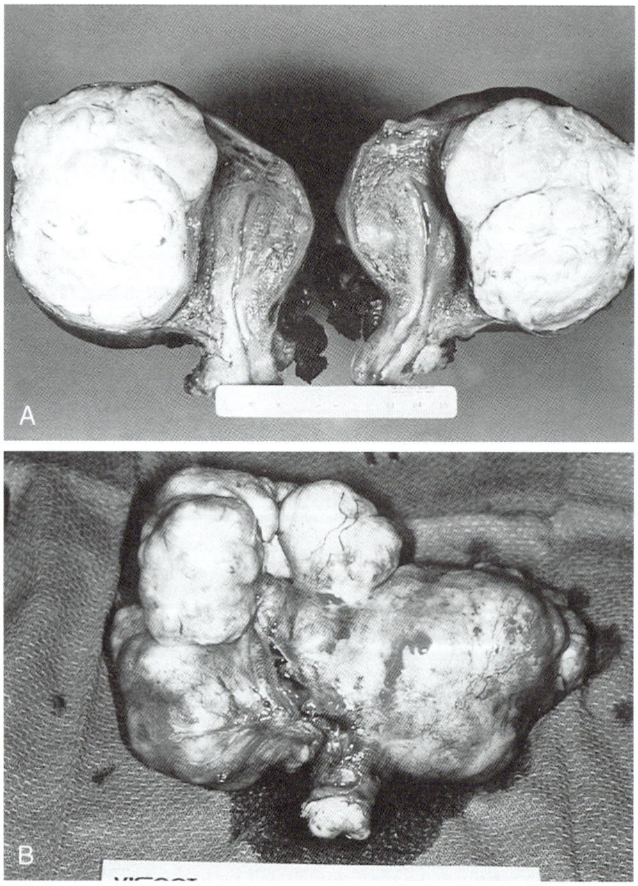


**Fig. 18.34 A,** Large subserosal myoma. **B,** Hysterectomy specimen of myomatous uterus. (Courtesy Vern L. Katz and William Droegemueller.)

myomas become submucosal, they usually are the most troublesome clinically (Fig. 18.35). These submucosal tumors may be associated with abnormal vaginal bleeding or distortion of the uterine cavity that may produce infertility or miscarriage. Rarely, a submucosal myoma enlarges and becomes pedunculated. The uterus will try to expel it, and the prolapsed myoma may protrude through the external cervical os (see Fig. 18.25).

Subserosal myomas give the uterus its knobby contour during pelvic examination. Further growth of a subserosal myoma may lead to a pedunculated myoma wandering into the peritoneal cavity. This myoma may outgrow its uterine blood supply and obtain a secondary blood supply from another organ, such as the omentum, and become a parasitic myoma. Growth of a myoma in a lateral direction from the uterus may result in a broad ligament myoma (see Fig. 18.24). The clinical significance of broad ligament myomas is that they are difficult to differentiate on pelvic examination from a solid ovarian tumor. Large, broad ligament myomas may produce a hydroureter as they enlarge.

Though the origin of uterine leiomyomas is incompletely understood, cytogenetic studies have yielded some clues to how and why myomas develop. Each tumor develops from a single muscle cell a progenitor myocyte, thus each myoma is monoclonal. Cytogenetic analysis has demonstrated that myomas have multiple chromosomal abnormalities. (Each myoma would have cells with the same abnormality.) Sixty percent are normal, 46XX. The larger the myoma, the more an abnormal karyotype will be detected. Interestingly, the chromosomal anomalies of myomata have a remarkable clustering of changes. Twenty percent of abnormalities involve translocations between chromosomes 12 and 14. Seventeen percent involve a deletion of chromosome 7. Twelve percent involve a deletion of chromosome 12, and some are trisomy 12. The affected regions on chromosome 12 are also abnormal in many other types of solid tumors. The regions of chromosome 12 and 7 involve genes that may regulate growth-inducing proteins and cytokines, including transforming growth factor beta (TGF-β), epidermal growth factor (EGF), insulin-like growth factors (IGF) 1 and 2, and platelet-derived growth factor (PDGF) (Fig. 18.36). Many of these cytokines have been found in significantly higher concentrations in myomas than in the surrounding myometrium. Current theory holds that the neoplastic transformation from normal myometrium to leiomyomata is the result of a somatic mutation in the single progenitor cell. The mutation then affects cytokines that affect cell growth. The growth may also be influenced by the relative levels of estrogen

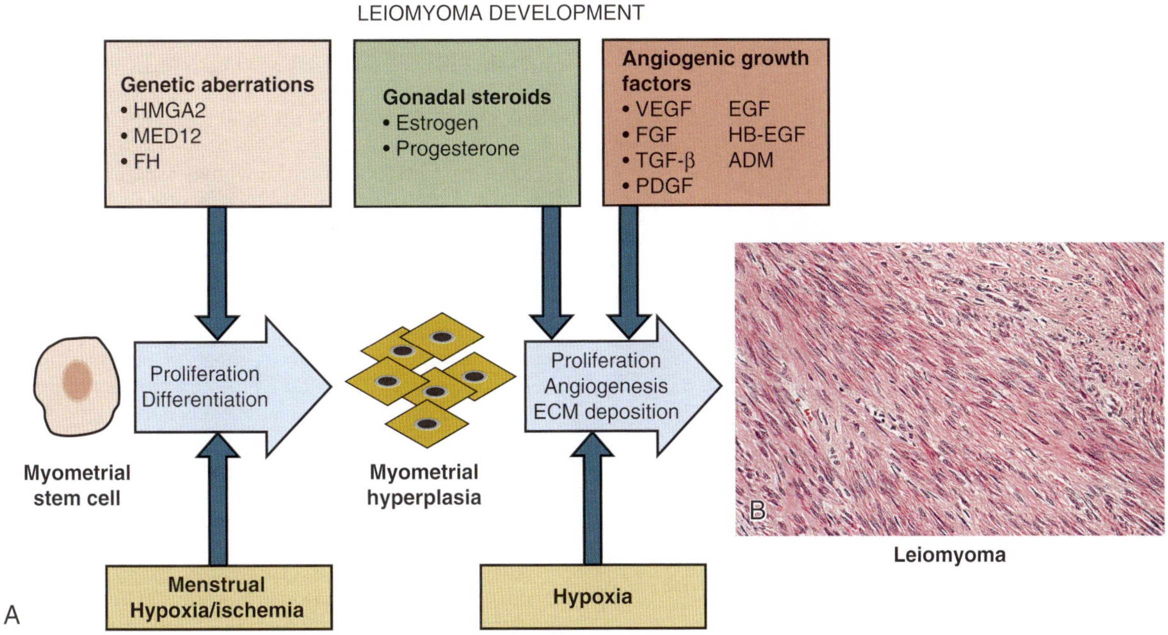


**Fig. 18.36 A,** Leiomyoma development. **B,** Leiomyoma. The smooth muscle cells are markedly elongated and have eosinophilic cytoplasm and elongated, cigar-shaped nuclei. The nuclei are uniform and mitotic figures absent or sparse. *EGF,* epidermal growth factor; *PDGF,* platelet-derived growth factor; *TGF-β*, transforming growth factor beta; *VEGF,* vascular endothelial growth factor. (**A,** Modified from Tal R, Segars JH. The role of angiogenic factors in fibroid pathogenesis: potential implications for future therapy. *Hum Reprod Update.* 2014;20(2):194-216. **B,** From Anderson MC, Robboy SJ, Russell P. Uterine smooth muscle tumors. In: Robboy SJ, Anderson MC, Russell P, eds. *Pathology of the Female Reproductive Tract.* Edinburgh: Churchill Livingstone; 2002.)

or progesterone. Both estrogen and progesterone receptors are found in higher concentrations in uterine myomas, as are other genomic changes that potentiate cellular proliferation. There also appear to be similarities between fibroids and keloid formation. Interestingly, Ishikawa and colleagues noted that myoma cells have an increased expression of aromatase, which further potentiates more local estrogen, and that African American women had the highest levels of aromatase in myoma cells (Ishikawa, 2009).

Myomas are rare before menarche, and most myomas diminish in size after menopause with the reduction of a significant amount of circulating estrogen. Myomas often enlarge during pregnancy and occasionally enlarge secondary to oral contraceptive therapy. Medically induced hypoestrogenic states produce reductions in the size of myomas. Many women, though, have small myomas that do not grow under the influence of high circulating estrogen levels. Thus the relationship between estrogen and progesterone levels and myoma growth is complex.

Grossly a myoma has a lighter color than the normal myometrium. On a cut surface, the tumor has a glistening, pearl-white appearance, with the smooth muscle arranged in a trabeculated or whorled configuration. Histologically there is a proliferation of mature smooth muscle cells. The nonstriated muscle fibers are arranged in interlacing bundles. Between bundles of smooth muscle cells are variable amounts of fibrous connective tissue, especially toward the center of any large tumor (see Fig. 18.36). The amount of fibrous tissue is proportional to the extent of atrophy and degeneration that has occurred over time. The intracellular structure of myoma cells is different from the surrounding normal myometrium. The abnormal cells contain more collagen and what has been described as a "stiffer" cytoskeleton secondary to the intracellular pressure generated by the densely packed surrounding myoma. Less than 5% of myomas exhibit hypercellularity, and these are termed *cellular leiomyomata.* Cellular leiomyomata tend to be larger in size and solitary. There is less accompanying adenomyosis or other uterine pathologic changes. The clinical presentation of cellular leiomyoma is more similar to that of a sarcoma (leiomyosarcoma). Other authors have noted a genomic expression that is similar, as well, to leiomyosarcomas. However, cellular leiomyomata are not precursors to sarcoma and have a benign prognosis.

The eventual fate of some myomas is determined by their relatively poor vascular supply. This supply is found in one or two major arteries at the base or pedicle of the myoma. The arterial supply of myomas is significantly less than that of a similarly sized area of normal myometrium. Thus with continued growth, degeneration occurs because the tumor outgrows its blood supply. The severity of the discrepancy between the myoma's growth and its blood supply determines the extent of degeneration: hyaline, myxomatous, calcific, cystic, fatty, or red degeneration and necrosis. The mildest form of degeneration of a myoma is hyaline degeneration (Fig. 18.37). Grossly in this condition the surface of the myoma is homogeneous with loss of the whorled pattern. Histologically, with hyaline degeneration, cellular detail is lost as the smooth muscle cells are replaced by fibrous connective tissue.

The most acute form of degeneration is red, or carneous, infarction (Fig. 18.38). This acute muscular infarction causes severe pain and localized peritoneal irritation. This form of degeneration occurs during pregnancy in approximately 5% to 10% of gravid women with myomas. The condition is best treated with nonsteroidal antiinflammatory agents for 72 hours, as long as the woman is less than 32 weeks' gestation. The ultrasound appearance of painful myomas is one of mixed echodense and echolucent areas. Serial ultrasound examinations have also demonstrated that most myomas (80%) do not change size during pregnancy; if a change in size does occur, it is usually not

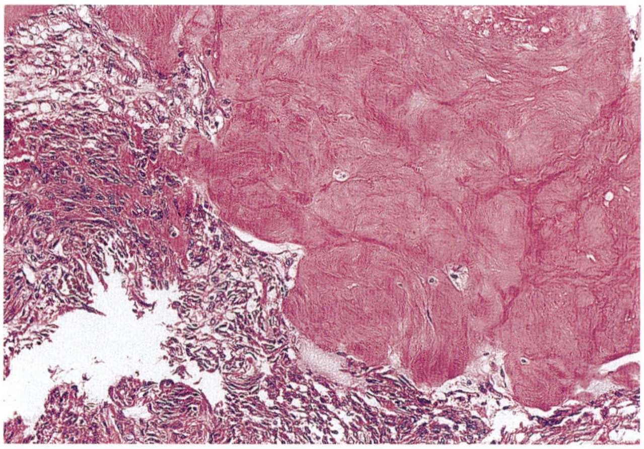

Fig. 18.37 Hyaline degeneration is a leiomyoma. There is an eosinophilic ground-glass appearance. (From Anderson MC, Robboy SJ, Russell P. Uterine smooth muscle tumors. In: Robboy SJ, Anderson MC, Russell P, eds. *Pathology of the Female Reproductive Tract.* Edinburgh: Churchill Livingstone; 2002.)

associated with painful symptomology. During pregnancy this complication should be treated medically because attempts at operative removal may result in profuse blood loss. If the patient is not pregnant, acute degeneration is not a contraindication to myomectomy. The more advanced forms of degenerating myomas may become secondarily infected, especially when large necrotic areas exist. The histologic changes of degeneration are found more commonly in larger myomas. However, two-thirds of all myomas show some degree of degeneration, with the three most common types being hyaline degeneration (65%), myxomatous degeneration (15%), and calcific degeneration (10%).

The literature emphasizes that the incidence of malignant degeneration is estimated to be between 0.3% and 0.7%. The term *malignant degeneration* is incorrect. It is unknown as to whether myomas degenerate into sarcomas. Given the very high prevalence of myomas, most investigators believe that sarcomas arise spontaneously in myomatous uteri. The possibility of a uterine tumor being a leiomyoma sarcoma is 10 times greater in a woman in her 60s than in a woman in her 40s.

The most common symptoms related to myomas are pressure from an enlarging pelvic mass; pain, including dysmenorrhea; and abnormal uterine bleeding. The severity of symptoms is usually related to the number, location, and size of the myomas. However, more than two-thirds of women with uterine myomas are asymptomatic.

One of three women with myomas experiences pelvic pain or pressure. Acquired dysmenorrhea is one of the most common complaints. Various forms of vascular compromise, either acute degeneration or torsion of the pedicle, produce severe pelvic pain. Mild pelvic discomfort is described as pelvic heaviness or a dull, aching sensation that may be secondary to edematous swelling in the myoma. An enlarged myoma or myomas often produce pressure symptoms similar to those of an enlarging pregnant uterus. Sometimes a woman will notice that her abdominal girth is increasing without appreciable change in weight. Alternatively, an anterior myoma pressing on the bladder may produce urinary frequency and urgency. In general, urinary symptoms are more common than rectal symptoms. Extremely large myomas and broad ligament myomas may produce a unilateral or bilateral hydroureter.

Abnormal bleeding is experienced by 30% of women with myomas. The most common symptom is menorrhagia, but intermenstrual spotting and disruption of a normal pattern are other common complaints. Wegienka and colleagues evaluated the bleeding pattern of 596 women with myomas. Compared with a control group, bleeding was more often described as gushing. Menses were longer in duration and heavier. In this study, symptoms of bleeding were related to the size of myomas. Interestingly, the location of the myomas, submucous versus intramural, was not related to bleeding symptoms (Wegienka, 2003). The exact cause-and-effect relationship between myomas and abnormal bleeding is difficult to determine and is poorly understood. The explanation is straightforward when there are areas of ulceration over submucous myomas. However, ulceration is a rare finding. The most popular theory is that myomas result in an abnormal microvascular growth pattern and function of the vessels in the adjacent endometrium. The older theory that the amount of menorrhagia is directly related to an increase of endometrial surface area has been disproved. One of three women with abnormal bleeding and submucous myomas also has endometrial hyperplasia, which may be the cause of the symptom.

Occasionally, myomas are the only identifiable abnormality after a detailed infertility investigation. Because the data relating

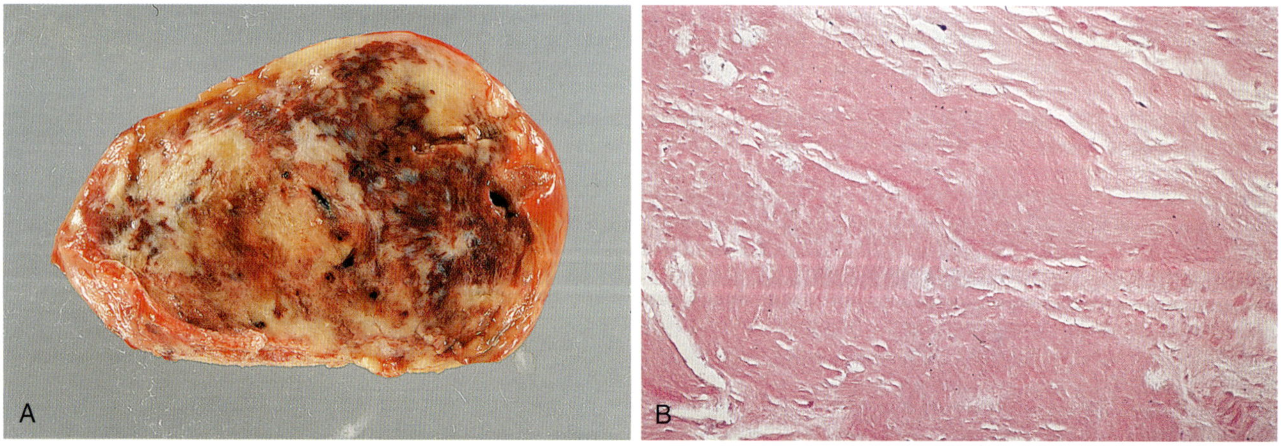


Fig. 18.38 **A,** Gross view of an infarcted leiomyoma. **B,** Red degeneration; the ghosts of the muscle cells and their nuclei remain. (**A,** From Anderson MC, Robboy SJ, Russell P. Uterine smooth muscle tumors. In: Robboy SJ, Anderson MC, Russell P, eds. *Pathology of the Female Reproductive Tract.* Edinburgh: Churchill Livingstone; 2002. **B,** From Voet RL. *Color Atlas of Obstetric and Gynecologic Pathology.* St. Louis: Mosby-Wolfe; 1997.)

myomas to infertility are weak, myomectomy is indicated only in long-standing infertility and recurrent abortion after all other potential factors have been investigated and treated. Studies suggest that submucous myomas that distort the uterine cavity are the myomas that may affect reproduction. Successful full-term pregnancy rates of 40% to 50% have been reported after a myomectomy. The success of an operation is most dependent on the age of the patient, the size of the myomas, and the number of compounding factors that affect the couple's fertility. A Cochrane review of the surgical treatment of fibroids for subfertility noted "insufficient evidence from randomized controlled trials to evaluate the role of myomectomy to improve fertility" (Metwally, 2012).

Rapid growth of a uterine myoma after menopause is a disturbing symptom. This is the classic symptom of a leiomyosarcoma; however, fibroids can have growth spurts, and most (but not all) guidelines suggest rapid growth is not necessarily an indication for treatment (Stewart, 2015). Rarely, a secondary polycythemia is noted in women with uterine myomas. This syndrome is related to elevated levels of erythropoietin. The polycythemia diminishes after removal of the uterus.

Clinically the diagnosis of uterine myomas is usually confirmed by physical examination. On palpation, an enlarged, firm, irregular uterus may be felt. The three conditions that commonly enter into the differential diagnosis are pregnancy, adenomyosis, and an ovarian neoplasm. The discrimination between large ovarian tumors and myomatous uteri may be difficult on physical examination because the extension of myomas laterally may make palpation of normal ovaries impossible during the pelvic examination. The mobility of the pelvic mass and whether the mass moves independently or as part of the uterus may be helpful diagnostically. Ultrasound is diagnostic; it can easily differentiate fibroids from a pregnant uterus or adnexal mass (Stewart, 2015). Submucosal myomas may be diagnosed by vaginal ultrasound, sonohysterography, hysteroscopy, or as a filling defect on hysterosalpingography. Occasionally an abdominopelvic radiograph will note concentric calcifications. Several reports promote CT and MRI studies of uterine myomas. However, these imaging techniques are more expensive than ultrasound is. Until CT and MRI can distinguish between benign and malignant myomas, they will rarely be ordered in routine clinical management of myomas. MRI is helpful in differentiating adenomyosis or an adenomyoma from a single, solitary myoma, especially in a woman desiring preservation of her fertility. MRI with gadolinium contrast can also provide information on devascularized (degenerated) fibroids and more detail on the location of fibroids with respect to endometrial, intramural, or serosal (Stewart, 2015). Serial ultrasound examinations have been used to evaluate progression in the size of myomas or response to therapy, although there is a strong correlation between pelvic examination results and ultrasound in determining the size of myomas.

The management of small, asymptomatic myomas is judicious observation. When the tumor is first discovered, it is appropriate to perform a pelvic examination at 6-month intervals to determine the rate of growth. The majority of women will not need surgery, especially those women in the perimenopausal period, where the condition usually improves with diminishing levels of circulating estrogens.

Cases of abnormal bleeding and leiomyomas should be investigated thoroughly for concurrent problems such as endometrial hyperplasia. If symptoms do not improve with conservative management, operative therapy may be considered. The choice between a myomectomy and hysterectomy is usually determined by the patient's age, parity, and, most important, future reproductive plans. Myomectomy is associated with longer hospital stays and more pelvic adhesions than hysterectomy. Studies suggest that myomectomy results in approximately 80% resolution of symptoms. Hysterectomy is associated with a greater than 90% patient satisfaction rate, though hysterectomy has a higher rate of urinary tract injuries, particularly abdominal hysterectomy. When myomectomies are performed to preserve fertility, care must be taken to avoid adhesions, which may compromise the goal of the operation. In the past, full-thickness myomectomies (surgeries that entered the endometrial cavity) were considered an indication for cesarean delivery before labor; however, most clinicians now recommend strong consideration for cesarean section for all degrees of myomectomy other than removal of a pedunculated leiomyomata or small hysteroscopic resection.

Classic indications for a myomectomy include persistent abnormal bleeding, pain or pressure, or enlargement of an asymptomatic myoma to more than 8 cm in a woman who has not completed childbearing. The causal relationship of myomas and adverse reproductive outcomes is poorly understood. Long-standing infertility or repetitive abortion directly related to myomas is rare. Contraindications to a myomectomy include pregnancy, advanced adnexal disease, malignancy, and a situation in which enucleation of the myoma would severely reduce endometrial surface so that the uterus would not be functional. The choice between the two operations is not always an easy one.

Within 20 years of the myomectomy operation, one in four women subsequently has a hysterectomy performed, the majority for recurrent leiomyomas. Myomectomy can be performed in select women using laparoscopic techniques. Similar to the open myomectomy, women undergoing a laparoscopic myomectomy should have a multilayer closure and consideration of the use of antiadhesive barriers. These myomas can be extirpated through extension of the umbilical incision, via minilaparotomy, or vaginally through a colpotomy. Submucous myomas may be resected via the cervical canal using the hysteroscope. Although preliminary studies using laser surgery have been reported, most investigators advocate using an operative resectoscope or tissue removal system. Three out of four women have long-term relief of their menorrhagia secondary to uterine myomas after hysteroscopic resection of the myomas.

The indications for hysterectomy for myomas are similar to indications for myomectomy, with a few additions. Some gynecologists selectively perform a hysterectomy for asymptomatic myomas when the uterus has reached the size of a 14- to 16-week gestation. The hypothesis is that most myomas of this size will eventually produce symptoms. However, it is impossible to predict which individual woman will develop symptoms. Rapid growth of a myoma after menopause warrants investigation and consideration for surgery. Prolapse of a myoma through the cervix is optimally treated by vaginal removal and ligation of the base of the myoma, with antibiotic coverage. Hysteroscopic resection aids the transvaginal removal of a prolapsed myoma.

There has been much controversy regarding the prevalence of undiagnosed uterine cancers among women with presumed benign fibroids at the time of hysterectomy. The risk of unexpected leiomyosarcoma at the time of hysterectomy has been reviewed in multiple publications, including the 2017 Agency for Healthcare Research and Quality report, and was found to be less than 1 in 770 to 1 in 10,000 surgeries for symptomatic leiomyomas (ACOG, 2019b). Morcellation is the process by which a large portion of tissue is divided into smaller pieces. The benefit of morcellation is the ability to perform a hysterectomy or myomectomy in a minimally invasive fashion, avoiding an open abdominal incision and the associated longer recovery time and higher mortality rate. This can be accomplished manually (i.e., with a scalpel or scissors) or via a rapidly rotating blade known as a *power morcellator*. The use of power morcellation may spread unsuspected cancer during surgery for treatment of symptomatic fibroids. The Food and Drug Administration (FDA) recommends against the use of laparoscopic power morcellators in the majority of women undergoing myomectomy or hysterectomy for treatment of fibroids, thereby significantly limiting the use of morcellation to hysterectomy in premenopausal women who are not candidates for en bloc resection, and only after counseling women about the risks of power morcellation and the potential spread of cancer and offering alternatives such as morcellation in a contained system, such as a laparoscopic retrieval bag (USFDA, 2014). The use of an intraperitoneal bag for morcellation has been proposed to reduce tissue dissemination. Unfortunately, the intraperitoneal bags are not designed for concurrent use with a power morcellator (ACOG, 2019b).

For women undergoing minimally invasive surgery for symptomatic fibroids, preoperative considerations must be made regarding age, menopausal status, hereditary factors, uterine size, rapid uterine growth, endometrial sampling, cervical cytologic test results, and pelvic imaging. Informed consent for these procedures should include a discussion of the risks and benefits of power morcellation. If after careful review malignancy is strongly suspected or known, then power morcellation must be avoided. The impact of the FDA warning on clinical practice has become quickly evident. A survey of American Association of Gynecologic Laparoscopists (AAGL) and American College of Obstetricians and Gynecologists (ACOG) members showed nearly half of the respondents had increased their rate of laparotomy and nearly three-quarters stopped using power morcellation during hysterectomy and myomectomy primarily because of hospital mandates, although they did not believe it resulted in improved patient outcomes (Lum, 2016). Ultimately the physician and the patient must participate in shared decision making about the route of hysterectomy, after detailed discussion of the rare risk of encountering a leiomyosarcoma with its associated mortality and the increased morbidity of the abdominal hysterectomy compared with minimally invasive approaches (ACOG, 2019b).

It is possible to treat leiomyomas medically by reducing the circulating level of estrogen and progesterone. GnRH agonists, medroxyprogesterone acetate (Depo-Provera), danazol, aromatase inhibitors, and the antiprogesterone RU 486 have undergone clinical trials. Randomized controlled trials of 5 and 10 mg of mifepristone (RU486) have shown significant reduction in size, bleeding, and improvement in quality of life. Mifepristone acts through inhibition of progesterone receptors. Daily administration of 5 mg and 10 mg has shown uterine volume reductions of 48% and 52% after 1 year for both doses. Amenorrhea occurred in 65% of the women in 6 months and in 705 within a year. However, long-term use is controversial because of the potential of inducing endometrial pathology (Eisinger, 2005). The use of GnRH agonists, sometimes with add-back hormonal therapy, has also been successful in treating myomas. A Cochrane review on add-back therapy with GnRH analogs for uterine fibroids concluded there was low or moderate evidence that tibolone, raloxifene, estriol, and ipriflavone help preserve bone density and medroxyprogesterone acetate (MPA) and tibolone may reduce vasomotor symptoms. The studies assessed only short-term (within 12 months) effectiveness and safety. Larger uterine volume was an adverse effect associated with some of the therapies (MPA, tibolone, and conjugated estrogens) (Moroni, 2015). Reductions in mean uterine volume and myoma size by 40% to 50% have been documented. However, individual responses vary greatly. With medical treatments, most of the size reductions occur within the first 3 months. After cessation of therapy, myomas gradually resume their pretreatment size. By 6 months after treatment, most myomas will have returned to their original size. During treatment, Doppler flow studies have demonstrated increased resistance in the uterine arteries and in the smaller arteries feeding the myoma. Also during treatment, the proliferative activity of the myoma and the binding of epidermal growth factor are reduced. The use of medical suppressive therapies such as GnRH agonists for women with large myomas and those with anemia may reduce blood loss at the time of hysterectomy or myomectomy. However, one study found that tourniquets at the time of myomectomy were as effective as pretreatment with GnRH agonists in decreasing blood loss.

### Therapies for Heavy Menstrual Bleeding

In women who have heavy menstrual bleeding as the primary symptom, limited data support the effectiveness of medical therapies, including tranexamic acid and the levonorgestrel-releasing intrauterine device (Stewart, 2015). Tranexamic acid is an oral fibrinolytic agent that may decrease bleeding when taken only during heavy menstrual bleeding. Because its mechanism of action is concerning for increased thrombotic risk, it should not be taken concomitantly with oral contraceptives. The levonorgestrel-releasing intrauterine device decreased menstrual bleeding while providing contraception; however, the rate of expulsion among women with submucosal fibroids may be as high as 12% (Stewart, 2015). Oral contraceptives reduce menstrual bleeding in women with fibroids according to observational data. In addition, nonsteroidal antiinflammatory drugs decrease heavy menstrual bleeding and menstrual pain. Oral progestogens have not been shown to reduce fibroid size or fibroid-related symptoms

### Future Options for Medical Treatment

No validated medical treatment is yet able to eliminate fibroids; therefore surgery is the most effective treatment for symptomatic fibroids. However, there are emerging medical treatments such as ulipristal acetate that may be an option for women who wish to avoid surgery or, before surgery, to reduce the extent of the operation by reducing the size of the fibroids.

Ulipristal acetate is a selective progesterone receptor modulator that on binding to the progesterone receptor in target tissues displays antagonist and partial agonist effects (McKeage, 2011). The efficacy of ulipristal acetate has been demonstrated in three European phase III studies evaluating PGL4001 (Ulipristal Acetate) Efficacy Assessment in Reduction of Symptoms Due to Uterine Leiomyomata (PEARL I, II, and III) (Donnez, 2014). It has been approved for medical treatment of fibroids in Canada and Europe, but it is not FDA approved for treatment of fibroids in the United States.

Aromatase inhibitors block the synthesis of estrogen. They have been shown to reduce uterine fibroid size (up to 71% in 2 months) and ameliorate uterine fibroid symptoms, including a reduction in menstrual volume and duration of menstruation, and urinary retention (Shozu, 2003). Table 18.3 summarizes the medical options for the management of patients with uterine leiomyomas.

### Uterine Artery Embolization

Uterine myomas may also be treated with uterine artery embolization (UAE) (Fig. 18.39). Multiple embolic materials have been used, including gelatin sponge (Gelfoam) silicone spheres, gelatin microspheres, metal coils, and most commonly polyvinyl alcohol (PVA) particles of various diameters. Postprocedural abdominal and pelvic pain is common for the first 24 hours and may last up to 2 weeks. Most patients remain overnight in the hospital for pain relief and observation; however, some women will go home a few hours after treatment. Large trials, including the EMMY trial (Uterine Artery Embolization for Treatment of Symptomatic Uterine Fibroid Tumors), have consistently documented shorter hospitalizations and shorter recoveries, with a similar complication rate to hysterectomy. Reviews of the large trials and reports find that the need for reoperation within the first few years after embolization is 20% to 30%, with an overall failure rate of 40%, *failure rate* being defined as a return of symptoms and decrement in quality-of-life measures. The 5-year failure rate from the EMMY trial as reported by van der Kooij and associates included

**TABLE 18.3** Summary of the Medical Management Options for Patients With Uterine Leiomyomas

| Drug Class | Action | Benefits | Risks | Side Effects (%) | Authors* |
|---|---|---|---|---|---|
| COC | Inhibits ovulation; inhibits sex steroid secretion | 17% decrease in the risk of leiomyoma growth; decreases bleeding and increases hematocrit | Thromboembolic events; hepatocellular adenoma (rare) | Spotting; mastalgia; headache; gastrointestinal upset | Qin et al; Orsini et al |
| Progestogens | May inhibit ovulation and sex steroid synthesis; decidualizes endometrium, inducing a "pseudopregnancy" state | Improves bleeding in up to 70%; amenorrhea in up to 30%; may decrease uterine volume in up to 50% | Loss of bone mass (prolonged use of depot MPA) | Irregular bleeding/ spotting; ovarian follicular cysts | Venkatachalam et al; Ichigo et al |
| LNG-IUS | Endometrial atrophy | Reduces bleeding intensity in up to 99%; decreases uterine volume in about 40% | Device expulsion | Ovarian cysts; acne | Kriplani et al; Sayed et al |
| GnRH-a | Hypoestrogenism due to gonadotrophin secretion inhibition | Uterine volume decrease in up to 50%; high rates of amenorrhea | Loss of bone mass with prolonged use | Hot flashes (>90%); vaginal atrophy; headache; mood disorders | Friedman et al; Tummon et al; Dawood et al |
| SPRM | Inhibits ovulation; inhibits progesterone action on fibroid tissue | Improves bleeding in up to 98% of patients; decreases fibroid volume in up to 53% | Long-term endometrial safety is unknown | Benign endometrial changes after short-term use | Donnez et al; Williams et al |

From Moroni RM, Vieira CS, Ferriani RA, et al. Pharmacological treatment of uterine fibroids. *Ann Med Health Sci Res.* 2014;4(Suppl 3):S185-S192.
*All citations are from the original source article.
*COC,* combined oral contraceptive; *GnRH-a,* gonadotropin-releasing hormone analog; *LNG-IUS,* levonorgestrel-releasing intrauterine system; *MPA,* medroxyprogesterone acetate; *SPRM,* selective progesterone receptor modulators.

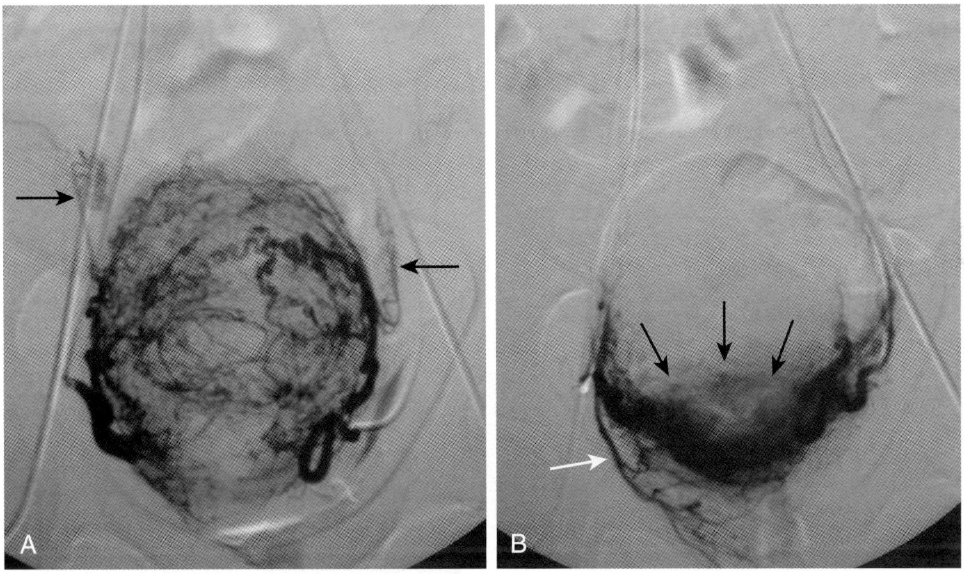


**Fig. 18.39** Uterine fibroid embolization. **A,** Angiographic image of uterine leiomyoma before uterine fibroid embolization. *Arrows* point to preembolization uterine artery. **B,** Postembolization image of same devascularized myoma with normal myometrial perfusion maintained *(black arrows). White arrow* points to patent cervicovaginal branch of uterine artery at completion of embolization. (From Spies JB, Czeyda-Pommersheim F. Uterine fibroid embolization. In Mauro MA, Murphy KPJ, Thomson KR, et al, eds. *Image-Guided Interventions.* 2nd ed. Philadelphia: Elsevier; 2014:542-546.)

a 28.4% subsequent hysterectomy rate (van der Kooij, 2010). Risk factors for failure with UAE included younger age at embolization, bleeding as an indication for therapy, multiple myomas, and the finding at the time of imaging of collateral ovarian vessels feeding the myoma. Thus the procedure itself, though a valuable alternative to hysterectomy, is not for all women, with a significant proportion of women needing follow-up procedures.

Fertility after arterial embolization is difficult to quantify. Higher than expected rates of intrauterine growth restriction, preterm delivery, and miscarriage have been reported. In general, women choosing a conservative approach to preserve fertility should have a surgical myomectomy rather than UAE.

Complications of UAE affect about 5% of patients and include postembolization fever; sepsis from infarction of the necrotic myometrium, which may occur several weeks to a few months post procedure; and ovarian failure, affecting up to 3% of cases in women younger than 45 and 15% in women older than 45. This is thought to occur from spread of emboli material into the ovarian circulation. There is, in general, a decreased ovarian reserve found in older women after embolization. Amenorrhea may

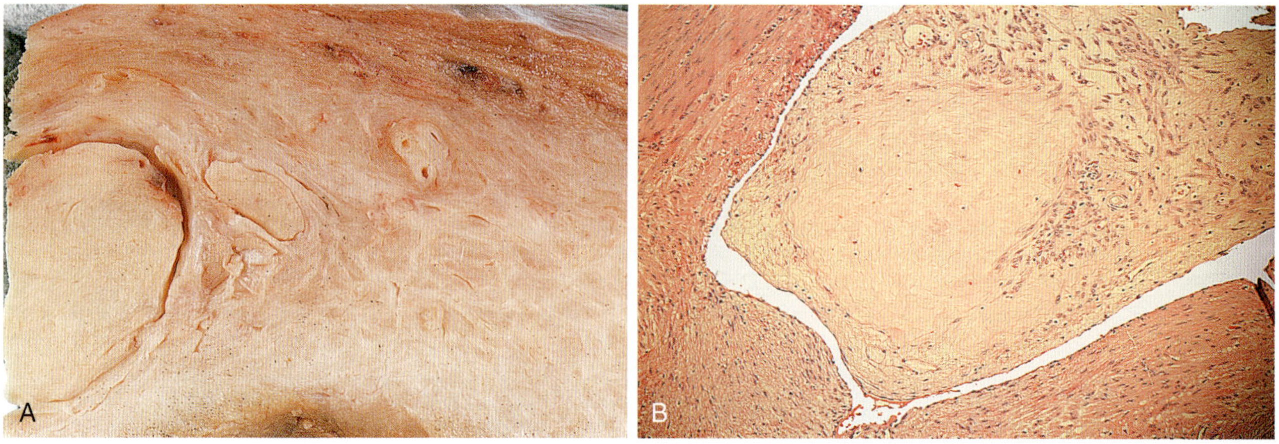


**Fig. 18.40** Intravenous leiomyomatosis. **A,** Tumor masses are present within distended blood vessels. **B,** This example shows hyaline degeneration of the intravascular element. (From Anderson MC, Robboy SJ, Russell P. Uterine smooth muscle tumors. In: Robboy SJ, Anderson MC, Russell P, eds. *Pathology of the Female Reproductive Tract.* Edinburgh: Churchill Livingstone; 2002.)

occur secondary to an endometrial hypoxic injury, as well. Rarely, necrosis of surrounding tissues may present as a complication of embolization.

Another complication of UAE is shedding of necrotic myomata or portions of myomata into the intrauterine cavity. Shedding may lead to infection or abdominal pain as the uterus tries to pass the material. This may require either a uterine curettage or hysteroscopic removal, although some authors have reported removing the necrotic material in the office. Because shedding of necrotic material is a relatively common complication, several authors have recommended that submucous myomata be removed hysteroscopically rather than attempted through UAE because these types of myomata are more at risk to be shed into the uterine cavity. Intraabdominal adhesions, particularly after embolization of larger myomata, are also an uncommon but not rare complication.

## Other Minimally Invasive Interventions

Endometrial ablation is used mainly to manage heavy uterine bleeding. It is limited to women with a normal-size uterus and uterine fibroids less than 3 cm in diameter. Compared with hysterectomy, endometrial ablation has a shorter intraoperative time, faster recovery, and fewer adverse events; however, it has inferior reduction in menstrual bleeding and lower patient satisfaction (Lethaby, 2000). Pregnancy after endometrial ablation is not recommended because of the high risk of miscarriage, ectopic pregnancy, and invasive placental disorders that may occur after this procedure.

Myolysis (the destruction of uterine fibroids or their blood supply via ultrasound, laser, cryotherapy, or other methods) has been studied as a conservative alternative for women who want to preserve their uterus but not fertility. Candidates are women with small fibroids (typically less than or equal to 5 cm) or the largest fibroid being less than 10 cm in diameter. Magnetic resonance–guided, focused ultrasound surgery appears to be the most effective and least aggressive; however, this technique is restricted by the need for costly equipment and the limited data regarding efficacy and safety (Marret, 2012).

Two associated but rare diseases should be noted: intravenous leiomyomatosis and leiomyomatosis peritonealis disseminata. *Intravenous leiomyomatosis* is a rare condition in which benign smooth muscle fibers invade and slowly grow into the venous channels of the pelvis (Fig. 18.40). The tumor grows by direct extension and grossly appears like a "spaghetti" tumor. Only 25% of tumors extend beyond the broad ligament. However, case series and reports document tumor growth into the vena cava and right heart. The tumors may present with cardiac symptomology and usually require surgical resection. Series from Zhang and colleagues and Worley and colleagues noted good results with single-stage surgeries. Most authors recommend antiestrogen therapy with aromatase inhibitors after resection of leiomyomatosis of any degree (Worley, 2009; Zhang, 2010).

*Leiomyomatosis peritonealis disseminata* (LPD) is a benign disease with multiple small nodules over the surface of the pelvis and abdominal peritoneum. Grossly, LPD mimics disseminated carcinoma (Fig. 18.41). However, histologic examination demonstrates benign-appearing myomas (Fig. 18.42). This disorder is often associated with a recent pregnancy. Also, the use of power morcellation increases the risk of LPD because of intraperitoneal spread of uterine tissue (Kumar, 2008). Therapies with progestogens, selective estrogen receptor modulators (SERMs), and aromatase inhibitors have all been used in management. A rare autosomal syndrome of uterine and cutaneous leiomyomata and renal cell carcinoma also exists. Consideration should be given to renal evaluation in families with this history and with cutaneous leiomyomas.

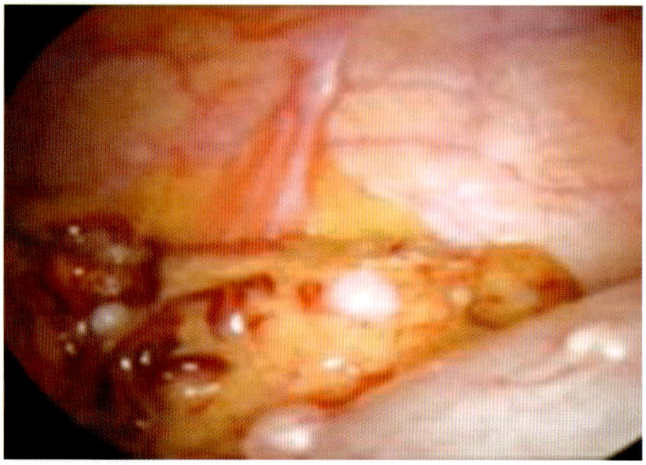

**Fig. 18.41** Laparoscopic image of the omental, peritoneal, and intestinal dissemination of leiomyomatosis peritonealis disseminata. (From Honemeyer U, Ross JR, Barnard JJ, et al. Recurrent leiomyomatosis peritonealis disseminata: sonographic and laparoscopic correlation. *Donald School J Ultrasound Obstet Gynecol.* 2012:6;327-332.)

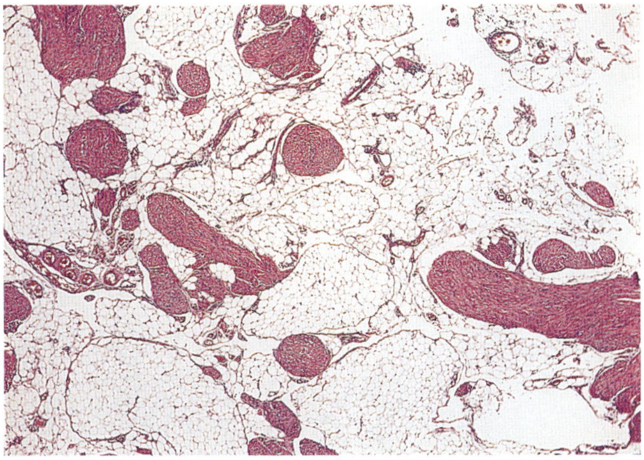

**Fig. 18.42** Peritoneal leiomyomatosis. Multiple tiny nodules of smooth muscle are scattered throughout the omentum. (From Anderson MC, Robboy SJ, Russell P. Uterine smooth muscle tumors. In: Robboy SJ, Anderson MC, Russell P, eds. *Pathology of the Female Reproductive Tract.* Edinburgh: Churchill Livingstone; 2002.)

In summary, leiomyomas are the most common tumor in women, and certainly one of the most common problems facing the gynecologist. Symptoms will present in 30% to 50% of women with myomata. Management is individualized to fit the patient's symptoms and reproductive desires.

## ADENOMYOSIS

Adenomyosis has often been referred to as *endometriosis interna*. This term is misleading because endometriosis and adenomyosis are discovered in the same patient in less than 20% of women. More important, endometriosis and adenomyosis are clinically different diseases. The only common feature is the presence of ectopic endometrial glands and stroma. Adenomyosis is derived from aberrant glands of the basalis layer of the endometrium. Therefore these glands do not usually undergo the traditional proliferative and secretory changes that are associated with cyclic ovarian hormone production. The disease is common and may be found in up to 60% of hysterectomy specimens in women in the late reproductive years. Most studies have documented an incidence closer to 30%, with greater than 50% of these women being relatively asymptomatic. The symptoms of menorrhagia and dysmenorrhea form a spectrum and are subjective, thus delineating an incidence of associated symptomology with adenomyosis is problematic.

Adenomyosis is usually diagnosed incidentally by the pathologist examining histologic sections of surgical specimens. The frequency of the histologic diagnosis is directly related to how meticulously the pathologist searches for the disease. Adenomyosis is also a common incidental finding during autopsy. Serial histologic slides confirm the continuity of benign growth of the basalis layer of the endometrium into the myometrium. Thus the histogenesis of adenomyosis is direct extension from the endometrial lining.

The disease is associated with increased parity, particularly uterine surgeries and traumas. The pathogenesis of adenomyosis is unknown but is theorized to be associated with disruption of the barrier between the endometrium and myometrium because one series noted a 1.7 RR (1.1 to 2.6) of a dilation and curettage with an SAB in women with adenomyosis versus control subjects (Parazzini, 1997). Other studies have found a higher rate of induced abortion with presumed curettage in women with adenomyosis versus controls. These studies and experimental work in animals strongly support the theory that trauma to the endometrial-myometrial interface is a significant factor in the cause of this condition. However, because adenomyosis was described well before uterine curettage and may occur (though uncommonly) in nulliparous women, the full pathogenesis is yet to be determined.

### Pathology

There are two distinct pathologic presentations of adenomyosis. The most common is a diffuse involvement of both anterior and posterior walls of the uterus. The posterior wall is usually involved more than the anterior wall (Fig. 18.43). The individual areas of adenomyosis are not encapsulated. The second presentation is a focal area or adenomyoma. This results in an asymmetric uterus, and this special area of adenomyosis may have a pseudocapsule. Diffuse adenomyosis is found in two-thirds of cases.

In the more common, diffuse type of adenomyosis the uterus is uniformly enlarged, usually two to three times normal size. It is often difficult to distinguish on physical examination from uterine leiomyomas. However, the ultrasound appearance of leiomyomata helps to distinguish the two. Similarly on visual inspection the two entities are quite different. When a knife transects the myometrium, the cut surface protrudes convexly and has a spongy appearance. The cut surface of a uterus with adenomyosis is darker than the white surface of a myoma. Sometimes there are discrete areas of adenomyosis that are not densely encapsulated and contain small, dark cystic spaces. There is not a distinct cleavage plane around focal adenomyomas as there is with uterine myomas.

Histologic examination will note benign endometrial glands and stroma are within the myometrium. These glands rarely undergo the same cyclic changes as the normal uterine endometrium. Studies have demonstrated both estrogen and progesterone receptors in tissue samples from adenomyosis.

The standard criterion used in diagnosis of adenomyosis is the finding of endometrial glands and stroma more than one low-powered field (2.5 mm) from the basalis layer of the endometrium. The small areas of adenomyosis have the same general appearance as the basalis layers of the endometrium. Histologically the glands exhibit an inactive or proliferative pattern. Rarely one can also see cystic hyperplasia or a pseudodecidual pattern. In general, there is a lack of inflammatory cells surrounding the fossae of adenomyosis. Although the areas do not undergo full menstrual-type changes, bleeding may occur in these ectopic areas, as evidenced by both gross and microscopic findings. It is not unusual to see histologic variability in several different areas

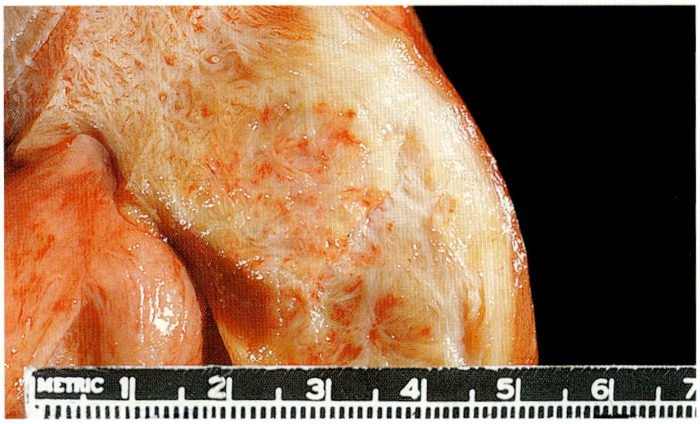


**Fig. 18.43** Adenomyosis. The myometrial wall is distorted and thickened by poorly circumscribed trabeculae that contain pinpoint hemorrhagic cysts. (From Anderson MC, Robboy SJ, Russell P. Uterine smooth muscle tumors. In: Robboy SJ, Anderson MC, Russell P, eds. *Pathology of the Female Reproductive Tract.* Edinburgh: Churchill Livingstone; 2002.)

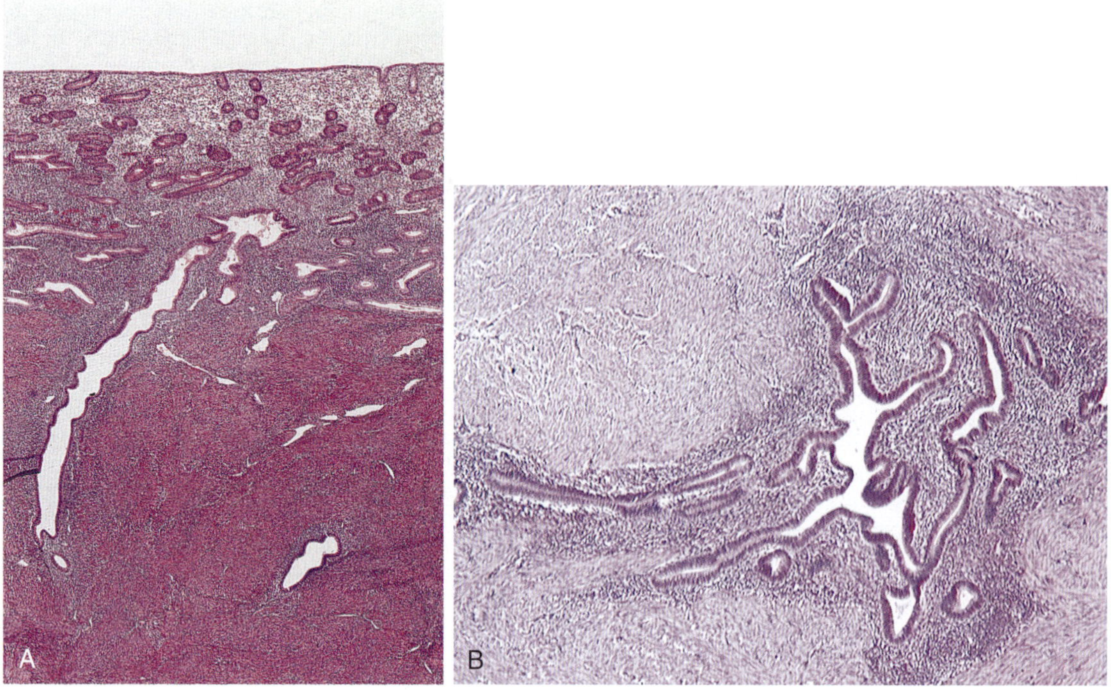

**Fig. 18.44** Adenomyosis, histologic appearance. **A,** Endometrial tissue infiltrates into the myometrium. **B,** The infiltrating islands of endometrium consist of both glands and stroma. The glands are inactive and of basal pattern. (From Anderson MC, Robboy SJ, Russell P. Uterine smooth muscle tumors. In: Robboy SJ, Anderson MC, Russell P, eds. *Pathology of the Female Reproductive Tract.* Edinburgh: Churchill Livingstone; 2002.)

deep in the walls of the myometrium from the same uterus. Some fossae of adenomyosis undergo decidual changes either during pregnancy or during estrogen-progestin therapy for endometriosis. The reaction of the myometrium to the ectopic endometrium is hyperplasia and hypertrophy of individual muscle fibers (Fig. 18.44; see 18.43). Surrounding most foci of glands and stroma are localized areas of hyperplasia of the smooth muscle of the uterus. This change in the myometrium produces the globular enlargement of the uterus (Fig. 18.45).

## Clinical Diagnosis

More than 50% of women with adenomyosis are asymptomatic or have minor symptoms that do not annoy them enough to seek medical care. They attribute the increase in dysmenorrhea or menstrual bleeding to the aging process and tolerate the symptoms. Symptomatic adenomyosis usually presents in women between the ages of 35 and 50. The severity of pelvic symptoms increases proportionally to the depth of penetration and the total volume of disease in the myometrium.

The classic symptoms of adenomyosis are secondary dysmenorrhea and menorrhagia. The acquired dysmenorrhea becomes increasingly more severe as the disease progresses. Occasionally the patient complains of dyspareunia, which is midline in location and deep in the pelvis. On pelvic examination the uterus is diffusely enlarged, usually two to three times normal size. It is most unusual for the uterine enlargement associated with adenomyosis to be larger than the size of a 14-week gestation unless the patient also has uterine myomas. The uterus is globular and tender immediately before and during menstruation (see Fig. 18.45).

The diagnosis of adenomyosis is usually confirmed after histologic examination of the hysterectomy specimen. Often the clinical diagnosis is inaccurately assigned to the patient who has chronic pelvic pain. Traditionally the patient will have endometrial sampling to rule out other organic causes of abnormal bleeding.

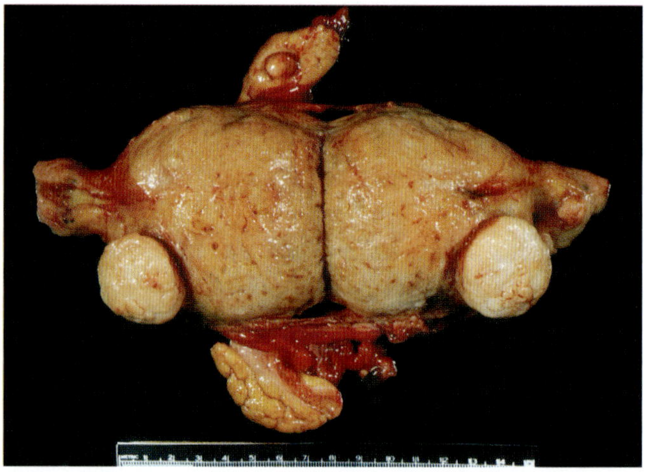

**Fig. 18.45** Hysterectomy with adenomyosis. The uterine corpus is thickened and shows prominent trabeculation of the myometrium with multiple small foci of hemorrhage. (From Oliva E. Endometrial stromal tumors, mixed müllerian tumors, adenomyosis, adenomyomas and rare sarcomas. In: Mutter GL, Prat J, eds. *Robboy's Pathology of the Female Reproductive Tract.* 3rd ed. Philadelphia: Elsevier; 2014:425-458.)

Many times adenomyosis is diagnosed retrospectively after a hysterectomy for other indications. Attempts have been made to establish the diagnosis preoperatively by transcervical needle biopsy of the myometrium. However, even with multiple needle biopsies, the sensitivity of the test is too low to be of practical clinical value. Adenomyosis may coexist with both endometrial hyperplasia and endometrial carcinoma. Approximately two of three women with adenomyosis have a coexistent pelvic pathologic condition, most commonly myomas but also endometriosis, endometrial hyperplasia, and salpingitis isthmica nodosa.

Ultrasound and MRI are both useful to help differentiate between adenomyosis and uterine myomas in a young woman desiring future childbearing. Diagnosing adenomyosis by transvaginal ultrasonography has a reported sensitivity between 53% and 89% and a specificity of 50% to 89%. In some series, MRI is more sensitive, ranging between 88% and 93%, and has a higher specificity (66% to 91%) than ultrasonography in the diagnosis of adenomyosis. Verma and associates reported the addition of sonohysterography with vaginal ultrasound, with an increase in sensitivity and specificity comparable with MRI. T2-weighted images are superior in making the diagnosis and documenting widened junctional zones (Verma, 2009). Studies indicate that three-dimensional transvaginal ultrasound is superior to two-dimensional transvaginal ultrasound and may allow for the diagnosis of early-stage disease (Struble, 2016). Findings of poorly defined junctional zone markings in the endometrial-myometrial interface help confirm the diagnosis. MRI is clinically useful in differentiating adenomyosis from uterine leiomyoma, especially preoperatively in women who desire future fertility or who may choose uterine artery embolization for treatment of myomata. The success of uterine artery embolization for adenomyosis is unproved.

## Management

There is no proven satisfactory medical treatment for adenomyosis. Patients with adenomyosis have been treated with GnRH agonists, progestogens, and progesterone-containing IUDs, cyclic hormones, or prostaglandin synthetase inhibitors for their abnormal bleeding and pain. Hysterectomy is the definitive treatment if this therapy is appropriate for the woman's age, parity, and plans for future reproduction. Size of the uterus, degree of prolapse, and presence of associated pelvic pathology determine the choice of surgical approach. Women who become pregnant with adenomyosis are at increased risk of pregnancy complications such as premature labor and delivery, low birthweight, and preterm premature rupture of membranes.

# OVIDUCT

## Leiomyomas

Both benign and malignant tumors of the oviduct are uncommon compared with other gynecologic neoplasms. Although these tumors are underreported, fewer than 100 women with myomas or leiomyomas of the oviduct are described in the literature. Tubal leiomyomas may be single or multiple and usually are discovered in the interstitial portion of the tubes. They usually coexist with the more common uterine leiomyomas. Myomas may originate from muscle cells in the walls of the tube or blood vessels or from smooth muscle in the broad ligament.

Leiomyomas of the tube present as smooth, firm, mobile, usually nontender masses that may be palpated during the bimanual examination. Similar to uterine myomas, they may be subserosal, interstitial, or submucosal. During laparoscopy the myomas appear as a spherical mass that protrudes from beneath the peritoneal surface. They vary from a few millimeters to 15 cm in diameter. Histologically they are identical to uterine leiomyomas.

The majority of the myomas of the oviduct are asymptomatic. Rarely they may undergo acute degeneration or be associated with unilateral tubal obstruction or torsion. Treatment of a symptomatic tubal leiomyoma is excision.

## Adenomatoid Tumors

The most prevalent benign tumor of the oviduct is the *angiomyoma* or *adenomatoid tumor* (Fig. 18.46), a small, gray-white, circumscribed nodule, 1 to 2 cm in diameter. These tumors are usually unilateral, present as small nodules just under the tubal serosa, and do not produce pelvic symptoms or signs. These benign tumors also are found below the serosa of the fundus of the uterus and the broad ligament. Microscopically they are composed of small tubules lined by a low cuboidal or flat epithelium. Histologic studies have established that the thin-walled channels that comprise these tumors are of mesothelial origin (Fig. 18.47). These tumors do not become malignant; however, they may be mistaken for a low-grade neoplasm when initially viewed during a frozen-section evaluation.

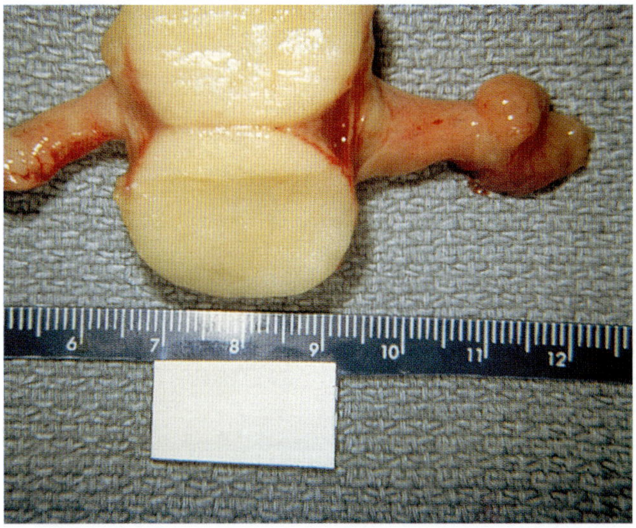


**Fig. 18.46** Adenomatoid tumor. (From Anderson MC, Robboy SJ, Russell P. The fallopian tube. In: Robboy SJ, Anderson MC, Russell P, eds. *Pathology of the Female Reproductive Tract.* Edinburgh: Churchill Livingstone; 2002.)

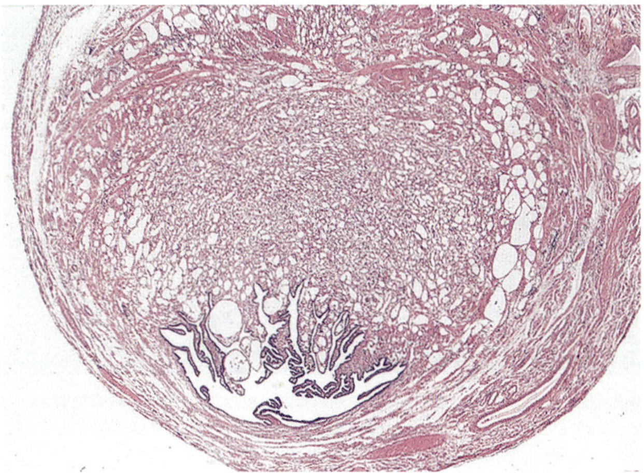

**Fig. 18.47** Adenomatoid tumor arising in the fallopian tube. (From Voet RL. *Color Atlas of Obstetric and Gynecologic Pathology*. St. Louis: Mosby-Wolfe; 1997.)

## Paratubal Cysts

Paratubal cysts are often incidental discoveries during gynecologic operations for other abnormalities. They are commonly multiple and may vary from 0.5 cm to more than 20 cm in diameter. Most cysts are small, asymptomatic, and slow growing and are discovered during the third and fourth decades of life. When

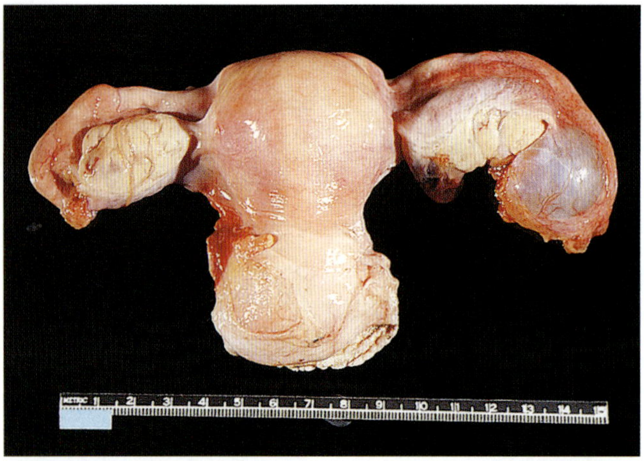

**Fig. 18.48** Broad ligament cyst. This parovarian, or paratubal cyst, is thin walled and contains clear watery fluid. (From Anderson MC, Robboy SJ, Russell P. The fallopian tube. In: Robboy SJ, Anderson MC, Russell P, eds. *Pathology of the Female Reproductive Tract.* Edinburgh: Churchill Livingstone; 2002.)

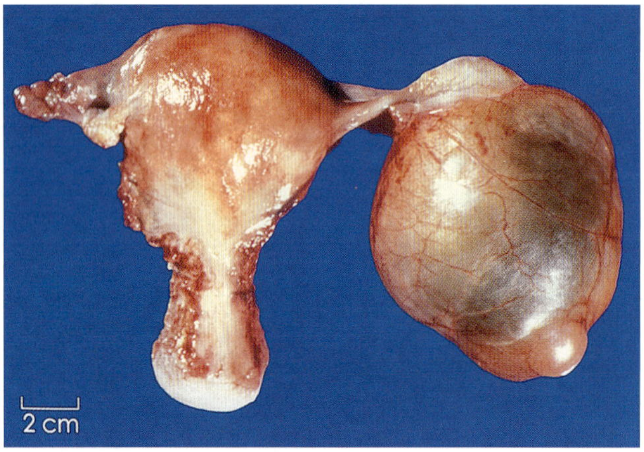


**Fig. 18.49** A nonneoplastic cyst with the broad ligament abuts the normal ovary. (From Clement PB, Young RH. *Atlas of Gynecologic Surgical Pathology.* Philadelphia: Saunders; 2000.)

paratubal cysts are *pedunculated* and near the fimbrial end of the oviduct, they are called hydatid cysts of Morgagni (Figs. 18.48 and 18.49). Cysts near the oviduct may be of mesonephric, mesothelial, or paramesonephric origin. Sometimes the histologic differentiation is difficult because of mechanically produced changes in the cells that line the cyst. These cysts are translucent and contain a clear or pale yellow fluid.

The histogenesis of the majority of paratubal cysts had been believed to be from the mesonephric duct, with the cysts arising from the main duct or accessory tubules. These latter cysts often develop between the leaves of the broad ligament in the mesosalpinx, with the ovary being separate. However, a histologic study of 79 paratubal cysts documented that 60 of the cysts were of tubal origin. Thus the majority of grossly identified "paratubal cysts" are in reality accessory lumina of the fallopian tubes. The remaining 19 cysts were of mesothelial origin. Paratubal cysts are thin walled and smooth and contain clear fluid. Often there are multiple small cysts, and occasionally there is a papillomatous proliferation on the internal wall of these cysts. Inflammatory cysts of the peritoneum may be found anywhere in the pelvis.

The majority of paratubal cysts are asymptomatic and are usually discovered incidentally during ultrasound or during gynecologic operations. When paratubal cysts are symptomatic, they generally produce a dull pain. During a pelvic examination it is difficult to distinguish a paratubal cyst from an ovarian mass. At operation the oviduct is often found stretched over a large paratubal cyst. The oviduct should not be removed in these cases because it will return to normal size after the paratubal cyst is excised. In one retrospective 10-year review of 168 women with parovarian tumors, three low-grade malignant neoplasms were found. These malignancies were in women of reproductive age who had cysts greater than 5 cm in diameter with internal papillary projections. The authors cautioned that the differentiation between benign and malignant parovarian masses cannot be made by external examination of the cyst. The practice of aspirating cysts via the laparoscope should be limited to cysts that are completely simple and associated with normal CA-125 levels. More recent theories of epithelial ovarian carcinogenesis suggest that serous, endometrioid, and clear cell carcinomas are derived from the fallopian tube and the endometrium rather than the ovarian surface epithelium (Erickson, 2013). ACOG supports the view that prophylactic salpingectomy may offer clinicians the opportunity to prevent ovarian cancer in their patients, and the surgeon should discuss the potential benefits of the removal of the fallopian tubes during hysterectomy in women at population risk for ovarian cancer. However, they do not encourage altering the planned route of hysterectomy merely to be able to perform an opportunistic salpingectomy (ACOG, 2019a).

Paratubal cysts may grow rapidly during pregnancy, and most of the cases of torsion of these cysts have been reported during pregnancy or the puerperium. Treatment is simple excision.

## Torsion

Acute torsion of the oviduct is a rare event; however, it has been reported with both normal and pathologic fallopian tubes. Pregnancy predisposes to this problem. Tubal torsion usually accompanies torsion of the ovary because they have a common vascular pedicle. (See the discussion of ovarian torsion presented later in this chapter.) Torsion of the fallopian tube is secondary to an ovarian mass in approximately 50% to 60% of patients. The right tube is involved more often than is the left (Fig. 18.50). The degree of tubal torsion varies from less than one turn to four complete rotations. Torsion of the oviduct is usually seen in women of reproductive age; however, it occurs also in preadolescent children, especially when part of the tube is enclosed in the sac of a femoral or inguinal hernia.

Tubal torsion may be divided into intrinsic and extrinsic causes. Prominent intrinsic causes include congenital abnormalities, such as increased tortuosity caused by excessive length of the tube, and

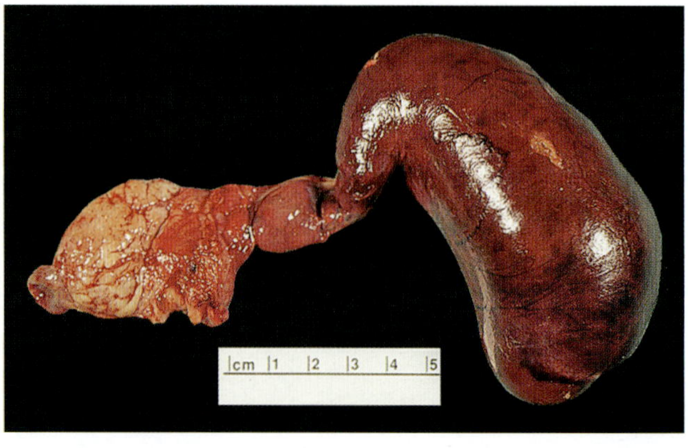


**Fig. 18.50** Hematosalpinx with torsion. (From Voet RL. Color Atlas of Obstetric and Gynecologic Pathology. St. Louis: Mosby-Wolfe; 1997.)

pathologic processes, such as hydrosalpinx, hematosalpinx, tubal neoplasms, and previous operation, especially tubal ligation. Torsion of the fallopian tube after tubal ligation is usually of the distal end. Extrinsic causes of tubal torsion are ovarian and peritubal tumors, adhesions, trauma, and pregnancy.

The most important symptom of tubal torsion is acute lower abdominal and pelvic pain. The onset of this pain is usually sudden, but it may also be gradual, and the pain is usually located in the iliac fossa, with radiation to the thigh and flank. The duration of pain is generally less than 48 hours, and it is associated with nausea and vomiting in two-thirds of the cases. Usually the pelvic pain, secondary to hypoxia, is so intense that it is difficult to perform an adequate pelvic examination. Unless there is associated torsion of the ovary, a specific mass is usually not palpable on pelvic examination.

The preoperative diagnosis of tubal torsion is made in less than 20% of reported cases. However, the number of cases diagnosed preoperatively has increased dramatically with the use of vaginal ultrasonography. Because of the severity of the pain, a wide differential diagnosis of abdominal and pelvic pathologic conditions must be considered. The differential diagnosis includes acute appendicitis, ectopic pregnancy, pelvic inflammatory disease, and rupture or torsion of an ovarian cyst.

Exploratory operation determines the extent of hypoxia and the choice of operative techniques. With tubal torsion, usually the tubes are gangrenous and must be excised. The twisted tube is usually filled with a bloody or serous fluid. It may be possible to restore normal circulation to the tube by manually untwisting it. The tube is usually sutured into a secure position to prevent recurrence.

## OVARY

Ovarian masses are a common finding on pelvic examination and pelvic imaging. The task of the clinician is to determine whether the mass should be removed or may be managed expectantly. The general factors used to consider removal include the symptoms produces by the mass, the chances that the mass is malignant, and the likelihood of spontaneous resolution.

### Functional Cysts

#### Follicular Cysts

Follicular cysts are by far the most common cystic structures in normal ovaries. They may be found as early as 20 weeks' gestation in female fetuses and throughout a woman's reproductive life. Follicular cysts are often multiple and may vary from a few millimeters to as large as 15 cm in diameter. A normal follicle may develop into a physiologic cyst. A minimum diameter to be considered as a cyst is generally considered to be between 2.5 and 3 cm. Follicular cysts are not neoplastic and are believed to be dependent on gonadotropins for growth. They arise from a temporary variation of a normal physiologic process. Clinically they may present with the signs and symptoms of ovarian enlargement and therefore must be differentiated from a true ovarian neoplasm. Functional cysts may be solitary or multiple. These cysts are found most commonly in young, menstruating women but may be found in postmenopausal women. Solitary cysts may occur during the fetal and neonatal periods and rarely during childhood, but there is an increase in frequency during the perimenarchal period. Large solitary follicular cysts in which the lining is luteinized are occasionally discovered during pregnancy and the puerperium. CA-125 may be used to evaluate such cysts in pregnancy. The values for CA-125 should be within the normal range past 12 weeks' gestation. Multiple follicular cysts in which the lining is luteinized are associated with either intrinsic or extrinsic elevated levels of gonadotropins. Interestingly, reproductive-age women with cystic fibrosis appear to have an increased propensity for developing individual follicular cysts.

Follicular cysts are translucent, thin-walled, and filled with a watery, clear to straw-colored fluid. If a small opening in the capsule of the cyst suddenly develops, the cyst fluid under pressure will squirt out. These cysts are situated in the ovarian cortex, and sometimes they appear as translucent domes on the surface of the ovary. Histologically the lining of the cyst is usually composed of a closely packed layer of round, plump granulosa cells, with the spindle-shaped cells of the theca interna deeper in the stroma. In many cysts the lining of granulosa cells is difficult to distinguish, having undergone pressure atrophy. All that remains is a hyalinized connective tissue lining. The temporary disturbance in follicular function that produces the clinical picture of a follicular cyst is poorly understood. Follicular cysts may result from either the dominant mature follicle's failing to rupture (persistent follicle) or an immature follicle's failing to undergo the normal process of atresia. In the latter circumstance, the incompletely developed follicle fails to reabsorb follicular fluid. Some follicular cysts lose their ability to produce estrogen, and in others the granulosa cells remain productive, with prolonged secretion of estrogens. Occasionally, follicular cysts are better termed *follicular hematomas* because blood from the vascular theca zone fills the cavity of the cyst.

Most follicular cysts are asymptomatic and are discovered during ultrasound imaging of the pelvis or a routine pelvic examination. Ultrasound cannot reliably differentiate a benign from a malignant process. However, several characteristics of ovarian masses correlate with malignancy, including internal papillations (echogenic structures protruding into the mass), loculations, solid lesions or cystic lesions with solid components, thick septations, and smaller cysts adjacent to or part of the wall of the larger cyst–daughter cysts (Fig. 18.51).

Because of their thin walls these cysts may rupture during examination. The patient may experience tenesmus, a transient pelvic tenderness, deep dyspareunia, or no pain whatsoever. Rarely is significant intraperitoneal bleeding associated with the rupture of a follicular cyst. However, women who are chronically anticoagulated or those with von Willebrand disease may bleed. Occasionally, menstrual irregularities and abnormal uterine bleeding may be associated with follicular cysts, which produce elevated blood estrogen levels. The syndrome associated with such follicular cysts consists of a regular cycle with a prolonged intermenstrual interval, followed by episodes of menorrhagia. Some women with larger follicular cysts notice a vague, dull sensation or heaviness in the pelvis.

The initial management of a suspected follicular cyst is conservative observation. The majority of follicular cysts disappear spontaneously by either reabsorption of the cyst fluid or silent rupture within 4 to 8 weeks of initial diagnosis. However, a persistent ovarian mass necessitates operative intervention to differentiate a physiologic cyst from a true neoplasm of the ovary. There is no way to make the differentiation on the basis of signs, symptoms, or the initial growth pattern during early development of either process. Endovaginal ultrasound examination is helpful in differentiating simple from complex cysts and is also helpful during conservative management by providing dimensions to determine whether the cyst is increasing in size. When the diameter of the cyst remains stable for greater than 10 weeks or enlarges, a neoplasia should be ruled out. Oral contraceptives may be prescribed for 4 to 6 weeks for young women with adnexal masses. This therapy removes any influence that pituitary gonadotropins may have on the persistence of the ovarian cyst. It also allows for several weeks of observation. In one series, 80% of cystic masses 4 to 6 cm in size disappeared during the time the patient was taking oral contraceptives. However, randomized prospective trials found no difference in the rate of disappearance of functional ovarian cysts between the group that received oral

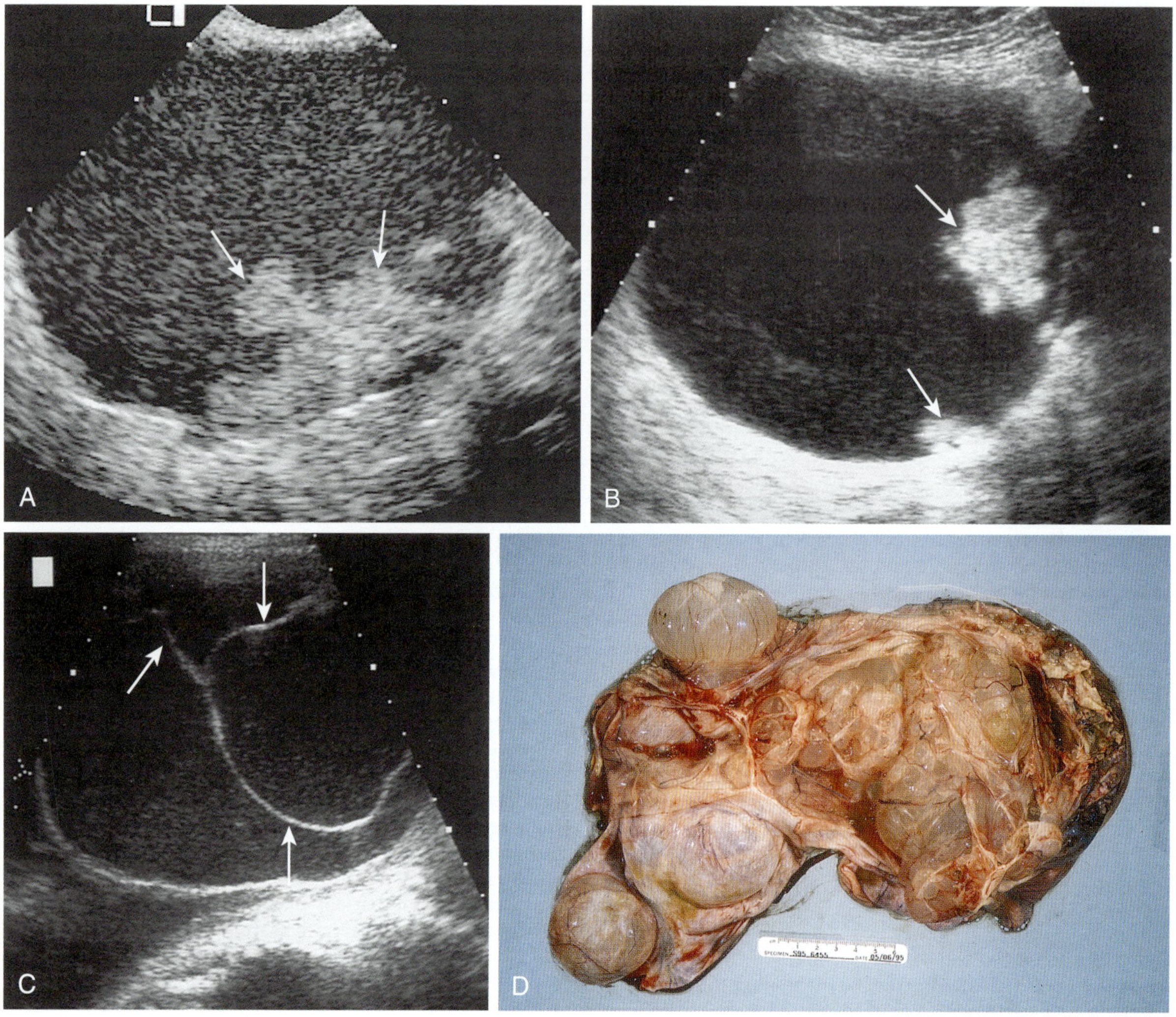

**Fig. 18.51** Serous cystadenocarcinoma, varying appearances. **A,** Transvaginal scan shows large cystic mass containing multiple low-level internal echoes and solid echogenic components *(arrows)*. **B,** Transabdominal scan shows large cystic mass with irregular solid echogenic mural nodules *(arrows)* and low-level internal echoes. **C,** Mucinous cystadenoma. Transabdominal scan shows large cystic mass with multiple thin septations *(arrows)* and fine low-level internal echoes. **D,** Gross pathologic specimen shows multiple cystic loculations. (From Salem S. The uterus and adnexa. In: Rumack CM, Wilson SR, Charboneau JW, eds. *Diagnostic Ultrasound.* St. Louis: Mosby; 1998:555-556.)

contraceptives and the control group, perhaps because so many cysts will resolve spontaneously.

The evaluation of an asymptomatic cyst, found incidentally, is based on the principle that the cyst should be removed if there is any suspicion of malignancy. Suspicion may develop because of history, including family history, patient age, and other nongynecologic signs and symptoms. The size and physical characteristics of the cyst are as important as are other laboratory parameters. CA-125 is helpful in evaluating the adnexal mass in postmenopausal women. In premenopausal women, CA-125 is rarely helpful unless the mass is extremely suggestive of malignancy. As discussed earlier, measurement of diastolic and systolic velocities provide indirect indices of vascular resistance. Muscular arteries have high resistance. Newly developed vessels, such as those arising in malignancies, have little vascular wall musculature and thus have low resistance. When a color flow Doppler scan demonstrates vascularity, the vascular resistance can be calculated. Low resistance is associated with malignancy, and high resistance usually is associated with normal tissue or benign disease. Although color flow Doppler has been shown to be sensitive in evaluating ovarian neoplasms, it is neither sensitive nor specific enough to be used as a determining study. In most cases, simple small cysts may be observed. In general, complex cysts or persistent simple cysts larger than 10 cm should be evaluated. In women with cysts in pregnancy, if the cyst is simple with a normal CA-125, conservative management is acceptable. (CA-125 is generally not obtained in pregnant women with cysts less than 5 cm if they are simple.)

A cyst in a perimenopausal or postmenopausal woman should be removed if it is anything other than a simple cyst, if the CA-125 is abnormal (>35), or if the cyst is persistent or large (>10 cm), although observation may be reasonable in select cases. A small simple cyst (<5 cm) in a perimenopausal or postmenopausal woman with a normal CA-125 may be observed with follow-up ultrasound and CA-125 testing every 6 months for 2 years. If unchanged at that point, routine monitoring can be stopped. Several studies, including a large prospective series from Greenlee and colleagues, examined the issue of simple cysts in postmenopausal women with simple cysts. These studies have noted that expectant management is safe and reasonable. In the series by Greenlee, the Prostate, Lung, Colorectal, and Ovarian Cancer Screening Trial, women were followed for 4 years with transvaginal ultrasound. Of 15,735 women, 2217 (14%) had at least one simple cyst. Cysts were more common in women in the 50- to 59-year-old age group and women with hysterectomies before age 40. Cysts were less common among smokers and older women. In all, 54% of cysts were present on scans 1 year later; 8% of women had more than one cyst. Only 0.4% of the entire population developed ovarian cancer, and half of the women who developed cancer did not have cysts. The 14% incidence of cysts in postmenopausal women is similar to rates of simple cysts in other large series. Thus women with simple cysts who are asymptomatic and with negative CA-125 may be reassured and, if desired, followed expectantly (Greenlee, 2010). Management of cysts between 5 and 10 cm that are otherwise not suggestive should be individualized. Cysts with internal structures have a much higher rate of malignancy.

In premenopausal women, operative management of nonmalignant cysts is cystectomy, not oophorectomy. Many clinicians will manage simple cysts laparoscopically. Because this procedure has an accompanying risk of spilling malignant cells into the peritoneal cavity if the cyst is an early carcinoma, strict preoperative criteria should be fulfilled before laparoscopy is attempted. These include the woman's age; size of the mass; and ultrasound characteristics, such as nonadherent, smooth, and thin-walled cysts, without papillae or internal echoes (simple). Higher rates of recurrence, up to 40%, have been reported for simple drainage of multiple types of benign cysts, the point being that drainage or fenestration is effective for follicular cysts and poorly effective for other cysts. When cysts are drained, it is essential to remember that cytologic examination of cyst fluid has poor predictive value and poor sensitivity in differentiating benign from malignant cysts. If there is any suspicion of malignancy, the cyst should be removed as carefully as possible and a histopathologic evaluation obtained. The size of the cyst is not a necessary reason to avoid laparoscopy. Most simple cysts, even those larger than 10 cm, can be managed via minimally invasive surgery.

## Corpus Luteum Cysts

Corpus luteum cysts are less common than follicular cysts, but clinically they are more important. This discussion collectively combines corpus luteum cysts and persistently functioning mature corpora lutea (Fig. 18.52). Pathologists are sometimes able to distinguish between a hemorrhagic cystic corpus luteum and a corpus luteum cyst, but at other times this difference cannot be established. All corpora lutea are cystic with gradual reabsorption of a limited amount of hemorrhage, which may form a cavity. Clinically, corpora lutea are not termed *corpus luteum cysts* unless they are a minimum of 3 cm in diameter. Corpus luteum cysts may be associated with either normal endocrine function or prolonged secretion of progesterone. The associated menstrual pattern may be normal, delayed menstruation, or amenorrhea.

Corpora lutea develop from mature graafian follicles. Intrafollicular bleeding does not occur during ovulation. However, 2 to 4 days later, during the stage of vascularization, thin-walled capillaries invade the granulosa cells from the theca interna. Spontaneous but limited bleeding fills the central cavity of the maturing corpus luteum with blood. Subsequently this blood is absorbed, forming a small cystic space. When the hemorrhage is excessive, the cystic space enlarges. If the hemorrhage into the central cavity is brisk, intracystic pressure increases, and rupture of the corpus luteum is a possibility. If rupture does not occur, the size of the resulting corpus luteum cyst usually varies between 3 and 10 cm. Occasionally a cyst may be 11 to 15 cm in diameter. If a cystic central cavity persists, blood is replaced by clear fluid, and the result is a hormonally inactive corpus albicans cyst (Fig. 18.53). A corpus luteum of pregnancy is normally 3 to 5 cm in diameter with a central cystic structure, occupying at least 50% of the ovarian mass.

Most corpus luteum cysts are small, the average diameter being 4 cm. Grossly they have a smooth surface and, depending on whether the cyst represents acute or chronic hemorrhage, are purplish red to brown. When a corpus luteum is cut, the convoluted lining is yellowish orange, and the center contains an organizing blood clot. Both the granulosa and the theca cells undergo luteinization. In chronic corpus luteum cysts, the wall becomes gray-white, and the polygonal luteinized cells usually undergo pressure atrophy.

Corpus luteum cysts vary from being asymptomatic masses to causing catastrophic and massive intraperitoneal bleeding associated with rupture. Many corpus luteum cysts produce dull, unilateral, lower abdominal and pelvic pain. The enlarged ovary is moderately tender on pelvic examination. Depending on the amount of progesterone secretion associated with cysts, the menstrual bleeding may be normal or delayed several days to weeks with subsequent menorrhagia. Halban, in 1915, described a syndrome of a persistently functioning corpus luteum cyst that has clinical features similar to an unruptured ectopic pregnancy. Halban's classic triad was a delay in a normal period followed by

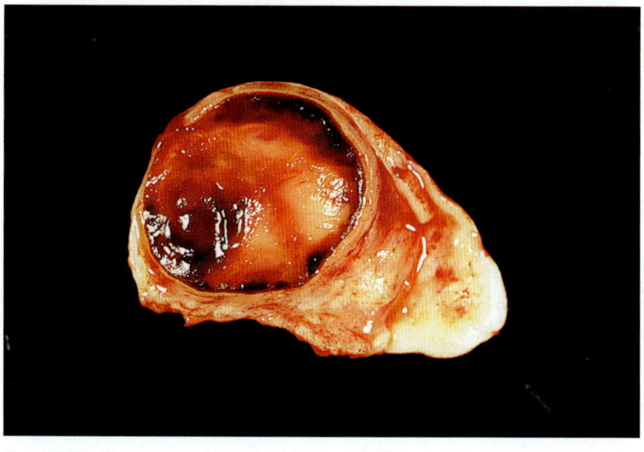

**Fig. 18.52** Hemorrhagic corpus luteum with an outer yellow rim and central hemorrhage. (From Voet RL. *Color Atlas of Obstetric and Gynecologic Pathology*. St. Louis: Mosby-Wolfe; 1997.)

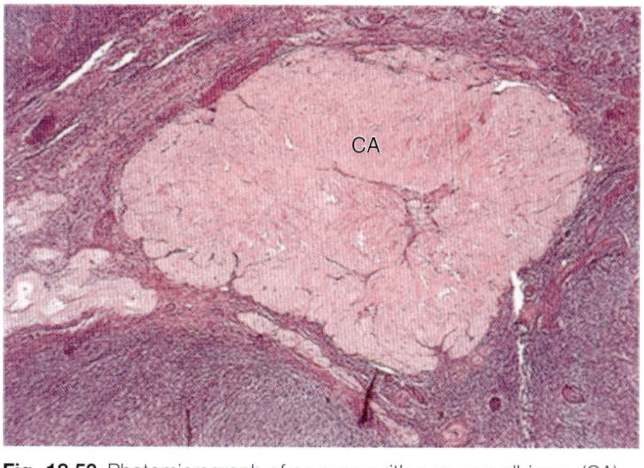


**Fig. 18.53** Photomicrograph of an ovary with a corpus albicans (CA) made up of a scar of dense connective tissue at the site of a prior corpus luteum. (From Basicmedical Key Online Library. Available at: https://radiologykey.com/wp-content/uploads/2016/03/B9781416032649500331_f29-07-9781416032649.jpg.)

**TABLE 18.4** Symptoms of 173 Women With Ruptured Corpus Luteum

| Location | Number | Percentage |
|---|---|---|
| Right ovary | 114 | 66 |
| Left ovary | 56 | 32 |
| Unknown | 3 | 2 |
| Abdominal pain | 173 | 100 |
| Right ovary | 21 | 72 |
| Left ovary | 8 | 28 |
| Duration | | |
| Less than 24 hours | 94 | 54 |
| 1-7 days | 40 | 23 |
| Over 7 days | 14 | 8 |
| Unknown | 25 | 15 |
| Nausea or vomiting or diarrhea | 60 | 35 |

From Hallatt JG, Steele CH Jr, Snyder M. Ruptured corpus luteum with hemoperitoneum: a study of 173 surgical cases. *Am J Obstet Gynecol.* 1984;149(1):5-9.

spotting, unilateral pelvic pain, and a small, tender, adnexal mass. This triad of symptomology is similar to the triad of an anomalous period or delay in a normal period, spotting, and unilateral pelvic pain that are exhibited by the classic ectopic pregnancy. The differential diagnosis between these two conditions without a sensitive pregnancy test is difficult.

Corpus luteum cysts may cause intraperitoneal bleeding. The amount of bleeding varies from slight to clinically significant hemorrhage, necessitating blood transfusion. Internal bleeding often follows coitus, exercise, trauma, or a pelvic examination. However, episodes of bleeding usually do not recur, which differs from an ectopic pregnancy. Women with a bleeding diathesis or those undergoing chronic anticoagulation therapy are especially at risk for developing ovarian hemorrhage from a corpus luteum cyst. Bleeding occurs usually between days 20 and 26 of their cycle, and these women have a 31% chance for subsequent hemorrhage from a recurrent corpus luteum cyst. Oral contraceptives are sometimes used to suppress ovulation and avoid recurrent hemorrhage.

Tang and coworkers have also reported a right-sided predominance in the incidence of hemorrhage from corpus luteum cysts. They postulated that the difference is related to a higher intraluminal pressure on the right side because of the differences in ovarian vein architecture (Tang, 1985). Most ruptures occur between days 20 and 26 of the cycle, although in the series of Hallatt and colleagues (Fig 18.4), 28% of the women had a delay in menses not explained by pregnancy.

The differential diagnosis of a woman with acute pain and suspected ruptured corpus luteum cyst includes ectopic pregnancy, a ruptured endometrioma, and adnexal torsion. A sensitive serum or urinary assay for human chorionic gonadotropin (HCG) will help differentiate a bleeding corpus luteum from ectopic pregnancy (see Chapter 17). Vaginal ultrasound is useful in establishing a preoperative diagnosis. Culdocentesis has been used in the past to establish the severity of the hemorrhage, but it is rarely used today. If the hematocrit of the fluid obtained from the posterior cul-de-sac is greater than 15%, operative therapy is recommended. Cystectomy is the operative treatment of choice, with preservation of the remaining portion of the ovary. Unruptured corpus luteum cysts may be followed conservatively. Raziel and coworkers reported on a series of 70 women with ruptured corpora lutea. Ultrasonic evidence of large amounts of peritoneal fluid and severe pain were indications for operative intervention. In 12 of 70 patients with small amounts of intraperitoneal fluid and mild to moderate pain, observation alone was associated with resolution of symptoms (Raziel, 1993).

## Theca Lutein Cysts

Theca lutein cysts are by far the least common of the three types of physiologic ovarian cysts (Fig. 18.54), arising from either prolonged or excessive stimulation of the ovaries by endogenous or exogenous gonadotropins or increased ovarian sensitivity to gonadotropins. Unlike corpus luteum cysts, theca lutein cysts are almost always bilateral and produce moderate to massive enlargement of the ovaries. The individual cysts vary in size from 1 cm to 10 cm or more in diameter. The condition of ovarian enlargement secondary to the development of multiple luteinized follicular cysts is termed *hyperreactio luteinalis*. Approximately 50% of molar pregnancies and 10% of choriocarcinomas have associated bilateral theca lutein cysts (see Chapter 35). In these patients the HCG from the trophoblast produces luteinization of the cells in immature, mature, and atretic follicles. The cysts are also discovered in the latter months of pregnancies, often with conditions that produce a large placenta, such as twin gestations, diabetes, and Rh sensitization. It is not uncommon to iatrogenically produce theca lutein cysts in women receiving medications to induce ovulation. Theca lutein cysts are occasionally discovered in association with normal pregnancy, as well as in newborn infants secondary to transplacental effects of maternal gonadotropins. Rarely these cysts are found in young girls with juvenile hypothyroidism.

Grossly the total ovarian size may be voluminous, 20 to 30 cm in diameter, with multiple theca lutein cysts. Bilateral ovarian enlargement is produced by multiple gray to bluish-tinged cysts. The bilateral enlargement is secondary to hundreds of thin-walled locules or cysts, producing a honeycombed appearance. Grossly the external surface of the ovary appears lobulated, and the small cysts contain a clear to straw-colored or hemorrhagic fluid. Histologically the lining of the cyst is composed of theca

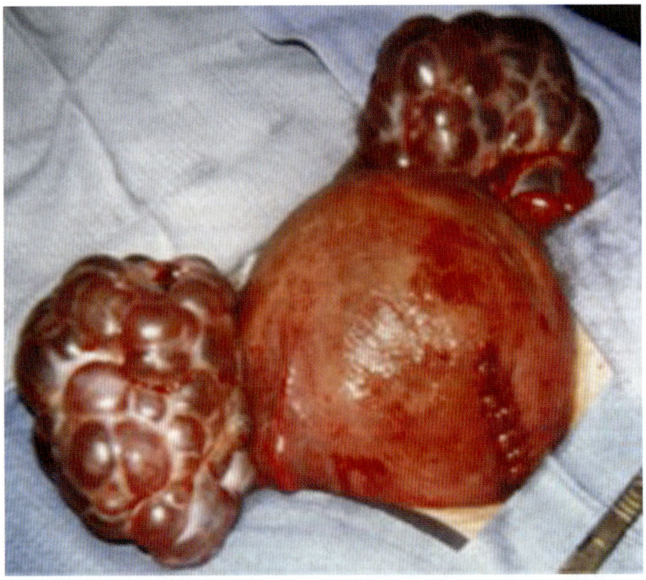

**Fig. 18.54** Postgravid uterus with bilateral theca lutein cysts. (From Peter Callen: *Ultrasonography in Obstetrics and Gynecology*, 5th Edition, 2007; Yee B, Tu B, Platt LD: Coexisting hydatidiform mole with a live fetus presenting as a placenta previa on ultrasound. *Am J Obstet Gynecol.* 144:726, 1982.)

lutein cells (paralutein cells), believed to originate from ovarian connective tissue. Occasionally there is also luteinization of granulosa cells. These voluminous and congested ovaries are slow growing, and the majority of women with smaller cysts are asymptomatic. Generally only the larger cysts produce vague symptoms, such as a sense of pressure in the pelvis. Ascites and increasing abdominal girth have been reported with hyperstimulation from exogenous gonadotropins. Associated adnexal torsion or bleeding may occur less than 1% of the time. Some theca lutein cysts persist for weeks after HCG levels normalize.

The presence of theca lutein cysts is established by palpation and often confirmed by ultrasound examination. Treatment is conservative because these cysts gradually regress. If these cysts are discovered incidentally at cesarean delivery, they should be handled delicately. No attempt should be made to drain or puncture the multiple cysts because of the possibility of hemorrhage. Bleeding is difficult to control in these cases because of the thin walls that constitute the cysts.

A condition related to theca lutein cysts is the luteoma of pregnancy. The condition is rare and not a true neoplasm but rather a specific, benign, hyperplastic reaction of ovarian theca lutein cells (Figs. 18.55 and 18.56). These nodules do not arise from the corpus luteum of pregnancy. Fifty percent of luteomas are multiple, and approximately 30% of those reported have bilateral nodules. In appearance they are discrete and brown to reddish brown and may be solid or cystic.

The majority of patients with luteomas are asymptomatic. The solid, fleshy, often hemorrhagic nodules are discovered incidentally at cesarean delivery or postpartum tubal ligation. Most cases have been reported in multiparous African American women. Masculinization of the mother occurs in 30% of cases, and masculinization of the external genitalia of the female fetus may sometimes occur. These tumors regress spontaneously after completion of the pregnancy.

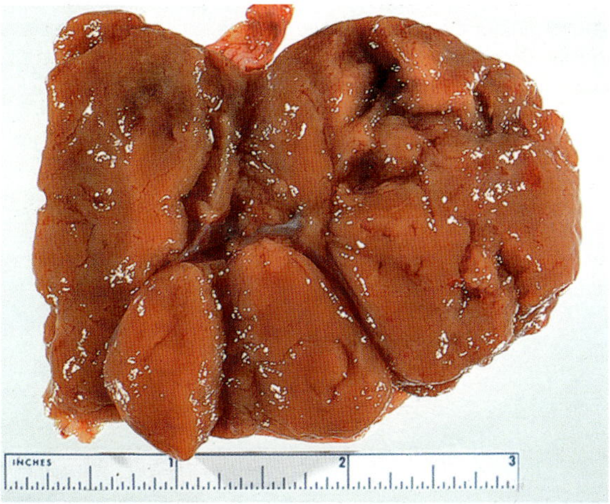


**Fig. 18.55** Luteoma of pregnancy with numerous solid brown nodules. (From Voet RL. *Color Atlas of Obstetric and Gynecologic Pathology.* St. Louis: Mosby-Wolfe; 1997.)

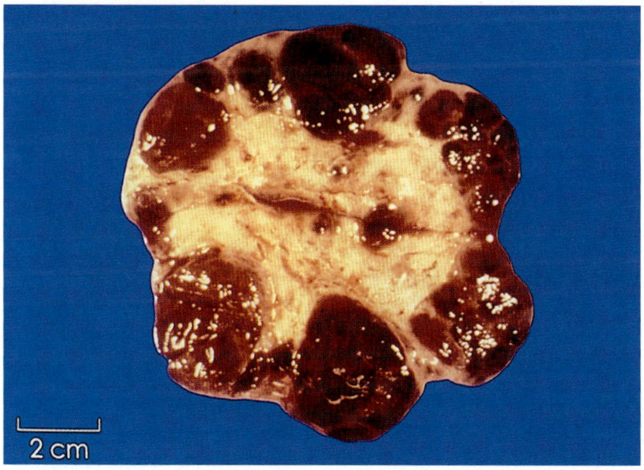


**Fig. 18.56** Luteoma with multiple reddish nodules. (From Clement PB, Young RH. *Atlas of Gynecologic Surgical Pathology.* Philadelphia: WB Saunders; 2000.)

## Benign Neoplasms of the Ovary

### Benign Cystic Teratoma (Dermoid Cyst, Mature Teratoma)

Benign ovarian teratomas are usually cystic structures that on histologic examination contain elements from all three germ cell layers. The word *teratoma* was first advanced by Virchow and translated literally means "monstrous growth." Teratomas of the ovary may be benign or malignant. Although *dermoid* is a misnomer, it is the most common term used to describe the benign cystic tumor, composed of mature cells, whereas the malignant variety is composed of immature cells (immature teratoma). *Dermoid* is a descriptive term in that it emphasizes the preponderance of ectodermal tissue with some mesodermal and rare endodermal derivatives. Malignant teratomas that are immature are usually solid with some cystic areas and histologically contain immature or embryonic-appearing tissue. (See Chapter 33, for further discussion of malignant teratomas.) Benign teratomas may contain a malignant component, usually in women older than 40 (mean age 48). The malignant component is generally a squamous carcinoma and is found in less than 1% of cases. Nonovarian teratomas may arise in any midline structure of the body where the germ cell has resided during embryonic life.

Benign teratomas are among the most common ovarian neoplasms. They account for more than 90% of germ cell tumors of the ovary. These slow-growing tumors occur from infancy to the postmenopausal years. Depending on the series, dermoids represent 20% to 25% of all ovarian neoplasms and approximately 33% of all benign tumors, if follicular and corpus luteum cysts are excluded. Dermoids are the most common ovarian neoplasm in prepubertal girls and are also common in teenagers. More than 50% of benign teratomas are discovered in women between the ages of 25 and 50 years. In one series of 118 women with dermoids, 86% of the women were younger than 40, and 3.4% had recurrences (Fig. 18.57). With routine obstetric ultrasound, the mean age at diagnosis is expected to fall. In most large series of benign tumors in postmenopausal women, dermoids account for approximately 20% of the neoplasms.

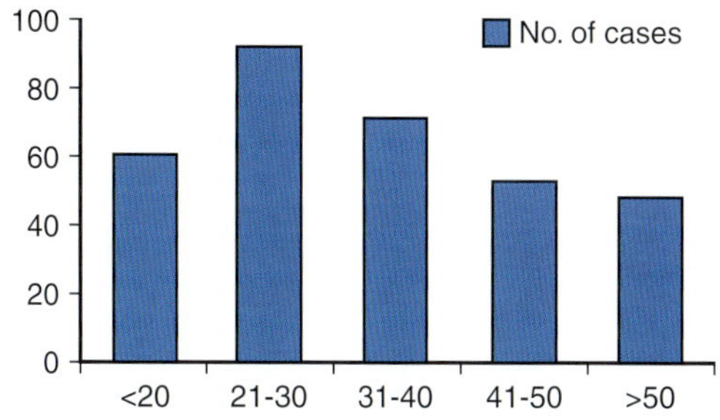


**Fig. 18.57** Age distribution of all the mature cystic teratoma in a study of 223 cases. (From Rathore R, Sharma S, Arora D. Clinicopathological evaluation of 223 cases of mature cystic teratoma, ovary: 25-year experience in a single tertiary care centre in India. *J Clin Diagn Res.* 2017;11(4):EC11-EC14.)

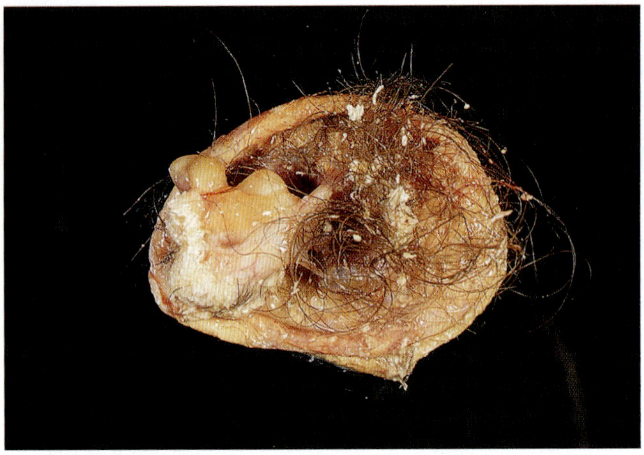

**Fig. 18.58** Mature cystic teratoma (dermoid cyst) filled with hair and keratinous debris with one solid nodular area (Rokitansky protuberance). (From Voet RL. *Color Atlas of Obstetric and Gynecologic Pathology.* St. Louis: Mosby-Wolfe; 1997.)

Dermoids vary from a few millimeters to 25 cm in diameter, although they have been reported to weigh as much as 7657 g in an asymptomatic woman. However, 80% are less than 10 cm. These tumors may be single or multiple, with as many as nine individual dermoids having been reported in the same ovary. Benign teratomas occur bilaterally 10% to 15% of the time. Often, dermoid cysts are pedunculated. These cysts make the ovary heavier than normal, and thus they are usually discovered either in the cul-de-sac or anterior to the broad ligament. On palpation these tumors, which have both cystic and solid components, have a doughy consistency.

The cysts are usually unilocular. The walls of the cyst are a smooth, shiny, opaque white color. When they are opened, thick sebaceous fluid pours from the cyst, often with tangled masses of hair and firm areas of cartilage and teeth (Figs. 18.58 and 18.59). The sebaceous material is a thick fluid at body temperature but solidifies when it cools in room air.

Benign teratomas are believed to arise from a single germ cell after the first meiotic division. Therefore they develop from totipotential stem cells, and they are neoplastic sequelae from a transformed germ cell. Dermoids have a chromosomal makeup of 46,XX and the chromosomes of dermoids were different from the chromosomes of the host, leading one to postulate that dermoids began by parthenogenesis from secondary oocytes. An alternative hypothesis was that the dermoid resulted from fusion of the second polar body with the oocyte. One thing is certain—dermoids do not arise from somatic cells nor from an oogonium before the first stage of meiosis. The first meiotic division occurs at approximately 13 weeks' gestation. Thus dermoids begin in fetal life sometime after the first trimester.

Histologically, benign teratomas are composed of mature cells, usually from all three germ layers (Fig. 18.60). A combination of skin and skin appendages, including sebaceous glands, sweat glands, hair follicles, muscle fibers, cartilage, bone, teeth, glial cells, and epithelium of the respiratory and gastrointestinal tracts, may be visualized. Teeth are predominantly premolar and molar forms. The fluid in dermoid cysts is usually sebaceous. Most solid elements arise and are contained in a protrusion or nipple (mammilla) in the cyst wall, termed the *prominence or tubercle of Rokitansky*. This prominence may be visualized by ultrasound as an echodense region, thus aiding in the sonographic diagnosis. If malignancy occurs, it is almost always found in this nest of cells. The wall of the cyst will often contain granulation tissue, giant cells, and pseudoxanthoma cells.

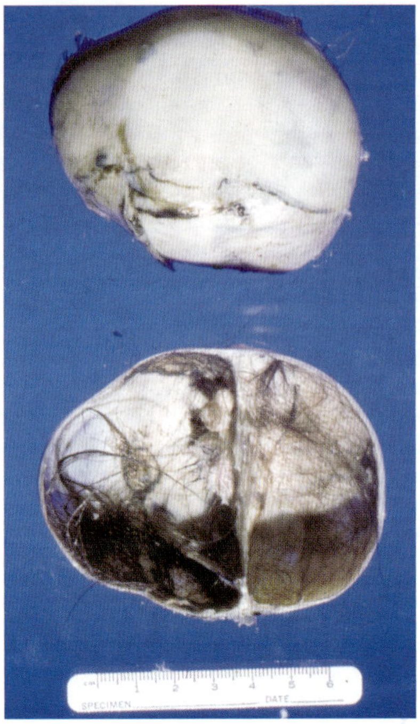

**Fig. 18.59** Bilateral mature cystic teratomas in pregnancy. The cyst is bilocular. Dermal papillae are noted. Teeth are also present in the left lobule. (From Russell P, Robboy SJ, Anderson MC. Germ cell tumors of the ovaries. In: Robboy SJ, Anderson MC, Russell P, eds. *Pathology of the Female Reproductive Tract.* Edinburgh: Churchill Livingstone; 2002.)

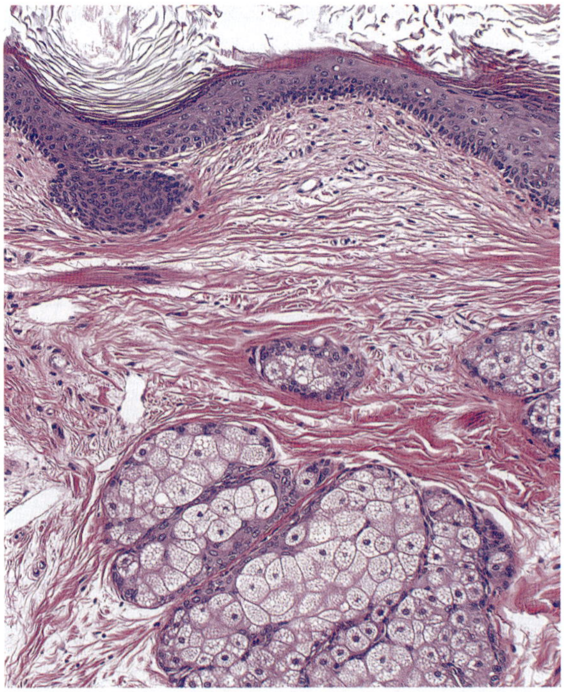

**Fig. 18.60** Mature cystic teratoma. This cyst is lined with mature epidermis and is subtended by connective tissue containing exuberant dermal appendages (pilosebaceous follicles). (From Russell P, Robboy SJ, Anderson MC. Germ cell tumors of the ovaries. In: Robboy SJ, Anderson MC, Russell P, eds. *Pathology of the Female Reproductive Tract.* Edinburgh: Churchill Livingstone; 2002.)

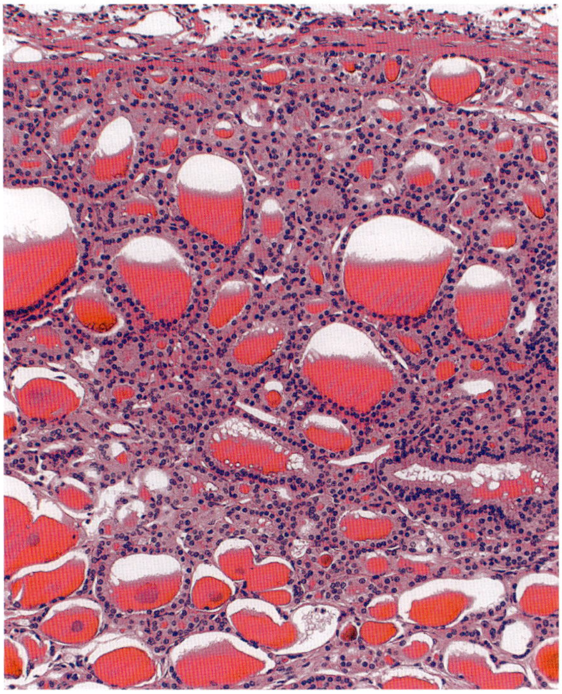

**Fig. 18.61** Struma ovarii. Variably sized banal thyroid follicles. (From Russell P, Robboy SJ, Anderson MC. Germ cell tumors of the ovaries. In: Robboy SJ, Anderson MC, Russell P, eds. *Pathology of the Female Reproductive Tract.* Edinburgh: Churchill Livingstone; 2002.)

From 50% to 60% of dermoids are asymptomatic and are discovered during a routine pelvic examination, coincidentally visualized during pelvic imaging, or found incidentally at laparotomy. Presenting symptoms of dermoids include pain and the sensation of pelvic pressure. Specific complications of dermoid cysts include torsion, rupture, infection, hemorrhage, and malignant degeneration. Three medical diseases also may be associated with dermoid cysts: thyrotoxicosis, carcinoid syndrome, and autoimmune hemolytic anemia, the latter two being quite rare.

Adult thyroid tissue is discovered microscopically in approximately 12% of benign teratomas. Struma ovarii is a teratoma in which the thyroid tissue has overgrown other elements and is the predominant tissue (Fig. 18.61). Strumae ovarii constitute 2% to 3% of ovarian teratomas. These tumors are usually unilateral and measure less than 10 cm in diameter. Less than 5% of women with strumae ovarii develop thyrotoxicosis, which may be secondary to the production of increased thyroid hormone by either the ovarian or the thyroid gland.

Another rare finding with dermoids is the presence of a primary carcinoid tumor from the gastrointestinal or respiratory tract epithelium contained in the dermoid. One of three of these tumors is associated with the typical carcinoid syndrome even without metastatic spread. If the carcinoid is functioning, it may be diagnosed by measuring serum serotonin levels or urinary levels of 5-hydroxyindoleacetic acid. The autoimmune hemolytic anemia associated with dermoids is the rarest of the three medical complications.

Rupture or perforation of the contents of a dermoid into the peritoneal cavity or an adjacent organ is a potentially serious complication. The incidence varies between 0.7% and 4.6%. However, most series report less than 1%. Rupture is more common in pregnancy. If a rupture occurs during surgery, the abdomen should be copiously irrigated with saline, with careful removal of any particulate matter. Chemical peritonitis is reported in less than 1% of ruptured dermoids. Rupture may occur either catastrophically, which produces an acute abdomen, or by a slow leak of the sebaceous material. The latter is clinically more common, with the sebaceous material producing a severe chemical granulomatous peritonitis. Some warn that this possibility should be considered and a frozen section obtained so that the true diagnosis is established. Thus a young woman will not be mistakenly treated for suspected ovarian carcinoma with metastasis because of the identical gross appearance of a slow-leaking dermoid cyst. Infection, hemorrhage, and malignant degeneration are all unusual complications of dermoids, occurring in less than 1% of patients.

Torsion of a dermoid is the most common complication, occurring in 3.5% to 11% of cases. Because of its weight, the benign teratoma is often pedunculated, which may predispose to torsion. Torsion is more common in younger women. Small dermoid cysts, less than 6 cm in diameter, grow slowly at an approximate rate of 2 mm per year.

The diagnosis of a dermoid cyst is often established when a semisolid mass is palpated anterior to the broad ligament. Approximately 50% of dermoids have pelvic calcifications on radiographic examination. Often an ovarian teratoma is an incidental finding during radiologic investigation of the genitourinary or gastrointestinal tract. Most dermoids have a characteristic ultrasound picture. These characteristics include a dense echogenic area within a larger cystic area, a cyst filled with bands of mixed echoes, and an echoic dense cyst. Unfortunately, only one of three dermoids has this "typical picture." In one series of 45 patients with 51 biopsy-proved dermoid cysts, 24% of the dermoid cysts were predominantly solid, 20% were almost entirely cystic, and 24% were not visible. Ultrasound has a more than 95% positive predictive value and a less than 5% false-positive rate (Laing, 1981).

Operative treatment of benign cystic teratomas is cystectomy with preservation of as much normal ovarian tissue as possible. Laparoscopic cystectomy is an accepted approach. Rates of spillage are comparable with that from open laparotomy. However, adequate irrigation in such cases is essential and often more time consuming. Many authors use a 10-cm diameter cutoff as the upper limit for a laparoscopic approach.

When a teratoma is diagnosed incidentally during pregnancy, conservative management is acceptable. Though dermoids have a higher incidence of torsion and potential for rupture during pregnancy, most large series have not shown that an aggressive approach to asymptomatic teratomas less than 10 cm confers any advantage for the mother or pregnancy. Though laparoscopy is safe during pregnancy, a small periumbilical minilaparotomy may be a faster, less traumatic approach. The treatment is cystectomy, and with the recommendation for reduced intraoperative time this approach may be preferable during pregnancy.

## Endometriomas

Endometriosis of the ovary is usually associated with endometriosis in other areas of the pelvic cavity. Approximately two out of three women with endometriosis have ovarian involvement. Interestingly, only 5% of these women have enlargement of the ovaries that is detectable by pelvic examination; however, because of the prevalence of the disease, endometriosis is one of the most common causes of enlargement of the ovary. Because most authors do not classify endometriosis as a neoplastic disease, the diagnosis of endometriosis may not be given due consideration in the differential diagnosis of an adnexal mass. Ovarian endometriosis is similar to endometriosis elsewhere and is described in greater detail in Chapter 19.

The size of ovarian endometriomas varies from small, superficial, blue-black implants that are 1 to 5 mm in diameter to large, multiloculated, hemorrhagic cysts that may be 5 to 10 cm in diameter (Fig. 18.62). Clinically, large ovarian endometriomas, greater than 20 cm in diameter, are extremely rare. Areas of ovarian endometriosis

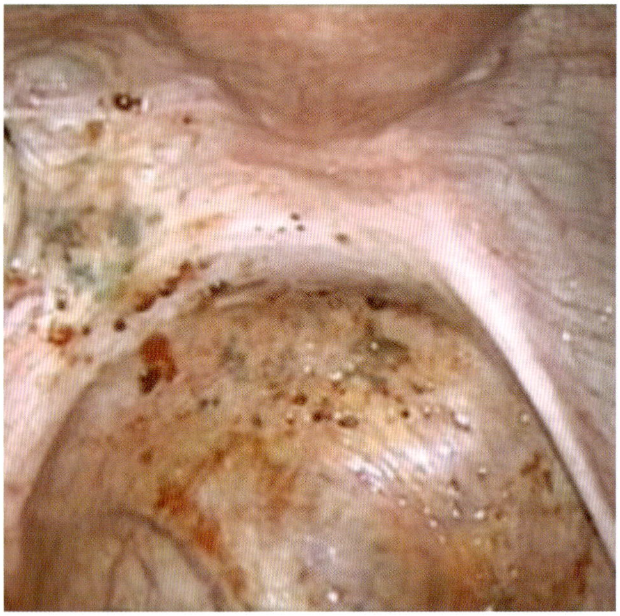

**Fig. 18.62** Scattered variable-appearing endometriosis lesions with severe disease in the left pelvis. (From Dun E, Kho K, Morozov V, Kearney S, Zurawin J, Nezhat C. Endometriosis in adolescents. *JSLS.* 2015;19(2):e2015.00019.)

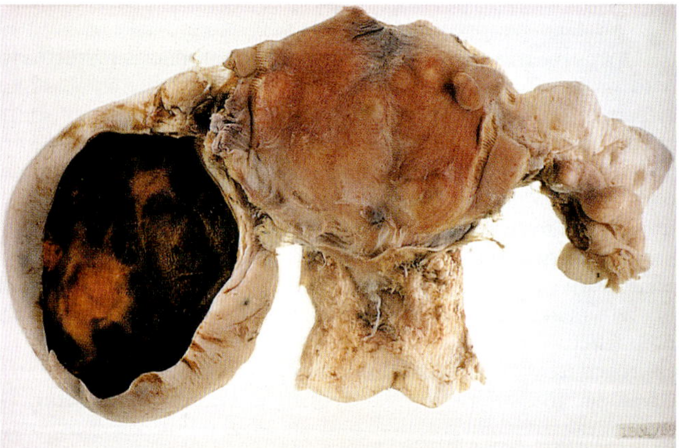

**Fig. 18.63** "Chocolate cyst" of the ovary. The endometrioma is large, but it has not yet completely replaced the ovary. (From Robboy SJ. Endometriosis. In: Robboy SJ, Anderson MC, Russell P, eds. *Pathology of the Female Reproductive Tract.* Edinburgh: Churchill Livingstone; 2002.)

that become cystic are termed *endometriomas.* Rarely, large chocolate cysts of the ovary may reach 15 to 20 cm (Fig. 18.63). Larger cysts are often bilateral. The surface of an ovary with endometriosis is often irregular, puckered, and scarred. Depending on their size, endometriomas replace a portion of the normal ovarian tissue.

Although most women with endometriomas are asymptomatic, the most common symptoms associated with ovarian endometriosis are pelvic pain, dyspareunia, and infertility. Approximately 10% of the operations for endometriosis are for acute symptoms, usually related to a ruptured ovarian endometrioma that was previously asymptomatic. Smaller cysts generally have thin walls, and perforation occurs commonly secondary to cyclic hemorrhage into the cystic cavity.

On pelvic examination the ovaries are often tender and immobile, secondary to associated inflammation and adhesions. Most commonly the ovaries are densely adherent to surrounding structures, including the peritoneum of the pelvic sidewall, the oviduct, the broad ligament, and sometimes the small or large bowel. Endometrial glands, endometrial stroma, and large phagocytic cells containing hemosiderin may be identified histologically (see Fig. 19.11). Pressure atrophy may lead to the loss of architecture of the endometrial glands. The ultrasound characteristics include a thick-walled cyst with a relatively homogeneous echo pattern that is somewhat echolucent. This appearance confers a greater than 95% positive predictive value in some studies.

The choice between medical and operative management depends on several factors, including the patient's age, future reproductive plans, and severity of symptoms. Medical therapy is rarely successful in treating ovarian endometriosis if the disease has produced ovarian enlargement. Often surgical therapy is complicated by formation of *de novo* and recurrent adhesions.

On pathologic examination, it is important to distinguish endometriosis from benign endometrial tumors, which are usually adenofibromas. The latter tumor is a true neoplasm, and there is a malignant counterpart.

## Fibroma

Fibromas are the most common benign, solid neoplasms of the ovary. Their malignant potential is low, less than 1%. These tumors make up approximately 5% of benign ovarian neoplasms and approximately 20% of all solid tumors of the ovary.

Fibromas vary in size from small nodules to huge pelvic tumors weighing 50 pounds. One of the predominant characteristics of fibromas is that they are extremely slow-growing tumors. The average diameter of a fibroma is approximately 6 cm; however, some tumors have reached 30 cm in diameter. In most series, less than 5% of fibromas are greater than 20 cm in diameter. The diameter of a fibroma is important clinically because the incidence of associated ascites is directly proportional to the size of the tumor. Many ovarian fibromas are misdiagnosed and are believed to be leiomyomas before operation. Ninety percent of fibromas are unilateral; however, multiple fibromas are found in the same ovary in 10% to 15% of cases. The average age of a woman with an ovarian fibroma is 48, and thus this tumor, which arises from the undifferentiated fibrous stroma of the ovary, often presents in postmenopausal women. Bilateral ovarian fibromas are commonly found in women with the rare genetic transmitted basal cell nevus syndrome.

The pelvic symptoms that develop with growth of fibromas include pressure and abdominal enlargement, which may be secondary to both the size of the tumor and ascites. Smaller tumors are asymptomatic because they do not elaborate hormones, and thus there is no change in the pattern of menstrual flow. Fibromas may be pedunculated and therefore easily palpable during one examination yet difficult to palpate during a subsequent pelvic examination. Sometimes on pelvic examination the fibromas appear to be softer than a solid ovarian tumor because of the edema or occasional cystic degeneration.

Meigs syndrome is the association of an ovarian fibroma, ascites, and hydrothorax. Both the ascites and the hydrothorax resolve after removal of the ovarian tumor. The ascites is caused by transudation of fluid from the ovarian fibroma; the incidence of ascites is directly related to the size of the fibroma. Fifty percent of patients have ascites if the tumor is greater than 6 cm; however, true Meigs syndrome is rare, occurring in less than 2% of ovarian fibromas. The hydrothorax develops secondary to a flow of ascitic fluid into the pleural space via the lymphatics of the diaphragm. Statistically the right pleural space is involved in 75% of reported cases, the left in 10%, and both sides in 15%. The clinical features of Meigs syndrome are not unique to fibromas, and a similar clinical picture is found with many other ovarian tumors.

Grossly, fibromas are heavy, solid, well encapsulated, and grayish white. The cut surface usually demonstrates a homogeneous

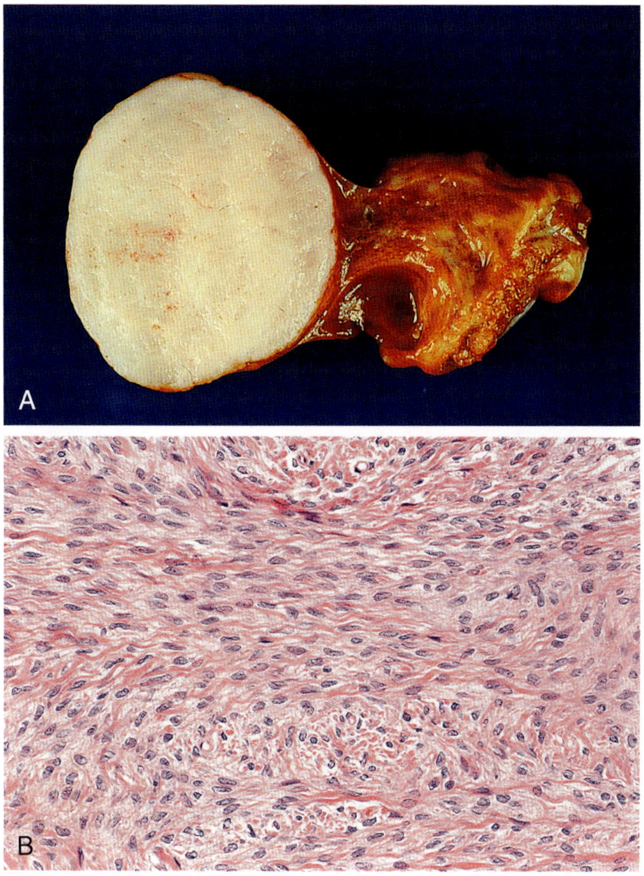


**Fig. 18.64 A,** Fibroma of the ovary with a well-circumscribed light tan mass. **B,** Histologic view of fibroma of the ovary demonstrating bland fibrous differentiation. (From Voet RL. *Color Atlas of Obstetric and Gynecologic Pathology.* St. Louis: Mosby-Wolfe; 1997.)

white or yellowish white solid tissue with a trabeculated or whorled appearance similar to that of myomas. The majority of fibromas are grossly edematous (Fig. 18.64). Less than 10% of fibromas have calcifications or small areas of hyaline or cystic degeneration. Histologically, fibromas are composed of connective tissue, stromal cells, and varying amounts of collagen interposed between the cells. The connective tissue cells are spindle-shaped, mature fibroblasts arranged in an imperfect pattern. A few smooth muscle fibers may be occasionally identified. It is sometimes difficult to distinguish fibromas from nonneoplastic thecomas. Histologically the pathologist must differentiate fibromas from stromal hyperplasia and fibrosarcomas and also look for epithelial elements of an associated Brenner tumor.

The management of fibromas is straightforward because any woman with a solid ovarian neoplasm should have an exploratory operation soon after the tumor is discovered. Simple excision of the tumor is all that is necessary. After excision of the tumor, there is resolution of all symptoms, including ascites. Because these tumors are commonly discovered in postmenopausal women, often a bilateral salpingo-oophorectomy and total abdominal hysterectomy are performed. Conversely, it is important to note that most women who preoperatively have the combination of a solid ovarian tumor and ascites are found to have ovarian carcinoma.

## Transitional Cell Tumors: Brenner Tumors

Brenner tumors are rare, small, smooth, solid, fibroepithelial ovarian tumors that are generally asymptomatic and usually occur in women ages 40 to 60 years. The semantic classification of neoplasms changes, and the current preferred term for benign Brenner tumor is *transitional cell tumor.* The benign, proliferative (low malignant potential), and malignant forms together constitute approximately 2% of ovarian tumors. Approximately 30% of transitional cell tumors are discovered as small, solid tumors in association with a concurrent serous cystic neoplasia, such as serous or mucinous cystadenomas of the ipsilateral ovary. Some are microscopic, with the entire tumor contained in a single low-powered microscopic field, and others may reach a diameter of 20 cm; the majority are less than 5 cm in diameter. The tumor is unilateral 85% to 95% of the time.

The Brenner tumor was first described in 1898. In 1932, Robert Meyer postulated that it was a distinct, independent neoplasm from granulosa cell tumors. Since that time there has been a controversy in the gynecologic pathology literature regarding the histogenesis of the neoplasm. Presently, most authorities accept the theory that most of these tumors result from metaplasia of coelomic epithelium into uroepithelium. Detailed three-dimensional histologic studies have demonstrated a downward growth in a cordlike fashion of epithelium from the surface of the ovary to deeper areas in the ovarian cortex. Others have postulated that sometimes the solid nests of epithelial cells of the tumor originate from the rete ovarii or Walthard rests. Electron microscopy confirmed the histologic and ultrastructural similarity between the epithelium in Brenner tumors and transitional epithelium. These authors argue that because of the histogenesis from coelomic inclusion cysts and also the mixture of müllerian-type epithelium in 30% of Brenner tumors, it might be appropriate to classify Brenner tumors in the epithelial group of ovarian neoplasms.

Approximately 90% of these small neoplasms are discovered incidentally during a gynecologic operation, although large tumors may produce unilateral pelvic discomfort. Postmenopausal bleeding is sometimes associated with Brenner tumors because endometrial hyperplasia is a coexisting abnormality in 10% to 16% of cases. It is postulated that luteinization of the stroma produces estrogen with resulting hyperplasia that leads to classic findings of ovarian Brenner tumors on CT or MRI. The extensive fibrous content of these tumors results in lower signal intensity in T2-weighted images. During CT scanning, Brenner tumors characteristically demonstrate a finding of extensive amorphous calcification within the solid components of the ovarian mass.

Grossly, Brenner tumors are smooth, firm, gray-white, solid tumors that grossly resemble fibromas, and similar to fibromas, transitional cell tumors are slow growing. On sectioning, the tumor usually appears gray; however, occasionally there is a yellowish tinge with small cystic spaces (Fig. 18.65). Approximately 1% to 2%

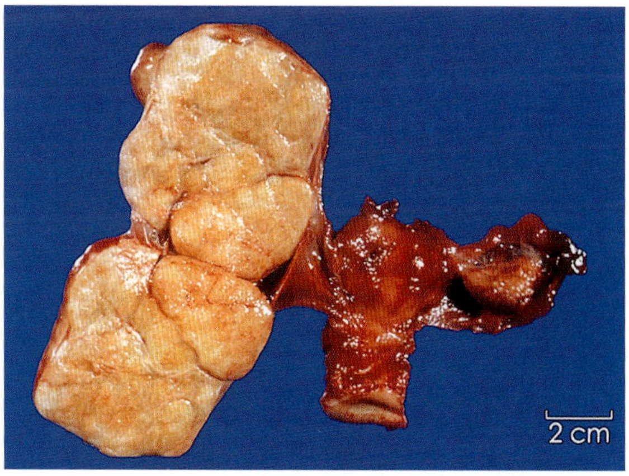


**Fig. 18.65** Brenner tumor. (From Clement PB, Young RH: *Atlas of Gynecologic Surgical Pathology.* Philadelphia: WB Saunders; 2000.)

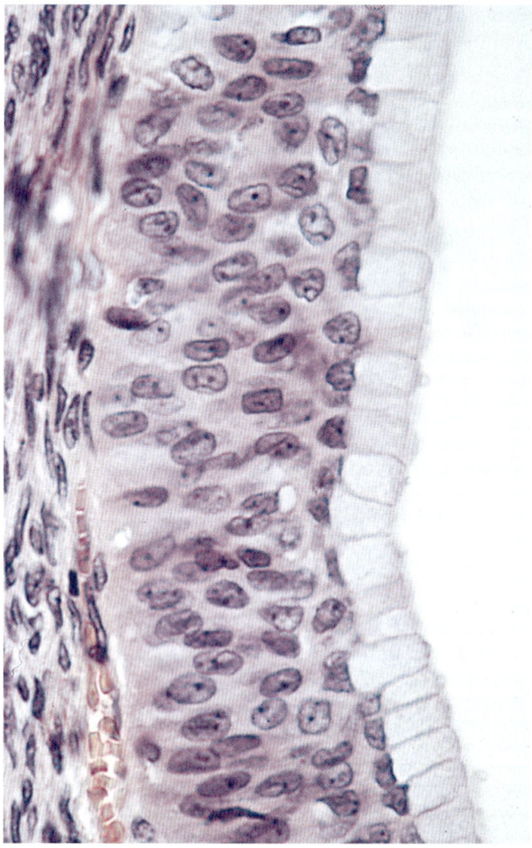

**Fig. 18.66** Benign Brenner tumor. A cyst in the Brenner tumor is lined by an inner layer of endocervical-type mucinous cells and an outer layer of stratified transitional cells, a few of which have grooved nuclei. (From Clement PB, Young RH. *Atlas of Gynecologic Surgical Pathology.* Philadelphia: WB Saunders, 2000.)

of these tumors undergo malignant change (see Chapter 33). Histologically, Brenner tumors have two principal components: solid masses or nests of epithelial cells and a surrounding fibrous stroma. The epithelial cells are uniform and do not appear anaplastic (Fig. 18.66). The histologic characteristics and ultrastructure of the epithelial cells of a Brenner tumor are similar to transitional epithelium of the urinary bladder. The pale epithelial cells have a coffee bean–appearing nucleus, which is also described as a longitudinal groove in the cell's nucleus.

Electron microscopy has demonstrated that the longitudinal groove during routine microscopy is produced by prominent indentation of the nuclear membrane. An additional ovarian neoplasm, such as a serous or mucinous cystadenoma or teratoma, is often found in association with Brenner tumors.

Management of Brenner tumors is operative, with simple excision being the procedure of choice. However, as with ovarian fibromas, the patient's age is often the principal factor in deciding the extent of the operation.

## Adenofibroma and Cystadenofibroma

Adenofibromas and cystadenofibromas are closely related. Both these benign firm tumors consist of fibrous and epithelial components. The epithelial element is most commonly serous but histologically may be mucinous and endometrioid or clear cell. They differ from benign epithelial cystadenomas in that there is a preponderance of connective tissue. Most pathologists emphasize that at least 25% of the tumor consists of fibrous connective tissue. Obviously, cystadenofibromas have microscopic or occasional macroscopic areas that are cystic. The varying degree of fibrous stroma and epithelial elements produces a spectrum of tumors, which have resulted in a confusing nomenclature with terms such as *papillomas*, *fibropapillomas*, and *fibroadenomas*.

Adenofibromas are usually small fibrous tumors that arise from the surface of the ovary. They are bilateral in 20% to 25% of women, usually occur in postmenopausal women, and are 1 to 15 cm in diameter. Grossly they are gray or white tumors, and it is difficult to distinguish them from fibromas. Papillary adenofibromas, which project from the surface of the ovary, at first glance may appear to be external excrescences of a malignant tumor. Histologically, small precursors of adenofibromas are identified in many normal ovaries. Under the microscope, true cystic gland spaces lined by cuboidal epithelium are characteristic. However, differing from serous cystadenomas, the fibrous connective tissue surrounding the cystic spaces is abundant and is the predominant tissue of the tumor.

Smaller tumors are asymptomatic and are only discovered incidentally during abdominal or pelvic operations. Large tumors may cause pressure symptoms or, rarely, undergo adnexal torsion. A small series of the MRI features of these tumors has been reported. Similar to Brenner tumors, the fibrous component produces a very low signal intensity on T2-weighted images. This interest in imaging results from an attempt to distinguish, before operation, whether a predominantly solid ovarian mass is benign or malignant. Because adenofibromas are usually discovered in postmenopausal women, the treatment of choice is bilateral salpingo-oophorectomy and total abdominal hysterectomy. Because these tumors are benign and because malignant transformation is rare, simple excision of the tumor and inspection of the contralateral ovary are appropriate in younger women.

## Torsion

Torsion of the ovary or both the oviduct and the ovary (adnexal torsion) is uncommon but an important cause of acute lower abdominal and pelvic pain. Torsion may cause up to 3% of all acute abdomens presenting to emergency departments. Torsion of the ovary may occur separately from torsion of the fallopian tube, but most commonly the two adnexal structures are affected together.

Adnexal torsion occurs most commonly during the reproductive years, with the average patient being in her mid-20s. However, adnexal torsion is also a complication of benign ovarian tumors in the postmenopausal woman. Pregnancy appears to predispose women to adnexal torsion. Approximately one in five women are pregnant when the condition is diagnosed. Most susceptible are ovaries that are enlarged secondary to ovulation induction during early pregnancy. The most common cause of adnexal torsion is ovarian enlargement by an 8- to 12-cm benign mass of the ovary, although smaller ovaries may also undergo torsion. Ovarian tumors are discovered in 50% to 60% of women with adnexal torsion. Torsion of a normal ovary or adnexum is also possible and occurs more commonly in children. Dermoids are the most commonly reported tumors in women with adnexal torsion. However, the relative risk of adnexal torsion is higher with parovarian cysts, solid benign tumors, and serous cysts of the ovary. The right ovary has a greater tendency to twist than does the left ovary. Torsion of a malignant ovarian tumor is comparatively rare.

Patients with adnexal torsion present with acute, severe, unilateral, lower abdominal and pelvic pain. Often the patient relates the onset of the severe pain to an abrupt change of position. A unilateral, extremely tender adnexal mass is found in more than 90% of patients. Approximately two-thirds of patients have associated nausea and vomiting. These associated gastrointestinal symptoms sometimes lead to a preoperative diagnosis of acute appendicitis or small intestinal obstruction. Many patients have

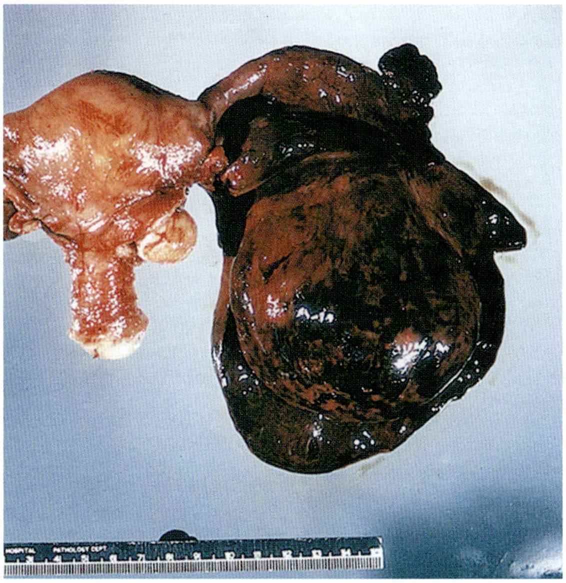

**Fig. 18.67** Adnexal torsion with hemorrhagic infarction. A benign cyst was found in the ovary. (From Clement PB, Young RH: *Atlas of Gynecologic Surgical Pathology.* Philadelphia: WB Saunders; 2000.)

noted intermittent previous episodes of similar pain for several days to several weeks. The hypothesis is that previous episodes of pain were secondary to partial torsion, with spontaneous reversal without significant vascular compromise. With progressive torsion, initially venous and lymphatic obstruction occurs. This produces a cyanotic, edematous ovary that on pelvic examination presents as a unilateral, extremely tender adnexal mass. Further progression of the torsion interrupts the major arterial supply to the ovary, resulting in hypoxia, adnexal necrosis, and a concomitant low-grade fever and leukocytosis. Fever is more common in women who have developed necrosis of the adnexa. Approximately 10% of women with adnexal torsion have a repetitive episode affecting the contralateral adnexa.

Most patients with adnexal torsion present with symptoms and signs severe enough to demand operative intervention (Fig. 18.67). Some authors have reported the successful use of Doppler ultrasound to evaluate ovarian arterial blood flow to help diagnose torsion. Abnormal color Doppler flow is highly predictive of torsion of the ovary. However, approximately 60% of women with surgically confirmed adnexal torsion will have a normal Doppler flow study (Sasaki, 2014). The false-negative rate is high enough that normal Doppler studies should never trump clinical suspicion. Women with ovarian torsion may be treated via laparoscopic surgery. The most common gynecologic conditions that may be confused with adnexal torsion are a ruptured corpus luteum or an adnexal abscess. In series emphasizing the early diagnosis of adnexal torsion, conservative operative management has been possible in 75% of cases.

Because the majority of cases of adnexal torsion occur in young women, a conservative operation is ideal. The clinician should maintain a high index of suspicion for adnexal torsion so that early and conservative surgery is possible. Even with severe vascular compromise, the appropriate operation in young women is to untwist the pedicle and preserve ovarian function. If unilateral salpingo-oophorectomy is to be performed, the vascular pedicle should be clamped with care so as not to injure the ureter, which may be tented up by the torsion.

Although salpingo-oophorectomy has been the routine treatment for ovarian torsion, large series of conservative management have been reported. Conservative surgery either through the laparoscope or via laparotomy entails gentle untwisting of the pedicle, possibly cystectomy, and stabilization of the ovary with sutures. The increasing use of detorsion may result in retorsion. A review noted that the risk of retorsion in pregnancy was as high as 19.5% to 37.5%; among fertile women it was 28.6%. Based on observational studies, detorsion and fixation of the ovary is a safe procedure that reduces the risk of recurrence (Hyttel, 2015).

The risk of pulmonary embolus (PE) with adnexal torsion is small, approximately 0.2%. One series noted the risk of PE to be similar when torsion was managed by conservative surgery with untwisting or adnexal removal without untwisting (McGovern, 1999).

## Ovarian Remnant Syndrome

Chronic pelvic pain secondary to a small area of functioning ovarian tissue after intended total removal of both ovaries is termed *ovarian remnant syndrome.* Most of the women who develop this condition had endometriosis or chronic pelvic inflammatory disease and extensive pelvic adhesions discovered during previous surgical procedures. A more recently described risk factor is laparoscopic oophorectomy.

The chronic pelvic pain is usually cyclic and exacerbated after coitus. Approximately half of women present with pain, and half with a pelvic mass. Usually the masses are small, approximately 3 cm in diameter, and most commonly located in the retroperitoneal space immediately adjacent to either ureter. Histologically the mass contains both ovarian follicles and stroma (Fig. 18.68). If the mass cannot be palpated during pelvic examination, imaging studies such as vaginal ultrasound or MRI are often helpful. Premenopausal levels of follicle-stimulating hormone or estradiol help establish the diagnosis in a woman who has a history of a bilateral salpingo-oophorectomy. However, sometimes a small area of ovarian tissue does not produce enough circulating estrogen to suppress gonadotropins. Difficult cases have been diagnosed by challenging and stimulating the suspected ovarian remnant with either clomiphene citrate or a GnRH agonist.

Once the diagnosis is suspected, the most effective treatment is surgical removal of the ovarian remnant. The tissue should be removed by laparoscopy or laparotomy with wide excision of the mass using meticulous techniques so as to protect the integrity of the ureter. Removal of an ovarian remnant is associated with a high complication rate. However, a retrospective review reported that laparoscopic and robotic surgery for the treatment of ovarian remnant syndrome had less blood loss, lower postoperative complications, and a shorter length of stay than laparotomy (Zapardiel, 2012).

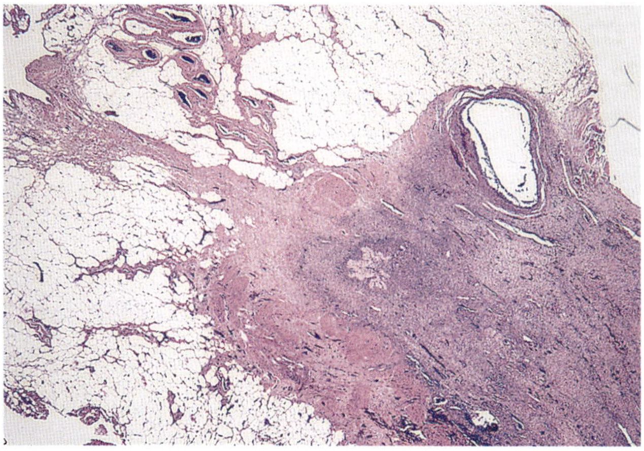

**Fig. 18.68** Ovarian remnant syndrome. Ovarian tissue that was left behind at the time of oophorectomy has regrown and is functional. (From Robboy SJ, Bentley RC, Russell P, et al. The peritoneum. In: Robboy SJ, Anderson MC, Russell P, eds. *Pathology of the Female Reproductive Tract.* Edinburgh: Churchill Livingstone; 2002.)

## KEY REFERENCES


American College of Obstetricians and Gynecologists (ACOG). Opportunistic salpingectomy as a strategy for epithelial ovarian cancer prevention. ACOG Committee Opinion No. 774. *Obstet Gynecol.* 2019a;133:e279-e284.

American College of Obstetricians and Gynecologists (ACOG). Uterine morcellation for presumed leiomyomas. ACOG Committee Opinion No. 770. *Obstet Gynecol.* 2019b;133:e238-e248.

Baird DD, Dunson DB, Hill MC, et al. High cumulative incidence of uterine leiomyoma in black and white women: ultrasound evidence. *Am J Obstet Gynecol.* 2003;188(1):100-107.

Baird DD, Hill MC, Schectman JM, et al. Vitamin D and the risk of uterine fibroids. *Epidemiology.* 2013;24(3):447-453.

Donnez J, Vazquez F, Tomaszewski J, et al. Long-term treatment of uterine fibroids with ulipristal acetate. *Fertil Steril.* 2014;101(6):1565-1573.

Edwards L, Lynch P. Skin-colored lesions. In: Edwards L, Lynch PJ, eds. *Genital Dermatology Atlas.* 2nd ed. Philadelphia: Lippincott Williams and Wilkins; 2011:197-227.

Eisinger SH, Bonfiglio T, Fiscella K, et al. Twelve-month safety and efficacy of low-dose mifepristone for uterine myomas. *J Minim Invasive Gynecol.* 2005;12(3):227-233.

Erickson BK, Conner MG, Landen Jr CN. The role of the fallopian tube in the origin of ovarian cancer. *Am J Obstet Gynecol.* 2013;209(5):409-414.

Foley CL, Greenwell TJ, Gardiner RA. Urethral diverticula in females. *BJU Int.* 2011;108(Suppl 2):20-23.Greenlee RT, Kessel B, Williams CR, et al. Prevalence, incidence, and natural history of simple ovarian cysts among women >55 years old in a large cancer screening trial. *Am J Obstet Gynecol.* 2010;202(4):373.e1-373.e9.

Hallatt JG, Steele CH, Snyder M. Ruptured corpus luteum with hemoperitoneum: a study of 173 surgical cases. *Am J Obstet Gynecol.* 1984; 149(1):5-9.

Heller DS. Benign papular lesions of the vulva. *J Low Genit Tract Dis.* 2012;16(3):296-305.

Hyttel TE, Bak GS, Larsen SB, et al. Re-torsion of the ovaries. *Acta Obstet Gynecol Scand.* 2015;94(3):236-244.

Ishikawa H, Reierstad S, Demura M, et al. High aromatase expression in uterine leiomyoma tissues of African-American women. *J Clin Endocrinol Metab.* 2009;94(5):1752-1756.

Jayi S, Laadioui M, El Fatemi H, et al. Vulvar lipoma: a case report. *J Med Case Rep.* 2014;8:203.

Kumar S, Sharma JB, Verma D, et al. Disseminated peritoneal leiomyomatosis: an unusual complication of laparoscopic myomectomy. *Arch Gynecol Obstet.* 2008;278(1):93-95.

Lee JW, Fynes MM. Female urethral diverticula. *Best Pract Res Clin Obstet Gynaecol.* 2005;19(6):875-893.

Lee SC, Kaunitz AM, Sanchez-Ramos L, et al. The oncogenic potential of endometrial polyps: a systematic review and meta-analysis. *Obstet Gynecol.* 2010;116(5):1197-1205.

Lethaby A, Shepperd S, Cooke I, et al. Endometrial resection and ablation versus hysterectomy for heavy menstrual bleeding. *Cochrane Database Syst Rev.* 2000;(2):CD000329.

Lum DA, Sokol ER, Berek JS, et al. Impact of the 2014 FDA warnings against power morcellation. *J Minim Invasive Gynecol.* 2016; 23(4):548-556.

Marret H, Fritel X, Ouldamer L, et al. Therapeutic management of uterine fibroid tumors: updated French guidelines. *Eur J Obstet Gynecol Reprod Biol.* 2012;165(2):156-164.

McKeage K, Croxtall JD. Ulipristal acetate: a review of its use in emergency contraception. *Drugs.* 2011;71(7):935-945.

Metwally M, Cheong YC, Horne AW. Surgical treatment of fibroids for subfertility. *Cochrane Database Syst Rev.* 2012;11:CD003857.

Raziel A, Ron-El R, Pansky M, et al. Current management of ruptured corpus luteum. *Eur J Obstet Gynecol Reprod Biol.* 1993;50(1):77-81.

Sasaki KF, Miller CE. Adnexal torsion: review of the literature. *J Minim Invasive Gynecol.* 2014;21(2):196-202.

Scurry J, Van der Putte SC, Pyman J, et al. Mammary-like gland adenoma of the vulva: review of 46 cases. *Pathology.* 2009;41(4):372-378.

Shozu M, Murakami K, Segawa T, et al. Successful treatment of a symptomatic uterine leiomyoma in a perimenopausal woman with a nonsteroidal aromatase inhibitor. *Fertil Steril.* 2003;79(3):628-631.

Stewart EA. Uterine fibroids. *N Engl J Med.* 2015;372(17):1646-1655.

Stockdale CK, Lawson HW. 2013 vulvodynia guideline update. *J Low Genit Tract Dis.* 2014;18(2):93-100.

Struble J, Reid S, Bedaiwy MA. Adenomyosis: a clinical review of a challenging gynecologic condition. *J Minim Invasive Gynecol.* 2016; 23(2):164-185.

Sugiyama VE, Chan JK, Shin JY, et al. Vulvar melanoma. A multivariable analysis of 644 patients. *Obstet Gynecol.* 2007;110(2 Pt 1):296-301.


**Full references and Suggested readings for this chapter can be found on ExpertConsult.com.**

# 19 Endometriosis

## Etiology, Pathology, Diagnosis, Management

*Arnold P. Advincula, Mireille Truong, Roger A. Lobo*

### KEY POINTS

- Endometriosis is a benign, usually progressive, and sometimes recurrent disease that invades locally and disseminates widely. Causes include retrograde menstruation, coelomic metaplasia, vascular metastasis, immunologic changes, iatrogenic dissemination, and a genetic predisposition.
- Endometriosis lesions produce estrogen locally and have increased secretion of prostaglandins and inflammatory cytokines, which can cause pain and contribute to infertility. There is also a relative resistance to progesterone in endometriosis lesions.
- There are several established treatments for endometriosis (such as oral contraceptives, gonadotropin-releasing hormone [GnRH] agonists, and danazol) and some novel therapies undergoing trials such as the use of oral antagonists, aromatase inhibitors, progesterone receptor modulators, and cytokine inhibitors. The recurrence rate after medical therapy is 5% to 15% in the first year and increases to 40% to 50% in 5 years.
- The recurrence rate after medical therapy is 5% to 15% in the first year and increases to 40% to 50% in 5 years.
- The incidence of endometriosis is 30% to 45% in women with infertility. There is probably some benefit to ablating endometriosis lesions when seen at laparoscopy. In patients with endometriosis, the success of in vitro fertilization–embryo transfer (IVF-ET) decreases only in women with severe disease.

- Endometriosis is a benign, usually progressive, and sometimes recurrent disease that invades locally and disseminates widely. Causes include retrograde menstruation, coelomic metaplasia, vascular metastasis, immunologic changes, iatrogenic dissemination, and genetic predisposition.
- Endometriosis lesions produce estrogen locally and have increased secretion of prostaglandins and inflammatory cytokines, which can cause pain and contribute to infertility. Endometriosis lesions also have a relative resistance to progesterone.
- There are several established treatments for endometriosis (such as oral contraceptives and gonadotropin-releasing hormone agonists and danazol) and some novel therapies undergoing trials, such as the use of oral antagonists, aromatase inhibitors, progesterone receptor modulators, and cytokine inhibitors. The recurrence rate after medical therapy is 5% to 15% in the first year, increasing to 40% to 50% in 5 years.
- The recurrence rate after medical therapy is 5% to 15% in the first year, increasing to 40% to 50% in 5 years.
- The incidence of endometriosis is 30% to 45% in women with infertility. There is probably some benefit to ablating endometriosis lesions when seen at laparoscopy. In patients with endometriosis, the success of IVF-ET decreases only in women with severe disease.

## ENDOMETRIOSIS: OVERVIEW

Endometriosis is a benign but, in many women, progressive and aggressive disease, with a major impact on the quality of women's lives and creating a significant economic burden of billions of dollars. The wide spectrum of clinical problems that occur with endometriosis has frustrated gynecologists, fascinated pathologists, and burdened patients for years. Although endometriosis was first described in 1860, the **classic studies by Sampson** in the 1920s were the first to emphasize the clinical and pathologic correlations of endometriosis (Sampson, 1927). Even today, many aspects of the disease remain enigmatic.

By definition, endometriosis is the presence and growth of the glands and stroma of the lining of the uterus in an aberrant or heterotopic location. **Adenomyosis** is the growth of endometrial glands and stroma into the uterine myometrium to a depth of at least 2.5 mm from the basalis layer of the endometrium. Adenomyosis is sometimes termed *internal endometriosis;* however, this is a semantic misnomer because most likely they are separate diseases.

It is often stated that the incidence of endometriosis has been increasing, but this is likely secondary to an enlightened awareness of mild endometriosis as diagnosed by the increasing use of laparoscopy. Delay in making the diagnosis is common; it has been estimated to take an average time of 11.7 years in the United States and 8 years in the United Kingdom to make the diagnosis. Evers has advanced a provocative hypothesis that endometrial implants in the peritoneal cavity are a physiologic finding secondary to retrograde menstruation, and their presence does not confirm a disease process (Evers, 1994). **The overall prevalence of endometriosis in reproductive-age women has been suggested to be as high as 11%** (Buck Louis, 2011). The age-specific incidence or prevalence of endometriosis is not known and has only been estimated. Many patients are diagnosed incidentally during surgery performed for a variety of other indications. Conservative estimates find that endometriosis is present in 5% to 15% of laparotomies performed on reproductive-age female patients. **Active endometriosis may be found in approximately three-quarters of women with chronic pelvic pain and in 30% to 45% of women with subfertility.** In subfertile women the diagnosis is not commonly made because diagnostic laparoscopy is rarely carried out. In a compilation of eight studies encompassing 162 patients with endometriosis, the natural course of endometriosis was **reported to increase or progress in 31% of cases**, to remain the same in 32%, and to regress in 38%.

The cause of endometriosis is uncertain and involves many mechanisms including retrograde menstruation, vascular dissemination, metaplasia, genetic predisposition, immunologic changes, and hormonal influences, as discussed later. In addition, there is increasing evidence that environmental factors may also play a role, including exposure to dioxin and other endocrine disruptors. Clinically it is most difficult to predict the natural course of endometriosis in any one individual.

The classic symptom of endometriosis is pelvic pain. However, in clinical practice the majority of cases are not "classic." The diagnosis and treatment of infertility associated with endometriosis is discussed in Chapter 40. Aberrant endometrial tissue grows under the cyclic influence of ovarian hormones and is particularly estrogen dependent; therefore the disease is most commonly found during the reproductive years. However, 5% of women with endometriosis are diagnosed after menopause. Postmenopausal endometriosis is usually stimulated by exogenous estrogen. Teenagers with endometriosis should be investigated for obstructive reproductive tract abnormalities that increase the amount of retrograde menstruation. Although previously thought to be rare in adolescents, endometriosis has been found in approximately half of teens with pelvic pain.

Endometriosis is a disease not only of great individual variability but also of contrasting pathophysiologic processes. **There is an inverse relationship between the extent of pelvic endometriosis and the severity of pelvic pain.** Women with extensive endometriosis may be asymptomatic, whereas other patients with minimal implants may have incapacitating chronic pelvic pain. However, as would be expected, women with deep infiltrating endometriosis (DIE), especially in retroperitoneal spaces, often experience severe episodes of pain. **Pelvic lesions of endometriosis have been found to have positive immune staining for smooth muscle and nerve cells** (Medina, 2009). The clinical variability in responses among women with endometriosis may relate to **differences in immunologic function and variations in cytokine production.**

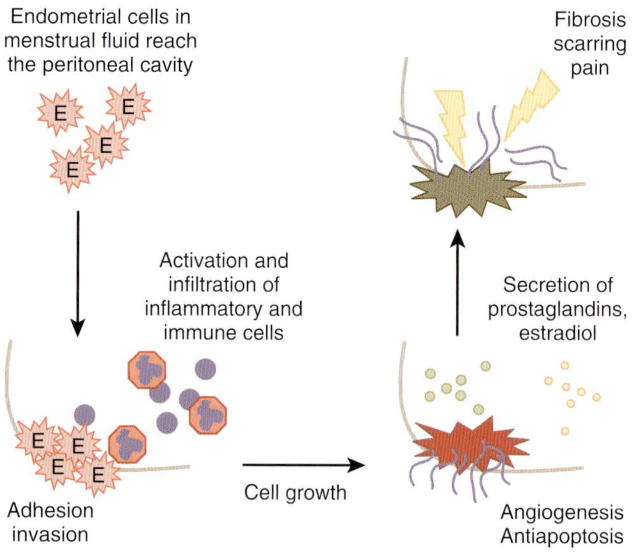


**Fig. 19.1** Proposed establishment of peritoneal endometriotic implants via retrograde menstruation, attachment, proliferation, migration, neovascularization, inflammation, and fibrosis. *E,* Endometrial cell. (From Flores I, Rivera E, Ruiz LA, et al. Molecular profiling of experimental endometriosis identified gene expression patterns in common with human disease. *Fertil Steril.* 2007;87(5):1180-1199.)

## Etiology

Several theories have been posited to explain the pathogenesis of endometriosis, but no single theory adequately explains all the manifestations of the disease. Most important, there is only speculation as to why some women develop endometriosis and others do not. One popular theory is that there is a complex interplay between a dose-response curve of the amount of retrograde menstruation and an individual woman's immunologic response (these in turn may depend on ethnic and genetic variability).

### Retrograde Menstruation

The most popular theory is that endometriosis results from retrograde menstruation. Sampson suggested that pelvic endometriosis was secondary to implantation of endometrial cells shed during menstruation (Sampson, 1927). **It has been suggested that the shedding of endometrial-based adult stem cells and mesenchymal cells may explain this phenomenon** (Gargett, 2010). These cells attach to the pelvic peritoneum and under hormonal influence grow as homologous grafts. Indeed, reflux of menstrual blood and viable endometrial cells in the pelvis of ovulating women has been documented. Endometriosis is discovered most often in areas immediately adjacent to the tubal ostia or in the dependent areas of the pelvis.

Endometriosis is commonly found in women with outflow obstruction of the genital tract. The attachment of the shed endometrial cells involves the expression of adhesion molecules and their receptors. This is thought to be an extremely rapid process as demonstrated in vitro. Figs. 19.1 and 19.2 depict the process of implants from retrograde menstruation and early invasion (Flores, 2007; Witz, 2001).

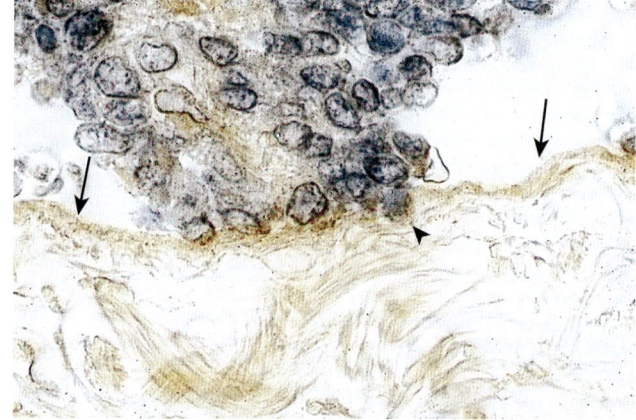

**Fig. 19.2** Early invasion of an endometrial implant through the mesothelium. The mesothelium is labeled with monoclonal antibody to cytokeratin and stained with diaminobenzidine *(arrows).* An endometrial stromal cell *(arrowhead)* passing through the mesothelium is thought to represent the initial step of invasion into the stroma of the peritoneum. Original magnification, ×31,000. Counterstained with hematoxylin. (From Witz CA, Monotoya-Rodrigueez I, Schenken RS. Whole explants of peritoneum and endometrium: a novel model of the early endometriosis lesion. *Fertil Steril.* 1999;71(1):56-60.)

### Metaplasia

In contrast to the theory of seeding from retrograde menstruation is the theory that **endometriosis arises from metaplasia of the coelomic epithelium or proliferation of embryonic rests.** The müllerian ducts and nearby mesenchymal tissue form the majority of the female reproductive tract. The müllerian duct is derived from the coelomic epithelium during fetal development. The metaplasia hypothesis postulates that the coelomic epithelium retains the ability for multipotential development. The decidual reaction of isolated areas of peritoneum during pregnancy is an example of this process. It is well known that the surface epithelium of the ovary can differentiate into several different histologic cell types. Endometriosis has been discovered in prepubertal girls, women with congenital absence of the uterus, and, rarely, in men. These examples support the coelomic metaplasia theory.

Metaplasia occurs after an "induction phenomenon" has stimulated the multipotential cell. The induction substance may be a combination of menstrual debris and the influence of estrogen and progesterone. It has been hypothesized that the histogenesis of endometriosis in peritoneal pockets of the posterior pelvis results from a congenital anomaly involving rudimentary duplication of the müllerian system (Batt, 1989). The peritoneal pockets that they describe are found in the posterior pelvis, the posterior aspects of the broad ligament, and the cul-de-sac (Fig. 19.3). Similarly, it has been postulated that metaplasia of the coelomic epithelium that invaginates into the ovarian cortex is the pathogenesis for the development of ovarian endometriosis (Nisolle, 1997).

## Lymphatic and Vascular Metastasis

The theory of endometrium being transplanted via lymphatic channels and the vascular system helps to explain rare and remote sites of endometriosis, such as the spinal column and nose. Endometriosis has been observed in the pelvic lymph nodes of approximately 30% of women with the disease. Hematogenous dissemination of endometrium is the best theory to explain endometriosis of the forearm and thigh, as well as multiple lesions in the lung.

## Iatrogenic Dissemination

Endometriosis of the anterior abdominal wall is sometimes discovered in women after a cesarean delivery. The hypothesis is that endometrial glands and stroma are implanted during the procedure. The aberrant tissue is found subcutaneously at the abdominal incision. Rarely, iatrogenic endometriosis may be discovered in an episiotomy scar.

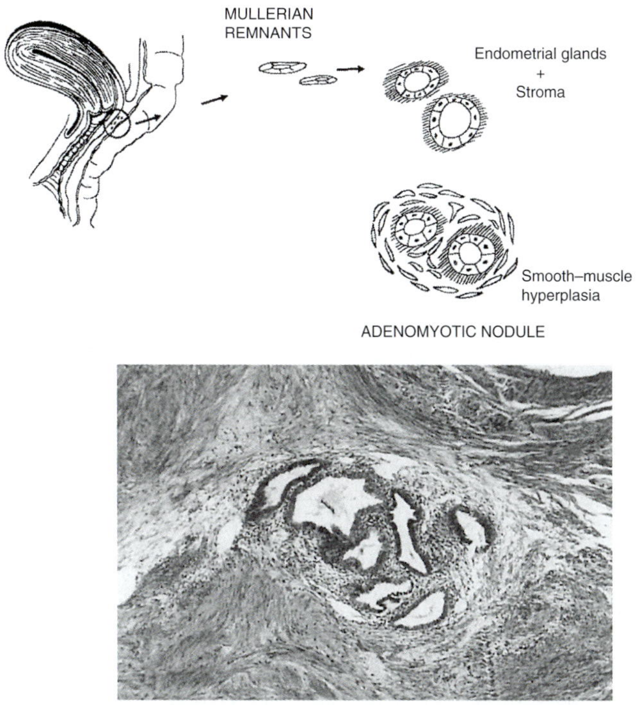


**Fig. 19.3** Proposed derivation of endometriotic lesion in the rectovaginal septum. (From Strauss JF, Barbieri R. *Yen & Jaffe's Reproductive Endocrinology.* 5th ed. Philadelphia: Saunders: 2004:692-693.)

## Immunologic Changes

One of the most perplexing, unanswered questions concerning the pathophysiology of endometriosis is that some women with retrograde menstruation develop endometriosis, but most do not. **Multiple investigations have suggested that changes in the immune system, especially altered function of immune-related cells, are directly related to the pathogenesis of endometriosis.** Whether endometriosis is an autoimmune disease has been intensely debated for many years. Studies have demonstrated abnormalities in cell-mediated and humoral components of the immune system in both peripheral blood and peritoneal fluid. Box 19.1 depicts various cytokines and growth factors that have been implicated in the pathogenesis of endometriosis (McLaren, 1997).

Most likely the primary immunologic change involves an alteration in the function of the peritoneal macrophages so prevalent in the peritoneal fluid of patients with endometriosis. It has been hypothesized that women who do not develop endometriosis have monocytic-type macrophages in their peritoneal fluid that have a short life span and limited function. Conversely, women who develop endometriosis have more peritoneal macrophages that are larger. **These hyperactive cells secrete multiple growth factors and cytokines that enhance the development of endometriosis.** The attraction of leukocytes to specific areas is controlled by chemokines, which are chemotactic cytokines. Changes in the expression of integrins also may be an important local factor. Following the theory of different macrophage populations in endometriosis is

### BOX 19.1 Cytokines and Growth Factors in Peritoneal Fluid

**CONCENTRATIONS INCREASED IN ENDOMETRIOSIS**

Complement
Eotaxin
Glycodelin
IL-1
IL-6
IL-8
MCP-1
PDGF
RANTES
Soluble ICAM-1
TGF-β
VEGF

**CONCENTRATIONS UNCHANGED IN ENDOMETRIOSIS**

EGF
Basic FGF
Interferon-γ
IL-2
IL-4
IL-12

**CONCENTRATIONS DECREASED IN ENDOMETRIOSIS**

IL-13

*EGF,* Epidermal growth factor; *FGF,* fibroblast growth factor; *ICAM,* intercellular adhesion molecule; *IL,* interleukin; *MCP,* membrane cofactor protein; *PDGF,* platelet-derived growth factor; *RANTES,* regulated on activation, normal T cell expressed and secreted; *TGF,* transforming growth factor; *VEGF,* vascular endothelial growth factor. References are from the original source.

*From McLaren J, Deatry G, Prentice A, et al. Decreased levels of the potent regulator of monocyte/macrophage activation, interleukin-13, in the peritoneal fluid of patients with endometriosis. Hum Reprod.* 1997;12(6):1307-1310.

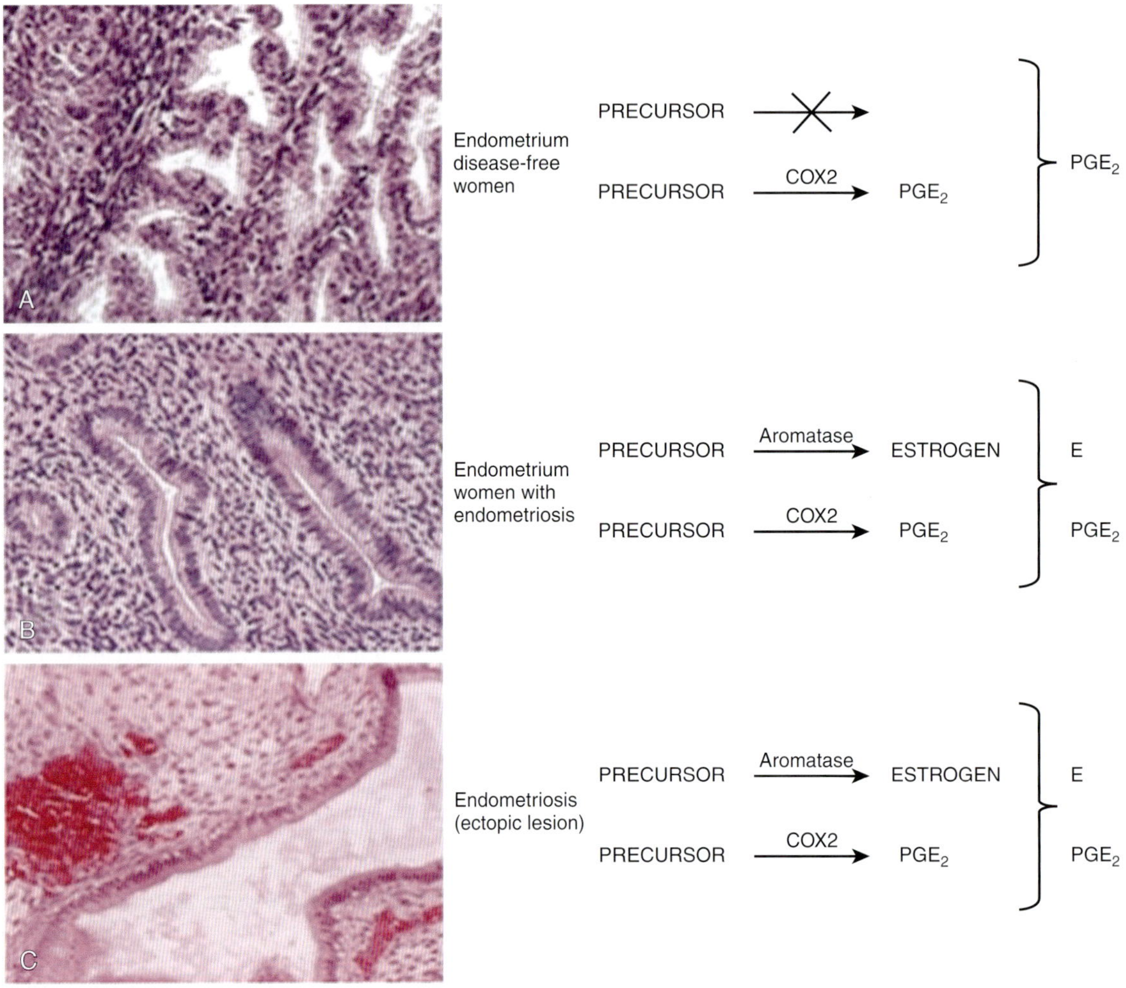


**Fig. 19.4** Molecular defects in endometrium and endometriosis. COX2, Cyclooxygenase-2; *E,* estrogen; *$PGE_2$,* prostaglandin E2; (From Strauss JF, Barbieri R. *Yen & Jaffe's Reproductive Endocrinology.* 5th ed. Philadelphia: Saunders: 2004:615.)

the finding that **the destroying of normally extruded endometrial cells in endometriosis may be deficient.** It has been shown that natural killer (NK) cells have decreased cytotoxicity against endometrial and hematopoietic cells in women with endometriosis. Also, **peritoneal fluid of women with endometriosis has less influence of NK activity than is found in fertile women without endometriosis.**

Another attractive theory is the finding of a protein similar to haptoglobin in endometriosis epithelial cells called endo-1. This chemoattractant protein–enhanced local production of interleukin-6 (IL-6) self-perpetuates lesion/cytokine interactions. Further compounding the proliferative activity of endometriosis lesions are angiogenic factors that are increased in lesions. Here the expression of basic fibroblast factor, IL-6, IL-8, platelet-derived growth factor (PDGF), and vascular endothelial growth factor (VEGF) are all increased (see Box 19.1).

Steroid interactions also enhance the progression of disease. **Estrogen production is enhanced locally, and there is evidence for upregulation of aromatase activity,** increased cyclooxygenase-2 (COX-2) expression, and dysregulation of 17β-dehydrogenase activity, where there is a deficiency in 17β-dehydrogenase II activity and possibly an enhancement of type II activity favoring local estradiol production (Bulun, 2009). Fig. 19.4 shows abnormalities of COX-2, aromatase, and 17β-hydroxysteroid dehydrogenase type 2 (HSD17B2) in disease-free women, and endometrium and ectopic

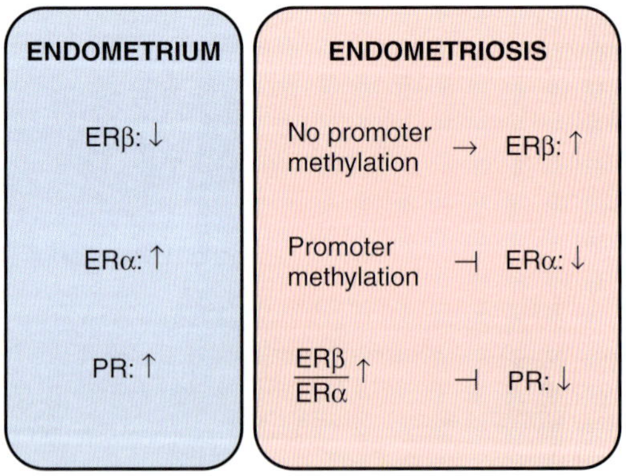


**Fig. 19.5** Steroid receptor expression in endometriosis. *ER,* Estrogen receptor; *PR,* progesterone receptor. (From Strauss JF, Barbieri R. *Yen & Jaffe's Reproductive Endocrinology.* 5th ed. Philadelphia: Saunders: 2004:622.)

lesions in women with endometriosis where high local concentrations of estrogen and prostaglandin $E_2$ predominate (Fig. 19.5). **Enhanced aromatase activity appears to be the result of overexpression of the orphan nuclear receptor steroidogenic factor-1 (SF-1) in lesions.** The local production of estrogen

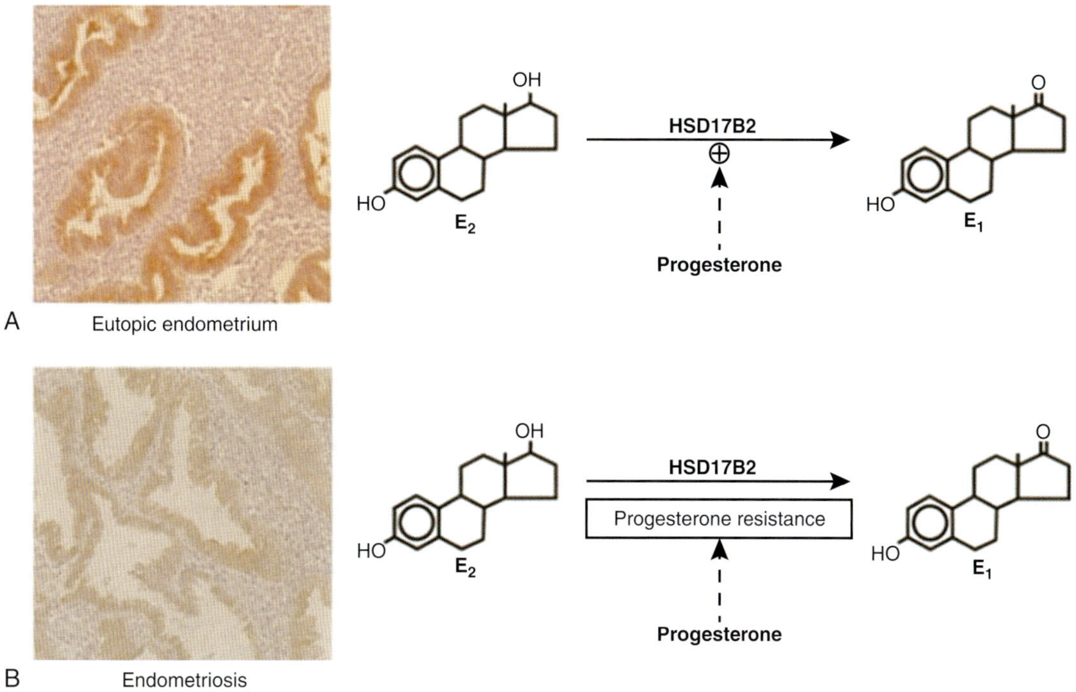


**Fig. 19.6** A 17β-hydroxysteroid dehydrogenase type 2 (HSD17B2) in endometriotic epithelium. (From Strauss JF, Barbieri R. *Yen & Jaffe's Reproductive Endocrinology*. 5th ed. Philadelphia: Saunders: 2004:626.)

through aromatase activity explains why progression of lesions may occur even with ovarian suppression. Further, there is evidence for **progesterone "resistance"** (Bulun, 2009) (Fig. 19.6). This is occasioned by a dysregulation of the isoform B of the progesterone receptor in most endometriotic lesions, where levels may be undetectable. The latter propensity may be on a genetic basis, as discussed later.

**Autoimmunity may well exist in women with endometriosis,** and although the findings of abnormalities of the histocompatibility locus antigen system have not been consistent, there are reports of increased B and T cells and serum immunoglobulin (IgG, IgA, and IgM) autoantibodies in endometriosis. **A survey from the U.S. Endometriosis Association has provided suggestive evidence of the higher prevalence of other autoimmune diseases.** The association of all these immune processes in the symptoms and signs of endometriosis is depicted in Fig. 19.7.

## Genetic Predisposition

Several studies have documented a **familial predisposition to endometriosis** with grouping of cases of endometriosis in mothers and their daughters. An investigation by Simpson and coworkers demonstrated a **sevenfold increase in the incidence of endometriosis in relatives** of women with the disease compared with controls (Simpson, 1980). One of 10 women with severe endometriosis will have a sister or mother with clinical manifestations of the disease. **The genetic heritability of endometriosis has been estimated at 52% based on twin studies** (Treloar, 1999). Women who have a family history of endometriosis are likely to develop the disease earlier in life and to have more advanced disease than women whose first-degree relatives are free of the disease.

Endometriosis is clearly not a single-gene disease but rather **polygenic, with various susceptibility factors** discovered. Studies have identified deletions of genes, most specifically increased heterogenicity of chromosome 17 and aneuploidy, in women with endometriosis compared with controls (Kosugi, 1999). Loci on 7p and 10q have also been found to increase the susceptibility for endometriosis. The expression of this genetic liability most likely depends on **an interaction with environmental and epigenetic factors**, with many factors being involved.

**Epigenetic factors** play a significant role and may be influenced by **environmental factors** (Bulun, 2009). The epigenetics involves **hypomethylation of genes** and may help explain, for example, the increased expression of SP1 leading to increased estrogen receptor (ER)β over ERα, which in turn leads to progesterone resistance in endometriosis.

**Preliminary data suggest some bilateral ovarian endometrial cysts may arise independently from different clones. Although no consistent abnormality has been found in women with endometriosis, there are several candidate genes.** Box 19.2 provides a partial list of genes and gene products aberrantly expressed in endometriosis.

**Several of these aberrantly expressed gene products, such as the matrix metalloproteinases (MMPs) and integrins, have important implications for endometrial lesion attachment and for implantation defects, which may exist in infertile women with endometriosis. Reflux of MMPs into the peritoneal cavity at menstruation may contribute to peritoneal attachment in susceptible women.**

**MicroRNAs have also been found to be involved** (particularly the 9 and 34 families) and may be implicated in the pathogenesis as well. Also, the measurement of certain microRNAs has been suggested as a test for endometriosis, although there are no data to support this.

Certain ethnic groups have an increased risk of endometriosis. This is particularly striking in **Asian women, in whom a ninefold increase** has been suggested.

## Pathology

The majority of endometrial implants are located in the **dependent portions of the female pelvis** (Fig. 19.8). The ovaries are the most common site, being involved in two of three women

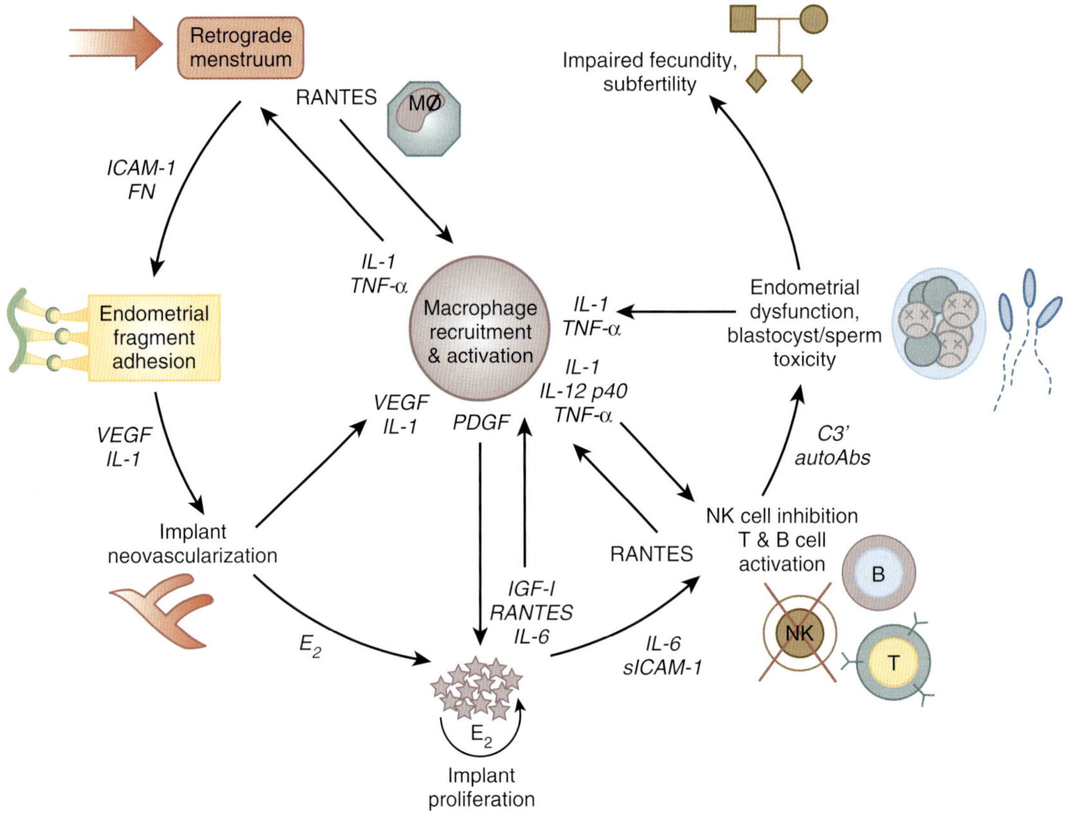


**Fig. 19.7** Schematogram depicting the network of chemokines, cytokines, and growth factors in the pathophysiology of endometriosis. *autoAbs,* Autoantibodies; *C3,* complement 3; *$E_2$,* estradiol; *FN,* fibronectin; *sICAM,* soluble intercellular adhesion molecule; *IGF-1,* insulin-like growth factor-1; *IL,* interleukin; *MØ,* macrophage; *NK cell,* natural killer cell; *PDGF,* platelet-derived growth factor; *RANTES,* regulated on activation, normal T cell expressed and secreted; *TNF,* tumor necrosis factor; *VEGF,* vascular endothelial growth factor.

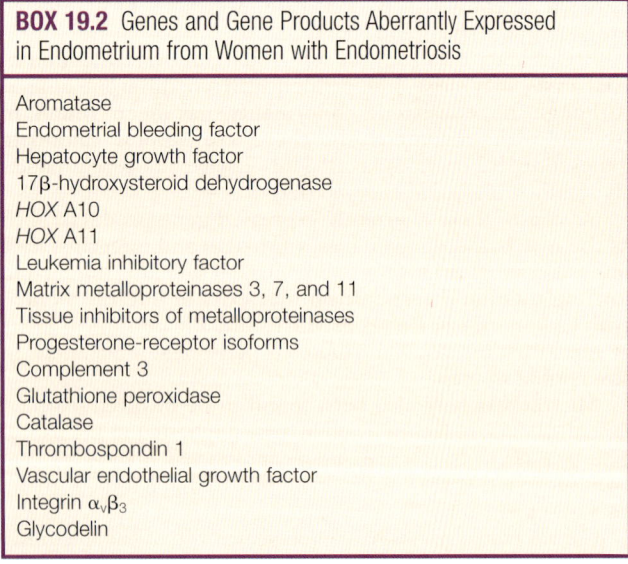

**BOX 19.2** Genes and Gene Products Aberrantly Expressed in Endometrium from Women with Endometriosis

Aromatase
Endometrial bleeding factor
Hepatocyte growth factor
17β-hydroxysteroid dehydrogenase
*HOX* A10
*HOX* A11
Leukemia inhibitory factor
Matrix metalloproteinases 3, 7, and 11
Tissue inhibitors of metalloproteinases
Progesterone-receptor isoforms
Complement 3
Glutathione peroxidase
Catalase
Thrombospondin 1
Vascular endothelial growth factor
Integrin $\alpha_v\beta_3$
Glycodelin

with endometriosis. In most of these women the involvement is bilateral. The pelvic peritoneum over the uterus; the anterior and posterior cul-de-sac; and the uterosacral, round, and broad ligaments are also common sites where endometriosis develops. Pelvic lymph nodes have been found to be involved in up to 30% of cases.

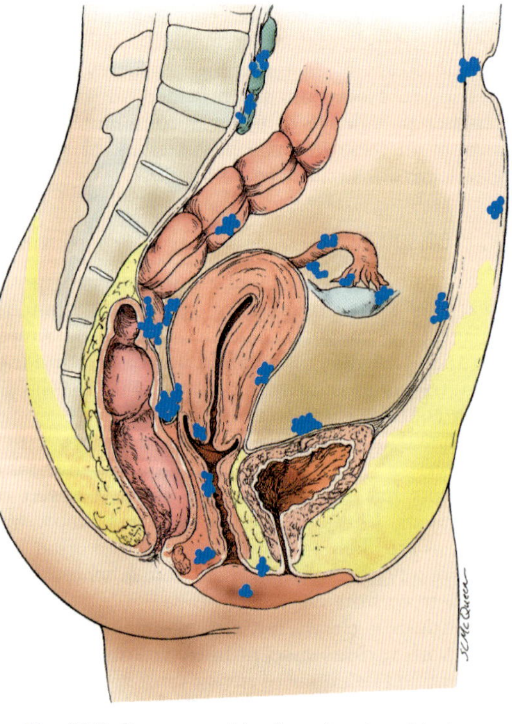

**Fig. 19.8** Common pelvic sites of endometriosis.

**TABLE 19.1** Anatomic Distribution of Endometriosis

| Common Sites | Rare Sites |
|---|---|
| Ovaries | Umbilicus |
| Pelvic peritoneum | Episiotomy scar |
| Ligaments of the uterus | Bladder |
| Sigmoid colon | Kidney |
| Appendix | Lungs |
| Pelvic lymph nodes | Arms |
| Cervix | Legs |
| Vagina | Nasal mucosa |
| Fallopian tubes | Spinal column |

**TABLE 19.2** Preoperative Symptoms in 130 Patients Undergoing Colorectal Resection for Endometriosis

| Symptom | No. of Patients | (%) |
|---|---|---|
| Pelvic pain | 111 | (85) |
| Rectal pain | 68 | (52) |
| Cyclic rectal bleeding | 24 | (18) |
| Diarrhea | 55 | (42) |
| Constipation | 53 | (41) |
| Diarrhea and constipation | 18 | (14) |
| Dyspareunia | 83 | (64) |

From Bailey HR, Ott MT, Hartendorp P. Aggressive surgical management for advanced colorectal endometriosis. *Dis Colon Rectum.* 1994; 37(8):747-753.

The cervix, vagina, and vulva are other possible pelvic locations. Brosens has emphasized the importance of distinguishing between superficial and deep lesions of endometriosis (Brosens, 2000). **Deep lesions, penetrations of greater than 5 mm, represent a more progressive form of the disease.** Distinguishing superficial implant lesions on peritoneal surfaces, including the ovary, from deep endometriotic ovarian cysts and cul-de-sac nodules is important for therapy because the latter abnormalities may suggest different causes of the disease (e.g., metaplasia), which require a surgical approach.

Approximately 10% to 15% of women with advanced disease have lesions involving the rectosigmoid. Depending on the amount of associated scarring, endometriosis of the bowel may be difficult to differentiate grossly from a primary neoplasm of the large intestine. Endometriosis may be found in a wide variety of sites, including the umbilicus, areas of previous surgical incisions of the anterior abdominal wall or perineum, the bladder, ureter, kidney, lung, arms, legs, and even the male urinary tract (Table 19.1).

Gross pathologic changes of endometriosis exhibit wide variability in color, shape, size, and associated inflammatory and fibrotic changes. The visual manifestations of endometriosis in the female pelvis are protean and have many appearances. Increased awareness and anticipation have focused on the subtle lesions of endometriosis. Clinicians closely inspect the pelvic peritoneum to identify abnormal areas and small, nonhemorrhagic lesions. More emphasis has been placed on biopsy confirmation of endometriosis because of increasing awareness of subtle lesions. The gross appearance of the implant depends on the site, activity, relationship to the day of the menstrual cycle, and chronicity of the area involved. The color of the lesion varies widely and may be red, brown, black, white, yellow, pink, clear, or a red vesicle. The predominant color depends on the blood supply and the amount of hemorrhage and fibrosis. The color also appears related to the size of the lesion, the degree of edema, and the amount of inspissated material (Table 19.2). Fig. 19.9 depicts the spectrum of lesions with black and white lesions reflecting older lesions with inflammatory and fibrotic changes. Other peritoneal lesions that grossly appear similar to endometriosis, but on histologic examination are not, include necrotic areas of an ectopic pregnancy, fibrotic reactions to suture, hemangiomas, adrenal rest, Walthard rest, breast cancer, ovarian cancer, epithelial inclusions, residual carbon from laser surgery, peritoneal inflammation, psammoma bodies, peritoneal reactions to oil-based hysterosalpingogram dye, and splenosis.

New lesions are small, bleblike implants that are less than 1 cm in diameter. Initially these areas are raised above the surrounding tissues. Red, blood-filled lesions have been shown, by histologic and biochemical studies, to be the most active phase of the disease (Fig. 19.9). With time, the areas of endometriosis become larger and assume a light or dark brown color, and they may be described

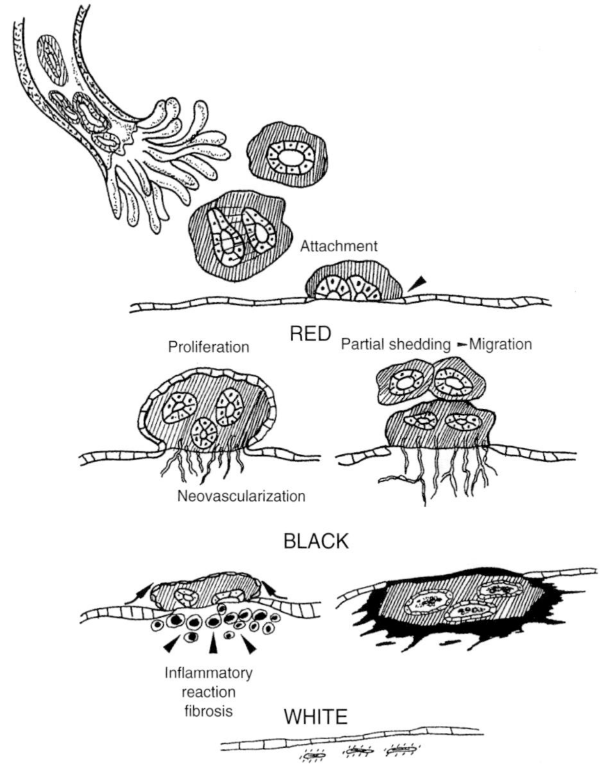


**Fig. 19.9** Proposed establishment of peritoneal endometriotic implants via retrograde menstruation and the like. (From Strauss JF, Barbieri R. *Yen & Jaffe's Reproductive Endocrinology.* 5th ed. Philadelphia: Saunders; 2004:692-693.)

as "powder burn" areas or "chocolate cysts." The older lesions are white, have more intense scarring, and are usually puckered or retracted from the surrounding tissue. White or mixed-colored lesions are more likely to provide histologic confirmation of endometriosis. Also, the progression from red to white lesions also seems to correlate with age.

The pattern of ovarian endometriosis is also variable. Individual areas range from 1 mm to large chocolate cysts greater than 8 cm in diameter (Fig. 19.10). The associated adhesions may be filmy or dense, and larger cysts are usually densely adherent to the surrounding pelvic sidewalls or broad ligament.

The three cardinal histologic features of endometriosis are ectopic endometrial glands, ectopic endometrial stroma, and hemorrhage into the adjacent tissue (Fig. 19.11). Previous hemorrhage

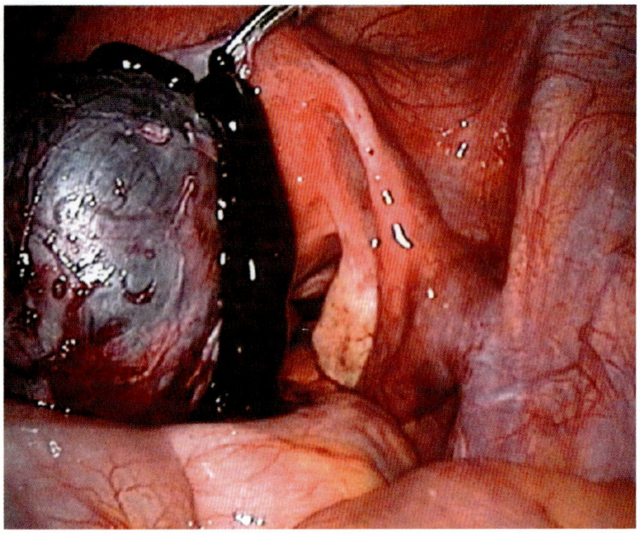

Fig. 19.10 Rupture of large endometrioma "chocolate cyst." (From Pathology Student. Available at: www.pathologystudent.com.)

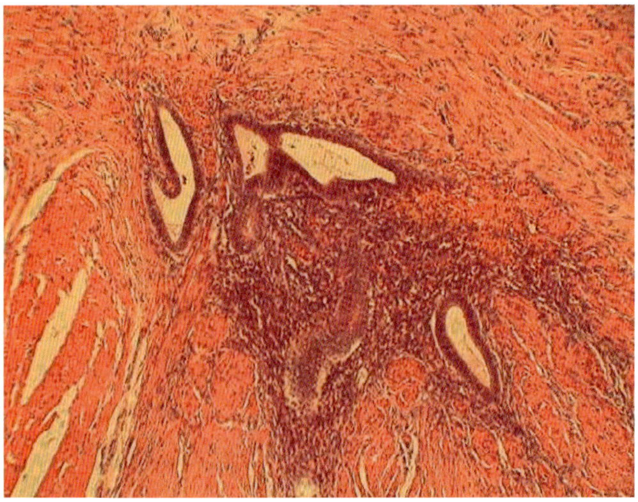

Fig. 19.11 Histologic examination of endometriosis involving the bowel. (From The Internet Journal of Pulmonary Medicine. Available at: www.ispub.com/journal.)

can be discovered by identifying large macrophages filled with hemosiderin near the periphery of the lesion. In the majority of cases, the aberrant endometrial glands and stroma respond in cyclic fashion to estrogen and progesterone. These changes may or may not be in synchrony with the endometrial lining of the uterus. The ectopic endometrial stroma will undergo classic decidual changes similar to pregnancy when exposed to high physiologic or pharmacologic levels of progesterone.

**In approximately 25% of cases of endometriosis, viable endometrial glands and stroma cannot be identified.** Repetitive episodes of hemorrhage may lead to severe inflammatory changes and result in the glands and stroma undergoing necrobiosis secondary to pressure atrophy or lack of blood supply. In these cases a presumptive diagnosis of endometriosis is made by visualizing the intense inflammatory reaction and the large macrophages filled with blood pigment.

The natural history of endometriosis has been discussed, and although clinicians usually think of endometriosis as a progressive disease, this is not always the case; it has been shown to be progressive only about one-third of the time. The pathophysiology of progression from subtle endometriosis to severe disease may be expected from the multiple mechanisms of potential disease acceleration discussed earlier, with immune function most likely involved.

## Clinical Diagnosis

### Symptoms

It is important to reemphasize that endometriosis has many clinical presentations, with **one in three women being asymptomatic**. Most important, the disease has an extremely unpredictable course. The classic symptoms of endometriosis are cyclic pelvic pain and infertility. The chronic pelvic pain usually presents as secondary dysmenorrhea or dyspareunia (or both). Secondary dysmenorrhea usually begins 36 to 48 hours before the onset of menses. However, approximately one-third of patients with endometriosis are asymptomatic, with the disease being discovered incidentally during an abdominal operation or visualized at laparoscopy for an unrelated problem. Conversely, **endometriosis is discovered in at least one of three women whose primary symptom is chronic pelvic pain**.

Clinicians have appreciated the paradox that the extent of pelvic pain is often inversely related to the amount of endometriosis in the female pelvis. Women with large, fixed adnexal masses sometimes have minor symptoms, whereas other patients with only a few small foci with deep infiltration may experience moderate to severe chronic pain. The cyclic pelvic pain is related to the sequential swelling and the extravasation of blood and menstrual debris into the surrounding tissue. The chemical mediators of this intense sterile inflammation and pain are believed to be prostaglandins and cytokines. Infiltrative endometriosis, which involves extensive areas of the retroperitoneal space, often is associated with moderate to severe pelvic pain. Studies of pain mapping by laparoscopy under minimal sedation have found that pelvic pain arises from areas of normal peritoneum adjacent to areas of endometriosis.

**Secondary dysmenorrhea is a common component of pain that varies from a dull ache to severe pelvic pain.** It may be unilateral or bilateral and may radiate to the lower back, legs, and groin. Patients often complain of pelvic heaviness or a perception of their internal organs being swollen. Unlike primary dysmenorrhea, the pain may last for many days, including several days before and after the menstrual flow.

The dyspareunia associated with endometriosis is described as pain deep in the pelvis. The cause of this symptom seems to be immobility of the pelvic organs during coital activity or direct pressure on areas of endometriosis in the uterosacral ligaments or the cul-de-sac. Sometimes patients describe areas of point tenderness. The acute pain, experienced during deep penetration, may continue for several hours after intercourse.

**Abnormal bleeding is a symptom noted by 15% to 20% of women with endometriosis.** The most common complaints are **premenstrual spotting and menorrhagia**. Usually this abnormal bleeding is not associated with anovulation and may be related to abnormalities of the endometrium. On the other hand, patients with endometriosis often have ovulatory dysfunction. Approximately 15% of women with endometriosis have coincidental anovulation or luteal dysfunction.

An increased incidence of first-trimester abortion in women with untreated endometriosis has been reported, although this notion has been challenged and remains an unproven association. Less common, yet troublesome, are the symptoms resulting from endometriosis influencing the **gastrointestinal and urinary tracts**. Cyclic abdominal pain, intermittent constipation, diarrhea, dyschezia, urinary frequency, dysuria, and hematuria are all possible symptoms. Bowel obstruction and hydronephrosis may occur. One rare clinical manifestation of endometriosis is **catamenial hemothorax**, which is bloody pleural fluid occurring during menses. Massive ascites is a rare symptom of endometriosis. This is important because the disease process initially masquerades as ovarian carcinoma.

## Clinical Findings (Physical Examination)

The classic pelvic finding of endometriosis is a fixed retroverted uterus, with scarring and tenderness posterior to the uterus. The characteristic nodularity of the uterosacral ligaments and cul-de-sac may be palpated on rectovaginal examination in women with this distribution of the disease. Advanced cases have extensive scarring and narrowing of the posterior vaginal fornix. The ovaries may be enlarged and tender and are often fixed to the broad ligament or lateral pelvic sidewall. The adnexal enlargement is rarely symmetric, as one may expect in some benign pelvic conditions. Speculum examination may demonstrate small areas of endometriosis on the cervix or upper vagina. Lateral displacement or deviation of the cervix is visualized or palpated by digital examination of the vagina and cervix in approximately 15% of women with moderate or severe endometriosis. Carrying out a pelvic examination during the first or second day of menstrual flow may aid in the diagnosis because it is the time of maximum swelling and tenderness in the areas of endometriosis. The diagnosis can be confirmed in most cases by direct laparoscopic visualization of endometriosis with its associated scarring and adhesion formation. In many patients, endometriosis was discovered for the first time during an infertility investigation, although routine laparoscopy is no longer being carried out in the infertility investigation. Biopsy of selected implants confirms the diagnosis.

### Imaging

Imaging can be a useful adjunct to the clinical presentation and physical examination for evaluation of endometriosis, especially with DIE.

Ultrasound examination shows no specific pattern to screen for pelvic endometriosis but may be helpful in differentiating solid from cystic lesions and may help distinguish an endometrioma from other adnexal abnormalities. Because the lesions are vascular, increased Doppler flow may be demonstrated in endometriosis (Fig. 19.12). More recent studies have demonstrated a fair sensitivity from 49% to 91%, with high specificity (93% to 100%) when using transvaginal ultrasound (TVUS) to detect DIE, with the greatest sensitivity and specificity for detection of rectosigmoid lesions. **Modified techniques such as rectal water contrast TVUS can increase the probability of detecting a DIE lesion and are now considered to be the more sensitive technique for the diagnosis of DIE.**

**Magnetic resonance imaging (MRI)** provides the best overall diagnostic tool for endometriosis but is not always a practical modality for its diagnosis. With a detection ratio and specificity of around 78% for implants, **MRI for endometriosis has a reported sensitivity and specificity of approximately 91% to 95%.** There is a characteristic hyperintensity on T1-weighted images and a hypointensity on T2-weighted images (de Venecia, 2015).

### Endometrial Biopsy

In part because the endometrium of women with endometriosis shows abnormal features such as enhanced aromatase expression and progesterone resistance, it has been suggested that an endometrial biopsy may aid in the outpatient diagnosis of endometriosis. One such candidate marker is **B-cell lymphoma 6 (BCL6),** which is only minimally expressed in the normal secretory endometrium of women without endometriosis; however, **enhanced expression of BCL6 has been found in the eutopic endometrium of women with endometriosis.** Using an immunochemical staining score for BCL6, the receive operating characteristic (ROC) curve showed a sensitivity of about 94% (Evans-Hoeker, 2016). Although there is a commercially available test for this marker, it is still not universally accepted.

### Diagnostic Laparoscopy

**Laparoscopy remains the gold standard for the diagnosis of endometriosis.** When laparoscopy is undertaken to establish the diagnosis of endometriosis, it is important to describe systematically the extent of the pathology. **The American Society for Reproductive Medicine (ASRM) developed a point-scoring system in 1996** designed primarily to record the extent of the disease in fertility patients (ASRM, 1997). The focus was intended to provide characterization of disease extent for fertility and not for pain assessment. Nevertheless, there are no data supporting this correlation of scoring with pregnancy rates. Another classification system, ENZIAN, is more recent and may be helpful for the classification of deep pelvic endometriosis (Johnson, 2017). In addition, the **Endometriosis Fertility Index (EFI),** a proposed scoring system by Adamson focused on the fertility potential of patients with endometriosis, has been shown in prospective evaluation to correlate with pregnancy rates (Adamson, 2010). For example, patients with a low score of 0.3 were shown to have a 3-year cumulative pregnancy rate of only 10% to 11%.

Figs. 19.13 and 19.14 illustrate ultrasound and MRI findings in retrocervical endometriosis and endometriosis infiltrating the bowel.

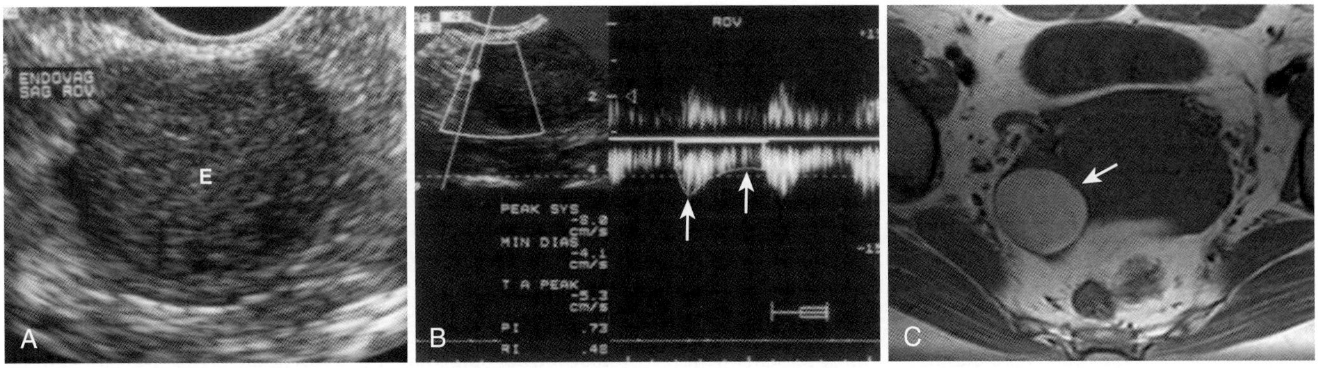


**Fig. 19.12** Ultrasound of endometriosis. **A,** Endovaginal ultrasound showing an endometrioma. Note low-level echoes. **B,** Doppler showing increased flow (RI = 0.48), which suggests a malignancy. **C,** T1-weighted magnetic resonance imaging showing an endometrioma *(arrow)* with a high-intensity similar to fat. (Modified from www.medscape.com.)

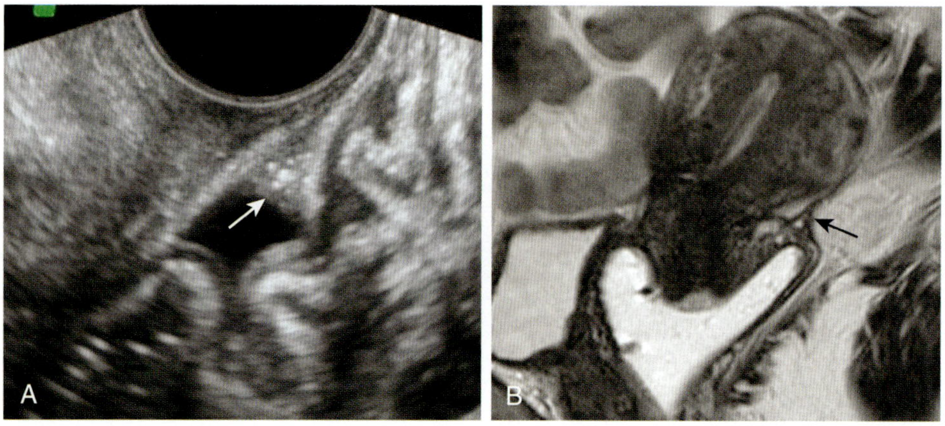


**Fig. 19.13** Retrocervical endometriosis attached to posterior vaginal fornix on vaginal ultrasound (**A**) and magnetic resonance imaging (**B**). *Arrows* show the lesions in different patients. (Courtesy Manoel Goncalves, MD, Clinica Medicina da Mulher and RDO Medicina Diagnostica, and Mauricio Abrão, MD, University of Sao Paulo, Sao Paulo, Brazil.)

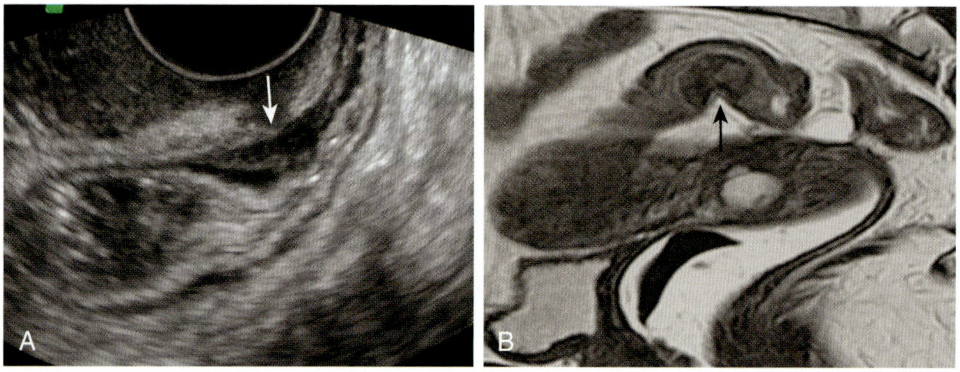


**Fig. 19.14** Rectal endometriosis infiltrating part of the muscular wall of the intestine on vaginal ultrasound (**A**) and sigmoid endometriosis infiltrating part of the muscular wall of the intestine on magnetic resonance imaging (**B**). *Arrows* show the lesions. (Courtesy Manoel Goncalves, MD, Clinica Medicina da Mulher and RDO Medicine Diagnostica, and Mauricio Abrão, MD, University of Sao Paulo, Sao Paulo, Brazil.)

Although a benign disease, endometriosis exhibits characteristics of both malignancy and sterile inflammation. Therefore the common considerations in the differential diagnosis include chronic pelvic inflammatory disease, ovarian malignancy, degeneration of myomas, hemorrhage or torsion of ovarian cysts, adenomyosis, primary dysmenorrhea, and functional bowel disease.

Occasionally a large endometrioma of the ovary may rupture into the peritoneal cavity. This results in an acute surgical condition of the abdomen and brings into the differential diagnosis conditions such as ectopic pregnancy, appendicitis, diverticulitis, and a bleeding corpus luteum cyst.

## MONITORING THE COURSE OF DISEASE: ARE THERE MARKERS?

Serial pelvic examinations are a poor indicator of progression of disease. Serum levels of CA-125 have been used as a marker for endometriosis. CA-125 levels are elevated in most patients with endometriosis and increases incrementally with advanced stages. However, assays for serum levels of CA-125 have a low specificity because they also increase with other pelvic conditions such as leiomyomas, acute pelvic inflammatory disease, and the first trimester of pregnancy. Similarly, serum CA-125 levels have a low sensitivity for the diagnosis of early or minimal endometriosis (Cheng, 2002).

Glycodelin, previously known as *placental protein 14*, has been shown to be elevated in endometriosis and is produced in endometriotic lesions. Levels also fall with removal of the disease. However, because of great variability in levels, glycodelin has not proved to be useful clinically. The most predictive markers appear to be IL-1, chemoattractant protein-1 and interferon gamma, with IL-1 being the most useful marker. There has been interest in proteomic analyses as well (Fassbender, 2012).

Although it is generally thought that endometriosis improves during pregnancy, this is not always the case, and an increase in lesions has been documented, although primarily in the first trimester. Ovarian endometriomas, which may have a different pathogenetic origin from surface implants of endometriosis on the ovary, may persist during pregnancy, and they are at risk for rupture during pregnancy as well.

**Endometriosis may be associated with ovarian cancer.** Not only are lesions found at the time of diagnosis of ovarian cancer, but the risk of developing ovarian cancer may increase fourfold in women with endometriosis. **Loss of heterozygosity and mutations in suppressor genes, such as *P53*, may explain**

**this association** (Dinulescu, 2005). These findings warrant caution in the long-term follow-up of women who have extensive disease and ovarian endometriomas, particularly with large masses and those that increase in size.

The association of other cancers with endometriosis, although suggested, has not been substantiated. However, cervical endometriosis is a particular condition that can produce abnormalities in cervical cytologic test results.

Endometriosis is dependent on ovarian hormones to stimulate growth. **With natural menopause, there is often a gradual relief of symptoms**, and after surgical menopause, areas of endometriosis rapidly disappear. However, it is important to note that **5% of symptomatic cases of endometriosis present after menopause.** The majority of cases in women in their late 50s or early 60s are related to the use of exogenous estrogen, which may stimulate existing lesions.

## TREATMENT

The two primary short-term goals in treating endometriosis are the relief of pain and promotion of fertility. The primary long-term goal in the management of endometriosis is attempting to prevent progression or recurrence of the disease process, but there is a paucity of definitive, evidence-based literature to select the most appropriate method of treatment. A Cochrane review of evidence-based therapies lists a variety of agents that may be helpful but does not specify a clearly preferred agent. This is because there have been few prospective head-to-head comparisons and because the disease is heterogeneous, with vast differences in the spectrum of clinical symptoms and extent of disease from one woman to another. Therefore **the treatment plan must be individualized**. Choice of therapy, for women whose primary symptom is pelvic pain, depends on multiple variables, including the patient's age, her future reproductive plans, the location and extent of her disease, the severity of her symptoms, and any associated pelvic pathologic conditions she may have. Although the gold standard for making a diagnosis is laparoscopy to establish the nature and extent of endometriosis, this is not always possible, particularly in a younger population. Imaging techniques may only be helpful if a mass is identified, and the suggestion of performing an endometrial biopsy may be too invasive for younger nulliparous woman. **If other gynecologic conditions such as chronic pelvic inflammatory disease or neoplasia have been ruled out, empiric medical therapy for 3 months is a reasonable option.** Various **suppressive treatments** (gonadotropin-releasing hormone [GnRH] analogs, oral contraceptives, progestins) and aromatase inhibitors and where they act in the pathophysiology of endometriosis may be found in Fig. 19.15.

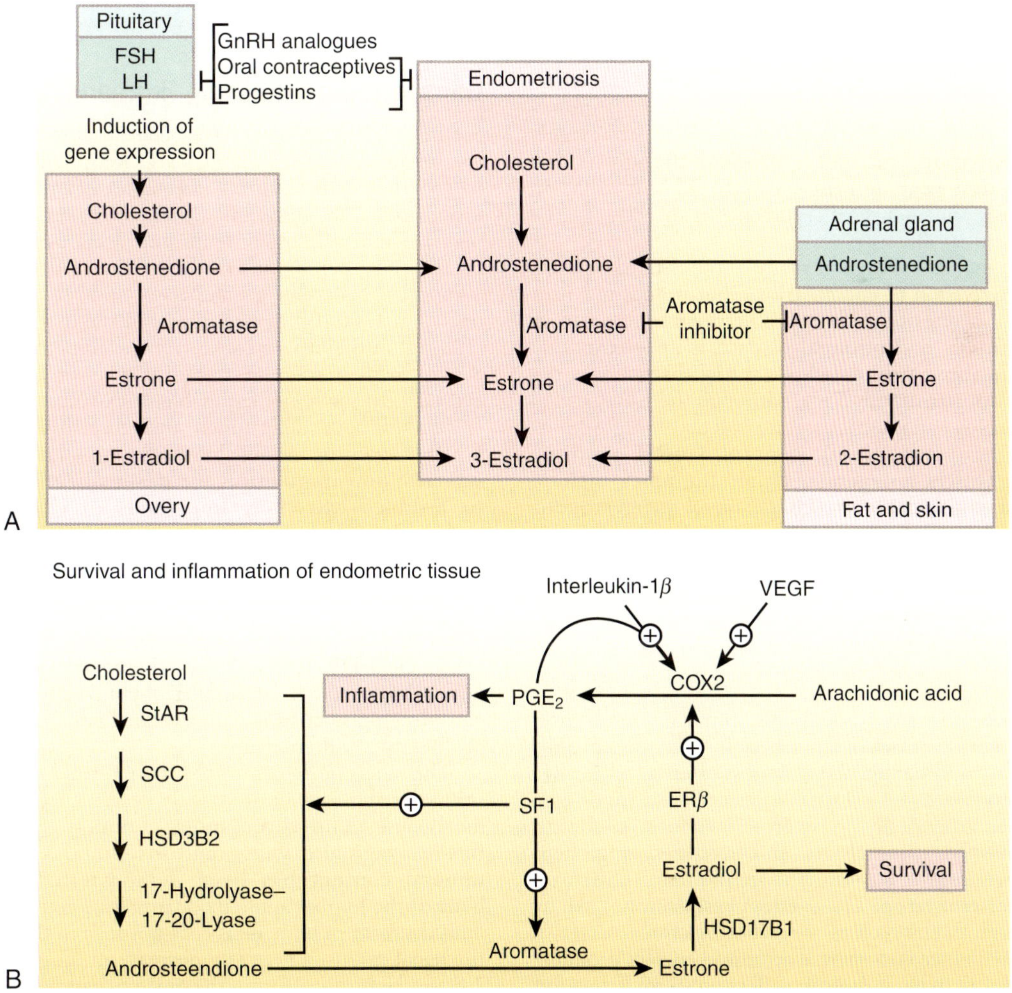


**Fig. 19.15** Molecular distinctions between endometriotic tissue and endometrium. *COX2,* cyclooxygenase-2; *FSH,* follicle-stimulating hormone; *HSD17B1,* 17β-hydroxysteroid dehydrogenase type 1; *LH,* luteinizing hormone; *PGE*$_2$, prostaglandin $E_2$; *SCC,* side chain cleavage enzyme; *SF1,* steroidogenic factor 1; *StAR,* steroidogenic acute regulatory protein; *VEGF,* vascular endothelial growth factor. (From Strauss JF, Barbieri R. *Yen & Jaffe's Reproductive Endocrinology.* 5th ed. Philadelphia: Saunders: 2004:623.)

Treatment of endometriosis can be medical, surgical, or a combination of both. Most of the sex steroids, alone or in combination, have been tried in clinical studies to suppress the growth of endometriosis. Optimal regression secondary to medical treatment is observed in small endometriomas that are less than 1 to 2 cm in diameter. **Response in larger areas of endometriosis may be minimal with medical therapy**. A poor therapeutic result may be governed by the reduction of blood supply to the mass caused by surrounding scar tissue. Some data have suggested that with certain suppressive therapies, such as the use of dienogest, there is **a decrease in nerve fiber density** in endometriosis lesions.

Surgical therapy is divided into conservative and definitive operations. Conservative surgery involves the resection or destruction of endometrial implants, lysis of adhesions, and attempts to restore normal pelvic anatomy. Definitive surgery involves the removal of both ovaries, the uterus, and all visible ectopic foci of endometriosis. This type of surgery is analogous to cytoreductive surgery in ovarian carcinoma.

## Medical Therapy

Medical therapy is aimed at suppression of lesions and associated symptoms, particularly pain. This is best achieved by menstrual suppression, ideally without inducing hypoestrogenism. Unfortunately, once suppressive therapy is stopped, symptoms tend to recur at variable rates. The choice of medical therapy should be individualized, weighing in potential adverse effects, side effects, cost of therapy, and expected patient compliance. The clinical effectiveness, as measured by relief of symptoms and recurrence rates of current medical therapies, are largely similar. The **recurrence rate after medical therapy is 5% to 15% in the first year and increases to 40% to 50% in 5 years**; obviously the chance of recurrence is directly related to the extent of initial disease.

In summary, medical therapy usually suppresses symptoms and prevents progression of endometriosis, but it does not provide a long-lasting cure of the disease. The **recurrence rate in women who initially had minimal disease is approximately 35%, whereas in those women whose initial disease was severe the rate is approximately 75%.** Although there are several medical therapies for endometriosis, the Food and Drug Administration (FDA) has approved only **danazol, GnRH agonists,** and **elagolix, a GnRH antagonist. Other therapies include traditional oral contraceptives (OCs), novel progestogens such as gestrinone and dienogest, an oral GnRH antagonist, the levonorgestrel-releasing intrauterine system (IUS), the aromatase inhibitor letrozole, and certain selective progesterone receptor modulators.**

### Danazol

Although approved for use in the 1970s, clinicians rarely prescribe danazol (because of lack of familiarity, its side effect profile, and the availability of other agents) and most often select GnRH agonists, progestogens, or OCs. Danazol, an attenuated androgen that is active when given orally, is also prescribed for women with benign cystic mastitis, menorrhagia, and hereditary angioneurotic edema. Chemically it is a synthetic steroid that is the isoxazole derivative of ethisterone (17-α-ethinyltestosterone). Many years ago, oral androgens such as methyltestosterone were also used because they induce endometrial atrophy. Danazol produces a hypoestrogenic and hyperandrogenic effect on steroid-sensitive end organs. The drug is mildly androgenic and anabolic, leading to its side effect profile.

Danazol induces atrophic changes in the endometrium of the uterus and similar changes in endometrial implants. It has been suggested to also modulate immunologic function. **Although doses of 400 to 800 mg of danazol have been prescribed, many clinicians reduce the total daily dosage of the drug to 200 mg, and even 100 mg, of danazol daily.** Danazol is usually begun during menses (days 1 to 5). Because the relief of the symptoms is directly related to the incidence of amenorrhea, the lower dosages of danazol are not as effective. **Side effects of the hormonal changes are encountered by 80%, and approximately 10% to 20% of women discontinue danazol because of side effects.** There have been reports of deepening of the voice that did not resolve after discontinuation. Mild elevation in serum liver enzyme levels has been reported in women treated for endometriosis, and women who take danazol for longer than 6 months should have serum liver enzyme determinations. An androgenic effect on lipids occurs, with reduction in high-density lipoprotein (HDL) cholesterol and triglycerides and an increase in low-density lipoprotein (LDL) cholesterol.

The standard length of treatment with danazol is 6 to 9 months. Approximately three of four patients note significant improvement in their symptoms, and about 90% have objective improvement discovered at a second-look laparoscopy. The uncorrected fertility rate after danazol therapy is approximately 40%. Unfortunately, symptoms will recur in 15% to 30% of women within 2 years after therapy.

Several randomized, double-blind clinical studies have compared the therapeutic effectiveness of danazol with GnRH agonists. The results do not show significant differences between the efficacies of these two drugs.

## Gonadotropin-Releasing Hormone Agonists

Several GnRH agonists have been developed and approved for the treatment of endometriosis. Representative agonists are leuprolide acetate (Lupron, injectable), nafarelin acetate (Synarel, intranasal), and goserelin acetate (Zoladex, subcutaneous implant). The usual dose of leuprolide acetate is 3.75 mg intramuscularly once per month or an 11.25-mg depot injection every 3 months. Nafarelin acetate nasal spray is given in a dose of one spray (200 μg) in one nostril in the morning and one spray (200 μg) in the other nostril in the evening up to a maximum of 800 μg daily. Goserelin acetate is given in a dosage of 3.6 mg every 28 days in a biodegradable subcutaneous implant.

Studies have determined the dose-response curve of the GnRH agonists, establishing the optimal dose to produce sufficient **downregulation and desensitization of the pituitary to produce extremely low levels of circulating estrogen and amenorrhea**. Chronic use of GnRH agonists produces a "medical oophorectomy." A dramatic reduction occurs in serum estrone, estradiol ($E_2$), testosterone, and androstenedione to levels similar to the hormonal levels in oophorectomized women. There are no significant changes in total serum cholesterol, HDL, or LDL levels during therapeutic periods as long as 6 months. Endometrial samples obtained after several months of chronic agonist therapy demonstrated either atrophic or an early proliferative endometrium.

The side effects associated with GnRH agonist therapy are primarily those associated with decreased estrogen, similar to menopause. **The three most common symptoms are hot flushes, vaginal dryness, and insomnia. A decrease in bone mineral content has been demonstrated** in the trabecular bone of the lumbar spine by quantitative computed tomography. This decrease in bone density is not seen in the compact bone of the distal radius. There is a decrease in measured bone mass of 2% to 7% during a 6-month course of agonist therapy. However, it has been established that **the decrease in bone density associated with 6 months of therapy is completely recovered between 12 and 24 months.**

The clinical response to agonist therapy depends on when the therapy is initiated as related to the menstrual cycle. If agonist therapy is begun during the follicular phase, an agonist phase results in an initial rapid rise in follicle-stimulating hormone (FSH) and $E_2$ for approximately 3 weeks. FSH levels fall to basal levels by the third to fourth week of therapy. **$E_2$ levels rapidly decline after 21 days of therapy.** The expected surge in luteinizing hormone (LH) does not occur, and serum progesterone levels do not become elevated. Amenorrhea is induced within 6 to 8 weeks. In contrast, when beginning agonist therapy during the luteal phase or if artificially manipulated by the concurrent administration of oral progestogen, **serum $E_2$** levels are suppressed within 2 weeks. Amenorrhea is induced in 4 to 5 weeks. It is important to ensure that the patient is not pregnant when beginning GnRH agonist therapy during the luteal phase.

**GnRH agonist therapy improves symptoms in 75% to 90% of patients with endometriosis**, depending on the extent of the disease in the study group. Growth of endometriosis is arrested, diminished, or eliminated. The greatest therapeutic effects are seen when areas of endometriosis are less than 1 cm in diameter. **Ovarian function usually returns to normal in 6 to 12 weeks after 6 months of GnRH agonist therapy**. Large ovarian endometriomas and severe adhesive disease have not responded to hormonal therapy.

Many clinicians "add back" hormone replacement therapy with dosages similar to those used in menopausal therapy in combination with chronic GnRH agonist regimens. The clinical hypothesis is that the add-back medication will reduce or eliminate the vasomotor symptoms and vaginal atrophy and also diminish or overcome the demineralization of bone. Barbieri has suggested that there is a therapeutic window that he estimates is a circulating level of approximately 30 pg/mL of $E_2$ (Barbieri, 1992). He postulated that this level of $E_2$ is enough to protect the body from substantial bone loss and is not high enough to interfere with the inhibition of growth of endometriosis (Fig. 19.16). **Multiple randomized trials have demonstrated that add-back therapy does not interfere with the effectiveness of agonists to relieve the pelvic pain from endometriosis.** The majority of studies have also demonstrated no diminished therapeutic efficacy when add-back therapy is initiated simultaneously with the GnRH agonist. Some clinicians additionally give bisphosphonates and calcium with the **low-dose progestins and estrogen,** but bisphosphonates are not recommended in younger women who may wish to become pregnant. **Add-back regimens** not only reduce or eliminate adverse clinical and metabolic side effects associated with hypoestrogenism but also facilitate safe and effective prolongation of GnRH agonist therapy for up to 12 months. Additional agents that have been used for add-back therapy are tibolone and raloxifene.

GnRH antagonists have also been considered an attractive option in that they have no "flare" effect. A direct effect on lesions has also been hypothesized. **Elagolix** has now been approved for the treatment of moderate to severe endometriosis. **Doses to 150 mg/day for less severe cases and doses of 200 mg twice daily for more severe cases** have been approved for use for 6 months. The flexibility of oral dosing offers some advantage and may result in less severe side effects such as hot flushes and bone loss compared with GnRH agonist therapy. In large randomized trials dysmenorrhea was improved in 46% and 76% of women with the lower and higher doses, respectively. Nonmenstrual pain was improved in about 50% of women with both doses (Taylor, 2017). Add-back therapy can also be considered as with GnRH agonist therapy. Elagolix was combined with 0.5 mg oral estradiol and 0.1 mg of norethindrone acetate or with 1 mg of estradiol and 0.5 mg of norethindrone acetate in a trial for the treatment of fibroids (Carr, 2018).

One concern of using elagolix is its price, which is approximately $850 per month.

For women not wishing to conceive, who predominantly have pain and no indication for surgery (which may include failed medical therapy), **stopping and starting various treatments and interchanging them is a reasonable approach to control symptoms.**

## Oral Contraceptives

In the late 1950s, very large doses of norethynodrel with mestranol daily were given to produce amenorrhea and a "pseudopregnancy." Most of the published studies involved the first-generation, high-estrogen OCs. However, more recent reports have established that the present low-estrogen monophasic combination pills, specifically the ones with a relatively high progestin potency, are equally effective when used in a continuous fashion. **It has been accepted that the most economical regimen for the treatment of women with mild or moderate symptoms of endometriosis has been continuous daily OCs for 6 to 12 months. Continuous-dose regimens are aimed at more complete suppression, with an advantage over cyclic use**, and the only concern is with breakthrough bleeding, which can be dealt with in a variety of ways as with contraceptive therapy.

One potential risk of using OCs or progestogens is that there is some risk of rupture if a large endometrioma is present. Rupture of large endometriomas may result in an acute surgical abdominal condition during the first 6 weeks of OC therapy. During prolonged therapy the endometrial glands atrophy and the stroma undergoes a marked decidual reaction. Some

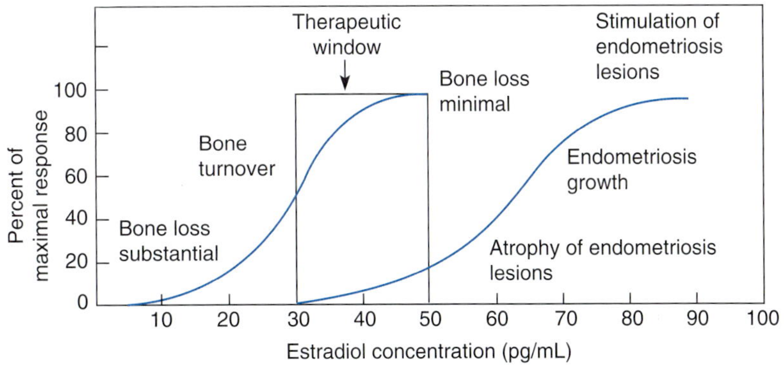


**Fig. 19.16** Estradiol therapeutic window. The concentration of estradiol required to cause the growth of endometriosis lesions may be greater than the concentration required to stabilize bone mineral density. (From Barbieri RL. Hormone treatment of endometriosis: the estrogen threshold hypothesis. *Am J Obstet Gynecol.* 1992;166(2):740-745.)

smaller endometriomas (~3 cm) can undergo necrobiosis and resorption.

The most common side effects of inducing amenorrhea with OCs include weight gain and breast tenderness. Approximately one in three women discontinues this therapy because of side effects.

The results of continuous OC therapy include a decrease in symptoms in approximately 80% of patients during therapy.

## Nonsteroidal Antiinflammatory Drugs

Nonsteroidal antiinflammatory drugs (NSAIDs) are beneficial for pain relief and as concomitant therapy may improve the bleeding control of patients on OCs. There may also be a direct therapeutic value in endometriosis. Although COX-2 inhibitors are now infrequently used because of cardiovascular concerns in older individuals, **this therapy for endometriosis has a rationale in that lesions of endometriosis have been found to express high levels of COX-2** (see Fig. 19.15). In summary, antiinflammatory agents may be beneficial for pain relief as well as potentially for the treatment of endometriosis, particularly when other suppressive therapy cannot be used.

### Other Hormonal Treatments

For women who cannot tolerate the high dosage of estrogen in an OC or who have a contraindication to estrogen therapy, treatment with progestogens only has been successful. **Medroxyprogesterone acetate (Provera)** in a dosage of 20 to 30 mg orally per day or **depo-medroxyprogesterone acetate (Depo-Provera)** in a dosage of 150 mg intramuscularly every 3 months to a maximum of 200 mg every month will produce a prolonged amenorrhea. The medication is most appropriate for older women who have completed childbearing. The timing of resumption of ovulation after discontinuation of injectable medroxyprogesterone is prolonged and extremely variable. Some women will not ovulate for more than a year after their last injection; therefore this form of therapy should not be prescribed for a young woman who is contemplating pregnancy in the near future. Oral medroxyprogesterone in a dosage of 30 mg/day is an alternative mode of therapy, as is norethindrone acetate (10 to 40 mg daily). This more androgenic progestogen, although quite effective, has a similar symptom profile to that for continuous medroxyprogesterone.

**Gestrinone** is a progestogen originally developed as a once-a-week OC. This drug has undergone clinical trials for endometriosis with dosages ranging from 2.5 to 7.5 mg/week. Gestrinone acts as an agonist-antagonist of progesterone receptors and an agonist of androgen receptors and also binds weakly to estrogen receptors. At completion of therapy in a randomized trial, a tendency for prolonged pain relief was observed for gestrinone compared with GnRH agonist and it showed similar efficacy (Gestrinone Italian Study Group, 1996).

**Dienogest** is a selective progestogen that causes anovulation, has an antiproliferative effect on endometrial cells, and may inhibit cytokine secretion. In clinical trials at 2 mg/day orally, it has been found to be as effective as GnRH agonists (Ferrero, 2015).

**The levonorgestrel IUS** has been shown to be beneficial for pain relief in women with endometriosis compared with expectant management. It is particularly suited for women who have rectocervical and cul-de-sac disease (Fedele, 2001).

**Aromatase inhibitors** (anastrozole 1 mg; letrozole 2.5 and 5 mg) have been found to be beneficial in that not only does estrogen tend to cause proliferation of the disease, but also endometriosis lesions have been found to contain the aromatase enzyme (Bulun, 2009). When given alone to premenopausal women it will cause stimulation of gonadotropins and has been used to induce ovulation, but **in postmenopausal women and in premenopausal women in combination with a progestogen or OCs, there is good promise that it will be beneficial for the treatment of endometriosis** (Attar, 2006).

## Other Possible Medical Therapies

There are several other less well-proved therapies. These include the peroxisome proliferator-activated receptor (PPAR) ligands, which have been shown to inhibit macrophage action in animal models (Lebovic, 2007); targeting haptoglobin because of structural similarity to endo-1; targeting MMPs; and tumor necrosis factor alpha and VEGF (Falconer, 2008). Newer antiprogestogens have also shown efficacy in small clinical trials (Chabbert-Buffet, 2005), and several compounds are being studied further. ERβ agonists may also play some role in the future trials in that some of the estrogen action involved in increasing VEGF and angiogenetic factors are mediated through ERβ (see Fig. 19.15). ERβ may also modulate immune function. It should be noted that selective estrogen receptor modulators, specifically tamoxifen and raloxifene, have not been shown to be beneficial. **Another antiinflammatory immunomodulator, pentoxifylline, has also shown promise.**

Various medicinal herbs have been suggested for use based on their antiproliferative, antiinflammatory, pain-relieving properties. However, no rigorous clinical trial data are available.

## Route of Administration

Delivering various progestogens or danazol locally (intrauterine as with the levonorgestrel IUS or vaginally) may also enhance effectiveness. Small clinical trials have suggested the benefit of using suppositories and local agents, particularly in those women with cul-de-sac disease.

## Surgical Therapy

Surgery therapy can serve as an adjunct or alternative to medical therapy and can help prevent or delay further disease progression. The main roles of surgical therapy in the management of endometriosis are to provide symptomatic relief (pain) and to improve fertility outcomes.

Surgical management includes conservative and definitive approaches that address three main categories of lesions: superficial endometriosis, endometriomas, and DIE.

Conservative surgery involves preservation of reproductive organs and restoration of normal pelvic anatomy while removing all macroscopic endometriotic lesions or endometriomas and performing lysis of adhesions. Definitive surgery involves removing the uterus and cervix along with any visible lesions while preserving or removing either one or both of the ovaries.

Minimally invasive surgical approaches such as laparoscopy and robotic surgery have largely replaced the need for laparotomy because of advantages such as improved visualization, shorter recovery period, decreased blood loss, and decreased risks of complications (Daraï, 2010). Laparoscopic and robotic surgery for surgical management of endometriosis have been found to have comparable perioperative outcomes and provide significant improvement in quality of life (Soto, 2017).

Surgical techniques for endometriosis may vary from surgeon to surgeon, but key surgical principles should be maintained. A survey of the abdomen and pelvis should always be performed which should include exploration of the subdiaphragmatic peritoneum, abdominal wall, ovarian fossa, uterosacral ligaments, posterior cul-de-sac, anterior cul-de-sac, bladder, appendix, and bowel. It is also important to identify key anatomic structures including the ureter. Restoring normal pelvic anatomy, preventing adhesions, and limiting tissue damage are essential for successful endometriosis surgery. It is often helpful to start dissections going from normal anatomy toward abnormal anatomy. Energy should be used judiciously and cautiously especially with difficult dissections with distorted anatomy and when adjacent to vital structures such as major blood vessels, the ureter, bladder, or bowel. Although both techniques of ablation and excision have shown improvement in outcomes compared with expectant management, there is still debate on which is most effective (Pundir, 2017; Riley, 2019).

## Surgical Management for Pain

In women suffering from chronic pelvic pain as a result of endometriosis for whom conservative medical therapy has failed, surgery can be an effective treatment, especially in cases of moderate or severe endometriosis in which pelvic adhesive disease is present along with the involvement of nonreproductive organs.

In a prospective randomized trial, Sutton compared the effect of laser laparoscopy over expectant management after diagnostic laparoscopy. Pain decreased by 62.5% compared with 22.6% with expectant management, and pain relief continued in 55% of women over 72 months. The placebo response was noted to be 22%. Another randomized trial demonstrated an 80% improvement in symptoms with a 30% placebo response rate from surgery. The median time to pain recurrence after surgery has been estimated to be 20 months and reported to be approximately 15% at 1 year, 36% at 5 years, and 50% by 7 years. It has been suggested that up to 25% of women are likely to undergo additional surgery for endometriosis within 4 years, and 10% will need a hysterectomy.

Definitive surgical treatment with hysterectomy is effective for symptomatic relief with reoperation free rates of 86% (with ovarian preservation) and 91% (without ovarian preservation) at 5 years; however, note that the evaluation of ovarian preservation compared with oophorectomy is based on limited retrospective data (Namnoum, 1995; Shakiba, 2008). **Although removal of the ovaries may decrease the risk of disease recurrence and reoperation, this should be balanced with the risks associated with removing the ovaries, such as premature menopause and increased mortality particularly in younger patients** (Parker, 2013). Approximately **one out of three women will develop recurrent symptoms and subsequently have a second operation involving oophorectomy**. In the study by Shakiba and colleagues, there was no difference between ovarian preservation and oophorectomy in the surgery-free interval for women between the ages of 30 to 39 (Shakiba, 2008). Given the available data and risks associated with oophorectomy, ovarian preservation is a reasonable option for patients younger than 40. Nevertheless, ovarian preservation or removal should be individualized based on the patient's age, clinical presentation, and goals. If bilateral oophorectomy is performed, hormonal replacement therapy should be considered. Whether a patient undergoes conservative or definitive surgery, postoperative hormonal suppression with progestins or OCs may be considered to decrease risks of recurrence, especially if there is any residual or unresectable disease at the time of surgery.

Another surgical treatment that has been considered for management of pain is **presacral neurectomy**. In select patients with midline pain, this procedure may be an option for short-term improvement in symptoms, but complications can include bowel and bladder dysfunction, and this type of surgery is generally ineffective for endometriosis-related pelvic pain.

## Surgical Management for Fertility

Management of patients with endometriosis undergoing assisted reproductive treatment can be challenging. Medical therapy may sometimes be required for symptomatic control while waiting for fertility treatment; however, this is generally not recommended. There have been studies suggesting improved fertility outcomes with prolonged GnRH agonist use when administered prior to assisted reproductive treatment. Surgical management in these women can be considered, though there has been debate about the timing and risks/benefits of surgery in the setting of in vitro fertilization (IVF). **Surgery is generally only recommended if the patient is symptomatic (such as having significant pain—visual analog scale [VAS] score > 7) or has failed two cycles of IVF** (Kho, 2018).

For stage I/II endometriosis, excision or ablation of endometriosis has been shown to increase live birth and ongoing pregnancy rates and is therefore recommended when visible lesions are present. Although there is lack of randomized trials, for patients with stage III/IV disease, surgical treatment has also been suggested to increase pregnancy rates (see Therapy for Subfertility later in this chapter).

There has been a movement to incorporate BCL6 marker positivity as an indicator for possible endometriosis and subsequent rationale for laparoscopy in patients with unexplained infertility.

### Endometriomas

Conservative management of endometriomas has potential risks, such as infection of the endometriomas, interfering with response to infertility treatments and oocyte retrieval, risks of complications in pregnancy, and malignancy. Despite these theoretic risks, surgical removal of endometriomas is not generally recommended before IVF. Evidence suggests that surgery for endometriomas does not necessarily increase fertility outcome, whereas it can further compromise ovarian reserve, increase the risk of premature ovarian failure, and induce early menopause. **Patients with endometriomas have lower antimüllerian hormone (AMH) levels compared with those without endometriosis and therefore may have diminished ovarian reserve at baseline**. Surgical excision of endometriomas may even further decrease ovarian reserve, though this effect may be temporary. On the other hand, surgical treatment of endometriomas can be beneficial for certain cases such as when endometriomas are larger than 3 cm in symptomatic patients (i.e., patients with pelvic pain) or in those with difficult access to follicles (Dunselman, 2014). Fig. 19.17 depicts significant endometriomas in a woman with stage IV disease. If there is decision to proceed with surgical

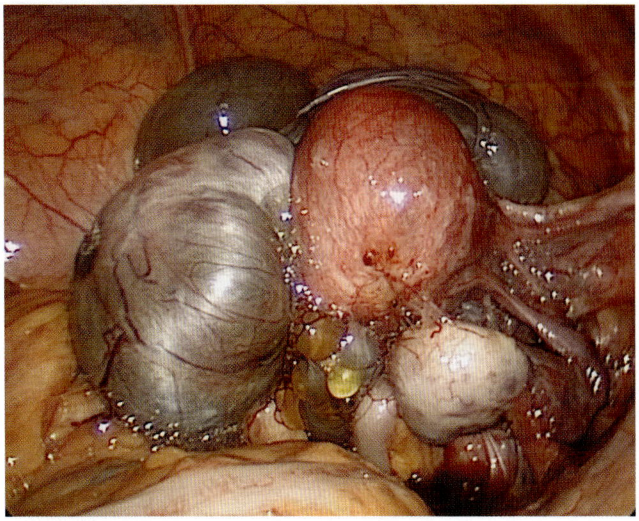

**Fig. 19.17** Significant large endometriomas in a woman with stage IV endometriosis. (Courtesy A. Advincula.)

management for endometrioma, though there is less decrease in AMH levels with ablation, cystectomy with removal of the capsule is preferable over ablation or drainage because of a high risk of recurrence (80% to 100%) (Giampaolino, 2015). Cystectomy has been shown to increase clinical pregnancy rates compared with ablation or drainage. It is important to avoid or minimize electrosurgery when attempting to achieve hemostasis because this can further affect ovarian reserve.

In patients failing to conceive spontaneously after the initial surgery, assisted reproductive therapy is recommended because it has been shown to be more effective than repeat surgery. Although controversial, repeat surgery can be considered after failed assisted reproductive treatments, but further studies are needed to determine optimal management of such patients.

## Therapy for Subfertility

The subfertility that occurs in women with endometriosis can be the result of multiple mechanisms (Fig. 19.18).

Medical therapy cannot be first-line treatment for endometriosis because suppression of ovulation interferes with the ability to conceive. Occasionally as an adjunct, more prolonged (than usual) GnRH agonist therapy may be used before IVF. In this section, surgical options are considered.

There has long been a debate as to whether treating *mild* endometriotic lesions or implants would improve fertility. Two prospective randomized trials have provided some guidance. Data from Canadian and Italian studies, taken together, suggest that pregnancy rates improve with implant ablation (Jacobson, 2002) (Fig. 19.19). Thus one additional pregnancy may be expected from eight surgical procedures. The way these data should be extrapolated into practice is that if a laparoscopy is being performed in a woman wishing to conceive, visible lesions should be ablated if technically possible rather than ignored.

Apart from the mechanical factors (endometriomas, adhesions, fibrosis) affecting pregnancy rates, in endometriosis, macrophage and cytokine abnormalities are thought to play a significant role in inhibiting fertility (see Fig. 19.18. These factors may affect oocyte quality, fertilization, and embryo quality as well as endometrial receptivity. Therefore in addition to ablating lesions when present, several strategies have been devised to enhance fecundity. **Controlled ovarian stimulation along with intrauterine insemination, an approach to enhance fecundity in women with unexplained infertility, has been found to be beneficial in women with endometriosis.** Finally, if IVF–embryo transfer (ET) is undertaken (because of mechanical factors or with other failed approaches), there has been controversy regarding whether pregnancy rates and live birth rates are affected by having the disease. Although an older meta-analysis suggested an approximate 20% reduction in pregnancy rates (Barnhart, 2002), data suggest that pregnancy rates are comparable unless endometriosis is severe (Hamdan, 2015). However, at the same time, prior suppressive therapy (before initiation of an IVF cycle) has been shown to be of benefit. **A Cochrane systematic review of three RCTs found that suppression of endometriosis with a GnRH agonist for 3 to 6 months before IVF-ET improves outcomes, with an odds ratio of 9.19** (Sallam, 2006). This reemphasizes the pathophysiologic consequences involved with having endometriosis (described earlier).

The role of surgical therapy in the management of endometriosis is very much dependent on the clinical presentation of the patient and her desire for future fertility. Although there can be a beneficial effect for fertility, a detrimental effect can also be seen.

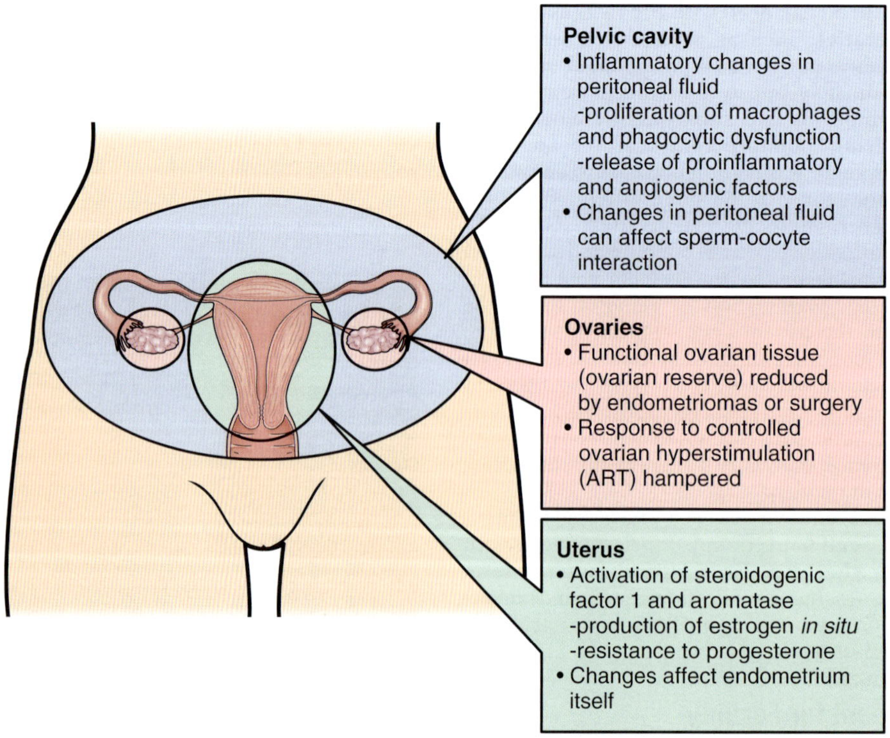
Pelvic cavity
• Inflammatory changes in peritoneal fluid
-proliferation of macrophages and phagocytic dysfunction
-release of proinflammatory and angiogenic factors
• Changes in peritoneal fluid can affect sperm-oocyte interaction
Ovaries
• Functional ovarian tissue (ovarian reserve) reduced by endometriomas or surgery
• Response to controlled ovarian hyperstimulation (ART) hampered
Uterus
• Activation of steroidogenic factor 1 and aromatase
-production of estrogen *in situ*
-resistance to progesterone
• Changes affect endometrium itself

**Fig. 19.18** Mechanisms of endometriosis associated infertility. *ART,* Assisted reproductive technologies. (Modified from de Ziegler, Borghese B, Chapron C. Endometriosis and infertility: pathophysiology and management. *Lancet.* 2010;376(9742):730-738. Data from Strauss J, Barbieri R. *Yen and Jaffe's Reproductive Endocrinology.* 7th ed. Philadelphia: Elsevier; 2014.)

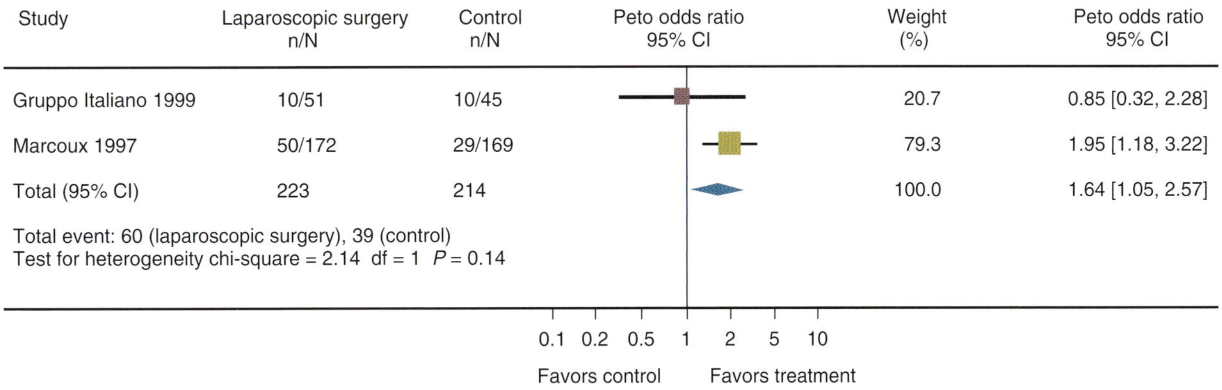
Study
Laparoscopic surgery n/N
Control n/N
Peto odds ratio 95% CI
Weight (%)
Peto odds ratio 95% CI
Gruppo Italiano 1999
10/51
10/45
20.7
0.85 [0.32, 2.28]
Marcoux 1997
50/172
29/169
79.3
1.95 [1.18, 3.22]
Total (95% CI)
223
214
100.0
1.64 [1.05, 2.57]
Total event: 60 (laparoscopic surgery), 39 (control)
Test for heterogeneity chi-square = 2.14 df = 1 P = 0.14
0.1 0.2 0.5 1 2 5 10
Favors control
Favors treatment

**Fig. 19.19** Meta-analysis of the two randomized trials assessing the efficacy of laparoscopic surgery in the treatment of subfertility associated with minimal-to-mind endometriosis. Combing live birth and ongoing pregnancy data from the two studies shows an improvement with laparoscopic surgical treatment (odds ratio, 1.64; 95% confidence interval [CI], 1.05 to 2.57). Df, Degrees of freedom. (From Jacobson TZ, Barlow DH, Koninckx PR, et al: Laparoscopic surgery for subfertility associated with endometriosis. *Cochrane Database Syst Rev*. 2002;4:CD001398.)

Advanced stages of disease, particularly those involving extrapelvic locations (discussed later), are often best managed in a multidisciplinary fashion.

## ENDOMETRIOSIS AT OTHER SITES

### Gastrointestinal Tract Endometriosis

The incidence of gastrointestinal (GI) tract involvement in women who have histologically proven endometriosis has been estimated to range from 3% to 37%. Most large series document an incidence of approximately 5%. Implants that involve the GI tract are the most common site of extrapelvic endometriosis but can be the most challenging to manage. The severity and extent of involvement of the bowel by ectopic endometrium varies from the incidental finding of a spot on the serosa of the bowel to obstruction of the rectosigmoid. In the majority of cases, endometriosis of the GI tract involves the sigmoid colon and the anterior wall of the rectum, accounting for approximately 90% of cases.

Involvement of the appendix is the next most common type of GI tract endometriosis with an incidence reported to be between 1% and 13% (Fig. 19.20). In a series of more than 100 consecutive patients with endometriosis, 13% had histologic evidence of endometriosis in the appendix, whereas only 60% of these cases are detected on gross examination. Endometriosis of the small bowel is rare, where only approximately 200 cases of endometriosis of the ileum have been reported in the literature. Of note, 48% of patients with rectosigmoid lesions will also have endometriosis of the ovaries, and 84% will have rectocervical lesions (Fig. 19.21).

In most cases the implants do not produce clinical symptoms. Classic symptoms of endometriosis of the large bowel include dysmenorrhea (cyclic pelvic cramping and lower abdominal pain) and dyschezia (rectal pain with defecation), especially during the menstrual period. Other associated symptoms include deep dyspareunia, change in bowel function, diarrhea or constipation (or both), and occasionally hematochezia. Studies have demonstrated that 25% to 35% of women with advanced endometriosis of the large bowel experience episodic rectal bleeding as a result of endometriosis extending into the submucosa. A distinct dysfunction of the enteric nervous system has been suggested to be the primary cause of the abnormalities of

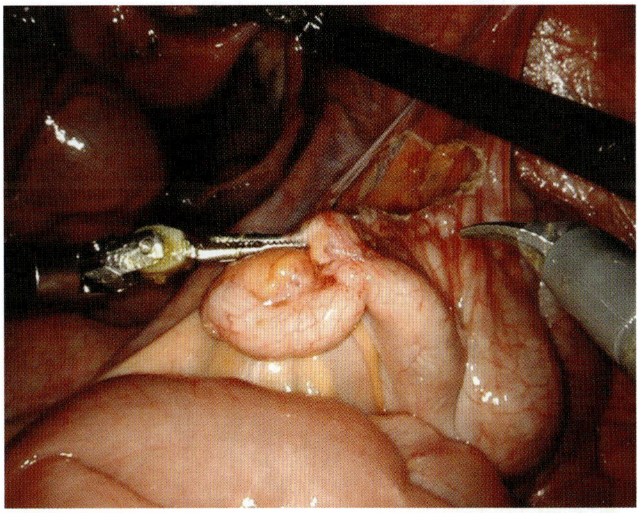

**Fig. 19.20** Endometriosis of the appendix. (Courtesy A. Advincula.)

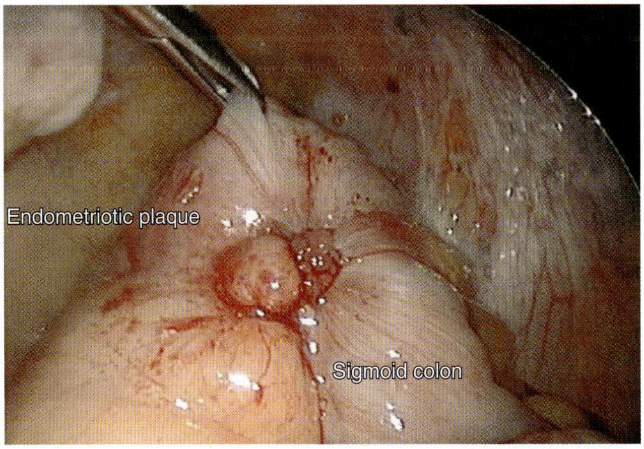


**Fig. 19.21** Endometriosis involving the sigmoid colon. (From Hemmings R, Falcone T. Endometriosis. In: Falcone T, Hurd WW. *Clinical Reproductive Medicine and Surgery.* Philadelphia: Mosby; 2007.)

bowel function in women with endometriosis. It is difficult to differentiate the symptoms associated with endometriosis from the overlapping constellation of symptoms associated with inflammatory disease of the colon or malignancy. Hence, early diagnosis of GI endometriosis and differentiation from other GI conditions are important. Women with a GI malignancy usually experience intermittent rather than cyclic intestinal bleeding. Although acyclic bowel symptoms can occur with GI endometriosis, cyclic GI symptoms generally occur up to 89% cases, and therefore suspicion of GI endometriosis should be high with this type of presentation.

Physical examination can also help with diagnosis of DIE invading the rectosigmoid, such as by palpation of a pelvic mass or "rectal shelf" on rectovaginal examination. Sigmoidoscopy usually demonstrates absence of a mucosal lesion in addition to fixation and immobility of the anterior rectal wall. Donnez and coworkers speculated that endometriosis of the rectovaginal septum is a disease process more closely related to foci of adenomyosis than endometriosis (Donnez, 1997).

Endometriosis involving the GI tract is usually unresponsive to medical therapy and often requires surgical excision. Surgery should generally be performed in coordination with a multidisciplinary team. Complete excision of these lesions sometimes necessitates bowel resection. Although no consensus exists, bowel resection generally is indicated in symptomatic women when lesions are greater than 2 cm, greater than 30% of the circumference is involved, or when there is invasion into the inner muscularis layer, which may require bowel resection. When surgery is indicated, although still unclear which is more effective, bowel resection can either be done via segmental or discoid resection. Parameters that should be considered in surgical planning include size, number and depth of lesions, extent of bowel circumference involvement, distance to anal verge, and presence of lymph node involvement. **A study by Abrão and colleagues suggests that surgical management should be performed only in patients with significant pain (VAS > 7)** and recommends a surgical approach as follows: (1) shaving resection with lesions that involve only the external muscularis of the bowel; (2) disc resection with solitary lesions smaller than 3 cm, invasion beyond the external muscularis, located between 5 and 9 cm from the anal verge, and with no more than 40% of the bowel circumference compromised; and (3) segmental resection and reanastomosis when the lesion is more than 3 cm and is located more than 5 cm from the anal verge or when multiple lesions are present (Abrão, 2020).

After surgical resection, up to 70% of patients have improvement of symptoms with a recurrence rate of 0% to 34%. Pregnancy rates have been reported to be between 24% to 66%.

## Urinary Tract Endometriosis

Endometriosis in the female pelvis occasionally produces dysfunction in adjacent pelvic organs. Approximately 10% of women with endometriosis have involvement of the urinary tract, which most commonly involves endometriotic implants and associated retroperitoneal fibrosis located in the peritoneum overlying the ureter or the bladder. In most cases an incidental finding of aberrant endometrial glands and stroma is discovered on the bladder peritoneum and anterior cul-de-sac. The most serious consequence of urinary tract involvement is ureteral obstruction, which occurs in about 1% of women with moderate or severe pelvic endometriosis. The pathogenesis of endometriosis of the bladder is controversial (Fig. 19.22). Interestingly, approximately 50% of women with endometriosis of the urinary tract have a history of previous pelvic surgery. The lesions may develop from implanted endometrium during cesarean delivery or may be an extension from adenomyosis of the anterior uterine wall.

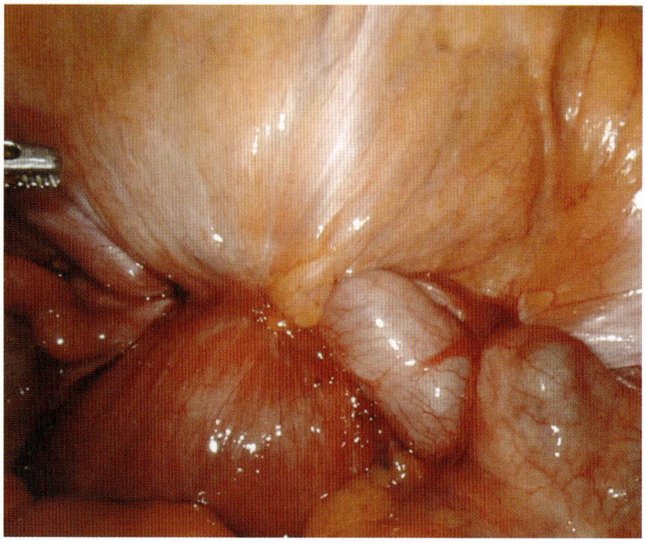

Fig. 19.22 Involvement of the bladder with endometriosis. (Courtesy A, Advincula.)

Patients with endometriosis involving the urinary tract have nonspecific clinical presentations. Hematuria and flank pain are experienced by less than 25% of women. One of three women with documented complete ureteral obstruction secondary to endometriosis has no pelvic symptoms whatsoever. The clinical challenge is to diagnose minimal ureteral obstruction at an early stage, before loss of renal function. The obstruction is almost always in the distal one-third of the course of the ureter. The importance of an imaging study to diagnose ureteral compromise in all women with retroperitoneal endometriosis cannot be overemphasized.

Endometriosis of the bladder is discovered most often in the region of the trigone or the anterior wall of the bladder. Bladder endometriosis produces midline, lower abdominal, and suprapubic pain; dysuria; and, occasionally, cyclic hematuria. Treatment of endometriosis of the peritoneum over the bladder can be accomplished by medical or surgical means. Ureteral obstruction may be intrinsic, from active endometriosis, or extrinsic, from long-standing fibrotic reactions to retroperitoneal inflammation. Extrinsic endometriosis is three to five times more common than the intrinsic form. There are few reports of endometriosis of the ureter responding to danazol or GnRH agonists. However, long-term follow-up with serial ultrasound imaging or intravenous pyelograms must be undertaken to ensure that the disease process does not recur.

Surgical therapy is the preferred treatment for ureteral obstruction secondary to endometriosis. The operations are rare and should be individualized. The most common surgical approaches include removal of the uterus and both ovaries and the relief of urinary obstruction by ureterolysis or by ureteroneocystostomy. Ureteral resection is often needed if hydronephrosis is present. If ureterolysis is performed, peristalsis in the involved segment of the ureter should be observed, along with adequate resection of the endometriosis and surrounding inflammation in the retroperitoneal space. Ureteroneocystostomy has the advantage of bypassing the urinary obstruction and making it technically easier to resect the area of endometriosis and associated retroperitoneal fibrosis.

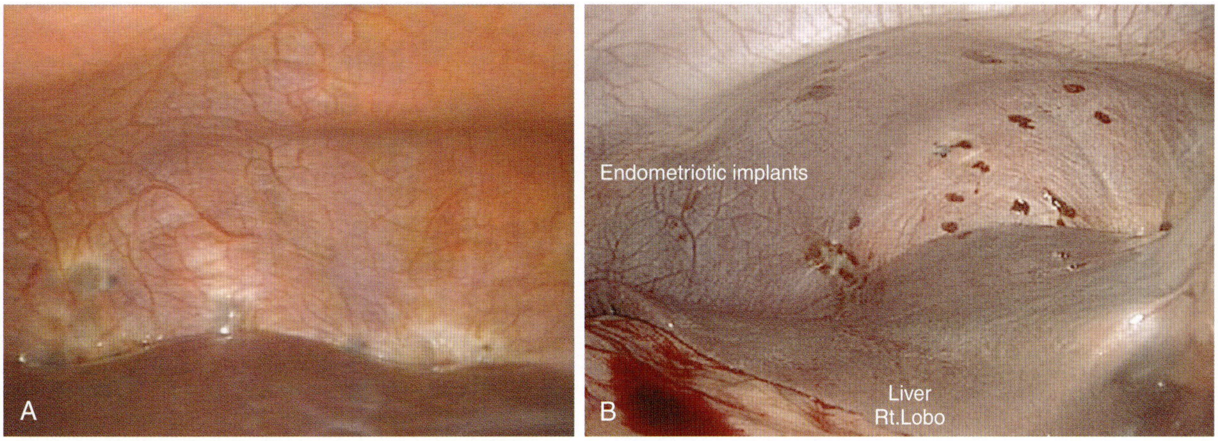


**Fig. 19.23 A,** Fibrotic-type endometriosis involving the right hemidiaphragm. The lesions are seen above the liver. Most are obscured by the liver. **B,** Hemorrhagic-type endometriosis lesions of the right hemidiaphragm. (From Hemmings RR, Falcone T. Endometriosis. In: Falcone T, Hurd WW. *Clinical Reproductive Medicine and Surgery.* Philadelphia: Mosby; 2007:741.)

## EXTRA PELVIC ENDOMETRIOSIS

Endometriosis can also involve the diaphragm (Fig. 19.23). This may be an incidental finding at laparoscopy and can be asymptomatic. However, if a patient is symptomatic, the most common presentation of diaphragmatic endometriosis is right-sided catamenial pneumothorax. Other signs and symptoms can include dyspnea, chest pain, shoulder pain, hemoptysis, and the presence of pulmonary nodules. Medical suppressive therapy is the first approach, although surgery, including pleurodesis, may be considered. These patients should be referred to a thoracic surgeon.

### KEY REFERENCES


Abrão MS, Andres MP, Barbosa RN, Bassi MA, Kho RM. Optimizing perioperative outcomes with selective bowel resection following an algorithm based on preoperative imaging for bowel endometriosis. *J Minim Invasive Gynecol.* 2020,27:883-891.

Adamson GD, Pasta DJ. Endometriosis fertility index: the new, validated endometriosis staging system. *Fertil Steril.* 2010;94:1609-1615.

Attar E, Bulun SE. Aromatase inhibitors: the next generation of therapeutics for endometriosis? *Fertil Steril.* 2006;85:1307-1318.

Barnhart K, Dunsmoor-su R, Coutifaris C. Effect of endometriosis on in vitro fertilization. *Fertil Steril.* 2002;77:1148-1155.

Batt RE, Smith RA. Embryologic theory of histogenesis of endometriosis in peritoneal pockets. *Obstet Gynecol Clin North Am.* 1989;16:15-28.

Brosens IA, Brosens JJ. Redefining endometriosis: Is deep endometriosis a progressive disease? *Hum Reprod.* 2000;15:1-3.

Buck Louis GM, Hediger ML, Peterson CM, et al. Incidence of endometriosis by study population and diagnostic method: the ENDO study. *Fertil Steril.* 2011;96:360-365.

Bulun SE. Mechanisms of disease: endometriosis. *N Engl J Med.* 2009; 360(3):268-279.

Carr BR, Stewart EA, Archer DF et al. Elagolix alone or with add-back therapy in women with heavy menstrual bleeding and uterine leiomyomas: a randomized controlled trial. *Obstet Gynecol.* 2018;132:1252-1264.

Chabbert-Buffet N, Meduri G, Bouchard P, et al. Selective progesterone receptor modulators and progesterone antagonists: mechanisms of action and clinical applications. *Hum Reprod Update.* 2005;11:293-307.

Cheng YM, Wang ST, Chou CY. Serum CA-125 in preoperative patients at high risk for endometriosis. *Obstet Gynecol.* 2002;99:375-380.

Daraï E, Dubernard G, Coutant C, Frey C, Rouzier R, Ballester M. Randomized trial of laparoscopically assisted versus open colorectal resection for endometriosis: morbidity, symptoms, quality of life, and fertility. *Ann Surg.* 2010;251(6):1018-1023.

de Venecia, Ascher SM. Pelvic endometriosis: a spectrum of magnetic resonance imaging findings. *Semin Ultrasound CT MR.* 2015;36(4):385-393.

Dinulescu DM, Ince TA, Quade BJ, et al. Role of K-ras and ten in the development of mouse models of endometriosis and endometrioid ovarian cancer. *Nat Med.* 2005;11:63-70.

Donnez J, Nisolle M, Gillerot S, et al. Rectovaginal septum adenomyotic nodules: a series of 500 cases. *Br J Obstet Gynaecol.* 1997;104:1014-1018.

Dunselman GA, Vermeulen N, Becker C, et al. ESHRE guideline: management of women with endometriosis. *Hum Reprod.* 2014;29(3):400-412.

Evans-Hoeker E, Lessey BA, Jeong JW et al . Endometrial BCL6 overexpression in eutopic endometrium of women with endometriosis. *Reprod Sci.* 2016;23:1234-1241.

Evers JL. Endometriosis does not exist; all women have endometriosis. *Hum Reprod.* 1994;9:2206-2209.

Ezzati M, Carr BR. Elagolix, a novel, orally bioavailable GnRH antagonist under investigation for the treatment of endometriosis-related pain. *Womens Health (Lond).* 2015;11:19-28.

Falconer H, Mwenda JM, Chai DC, et al. Effects of anti-TNF-mAb treatment on pregnancy in baboons with induced endometriosis. *Fertil Steril.* 2008;89(Suppl 5):1537-1545.

Fassbender A, Waelkens E, Verbeeck N, et al. Proteomics analysis of plasma for early diagnosis of endometriosis. *Obstet Gynecol.* 2012;119:276-285.

Fedele L, Bianchi S, Zanconato G, et al. Use of a levonorgestrel-releasing intrauterine device in the treatment of rectovaginal endometriosis. *Fertil Steril.* 2001;75:485-488.

Ferrero S, Remorgida V, Venturini PL, et al. Endometriosis: the effects of dienogest. *BMJ Clin Evid.* 2015.

Flores I, Rivera E, Ruiz LA, et al. Molecular profiling of experimental endometriosis identified gene expression patterns in common with human disease. *Fertil Steril.* 2007;87:1180-1199.

Gargett CE, Masuda H. Adult stem cells in the endometrium. *Mol Hum Reprod.* 2010;16:818-834.

Gestrinone Italian Study Group. Gestrinone versus a gonadotropin-releasing hormone agonist for the treatment off pelvic pain associated with endometriosis: a multicenter, randomized, double-blind study. *Fertil Steril.* 1996;66:911-919.

Giampaolino P, Bifulco G, Di Spiezio Sardo A, Mercorio A, Bruzzese D, Di Carlo C. Endometrioma size is a relevant factor in selection of the most appropriate surgical technique: a prospective randomized preliminary study. *Eur J Obstet Gynecol Reprod Biol.* 2015;195:88-93.

Hamdan M, Omar SZ, Dunselman G, et al. Influence of endometriosis on assisted reproductive technology outcomes: a systematic review and meta-analysis. *Obstet Gynecol.* 2015;125(1):79-88.

Healey M, Cheng C, Kaur H. To excise or ablate endometriosis? A prospective randomized double-blinded trial after 5-year follow-up. *J Minim Invasive Gynecol.* 2014;21(6):999-1004.

Jacobson TZ, Barlow DH, Konincks PR, et al. Laparoscopic surgery for subfertility associated with endometriosis. *Cochrane Database Syst Rev.* 2002;4:CD001398.


**Full references and Suggested readings for this chapter can be found on ExpertConsult.com.**

# 20 Pelvic Organ Prolapse, Abdominal Hernias, and Inguinal Hernias

## Diagnosis and Management

*Anna C. Kirby, Gretchen M. Lentz*

### KEY POINTS

- Pelvic organ prolapse is defined as the descent of one or more compartments of the vagina: the anterior vaginal wall, posterior vaginal wall, uterus (cervix), or apex (vaginal vault or cuff scar after hysterectomy). Pelvic organ prolapse often includes a mixture of anterior, posterior, and apical prolapse, and each compartment should be evaluated under strain before determining the appropriate operative treatment.
- Pelvic organ prolapse is more likely to be symptomatic when the leading edge protrudes past the hymen; it can be managed expectantly if asymptomatic.
- Pessaries should be offered to all women with symptomatic pelvic organ prolapse. Renal function should be evaluated in women with advanced pelvic organ prolapse if the patient declines treatment to reduce the prolapse (because of concern for ureteral obstruction).
- Surgery for pelvic organ prolapse is usually effective at decreasing a vaginal bulge, but the effects on urinary, bowel, and sexual function can vary. It is important to elicit patients' goals before surgery.
- The cardinal and uterosacral ligaments normally hold the uterus and upper vagina in the proper location. Uterosacral and sacrospinous ligaments are the best surgical support structures for apical transvaginal, native tissue pelvic organ prolapse surgery.
- Vaginal vault prolapse can be repaired abdominally or vaginally. An abdominal sacral colpopexy with synthetic mesh appears to have a higher long-term success rates than vaginal surgery without mesh but with higher surgical complication rates.
- All women with significant apical prolapse, anterior prolapse, or both should have a preoperative evaluation for occult stress urinary incontinence, with full bladder cough stress testing or urodynamic testing with the prolapse reduced.

The structural supports of the abdomen and pelvis are susceptible to a number of stresses. **The development of defects might be affected by congenital anatomic predispositions, pregnancy, childbirth injuries, surgical damage, aging, and chronic stresses such as heavy lifting, chronic cough, and straining to defecate. Descent of the pelvic organs is called pelvic organ prolapse. It manifests as a vaginal bulge and is often associated with concurrent urinary, sexual, and bowel symptoms.** It is rarely medically dangerous unless it is associated with evisceration or urinary obstruction, and it can range from asymptomatic or mildly symptomatic to severely debilitating.

## ABDOMINAL WALL HERNIAS

**A hernia is a protrusion or bulge of an organ or part of an organ through the body wall.** The abdominal wall is made up of the following structures, beginning externally: skin; subcutaneous connective tissue; external oblique, internal oblique, and transversus abdominis muscles with their investing fascia; and parietal peritoneum. The rectus abdominis muscles run longitudinally in the midline from the xiphoid to the pubic symphysis. The investing fasciae of the external oblique, internal oblique, and transversus abdominis muscles completely encase the rectus abdominis muscles cephalad to the semilunar line. Caudally from the semilunar line the muscle is completely behind the aponeurosis of the fasciae of these muscles and lies directly on the peritoneum (Fig. 20.1). Normally the investing fasciae join in the midline after surrounding the rectus abdominis muscles.

In the male, the descent of the testes from their original retroperitoneal site to the scrotum necessitates passing through the abdominal wall to the inguinal region. At the level of the transversalis fascia where the descent begins, the internal inguinal ring is formed. The inferior epigastric artery defines the medial margin of this ring as it courses from the external iliac artery medially and superiorly into the rectus sheath. The inguinal canal runs from the internal inguinal ring obliquely downward, emerging through the external inguinal ring and opening in the external oblique aponeurosis just above the pubic spine, and then continuing into the scrotum. This allows for passage of the testes and for the presence of part of the spermatic cord. In the female, the round ligament courses in the same direction but ends short of the labia.

Common hernias are ventral (incisional and umbilical) and groin (inguinal and femoral). Rarer hernias are Spigelian and parastomal. An inguinal hernia—that is, a bulge of peritoneum through the internal inguinal ring and into the inguinal canal—is less common in the female than in the male and is often identified after stretching of the abdominal wall during or after pregnancy. It may be related to a congenital weakness of this area. Occasionally a femoral-type groin hernia may develop. In this case the defect in the transversalis fascia occurs in the Hesselbach triangle, which is an area bounded laterally by the inferior epigastric artery, inferiorly by the inguinal ligament, and medially by the lateral margin of the rectus sheath (Fig. 20.2). The hernia sac passes under the inguinal ligament into the femoral triangle rather than coursing through the inguinal canal. Femoral hernias are more common in females than in males and have higher risk of strangulation (Fitzgibbons, 2015).

A ventral hernia occurs in the abdominal wall away from the groin. Examples include umbilical hernias, which are caused by congenital relaxation of the umbilical ring, and incisional hernias, which are herniations through separation of fascial planes after operative incision. Umbilical hernias are more common in women than men. Incisional hernias generally involve the separation of

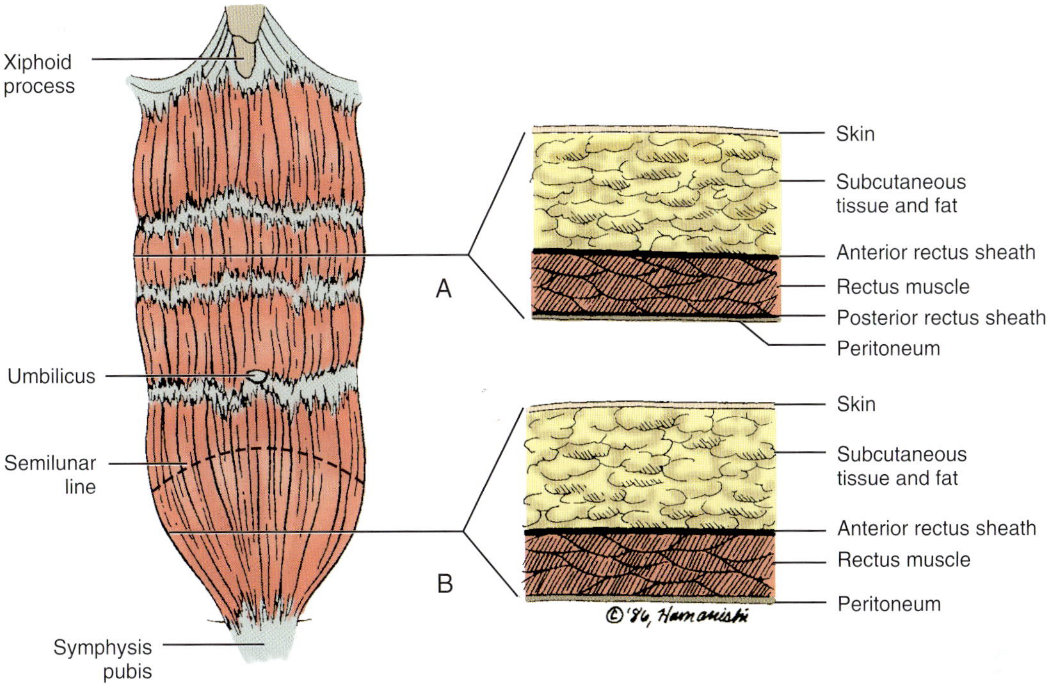


**Fig. 20.1** Layers of the abdominal wall. **A,** Above semilunar line. **B,** Below semilunar line.

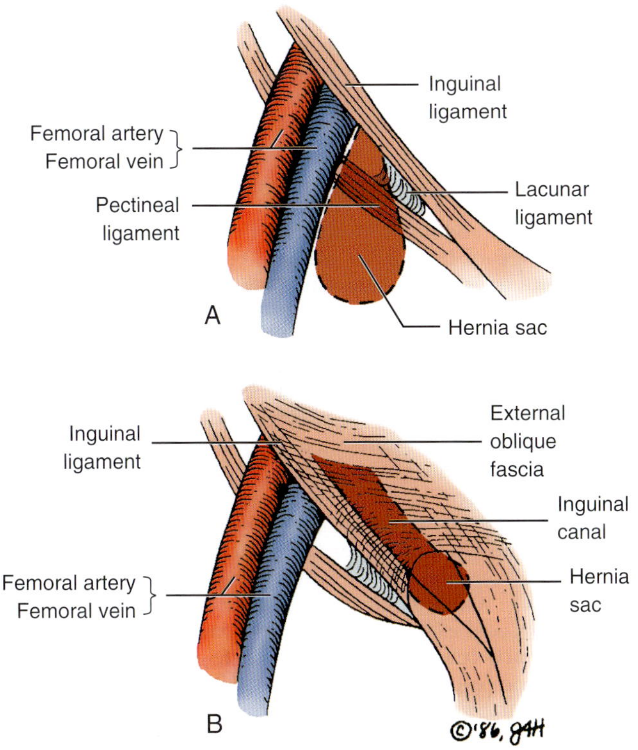


**Fig. 20.2** Right femoral (**A**) and right inguinal (**B**) hernias in the female.

the fascia of the abdominal wall with the hernia sac palpated beneath the skin and subcutaneous tissue. The sac wall is composed of peritoneum. Because the umbilicus consists of a fusion of skin, fascia, and peritoneum, an umbilical hernia generally occurs because the fascial ring is grossly separated, allowing the hernia sac to protrude. This occurs most often in obese women. The hernia sac itself is made up of peritoneum and subcutaneous tissue beneath the skin (Fig. 20.3). Two special ventral hernias include the epigastric hernia, which occurs in a defect of the linea alba above the umbilicus, and spigelian hernia, which is a herniation at a point where the vertical linea semilunaris joins the lateral border of the rectus muscle. Spigelian hernias are rare (<2% of all hernias).

With a reducible hernia, the contents can be returned to the abdominal cavity. If the contents cannot be reduced, the hernia is said to be incarcerated. An incarcerated hernia may be acute, accompanied by pain, or long-standing and asymptomatic. If the blood supply to the incarcerated structure is compromised, the hernia is said to be *strangulated.* Because the hernia sac is primarily prolapsed peritoneum, the hernia itself is not strangulated but only its contents. On rare occasions, a portion of the wall of the hernia sac is composed of an organ such as the sigmoid colon or the cecum.

**Rectus abdominis diastasis is an acquired abdominal wall defect in which the rectus muscles on either side of the midline separate. This is not a true hernia because there is no fascial defect,** but it is mentioned here for differential diagnosis purposes. Pregnancy is a common risk factor for rectus diastasis.

## Etiology

**Hernias may be the result of a congenital malformation. The umbilical hernia is the best example.** Before 10 weeks' gestation, the abdominal contents are partially herniated through the umbilicus into the extra embryonic coelomic cavity; however, after 10 weeks the viscera normally return to the abdominal cavity, and the defect in the abdominal wall closes during subsequent fetal growth. Generally at birth only the space occupied by the umbilical cord remains patent. After the cutting of the cord, the area heals so that the skin in the area of the umbilicus fuses above the closed fascial layer. Some infants at birth will show a small umbilical hernia, but in most instances the fascial defect closes during the first 3 years of life. If it does not close, an umbilical hernia will form. Black infants have umbilical hernias more often than do white infants. Occasionally, umbilical hernias are acquired in adults after the distention of the abdominal cavity with pregnancy or with ascites.

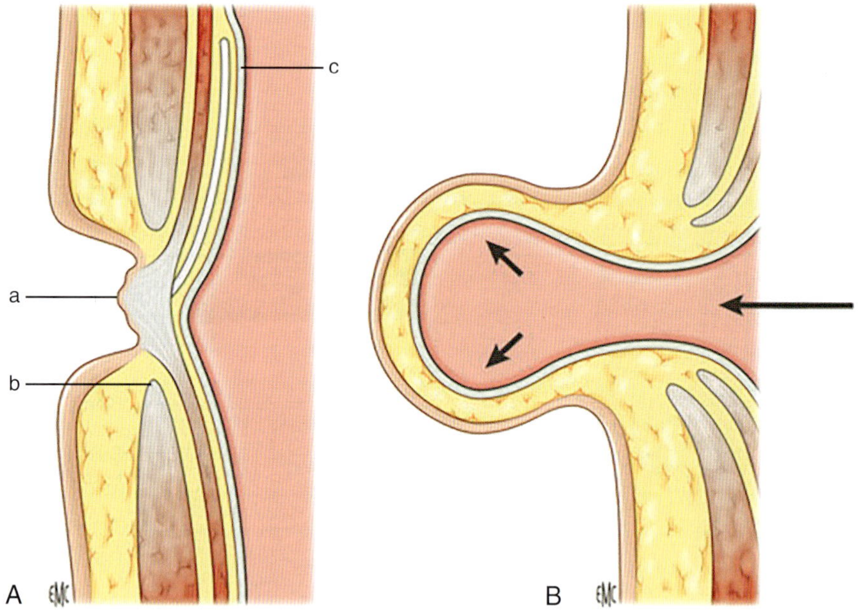


**Fig. 20.3** Umbilical hernia. Schemas depicting the normal umbilicus: **A,** normal anatomy; **B,** in a cirrhotic patient with umbilical hernia. a, umbilicus; b, rectus abdominus muscle, and c parietal peritoneum. (From Dokmak S, Aussilhou B, Belghiti J. Umbilical hernias and cirrhose. *J Visc Surg.* 2012;149(5):e32-e39.)

In rare cases the abdominal wall closure process is less complete during gestation, leading to an omphalocele, which is a hernia sac at the umbilicus covered only by peritoneum and including bowel and other abdominal contents. Omphaloceles are usually seen in infants with other malformations and possibly chromosome anomalies, such as trisomy 13.

Hernias that occur in adults are often associated with trauma or injury. In many instances, the hernia bulge develops slowly after years of heavy labor. It is likely that a congenital anatomic defect was always present but became exaggerated over time, leading to the development of a hernia. It has been suggested that inguinal lesions resulted from inadequate muscle support at the lower area of the inguinal canal, primarily caused by a defect in the internal oblique muscle. Stretching of this area in pregnancy may initiate a hernia, but multifactorial reasons are likely responsible.

**Summarized risk factors for hernia development are:**

History of prior hernia
Male sex
Caucasian race
Chronic cough
Chronic constipation
Abdominal wall injury
Smoking
Family history of hernia

**Incisional hernias generally occur because of poor healing of the fascia after surgery. Risks factors for incisional hernias are usually multifactorial:**

Vertical midline incision
Upper abdominal incision
Older age
Obesity
Smoking
Connective tissue diseases
Malnutrition
Wound infection
Excessive tension on the fascial closure with resultant necrosis of the fascia secondary to suturing

Incisional hernias may also occur because absorbable suture loses its tensile strength before healing is complete. Stress and strain secondary to chronic cough or vomiting in the postoperative period may contribute to the process. Emergency surgery increases the risk of incisional hernia. Incisional hernias develop in 10% to 15% of patients after abdominal laparotomy incisions.

## Symptoms, Signs, and Diagnosis

**Bulges in the abdominal wall lead to the discovery of most ventral or groin hernias in women, either by a physician at the time of physical examination or by the patient.** Occasionally, excessive straining or trauma will be implicated, and the patient may experience a feeling of tearing of tissue. Often the bulges are noted during an increase in intraabdominal pressure such as with coughing, pregnancy or lifting. Most hernias are asymptomatic, but in some cases, particularly with larger ones, there may be aching or discomfort. Should intraabdominal organs move into the sac, the patient may experience some discomfort. Organs that strangulate within the sac cause acute pain and discomfort. Incarcerated organs may give nonspecific visceral pain, which is most likely the result of mesenteric stretching. An incisional hernia with incarceration may present with a bowel obstruction.

**In cases in which a hernia exists but no contents are within the sac, physical examination reveals a weakening at the site of the hernia. It is often possible to feel the "ring" of the hernia as one palpates the defect through the skin and subcutaneous tissue. The patient's straining will generally accentuate the hernia, making it more palpable and visible. In the case of inguinal and femoral hernias, it may be necessary for the patient to be standing for one to palpate the hernia.**

When there are intraabdominal contents within the hernia sac, the hernia is more easily palpated. The physician should then decide, based on his or her attempts to gently milk the contents from the sac back through the defect ring, whether the contents are reducible. For a hernia that does not reduce easily but in which there is no evidence of vascular compromise, it is sometimes useful to apply ice packs to the abdomen in the area of the incarcerated hernia before additional attempts are made to reduce it. In cases of strangulated hernia, evidence of devitalization of an organ, such as fever, leukocytosis, and evidence for an acute abdomen, may be noted.

With classic presentation of strangulated hernia on history and physical examination, surgical management should be pursued without imaging confirmation. If symptoms are present but the examination cannot confirm a hernia, ultrasonography can be ordered. Computed tomography (CT) and magnetic resonance imaging (MRI) provide more anatomic detail and accuracy, but at increased cost and radiation exposure with CT. CT imaging is often recommended for complex, large ventral hernias.

**Although not a hernia, rectus abdominis diastasis is usually quite apparent on physical examination. Having the patient raise her head and begin a sit up, which increase in intraabdominal pressure as the two rectus muscles contract, can make the defect apparent as a vertical, midline bulge.** This can appear as a long prominent ridge extending from the xiphoid to the umbilicus.

## Management of Hernias

**Nonoperative management of ventral wall and incisional hernias in women is often feasible.** Umbilical hernias in little girls generally close by age 3 or 4 years and rarely become incarcerated. Unincarcerated groin hernias are often small and become uncomfortable only with an increase in intraabdominal pressure, such as occurs with pregnancy. Watchful waiting might be appropriate, but surgical repair is often offered. With pregnancy, the opportunity for incarceration is reduced because the increasing size of the uterus pushes bowel contents away from the area of the herniation. Trusses and other supports are generally difficult to fit and are of little value in women. There is no need to restrict physical activities.

**Larger hernias, hernias that continuously contain intraabdominal contents, hernias that cause continuing discomfort, and those that have been incarcerated should be repaired.** Some general principles of operative repair can be stated. Open and laparoscopic inguinal hernia repairs have been compared in randomized trials. The laparoscopic approach is favored because of decreased pain in the short run and long term. Femoral hernias are often repaired laparoscopically. In many cases the fascial defect is large, and the degree of mobilization that is required may be impossible for a tension-free, simple suture repair. In such instances, patching with inert material, such as polypropylene mesh is necessary. Mesh repairs for uncomplicated groin hernia repairs have become the preferred technique because the recurrence rate is lowered; however, the infection risk is higher. Nonmesh repair techniques may be required for patients with active groin infection or contamination (e.g., as a result of bowel perforation from a strangulated hernia),

Umbilical hernia repair can be done open or laparoscopically. In open repair a curved incision is made at the inferior margin of the umbilicus (Fig. 20.4). The umbilicus is dissected free of the sac and reflected upward. The sac is then dissected free of the fascial defect and either reduced or excised, depending on the circumstances. The fascial edges are freshened and either closed by direct approximation anterior to posterior using nonabsorbable sutures or mobilized and closed in a "vest over pants" manner, suturing the anterior edge to the posterior edge in an overlapping fashion. The umbilicus is then tacked to the fascial defect and the skin margin approximated to recreate a normal appearing umbilicus. Large defects or defects where it is not possible to close the fascial edges without tension will require mesh placement. Laparoscopic repair is also possible and useful to assess viability of incarcerated bowel or in larger defects where mesh is needed. Open mesh repair was associated with significant reduction in the recurrence rate compared with suture repair of umbilical hernia in a meta-analysis of four randomized controlled trials (odds ratio [OR], 0.22; 95% confidence interval (CI), 0.10 to 0.48; $P = .0001$) (Shrestha, 2019). A separate multicenter randomized trial showed a high-level evidence for mesh repair even in patients with small hernias of diameter 1 to 4 cm (Kaufmann, 2018).

Incisional hernia surgical repair is too large of a topic to cover here; however, laparoscopic approaches are increasingly common, as is mesh use. In a meta-analysis of five randomized controlled trials involving 611 patients, the recurrence risk and length of hospital stay were similar, but laparoscopic repairs had reduced risk of wound infection compared with open repairs (Al Chalabi, 2015).

For rectus abdominis diastasis, there is evidence that antenatal exercises reduce this risk of developing this condition; however, it is unclear if exercise postpartum helps. Surgical repair can be considered.

### Incisional Hernia Prevention

**Prevention of incisional hernias bears mention because a hernia will develop in 10% to 15% of patients with abdominal incisions.** Preventing wound infection with appropriate antibiotic prophylaxis if indicated and careful surgical technique is worthwhile because the hernia rate increases to 23% with postoperative wound infection. Choosing an off-midline incision has been shown to have fewer incisional hernias than midline incisions. A meta-analysis of abdominal fascial closure concluded that a continuous, slowly absorbing, monofilament suture closure resulted in the lowest rates of incisional hernia. A randomized trial comparing long stitch width (>10 mm) with shorter stitch width (5 to 8 mm) identified longer stitch width as an independent risk factor for the development of both incisional hernia (18% vs. 5.6%) and surgical site infection.

Weight loss and smoking cessation should be recommended because these are risk factors for hernia development.

# PELVIC ORGAN PROLAPSE

**Pelvic organ prolapse (POP) is a condition characterized by the failure of various anatomic structures to support the pelvic viscera. It is defined as the descent of one or more of the vaginal walls or cervix: anterior vaginal wall prolapse (cystocele, urethrocele, paravaginal defect), posterior vaginal wall prolapse (rectocele or enterocele), uterine/cervical prolapse, or vaginal vault prolapse (after hysterectomy, often with an enterocele) (Fig. 20.5). Symptoms can include vaginal bulging, pelvic pressure, need to replace the prolapse (splint) to void or defecate, sexual dysfunction, vaginal bleeding or discharge, and low backache, or POP can be asymptomatic. Symptoms are more common when the prolapse extends beyond the hymen (Fig. 20.6)** (Tan, 2005). **POP usually involves more than one wall of the vagina.**

Present terminology for prolapse refers to ***anterior vaginal wall, posterior vaginal wall,*** and ***vaginal vault prolapse,*** making no assumptions regarding the organs behind the walls. This system has replaced terms such as *cystocele, rectocele,* and *enterocele,* which technically refer to the organs behind the walls of the vagina that are prolapsing. *Cystocele, rectocele,* and *enterocele* are still in wide clinical use and are appropriate with when it is known which organs are prolapsing behind the vaginal walls.

## Epidemiology of Pelvic Organ Prolapse

**POP is common, particularly in parous women, although many are asymptomatic.** The prevalence of POP is 30% to 50% (Nygaard, 2008). **The lifetime risk of undergoing prolapse surgery in the United States is 13%** (Wu, 2014), but most POP does not require treatment (Fig. 20.7). The average age of women having surgery for prolapse is the mid-50s.

**Pelvic support structure defects have been associated with age, parity, vaginal childbirth (neurologic or muscular injury or both), obesity, larger genital hiatus, menopausal status, chronic constipation, connective tissue disorders, genetics/family history, and neurologic diseases** (Blomquist, 2018; Cartwright, 2014) (Box 20.1). **A single vaginal childbirth is associated with up to 10-fold higher odds of POP, and the**

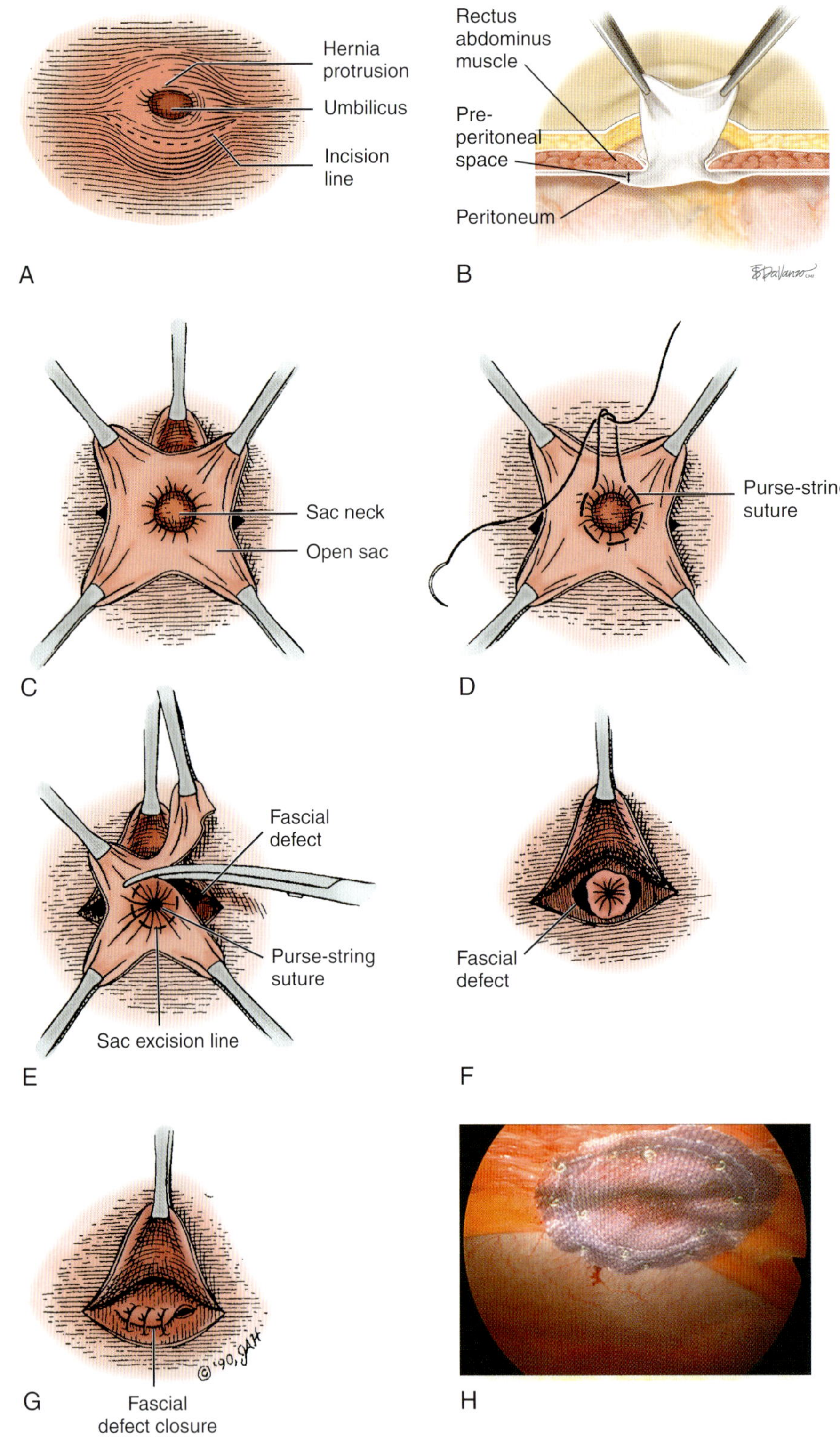


**Fig. 20.4** Repair of umbilical hernia. **A,** Site of incision. **B,** Umbilicus dissected free of sac and reflected upward. **C,** Appearance of sac that is cut open. **D,** Placement of purse-string suture at neck of sac. **E,** Sac dissected free of fascial defect after suture is tied. **F,** Appearance of fascial defect after sac has been excised. **G,** Fascial defect closed; umbilicus will be tacked to it. **H,** Umbilical hernia repair laparoscopically with mesh. Many umbilical hernia repairs are now done with mesh grafts. (From Blair LJ, Kercher KW. Umbilical hernia repair. In *Atlas of Abdominal Wall Reconstruction.* Philadelphia: Elsevier; 2017:360-381.)

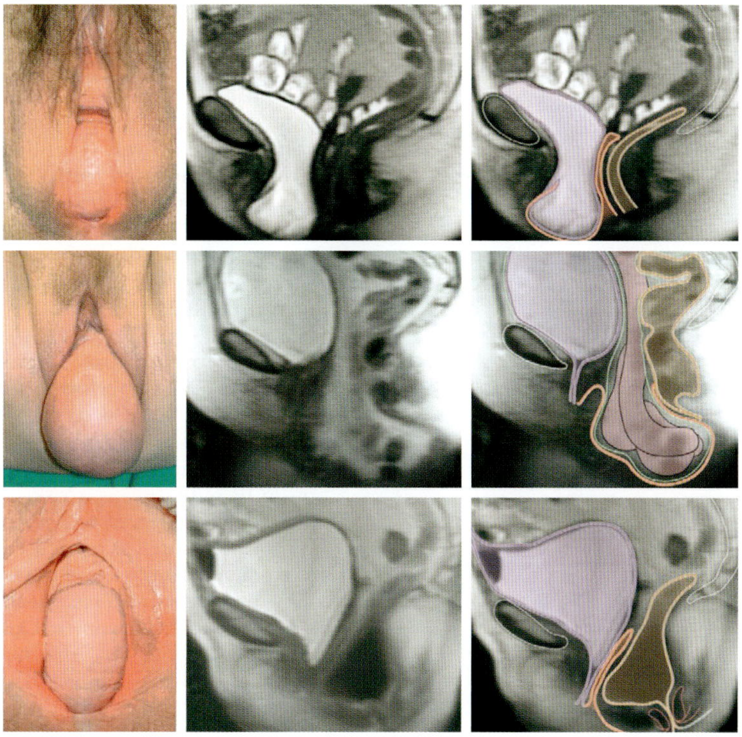

Fig. 20.5 Photographs in lithotomy position and sagittal magnetic resonance images showing vaginal wall prolapse. Prolapse might include *(top to bottom):* bladder (cystocele), small bowel (enterocele) or rectum (rectocele). Purple: bladder; orange: vagina; brown: colon, and rectum; green: peritoneum. (From Jelovsek JE, Maher C, Barber MD. Pelvic organ prolapse. *Lancet.* 2007;369:1027-1038.)

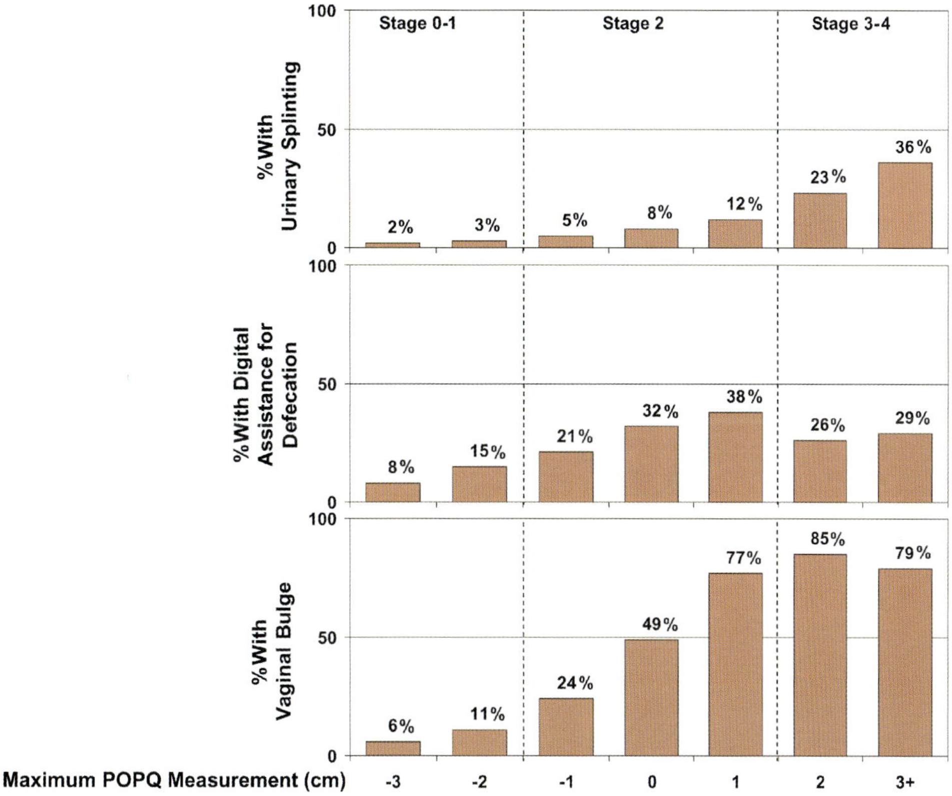


Fig. 20.6 Prevalence of prolapse symptoms per the pelvic organ prolapse quantification (POPQ) system. The percentage of patients who report urinary splinting, digital assistance, and vaginal bulge is demonstrated for each relevant POPQ measurement. (Modified from Tan JS, Lukacz ES, Menefee SA, et al. Predictive value of prolapse symptoms: a large database study. *Int Urogynecol J Pelvic Floor Dysfunct.* 2005;16:203-209.)

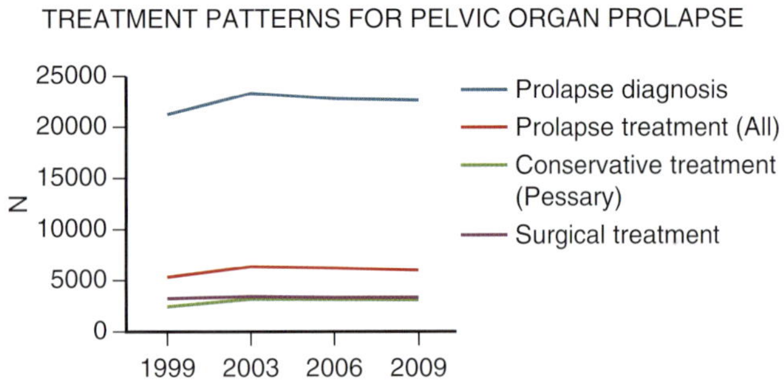


**Fig. 20.7** Prolapse diagnosis and rates of different management patterns among female Medicare beneficiaries. (From Khan AA. Trends in management of pelvic organ prolapse among female Medicare beneficiaries. *Am J Obstet Gynecol.* 2015;212(4):463.e1-463.e8.)

**BOX 20.1** Risk Factors for Development of Pelvic Organ Prolapse

Vaginal childbirth
Increasing parity
Aging
Obesity
Enlarged genital hiatus
Menopausal status
Chronic constipation/straining
Genetic component and family history
Connective tissue disorders (Ehlers-Danlos)
Neurologic injury

**POSSIBLE ASSOCIATIONS WITH PELVIC ORGAN PROLAPSE**

Prior pelvic surgery
Hysterectomy
Race and ethnicity
Irritable bowel syndrome
Episiotomy
Higher weight of the largest infant delivered vaginally
Chronic cough and respiratory diseases
Heavy lifting

**risk of surgery for POP may increase with each additional vaginal delivery** (Larsson, 2009). In some cases, the injury from childbirth is subtle, but sometimes it is readily apparent, as shown in the images of this woman who had complete right-sided avulsion of her puborectalis (one of the levator ani muscles) after a normal vaginal delivery (Fig. 20.8). **Obstetric levator avulsion is strongly associated with POP.** Of 453 participants who were 6 to 17 years from first delivery (median, 11 years), levator avulsion was identified in 15% and was more common among those who had undergone forceps-assisted delivery ($P < .001$). Levator avulsion was strongly associated with prolapse beyond the hymen (OR, 2.7; 95% CI, 1.3 to 5.7) and with symptoms of prolapse (OR, 3.0; 95% CI, 1.2 to 7.3) (Handa, 2019). **Approximately 98% of prolapse surgery is performed on parous women, and 2% is performed on women who have never been pregnant.** Compared with spontaneous vaginal delivery, cesarean delivery was associated with significantly lower hazard for POP (Blomquist, 2018). It is unclear if prior hysterectomy for a non-POP indication is a risk factor for developing prolapse. White women appeared to have more overall symptom bother from prolapse, as well as more urinary symptoms, compared with black women, when assessed by validated questionnaire tools in a cohort of patients who underwent prolapse surgery. Compared with African American women, Latina and white women had four to five times higher risk of symptomatic prolapse, and white women had 1.4-fold higher risk of objective prolapse with leading edge of prolapse at or beyond the hymen.

**Recurrent POP after surgery remains a challenge, especially for the anterior vaginal wall. Risk factors for recurrent POP include age younger than 60 years in women who had vaginal surgery, obesity, and stage III or IV prolapse.** Addressing modifiable risk factors before initial surgery might be important (e.g., obesity, chronic constipation). Suspension of the vaginal apex is associated with a decreased reoperation rate (Eilber, 2013).

Often, damage to the pelvic floor results in urinary incontinence instead of or in addition to POP. Urinary incontinence is discussed in detail in Chapter 21.

## Normal Pelvic Anatomy

**Normal support of pelvic organs is provided by several key anatomic structures, including the pelvic floor muscles and**

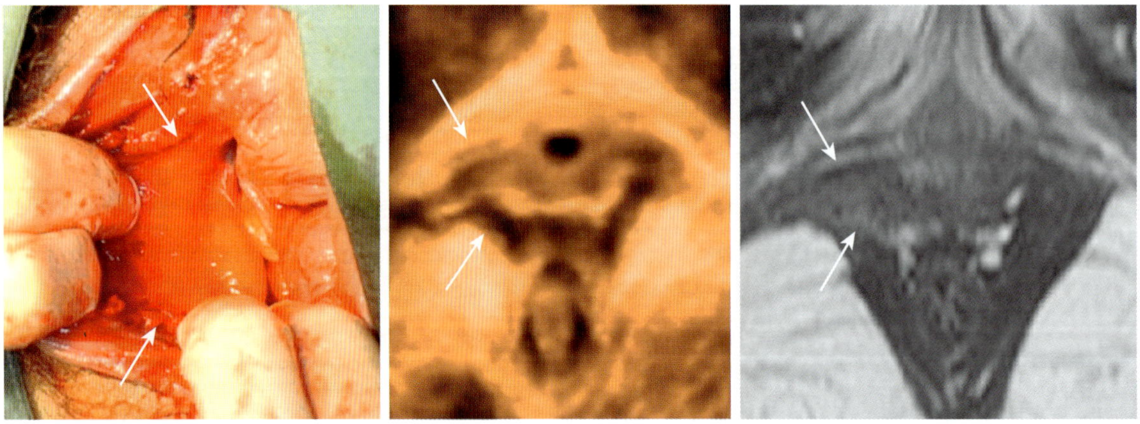

**Fig. 20.8** Right-sided puborectalis avulsion after normal vaginal delivery at term. The *left image* shows appearances immediately postpartum, with the avulsed muscle exposed by a large vaginal tear. The middle image shows a rendered volume (axial plane, translabial three-dimensional ultrasound scan) 3 months postpartum, and the *right image* shows magnetic resonance imaging findings (single slice in the axial plane) at 3.5 months postpartum. *Top arrows* indicate the site of avulsion on the inferior pubic ramus, and *bottom arrows* show the retracted stump of puborectalis. (From Dietz HP, Gillespie A, Phadke P. Avulsion of the pubovisceral muscle associated with large vaginal tear after normal vaginal delivery at term: a case report. *Aust N Z J Obstet Gynaecol.* 2007;47:341-344.)

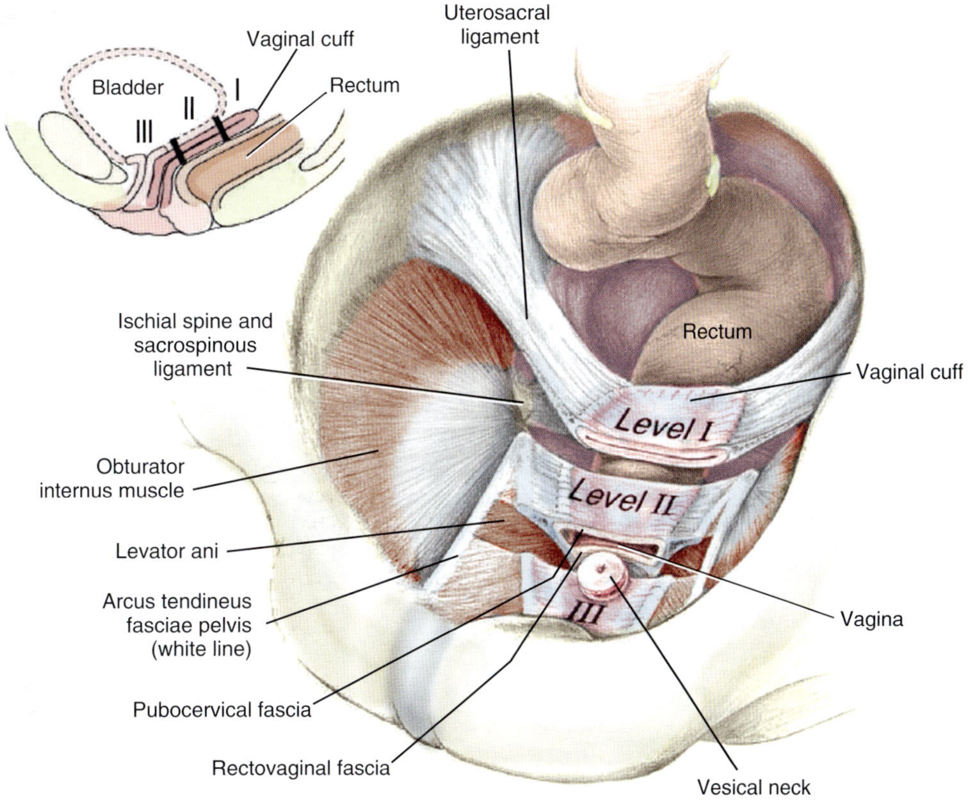


**Fig. 20.9** Level I (suspension) and level II (attachment) support of the vagina. In level I the paracolpium (uterosacral ligaments) suspends the vagina from the lateral pelvic walls. Fibers of level I extend both vertically and posteriorly toward the sacrum. In level II support, the vagina is attached to the arcus tendineus fasciae pelvis and superior fascia of the levator ani by condensations of the levator fascia (e.g., endopelvic and pubocervical fascia). In level III support, the vaginal wall is attached directly to adjacent structures without intervening paracolpium (i.e., urethra anteriorly, perineal body posteriorly, and levator ani muscles laterally). (From Biggs GY, Nitti VW, Karram M. Pelvic organ prolapse. In: Nitti VW, ed. *Vaginal Surgery for the Urologist.* Philadelphia: Elsevier; 2012:17-22. Data modified from DeLancey J. Anatomic aspects of vaginal eversion after hysterectomy. *Am J Obstet Gynecol.* 1992;166(6 Pt 1):1717-1728.)

**connective tissue attachments** (Fig. 20.9). Level I support of the vaginal apex and cervix is provided by the uterosacral and cardinal ligaments and associated connective tissue, level II support of the midvagina is provided by connective tissue attachments to the arcus tendineus fasciae pelvis on the lateral pelvic side walls, level III support of the distal (inferior) vagina is provided by the perineal membrane and muscles (DeLancey, 1992), and all of the attachments are connected through endopelvic connective tissue.

**The vagina is a hollow, fibromuscular tube composed of three layers: nonkeratinizing stratified epithelium, lamina propria (loose connective tissue), and muscularis (fibromuscular tissue with collagen and elastin). It is supported by attachments to the sacrum, coccyx, and lateral pelvic sidewalls. In young, nulliparous women, the distal one-third of the vagina is oriented vertically and the upper two-thirds is oriented horizontally** (Fig. 20.10). Anteriorly the vagina supports the base of the bladder and urethra, posteriorly it supports the rectum, and superiorly it supports the small bowel. The vagina is fused with the vaginal muscularis inferiorly.

## Pathophysiology of Pelvic Organ Prolapse

**The pathophysiology of POP is probably multifactorial.** Bump and Norton outlined a useful concept for looking at risk factors as predisposing, inciting, promoting, or decompensating (Fig. 20.11). Although imaging is not usually necessary in the clinical evaluation of POP, imaging techniques, including ultrasonography and MRI, in research studies have improved our understanding of support defects. In one study, MRI three-dimensional (3D) color thickness mapping was used to compare the levator ani of 30 women: 10 asymptomatic, 10 with urodynamic stress incontinence, and 10 with POP. Loss of levator muscle bulk was found in women with POP and stress incontinence (Fig. 20.12) (Hoyte, 2004). Theoretic explanations for these findings include muscle atrophy from denervation from childbirth injuries, muscle wasting from muscle insertion detachment from childbirth injuries, or both. Remarkably, the pelvic floor muscles and pelvic support structures usually recover to a large extent after childbirth so that most women do not have symptomatic prolapse until later in life when the effects of aging combine with the childbirth injuries to result in clinically significant prolapse.

MRI studies of POP have also shown that women with POP have a more vertical vaginal axis and urogenital hiatus than women without POP. In young, healthy women without POP, the upper two-thirds of the vagina is nearly horizontal (see Fig. 20.10).

## Pelvic Organ Prolapse Symptoms

**Symptoms of POP are often not specific to the area that is prolapsing, and many women have no symptoms. The classic symptoms of prolapse include vaginal heaviness, pressure and vaginal bulging. Because more than one pelvic floor disorder**

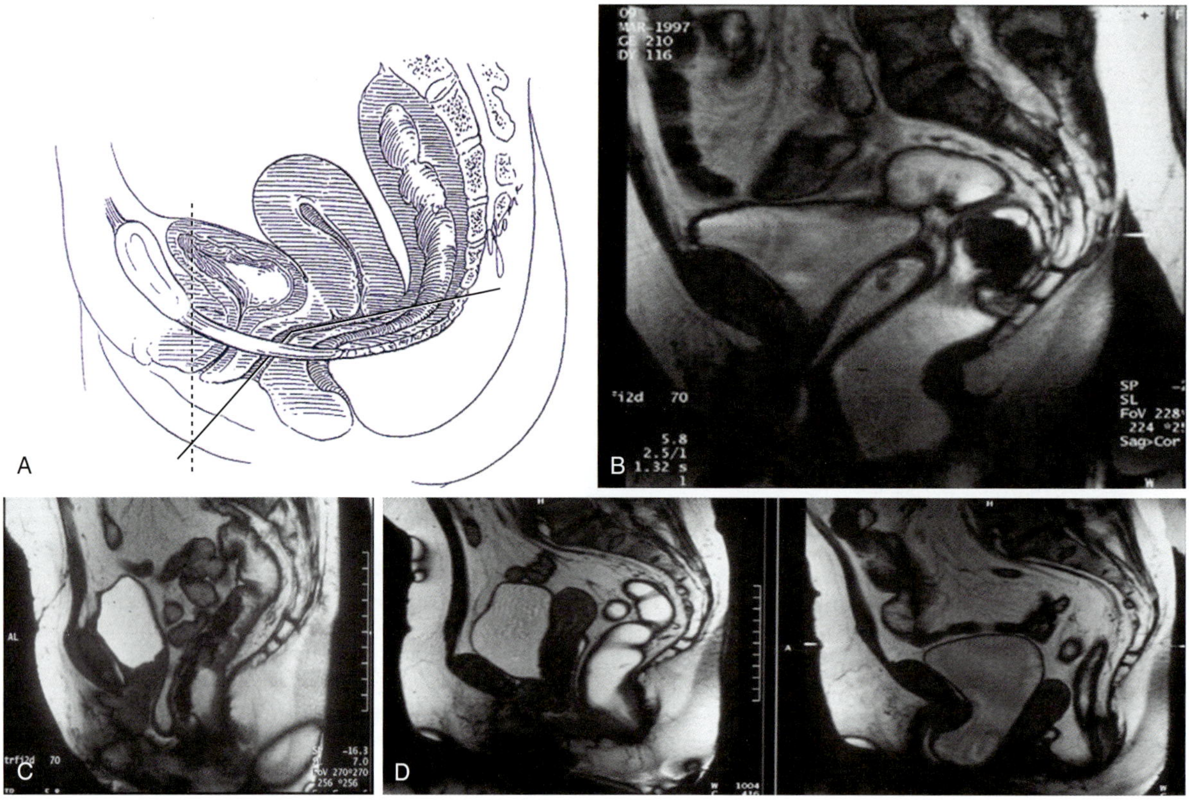

**Fig. 20.10** **A** and **B,** In the nulliparous patient, the lower one-third of the vagina is oriented more vertically, whereas the upper two-thirds deviate horizontally, thereby maintaining the vaginal axis in an almost horizontal position. **C,** During stressful maneuvers such as coughing or straining, the levator hiatus is shortened anteriorly by contraction of the pubococcygeus muscles. **D,** In the case of genital prolapse when the levator ani support is lost, the vaginal axis becomes more vertical, the urogenital hiatus broadens, and fascial supports are strained. (From Chapple CR, Milsom I. Urinary incontinence and pelvic prolapse. In: Wein AJ, Kavoussi LR, Novick AC, et al. *Campbell-Walsh Urology.* 10th ed. Philadelphia: Elsevier; 2012:1871-1895.e7.)

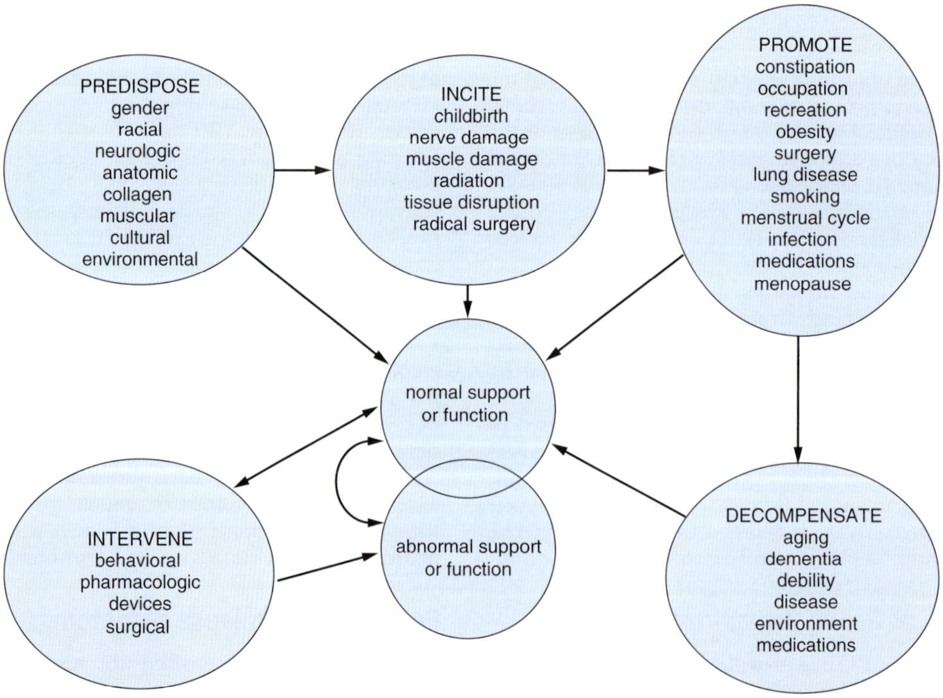


**Fig. 20.11** Model for the development of pelvic floor dysfunction in women. (From Bump RC, Norton PA. Epidemiology and natural history of pelvic floor dysfunction. *Obstet Gynecol ClNA.* 1998;25(4):723.)

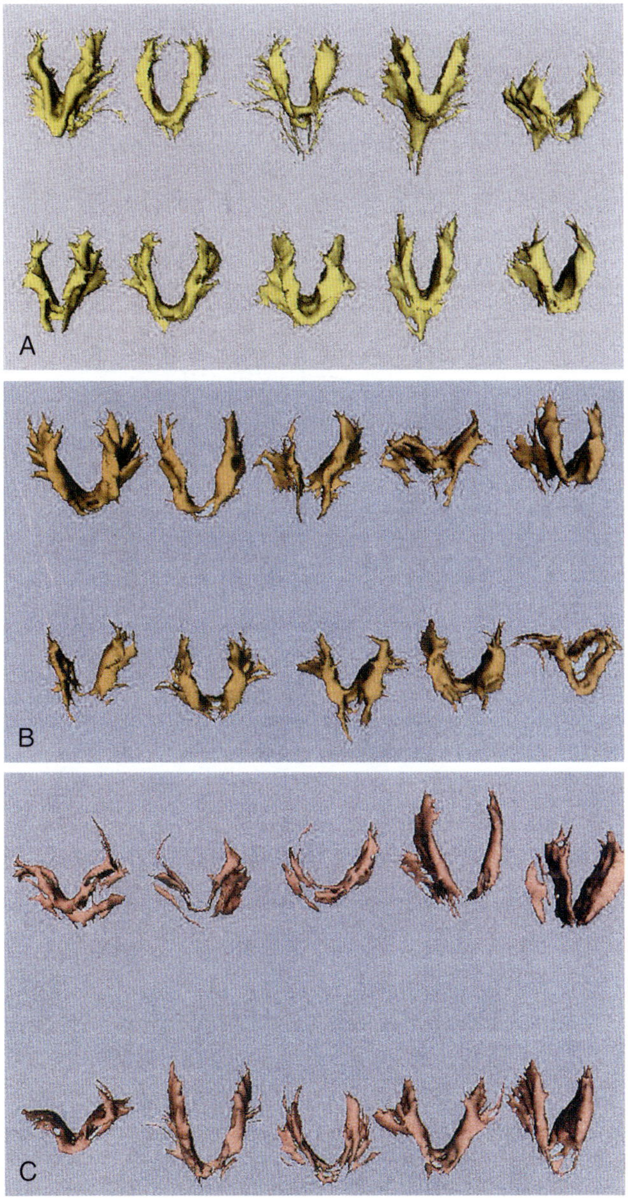


**Fig. 20.12** Color images of reconstructed levator ani muscles from three subject groups: (**A**) asymptomatic group, (**B**) stress incontinence group, and (**C**) prolapse group. (From Hoyte L, Jakab M, Warfield SK. Levator ani thickness variations in symptomatic and asymptomatic women using magnetic resonance-based 3-dimensional color mapping. *Am J Obstet Gynecol.* 2004;191:856.)

**is often present, urinary, bowel, and sexual symptoms should be assessed in addition to prolapse symptoms in any woman with POP** (Box 20.2). Urinary symptoms associated with prolapse can include urinary incontinence, difficulty voiding, urinary urgency, slow urinary stream, splinting (reducing the prolapse) to void, or a sensation of incomplete bladder emptying. Bowel symptoms associated with prolapse can include constipation, straining, incomplete evacuation, fecal incontinence, or splinting to achieve bowel movements. Associated sexual symptoms may include discomfort, irritation, and decreased sexual desire. Vaginal bleeding might occur from erosions of exposed vaginal epithelium. Note that if a postmenopausal woman with prolapse has vaginal bleeding and there are no obvious erosions, a uterine source must also be considered. Back pain and pelvic pain are not reliably associated with prolapse.

**BOX 20.2** Pelvic Organ Prolapse Symptom Categories for Clinical Evaluation

Lower urinary tract symptoms
Urinary incontinence
Frequency, urgency, nocturia
Voiding difficulty: slow stream, incomplete emptying, obstruction
Urinary splinting

**BOWEL SYMPTOMS**

Constipation
Straining
Incomplete evacuation
Bowel splinting
Anal incontinence

**SEXUAL SYMPTOMS**

Interference with sexual activity
Dyspareunia
Decreased sexual desire
Urinary incontinence with intercourse, orgasm

**OTHER SYMPTOMS**

Pelvic pressure, heaviness, pain
Presence of vaginal bulge/mass
Low back pain
Tampon not retained
Quality-of-life effects

**A patient with POP should also be asked about how her prolapse symptoms affect her quality of life, emotional health, and social interactions as well as whether or not they affect her ability to do usual daily chores, exercise, and participate in social events.** Validated, self-administered questionnaires are available, such as the Pelvic Organ Prolapse Quality of Life (P-QOL) scale and the Pelvic Floor Distress Inventory, which cover these categories. Understanding the woman's goals for treatment is important because often there are multiple symptoms in each of these areas that cause varying degrees of bother and distress.

If a woman with objective prolapse does not have any bothersome symptoms or evidence of associated medical risks such as urinary retention or renal impairment from urethral or ureteral kinking, she does not need treatment.

## Measuring Pelvic Organ Prolapse

**POP is best measured with a patient straining in the lithotomy position, although the physician should ask the patient if this reproduces her maximum bulge and, if not, repeat the examination in the standing position.** Maximum prolapse is more likely to be observed with a full bladder in the standing position at the end of the day. **All three compartments (anterior, posterior, and apical) should be individually assessed in all patients with prolapse.** To observe and measure anterior vaginal wall prolapse, a retractor or posterior wall blade of a Pederson or Graves speculum is used to depress the posterior vaginal wall without artificially supporting the apex. The patient is then asked to strain, and the amount of anterior vaginal wall prolapse is noted. This is repeated by using one blade of the speculum to depress the anterior vaginal wall to evaluate the posterior vaginal wall. To assess apical descent, a measuring device such a uterine sound or POPQ (Pelvic Organ Prolapse Quantification) stick can be placed in the apex or the examiner's finger can be placed on the vaginal vault or cervix while the patient strains.

**It is important to measure or at least qualitatively assess all of the vaginal walls because often more than one compartment is affected. For instance, at least 85% of patient with anterior vaginal wall prolapse more than 1 cm outside the hymen have**

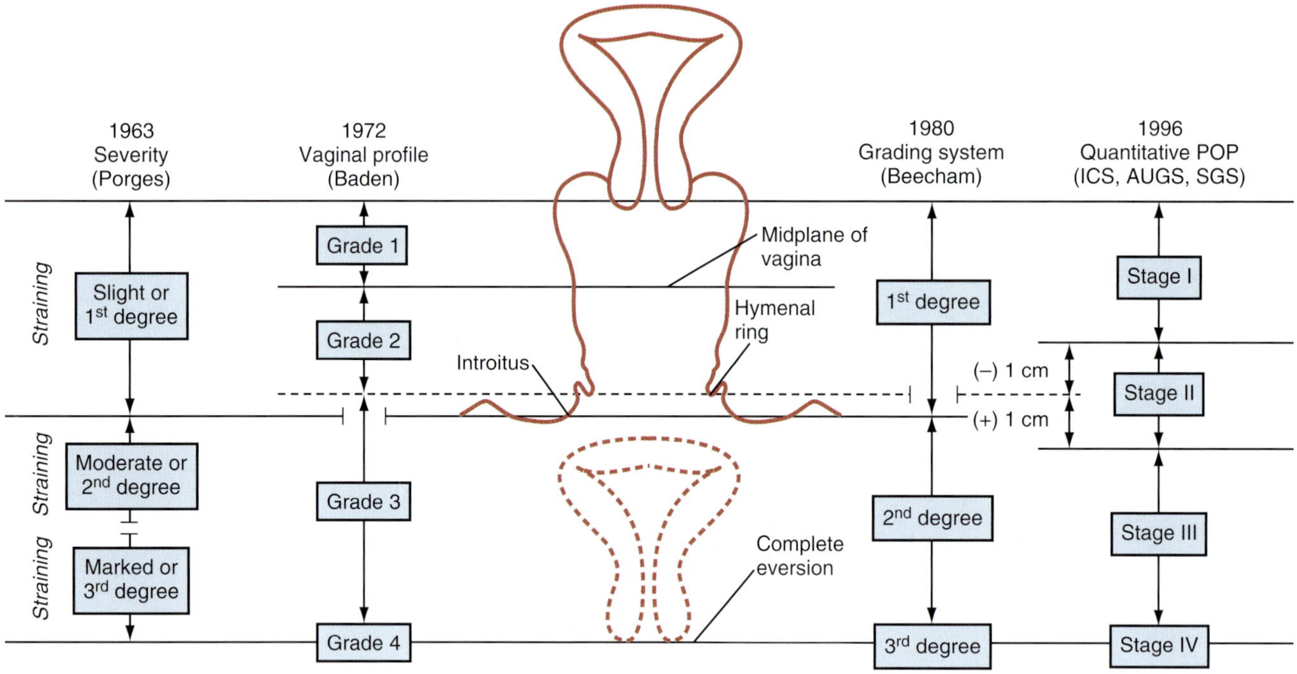


**Fig. 20.13** Visual comparison of systems used to quantify pelvic organ prolapse (POP). *AUGS,* American Urogynecologic Society; *ICS,* International Continence Society; *SGS,* Society of Gynecologic Surgeons. (From Theofrastous JP, Swift SE. The clinical evaluation of pelvic floor dysfunction. *Obstet Gynecol Clin North Am.* 1998;25(4):783-804.)

**associated apical descent** (Elliott, 2013). This is important to know for planning surgical correction because failure to address all areas of descent increases the risk of prolapse recurrence.

There are several systems for objectively measuring POP. In one system, prolapse into the upper barrel of the vagina is called **first degree**, prolapse is to the introitus is **second degree**, prolapse past the introitus is **third degree**, and complete eversion of the vagina is **fourth degree** prolapse. In the Baden-Walker system, **grade 0** is normal position, **grade 1** is descent halfway to the hymen, **grade 2** is descent to the hymen, **grade 3** is descent halfway past the hymen, and **grade 4** is maximum possible descent (Baden, 1972). Although these systems are commonly used and reasonable, they provide no information regarding which walls of the vagina are prolapsed and are rather imprecise regarding the severity of the prolapse, so in 1996 the Pelvic Organ Prolapse Quantification (**POP-Q**) system was developed (see the next section of this chapter) (Bump, 1996). A comparison of these measurement systems is shown in Fig. 20.13. Whatever system is used, it is important to measure all three compartments (anterior, posterior, and apical) and document the level of prolapse compared with the introitus or hymen while the patient strains.

The degree of prolapse can vary by day depending on time of day and recent activities, so it is helpful to ask a patient if what you are seeing in clinic is what she experiences at home. In addition, if the prolapse measured while she is supine on an examination table does not reproduce the prolapse she reports, the examination should be repeated with the patient straining in a standing rather than supine position.

Vaginal tissues should also be checked for ulceration and bleeding. Pelvic floor muscle bulk, symmetry, and function should be assessed during the bimanual examination by asking the woman to tighten her muscles like she is trying to inhibit voiding or flatus. A bimanual examination of the uterus and adnexa, if present, should always be performed to screen for masses and help with surgical planning if indicated.

## Pelvic Organ Prolapse Quantification (POP-Q)

In 1996 the International Continence Society (ICS), the American Urogynecologic Society (AUGS), and the Society of Gynecologic Surgeons (SGS) adopted a standardized terminology for the description of female POP (anterior, posterior, and uterine/cervical or vault prolapse, as mentioned earlier) and a standard measurement system for POP: the POP-Q (Bump, 1996). POP-Q is an objective, site-specific system for describing, quantifying, and staging pelvic support and was developed to enhance clinical and academic communication with respect to individual patients and populations of patients.

In the POP-Q system, as shown in Fig. 20.14, all measurements except for total vaginal length (TVL) are performed while the patient strains (bears down). Point Aa is a point located in the midline of the anterior wall 3 cm proximal to the external urethral meatus and is roughly the location of the urethrovesical crease (Fig. 20.15). Point Ba represents the most distal position of the anterior vaginal wall between Aa and the cervix or cuff. Point C represents either the most distal edge of the cervix or the leading edge of the vaginal cuff if a hysterectomy has been performed. Point D represents the location of the posterior fornix (pouch of Douglas) or the posterior point of attachment of the uterosacral ligaments (there is debate among the experts) in a woman with a cervix. In a patient who has no cervix, no D point is measured. Point Bp is the most distal of any part of the upper posterior vaginal wall between Ap and the cervix or cuff, and point Ap is a point located in the midline of the posterior vaginal wall 3 cm proximal to the hymen. These points should be expressed in centimeters above or below the hymen (i.e., negative measurements are above the hymen and positive measurements are below the hymen). PB, which is the length of the perineal body between the posterior vagina and rectum, and GH, which is the genital hiatus measurement from the urethra to the posterior vagina, are measured during strain and do not have positive or negative values because they are not compared with the hymen.

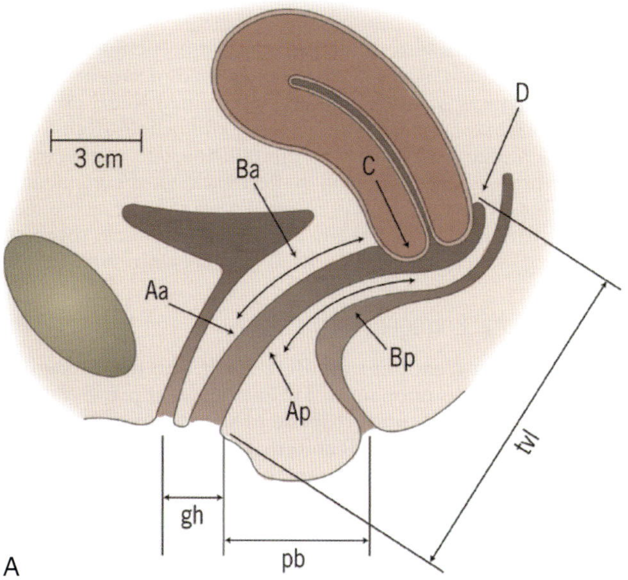


B

| Point | Description | Range of values |
|---|---|---|
| Aa | Anterior vaginal wall 3 cm proximal to the hymen | –3 cm to +3 cm |
| Ba | Most distal position of remaining upper anterior vaginal wall | –3 cm to +tvl |
| C | Most distal edge of cervix or vaginal cuff scar | – |
| D | Posterior fornix (N/A if post-hysterectomy) | – |
| Ap | Posterior vaginal wall 3 cm proximal to the hymen | –3 cm to +3 cm |
| Bp | Most distal position of remaining upper posterior vaginal wall | –3 cm to +tvl |
| gh (genital hiatus) | Measured from middle of external urethral meatus to posterior midline hymen | – |
| pb (perineal body) | Measured from posterior margin of gh to middle of anal opening | – |
| tvl (total vaginal length) | Depth of vagina when point D or C is reduced to normal position | – |

**Fig. 20.14 A,** Landmarks for the Pelvic Organ Prolapse Quantification System (POP-Q) system. **B,** POP-Q points of reference. (**A,** from Bump RC, Mattiasson A, Bo K, et al. The standardization of terminology of female pelvic organ prolapse and pelvic floor dysfunction. *Am J Obstet Gynecol.* 1996;175(1):10–17. **B** from and **A** also modified from Kobashi KC. Evaluation of patients with urinary Incontinence and pelvic prolapse. In: Wein AJ, Kavoussi LR, Novick AC, et al. *Campbell-Walsh Urology.* 10th ed. Philadelphia: Elsevier; 2012:1896-1908.e30.)

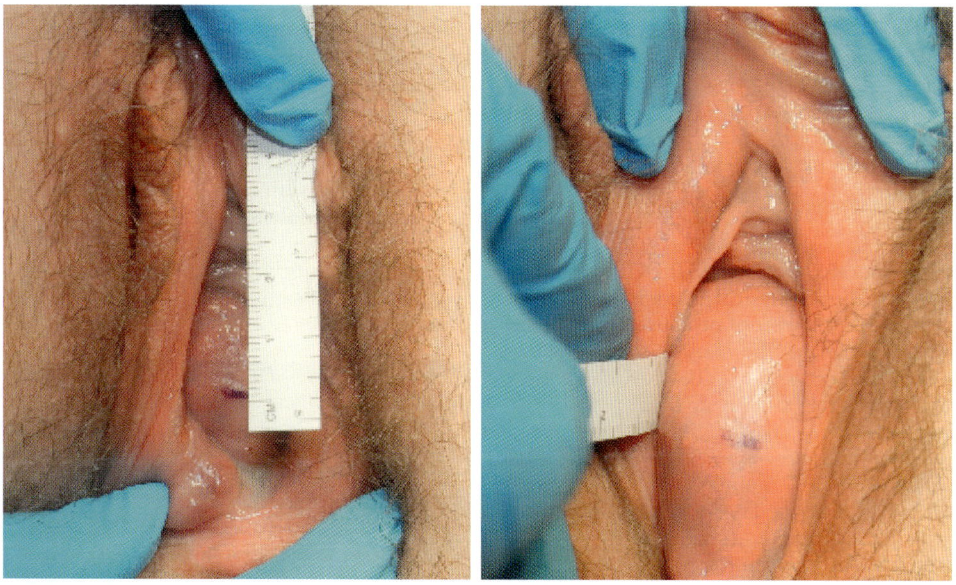

**Fig. 20.15** Measuring point Aa. At rest, the Aa point is marked 3 cm proximal to the urethral meatus along the anterior vaginal wall *(left).* Then the patient is asked to strain, and the location of this point is measure in relation to the plane of the hymenal remnant *(right).* In this case Aa is equal to +2 cm (2 cm past the hymen). In clinical practice, an imaginary mark is used. (From Reid F. Assessment of pelvic organ prolapse. *Obstet Gynaecol Reprod Med.* 2011;21(7):190-197.)

## Stage

The most severe prolapse measurement on any of the vaginal walls can then be used to assign the **stage** of prolapse, as described in Box 20.3: **Stage 0**: no prolapse; **stage I**: the most distal prolapse is more than 1 cm above (inside) the hymen; **stage II**: prolapse between 1 cm above and 1 cm below (outside) the hymen; **stage III**: prolapse more than 1 cm beyond the hymen but no farther than TVL − 2 cm; and **stage IV**: complete eversion/procidentia.

The POP-Q provides a clear and complete description of a patient's prolapse that facilitates effective communication between physicians and reproducible, meaningful measures for research.

**BOX 20.3** Staging of Pelvic Floor Prolapse Using International Continence Society Terminology

**STAGE 0**

No prolapse is demonstrated. Points Aa, Ap, Ba, and Bp are all at −3 cm, and either point C or D is between total vaginal length −2 cm.

**STAGE I**

Criteria for stage 0 are not met, but the most distal portion of the prolapse is more than 1 cm above the level of the hymen.

**STAGE II**

The most distal portion of the prolapse is 1 cm or less proximal or distal to the plane of the hymen.

**STAGE III**

The most distal portion of the prolapse is more than 1 cm below the plane of the hymen but protrudes no farther than 2 cm less than the total vaginal length in centimeters.

**STAGE IV**

Essentially complete eversion of the total length of the lower genital tract.

## Conservative Management of Pelvic Organ Prolapse

### Expectant Management

**If the patient is not bothered by the prolapse, it can be left alone and managed expectantly unless it causes urinary retention or hydronephrosis no matter what degree or stage it is.** Patients can be advised to do pelvic floor strengthening exercises (i.e., Kegels, discussed in Chapter 21) with or without a pelvic floor physical therapist to decrease the risk that mild POP will progress and become symptomatic.

Treatment of vaginal wall prolapse may be nonoperative or operative depending on patient preferences and goals.

### Pelvic Floor Strengthening

**Women with mild to moderate (e.g., stage II) POP may elect for treatment with pelvic floor physical therapy and Kegel exercises, which can decrease the risk of prolapse progression and can be effective at improving the sensation of pressure from mild POP** (Kegel exercises are described in Chapter 21). Pelvic floor physical therapy can also treat associated urinary, bowel, and sexual dysfunction.

There is reasonable evidence to recommend pelvic floor exercises. In one multicenter study, 447 women were randomly assigned to receive individualized pelvic floor muscle training or a prolapse lifestyle advice leaflet with no muscle training (control group). At 6 and 12 months, the women assigned to pelvic floor muscle training had fewer prolapse symptoms as measured by a prolapse symptom questionnaire (the Pelvic Organ Prolapse Symptom Score [POP-SS]) than the control group (Hagen, 2014). Another randomized controlled trial investigated morphologic and functional changes after pelvic floor muscle training in 109 women with stage I to III POP (Braekken, 2010). This supervised training led to a 44% increase in muscle strength, a 15% increase in muscle thickness, a decreased levator hiatus area, shortened muscle length, and elevation of the bladder and rectum positions. It took 6 months of muscle training to achieve these results, so this option requires motivated patients. A follow-up study by the same group reported that 11 (19%) of women in the exercise group improved one stage on the POP-Q system compared with 4 controls (8%). This improvement in stage corresponded with reduced frequency and bother of vaginal bulging and heaviness by 74% and 67%, respectively.

About half of patients cannot isolate their pelvic floor muscles to do Kegel exercises and need to be coached or taught how to do these exercises. Women who have performed Kegel exercises on their own and have not improved may still benefit from working with a physical therapist who can individualize muscle training and provide feedback and biofeedback to these patients. Pelvic floor strengthening has essentially no risks or side effects (unless a patient does too many and develops muscle soreness) and so should be offered to nearly all patients with POP.

### Topical Vaginal Estrogen

**Although not a treatment for POP itself, the use of vaginal estrogen in postmenopausal patients may improve vaginal atrophy and patient comfort if the prolapsed vaginal epithelium is dry, irritated, or ulcerated.** There is no evidence that estrogen therapy will prevent or treat POP, but it can often make existing POP less uncomfortable.

The use of vaginal estrogen can also make vaginal intercourse more comfortable; for patients with dyspareunia (with or without prolapse), vaginal estrogen should always be considered because atrophic vaginitis caused by lack of estrogen is much more likely to cause pain with vaginal intercourse than prolapse. Vaginal estrogen can improve the comfort and decrease the risk of irritation and erosions from pessaries (described later), and it can decrease irritative bladder symptoms including frequency, urgency, nocturia, and frequent urinary tract infections.

There are several ways to apply topical vaginal estrogens (vaginal creams, vaginal tablets, and a vaginal ring), and they all have similar efficacy. Because the dose of vaginal estrogen is very low, using vaginal estrogen is not associated with the development of cancers or blood clots and can be offered to almost all women, even many of those with a personal history of breast cancer or deep venous thrombosis.

### Pessaries

**Nonoperative support of the POP can also be achieved with a silicone vaginal support device called a pessary** (Fig. 20.16). If silicone pessaries are not available, a woman can support her prolapse with intermittent use of a large tampon, although support objects with absorptive properties may be associated with

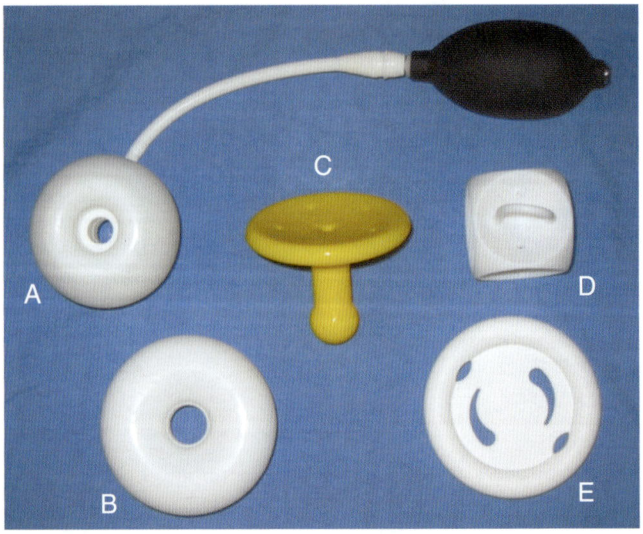


**Fig. 20.16** Examples of pessaries: **A,** inflatable; **B,** donut; **C,** Gellhorn; **D,** cube; **E,** ring with support.

toxic shock syndrome if left in for prolonged periods and so need to be removed more often.

**All women should be offered pessary management for symptomatic prolapse, regardless of the age of the patient or stage of the prolapse. Approximately 85% of patients can be successfully fit with a pessary.** Pessary management should be particularly encouraged as an alternative to surgery in women with medical conditions that make surgery dangerous and in women who have not completed childbearing.

Pessaries support the vagina in its normal position in the pelvis, thus supporting the surrounding structures including the uterus, bladder, small bowel, and rectum. Pessaries are available in varying shapes and sizes and need to be fitted for each individual patient. There are limited data to direct the selection of the pessary based on patient factors or type of prolapse, and pessary fitting is largely trial and error. When trying a new pessary, the patient is asked if the pessary feels comfortable; if it is comfortable, she is asked to bear down. If the pessary falls down or out, then a different size or shape should be tried.

**The ring pessary is the most commonly used shape, partly because it is the easiest for the patient to place and remove.** Space-occupying pessaries such as the cube, Gelhorn, donut, and Inflatoball, are common second options if the rings turn sideways or falls down. Gelhorn pessaries may have a higher chance of adequate support than rings in patients who have undergone hysterectomy or have advanced prolapse, but it is reasonable to start with the smallest and easiest to use shapes first. In a postmenopausal woman, estrogen replacement for at least 30 days with vaginal estrogen cream before pessary fitting may help improve atrophic vaginitis and make fitting of a pessary more comfortable.

**Pessaries often successfully reduce the prolapse and symptoms associated with prolapse, but they do not always adequately control patients' symptoms or work for her lifestyle.** One prospective trial found that 75% of 203 women fitted with a pessary successfully retained the device at 2 weeks (Fernando, 2006). Failure to retain the pessary was significantly associated with increasing parity, prior POP surgery, large genital hiatus, and past hysterectomy. At 4 months the pessaries reduced symptoms associated with POP, including voiding problems (40%), urinary urgency (38%), urgency urinary incontinence (29%), bowel evacuation (28%), fecal urgency (23%), and urge fecal incontinence (20%). There was no improvement in stress urinary incontinence, and in fact sometimes reducing the prolapse (either with a pessary or surgery) can unmask stress urinary incontinence by supporting the bladder and unkinking the urethra. **Women are unlikely to continue wearing a pessary if it causes or worsens stress incontinence. Sometimes a ring pessary with a knob or incontinence dish pessary with knob, positioned correctly under the urethra, can improve urethral support and reduce stress incontinence.**

### Complications

**Complications from vaginal pessaries are rare with proper use.** This includes regular removal, cleaning, and replacement, as well as use of vaginal estrogen cream for postmenopausal women with vaginal atrophy if possible. Complications include bleeding, discomfort, vaginal erosions (2% to 9%), and difficulty removing a pessary. Rare, serious complications such as erosion into the bladder and rectum have been reported, usually from neglect. Though not a complication, and usually not a sign of infection, many patients notice increased vaginal discharge while using pessaries, and this is one reason some patients eventually elect for surgery instead of pessary management.

### Pregnancy

If a woman with advanced prolapse is pregnant, it is important to replace the uterus before it enlarges and becomes trapped in the lower pelvis or vagina around the beginning of the second trimester. If this happens, edema may cause incarceration and even loss of blood supply to the uterus, resulting in loss of the pregnancy.

### Surgery

If pelvic floor strengthening or pessaries do not adequately control the prolapse symptoms or if a patient declines these options, then surgery can be considered. A young woman should be encouraged to avoid operative repair until she has completed her family. Surgical options including vaginal, laparoscopic, robotic, and open approaches, with and without mesh augmentation. **Shared decision making is optimal with these quality-of-life procedures, and the effectiveness of surgery, risks, recovery time, and patient goals all factor into the decision making. It is worth stating that hysterectomy alone is NOT a surgical treatment for prolapse**; all this does is trade uterine prolapse for vault prolapse, and the patient's symptoms and bother do not improve. Several specific surgical treatments to address the various types of prolapse are discussed later.

## Anterior Vaginal Wall Prolapse

**The anterior vaginal wall is the most common site of POP.** Anterior vaginal wall prolapse most commonly involves a cystocele, in which the bladder descends with the vaginal wall relaxation, and it can less commonly include an enterocele, in which the small bowel descends behind the upper vagina. Anterior compartment defects may also allow the descent of the urethra (urethrocele) and bladder neck. Normal support of the anterior vaginal wall depends on level I apical support and level II support from the endopelvic connective tissue and its attachments to the bony pelvis and pelvic muscles. The trapezoidal anterior vaginal wall has distal and medial attachments near the pubic symphysis, lateral attachments to the arcus tendineus fascia pelvis, and proximal and lateral attachments near the ischial spines. Anatomic studies have identified breaks in these attachments in women with POP. Distal detachments from near the pubic symphysis may result in urethroceles or urethral hypermobility. Anterior vaginal wall prolapse can be associated with stress urinary incontinence from urethral hypermobility, urgency urinary incontinence, or urinary retention from urethral kinking obstructs the flow of urine (Fig. 20.17). Although urethroceles and cystoceles almost always occur in parous women, they have been noted in nulliparous women who have poor structural supports. This is particularly true in women who have congenital malformations or weaknesses of the endopelvic connective tissue and musculature of the pelvic floor. Most parous women demonstrate some degree of cystocele, and when asymptomatic, they do not require therapy.

### Symptoms

**Symptoms of prolapse of any compartment can include a sensation of fullness, pelvic pressure, vaginal bulge, and a feeling that organs are falling out. With anterior vaginal wall prolapse, the woman may also report a feeling of incomplete bladder emptying, a slow urinary stream, or urinary urgency.** The patient may note a bulging of her vagina. She may feel her vagina descend within the vagina or to or beyond the introitus. In some patients this mass must be replaced manually before the patient can void, which is called splinting. Strain, cough, and prolonged standing often accentuate the bulge. Often POP symptoms are less bothersome in the morning and worsen later in the day after upright activities.

Women with anterior vaginal wall prolapse often have concurrent urinary symptoms. Some women have stress incontinence caused by urethral hypermobility or weak urethral sphincter, but others are continent despite a lack of urethral support. Some women with anterior vaginal wall prolapse may have occult or

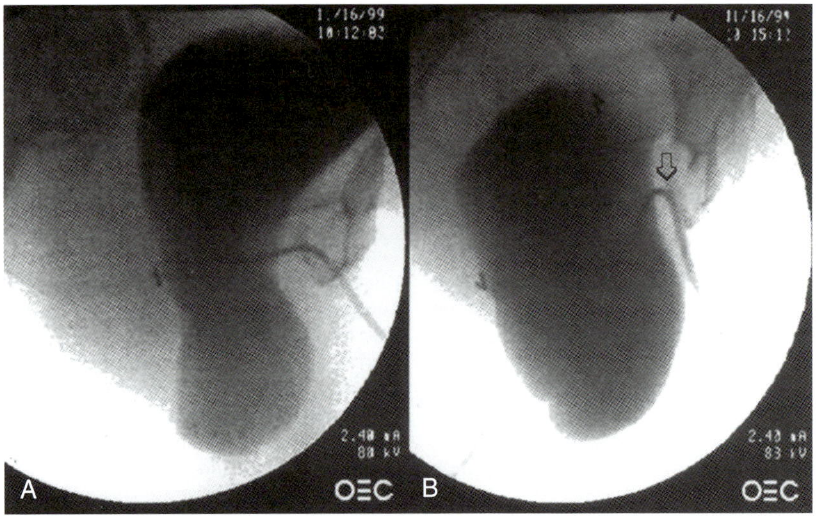


**Fig. 20.17** Urethral kinking caused by large cystocele. Fluorodynamic study shows a large cystocele before (**A**) and after (**B**) strain maneuver was performed. The urethra *(arrow)* clearly can be seen to "kink off" during the strain maneuver. The patient demonstrated severe stress incontinence after prolapse reduction. (From Gallentine ML, Cespedes RD. Occult stress urinary incontinence and the effect of vaginal vault prolapsed on abdominal leak point pressures. *Urology.* 2001;57(1):40-44.)

latent stress incontinence (stress incontinence on prolapse reduction) because their continence depends on urethral kinking or obstruction from severe prolapse.

**Sexual function symptoms should be considered.** Dyspareunia is uncommon from mild prolapse and is more likely caused by atrophic vaginitis as a result of hypoestrogenism or levator spasm than the prolapse itself. These causes are best addressed by topical vaginal estrogen and relaxation of the pelvic floor muscles—for example, with training from a pelvic floor physical therapist. Painful intercourse can also occur if vaginal epithelium that is exteriorized because of prolapse becomes irritated and even ulcerated.

## Diagnosis

**Urethroceles should be differentiated from inflamed and enlarged Skene glands and urethral diverticula. Cystoceles must be differentiated from bladder tumors and bladder diverticula, both of which are rare but may occur. Urethroceles and cystoceles are generally soft, pliable, and nontender.** Although diverticula may be reducible, a sensation of a mass is usually present. Inflamed Skene glands are generally tender (Fig. 20.18). With diverticula or Skene glands, it may be possible to express pus from the urethra or gland when they are palpated. In such cases, gonococcal, chlamydial, and other bacterial infections should be considered.

As described earlier, anterior vaginal wall prolapse is diagnosed by physical examination with the patient in dorsal lithotomy position using half a speculum or a retractor to depress the posterior vagina. If the amount of prolapse seen in this position does not reproduce what the patient notes at home, the examination can be repeated standing and/or later in the day when gravity makes the prolapse worse. The apex and posterior vagina must also be evaluated for prolapse if a surgical repair is being considered. Sometimes what manifests as anterior vaginal prolapse clinically is more caused by uterine or vault prolapse, and this is important to know because surgical correction of the anterior vaginal wall prolapse often requires repair of the apical support plus or minus an anterior repair.

**For patients with prolapse associated with any bladder complaints such as urinary incontinence, urinary urgency, slow stream, hesitancy, or difficulty emptying the bladder, an assessment of postvoid residual should be considered.** This

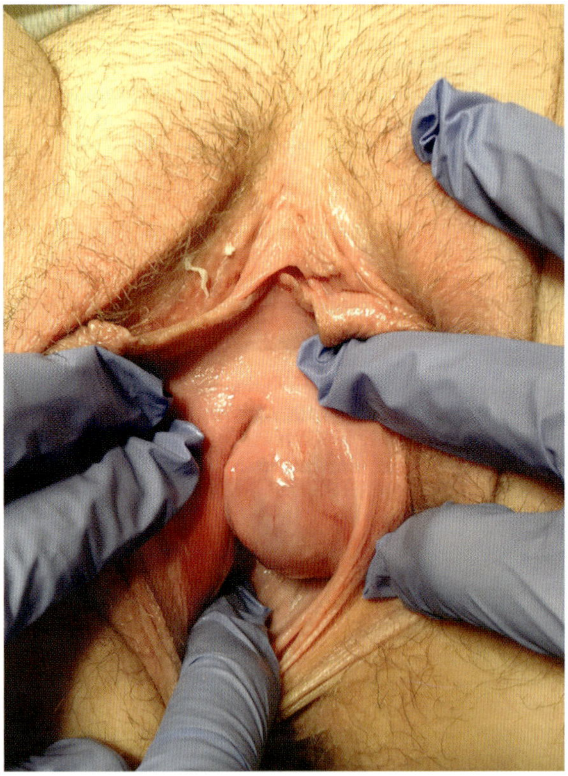

**Fig. 20.18** Left Skene gland cyst.

can be estimated with a bimanual examination to assess for bladder fullness or measured more precisely with an ultrasound or bladder drainage with nonindwelling small catheter.

Particularly for patients with anterior vaginal wall prolapse and arguably for all patients with prolapse, **if surgical management of prolapse is being considered and the patient does not complain of stress urinary incontinence, the physician may want to perform a preoperative prolapse reduction standing stress test to help estimate the risk of developing de novo**

**stress urinary incontinence after prolapse surgery.** With a comfortably full bladder (or with a bladder is backfilled approximately 300 mL as in research studies), ideally in the standing position, the patient is asked to cough while the prolapse is replaced in its normal anatomic position using a pessary, speculum, or large cotton swab. If she leaks during this test, she has latent or occult stress urinary incontinence that is likely to present after surgical repair of the prolapse. Based on one large study of women undergoing surgery for POP who were randomly allocated to surgery with or without an antiincontinence procedure, women with positive preoperative prolapse reduction stress tests have a 71.9% chance of urinary incontinence after surgery without a sling compared with a 29.6% chance of urinary incontinence without a sling. Women with negative preoperative prolapse reduction stress tests in this trial had a 38.1% chance of urinary incontinence without a sling and a 20.6% chance with a sling (Wei, 2012). A tool to estimate the risk of developing de novo stress incontinence is the Cleveland Clinic risk calculator. This calculator accounts for age, parity, body mass index (BMI), diabetes, urge incontinence, and whether the stress test was positive or negative. With this information, the patient and physician can decide whether or not to do an antiincontinence procedure at the time of prolapse repair. **She should be counseled regarding the risks of postoperative incontinence and advised of the risks and benefits of a concurrent continence procedure at the time of prolapse surgery.**

### Surgical Treatment

Pelvic floor strengthening and pessary use are first-line treatments for all types of prolapse (as described earlier). Vaginal estrogen can decrease discomfort and rubbing associated with the prolapse and may improve the vaginal tissues before surgery. Operative repair of anterior vaginal wall prolapse is generally performed in conjunction with the repair of all other pelvic support defects. It is unusual for anterior supports of the vagina to relax without an accompanying relaxation of the apical compartment; in one series 42%, 85%, and 100% of patients with stage II, III and IV anterior vaginal wall prolapse had apical descent, respectively (Elliott, 2013). Repair therefore usually consists of an anterior colporrhaphy and correction of uterine descensus or apical defect posthysterectomy. If noted, posterior vaginal wall prolapse may also be repaired at the same time.

### Anterior Colporrhaphy

In cases of anterior vaginal wall prolapse caused by uterine/cervical or vault prolapse, the most important part of the surgical repair is the apical suspension procedure (discussed later). In some cases the apical suspension may correct the anterior vaginal wall prolapse without a separate anterior colporrhaphy, and in some cases both are necessary.

Anterior wall repair (colporrhaphy) is performed by a midline plication of the fibromuscular layer of the anterior vagina wall. After placement of a Foley catheter, the vaginal epithelium is incised longitudinally from just distal to the anterior lip of the cervix or cuff to just proximal to the urethrovesical junction or bladder neck, which can be identified using the inflated bulb of a Foley catheter (see Fig. 20.19). The longitudinal incision is made through the vaginal epithelium to but not through the underlying fibromuscular tissue. When the longitudinal incision is complete, the cut edge of the vagina is held under tension, and the fibromuscular tissue underneath (sometimes called *pubocervical fascia*) is separated from it using sharp and blunt dissection to the lateral anterior vaginal wall, often to the arcus tendineus fascia pelvis or the inferior pubic rami. This is repeated on each side. The fibromuscular layer is imbricated in the midline by placing absorbable or delayed absorbable 0 or 2-0 sutures laterally on each side of the defect and tying them in the midline. For larger cystoceles, a two-layer plication may be needed to reduce the prolapse. The excess vaginal epithelium can be trimmed as needed and then the two edges closed over the repair using absorbable suture such as 2-0 polyglycol. Cystoscopy should be performed to assess bladder and ureteral integrity after the procedure is completed.

### Concomitant Apical Support Procedure

**The addition of an apical support procedure decreases the rate of reoperation for recurrent anterior vaginal wall prolapse from approximately 20% to 12% within 10 years after surgery** (Eilber, 2013).

### Concomitant Antiincontinence Surgery

**Midurethral sling surgery for associated stress urinary incontinence or stress urinary incontinence on prolapse reduction (occult or latent stress incontinence) can then performed after anterior colporrhaphy through a separate incision over the midurethra.** Placing the sling in the same incision as the anterior colporrhaphy is associated with decreased efficacy because the sling is more likely to be placed too proximal under the urethra. Alternatively, if midurethral slings are not available, or depending on physician comfort, a native tissue repair can be performed, such as Burch urethropexy or autologous fascial sling. Historically a Kelly plication suburethral plication was done at the time of anterior colporrhaphy or colpocleisis to treat or prevent stress urinary incontinence (SUI); however, this procedure is often unsuccessful in both situations. Randomized trial data show that anterior colporrhaphy alone or with a Kelly (or Kelly-Kennedy) plication is not an effective antiincontinence procedure.

## Postoperative Voiding Dysfunction

Postoperatively the bladder should be drained as long as there is a vaginal packing in place, usually for about 1 day, normally with a 16F urethral catheter. Because there is a risk of urinary retention immediately after surgery, a voiding trial should be performed after removing the vaginal pack and before discharging the patient. **There are two common ways to perform a voiding trial: backfill and autofill.** For the backfill, the bladder is retrograde filled with 300 mL of sterile saline until the patient feels an urge to void or to a maximum of 600 mL, and then the catheter is removed. The volume voided is recorded, and the residual volume can be calculated by subtracting the volume voided to the volume filled, or it can be measured using straight catheterization or bladder ultrasound. For autofill, the catheter is removed and the bladder is allowed to fill spontaneously. The voided volume is measured, and the residual volume is measured with a bladder ultrasound or straight catheterization. The patient can be considered to have passed the voiding trial if she voids at least two-thirds of the total bladder volume (e.g., a postvoid residual of less than 100 mL after voiding 200 mL of a 300-mL total bladder volume). Two randomized trials of the two voiding trial techniques revealed that the backfill technique was a better predictor of adequate postoperative bladder emptying than the autofill technique, and it was also preferred by patients (Geller, 2011; Pulvino, 2010). The chance of an unsuccessful voiding trial the day of surgery or the day after surgery is high, and as many as 40% of patients might be discharged home with a catheter. It is helpful to counsel women on this high chance of going home with a catheter before surgery so they can plan on it and not be too disappointed if it happens to them. One study found women reported going home with a Foley catheter to be the most negative aspect of the surgery and they considered it a surgical complication. If bladder function does not return before hospital discharge, the woman may be treated with a Foley catheter for continuous drainage for 1 to 7 days and then

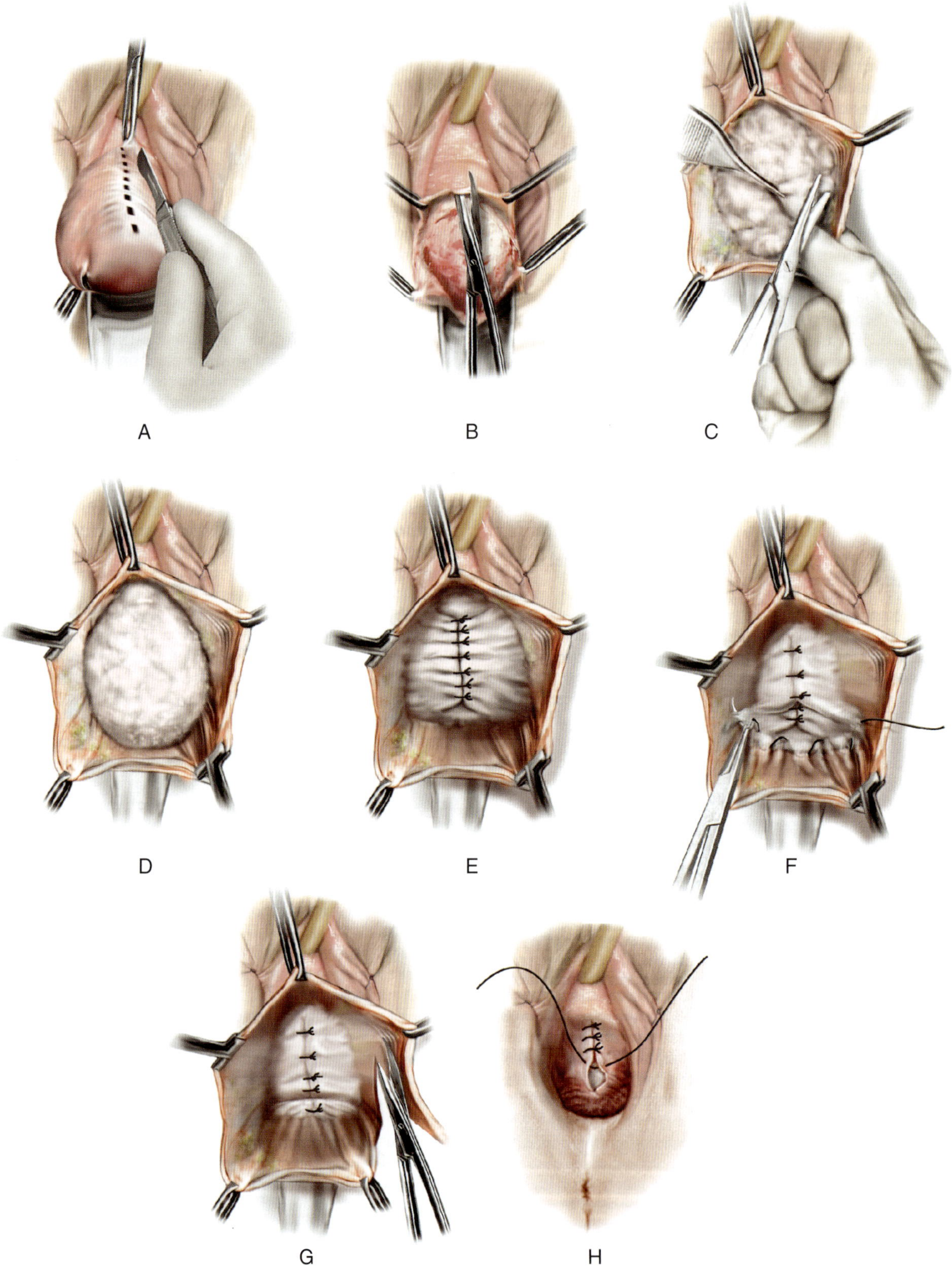


**Fig. 20.19** Classic anterior colporrhaphy. **A,** The initial midline anterior vaginal wall incision is demonstrated. **B,** The midline incision is extended using scissors. **C,** Dissection of the vaginal epithelium off the underlying connective tissue and fibromuscular layer. **D,** The dissection is complete. **E,** The initial plication layer is placed. **F,** The second plication layer is placed, if needed. **G,** Trimming of excess vaginal epithelium. **H,** Closure of vaginal epithelium. (From Maher CF, Karram MM. Surgical management of anterior vaginal wall prolapse. In: Karram MM, Maher CF, eds. *Surgical Management of Pelvic Organ Prolapse.* Philadelphia: Elsevier; 2013:117-137.)

another voiding trial can be performed as an outpatient. Alternatively, to decrease risk of infection, the patient can be taught clean intermittent self-catheterization (CISC) and asked to continue until her bladder function returns. Prophylactic antibiotics are rarely recommended for either indwelling catheterization or CISC; however, symptomatic lower urinary tract infections are common after surgery and should be treated as they occur.

Alternatives to voiding trials include suprapubic catheter drainage or teaching all patients how to perform CISC. With a suprapubic catheter, the drainage tube can be clamped, allowing the patient to void when she can and allowing residual urine to be easily measured. The suprapubic technique is simple to use and seems to have a lower incidence of infection than does transurethral catheterization, but patients may complain of extravasation of urine around the site and occasionally of hematoma formation. CISC can be intimidating for patients to learn, but once learned, many patients prefer not having an indwelling catheter, and they can measure their own postvoid residual urine volumes. The surgeon and patient should decide which method is best suited to the patient's needs and develop systems that the surgeon, nursing team, and patient understand and can follow.

## Postoperative Restrictions

Although there are little data regarding postoperative restrictions, in general patients are advised to avoid straining from constipation, heavy lifting, and strenuous activity for about 6 to 12 weeks while scarring takes place (Nygaard, 2013). One randomized trial failed to find differences in short-term outcomes in groups with activity restriction compared with those with liberal activity (Mueller, 2017). It is likely that the largest increases in intraabdominal pressure are from involuntary actions such as coughing or sneezing rather than activities of daily living. Nothing should be placed in the vagina until it heals with the possible exception of vaginal estrogen, which can be resumed after about 2 to 4 weeks or after the surgical site is no longer bleeding or spotting. Women should be able to resume other nonstrenuous normal activities as soon as they feel ready. Patients may drive when they are off narcotic pain medications.

### Recurrent Anterior Vaginal Wall Prolapse

Recurrent anterior vaginal wall prolapse remains a frustrating problem for gynecologic surgeons and patients. In 1909 George R. White was quoted as saying, "Ahlfet states that the only problem in plastic gynecology left unsolved by the gynecologist is that of permanent cure of cystocele." It remains a problem even now, with reported failure rates of 30% to 46% after anterior colporrhaphy based on strict anatomic criteria: POP-Q stage 0 or I, which was consistent with a 2001 National Institutes of Health (NIH) Standardization Workshop's recommendations at the time (Weber, 2001); however, it is increasingly recognized that strict anatomic "success" may not be clinically relevant for patients with POP. When the Weber 2001 study was reanalyzed with the more patient-centered outcomes (no POP beyond the hymen, no symptoms, and no retreatment), the success rate was 89% (Chmielewski, 2011). **Notably, the rate of recurrence has been found to significantly decrease with the addition of apical vaginal support** (Eilber, 2013). In the setting of apical support defects associated with anterior vaginal wall prolapse, repairs such as uterosacral ligament suspension, sacrospinous ligament suspension, and sacral colpopexy may be indicated. These procedures are discussed later in this chapter.

### Mesh-Augmented Surgery

Because recurrent POP is common, particularly in the anterior compartment, augmentation of anterior vaginal wall prolapse repairs with graft materials has been proposed; however, data suggest that, although transvaginal synthetic mesh may improve the anatomic result compared with traditional native tissue anterior colporrhaphy, it is associated with increased complications such as mesh exposure, pelvic pain, and dyspareunia, and it does not appreciably decrease subjective prolapse symptoms. Mesh augmentation in the anterior compartment is associated with increased operative times, blood loss, prolapse in other compartments, stress incontinence, and reoperation rates, including mesh complications (Jonsson, 2013; Maher, 2016). Fig. 20.20 shows the excision of exposed vaginal mesh that had been placed in a prior POP surgery. Certainly careful patient selection, detailed patient counseling, and a skilled surgeon with proper training are needed for these procedures and to manage the complications. The Food and Drug Administration (FDA) has removed vaginal mesh kits for POP from the U.S. market. Unlike mesh for anterior vaginal wall prolapse, mesh for abdominal apical suspensions, specifically sacral colpopexy (discussed later in this chapter) and stress incontinence (discussed in Chapter 21), remain more widely accepted and benefits are clearly supported by evidence.

Biologic grafts and paravaginal repairs have not been shown to improve outcomes after anterior vaginal wall prolapse surgery; anterior colporrhaphy remains the procedure of choice for isolated anterior vaginal wall prolapse.

## Posterior Vaginal Wall Prolapse (Rectocele)

The prevalence of posterior vaginal wall prolapse in community-dwelling women in the United States ranges from 18% to 40% and 9% to 76% in urogynecology clinics, depending on the definition used.

### Symptoms and Signs

As with other forms of POP, the patient with a rectocele often complains of pelvic pressure, a "falling out" feeling in the vagina, a vaginal bulge, or disruption in sexual activity. Protrusion of the prolapse may worsen later in the day and be aggravated by prolonged standing or exertion. **With a rectocele, the woman may also complain of constipation, difficulty with bowel movements, a feeling of incomplete emptying of the rectum, and the need to push on the vagina or perineum (splint) to have a bowel movement**. Obstructed defecation symptoms may be reported by 9% to 60% of women with pelvic floor disorders, with 18% to 25% splinting, 27% straining, and 26% incompletely evacuating. **Although reported symptoms might be related to the rectocele, there are many other potential causes of evacuation problems that are not (constipation, dysmotility, sigmoidocele, rectal prolapse, rectal intussusception)**. Defecatory symptoms often but not always improve after rectocele repair, and women should be counseled appropriately.

### Diagnosis

**Posterior vaginal wall prolapse is descent of the posterior vaginal wall and may include an enterocele (small bowel), a rectocele (rectum), or both**. Posterior vaginal wall prolapse may be identified by retracting the anterior vaginal wall upward with one-half of a Graves or Pederson speculum and asking the patient to strain (Fig. 20.21). POP-Q measurements should be performed of all compartments of the vagina. An example POP-Q for a women with isolated posterior vaginal wall prolapse is shown, although in reality POP usually involves more than one compartment, particularly after hysterectomy (Fig. 20.22).

**To assess for rectocele, the physician should place one finger in the rectum and one in the vagina and palpate the defect**. Often the rectovaginal septum is paper thin, and the rectocele can be palpated to its upper margin. One finger

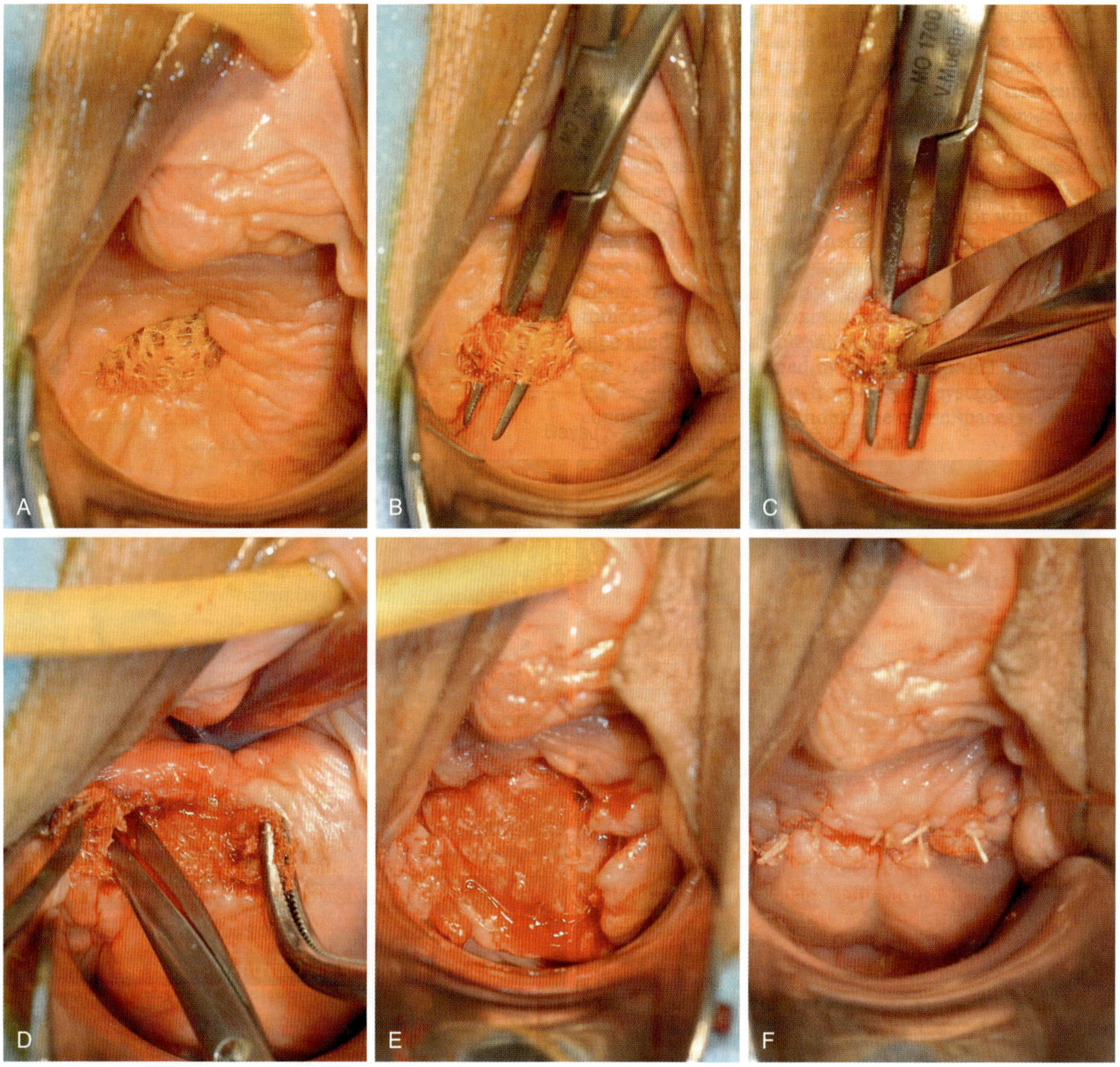


**Fig. 20.20** Surgical technique of mesh excision. **A,** Anterior vaginal wall with 2- × 2-cm perigee mesh exposure. **B,** Undermining the mesh. **C,** Transecting the mesh, which has folded over on itself. **D,** Dissecting between mesh and bladder. **E,** Most of the mesh has been excised. **F,** Closure with interrupted suture. (From Margulies RU. Complications requiring reoperation following vaginal mesh kit procedures for prolapse. *Am J Obstet Gynecol.* 2008;199(6):678.e1-678.e4.)

in the rectum can also evaluate for the presence of a "pocket" or bulge into the vaginal canal where stool may get trapped. If an enterocele is present, it may be possible to differentiate it from the rectocele by having the patient strain. Often, however, the diagnosis of a small enterocele is established only at the time of operation. **Evacuation symptoms that are out of proportion to the degree of rectocele bear further investigation by an expert such as gastroenterologist or colorectal surgeon, possibly with anal manometry, defecography, or dynamic MRI.**

## Management

Nonoperative management of a rectocele is similar to that mentioned for a cystocele. Pessaries, Kegel exercises, pelvic floor physical therapy, and vaginal estrogen may be offered. Gastrointestinal symptoms must be thoroughly evaluated, including screening for colorectal cancer if appropriate. If constipation and straining are issues, dietary fiber and fluid intake should be reviewed. At least 25 g of fiber, adequate hydration, regular exercise, and allowing time for defecation after meals can be recommended to regulate bowel habits as first-line therapy. Polyethylene glycol can be used nightly or as needed if these first-line therapies do not adequately normalize stool consistency.

### Posterior Repairs

**Although anatomic position is often corrected by a posterior repair, function may not be corrected.** Defecatory problems may remain, so patients should be forewarned. Posterior wall prolapse is associated with the loss of fibromuscular support overlying the rectum, laxity and separation of the levator ani place and tearing or separation of the perineal musculature. These are the deficiencies that need to be repaired. Therefore

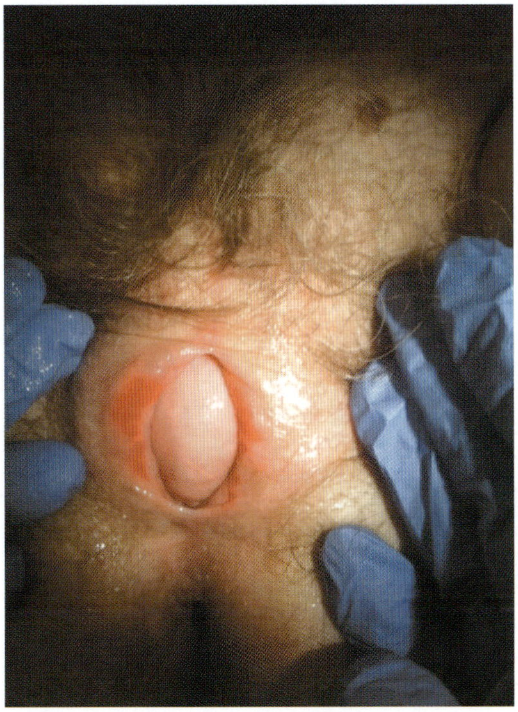

**Fig. 20.21** Rectocele. Although this may appear to be a cystocele, split speculum examination revealed a rectocele.

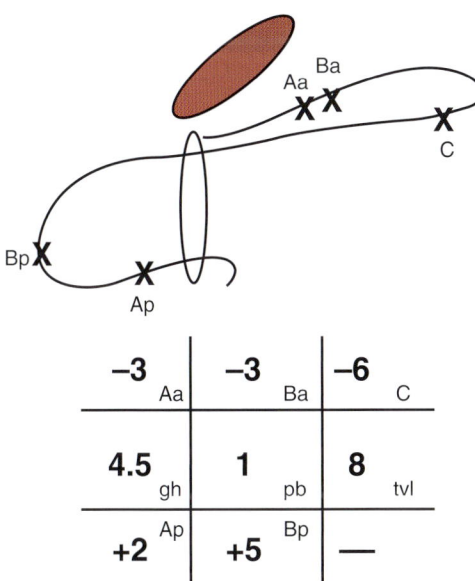

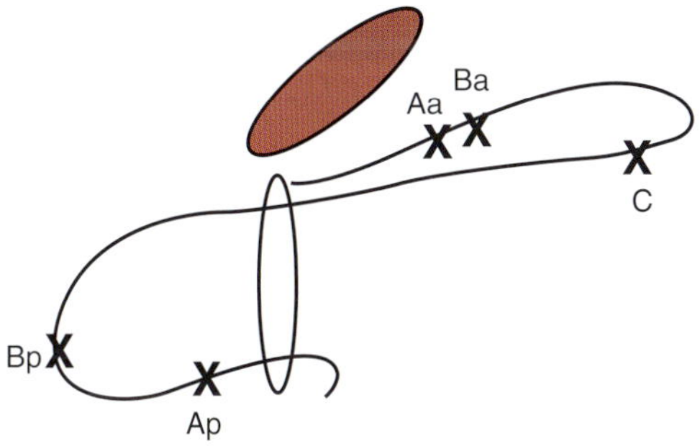


| | | |
|---|---|---|
| −3 Aa | −3 Ba | −6 C |
| 4.5 gh | 1 pb | 8 tvl |
| Ap +2 | Bp +5 | — |

**Fig. 20.22** Line drawing example of posterior support defect. The anterior compartment is well supported. The leading point of the prolapse is point Bp (+5), which is 5 cm beyond the hymen. Total vaginal length is 8 cm, and point C (−6), the cuff position, has descended 2 cm. (From Bump RC, Mattiasson A, Bo K, et al. The standardization of terminology of female pelvic organ prolapse and pelvic floor dysfunction. *Am J Obstet Gynecol.* 1996;175(1):10-17.)

operative management of posterior vaginal wall prolapse usually involves posterior colporrhaphy or a site-specific repair, plus or minus perineorrhaphy to treat a perineal body defect or enlarged genital hiatus (discussed later). Of course, surgical correction of apical prolapse and/or anterior vaginal wall prolapse if present needs to be repaired.

## Posterior Colporrhaphy

To perform a posterior colporrhaphy transvaginally, the vaginal epithelium is incised longitudinally in the midline to the top of the bulge (Fig. 20.23). The vaginal edges are grasped and placed under tension and the fibromuscular tissue is separated from the vaginal epithelium by blunt and sharp (if necessary) dissection bilaterally. Usually this dissection is carried out laterally to the medial aspect of the levator ani muscles, proximally toward the apex of the vagina above the limit of the rectocele, and inferiorly to the perineal body. At this point, a site-specific repair, posterior colporrhaphy, or a combination of both can be performed to reduce the bulge. Both methods have high success rates.

**The surgeon then places a delayed absorbable suture (0 or 2-0) into the perirectal fibromuscular tissue on either side and the posterior vaginal wall is plicated across the midline and/or site-specific defects in this layer are repaired with suture.** The surgeon may choose to place these sutures with one finger in the rectum and, if not, should check the rectum after the completion of the repair to ensure that no suture is placed into the rectum. When the sutures are tied, these tissues are interposed between rectum and vagina, thereby reducing the rectocele.

**Levator ani plication involves plication of the levator ani muscle toward the midline.** Sutures are placed laterally in the levator ani muscles incorporating a portion of the lateral fibromuscular layer of the posterior vaginal wall. The sutures are tied down in the midline to draw the muscles together to create a muscular shelf. **Creating a "shelf" in the posterior vaginal wall or constricting the wall may narrow the vagina too much and lead to dyspareunia, so it is relatively contraindicated in sexually active women.** Plication of the levator ani muscle in the midline was formerly considered part of the posterior colporrhaphy; it is now considered a separate procedure.

## Site-Specific Posterior Repair

A site-specific repair is limited to reapproximation of breaks in the fibromuscular layer (Fig. 20.24). There are two ways to perform a **site-specific posterior vaginal repair**. In the first, the fibromuscularis is examined after the dissection is performed and any defects individually isolated and repaired with delayed absorbable suture. The second approach is to approximate the strong connective tissue between the distal aspect of the rectovaginal septum to the proximal extent of the dissection. The edges of the vaginal epithelium are then trimmed and the vagina closed with a row of either continuous or interrupted absorbable sutures.

## Perineorrhaphy

Some women with posterior vaginal wall prolapse also have a gaping genital hiatus and a defect in their perineal body. Therefore a perineorrhaphy to rebuild the perineal body is sometimes performed at the same time, as shown in Fig. 20.23 and Fig. 20.25. Some data suggest that genital hiatus size may normalize after prolapse surgery even without perineorrhaphy (Carter-Brooks, 2019). Perineorrhaphy is performed to address a defect or attenuation of the perineal body, and it must approximate muscles of the perineal body. It generally results in a decrease in genital hiatus and an increase in the length of the perineal body. A perineorrhaphy incorporates structures that are caudad to the hymenal remnant. The components reapproximated can include the deep and superficial transverse perineal muscles; the fibromuscular layer of the posterior vaginal wall; the bulbospongiosus muscles; the anterior fibers of the external anal sphincter (EAS) or its capsule, the puborectalis muscle, which contributes fibers to the superior EAS; and/or the perineal membrane.

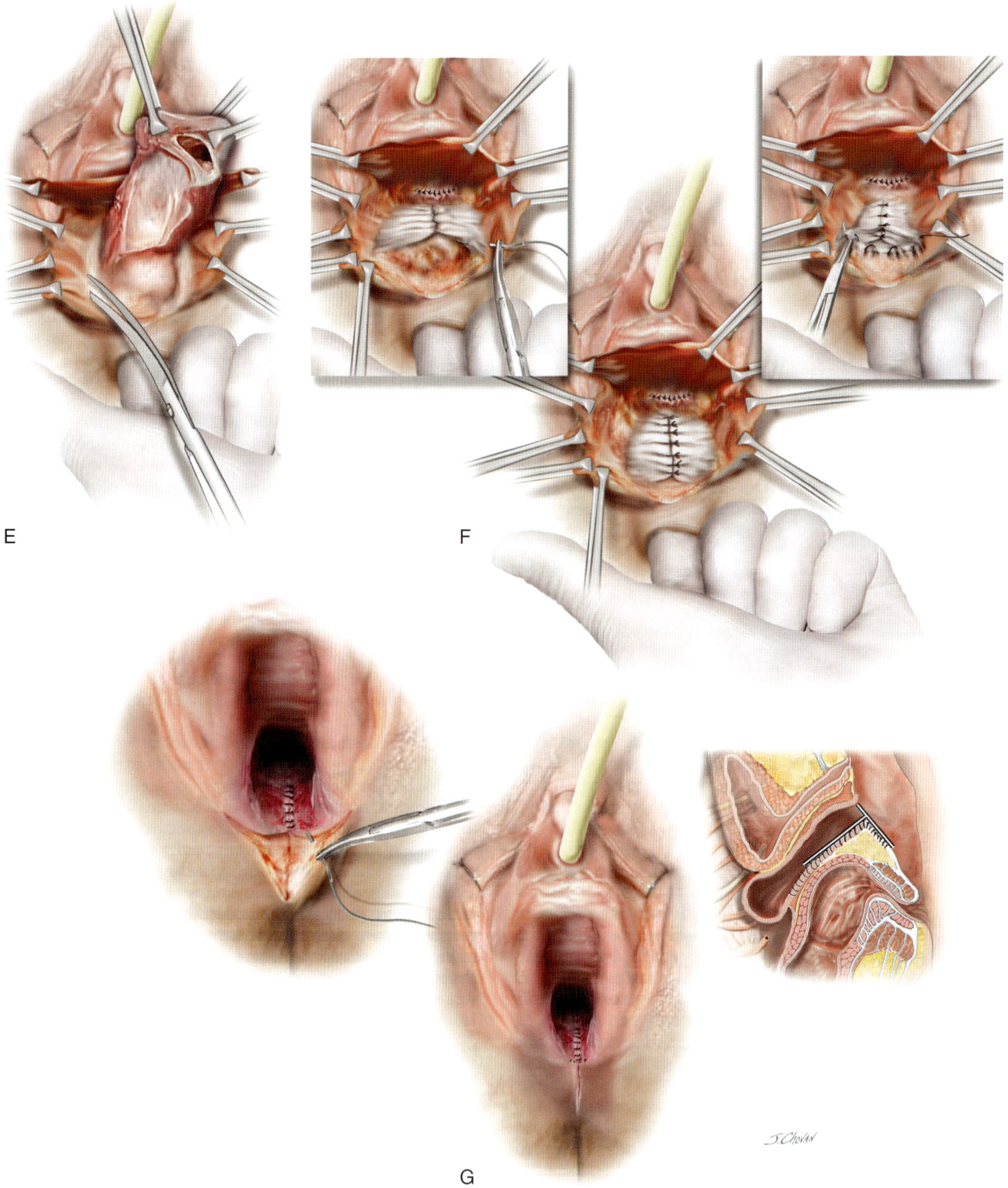


**Fig. 20.23** Posterior colporrhaphy. Repair of posterior vaginal wall prolapse, including the repair of a rectocele and a posterior enterocele, and perineoplasty. **A,** Built-up perineal skin is incised in the midline. **B,** With a finger in the rectum, sharp dissection is used to mobilize the anterior wall of the rectum off the posterior vaginal wall. **C,** The enterocele sac is mobilized off the anterior wall of the rectum. **D,** Sharp dissection is used to enter the enterocele sac. **E,** Fibromuscular layer of the vagina is mobilized off the vaginal epithelium and plicated across the midline. The enterocele sac is addressed. **F,** A second layer is mobilized and plicated across the midline. **G,** Perineoplasty is performed; the perpendicular relationship between posterior vaginal wall and perineum is noted. (From Karram MM, Maher CF. *Surgical Management of Pelvic Organ Prolapse: Female Pelvic Surgery Video Atlas Series.* Philadelphia: Saunders; 2012.) From: Karram, MM. Native tissue vaginal repair of cystocele, rectocele, and enterocele. *Atlas of Pelvic Anatomy and Gynecologic Surgery*. 2016. Pages 599-646. Figure 54-37.

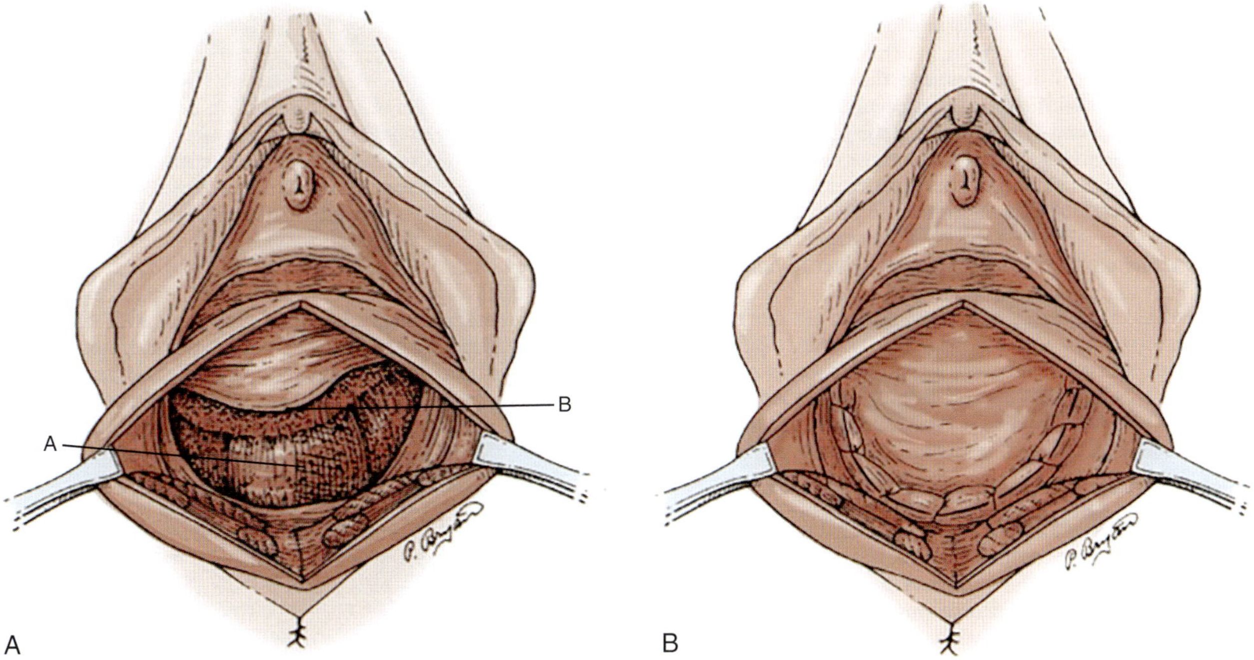


**Fig. 20.24 A** and **B,** Site-specific rectocele repair. A low transverse defect is identified and repaired primarily. (From Richardson AC. The rectovaginal septum revisited: its relationship to rectocele and its importance in rectocele repair. *Clin Obstet Gynecol.* 1993;36:976-983.)

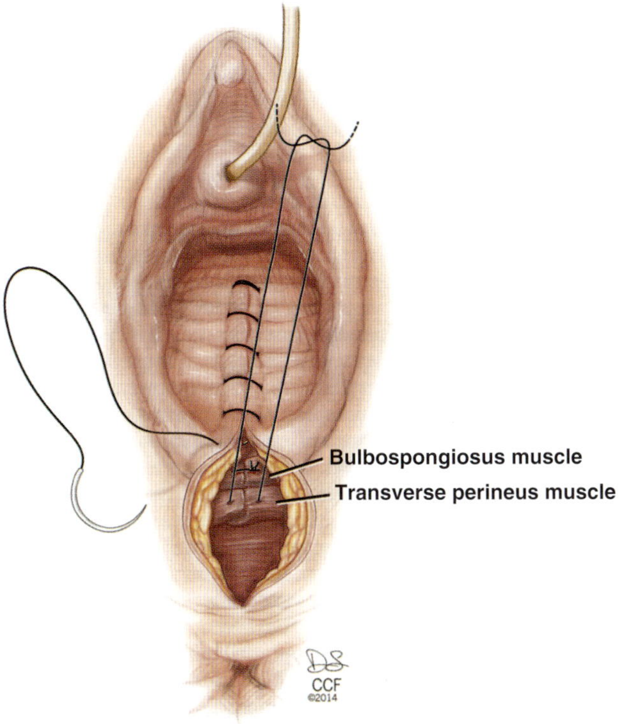


**Fig. 20.25** Perineorrhaphy. After the completion of the repair of the rectocele, the perineal body may need to be reconstructed. The bulbospongiosus and the superficial transverse peroneus muscles a re plicated in the midline with absorbable sutures. (From Muir TW. Surgical treatment of rectocele and perineal defects. In Walters MD, Karram MM. *Urogynecology and Reconstructive Pelvic Surgery.* 4th ed. Philadelphia: Elsevier: 2015;342-359.)

To perform a perineorrhaphy, either for an isolated perineal body defect or uncomfortably wide genital hiatus or at the time of posterior repair, the surgeon first estimates the degree of perineorrhaphy by placing Allis clamps on each side the posterior hymen such that reapproximating the clamps results in a normal genital hiatus (Fig. 20.25). **Overtightening the introitus may** cause dyspareunia. Often a diamond-shaped wedge is excised in the perineal skin and distal vaginal epithelium with a scalpel or curved Mayo scissors. It is closed in the following fashion according to what defects are found in the perineal body. Usually, absorbable sutures such as 0 polyglycol sutures are placed in the lateral margins of the transverse incision, essentially bringing bulbospongiosus and deep and superficial transverse perineal muscles together from either side to the midline. The operator can be sure that the bulbospongiosus muscle insertions are included in the sutures by pulling on the suture and noting whether the tension identifies the muscle bundles. The remainder of the perineal incision is then closed with a row of 2-0 polyglycol sutures to the deep tissue, and the skin of the perineum is closed with either interrupted or continuous subcuticular suture of 3-0 absorbable suture.

## Recurrent Posterior Vaginal Wall Prolapse

Successful repair of posterior vaginal wall prolapse may be slightly higher for posterior colporrhaphy (96%) than site-specific repair (89%) when defined as no prolapse beyond the hymen, but overall recurrence is uncommon. **Because of low recurrence rates of posterior vaginal wall prolapse and the increased risks of augmenting posterior repairs with grafts, the evidence does not support the use of any mesh or grafts at the time of posterior vaginal repair** (ACOG, 2019). Surgical correction of apical prolapse at the time of posterior vaginal wall prolapse should be performed when there is concurrent apical prolapse because this decreases recurrence.

## Enterocele

An **enterocele** is a herniation of the pouch of Douglas (cul-de-sac) between the uterosacral ligaments into the rectovaginal septum containing small bowel. It most often occurs after an abdominal or vaginal hysterectomy and generally is the result of a weakened support for the pouch of Douglas and the loss of vaginal apical support by the uterosacral ligaments. To decrease the risk of developing an enterocele after a hysterectomy, the uterosacral and cardinal ligaments, which are the most important support structures for the vagina, should be incorporated into the vault repair as described later under Management.

### Diagnosis

An enterocele is not always easy to diagnose. It is a true hernia of the peritoneal cavity emanating from the pouch of Douglas between the uterosacral ligaments and into the rectovaginal septum (Figs. 20.26 and 20.27). It may be noticed as a separate bulge above the rectocele, and at times it may be large enough to prolapse through the vagina (Figs. 20.28 and 20.29). If such is the case, it may be possible to make the specific diagnosis of enterocele by transilluminating the bulge and seeing small bowel shadows within the sac. It may also be possible to differentiate the enterocele from a rectocele by rectovaginal examination. The contents of an enterocele are always small bowel and may also include omentum; they may be easily reducible or may be fixed to the peritoneum of the sac by adhesions.

### Management

Like other types of prolapse, enteroceles may be managed expectantly if asymptomatic, or they can be treated with pessaries or surgery. They rarely occur in isolation, so surgical management usually also involves vaginal vault suspension, as described later in this chapter, with or without anterior and posterior repairs if indicated.

### Surgical Enterocele Repair: Abdominal

When repairing an enterocele transabdominally, the sac should be reduced upward if possible and dissected free from the bladder and rectum. If the uterosacral ligaments are present, these may be

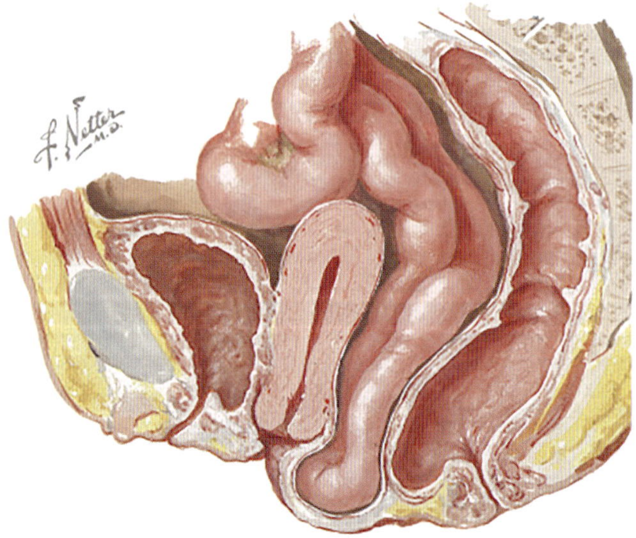

**Fig. 20.26** Enterocele and uterine prolapse. (Smith RP. Enterocele. In: *Netter's Obstetrics and Gynecology.* 3rd ed. Philadelphia: Elsevier; 2018:212-213.)

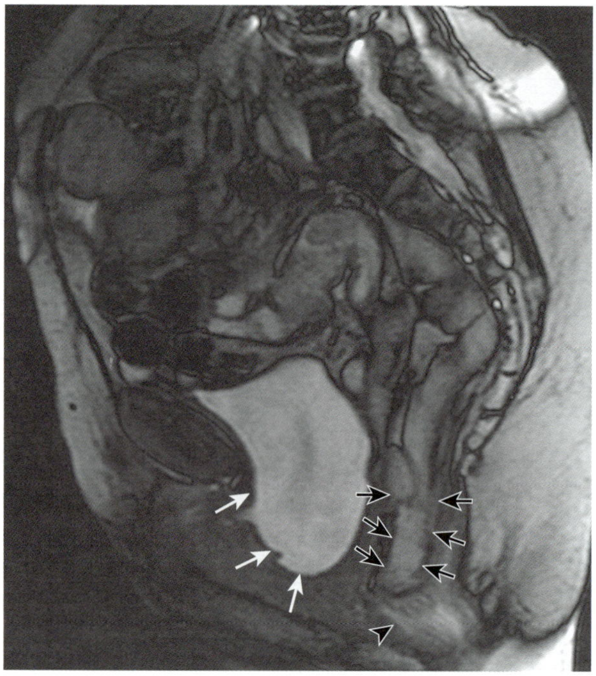

**Fig. 20.27** Sagittal imaging though the midline of the pelvis in a female patient during magnetic resonance imaging proctography. A loop of small bowel has descended anterior to the rectum to form a large enterocele *(black arrows).* Note the coexistent cystocele *(white arrows)* and small collapsed rectocele *(arrowhead).* (From Taylor SA. Imaging pelvic floor dysfunction. *Best Pract Res Clin Gastroenterol.* 2009; 23(4):487-503.)

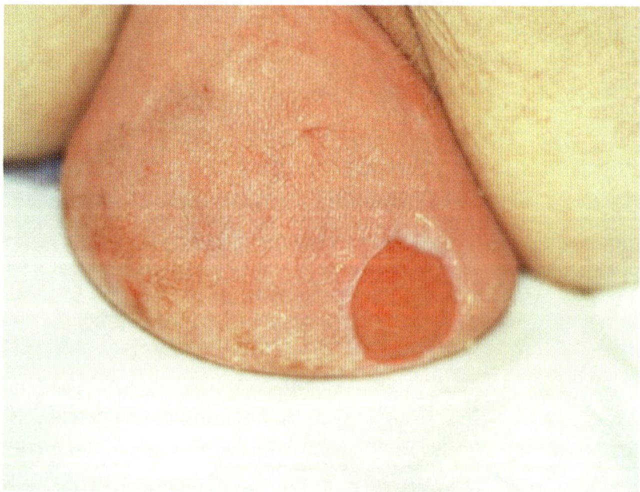

**Fig. 20.28** Elderly patient with stage IV apical eversion and enterocele with vaginal ulcers.

brought together in the midline and attached to the vaginal cuff. If the uterosacral ligaments cannot be identified, as with large enteroceles after previously performed hysterectomy, concentric purse-string sutures in the connective tissue over the vagina and rectum may obliterate the cul-de-sac. Care must be taken to avoid damaging the ureters, rectum, and sigmoid colon. It is best to perform this procedure with permanent sutures. Because the enterocele has probably occurred because of weakening of the apical supports (uterosacral ligaments), an apical suspension surgery such as abdominal sacral colpopexy is often necessary to suspend the vagina and close the enterocele defect.

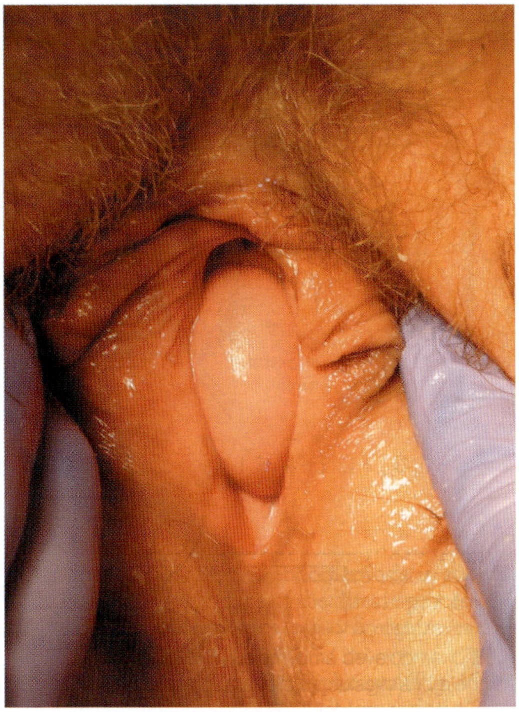

**Fig. 20.29** Enterocele with vaginal apical prolapse. Split speculum and digital examinations with palpation of bowel in the sac helped define this defect.

### Surgical Enterocele Repair: Transvaginal

Repair of an enterocele can be carried out transvaginally at the time of the apical repair with or without anterior or posterior vaginal wall repair. The sac will be visualized as the vagina is separated from the rectum. The sac can then be dissected free of underlying tissue and isolated at its neck. It should be opened to ensure that all contents are replaced. The neck of the hernia is then sutured with a purse-string permanent suture ligature and the sac excised (Fig. 20.30). It is important to support the neck of the enterocele sac as much as possible. Approximating the anterior and posterior vaginal connective tissue is also important to close the defect. Usually with an enterocele, support of the vaginal apex such as a sacrospinous ligament suspension is needed for optimal repair.

### Recurrent Enterocele

Correctly repaired enteroceles rarely recur. Enteroceles may recur when repaired without proper attention to ligation of the neck of the sac, closure of the anterior and posterior vaginal connective tissue of the vaginal cuff, or supporting the vaginal apex and when performed with concurrent rectocele repair. In such cases a subsequent operation with special attention to these surgical principles is indicated.

### Prevention: McCall Culdoplasty

If uterosacral ligaments can be identified at the time of a vaginal hysterectomy, they can be used to repair and prevent enterocele formation. This can be accomplished by fixing the uterosacral ligaments to the peritoneum of the sac and the vaginal vault connective tissue using a suture of absorbable or delayed absorbable suture, beginning on one side of the vagina and continuing through the uterosacral ligament of that side, the peritoneum, and the uterosacral ligament and then vagina on the opposite side. Multiple sutures can be placed if space allows. This technique, which effectively shortens the cul-de-sac and supports the enterocele neck, was described by McCall and is often called the *McCall stitch* or *McCall culdoplasty*.

## Uterine Prolapse

Prolapse of the uterus and cervix into or through the barrel of the vagina is associated with injuries of the endopelvic connective tissue and level I support structures, including the cardinal and uterosacral ligaments (Fig. 20.31). Uterine prolapse is often associated with anterior and posterior vaginal wall prolapse and, at times, enterocele.

### Symptoms and Signs

**Common symptoms noted by patients with uterine prolapse are a feeling of pelvic pressure and heaviness, fullness, bulge or "falling out" in the perineal area. Because uterine prolapse is often associated with anterior and posterior vaginal wall prolapse, symptoms that were reported earlier for cystocele and rectocele such as voiding or defecatory dysfunction may be present as well.** In cases in which the cervix and uterus are low in the vaginal canal, the cervix may be seen protruding from the introitus, giving the patient the impression that a tumor is bulging out of her vagina. Where stage III or IV prolapse has occurred, the patient may be aware that a mass has actually prolapsed out of the introitus. In stage IV prolapse the vagina is everted around the uterus and cervix and completely exteriorized. When prolapse occurs beyond the hymen, the epithelium and cervix can become dry, thickened, and chronically inflamed. The patient may also have pain and bleeding from ulcerations. There is often discharge, and secondary infection can occasionally occur. Stasis ulcers may result from edema and interference with blood supply to the vaginal wall. Evisceration of abdominal contents is a rare complication and a surgical emergency.

### Management

As with other forms of prolapse, mild or asymptomatic uterine prolapse does not need treatment or can be treated with pelvic floor muscle strengthening. If the prolapse is causing symptoms, infection, urinary retention (from outlet obstruction), or hydronephrosis (from ureteral kinking), it can be treated with a pessary or surgery.

### Surgery for Uterine Prolapse

**Operative repair for prolapse of the uterus and cervix can be transabdominal or transvaginal and must involve a suspension procedure to support the uterus or to support the vagina after hysterectomy. It must be emphasized that hysterectomy alone does not treat prolapse;** it simply changes the patient's condition from uterine prolapse to vaginal vault prolapse without improving her quality of life or pelvic function.

The surgical approach will depend on patient comorbidities, patient preferences regarding risks and durability, and surgeon expertise. Common surgical options to treat uterovaginal prolapse include vaginal hysterectomy with vault suspension to the uterosacral or sacrospinous ligaments, abdominal (open, laparoscopic, or robotic) supracervical hysterectomy with sacral colpopexy, and colpocleisis. Other surgeries, including abdominal (open laparoscopic, or robotic) uterosacral ligament suspension with or without hysterectomy, transvaginal hysteropexy with or without mesh, sacrohysteropexy, and Manchester procedures, can be appropriate for some patients. Sacral colpopexy, which is described in more detail in the Vaginal Vault Prolapse (Apical Prolapse after Hysterectomy) section, is the most durable surgery for

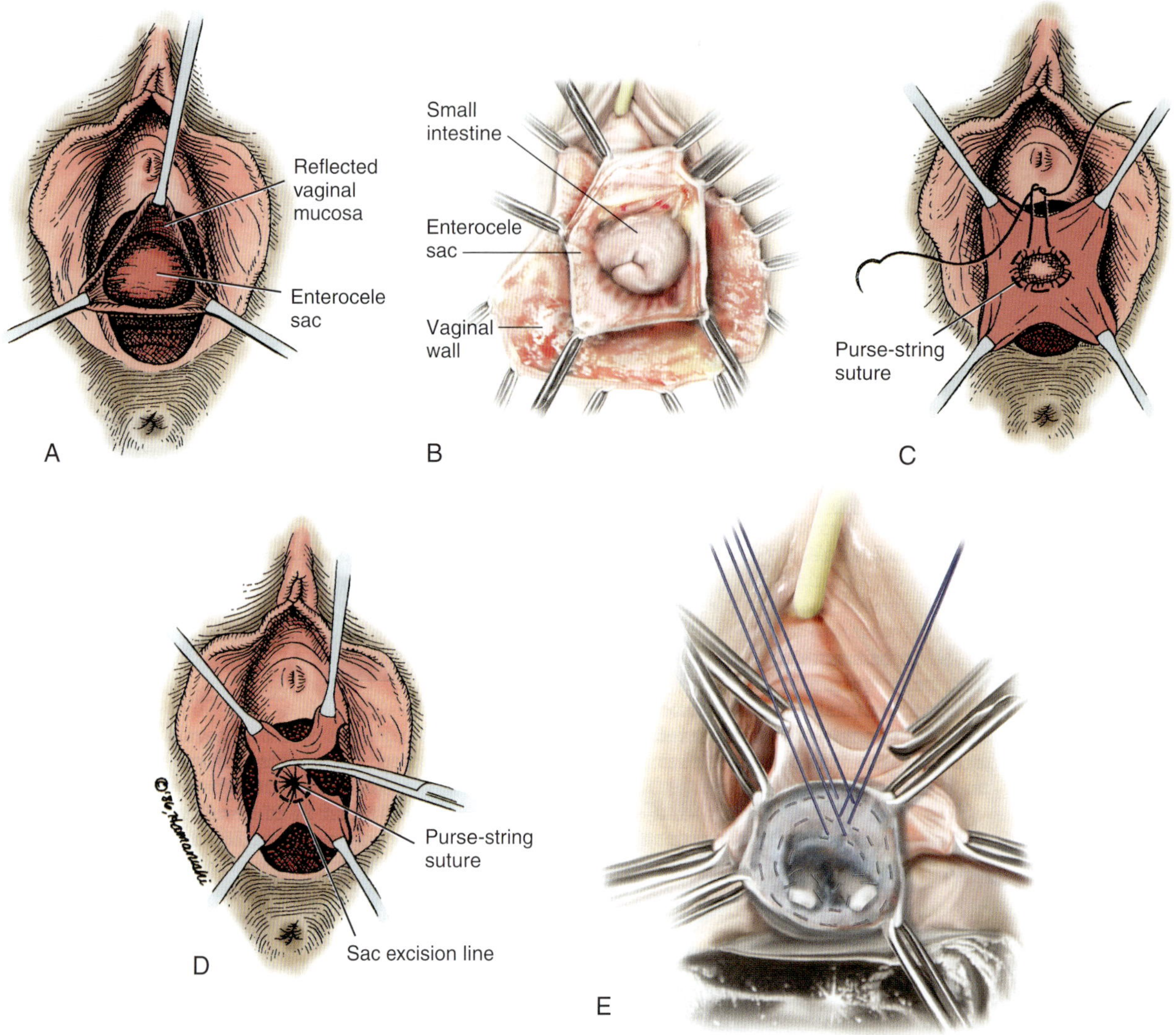


**Fig. 20.30** Repair of enterocele. **A,** Appearance of enterocele sac with vaginal wall reflected. **B,** Appearance of open enterocele sac with sac neck identified. **C,** Placing of purse-string suture at the neck of the enterocele sac. **D,** Excision of enterocele sac. **E,** Enterocele repair. (From Karram MM. *Native Tissue Vaginal Repair of Cystocele, Rectocele, and Enterocele. Atlas of Pelvic Anatomy and Gynecologic Surgery.* Philadelphia: Elsevier; 2016:599-646.)

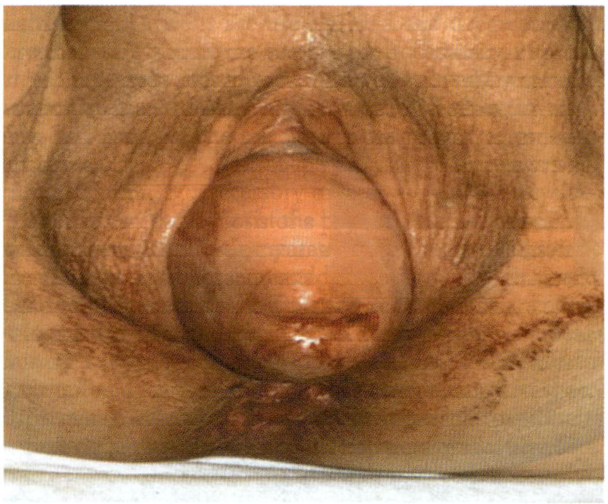

**Fig. 20.31** Uterine prolapse.

apical prolapse but has more surgical risks than vaginal surgeries. Transvaginal repair usually involves a vaginal hysterectomy followed by a vaginal vault suspension to the uterosacral or sacrospinous ligaments. The uterosacral ligaments can be sutured together so that the cul-de-sac is shortened or obliterated as in a McCall culdoplasty (described previously), or the vaginal vault can supported high up to the uterosacral ligament at the level of the ischial spines or to the sacrospinous ligament. High uterosacral ligament and sacrospinous ligament suspensions are described in the Vaginal Vault Prolapse (Apical Prolapse after Hysterectomy) section presented later in this chapter.

The American College of Obstetricians and Gynecologists' (ACOG's) committee opinion and a Cochrane systematic review (2015) suggest that vaginal hysterectomy is associated with better outcomes and fewer complications than laparoscopic or abdominal hysterectomy (ACOG, 2017; Aarts, 2015); however, the optimal route of hysterectomy depends on many factors, including the size and shape of the uterus, accessibility to the uterus, surgeon training and experience, and planned concurrent surgical procedures, including prolapse surgeries and intraabdominal surgeries. In cases in which an abdominal, laparoscopic-assisted vaginal, or total laparoscopic hysterectomy is preferable, an apical suspension can be performed vaginally or abdominally, and anterior and posterior colporrhaphies can be performed vaginally if needed.

## Surgery for Cervical Elongation

In some women (possibly up to one-third), the cervix is hypertrophied and elongated to the area of the introitus, but the supports of the uterus itself are intact. A cystocele and rectocele may be present, and operative repair can consist of a Manchester (Donald or Fothergill) operation. This operation combines an anterior and posterior colporrhaphy with the amputation of the cervix and the use of the cardinal ligaments to support the anterior vaginal wall and bladder. Although it was suggested for repair in young women who wish to maintain their reproductive abilities, the loss of the cervix may interfere with fertility or lead to incompetence of the internal cervical os. The operation has value in elderly women with comorbid medical conditions who have an elongated cervix and well-supported uterus because it is technically easier and has a shorter operative time than the vaginal hysterectomy, and the entering of the peritoneal cavity is avoided.

## Obliterative Prolapse Procedures

**In elderly women who are no longer sexually active, a simple and effective procedure for reducing prolapse is an obliterative procedure called a colpocleisis.** The classic partial colpocleisis procedure was described and popularized by Le Fort in 1877 (Fig. 20.32) and involves the removal of a strip of anterior and posterior vaginal epithelium with suturing of the fibromuscular layers anterior and posterior walls to each other. This "obliterates" the vaginal canal. This procedure may be performed with uterine preservation (Le Fort) or without the presence of a uterus and cervix. When it is completed, the vaginal cavity is nearly

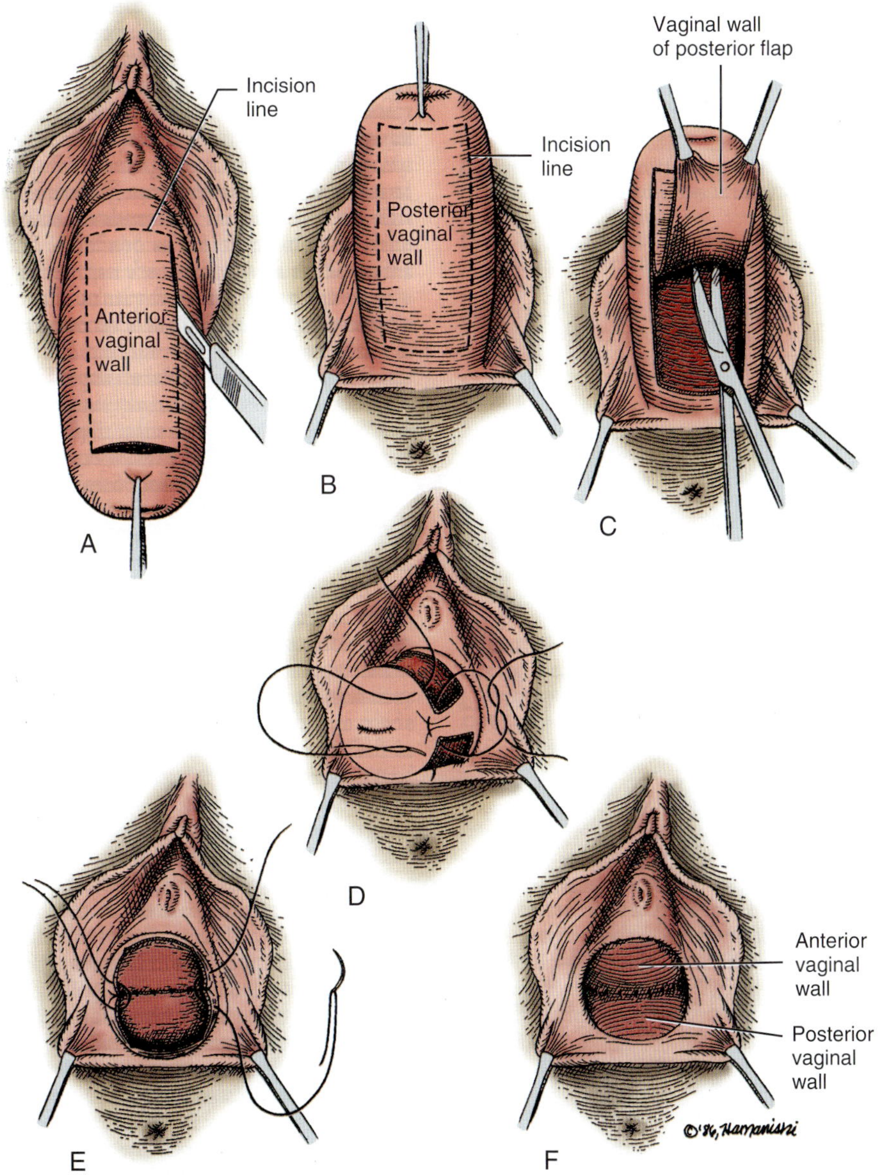


**Fig. 20.32** Le Fort procedure. **A,** Incision of anterior vaginal wall strip. **B,** Incision of posterior wall strip. **C,** Removal of vaginal strip. **D** and **E,** Placement of sutures. **F,** Appearance of vagina after procedure is completed but before perineorrhaphy is performed.

completely closed, with small vaginal canals epithelized on either side of the opposed vaginal walls to allow drainage of any fluid from the cuff or uterus. To perform, dissection of the vaginal epithelium is carried to the level of the bladder neck anteriorly and to the reflection of bladder onto the cervix at the upper margin of the vagina. Posteriorly the dissection is carried from just inside the introitus to a position just posterior to the cervix. If a hysterectomy has been previously performed, the dissection may begin approximately 1 cm on either side of the vaginal scar and canals may be left, or all the epithelium can be removed. If tunnels are being created in a colpocleisis without hysterectomy, a vessel loop or small catheter may be used to ensure patency and removed at the end of the surgery. Multiple layers of sutures are placed placating the posterior to the anterior fibromuscular layer of the vaginal walls. This can be either with horizontal rows of interrupted, absorbable sutures or with a purse-string absorbable suture. If the cervix and uterus are still present and intrauterine pathologic changes occur, bleeding through these canals can alert the physician to a potential problem. In low-risk women, no evaluation for uterine pathologic conditions is necessary before colpocleisis. In women with risk factors, however, a cervical or endometrial evaluation should be completed before colpocleisis because colpocleisis makes access to these organs difficult. If there is a cervical or uterine pathologic condition, the uterus and cervix should not be left in situ. Cystoscopy should be performed to assess bladder and ureteral integrity after the procedure is completed.

A large perineorrhaphy is usually performed in association with the colpocleisis. A levator plication may be necessary to decrease the size of the genital hiatus. Together, these procedures result in a short vagina of approximately 3 cm and a small genital hiatus of about 1 to 2 cm. The patient can be reassured that her external genitalia look completely normal, and her sensation and clitoral function are unchanged, although intercourse is not generally possible. Rectal examination is important to ensure no rectal injury after prolapse surgery.

An antiincontinence operation such as a midurethral synthetic sling may be carried out if the patient has stress urinary incontinence or stress urinary incontinence on prolapse reduction, either at the time of surgery or as an interval procedure.

The Goodall-Power modification of the Le Fort operation (Fig. 20.33) allows for the removal of a triangular piece of vaginal wall beginning at the cervical reflection or 1 cm above the vaginal scar at the base of the triangle, with the apex of the triangle just beneath the bladder neck anteriorly and just at the introitus posteriorly. The cut edge of vaginal wall making up the base of the triangle anteriorly is sutured to the similar wall posteriorly, and the vaginal incision is then closed with a row of interrupted sutures beginning beneath the bladder neck and carried side to side to the area of the introitus. This procedure works well for relatively small prolapses, whereas the Le Fort is best for larger ones.

Prognosis for a colpocleisis procedure to reduce the prolapse and prevent recurrence is generally excellent. Case series report 91% to 100% success rates. **Careful counseling must be done preoperatively to be sure the woman will never desire coital activity because occasional regret over closure of the vagina has been reported. Overall, patient satisfaction is high and regret is low** (Vij, 2014).

## Fertility-Sparing Surgery for Uterine Prolapse: Hysteropexy

If a young woman wishes to maintain her fertility and has symptomatic uterine prolapse, first-line treatment is pessary management until she completes childbearing; however, there are small studies suggesting surgical treatment may be an option. **There are more women with uterine prolapse who are done with childbearing and are requesting uterine preservation**

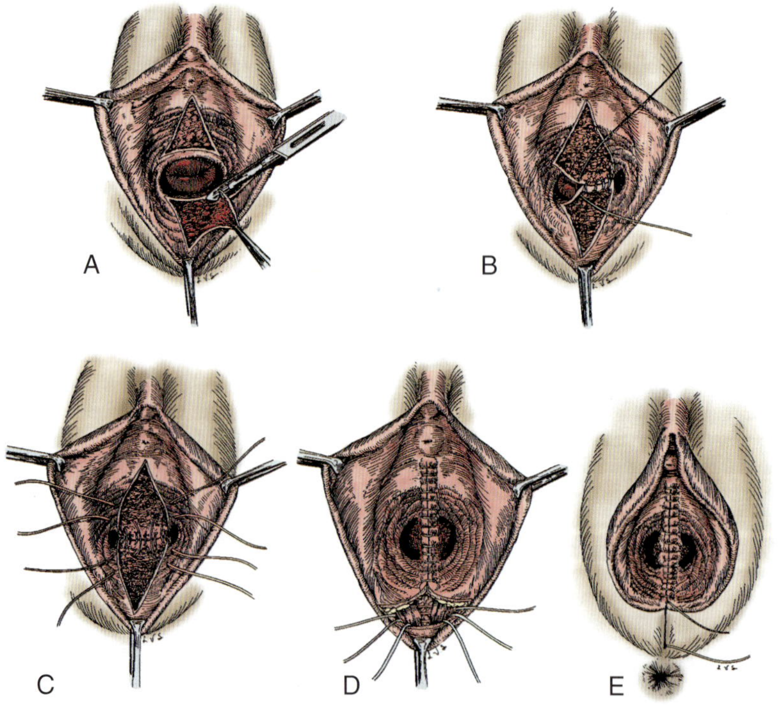


**Fig. 20.33** Goodall-Power modification of Le Fort operation. **A,** Representation of vaginal incision on anterior and posterior wall. **B,** Early placement of sutures. **C,** Later placement of sutures. **D,** Vaginal incision completely closed; perineorrhaphy being performed. **E,** Appearance at completion of procedure. (From Symmonds RE. Relaxation of pelvic supports. In: Benson RC, ed. *Current Obstetric and Gynecologic Diagnosis and Treatment,* 5th ed. Los Altos, CA: Lange Medical; 1984.)

**(hysteropexy). Uterine preservation is possible with the following approaches:**

- Transvaginal sacrospinous hysteropexy (sutured or with graft)
- Transvaginal or laparoscopic uterosacral ligament suspension
- Abdominal/laparoscopic/robotic sacrohysteropexy with graft (Fig. 20.34)
- Anterior abdominal wall hysteropexy
- Manchester procedure (although this might affect fertility and pregnancy)

A multicenter study, enrolling 150 women, compared laparoscopic sacral hysteropexy versus vaginal mesh hysteropexy. No differences in anatomic (77% vs. 80%; adjusted OR, 0.48; $P = .20$), symptomatic (90% vs. 95%; adjusted OR, 0.40; $P = .22$), or composite (72% vs. 74%; adjusted OR, 0.58; $P = .27$) cure were noted (*cure* was defined as no prolapse beyond the hymen and cervix above midvagina (anatomic), no vaginal bulge sensation (symptomatic), and no reoperations). Mesh exposures occurred in 2.7% laparoscopic versus 6.6% vaginal hysteropexy cases. A total of 95% of each group were very much better or much better. Pelvic floor symptom and sexual function scores improved for both groups with no difference among groups (Gutman, 2017). Another cohort study compared transvaginal uterosacral hysteropexy versus hysterectomy plus uterosacral ligament suspension. Similar objective and subjective cure rates and patient satisfaction were noted; however, postoperative cervical elongation lead to higher central prolapse recurrence rates and need for reoperation by 35 months (Milani, 2019). A randomized study comparing vaginal hysterectomy with uterosacral ligament suspension (absorbable sutures) to unilateral sacrospinous hysteropexy (without mesh, but with permanent Prolene suture) found hysteropexy noninferior at 1 year (Detollenaere, 2015). The 5-year follow-up of that study reported uterine preservation was slightly more effective, with 3% undergoing surgery for recurrent prolapse in the sacrospinous hysteropexy group versus 7% in the vaginal hysterectomy group (Schulten, 2019); however, overall anatomic failure, functional outcome, repeat surgery and sexual functioning did not differ significantly between the two procedures. A multicenter, randomized trial of vaginal hysterectomy with uterosacral apical suspension (one permanent and one absorbable suture each side) versus transvaginal mesh hysteropexy found no significant differences in the composite prolapse outcome (retreatment for prolapse, prolapse beyond the hymen or symptomatic outcomes) after 3 years (Nager, 2019). A large population-based cohort that hysterectomy at the time of prolapse repair is associated with a decreased risk of future POP surgery by 1-3% and is independently associated with higher perioperative morbidity (Dallas, 2018). More

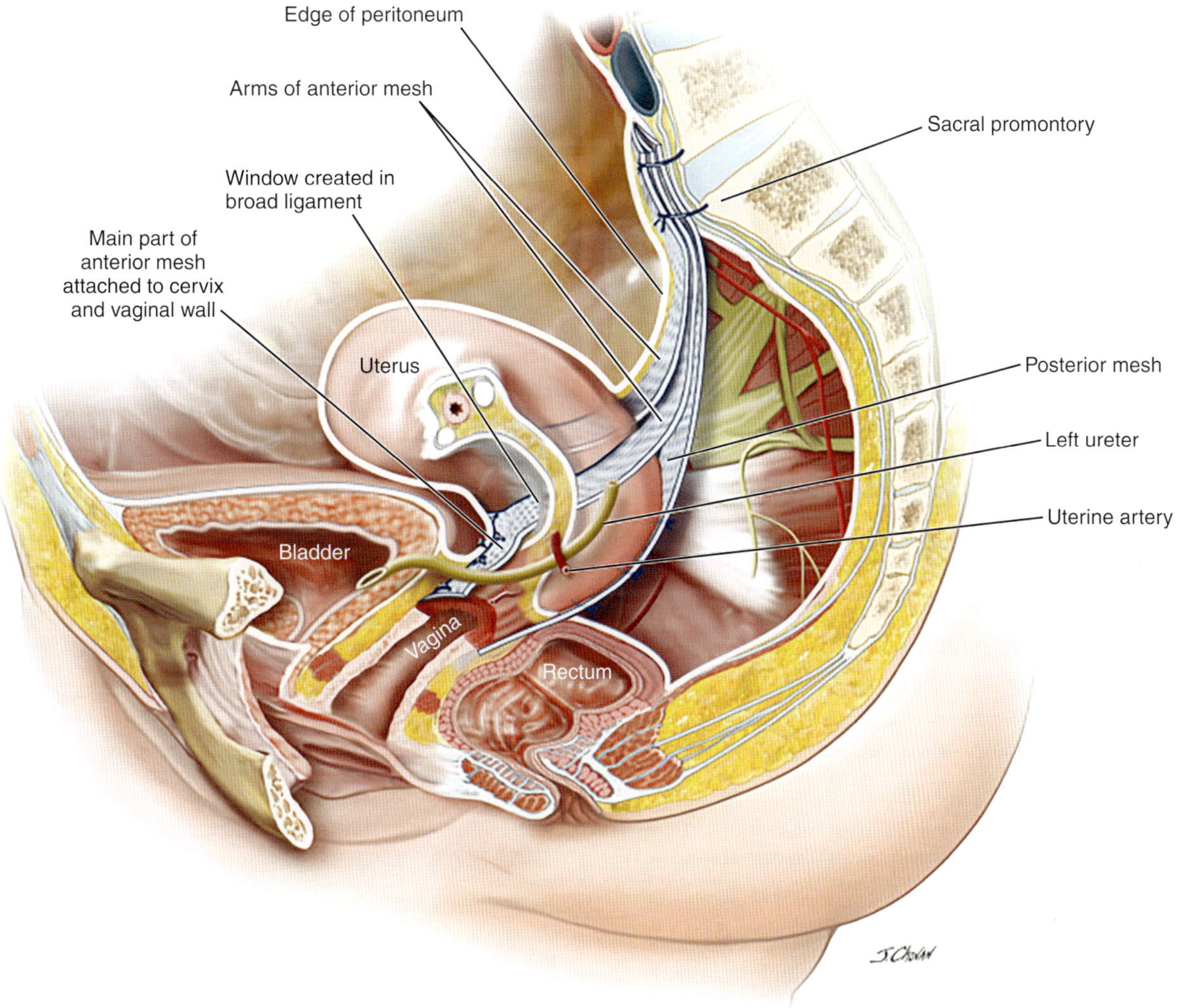


**Fig. 20.34** Dual-leaf sacral colpohysteropexy is represented. (From Karram MM, Maher CF. *Surgical Management of Pelvic Organ Prolapse: Female Pelvic Surgery Video Atlas Series.* Philadelphia: Saunders; 2012.)

long-term data are needed before hysteropexy becomes routine and to determine whether hysterectomy is necessary component of prolapse repair. Importantly, studies suggest about a third of women wish for uterine preservation even when done with childbearing, so patient choice and shared decision-making discussions are needed. Women with cervical or uterine cancer risk, elongated cervix, enlarged uterus, or abnormal uterine bleeding are not good candidates for uterine preservation.

If the uterus is well supported, isolated anterior colporrhaphy and/or posterior colporrhaphy can also be performed without affecting fertility. Data are limited regarding recommended route of delivery after prolapse surgery.

## Vaginal Vault Prolapse (Apical Prolapse after Hysterectomy)

Prolapse of the vaginal apex at some time remote to the performance of either abdominal or vaginal hysterectomy has been reported as occurring in 0.1% to 18.2% of patients, with 5% of women having surgery for posthysterectomy POP. Apical prolapse may be accompanied by a cystocele, a rectocele, an enterocele, or some combination thereof. It is rare to find isolated support defects of the anterior or posterior vaginal walls or an isolated apical defect (Rooney, 2006). **Vaginal vault prolapse is probably the result of continuing pelvic support defects in the connective tissues—namely, the cardinal and uterosacral ligaments attachments to the vaginal cuff. Multiple vaginal wall defects are usually found because the connective tissue, the pelvic floor muscles, and innervation are globally affected and usually not isolated damage to one site.**

### Symptoms and Signs

Symptoms and signs of vaginal apex prolapse are similar to those delineated for uterine and other types of vaginal prolapse. They include pelvic heaviness, a mass protruding through the introitus, vaginal bleeding or discharge, and discomfort sitting or walking. Bladder and rectal symptoms can include stress incontinence, urinary urgency, urinary frequency, incomplete bladder emptying, difficult bowel movements, and splinting to void or defecate.

### Diagnosis

POP-Q or other quantitative measurements should be performed, as with other forms of prolapse, to ensure that all three compartments are considered: anterior, apical, and posterior. Examination may help determine the contents of the herniation depending on where the vaginal scar is located in relation to the protruding mass and the extent to which the supports of the pelvis are lost. Rectovaginal examination is often helpful in delineating an enterocele from a rectocele.

### Management

As with other POP, if not bothersome and not causing excessive kinking of the urethra or ureters, vaginal vault prolapse can be managed expectantly or with pelvic floor muscle strengthening. Vaginal estrogen can be used to treat ulcerations. Pessaries should be offered even though prior hysterectomy makes successful pessary fitting difficult because the pessaries are more likely to fall out.

### Surgery for Uterine/Cervical or Vaginal Vault Prolapse

**Surgery for apical prolapse can be vaginal, abdominal, laparoscopic, robotic, or some combination thereof. Benefits of vaginal surgery include generally shorter operative times, fewer complications, and quicker return to daily activities. Abdominal sacral colpopexy (including open, laparoscopic, or robotic-assisted laparoscopic) appears to provide improved durability but with increased operative time, cost, and surgical risks including mesh complications. The material of choice for sacral colpopexy is type 1 wide-pore, monofilament polypropylene mesh.**

### Transvaginal Surgery for Apical Prolapse

**The most common transvaginal surgeries for prolapse are uterosacral ligament and sacrospinous ligament suspensions. These procedures can be performed with uterine preservation or concurrent hysterectomy and for posthysterectomy vaginal vault prolapse. A randomized controlled trial of 374 women assigned to transvaginal fixation to the uterosacral ligaments or the sacrospinous ligaments found comparably good success rates: 15% of women in the trial had prolapse beyond the hymen 2 years after surgery, and 5% required treatment for recurrent prolapse with pessary or surgery** (Barber, 2014). The overall rate of perioperative adverse events was comparable between the procedures, including less than 1% risk of urethral, major vascular, or rectal injury and a 3% risk of blood transfusion. Vaginal granulation and suture exposures were seen in approximately 15% of patients. Neurologic pain was higher in the sacrospinous ligament group (12%) than in the uterosacral group (7%). Ureteral obstruction was only seen in the uterosacral group (3%), and all but one was recognized and successfully managed intraoperatively. Mesh augmentation for vaginal vault prolapse is an alternative with some evidence to support it in terms of anatomic outcomes; however, as noted previously, it has higher complication rates and should only be placed by surgeons with adequate training and after careful patient counseling.

**For operative management, the first guiding principle is that the normal position of the vagina in the standing position is against the rectum and no more than 30 degrees from the horizontal** (Fig. 20.35). **The second principle is that all areas of prolapse need to be addressed as correction of the apical defect may not reduce all the prolapsed compartments. The third principle acknowledges that the perineal body is almost always defective in such patients and must therefore be reconstructed as well. For transvaginal procedures, goals include maintaining adequate vaginal length and width.**

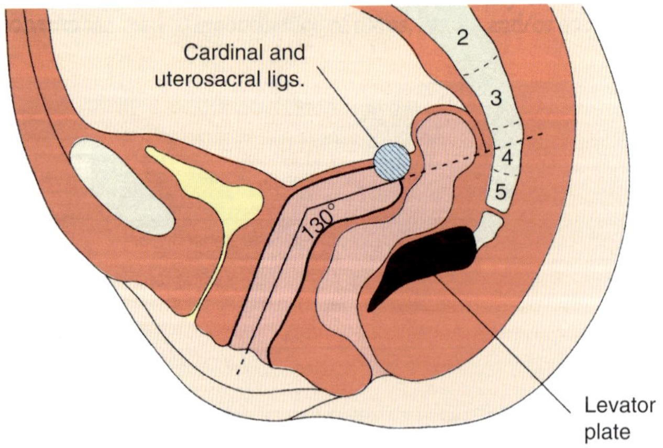


**Fig. 20.35** Normal vaginal axis of nulliparous woman in the standing position. Note that the upper third of the vagina is nearly horizontal and is directed toward the S3 and S4 sacral vertebrae. (From Funt MI, Thompson JD, Birch H. Normal vaginal axis. *South Med J.* 1978;71(12):1534.)

## Sacrospinous Ligament Suspension

Sacrospinous ligament suspension is performed by dissecting the vaginal epithelium off the underlying fibromuscular tissue all the way down through the perirectal space to the right ischial spine and then clearing off the sacrospinous ligament medial to the ischial spine toward the sacrum. The surgeon must first identify the apex of the vagina and ensure that it will reach the ligament without tension. The vaginal incision can be in the anterior, apical, or posterior vaginal wall. After the dissection is complete, sutures are placed through the sacrospinous ligament approximately 1.5 fingerbreadths medial to the ischial spine while the rectum is manually deflected medially. **Care must be taken to place the sutures sufficiently medially to avoid pudendal and sciatic nerve injury. Sutures should be placed through the inferior portion of the sacrospinous ligament to decrease the risk of injuring the inferior gluteal vessels.**

The sacrospinous ligament is deep in the pelvis, and several techniques and devices have been designed to assist with passage of the sutures through the sacrospinous ligament. The Miyazaki hook ligature carrier and Deschamps ligature carrier with nerve hook require direct visualization of the ligament using Breisky-Navratil retractors (Fig. 20.36). Other systems adopted from other fields include the Shutt suture punch system from orthopedics (Sharp, 1993) and the Endo Stitch (Covidien; Dublin, Ireland) autosuturing device from laparoscopic surgery. The Capio (Boston Scientific, Marlborough, MA, USA) was specifically designed to place sutures through the sacrospinous ligament without the need for direct visualization, which may minimize dissection and bleeding. Transvaginal mesh kits for apical support procedures often have their own methods of attachment to the sacrospinous ligaments. Transvaginal mesh for prolapse surgery is currently not available in the United States.

**Operative risks of sacrospinous colpopexy include injury to the pudendal and inferior gluteal arteries and the pudendal and sciatic nerves. Rectal injury is rare, although care must be taken when dissecting the rectal pillars to reach the ligament and to avoid the rectum while placing the sutures.** The iliococcygeal ligament can be used in cases in which the vagina is not long enough to reach the sacrospinous ligament without excessive tension and in cases in which sacral colpopexy is not desirable. It has a similar risk profile with respect to recurrent cystocele, buttock pain, and hemorrhage and only slightly inferior subjective success rates (91% compared with 94%) and patient satisfaction (71% compared with 91% on a 0 to 100 visual analog scale) (Maher, 2001).

## Uterosacral Ligament Suspension

To perform a uterosacral ligament suspension procedure, the anterior and posterior vaginal walls are opened in the midline and the enterocele sac is opened to enter the peritoneal cavity (Shull, 2000). It is commonly performed after vaginal hysterectomy, when the peritoneal cavity is already open, and it can be performed abdominally at the time of other abdominal open, robotic, or laparoscopic procedures. It can also be performed for vaginal vault prolapse. After packing the bowel out of the field, the uterosacral ligaments are identified by putting the ligaments under tension with traction of the vaginal apex. The ligaments are then grasped with Allis clamps, or sutures placed directly without grasping them with clamps, at the level of the ischial spines or the sutures. Sutures must be superficial and care must be taken to avoid the ureter. A series of two or three sutures placed high in each uterosacral ligament near the level of the ischial spine and then used to resupport the vaginal apex. Any enterocele defect is closed with this technique, and any residual anterior or posterior vaginal wall prolapse can be further reduced with colporrhaphy.

**Cystoscopy must be performed at the end of the procedure to ensure ureteral patency by looking for brisk efflux of urine from each ureteral orifice because there is as high as 11% rate of intraoperative ureteral kinking that requires removal and replacement of the offending sutures (3% in the trial described earlier).** Some surgeons prefer to perform cystoscopy midprocedure with the uterosacral sutures on tension before they are placed through the vaginal apex because they are easier to remove and replace at that time. They must repeat cystoscopy to ensure ureteral patency at the end of the procedure as well. Injury to the sacral nerves from sutures that are placed too deeply in the sidewall has been reported and usually presents as pain.

## Abdominal Surgery for Vaginal Vault Prolapse

For the abdominal surgical treatment of vaginal vault prolapse, a variety of procedures have been tried, and sacral colpopexy appears to be the most successful. Other methods of transabdominal apical support include fixation of the vaginal vault to the anterior abdominal wall, the lumbar spine, the sacral promontory, the uterosacral ligaments, and various tendinous lines in the musculature of the true pelvis (e.g., paravaginal repair to the arcus tendineus) and to the sacrospinous ligament. The anterior abdominal wall fixation increases the diameters of the pouch of Douglas and often adds to the risk of subsequent enterocele development, commonly creating a recurrence in short order. **Fixation to the lumbar spine or the sacral promontory is often difficult to achieve directly and requires the interposition of a graft to perform a sacral colpopexy.** Wide-pore, monofilament, light weight polypropylene mesh is most commonly used today because it has fewer complications compared with braided mesh with small pores and reduced recurrence rates compared with biologic materials such as cadaveric fascia and fascial aponeurosis harvested from the patient.

The technique for performing a sacral colpopexy is essentially the same whether it is performed through a laparotomy, via laparoscopy, or with robotic-assisted laparoscopy. The retroperitoneal space over the bony sacral promontory is entered and a window overlying the anterior longitudinal ligament at the level of S1-S2 is developed. Care must be taken when performing the dissection to access the anterior longitudinal ligament to avoid the middle sacral artery and the plexus of veins in its vicinity (Fig. 20.37). The peritoneum is either divided from this dissection along the right pelvic sidewall down to the vagina or a retroperitoneal tunnel under the peritoneum is created along the same course. Care must be taken to identify and avoid the right ureter and the rectosigmoid and bowel mesentery. The vaginal wall is dissected away from the bladder and rectum, and then the mesh graft is sutured to the anterior and posterior vaginal walls. Delayed absorbable sutures can be used to attach the mesh and decrease the rate of suture erosion into the bladder compared with permanent sutures (Tan-Kim, 2014). A bridge of mesh extends to the sacrum, where it is affixed to the anterior longitudinal ligament over first sacral vertebral body (S1-S2) in a tension-free manner. The level of S1-S2 is thought to minimize the bleeding risk and avoid the intervertebral disc and risk of discitis. The mesh graft can be made retroperitoneal by closing the peritoneum over it (or putting it through the tunnel before suturing to the anterior longitudinal ligament), theoretically to reduce internal hernias and adhesions that could result in small bowel obstruction, which nonetheless can occur. After sacral colpopexy, the pouch of Douglas may still be large enough to allow an enterocele to develop. Therefore some surgeons also perform a culdoplasty to obliterate the cul-de-sac.

**There are variations to sacral colpopexy. If a supracervical hysterectomy is done before the mesh attachment, the procedure is called a *sacrocervicopexy* and the uterine cervix**

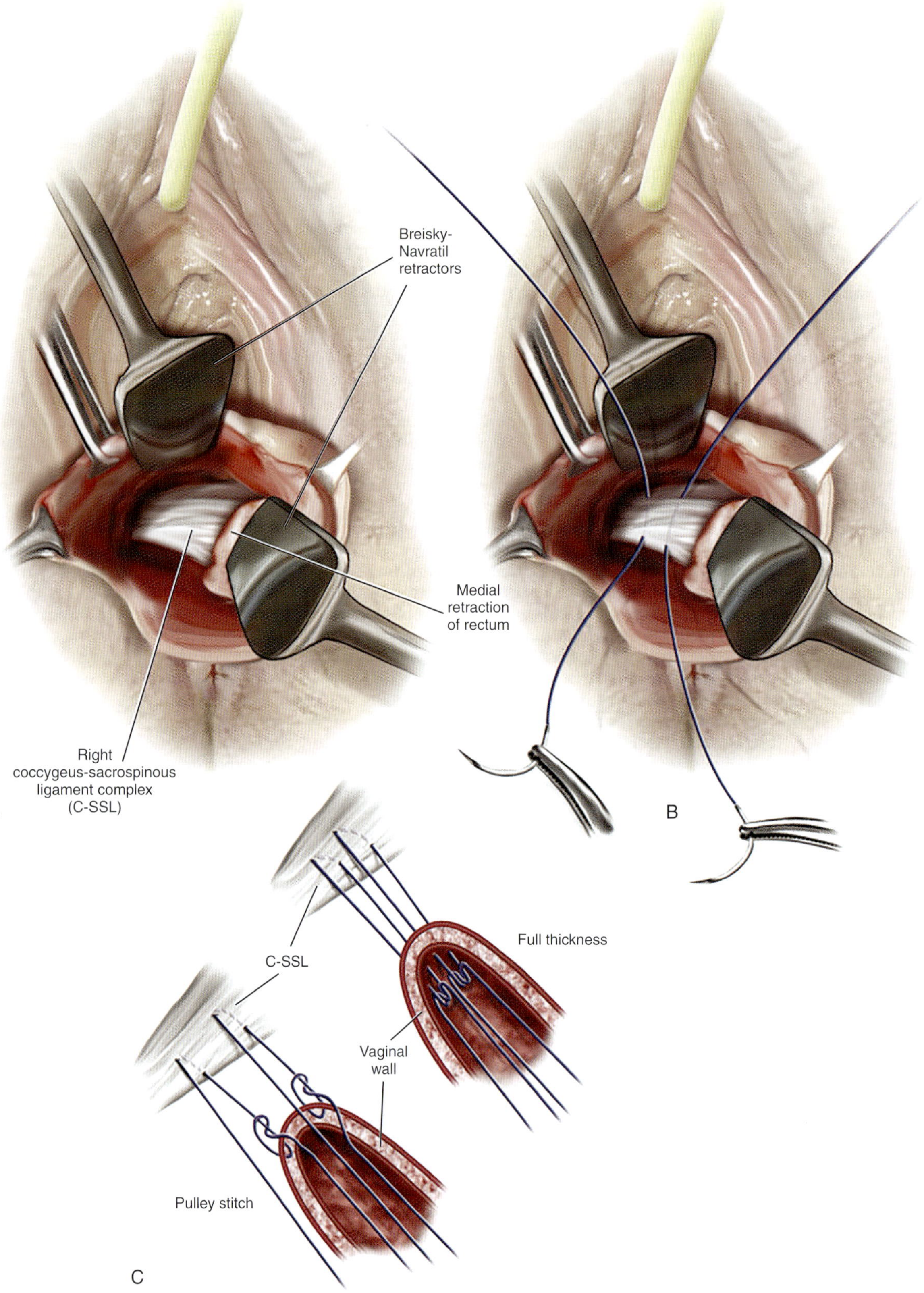


**Fig. 20.36** Sacrospinous ligament fixation. **A,** After the rectal pillar is perforated, retractors are used to help identify the coccygeus muscle–sacrospinous ligament complex. **B,** Two sutures are placed in the sacrospinous ligament 2 cm medial to the ischial spine. **C,** The vaginal apex can be fixed to the sacrospinous ligament using a pulley-stitch technique for nonabsorbable suture or a full-thickness technique for delayed absorbable suture. Nitti, VW, Karam M. Vaginal Repair of Enterocele and Apical Prolapse. Vaginal Surgery for the Urologist, Chapter 6, 49-70. Copyright © 2012 by Saunders, an imprint of Elsevier Inc.

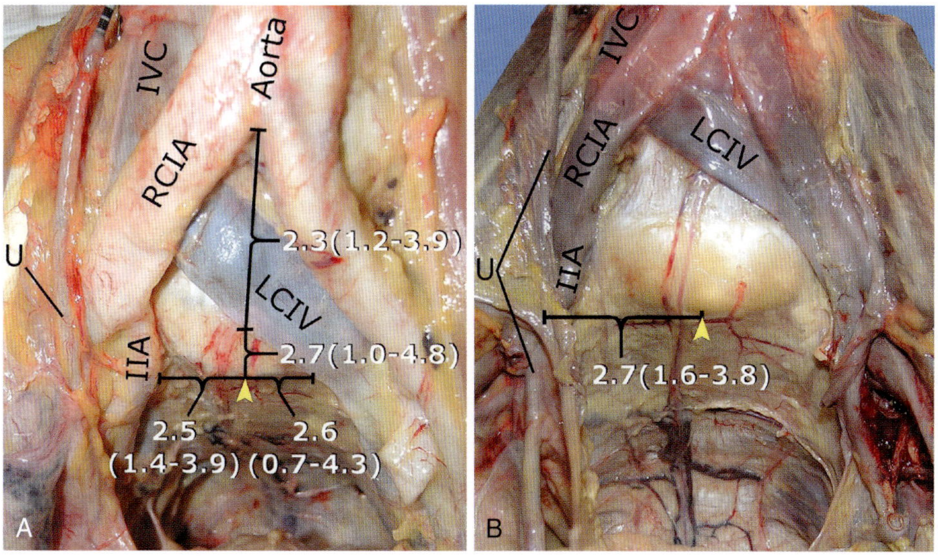


**Fig. 20.37** Exposed presacral space in two unembalmed cadavers. These exposed presacral space illustrate the average distances (in centimeters) and range from midsacral promontory *(yellow arrowhead)* to (**A**) the vascular structures and (**B**) the right ureter. Note the proximity of LCIV to the midsacral promontory in the cadaver on **A**. *IIA,* Internal iliac artery; *IVC,* inferior vena cava; *LCIV,* left common iliac vein; *RCIA,* right common iliac artery; *U,* ureter. (From Good MM, Abele TA, Balgobin S, et al. Vascular and ureteral anatomy relative to the midsacral promontory. *Am J Obstet Gynecol.* 2013;208(6):486.e1-486.e7.)

**is suspended to the anterior longitudinal ligament of the sacrum using a bridging graft, with incorporation of graft into the fibromuscular layer of the anterior and/or posterior vaginal walls.** Depending on the extent of prolapse, the location of graft attachment on the anterior vaginal wall might be from just the apex to running most of the length of the anterior vaginal wall to the bladder neck. Similarly, posteriorly the graft can run inferiorly along the vaginal wall to the perineal body if necessary.

Operative complications from abdominal sacral colpopexy include cystotomy (3.1%), enterotomy (1.6%), wound problems (4.6%), ileus (3.6%), thromboembolic event (3.3%), ureteral injury (1%), hemorrhage or transfusion (4.4%), and small bowel obstruction (1% to 5%). As with vaginally placed mesh, synthetic mesh for sacrocolpopexies can result in vaginal exposures or bladder or bowel erosions, although the rates of mesh complications for mesh placed abdominally is less than that for mesh placed vaginally. Some operative risks such as wound problems are decreased with minimally invasive techniques (laparoscopy, robot) compared with laparotomy (Fig. 20.36). Care must be taken to visualize the blood vessels and be prepared in the event of hemorrhage.

**As with other POP surgeries, abdominal sacral colpopexy can unmask stress urinary incontinence.** A multicenter study of 322 women with no preoperative stress incontinence symptoms were randomized to have a concomitant Burch colposuspension or not (controls). Three months after surgery, 24% of women in the Burch group and 44% of controls had stress incontinence, even though none reported stress incontinence preoperatively. Burch colposuspension significantly reduced postoperative stress incontinence when performed at the time of abdominal sacral colpopexy, without an increase in other urinary problems (Brubaker, 2006). Now that midurethral slings have largely replaced Burch colposuspensions, it is less imperative to preemptively treat stress incontinence at the time of a sacral colpopexy. Surgeons and patients have the option of concomitant antiincontinence surgery in the form of a midurethral sling or Burch at the time of sacral colpopexy or performing an interval midurethral sling surgery if indicated postoperatively.

In elderly women who are no longer sexually active, and particularly in those who have medical reasons to avoid a longer procedure, a Le Fort–type colpocleisis operation may be performed with low complication and recurrence rate. This procedure was discussed in detail in the uterine prolapse section of this chapter.

## RECTAL PROLAPSE

Rectal prolapse or rectal procidentia is partial or full-thickness protrusion of the rectum through the anus. It is uncommon but shares many of the same risk factors with POP, including prior pelvic surgery. General or colorectal surgeons usually manage this surgically.

## CONCLUSION

POP is common, particularly in parous women. In women with symptomatic POP, several areas of pelvic function should be discussed and potentially addressed, including urinary, bowel, and sexual concerns. Nonsurgical treatments are often effective, and women do not need any treatment if they have no symptoms or bother. Symptomatic women with mild prolapse should be offered pelvic muscle strengthening, with pelvic floor physical therapy if available. Symptomatic women with any stage of prolapse should be offered a pessary fitting.

If surgical treatment is desired, there are many factors to consider, including which walls of the vagina are prolapsing, patient values and goals, patient comorbidities, and surgeon skill. Recurrent POP after surgery is a substantial problem. Causes of POP and long-term treatments are areas of ongoing research.

## KEY REFERENCES

Al Chalabi H, Larkin J, Mehigan B, McCormick P. A systematic review of laparoscopic versus open abdominal incisional hernia repair, with meta-analysis of randomized controlled trials. *Int J Surg.* 2015;20:65-74.

American College of Obstetricians and Gynecologists (ACOG). ACOG Practice Bulletin. Pelvic Organ Prolapse. No. 214. *Obstet Gynecol.* 2019; 1334:3126-3142.

American College of Obstetricians and Gynecologists (ACOG). ACOG Committee Opinion No. 701: choosing the route of hysterectomy for benign disease. *Obstet Gynecol.* 2017;129(6):e155-e159.

Baden WF, Walker TA. Genesis of the vaginal profile: a correlated classification of vaginal relaxation. *Clin Obstet Gynecol.* 1972;15(4):1048-1054.

Barber MD, Brubaker L, Burgio KL, et al. Comparison of 2 transvaginal surgical approaches and perioperative behavioral therapy for apical vaginal prolapse: the OPTIMAL randomized trial. *JAMA.* 2014; 311(10):1023-1034.

Blomquist JL, Muñoz A, Carroll M, Handa VL. Association of delivery mode with pelvic floor disorders after childbirth. *JAMA.* 2018; 320(23):2438-2447. doi: 10.1001/jama.2018.18315.

Braekken IH, Majida M, Engh ME, Bo K. Morphological changes after pelvic floor muscle training measured by 3-dimensional ultrasonography: a randomized controlled trial. *Obstet Gynecol.* 2010;115(2 Pt 1): 317-324.

Brubaker L, Cundiff GW, Fine P, et al. Abdominal sacrocolpopexy with Burch colposuspension to reduce urinary stress incontinence. *N Engl J Med.* 2006;354(15):1557-1566.

Bump RC, Mattiasson A, Bo K, et al. The standardization of terminology of female pelvic organ prolapse and pelvic floor dysfunction. *Am J Obstet Gynecol.* 1996;175(1):10-17.

Carter-Brooks CM, Lowder JL, Du AL, Lavelle ES, Giugale LE, Shepherd JP. Restoring Genital Hiatus to Normative Values After Apical Suspension Alone Versus With Level 3 Support Procedures. *Female Pelvic Med Reconstr Surg.* 2019 May/Jun;25(3):226-230. doi:10.1097/ SPV.0000000000000528.PMID: 29210807

Cartwright R, Kirby AC, Tikkinen KA, et al. Systematic review and metaanalysis of genetic association studies of urinary symptoms and prolapse in women. *Am J Obstet Gynecol.* 2014;212(2):199.e1-199.e24.

Chmielewski L, Walters MD, Weber AM, Barber MD. Reanalysis of a randomized trial of 3 techniques of anterior colporrhaphy using clinically relevant definitions of success. *Am J Obstet Gynecol.* 2011; 205(1):69.e61-e68.

DeLancey JO. Anatomic aspects of vaginal eversion after hysterectomy. *Am J Obstet Gynecol.* 1992;166(6 Pt 1):1717-1724; discussion 1724-1728.

Detollenaere RJ, den Boon J, Stekelenburg J, et al. Sacrospinous hysteropexy versus vaginal hysterectomy with suspension of the uterosacral ligaments in women with uterine prolapse stage 2 or higher: multicentre randomised non-inferiority trial. *BMJ.* 2015;351:h3717.

Eilber KS, Alperin M, Khan A, et al. Outcomes of vaginal prolapse surgery among female Medicare beneficiaries: the role of apical support. *Obstet Gynecol.* 2013;122(5):981-987.

Elliott CS, Yeh J, Comiter CV et al. The predictive value of a cystocele for concomitant vaginal apical prolapse. *J Urol.* 2013;189(1):200-203.

Fernando RJ, Thakar R, Sultan AH, et al. Effect of vaginal pessaries on symptoms associated with pelvic organ prolapse. *Obstet Gynecol.* 2006; 108(1):93-99.

Fitzgibbons Jr RJ, Forse RA. Clinical practice. Groin hernias in adults. *N Engl J Med.* 2015;372(8):756-763.

Geller EJ, Hankins KJ, Parnell BA, et al. Diagnostic accuracy of retrograde and spontaneous voiding trials for postoperative voiding dysfunction: a randomized controlled trial. *Obstet Gynecol.* 2011;118(3):637-642.

Gutman RE, Rardin CR, Sokol ER, et al. Vaginal and laparoscopic mesh hysteropexy for uterovaginal prolapse: a parallel cohort study. *Am J Obstet Gynecol.* 2017;216:38.e1-e38.

Hagen S, Stark D, Glazener C, et al. Individualised pelvic floor muscle training in women with pelvic organ prolapse (POPPY): a multicentre randomised controlled trial. *Lancet.* 2014;383(9919):796-806.

Handa VL, Blomquist JL, Roem J, Muñoz A, Dietz HP. Pelvic floor disorders after obstetric avulsion of the levator ani muscle. *Female Pelvic Med Reconstr Surg.* 2019;25(1):3-7.

Hoyte L, Jakab M, Warfield SK, et al. Levator ani thickness variations in symptomatic and asymptomatic women using magnetic resonance-based 3-dimensional color mapping. *Am J Obstet Gynecol.* 2004;191(3): 856-861.

Jonsson Funk M, Visco AG, Weidner AC, et al. Long-term outcomes of vaginal mesh versus native tissue repair for anterior vaginal wall prolapse. *Int Urogynecol J.* 2013;24(8):1279-1285.

Kaufmann R, Halm JA, Eker HH, et al. Mesh versus suture repair of umbilical hernia in adults: a randomised, double-blind, controlled, multicentre trial. *Lancet.* 2018;391(10123):860-869.

Larsson C, Kallen K, Andolf E. Cesarean section and risk of pelvic organ prolapse: a nested case-control study. *Am J Obstet Gynecol.* 2009; 200(3):243.e241-e244.

**Full references and Suggested readings for this chapter can be found on ExpertConsult.com.**

# 21 Lower Urinary Tract Function and Disorders

## Physiology of Micturition, Voiding Dysfunction, Urinary Incontinence, Urinary Tract Infections, and Painful Bladder Syndrome

*Gretchen M. Lentz, Jane L. Miller*

### KEY POINTS

- Continence is determined by the balance between forces that maintain urethral closure and those that affect detrusor function. Parasympathetic nervous system activity via the neurotransmitter acetylcholine stimulates receptors in the bladder wall to activate detrusor contraction. Sympathetic nervous system activation leads to bladder relaxation. Nearly 50% of all women may suffer from some degree of urinary incontinence during their lifetime. Being obese or overweight increases the risk of urinary incontinence, and weight loss can reduce stress and urge incontinence.
- Approximately 20% of women with urinary incontinence suffer from detrusor overactivity. Behavioral changes and oral medications are first-line treatments, although often they have disappointing cure rates. Neuromodulation and surgical procedures are available and effective for refractory symptoms.
- The midurethral synthetic tape slings appear to have similar efficacy for the surgical treatment of stress incontinence, with a shorter surgery and recovery time than a Burch colposuspension. Retropubic and transobturator midurethral slings have similar success rates for stress incontinence, although with different risk profiles. The retropubic approach has a significantly higher risk of bladder perforation, bleeding, and voiding dysfunction, and the obturator approach has a higher risk of groin and leg pain.
- Approximately 50% of all women will develop urinary infections at some point in their lifetime, and by age 70 years, as many as 10% of women will have recurrent urinary tract infections.
- Painful bladder syndrome–interstitial cystitis is a painful, chronic bladder condition that is not related to infection and is associated with symptoms of bladder and pelvic pain, urinary frequency, urgency, or nocturia, and often dyspareunia.

A 48-year-old woman, gravida 2, para 2 (G2P2) and otherwise healthy, reports poorly defined perineal dampness, pelvic pain, and urinary frequency. Which provider does she make an appointment to see? Lower urinary tract complaints are very common in women, and their presentation is often similar to gynecologic disorders, present concurrently with gynecologic disorders, and occasionally are a result of gynecologic procedures. The provider that the majority of women with lower urinary tract disorders see first for evaluation of their symptoms is their gynecologist. **There is considerable overlap in symptoms with urinary tract infections, overactive bladder, endometriosis, dyspareunia, and bladder pain syndrome, so the gynecologist should be familiar with these conditions.** This chapter will review the anatomy and physiology, as well as the evaluation and treatment, of some of the more common disorders of the female lower urinary tract.

## PHYSIOLOGY OF MICTURITION

**The normal lower urinary tract has two functions: the storage of urine at low bladder pressures without leakage; and the voluntary and complete emptying of urine from the bladder.** These functions are achieved through complex anatomic, physiologic, and neurologic interactions. Much of our current understanding is obtained from animal models; the relevance to human physiology is not always clear, and opinions differ.

### Neurophysiology

In review, the central nervous system (CNS) consists of the brain and the spinal cord, with the peripheral nervous system (PNS) divided into the somatic and autonomic nervous systems, which are made up of afferent (sensory) and efferent (motor) neurons that communicate with the CNS. **The somatic system regulates structures that are under voluntary control, such as the striated external urethral sphincter and levator ani muscles. The autonomic system regulates visceral functions such as detrusor (bladder muscle) contraction and relaxation. The autonomic system consists of the parasympathetic system (cranial and sacral segments of the spinal cord) and the sympathetic system (thoracic and lumbar segments)** (Clemons, 2010) (Fig. 21.1).

During storage, bladder pressures rise slowly despite large increases in volume. Bladder filling activates afferent nerve fibers in the bladder wall, which results in stimulation of sympathetic efferent activity in the hypogastric nerve, which leads to contraction of the smooth muscles in the bladder base and proximal urethra as well as relaxation of the detrusor from activation of beta-adrenergic receptors in the bladder wall. After a certain bladder pressure is reached, there is a gradual increase in somatic efferent nerve activity through the pudendal nerve and possibly the pelvic nerve, which causes increased activity in the striated external urethral sphincter. These are spinal reflexes located in the lumbosacral spinal cord and promote continence. At the same time, the sympathetic system inhibits parasympathetic activity at the ganglia level, further promoting bladder relaxation. The result of all these actions is filling of the bladder with low pressures without any active bladder contractions (Fig. 21.2).

**Voiding depends on the coordinated activity of the bladder outlet (external sphincter, proximal urethra/bladder base) and detrusor muscle.** Bladder emptying is initiated voluntarily by signals from the cerebral cortex, which are a result of intravesicle pressure producing the sensation of distention. The first step in emptying is inhibition of somatic efferent activity, resulting in relaxation of the striated external urethral sphincter. This is closely followed by a detrusor contraction, as a result of

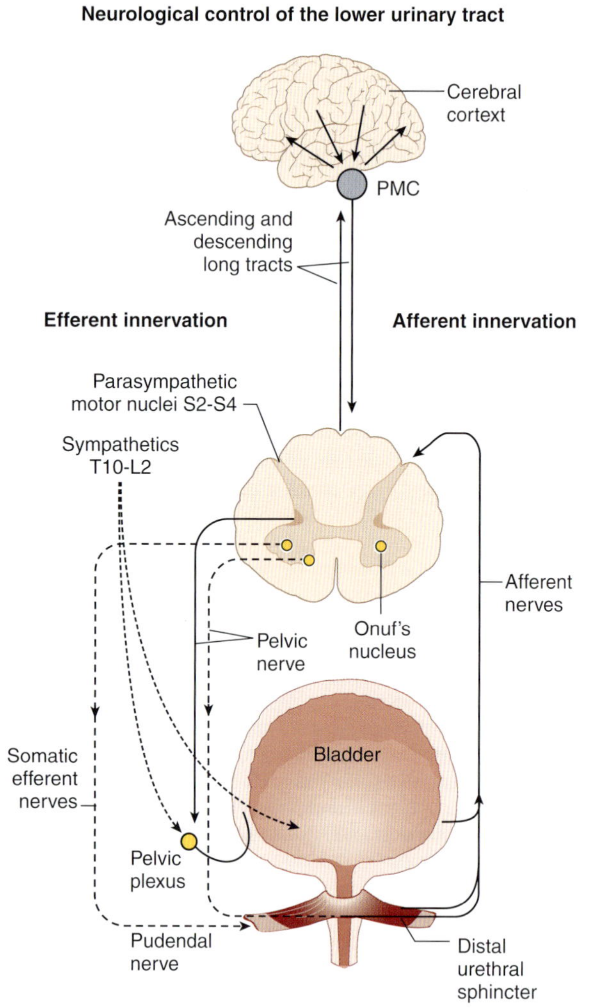


**Fig. 21.1** Neurologic control of the lower urinary tract. (From Zacharzewski A, Davies S. Micturition. *Anaesth Intensive Care Med.* 2018;19(5):258-262.)

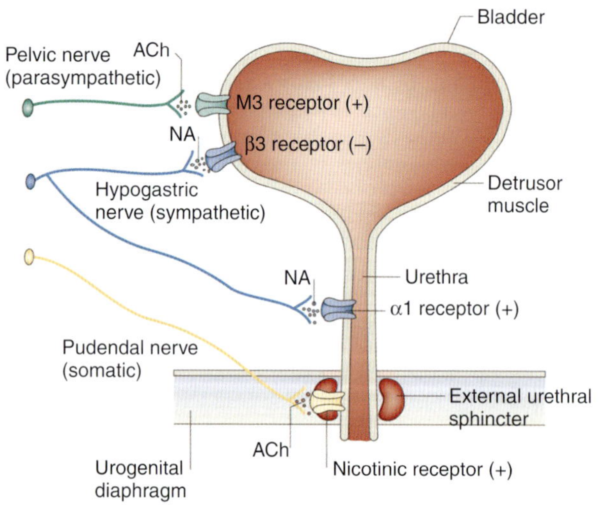


**Fig. 21.2** Efferent pathways and neurotransmitter mechanisms that regulate the lower urinary tract. *ACh,* Acetylcholine; *NA,* noradrenaline. From Li LF, Leung GKK, Lui WM. Sacral nerve Stimulation for neurogenic bladder. *World Neurosurg.* 2016;90:236-243. Copyright © 2016 Elsevier Inc. Figure 1. Reprinted from Fowler CJ, Griffiths D, de Groat WC. The neural control of micturition. *Nat Rev Neurosci.* 2008;9:453-466.)

inhibition of sympathetic efferent activity with concomitant activation of parasympathetic outflow through the pelvic nerve to the bladder and urethra. **Bladder contraction is mediated via muscarinic receptors in the bladder wall.** Superimposed on these autonomic and somatic reflexes are complex supraspinal (the midbrain, cerebellum, and cerebral cortex) inputs mediated through the pons (spinobulbospinal reflex), which allows for full conscious control of voiding and maintenance of the reflex until the bladder is empty (Table 21.1, Fig. 21.3).

Acetylcholine (Ach) is released from postganglionic parasympathetic neurons, preganglionic autonomic neurons, and somatic neurons. There are two main types of cholinergic receptors-nicotinic and muscarinic. Nicotinic receptors have little role in the lower urinary tract. The five muscarinic receptors (M1 to M5) play a significant role, with the M2-M3 most abundant in the detrusor. M3 receptors are responsible for bladder contraction. Norepinephrine and epinephrine released from postganglionic sympathetic neurons bind to adrenergic (alpha and beta) receptors. There are multiple adrenergic receptor subtypes. The alpha 1A subtype predominates in the urethra, where it plays a role in bladder outlet contraction. Beta 2 and 3 receptors cause detrusor relaxation. Location of these receptors plays a role in function as well. Parasympathetic activation via M3 muscarinic receptors located more densely in the bladder body than base results in detrusor contraction and voiding. Sympathetic activation via alpha-adrenergic receptors in the bladder base and urethra (contraction) and beta-adrenergic receptors in the bladder body (relaxation) result in storage (see Fig. 21.2).

Multiple other neurotransmitters and receptors have been found in the lower urinary tract. These include adenosine triphosphate (ATP), nitric oxide (NO), vanilloids, substance P, prostanoids, and estrogen. The roles of most of these have not been defined. Many drugs affect these receptors and therefore lower urinary tract function (Table 21.2).

**In light of the complexity and extensive involvement of the nervous system, a host of systemic disease processes, including neurologic disease, and direct trauma, in addition to medications, can affect lower urinary tract function.** Diabetes can result in sensory neuropathy with resultant bladder overdistention and detrusor injury with resultant urinary retention. Detrusor overactivity or involuntary detrusor contractions is commonly seen in patients with diabetes as well. Processes involving the brain and CNS such as stroke or traumatic brain injury often result in loss of bladder inhibition with detrusor overactivity as a result. Obviously a spinal cord injury with disruption of the spinal neural pathways will result in change in bladder function; what change is seen depends on the level of injury, degree of injury (partial vs. complete), and age of the injury. Approximately 15% of patients with multiple sclerosis will have a voiding complaint as their first reported symptom. Pelvic surgery with direct injury to pelvic or pudendal nerves can cause dysfunction. Pelvic nerve injury with resultant urinary retention is a known complication of radical hysterectomy.

**In summary, normal bladder function requires the bladder to accommodate increasing volumes of urine at low pressure with appropriate sensation and no involuntary contractions. The bladder outlet has to be closed at rest and stay closed with increase in intraabdominal pressures. The bladder must then contract in a coordinated manner of adequate strength as the bladder outlet resistance at the level of the smooth muscle sphincter and striated sphincter lowers. This requires intact local and spinal reflexes and an intact CNS.**

## Lower Urinary Tract Anatomy and Physiology (Female Continence)

**The bladder consists of the bladder body—the bladder above the ureteral orifices—and a bladder base consisting of the trigone and bladder neck. The bladder neck, urethra, and pelvic floor musculature make up the bladder outlet** (Fig. 21.4, A).

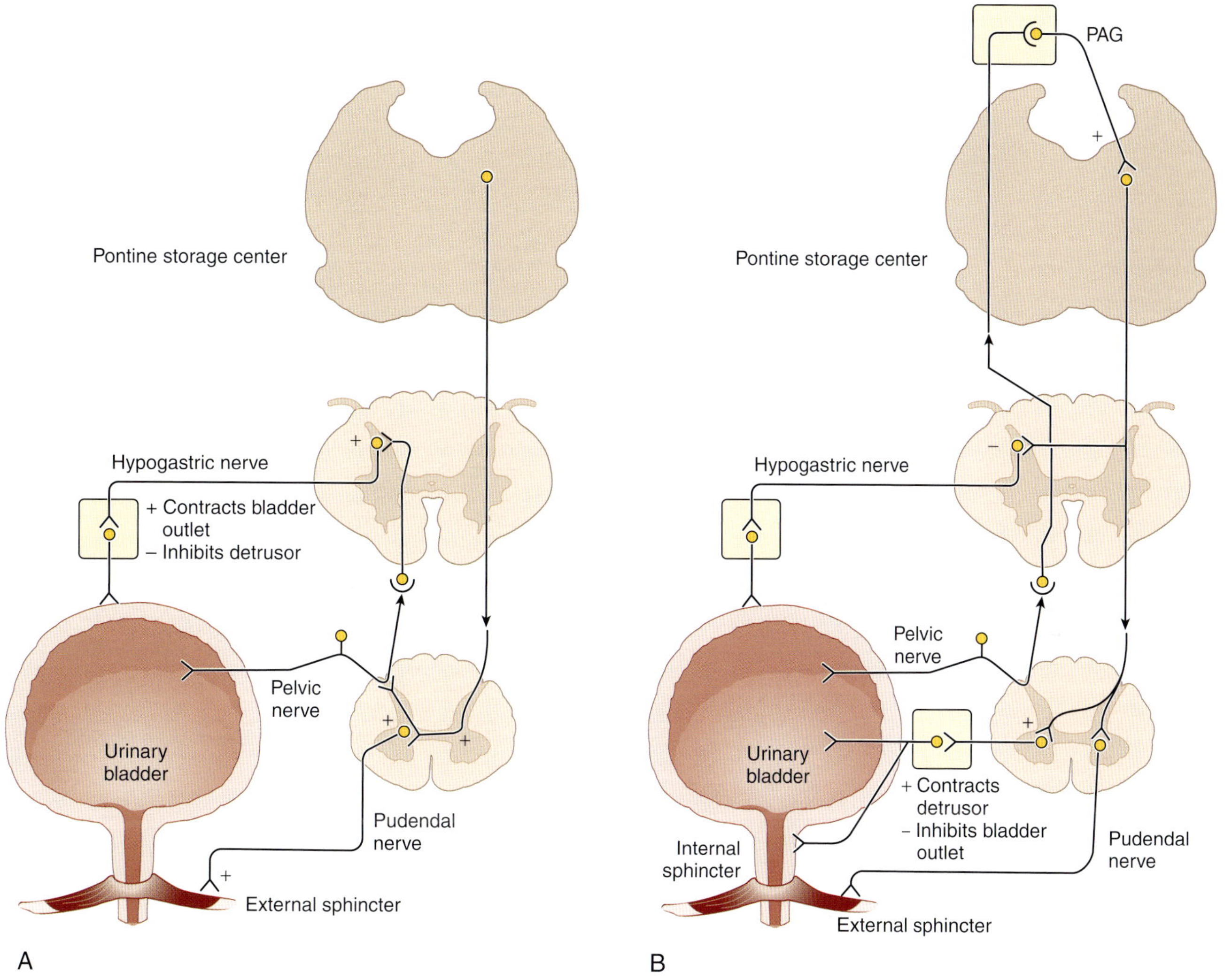


**Fig. 21.3** Neural circuits that control continence and micturition. *PAG,* periaqueductal gray. (From De Groat WC. Neurophysiology and neuroanatomy of the genitourinary organs. In: Krames ES, Peckham PH, Rezai AR, eds. *Neuromodulation: Comprehensive Textbook of Principles, Technologies, and Therapies.* 2nd ed. London: Elsevier; 2018:1437-1449.)

**TABLE 21.1** Neurologic Control of Micturition: Clinical Considerations on Central Nervous System Reflex Loops

| Loop | Origin | Termination | Function | Associated Conditions |
|---|---|---|---|---|
| I | Frontal lobe | Brainstem | Coordinates volitional control of micturition | Parkinson disease, brain tumors, trauma, micturition |
| II | Brainstem<br>Bladder wall | Brainstem | Detrusor muscle contraction to empty bladder | Spinal cord trauma, multiple sclerosis (MS), spinal cord tumors, neuropathy, local urinary tract disease |
| III | Sensory afferents of tumors, diabetic detrusor muscle disease | Striated muscle of urethral sphincter via pudendal motor neurons and sacral micturition center | Allows relaxation of urethral sphincter in synchrony with detrusor contraction | MS, spinal cord trauma or neuropathy, local urinary tract |
| IV | Frontal lobe | Pudendal nucleus | Volitional control of striated external urethral sphincter | Cerebral or spinal trauma or tumor, MS, cerebrovascular disease, lower urinary tract disease |

Modified from Ostergard DR. The neurological control of micturition and integral voiding reflexes. *Obstet Gynecol Surv.* 1979;34:417-423.

The bladder body and base includes a multilayered epithelium that is in contact with urine, including the following:

- Lamina propria with a diffuse plexus of unmyelinated nerve fibers making contact and regulating interactions between urothelium
- Detrusor smooth muscle and the wall made up of smooth muscle arranged in random directions, collagen, and elastin, resulting in the viscoelastic properties of the bladder.

These properties contribute to a low-pressure reservoir, which is needed for continence.

**TABLE 21.2** Drugs That Affect Continence and Micturition

| Classification | Examples | Pharmacologic Action |
|---|---|---|
| Anticholinergic agents | Atropine<br>Glycopyrrolate<br>Oxybutynin<br>Propantheline<br>Tolterodine | Inhibit muscarinic receptors, thus reducing the response to cholinergic stimulation; used to reduce pressure during bladder filling and for the treatment of unstable bladder contractions. |
| Smooth muscle relaxants | Dicyclomine<br>Flavoxate | Direct smooth muscle relaxation reduces intravesical pressure during filling and reduces severity and presence of unstable bladder contractions; most of these agents have some degree of anticholinergic action. |
| Calcium antagonists | Diltiazem<br>Nifedipine<br>Verapamil | Used in the treatment of unstable bladder contractions to reduce the magnitude of the spikes by reducing the entrance of calcium during an action potential. |
| Potassium channel openers | Cromakalim<br>Pinacidil | Act to increase the membrane potential and thus reduce the myogenic initiation of unstable bladder contractions. |
| Prostaglandin synthesis inhibitors | Flurbiprofen | Prostaglandins have been implicated in increased smooth muscle tone and in the induction of spontaneous activity. Inhibition of prostaglandin synthesis could promote relaxation of the bladder during filling and decrease spontaneous activity of the bladder. |
| β-Adrenergic agonists | Isoproterenol<br>Terbutaline | Stimulation of β receptors induces relaxation of the bladder body, resulting in a decrease in intravesical pressure during filling. |
| Tricyclic antidepressants | Amitriptyline<br>Imipramine | These agents have anticholinergic, direct smooth muscle relaxant, and norepinephrine reuptake inhibition properties. |
| α-Adrenergic agonists | Ephedrine<br>Phenylpropanolamine<br>Midodrine<br>Pseudoephedrine | Increase urethral tone and closure pressure by direct stimulation of α-adrenergic receptors. |
| Afferent nerve inhibitors | DMSO<br>Capsaicin<br>Resiniferatoxin | Reduce the sensory input from bladder and thereby increase bladder capacity and reduce detrusor overactivity. |
| Estrogen | Estradiol | Direct application to the vagina or oral therapy may increase the thickness of the urothelial mucosa, making a better seal and reducing the incidence of incontinence. Other actions may include increasing adrenergic effects on the urethra and increasing blood flow. |

From Chai TC, Birder LA. Physiology and pharmacology of the bladder and urethra. In: Wein A, Kavoussi L, Partin A, Peters C, eds. *Campbell-Walsh Urology*. 11th ed. Philadelphia: Elsevier; 2016:1631-1684.e14.
*DMSO,* Dimethyl sulfoxide.

The continence mechanism in women centers on the proximal urethra and urethrovesical junction. **Continence is maintained by multiple structural and physiologic mechanisms that promote a low-pressure reservoir and higher than storage pressure outlet, regulate closure of the urethra, and support of the bladder and urethrovesical junction. Actual closure of the urethra is produced by the involuntary internal sphincter at the bladder neck, the voluntary external sphincter muscles of the urethra, and mucosal coaptation produced by the urethral submucosal vascular plexus and anatomic attachments of the urethra and anterior vagina (hammock hypothesis).**

The internal sphincter is formed by a ring of involuntary smooth muscle from the bladder trigone and 2 u-shaped loops from the detrusor. Unlike the male internal sphincter, it is fairly common for the female internal sphincter or bladder neck to be incompetent but still continent. The bulk of the muscle responsible for sphincteric control in women is the external sphincter—the circular striated muscles located in the proximal urethra and midurethra. These muscles create a nearly complete circumferential compression of the midurethra under the influence of tonic pudendal (sympathetic) innervation. Pudendal nerve injury as a result of prolonged labor with resultant sphincteric weakness is one way incontinence may occur after vaginal childbirth.

The submucosal arteriovenous complex of the urethra plays a significant role in female continence as well. It has been estimated to contribute 30% of the forces responsible for continence as a result of the seal of mucosal folds supported by the spongy nature of this estrogen rich plexus. This plexus is thicker walled and less elastic in older women, which likely contributes to lower urethral pressures and greater risk of incontinence (Fig. 21.4, B).

**Musculofascial support for the urethra is also important for continence. Attachment of the midurethra anteriorly to the symphysis by the pubourethral ligaments and laterally to the arcus tendineus by the urethropelvic ligaments helps prevent transmission of intraabdominal pressure to the remainder of the urethra. The anterior vaginal wall, when intact, provides posterior support and compression of the midurethra, particularly with increased intraabdominal pressure.**

**The zone with the highest pressure in the urethra is approximately at the midpoint of the functional urethral length.**

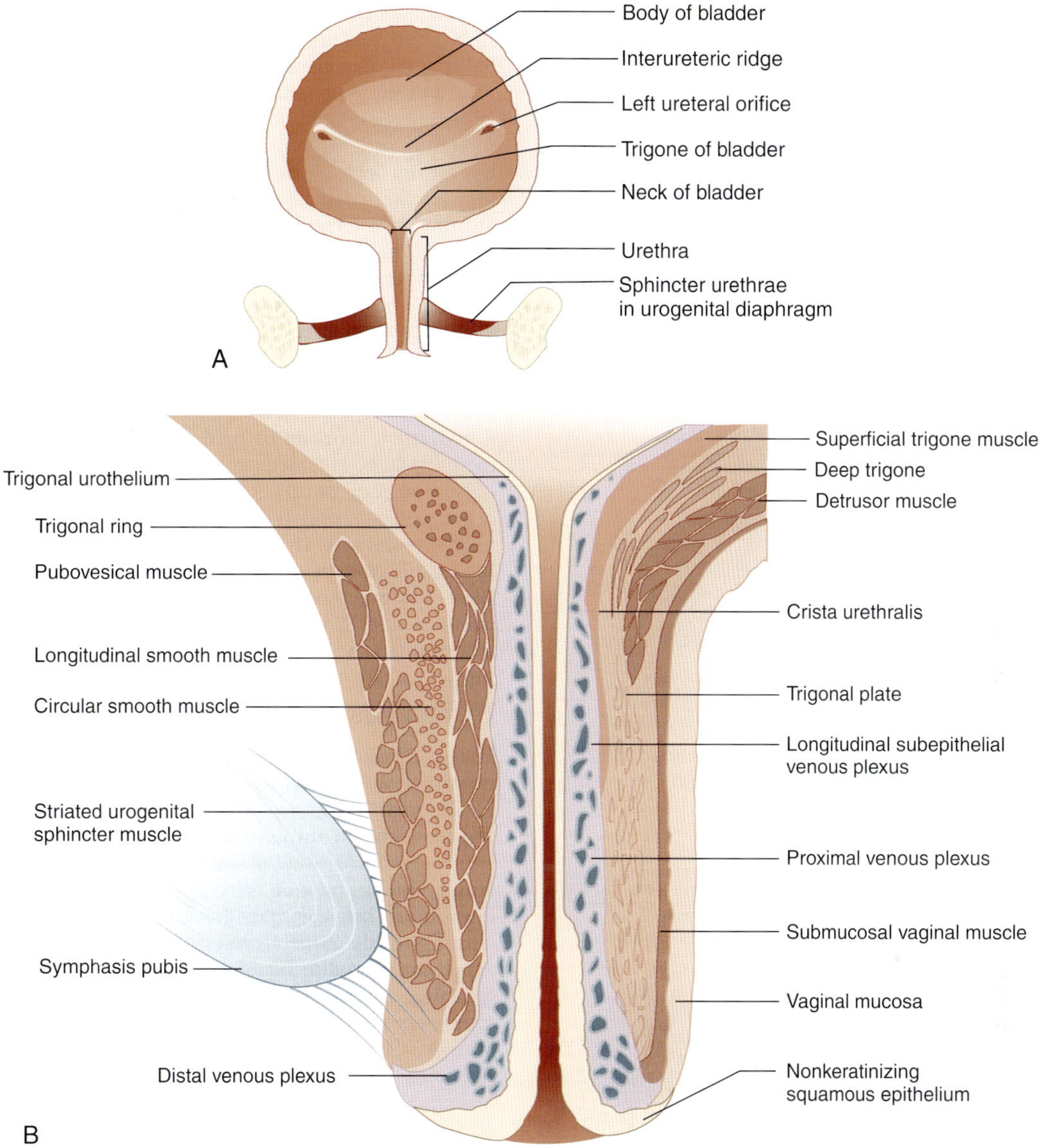


**Fig. 21.4 A,** Anatomy of the bladder and urethra in relationship to the perivesical structures. **B,** Female urethra showing importance of the multiple tissues in aid of continence including striated sphincter, smooth sphincter, and subepithelial venous plexus. (**A,** From Occhino JA, Heisler CA. Anatomy of the female urinary tract. In: Gebhart JB. *Urologic Surgery for the Gynecologist and Urogynecologist.* Philadelphia: Saunders; 2010:1-16. **B,** From Chai TC, Birder LA. Physiology and pharmacology of the bladder and urethra. In: Wein A, Kavoussi L, Partin A, Peters C, eds. *Campbell-Walsh Urology.* 11th ed. Philadelphia: Elsevier; 2016:1631-1684.)

The anatomic urethral length is approximately 3 to 4 cm. This high-pressure zone is located approximately 0.5 cm proximal to the urogenital diaphragm. Most of the functional urethral length is actually above the urogenital diaphragm (Fig. 21.5). The submucosal cavernous plexus of vessels, the bulk of the smooth and striated muscle, and the bulk of the autonomic nerve supply are most prominent in the area in which they record the maximum urethral pressure.

The combined effect of these anatomic attachments (Fig. 21.6), urethral attributes, and muscular and neurologic functions promote continence, and the loss of any one, though often there is loss of several, can result in female urinary incontinence.

## DIAGNOSTIC PROCEDURES

**The clinical history is very useful in the diagnosis of urinary incontinence.** A history consistent with urge-associated urinary incontinence—"I get an urge to go and I can't get to the bathroom on time"—is more sensitive than urodynamics for making such a diagnosis. Several validated scales are available, such as the Urogenital Distress Inventory (UDI), Incontinence Impact Questionnaire (IIQ), Bristol Female Lower Urinary Tract Questionnaire, and King's Health Questionnaire, although not one has become the preferred instrument. Useful testing can be done in the gynecologist's office without the need for sophisticated equipment. These procedures are described and their benefits noted. The description is followed by a discussion of more sophisticated diagnostic techniques requiring specialized equipment.

### Urinalysis and Culture

**A simple urinalysis and urine culture may provide much information.** The presence of white or red blood cells (RBCs) and

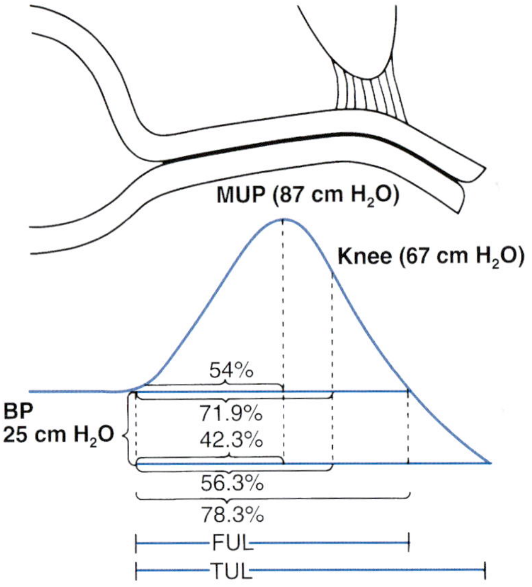


**Fig. 21.5** Location of maximum urethral pressure in relation to the urogenital diaphragm (average value of 25 normal women). Knee indicates the location of the urogenital diaphragm seen on x-ray film and transformed to the pressure curve. *BP,* Blood pressure; *FUL,* functional urethral length; *MUP,* maximal urethral pressure; *TUL,* total urethral length. (From Asmussen M, Ulmsten U. On the physiology of continence and pathophysiology of stress incontinence in the female. *Contrib Gynecol Obstet.* 1983;10:32-50.)

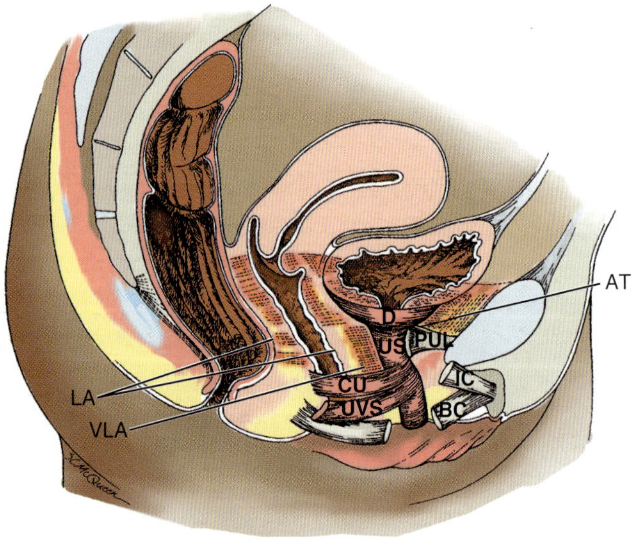


**Fig. 21.6** Interrelationships of approximate location of paraurethral structures. Levator ani muscles are shown as light lines running deep to the pelvic viscera. The vaginal levator attachment is shown as a darker area. *AT,* Arcus tendineus fasciae pelvis; *BC,* bulbocavernosus muscle; *CU,* compressor urethrae; *D,* detrusor muscle; *IC,* ischiocavernosus muscle; *LA,* levator ani muscles; *PUL,* pubourethral ligament; *US,* urethral sphincter; *UVS,* urethrovaginal sphincter; *VLA,* vaginal levator attachment. (Modified from DeLancey JO. Correlative study of paraurethral anatomy. *Obstet Gynecol.* 1986;68:91-97.)

bacteria in a catheterized or clean voided sample, in which the perineum around the urethra has been appropriately prepared with an antiseptic solution, may suggest a urinary tract infection (UTI), nephrolithiasis, kidney disease, or even urinary tract malignancy in rare cases. UTI may be associated with urgency, frequency, dysuria, suprapubic pain, and even incontinence. In such cases the urinalysis and urine culture may be diagnostic. Several dipstick methods are available to detect bacteriuria, pyuria, and the presence of nitrites and leukocyte esterase. The accuracy of these methods is variable, but they do have some use in screening patients who are incontinent or have symptoms suggestive of infection. In some cases, a culture should be obtained to identify the specific organism involved and verify the presence of an infection. Urinalysis is also useful to screen for microscopic hematuria (RBCs) in women with new-onset urgency and frequency because underlying pathologic conditions of the urinary tract may be present. **A formal microscopic urinalysis should be carried out to confirm screening results because urine dipstick tests can often yield a false-positive result (such as a urine dipstick test positive for occult blood), and actual RBCs need to be identified microscopically before proceeding with a hematuria workup or urologic referral.** A catheterized specimen should be obtained if abnormal results are questioned because of vaginal contamination. This is common in women with pelvic organ prolapse, obesity, postmenopausal bleeding, or menses or in older women with arthritis and poor hand function. With a goal of limiting unnecessary use of antibiotics and thus antibiotic resistance, routine treatment of bacteruria without symptoms even in patients with diabetes is no longer recommended except for pregnant women and women planning to undergo urologic procedures.

## Test for Residual Urine/Postvoid Residual

**Postvoid residual (PVR) testing is a simple procedure can be extremely helpful in the evaluation of a woman with incontinence with pelvic organ prolapse, voiding symptoms such as frequency or incomplete bladder emptying, or recurrent UTIs.** The woman with a full bladder is asked to void. Then within 10 to 15 minutes the residual urine in her bladder is measured either by inserting a catheter into the bladder (after which the urine collected may be sent for urinalysis and culture if needed) or noninvasively by using ultrasound or bladder scan ultrasound. The bladder ultrasound scan devices can occasionally result in false positives because of other pelvic conditions like ascites, a large ovarian cyst, or uterine fibroids. Confirmation is necessary with catheterization if this is suspected. Definitions of normal PVR volumes vary, but under normal circumstances the amount of residual urine should be less than 20% of the total bladder volume (e.g., 100 mL after voiding 400 mL). Postoperative patients have an 85% chance of avoiding retention if their initial postoperative PVR is a third of their total volume. **A large PVR suggests urinary retention resulting from inadequate bladder emptying as a result of detrusor underactivity, bladder outlet obstruction, or a combination of the two.**

## Bladder Diary

In many cases, stress and urge urinary incontinence can be correctly diagnosed from the clinical history alone. The bladder diary appears to be a cost-effective adjunct to clinical history for diagnosing overactive bladder. **Asking the woman to complete a bladder diary is a simple, inexpensive way to obtain information about her fluid intake, voiding habits, voided volumes, and incontinence episodes.** An example diary form is shown in Fig. 21.7.

## Office Cystometrics

It is possible to gain a great deal of information about bladder capacity and bladder function with relatively simple tools. Once a catheter is inserted to check for residual urine, the catheter is left in place and attached to a graduated Asepto syringe without a bulb. It is possible to pour sterile saline (or sterile water) into the syringe by gravity and measure the amount of saline that first

**Your Daily Bladder Diary**

This diary will help you and your health care team. Bladder diaries help show the causes of bladder control trouble. The "Example" line (below) will show you how to use the diary.

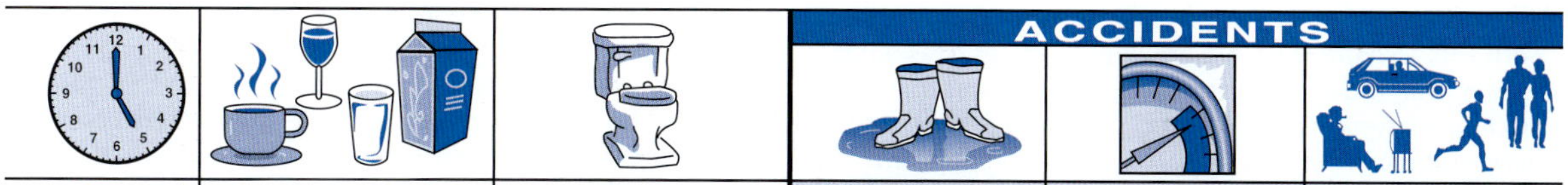

| Time | Drinks | | Urine | | ACCIDENTS | | |
|---|---|---|---|---|---|---|---|
| | *What kind?* | *How many?* | *How many times?* | *How much?* *sm med lg* | Accidental leaks *sm med lg* | Did you feel a strong urge to go? | What were you doing at the time? *Sneezing, exercising, driving, lifting, etc.* |
| Example | coffee | 2 cups | // | ☐ ☒ ☐ | ☐ ☒ ☐ | ☒ Yes ☐ No | Running |
| 6–7 am | | | | ☐ ☐ ☐ | ☐ ☐ ☐ | ☐ Yes ☐ No | |
| 7–8 am | | | | ☐ ☐ ☐ | ☐ ☐ ☐ | ☐ Yes ☐ No | |
| 8–9 am | | | | ☐ ☐ ☐ | ☐ ☐ ☐ | ☐ Yes ☐ No | |
| 9–10 am | | | | ☐ ☐ ☐ | ☐ ☐ ☐ | ☐ Yes ☐ No | |
| 10–11 am | | | | ☐ ☐ ☐ | ☐ ☐ ☐ | ☐ Yes ☐ No | |
| 11–12 noon | | | | ☐ ☐ ☐ | ☐ ☐ ☐ | ☐ Yes ☐ No | |
| 12–1 pm | | | | ☐ ☐ ☐ | ☐ ☐ ☐ | ☐ Yes ☐ No | |
| 1–2 pm | | | | ☐ ☐ ☐ | ☐ ☐ ☐ | ☐ Yes ☐ No | |
| 2–3 pm | | | | ☐ ☐ ☐ | ☐ ☐ ☐ | ☐ Yes ☐ No | |
| 3–4 pm | | | | ☐ ☐ ☐ | ☐ ☐ ☐ | ☐ Yes ☐ No | |
| 4–5 pm | | | | ☐ ☐ ☐ | ☐ ☐ ☐ | ☐ Yes ☐ No | |
| 5–6 pm | | | | ☐ ☐ ☐ | ☐ ☐ ☐ | ☐ Yes ☐ No | |
| 6–7 pm | | | | ☐ ☐ ☐ | ☐ ☐ ☐ | ☐ Yes ☐ No | |

**Your name:** ______________________________ **Date:** ______________

**Fig. 21.7** Daily bladder diary. (From Vasavada SP, Appell R, Sand PK, et al, eds. *Female Urology, Urogynecology, and Voiding Dysfunction.* New York: Marcel Dekker; 2005:127.)

causes the woman to have the urge to void. This first urge should normally occur after 150 to 200 mL of saline has been infused. Women with normal bladder function should be able to continue to maintain continence at that level. Similarly, a strong, normally controllable urge to void usually occurs when 400 to 500 mL has been instilled. Thus a normal bladder first transmits an urge to void at 150 to 200 mL, and functional capacity is reached at 400 to 600 mL. Larger volumes can be reached without incontinence, but this is usually accomplished with a great deal of conscious effort. If, during filling, the woman reports urgency and the column of fluid in the Asepto syringe rises, leakage may be seen around the catheter and detrusor overactivity confirmed.

## Cough Stress Test and Pad Weight Test

If a bladder has been previously filled to measure capacity, it should then be emptied to approximately 250 to 300 mL of saline, or if the bladder is empty, 250 to 300 mL of saline should be instilled. The catheter is then removed and the woman is asked to cough while in the recumbent position. If urine spurts from the urethral meatus, stress incontinence may be present and a positive cough stress test (CST) is noted. The CST should be repeated with the woman standing if no leakage is seen recumbent. Often she will appear to be continent with stress while lying down but may demonstrate incontinence when the influence of gravity on the pelvic organs is brought into play in the standing position. For research studies, 250 or 300 mL of saline is instilled, the woman is asked to cough 10 times, and any leakage is considered a positive CST. In clinical practice, if the patient has a comfortably full bladder, it is also reasonable to perform the standing CST and then calculate the volume in the bladder afterward by adding the voided volume and the PVR. If around 250 mL, the volume was adequate. If the volume in the bladder was low during a negative CST, it should be repeated with around 250 mL. The clinical stress test is effective in diagnosing stress incontinence.

Because urine loss with cough should be immediate if stress incontinence is the problem, it may be possible to detect evidence of detrusor overactivity by observing the time of the spurt of urine in the stress test. Typically the detrusor reacts a few seconds after the stimulus; therefore a spurt that occurs after a delay after a cough suggests the presence of a cough-induced involuntary detrusor contraction.

If no leakage is seen and anterior vaginal wall prolapse is present, occult stress incontinence is possible. It can be challenging to determine whether a woman with anterior vaginal wall relaxation is likely to develop overt stress incontinence after a pelvic organ prolapse repair. The CST can be repeated with the prolapse reduced with lubricated procto swabs or with a pessary. A positive prolapse reduction CST is associated with increased risk of de novo stress incontinence compared with a negative test, but it is not a perfectly accurate predictor.

A 1-hour pad weight test is another research tool for documenting pre- and postintervention urinary leakage volumes.

Again, with a 250-mL bladder volume, a pad is given to the woman and she is asked to complete a series of activities over the hour, including walking, climbing stairs, coughing, and other events. If the pad weighs more than 2 to 3 g, the test is considered positive. Both this test and the CST are commonly used as objective measures of outcome for surgical incontinence trials.

Thus with urinalysis, urine culture, measuring PVR urine, bladder diary, documented first urge to void, bladder capacity, and the CST, the physician will have a great deal of information concerning the cause of the woman's urinary complaints. More sophisticated urodynamic evaluations should be performed when these tests do not reveal an accurate diagnosis and further information is needed for treatment. A short discussion of these procedures and the equipment involved follows.

## Urodynamics

**Urodynamic investigation attempts to measure bladder and urethral function and voiding function. Cystometry, part of the urodynamic test, measures the pressure/volume relationship of the bladder during the filling (storage) phase of the micturition cycle.** Bladder sensations, first urge to void, normal desire to void, bladder pain, strong urge, and bladder capacity are noted. The woman can cough and perform the Valsalva maneuver to detect stress incontinence in the absence of a detrusor contraction. Detrusor overactivity may be noted with the symptom of urgency, with or without leakage, in association with a detrusor pressure rise. Poor compliance from a nonelastic bladder is noted with a gradual pressure rise of more than 15 cm $H_2O$ from baseline rather than phasic contractions of detrusor overactivity. **Pressure flow studies measure the relationship between pressure in the bladder and urine flow rate during voiding.** The ideal means of evaluating a woman for incontinence is to use a multichannel recorder that permits pressure determinations at two points within the urethra (proximal and midpoint to distal), one within the bladder, and one intraabdominally as recorded by an intrarectal sensor or by a sensor within the vagina if the vagina is in a relatively normal position (not prolapsed). Fig. 21.8, *A*, shows a multichannel urodynamic study during the pressure/flow or voiding phase and highlights a woman with a voiding disorder, which was the main reason the study was ordered.

Several authors have described the concept of leak point pressure tests for evaluating urethral function in stress incontinence. The International Continence Society defines an abdominal leak point pressure (ALPP) as the lowest of the intentional or actively increased intravesical pressure that provokes urinary leakage in the absence of a detrusor contraction. This test measures urethral function or outlet competence. Increased pressure from Valsalva or cough maneuvers are called the Valsalva leak point pressure (VLPP) and cough leak point pressure (CLPP). The ALPP has been used to separate urinary stress incontinence as related to either an anatomic defect (hypermobility of the urethra) or an intrinsic sphincter deficiency; however, it has become clear there is significant overlap in these conditions and using a cutoff of less than 60 cm $H_2O$ to define intrinsic sphincter deficiency is too simplistic. The woman's history and clinical picture must be considered carefully, not just an arbitrary cutoff point.

Maximal urethral closure pressure (MUCP) is another measure of urethral function in stress incontinence. MUCP is the maximum difference between the urethral pressure and the intravesical pressure. Less than 20 cm $H_2O$ is the criteria used to define intrinsic sphincter deficiency. Using the MUCP for choosing therapy in subtypes of stress incontinence or for outcome results in surgical trials has been criticized because, unlike the VLPP, the test is not performed during stress. A 2010 randomized controlled trial by Nager and colleagues studied the relationship between various measurements of urethral function and subjective scores of urinary incontinence (Nager, 2010). They found that VLPP and MUCP have moderate correlation with each other, but each had little or no correlation with the woman's subjective scores of incontinence severity or objective tests such as the supine empty bladder stress test. These data call into question the use of urodynamic measures of urethral function when they do not correlate with urinary incontinence severity; however, many stress incontinence surgical trials use the MUCP and leak point pressures to categorize incontinence and to predict risk of surgical failure, so being familiar with the tests is useful. In general, poor urethral function as found with lower ALPP and MUCP tends to predict less optimal outcomes with some types of therapy.

Other studies have called into question the usefulness of urodynamics for stress or urge incontinence symptoms in uncomplicated cases. The test correlates poorly with symptoms and often does not affect the outcome of treatment, even with stress incontinence surgery (Nager, 2012). When urodynamic testing is done, it must be correlated with the woman's symptoms and examination results because those factors may be more revealing than the test.

Multichannel devices involve more expensive equipment and require continuous maintenance. It is possible to add a video urodynamic system to the multichannel recorders, making it possible via fluoroscopy to identify reflux into the ureters in high-risk patients. The video system also makes it possible to actually observe the act of micturition (Fig. 21.8, B), any anatomic changes, the bladder neck opening, and the effect of stress. Because the data obtained by multichannel pressure recordings plus the ability to actually visualize the woman voiding offer the most accurate diagnostic information that the clinician can obtain, this technique is considered the standard against which other tests are measured.

**Urodynamic testing is not necessary for beginning a conservative treatment program for stress, urge, or mixed incontinence symptoms or for routine evaluation.** Urodynamics may be helpful in the following circumstances:

- Diagnosis is unclear and more invasive treatments are planned
- Conservative therapy has failed
- Prior incontinence surgery has failed
- The patient has expressed voiding complaints, especially after stress incontinence surgery
- Pelvic organ prolapse is present beyond the hymen
- The patient has a complicated medical history (e.g., neurologic disease, diabetes mellitus) or there is concern for upper urinary tract disease

## Cystourethroscopy

Diagnostic endoscopic inspection of the urethra, bladder, and ureteral orifices may be done in the office setting. It requires a cystoscope and irrigating fluid. The cystoscope can be rigid or flexible; studies in women, unlike those in men, have shown no difference in pain between the two. The bladder cannot be easily drained (e.g., for urine specimen or PVR measurement) or irrigated through the flexible scope, unlike the rigid scope. Sterile saline or water is used as irrigant and to expand the bladder and allow complete visualization of the bladder and urethra. Use of a camera allows the patient to visualize cystoscopic findings and better understand their pathologic condition. A 2% lidocaine jelly is often inserted into the urethra before the procedure, which is a good lubricant and may provide some analgesia. With rigid cystoscopy, the small 17 French (Fr) sheath is commonly used for routine inspection and larger sheaths (21, 22, 24 Fr) for operative procedures. Examination of the bladder is best accomplished using a 70-degree lens, which offers the angles needed to examine

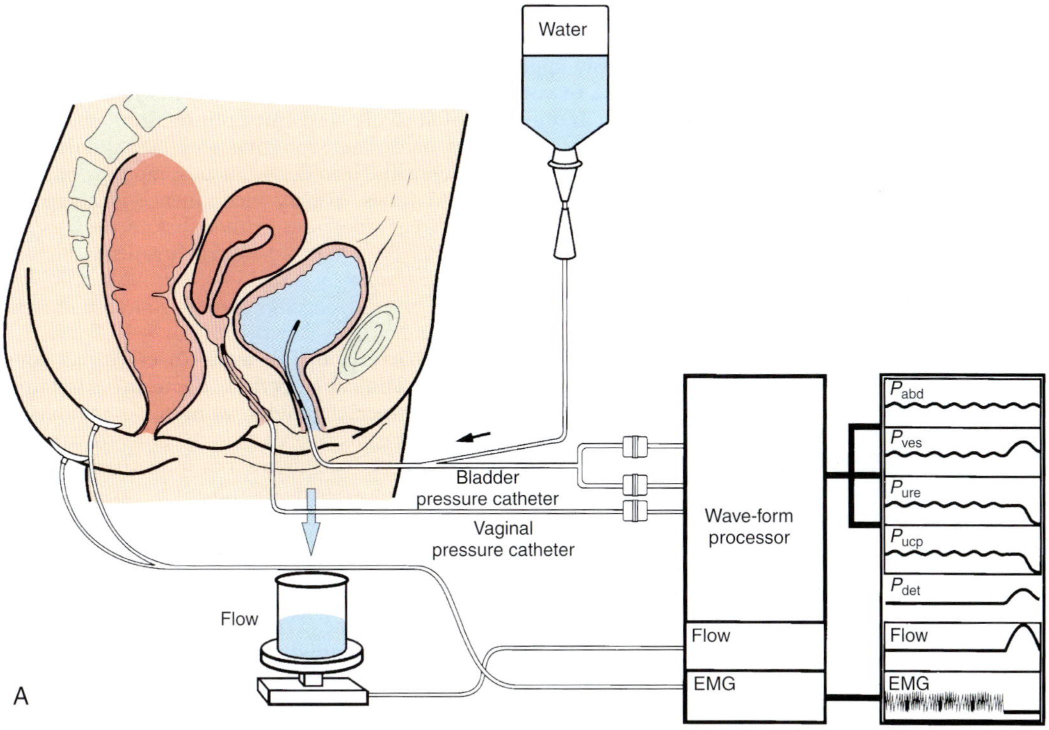


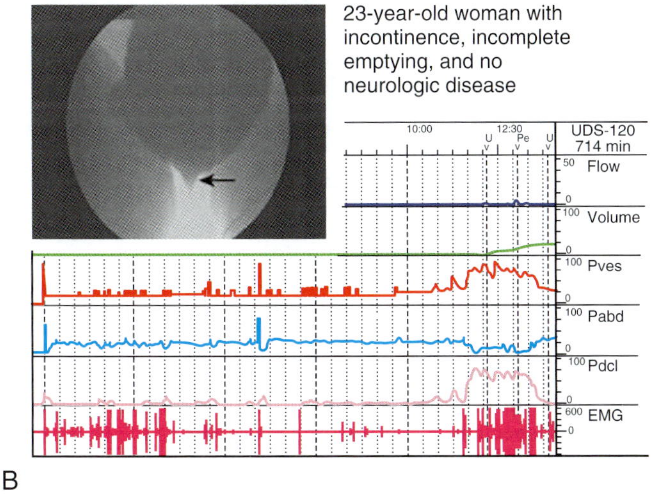


**Fig. 21.8 A,** Multichannel urodynamics. **B,** Urodynamic test showing dysfunctional voiding. *EMG,* Electromyography; $P_{abd}$, abdominal pressure; $P_{det}$, true detrusor pressure; $P_{ure}$, urethral pressure; $P_{ucp}$, urethral closure pressure; $P_{ves}$, bladder pressure. (**A,** From Karam MM, Mahdy A. *Urogynecology and Reconstructive Pelvic Surgery. Urodynamics: Indications, Techniques, Interpretation, and Clinical Utility.* 4th ed. Philadelphia: Saunder; 2015:130-136. **B,** From Nitti VW, Bruckner BM. Urodynamic and video-urodynamic evaluation of the lower urinary tract. In: Wein A, Kavoussi L, Partin A, Peters C, eds. *Campbell-Walsh Urology.* 11th ed. Philadelphia: Elsevier; 2016:1718-1742.e3.)

the bladder in its entirety. The 30-degree lens is used when performing procedures such as catheterizing a ureteral orifice or taking a biopsy. A 0- or 12-degree lens is best for examining the urethra. The bladder may have to be flushed for optimal viewing if blood or debris obscures the view; this can easily be done with a rigid scope by filling, emptying, and refilling the bladder. A systematic survey should be done inspecting the trigone, ureteral orifices, bladder walls and dome and should be evaluated at different levels of filling. It is only after full distension that some eroded foreign bodies such as suture or mesh can be seen. The urethra is most easily inspected with irrigating fluid running as the small sheath cystoscope is removed from the bladder, rather than on initial introduction into the bladder. Endoscopic findings on cystourethroscopy include anatomic abnormalities, such as bladder and urethral diverticulum, urethral strictures, and duplicated ureters (Fig. 21.9), and the presence of inflammation, foreign bodies, urinary tract stones, Hunner lesions, and malignant lesions (Box 21.1).

## LOWER URINARY TRACT PAIN: ACUTE BACTERIAL CYSTITIS, BLADDER PAIN SYNDROME/ INTERSTITIAL CYSTITIS, URETHRAL DIVERTICULUM

### Acute Bacterial Cystitis

Although the term *urinary tract infection* formally includes both upper tract (i.e., pyelonephritis) and lower urinary tract infections, it is most commonly used for bacterial infections of the

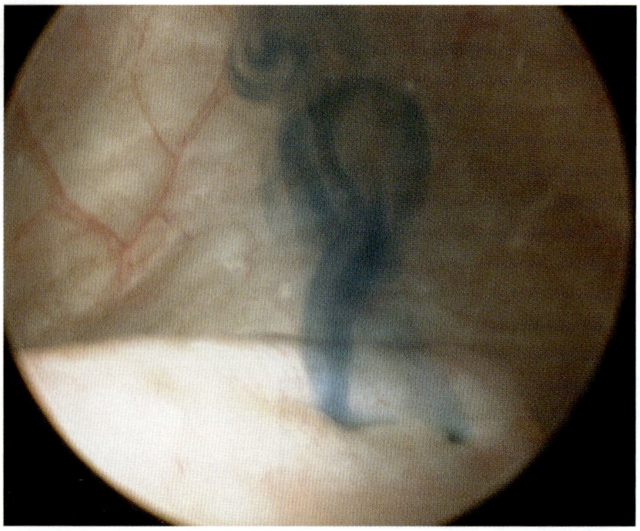

**Fig. 21.9** Cystoscopy after indigo carmine was infused intravenously to confirm the duplicated ureters on the left side and that both were functioning. (Courtesy Gretchen Lentz, MD.)

**BOX 21.1** Common Findings on Urethrocystoscopy

**NORMAL UROTHELIUM—PALE, FINE BLOOD VESSELS**

- Normal—squamous metaplasia in trigone (benign overgrowth)
- Abnormal—hypervascularity
- Abnormal—cystic lesions in the trigone; could be benign cystitis (UTI)
- Abnormal—stitch or mesh from incontinence surgery
- Abnormal—bladder stone or kidney stone that has passed
- Abnormal—lesion growing from wall; biopsy, could be carcinoma
- Abnormal—grapelike clusters; biopsy, could be transitional cell carcinoma
- Abnormal—trabeculations (hypertrophied detrusor muscle), benign; seen in OAB or outlet obstruction
- Abnormal—Hunner ulcer; pathognomonic for interstitial cystitis

**NORMAL URETHRA—COLLAPSED IN ABSENCE OF FLUID FLOW**

- Abnormal—fronds or pseudopolyps, benign response to inflammation
- Abnormal—stricture; prior surgery, especially urethral diverticulum excision

**URETERAL ORIFICES WITH BILATERAL JETS OF URINE FLOW**

- Abnormal—sluggish flow, could mean partial obstruction
- Abnormal—no flow, could mean obstruction from current or past surgery, stone, or stricture

*OAB*, Overactive bladder; *UTI*, urinary tract infection.

bladder and will be used in this section to refer to only bacterial infections of the bladder. Other commonly used terms are *acute, uncomplicated cystitis (AUC)* and *acute bacterial cystitis*. UTI is the most common bacterial infection seen in an outpatient setting. **As many as 50% of all women develop UTIs at some time during their life and, by age 70, as many as 10% of women will have recurrent UTIs. About 40% of all nosocomial infections are UTI's and usually related to urinary catheters. Lower urinary tract infections are almost always associated with some combination of the following: frequency, urgency, dysuria, suprapubic pain, pyuria, and hematuria. Dysuria is a highly specific symptom with more than 90% accuracy for UTI in young women without vaginal discharge and irritation and no risk of sexually transmitted infection.** Symptoms of flank pain, rigors, nausea and vomiting, and fever should raise concern for pyelonephritis. In older women, symptoms of UTI may be less clear. At times, urinary incontinence is associated with acute and recurrent infections. Although *Escherichia coli* is the cause of most UTIs (80% to 85%), myriad organisms, including *Staphylococcus saprophyticus* (5% to 15%), *Enterobacter, Klebsiella, Pseudomonas, Proteus, Streptococcus faecalis, Enterococcus*, and *Chlamydia*, can be found.

**The presence of bacteria in the urine (bacteriuria) does not necessarily prove clinical infection. Bacteriuria is fairly common in women, especially older women.** Asymptomatic bacteriuria is defined as organisms present in the urine that are not causing symptoms or illness. Cumulative data from several studies have suggested that 20% of women older than 65 years will demonstrate bacteriuria, but the percentage increases from approximately 15% in the 65- to 70-year group to 20% to 50% for women older than 80 years. Bacteriuria is present in women who perform chronic catheterization and common in women in nursing homes who are chronically incontinent. **Treatment for asymptomatic bacteriuria is not recommended, even in older women or people with diabetes, with no change in their morbidity or mortality** (Mody, 2014). Exceptions exist to this recommendation if the woman is undergoing an invasive genitourinary procedure, is pregnant, has a renal transplant, or is incontinent and her incontinence resolves with treatment. If a woman with asymptomatic bacteriuria becomes symptomatic, treatment is appropriate.

**Many explanations have been offered as to why the female urinary tract is vulnerable to infection:**

- Short female urethra, allowing easier access of bacteria to the bladder
- Proximity of the vulva, vagina, and rectum to the opening of the urethra
- Effects of sexual intercourse, with increased inoculation
- Contraception (e.g., spermicide)
- Effects of estrogen loss on the genitourinary tract of older women

**After menopause, the vaginal pH rises and may alter vaginal flora, allowing for the loss of the protective species *Lactobacillus crispatus* and the colonization of uropathogenic species, especially *E. coli*.** Estrogen also affects the maturation of the urethral and trigone mucosa, which can play a role in limiting bacterial infection. Genetic and immunologic factors (e.g., nonsecretors of certain blood group antigens are at increased UTI risk) also play a role in UTI susceptibility, but these are not specific to women.

The definition of a symptomatic UTI is a woman with dysuria, frequency, urgency, or suprapubic pain with pyuria. Uncomplicated UTIs occur in healthy women with normal urinary tract function. UTIs are classified as complicated when there are comorbid conditions with factors that increase colonization and that may require longer treatment courses:

- Underlying urologic abnormalities
- Presence of a foreign body (e.g., catheter), urinary calculi
- Obstruction of urine flow
- Diabetes mellitus
- Spinal cord injury (neurogenic bladder)
- Pregnancy
- Renal transplantation or other immunocompromise
- Multidrug-resistant bacteria

UTIs can often be diagnosed successfully with symptom assessment. **In outpatient settings, women with at least two of**

**three acute symptoms (dysuria, urgency, frequency) in the absence of vaginal discharge (or risk for sexually transmitted infection) have a greater than 90% probability of having AUC.** Additional urine testing does not aid in the diagnostic accuracy; however, outside of those criteria, a clean-catch midstream urine sample for chemical analysis (dipstick) testing for leukocyte esterase and nitrites or a microscopic unspun urine evaluation for white blood cells (pyuria) can be helpful. Pyuria should always be seen in the urine when UTI is present. Leukocyte esterase means there are white blood cells (WBCs) present and has a roughly 75% to 80% specificity and 85% sensitivity for UTI. **Nitrites indicate that certain gram-negative bacteria have converted nitrate to nitrite and is highly specific but not sensitive because it only occurs with gram-negative bacteria present.** Urine microscopy with pyuria (>10 WBC/high-power field [HPF] on spun specimen) is a very sensitive test (95%) but less specific for UTI. Hematuria, microscopic or gross, is common in acute infections, and infection is the most common cause of hematuria. Gross hematuria does not indicate a more severe infection but rather a more significant host response. If hematuria persists after UTI treatment (microscopic after 6 to 8 weeks), it should be evaluated. A contaminated specimen comes from organisms or cells collected while obtaining the clean catch urine. More than 15 to 20 squamous epithelial cells/HPF suggests contamination and a sterile straight catheterization for a urine specimen might be needed.

The pathogens are predictable in AUC, so culture is generally unnecessary and can be reserved for recurrent UTIs (two or more episodes in 6 months or three in a year) and complicated UTIs or when patients are at risk for multidrug-resistant bacterial infection such as a patient who has recently been hospitalized or institutionalized. When a urine culture is done, to be considered consistent with infection, or positive, a single uropathogenic organism grows. The number of organisms per milliliter is not important.

The American Urogynecologic Society (AUGS) and the American Urological Association (AUA) have developed **evidence-based guidelines for the treatment of acute uncomplicated cystitis (AUC)** and should be routinely referenced for appropriate antibiotic management in light of developing bacterial resistance. Following are current recommendations for empiric treatment of AUC-UTIs in nonpregnant, premenopausal women without pyelonephritis:

- Nitrofurantoin monohydrate/macrocrystals twice a day for 5 days (resistance rates of *E. coli* to nitrofurantoin have remained low).
- Trimethoprim-sulfamethoxazole (TMP-SMX) double strength, twice a day for 3-day therapy (if local *E. coli* bacterial resistance rates are less than 20%). Short-course (3-day) therapy improves patient tolerability and compliance. This treatment strategy results in more than a 90% cure rate.
- Fosfomycin trometamol, 3 g given as a single dose. This may have slightly lower efficacy than the other two options.

**Fluoroquinolones, although highly efficacious, should be avoided in AUC because resistance is rising and more concerning side effects have occurred.** The Food and Drug Administration (FDA) has issued several updates on safety labeling changes, including risk of tendonitis and tendon rupture, mental health side effects, serious blood sugar disturbances (hypoglycemia), aortic dissections, and aortic aneurysm rupture. It is recommended that these medications be reserved for more serious infections. Because of high resistance and relatively poor efficacy, amoxicillin and ampicillin should not be used for empiric treatment. Progression from cystitis to pyelonephritis is uncommon. Cystitis patients should remain adequately hydrated and be encouraged to complete antibiotics, even though symptoms generally disappear within 48 hours. Infections can recur because they are not adequately eradicated. This may result from physician error (treating with too low a dose of antibiotic, the wrong antibiotic, or for too short a period), patient error (not taking the medication as prescribed), or undiagnosed complicating factors and may require imaging, cystoscopy, or other further investigation for bacterial nidus. These patients who relapse (the same pathogen within 2 weeks of an appropriate course of antibiotics) are differentiated from patients with recurrent UTIs (a subsequent UTI occurred beyond the initial 2 weeks or with a different pathogen). For complicated UTIs, urine culture should be done. A 7- to 14-day course of an antibiotic is recommended, and often TMP-SMX double strength, fluoroquinolones, and sometimes a one-time intravenous (IV) antibiotic to initiate treatment (ceftriaxone, aminoglycoside, or fluoroquinolones). When urine culture and sensitivity results return, the antibiotic may be changed if the organisms noted are not sensitive to the antibiotic in use.

Thirty percent to 40% of women will have a recurrent UTI after a single UTI; 50% of these women will have a third episode if they have had two UTIs in 6 months (Gupta, 2013). **Women with recurrent UTIs (rUTI), defined as three or more UTIs in a year or two or more UTIs in 6 months,** do not generally need routine radiographic imaging—seeking structural abnormalities of the bladder, kidney, or ureters—for it is rarely useful in otherwise healthy women. More than 90% of recurrences in young women are exogenous reinfection with new isolates arising from local flora.

There are several strategies for managing recurrent UTIs (Fig. 21.10). Behavioral modification has become popular for preventing rUTIs. Recommended modifications in lifestyle include increasing water intake in premenopausal women (Hooton, 2018), which dropped rUTIs about 50%. Another strategy is eliminating risk factors, such as discontinuing use of spermicide for contraception; use of nonoxynol-9 has been associated with an increased risk of UTIs in women (Fihn, 1996). **Correcting vaginal atrophy in postmenopausal women with rUTIs is often successful. Vaginal estrogen therapy restores the acidic environment of the vagina and protective microbiome** (Raz, 1993).

There are other nonantibiotic prevention strategies, such as cranberry supplements, vitamin C, probiotics, D-mannose, and methenamine salts. Strong evidence of benefit is lacking for these options, but some women wish to try these instead of antibiotics. Most evidence exists for cranberry supplements, but the correct dosage and formulation is unknown, studies are contradictory and not conclusive. Cranberries seem biologically plausible, with the active ingredient being proanthocyanidins (PACs), which is thought to prevent binding of *E. coli* to urothelial cells. Women can try a cranberry supplement, but evidence is less effective than previously thought when 14 more studies were added to the Cochrane review. There is some evidence in a 2012 Cochrane review supporting methenamine hippurate for short-term use (1 week or less). It is metabolized via the production of formaldehyde from hexamine in acidic urine and is bacteriostatic. This does not induce resistance and has minimal side effects. Delaying treatment with antibiotics and trying ibuprofen and increased water has been studied, but it increased the duration of symptoms; furthermore, the majority of women needed antibiotics (Grigoryan, 2014). Oral probiotics have not shown clinical efficacy in randomized trials. Vaginal delivery of *Lactobacillus crispatus* may be a more promising strategy, but at present, routine use is not recommended. D-mannose is a natural sugar, thought to bind competitively to bacteria to decrease bacteria attaching to urothelial receptors. The clinical research is scant, but again, some women wish to try nonantibiotics strategies for rUTIs. Vitamin C to acidify the urine has limited data to recommend.

**Many episodes of recurrent UTIs in young women occur within 24 hours of coitus.** Although eliminating coitus is an option, it is not a widely accepted one. **These women are excellent candidates to be treated with postcoital single-dose prophylactic antibiotics.** The antibiotics most commonly

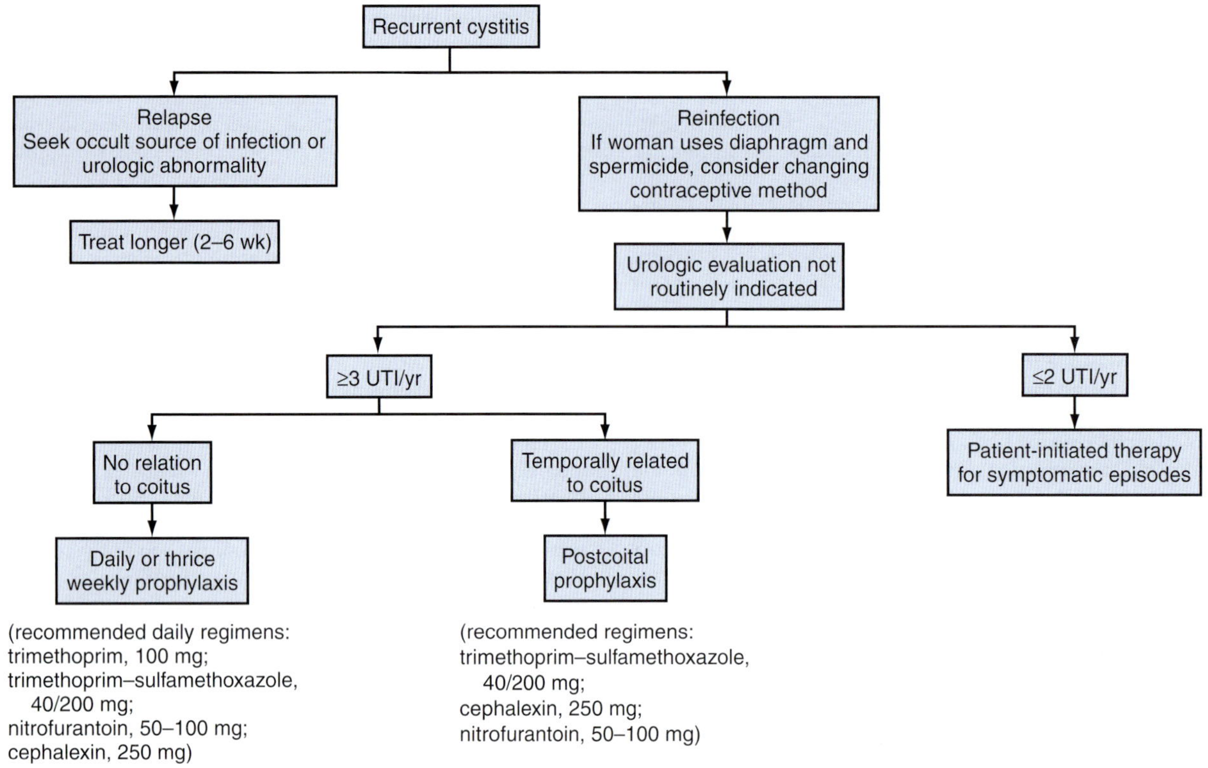


**Fig. 21.10** Strategies for managing recurrent cystitis in women. (From Stamm WE, Hooton TM. Management of urinary tract infections in adults. *N Engl J Med.* 1993;329:1328-1334.)

chosen for low-dose antibiotic prophylaxis include TMP-SMX single strength, nitrofurantoin (50 to 100 mg), and cephalexin (125 to 250 mg).

Often women with recurrent UTIs at unpredictable times prefer self-initiated treatment with the onset of symptoms. Clinicians must document positive urine cultures associates with prior symptomatic episodes before ordering self-initiated treatment antibiotics. Using the antibiotics presented earlier for uncomplicated UTI is reasonable. Continuous prophylactic antibiotics are needed in some situations. Continuous daily prophylaxis is considerably more effective than other options but may increase the risk of bacterial resistance and drug complications. Daily prophylaxis regimens have been reported up to 5 years; however, it is rarely continued beyond 6 months. Evaluation for efficacy and side effects is reasonable at 3 months.

**In summary, recommendations for rUTI management as outlined in the American Urogynecologic Society (AUGS) best practice statement include the following** (Brubaker, 2018):

Diagnosis:

- Urine culture should be performed before initiating antibiotic therapy.
- Urine culture after therapy may help define a distinct episode.

Antibiotic choice:

- Nitrofurantoin is a key first-line agent (50 to 100 mg daily).
- Fosfomycin is effective (3 g every 10 days) but sensitivity testing may be needed.
- TMP-SMX can also be used if resistance is less than 20% in the community.
- Fluoroquinolones are not a first-line treatment of acute cystitis without complicating factors.

Prevention:

- Postcoital antibiotic suppression is effective in women with coitally related rUTI.
- Low-dose daily antibiotic suppression (3 to 6 months) is effective in women with noncoitally related rUTI.
- Effective nonantibiotic measures are cessation of spermicides, vaginal estrogen in atrophic women, and methenamine.

Although the focus of this section was UTIs in patients with no complicating factors, there are gynecologic reasons for some women to present with complicated UTIs. These include the presence of an indwelling Foley catheter or need for clean intermittent catheterization after gynecologic surgery, pregnancy and physiologic hydronephrosis of pregnancy, pelvic prolapse with incomplete bladder emptying, urethral diverticulum or obstructed Skene gland, and eroded mesh or suture creating a bladder foreign body and stones. An indwelling catheter for 24 hours leads to bacteriuria in as many as 50% of patients. **When left in place for 96 hours, an indwelling catheter causes bacteriuria in almost 100% of patients. There is no good evidence supporting the use of prophylactic antibiotics in patients who must continue catheter use. A woman with an indwelling catheter should be monitored for the possibility of a symptomatic UTI,** be kept adequately hydrated, have a urine culture if symptoms occur, and be treated with the appropriate antibiotic; however, it is difficult to eradicate infection in the presence of an indwelling catheter. Removing the catheter or switching to clean intermittent self-catheterization is optimal if possible. Postoperative and debilitated patients are at greatest risk.

UTI with hydronephrosis in pregnancy may require improved drainage with ureteral stent or nephrostomy tube. Patients with prolapse and a UTI and incomplete bladder emptying may require urethral catheter drainage and ultimately prolapse reduction with pessary or surgery. Patients with a urethral diverticulum may need surgical repair, and patients with eroded mesh or suture with stone formation need surgical correction as well. Being aware of these complicating factors in patients with UTIs allows appropriate and timely care of these complicated patients.

## Bladder Pain Syndrome (Interstitial Cystitis)

**Bladder pain syndrome, originally called interstitial cystitis (IC/BPS), is a poorly understood chronic pain syndrome of unknown cause characterized by genitourinary pain and voiding symptoms. IC/BPS is a clinical diagnosis—one of exclusion.** Once thought of primarily as a disease of the bladder and of women, IC/BPS and its association with other chronic pain syndromes suggest that its cause in at least a subset of patients extends well beyond the bladder. The prevalence in men has approached that of women in some studies (Suskind, 2013). The diagnosis of IC/BPS should be considered in patients with chronic pelvic pain.

### Definitions of IC/BPS

Definitions of IC/BPS include the following:

- The International Continence Society (2018): "IC/BPS is a persistent or recurrent chronic pelvic pain, pressure or discomfort perceived to be related to the urinary bladder accompanied by at least one other urinary symptom such as an urgent need to void or urinary frequency, diagnosed in the absence of any identifiable pathology which could explain these symptoms. Interstitial cystitis/Hunner lesion is used when cystoscopic findings identify a Hunner lesion in conjunction with the same symptoms as IC/BPS."
- Society for Urodynamics and Female Urology (SUFU) (2011)/AUA (2014) IC/PBS Guidelines: "ICPBS is an unpleasant sensation (pain, pressure, discomfort) perceived to be related to the urinary bladder, associated with lower urinary tract symptoms of more than 6 weeks duration in the absence of infection or other identifiable causes."

The prevalence of IC/BPS varies widely, with more some studies estimating up to 3000 per 100,000 women, with about 3% of patients in Canadian urologist offices having IC/BPS. The BACH Survey (Clemens, 2007) showed nearly twice as many women as men are affected. Symptoms tend to fluctuate, with most patients experiencing no worsening of symptoms over time. It does not seem to complicate pregnancy. **Patients' quality of life is significantly decreased in all domains, and there is a high incidence of comorbidities, including depression, chronic pain, and anxiety.** These patients also have a higher rate of emotional, physical, and sexual abuse (nearly 30% in some studies), and practitioners should be aware of the possibility. Many patients with IC/BPS (maybe 50%) have associated nonbladder pain syndromes, including irritable bowel syndrome, fibromyalgia, and chronic fatigue syndrome. Notably, rates of vulvodynia and endometriosis in patients with IC/BPS were similar to those in the general population. Several studies have noted an association with systemic lupus erythematous, supporting an autoimmune cause. IC/BPS does not predispose patients to bladder cancer, a worry many patients carry.

### Etiology

**There is no known cause for IC/BPS, but most likely it has a multifactorial cause that eventually works through one pathway, resulting in the presenting symptoms.** Theories include the following:

- Epithelial permeability
  Defects in the bladder lining or glycosaminoglycan (GAG) layer allowing urinary irritants to penetrate the urothelium and activate underlying nerve and muscle tissue.
- Infection
  There are little data to support this, and although the concept that a UTI might trigger IC/BPS in some patients is appealing, it is unlikely that active infection is involved in the ongoing pathologic process or that antibiotics have a role in treatment.
- Autoimmunity and Inflammation
  Mast cells are often associated with IC/BPS. They have been reported as both a mechanism and marker in many studies, and they may serve as a common pathway.
  Although the immune system is a target for therapy for some IC patients, autoimmunity as the primary cause of IC has not been observed.
- Inhibition of uroepithelial cell proliferation: antiproliferative factor (APF)
  Cells from the bladder lining of normal controls grow significantly more rapidly in culture cells from patients with IC/BPS as a result of APF produced by the cells of these patients (Keay, 1997).
- Neurogenic inflammation
  Numerous studies of patients with IC/BPS show increase sympathetic activity.
- Pelvic organ cross-sensitization
  Neural pathways from two or more organs, one or both carrying noxious stimuli, may converge and lead to changes in function and pain sensation.

### Diagnosis

**The diagnosis of IC/BPS can be difficult, often resulting in misdiagnosis and delayed diagnosis. It is a diagnosis of exclusion, and many conditions present with similar symptoms,** as outlined in Table 21.4. The current definition from the AUA guidelines, as stated earlier, is typically used as the criteria for diagnosis.

Per the AUA guidelines, a basic assessment of a patient should include a thorough history, physical examination, urinalysis, and urine culture; if there is a history of smoking and/or the patient presents with unevaluated microhematuria, urine cytologic testing may be considered, given the risk of bladder cancer. The history should focus on factors that would exclude some of the other causes of urinary frequency and pelvic pain. Differentiating patients with overactive bladder (OAB) and IC/BPS can be done by simply asking them what happens when they have to delay voiding. Do they void often because they will experience marked urgency/urge incontinence or will they experience pain? (Table 21.3) Patients with IC/BPS have pain or worsening of their baseline pain and often some decrease in their pain with voiding. On physical examination, findings of anterior vaginal wall tenderness and pelvic floor muscle tenderness are more often found in patients with IC/BPS (Paulson, 2011; FitzGerald, 2012).

Other tests that can be useful in these patients include a frequency-volume chart and PVR measurement. Urodynamics, imaging, laparoscopy and specialist referral should be considered in more complex patients. These patients include those with the following:

- Hematuria
- Pain and urinary incontinence
- Incomplete bladder emptying
- Neurologic disorder that can affect bladder function
- History of prior radiation or trauma
- Pelvic prolapse beyond the hymen
- No response to treatment

Although routine use of cystoscopy for diagnosis, cystoscopy and bladder hydrodistention, and biopsy are not recommended by the AUA, they are recommended by the Japanese Urological Association (Homma, 2009). Hunner lesions are erythematous, often stellate bladder lesions proximal to the trigone that are thought by many to be pathognomonic for a distinct subtype of IC/BPS. They can tear, exposing underlying bladder muscle on bladder hydrodistension. This IC/Hunner subtype is distinct

**TABLE 21.3** Pelvic Pain, Urgency, Frequency (PUF) Patient Symptom Scale

| | Points | | | | | |
|---|---|---|---|---|---|---|
| **Question** | **0** | **1** | **2** | **3** | **4** | **Score** |
| 1. How many times do you go to the bathroom during the day? | 3-6 | 7-10 | 11-14 | 15-19 | 20+ | |
| 2. a. How many times do you go to the bathroom at night?<br>b. If you get up at night to go to the bathroom, does it bother you? | 0<br>Never | 1<br>Occasionally | 2<br>Moderate | 3<br>Severe | 4+ | |
| 3. Are you currently sexually active?<br>Yes/no | | | | | | |
| 4. a. If you are sexually active, do you now or have you ever had pain or symptoms during or after sexual intercourse?<br>b. If you have pain, does it make you avoid sexual intercourse? | Never<br>Never | Occasionally<br>Occasionally | Usually<br>Usually | Always<br>Always | | |
| 5. Do you have pain associated with your bladder or in your pelvis (vagina, labia, lower abdomen, urethra, perineum)? | Never | Occasionally | Usually | Always | | |
| 6. Do you still have urgency after you go to the bathroom? | Never | Occasionally | Usually | Always | | |
| 7. a. If you have pain, is it usually mild, moderate, or severe?<br>b. Does your pain bother you? | Never | Mild<br>Occasionally | Moderate<br>Usually | Severe<br>Always | | |
| 8. a. If you have urgency, is it usually mild, moderate, or severe?<br>b. Does your urgency bother you? | Never | Mild<br>Occasionally | Moderate<br>Usually | Severe<br>Always | | |
| Total Score: | | | | | | |

**TABLE 21.4** Diseases That May Be Mistaken for Bladder Pain Syndrome

| **Confusable Disease** | **Excluded or Diagnosed By** |
|---|---|
| Carcinoma and carcinoma in situ | Cystoscopy and biopsy |
| Infection with: | |
| Common intestinal bacteria | Routine bacterial culture |
| *Chlamydia trachomatis, Ureaplasma urealyticum, Mycoplasma hominis, Mycoplasma genitalium, Corynebacterium urealyticum, Candida species, Mycobacterium tuberculosis* | Special cultures<br>Dipstick; if "sterile" pyuria, culture for *M. tuberculosis* |
| Herpes simplex and human papillomavirus | Physical examination |
| Radiation | Medical history |
| Chemotherapy, including immunotherapy with cyclophosphamide | Medical history |
| Antiinflammatory therapy with tiaprofenic acid | Medical history |
| Bladder neck obstruction and neurogenic outlet obstruction | Uroflowmetry and ultrasonography |
| Bladder stone | Imaging or cystoscopy |
| Lower ureteral stone | Medical history and/or hematuria; upper urinary tract imaging (CT or IVP) |
| Urethral diverticulum | Medical history and physical examination |
| Urogenital prolapse | Medical history and physical examination |
| Endometriosis | Medical history and physical examination |
| Vaginal candidiasis | Medical history and physical examination |
| Cervical, uterine, and ovarian cancer | Physical examination |
| Incomplete bladder emptying (retention) | Postvoid residual urine volume measured by ultrasound evaluation |
| Overactive bladder | Medical history and urodynamics |
| Prostate cancer | Physical examination and PSA test |
| Benign prostatic obstruction | Uroflowmetry and pressure-flow studies |
| Chronic bacterial prostatitis | Medical history, physical examination, culture |
| Chronic nonbacterial prostatitis | Medical history, physical examination, culture |
| Pudendal nerve entrapment | Medical history, physical examination; nerve block may prove diagnosis |
| Pelvic floor muscle–related pain | Medical history, physical examination |

From Hanno PM. Bladder pain syndrome (interstitial cystitis) and related disorders. In: Wein A, Kavoussi L, Partin A, Peters C, eds. *Campbell-Walsh Urology.* 11th ed. Philadelphia: Elsevier; 2016:334-370.e18; and van de Merwe JP, Nordling J, Bouchelouche P, et al. Diagnostic criteria, classification, and nomenclature for painful bladder syndrome/interstitial cystitis: an ESSIC proposal. *Eur Urol.* 2008;53:60-67.

*CT,* Computed tomography; *IVP,* intravenous pyelogram; *PSA,* prostate-specific antigen.

enough—features commonly include less pain, decreased bladder capacity under anesthesia, and greater likelihood of response to certain therapies—that many think these patients should be considered their own IC phenotype.

## Treatment

**Because IC/BPS is a chronic pain syndrome with no clear cause, there is no cure. The goal of patient management is symptomatic relief and improvement in patient's quality of life and functionality.** Some patients have to void every 30 to 60 minutes, keeping them from participating in family life, maintaining a job, and getting adequate sleep. There are multiple approaches to management of IC/BPS but no one best approach. Generally an approach should involve working together with the patient, taking into account her most bothersome symptoms, limitations (e.g., too much urethral pain with catheterizations excludes bladder instillations as an option), and primary goals, works best. **Often multimodal therapy—directing therapy to limiting urothelial irritation, neuropathic pain (Fig. 21.11), associated pelvic floor dysfunction, and stress of a chronic illness—has a greater chance of symptom improvement (Pazin, 2016).**

Current therapies included here are from the AUA (Hanno, 2015) treatment guidelines and are organized in order of increasing risk. Patient referral for directed pain management is appropriate at any point.

- First-line treatments:
  - General relaxation/stress management
  - Patient education
  - Self-care/behavioral modification
- Second-line treatments:
  - Physical therapy techniques
  - Oral medications: amitriptyline, cimetidine, hydroxyzine, pentosan polysulfate sodium
  - Bladder instillations: dimethyl sulfoxide (DMSO), heparin lidocaine
- Third-line treatments:
  - Cystoscopy under anesthesia with hydrodistension
  - Treatment of Hunner lesions if found (i.e., fulguration, injection with steroids)
- Fourth-line treatments:
  - Intradetrusor botulinum toxin A
  - Neuromodulation
- Fifth-line treatments:
  - Cyclosporine A
- Sixth-line treatments:
  - Urinary diversion with or without cystectomy
  - Substitution cystoplasty

**Self-care and behavioral modification include avoidance of activities that exacerbate symptoms, application of heat or cold over the bladder or perineum, and, perhaps most often discussed, diet and fluid modification.** Some patients find that concentrated urine can worsen symptoms and increasing fluids may help. Others find that frequent bladder filling worsens symptoms and moderate fluid restriction may be beneficial. There are many "IC diets" available, but there are little if any data to support them (Box 21.2). Many patients, however, do report their symptoms to be exacerbated by specific foods, and if identified, it is reasonable to avoid them (Koziol, 1994; Shorter, 2007). Caffeine, alcohol, artificial sweeteners, hot peppers, and beverages that might acidify the urine such as cranberry juice are among those identified. In a patient survey of 136 patients' dietary changes, application of heat or cold and stress reduction all had positive response rates in more than 80% of responders (O'Hare, 2013).

**Patients who have a history suggestive of pelvic floor dysfunction or are found to have tenderness, especially reproduction of their pain, on palpation of their pelvic floor muscles have been shown to benefit from pelvic floor physical therapy.** In a multicenter, prospective randomized trial comparing traditional therapeutic full body massage to directed pelvic floor physical therapy in women, 29% versus 59% showed symptom improvement (Fitzgerald, 2012).

A heparin analog, pentosan polysulfate sodium (PPS, Elmiron), has been given orally 100 mg three times daily, with some

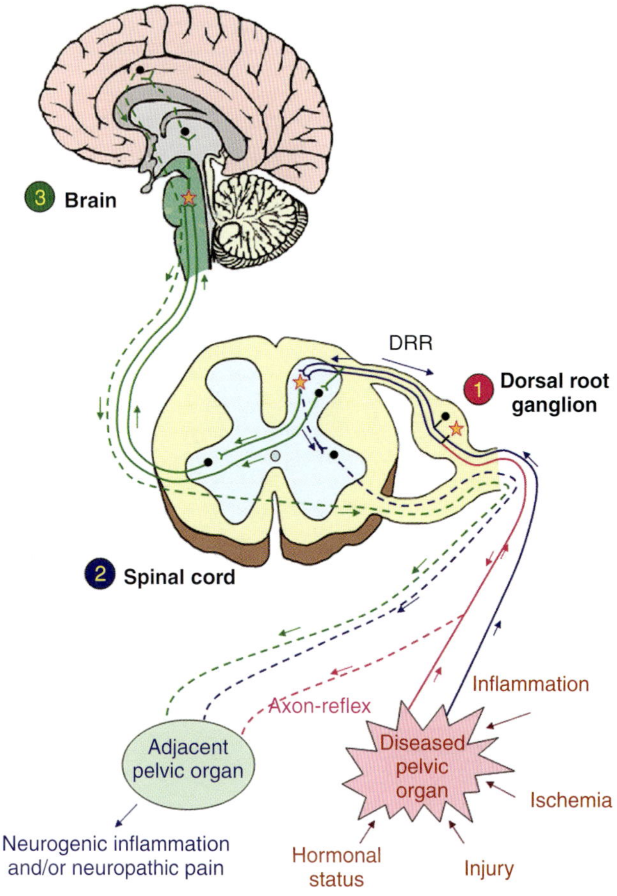


**Fig. 21.11** (From Wein A, Kavoussi L, Partin A, Peters C, eds. *Campbell-Walsh Urology.* 11th ed. Philadelphia: Elsevier; 2016.) Schematic representation of convergent afferent pathways. *1,* Convergence of sensory neural pathways within a dorsal root ganglion (red route). The propagation of noxious stimulus from a diseased pelvic organ to a normal adjacent structure occurs via dichotomizing afferents as a result of an "axon-reflex" mechanism. Axon-reflex–antidromic propagation of action potentials (APs) from dorsal root ganglion to the periphery. *2,* Convergence of afferent information in the spinal cord (blue route). *DRR* refers to dorsal root reflexes (antidromic conductance via sensory fibers from the spinal cord to the periphery). Note that an output neuron belongs to the population of intermediolateral neurons (not motoneurons) localized mostly in laminae VI to VII. *3,* Convergence of afferent inputs from two different pelvic organs in the brain (green route). Convergent neurons within the dorsal root ganglion, in the spinal cord, and in the brain are shown by star symbol. Orthodromic propagation of APs from pelvic organs to the points of convergence is depicted by *solid lines* and *arrows* in respective color for each route. Anterograde AP propagation from the brain, the spinal cord, and the dorsal root ganglion to the periphery is shown by *dotted lines.* (From Malykhina AP. Neural mechanisms of pelvic organ cross-sensitization. *Neuroscience* 2007;149:660–72.)

**BOX 21.2** Interstitial Cystitis Association Recommendations of Foods to Avoid

- Milk and dairy products
  - Aged cheeses
  - Sour cream
  - Yogurt
  - Chocolate
- Vegetables
  - Fava beans
  - Lima beans
  - Onions
  - Tofu
  - Soybeans
  - Tomatoes
- Fruits
  - Apples
  - Apricots
  - Avocados
  - Bananas
  - Cantaloupes
  - Citrus fruits
  - Cranberries
  - Grapes
  - Nectarines
  - Peaches
  - Pineapples
  - Plums
  - Pomegranates
  - Rhubarb
  - Strawberries
  - Juices from above fruits
- Carbohydrates and grains
  - Rye bread
  - Sourdough bread
- Meats and fish
  - Aged, canned, cured processed, smoked meats and fish
- Nuts
- Beverages
  - Alcoholic beverages including beer and wine
  - Carbonated drinks
  - Coffee
  - Tea
  - Fruit juices
- Seasonings
  - Mayonnaise
  - Ketchup
  - Mustard
  - Salsa
  - Spicy foods (Chinese, Mexican, Indian, Thai)
  - Soy sauce
  - Miso
  - Salad dressing
  - Vinegar
- Preservatives and additives
  - Benzyl alcohol
  - Citric acid
  - Monosodium glutamate
  - Artificial sweeteners
  - Preservatives
  - Artificial ingredients
  - Food coloring
- Miscellaneous
  - Tobacco
  - Caffeine
  - Diet pills
  - Junk foods
  - Recreational drugs
  - Allergy medications with ephedrine or pseudoephedrine
  - Certain vitamins

Modified from Interstitial Cystitis Association. Understanding the interstitial cystitis/painful bladder syndrome diet. Available at: http://www.ichelp.org/. Accessed March 7, 2021; and Hanno PM. Bladder pain syndrome (interstitial cystitis) and related disorders. In: Wein A, Kavoussi L, Partin A, Peters C, eds. *Campbell-Walsh Urology.* 11th ed. Philadelphia: Elsevier; 2016:352.

reported improvement. PPS is the only FDA-approved oral drug for IC and may help repair the GAG layer of the bladder epithelium. It can take 6 months to be effective, and improvements are modest; 38% of patients have a more than 50% improvement at 12 weeks. Tricyclic antidepressants may also be helpful because they can inhibit the neural activation that leads to pain. Amitriptyline is not FDA approved for IC, but doses of 10 to 75 mg nightly have produced pain relief in two-thirds of women and decreases in urgency and frequency. Unfortunately, in another trial, when reviewing all randomly allocated participants, amitriptyline with education and behavioral modification did not significantly improve symptoms; however, in this study it was found that amitriptyline might benefit those who can tolerate a daily dose of 50 mg or more, although this subgroup comparison was not specified in advance. Antihistamines such as hydroxyzine may be of benefit for patients with concurrent allergies and for decreasing mast cell degranulation, but most studies have not shown benefit. More study on cimetidine, used in these patients for its antiinflammatory effect, needs to be done. One randomized trial of 36 patients reported a significant improvement in symptom scores with cimetidine versus placebo.

Bladder instillations with various solutions have been tried. FDA-approved therapy includes DMSO bladder instillation. DMSO is an antiinflammatory agent that acts as a bladder anesthetic, relaxes muscles, causes mast cell inhibition, and may dissolve collagen. Because of its side effects of flulike symptoms and bladder pain, other bladder instillations are now used more often. These include heparin, lidocaine, steroids, and combinations, but trials are insufficient to show a benefit. With pain flares, heparin and lidocaine may be of benefit (though not FDA approved). In many practices patients are taught how to do these instillations themselves so that they can be done at home as needed.

Hydrodistention of the bladder under anesthesia in some practices is used for diagnosis, but in the AUA guidelines it is considered therapeutic. Hydrodistension can be temporarily (3 to 12 months) therapeutic in up to 30% of patients, particularly those with Hunner lesions; however, there is a risk of bladder rupture, and patients need to be made aware of this. There does not seem to any long-term bladder dysfunction. The mechanism of benefit is unclear but probably related to damage to mucosal afferent nerve endings.

Additional fourth- and fifth-line therapies, as noted earlier, can be tried if basic strategies have not been successful, including neuromodulation, intradetrusor Botox injections (Kuo, 2016), and even urinary diversion, though this is typically reserved for extremely severe, unresponsive disease and has been most successful in patient with small-capacity bladders (<300 mL) under anesthesia and those with Hunner lesions. Although IC/BPS is a challenging syndrome, the initial management and evaluation of most patients may be performed by a primary care clinician. Many patients, as noted earlier, may require referral to a specialist, such as an urologist or urogynecologist, ideally those with a particular interest in these patients.

## Urethral Diverticulum

**A urethral diverticulum (UD) is a periurethral cystic structure filled with urine connected to the urethra. UD can be difficult to diagnose without a high level of suspicion because of the many ways it can present,** from an asymptomatic anterior vaginal wall mass incidentally noted on pelvic examination to a history of years of poorly defined pelvic pain, incontinence, and dyspareunia. True UD prevalence is unknown, but series have reported occurrence ranging from 1% to 6% of women. There have been reports of congenital UD in young children, but UD is more commonly found in patients between ages 20 and 60 years. Some data suggest that UD may occur more often in African American women than in Caucasian women.

### Etiology

**A variety of causes for UD have been suggested, including congenital, traumatic, and inflammatory.** The exact cause of UD is still unknown, but most are thought to be acquired from infection, inflammation, and obstruction of the periurethral glands. Evidence for this comes from anatomic observations noting that the periurethral glands are located primarily dorsolateral to the urethra with their ducts located in the distal one-third of the urethra; periductal and interductal inflammation is common. In more than 90% of UD cases the ostium is located posterolaterally in the mid- or distal urethra, which corresponds to the anatomic location of the periurethral glands. Several authors have suggested that gonococcus is the cause of this condition, but *E. coli* and other organisms have been found in such processes. Reinfection, inflammation, and recurrent obstruction of the gland ostia are thought to result in patient symptoms and enlargement of the gland sac with eventual rupture of the now abscessed cavity into the urethral lumen and UD formation. UD can be fairly small and simple or markedly complex, multiple, and large, extending up to the bladder neck dorsally or wrapped around the entire urethra with the urethral connection, tiny, tortuous, and difficult to find. Because of the location and size of the UD (i.e., near or involving urinary sphincter), varying degrees of urinary sphincteric compromise may occur, which needs to be considered before surgical repair.

### Symptoms and Signs

Historically the classic patient with UD has been said to present with the "three Ds," dribbling (postvoid), dysuria, and dyspareunia; however, **the most common symptoms associated with UD are bladder or urethral pain, urinary frequency, urgency, and infection.** One-third of patients present with recurrent cystitis; thus the presence of a urethral diverticulum should be considered in those patients with recurrent cystitis. Hematuria, vaginal mass, vaginal discharge, urinary incontinence (often without activity or urge to void), slow urinary stream, and even urinary retention may be presenting complaints. As many as 20% of patients with UD may be asymptomatic, with the UD found incidentally on examination or on imaging. On occasion stones may be found in the diverticulum from urinary stasis, and there have been rare reports of cancer involving a UD.

### Diagnosis

With its wide range of presenting symptoms, UD diagnosis is often not suspected until a physical examination is performed, when, with **careful palpation of the anterior vaginal wall, tenderness or a mass is found.** UD is most often found at the mid- and proximal portions of the urethra. More distal cystic masses, often distorting the urethral meatus, are more likely Skene gland cysts or abscesses. Purulent material, blood, or cloudy urine may be expressed as the urethra and mass are massaged. Imaging for UD includes the double-balloon positive pressure urethrogram (more historic, rarely used because of the availability of specialized catheters and because of patient discomfort), voiding cystourethrogram (VCUG), transvaginal ultrasound, and magnetic resonance imaging (MRI) (Fig. 21.12, *A*). **MRI is typically the preferred study for UD** because it is relatively noninvasive, does not require the patient to void, and, with cross-sectional imaging, offers the most detailed anatomic study of the diverticulum, urethra, and surrounding anatomy. Other tests that can aid in diagnosis and treatment planning include urine analysis and culture; cystourethroscopy, which can eliminate other causes of urinary symptoms and at times allow visualization of the UD ostium; and urodynamics because 35% to 50% of patients have urinary incontinence.

### Treatment

**Asymptomatic UDs do not require treatment, although little is known about the natural history of untreated UD.** Carcinoma arising in UD has been reported, so patients should be counseled appropriately. Mild symptoms of frequency and urgency can be treated with anticholinergics and infections with antibiotics. A variety of procedures have been described for the management of UDs, including transurethral and open marsupialization, fulguration, and, most commonly, excision of the diverticulum with reconstruction. An open marsupialization technique, in which the diverticulum is opened and sutured to the vaginal epithelial surface, generally leads to a fistula, making this technique useful only in rare circumstances such as a grossly infected diverticulum with possible need to return for secondary closure of the fistula or with a distal diverticulum, where vaginal voiding is not a significant issue.

**Transvaginal diverticulectomy is the more common procedure.** An incision is made in the anterior vaginal wall; many surgeons prefer an inverted U-shaped incision (with the apex of the U at the distal urethra), which prevents overlapping suture lines and can be extended proximally as needed. A transverse incision is made in the periurethral fascia, preserving it to be an intervening layer between the urethra and vaginal wall. The diverticular sac is dissected free from the periurethral fascia. Dissection is carried to the diverticular neck, which is then excised. Often the Foley catheter is seen through the defect in the urethra. The urethra is closed with absorbable suture, usually in a longitudinal direction. The periurethral fascia is then closed transversely, often overlapping edges to take up redundancy and close dead space. Next the vaginal incision is closed (Fig. 21.12, *B*). The bladder is drained with a urethral Foley catheter. Some surgeons place a suprapubic tube for drainage as well, but this should be placed at the start of the case to prevent disruption of the repaired urethra.

Postoperative bladder spasms are common and treated aggressively with antispasmodics. Catheters are usually left in place

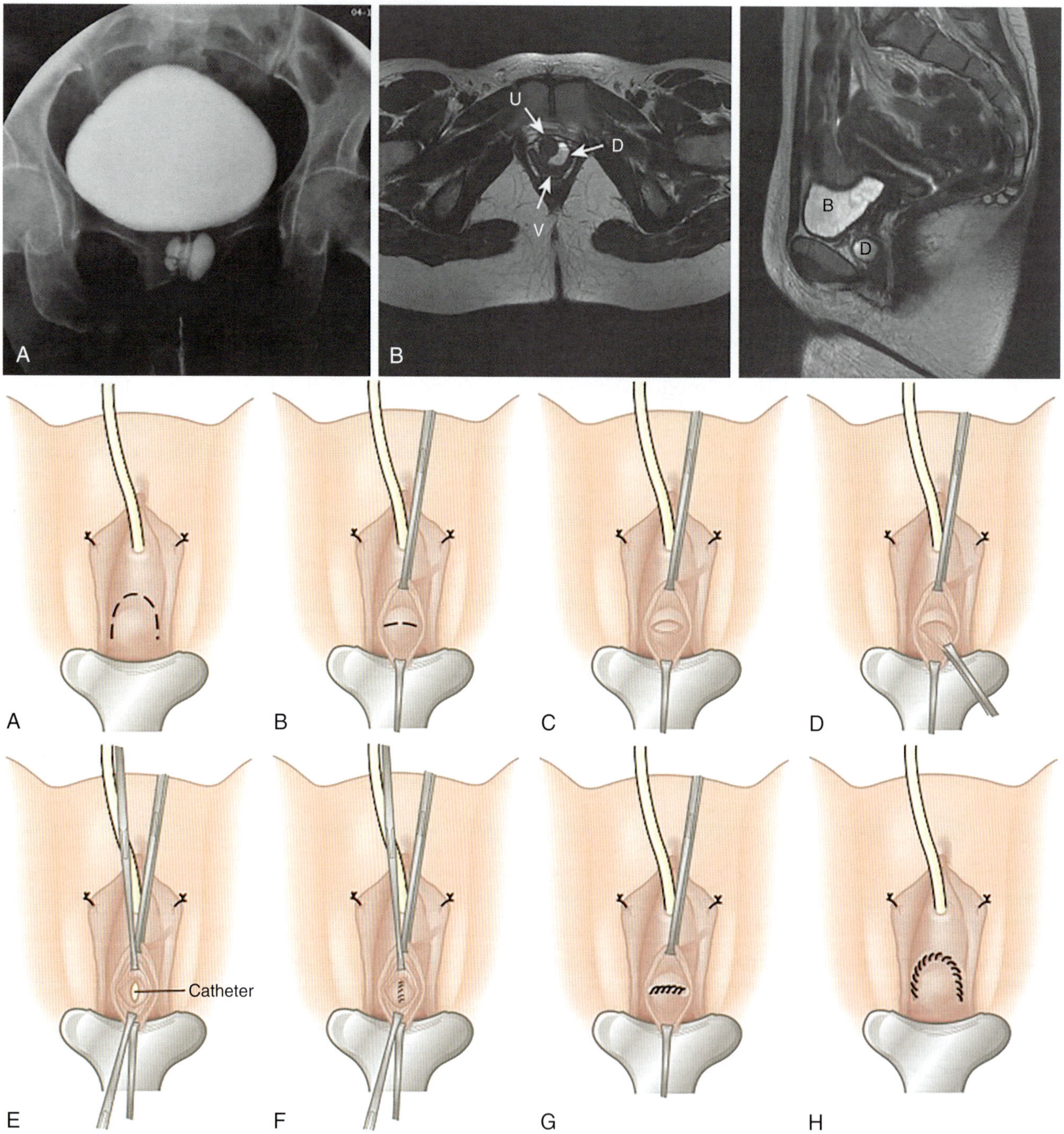


**Fig. 21.12 A,** Imaging of urethral diverticula. **B,** MRI of urethral diverticula. **Lower-level A–H,** Repair of urethral diverticula. *B,* Bladder; *D,* diverticulum; *U,* urethra; *V,* vagina. (From Rovner ES. Bladder and urethral diverticula. In: Wein A, Kavoussi L, Partin A, Peters C, eds. *Campbell-Walsh Urology.* 11th ed. Philadelphia: Elsevier; 2016:2140-2168.e5.)

for 14 to 21 days. A VCUG can be performed to ensure that there are no urethrovesical fistulas before discontinuing catheter drainage.

## Complications

**Complications from urethral diverticulectomy include recurrent UTIs, urinary incontinence, urethral stricture, urethrovaginal fistula, and recurrent UD.** Reported urethrovaginal fistula rates range from 0.9% to 8.3%. A distal urethrovaginal fistula generally results in few bothersome symptoms such as vaginal voiding; however, proximal fistulas, involving the sphincter or proximal to the sphincter, usually result in marked urinary incontinence and require repair, often using a Martius flap (labial fat flap) to provide a well-vascularized intervening layer. Recurrent diverticula are likely underestimated but have been reported to occur 10% to 20% of the time, although often this is not a new diverticulum but failure of the initial repair. Risk factors for recurrence included proximal diverticulum, multiple diverticula, and previous pelvic or vaginal surgery, excluding previous diverticulectomy. Some with recurrent diverticulum have persistent pain or discomfort with urination, and even with complete excision those symptoms can remain. Stricture of the urethra has been reported less than 5% of the time. Urinary incontinence rates range from 1.7% to 16.1%. Stress incontinence development may be related to the dissection of the bladder neck and proximal urethra with injury to the urethral sphincter mechanism. If intrinsic sphincter deficiency results, the incontinence can be difficult to treat because of tissue compromise from the diverticulectomy.

## URINARY INCONTINENCE

**Urinary incontinence (UI) is simply the involuntary loss of urine.** Even though UI results in significant economic, social, and health costs for women, it continues to be underdiagnosed and often undertreated. Some organizations recommend screening women annually for urinary incontinence (O'Reilly, 2018). The prevalence of UI varies significantly depending on the study and age of the population but usually ranges between 20% to 40% of women, with approximately 10% of these women experiencing UI at least weekly. One in six women report moderate to severe incontinence. There are several types of incontinence, including stress incontinence, urgency UI, mixed UI, overflow incontinence, continuous incontinence, and nocturnal enuresis. Identifying patients with UI and determining their type of incontinence and their treatment goals allows for appropriate patient and provider discussion of available treatment options.

### Risk Factors

Box 21.3 lists known risk factors associated with incontinence, summarizing the work of several authors. Some of the factors will be highlighted in this section. Although UI should not be considered an inevitable part of aging, age has been identified as an independent risk factor for UI. In a large survey of community-dwelling women older than 65 years, 28% reported urge incontinence and 21% reported stress incontinence (Sims, 2011). This study illustrates the fact that incontinence type tends to shift from stress incontinence to mixed and urge incontinence with age. One study compared risk factors and determinants of stress incontinence between smokers and nonsmokers using a case-control method (Bump, 1994). In this study, 71 smokers and 118 nonsmokers were compared after a complete urogynecologic evaluation. Smokers were found to have stronger urethral sphincters and generated a greater increase in bladder pressure with coughing, but similar findings with respect to urethral mobility and pressure transmission ratios were found compared with nonsmokers. Urodynamic stress incontinence developed in smokers despite their stronger urethral sphincter findings, probably because of more violent coughing leading to earlier development of anatomic defects.

Race and ethnicity also appear to be factors associated with the presence of UI. Caucasian women have an increased prevalence of UI and an increased risk for developing stress UI (SUI) compared with African American women and Asian women (Townsend, 2010). The findings may possibly relate to differences in collagen, connective tissue and pelvic floor muscle bulk and strength. Several other studies have found a higher prevalence of UI in non-Hispanic Caucasian women and Mexican American woman compared with rates in Asian and African American women, although at least two studies have found no difference between racial or ethnic groups.

**Obesity has a strong association with incontinence, and for every 5-unit increase in body mass index (BMI), the risk increases.** BMI greater than 30 can more than double a woman's risk of UI. Increasing adiposity, as measured by BMI, abdominal fatness, and weight gain, was associated with an increased risk of UI overall and with different subtypes of UI. Depression and anxiety are associated with incontinence. These women reported a higher number of weekly incontinence episodes than women without depressive symptoms, as well as more bothersome symptoms and poorer quality of life (Melville, 2009).

Several largely epidemiologic studies have suggested an increased risk of UI after hysterectomy, particularly radical hysterectomy, with findings of 40% of women developing UI in one study (Aoun, 2015); however, in a twin study, excluding concurrent pelvic floor defect surgeries, no relationship was found between hysterectomy and risk of UI. More research is needed to clarify this factor.

**Vaginal childbirth and higher fetal weight are risk factors in younger women. Compared with spontaneous vaginal delivery, cesarean delivery was associated with significantly lower hazard for SUI, OAB, and pelvic organ prolapse** (Blomquist, 2018). Although obstetric levator avulsion is strongly

**BOX 21.3 Factors Independently Associated With Urinary Incontinence in Women**

**MODIFIABLE FACTORS**

**Gynecologic**
- Cystocele
- Uterine prolapse
- Nonnormal gynecologic examination
- Poor pelvic floor muscle contraction

**Medications**
- Diuretics
- Estrogen
- Benzodiazepines
- Tranquilizers
- Antidepressants
- Hypnotics
- Laxatives

**Urologic and Gastrointestinal**
- Antibiotics
- Recurrent urinary tract infections
- Dysuria
- Fecal incontinence
- Constipation
- Bowel problems

**Other Factors**
- Smoking
- High caffeine intake
- Obesity
- Functional impairment
- Inactivity

**COMORBID DISEASES**
- Diabetes
- Stroke
- Depression
- Cognitive impairment
- Parkinsonism
- Arthritis
- Back problems
- Hearing and visual impairment

**NONMODIFIABLE FACTORS**

**Gynecologic Factors**
- Hysterectomy in older women
- Prolapse surgery
- Genitourinary syndrome of menopause

**Other Factors**
- Age
- White race
- Higher education
- Childhood enuresis
- Family history
- Presence of two or more comorbid diseases

**PREGNANCY-RELATED FACTORS**
- Vaginal delivery
- Forceps delivery—increased risk
- Cesarean section—decreased risk
- Higher parity
- Fetal birth weight

Modified from Holroyd-Leduc JM, Straus SE. Management of urinary incontinence in women: clinical applications. *JAMA*. 2004;291(8):996-999.

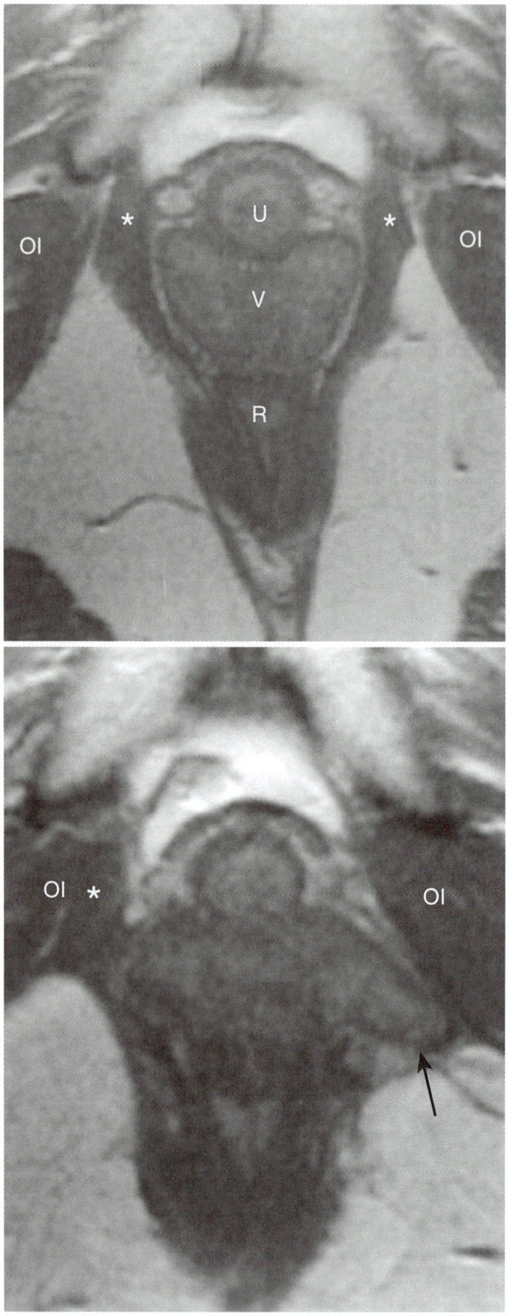


Fig. 21.13 Axial magnetic resonance imaging scan at the level of the midurethra in a normal nullipara *(left)* and a woman 9 months after vaginal birth *(right)* in whom the pubovisceral portion of the levator ani muscle has been lost. The pubovisceral muscle (*) is seen between the urethra *(U)* and obturator internus *(OI)* muscle in the normal woman but is missing in the woman on the right. *R,* Rectum; *V,* vagina. (From DeLancey JO, Ashton-Miller JA. Pathophysiology of adult urinary incontinence. *Gastroenterology.* 2004;126[Suppl 1]:S23-S32.)

associated with pelvic organ prolapse, it may not be associated with incontinence (Handa, 2019); however, this is still uncertain (Fig. 21.13).

The effect is larger in younger women and decreases as time passes from the delivery, possibly because the neuromuscular decline with aging becomes a more important factor. The prevalence of incontinence is significantly higher for women in nursing homes and women with cognitive impairment and poor mobility.

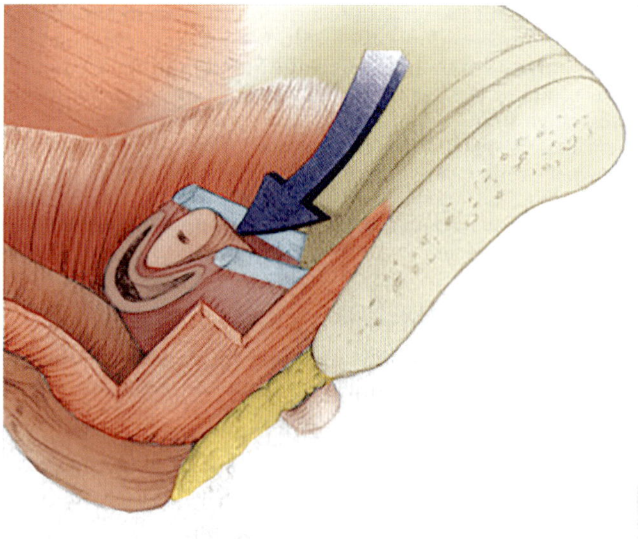

Fig. 21.14 (From Whiteside JL, Walters MD. *Pathophysiology of Urinary Incontinence. Urogynecology and Reconstructive Pelvic Surgery.* Philadelphia: Saunders; 2015:215-223.)

## Stress Urinary Incontinence

**Stress UI, a common condition for which nearly 14% of U.S. women will undergo surgery** (Wu, 2014), **is the involuntary loss of urine with physical exertion that causes an increase in intraabdominal pressure, such as exercise, cough, or sneeze.** This type of leakage is a result of a weakened bladder outlet from compromised urethral support or urethral coaptation. DeLancey's hammock theory suggests that the urethra is supported by the endopelvic fascia and anterior vaginal wall (DeLancey, 1994). Because that support layer is attached to the pelvic wall via the arcus tendineus fascia pelvis and levator ani, the urethra is compressed by increases in abdominal pressure. This maintains urethral pressure above bladder pressure and prevents urinary leakage (Fig. 21.14). Urethral coaptation is affected by the urethral mucosa and vasculature, adjacent connective tissue structures, striated and smooth muscles, and involuntary and voluntary muscles that contract in response to stress.

**Injury, particularly trauma from obstetric delivery, has been implicated in stress incontinence.** The odds ratio of SUI in parous compared with nulliparous women is threefold (Hansen, 2012); the odds ratio after vaginal compared with cesarean delivery is twofold (Lukacz, 2006). Results from a European meta-analysis show vaginal delivery is associated with an almost twofold increase in the risk of SUI, with an absolute risk increase of 8% compared with cesarean section. One study on forceps operative delivery found that 36% of women versus 21% who delivered spontaneously suffered from UI. Bladder neck mobility was significantly increased after all vaginal births, but bladder neck position at rest was only lowered in the forceps group. Women who underwent cesarean delivery were unaffected. DeLancey and coworkers have reported MRI studies showing levator ani injuries in 10% to 15% of primiparous women, which might later lead to incontinence (DeLancey, 2003) (see Fig. 21.13). Considering other forms of pelvic floor trauma, female American Olympic athletes were studied, and researchers could not find a difference between the low-impact (swimmers) and high-impact (gymnasts, track and field performers) athletes with respect to the development of stress incontinence later in life (Nygaard, 1997).

## Evaluation of Incontinence

**Urethral support and coaptation are both important for maintaining continence. Urethral hypermobility corresponds to the loss of the backstop support of the urethra.** This can be assessed by simply asking the patient to cough or Valsalva during pelvic examination with a single posterior speculum blade retracting the posterior vaginal wall or by palpating the anterior vaginal wall at level of the urethra. Often UI will be seen as well. If hypermobility is not seen in the supine position, palpation of the urethra at time of Valsalva can also be done in the standing position. If the patient has a cystocele, urethral hypermobility may be masked, with the cystocele supporting the urethra. In these patients, reducing the cystocele with a sponge stick or lubricated procto swabs and then performing Valsalva often allows demonstration of hypermobility and incontinence. Most incontinence procedures are thought to work by providing a new backstop with either vaginal wall, mesh, or tissue graft, resulting in compression of or limits on a hypermobile urethra during increases in intraabdominal pressure.

Urethral coaptation cannot be appreciated on physical examination; however, if UI is seen at the time of examination without urethral hypermobility, a diagnosis of intrinsic sphincter deficiency (ISD) or poor urethral coaptation should be considered. Women with stress incontinence without urethral hypermobility have a 1.9-fold risk of failure after midurethral sling and may be better served by a urethral bulking agent, which improves urethral coaptation at rest and during strain (Richter, 2011).

As stated earlier, stress incontinence may occur with loss of urethral support or urethral sphincter mechanism, and most women with incontinence have elements of both. Because treatment options and outcomes may differ, we often try to classify women with stress incontinence as having either urethral hypermobility or the often more severe leakage associated with urethral ISD. There is actually great overlap. The diagnosis of ISD is somewhat debatable but is given to women with low VLPP or low maximum urethral closure pressures as measured during urodynamic testing. These women may have more severe continence and higher failure rates after midurethral sling surgery as well (Nager, 2011).

**Evaluation of patients with SUI, particularly those who want to pursue surgical intervention, should include the following:**

- Patient's goals for treatment
- Complete history with indication of incontinence bother to her
- Urinalysis (to exclude UTI and hematuria)
- Physical examination, including pelvic examination with urethral observations described earlier, assessment of urethral mobility, and prolapse evaluation
- Demonstration of SUI by any objective method (e.g., urinary leakage with a CST, pad weight test)
- Measurement of PVR volume

Additional evaluations such as imaging or cystoscopy and/or urodynamic testing should be reserved for women with the following (Kobashi, 2017):

- An unclear diagnosis after the previously described evaluation
- Inability to demonstrate SUI
- Known or suspected neuropathic or significant voiding dysfunction
- Abnormal urinalysis
- Urgency-predominant mixed UI
- Elevated PVR
- Failure of prior antiincontinence or prolapse surgery

**All women should be offered conservative treatments first, and then surgery can be pursued if the treatment fails or the patient declines nonoperative treatments.**

**BOX 21.4** Methods of Pelvic Floor Muscle Training

Kegel exercises with or without referral to a pelvic floor physical therapist
Biofeedback
Isometric with vaginal cones (weights)
Electrical stimulation of pelvic floor

## Treatment

### Conservative Management: Pelvic Floor Muscle Strengthening

Conservative measures should be discussed and offered to all women with stress incontinence (Box 21.4). **The first-line treatment is pelvic floor muscle training (PFMT) directed toward the strengthening of the levator ani and pubococcygeal muscles, which affect the urethral closure mechanism.** This can be affected by isometric exercises—pelvic floor muscle strengthening—as described by Kegel. A Cochrane Database review of PFMT analyzed 31 trials involving 1817 women (Dumoulin, 2018). Women who did PFMT for stress incontinence were eight times more likely to be cured compared with the control group (56% vs. 6%; relative risk [RR], 8.28; 95% confidence interval (CI), 3.68 to 19.07). These exercises also helped women with several types of incontinence (urge and mixed UI), but women with stress incontinence enjoyed more benefit. Specifically, women with stress urinary incontinence in PFMT groups were, on average, six times more likely to report they were cured or improved. Women with all type of urinary incontinence in the PFMT group were roughly twice as likely to report they were cured or improved (Dumoulin, 2018). PFMT reduced the number of leakage episodes, the quantity of leakage on pad test, and incontinence symptoms on validated questionnaires for all these types of incontinence. Limited information from trials indicates that the benefit of PFMT seemed to persist for up to 1 year after treatment stopped in women with all types of UI (38.9%) with PFMT versus (1.6%) with control.

**Patients, however, must be able to localize their pelvic floor muscles and exercise them correctly and regularly to see benefit.** In a study in which 47 women were given simple verbal or written instructions, 23 (49%) had an ideal Kegel effort signified by an increase in force of the urethral closure; however, 12 participants (25%) were performing the technique poorly and in such a way that incontinence might be promoted (Bump, 1991). The authors recommended a demonstration approach rather than a written or verbal approach. Adequate and appropriate pelvic muscle contraction can be assessed at the time of pelvic examination by the examiner placing one or two fingers within the vagina and asking the patient to contract her pelvic floor by contracting the muscles she would use to stop herself from voiding or passing flatus. If she is able to contract her pelvic floor muscles, instructions on timing and frequency of the exercises is usually adequate. One useful technique is to teach women to contract these muscles slowly, 10 times, for a count of 3 seconds each, and to repeat this series for three sets daily. Then she can increase the hold of the muscle contraction by 1 second each week until 10-second holds can be accomplished. A meta-analysis of 12 randomized controlled trials found that at least 24 contractions a day for 6 weeks resulted in decreased incontinence episodes; more contractions did not result in additional improvement (Choi, 2007). Better efficacy was noted in younger women with stress incontinence than older women and women with mixed or urgency incontinence.

If unable to localize and contract their pelvic floors, additional therapies can help patients be successful and see improvement in their incontinence. These therapies for PFMT include pelvic floor physical therapy, biofeedback, weighted vaginal cones, and electrical stimulation. Supervised pelvic floor physiotherapy can be effective for women who have difficulty performing the exercises or have no improvement on their own. Studies have shown most successful physiotherapy includes an individualized plan with standard physiotherapy interventions with weekly sessions for at least 3 months. Biofeedback, usually under the direction of a physical therapist or continence nurse, involves a vaginal pressure sensor in the vagina that measures pressure and provides a visual or audible signal of muscle contraction strength. A Cochrane study found that women who received biofeedback were more likely to report improvement or cure of their UI than those women who received pelvic floor muscle exercises alone (Herderschee, 2011).

A variation in pelvic muscle training is the use of weighted vaginal cones. This involves a set of cones of increasing weight that require pelvic muscle contraction to hold them within the vagina. One study demonstrated an improvement in 70% of 30 premenopausal women with stress incontinence after only 1 month of exercise. A correlation was noted between decreased urine loss and the ability to retain cones of increased weight (Peattie, 1988). A Cochrane review reported some evidence that weighted vaginal cones are better than no active treatment and have similar effectiveness to PFMT and electrical stimulation (Herbison, 2013).

Pelvic floor electrical stimulation can also be used. Electrical stimulation delivers electrical impulses directly to striated pelvic floor muscles, usually via a small, removable vaginal or anal electrode. This activates a pelvic muscle contraction and may indirectly cause inhibition of a detrusor contraction. Studies have shown some to no benefit over sham stimulation.

### Conservative Management: Devices

**An incontinence pessary (Fig. 21.15, *A*) is a silicone ring device with a knob placed in the vagina, with the goal of stabilizing the urethra to eliminate hypermobility and increase urethral pressure during increases in intraabdominal pressure.** This is a safe and effective conservative treatment, with 40% of women reporting their stress incontinence was "much better" or "very much better" (Richter, 2010). Some patients can achieve improved incontinence with the use of a tampon or an over-the-counter device called Impressa Bladder Support (Fig. 21.15, *B*). Urethral inserts (see Fig. 21.15, *A*) have been used but are no longer available. Their use was limited by patients, which is believed to have been because of the need to remove the device with each void and because of high rates of UTIs associated with them.

### Conservative Management: Weight Loss

**Weight loss in women who are overweight or obese significantly reduces urinary leakage, as shown in a randomized controlled trial** (Subak, 2009). Women were randomly assigned to a 3-month liquid diet weight reduction program or a wait-list delayed intervention group. The women in the intervention group lost 16 kg compared with 0 kg in the control group. Weekly incontinence episodes declined by 60% and 15%, respectively ($P$ = .0005). **Improvement in stress and urge incontinence was seen.**

### Conservative Management: Others

The role of estrogen therapy in the treatment of UI has been unclear. The confusion, however, seems to be related to the different effects of systemic versus topical estrogen. Evidence such as that from a Cochrane review (Cody, 2012) suggests that systemic estrogen in postmenopausal women may worsen UI; however, topical vaginal estrogen for women with UI and genitourinary syndrome of menopause has been associated with improved continence. The type of vaginal estrogen—cream, tablet, or ring—does not seem to matter, but it may take 3 months of use for patients to appreciate benefit.

Other non–FDA-approved drugs and combinations of drugs have been studied to determine whether pharmacologic therapy can aid stress-incontinent women. Imipramine, a tricyclic antidepressant, has alpha-adrenergic enhancement characteristics. Its action on the alpha receptors in the bladder neck and urethra may cause muscle contraction and could theoretically lessen stress incontinence; however, imipramine has limited benefit for treating stress incontinence, and there is weak evidence to suggest that any adrenergic drugs are better than placebo treatment.

Duloxetine is not FDA approved for treating stress incontinence in the United States but has been approved in Europe. Duloxetine is a serotonin and norepinephrine reuptake inhibitor that stimulates pudendal motor neuron activity in the Onuf nucleus in the spinal cord and causes rhabdosphincter contraction in the urethra. Several large randomized trials have compared duloxetine to placebo, but the reduction in incontinence is modest and cure rates are no different than placebo. Nausea is a frequent side effect. For a woman considering treatment for depression who also has bothersome stress incontinence, duloxetine is a reasonable medication to consider many drugs may affect urinary function.

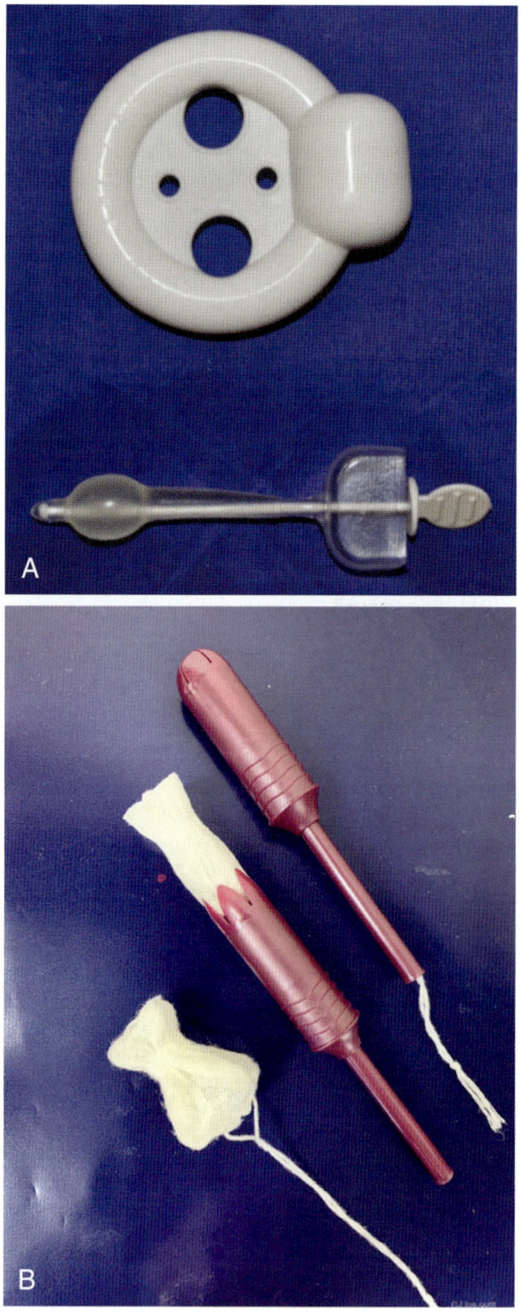


**Fig. 21.15 A,** Incontinence ring pessary and FemSoft urethral insert. **B,** Impressa vaginal support device. (Courtesy Gretchen Lentz, MD.)

**TABLE 21.5** Typical Symptom Differences in Stress and Urge Incontinence

| Symptom | Stress Incontinence | Urge Incontinence |
|---|---|---|
| Leakage with exertion, cough, sneeze, activity | Yes | No |
| Leakage with sensation or urgency | No | Yes |
| Frequency, nocturia | No | Yes |
| Large volume urine loss | No | Yes |
| Leakage with running water, key in the door | No | Yes |
| Leakage with position change from sitting to standing | Possible | Yes |
| Leakage while recumbent | No | Possible |
| History of childhood bedwetting | No | Yes |

### Surgical Management

**Surgery is thought to be the most effective and durable long-term therapy for SUI; however, it is associated with significant potential complications. Treatment for SUI is elective, and often the patient's goal is to be better but not perfect.** Patient preference and therapeutic considerations such as cost, convenience, and particularly morbidity are important. For patients who have inadequate improvement after conservative therapy or decline conservative therapy, several surgical options are available. More than 100 surgical procedures for SUI have been described, and no one surgery is optimal for all patients. Current guidelines (AUA/SUFU, 2017) for surgical treatment of SUI include urethral bulking agents, Burch colposuspension, autologous fascial pubovaginal sling, and midurethral synthetic/mesh sling (retropubic, transobturator, single incision).

### Surgical Management: Bulking Agents

Periurethral injectable agents, of which there are several, are typically injected transurethrally into the urethral submucosa about 1 cm distal to the bladder neck under direct vision with a cystoscope (Fig. 21.16). The reason for improved continence associated with these agents is thought to be augmentation or restoration of urethral mucosal coaptation, but it is not well understood. The mechanism of eventual failure for most of these agents is not well understood either; possibilities include reabsorption, migration, and degeneration. These agents were initially used primarily in patients with ISD alone; however, some studies have suggested improvement in patients with urethral hypermobility as well (Steele, 2000). From noninferiority studies with collagen, the efficacy of these agents has been reported at about 50% at 1 year, with decline to 32% at 3 years (Sokol, 2014). Many providers will consider these agents for certain patients in the following situations:

- Inadequate continence after midurethral sling surgery
- Older women who do not wish for invasive surgery
- Women at high anesthetic risk
- Women with poor bladder emptying

A number of substances have been used as periurethral bulking agents. Agents rarely used include the patient's own fat or blood and autologous muscle-derived cells. Agents no longer used include polytetrafluoroethylene (Teflon) and glutaraldehyde cross-linked (GAX) collagen. Currently available agents include calcium hydroxyapatite (Coaptite); pyrolytic carbon, which are carbon-coated beads (Durasphere); polydimethylsiloxane, which is a silicone polymer (Macroplastique). Nonanimal hyaluronic acid/dextranomer gel (Deflux) is approved for management of vesicoureteral reflux and has been approved for use in incontinence in some countries. Polyacrylamide hydrogel (Bulkamid) became available in the United States in 2020.

### Surgical Management: Burch Colposuspension

Understanding retropubic anatomy is critical when any incontinence operation is performed (Fig. 21.17). In 1961 Burch advocated a modification of the earlier MMK (Marshall-Marchetti-Krantz) retropubic bladder neck suspension by suspending the vaginal wall to Cooper's ligament, now referred to as a *Burch colposuspension* or *Burch procedure* (Fig. 21.18). The bladder neck and proximal urethra are mobilized in the retropubic space; suspending sutures are placed laterally into the tissue on either side of the bladder neck. These sutures are then placed through the ipsilateral Cooper ligament and tied, thereby supporting the vesicourethral junction within the retropubic space. This limits movement and creates a "backboard" of support for urethral compression with the anterior vaginal wall during times of increased abdominal pressure. Intraoperative cystoscopy is recommended to ensure no suspending sutures are placed through the bladder. A 2017 Cochrane Database review of 55 trials of open Burch procedure, including 5417 women, noted that the success rate reported ranged from 85% to 90% at 1 year, and 70% were dry at 5 years (Lapitan, 2017). Follow-up urodynamic studies performed 10 years later in one study reported a surgical cure rate of 90.3%, but five of seven patients who were considered failures reported their symptoms had improved. Complications have included 10% voiding dysfunction, 17% de novo urgency UI, and 13% prolapse at 5 years.

The Burch procedure can also be performed laparoscopically. Reports back to 1998 found roughly a 90% success rate at 1 to 2 years, with one study using multichannel urodynamic studies for outcomes. The laparoscopic procedures have a somewhat longer

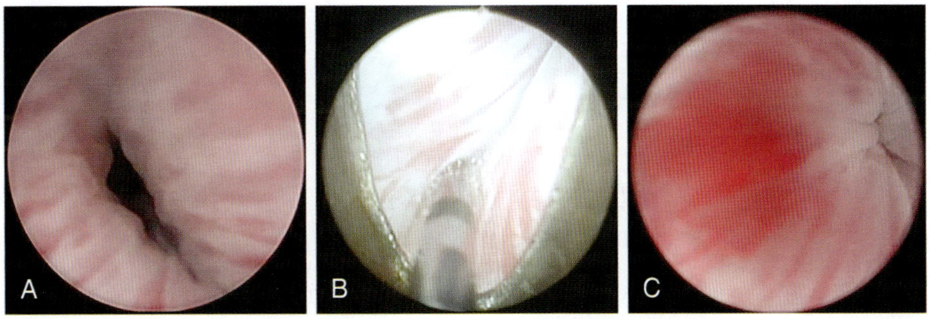


**Fig. 21.16** Endoscopic view of before, during, and after urethral injection. A patient with previous urethral injection is noted to have incomplete coaptation of the urethra with residual bulge on the left side of the urethra (A). After injecting the right side of the urethra (B), coaptation is noted (C). (From Li H, Westney OL. Injection of urethral bulking agents. *Urol Clin North Am.* 2019;46(1):1–15.)

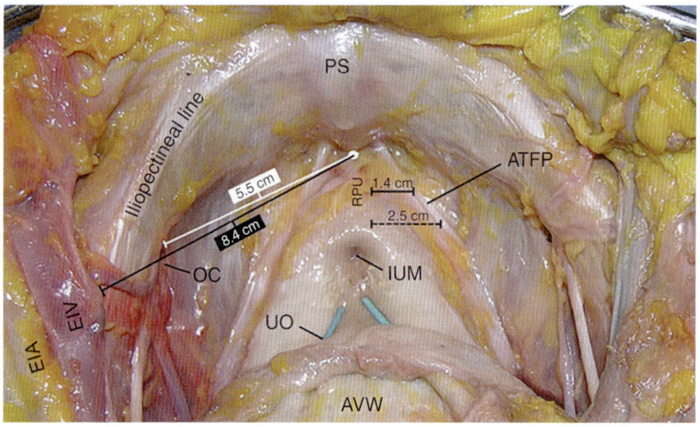


**Fig. 21.17** Retropubic urethra anatomy. Shown is retropubic urethra to arcus tendineus fascia pelvis at level of urethrovesical junction (dashed line) and 1 cm distal (solid line). Also shown are median distances from distal portion of RPU (white circle) to distal margin of obturator canal and to medial border of external iliac vein. *ATFP,* arcus tendineus fascia pelvis; *AVW,* anterior vaginal wall; *EIA,* external iliac artery; *EIV,* external iliac vein; *IUM,* internal urethral meatus; *PS,* pubic simphysis; *OC,* obturator canal; *RPU,* retropubic urethra; *UO,* Ureteric orifice. (From Hamner JJ, Carrick KS, Ramirez DMO, Corton MM. Gross and histologic relationships of the retropubic urethra to lateral pelvic sidewall and anterior vaginal wall in female cadavers: clinical applications to retropubic surgery. *Am J Obstet Gynecol.* 2018;219(6):597.)

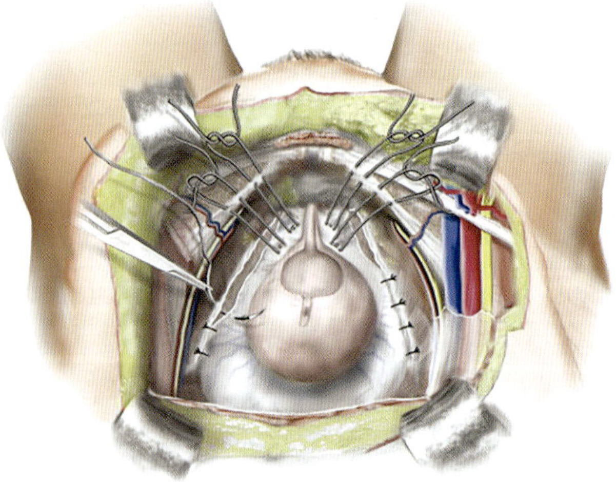

**Fig. 21.18** Burch colposuspension. Sutures have been appropriately placed on each side of the proximal urethral and bladder neck. Figure-of-eight bites are taken through the vagina. Double-armed sutures are used so that the end of each suture can be brought up through the ipsilateral Cooper ligament, allowing the sutures to be tied above the ligament. (From Walters MD. Retropubic operations for stress urinary incontinence. In: Surgery *for Urinary Incontinence.* Philadelphia: Saunders; 2013:33-50.)

operative time in several studies but a shorter hospital stay. A recent retrospective, single-institution center reported a 90.5% outcome success using a standardized questionnaire, with 10% developing new or worsened OAB and 9% having voiding dysfunction (Conrad, 2019). A Cochrane review about laparoscopic colposuspension included 22 randomized controlled trials and found that cure rates of laparoscopic and open Burch colposuspension were similar. Numerous trials have compared laparoscopic Burch colposuspension with midurethral sling (MUS) with no statistically significant difference in subjective cure rates within 18 months; however, objective cure rates tended to be higher for MUS.

For patients who want a native tissue repair, to avoid the unique complications of a mesh sling, the Burch colposuspension is an appropriate incontinence operation. This approach can also facilitate correction of a cystocele by simply placing more suspending sutures proximally, approaching the ischial spine.

### Surgical Management: Midurethral Slings

**Minimally invasive midurethral synthetic slings have become the surgical procedure of choice for most women with SUI and their surgeons as a result of their excellent cure rates, overall low complication rates, minimal recovery time, and high patient satisfaction** (Chapple, 2017). Three types of midurethral slings are available: retropubic, transobturator, and single-incision slings. Concerns regarding mesh used in transvaginal prolapse operations have created confusion and concern for some patients, cessation of mesh sling surgeries in the UK for now, and greater oversight of their use in most countries.

The first midurethral sling introduced was the retropubic tension-free vaginal tape sling (TVT). It was developed based on the theory that the tension on the pubourethral ligaments interacts with muscles of the pelvic floor and suburethral vaginal support structure. Ulmsten and coworkers published a 1996 article on 75 women treated with a midurethral sling made of permanent mesh (Fig. 21.19) (Ulmsten, 1996). The sling was placed under local anesthesia with sedation. A small vaginal incision was made under the midurethra. Small tunnels were made bilaterally to aid in passage of the trocar from the vaginal area through the retropubic space against the pubic bone and exiting through abdominal skin punctures suprapubically. Cystoscopy was performed to evaluate for bladder perforation before the sling was brought into place. The sling was a monofilament polypropylene synthetic mesh, 1 cm wide and 40 cm long. An 84% cure rate was reported, an additional 8% of patients experienced improvement, and 8% of surgeries failed. At 3 years after surgery, Ulmsten and colleagues reported an 86% cure rate.

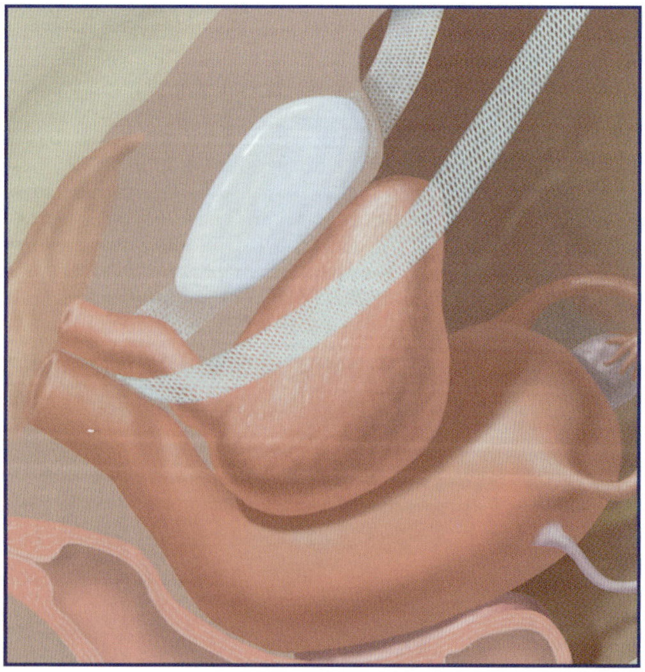

**Fig. 21.19** Tension-free vaginal tape (TVT) sling with Prolene mesh placed midurethrally, without the need for fixation. (Courtesy Gynecare, Ethicon, Somerville, NJ.)

Many other researchers worldwide have published similar success rates. Complications have included retropubic hematoma, bladder perforation, intraoperative bleeding, urinary retention, mesh exposure, and, rarely, bowel and urethral injuries. Ward, Hilton, and the UK and Ireland TVT trial group published a prospective randomized study comparing TVT with Burch colposuspension for primary urodynamic stress incontinence (Ward, 2004). With strict outcome data, the TVT procedure appears to be as effective as the Burch procedure at 2 years, with 63% and 51% cured by objective outcome data, respectively. The lower cure rates in this trial are likely because of the strict outcome criteria. Although the Burch procedure is often successful, the 1- to 3-day hospital stay, 4- to 6-week recovery, and additional risks are much less attractive than a short outpatient procedure (usually less than 30 minutes) with three small incisions and a 2-week recovery time; however, the placement of a permanent mesh has additional risks of mesh erosion and infection not seen with the Burch procedure.

Delorme introduced the transobturator tape (TOT) sling approach in 2001 with the hope of avoiding vascular, bladder, and bowel injuries (Delorme, 2001). TOT sling trocars traverse the obturator canal instead of the retropubic space and enter through small groin incisions at the level of the clitoris bilaterally. Delorme described an out-to-in passage through the obturator membrane along the inferior pubic ramus. Two years later, an in-to-out passage was described and touted to reduce urethral injury. Complications include bleeding, groin or leg pain, and urethral injuries. Objective and subjective cure rates were similar in a randomized trial comparing a TOT sling with a Burch colposuspension. In the largest multicenter randomized trial comparing retropubic TVT with TOT sling, 597 women were randomly allocated, and 95% completed 12-month follow-up for treatment success analysis (Richter, 2010). Objective treatment success required a negative CST, negative pad test, and no retreatment. Objective success was 80.8% for the retropubic sling and 77.7% for a TOT sling; subjective success rates were 62.2% and 55.8%, respectively. Voiding dysfunction was significantly more common in the retropubic sling group (2.7% vs. 0%; $P = .004$). Neurologic symptoms of thigh and groin pain were higher in the TOT group (9.4% vs. 4%; $P = .01$). Results from the 5-year follow-up included decline in efficacy (51.3% in the retropubic sling vs. 43.4% in the TOT group), though patient satisfaction remained high in both groups. TOT patients reported more sustained improvement in urinary symptoms, quality of life, and sexual function despite lower treatment success. New vaginal mesh exposures continued in both groups over time, with a low overall rate of 1.7% (Kenton, 2015).

Some studies suggest that the retropubic sling is more effective in patients with ISD and that reoperation rate for recurrent SUI is less likely with the retropubic sling approach. Without data to support a clearly superior procedure, the choice of TVT versus TOT sling should be made with the patient after discussion regarding the efficacy and potential complications of these procedures. Patients should be informed about increased BMI and poorer outcomes after midurethral slings (Fig. 21.20), although the literature does not agree on this risk.

Single-incision slings are the newest type of synthetic midurethral sling and were designed to avoid both the retropubic space and the groin by anchoring to the obturator membrane through a single vaginal incision. The amount of mesh is much less (approximately 8 cm vs. 40 cm). Most small studies regarding single-incision slings report a subjective cure rate of 74% to 95% at 6 to 12 months. A 3-year follow-up study of 173 patients with single-incision slings reported an 83% objective cure, 6.4% subjective cure, and 9.8% failure rate. A total of 6.4% of patients had de novo urge incontinence; no patients had urinary retention, and the vaginal mesh exposure rate was 5.2% (Yildiz, 2016). Although there are systemic review and meta-analysis comparing single-incision with full-length midurethral slings, much of the data are obscured by the early TVT-Secur sling, which had an inferior anchoring system and worse outcomes. It has been removed from the market. At this time there are not enough data to reliably compare single- incision slings to the transobturator or retropubic slings.

## Risks of Mesh

**Frank discussions must be offered regarding the use of surgical mesh for slings.** Synthetic mesh is a permanent implant. In 2008 the U.S. FDA issued a public health notification regarding complications from the transvaginal use of mesh for prolapse and incontinence (FDA, 2008). Further notifications came out suggesting that the risks from transvaginal mesh for prolapse is more of a concern than transvaginal mesh for incontinence, so the 2011 U.S. FDA advisory refers to prolapse only (FDA, 2011). With the withdrawal of vaginal mesh kits for pelvic organ prolapse and midurethral mesh slings in some countries, AUGS/SUFU came out with a joint position statement on mesh sling use for SUI in 2014, which was updated in 2018 and has the support of many other organizations. Mesh complications from midurethral slings are possible and can include mesh erosions into the bladder or urethra, mesh exposures in the vagina, pain, dyspareunia, and urinary retention as well as rare complications such as severe infections. Despite the risks associated with using a permanent im-

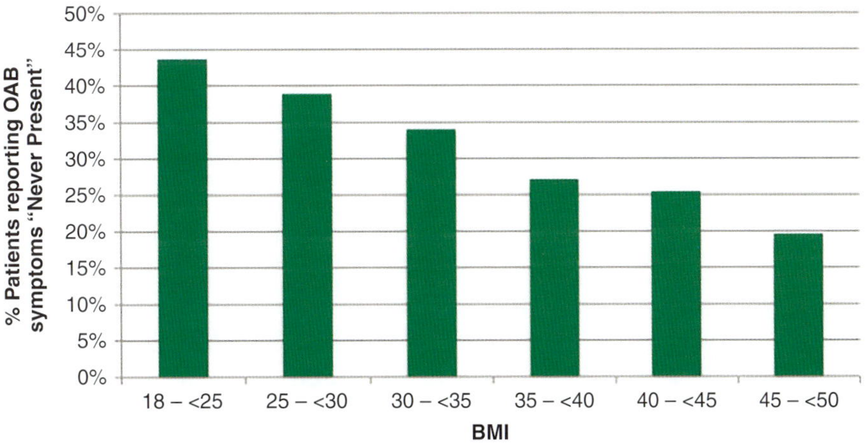


**Fig. 21.20** Effect of body mass index (BMI) on sling outcomes. *OAB,* Overactive bladder. (From Bach F, Hill S, Toozs-Hobson P. The effect of body mass index on retropubic midurethral slings. *Am J Obstet Gynecol.* 2019;220:371.e1-9.)

plant, midurethral slings are the most studied antiincontinence surgery in medical history and remain the most commonly performed surgeries for stress incontinence. A 2018 review of 95,057 midurethral mesh sling insertions found the rate of mesh sling removal at 9 years was 3.3% (Gurol-Urganci, 2018). The rate of reoperation for stress incontinence was 4.5% at 9 years.

## Surgical Management: Autologous Fascia Pubovaginal Sling

In patients who want to or should avoid mesh slings (e.g., patients with an irradiated field in the area of placement), the pubovaginal fascial sling is an appropriate operation. The fascial sling is created from the patient's rectus fascia or fascia lata. Rectus fascia is typically used because it is in the operative field; however, fascia lata is a good alternative if the rectus fascia is compromised. The specific technique (Fig. 21.21) varies between surgeons, but an incision is made in the anterior vaginal wall such that the sling can be placed underneath the urethrovesical junction, providing a "backstop" or compression for the proximal urethra. The limbs of the sling are passed retropubically alongside the bladder neck and through the rectus muscle and the reapproximated rectus fascia. Either the ends of the sling if long enough or the suspending sutures are then tied across the intervening rectus or anchored to the pubic tubercles, securing the sling such that there is no tension on the urethrovesical junction. Cystoscopy is carried out to ensure no bladder or urethral injuries occurred during passage of the sling.

Reported cure rates range from 73% to 89% at 4 years. Complications include voiding dysfunction ranging from 2% to 20%; long-term urinary retention, 1.5% to 7.8%; and de novo urgency UI, 3% to 23% (Haab, 1997). A 2007 multicenter randomized controlled trial compared 655 women assigned to have an autologous fascial sling or Burch procedure (Albo, 2007). At 24 months, the success rates were higher for women who had the fascial sling than the Burch procedure, 44% versus 38% ($P = .01$), using the strictest outcome criteria, and 66% versus 49% ($P < .001$), respectively, if specifically considering stress incontinence outcomes; however, the fascial sling group had more complications with UTIs, voiding difficulty, and postoperative urge incontinence.

## Choosing a Surgical Procedure

Without definitive data to support a clearly superior surgery for stress incontinence, how is a specific operation selected for a specific patient? Factors to consider when making this decision include the following:

- Patient preference
- Mesh or native tissue
- Vaginal or abdominal approach
- Risk tolerance (i.e., some patients want to limit their risk of postoperative urinary urgency or retention)
- Patient factors, such as previous radiation, medical infirmity (most experts would avoid placing mesh in a patient with previous pelvic radiation or severe scarring), obesity, and whether the patient is planning a pregnancy in the future
- Surgeon experience
- Expert opinion

At this time, most experts recommend full-length (retropubic or TOT) midurethral slings for most healthy women who desire surgical treatment of SUI and accept the use of synthetic surgical materials; however, as more long-term follow-up is available for the single-incision sling, this may change. In patients with SUI with a fixed, immobile urethra (possibly ISD), a pubovaginal sling, retropubic midurethral sling, or urethral bulking agent might be best considered. Bulking agent injections can be performed in patients who could not tolerate more invasive procedures.

Although the optimal surgery women with obesity is not known, they are, for example, more likely to have wound complications from harvesting a fascial sling. Several different stress incontinence surgeries appear to be effective in women with obesity, although increasing BMI has been associated with somewhat reduced efficacy of the midurethral sling compared with women of normal BMI (Bach, 2019) (see Fig. 21.20). Furthermore, when only patients with no preoperative OAB symptoms were studied, the rate of patient-reported "new OAB" cases increased with increasing BMI (Bach, 2019). The information should not preclude patients with high BMI from receiving surgical interventions; however, individualized patient counseling is of vital importance before placement of a midurethral sling; weight loss referral can be made if desired, and patients who are overweight should be made aware of the possibility of a lower success rate.

## Postoperative Voiding Trial

**It is usual postoperatively to check a woman for residual urine after she voids because she has a 24% chance of needing a catheter for temporary urinary retention after surgery** (Richter, 2010). After a retrograde fill of 300 mL, she should be able to void about 200 mL, and if not, the catheter should be replaced for 1 to 3 days or the patient should be instructed on clean intermittent self-catheterization. The risk of continued catheterization is 6% 2 weeks after sling surgery and 2% after 6 weeks. In these circumstances, loosening or cutting the sling may be indicated. Voiding trials are discussed in more detail in Chapter 20.

## Intrinsic Sphincter Deficiency

In 1981, McGuire noted the loss of intrinsic urethral tone in a number of women, particularly those with a history of pelvic trauma, radiation, underlying neurologic conditions, or scarring of the urethral sphincter. This has been termed *intrinsic sphincter deficiency*. Currently the two types of stress incontinence, hypermobility and ISD, are thought to be interdependent and not separate entities, as mentioned earlier; however, it is still useful to discuss severe stress incontinence in women with a fixed and poorly functioning urethra. ISD may be why at least some retropubic urethropexies and midurethral sling operations fail. At present, treatment for SUI caused by ISD consists of one of the following: urethral bulking injections, autologous pubovaginal sling procedure, midurethral retropubic synthetic sling, or, rarely, use of an artificial sphincter device.

Midurethral synthetic slings have been studied for ISD. The differing definitions of ISD with urethral hypermobility versus a fixed, nonmobile urethra have made comparisons difficult. In published trials of a retropubic midurethral sling with hypermobility and a low maximum urethral closure pressure (MUCP), the low MUCP did not seem to affect the outcome. Reported cure rates range from 73% to 86%. One study with a 5-year follow-up found that 57% of the women were very satisfied and another 17% had improved continence. In contrast, using a TOT approach in this circumstance resulted in more failures. In the setting of a fixed urethra, only 33% of women reported being cured of incontinence. An anterior rectus sheath fascial sling procedure is now generally reserved for women whose previous antiincontinence procedure failed and a fixed, immobile urethra is found.

# URGENCY URINARY INCONTINENCE/OVERACTIVE BLADDER

**Overactive bladder is a syndrome defined by the symptoms of urinary urgency, with or without urge incontinence, usually with frequency and nocturia in the absence of UTI or other pathologic condition. Urgency is the complaint of a sudden compelling desire to pass urine, which is difficult to defer,**

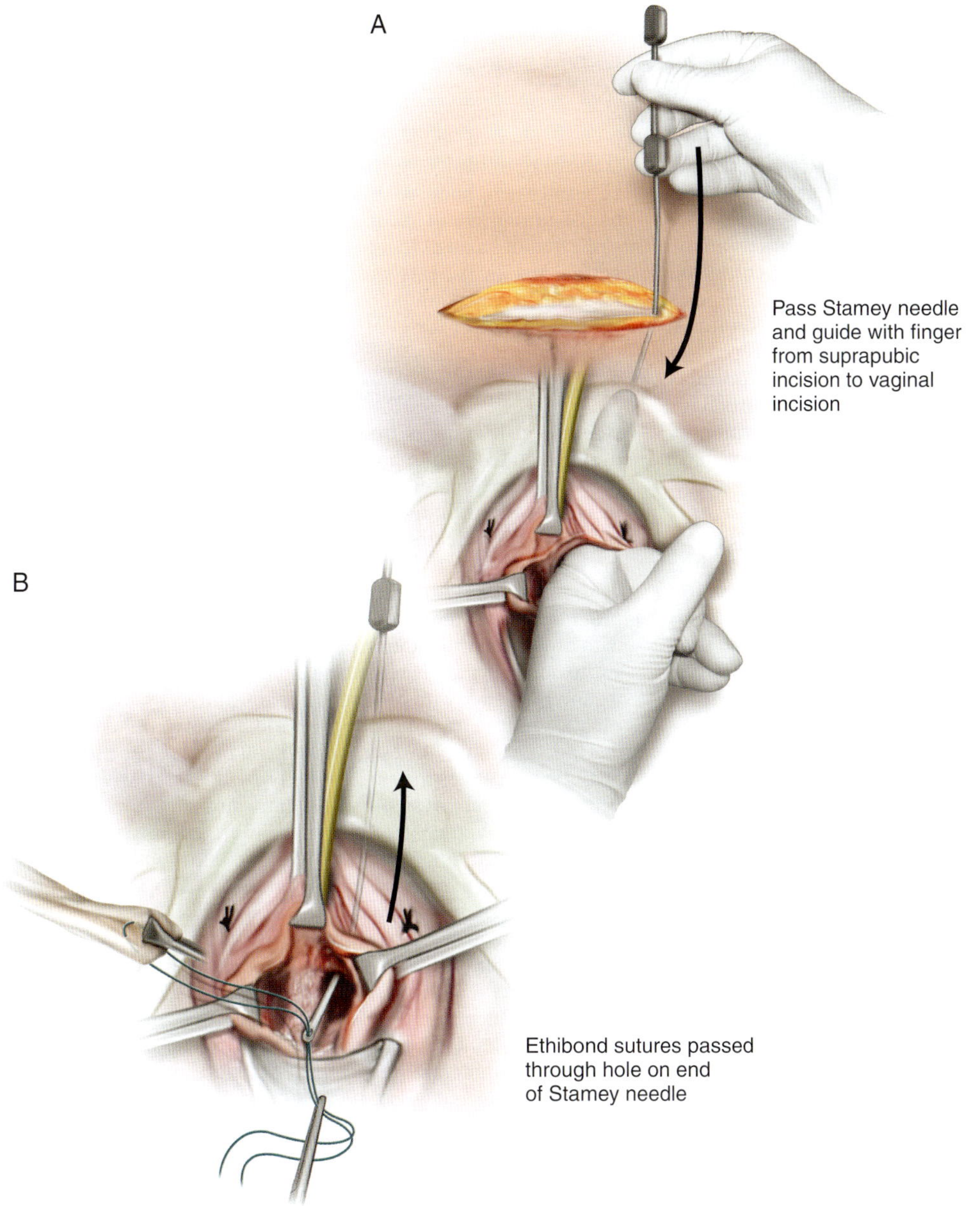
A
Pass Stamey needle and guide with finger from suprapubic incision to vaginal incision
B
Ethibond sutures passed through hole on end of Stamey needle

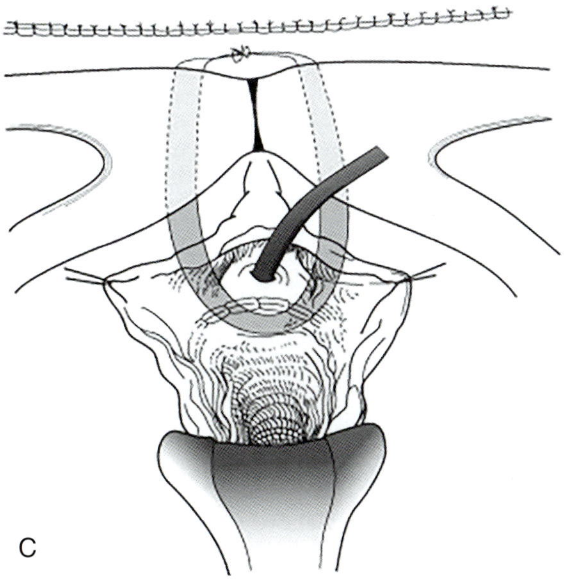
C

**Fig. 21.21** The completed procedure. The sling is beneath the urethra, and each end is tied to the other over the rectus fascia. (**A, B,** From Karam, MM, Zoorob D. Biologic bladder neck pubovaginal slings. In: Walters MD, Karram MM (eds), Urogynecology *and Reconstructive Pelvic Surgery.* Philadelphia: Saunders; 2013:51-63. **C,** From Blavias JG, Chaikin DC. Pubovaginal fascial sling for the treatment of all types of stress urinary incontinence: surgical technique and long-term outcome. *Urol Clin North Am*. 2011;38(1):7-15.)

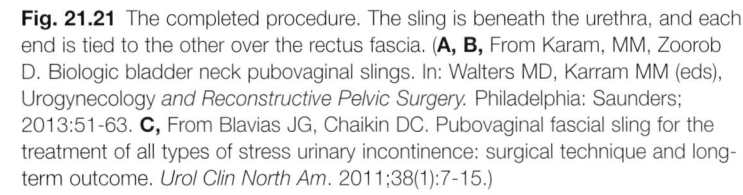

usually because of a fear of leakage if not actual leakage. Urgency UI (UUI, or simply urge incontinence) is the complaint of involuntary leakage of urine accompanied by or immediately preceded by urgency. **OAB is generally chronic, and symptoms may wax and wane.** OAB is often slowly progressive and associated with an urgency-frequency problem that is usually accompanied by painless, involuntary, large-volume urine loss. Rarely an event usually associated with stress incontinence, such as coughing, triggers this urge incontinence, but it is generally delayed until seconds after the increase in abdominal pressure has occurred. Large-volume urine loss is more characteristic of urge incontinence compared with stress incontinence. Stress incontinence often disappears when the woman is recumbent, but urge incontinence continues, often with nocturia. Table 21.5 summarizes the differences in symptoms. **OAB occurs in approximately 17% of the population, and the incidence increases with age. OAB patients have a lower quality of life than women with stress incontinence.** Differential diagnoses include pathologic conditions of the urinary tract, IC/BPS, polydipsia, polyuria, nocturnal polyuria syndrome, diabetes insipidus, atrophic vaginitis, and medical conditions that are associated with nocturia (e.g., vascular or sleep disorders).

Detrusor overactivity is a urodynamic observation; it is the result of sudden, spontaneous (involuntary) detrusor contraction and has previously been termed *detrusor hyperreflexia*, *unstable bladder*, and *detrusor instability*. The term *idiopathic detrusor overactivity* is used as a urodynamic definition when there is no defined cause of the condition. If a neurologic disorder, such as stroke, Parkinson disease, multiple sclerosis, spinal cord injury, or another CNS pathologic condition is present, the term *neurogenic detrusor overactivity* is appropriate. In older women, urgency and incomplete bladder emptying can coexist. Dribbling often results. This condition is termed *detrusor hyperactivity with impaired contractile function* (DHIC), and these two conditions may have different causative factors.

## Etiology

**The increased bladder sensation in OAB is likely increased sensory activity in the afferent nerve endings in the bladder wall.** The involuntary loss of urine with UUI/OAB explained by the neurogenic hypothesis is a result emergence of inappropriate excitation of bladder muscle during storage, which implies a loss of inhibition from the CNS, reemergence of primitive spinal reflexes, acquisition of new reflexes, or sensitization of sensory afferent nerves (de Groat, 1997). The integrative hypothesis suggests that a range of triggers can generate localized detrusor contractions ("micromotions") that spread in the bladder wall and, if they become coordinated, can result in involuntary bladder contractions.

**Aging, neurologic disease, female gender, bladder outlet obstruction, and metabolic diseases are associated with a higher prevalence of OAB** and thus potential influences on OAB etiology. OAB prevalence has been reported as 11.8%, with UUI prevalence estimated at 1.7% to 36.4% in U.S. populations (Milsom, 2014). In women the prevalence of UUI rose from 2% in those aged 18 to 24 to 19.1% in those aged 65 to 74 years.

## Diagnosis

The AUA/SUFU 2019 guidelines for OAB recommend that clinicians engage in a diagnostic process to document symptoms and signs that characterize OAB and exclude other disorders that could be the cause of the patient's symptoms. Minimum requirements include a careful history, physical examination, and urinalysis. Other procedures and workups could include a urine culture, PVR urine measurement, and home, patient collected. Urodynamics, cystoscopy, and ultrasound imaging should not be used in the initial workup of a patient with an uncomplicated situation. A bladder diary such as that shown in Fig. 21.7 can be useful in diagnosing OAB because it can document frequency (more than eight daytime voids), nocturia (more than one nighttime void), and episodes of incontinence preceded by urgency. Additional information can be obtained about incontinence related to activity (stress incontinence), fluid intake, types of fluids ingested, pad usage, and voided volumes (a measure of bladder capacity). The ideal diary duration has yet to be established, but 1 to 3 days is generally recommended. Urodynamic testing is not recommended for the uncomplicated patient suspected of having OAB because 30% to 40% of these studies will be negative in patients with known idiopathic OAB, possibly as a result of increased inhibition in the test situation. History is the most sensitive indicator for UUI/OAB in these patients.

## Treatment: Behavioral—First Line

**Behavioral therapy is first-line treatment. Behavioral management includes fluid management, avoidance of bladder irritants (caffeine, carbonated beverages, diet beverages, and alcohol), weight loss, smoking cessation, PFMT, and bladder training.** Because most patients with detrusor overactivity have abnormal voiding habits, bladder training is useful (also called bladder drill or bladder retraining). This program consists of patient education and a programmed progressive lengthening of the period between voiding, with or without the addition of biofeedback techniques. Specific goals are to correct faulty habits with voiding frequently, to improve control over urgency with prolonging voiding intervals, increase bladder capacity, reduce urge incontinence, and improve confidence in bladder function. This, however, is not useful in those patients with urge incontinence unless they are able to prevent leakage with pelvic floor contractions (suppression of the contraction and physically closing the urethra). Women need to be taught urge suppression using distraction, relaxation techniques, and pelvic floor muscle contractions. The goal is to increase the voiding interval to 2 to 3 hours with normal fluid intake. In their study, Millard and Oldenburg demonstrated improvement in 74% of women with detrusor overactivity using these techniques (Millard, 1983). Cystometric studies performed on these patients revealed a reversion to stable bladder function; however, compliance with bladder retraining by patients is often a problem. Visco and associates studied 123 women who were offered bladder retraining and found that 55% never started treatment or were noncompliant (Visco, 1999). They noted that women who were given concurrent pharmacologic therapy had a higher (87%) compliance rate. Other scheduled voiding regimes include habit training (voiding at an interval before they would usually get an urge to void to preempt incontinence), prompted voiding (caregivers help with scheduled voiding regimen and give positive reinforcement), and timed voiding (caregivers initiate a fixed voiding schedule). Fluid consumption or restriction and elimination of dietary irritants are part of this program. A bedside commode may be particularly helpful for older women with mobility issues (e.g., arthritis) with OAB.

**Although women with urge incontinence may experience less benefit from PFMT than women with stress incontinence, there did appear to be improvement and few adverse effects.** The program is same as described under stress incontinence earlier. Women also need a strategy for urge suppression to prevent leakage, and a few quick Kegel exercises followed by deep breathing and relaxation may help reduce urge. Perineal pressure such as sitting on a hard chair, toe curling, or plantar flexion of the ankle sometimes helps suppress urge. Given the noninvasive nature of muscle training, it makes sense as initial therapy for all stress, urge, and mixed UI.

## Treatment: Pharmacologic—Second Line

**Anticholinergic (antimuscarinic) or beta$_3$-adrenergic receptor agonist drugs may be useful;** Table 21.6 shows currently available drugs. These medications, in conjunction with bladder

**TABLE 21.6** Medications for Overactive Bladder

| Drug | Dosage* |
|---|---|
| Oxybutynin (Ditropan IR)† | 5 mg bid, tid, qid |
| Oxybutynin (Ditropan XL)‡ | 5-30 mg daily |
| Tolterodine (Detrol IR)† | 1 or 2 mg bid |
| Tolterodine (Detrol LA)§ | 4 mg daily |
| Oxybutynin transdermal (Oxytrol) | 3.9-mg patch (twice weekly) |
| Darifenacin (Enablex) | 7.5 or 15 mg daily |
| Solifenacin (VESIcare) | 5 or 10 mg daily |
| Trospium (Sanctura) | 20 mg bid or 60 mg daily (ER)‡ |
| Fesoterodine (Toviaz) | 4-8 mg daily |
| Mirabegron (Myrbetriq) | 25-50 mg daily |

**bid,* Twice per day; *tid,* three times per day; *qid,* four times per day.
†Intermediate release (IR).
‡Extended release (XL, ER).
§Long acting (LA).

retraining, have greater efficacy than either alone. In one trial, combination therapy yielded better outcomes over time on the UDI and Overactive Bladder Questionnaire ($P < .001$), at both time points studied, for patient satisfaction and perceived improvement but not health-related quality of life (Burgio, 2000).

**Overall, in clinical studies, antimuscarinic drugs reduce incontinence episodes by 60% to 75%, but only 20% to 40% of patients have no incontinent episodes. Although efficacy has been proven in many randomized trials, poor patient compliance is often found with these medications because of continued incontinence, expense without cure, and anticholinergic side effects.** The most common side effect is dry mouth. Flexible dosing schedules of several drugs, changing to a different drug, or using a drug patch delivery system are options for finding a tolerable drug for this chronic condition. Salvatore found that two-thirds of women discontinued therapy within 4 months, likely because the therapy did not provide long-lasting symptom relief (Salvatore, 2005). A randomized trial that examined adding behavioral training to medication therapy found reduced incontinence frequency, but when they stopped the medication, they did not maintain improvement (Burgio, 2008). Caution must be advised in elderly patients because antimuscarinics can have more adverse effects (dizziness) and cognitive effects. Several studies have linked higher cumulative anticholinergic use with an increased risk of dementia (Gray, 2015). Contraindications include narrow-angle glaucoma, gastric retention, and urinary retention; in addition, these medications may aggravate existing cardiac arrhythmias.

**The newer beta$_3$-adrenergic agonist drug mirabegron has similar efficacy** (symptom control of 44% to 46%) to the anticholinergics, but instead of inhibiting detrusor contraction like the antimuscarinics, it promotes detrusor relaxation and facilitates urine storage. It appears to have fewer side effects than anticholinergic medications but is contraindicated in women with uncontrolled hypertension. If patients have inadequate symptom control with one medication, combination therapy with these two types of drugs may be considered.

**Low-dose vaginal estrogens are approved for vaginal atrophy, and studies do suggest improvement of urinary frequency, urgency, and possibly urge incontinence.** Systemic estrogens may worsen incontinence.

## Treatment: Procedures—Third Line

Women for whom behavioral and pharmacologic therapies have failed have procedural and surgical options. Fig. 21.22 shows a therapeutic pathway for OAB that demonstrates first-line through third-line options.

Pelvic floor electrical stimulation has been studied for improving a woman's ability to inhibit involuntary detrusor contractions and decreasing symptoms of urge incontinence but has produced mixed results. A small, removable vaginal probe is placed in the vagina or anus; electrical stimulation activates a pelvic muscle contraction. This transvaginal neuromodulation appears to be of benefit compared with placebo, although data are limited.

**Neuromodulation is increasingly recognized as beneficial for women with refractory symptoms** (failed behavioral treatments and medications over roughly 3 months). It includes direct sacral neuromodulation of S3 or neuromodulation through the peripheral tibial nerve. In practice, percutaneous tibial nerve stimulation (PTNS) is done weekly for 30 minutes for 12 weeks and then every 3 to 4 weeks for maintenance therapy if the patient desires. There are few reported side effects except for possible discomfort during the stimulation. Many women prefer this to long-term medication use. Many trials and even a randomized trial with a sham treatment group support the efficacy of this treatment (Peters, 2010). Systematic reviews evaluating PTNS generally demonstrate a benefit, with an approximate efficacy of about 60%, similar to pharmacologic benefits. Most studies are small with short-term outcomes; however, in 2017 a prospective study of 200 women showed persistence of the improvement of their daytime frequency after 12 weeks of PTNS for at least 24 months. One randomized crossover trial compared PTNS with solifenacin (Vecchioli-Scaldazza, 2013). There were fewer daily voids, nocturia episodes, and urge incontinence events in both groups, but PTNS showed greater effectiveness than solifenacin. The PTNS group also reported better quality of life and perceived effectiveness of urgency control. Much remains to be learned about patient selection criteria and long-term effects.

Another route of neuromodulation involves an implantable device, which continuously stimulates the sacral nerves and reduces symptoms. In 1997 the FDA approved InterStim (Medtronic, Minneapolis, MN) for sacral neuromodulation (SNS) for urgency and urge incontinence and later for urinary retention and fecal incontinence (Fig. 21.23). Patients have a stimulation trial or test phase to determine whether the therapy is beneficial. The trial is done with either a temporary percutaneous lead, usually placed in the office, though lead migration can be an issue, or a potentially permanent tined-lead wire that is put in place in the operating room under fluoroscopy. If the therapy results in a 50% or greater improvement in symptoms and the patient desires, the permanent pacemaker-like stimulator is implanted. The device complication rate has decreased with improvement in the wire lead that is placed (Fig. 21.24), along with other improvements in standardizing the implantation procedure; however, infection, failure to provide long-term symptom improvement, and the need for explantation problems remain. One randomized trial of SNS versus standard antimuscarinic medication in 147 patients found that at 6 months the success rate was 61% in the SNS group versus 42% in the medication group ($P = .02$) (Siegel, 2015). There were significant improvements in the quality-of-life scores in the SNS group. Furthermore, the improved or greatly improved urinary symptom scores were 86% for SNS versus 44% in the medication group. The complication rate for the SNS device was 30.5% compared with a 27.3% adverse event rate for medication. Multiple long-term outcome studies have been published confirming that this is a feasible option for many women with refractory urge incontinence. A 2015 review noted that as many as one in three patients required subsequent surgeries. Women must have good cognitive function to consider this option. The current Medtronic InterStim device

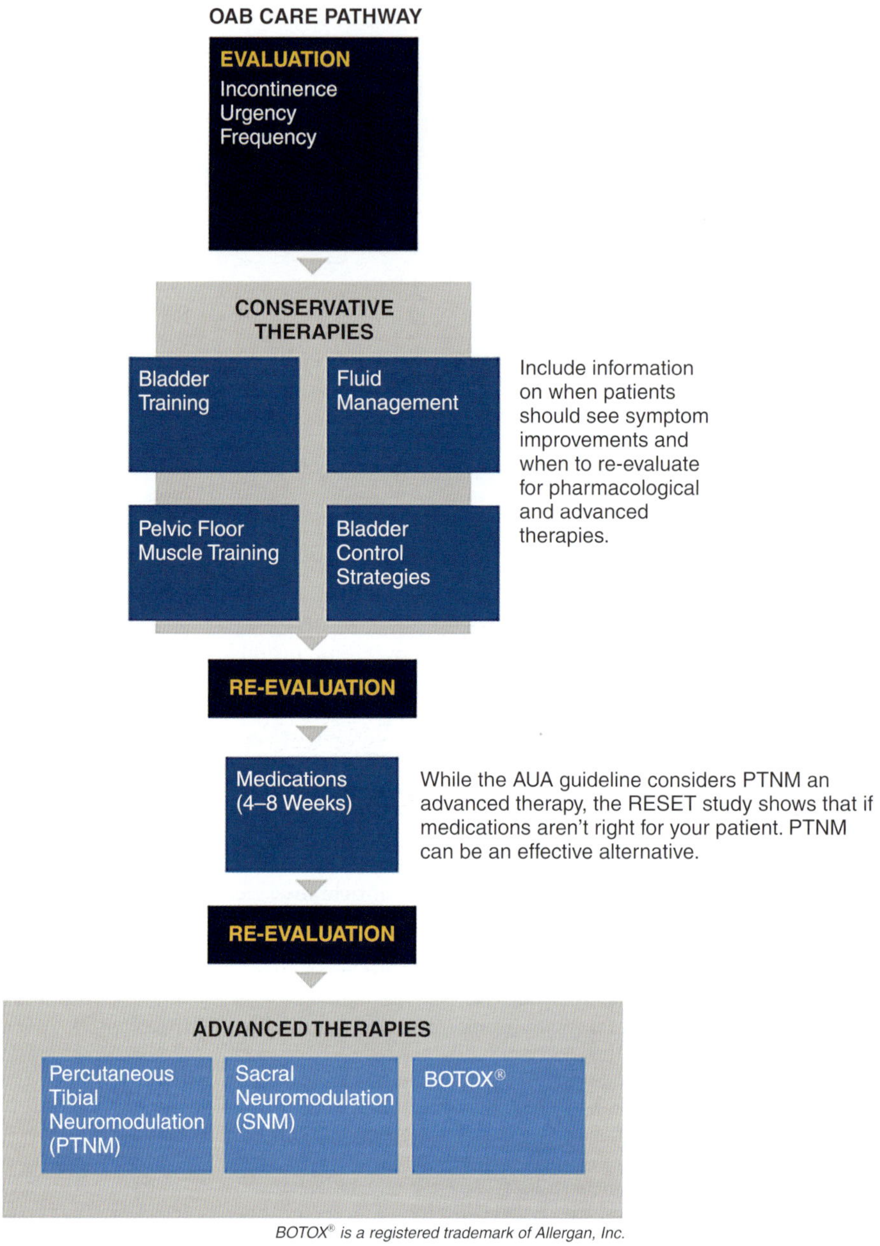
OAB CARE PATHWAY
EVALUATION
Incontinence
Urgency
Frequency
CONSERVATIVE THERAPIES
Bladder Training
Fluid Management
Pelvic Floor Muscle Training
Bladder Control Strategies
Include information on when patients should see symptom improvements and when to re-evaluate for pharmacological and advanced therapies.
RE-EVALUATION
Medications (4–8 Weeks)
While the AUA guideline considers PTNM an advanced therapy, the RESET study shows that if medications aren't right for your patient. PTNM can be an effective alternative.
RE-EVALUATION
ADVANCED THERAPIES
Percutaneous Tibial Neuromodulation (PTNM)
Sacral Neuromodulation (SNM)
BOTOX®
BOTOX® is a registered trademark of Allergan, Inc.

**Fig. 21.22** Treatment algorithm for urge incontinence. *AUA,* American Urological Association; *OAB,* Overactive bladder. (Courtesy Medtronic, Minneapolis, MN.)

is not MRI compatible, and the battery lasts about 5 years. In 2019 an MRI-compatible device was approved by the FDA for fecal incontinence, and it has a rechargeable battery.

**Botulinum toxin (BoNT), specifically onabotulinumtoxinA, is a potent neurotoxin with many medical uses. Injections into the bladder are used to treat patients with both idiopathic detrusor overactivity and neurogenic overactivity.** It is also used in patients with BPS and pelvic floor hypertonus/vaginismus. In the bladder, BoNT blocks presynaptic Ach from parasympathetic nerves, causing paralysis of the detrusor smooth muscle, although it may also affect bladder afferent or urothelial cell neurotransmitters. Botulinum toxin A, generally 100 to 200 units reconstituted in 10 to 20 mL sterile injectable saline, is injected into 5 to 30 sites in the bladder wall via cystoscopy either in the office or in an outpatient surgery setting (Fig. 21.25). It is FDA approved, and published studies show 60% to 70% cure or improvement rates. Temporary urinary retention was reported as high as 40% with early studies using higher doses but is 2% to 6% in newer studies with a definition of retention including only symptomatic patients. Women should return for PVR urine testing and be prepared to learn clean intermittent self-catheterization if needed until the drug wears off, usually no longer than 3 months. Dose-finding studies compared with placebo have found that 100 units and 150 units are superior to placebo. UTIs are more common after injection, with rates ranging from 21% to 35% in the first year after injection (Dowson, 2012). Long-term efficacy data show that reinjection is usually necessary, but repeat injections remain as effective as initial injections. The benefit is maintained for 3 to 12 months. The anticholinergic versus Botox comparison trial (Visco, 2012) showed that 100 units of Botox may only work marginally better than higher doses of anticholinergics. A randomized trial comparing onabotulinumtoxinA, 200 units, with SNS reported a small but statistically significant superiority for onabotulinumtoxinA in the reduction of urinary urge incontinence episodes at 6 months (72% vs. 63%) (Amundsen, 2016).

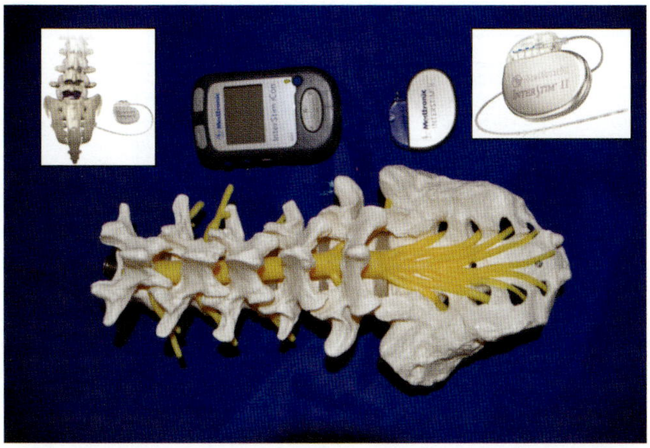

**Fig. 21.23** InterStim test generator and permanent implantable generator, along with spinal cord model. (Courtesy Medtronic, Minneapolis, MN, and Gretchen M. Lentz, MD.)

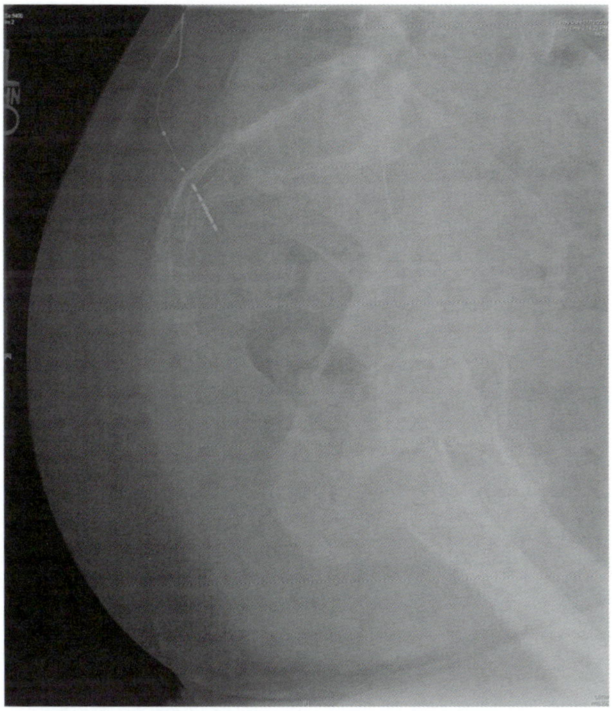

**Fig. 21.24** Lateral radiograph showing the lead wire in the final implantation site at S3. (Courtesy Dr. Jane L. Miller, Department of Urology, School of Medicine, University of Washington, Seattle, WA.)

It appears that third-line therapies are underused because only 3.5% of patients received these treatments compared with 10% to 14% who were seen by specialists. When more comparative data are available, hopefully the ideal treatment for an individual women will be evident.

Table 21.7 summarizes the treatment options for the two most common types of UI. Fig. 21.26 shows an evaluation and treatment algorithm for stress, urge, and mixed incontinence.

## Mixed Urinary Incontinence

As the term implies, ***mixed urinary incontinence*** **means that a woman complains of both stress and urge incontinence—** involuntary loss of urine with urgency and with physical exertion, sneezing or coughing. Mixed incontinence may be urge predominant, stress predominant, or equal. The pathophysiology and treatment of mixed incontinence have not been well studied despite the fact that it accounts for one-third of incontinence complaints. Pelvic floor muscle exercises and behavioral training are appropriate first-line therapies for both types of incontinence (see the stress and urge incontinence sections presented earlier). Usually women can articulate which problem is worse, and treatment can begin for their more bothersome symptom, stress or urgency. The literature supports trying antimuscarinic drugs in urge-predominant mixed incontinence, which in one trial significantly reduced incontinence episodes similar to those with pure urgency incontinence. A systematic review and meta-analysis of midurethral slings in women with

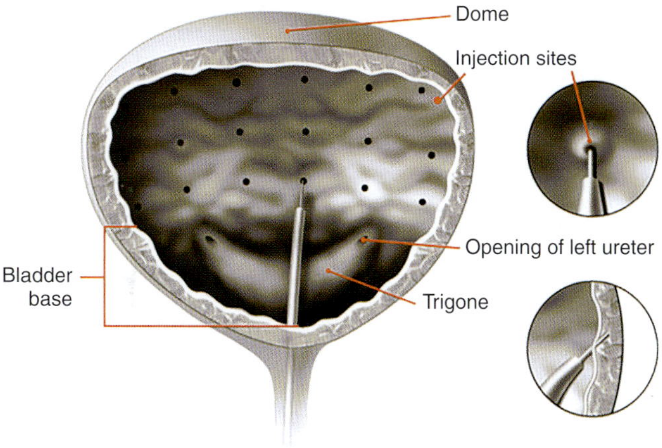


**Fig. 21.25** Injection-site pattern for the administration of onabotulinumtoxinA in the detrusor. (From Fowler CJ, Auerbach S, Ginsberg D, et al. OnabotulinumtoxinA improves health-related quality of life in patient with urinary incontinence due to idiopathic overactive bladder: a 36-week, double-blind, placebo-controlled, randomized, dose-ranging trial. *Eur Urol.* 2012;62(1):148-157.)

**TABLE 21.7** Effective Treatment Options for Women With Urinary Incontinence by Type of Incontinence

| Treatment Option | Stress Incontinence | Urge Incontinence |
|---|---|---|
| Nonpharmacologic | Pelvic floor muscle training<br>Bladder training<br>Prompted voiding<br>Incontinence pessary<br>Impressa<br>Weight loss | Pelvic floor muscle training<br>Bladder training<br>Prompted voiding<br>Weight loss<br>Posterior tibial nerve stimulation |
| Pharmacologic | | Anticholinergic drugs (antimuscarinic)<br>Beta agonist<br>Vaginal estrogen (possibly) |
| Surgical | Midurethral synthetic sling<br>Retropubic colposuspension<br>Suburethral fascial sling | Botulinum toxin A injection<br>Sacral neuromodulation |

Modified from Holroyd-Leduc JM, Straus SE. Management of urinary incontinence in women: clinical applications. *JAMA.* 2004;291(8):996-999.

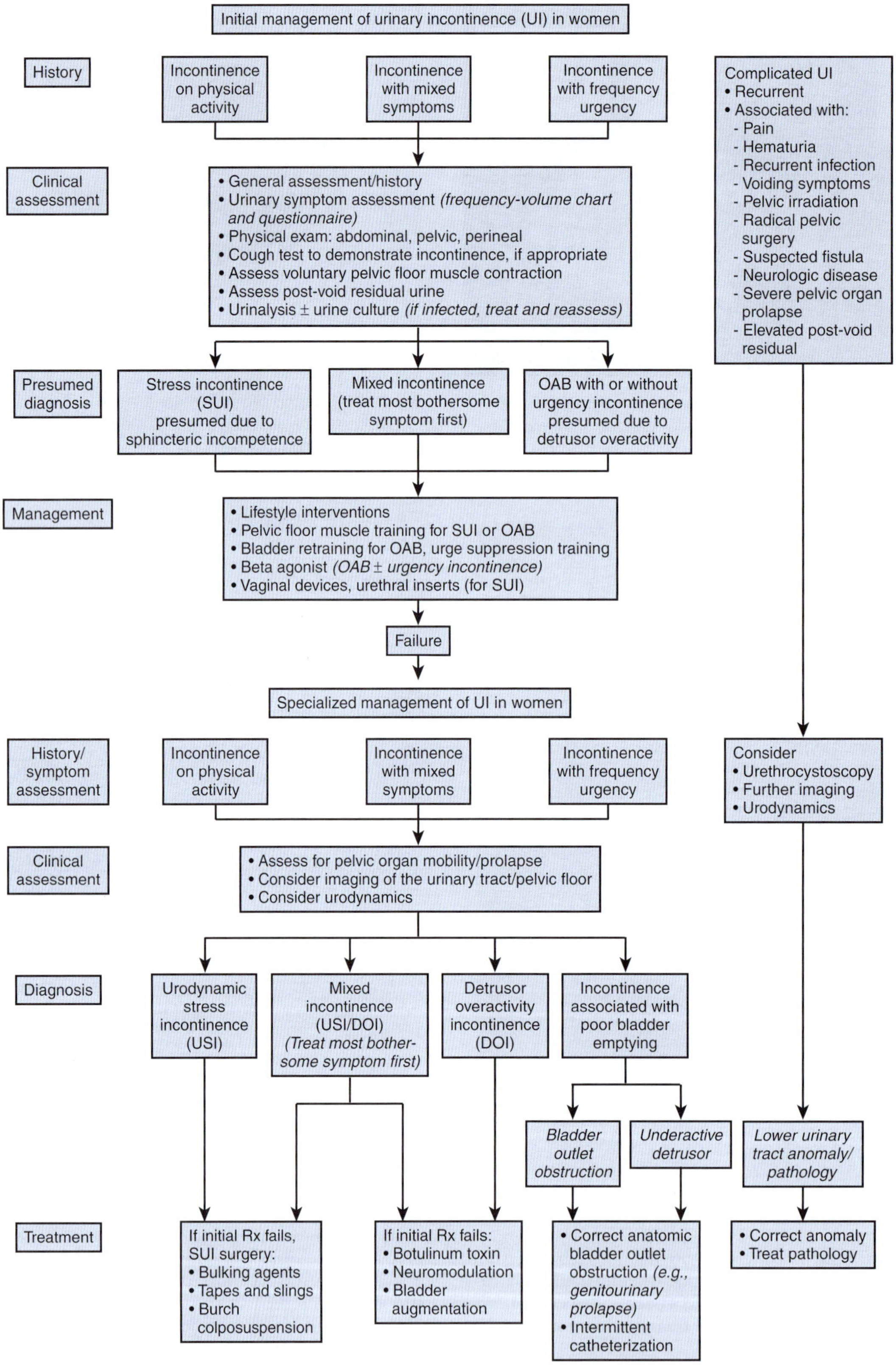


**Fig. 21.26** Summary treatment algorithm for stress, urge, and mixed incontinence.

mixed UI showed an overall subjective incontinence cure rate of 56% among women, with a follow-up of 3 years. Overall success rates were 50% for urge predominant, 60% for equal mixed incontinence, and 80% for stress predominant. Although the success rate in stress-predominant incontinence patients is good, the durability of this improvement may be limited (Welk, 2017). In a randomized trial of 464 women with mixed incontinence, behavioral and pelvic floor muscle therapy combined with a midurethral sling surgery was compared with surgery alone. While there was a small statistically significant difference in urinary incontinence symptoms at 1 year, it was of questionable clinical importance (Sung, 2019). The patient with mixed incontinence who undergoes surgery for her incontinence is often disappointed to still be leaking because the urge component has not improved. The risk of having persistent detrusor overactivity after surgery must be discussed and emphasized during preoperative counseling.

## Other Types of Urinary Incontinence

Nocturnal enuresis is the complaint of loss of urine during sleep. The term *continuous urinary incontinence* is the complaint of continuous urine loss, day and night. This type of incontinence is typically seen with fistula of the lower urinary tract. Insensible UI is the complaint of urine loss when the patient is unaware of how or precisely when the urine loss occurred. Postural UI occurs with change in body position, such as going from sitting to standing or getting out of bed from being supine. Coital UI can occur with penetration or intromission and/or at orgasm. Extraurethral incontinence is a sign rather than a symptom and is defined as the observation of urine leakage through channels other than the urethra, such as the vagina or colon, and may be seen with urinary fistulas or ectopic ureters.

*Overflow incontinence* is the complaint of UI in the symptomatic presence of an excessively full bladder with no cause identified. Overflow incontinence usually occurs in the face of chronic (typically not painful) retention rather than acute retention, because these latter patients are typically in pain and are unable to void at all. Overflow incontinence occurs when a bladder does not empty well either because the bladder is not contracting (detrusor underactivity) or the bladder outlet is obstructed or some combination of both, resulting in a full bladder. The problem may be caused by a neurologic disorder that interferes with normal bladder reflexes, neuropathy, myogenic failure, or obstruction of the urethra. Typically a woman with overflow incontinence complains of small, poorly defined leakage episodes and small voids, possibly with increased frequency, a slow stream, and still feeling that there is urine in her bladder. The bladder usually is not painful and may be palpable after the woman has voided. The diagnosis is made when there is persistence of a significant amount of urine left in the bladder after voiding (PVR), as confirmed with ultrasound bladder scanning or catheterization.

In women this is most often seen after incontinence surgery; the patient's outlet resistance now too great for her detrusor muscle action, resulting in bladder outlet obstruction and thus retention. This can also be seen in female patients with a neurologic disease such as multiple sclerosis, diabetes, with certain medications, and trauma or tumors of the CNS and PNS. A complete general medical and urologic workup is necessary to clarify the patient's condition. Therapy directed at the primary cause may be beneficial, such releasing a suburethral sling that is obstructive. If the cause is unclear or irreversible, the patient will need bladder drainage, which can be achieved by mechanical drainage with either intermittent self-catheterization or an indwelling catheter—preferably a suprapubic tube if it will be chronic, to prevent the risk of urethral erosion with urethral catheters. Sacral neuromodulation is FDA approved for women with idiopathic urinary retention. Alpha-blockers used for men with prostatic hypertrophy are not FDA approved for women and rarely work.

## KEY REFERENCES


Albo ME, Richter HE, Brubaker L, et al. Burch colposuspension versus fascial sling to reduce urinary stress incontinence. *N Engl J Med.* 2007;356(21):2143–2155.

Amundsen CL, Richter HE, Menefee SA, et al. OnabotulinumtoxinA vs Sacral neuromodulation on refractory urgency urinary incontinence in women: a randomized clinical trial. *JAMA.* 2016:316(13):1366–1374.

Bach F, Hill S, Toozs-Hobson P. The effect of body mass index on retropubic midurethral slings. *Am J Obstet Gynecol.* 2019;220:371.e1–e9.

Blomquist JL, Munoz A, Carroll M, Handa VL. Association of delivery mode with pelvic floor disorders after childbirth. *JAMA.* 2018;320(23):2438.

Brubaker L, Carberry C, Nardos R, Carter-Brooks C, Lowder JL. American Urogynecologic Society Best-Practice Statement: Recurrent urinary tract infection in adult women. *Female Pelvic Med Reconstr Surg.* 2018;24(5):321.

Burgio KL, Kraus SR, Menefee S, et al and the Urinary Incontinence Treatment Network. Behavioral therapy to enable women with urge incontinence to discontinue drug treatment: a randomized trial. *Ann Intern Med.* 2008;149(3):161–169.

Clemens JQ. Basic bladder neurophysiology. *Urol Clin North Am.* 2010; 37:487.

Conrad DH, Pacquee S, Saar TD, et al. Long-term patient-reported outcomes after laparoscopic Burch colposuspension. *Aust N Z J Obstet Gynaecol.* 2019;59(6):850–855.

DeLancey JO. Correlative study of paraurethral anatomy. *Obstet Gynecol.* 1986;68(1):91–97.

DeLancey JO. Structural support of the urethra as it relates to stress urinary incontinence: the hammock hypothesis. *Am J Obstet Gynecol.* 1994;170(6):1713–1720; discussion 1720–1723.

Delorme E. Transobturator urethral suspension: mini-invasive procedure in the treatment of stress urinary incontinence in women. *Prog Urol.* 2001;11(6):1306–1313.

Dumoulin C, Cacciari LP, Hay-Smith EJC. Pelvic floor muscle training versus no treatment, or inactive control treatments, for urinary incontinence in women. *Cochrane Database Syst Rev.* 2018;(10):CD005654.

Fitzgerald MP, Payne CK, Lukacz ES, et al. Randomized multicenter clinical trial of myofascial physical therapy in women with interstitial cystitis/painful bladder syndrome and pelvic floor tenderness. *J Urol.* 2012;187(6):2113–2118.

Gomelsky A, Athanasiou S, Choo MS, et al. Surgery for urinary incontinence in women: Report from the 6th international consultation on incontinence. *Neurourol Urodyn.* 2019;38(2):825.

Gray SL, Anderson ML, Dublin S, et al. Cumulative use of strong anticholinergics and incident dementia: a prospective cohort study. *JAMA Intern Med.* 2015;175(3):401–407.

Gurol-Urganci I, Geary RS, Mamza JB, et al. Long-term rate of mesh sling removal following midurethral mesh sling insertion among women with stress urinary incontinence. *JAMA.* 2018;320(16): 1659–1669.

Haab F, Trockman BA, Zimmern PE, Leach GE. Results of pubovaginal sling for the treatment of intrinsic sphincteric deficiency determined by questionnaire analysis. *J Urol.* 1997;158(5):1738–1741.

Handa VL, Blomquist JL, Roem J, Muñoz A, Dietz HP. Pelvic floor disorders after obstetric avulsion of the levator ani muscle. *Female Pelvic Med Reconstr Surg.* 2019;25(1):3–7.

Hanno PM, Erickson D, Moldwin R, et al. Diagnosis and treatment of interstitial cystitis/bladder pain syndrome. AUA guideline amendment. *J Urol.* 2015;193:1545–1553.

Hansen BB, Svare J, Viktrup L, Jorgensen T, Lose G. Urinary incontinence during pregnancy and 1 year after delivery in primiparous women compared with a control group of nulliparous women. *Neurourol Urodyn.* 2012;31(4):475–480.

Herbison GP, Dean N. Weighted vaginal cones for urinary incontinence. *Cochrane Database of Systematic Reviews* 2013;7:CD002114.

Herderschee R, Hay-Smith EJ, Herbison GP, Roovers JP, Heineman MJ. Feedback or biofeedback to augment pelvic floor muscle training for urinary incontinence in women. *Cochrane Database Syst Rev.* 2011;7: CD009252.

Homma Y, Ueda T, Tomoe H, Lin AT, Kuo HC, Lee MH, Lee JG, Kim DY, Lee KS; Interstitial Cystitis Guideline Committee. Clinical guidelines for interstitial cystitis and hypersensitive bladder syndrome. *Int J Urol.* 2009;16(7):597–615.

Kenton K, Stoddard AM, Zyczynski H, et al. 5-year longitudinal follow up after retropubic and transobturator mid urethral slings. *J Urol.* 2015;1993(1):203.

Kobashi KC, Albo ME, Dmochowski RR, et al. Surgical treatment of female stress urinary incontinence: AUA/SUFU Guideline. *J Urol.* 2017;198(4):875.
Koziol JA. Epidemiology of interstitial cystitis. *Urol Clin North Am.* 1994;21(1):7–20.
Kuo HC. Jiang YH, Tsai YC, Kuo YC. Intravesical botulinum toxin-A injections to reduce bladder pain of interstitial cystitis/bladder pain syndrome refractory to conventional treatment-A prospective, multicenter, randomized, double-blind, placebo-controlled clinical trial. *Neurourol Urodyn.* 2016;35:609
Nager CW, Brubaker L, Litman HJ, et al. A randomized trial of urodynamic testing before stress-incontinence surgery. *N Engl J Med.* 2012;366(21):1987–1997.
O'Hare PG 3rd, Hoffmann AR, Allen P, Gordon B, Salin L, Whitmore K. Interstitial cystitis patients' use and rating of complementary and alternative medicine therapies. *Int Urogynecol J.* 2013;24(6):977–982.
O'Reilly N, Nelson HD, Conry JM, Frost J, Gregory KD, Kendig SM, Phipps M, Salganicoff A, Ramos D, Zahn C, Qaseem A; Women's Preventive Services Initiative. Screening for urinary incontinence in women: a recommendation from the Women's Preventive Services Initiative. *Ann Intern Med.* 2018;169(5):320–328. Erratum in: Ann Intern Med. 2019 Sep 3;171(5):388.

**References and Suggested readings for this chapter can be found on ExpertConsult.com.**

# 22 Anal Incontinence

## Diagnosis and Management

*Gretchen M. Lentz, Michael Fialkow*

### KEY POINTS

- Estimates of fecal incontinence range from 11% to 20% of community-dwelling women older than 64 years. More than 30% of women reporting urinary incontinence also report fecal incontinence, known as *dual incontinence*.
- The internal anal sphincter, under autonomic control, maintains the high-pressure zone or continence zone, whereas the external anal sphincter (EAS) provides the voluntary squeeze pressure that prevents incontinence with increasing rectal or abdominal pressure. The EAS is innervated by the hemorrhoidal branch of the pudendal nerve from the S2-S4 nerve roots.
- A common cause of fecal incontinence is damage to the anal sphincter at the time of vaginal delivery, with or without neuronal injury. Prevention of these injuries is critical. The incidence of occult external anal sphincter disruption after vaginal delivery determined by endoanal ultrasound ranges from 11% to 35%. The chance of muscular injury is increased with midline episiotomy, instrumented delivery, and vaginal delivery of larger infants.
- Approximately 1 in 10 women will develop some fecal incontinence or fecal urgency after one vaginal delivery.
- Conservative treatments of fecal incontinence can help. Biofeedback for women with FI shows a similar reduction in incontinence episodes after intense education with a nurse specialist on the subjects of bowel care, medications, and dietary and fluid management. This highlights the importance of conservative management techniques. Additionally, for women with dual incontinence, this single therapy may improve both conditions. Fiber, laxatives, and antimotility medications can be recommended as effective treatment options for FI.
- Overlapping anterior anal sphincteroplasty provides symptomatic control of incontinence in 60% to 80% of women initially, but long-term outcomes are not nearly as successful. According to the American College of Colorectal and Anal Surgeons, sacral neuromodulation is a first-line surgical treatment for women with or without sphincter disruption.

Anal incontinence is a common, distressing condition. *Anal incontinence* is a general term that refers to loss of gas or fecal material via the anus, whereas *fecal incontinence (FI)* is the inability to prevent loss of stool from the anus until desired. Women are often reluctant to discuss this problem with their physician because of embarrassment. *Accidental bowel leakage* is a newer term being used and may be a more acceptable term to women. Obstetrician-gynecologists are often the first provider a woman sees because of the contribution of pregnancy and delivery to the development of FI. **Prevalence also increases with age, with nearly 1 in 5 U.S. women 65 and older suffering from anal incontinence at an estimated pretreatment cost of approximately $300 per year (Patton, 2018). As women age, FI becomes the second leading cause of nursing home placement.** Because of the significant effects that these disorders can have on a woman's self-sufficiency and ability to carry out activities of daily living, it is imperative that physicians are equipped to screen and address these problems for women. This chapter addresses the causes, diagnosis, and treatment of FI.

## EPIDEMIOLOGY OF INCONTINENCE

FI is one of the most devastating of all physical disabilities, but most women fail to report their symptoms and many physicians do not ask. For example, a study of primary care physicians found that 75% screened for urinary incontinence but only 35% for FI, even though more than 30% of women reporting urinary incontinence also report FI (known as *dual incontinence*). Prevalence estimates range from 9% to 16% of community-dwelling women with an average age of onset between 47 and 55 years. Although little is known about racial differences, a 2010 study found a prevalence of 6.1% in noninstitutionalized African Americans aged 52 to 68 years. Approximately 10% of women will report some change in bowel habits after one vaginal delivery, but late-onset FI may have a different set of risk factors. For example, in one case-control study, bowel disturbances were a more important contributor to FI than obstetric events. Box 22.1 lists common risk factors.

FI can be subdivided into three groups:

1. Fecal urge incontinence
2. Passive incontinence
3. Fecal seepage

***Fecal urge incontinence* is the loss of fecal contents despite attempts to avoid defecation. *Passive incontinence* refers to the involuntary discharge of feces without awareness or sensation. *Fecal seepage* is most often defined as the involuntary leakage of small amounts of stool.**

FI affects each woman's life in a different manner. What may be acceptable for one woman may be intolerable to another. During a woman's evaluation it is important to understand her symptoms, type of loss (i.e., flatus or liquid/solid stool), frequency of incontinence, impact on quality of life, and concurrent pelvic floor derangements. Evaluation and treatment should be directed by the severity of the woman's symptoms and the expected goals of therapy.

### Physiology of Fecal Continence

Fecal continence is a complex physiologic process that requires a person's ability to perceive the type of fecal bolus, store or retain when necessary, and excrete when desirable. Continence is affected by the following:

- Stool consistency and volume
- Colonic transit time
- Rectal compliance

**BOX 22.1 Common Risk Factors for Fecal Incontinence**

General
- Aging
- Current smoking
- Obesity

Obstetric/gynecologic
- Obstetric anal sphincter laceration
- Midline episiotomy
- Operative vaginal delivery with forceps
- Rectocele
- Urinary incontinence

Gastrointestinal bowel motility disorders
- Irritable bowel syndrome
- Diarrhea
- Fecal impaction
- Hemorrhoids

Medical
- Neuropathy, including diabetes
- Dementia
- Pelvic radiation
- Medication side effects
- Dietary

Surgical
- Hemorrhoidectomy
- Cholecystectomy
- Bariatric surgery
- Anorectal surgery

- Innervation of the pelvic floor and anal sphincter
- The interplay among the puborectalis muscle, rectum, and anal sphincters.

Dysfunction of one or more of these components can lead to FI (Table 22.1).

As a bolus of stool and/or gas passes from the sigmoid colon to the rectal canal, receptors in the wall of the puborectalis sense the distention of the rectum. As long as the pressure in the anal canal is maintained at a higher level than the rectal pressure, continence is maintained. Anal canal pressure depends on a competent internal and external anal sphincter (IAS and EAS). **The IAS, under autonomic control, is a thickened continuation of the circular muscle of the colon and provides 75% to 85% of the resting tone of the anal canal high-pressure zone.** The EAS, innervated by the hemorrhoidal branch of the pudendal nerve from the S2-S4 nerve roots, provides the voluntary squeeze pressure that prevents incontinence with increasing rectal or abdominal pressure. The shape of the combined IAS and EAS is almost cylindrical, encircling and keeping the anal canal closed. Magnetic resonance imaging (MRI) scans from nulliparous women have shown that the EAS also has lateral winged projections, but their function is not understood. The sphincter complex averages 18.3 mm in thickness and 2.8 cm in length in the midline anteriorly; 54% of the anterior thickness is attributable to the IAS and the remainder to the EAS. **Contraction of the EAS increases the anal canal pressure by approximately 25%, but this tone cannot be maintained indefinitely because these are fatigable, fast-twitch muscles.** Disruption or dysfunction of the IAS may lead to passive incontinence, whereas dysfunction of the EAS typically results in fecal urge incontinence.

The third muscular component of the sphincter complex is the puborectalis muscle, which is innervated by direct branches from S3 and S4 and, to a lesser degree, the pudendal nerve (Fig. 22.1). The puborectalis, part of the levator ani muscle complex, originates from the pubic bone on either side of the midline, passes beside the vagina and rectum, and fuses posteriorly behind the anorectal junction to form a U-shaped sling that cradles the rectum. Like the IAS, the puborectalis maintains a constant muscle tone proportional to the volume of the rectal contents and pressure and relaxes for defecation. The puborectalis and EAS are primarily type I, or slow-twitch, muscle fibers ideally suited for maintaining a constant contraction or tone. The small proportion of type II, or fast-twitch, fibers allows for quick responses to rapid increases in intraabdominal pressure such as coughing or sneezing. The constant contraction of the puborectalis creates a roughly 90-degree angle, known as the *anorectal angle*, between the rectum and anal canal. The role of this angle and potentially pathologic changes to it in the maintenance and failure of continence has long been debated; however, no conclusions have been reached (Fig. 22.2).

**When a bolus of stool or gas is sensed in the rectum, the IAS reflexively relaxes, allowing for colonic contents to be sampled by the anal canal to distinguish solid, liquid, and gas forms of fecal material. This is known as the *rectoanal inhibitory reflex (RAIR)*.** After sampling, the IAS contracts and the fecal material is pushed back into the rectum. The RAIR can be inhibited by fecal impaction and chronic dilation of the anus, which can lead to incontinence, but if the impaction is cured, the reflex and anal tone can return to normal. The RAIR is also absent in women with Hirschsprung disease.

If the rectum has normal compliance and the person chooses to defer defecation, the IAS, EAS, and puborectalis remain contracted until the appropriate time to eliminate. Loss of any of these components can lead to incontinence of flatus, liquid, and/or solid stool.

**TABLE 22.1** Anal Incontinence: Components of the Continence Mechanism

| Component | Function | Symptoms of Deficit |
|---|---|---|
| External anal sphincter | Provides emergency control for liquid stool and flatus | Fecal urgency; urge-related incontinence of liquid stool and flatus |
| Puborectalis | Maintains continence of solid stool | Incontinence of solid stool |
| Internal anal sphincter | Keeps anal canal closed at rest; allows sampling of stool content and enhances continence of liquid stool and flatus | Fecal soiling<br>Incontinence of liquid stool and flatus |
| Anal sensation | Allows discrimination of gas, liquid, and solid stool; provides warning of impending incontinence | Fecal soiling; fecal leakage that is promptly halted by voluntary contraction on conscious detection |
| Colonic motility | Controls stool volume, consistency, and delivery rate to the rectum | Incontinence of liquid or loose stools during prolonged or severe diarrheal states |
| Rectal reservoir | Maintains adequate reservoir under low pressure | Incontinence of solid stool associated with sudden rectal distention; fecal urgency and urge-related incontinence |

From Toglia M. Anal incontinence: an underrecognized, undertreated problem. *Female Patient.* 1996;21:27.

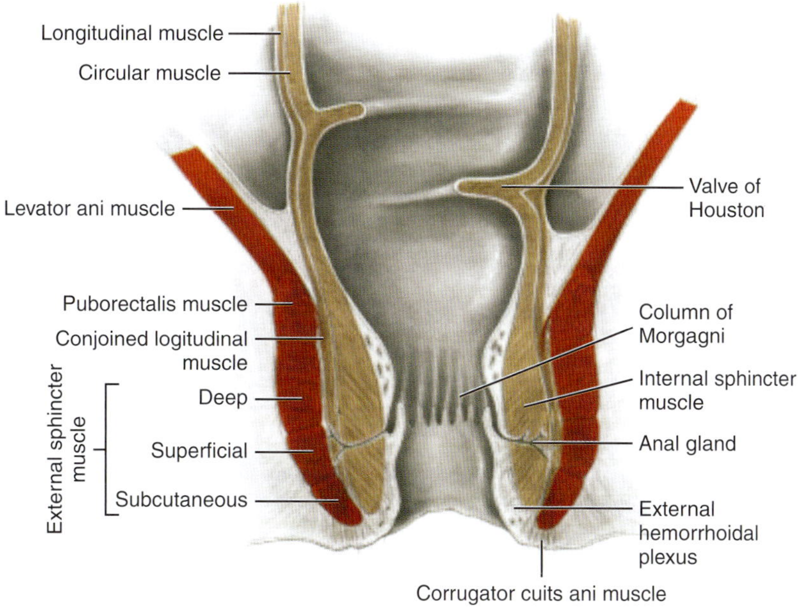


**Fig. 22.1** Coronal section of the anal canal and lower rectum. (From Gordon PH, Nivatvongs S. *Principles and Practice of Surgery for the Colon, Rectum and Anus.* 3rd ed. New York: Informa Healthcare USA; 2007.)

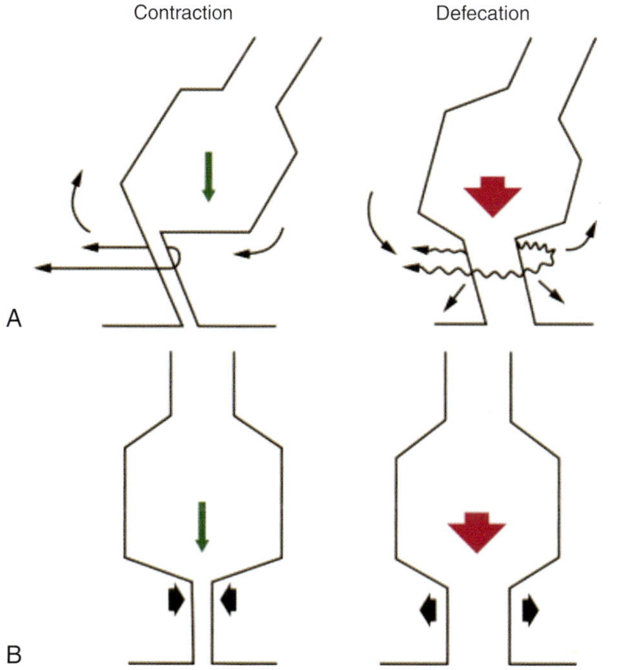


**Fig. 22.2** Angulation between the rectum and the anal canal. **A,** Lateral view. **B,** Anteroposterior view. (From Gordon PH, Nivatvongs S. *Principles and Practice of Surgery for the Colon, Rectum and Anus.* 3rd ed. New York: Informa Healthcare USA; 2007.)

## Causes and Pathophysiology

Categorizing the many causes of FI (Box 22.2) can be done by separating the initial cause into those that start outside the pelvis in a woman with a normal pelvic floor from those that start with an abnormal pelvic floor. Causes that start outside the pelvis

**BOX 22.2** Common Causes of Fecal Incontinence

- Obstetric injury
  - Disruption of internal anal sphincter
  - Disruption of external anal sphincter
  - Pelvic floor denervation
- Trauma
  - Pelvic fracture
  - Accidental injury
  - Anal intercourse
  - Anorectal surgery
  - Rectovaginal fistula
- Diarrheal states
  - Irritable bowel syndrome
  - Infectious diarrhea
  - Inflammatory bowel disease
  - Short gut syndrome
  - Laxative abuse
  - Radiation
- Malabsorption
- Rectal neoplasia
- Rectal prolapse
- Rectocele
- Hemorrhoids
- Overflow
  - Impaction
  - Encopresis
- Neurologic disease
  - Congenital anomalies (e.g., myelomeningocele)
  - Multiple sclerosis
  - Diabetic neuropathy
  - Neoplasms or injury of brain, spinal cord, cauda equina
  - Pudendal neuropathy (e.g., from childbirth, chronic straining, perineal descent)
- Congenital anomalies of the anorectum or pelvis

include all the pathologic conditions that cause diarrhea or increased intestinal motility, overflow incontinence from fecal impaction, and rectal neoplasms. Known or diagnosable neurologic conditions such as multiple sclerosis, diabetic neuropathy, trauma, and neoplasms in the spinal cord or cauda equina initially begin as pathologic processes outside the pelvis, and the pelvic floor is presumed to be normal. As these neuropathies progress, typically there is damage to the pelvic floor musculature or rectal sensation, resulting in FI. People with diabetes, in particular, can develop autonomic neuropathy resulting in decreased IAS resting pressure, which can contribute to FI. Research on efferent brain-anorectal and spinoanorectal motor-evoked potentials identified the possibility that spinoanal and spinorectal neuropathy may play a role in the pathophysiology of FI.

FI secondary to an abnormal pelvic floor is caused by congenital anorectal malformations, surgery, obstetric injury, aging, or pelvic floor denervation without a known neurologic disease. **FI secondary to denervation has typically been designated as idiopathic and is thought to represent more than 80% of patients.** Pelvic floor nerve injury has been studied extensively in women with pelvic floor disorders. Denervation has been attributed to vaginal delivery, chronic straining with constipation, rectal prolapse, and descending perineal syndrome. In women with idiopathic FI, histologic studies of the EAS and puborectalis show fibrosis, scarring, and fiber-type grouping consistent with nerve damage and reinnervation. Pelvic floor electromyography (EMG) studies have also demonstrated increased fiber density consistent with reinnervation.

**Injury to the anal sphincters at the time of vaginal delivery is the most common cause of FI in otherwise healthy women.** Compared with spontaneous vaginal delivery, an operative vaginal delivery has consistently been associated with a significantly higher hazard of anal incontinence. A population-based survey of nearly 13,000 women in Norway identified that 1 in 4 women with a history of obstetric sphincter injury complained of anal incontinence as opposed to 1 in 6 in those who did not. During vaginal delivery, the EAS and/or the IAS can be disrupted, or stretching or crushing can injure the sphincter innervation. Sultan's landmark study of normal spontaneous vaginal delivery showed by endoanal ultrasound that the incidence of occult EAS disruption ranged from 11% to 35%. This study found that 13% of primiparas and 23% of multiparas developed FI or fecal urgency by 6 weeks postpartum, and all but one of these women had evidence of anal sphincter disruption. Because anal sphincter injury correlated with the development of symptoms, reducing anal sphincter injury and understanding risk factors are critical to prevention. **The first vaginal delivery appears to have the greatest effect on pelvic floor function and risk of EAS disruption, but subsequent deliveries can increase the risk of permanent damage, especially in women with transient symptoms of FI after their first delivery.** Risk factors for anal sphincter injury include the following:

- Midline episiotomy
- Instrumented delivery
- Vaginal delivery of larger infants
- Persistent occiput posterior presenting head position
- Older maternal age

## Diagnosis and Assessment

For FI, even more than urinary incontinence, if the physician does not ask, women will typically not volunteer this information. Several reports have shown that twice as many women report fecal or flatal incontinence when given a written questionnaire rather than answering verbal questioning. A question such as "How often do you leak gas, liquid, or solid stool?" should be placed on standard office intake questionnaires. Of note, one study identified that women prefer the term *accidental bowel leakage* to *fecal incontinence.*

**BOX 22.3 History in a Patient With Suspected Fecal Incontinence**

Onset and precipitating event(s)
Duration, severity, and timing
Stool consistency and urgency
Coexisting problems, surgery, urinary incontinence, back injury, diabetes or other neurologic problem
Medications contributing to diarrhea or constipation
Obstetric history—forceps, tears, presentation, repair
Drugs, caffeine, diet
Clinical subtypes—passive or fecal urge incontinence or fecal seepage
Possibility of impaction
Clinical grading of severity
History of pelvic surgery or radiation

Because approximately 1 in 10 or more women will develop FI or fecal urgency after one vaginal delivery, it is important to incorporate open-ended questions concerning these problems as part of the 6-week postpartum visit. But the chance of developing FI also increases with age, so it is also important to target older women for questioning.

### Evaluation

Assessment of the woman with FI must include a thorough history because the origin of the problem may be the single most important criterion of therapy. Box 22.3 lists some questions to consider when taking an FI history.

The history should elicit the onset, duration, and severity of the condition; effect on the woman's daily activities; pad use; frequency and consistency of bowel movements; use of laxatives; fiber intake; and dietary habits. Specific questions concerning diarrhea, amount of flatus, average number of stools per day, passage of mucus, and bloating should be asked. Physicians and patients can define normal bowel function differently. *Diarrhea* may mean frequent bowel movements to one person but loose and watery bowel movements to another. It is best to have the woman quantitate the number of bowel movements and incontinent episodes and describe the stool consistency. **A diary of bowel habits and incontinent episodes can be useful, particularly in women who struggle to provide a clear history (Fig. 22.3).** In women who wear pads, these can be inspected to see if that represents her normal amount of leakage. Table 22.2 gives a commonly used scoring system developed by Jorge and Wexner (1993), although there are several other options to consider. The woman circles the appropriate number on each line of the scale. The sum of the lines indicates the severity of FI, with 0 indicating no incontinence and a score of 20 indicating complete incontinence. A score of 4 or more is typically considered significant. The value of this continence grading scale is that it can be used before and after treatment to determine the efficacy of the intervention. **A standardized questionnaire should be used whenever possible to assess baseline FI severity and efficacy of treatment.**

The history should identify complaints such as feelings of incomplete emptying, straining with bowel movements, fecal urgency, pain with defecation, and insensible loss of stool. **It is particularly important to determine whether the woman has FI when she is aware of the need to defecate or if she is unaware and simply finds stool in her undergarments. When stool leakage occurs without warning, a sensory impairment or hygiene problem is implied, whereas if the woman is aware but cannot prevent the passage of stool, a motor impairment is more likely.** Soiling may also be due to prolapsing hemorrhoids or rectovaginal or anovaginal fistulas.

Women should be questioned about other pelvic floor pathologic conditions, particularly rectal prolapse, rectovaginal fistulas,

## BOWEL DIARY

colon& rectal surgery associates — Pelvic Floor Center®

PATIENT NAME: ______________________

PATIENT DATE OF BIRTH: ______________________

**Instructions:** Use this form to document all bowel movements for 14 consecutive days. Please use a spearate line for each bowel movement. Also use a separate line to record any time you have leakage the occurs at time other than when you have a bowel movement. Please bring this diary with you to your next appointment.

| DATE | TIME | URGENCY "HAD TO RUSH" Y = YES N = NO | QUANTITY (BM) S = SMALL M = MEDIM L = LARGE | ACCIDENTAL BOWEL LEAKAGE QUANTITY S = SMALL M = MEDIM L = LARGE | STOOL CONSISTENCY SCORE (See key in right column) | MEDICATION TAKEN FOR BOWELS Laxitives, enemas, suppositories, stool softerners, (fiber, anti-diarrhea, etc.) | COMMENTS |
|---|---|---|---|---|---|---|---|
| **Example** *10/1/20* | *7 am* | *Y* | *M* | *S* | *5* | *Metamucil (fiber), Imodium* | *Ill, bad day, not what it's normally like for me.* |
| | | | | | | | |
| | *11 am* | *N* | *S* | *L* | *7* | | |
| | | | | | | | |
| | | | | | | | |
| | | | | | | | |
| | | | | | | | |
| | | | | | | | |
| | | | | | | | |
| | | | | | | | |
| | | | | | | | |
| | | | | | | | |
| | | | | | | | |
| | | | | | | | |
| | | | | | | | |
| | | | | | | | |
| | | | | | | | |
| | | | | | | | |
| | | | | | | | |
| | | | | | | | |
| | | | | | | | |
| | | | | | | | |
| | | | | | | | |
| | | | | | | | |
| | | | | | | | |
| | | | | | | | |
| | | | | | | | |
| | | | | | | | |

**STOOL CONSISTENCY SCALE**

**Type 1:** Separate hard lumps (hard to pass)

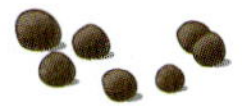

**Type 2:** Sausage shaped, but lumpy

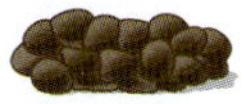

**Type 3:** Like a sausage, but with cracks on surface

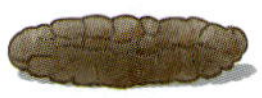

**Type 4:** Like a sausage or snake, smooth and soft

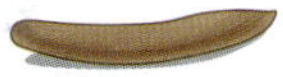

**Type 5:** Soft blobls with clear edges, passed easily

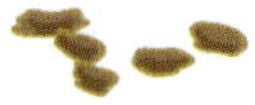

**Type 6:** Fluffy pieces with ragged edges, a mushy stool

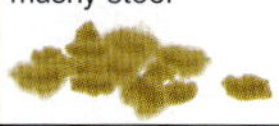

**Type 7:** Watery, no solid pieces, entirely liquid stool

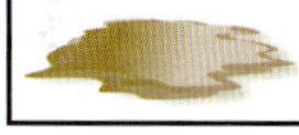

**Fig. 22.3** Stool diary. This is a sample stool diary for assessing patients with fecal incontinence. (From Lee JT. *Shackelford's Surgery of the Alimentary Tract.* St. Paul, MN: Colon & Rectal Surgery Associates, Ltd.:1721-1732.)

**TABLE 22.2** Continence Grading Scale*

| Type of Incontinence | Frequency: Never | Rarely | Sometimes | Usually | Always |
|---|---|---|---|---|---|
| Solid | 0 | 1 | 2 | 3 | 4 |
| Liquid | 0 | 1 | 2 | 3 | 4 |
| Gas | 0 | 1 | 2 | 3 | 4 |
| Wears pad | 0 | 1 | 2 | 3 | 4 |
| Lifestyle alteration | 0 | 1 | 2 | 3 | 4 |

From Jorge JM, Wexner SD. Etiology and management of fecal incontinence. *Dis Colon Rectum.* 1993;36:77-97.

*The continence score is determined by adding points from this table, which takes into account the type and frequency of incontinence and the extent to which it alters the patient's life.

0 = perfect, 20 = complete incontinence; never = 0 (never); rarely = <1/month; sometimes = <1/week, ≥1/month; usually = <1/day, ≥1/week; always = ≥1/day.

and urinary incontinence. Review of systems should include abdominal pain or cramping, lower back or pelvic pain, and changes in sexual response. **Changes in pelvic or lower extremity neurologic function or acute onset of FI, in particular, should prompt evaluation for a neurologic disease, such as multiple sclerosis or a neoplasm of the brain or lumbosacral spinal cord.**

The medical history is important to establish the state of the woman's pelvic floor and anal sphincters. It should, when possible, include a detailed history of vaginal deliveries, including birthweights, length of second stage, episiotomies or lacerations, and use of forceps. Any breakdown or complications of episiotomy healing should be noted. Any history of abdominal or pelvic surgeries and/or trauma to the back or pelvis should be reviewed. The operative reports of any rectal or vaginal surgeries should be obtained and reviewed in particular for complications. The results of flexible sigmoidoscopies, colonoscopies, barium enemas, and defecography should be documented. Family history of colon cancer, inflammatory bowel disease, or familial polyposis should be elicited.

Many medications also affect bowel function (Table 22.3). The woman should not only be asked about laxatives and bowel stimulants, but a complete list of all prescription and over-the-counter

**TABLE 22.3** Medications That Can Contribute to or Worsen Fecal Incontinence

| Drug | Mechanism of Action |
|---|---|
| Nitrates, calcium channel blockers, beta-blockers, sildenafil, selective serotonin reuptake inhibitor | Reduce sphincter tone |
| Glyceryl trinitrate ointment, diltiazem gel, bethanechol cream, botulinum A toxin injection | Reduce sphincter tone via application of topical medications to the anus |
| Antibiotics, laxatives, metformin, orlistat, selective serotonin reuptake inhibitor, magnesium-containing antacids, digoxin, proton pump inhibitor | Cause loose stools or diarrhea |
| Benzodiazepines, selective serotonin reuptake inhibitor, antipsychotics | Relaxant, hypnotic |

From Freeman A, Menees S. Fecal incontinence and pelvic floor dysfunction in women: a review. *Gastroenterol Clin North Am*. 2016;45(2):217-237.

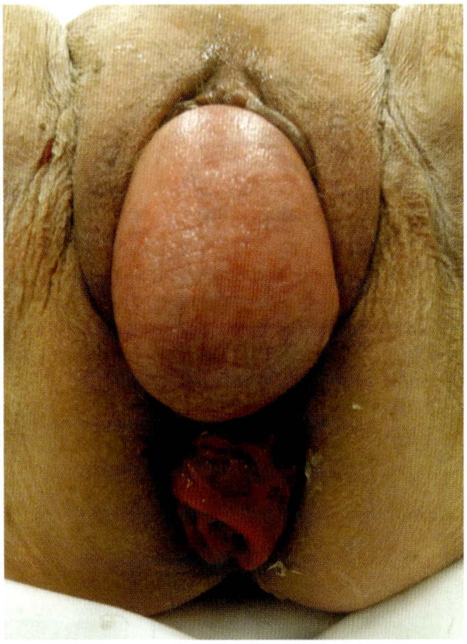

**Fig. 22.4** Combined severe rectal prolapse and vaginal pelvic organ prolapse. Note the protrusion of the rectal mucosa from the anus.

medications, as well as any dietary or herbal supplements, should be reviewed. Many drugs, including anticholinergics, antidepressants, iron, narcotics, nonsteroidal antiinflammatory drugs (NSAIDs), and pseudoephedrine, can cause chronic constipation that may contribute to overflow incontinence or pelvic floor neuropathy secondary to straining.

## Physical Examination

The physical examination begins with inspection of the perineum and anal region. Pruritus ani, or discoloration and irritation of the perianal skin, is commonly seen with FI of liquid stool and chronic diarrhea. Perianal skin creases or folds should completely encircle the anus. Note the presence of protruding tissue around or from the anus and determine whether there are external hemorrhoids or mucosal or full-thickness rectal prolapse (Fig. 22.4).

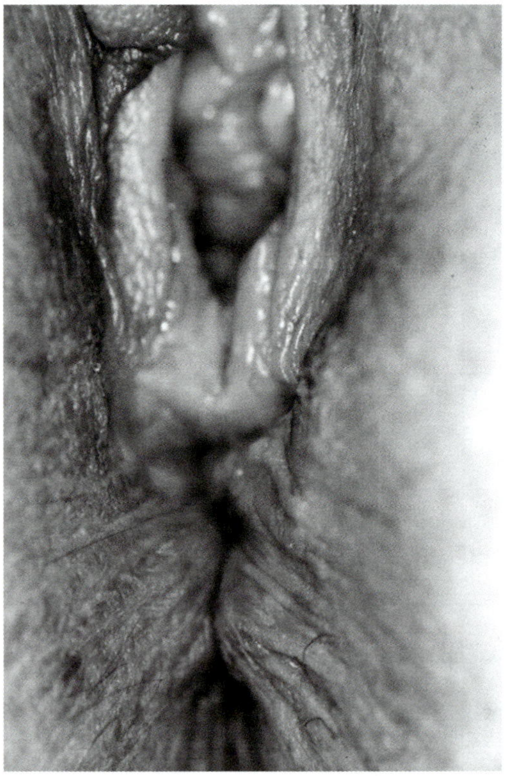

**Fig. 22.5** Perineum with chronic laceration of external anal sphincter (EAS). Inspection of the perineum shows the classic dovetail sign with loss of the anal skin creases anteriorly because of a chronic third-degree laceration of the EAS. Normally, with an intact sphincter, the skin creases are arranged radially around the anus. (From Stenchever MA, Benson JT, eds. *Atlas of Clinical Gynecology.* New York: McGraw-Hill; 2000.)

**The dovetail sign, or loss of anterior perineal folds, indicates a defect in the EAS or chronic third-degree laceration (Fig. 22.5).** Previous episiotomy, laceration, or surgical scars should be noted. The size of the genital hiatus and presence of genital prolapse should be assessed as an indicator of pelvic floor neuromuscular function. Eliciting the clitoral-anal or bulbocavernosus reflex can grossly test the innervation of the EAS. Using a cotton swab, a gentle, quick touch beside the clitoris or over the bulbocavernosus muscle should elicit a contraction of the EAS. If intact, the reflex implies that the pudendal afferent nerves and rectal or external hemorrhoidal branch of the pudendal efferent nerves are functional; however, 10% of women lack this reflex naturally. If absent in the presence of FI, though, further neurologic testing is suggested. Sensation in the S2-S4 dermatomes should be screened by dull and pinprick discrimination when touching the perineum. The same wooden cotton swab used to elicit bulbocavernosus reflexes can be broken and then used for pinprick (broken end) and dull (cotton end) sensation testing. Loss of sensation should direct the clinician to further neurologic or radiologic assessment of the nervous system.

Next the woman should be asked to squeeze as if trying not to pass gas. The perianal folds should be evaluated for a concentric contraction and some upward movement of the perineal body as she contracts the EAS and levator ani; the patient should be instructed not to compensate by using contraction of the buttocks, upper thighs, or abdomen. The woman should then be asked to bear down as if trying to have a bowel movement. She should be reassured that it is expected that she might pass flatus during this part of the examination. The degree of perineal descent and any prolapse of the vagina, pelvic viscera, or rectum should be noted.

If there appears to be any pelvic organ prolapse or if the degree or type of prolapse the woman complains of cannot be seen in the supine position, the examination should be performed with the woman in the standing position or after straining on a commode to maximize the prolapse.

Rectal examination is used to assess resting and squeeze tones of the anal canal. The resting tone of the anal canal is an indicator of IAS function. During squeezing of the EAS the examiner should feel circumferential contraction and tightening. An upward movement of the rectum and posterior compartment of the pelvis should be seen as the levator ani muscles contract. Because these muscles also play an important role in anal continence, evaluation of the levators for strength and symmetry should be performed by palpating the muscles on each side of the vagina at the introitus. Women with a history of vaginal delivery will often have a noticeable asymmetry because this portion of the levator is the most commonly injured. While doing the rectal examination, the presence of a rectocele, enterocele, rectal prolapse, or bowel intussusception should also be assessed as the woman strains. With a finger in the rectum and another in the vagina, the integrity of the rectovaginal septum, posterior vaginal wall, and perineal body can also be evaluated.

The anal canal and rectum should also be palpated for masses, a dilated rectum, and the presence of stool in the rectal vault. As noted earlier, a rectum chronically distended with stool, a tumor, or an intussuscepting bowel will disrupt the RAIR. If this reflex is suppressed, the anal canal remains dilated, the EAS fatigues, and incontinence can occur.

## Testing

**Clinical diagnosis based on physical examination and history alone will be sufficient in most women; however, a prospective study at a tertiary colorectal referral clinic found that further evaluation, including radiologic and physiologic tests, altered the final FI diagnosis in 19% of cases.** The algorithm outlined in Fig. 22.6 recommends further evaluation based on history and the rectal tone. Normal rectal tone directs the clinician away from anal incontinence and toward a metabolic or colonic origin. Common metabolic tests include thyroid-stimulating hormone and glucose levels. If chronic diarrhea is present with normal rectal sphincter tone, stool cultures, colonoscopy, and diarrhea evaluation are suggested. The differential diagnosis for a diarrhea workup includes the following:

- Lactose intolerance
- Celiac sprue
- Inflammatory bowel disease
- Irritable bowel syndrome
- Bacterial overgrowth from diabetic gastroparesis

In cases of FI with normal rectal sphincter tone without diarrhea, anal manometry to evaluate rectal sensation may be useful to assess for peripheral neuropathy causes.

Poor resting tone on rectal examination directs the clinician to a neuromuscular cause. A normal resting tone, but with poor squeeze, suggests an anterior sphincter defect and chronic third-degree laceration of the EAS. If poor rectal squeeze is detected, endoanal ultrasonography is the considered the best method to assess for a disrupted EAS.

Evaluation or further testing is performed not only for diagnostic purposes but also to determine which nonsurgical and surgical therapies are most likely to benefit the woman. Whenever the woman's history does not match her physical examination findings, further testing should be considered. In addition, if the woman has had prior surgery or has other pelvic floor dysfunction, testing before treatment, especially surgical, may help clarify the optimal care plan. It is important to remember that the woman may have more than one pathologic process contributing to her FI, such as pudendal neuropathy and an anal sphincter defect in combination with a weakened pelvic floor and diarrheal state (Table 22.4).

## Diagnostic Procedures

### Colonoscopy

**A colonoscopy is indicated for any woman with chronic diarrhea to evaluate for inflammatory bowel disease or infectious diarrhea.** It is also appropriate screening for any woman older than 50 years, particularly if an acute change in bowel habits is reported. Endoscopic evaluation detects mucosal disease or neoplasia effectively. In addition, any woman presenting with FI in the setting of rectal prolapse should undergo a colonoscopy to ensure that a rectal mass is not the cause of the prolapse.

### Endoanal Ultrasound

Endoanal ultrasound (EAUS) has significantly enhanced the ability to delineate defects of the IAS and EAS. It is one of the simplest and least expensive tests for imaging sphincter defects; however, it is user dependent and requires significant training. EAUS is generally performed with a 10-MHz rigid probe that creates a 360-degree circular image of the anal sphincter complex, allowing assessment of the integrity, thickness, and length of the anal sphincter complex. The IAS is visible as a hypoechoic circle, and the EAS is seen as a hyperechoic or mixed echogenic circle (Fig. 22.7). The distal anal canal is characterized by the presence of the EAS but a thin or absent IAS. In the mid–anal canal the IAS and EAS are both robust, whereas the proximal anal canal is characterized by the posterior sling of the puborectalis. EAUS can also be used to determine the size of the perineal body by using a gloved finger inserted into the vagina to oppose the rectovaginal septum against the probe.

**EAUS is most useful in the evaluation of women with chronic third-degree lacerations or for suspicion of occult sphincter tears (Fig. 22.8).** Knowing the boundaries of the sphincter defect and whether both the EAS and IAS are disrupted can direct the surgeon at the time of anal sphincteroplasty if that is indicated.

### Magnetic Resonance Imaging

Although not routinely used for imaging anal sphincter anatomy, a 2019 paper comparing prepregnancy to postdelivery anal sphincters in primiparous women has challenged conventional thinking. In this small trial of 19 women, 15 became pregnant and 10 returned for postdelivery MRI. Anal sphincter measurements did not change significantly regardless of mode of delivery, and the EAS was not measurable at 12 o'clock in any women. It may be that anal sphincter damage from delivery is not visible with imaging, and neurologic or microscopic damage is more important than muscle injury. This may explain the poor outcomes discussed later with anal sphincter repairs for FI.

### Anal Manometry

Anal manometry is a commonly used test that objectively assesses several parameters of rectal function (Fig. 22.9). Anal manometry is particularly helpful for women who could have altered rectal storage function as a result of prior anorectal surgery or radiation therapy.

Anal manometry uses a rectal balloon to assess rectal sensation, rectal compliance, the RAIR, and maximal tolerable rectal volume (Fig. 22.10). Resting and squeeze pressures in the anal canal are obtained by pulling a perfusion catheter with radial ports through the anal canal, although there are slight variations depending on the equipment and technique used. The squeeze pressure is attributed to voluntary contraction of the EAS and assessed by the force (known as the maximum pressure) and duration of the squeeze. A normal squeeze pressure is in the 120 to 180 mm Hg range and can be sustained for

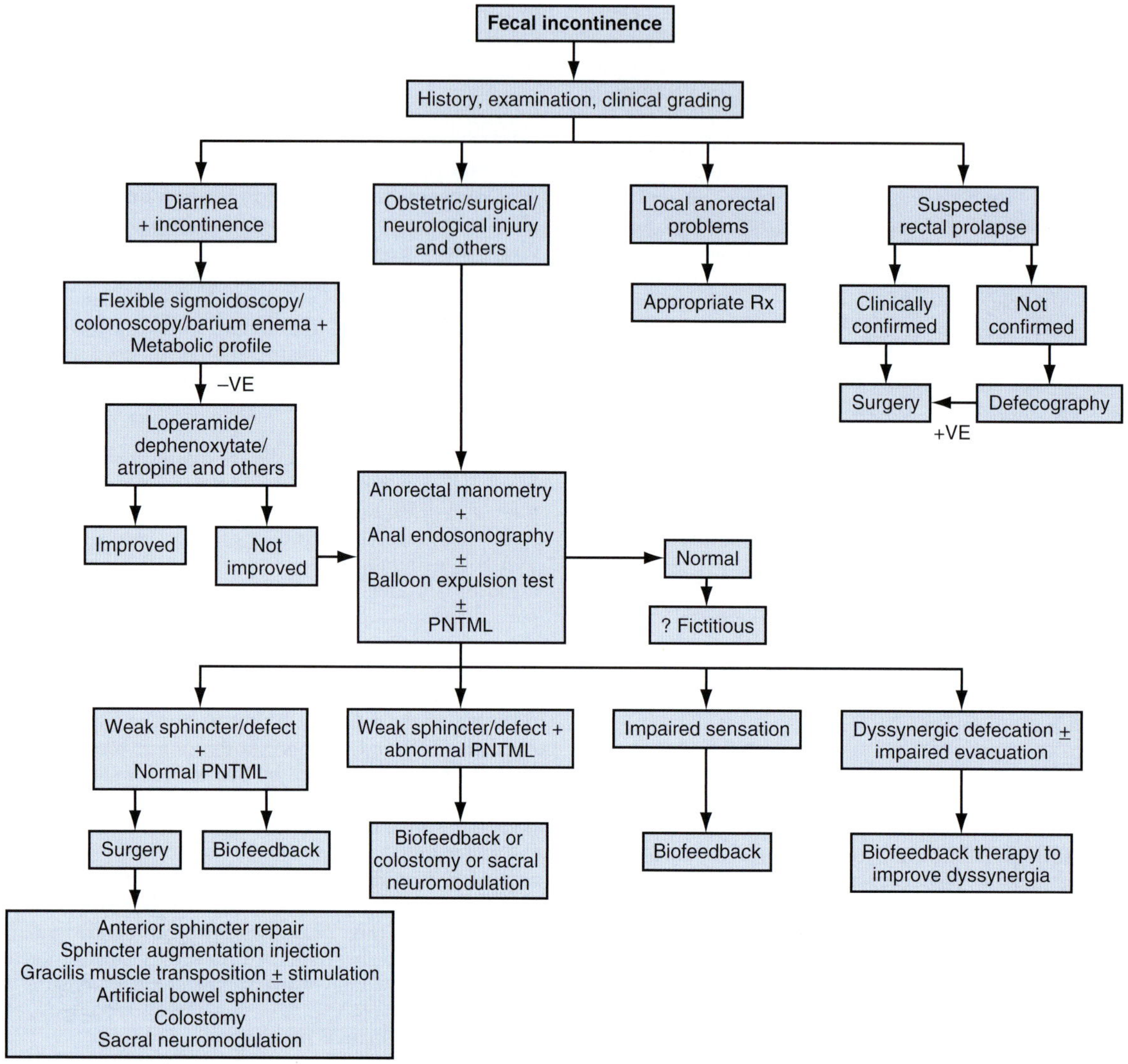


**Fig. 22.6** Algorithmic approach to the evaluation and management of fecal incontinence. A detailed history differentiates incontinence of gas, liquid, or solid stool, along with frequency, onset, and effect on the patient's quality of life. The history should assess the possibility of Crohn disease, ulcerative colitis, irritable bowel syndrome, radiation to the pelvis, neurologic diseases such as multiple sclerosis, and prior anorectal surgeries. A detailed obstetric history should include type of delivery, weight of largest infant, length of second stage, episiotomy or lacerations, and use of forceps or vacuum extraction. Rectal examination should assess resting and squeeze tone, presence of a rectocele or rectal mass, and fecal impaction. Inspection of the rectum and vagina should evaluate for a rectovaginal fistula, prolapsing hemorrhoids, or rectal prolapse. In a prospective study at a tertiary colorectal referral clinic, further evaluation, including radiologic and physiologic tests, was shown to alter the final diagnosis of the cause of fecal incontinence in 19% of cases. *PNTML,* Pudendal nerve terminal motor latency; *Rx,* prescription. (From Rao SS. American College of Gastroenterology Practice Parameters Committee: diagnosis and management of fecal incontinence. American College of Gastroenterology Practice Parameters Committee. *Am J Gastroenterol.* 2004;99:1585.)

20 seconds (Fig. 22.11). Both resting and anal squeeze pressures are reduced in women with anorectal incontinence.

**The utility of anal manometry is debatable because studies have demonstrated that manometry poorly predicts response to surgical intervention, may not correlate well with incontinence scores after intervention, and rarely determines treatment decisions.**

### Electromyography

EMG can be used to map an EAS defect to determine the presence and degree of neuropathy, denervation, and reinnervation. EMG tests the action potentials generated by the depolarization of skeletal striated muscle to assess the spontaneous activity, recruitment patterns, and waveforms of the motor unit action potentials (MUAPs).

Performing and interpreting an EMG of the EAS requires special training. Typically a needle electrode is inserted into the skeletal muscle of the EAS, after which spontaneous activity is heard and seen. Next the woman voluntarily squeezes her pelvic floor to assess recruitment activity in that muscle group. Typically, straining decreases activity and coughing increases recruitment to increase resistance to incontinence. The final step is evaluation of the MUAP waveform. After sphincter injury with nerve damage, reinnervation of the muscle fibers leads to a single

**TABLE 22.4** Tests of Anorectal Function for Patients With Fecal Incontinence

| Test | Measures | Indication | ASCRS Recommendation |
|---|---|---|---|
| Anal manometry | Resting anal pressures<br>Maximum squeeze pressure<br>Rectoanal inhibitory reflex<br>Rectal sensation | Low resting and squeeze pressure on rectal examination<br>Prior radiation treatment<br>Fecal urgency<br>Fecal impaction | Can be considered to help define the elements of dysfunction and guide management. Strong recommendation based on low- or very-low-quality evidence, 1C |
| Single-fiber EMG | Fiber density<br>Muscle activity | Denervation<br>Reinnervation injury<br>Map EAS defect | No recommendation |
| Pudendal nerve motor latency | Speed of signal along pudendal nerve | Pudendal nerve damage from childbirth or straining | May be performed but has limited impact in the diagnosis and management of patients with FI, and is not routinely recommended. Strong recommendation based on moderate-quality evidence,1B |
| Endoscopic ultrasound | IAS and EAS defect | Obstetric or traumatic sphincter injuries | Useful to confirm sphincter defects in patients with suspected sphincter injury. Strong recommendation based on moderate-quality evidence, 1B |
| Defecating proctography or MRI defecography | Movement of pelvic floor<br>Pelvic floor defects | Perineal descent<br>Posterior compartment deficits | |

From Paquette IM, Madhulika V, Kaiser AM, et al. The American Society of Colon and Rectal Surgeons' clinical practice guideline for the treatment of fecal incontinence. *Dis Colon Rectum.* 2015;58(7):623-636.

*ASCRS,* American Society of Colon and Rectal Surgeons; *EAS,* External anal sphincter; *EMG,* electromyography; *FI,* fecal incontinence; *IAS,* internal anal sphincter; *MRI,* magnetic resonance imaging.

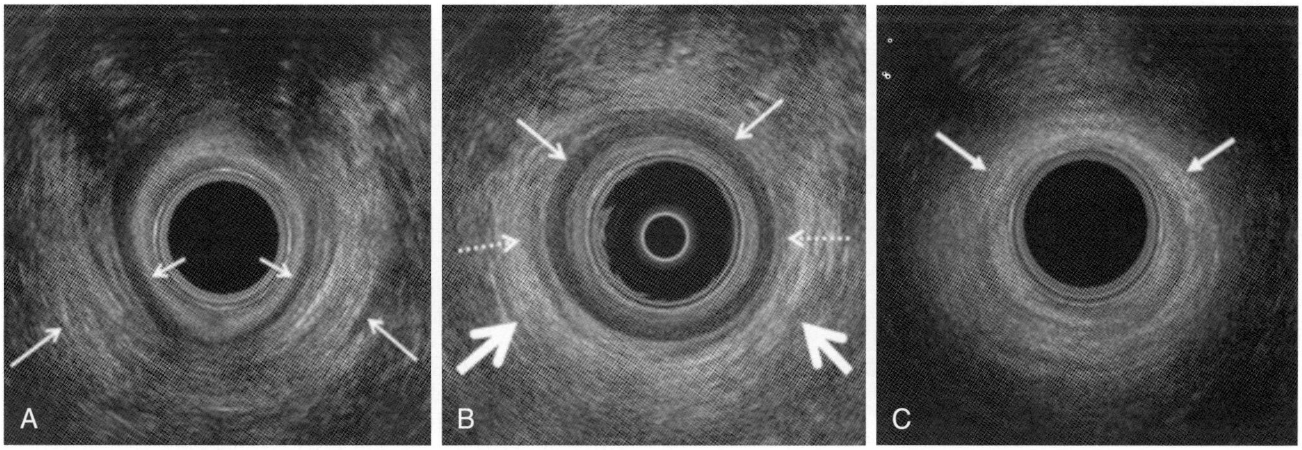


**Fig. 22.7** Anal ultrasound. Transverse ultrasound images of the normal anal sphincter. Endoanal ultrasound images at three levels (upper sphincter, midsphincter, and caudal sphincter) at the level of the puborectalis muscle (PRM) shows the internal sphincter, intersphincteric fat, and external sphincter as separate structures. **A,** Endoanal ultrasound image: transverse image of the cephalad (upper) anal sphincter demonstrating the striated relatively echogenic U-shaped sling of the posterior PRM *(long arrows)* and the hypoechoic internal anal sphincter (IAS) *(short arrows).* Note that at this level the external anal sphincter (EAS) is absent. The innermost echogenic ring represents the rectal mucosa and interface with the transducer (central round black structure). **B,** Normal appearance on endoanal ultrasound of the anal sphincters at the midsphincteric level demonstrating the characteristic target or layered appearance. The inner echogenic ring represents the mucosa and interface with the transducer; the IAS is the subjacent markedly hypoechoic ring *(thin arrows),* and the outermost ring represents the EAS *(thick arrows)* and is typically either hyperechoic or of mixed echogenicity. Wispy hypoechoic curvilinear strands with a striated appearance *(dotted arrows)* between the IAS and EAS represent the longitudinal muscle layer. **C,** Endoanal ultrasound image: transverse image of the normal caudal or distal anal sphincter image where the echogenic EAS *(arrows)* extends beyond the IAS, representing the superficial portion of the EAS. (From Weinstein MM, Lockhart ME. Ultrasound and magnetic resonance imaging in urogynecology. In: Norton ME, Scoutt LM, Feldstein VA, eds. *Callen's Ultrasonography in Obstetrics and Gynecology.* 6th ed. Philadelphia: Elsevier: 1025-1044.)

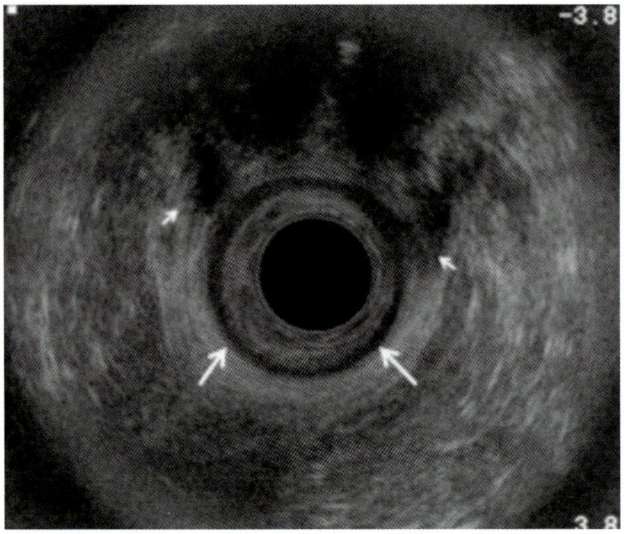


**Fig. 22.8** Anal ultrasound: sphincter tear. Endorectal axial ultrasound image demonstrating an intact hypoechoic internal anal sphincter *(arrows)* but disruption of the anterior aspect of the external anal sphincter *(arrowheads)* from the 11 o'clock to the 3 o'clock position. (From Weinstein MM, Lockhart ME. Ultrasound and magnetic resonance imaging in urogynecology. In: Norton ME, Scoutt LM, Feldstein VA, eds. *Callen's Ultrasonography in Obstetrics and Gynecology.* 6th ed. Philadelphia: Elsevier: 1025-1044.)

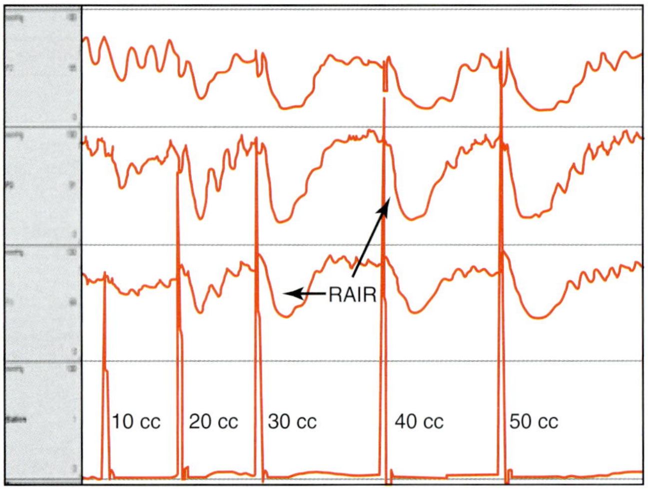


**Fig. 22.10** Normal anorectal manometry. Anorectal manometry tracing that shows the presence of the rectoanal inhibitory reflex (RAIR) after balloon distention. The lower channel shows the balloon distention. The upper three channels reflect the measurements obtained in the high-pressure zone of the anal canal. There is a normal dose–response curve, with a progression in the degree of relaxation as the balloon volume is increased. (From Rodriguez L, Nurko S. Gastrointestinal motility procedures. In *Pediatric Gastrointestinal and Liver Disease,* 5th ed. Philadelphia: Elsevier, 2016;748-765.)

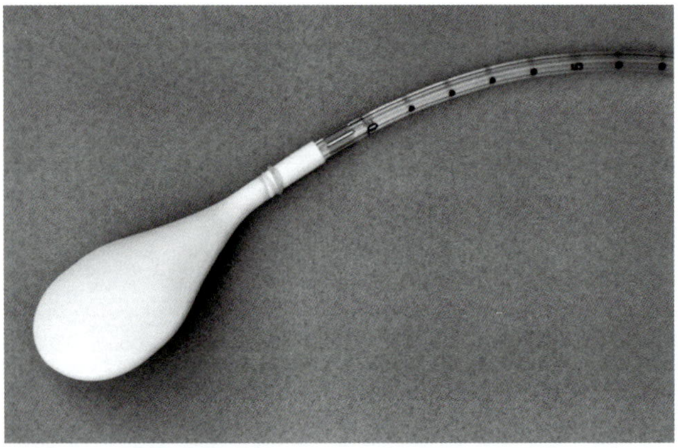

**Fig. 22.9** Anal manometer, a four-channel perfusion catheter with balloon tip. There are many different types of manometers and methods for performing anal manometry. A balloon or probe is inserted into the rectum, and a pressure transducer relays information to a recorder or computer. Important manometric parameters include sphincter length, resting and squeeze pressures, rectal sensation, and presence of the anorectal inhibitory reflex (RAIR). The balloon is placed in the rectum and inflated in 10-$cm^3$ increments to determine rectal sensation and compliance. The presence of the RAIR is determined with balloon inflation and observing the internal anal sphincter relax and the external anal sphincter contract to allow for the sampling of rectal contents. The four radical ports are perfused with sterile water, and resting and squeeze pressures around the anal canal are measured at 1-cm intervals along the anal canal. The catheter can be pulled at a constant rate to determine the length of the sphincter and the high-pressure or continence zone.

motor unit innervating multiple muscle fibers. On single-fiber EMG, the MUAPs will have larger amplitudes, longer duration, and more phases or crossings of the baseline. Despite the benefit of these data, because of the need for specialty training and the discomfort for the woman from the EMG needles, EAUS has essentially replaced EMG for anatomic evaluation of the anal sphincter.

### Pudendal Nerve Terminal Motor Latency

Nerve conduction studies measure the time from stimulation of a nerve to a response in the muscle it innervates. The pudendal nerve terminal motor latency (PNTML) is determined by using a glove-mounted electrode known as a *St. Mark pudendal electrode,* connected to a pulsed stimulus generator; with the examiner's index finger in the vagina or anus, the pudendal nerve is stimulated around the ischial spine.

The latent period between the pudendal nerve stimulation and the electromechanical response of the muscle is measured. Prolonged PNTMLs have been found in women with idiopathic FI and in women with rectal prolapse and at one point were thought to be predictive of continence after surgical repair. These tests are rarely performed now, however, because research shows poor correlation of prolonged pudendal terminal latencies with clinical symptoms, and PNTML does not seem to directly reflect nerve function in the way that quantitative EMG can.

### Defecography

Dynamic cystoproctography, or defecography, is an imaging technique that has been widely used in the evaluation of anorectal function and anatomy. Defecography may be used as an adjunct to physical examination in women with chronic constipation and pelvic floor defects that may be contributing to their FI. Rectal intussusception, rectal prolapse, enterocele, and sigmoidocele can be seen on defecography, along with rectoceles that do not empty at the time of defecation. Stool retained in a rectocele can cause chronic distention of the rectum and loss of rectal sensation. Loss of rectal sensation can lead to chronic constipation or impaction, causing further neuromuscular damage to the pelvic floor and ultimately FI.

Fluoroscopic defecography usually involves the insertion of radiopaque contrast transanally, after which the woman is seated on a special commode and asked to perform a variety of maneuvers including straining, contracting and of course defecating. From the

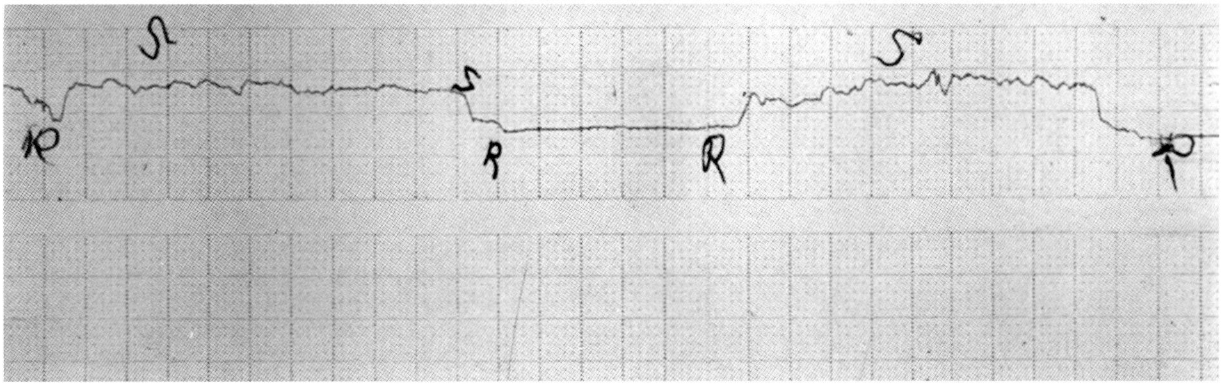


**Fig. 22.11** A single-channel recording of the resting pressure of the anal canal *(R)* and the squeeze pressure *(S)*. The internal anal sphincter contributes 80% of the resting pressure. Voluntary contraction or squeezing of the external anal sphincter should double the resting pressure.

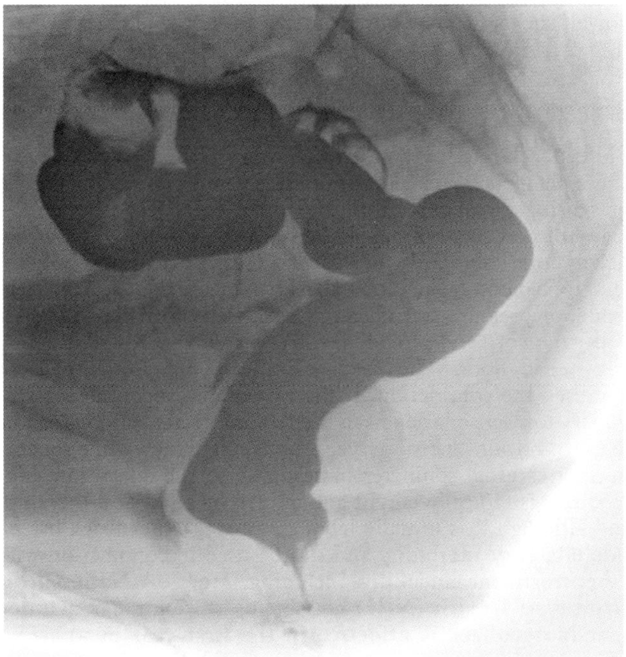

**Fig. 22.12** Cinedefecography. Sagittal pelvic view with moderate anterior rectocele. (From Wolf JH, Weiss EG. *Current Surgical Therapy,* 12th ed. Philadelphia: Elsevier, 2017.)

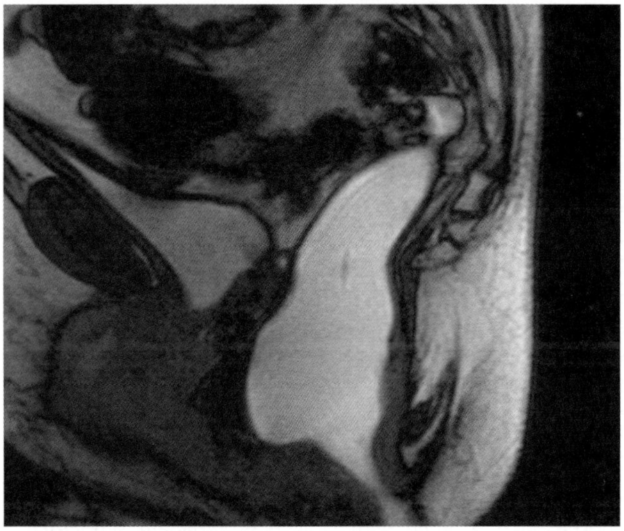

**Fig. 22.13** MRI defecography. Diffusely abnormal descent of the pelvic floor with associated rectocele.

real-time fluoroscopic images obtained, perineal descent and the anorectal angle, among other findings, can be objectively measured (Fig. 22.12). Defecography is user dependent, and there can be significant interobserver differences in the interpretation of these images. Fluoroscopic defecography, however, has begun to be steadily replaced by MRI for the evaluation of the pelvic floor and defecation disorders. **Unlike fluoroscopy, specialized dynamic MRI is capable of evaluating other pelvic anatomy, such as pelvic organ prolapse, as well as muscular defects and perineal descent (Fig. 22.13). Detractors of MRI defecography point out, however, that it is performed in a nonphysiologic supine position.** Although open MRI technology addresses this issue, it is not widely available.

### Transit Study

A colonic transit study is used to evaluate colonic motility, typically for the evaluation of chronic constipation. If fecal impaction or overflow incontinence is high on one's differential, a transit study may also be indicated. For a common approach to this study, a woman ingests a Sitzmark capsule containing 20 or 25 radiopaque rings. She does not take any laxatives or bowel stimulants. On days 1, 3, and 5 after taking the capsule, an abdominal flat-plate radiograph is obtained. Eighty percent of the capsules will have been passed by day 5 in women with normal colonic transit time. Diffuse or global colon dysfunction is indicated if the rings are dispersed throughout the colon, and segmental abnormalities can be seen if the rings are clustered in one area or trapped in a rectocele (Fig. 22.14).

## Treatment

Treatment of FI includes lifestyle changes, dietary management, biofeedback, electrical stimulation, medications, devices, and surgery (Table 22.5); however, treatment of any underlying conditions that may be causing FI, such as medications or surgery for inflammatory bowel disease, abnormal bowel motility or surgery for a neoplasm of the cauda equina, is the first step in management. For women with liquid or watery stools, dietary modifications and medications are first-line therapies. Similarly, for women with constipation there is strong evidence supporting several medication options, including stimulant and osmotic laxatives, intestinal secretagogues, and peripherally restricted

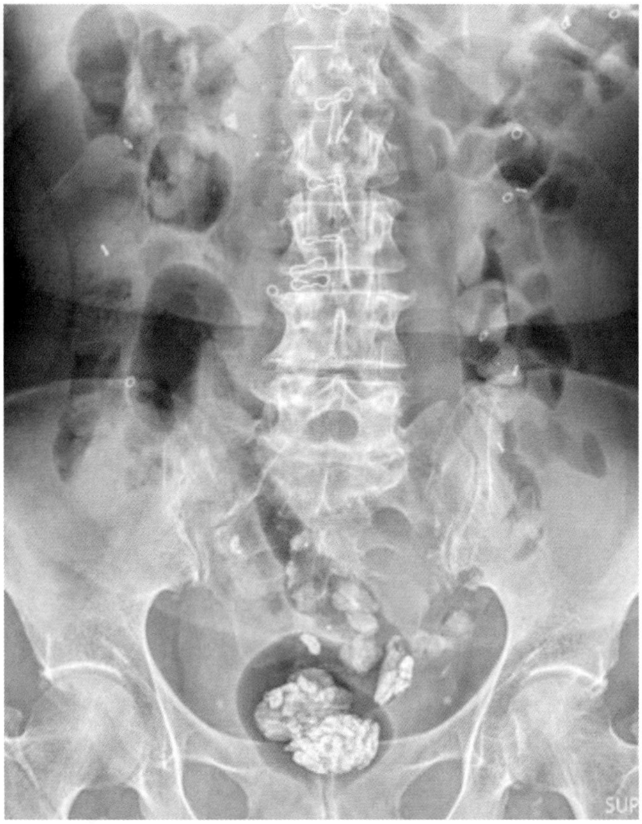

Fig. 22.14 Colonic transit study on day 5. Follow-up radiograph showing retention of markers at 5 days, suggestive of slow-transit constipation. (From Wolf JH, Weiss EG. *Current Surgical Therapy.* 2017.)

mu-opiate antagonists (Table 22.6). Consider a gastroenterology referral when women with constipation remain refractory to medical management, in particular if it is believed to be a principal cause of their FI.

## Education, Diet, Lifestyle Interventions, and Devices

Education regarding good bowel function and a regular bowel evacuation program is sensible for all women. **For those with FI, optimizing normal stool consistency and frequency is essential first-line treatment.** Loose stool or frank diarrhea taxes the system, whereas predictable larger formed stool allows for rectal distention and sensation that may provide earlier warning and better emptying.

Adding dietary fiber through diet changes, bulking agents, or fiber supplements such as methylcellulose or psyllium increases stool size. There is low-strength evidence that psyllium decreases weekly FI frequency by 2.5 occurrences after 1 month of use, although this change did not affect the participants' quality of life (QOL). Eating high-fiber cereals and drinking hot coffee or tea at breakfast can stimulate the gastrocolic reflex, leading to elimination before leaving home. **Evidence suggests that, compared with placebo, adding soluble dietary fiber reduces the rate of FI in women with or without loose stools.** An analysis of nearly 200,000 person-years (60,000 older women) from the Nurses' Health Study found that women in the quintile with an intake of 25 g of fiber per day had an 18% reduction in risk of FI; however, women must be warned that these supplements can worsen diarrhea and cause bloating. In some women, diet contributes to stool consistency problems, and by keeping a food diary, they may identify and eliminate offending foods (e.g., lactose, fructose) that aggravate their FI. A 2019 study researched foods high in fermentable oligo-, di-, and monosaccharides and polyols (FODMAP), because they cause symptoms of diarrhea and urgency. About 64.6% of the 42 patients reported a reduction in their FI symptoms with the low-FODMAP diet. A low-FODMAP diet might be a useful tool to treat patients who suffer from FI as a result of loose stools. Nicotine affects rectosigmoid transit time by stimulating distal colonic motility, contributing to fecal urgency in smokers.

Brisk exercise, particularly after meals, may precipitate FI because of increased colonic activity; however, in a nursing home study, the daily exercise program with education around toileting opportunities improved FI. An additional analysis of 175,000 person-years from the Nurses' Health Study suggested higher levels of physical activity was associated with a modest reduction of incident FI. Obstructive devices, including transanal plugs, have been marketed but are not widely used. A vaginal pessary (detailed later) for bowel control, which uses a balloon that inflates posteriorly to obstruct the bowel, shows promise for women who can tolerate a pessary (Fig. 22.15).

## Biofeedback

Biofeedback requires a motivated woman, the feedback device, and a planned exercise program. It is based on hearing, seeing, or sensing a response from a planned exercise. Although she may not perceive normal sensation or be able to contract her pelvic floor voluntarily, the patient must be neurologically intact to benefit from biofeedback. A measuring device, electrode, or pressure transducer is used transvaginally or transanally to record and provide feedback on how she is contracting her pelvic floor. The feedback allows her to increase or lengthen the contraction. If the woman has incontinence secondary to a sensory deficit in the rectum, rectal balloons can be used to "retrain" her to perceive rectal distention while squeezing her external sphincter in response to the distention. Biofeedback is typically taught and guided by a physical therapist, and although it is initially labor intensive, biofeedback has no side effects or morbidity and can be used in conjunction with other treatment modalities, including surgery. **A National Institutes of Health (NIH) consensus statement concluded that biofeedback is effective in the first year postpartum for reversing some pregnancy-related FI.** The American College of Gastroenterology recommends biofeedback therapy despite imperfect evidence to support its use.

One trial reported approximately 65% of patients with an abnormal pelvic floor and FI had a 90% reduction in incontinence through biofeedback; however, success rates can vary from 38% to 100% in other studies. For example, in a single-center randomized controlled trial, the addition of biofeedback to a regimen of pelvic floor exercises resulted in 44% of patients reporting complete continence at 3 months compared with 21% in patients undergoing pelvic floor exercises alone ($P$ = .008). The largest prospective study compared standard care with biofeedback. The standard group received nine 40- to 60-minute sessions with a nurse specialist on diet, fluid management, bowel evacuation techniques, bowel training, and use of antidiarrheal medications. The biofeedback group experienced 54% improvement compared with 53% in the standard care group. Although this result calls the benefit of biofeedback into question, the key takeaway from this trial was that more than 50% of patients improved with conservative measures. A 2019 study randomly assigned 98 adults with FI to either pelvic floor muscle training and biofeedback plus conservative treatment measures or attention-control treatment plus conservative measures. The pelvic floor muscle training and biofeedback group

**TABLE 22.5** Recommendations for Treatments for Fecal Incontinence From Professional Society Guidelines

| Treatment | American College of Gastroenterology (ACG) | American Society of Colon and Rectal Surgeons (ASCRS) | American College of Obstetrics and Gynecology (ACOG) |
|---|---|---|---|
| **NONSURGICAL** | | | |
| Dietary fiber | Not separately addressed. | Not separately addressed. | Can be recommended as useful treatment for FI (level B). |
| Antidiarrheal drugs | Gastroenterologists and other providers should prescribe antidiarrheal agents for FI in patients with diarrhea (strong recommendation, low quality of evidence). | Not separately addressed. | Can be recommended as useful treatment for FI (level B). |
| Combined: diet, medications, education, etc. | Gastroenterologists and other providers should manage patients with FI using education, dietary modifications, skin care, and pharmacologic agents to modify stool delivery and liquidity before diagnostic testing, particularly when symptoms are mild and not bothersome (strong recommendation, moderate quality of evidence). | Dietary and medical management are recommended as first-line therapy for patients with FI (strong recommendation, low- or very-low-quality evidence). | Based on expert opinion, dietary manipulation and bowel schedules, along with other treatments, should be offered because they may help and have few adverse events (level C). |
| PFMT-BF (any/all comparators) | Not addressed. | Biofeedback should be considered as an initial treatment for patients with incontinence and some preserved voluntary sphincter contraction (strong recommendation, moderate-quality evidence). | PFMT (with or without BF) is recommended because most studies report improvement without adverse events. Insufficient data are available on the most effective treatment protocol (level B). |
| PFMT-BF vs. PFMT alone | Pelvic floor rehabilitative techniques are effective and superior to pelvic floor exercises alone in patients with FI who do not respond to conservative measures (strong recommendation, moderate quality of evidence). | Not separately addressed. | PFMT (with or without BF) is recommended because most studies report improvement without adverse events. Insufficient data are available on the most effective treatment protocol (level B). |
| Bowel management program (enema, suppository) | Not addressed. | Bowel management programs to aid in rectal evacuation are useful in select patients (weak recommendation, low- or very-low-quality evidence). | No recommendation. |
| Injectable anal sphincter tissue bulking agents | Minimally invasive procedures such as injectable anal bulking agents may have a role in treatment of patients with FI who do not respond to conservative therapy (weak recommendation, moderate quality of evidence). | Injection of biocompatible bulking agents into the anal canal may help decrease episodes of passive FI (weak recommendation, moderate-quality evidence). | Can be considered as a short-term option but data only support efficacy to 6 months (level B). |
| Percutaneous tibial nerve stimulation (FDA approved for UI not FI) | Not addressed. | Percutaneous tibial nerve stimulation may be considered because it provides short-term improvement in episodes of fecal incontinence (weak recommendation, low- or very-low-quality evidence). | Should not be offered routinely to patients because of insufficient evidence supporting its use. |
| **SURGICAL** | | | |
| Sacral neurostimulation (SNS) | Sacral nerve stimulation should be considered in patients with FI who do not respond to conservative therapy (strong recommendation, moderate quality of evidence). | Sacral neuromodulation may be considered as a first-line surgical option for incontinent patients with and without sphincter defects (strong recommendation, moderate-quality evidence). | Can be considered for women with or without anal sphincter disruption for whom conservative options have failed (level B). |
| Anal sphincter repair (sphincteroplasty) | Anal sphincteroplasty should be considered in patients with FI who do not respond to conservative therapy and who have an anatomic sphincter defect (weak recommendation, low quality of evidence). | Sphincter repair (sphincteroplasty) may be offered to symptomatic patients with a defined defect of the external anal sphincter. (Strong recommendation, moderate-quality evidence.) | Can be considered for women with anal sphincter disruption who have failed conservative options (level B). |

*Continued*

**TABLE 22.5** Recommendations for Treatments for Fecal Incontinence From Professional Society Guidelines—cont'd

| Treatment | American College of Gastroenterology (ACG) | American Society of Colon and Rectal Surgeons (ASCRS) | American College of Obstetrics and Gynecology (ACOG) |
|---|---|---|---|
| Repeat anal sphincter repair | Not addressed | Repeat anal sphincter reconstruction after a failed overlapping sphincteroplasty should generally be avoided unless other treatment modalities are not possible or have failed (strong recommendation, low- or very-low-quality evidence). | No recommendation. |
| Artificial anal sphincter replacement | Artificial anal sphincter may possibly allow the occasional patient with FI to avoid colostomy (weak recommendation, insufficient evidence). | Implantation of an artificial bowel sphincter remains an effective tool for select patients with severe fecal incontinence (strong recommendation, low- or very-low-quality evidence). | No recommendation. |
| Anatomic defect correction (prolapse, fistula, etc.) | Not addressed. | Obvious anatomic defects such as rectovaginal fistula, rectal or hemorrhoidal prolapse, fistula in ano or cloaca-like deformity should be corrected as part of the treatment of fecal incontinence (strong recommendation, low- or very-low-quality evidence). | Surgical treatment should be considered in advance of conservative options. |
| Radiofrequency anal sphincter remodeling (SECCA) | There is insufficient evidence to recommend radiofrequency ablation treatment to the anal sphincter (SECCA) at this time (no recommendation, insufficient evidence). | Application of temperature-controlled radiofrequency energy to the sphincter complex may be used to treat fecal incontinence (weak recommendation, moderate-quality evidence). | This procedure should not be offered routinely to patients because there are currently no data from high-quality studies to support its use. |
| Non–FDA-approved surgeries | Dynamic graciloplasty may possibly allow the occasional patient with FI to avoid colostomy (weak recommendation, insufficient evidence). | Current data are insufficient to support the use of the magnetic sphincter for fecal incontinence (weak recommendation, low- or very-low-quality evidence). | No recommendation. |
| Colostomy | Colostomy is a last-resort procedure that can markedly improve the quality of life in a patient with severe or intractable FI (strong recommendation, low quality of evidence). | Creation of a colostomy is an excellent surgical option for patients in whom other therapies have failed or who do not wish to pursue other therapies for fecal incontinence (low- or very-low-quality evidence). | No recommendation |

Modified from Wald A, Bharucha AE, Cosman BC, et al. ACG clinical guideline: management of benign anorectal disorders. *Am J Gastroenterol.* 2014;109(8):1141-1157; Paquette IM, Madhulika V, Kaiser AM, et al. The American Society of Colon and Rectal Surgeons' Clinical Practice Guideline for the Treatment of Fecal Incontinence. *Dis Colon Rectum.* 2015;58(7):623-636.; and American College of Obstetricians and Gynecologists' Committee on Practice Bulletins—Gynecology. ACOG Practice Bulletin No. 210: fecal incontinence. *Obstet Gynecol.* 2019;133(4):e260-e273.

*BF,* Biofeedback; *FDA,* Food and Drug Administration; *FI,* fecal incontinence; *PFMT,* pelvic floor muscle training; *UI,* urinary incontinence.

**TABLE 22.6** Medications for the Treatment of Constipation

| Medication | Usual Dose | Comments |
|---|---|---|
| **Bulk-Forming Laxatives** | | |
| Psyllium | Up to 1 tablespoon (≅3.5 g fiber) 3 times per day | Start with low dose and gradually increase<br>May cause fluid overload, gas, and bloating |
| Methylcellulose | Up to 1 tablespoon (≅2 g fiber) or 4 caplets (500 mg fiber per caplet) 3 times per day | |
| Polycarbophil | 2-4 tabs (500 mg fiber per tab) per day | |
| Wheat dextrin | 1-3 caplets (1 g fiber per caplet) or 2 teaspoonsful (1.5 g fiber per teaspoon) up to 3 times per daily | |
| **Stimulant Laxatives** | | |
| Bisacodyl | 5-15 mg tabs 1 time per day or 10 mg suppository per rectum 1 time per day | Suppository preferably administered 30 minutes after breakfast<br>May cause gastric or rectal irritation |
| Senna | 2-4 tabs (8.6 mg sennosides per tab) or 1-2 tabs (15 mg sennosides per tab) as a single daily dose or divided twice daily | Widely used anthraquinone laxative. May cause melanosis coli |
| **Stool Softeners** | | |
| Docusate sodium | 50-360 mg once daily or in divided doses | Use lower dose if taken with another laxative<br>Contact dermatitis reported |
| Docusate calcium | 240 mg 1 time per day | |
| **Osmotic Agents** | | |
| Polyethylene glycol | 8.5-34 g in 240 mL (8 oz) liquids | More data for chronic constipation patients than in IBS patients with constipation<br>May cause nausea, bloating and cramping |
| Glycerin | One suppository (2 or 3 g) per rectum for 15 minutes 1 time per day | May cause rectal irritation |
| Lactulose | 10-20 g (15-30 mL) daily<br>May increase up to 2 times per day | May cause bloating, distension and flatulence |
| Sorbitol | 30-45 mL (as 70% solution) 1 time per day | May cause bloating and flatulence |
| Magnesium sulfate | 2 to 4 level teaspoonsful (≅10-20 g) dissolved in 240 mL (8 oz) water 1 time per day | May cause watery stools and urgency<br>Concern in renal insufficiency because of magnesium toxicity |
| Magnesium citrate | 200 mL (11.6 g) 1 time per day | Magnesium toxicity |
| **Other** | | |
| Prucalopride | 2 mg 1 time per day | Recently approved in the United States |
| Linaclotide | 145 μg 1 time per day | Improves pain, bloating, and global symptoms in patients with IBS<br>May cause diarrhea and bloating |
| Lubiprostone | 24 μg 2 times per day | Improves bloating, discomfort, and constipation severity in opioid-induced constipation<br>May cause nausea and diarrhea |
| Plecanatide | 3 mg 1 time per day | Improves pain, bloating, and global symptoms in patients with IBS<br>May cause diarrhea |

Modified from Wald A. Medications for treatment of constipation. 2019 UpToDate. Additional data from Lexicomp Online; 2019, https://www.uptodate.com/contents/image?imageKey=GAST%2F59746&topicKey=GAST%2F2636&search=constipation&source=outline_link&selectedTitle=1~150; and Bharucha AE, Wald A. Chronic constipation. *Mayo Clin Proc.* 2019;6196(19)30123-30125.

*IBS,* Irritable bowel syndrome.

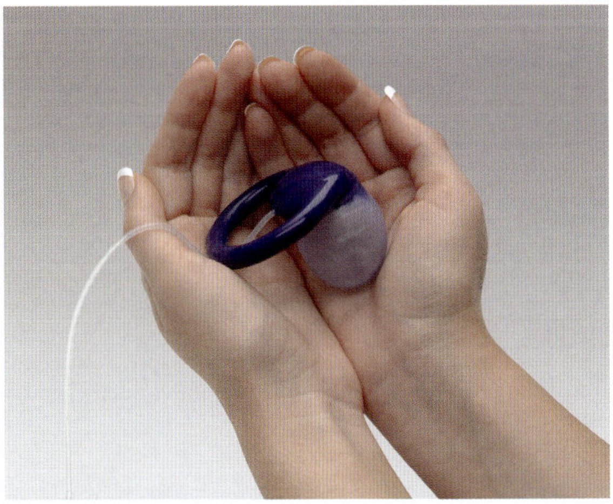

**Fig. 22.15** Pelvalon Eclipse vaginal pessary for fecal incontinence.

had fivefold higher odds of reporting improvements in FI symptoms and, on a validated scale, larger mean reductions of incontinence compared with the attention-control massage treatment. **The American Society of Colon and Rectal Surgeons (ASCRS) Clinical Practice Guidelines recommend that first-line therapy for FI include dietary modifications, medical management with antidiarrheal or fiber supplement (or both) to bulk the stool, and biofeedback exercises for women with mild FI.**

## Electrical Stimulation Therapy

Electrical stimulation therapy has been shown to improve FI in women with a weakened pelvic floor who are unable to voluntarily contract their EAS or puborectalis; however, because of the expense and limited data supporting its benefit, electrical stimulation is generally reserved for women who have failed traditional biofeedback protocols. Most protocols recommend using a transvaginal or transrectal probe, 15 to 20 minutes of maximum tolerable high-frequency stimulation (50 Hz max) twice daily. Response to therapy is usually seen in 6 weeks, with maximum improvement by 12 weeks. A 2010 randomized trial of 158 patients' new stimulation protocols combining biofeedback with electrical stimulation reported a 50% continence rate at 3 months.

### Devices

A vaginal device that is fit like a pessary controls FI through the pressure generated by an inflatable balloon directed toward the rectum. One multicenter study found, if successfully fitted, a success rate at 3 months of 86% and durable efficacy at 6 and 12 months (77.6% and 79.6%, respectively) (Richter, 2020). Success was defined as women who considered their bowel symptoms to be "much better" or "very much better." Of note, 56% of the 110 women enrolled were successfully fit with the device. The primary adverse event was a complaint of pelvic cramping or discomfort in 23%.

### Anal Plugs

Anal plugs are another device available for managing FI. They simply block the involuntary loss of stool. A small study of 31 patients FI over an 11-week median follow-up found that patients used one to three devices per day and 80% of the participants "liked them." At completion 57% of participants wanted to continue this approach for the long term.

### Stem Cells

The use of stem cells for FI has been postulated as a means of providing recovery of sphincter function through regeneration of damaged striated sphincter muscle and allowing reinnervation of newly formed myofibers. In 2018, a randomized, double-blind, placebo-controlled study of 24 patients was conducted. At 6 months, both groups demonstrated reduction in the Cleveland Clinic Incontinence (CCI) score, but at 12 months, the treatment group continued to show improvement in the CCI score, whereas the control arm did not. Further studies are underway, but this is not currently approved by the Food and Drug Administration (FDA) in the United States.

### Percutaneous Tibial Nerve Stimulation

Data support percutaneous tibial nerve stimulation (PTNS) as an effective option for the management of urge urinary incontinence (see Chapter 21) and is hypothesized to help with FI because of the shared sacral segmental innervation for anorectal neuromuscular function. **Although initial trials were promising, a randomized controlled trial of PTNS in 227 patients showed no significant benefit over sham stimulation; 38% of the PTNS group had a greater than 50% reduction in episodes of FI per week compared with 31% in the sham stimulation group.** At this point FI is not an indication for PTNS, but studies are ongoing.

## Medications

No specific medication is approved for FI except for antidiarrheal medications. A Cochrane review concluded that there is limited evidence to guide clinicians in the selection of pharmacologic agents. Because the majority of women with FI have soft to loose stools, a common initial management option is to firm the woman's stools. To slow intestinal transit and allow for increased water absorption, several options (Table 22.7) are available. **Loperamide is an antidiarrheal agent that slows small and large bowel peristalsis, decreasing transit time through the gastrointestinal tract. It appears more effective than diphenoxylate for fecal urgency–related incontinence because it also increases IAS tone and decreases sensitivity of the RAIR.** Loperamide is almost completely metabolized in the liver, resulting in minimal levels entering the systemic circulation. Also, unlike diphenoxylate, it does not cross the blood-brain barrier and therefore has fewer central nervous system (CNS) side effects. Amitriptyline, a tricyclic antidepressant, has also been shown in a small study to significantly improve symptoms of FI, likely by increasing colonic transit time. For women with loose stools after cholecystectomy, cholestyramine, which helps bile acid malabsorption, has proven to be effective. Hyoscyamine, taken before meals, is recommended for women with FI after meals. Some women benefit from a cleansing of the rectum with an enema, which can provide several hours or more of freedom from their incontinence.

**TABLE 22.7** Medications for Treatment of Diarrhea

| Drug | Dosage | Mechanism of Action |
|---|---|---|
| Loperamide | 2 mg tid or 4 mg followed by 2 mg after loose bowel movement<br>Maximum, 16 mg/day | Inhibits circular and longitudinal muscle contraction |
| Diphenoxylate with atropine | 5 mg qid initial dose | Direct action of circular smooth muscle to decrease peristalsis |
| Hyoscyamine sulfate | 0.375 mg bid (extended release) | Anticholinergic |
| Cholestyramine | 4 - 36 g/day in 1 to 4 divided doses. Increase by 4 g at weekly intervals | Binds bile acids after cholecystectomy |

*bid,* Twice a day; *tid,* three times per day; *qid,* four times per day.

## Surgery

A variety of surgical options are available to treat FI; however, if the woman has an anatomic defect that may be contributing to FI, such as full-thickness or hemorrhoidal prolapse, rectal prolapse, or ano- or rectovaginal fistula, these should addressed first. For women with idiopathic FI or those with sphincter injury, options include sacral neuromodulation, anal sphincteroplasty, radiofrequency treatment, injectable bulking materials, anal neosphincter muscular flaps, and artificial sphincters. Postanal repair and posterior levatorplasty have not been shown to be effective in most patients.

### Injectables

Injection of perianal bulking agents for FI has been done with several materials, including silicone, collagen, and carbon-coated microbeads. The objective is to augment the anal canal IAS closing pressure. Graf performed a double-blinded randomized trial of patients for whom conservative measures had failed, assigned participants to either nonanimal stabilized hyaluronic acid/dextranomer gel (NASHA/Dx) ($n = 136$) or sham treatment ($n = 70$). At 6 months, 52% of the treatment group compared with 31% of the sham group reported 50% or greater improvement from baseline in the number of FI episodes ($P = .0089$); however, incontinence scores were not significantly different between the two groups, despite the fact that the patients in the treatment group reported a higher number of incontinence-free days. A 2-year QOL study found that patients who received two injections were more likely to achieve 50% improvement compared with those receiving one injection; however, only patients who achieved at least 75% improvement in symptoms reported a benefit in terms of QOL. A 2013 Cochrane review concluded that although several studies demonstrated short-term benefits, the overall quality of the data is poor and long-term follow-up is still needed. Bulking agents are contraindicated in women with full-thickness rectal prolapse, rectocele, anorectal malformations, active inflammatory bowel disease, and a history of anorectal radiation.

### SECCA Procedure

The SECCA procedure delivers temperature-controlled radiofrequency waves to the anal canal, which denatures collagen and

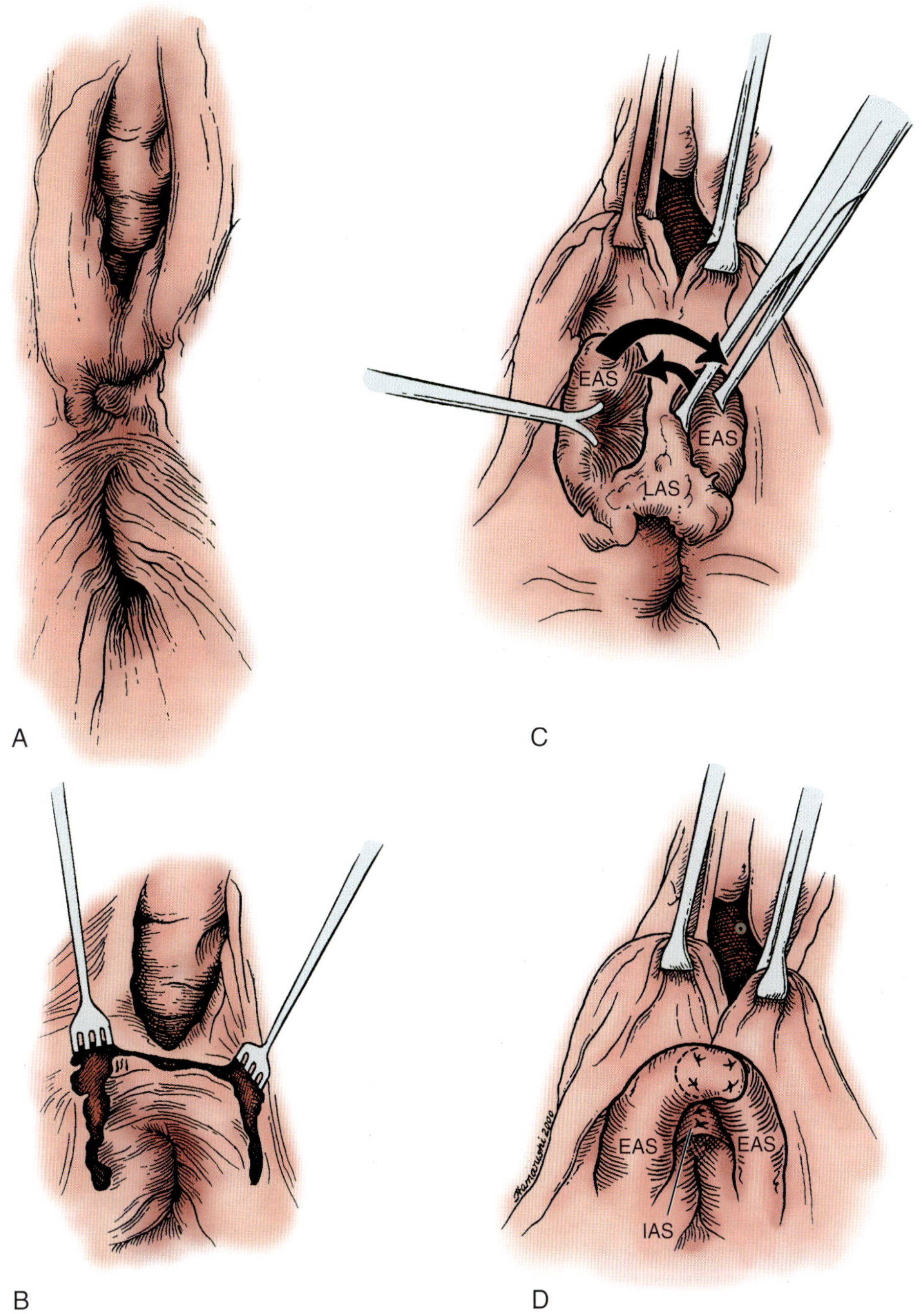


**Fig. 22.16** Sphincter drawing. **A**, Dovetail sign with loss of anal skin creases anteriorly. **B,** Transperineal incision. **C,** external anal sphincter (EAS) identified. **D,** Overlapping sphincteroplasty and internal anal sphincter (IAS) repaired.

changes to tissue compliance to narrow the anal canal. Most studies of SECCA are small, single-institution series with short to at most 1-year follow-up. One small randomized trial with 12-month follow-up showed modest improvement, but most of the series failed to demonstrate a 50% improvement in Cleveland Clinic Florida Fecal Incontinence Scale. Complications, such as pain, bleeding, and ulceration, are rare. The procedure is contraindicated in women previously treated with injection of a bulking agent.

### Anterior Sphincteroplasty

Sphincteroplasty has long been performed for FI in the setting of chronic anal sphincter lacerations, but the long-term results remain disappointing. The literature is conflicting regarding overlapping versus end-to-end sphincteroplasty techniques. The hypothetical advantage of the overlapping sphincteroplasty over the traditional end-to-end repair is decreased tension to prevent separation of the suture line once anesthesia no longer prevents sphincter contraction. Repair of an anal sphincter laceration includes not only repair of the EAS but also identification and repair of any IAS defects. Because the IAS maintains the resting tone of the anus, it is important to restore sphincter integrity, especially for control of flatus (Fig. 22.16).

**In the short term an overlapping sphincteroplasty provides symptomatic control of incontinence in 60% to 80% of**

**patients with anatomic EAS defects. These results are, unfortunately, not durable, and cure rates 5 to 10 years after surgery may be as low as 1% to 28%.** A number of studies have attempted to identify factors associated with sphincteroplasty outcomes, but no single variable has proved predictive. As a result, the use of overlapping sphincteroplasty as the primary surgical treatment for FI in women who develop symptoms years after their initial sphincter injury is discouraged.

When anal sphincter injury occurs during vaginal delivery, the type of repair needed has been debated. To date, according to conflicting small studies with short-term follow-up, there is no significant difference between end-to-end and overlapping anal sphincteroplasties. The outcome of anal sphincteroplasties after delivery is unacceptably poor, with 47% to 67% of women complaining of defecatory symptoms such as flatus incontinence, fecal urgency, and FI. Although frank FI is reported at a much lower rate, 2% to 9%, the other defecatory symptoms are nonetheless bothersome to women. Furthermore, EAUS examinations after sphincteroplasty show persistent anatomic defects in 40% to 85% of repairs. Anal sphincter injury during vaginal childbirth is a common cause of FI; therefore providers should avoid midline episiotomy because it has been shown repeatedly in various studies to be strongly associated with anal sphincter damage. If absolutely necessary, a mediolateral episiotomy has been shown to be less injurious to the sphincter.

## Sacral Nerve Stimulation

The FDA approved sacral nerve stimulation (SNS, also referred to as sacral neuromodulation) for FI in 2011. The stimulation is targeted at the S3 nerve root, and although the mechanism of action is unknown, the data supporting its benefit in this population have been consistent. The procedure is typically outpatient and performed in two steps because of the cost of the generator. If a woman has a 50% or greater improvement in symptoms during the test phase, she is typically approved for implantation of the generator. **A 2008 study randomly assigned participants to maximal medical management, including pelvic floor physical therapy (PT), versus SNS. The group averaged nine episodes of FI per week. By 1 year the medical group remained effectively unchanged, whereas the SNS group was averaging only 3.1 episodes per week. Additionally a majority of the SNS group (20% at baseline vs. 60% at 1 year) had significant improvement in their ability to defer defecation.** A systematic review reported that 79% of patients experienced at least 50% improvement in weekly FI episodes in the short term and 84% in the long term (>36 months) based on a pooled analysis of all current studies in the literature. When these pooled data were analyzed on an intention-to-treat basis, 63% of patients achieved improvement of at least 50% in the short term and 35% reported 100% continence in the long term. A 2019 randomized trial of urinary urge incontinence compared bladder Botox injections versus sacral neuromodulation (Andy, 2019). They reported the FI symptoms prospectively in this trial. Because of the clinically important improvement in FI symptoms with neuromodulation, the authors pointed out women with both urinary and FI may wish to consider neuromodulation in this situation. The challenges associated with SNS include an infection rate of 10.8%, and at 5 years, 24.4% of patients had undergone at least one revision or replacement.

Sacral neuromodulation was initially viewed as a treatment for women who had failed an anterior sphincteroplasty or did not have a sphincter defect. **One study that included 91 women with no sphincter defect and 54 with a complete external sphincter defect confirmed with ultrasound showed that the presence of a sphincter defect did not affect the outcome of sacral neuromodulation.** A later study of 237 participants, some of whom had undergone sphincter repair, found that the state of the sphincter did not influence the results of the SNM test phase. Significant improvements in FI scores have been seen in patients with up to a 120-degree sphincter defect. **Although there have been no randomized controlled trials comparing sacral neuromodulation with overlapping sphincteroplasty, the latest practice parameters of the ASCRS include SNS as a first-line surgical treatment for FI.**

### Neosphincters

Artificial sphincters are indicated for women with anal incontinence caused by neuromuscular disease, congenital malformations, and sphincter defects greater than 180 degrees and women for whom all other treatments have failed. Of the two types of neosphincters, one uses the woman's own skeletal muscle, typically the gracilis, and the other uses an artificial Silastic cuff connected to a fluid reservoir. The gracilis muscle wrap was described by Pickrell and involves mobilization of the entire muscle, wrapping the distal portion around the anus and anchoring it to the contralateral ischial tuberosity. The results of the gracilis muscle wrap have been inconsistent, but the addition of chronic, low-frequency electrical stimulation of the nerve or muscle has been applied to try to convert fatigue-prone type II to fatigue-resistant type I muscle fibers. Once converted, the muscle may then be continuously stimulated, resulting in prolonged closure of the anal canal. A report from the Dynamic Graciloplasty Therapy Study Group about 123 adults treated at 20 institutions found that 63% of patients reported a 50% or greater improvement in incontinent events 1 year after surgery. Another 11% noted some improvement, and 26% reported no improvement or worsened incontinence; 74% of patients experienced an adverse event related to the treatment, however, including one death, and 40% required additional surgery. Despite these frequent complications, most patients reported a significant improvement in QOL.

For the Silastic cuff neosphincters, a fluid reservoir encircles the anal canal to cause closure. The cuff is deflated before defecation. Studies of the silastic neosphincter are small and retrospective; a few prospective studies have shown improvement in symptoms if the device is retained without complication. Of the surgical options for FI, sphincter replacement has the highest number of reported complications, including infection, anorectal ulceration, device migration, pain, device erosion, and mechanical breakdown.

### Stoma Creation

A stoma may be offered if all other acceptable treatments have failed or the woman does not want to pursue other surgical options. **Although this sounds extreme, it can greatly improve the QOL for women with severe FI. One study of patients undergoing stoma for FI reported that 84% would "probably or definitely" have their stoma again, whereas only 7% reported they would "probably or definitely not."**

# RECTOVAGINAL FISTULAS

Although not FI by definition, rectovaginal fistulas (RVFs) are a common enough cause of fecal loss to be addressed under this heading. An RVF is an abnormal connection between the vagina and rectum and is typically caused by a vaginal birth complication. It is estimated that 0.1% of vaginal births will result in an RVF. Whenever a woman presents with complaints of fecal or flatal incontinence, an RVF should be included in the differential diagnosis. Depending on the size and location of the fistula, a woman's symptoms may range from a small amount of flatus passing into her vagina to a complaint of formed stool through the vagina with every bowel movement. The causes of RVF are outlined in Table 22.8 and include traumatic, inflammatory, and neoplastic origins in addition to obstetric injuries.

True RVFs occur more than 3 cm above the anal verge, whereas a fistula occurring caudad or adjacent to the EAS is termed an *anovaginal fistula* and is managed differently from an

**TABLE 22.8** Origin of Rectovaginal Fistula

| Category | Condition | Mechanism |
|---|---|---|
| **TRAUMATIC** | | |
| Obstetric | Prolonged second stage of labor<br>Midline episiotomy<br>Perineal lacerations<br>Perineal lacerations | Pressure necrosis of rectovaginal septum<br>Extension directed into rectum |
| Foreign body | Vaginal pessaries<br>Violent coitus<br>Sexual abuse | Pressure necrosis<br>Mechanical perforation<br>Mechanical perforation |
| Iatrogenic | Hysterectomy<br>Stapled colorectal anastomosis<br>Transanal excision of anterior rectal tumor<br>Enemas<br>Anorectal (e.g., incision and drainage of intramural abscesses) | Injury to anterior rectal wall<br>Staple line includes vagina<br>Deep margin of resection into vagina<br>Mechanical perforation<br>Mechanical perforation |
| Inflammatory | Crohn disease<br>Pelvic radiation<br>Pelvic abscess<br>Perirectal abscess | Transmural inflammation-perforation<br>Early tumor necrosis<br>Late transmural inflammation<br>Late transmural inflammation |
| Neoplastic | Rectal<br>Cervical<br>Uterine<br>Vaginal<br>Primary or recurrent tumors | Local tumor growth into neighboring structure |

From Stenchever MA, Benson JT, eds. *Atlas of Clinical Gynecology.* New York: McGraw-Hill; 2000.

RVF. Most RVFs secondary to obstetric injury occur in the lower third of the vagina and may be associated with a sphincter defect in the EAS. It is important to evaluate the EAS (discussed earlier) with transanal ultrasound or EMG to map any defects before surgical treatment.

Fistulas secondary to surgical trauma, malignancy, or an inflammatory process may occur at any point along the vaginal wall and may involve multiple tracts, so it is important to check for more than one fistula before repair. If the woman has a history of malignancy, examination with biopsy specimens should be performed to rule out cancer as the cause of the fistula. Rectal bleeding is more likely to be reported with a neoplastic process or after pelvic radiation.

If there is suspicion of inflammatory bowel disease, a colonoscopy is warranted. Perineal skin and rectal examinations are important to determine the integrity of the anal sphincters and quality of the tissues surrounding the fistula, as well as to palpate for abscesses and other masses. An office anoscopy or proctoscopy may also help evaluate the surrounding tissues. Most obstetric-related RVFs will be found along the scar line. If the RVF tract cannot be identified on examination, methylene blue mixed in lubricant and placed in the rectum or a dilute methylene blue enema with a tampon in the vagina may help isolate the fistula. If the vaginal orifice is found but not the rectal opening, insertion of an angiocatheter with a squirt of hydrogen peroxide can show bubbling on the rectal side, or a small lacrimal duct probe may allow passage through the vaginal tract to identify the rectal exit site.

In general, a mature epithelialized fistula that is not infected will not be painful on digital examination. If the office examination is not successful in locating the fistula or is too painful for the woman, she should be taken to the operating room (OR) for examination under anesthesia. In the OR one can fill the vagina with water and insufflate the rectum to produce bubbling in the vagina that can be traced to the fistula opening. For high fistulas, a barium enema or vaginography using dilute barium solution may be helpful.

Surgical management of an anovaginal or anoperineal fistula is accomplished by opening the fistula tract, curetting the tract, and leaving the tract open to heal secondarily. Excision of the tract and primary closure will result in recurrent fistula formation in most cases.

Many surgical procedures have been described for the treatment of a true RVF. Because the tissue must be healthy, well vascularized, and most importantly free of infection, women may need to wait up to 3 months or more after the original trauma, surgery, or infection for complete healing. If there is significant fecal contamination, prior radiation, or persistent abscess, a diverting colostomy should be considered in advance. Preoperatively the woman should have a complete mechanical bowel preparation starting several days before the surgery to prevent liquid stool from contaminating the field. Some surgeons place the woman on a liquid diet several days before surgery with no mechanical bowel preparation except enemas until clear the night before surgery. The goal is to have no liquid stool in the rectum and to have the woman's first postoperative bowel movement, several days after surgery, be soft but formed. Antibiotic bowel prophylaxis is warranted.

Other surgical principles include excision of the entire fistulous tract, wide mobilization of the rectal tissue, broad tissue-to-tissue closure without tension, and possible use of a Martius flap. The rectal side is the high-pressure side and requires attention to repair. The vaginal side may be closed or left open to drain, if indicated, and should close spontaneously. Monofilament delayed absorbable suture such as Maxon (monofilament polyglyconate) or PDS (polydioxanone) may lower the risk of infection over a braided suture, but permanent sutures should not be used.

Transvaginal, transperineal (Wiskind, 1992), and transrectal repairs have been described, but gynecologists generally prefer the transvaginal approach. Transrectal repairs, preferred by many colorectal surgeons, generally involve the development of rectal mucosal flaps that are mobilized and brought down or lateral to cover the excised fistula site. In 23 patients treated at the Cleveland Clinic with rectal advancement flaps, fistulas were successfully cured in 77% of patients with obstetric or surgical injury and 60% of patients with Crohn disease.

Postoperatively the woman's diet and medications should be managed to keep her bowel movements soft but formed. Classically a clear liquid diet is continued for the first 3 days after surgery, followed by a low-residue diet. Broad-spectrum antibiotics should be continued for 2 weeks. Sitz baths, two or three times daily, followed by the use of a blow dryer or heat lamp to keep the area clean and dry, are recommended.

## REFERENCES


ACOG Practice Bulletin No. 210: Fecal Incontinence. *Obstet Gynecol.* 2019;133(4):e260–e273.

Andy UU, Amundsen CL, Honeycutt E, et al. Sacral Neuromodulation versus OnabotulinumtoxinA for refractory urgency urinary incontinence: impact on fecal incontinence symptoms and sexual function. *Am J Obstet Gynecol.* 2019;221(5):513.e1–513.e15.

Baeten CG, Bailey HR, Bakka A, et al. Safety and efficacy of dynamic graciloplasty for fecal incontinence: report of a prospective, multicenter trial. Dynamic Graciloplasty Therapy Study Group. *Dis Colon Rectum.* 2000;43:743–751.

Bharucha AE, Wald A. Chronic constipation. *Mayo Clin Proc.* 2019;94(11): 2340–2357.

Blomquist JL, Muñoz A, Carroll M, Handa VL. Association of delivery mode with pelvic floor disorders after childbirth. *JAMA.* 2018;320(23):2438–2447.

Brouwer R, Duthie G. Sacral nerve neuomodulation is effective treatment for fecal incontinence in the presence of a sphincter defect, pudendal neuropathy, or previous sphincter repair. *Dis Colon Rectum.* 2010;53:273–278.
Brown SR, Wadhawan H, Nelson RL. Surgery for faecal incontinence in adults. *Cochrane Database Syst Rev.* 2013;(7):CD001757.
De Ligny WR, Kerkhof MH, Ruiz-Zapata AM. Regenerative medicine as a therapeutic option for fecal incontinence: a systematic review of preclinical and clinical studies. *AJOG.* 2019;220(2):142–154.e2.
Deutekom M, Dobben A. Plugs for containing faecal incontinence. *Cochrane Database Syst Rev.* 2015;(3):CD005086.
Forte ML, Andrade KE, Butler M, et al. *Treatments for Fecal Incontinence. Comparative Effectiveness Review No. 165.* (Prepared by the Minnesota Evidence-based Practice Center under Contract No. 290-2012-00016-I.) AHRQ Publication No. 15(16)-EHC037-EF.
Frascio M, Mandolfino F, Imperatore M, et al. The SECCA procedure for faecal incontinence: a review. *Colorectal Dis.* 2014;16:167–172.
Freeman A, Menees S. Fecal incontinence and pelvic floor dysfunction in women: a review. *Gastroenterol Clin North Am.* 2016;45(2):217–237.
Gilliland R, Altomare DF, Moreira Jr H, et al. Pudendal neuropathy is predictive of failure following anterior overlapping sphincteroplasty. *Dis Colon Rectum.* 1998;41:1516–1522.
Graf W, Mellgren A, Matzel KE, et al. Efficacy of dextramomer in stabilised hyaluronic acid for treatment of faecal incontinence: a randomised, sham-controlled trial. *Lancet.* 2011;377:997–1003.
Hay-Smith J, Mørkved S, Fairbrother KA, et al. Pelvic floor muscle training for prevention and treatment of urinary and faecal incontinence in antenatal and postnatal women. *Cochrane Database Syst Rev.* 2015;(4): CD007471.
Heilbrun ME, Nygaard IE, Lockhart ME, et al. Correlation between levator ani muscle injuries on magnetic resonance imaging and fecal incontinence, pelvic organ prolapse, and urinary incontinence in primiparous women. *Am J Obstet Gynecol.* 2010;202(5):488.e1–e6.
Inadomi JM. Screening for colorectal neoplasia. *N Engl J Med.* 2017; 376(16):1599-1600.
Jangö H, Langhoff-Roos J, Rosthøj S, Saske A. Long-term anal incontinence after obstetric anal sphincter injury-does grade of tear matter? *Am J Obstet Gynecol.* 2018;218(2):232.e1–e232.
Jelovsek JE, Markland AD, Whitehead WE, et al. Controlling faecal incontinence in women by performing anal exercises with biofeedback or loperamide: a randomised clinical trial. *Lancet Gastroenterol Hepatol.* 2019;4(9):698–710.
Jorge JM, Wexner SD. Etiology and management of fecal incontinence. *Dis Colon Rectum.* 1993;36:77–97.
Kirss Jr J, Pinta T, Rautio T, et al. Impact of sphincter lesions and delayed sphincter repair on sacral neuromodulation treatment outcomes for faecal incontinence: results from a Finnish national cohort study. *Int J Colorectal Dis.* 2018;33(12):1709–1714.
Knowles CH, Horrocks E, Bremner SA, et al. Percutaneous tibial nerve stimulation versus sham electrical stimulation for the treatment of faecal incontinence in adults (CONFIDeNT): a double-blind, multicentre, pragmatic, parallel-group, randomised controlled trial. *Lancet.* 2015;386(10004):1640–1648.
Larsson C, Hedberg CL, Lundgren E, Söderström L, Tunón K, Nordin P. Anal incontinence after caesarean and vaginal delivery in Sweden: a national population-based study. *Lancet.* 2019;393(10177):1233–1239.
Menees SB, Chandhrasekhar D, Liew EL, Chey WD. A low FODMAP diet may reduce symptoms in patients with fecal incontinence. *Clin Transl Gastroenterol.* 2019;10(7):e00060.
Meriwether KV, Lockhart ME, Meyer I, Richter HE. Anal sphincter anatomy prepregnancy to postdelivery among the same primiparous women on dynamic magnetic resonance imaging. *Female Pelvic Med Reconstr Surg.* 2019;25(1):8–14.
Norton C, Chelvanayagam S, Wilson-Barnett J, et al. Randomized controlled trial of biofeedback for fecal incontinence. *Gastrenterology.* 2003;125:1320–1329.
Paquette IM, Varma MG, Kaiser AM, et al. The American Society of Colon and Rectal Surgeons' clinical practice guideline for the treatment of fecal incontinence. *Dis Colon Rectum.* 2015;58:623–636.
Richter HE, Dunivan G, Brown HW, et al. A 12-month clinical durability of effectiveness and safety evaluation of a vaginal bowel control system for the nonsurgical treatment of fecal incontinence. *Female Pelvic Med Reconstr Surg.* 2019;25(2):113–119.
Schei B, Johannessen HH, Rydning A, Sultan A, Mørkved S. Anal incontinence after vaginal delivery or cesarean section. *Acta Obstet Gynecol Scand.* 2019;98(1):51–60.
Staller K, Song M, Grodstein F, et al. Physical activity, BMI, and risk of fecal incontinence in the nurses' health study. *Clin Transl Gastroenterol.* 2018;9(10):200.
Sultan AH, Kamm MA, Hudson CN, et al. Anal-sphincter disruption during vaginal delivery. *N Engl J Med.* 1993;329:1905–1911.
Thin NN, Horrocks EJ, Hotouras A, et al. Systematic review of the clinical effectiveness of neuromodulation in the treatment of faecal incontinence. *Br J Surg.* 2013;100:1430–1447.
Tjandra JJ, Chan MK, Yeh CH, et al. Sacral nerve stimulation is more effective than optimal medical therapy for severe fecal incontinence: a randomized, controlled study. *Dis Colon Rectum.* 2008;51:494–502.
Ussing A, Dahn I, Due U, Sørensen M, Petersen J, Bandholm T. Efficacy of supervised pelvic floor muscle training and biofeedback vs attention-control treatment in adults with fecal incontinence. *Clin Gastroenterol Hepatol.* 2019;17(11):2253–2261.
Wong MT, Meurette G, Wyart V, et al. The artificial bowel sphincter: a single institution experience over a decade. *Ann Surg.* 2011;254:951–956.

**Suggested readings for this chapter can be found on ExpertConsult.com.**

# 23 Genital Tract Infections

## Vulva, Vagina, Cervix, Toxic Shock Syndrome, Endometritis, and Salpingitis

*Linda O. Eckert, Gretchen M. Lentz*

23

### KEY POINTS

- The Centers for Disease Control and Prevention regularly revises its treatment protocols for sexually transmitted infections (STIs). This information may be accessed online at www.cdc.gov/publications.
- Pediculosis pubis, an infestation by the crab louse *Phthirus pubis,* is characterized by constant itching, predominantly vulvar involvement, and the finding of eggs and lice by visual inspection. It may be treated by topical application of 1% permethrin cream rinse (Nix) or 1% lindane shampoo (Kwell).
- Scabies, an infection by the itch mite *Sarcoptes scabiei,* is characterized by intermittent pruritus, most commonly in the hands, wrists, breasts, vulva, and buttocks. It may be treated by a topical application of 5% permethrin cream or 1% lindane lotion or 30 g of cream.
- Genital herpes is a recurrent incurable STI. Approximately 80% of individuals are unaware that they are infected. It is usually transmitted by individuals who are asymptomatic and unaware that they have the infection at the time of transmission.
- Nonspecific tests for syphilis, the VDRL and rapid plasma reagin, have a 1% false-positive rate; therefore specific tests such as the *Treponema pallidum* immobilization, fluorescent-labeled *Treponema* antibody absorption, and microhemagglutination assay for antibodies to *T. pallidum* must be used when a positive nonspecific test result is encountered.
- In women in the reproductive age range, bacterial vaginosis represents approximately 50% of vaginitis cases and *Candida* and *Trichomonas* infections represent approximately 25% each. HIV acquisition is increased in women with bacterial vaginosis and *Trichomonas vaginalis* infection.
- *T. vaginalis* is a highly contagious STI. It is the most prevalent nonviral, nonchlamydial STI in women. An asymptomatic female patient in whom *Trichomonas* has been identified in the lower female genital urinary tract should definitely be treated.
- Symptoms that suggest cervical infection include vaginal discharge, deep dyspareunia, and postcoital bleeding. Most women who have lower reproductive tract infections caused by *Chlamydia trachomatis* or *Neisseria gonorrhoeae* do not have mucopurulent cervicitis. The corollary is that most women who have mucopurulent cervicitis are not infected by *C. trachomatis* or *N. gonorrhoeae.*
- Acute pelvic inflammatory disease (PID) is usually caused by a polymicrobial infection of organisms ascending from the vagina and cervix, traveling along the mucosa of the endometrium to infect the mucosa of the oviduct. It should be diagnosed with a minimum of suspicion and treated with broad-spectrum antibiotics with the knowledge that overtreatment is preferable to missed diagnosis.
- Approximately one in four women with acute PID experiences further medical sequelae, including recurrent acute PID, ectopic pregnancy, and chronic pelvic pain.

For clarity of presentation, discussion of infectious diseases of the female genital tract is divided into those of the lower genital tract, the vulva, vagina, and cervix, and those of the upper genital tract, the endometrium and fallopian tubes; however, the female genital tract has anatomic and physiologic continuity. One must keep in mind that infectious agents that colonize and involve one organ often infect adjacent organs to understand the pathophysiology and natural history of infectious diseases of the genital tract.

The symptoms caused by infections of the lower genital tract produce the most common conditions seen by gynecologists. Therefore the initial focus of this chapter is on clinical presentation and the differential diagnosis of vulvitis, vaginitis, and cervicitis.

Toxic shock syndrome (TSS) and syphilis are also discussed in this chapter. Although the most devastating pathologic processes from these diseases occur in sites other than the genital tract, they often obtain entry into the body through the vulvar, rectal, vaginal, or cervical epithelium.

Many of the infections discussed in this chapter may be acquired through sexual contact and are termed *sexually transmitted infections* (STIs). STIs often coexist—for example, *Chlamydia trachomatis* and *Neisseria gonorrhoeae.* When one disease is suspected, appropriate diagnostic methods must be used to detect other infections.

> The Centers for Disease Control and Prevention (CDC) regularly revises management protocols for infections of the female genital tract. Recommendations and medications in this edition are based on the 2015 CDC guidelines. Readers are urged to consult updates in the online CDC guidelines (http://www.cdc.gov) because bacterial sensitivities and epidemiologic concerns may lead to changes in treatment protocols.

## INFECTIONS OF THE VULVA

Similar to skin elsewhere on the body, the vulvar area is subject to primary and secondary bacterial, viral, parasitic, or fungal infections and is sensitive to hormonal and allergic influences. The skin of the vulva is composed of a stratified squamous epithelium containing hair follicles and sebaceous, sweat, and apocrine glands. The subcutaneous tissue of the vulva also contains specialized structures such as the Bartholin glands. **Vulvar pruritus accounts for approximately 10% of outpatient gynecology visits.** Pruritis may be infectious or have other causes.

- Short-duration vulvar pruritis: causes include infection or contact dermatitis.

- Long-duration vulvar pruritis: causes infection or contact dermatitis and vulvar dystrophies such as lichen sclerosis, lichen planus, lichen simplex chronicus, and psoriasis.

## Infections of Bartholin Glands

Mucinous secretions from Bartholin glands provide moisture for the epithelium of the vestibule and open the vagina at 5 and 7 o'clock, in the groove between the hymen and the labia minora. Because they drain via narrow ducts approximately 2 cm long, approximately **2% of adult women develop enlargements of one or both glands. The most common cause is cystic dilation of the Bartholin duct typically caused by distal obstruction secondary to nonspecific inflammation or trauma with subsequent continued glandular fluid secretion resulting in the cystic dilation.**

Most women with Bartholin duct cysts are asymptomatic. The cysts vary in size and can be up to 8 cm in diameter; they are usually unilocular, unilateral, tense, and nonpainful. In chronic or recurrent cysts there occasionally are multiple compartments.

**In contrast, an abscess of a Bartholin gland (Fig. 23.1) tends to develop rapidly over 2 to 4 days with significant acute pain and tenderness with signs of a classic abscess**: erythema, acute tenderness, edema, and, occasionally, cellulitis of the surrounding subcutaneous tissue. Without therapy, most abscesses tend to rupture spontaneously by the third or fourth day. **Bartholin gland abscesses are often polymicrobial, reflecting the normal flora of the vagina, and rarely are caused by an STI.**

Treatment depends on symptoms. Asymptomatic cysts in women younger than 40 years do not need treatment. Simple incision and drainage often leads to recurrence; hence, marsupialization to develop a fistulous tract from the dilated duct to the vestibule is the surgical treatment of choice, with a 5% to 10% recurrence rate. An alternative surgical approach is to insert a Word catheter, a short catheter with an inflatable Foley balloon, through a stab incision into the abscess and leave it in place for 4 to 6 weeks (Fig. 23.2), enabling a tract of epithelium to form. All the procedures mentioned may be performed with local anesthesia. Antibiotics are not necessary unless there is an associated cellulitis surrounding the Bartholin gland abscess.

Excision of a Bartholin duct and gland is indicated for persistent deep infection, multiple recurrences of abscesses, or recurrent enlargement of the gland in women older than 40 years. Excision requires regional block or general anesthesia and can be challenging because of the rich vascular supply to the region and risk for intraoperative hemorrhage, hematoma formation, fenestration of the labia, postoperative scarring, and associated dyspareunia. Excision of a Bartholin gland for recurrent infection should be performed when the infection is quiescent. Bartholin's gland carcinoma is exceedingly rare; hence, routine recommendation for excision in women older than 40 with persistent enlargement may not be merited. Drainage and biopsy may be sufficient.

The differential diagnosis of vulvar cysts includes mesonephric cysts of the vagina (generally more anterior and cephalad in the vagina) and epithelial inclusion cysts (more superficial). Rarely, a lipoma, fibroma, hernia, vulvar varicosity, or hydrocele may be confused with a Bartholin duct cyst.

## Pediculosis Pubis and Scabies

Vulvar pruritis may be caused by animal parasites, the two most common being the crab louse and the itch mite. Ideally, early diagnosis and treatment are of the utmost importance in controlling parasitic infection.

Pediculosis pubis is an infestation by the crab louse, *Phthirus pubis*, which is a different species from the body or head louse. **Lice in the pubic hair are the most contagious of all STIs, with more than 90% of sexual partners becoming infected after a single exposure,** and although usually transmitted by close contact, nonsexual transmission of pubic lice via towels or bedding has been documented. *P. pubis* is generally confined to the hairy areas of the vulva. The incubation period for pediculosis is approximately 30 days.

The predominant clinical symptom is constant pubic pruritus caused by allergic sensitization. Initial sensitization typically takes several weeks to develop but may occur as rapidly as 5 days after initial infection. After a reinfection, pruritus may occur within 24 hours. Examination of the vulvar area without magnification demonstrates eggs and adult lice and pepper grain feces adjacent to the hair shafts (Fig. 23.3). The vulvar skin may become secondarily irritated or infected by constant scratching. For definitive diagnosis, one can make a microscopic slide by scratching the skin papule with a needle and placing the crust under a drop of mineral oil. The louse's body looks like that of a miniature crab, with six legs that have claws on them (Fig. 23.4).

**Scabies is a parasitic infection of the itch mite, *Sarcoptes scabiei*, also transmitted by close contact. Scabies is widespread over the body, without a predilection for hairy areas.** Unlike the crab louse, an itch mite travels rapidly over skin and may move up to 2.5 cm in 1 minute. Mites are able to survive for only a few hours away from the warmth of skin.

The predominant clinical symptom of scabies is severe but intermittent itching. Generally, more intense pruritus occurs at night. Initial symptoms usually present approximately 3 weeks after primary infestation. Scabies may present as papules, vesicles, with the pathognomonic sign of scabies the burrow in the. Although any area of the skin may be infected, the hands, wrists, breasts, vulva, and buttocks are the most common (Fig. 23.5). A handheld magnifying lens is helpful for examining suspicious areas. Microscopic slides may be made using mineral oil and a scratch technique Mites lack lateral claw legs but have two anterior triangular hairy buds. Scabies has been termed the *great dermatologic imitator*, and the differential diagnosis includes almost all dermatologic diseases that cause pruritus. The treatment of pediculosis pubis or scabies involves an agent that kills both the adult parasite and the eggs.

**Treatment for pediculosis pubis and scabies can change, so consult the CDC treatment guidelines for updates.** The therapy recommended by the CDC's 2015 guidelines for pediculosis pubis involves the use of permethrin 1% cream rinse, applied to affected areas and washed off after 10 minutes, or pyrethrins, with piperonyl butoxide applied to the affected area and washed off after 10 minutes. None of these should be applied to the eyelids. Retreatment may be necessary if lice are found or if eggs are observed at the hair-skin junction. Patients with pediculosis pubis should be evaluated for other STIs and evaluated after 1 week if symptoms persist. Those who do not respond to one of the recommended regimens should be retreated with an alternative regimen.

To treat scabies, the CDC recommends permethrin 5% cream applied to all areas of the body from the neck down and washed off after 8 to 14 hours or ivermectin, 200 μg/kg orally, repeated in 2 weeks, if necessary. Alternative regimens include lindane 1%, 1 oz of lotion or 30 g of cream applied thinly to all areas of the body from the neck down and thoroughly washed off after 8 hours. Resistance to lindane has been reported in some parts of the United States. Lindane is not recommended as first-line therapy because of toxicity. It should only be used as an alternative if the woman cannot tolerate other therapies or if they have failed. Lindane should not be used immediately after a bath or shower and should not be used by persons who have extensive dermatitis, women who are pregnant or lactating, or children younger than 2 years. Patients with scabies have intense pruritus that may persist for many days after effective therapy. An antihistamine will help alleviate this symptom. Similar to pediculosis pubis, women should be examined 1 week after initial therapy and retreated with an alternative regimen if live mites are observed.

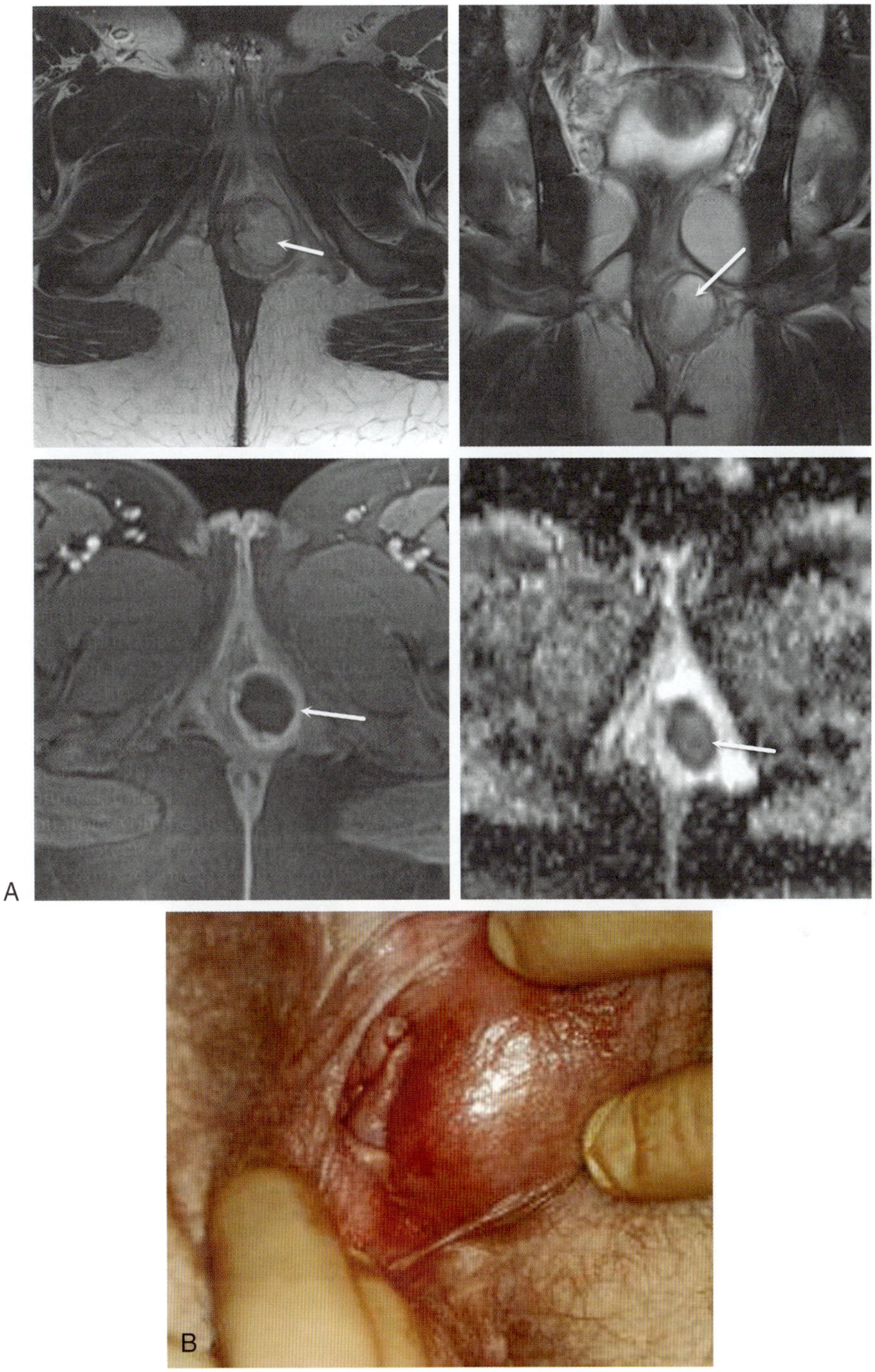


**Fig. 23.1** Bartholin Gland Abscess (From Fowler GC. *Pfenninger and Fowler's Procedures for Primary Care.* 4th ed. Philadelphia: Elsevier; 2020.)

To avoid reinfection by pediculosis pubis or scabies, treatment should be prescribed for sexual contacts within the previous 6 weeks and other close household contacts. Those with close physical contact should be treated at the same time as the infected woman, regardless of whether they have symptoms. Bedding and clothing should be decontaminated (i.e., machine washed, machine dried using the heat cycle, or dry cleaned) or removed from body contact for at least 72 hours. Fumigation of living areas is not necessary. **Importantly, women and physicians should not confuse the 1% cream rinse of permethrin dosage recommended for pubic lice with the 5% permethrin cream recommended for scabies.**

## Molluscum Contagiosum

Molluscum contagiosum is a poxvirus spread by direct skin-to-skin contact resulting in flesh-colored, dome-shaped papules with an umbilicated center. Lesions can be spread by autoinoculation, during contact sports, or by fomites on bath sponges or towels. The incubation period is 2 to 7 weeks. In adults it is primarily an

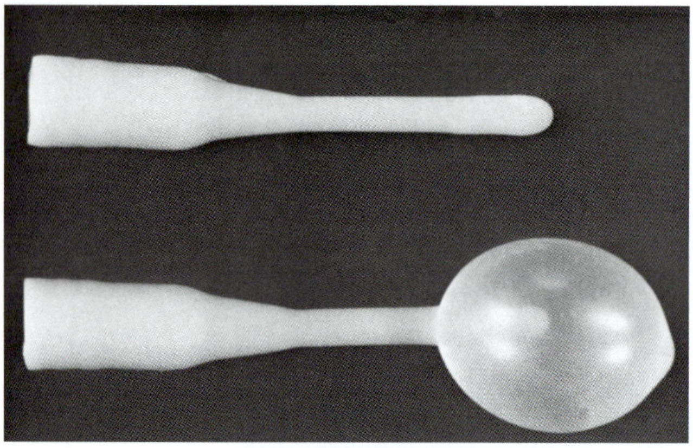

**Fig. 23.2** Word catheters before and after inflation. They are used to develop a fistula from a Bartholin cyst or abscess to the vestibule. (From Friedrich EG. *Vulvar Disease.* 2nd ed. Philadelphia: WB Saunders; 1983.)

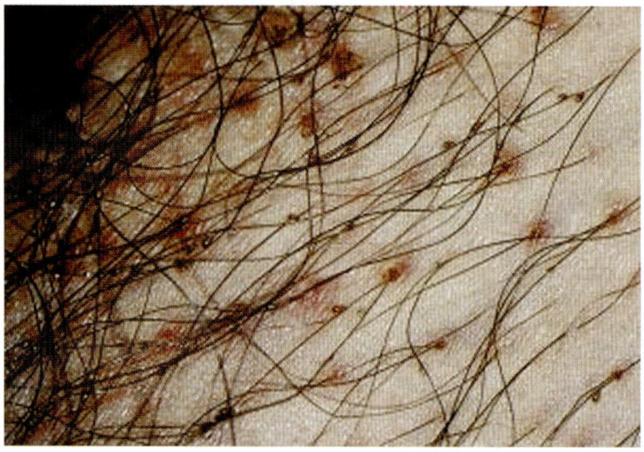

**Fig. 23.3** Crab lice of pediculosis pubis. (Adapted from Ko CJ, Elston DM: Pediculosis. J Am Acad Dermatol. 50:1-12, 2004.)

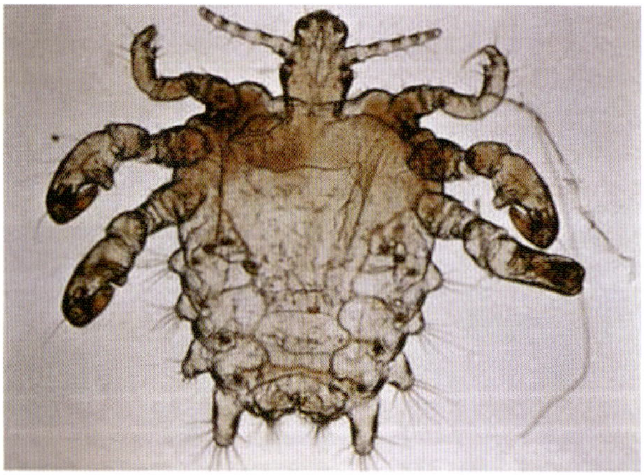

**Fig. 23.4** Public louse. (From Centers for Disease Control and Prevention [CDC], Atlanta, GA. CDC Public Health Image Library, image 4077.)

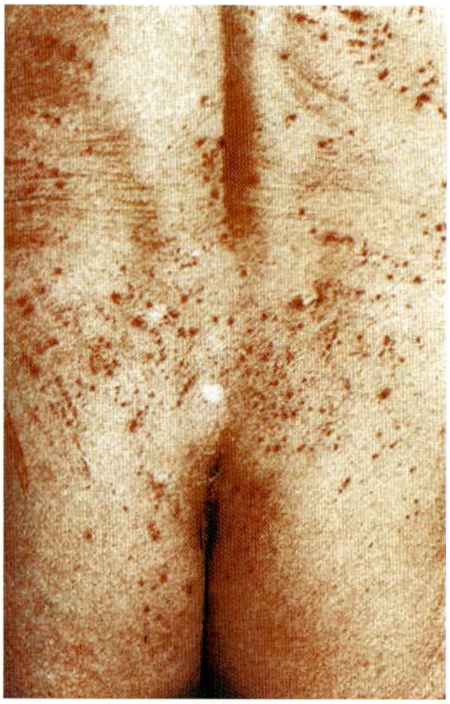

**Fig. 23.5** Scabies.

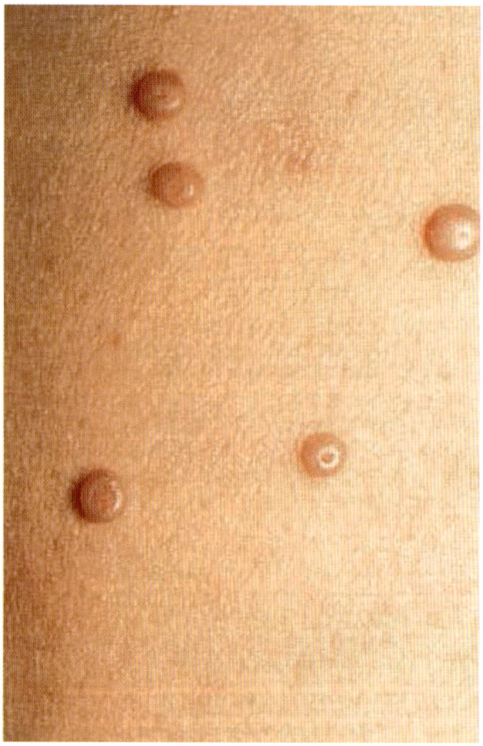

**Fig. 23.6** Molluscum contagiosum. (From Nodules and tumors. In: Cohen BA, ed. *Pediatric Dermatology.* Philadelphia: Saunders; 2013.)

asymptomatic disease of the vulvar skin, and, unlike most STIs, it is only mildly contagious. Widespread infection in adults is most closely related to underlying cellular immunodeficiency, such as in human immunodeficiency virus (HIV) infection. It can also occur in the setting of chemotherapy or corticosteroid administration.

Diagnosis is made by the characteristic appearance of the lesions: The small nodules or domed papules of molluscum contagiosum are usually 1 to 5 mm in diameter (Fig. 23.6). Close inspection reveals that many of the more mature nodules have an umbilicated center. The major complication of molluscum contagiosum is bacterial superinfection. The umbilicated papules may resemble furuncles when secondarily infected.

**Molluscum contagiosum is usually a self-limiting infection and spontaneously resolves after a few months** in immunocompetent individuals; however, treatment of individual papules will decrease sexual transmission and autoinoculation of the virus. After injection of local anesthesia, the caseous material is evacuated and the nodule excised with a sharp dermal curette. The base of the papule is chemically treated with ferric subsulfate (Monsel solution) or 85% trichloroacetic acid. Alternative methods are cantharidin, a chemical blistering agent; imiquimod; or cryotherapy.

In immunocompromised individuals, treatment is more difficult. In women with HIV, there have been multiple reports of recalcitrant molluscum lesions resolving only after initiating highly active antiretroviral therapy (HAART).

## Genital Ulcers

Herpes, granuloma inguinale (donovanosis), lymphogranuloma venereum, chancroid, and syphilis may all present as ulcerations in the genital area; however, their causes, disease courses, and treatments are different. Table 23.1 lists some of their major characteristics. Physicians must always consider the possibility of more than one STI concurrently infecting an individual.

### Genital Herpes

**Genital herpes is a recurrent viral infection that is incurable and highly contagious, with 75% of sexual partners of infected individuals contracting the disease. Although among the most prevalent STIs, 80% of infected individuals are unaware that they are infected. Asymptomatic shedding that leads to transmission may occur as frequently as once in 5 days.** Excellent online patient education and support can be found www.ashastd.org.

There are two distinct types of herpes simplex virus (HSV), type 1 (HSV-1) and type 2 (HSV-2). Genital HSV-1 transmitted from orolabial lesions to the vulva during oral-genital contact or from genital to genital to contact with a partner with genital HSV-1, is the most commonly acquired genital herpes in women younger than 25 years.

Although subclinical primary herpes infection is common, when the primary infection is symptomatic, both local and systemic disease manifestations occur. Local effects include vulvar skin paresthesia preceding eruption of multiple painful vesicles, which progress to shallow, superficial ulcers over a large area of the vulva. Patients may experience multiple ulcer crops for 2 to 6 weeks, which heal without scarring (Fig. 23.7). Viral shedding may occur for 2 to 3 weeks, and during primary infections, positive cultures for herpesvirus may be obtained from lesions in 80% of women. Severe vulvar pain, tenderness, and inguinal adenopathy and simultaneous involvement of the vagina and cervix are common (Fig. 23.8).

Systemic symptoms, including general malaise and fever, are experienced by 70% of women during the primary infection. Primary infections of the urethra and bladder may result in acute urinary retention, necessitating catheterization. The symptoms of vulvar pain, pruritus, and discharge peak between days 7 and 11 of the primary infection. The typical woman experiences severe symptoms for approximately 14 days.

Recurrent genital herpes is a local disease with less severe symptoms typically with unilateral involvement lasting an average of 7 days. In the first year of HSV-2 infection, 80% of women experience a recurrence, and if the primary HSV-2 infection was severe, the recurrences will occur approximately twice as often. With an initial HSV-1 pelvic infection, there is a 55% chance of a recurrence within 1 year, with the average rate of recurrence slightly less than one episode per year.

A common feature of recurrence is a prodromal phase of sacroneuralgia, vulvar burning, tenderness, and pruritus for a few hours to 5 days before vesicle formation. Extragenital sites of recurrent infection are common. The herpesvirus resides in a latent phase in the dorsal root ganglia of S2, S3, and S4.

**The diagnosis of genital herpes is often made clinically by simple inspection. Viral cultures are useful in primary episodes, when culture sensitivity is 80%, but less useful in recurrent episodes. The most accurate and sensitive technique for identifying herpesvirus is the polymerase chain reaction (PCR) assay. Serologic tests determine whether a woman was infected with herpesvirus in the past.** The Western blot assay

**TABLE 23.1** Clinical Features of Genital Ulcers

| | Type | | | | |
|---|---|---|---|---|---|
| **Parameter** | **Syphilis** | **Herpes** | **Chancroid** | **Lymphogranuloma Venereum** | **Donovanosis** |
| Incubation period | 2-4 wk (1-12 wk) | 2-7 days | 1-14 days | 3 days-6 wk | 1-4 wk (up to 6 mo) |
| Primary lesion | Papule | Vesicle | Papule or pustule | Papule, pustule, or vesicle | Papule |
| Number of lesions | Usually one | Multiple, may coalesce | Usually multiple, may coalesce | Usually one | Variable |
| Diameter (mm) | 5-15 | 1-2 | 2-20 | 2-10 | Variable |
| Edges | Sharply demarcated Elevated, round or oval | Erythematous | Undermined, ragged, irregular | Elevated, round or oval | Elevated, irregular |
| Depth | Superficial or deep | Superficial | Excavated | Superficial or deep | Elevated |
| Base | Smooth, nonpurulent | Serous, erythematous | Purulent | Variable | Red and rough (beefy) |
| Induration | Firm | None | Soft | Occasionally firm | Firm |
| Pain | Unusual | Common | Usually very tender | Variable | Uncommon |
| Lymphadenopathy | Firm, nontender Pseudoadenopathy bilateral | Firm, tender, often bilateral | Tender, may suppurate, usually unilateral | Tender, may suppurate, loculated, usually unilateral | |

From Holmes KK, Mårdh PA, Sparling PF, et al, eds. *Sexually Transmitted Diseases*. 2nd ed. New York: McGraw-Hill; 1990.

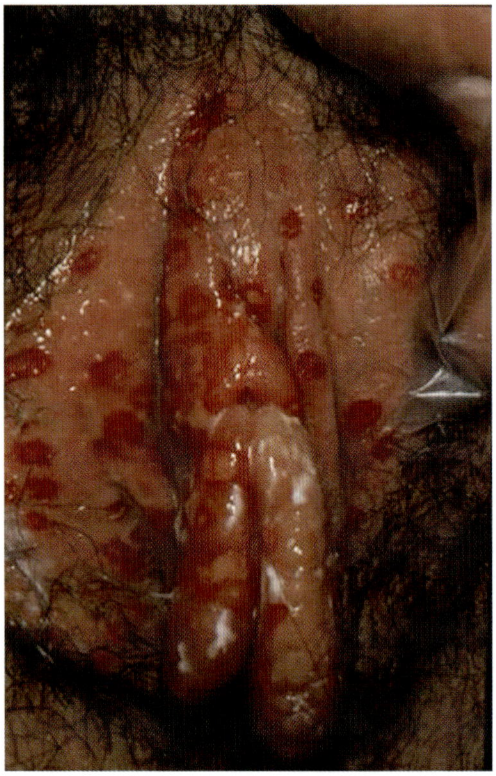

**Fig. 23.7** Herpes genitalis. Superficial ulcers are noted following rupture of vesicles.

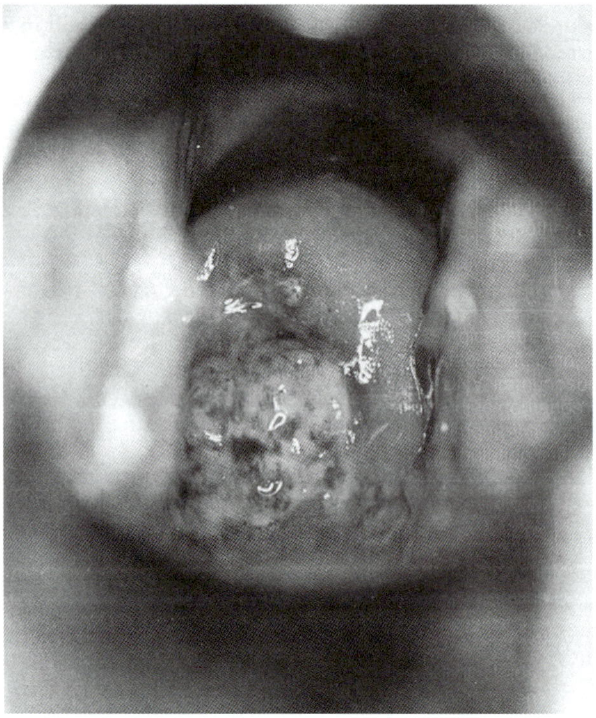

**Fig. 23.8** Primary herpes involving the cervix. A necrotic exophytic mass is seen on posterior lip. This was clinically thought to be invasive carcinoma. Herpes simplex virus culture was positive. The lesion spontaneously disappeared. (From Kaufman RH, Faro S. Herpes genitalis: clinical features and treatment. *Clin Obstet Gynecol.* 1985;28:152-163.)

for antibodies to herpes is the most specific method but is not widely available and is difficult to perform. HSV serologic testing should be considered for persons presenting for an STI evaluation, especially for those with multiple sex partners or HIV infection and at increased risk for HIV acquisition. **Screening for HSV-1 or HSV-2 in the general population is not indicated.**

Enzyme-linked immunoassay (ELISA) and immunoblot tests are available for HSV-1 and HSV-2. Rapid serologic point-of-care tests are available for HSV-2 antibodies. Appropriate screening tests for other STIs should be obtained because they may coexist with herpes.

**Treatment of HSV-1 or HSV-2 may be used for three different clinical scenarios summarized in Table 23.2**: primary episode, recurrent episode and daily suppression. Daily suppressive therapy is recommended when the woman has six or more episodes annually or for psychological distress. It is important for patients to be aware that asymptomatic viral shedding can occur even when on daily suppressive therapy.

In serodiscordant couples a prospective placebo-controlled randomized trial has demonstrated that daily use of valacyclovir for suppression in the seropositive partner results in significantly fewer cases of HSV acquisition in the seronegative partner. Regular use of condoms in serodiscordant couples also decreases transmission but is not 100% protective. Women who are HSV seronegative are three times as likely to acquire HSV infection from seropositive male partners compared with seronegative males acquiring HSV from infected female partners.

The CDC recommends that acyclovir or other suppressive drugs be discontinued after 12 months to determine the subsequent rate of recurrence for each individual woman. Acyclovir is a drug with minimal toxicity, and reports have documented its safety in patients receiving daily therapy for as long as 6 years and with valacyclovir or famciclovir for 1 year; however, even without HSV suppressive treatment, clinical recurrences tend to dramatically decrease in number.

A vaccine would be the logical approach for optimum prevention of herpes. Research is ongoing.

## Granuloma Inguinale (Donovanosis)

Granuloma inguinale, also known as *donovanosis*, is a chronic, ulcerative, bacterial infection of the skin and subcutaneous tissue of the vulva. **Granuloma inguinale is common in tropical climates** such as New Guinea and the Caribbean Islands, but fewer than 20 cases are reported each year in the United States. **Spread through both sexual and close nonsexual contact, it is not highly contagious, and chronic exposure is usually necessary with a variable incubation period** from 1 to 12 weeks. It is caused by an intracellular, gram-negative, nonmotile, encapsulated rod, *Klebsiella granulomatis*, which is difficult to culture on standard media. There are no U.S. Food and Drug Administration (FDA)–approved molecular tests for the detection of *K. granulomatis* DNA. Serologic tests are nonspecific.

The disease course is as follows:

- The initial nodule progresses into a painless, slowly progressing ulcer surrounded by granulation tissue.
- The ulcer has a beefy red appearance, bleeds easily when touched, and is painless and without regional adenopathy.
- Multiple nodules are typically present, resulting in ulcers that grow and coalesce.
- Chronic disease eventually destroys the normal vulvar architecture with scarring and lymphatic obstruction, producing marked enlargement of the vulva.

The disease is usually clinically diagnosed in endemic areas but may also be established by identifying Donovan bodies in smears and specimens taken from the ulcers (Fig. 23.9). Donovan bodies appear as clusters of dark-staining bacteria with a bipolar

**TABLE 23.2** Antiviral Treatment for Herpes Simplex Virus in the Nonpregnant Patient

| | Antiviral Agent | | |
|---|---|---|---|
| **Indication** | **Valacyclovir** | **Acyclovir** | **Famciclovir** |
| First clinical episode | 1000 mg bid, 7–10 days | 400 mg tid; or 200 mg five times/day, 7–10 days | 250 mg tid, 7–10 days |
| Recurrent episodes | 1000 mg daily, 5 days; or 500 mg bid, 3 days | 400 mg tid, 5 days; 800 mg bid, 5 days; or 800 mg tid, 2 days | 125 mg bid, 5 days<br>500 mg once then 250 mg bid, 2 days; 1000 mg bid, 1 day |
| Daily suppressive | 1000 mg daily (≥10 recurrences/year) or 500 mg daily (≤9 recurrences/year) | 400 mg bid | 250 mg bid |

Data from Workowski KA, Bolan GA, Centers for Disease Control and Prevention. Sexually transmitted diseases treatment guidelines, 2015. *MMWR Recomm Rep.* 2015;64(RR-03):1-137.
*bid,* Twice per day; *tid,* three times per day.

(safety pin) appearance found in the cytoplasm of large mononuclear cells. The differential diagnosis includes lymphogranuloma venereum, vulvar carcinoma, syphilis, chancroid, genital herpes, amebiasis, and other granulomatous diseases.

A wide range of oral broad-spectrum antibiotics may be used to manage granuloma inguinale. The CDC recommends azithromycin 1 g orally once a week or 500 mg daily for 3 weeks and until all lesions have healed. See guidelines for alternative antibiotic regimens. Rarely, medical therapy fails and surgical excision is required. Coinfection with another sexually transmitted pathogen is a distinct possibility. Sex partners of women who have granuloma inguinale should be examined if they have had sexual contact during the 60 days preceding the onset of symptoms.

## Lymphogranuloma Venereum

**Lymphogranuloma venereum (LGV) is a chronic infection of lymphatic tissue produced by *Chlamydia trachomatis* found most commonly in the tropics with fewer than 150 new cases reported each year in the United States, most of which occur in men.** In women the vulva is the most common site of infection, but the urethra, rectum, and cervix may also be involved. This STI is caused by serotypes L1, L2, and L3 of *C. trachomatis*. Serologic studies in high-risk populations have found that subclinical infection is common. The incubation period is between 3 and 30 days.

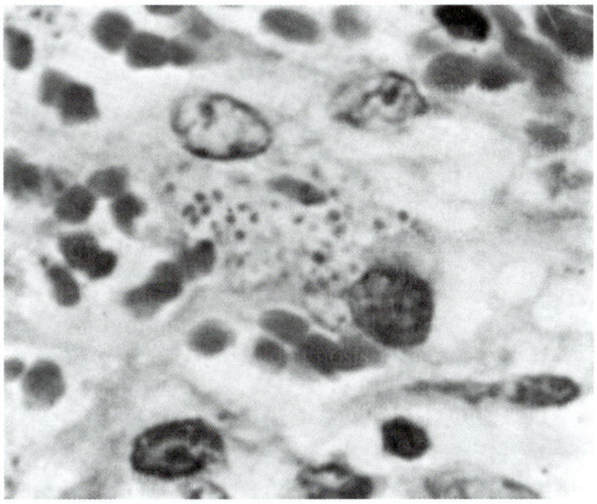

**Fig. 23.9** Donovanosis. Biopsy specimen shows intracytoplasmic Donovan bodies (hematoxylin-eosin stain). (From Hart G. Donovanosis. In: Holmes KK, Mårdh PA, Sparling PF, et al, eds. *Sexually Transmitted Diseases.* New York: McGraw-Hill; 1984.)

There are three distinct phases of vulvar and perirectal LGV.

- Primary infection: A shallow, painless ulcer is present that heals rapidly without therapy typically located on the vestibule or labia but occasionally in the periurethral or perirectal region.
- Secondary phase: 1 to 4 weeks later, painful inguinal and perirectal adenopathy is present, with 50% of patients developing systemic symptoms, including general malaise and fever. Without treatment, the infected nodes become increasingly tender, enlarged, matted together, and adherent to overlying skin, forming a bubo (Fig. 23.10) (tender lymph nodes), which is a double genitocrural fold, or groove sign.
- Tertiary phase: Extensive tissue destruction of the external genitalia and anorectal region may occur during the tertiary phase. This tissue destruction and secondary extensive scarring and fibrosis may result in elephantiasis, multiple fistulas, and stricture formation of the anal canal and rectum.

Diagnosis is established by detecting *C. trachomatis* by culture, direct immunofluorescence, or nucleic acid detection from the pus or aspirate from a tender lymph node. *Chlamydia* serologic testing (complement fixation titers >1:64) can support the diagnosis in the appropriate clinical context. In the absence of specific LGV diagnostic testing, patients should be treated based on the clinical presentation, including proctocolitis or genital ulcer disease with lymphadenopathy. The differential diagnosis of LGV includes syphilis, chancroid, granuloma inguinale, bacterial lymphadenitis, vulvar carcinoma, genital herpes, and Hodgkin disease.

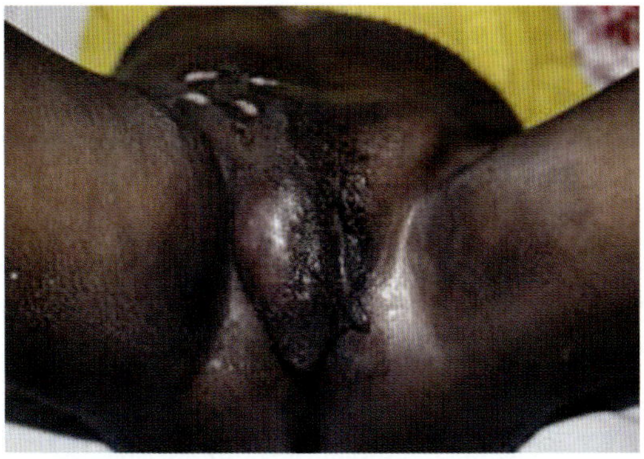

**Fig. 23.10** Lymphogranuloma venereum bubo.

The CDC recommends doxycycline, 100 mg twice daily for at least 21 days, as the preferred treatment, with alternative treatments listed on CDC website. Antibiotic therapy cures the bacterial infection and prevents further tissue destruction, but fluctuant nodes should be aspirated to prevent sinus formation. Rarely, incision and drainage of infected nodes are necessary to alleviate inguinal pain. The late sequelae of the destructive tertiary phase of LGV often require extensive surgical reconstruction. It is important to administer antibiotics during the perioperative period.

## Chancroid

**Chancroid is a sexually transmitted, acute, ulcerative disease of the vulva, common in developing countries but infrequent in the United States**, caused by *Haemophilus ducreyi*, a highly contagious, small, nonmotile, gram-negative rod. Epidemiologic studies have suggested that chancroid tends to occur in clusters and may account for a substantial portion of genital ulcer cases when present; however, difficulty in making the diagnosis may cause underreporting. **The clinical importance of chancroid has been enhanced by reports that the genital ulcers of chancroid facilitate the transmission of HIV infection**. The incubation period is short, usually 3 to 6 days. Tissue trauma and excoriation of the skin must precede initial infection because *H. ducreyi* is unable to penetrate and invade normal skin.

### Clinical Manifestations

- The initial lesion is a small papule and is always painful and tender.
- Within 48 to 72 hours, the papule evolves into a pustule and subsequently ulcerates.
- Ulcers are usually in the vestibule, shallow, extremely painful, with a characteristic ragged edge, and have a dirty, gray, necrotic, foul-smelling exudate and lack induration at the base (the soft chancre).
- Within 2 weeks of an untreated infection, 50% of women develop acutely tender inguinal adenopathy, a bubo, which is typically unilateral.
- Fluctuant nodes should be treated by needle aspiration to prevent rupture or by incision and drainage if larger than 5 cm.

A definitive diagnosis requires the identification of *H. ducreyi* on special culture media that are not widely available and no FDA-approved PCR test for *H. ducreyi* is available in the United States, but this testing can be performed by clinical laboratories that have developed their own PCR test and conducted a Clinical Laboratory Improvement Amendments (CLIA) verification study. Chancroid can be diagnosed clinically in a woman with painful vulvar ulcers after excluding other common STIs that produce vulvar ulcers, including genital herpes, syphilis, LGV, and donovanosis.

Because of antibiotic resistance to tetracyclines and sulfonamides, the CDC recommends the following: azithromycin, 1 g orally in a single dose, or ceftriaxone, 250 mg intramuscularly (IM) in a single dose or ciprofloxacin, 500 mg orally twice daily for 3 days; or erythromycin base, 500 mg orally three times daily for 7 days. **Sexual partners should be treated in a similar fashion.** Approximately 10% of women whose ulcers initially heal have a recurrence at the same site. Women with HIV infection have an increased rate of failure of the standard treatments for chancroid and therefore often require more prolonged therapy. **Coinfection with another ulcer causing an STI should be considered, especially in women lacking an appropriate response to treatment.**

## Syphilis

**Syphilis is a chronic, complex systemic disease that is commonly underreported. It remains one of the most important STIs in the United States. Early syphilis is a cofactor in the transmission and acquisition of HIV, and 25% of new syphilis cases occur in persons coinfected with HIV.** Even with mandatory screening, congenital syphilis continues to be a public health problem. Syphilis should be included in the differential diagnosis of all genital ulcers and cutaneous rashes of unknown origin, and all women diagnosed with syphilis should be screened for HIV.

Syphilis facts include the following:

- Etiologic agent: the spirochete *Treponema pallidum*, which penetrates skin or mucous membranes
- Detection: noncultivable. Can be diagnosed via dark-field microscopy, direct fluorescent antibody tests (Fig. 23.11), or serologic testing.
- Incubation period: 10 to 90 days, with an average of 3 weeks.
- Moderately contagious: 3% to 10% of patients contract the disease from a single sexual encounter with an infected partner; 30% of individuals become infected during a 1-month exposure to a sexual partner with primary or secondary syphilis. Patients are contagious during primary and secondary stages and probably for the first year of latent syphilis.
- Transmission: via kissing or touching a person who has an active lesion on the lips, oral cavity, breast, or genitals. Case transmission can occur with oral-genital contact.

**Presumptive diagnosis and screening of syphilis rely on two types of serologic tests: the nonspecific nontreponemal and the specific antitreponemal antibody tests.** The nontreponemal tests, such as the Venereal Disease Research Laboratory (VDRL) slide test and the rapid plasma reagin (RPR) card test, are inexpensive and easy to perform and are used as screening tests for the disease. They become positive 4 to 6 weeks after exposure and also are a useful index of treatment response because quantitative nontreponemal antibody titers usually correlate with the activity of the disease. Approximately 1% of patients have technical or biologic false-positive results, usually associated with extremely low titers (<1:8). A false-negative result also is a possibility, occurring in approximately 1% to 2% of tests. This negative reaction occurs in women in whom there is an excess of anticardiolipin antibody in the serum, termed the *prozone phenomenon*. Because serologic testing relies on a humoral immune response to infection, women with immunocompromise also may have false-negative tests.

**A nonspecific positive test result is confirmed by a specific antitreponemal test, which is more sensitive but may produce false-positive results, especially in women with lupus erythematosus** (Table 23.3). The standard for antitreponemal

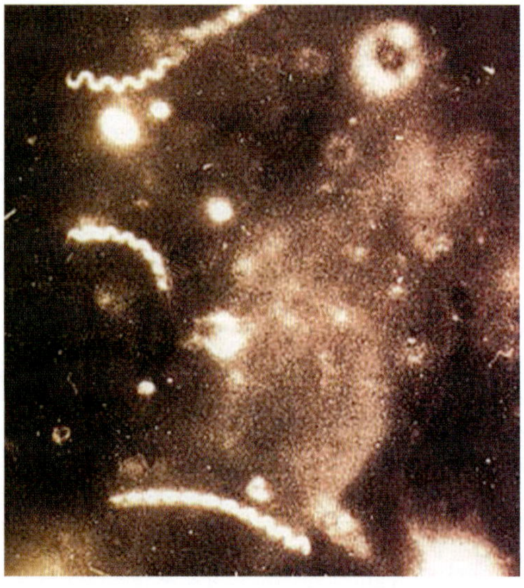

**Fig. 23.11** Dark-field microscopic appearance of *Treponema pallidum*.

**TABLE 23.3** Potential Causes of Biologic False-Positive Results in Syphilis Serology

| | Biologic False-Positive Reaction | |
|---|---|---|
| **Cause** | **Acute** | **Chronic** |
| Physiologic | Pregnancy | Advanced age, multiple blood transfusions |
| Infectious | Varicella, vaccinia, measles, mumps, infectious mononucleosis, herpes simplex, viral hepatitis, HIV seroconversion illness, cytomegalovirus, pneumococcal pneumonia, *Mycoplasma pneumoniae,* chancroid, lymphogranuloma venereum, psittacosis, bacterial endocarditis, scarlet fever, rickettsial infections, toxoplasmosis, Lyme disease, leptospirosis, relapsing fever, rat bite fever | HIV, tropical spastic paraparesis, leprosy,* tuberculosis, malaria,* lymphogranuloma venereum, trypanosomiasis,* kala-azar* |
| Vaccinations | Smallpox, typhoid, yellow fever | |
| Autoimmune disease | | Systemic lupus erythematosus, discoid lupus, drug-induced lupus, autoimmune hemolytic anemia, polyarteritis nodosa, rheumatoid arthritis, Sjögren syndrome, Hashimoto thyroiditis, mixed connective tissue disease, primary biliary cirrhosis, chronic liver disease, idiopathic thrombocytopenic purpura |
| Other | | IV drug use, advanced malignancy hypergammaglobulinemia, lymphoproliferative disease |

Data from Nandwani R, Evans DTP. Are you sure it's syphilis? A review of false-positive serology. *Int J STD AIDS.* 1995;6:241; Hook EW III, Marra CM. Acquired syphilis in adults. *N Engl J Med.* 1992;326:1062.
*Biologic false-positive reaction resolves with resolution of infection.
*HIV,* Human immunodeficiency virus; *IV,* intravenous.

tests are the fluorescent-labeled *Treponema* antibody absorption (FTA-ABS) test and the microhemagglutination assay for antibodies to *T. pallidum* (MHA-TP). A woman with a positive reactive treponemal test usually will have this positive reaction for her lifetime, regardless of treatment or activity of the disease.

Clinically, syphilis is divided into primary, secondary, latent, and tertiary stages.

### Primary Syphilis

**Approximately 2 to 3 weeks after exposure painless papule appears at inoculation site and soon ulcerates to produce the classic chancre—a painless ulcer,** 1 to 2 cm, with a raised indurated margin and a nonexudative base (Fig. 23.12). The chancre is typically solitary, painless, and found on the vulva, vagina, or cervix, with nontender and firm regional adenopathy during the first week of clinical disease. Within 2 to 6 weeks, the painless ulcer heals spontaneously; hence, many women do not seek treatment, a feature that enhances the likelihood of transmission. **Syphilis is not often diagnosed in the primary stage in women.**

### Secondary Syphilis

**Hematogenous dissemination of the spirochetes leads to systemic disease that develops in approximately 25% of patients between 6 weeks and 6 months** (average, 9 weeks) after the primary chancre if primary syphilis is untreated. **An untreated attack of secondary syphilis lasts 2 to 6 weeks and produces a multitude of systemic symptoms,** such as rash, fever, headache, malaise, lymphadenopathy, and anorexia. The classic rash of secondary syphilis is red macules and papules over the palms of the hands and the soles of the feet (Fig. 23.13). Vulvar lesions of condyloma latum are large, raised, flattened, grayish white areas (Fig. 23.14). On wet surfaces of the vulva, soft papules often coalesce to form ulcers that are larger than herpetic ulcers and are not tender unless secondarily infected. **A woman with syphilis is most infectious during the first 1 to 2 years of disease, with decreasing infectivity thereafter.**

### Latent-Stage Syphilis

Positive serologic testing without symptoms or signs of disease follows the secondary stage and varies in duration from 2 to 20 years. This is when most women are diagnosed with syphilis, which is detected via positive blood tests. **Early latent syphilis is an infection of 1 year or less and women are infectious during the first year of latent syphilis. All other cases are referred to as *late latent* or *latent syphilis of unknown duration.*** Women with latent syphilis who have been sexually active should have a pelvic examination to discover potential lesions involving the vagina or cervix.

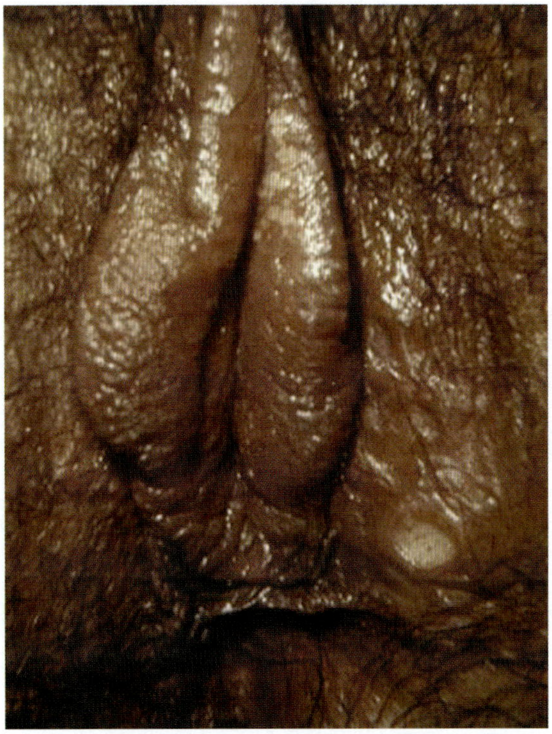

**Fig. 23.12** Primary chancre of syphilis.

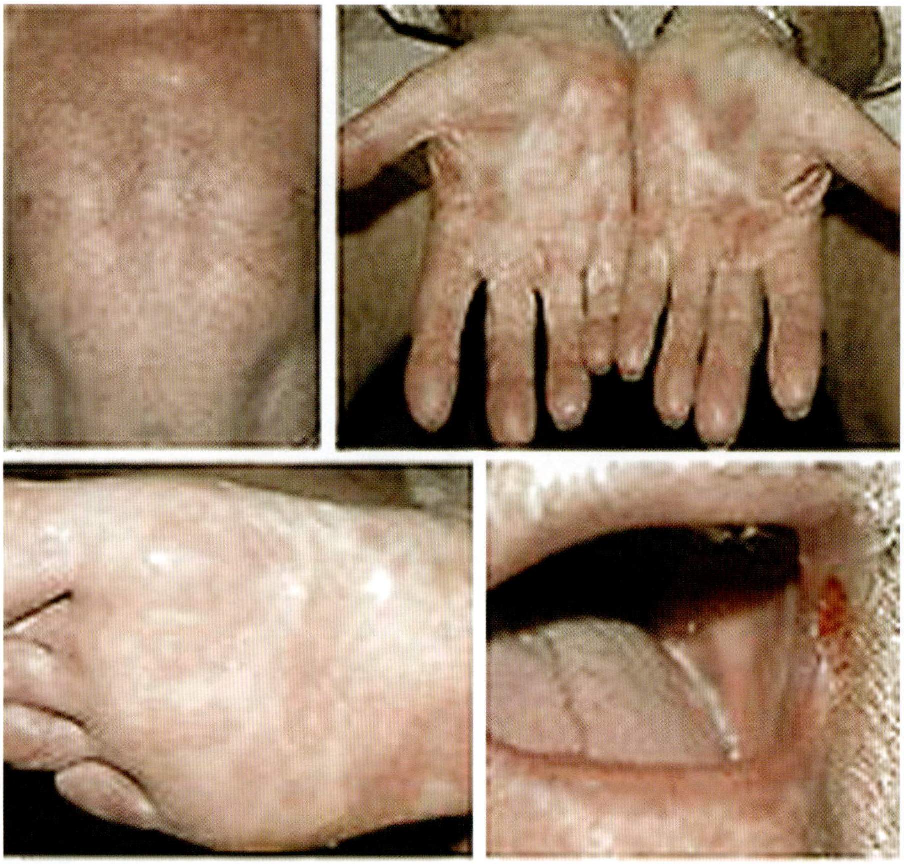

**Fig. 23.13** Secondary syphilis: maculopapular rash. Characteristic maculopapular rash of secondary syphilis affecting the trunk (A), palms (B), and soles (C). (D) Angular mouth ulcer in the same patient. (From Wickremasinghe S, et al. Syphilitic punctate inner retinitis in immunocompetent gay men. *Ophthalmology.* 2009;116(6): 1195-200.)

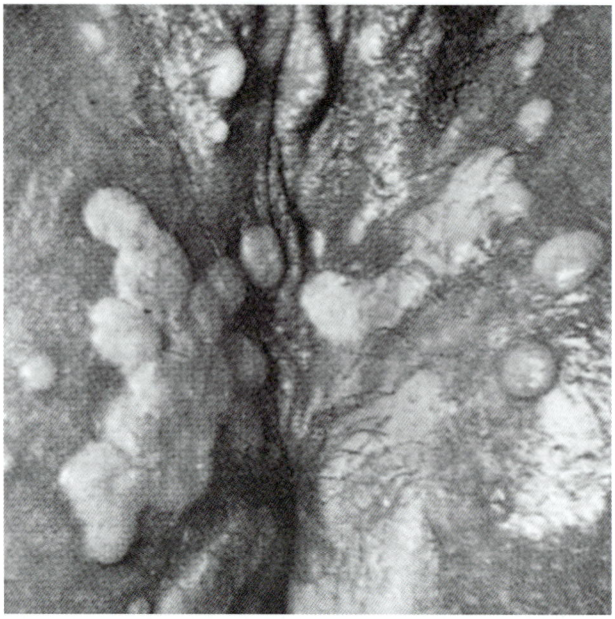

**Fig. 23.14** Multiple lesions of condylomata lata on vulva and perineum. Dark-field microscopic findings were positive. (From Faro S. Sexually transmitted diseases. In: Kaufman RH, Faro S, eds. *Benign Diseases of the Vulva and Vagina.* 4th ed. St. Louis: Mosby–Year Book; 1994.)

### Tertiary Syphilis

**Tertiary syphilis develops in approximately 33% of patients who are not appropriately treated during the primary, secondary, or latent phases of the disease (Fig. 23.15) and is devastating** in its potentially destructive effects on the central nervous, cardiovascular, and musculoskeletal systems. The manifestations of late syphilis include optic atrophy, tabes dorsalis, generalized paresis, aortic aneurysm, and gummas of the skin and bones. A gumma is similar to a cold abscess, with a necrotic center and the obliteration of small vessels by endarteritis.

### Treatment

***T. pallidum*** **is exquisitely sensitive to penicillin; parenteral penicillin G is the drug of choice for syphilis.** Because of the slow replication time of the spirochete, blood levels must be maintained for 7 to 14 days. Box 23.1 lists CDC standard treatment protocols for syphilis. **Approximately 60% of women develop an acute febrile reaction associated with flulike symptoms such as headache and myalgia within the first 24 hours after parenteral penicillin therapy for early syphilis. This response is known as the *Jarisch-Herxheimer reaction.***

### Follow-up

Following are guidelines for follow-up:

- Early syphilis: reexamine clinically and serologically at 6 and 12 months after therapy; titer should decline fourfold in 6 months and become negative within 12 months.
- Latent syphilis: quantitative nontreponemal serologic tests 6, 12, and 24 months after therapy. With successful treatment, the

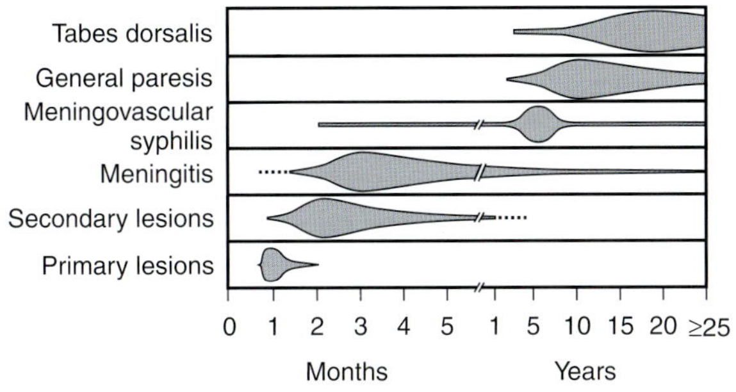


**Fig. 23.15** Approximate time course of the clinical manifestations of early syphilis and neurosyphilis. Shaded areas corresponding to each syndrome represent the approximate proportion of patients with the syndrome specified and do not indicate the proportion of all patients with syphilis who have that syndrome. (From Hook EW 3rd, Marra CM. Acquired syphilis in adults. *N Engl J Med.* 1992;326(16):1060-1069.)

**BOX 23.1** Centers for Disease Control and Prevention Recommended Treatment of Syphilis (2014)

**EARLY SYPHILIS (PRIMARY, SECONDARY, AND EARLY LATENT SYPHILIS OF LESS THAN 1 YEAR IN DURATION)**

Recommended regimen: Benzathine penicillin G, 2.4 million U IM, one dose

Alternative regimen (penicillin-allergic nonpregnant patients): Doxycycline, 100 mg orally bid for 2 wk *or* tetracycline, 500 mg orally qid for 2 wk

**LATE LATENT SYPHILIS (>1 YEAR IN DURATION, GUMMAS, AND CARDIOVASCULAR SYPHILIS)**

Recommended regimen: Benzathine penicillin G, 7.2 million U total, administered as three doses of 2.4 million U IM at 1-wk intervals

Alternative regimen (penicillin-allergic nonpregnant patients): Doxycycline 100 mg orally 2 times a day for 2 wk if <1 year, otherwise, for 4 wk; *or* tetracycline, 500 mg orally qid for 2 wk if <1 year; otherwise, for 4 wk

**NEUROSYPHILIS**

Recommended regimen: Aqueous crystalline penicillin G, 18-24 million U daily, administered as 3-4 million U IV every 4 hr, for 10-14 days

Alternative regimen: Procaine penicillin, 2.4 million U IM daily, for 10-14 days plus probenecid, 500 mg PO qid for 10-14 days

**SYPHILIS IN PREGNANCY**

Recommended regimen: Penicillin regimen appropriate for stage of syphilis. Some experts recommend additional therapy (e.g., second dose of benzathine penicillin, 2.4 million U IM) 1 wk after the initial dose for those who have primary, secondary, or early latent syphilis

Alternative regimen (penicillin allergy): Pregnant women with a history of penicillin allergy should be skin-tested and desensitized

**SYPHILIS IN HIV-INFECTED PATIENTS**

Primary and secondary syphilis: Benzathine penicillin G, 2.4 million U IM. Some experts recommend additional treatments, such as three weekly doses of benzathine penicillin G. Penicillin-allergic patients should be desensitized and treated with penicillin

Latent syphilis (normal CSF examination): Benzathine penicillin G, 7.2 million U as three weekly doses of 2.4 million U each

Data from Workowski KA, Bolan GA, Centers for Disease Control and Prevention. Sexually transmitted diseases treatment guidelines, 2015. *MMWR Recomm Rep.* 2015;64(RR-03):1-137.

*bid,* Twice per day; *CSF,* cerebrospinal fluid; *HIV,* human immunodeficiency virus; *IM,* intramuscularly; *PO,* per os (orally) *qid,* four times per day.

VDRL titer will become nonreactive or at most be reactive, with a lower titer within 1 year. There is a 1% to 2% chance that the woman will not exhibit a fourfold titer decline, and these cases are considered therapeutic failures. Women who have a sustained fourfold increase in nontreponemal test titers have experience treatment failure or become reinfected; they should be retreated with three weekly injections of benzathine penicillin G, 2.4 million units IM, and evaluated for concurrent HIV infection. Patients with syphilis lasting longer than 1 year should have quantitative VDRL titers for 2 years after therapy because their titers will decline more slowly. A specific test for syphilis, such as the FTA-ABS, remains reactive indefinitely.

- **Summary: All women with a first attack of primary syphilis should have a negative nonspecific serologic test within 1 year, and women treated for secondary syphilis should have a negative serologic test within 2 years. If they do not, treatment failure, reinfection, and concurrent HIV infection should be investigated.**

**Syphilis often involves the CNS and this may occur during any stage of syphilis.** Diagnosis is based on a combination of clinical findings, reactive serologic tests, and abnormalities of cerebrospinal fluid, serology, cell count, or protein. **Women should undergo a cerebrospinal fluid examination if they develop neurologic or ophthalmologic signs or symptoms, evidence of active tertiary syphilis, treatment failures, and HIV infection with late latent syphilis or syphilis of an unknown duration. Treatment is reviewed in Box 23.1.**

**It is important for all women with syphilis to be tested for HIV infection.** Simultaneous syphilis and HIV infections alter the natural history of syphilis, with earlier involvement of the CNS. Women with HIV infection may have a slightly increased rate of treatment failure with currently recommended regimens. Similarly, they may exhibit unusual serologic responses. Usually, serologic titers are higher than expected; however, false-negative serologic tests or delayed appearance of seroreactivity has been reported. Nevertheless, the CDC's recommendation for treating early syphilis in women is the same whether or not they are concurrently infected with HIV. After penicillin treatment for syphilis, women with HIV should be followed with quantitative titers at more frequent intervals—for example, at 3, 6, 9, 12, and 24 months after therapy.

Partner treatment:

- Evaluate all partners clinically and serologically.
- Identify an at-risk sex partner: 3 months plus duration of symptoms for primary or secondary syphilis, and 1 year for early latent syphilis.
- Those exposed within the 90 days preceding the diagnosis of a partner with primary, secondary, or early latent syphilis should be treated presumptively because they may be infected, even if seronegative.

## VAGINITIS

**Vaginal discharge is the most common symptom in gynecology**; dyspareunia, dysuria, odor, and vulvar burning, and pruritus are other symptoms associated with vaginal infection. The three common causes of vaginitis are (1) a fungus (candidiasis), (2) a protozoon *(Trichomonas)*, and (3) a disruption of the vaginal bacterial ecosystem leading to bacterial vaginosis. The relative prevalence of vaginitis causes differs depending on the population studied. In a group of mid–socioeconomic class women in the reproductive range, bacterial vaginosis represents approximately 50% of cases, whereas candidiasis and *Trichomonas* infection each constitute approximately 25% of cases.

The vaginal environment is a dynamic ecosystem. The normal vaginal pH, approximately 4.0 in premenopausal women, is maintained by a complex interplay of hormonal, microbiologic, and other unknown factors.

***Lactobacillus* is the regulator of normal vaginal flora:**

- The aerobic, gram-positive rod is found in 62% to 88% of asymptomatic women.
- It makes lactic acid, which maintains the normal vaginal pH of 3.8 to 4.5 and inhibits the adherence of bacteria to vaginal epithelial cells.
- Approximately 60% of vaginal lactobacilli strains make hydrogen peroxide, which inhibits the growth of bacteria and destroys HIV in vitro.
- Estrogen improves lactobacilli concentration by enhancing the vaginal epithelial cell production of glycogen, which breaks down into glucose and acts as a substrate for the bacteria.

Normal physiologic vaginal discharge consists of cervical and vaginal epithelial cells, normal bacterial flora, water, electrolytes, and other chemicals. The quantitative concentration of bacterial organisms is $10^8$ to $10^9$ colonies/mL of vaginal fluid, varying considerably during the menstrual cycle, with the concentrations of anaerobic bacteria five times more common than aerobic bacteria and aerobic bacteria.

In addition to lactobacilli, other common aerobic bacteria found in the vagina are diphtheroids, streptococci, *Staphylococcus epidermidis*, and *Gardnerella vaginalis*. The most common gram-negative bacillus is *Escherichia coli*. Anaerobic bacteria have been detected in approximately 80% of women, with the most prevalent being *Peptococcus*, *Peptostreptococcus*, and *Bacteroides* spp. (Table 23.4). *Candida* spp. and mycoplasmas are also common inhabitants of asymptomatic women. Our knowledge of vaginal flora has traditionally relied on classic microbiology. Newer molecular techniques are demonstrating even greater complexity in vaginal flora.

**TABLE 23.4** Bacterial Vaginal Flora in Asymptomatic Women without Vaginitis

| Organism | Range of Recovery (%) |
|---|---|
| **FACULTATIVE ORGANISMS** | |
| **Gram-Positive Rods** | |
| Lactobacilli | 50-75 |
| Diphtheroids | 40 |
| **Gram-Positive Cocci** | |
| *Staphylococcus epidermidis* | 40-55 |
| *Staphylococcus aureus* | 0-5 |
| Beta-hemolytic streptococci | 20 |
| Group D streptococci | 35-55 |
| **GRAM-NEGATIVE ORGANISMS** | |
| *Escherichia coli* | 10-30 |
| *Klebsiella* spp. | 10 |
| Other organisms | 2-10 |
| **ANAEROBIC ORGANISMS** | |
| *Peptococcus* spp. | 5-65 |
| *Peptostreptococcus* spp. | 25-35 |
| *Bacteroides* spp. | 20-40 |
| *Bacteroides fragilis* | 5-15 |
| *Fusobacterium* spp. | 5-25 |
| *Clostridium* spp. | 5-20 |
| *Eubacterium* spp. | 5-35 |
| *Veillonella* spp. | 10-30 |

From Eschenbach DA. Vaginal infection. *Clin Obstet Gynecol.* 1983;26(1):186-202.

Normal vaginal secretions are white, floccular or curdy, and odorless. In a woman with a normal or physiologic discharge, vaginal discharge is typically present only in the dependent portions of the vagina. Pathologic discharges usually involve the anterior and lateral walls of the vagina. **Vaginal discharge characteristics, especially the amount of discharge, are insensitive and nonspecific diagnostic criteria for vaginitis**; however, thick, white, curdy, patchy discharge, when present, is highly associated with fungal infections. Gray-white discharges that are thin and usually profuse suggest a differential diagnosis of *Trichomonas* or bacterial vaginosis, as do vaginal discharges that have a foul odor. The clinical diagnosis of vaginitis depends on the examination of the vaginal secretions under the microscope and measurement of the vaginal pH. Nevertheless, it is helpful to generalize about the characteristics of normal secretions and the three common vaginal infections (Table 23.5). Table 23.6 lists the diagnostic tests available for vaginitis.

**Vaginal acidity measured with pH indicator paper is one of the most helpful diagnostic aids in the differential diagnosis of vaginitis.** A vaginal pH higher than 5.0 indicates bacterial vaginosis or *Trichomonas* infection, or possibly an atrophic vaginal discharge. A vaginal pH less than 4.5 represents a physiologic discharge or fungal infection, although fungal infection can occur concurrently with bacterial vaginosis or *Trichomonas.* Cervical mucus and semen have neutral or basic pH and may temporarily change the normal acidity. Semen has been found to buffer vaginal acidity for 6 to 8 hours after intercourse. The vaginal pH is slightly higher in postmenopausal than in premenopausal women.

## Bacterial Vaginosis

- **Most prevalent cause of symptomatic vaginitis: 15% to 50% of vaginitis.**
- Most common symptom is an unpleasant vaginal odor, "musty or fishy." The odor is often stronger after intercourse, when the alkaline semen results in a release of aromatic amines.
- Represents a shift in vaginal flora—marked decrease in lactobacilli-dominant flora. Several-fold increase in mixed flora, including genital mycoplasmas, *G. vaginalis*, and anaerobes, such as peptostreptococci, and *Prevotella* and *Mobiluncus* spp.
- Origin of bacterial vaginosis (BV) is elusive. No causative agent has been identified. Because of the inability to find a transmissible agent, bacterial vaginosis has not been classified as an STI. BV is described as a "sexually associated" infection rather than a true STI.
- Clinically diagnosed. Three of these four criteria are sufficient for a presumptive diagnosis; % of women who have three of the four clinical criteria for bacterial vaginosis are asymptomatic: (1) a homogeneous vaginal discharge—thin and gray-white, mildly adherent to the vaginal walls, in contrast to a physiologic discharge, which is in the most dependent areas of the vagina; vaginal discharge is frothy in approximately 10% of women, and it is rare to have associated pruritus or vulvar irritation; (2) discharge has a pH of 4.5 or higher; (3) discharge has an amine-like odor when mixed with potassium hydroxide, the whiff test; and (4) a wet smear of the vaginal discharge demonstrates clue cells (vaginal epithelial cells with clusters of bacteria adherent to their external surfaces) (Fig. 23.16) more than 20% of the number of the vaginal epithelial cells.
- **Vaginal bacterial culture has no role in the evaluation of bacterial vaginosis.**
- Histologically there is an absence of inflammation in biopsy specimens of the vagina and few leukocytes on wet mount—thus the term *vaginosis* rather than *vaginitis.*
- Associated with upper tract infections, including endometritis, pelvic inflammatory disease, postoperative vaginal cuff cellulitis, and multiple complications of infection during pregnancy, such as preterm rupture of the membranes, endomyometritis,

**TABLE 23.5** Typical Features of Vaginitis

| Condition | Symptoms and Signs* | Findings on Examination* | pH | Wet Mount | Comment |
|---|---|---|---|---|---|
| Bacterial vaginosis[†] | Increased discharge (white, thin) Increased odor | Thin, whitish gray, homogeneous discharge, cocci, sometimes frothy | >4.5 | Clue cells (>20%) shift in flora<br>Amine odor after adding potassium hydroxide to wet mount | Greatly decreased lactobacilli<br>Greatly increased cocci<br>Small curved rods |
| Candidiasis | Increased discharge (white, thick)[‡]<br>Dysuria<br>Pruritus<br>Burning | Thick, curdy discharge<br>Vaginal erythema | <4.5 | Hyphae or spores | Can be mixed infection with bacterial vaginosis, *T. vaginalis,* or both, and have higher pH |
| Trichomoniasis[§] | Increased discharge (yellow, frothy)<br>Increased odor<br>Dysuria<br>Pruritus | Yellow, frothy discharge, with or without vaginal or cervical erythema | >4.5 | Motile trichomonads<br>Increased white cells | More symptoms at higher vaginal pH |

From Eckert LO. Clinical practice: acute vulvovaginitis. *N Engl J Med.* 2006;355(12):1244-1252.

*Although these features are typical, their sensitivity and specificity are generally inadequate for diagnosis.

[†]For a diagnosis of bacterial vaginosis, a report of increased discharge has a sensitivity of 50% and a specificity of 49%; odor, a sensitivity of 49% and a specificity of 20%; and pH >4.7, a sensitivity of 97%, and a specificity of 65%, compared with the use of a Gram stain.

[‡]Of patients presenting with symptoms of vaginitis, 40% report increased (white) discharge, but this discharge is not related to *Candida albicans* in many studies.

[§]A report of a yellow discharge has a sensitivity of 42% and a specificity of 80%; a frothy discharge on examination has a sensitivity of 8% and a specificity of 99%.

**TABLE 23.6** Diagnostic Tests Available for Vaginitis

| Test | Sensitivity (%) | Specificity (%) | Comments |
|---|---|---|---|
| **BACTERIAL VAGINOSIS** | | | |
| pH >4.5 | 97 | 64 | |
| Amsel's criteria | 92 | 77 | Must meet three of four clinical criteria (pH >4.5, thin watery discharge, >20% clue cells, positive whiff test), but similar results achieved if two of four criteria meet Nugent criteria; Gram stain morphology score (1-10) based on lactobacilli and other morphotypes; score of 1-3 indicates normal flora, score of 7-10 bacterial vaginosis; high interobserver reproducibility |
| Pap smear | 49 | 93 | |
| **Point-of-care tests** | | | |
| Affirm VP III Test | 95 | 99 | Positive if pH >4.7 |
| Molecular BD MAX | 90 | 85 | FDA approved vaginal microbiome test. Not widely used if microscopy available. |
| OSOM BV blue | 90 | <95 | Tests for vaginal sialidase activity |
| **CANDIDA** | | | |
| Wet mount | | | |
| Overall | 50 | 97 | |
| Growth of 3-4+ on culture | 85 | | *C. albicans* a commensal agent in 15%-20% of women |
| Growth of 1+ on culture | 23 | | |
| pH ≤4.5 | Usual | | If symptoms present, pH may be elevated if mixed infection with bacterial vaginosis or *Trichomonas vaginalis* present |
| Pap smear | 25 | 72 | |
| **TRICHOMONAS VAGINALIS** | | | |
| Wet mount | 45-60 | 95 | Increased visibility of microorganisms with a higher burden of infection |
| Culture | 85-90 | >95 | |
| pH >4.5 | 56 | 50 | |
| Pap smear | 92 | 61 | False-positive rate of 8% for standard Pap test and 4% for liquid-based cytologic test |
| Point-of-care test: OSOM | 83 | 98.8 | 10 min required to perform tests for *T. vaginalis* antigens |
| Nucleic acid test | 95-100 | 95-100 | Recommended by CDC as first choice method for testing. Vaginal swab or first-void urine may be used. |

Modified from Eckert LO. Clinical practice: acute vulvovaginitis. *N Engl J Med.* 2006;355(12):1244-1252.

*CDC,* Centers for Disease Control and Prevention; *FDA,* Food and Drug Administration; *Pap,* Papanicolaou.

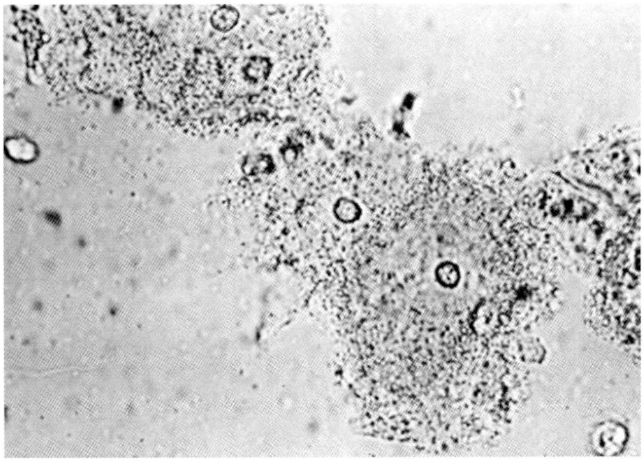

**Fig. 23.16** Bacterial vaginosis. Typical clue cells of vaginal epithelium are heavily covered by coccobacilli, with loss of distinct cell margins (magnification ×400). (From Holmes KK. Lower genital tract infections in women: cystitis/urethritis, vulvovaginitis, and cervicitis. In Holmes KK, Mårdh PA, Sparling PF, et al, eds. *Sexually transmitted diseases*. New York: McGraw-Hill; 1984.)

decreased success with in vitro fertilization, and increased pregnancy loss of less than 20 weeks' gestation.

- If available, Gram staining of vaginal secretion is an excellent diagnostic method. A colorimetric test that detects proline aminopeptidase has been developed for office use. Molecular diagnostic test is now FDA approved for use.
- Enzyme levels in vaginal fluid are elevated in women with bacterial vaginosis.

Risk factors include new or multiple sexual partners and women who have sex with women; genotyping has revealed identical bacterial strains between monogamous lesbian partners. BV is more common in lesbian couples who share sex toys with each other without cleaning the toys between use. Other risk factors include douching at least monthly or within the prior 7 days and social stressors (e.g., homelessness, threats to personal safety, insufficient financial resources). A lack of hydrogen peroxide–producing lactobacilli is also a recognized risk factor for bacterial vaginosis and may explain, in part, the higher prevalence of bacterial vaginosis in black women independent of other risk factors.

### Treatment

See the CDC Treatment guidelines for the latest regimens for acute and recurrent BV. Because there are no effective means of replacing lactobacilli, the treatment for bacterial vaginosis is to decrease anaerobes with antibiotic therapy and hope the woman will then regenerate her own lactobacilli. Table 23.7 provides treatment options. Cure rates are comparable; the agent used should depend on the woman's preference and cost factors. **Concurrent treatment of the male partner is not recommended at this time. Alternative therapies such as the use of oral or vaginal *Lactobacillus* are not efficacious.** Recurrent BV (3 or more episodes in the previous year) occurs in up to 20% of women, and specific treatment regimens are indicated (see CDC Treatment Guidelines).

## *Trichomonas* Vaginal Infection

- Caused by the anaerobic flagellated protozoon *Trichomonas vaginalis* (Fig. 23.17, A).
- **The most prevalent nonviral, nonchlamydial STI of women with 5 million new cases of trichomoniasis annually in the United States.**
- Cause of acute vaginitis in 5% to 50% of cases, depending on the population studied.
- Highly contagious STI; after a single sexual contact, at least two-thirds of male and female sexual partners become infected.
- Incubation period is 4 to 28 days.
- *Trichomonas* is a hardy organism and will survive for up to 24 hours on a wet towel and up to 6 hours on a moist surface; however, experimental studies have established that successful vaginal infection depends on the deposition of an inoculum of several thousand organisms. Hence, it is unlikely that infection may be related to exposure from infected towels or swimming pools.
- Primary symptom is profuse vaginal discharge. (Patients often complain that the copious discharge makes them feel "wet.") (Fig. 23.17, B).
- Approximately 50% of symptomatic women also detect an abnormal vaginal odor and experience vulvar pruritus; dysuria is a symptom in approximately one of five women with symptomatic *Trichomonas* infection. Women with chronic infection may have a malodorous discharge as their only complaint.
- Many women with *Trichomonas* are symptom free and can remain so for years.
- On physical examination a woman with *T. vaginalis* may have erythema and edema of the vulva and vagina. Vulvar skin involvement is limited to the vestibule and labia minora, which helps distinguish it from the more extensive vulvar involvement of *Candida* vulvovaginitis. The discharge color may be white, gray, yellow, or green, and the classic discharge of *Trichomonas* infection is termed *frothy* (with bubbles) and often has an unpleasant odor. The classic sign of a strawberry appearance of the upper vagina and cervix is rare and is noted in less than 10% of women.
- Diagnosis: the CDC encourages use of highly sensitive tests nucleic acid amplification tests (NAATs), which can be performed on vaginal secretions or urine, to detect *T. vaginalis* in both symptomatic and asymptomatic women. NAATs are three to five times more sensitive than wet preparations. Attempts to diagnose *T. vaginalis* infection by Papanicolaou (Pap) smear results in an error rate of at least 50%. There have been a large number of false-positive and false-negative reports.
- Similar to bacterial vaginosis, *T. vaginalis* is associated with upper genital tract infections, including infections after delivery, surgery, abortion, pelvic inflammatory disease, preterm delivery, infertility, and cervical dysplasia treatment. Because all STIs have common epidemiologic backgrounds, finding one dictates carrying out appropriate studies to rule out colonization or infection with another STI.

### Treatment

**Nitroimidazoles are the only class of drugs recommended for treatment of *Trichomonas* vaginitis.** (See CDC Treatment guidelines.) Other treatment guidelines are as follows:

- Primary regimen is a single oral dose (2 g) of metronidazole or tinidazole.
- An alternate regimen is metronidazole, 500 mg orally, twice daily for 7 days.
- Patients should be warned that nitroimidazoles inhibit ethanol metabolism (avoid alcohol for 24 hours after metronidazole and 72 hours after tinidazole therapy to avoid a disulfiram-like reaction.
- **Topical therapy for *Trichomonas* vaginitis is not recommended because it does not eliminate disease reservoirs in Bartholin and Skene glands.**
- **Asymptomatic women with *Trichomonas* identified in the lower genital urinary tract should be treated** (one of three

**TABLE 23.7** Centers for Disease Control and Prevention Recommendations for Treatment of Acute Vaginitis (2015)

| Disease | Drug | Dose |
|---|---|---|
| **Bacterial vaginosis*** | Metronidazole (Flagyl) | 500 mg PO, bid for 7 days† |
| | Tinidazole | 2-g dose PO daily for 2 days |
| | Tinidazole | 1-g dose PO daily for 5 days |
| | 0.75% metronidazole gel | One 5-g application intravaginally daily for 5 days‡ |
| | 2% clindamycin cream | One 5-g application intravaginally every night for 7 days |
| | Clindamycin | 300 mg PO, bid for 7 days |
| | Clindamycin ovules | 100 mg intravaginally every night for 3 days |
| Fungal Vulvovaginitis uncomplicated vaginal therapy uncomplicated Intravaginal therapy‡,§ | Azoles | |
| | 2% sustained-release butoconazole cream (Gynazole) | One 5-g dose |
| | 1% clotrimazole cream (Mycelex-7) | 5 g for 7-14 days§ |
| | 2% Clotrimazole cream | 5 gm intravaginally for 3 days§ |
| | 2% Miconazole cream | 5 g/day for 7 days§ |
| | 4% Miconazole cream | 5 gm intravaginally × 3 days§ |
| | Miconazole (Monistat-7) | One 100-mg vaginal suppository/day for 7 days§ |
| | Miconazole (Monistat-3) | One 200-mg vaginal suppository/day for 3 days |
| | Miconazole (Monistat-1) | One 1200-mg vaginal suppository§ |
| | 0.4% Terconazole cream (Terazol 7) | 5 g/day for 7 days |
| | 0.8% Terconazole cream (Terazol 3) | 5 g/day for 3 days |
| | Terconazole vaginal | One 80-mg vaginal suppository/day for 3 days |
| Uncomplicated Oral therapy | Fluconazole (Diflucan) | One 150-mg dose PO |
| Complicated Intravaginal therapy‡ | Azole | 7-14 days |
| Complicated Oral therapy¶ | Fluconazole (Diflucan) | Two 150-mg doses PO, 72 hr apart |
| **Trichomoniasis** | Metronidazole (Flagyl) | One 2-g dose PO, 500 mg orally bid for 7 days |
| | Tinidazole (Tindamax) | One 2-g dose PO** |

Modified from Eckert LO. Clinical practice: acute vulvovaginitis. *N Engl J Med.* 2006;355(12):1244-1252.
*,†Oral therapy is recommended for pregnant women.
†,‡Drug may cause gastrointestinal upset in 5% to 10% of patients; a disulfiram reaction is possible; alcohol should be avoided for 24 hr after ingestion.
‡,§Vaginal treatments cause local vaginal irritation in 2% to 5% of patients.
§This agent is available over the counter.
Complicated vulvovaginitis refers to disease in women who are pregnant, women who have uncontrolled diabetes, women who are immunocompromised, or women who have severe symptoms, non–*Candida albicans* candidiasis, or recurrent episodes (four or more per year).
¶Oral therapy is not recommended for pregnant women.
**Drug may cause gastrointestinal upset in 2% to 5% of patients; disulfiram reaction is possible; alcohol should be avoided 72 hr after ingestion.
*Bid,* Twice per day.

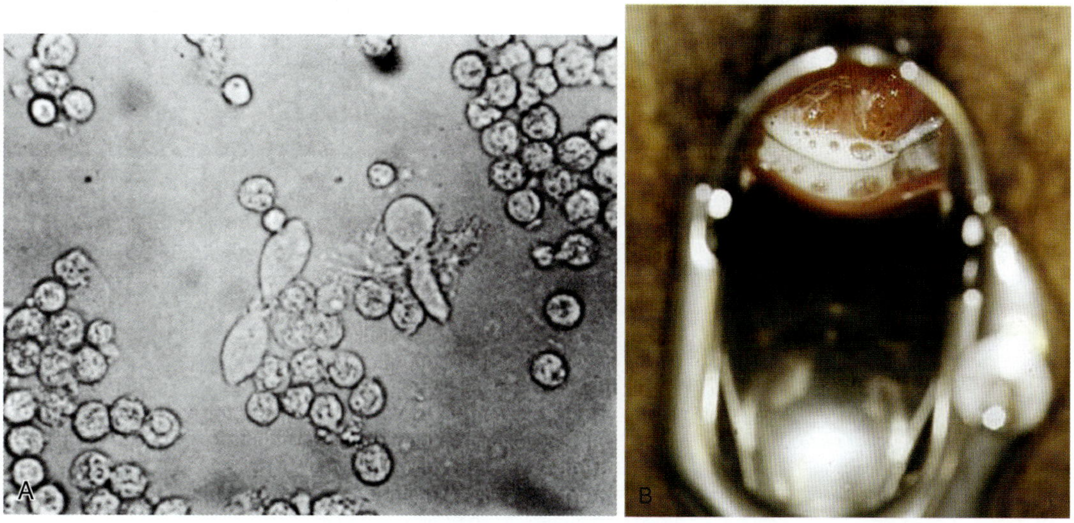


**Fig. 23.17** (Part A From Faro S. Trichomoniasis. In: Kaufman RH, Faro S, eds. Benign Diseases of the Vulva and Vagina. 4th ed. St. Louis: Mosby–Year Book; 1994.) B, From Jane R. Schwebke: Trichomonas vaginalis. In John E. Bennett, Raphael Dolin and Martin J. Blaser: Mandell, Douglas, and Bennett's Principles and Practice of Infectious Diseases, Vol: 2, Page: 3161-3164.e1. Publication Year 2015. FIGURE 282-2 Vaginal discharge in a patient with trichomoniasis. Note the bubbles, which give the discharge a "frothy" appearance.

asymptomatic women will become symptomatic within 3 months).

- **HIV acquisition is increased in women with *Trichomonas* infection.**
- In women with HIV infection, 500 mg twice daily for 7 days for trichomoniasis is more effective.
- The prevalence of low-level metronidazole resistance in *T. vaginalis* is 2% to 5% (in case series, prolonged treatment with higher doses of metronidazole and tinidazole has been successful).
- **Because *T. vaginalis* is sexually transmitted, treatment of the woman's partner is important and increases cure rates.**

Patients should be rescreened with a NAAT in 3 months because of high reinfection rates. If reexposure is not an issue and the infection is not cleared after adequate therapy, consult the CDC treatment guidelines for further therapeutic options or for assistance in performing susceptibility testing.

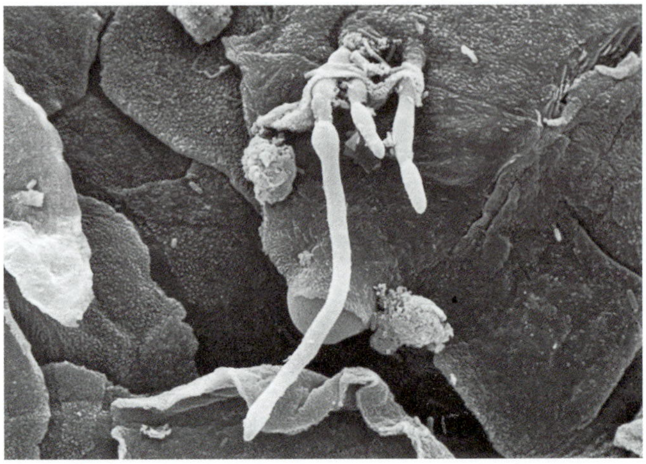

**Fig. 23.19** Scanning electron micrograph of intraluminal debris of specimen of vaginal wall taken from patient with vaginal candidiasis (× 3500). The hyphae of *Candida albicans* penetrate the epithelial layers of vaginal surface. (From Merkus JM, Bisschop MP, Stolte LA. The proper nature of vaginal candidosis and the problem of recurrence. *Obstet Gynecol Surv.* 1985;40:493-504.)

## *Candida* Vaginitis

***Candida vaginalis* is produced by a ubiquitous, airborne, gram-positive fungus. In most populations, more than 90% of cases are caused by *Candida albicans*** (Fig. 23.18), with 5% to 10% of vaginal fungal infections produced by *Candida glabrata* or *Candida tropicalis*. *Candida* spp. are part of the normal flora of approximately 25% of women, being a commensal saprophytic organism on the mucosal surface of the vagina. *Candida* prevalence in the rectum is three to four times greater and in the mouth two times greater than in the vagina. *Candida* organisms develop filamentous (hyphae and pseudohyphae) and ovoid forms, termed *conidia*, *buds*, or *spores*. The filamentous forms of *C. albicans* have the ability to penetrate the mucosal surface and become intertwined with the host cells (Fig. 23.19). This results in secondary hyperemia and limited lysis of tissue near the site of infection. In contrast, *C. glabrata* does not produce filamentous forms. Some women with recurrent vulvovaginal candidiasis have tissue infiltration with polymorphonuclear (PMN) leukocytes. This high density of PMNs correlates with symptoms but does not result in clearance of *Candida*.

Risk factors for *C. albicans* can enhance its ability to become an opportunistic pathogen and include common influences on the vaginal ecosystem:

- Hormonal factors (pregnancy, immediately preceding and after menses)

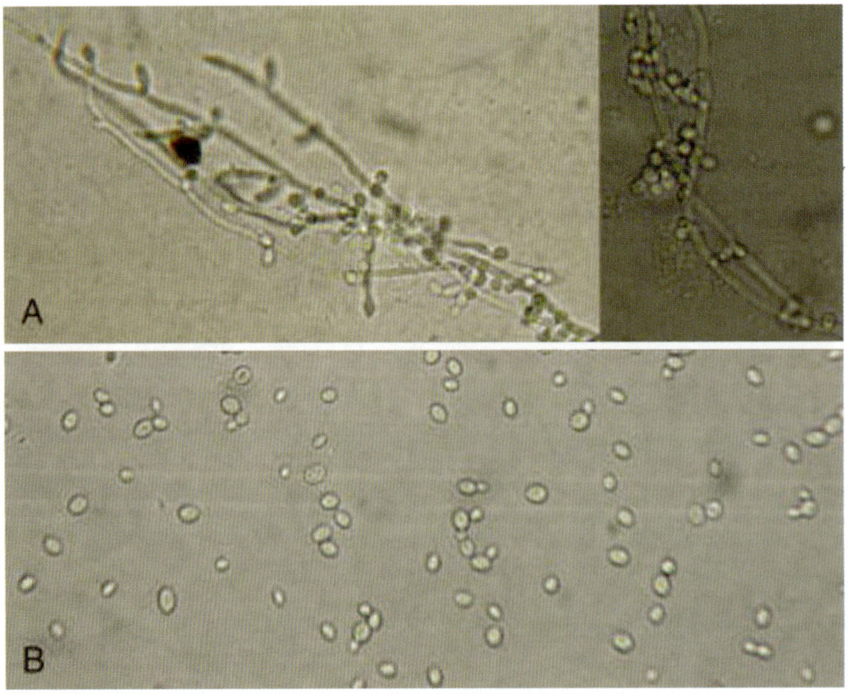


**Fig. 23.18** Candida spp. in clinical specimens. A, Candida albicans, and B, glabrata from the oral cavity showing budding yeast. Note the absence of pseudohyphae, which is typical for this species (unstained wet mount). (Courtesy Service de Parasitologie-Mycologie, Hôpital Universitaire Pitié-Salpêtrière, Paris, France.)

- Depressed cell-mediated immunity (e.g., corticosteroid users, HIV)
- Antibiotic use, especially those that destroy lactobacilli (e.g., penicillin, tetracycline, cephalosporins)

Obesity and debilitating disease are other predisposing factors.

## Fungal Vulvovaginitis

- Primarily a disease of the childbearing years.
- Common: three of four women will have at least one episode.
- Recurrence rate after an apparent cure varies from 20% to 80%.
- Approximately 3% to 5% of women experience recurrent vulvovaginal candidiasis (RVVC), which is defined as four or more documented episodes in 1 year.
- Pruritus is the predominant symptom; may have vulvar burning, external dysuria, and dyspareunia.
- Vaginal signs: vaginal pH associated with this infection is less than 4.5; discharge is variable in amount, white or whitish gray, highly viscous, granular or floccular, with no odor. With speculum, a cottage cheese–type discharge is often visualized, with adherent clumps and plaques (thrush patches) (Fig. 23.20, *A*).
- Vulvar signs include erythema, edema, and fissuring (Fig. 23.20, *B*).
- For diagnosis: wet smear mixed with potassium hydroxide; the ability to detect *C. albicans* on a wet mount is 80% when semiquantitative culture growth is 3 to 4+, but only 20% when culture growth is 2+; hence, a negative smear does not exclude *Candida* vulvovaginitis.
- **Vaginal fungal culture is particularly useful** when a wet mount is negative for hyphae but the patient has symptoms and discharge or other signs suggestive of vulvovaginal candidiasis on examination, or for women who have recently treated themselves with an antifungal agent; up to 90% have a negative culture within 1 week after treatment.
- Over-the-counter (OTC) availability of vaginal antifungal therapy makes self-treatment an option for many women, though the nonspecific symptoms of fungal infections may reflect an alternative diagnosis; hence, if a woman chooses self-treatment, she should be advised to come in for examination if the symptoms are not eliminated with a single course of OTC therapy.
- Also consider noninfectious conditions such as allergic reactions, contact dermatitis, chemical irritants, and rare diseases such as lichen planus.

For treatment of vulvovaginal candidiasis, the CDC recommends placing the woman into an uncomplicated or complicated category to guide treatment (Box 23.2).

- Uncomplicated vulvovaginal candidiasis: topical antifungal agents for 1 to 3 days, or a single oral dose of fluconazole.
- Complicated vaginitis: topical azoles for 7 to 14 days or for oral therapy; a second fluconazole dose (150 mg) given 72 hours after the first dose.
- If RVVC: longer duration of therapy; 7 to 14 days of topical therapy or three doses of oral fluconazole 3 days apart (e.g., days 1, 4, and 7) are options. Then maintenance therapy such as oral fluconazole (e.g., 100-, 150-, or 200-mg dose) weekly for 6 months or topical treatments used intermittently as a maintenance regimen may be considered.
- **Women with recurrent vulvovaginitis should receive a vaginal fungal culture to determine species and sensitivities.**
- **Infections with *Candida* spp. other than *C. albicans* are often azole resistant**; however, one study of terconazole for non–*C. albicans* fungal vaginitis resulted in a mycologic cure in 56% of patients and a symptomatic cure in 44% of women. **Vaginal boric acid capsules (600 mg in 0 gelatin capsules) for a minimum of 14 days resulted in a symptomatic cure rate of 70% for women with non–*C. albicans* infection.** Boric acid inhibits fungal cell wall growth. It may also be used for suppression in women with RVVC. After 10 days of therapy, one 600-mg capsule intravaginally twice weekly for 4 to 6 months decreases symptomatic recurrences. Boric acid is toxic

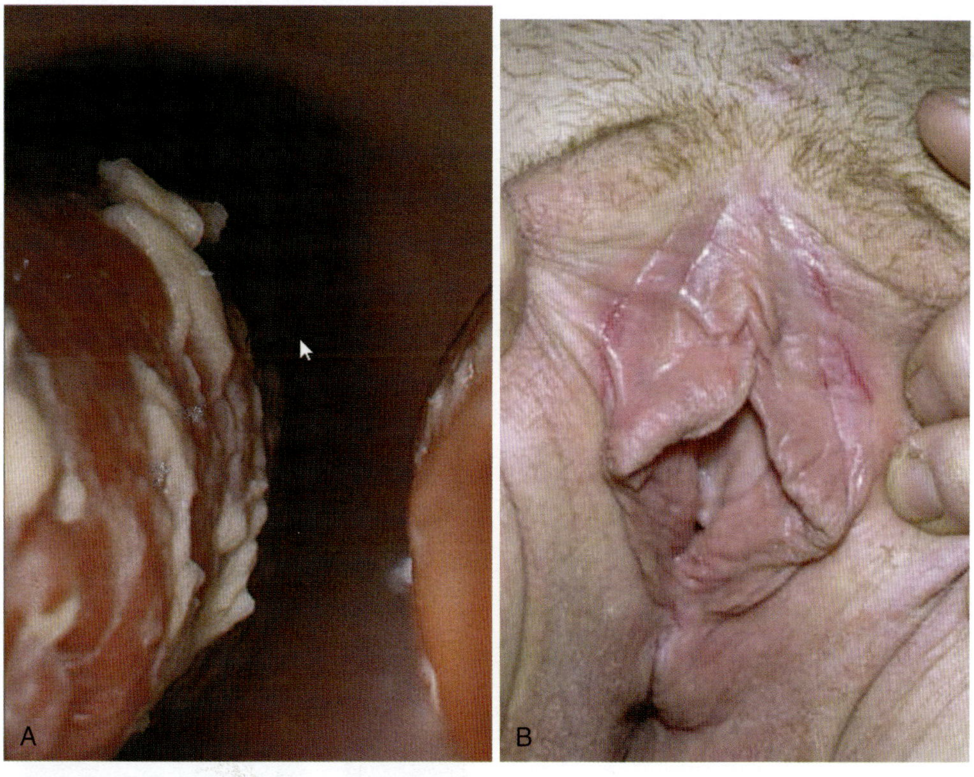


**Fig. 23.20** (**A** from McMillan A, Young H, Ogilvie MM, Scott GR, eds. *Clinical Practice in Sexually Transmissible Infections.* Philadelphia: Saunders; 2003.)

**BOX 23.2** Classification of Vulvovaginal Candidiasis (VVC)

| Uncomplicated VVC | Complicated VVC |
|---|---|
| Sporadic or infrequent vulvovaginal candidiasis | Recurrent vulvovaginal candidiasis |
| *and* | *or* |
| Mild to moderate vulvovaginal candidiasis | Severe vulvovaginal candidiasis |
| *and* | *or* |
| Likely to be *Candida albicans* | Non-*albicans* candidiasis |
| *and* | *or* |
| Nonimmunocompromised women | Women with uncontrolled diabetes, debilitation, or immunosuppression |

Modified from Workowski KA, Bolan GA, Centers for Disease Control and Prevention. Sexually transmitted diseases treatment guidelines, 2015. *MMWR Recomm Rep.* 2015;64(RR-03):1-137.

if ingested, so it should be stored in a safe manner (Eckert, 1998; Sobel, 2001, 2003).

- **Studies of alternative therapies for vulvovaginal candidiasis (such as oral or vaginal *Lactobacillus*, garlic, or diet alterations such as yogurt ingestion) do not show efficacy.**
- A summary of diagnostic tools for determining the cause of vaginitis is given in Table 23.6 and a list treatment options is provided in Table 23.7.

## TOXIC SHOCK SYNDROME

TSS is an acute febrile illness produced by a bacterial exotoxin, with a fulminating downhill course involving dysfunction of multiple organ systems. The cardinal features of the disease are its abrupt onset and rapidity with which the clinical signs and symptoms may present and progress. It is not unusual for the syndrome to develop from a site of bacterial colonization rather than from an infection. There are three requirements for the development of classic TSS: (1) The woman must be colonized or infected with *S. aureus*, (2) the bacteria must produce TSS toxin 1 (TSST-1) or related toxins, and (3) the toxins must have a route of entry into the systemic circulation. Most strains of *S. aureus* are unable to produce TSST-1. With the withdrawal of high-absorbency tampons from the market, the number of cases of TSS has markedly decreased; however, tampon use remains a risk factor for TSS, and women should be encouraged to change tampons every 4 to 6 hours. The intermittent use of external pads is also good prevention for TSS.

Approximately 50% of cases of TSS are not related to menses. Nonmenstrual TSS may be a sequela of focal staphylococcal infection of the skin and subcutaneous tissue, often after a surgical procedure. The signs and symptoms of TSS are produced by the exotoxin named *toxin 1*, which acts as a superantigen, activating up to 20% of T cells at once, resulting in massive cytokine production. The primary effects of toxin 1 are to produce increased vascular permeability, thus resulting in profuse leaking of fluid (capillary leak) from the intravascular compartment into the interstitial space and an associated profound loss of vasomotor tone, causing decreased peripheral resistance. Because of the severity of the disease, gynecologists should have a high index of suspicion for TSS in a woman who has an unexplained fever and a rash during or immediately after her menstrual period. The management of a classic case of severe TSS demands an intensive care unit and the skills of an expert in critical care medicine.

## CERVICITIS

The cervix acts as a barrier between the abundant bacterial flora of the vagina and the bacteriologically sterile endometrial cavity and oviducts. Cervical mucus exerts a bacteriostatic effect, contains antibodies and inflammatory cells that are active against various sexually transmitted organisms, and also may act as a competitive inhibitor with bacteria for receptors on the endocervical epithelial cells.

Cervicitis, an inflammatory process in the cervical epithelium and stroma, can be associated with trauma, inflammatory systemic disease, neoplasia, and infection. Although it is clinically important to consider all causes of inflammation, this section focuses on infectious origins.

Cervical infection can be ectocervicitis or endocervicitis. Ectocervicitis can be viral (HSV) or from a severe vaginitis (e.g., strawberry cervix associated with *T. vaginalis* infection) or *C. albicans.* Endocervicitis may be secondary to infection with *C. trachomatis* or *N. gonorrhoeae.* Bacterial vaginosis and *Mycoplasma genitalium* have also been associated with endocervicitis. Primary endocervical infection may result in secondary ascending infections, including pelvic inflammatory disease and perinatal infections of the membranes, amniotic fluid, and parametria. Chronic cervicitis, when found on a cervical biopsy as a histologic diagnosis, is so prevalent that it should be considered the norm for parous women of reproductive age and does not merit empiric therapy.

This section focuses on mucopurulent cervicitis and techniques to diagnose common cervical infections.

### Mucopurulent Cervicitis

Mucopurulent cervicitis (MPC) is diagnosed clinically with any of the following physical examination manifestations:

- Yellow mucopurulent cervical discharge (Fig. 23.21) and/or the presence of 10 or more PMN leukocytes per microscopic field (magnification, × 1000) on endocervical Gram-stained smears.
- Hypertrophy or edema or increased erythema in cervical ectropion
- Bleeding secondary to endocervical ulceration
- Friability when the endocervical smear is obtained

Symptoms of MPC include the following:

- Increased vaginal discharge
- Intermenstrual or postcoital vaginal bleeding
- Deep dyspareunia

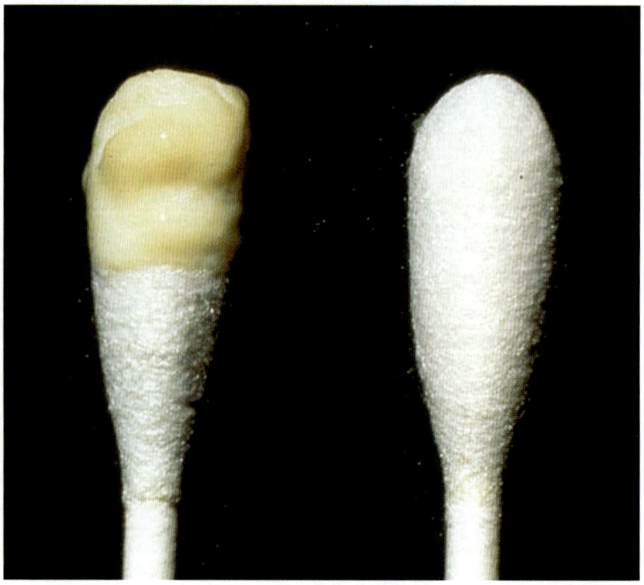

**Fig. 23.21** Mucopurulent cervicitis demonstrated by a cotton swab test.

The prevalence of MPC depends on the population being studied. Approximately 30% to 40% of women attending clinics for STIs and 8% to 10% of women in university student health clinics have the condition. More than 60% of women with this disease are asymptomatic.

### Etiology

**MPC is present in approximately 40% to 60% of women in whom no cervical pathogen can be identified**. When a cause is found, *C. trachomatis* (Fig. 23.22) or *N. gonorrhoeae* are important causes; however, most women who have cervical infections caused by *C. trachomatis* or *N. gonorrhoeae* do not have MPC, and most women who have mucopurulent cervicitis are not infected by *C. trachomatis* or *N. gonorrhoeae*.

*Mycoplasma genitalium*, which is noncultivable, has been associated with mucopurulent cervicitis by DNA testing. FDA-approved NAATs are now available for testing. Treatment is with moxifloxacin or azithromycin. Resistance has been found, so in women with persistent cervicitis with a positive NAAT for *M. genitalium* after moxifloxacin and azithromycin treatment, consider consulting a specialist.

Bacterial vaginosis has also been associated with mucopurulent cervicitis; cervicitis resolved with bacterial vaginosis treatment.

### Treatment

When clinically diagnosed, empirical therapy for *C. trachomatis* is recommended for women at increased risk of this common STI (age younger than 25 years, new or multiple sex partners, unprotected sex). Concurrent therapy for *N. gonorrhoeae* is indicated if the prevalence of *N. gonorrhoeae* is more than 5% in the population. Concomitant trichomoniasis should also be treated if detected, as should bacterial vaginosis. If presumptive treatment is deferred, the use of a sensitive nucleic acid test for *C. trachomatis* and *N. gonorrhoeae* is needed with consideration of adding a NAAT for *Trichomonas*.

Recommended regimens for presumptive cervicitis therapy include azithromycin, 1 g orally in a single dose, or doxycycline, 100 mg orally twice daily for 7 days, adding gonococcal treatment if the prevalence is more than 5% in the population assessed. Because resistance patterns and recommendations may change, please consult the CDC Treatment Guidelines for recommended treatment. **Women treated for cervicitis should be instructed to abstain from sexual intercourse for 7 days after single-dose therapy or until completion of the 7-day regimen.**

## Detection of Cervical Bacteria

### Neisseria Gonorrhoeae

- NAAT of the urine or vaginal secretions are over 95% sensitive and specific and are the most sensitive and specific diagnostic tool for identifying gonorrheal infections.
- Urine tests should be first void (either the first void in morning or at least 1 hour since last void).
- Most women who are colonized with *N. gonorrhoeae* are asymptomatic.
- Screening of high-risk individuals is the primary modality to control the disease.
- **Antibiotic-resistant gonorrhea (GC) is problematic. The CDC STD Treatment Guidelines** (2015) recommend dual **therapy with ceftriaxone** 500 mg **once IM as solo therapy for all GC infections** (Box 23.3).

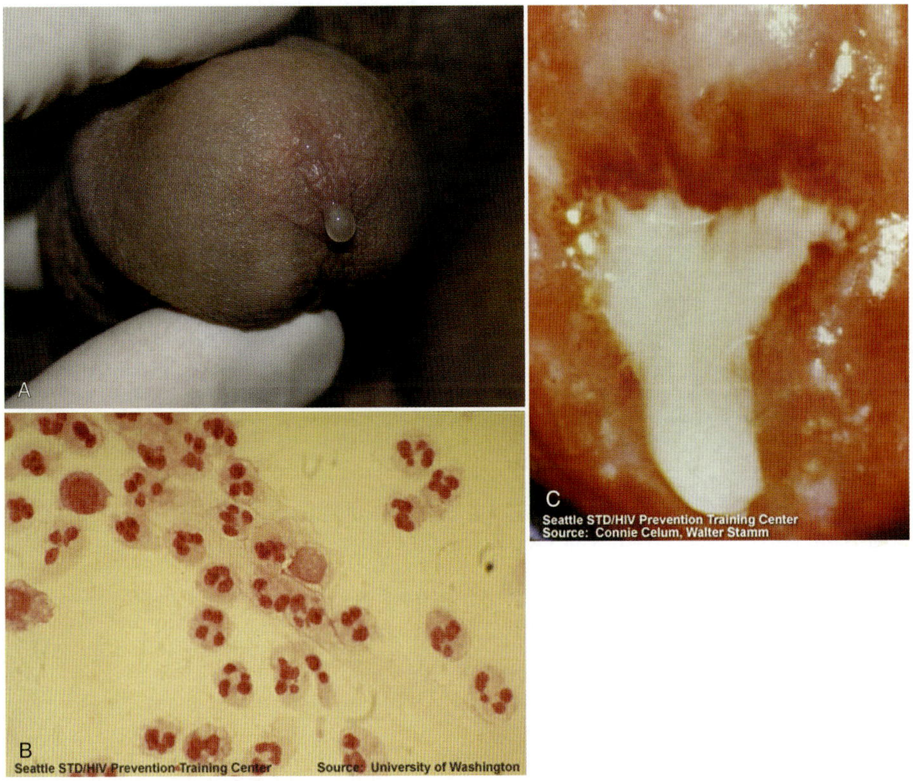


**Fig. 23.22** (From *Practitioner's Handbook for the Management of Sexually Transmitted Disease.* University of Washington STD Prevention Training Center. http://depts.washington.edu/handbook. Accessed March 18, 2015.)

**BOX 23.3** Centers for Disease Control and Prevention Recommended Dual Treatment of Uncomplicated Gonococcal Infections of the Cervix, Urethra, and Rectum in Adults (2020)

Ceftriaxone, 500 mg IM, single dose

Modified from St. Cyr S, Barbee L, Workowski KA, et al. Update to Treatment guidelines for gonococcal infection, 2020. *MMWR Morb Mortal Wkly Rep*. 2020;69:1911–1916.
*IM,* Intramuscularly.

- The CDC no longer recommends follow-up test of cure, but because of a high rate of reinfection, frequent rescreening is prudent.
- Women with positive test for gonorrhea should have a serologic test for syphilis in 4 to 6 weeks
- *N. gonorrhoeae* attaches to the columnar epithelium, so a vaginal cuff swab in women with prior hysterectomies is not recommended

**BOX 23.4** Recommended Regimens for Treatment of Chlamydial Infection

Azithromycin, 1 g PO, single dose*
*or*
Doxycycline, 100 mg PO bid for 7 days

**ALTERNATIVE REGIMENS**

Erythromycin base, 500 mg PO qid for 7 days
*or*
Erythromycin ethylsuccinate, 800 mg PO qid for 7 days
*or*
Ofloxacin, 300 mg PO bid for 7 days
*or*
Levofloxacin, 500 mg PO once daily for 7 days

Modified from Workowski KA, Bolan GA, Centers for Disease Control and Prevention. Sexually transmitted diseases treatment guidelines, 2015. *MMWR Recomm Rep*. 2015;64(RR-03):1-137.
*Consider concurrent treatment for gonococcal infection if prevalence of gonorrhea is high in the patient population under assessment.
*bid,* Twice per day; *PO,* per os (orally); *qid,* four times per day.

### Chlamydia Trachomatis

- The gold standard test is NAAT.
- Similar to *N. gonorrhoeae*, *C. trachomatis* attaches to the columnar epithelium; hence, vaginal cuff specimens from women who have had a hysterectomy are not appropriate.
- ***C. trachomatis* is often asymptomatic**. The CDC recommends annual screening of all sexually active women 25 years of age or younger and screening of older women with risk factors (e.g., those who have a new sex partner or multiple partners).
- **For all women with a chlamydial or gonorrheal infection, partners should be treated. Instruct patients to refer all sex partners of the past 60 days for evaluation and treatment and to avoid sexual intercourse until therapy is completed and they and their partner have resolution of symptoms.**
- Studies have demonstrated that patient-delivered partner therapy results in lower rates of chlamydial persistence or recurrence.
- All women with *C. trachomatis*, *N. gonorrhoeae*, or mucopurulent cervicitis of unknown origin need evaluation to rule out pelvic inflammatory disease.
- The preferred CDC treatment for *C. trachomatis* is azithromycin, 1 g orally, single dose (Box 23.4).

## ENDOMETRITIS

Endometritis is an upper genital tract infection of the uterine lining and occurs once an infection ascends through the cervix into the endometrium or into the salpinx. Although endometritis commonly coexists with salpingitis, several studies support endometritis as a distinct clinical syndrome with distinct risk factors (douching in past 30 days, current intrauterine device [IUD] in place, and douching in days 1 to 7 of the menstrual cycle) and clinical manifestations intermediate in frequency between women with salpingitis and those with neither salpingitis nor endometritis. An endometrial biopsy (EMB) is the diagnostic gold standard for endometritis with a histopathologic criterion of at least one plasma cell per ×120 field of endometrial stroma combined with five or more neutrophils in the superficial endometrial epithelium per ×400 field. **Because many of the symptoms and signs associated with endometritis are subtle, a clinician needs to have a low threshold for performing an endometrial biopsy to aid in the diagnosis.** As many as 40% of women with cervicitis without upper tract symptoms will have endometritis noted on endometrial biopsy.

Many women with tubal infertility have no history of clinical symptoms consistent with prior PID; hence, the concept of subclinical endometritis has evolved. Large, cross-sectional studies of women without symptoms or signs of acute salpingitis have defined subclinical endometritis further. These studies, mostly conducted in STI clinics or emergency rooms in women at risk for PID, found endometritis associated with young age (20 to 22 years old in most studies), abnormal uterine bleeding (menorrhagia or metrorrhagia or mid-cycle spotting), menstrual cycle day less than 14, douching in the past 30 days, and a history of prior PID.

Lower genital tract infections with *C. trachomatis*, *N. gonorrhoeae*, bacterial vaginosis, *M. genitalium*, and *T. vaginalis* and mucopurulent cervicitis are associated with histologic endometritis with an odds ratio (OR) of 1.5 to 3.0, depending on the study. One study demonstrated that in women with current *N. gonorrhoeae* or *C. trachomatis* infection, endometritis was apparent in 43% of those with a history of prior PID and 23% of those without prior PID. This is suggestive of possible immunologic memory. Some women with endometritis do not have an isolated pathogen.

Antimicrobial therapy for endometritis is effective, with studies demonstrating reduction in abnormal bleeding, cervicitis, uterine tenderness, and histologic endometritis after broad-spectrum outpatient treatment. Endometritis in HIV-seropositive women has not been well characterized, but in one series of 42 seropositive women, none of whom had *C. trachomatis* or *N. gonorrhoeae*, 38% had endometritis and 50% had histologic resolution after outpatient therapy. Women with endometritis found on EMB should be treated using one of the CDC recommended treatment regimens for PID. In one large treatment study of women with endometritis (the PEACH study), the group with clinically suspected mild PID, endometritis, or upper genital tract infection treated with standard antimicrobial therapy did not have increased reproductive morbidity. **This supports routine use of outpatient therapy when the patient is able to tolerate oral medication.**

## PELVIC INFLAMMATORY DISEASE

PID is an infection in the upper genital tract not associated with pregnancy or intraperitoneal pelvic operations. Thus it may include infection of any or all of the following anatomic locations: endometrium (endometritis; see the previous section), oviducts (salpingitis), ovary (oophoritis), uterine wall (myometritis), uterine serosa and broad ligaments (parametritis), and pelvic peritoneum. Many authors prefer the term *salpingitis* because infection of the oviducts is the most characteristic and common component of PID. Importantly, most long-term sequelae of PID result from destruction of the tubal architecture by the infection. In most clinical situations, the terms *acute salpingitis* and *pelvic inflammatory disease* are used synonymously to describe an acute infection. Acute PID results from ascending infection from the bacterial flora of the vagina and cervix in more than 99% of cases; it is rare in the woman without menstrual periods, such as the pregnant, premenarcheal, or postmenopausal woman. In less than 1% of cases, acute PID results from transperitoneal spread of infectious material from a perforated appendix or intraabdominal abscess.

- The incidence of PID in the United States is decreasing; however, the prevalence of STIs and corresponding PID remains a major public health concern. Annually, acute PID occurs in 1% to 2% of all young, sexually active women. It is the most common serious infection of women ages 16 to 25 years. Reduction of the medical impact of acute PID requires aggressive therapy for lower genital tract infection and early diagnosis and treatment of upper genital tract infection.
- Public health emphasis also must be placed on primary prevention of PID involving attempts to prevent exposure and acquisition of STIs such as safe sex practices and promoting the use of condoms.
- Secondary prevention of PID involves the universal screening of women at high risk for chlamydia and gonorrhea, screening for active cervicitis, increasing use of sensitive tests to diagnose lower genital infection, treatment of sexual partners, and education to prevent recurrent infection.

Although specific disease aspects of PID are discussed later, the CDC has emphasized that **physicians should treat women aggressively if there is any suspicion of the disease because the sequelae are so devastating and the clinical diagnosis made from symptoms, signs, and laboratory data is imprecise and often incorrect.**

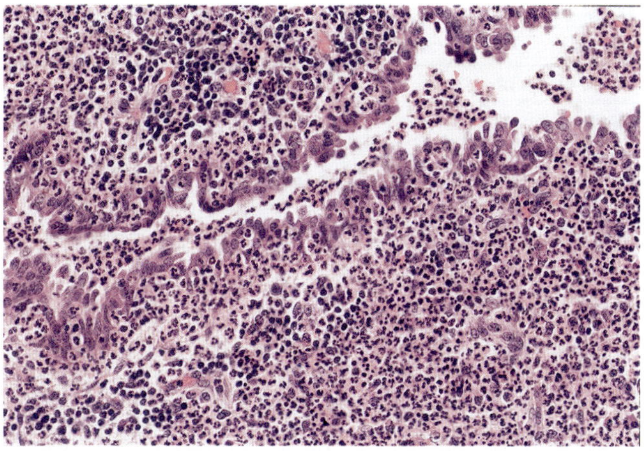

**Fig. 23.23** Acute salpingitis with a mixture of neutrophils, lymphocytes, and plasma cells in the fallopian tube destroying some of the epithelial lining. (From Voet RL. *Color Atlas of Obstetric and Gynecologic Pathology.* St. Louis: Mosby; 1997:107.)

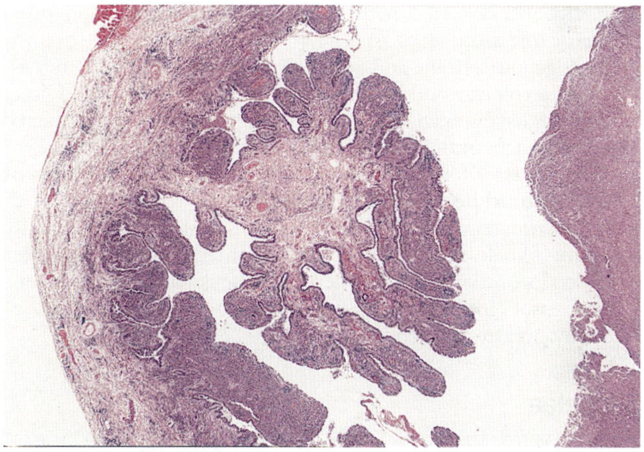

**Fig. 23.24** Acute salpingitis showing dilation of the fallopian tube and blunting of the papillary fronds. (From Voet RL. *Color Atlas of Obstetric and Gynecologic Pathology.* St. Louis: Mosby; 1997:102.)

### Etiology

The two classic sexually transmitted organisms associated with PID, *N. gonorrhoeae* and *C. trachomatis*, cause acute PID in many cases.

- **Approximately 15% of women with cervical infection by *N. gonorrhoeae* subsequently develop acute PID.** The virulence of the strain or colony type of *N. gonorrhoeae* helps predict the incidence of upper genital tract infection. Antibodies against the outer membrane protein of the gonococcus develop in approximately 70% of women after severe pelvic infection. The lack of significant antibody titers may help explain why teenagers are more likely to develop upper genital tract disease than women in their late 20s.
  - The gonococcus ascends to the fallopian tube, and damage occurs to the ciliated cells, most likely because of an acute complement-mediated inflammatory response with the migration of PMN leukocytes, vasodilation, and transudation of plasma into the tissues (Figs. 23.23 and 23.24).
  - This robust inflammatory response causes cell death and tissue damage. The process of repair with removal of dead cells and fibroblast presence results in scarring and tubal adhesions.
  - *N. gonorrhoeae* remains in the fallopian tubes for at most a few days in untreated patients.
- **Approximately 30% of women with documented acute cervicitis secondary to chlamydia subsequently develop acute PID.** From 10% to 30% of women with acute PID who do not have cultures positive for *Chlamydia* have evidence of acute chlamydial infection by serial antibody titer testing.
  - Upper tract chlamydial infection increases the risk of an ectopic pregnancy by three to six times compared with women without chlamydial infection.
  - *Chlamydia* may remain in the fallopian tubes for months after initial colonization of the upper genital tract.
  - Cell-mediated immune mechanisms appear to be important in tissue destruction associated with *C. trachomatis* infection.
  - Because chlamydial 57-kDa protein and human 60-kDa heat shock protein have homologous regions, repeated exposures to *Chlamydia*, such as may occur in asymptomatic untreated *C. trachomatis* cervical infection, may lead to an autoimmune response that causes severe tubal damage, even if *C. trachomatis* is no longer present.
  - The specific chlamydial strain also may be an important variable.

**TABLE 23.8** Microorganisms Isolated from Fallopian Tubes of Patients with Acute Pelvic Inflammatory Disease

| Type of Agent | Organism |
|---|---|
| Sexually transmitted disease | *Chlamydia trachomatis*<br>*Neisseria gonorrhoeae*<br>*Mycoplasma hominis* |
| Endogenous agent aerobic or facultative | *Streptococcus* species<br>*Staphylococcus* species<br>*Haemophilus*<br>*Escherichia coli* |
| Anaerobic | *Bacteroides* species<br>*Peptococcus* species<br>*Peptostreptococcus* species<br>*Clostridium* species<br>*Actinomyces* species |

From Weström L. Introductory address: treatment of pelvic inflammatory disease in view of etiology and risk factors. *Sex Transm Dis.* 1984; 11(4 Suppl):437-440.

- The role of genital mycoplasmas *Mycoplasma hominis* and *Ureaplasma urealyticum* as the cause of acute PID is unclear.
- *M. genitalium*, which is noncultivable and identified by PCR, has been associated with cervicitis, endometritis, and tubal factor infertility.
- Endogenous aerobic and anaerobic flora of the vagina often ascend to colonize and infect the upper reproductive tract. Direct cultures have shown that tubal infections are usually polymicrobial throughout the active infectious process (Table 23.8).
- **Regardless of the initiating event, the microbiology of PID should be treated as mixed.**
- Approximately 85% of infections are spontaneous in sexually active females. The other 15% of infections develop after procedures that break the cervical mucus barrier, such as endometrial biopsy, curettage, IUD insertion, hysterosalpingography, and hysteroscopy.

## Sequelae

**One in four women with acute PID experiences medical sequelae.**

- After acute PID, the rate of ectopic pregnancy increases 6- to 10-fold.
- Approximately 10% to 15% of pregnancies will be ectopic after laparoscopically mild to moderate PID, and almost 50% after severe PID.
- The chance of developing chronic pelvic pain increases fourfold after acute PID.
- In the United States each year 26,100 ectopic pregnancies and 90,000 new cases of chronic abdominal pain are directly related to PID.
- Infertility incidence after acute PID varies widely (6% to 60%), depending on the severity of the infection, number of episodes of infection, and age of the woman. Weström reported that hospitalized patients have an incidence of infertility caused by tubal obstruction of 11.4% after one episode of PID, 23.1% after two episodes, and 54.3% after three or more episodes (Fig. 23.25).
- Approximately 25% of women with acute PID subsequently develop another acute tubal infection.
  See Tables 23.9 to Table 23.12.

## Diagnosis

- The diagnosis of acute PID, even by experienced clinicians, is imprecise. The differential diagnosis of acute PID includes lower genital tract pelvic infection, ectopic pregnancy, torsion or rupture of an adnexal mass, acute appendicitis, gastroenteritis, and endometriosis.
- CDC treatment guidelines state that empirical therapy for PID should be initiated in sexually active young women and other women at risk for STIs with pelvic or lower abdominal pain if cervical motion tenderness, uterine tenderness, or adnexal tenderness is present. The CDC 2015 diagnostic criteria are summarized in Box 23.5.
- The most common symptom of acute PID is new-onset lower abdominal and pelvic pain.
- On pelvic examination, bilateral tenderness of the parametria and adnexa is present and may be exacerbated with movement of the uterus or cervix.
  - If the pain has been present for longer than 3 weeks, it is unlikely that the woman has acute PID.

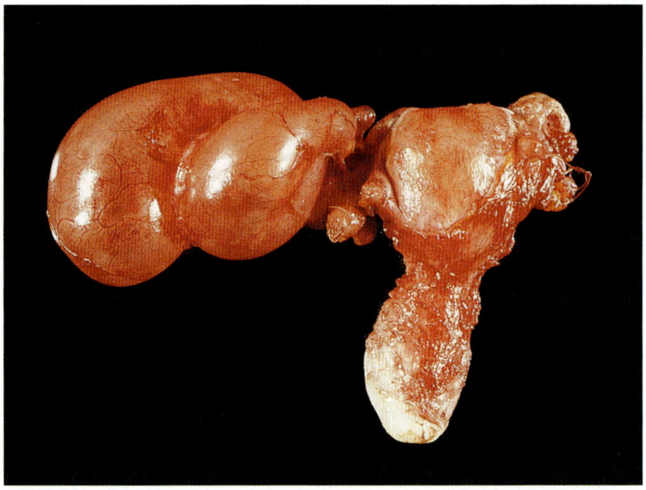

**Fig. 23.25** Hydrosalpinx with marked dilation of the fallopian tube and blunting of the fimbriated end. (From Voet RL. *Color Atlas of Obstetric and Gynecologic Pathology.* St. Louis: Mosby; 1997:107.)

**TABLE 23.9** Summary of Reproductive Events after Index Laparoscopy in the Total Sample of 1732 Patients and 601 Control Subjects

| Category | No. of Patients (%) | No. of Control Subjects (%) |
|---|---|---|
| Total no. followed | 1732 | 601 |
| Avoiding pregnancy | 370 (21.4) | 144 (24.0) |
| Not pregnant for unknown reasons* | 53 (3.1) | 6 (1.0) |
| Attempting pregnancy | 1309 | 451 |
| Pregnant | 1100 (80.8) | 439 (96.1) |
| First pregnancy ectopic | 100 (9.1) | 6 (1.4) |
| Not pregnant | 209 (16.0) | 12 (2.7) |
| Completely examined | 162 | 3 |
| With proved TFI | 141 | 0 |
| With nTFI (other cause of infertility) | 21 | 3 |
| Incompletely examined | 47 | 9 |

From Weström L, Joesoef R, Reynolds G, et al. Pelvic inflammatory disease and fertility: a cohort study of 1,844 women with laparoscopically verified disease and 657 control women with normal laparoscopic results. *Sex Transm Dis.* 1992;19(4):185-192.

*Reporting no use of contraceptive and not consulting for infertility.
*nTFI,* Nontubular factor infertility; *TFI,* tubal factor infertility.

**TABLE 23.10** Frequency and Predictors of Long-Term Sequelae of Acute Pelvic Inflammatory Disease

| | | | Univariate Analysis | | |
|---|---|---|---|---|---|
| **Sequela** | **Frequency (No. and %)** | **Risk Factor** | ***P*** | **Relative Risk and 95% Confidence Interval** | **Multivariate Analysis *P* Value** |
| Involuntary infertility | 17/42 (40%) | History of PID | 0.05 | 1.8 (1.0-3.3) | 0.05 |
| | | Age at time of first sex | 0.04 | 0.39 | 0.07 |
| | | ≥2 days of pain before therapy | 0.02 | 2.0 (1.1-3.6) | |
| Chronic pelvic pain | 12/51 (24%) | History of PID | 0.03 | 1.5 (1.0-2.2) | |
| PID after index episode | 22/51 (43%) | History of PID | 0.06 | 1.7 (0.9-3.1) | 0.02 |
| | | Mean no. of days of pain before therapy | 0.04 | — | 0.04 |
| | | Age at time of first sex | 0.0008 | — | 0.01 |
| Ectopic pregnancy | 2/51 (2.4%) | * | | | |

From Safrin S Schacter J, Dahrouge D, Sweet RL. Long-term sequelae of acute inflammatory disease: a retrospective cohort study. *Am J Obstet Gynecol.* 1992;166(4):1300-1305.
*Risk analysis not performed because of small numbers involved.
*PID,* Pelvic inflammatory disease.

**TABLE 23.11** Standardized (Indirect Standardization) First Event Rates per 1000 Woman-Years for Specified Outcomes*

| Outcome Condition | Women with PID (N = 1,200) | Women with Control Conditions (N = 10,507) | Relative Risk |
|---|---|---|---|
| Nonspecific abdominal pain | 16.7 (155) | 1.7 (158) | 9.8 |
| Gynecologic pain | 3.6 (38) | 0.8 (70) | 4.5 |
| Endometriosis | 2.2 (18) | 0.4 (34) | 5.5 |
| Hysterectomy | 18.2 (152) | 2.3 (204) | 7.9 |
| Ectopic pregnancy | 1.9 (19) | 0.2 (14) | 9.5 |

From Buchan H, Vessey M, Goldacre M, et al. Morbidity following pelvic inflammatory disease. *Br J Obstet Gynaecol.* 1993;100(6):558-562.
*After admission with acute pelvic inflammatory disease or a control event in cohorts of women in the Oxford Record Linkage Study followed from 1970 to 1985. Number of women shown in parentheses.

**TABLE 23.12** Percentage and Number of Patients Attempting to Conceive*

| | Age (Years) | | |
|---|---|---|---|
| **No. of Episodes of PID** | **<25 % (n/N)** | **≥25 % (n/N)** | **Total % (n/N)** |
| One | 7.7 (59/771) | 9.1 (20/220) | 8.0 (79/991) |
| Mild | 0.8 (2/241) | 0.0 (0/71) | 0.6 (2/312) |
| Moderate | 6.4 (23/361) | 5.6 (5/89) | 6.2 (28/452) |
| Severe | 20.1 (34/169) | 25.0 (15/60) | 21.4 (49/229) |
| Two | 18.4 (29/158) | 25.9 (7/27) | 19.5 (36/185) |
| Three or more | 37.7 (23/61) | 75.0 (3/4) | 40.0 (26/65) |
| Total | 11.2 (111/990) | 12.0 (30/251) | 11.4 (141/1241) |

From Weström L, Joesoef R, Reynolds G, et al. Pelvic inflammatory disease and fertility: a cohort study of 1,844 women with laparoscopically verified disease and 657 control women with normal laparoscopic results. *Sex Transm Dis.* 1992;19(4):185-192.
*Women had tubal factor infertility by age, number of acute PID episodes, and severity of PID, excluding those with nontubal factor infertility and with incomplete infertility examinations.
*n,* Total number of cases followed; *N,* total number of evaluable cases; *PID,* pelvic inflammatory disease.

- Approximately 75% of patients with acute PID have an associated endocervical infection or coexistent purulent vaginal discharge.
- **Abnormal uterine bleeding, especially spotting or menorrhagia, is noted in approximately 40% of patients.**
   - Acute pelvic infection secondary to *N. gonorrhoeae* is of rapid onset, and the pelvic pain usually begins a few days after the start of a menstrual period.
   - Acute pelvic infection caused by *C. trachomatis* alone often may have an indolent course with slow onset, less pain, and less fever.
   - Approximately 5% to 10% of women with acute PID develop symptoms of perihepatic inflammation, Fitz-Hugh–Curtis syndrome (Fig. 23.26), with right upper quadrant pain, pleuritic pain, and tenderness in the right upper quadrant when the liver is palpated. The pain may radiate to the shoulder or into the back. Liver transaminase levels may be elevated.
- The incidence of true adnexal abscess is approximately 10% in women with acute PID.
- **It is important to remember that up to 50% of women with tubal damage never experience any symptoms consistent with PID.**
- Laparoscopy with direct visualization of the internal female organs improves diagnostic accuracy and presents an opportunity for direct culture of purulent material. In practice, most women with acute PID do not undergo laparoscopy because of the invasiveness and expense of this technique. **Endometrial biopsy is more readily available as a diagnostic tool.**
- Laparoscopic studies of women with a clinical diagnosis of acute PID have established the inadequacy of diagnosis by the usual criteria of history, physical examination, and laboratory studies. In these studies, approximately 20% to 25% of women had no identifiable intraabdominal or pelvic disease. Another 10% to 15% of patients were found to have other pathologic conditions, such as ectopic pregnancy, acute appendicitis, or torsion of the adnexa (Tables 23.13 and 23.14).

**BOX 23.5** Centers for Disease Control and Prevention Guidelines for Diagnosis of Acute Pelvic Inflammatory Disease: Clinical Criteria for Initiating Therapy

**MINIMUM CRITERIA**

Empirical treatment of PID should be initiated in sexually active young women and others at risk for STIs if the following minimum criteria are present and no other causes(s) for the illness can be identified:
Lower abdominal tenderness *or*
Adnexal tenderness *or*
Cervical motion tenderness

**ADDITIONAL CRITERIA FOR DIAGNOSING PID**

Oral temperature >38° C
Abnormal cervical or vaginal discharge (mucopurulent)
Presence of abundant WBCs on microscopy of vaginal secretions
Elevated erythrocyte sedimentation rate
Elevated C-reactive protein
Laboratory documentation of cervical infection with *Neisseria gonorrhoeae* or *Chlamydia trachomatis*

**DEFINITIVE CRITERIA FOR DIAGNOSING PID**

Histopathologic evidence of endometritis on endometrial biopsy
Transvaginal sonography or MRI showing thickened fluid-filled tubes, with or without free pelvic fluid or tubo-ovarian complex
Laparoscopic abnormalities consistent with PID
Although initial treatment can be made before bacteriologic diagnosis of *C. trachomatis* or *N. gonorrhoeae* infection, such a diagnosis emphasizes the need to treat sex partners.

Data from Workowski KA, Bolan GA, Centers for Disease Control and Prevention. Sexually transmitted diseases treatment guidelines, 2015. *MMWR Recomm Rep.* 2015;64(RR-03):1-137.
*MRI,* Magnetic resonance imaging; *PID,* pelvic inflammatory disease; *STIs,* sexually transmitted infections; *WBCs,* white blood cells.

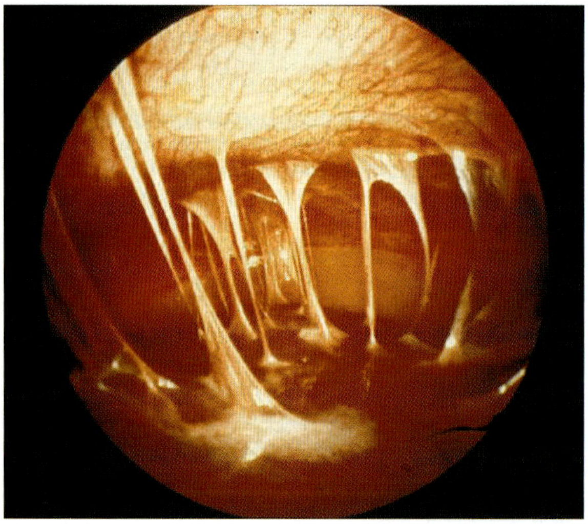

**Fig. 23.26** Classic violin string sign of Fitz-Hugh–Curtis syndrome in pelvic inflammatory disease.

- Laparoscopic studies also demonstrate a lack of correlation among the number and intensity of symptoms, signs, and degree of abnormality of laboratory values and the severity of tubal inflammation.
- Other factors that improve the likelihood of diagnosis but are insensitive and nonspecific include elevated temperature, elevated white blood cell (WBC) count, and elevated erythrocyte sedimentation rate. The presence of an increased number of vaginal WBCs is the most sensitive laboratory indicator of acute PID.
- Ultrasonography is of limited value for patients with mild or moderate PID because of its low sensitivity, but vaginal ultrasonography is helpful in documenting an adnexal mass (Fig. 23.27).
- **If the cervical discharge appears normal and no WBCs are found on the wet preparation of vaginal fluid, the diagnosis of PID is unlikely, and alternative causes of pain should be considered.**

**TABLE 23.13** Laparoscopic Findings in Patients with False-Positive Clinical Diagnosis of Acute Pelvic Inflammatory Disease (PID) but with Pelvic Disorders Other Than PID

| Laparoscopic Finding | Number |
|---|---|
| Acute appendicitis | 24 |
| Endometriosis | 16 |
| Corpus luteum bleeding | 12 |
| Ectopic pregnancy | 11 |
| Pelvic adhesions only | 7 |
| Benign ovarian tumor | 7 |
| Chronic salpingitis | 6 |
| Miscellaneous | 15 |
| Total | 98 |

From Jacobson LJ. Differential diagnosis of acute pelvic inflammatory disease. *Am J Obstet Gynecol.* 1980;138(7 Pt 2):1006-1011.

**TABLE 23.14** Preoperative Diagnoses in Patients with False-Negative Clinical Diagnosis of Acute Pelvic Inflammatory Disease Prior to Laparoscopy/Laparotomy

| Clinical Diagnosis | Visual Diagnosis: Acute PID (Number) |
|---|---|
| Ovarian tumor | 20 |
| Acute appendicitis | 18 |
| Ectopic pregnancy | 16 |
| Chronic salpingitis | 10 |
| Acute peritonitis | 6 |
| Endometriosis | 5 |
| Uterine myoma | 5 |
| Uncharacteristic pelvic pain | 5 |
| Miscellaneous | 6 |
| Total | 91 |

From Jacobson LJ. Differential diagnosis of acute pelvic inflammatory disease. *Am J Obstet Gynecol.* 1980;138(7 Pt 2):1006-1011.
*PID,* Pelvic inflammatory disease.

## Risk Factors

- In epidemiologic studies, age at first intercourse, marital status, and number of sexual partners are all gross indicators of the frequency of exposure to STIs and PID.
  - The age distribution of uncomplicated STI is usually the same as that for acute PID. It is a condition of young women, with 75% of cases occurring in women younger than 25 years.

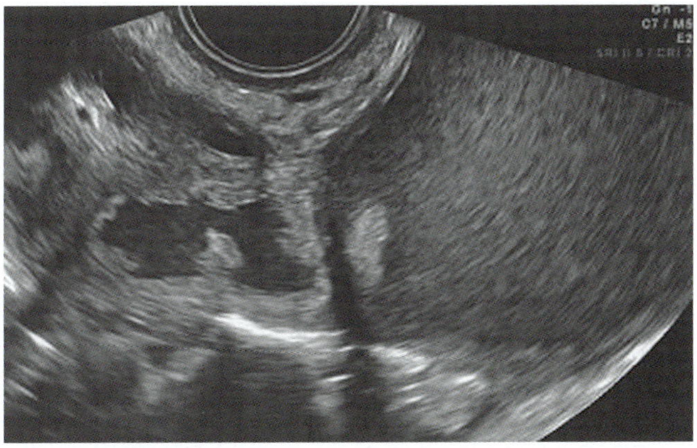

**Fig. 23.27.** Pyosalpinx ultrasound: hydrosalpinx.

- The risk that a sexually active adolescent female will develop acute PID is 1 in 8, which decreases to 1 in 80 for women older than 25 years.
- Multiple sexual partners increase the chance of acquiring acute PID by approximately fivefold.
- Condom use prevents the deposition and transmission of infected organisms from the semen to the endocervix.
- Women with frequent vaginal douching have a threefold to fourfold increased relative risk of PID compared with women who douche less frequently than once a month.
- Increased PID with IUD use occurs only at time of insertion. An analysis from the World Health Organization (WHO) has found the rate of PID to be 9.7 in 1000 woman-years for the first 20 days after insertion compared with 1.4 in 1000 woman-years for the next 8 years of follow-up.
- Social factors such as involvement with a child protective agency, prior suicide attempt, and alcohol use before intercourse have also been identified in case-control studies as risk factors for PID.
- The frequency of intercourse with a monogamous partner is not a risk factor.
- Acute salpingitis occurring in a woman with a previous tubal ligation is extremely rare and, when it does occur, the symptoms of the infection are less severe.
- The incidence of upper genital tract infection associated with first-trimester terminations is approximately 1 in 200 cases. Clinical practice has emphasized the use of prophylactic antibiotics to decrease the incidence of associated acute PID. Women with concurrent bacterial vaginosis have a higher risk for postabortal infection and thus should be treated with oral antibiotics with anaerobic coverage.
- Women with HIV and PID have a higher incidence of adnexal masses but respond to antibiotic therapy in a similar fashion to that in women who are not infected with HIV.

## Treatment

**The two most important goals of the medical therapy of acute PID are the resolution of symptoms and preservation of tubal function.**

- **Timely initiation of antibiotic therapy as soon STI screening results have been obtained and the diagnosis has been suggested.**
  - Women who are not treated in the first 72 hours after the onset of symptoms are three times as likely to develop tubal infertility or ectopic pregnancy as those who are treated early in the disease process.
  - Determining the need for hospitalization, patient education, treatment of sexual partners, and careful follow-up are key issues.

**BOX 23.6** Centers for Disease Control and Prevention Recommendations for Ambulatory Management of Acute Pelvic Inflammatory Disease

Ceftriaxone, 250 mg IM, single dose
*or*
Cefoxitin, 2 g IM, single dose, and probenecid, 1 g PO administered concurrently in a single dose
*or*
Other parenteral third-generation cephalosporin (e.g., ceftizoxime, cefotaxime)
*plus*
Doxycycline, 100 mg PO bid for 14 days
*with or without*
Metronidazole, 500 mg PO bid for 14 days

Modified from Workowski KA, Bolan GA, Centers for Disease Control and Prevention. Sexually transmitted diseases treatment guidelines, 2015. *MMWR Recomm Rep.* 2015;64(RR-03):1-137.
*bid,* Twice daily; *IM,* intramuscularly; *PO,* per os (orally).

Treatment and education of the male partner for the prevention of the disease, including the use of proper contraceptives, which help reduce the rate of upper genital tract infection. **Because most cases of PID are polymicrobial, broad-spectrum antibiotic coverage is indicated.**

**Outpatient treatment is appropriate if the patient can tolerate oral therapy.** The CDC has published recommendations for the outpatient treatment of PID (Box 23.6).

- Ceftriaxone, 250 mg IM once, or cefoxitin, 2 g IM, plus probenecid, 1 g orally in a single dose, concurrently once, or another parenteral third-generation cephalosporin such as ceftizoxime or cefotaxime together with doxycycline, 100 mg orally twice daily for 14 days, is the recommended outpatient regimen.
- The optimal cephalosporin choice is not known. Importantly, if the woman has BV, adding prolonged coverage with metronidazole, 500 mg orally twice daily for 14 days, is preferable. Other regimens with at least one trial include amoxicillin–clavulanic acid and doxycycline. Azithromycin has demonstrated short-term effectiveness in one randomized trial; another trial used azithromycin combined with ceftriaxone, 250 mg IM single dose, with azithromycin, 1 g orally once weekly for 2 weeks. Also, with these regimens, consider the addition of metronidazole, because anaerobic organisms are suspected in the cause of PID and metronidazole will also treat BV, which is often associated with PID.
- Quinolone-containing regimens are no longer routinely recommended because of gonorrhea resistance; however, if parenteral cephalosporin therapy is not feasible, the use of fluoroquinolones (levofloxacin, 500 mg orally once daily, or ofloxacin, 400 mg twice daily for 14 days), with or without metronidazole, may be considered if the community prevalence and individual risk of gonorrhea are low, or if the diagnostic test result for gonorrhea performed before instituting therapy is negative.
- Reexamine the women within 48 to 72 hours of initiating outpatient therapy to evaluate the response of the disease to oral antibiotics.
- If a patient develops PID with an IUD in place, outpatient therapy leaving the IUD in situ may be attempted if close follow-up of the woman is possible. If the pelvic infection worsens or does not improve, the IUD should be removed.

The CDC has established criteria for hospitalization (Box 23.7) These include unsure diagnosis, being too ill to tolerate oral therapy, no improvement with oral therapy, and presence of a tubo-ovarian abscess or pregnancy. In the past, many practitioners

**BOX 23.7** Indications for Hospitalizing Patients With Acute Pelvic Inflammatory Disease

The patient is pregnant.

Surgical emergencies (e.g., appendicitis) cannot be excluded.
The patient is pregnant.
The patient does not respond clinically to oral antimicrobial therapy.
The patient is unable to follow or tolerate an outpatient oral regimen.
The patient has severe illness, nausea and vomiting, or high fever.
The patient has a tubo-ovarian abscess.

Data from Workowski KA, Bolan GA, Centers for Disease Control and Prevention. Sexually transmitted diseases treatment guidelines, 2015. *MMWR Recomm Rep.* 2015;64(RR-03):1-137.

**BOX 23.8** Inpatient Management of Acute Pelvic Inflammatory Disease

**PARENTERAL REGIMEN A**

Cefotetan, 2 g IV every 12 hours
*or*
Cefoxitin, 2 g IV every 6 hours
*plus*
Doxycycline, 100 mg PO or IV every 12 hours

Note: Because of pain associated with infusion, doxycycline should be administered orally when possible, even when the patient is hospitalized. PO and IV administration of doxycycline provide similar bioavailability.

**Parenteral Regimen B**

Clindamycin, 900 mg IV every 8 hours
*plus*
Gentamicin, loading dose IV or IM (2 mg/kg of body weight) followed by a maintenance dose (1.5 mg/kg) every 8 hours; single daily dosing (3–5 mg/kg) may be substituted

**ALTERNATIVE PARENTERAL REGIMENS**

Limited data support the use of other parenteral regimens. The following regimen has been investigated in a least one clinical trial and has broad-spectrum coverage:
Ampicillin-sulbactam, 3 g IV every 6 hours
*plus*
Doxycycline, 100 mg PO or IV every 12 hours

One trial has demonstrated high short-term clinical cure rates with azithromycin, either as monotherapy for 1 week (500 mg IV × one or two doses followed by 250 mg PO for 5-6 days) or combined with a 12-day course of metronidazole.

Modified from Workowski KA, Bolan GA, Centers for Disease Control and Prevention. Sexually transmitted diseases treatment guidelines, 2015. *MMWR Recomm Rep.* 2015;64(RR-03):1-137.
*IM*, Intramuscularly; *IV*, intravenously; *PO*, per os (orally).

preferred to hospitalize nulliparous women for the treatment of PID, but this is no longer recommended because **studies have not shown future fertility advantage with inpatient treatment.**

The CDC guidelines for inpatient treatment of acute PID with parenteral therapy are listed in Box 23.8. **The protocols stress the polymicrobial origin of acute pelvic infection**, increasing importance of *C. trachomatis*, and emergence of penicillin-resistant *N. gonorrhoeae*. With intravenous (IV) protocols, the CDC recommends that IV antibiotics be continued for at least 24 hours after substantial improvement in the patient. When the woman has a mass, we add ampicillin to clindamycin and gentamicin; however, for patients without a mass, we switch to oral antibiotics when the symptoms have diminished and the woman has been afebrile for 24 hours. In both regimens, doxycycline is continued for a total of 14 days.

**Regimen A is a combination of doxycycline and IV cefoxitin. It is excellent for community-acquired infection.** Doxycycline and cefoxitin provide excellent coverage for *N. gonorrhoeae*, *C. trachomatis*, and penicillinase-producing *N. gonorrhoeae*. Cefoxitin is an excellent antibiotic against *Peptococcus* and *Peptostreptococcus* spp. and *E. coli*. The disadvantage of this combination is that the two drugs are less than ideal for a pelvic abscess or anaerobic infections. To date, cefotetan has been found to be as effective as cefoxitin. **There is no clinically significant difference in the bioavailability of doxycycline whether it is given by the oral or IV route. Thus doxycycline should be administered orally whenever possible because of the marked superficial phlebitis produced by IV infusion.**

Doxycycline should be included in the regimen of follow-up oral therapy; prolonged therapeutic levels of the antichlamydial antibiotic are imperative.

**Regimen B is a combination of clindamycin and an aminoglycoside (gentamicin).** It has the advantage of providing excellent coverage for anaerobic infections and facultative gram-negative rods. **Therefore it is preferred for patients with an abscess, IUD-related infection, and pelvic infection after a diagnostic or operative procedure.** Studies have demonstrated that high IV levels of clindamycin, such as 900 mg every 8 hours, provide activity against 90% of bacterial strains of *Chlamydia*. Most infectious disease experts recommend the use of a single daily dose of gentamicin rather than a dose given every 8 hours. The initial once-daily aminoglycoside dosage is based on nomograms that take body weight into consideration. The advantages of a once-daily aminoglycoside program are decreased toxicity, increased efficacy, and decreased cost. Also, no serum drug levels must be measured. Parenteral antibiotic therapy may be discontinued when the woman has been afebrile for 24 hours, and oral therapy with doxycycline (100 mg twice daily) should continue to complete 14 days of therapy.

Alternative inpatient regimens include ampicillin-sulbactam plus doxycycline because they have excellent anaerobic coverage and would be a good choice for women with a tubo-ovarian complex. The alternative regimen has less extensive clinical trials.

**In summary, no regimen is uniformly effective for all patients. To date, there are insufficient clinical data to suggest the superiority of one regimen over another with respect to initial response or subsequent fertility.**

Operative treatment of acute PID are restricted to life-threatening infections, ruptured tubo-ovarian abscesses, laparoscopic drainage of a pelvic abscess, persistent masses in some older women for whom future childbearing is not a consideration (Fig. 23.28), and removal of a persistent symptomatic mass. Because of the techniques of in vitro fertilization, every effort is made to perform conservative surgery and preserve ovarian and uterine function in women who are not done with childbearing. Unilateral removal of a tubo-ovarian complex or an abscess is a common conservative procedure for acute PID. Similarly, drainage of a cul-de-sac abscess via percutaneous drainage or a colpotomy incision results in preservation of the reproductive organs. Operative intervention in a postmenopausal woman should be considered early in the disease, especially if the condition does not improve rapidly with medical treatment.

## Abscess Treatment

A tubo-ovarian complex is a collection of pus within an anatomic space created by the adherence of adjacent organs. Abscesses caused by acute PID contain a mixture of anaerobes and facultative or aerobic organisms. Clindamycin penetrates the human

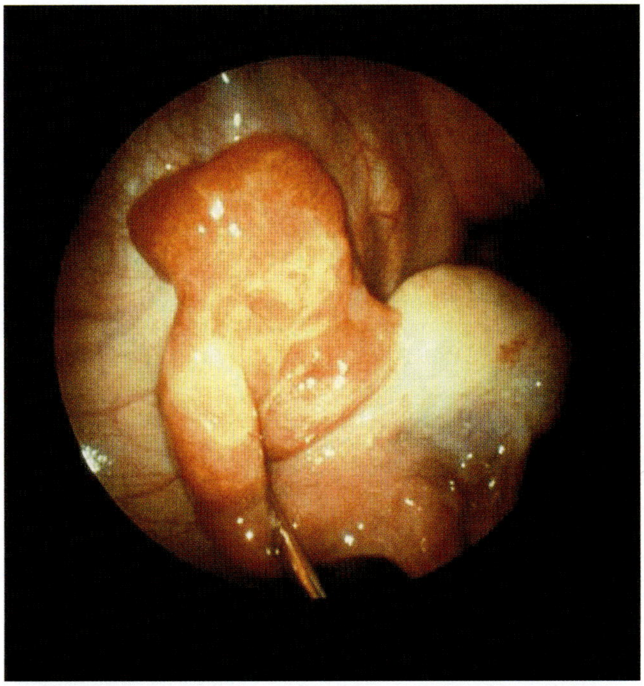

**Fig. 23.28** Laparoscopic view of acute pelvic inflammatory disease and a tubo-ovarian abscess.

neutrophil, and it is possible that this property facilitates the level of clindamycin within the abscess. Clindamycin is also stable in the abscess environment, which is not true of many other antibiotics. Thus a combination of clindamycin and an aminoglycoside is considered the standard for treatment of a tubo-ovarian abscess. This combination does not treat *Enterococcus*, and ampicillin should be added if there is suspicion that this organism is involved. Metronidazole alone is an effective alternative to clindamycin for anaerobic infections but does not provide gram-negative coverage. **If abscesses do not respond to parenteral broad-spectrum antibiotics, drainage is imperative**. Transvaginal or transabdominal percutaneous aspiration or drainage of pelvic abscesses may be accomplished under ultrasonic or computed tomography (CT) guidance. This technique has shown excellent results.

## ACTINOMYCES INFECTION

*Actinomyces* is a rare cause of upper genital tract infection. Most cases described have been in women chronically wearing an IUD for an average of 8 years. Usually, *Actinomyces israelii* is part of a polymicrobial infection, and whether its role is primary or secondary in the infectious process is unknown.

There is controversy about the significance of discovering actinomycetes on a Pap smear of women wearing an IUD. The contrasting, relatively high detection rate of actinomycetes observed on Pap smears from IUD users and the extreme rarity of subsequent development of pelvic actinomycosis has led most experts to conclude that progression to upper tract infection is highly unlikely to be related. Unless there are associated symptoms, such as fever, abdominal pain, or abnormal uterine bleeding, the identification of the organism in any cervical smear should not prompt antibiotic therapy or IUD removal.

## TUBERCULOSIS

Tuberculosis of the upper genital tract, primarily chronic salpingitis and chronic endometritis, is a rare disease in the United States. Most gynecologists may never encounter a single case. Tuberculosis is a common cause of chronic PID and infertility in other parts of the world, and thus it should be suspected in patients who are immigrants, especially those from Asia, the Middle East, and Latin America. Although the disease is usually found in premenopausal women, it occurs in postmenopausal women 10% of the time. The diagnosis may be established by performing an endometrial biopsy late in the secretory phase of the cycle. A portion of the endometrial biopsy should be sent for culture and animal inoculation and the remaining portion should be examined histologically. The findings of classic giant cells, granulomas, and caseous necrosis confirm the diagnosis. Approximately two of three women with tuberculous salpingitis will have concomitant tuberculous endometritis.

The predominant presentations of this chronic infection are infertility and abnormal uterine bleeding. Mild to moderate chronic abdominal and pelvic pain occur in 35% of women with the disease. Advanced cases are often accompanied by ascites. Some women may be asymptomatic. The findings at pelvic examination are normal in approximately 50% of cases. The remaining patients have mild adnexal tenderness and bilateral adnexal masses, with an inability to manipulate the adnexa because of scarring and fixation.

Tuberculous salpingitis may be suspected when a woman is not responding to conventional antibiotic therapy for acute bacterial PID. Results of a tuberculin skin test will be positive. Approximately two of three women with tuberculous salpingitis will have concomitant tuberculous endometritis. The treatment of pelvic tuberculosis is medical. The CDC has recommended starting a woman on a multidrug regimen until the culture results yield specific sensitivity. At that time, medications may be decreased to two or three agents. Patients who have infection from MDR strains are usually kept on a five-drug regimen. Operative therapy for pelvic tuberculosis is reserved for women with persistent pelvic masses, some women with resistant organisms, women older than 40 years, and women whose endometrial cultures remain positive. Although the major sequela of pelvic tuberculosis is infertility, occasionally a woman will become pregnant after medical therapy.

## REFERENCES


Allsworth JE, Peipert JF. Prevalence of bacterial vaginosis: 2001-2004 National Health and Nutrition Examination Survey data. *Obstet Gynecol.* 2007;109(1):114-120.

Bavaro JB, Drolette L, Koelle DM, et al. One-day regimen of valacyclovir for treatment of recurrent genital herpes simplex virus 2 infection. *Sex Transm Dis.* 2008;35(4):383-386.

Bernstein DI, Bellamy AR, Hook EW III, et al. Epidemiology, clinical presentation, and antibody response to primary infection with herpes simplex virus type 1 and type 2 in young women. *Clin Infect Dis.* 2013; 56(3):344-351.

Binstock M, Muzsnai D, Apodaca L, et al. Laparoscopy in the diagnosis and treatment of pelvic inflammatory disease: a review and discussion. *Int J Fertil.* 1986;31(5):341-351.

Chen X, Anstey AV, Bugert JJ. Molluscum contagiosum virus infection. *Lancet Infect Dis.* 2013;13(10):877-888.

Chow TW, Lim BK, Vallipuram S. The masquerades of female pelvic tuberculosis: case reports and review of literature on clinical presentations and diagnosis. *J Obstet Gynaecol Res.* 2002;28(4):203-210.

Eckert LO, Hawes SE, Stevens CE, et al. Vulvovaginal candidiasis: clinical manifestations, risk factors, management algorithm. *Obstet Gynecol.* 1998;92:757.

Evans DT. Actinomyces israelii in the female genital tract: a review. *Genitourin Med.* 1993;69(1):54-59.

Fredricks DN, Fiedler TL, Marrazzo JM. Molecular identification of bacteria associated with bacterial vaginosis. *N Engl J Med.* 2005;353(18): 1899-1911.

Gaydos CA, Beqaj S, Schwebke JR, et al. Clinical validation of a test for the diagnosis of vaginitis. *Obstet Gynecol.* 2017;130(1):181.

Gupta R, Wald A, Krantz E, et al. Valacyclovir and acyclovir for suppression of shedding of herpes simplex virus in the genital tract. *J Infect Dis.* 2004;190(8):1374-1381.

Heller DS, Bean S. Lesions of the Bartholin gland: a review. *J Low Genit Tract Dis.* 2014;18(4):351-357.
Hillier SL. The complexity of microbial diversity in bacterial vaginosis. *N Engl J Med.* 2005;353(18):1886-1887.
Hu S, Bigby M. Treating scabies: results from an updated Cochrane review. *Arch Dermatol.* 2008;144(12):1638-1640; discussion 1640-1631.
Ilhan AH, Durmusoglu F. Case report of a pelvic-peritoneal tuberculosis presenting as an adnexal mass and mimicking ovarian cancer, and a review of the literature. *Infect Dis Obstet Gynecol.* 2004;12(2):87-89.
Kessous R, Aricha-Tamir B, Sheizaf B, et al. Clinical and microbiological characteristics of Bartholin gland abscesses. *Obstet Gynecol.* 2013;122(4):794-799.
Leone PA. Scabies and pediculosis pubis: an update of treatment regimens and general review. *Clin Infect Dis.* 2007;44(Suppl 3):S153-S159.
LeRiche T, Black AY, Fleming NA. Toxic shock syndrome of a probable gynecologic source in an adolescent: a case report and review of the literature. *J Pediatr Adolesc Gynecol.* 2012;25(6):e133-e137.
Marrazzo JM, Thomas KK, Fiedler TL, et al. Risks for acquisition of bacterial vaginosis among women who report sex with women: a cohort study. *PLoS One.* 2010;5(6):e11139.
Phillips AJ, d'Ablaing G III. Acute salpingitis subsequent to tubal ligation. *Obstet Gynecol.* 1986;67(Suppl 3):55S-58S.
Phipps W, Saracino M, Magaret A, et al. Persistent genital herpes simplex virus-2 shedding years following the first clinical episode. *J Infect Dis.* 2011;203(2):180-187.
Prabhu A, Gardella C. Common vaginal and vulvar disorders. *Med Clin North Am.* 2015;99(3):553-574.
Risser WL, Risser JM. The incidence of pelvic inflammatory disease in untreated women infected with Chlamydia trachomatis: a structured review. *Int J STD AIDS.* 2007;18(11):727-731.
Rosumeck S, Nast A, Dressler C. Ivermectin and permethrin for treating scabies. *Cochrane Database Syst Rev.* 2018;(4):CD012994. doi:10.1002/14651858.CD012994.
Sobel JD, Brooker D, Stein GE, et al. Single oral dose fluconazole compared with conventional clotrimazole topical therapy of Candida vaginitis. Fluconazole Vaginitis Study Group. *Am J Obstet Gynecol.* 1995;172(4 Pt 1):1263-1268.
Sobel JD, Chaim W, Nagappan V, et al. Treatment of vaginitis caused by Candida glabrata: use of topical boric acid and flucytosine. *Am J Obstet Gynecol.* 2003;189(5):1297-1300.
Sobel JD, Kapernick PS, Zervos M, et al. Treatment of complicated Candida vaginitis: comparison of single and sequential doses of fluconazole. *Am J Obstet Gynecol.* 2001;185(2):363-369.
Tronstein E, Johnston C, Huang ML, et al. Genital shedding of herpes simplex virus among symptomatic and asymptomatic persons with HSV-2 infection. *JAMA.* 2011;305(14):1441-1449.

# 24 Preoperative Counseling and Management

## Preoperative Evaluation, Informed Consent, Perioperative Planning, Surgical Site Infection Prevention, and Avoidance of Complications

*Jamie N. Bakkum-Gamez, Sean C. Dowdy, Fidel A. Valea*

### KEY POINTS

- Optimal preparation for an operation facilitates a successful result and protects the patient and physician.
- The most significant risk factors for postoperative morbidity are preoperative conditions. They may affect the operation, anesthesia, and postoperative course and may preclude the procedure altogether.
- Approximately 0.5% of the general population and 1.5% of women older than 55 years are receiving continuous glucocorticoids.
- Latex allergy is directly responsible for 12% of the perioperative anaphylactic reactions in adult women and for 70% in children. Health care workers, women with spinal cord injuries, or those who have had to perform self-catheterization are at higher risk for latex allergy.
- The preoperative physical examination should answer three basic questions:
  - Has the primary gynecologic disease process changed since the initial diagnosis?
  - What is the effect of the primary gynecologic disease on other organ systems?
  - What deficiencies in other organ systems may affect the proposed surgery and hospitalization?
- An examination while the patient is under anesthesia may provide additional information, help avoid intraoperative surprises, and affect the surgical plan.
- It is estimated that 60% of routinely ordered tests would not have been performed if tests had been ordered only for an indication discovered by history or physical examination.
- The American Society of Anesthesiologists (ASA) Practice Advisory for Preanesthesia Evaluation states that routine preoperative tests, defined as a test ordered in the absence of a clinical indication or purpose, should not be ordered.
- A preoperative complete blood cell count and blood type and antibody screen should be performed before most major gynecologic surgeries.
- Other individualized preoperative laboratory testing should be determined based on the age of the woman, extent of the surgical procedure, and findings at the time of complete history and physical examination.
- Determining the preoperative creatinine or blood urea nitrogen level is especially important if the woman is going to be treated with antibiotics excreted by the kidneys.
- A pregnancy test may be appropriate, depending on contraceptive and sexual history. The PREG criteria can be used to optimize screening for pregnancy in women 18 years and older. A pregnancy test should almost always be performed if the patient is a teenager, as menstrual history is at best an imperfect indication of an early pregnancy.
- Serum electrolyte levels are ordered for women taking diuretics or those with a history of renal disease or heart disease. Also, serum electrolyte levels should be evaluated in women with vomiting, diarrhea, ileus, bowel obstruction, or any condition that affects electrolyte balance.
- Routine radiographs on all patients often do not affect perioperative management in elective gynecologic surgery, but they should be ordered for women who are current or former smokers, women with cardiac or pulmonary symptoms, immigrants who have not had a recent chest film, and women older than 70 years.
- A baseline preoperative electrocardiogram has been found to be cost effective in asymptomatic women 60 years and older without a history of cardiac disease or significant risk factors.
- In the present medicolegal climate, the absence of informed consent is cited as a major problem in many lawsuits.
- Preoperative orders should be standardized to avoid omissions, and electronic order sets are standard at most institutions.
- If an enhanced recovery pathway is being used, the patient can usually eat solid food up until midnight and clear liquids until 30 minutes before presenting to the hospital.
- To avoid hypoglycemia, most enhanced recovery after surgery (ERAS) protocols allow patients to eat solid food up to 6 hours before surgery.
- Anesthesiologists classify surgical procedures according to the patient's risk of mortality using the ASA risk class stratification (classes 1 to 5).
- An emergency operation doubles the mortality risks for ASA classes 1, 2, and 3; produces a slightly increased risk in class 4; and does not change the risk in class 5.
- *Enhanced recovery* refers to a bundled process with the aim of attenuating pathophysiologic changes and the stress response occurring with surgery. These processes replace traditional but untested practices of perioperative care with the primary goal of hastening recovery.
- Adoption of enhanced recovery has resulted in an average reduction in length of stay of 2.5 days and a decrease in complications by as much as 50%.
- Enhanced recovery achieved the greatest benefit in patients undergoing complex cytoreduction for ovarian cancer, of whom 57% underwent colonic or small bowel resection.
- The popularity of thoracic epidural anesthesia (TEA) after major open gynecologic surgery is due to its effectiveness in controlling pain and the quicker return of bowel function seen in patients with epidural anesthetics.
- The role of TEA in an ERAS care plan is less clear because it can compete at times with some of the ERAS goals and its use. TEA has been associated with more interventions to treat

*Continued*

KEY POINTS—cont'd

hypotension, longer length of hospital stay, and more complications in one series of early stage endometrial cancer patients.

- A surgical site infection (SSI) is one of the most common complications after surgery. SSIs dissatisfy patients and providers, but they also increase the cost of surgical care, increase morbidity, and can increase mortality.
- There are three classifications of SSIs according to the Centers for Disease Control and Prevention and the American College of Surgeons National Surgical Quality Improvement Program: (1) superficial incisional, (2) deep incisional, and (3) organ/space.
- Elements shown to decrease SSI that are often included in reduction bundles include preoperative nicotine cessation, preoperative antiseptic showering and chlorhexidine preparation, using hair clippers instead of a razor, appropriate preoperative antibiotic selection, normothermia, and glycemic control.
- There is abundant literature supporting the use of prophylactic antibiotics in gynecology. The incidence of febrile morbidity may be reduced from 40% to 15% and the incidence of pelvic infection decreased from 25% to 5%.
- The current guidelines for antimicrobial prophylaxis for vaginal or abdominal hysterectomy include the first- or second-generation cephalosporins of cefazolin, cefotetan, cefoxitin, or ampicillin-sulbactam.
- Among women with a β-lactam allergy, the recommended combinations are (1) clindamycin or vancomycin plus an aminoglycoside, or (2) aztreonam, or (3) a fluoroquinolone, metronidazole, and aminoglycoside, or (4) a fluoroquinolone alone.
- Comparative studies have documented that single-dose therapy is as effective as 24 hours of antibiotics. No advantage exists to continuing prophylactic antibiotics beyond the immediate operative period.
- Vaginal surgery continues to carry the lowest risks of SSI and should remain the preferred surgical approach when feasible. However, when minimally invasive approaches to hysterectomy replace laparotomy, the risk of SSI can be reduced by up to 16-fold.
- Multiple studies have documented a two- to threefold increase in the SSI rate directly related to perioperative shaving; if the hair is mechanically in the way, it should be clipped just before the operation.
- The use of chlorhexidine gluconate with 70% isopropyl alcohol as a skin preparation demonstrated a 40% reduction in SSIs in clean contaminated (type II) wound types compared with a 10% povidone-iodine solution.
- The risk of an SSI is significantly increased in the setting of smoking, and patients should be encouraged to stop as patients in a smoking cessation program had perioperative complication rates of 21% versus 41% in controls.
- Hypothermia has been shown to increase the incidence of wound infections, postoperative myocardial events, and perioperative blood loss; impair drug metabolism; and prolong postoperative recovery. Preventing intraoperative hypothermia improves surgical outcomes.
- Glucose levels greater than 180 mg/dL among patients with and without diabetes increase the risk of SSI by twofold. Perioperative blood glucose levels should be maintained at less than 200 mg/dL for all patients.
- Category 1A evidence has demonstrated that strict glucose control (80 to 130 mg/dL) in both patients with diabetes and those without does not improve SSI rates over glucose levels less than 200 mg/dL. Strict control may have detrimental effects on postoperative outcomes.
- Approximately 25% of all SSIs are caused by *Staphylococcus aureus.*
- Approximately 40% of deaths after gynecologic surgery are related to pulmonary emboli. Although the initial venous injury most often occurs at the time of the operation, approximately 15% of symptomatic emboli do not present until the first week after discharge from the hospital.
- Using the Caprini score, women in the very-low-risk group have less than a 3% risk of venous thromboembolism (VTE), women in the moderate group have a 10% to 30% risk, and women in the high-risk groups have a more than 30% risk of a VTE.
- Low-molecular-weight heparin (LMWH) is superior to standard unfractionated heparin because it has a longer half-life, almost 100% bioavailability, dose-independent clearance, and a more consistent anticoagulation effect from dose to dose.
- A meta-analysis of studies evaluating high-risk procedures found perioperative and postoperative LMWH administration to be equally effective.
- In general, warfarin should be held for at least 5 days before surgery and the international normalized ratio should be less than 1.5 before incision.
- Therapeutic dose aspirin should be held for 7 days before surgery. Once-daily dosing of baby aspirin (81 mg/day) can usually be continued.
- Factor Xa inhibitors should be held for 2 to 3 days before surgery, depending on the individual drug's half-life. Direct thrombin inhibitors should be held for 2 to 4 days before surgery, depending on renal function.
- Patients with bleeding disorders usually present early in their lives with bleeding. It is estimated that approximately 1% to 2% of patients in the United States have some type of bleeding diathesis, the most common of which is von Willebrand disease.
- Patients on chronic steroid therapy should receive their usual preoperative dose of steroids on the day of surgery. Any further administration of steroids should be done using a risk-assessment model. If there is a clinical concern of adrenal insufficiency, perioperative stress-dose steroid administration appears to carry minimal risk compared with the risk of adrenal crisis.
- Pulmonary function tests of lung volumes and flow rates are only indicated to evaluate women with a history or physical findings suggestive of restrictive or obstructive pulmonary disease.
- Predisposing factors that increase the incidence of atelectasis include morbid obesity, smoking, pulmonary disease, and advanced age. Increased pain, the supine position, abdominal distention, impaired function of the diaphragm, and sedation also contribute to decreased lung volumes and reduced dynamic measurements of pulmonary function postoperatively.
- The excessive mortality rate associated with a noncardiac operative procedure within 3 months of an acute myocardial infarct is 27% to 37%. After a 6-month interval, the chance of a reinfarction is 4% to 6% with elective operations.
- The routine use of beta-blockers perioperatively to reduce the risk of nonfatal myocardial infarction is no longer practiced because of the increased risk of death, nonfatal stroke, hypotension, and bradycardia. As a result, the common practice of perioperative beta-blockade has given way to its selective use.
- The administration of prophylactic antibiotics solely to prevent endocarditis is no longer recommended for patients who undergo genitourinary or gastrointestinal tract procedures.

Preoperative evaluation can involve both the art and science of clinical medicine. Optimal preparation for the operation facilitates a successful result and protects the patient and the physician.

The task of obtaining preoperative information serves two goals. The first is to ensure that the procedure is appropriate for the patient's diagnosis, relying heavily on the physician-patient relationship. The second goal, just as crucial as the first, is ensuring that the patient is safe for the procedure and that comorbidities are appropriately addressed. Some comorbidities will require further consultation with other specialists, and it is important for the gynecologic surgeon to recognize when consultation is needed.

The gynecologic surgeon, as leader of the surgical team, has a responsibility to prepare the patient, her family, and the surgical team for the surgical procedure. Even in emergency situations, preoperative preparation should be detailed and complete. Most surgical procedures are major events in a patient's life and can be accompanied by anxiety and apprehension in anticipation of surgery. It is not uncommon for patients to experience ambivalence when deciding to have an operation, elective or emergent. In all cases it is important for the surgeon to outline the natural history of the gynecologic disease and options for management. The risks, benefits, and alternatives must be discussed. The impact of a surgical intervention on normal body function, sexuality, and cosmesis should also be addressed. If the patient is ambivalent about the need for a surgical procedure, a second opinion may be warranted and should be offered. Some third-party payer programs may require patients to obtain a second opinion before elective gynecologic surgery.

It is the surgeon's responsibility to protect the patient's privacy and dignity throughout the perioperative period. The surgeon must appreciate that the preoperative period may be one of great psychological stress for the patient and her support team. Emotional responses may include vulnerability, helplessness, and grief associated with loss of a reproductive organ. The surgeon-patient relationship extends beyond the legal obligations. An important aspect of this relationship is that the surgeon and patient partner in shared decision making. Trust is established via mutual respect and open communication.

Preoperative consultation with the surgeon is a crucial first step in successful surgery. Ideally, the surgeon, patient, and her selected support team meet for a confidential consultation. A thorough and detailed history and physical examination should be performed during the surgical consultation. A number of studies have demonstrated that the most significant risk factors for postoperative morbidity are preoperative conditions. Known or unsuspected medical illnesses may affect the operation, anesthesia, and postoperative course and may preclude the procedure altogether. It is also important to evaluate the impact of the gynecologic diagnosis on other organ systems, such as a pelvic mass on the ureters or menorrhagia on hemoglobin level.

This chapter outlines the preoperative preparations for gynecologic surgery and perioperative management considerations. The preparations and plans for surgery extend into the postoperative period in a continuous spectrum. Thus several topics will be introduced here and discussed further in Chapter 25. **Emphasis is placed on obtaining a complete history, performing an adequate physical examination, counseling the patient, establishing informed consent, and perioperative planning to reduce complications associated with gynecologic surgery.**

## PREOPERATIVE HISTORY

**A detailed complete history not only obtains information but may also help relieve the patient's fears and anxieties.** When the history is obtained in an unhurried manner, the process can be reassuring. The extent and depth of the general history should be tailored to the age and general health of the woman and the surgical procedure that is being recommended. However, even minor operations may have major complications, so it is important to be prepared for all possibilities.

Obtaining a detailed and comprehensive preoperative history includes the use of open-ended questions and directed questions to complete the preoperative picture. A standardized historical questionnaire before the initial consultation is often requested by the surgeon or even required by the surgeon's institution. With the broadening use of electronic medical records, a patient's collated medical history may also be available. Regardless, each surgeon develops his or her method of preparation for consultation. Review of the patient's medical record, obtaining outside records and prior operative reports, and pertinent imaging and pathology reports can be done before the in-person consultation. This can allow for efficient evaluation, consultation, and preoperative referrals if needed.

Although this chapter does not review all the components of a complete history, it may be advantageous to group questions under the specific organ systems. Specific questions should be included to cross-check the review of symptoms. Questions should be included that address prior problems with surgery, anesthesia, or bleeding in the woman or her family. Medication allergies and current medications should be reviewed. Reconciliation of prescribed and over-the-counter (OTC) medications as well as vitamins, herbal medications, and supplements is critical because side effects and interactions with other medications can adversely affect coagulation and wound healing. **Approximately 0.5% of the general population and 1.5% of women older than 55 years are receiving continuous glucocorticoids.** Thus a specific question about glucocorticoid therapy for chronic medical problems should be included. The patient's primary care physician (PCP), or subspecialty medical provider, depending on the medication, should be involved in the decision to temporarily stop certain medications before surgery. The patient's PCP may also be able to provide guidance regarding anticoagulation bridging and stress-dose steroid dosing if either are needed.

**Patients often do not recognize aspirin or oral contraceptives as medication; therefore specific questions regarding these medications are needed.** General questions regarding smoking, alcohol, exercise tolerance, and recent upper respiratory infections should also be included. Specific questions should be directed toward sensitivity to iodine or latex. **Latex allergy is directly responsible for 12% of the perioperative anaphylactic reactions in adult women** and for 70% in children. Health care workers are particularly at risk for latex allergy. Women with spinal cord injuries, or those who have had to perform self-catheterization, are at higher risk for latex allergy.

The patient's contraceptive history, including any recent change, must be known. Ensuring that pregnancy is excluded either through the preoperative history or a pregnancy test is critical before gynecologic surgery. Included with the contraceptive history are key questions concerning possible exposure to viruses such as hepatitis B, hepatitis C, and human immunodeficiency virus (HIV). Also, the surgeon should discuss the possibility and risks of blood transfusion and learn whether there are religious objections if a blood transfusion is needed during surgery.

## PHYSICAL EXAMINATION

The preoperative physical examination should answer three basic questions:

1. Has the primary gynecologic disease process changed since the initial diagnosis?
2. What is the effect of the primary gynecologic disease on other organ systems?
3. What deficiencies in other organ systems may affect the proposed surgery and hospitalization?

Observations and findings in the physical examination may prompt further laboratory and diagnostic tests. One of the most important features of the preoperative physical examination is that it should be performed in a thorough and compulsive manner. One should use the same sequence every time to help focus attention on the evaluation of each organ system and to prevent omissions. Two important axioms should be stressed. First, even in emergency situations, it is imperative to perform a thorough physical examination. This should include an evaluation of blood pressure and pulse in the recumbent and sitting positions; orthostatic hypotension and tachycardia are crude indicators of hypovolemia. Second, although it is important to perform a pelvic examination during the initial consultation, it can also be informative to perform a pelvic examination in the operating room immediately before the surgical incision. An exam while the patient is under anesthesia may provide additional information, help avoid intraoperative surprises, and guide the surgical plan.

## LABORATORY AND PREOPERATIVE DIAGNOSTIC PROCEDURES

The general purpose of preoperative laboratory testing is to identify conditions that will alter or aid in perioperative management. Screening tests are used to find unsuspected asymptomatic conditions that may affect the anticipated surgical procedure. Preoperative laboratory tests may also help establish the extent of known disease and may influence the scheduling of elective surgery. **Being selective in ordering preoperative test avoids unnecessary costs associated with test results that would otherwise not affect the surgical plan.** Additionally, special imaging procedures may be needed to determine the effects of pelvic disease on other organ systems.

Age-appropriate screening tests should be reviewed with each patient before gynecologic surgery. Papanicolaou (Pap) tests should be up to date before elective gynecologic surgery. Mammograms should at least be discussed with women 40 years and older, and colonoscopy should be discussed with women older than 50 years.

There is debate over which preoperative laboratory procedures should be standard. Attention has been drawn to the cost-benefit ratio of preoperative screening. Although the cost of each individual test is usually low, the aggregate costs can be substantial. In a classic study, Kaplan and colleagues retrospectively studied the usefulness of preoperative laboratory procedures. They estimated that 60% of routinely ordered tests, such as differential cell count, platelet count, and 12-factor automated body chemistry analyses, would not have been performed if tests had been ordered only for an indication discovered by history or physical examination. Most important, only 0.22% of these tests demonstrated an abnormality that might influence perioperative management (Fig. 24.1). The final conclusion in their assessment of 2000 patients undergoing elective operations was that in the absence of specific indications, **most routine preoperative laboratory tests do not significantly contribute to patient care and could be eliminated** (Kaplan, 1985). Additionally, the current American Society of Anesthesiologists (ASA) Practice Advisory for Preanesthesia Evaluation states that routine preoperative tests, defined as a test ordered in the absence of a clinical indication or purpose, should not be ordered. Preoperative tests should be ordered for indicated purposes that guide or optimize perioperative care (Committee on Standards and Practice Parameters, Reaffirmed 2018).

However, a preoperative complete blood cell count and blood type and antibody screen should be performed before most major gynecologic surgeries. In the setting of anemia, the risks and benefits of proceeding with gynecologic surgery should be considered. It is important that the blood bank have the capability of providing cross-matched blood within a reasonable period if serious intraoperative bleeding were to occur. Routine preoperative

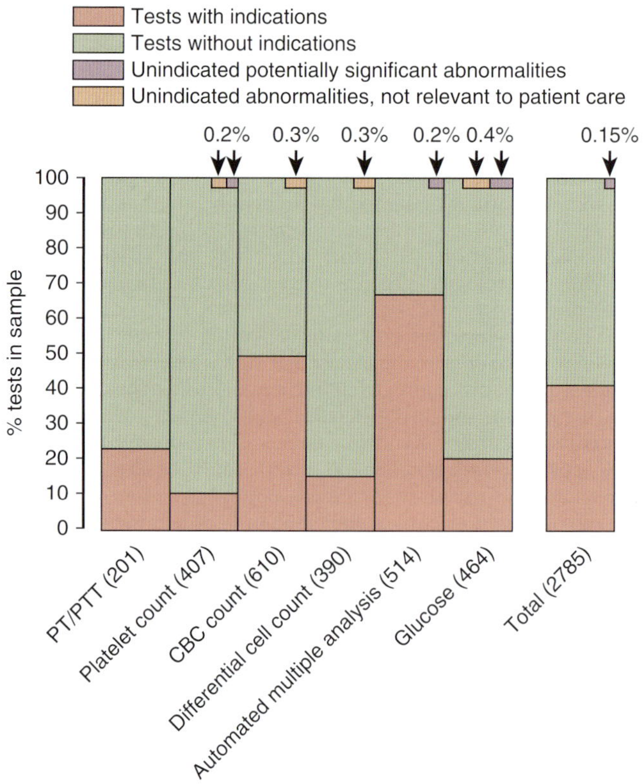


**Fig. 24.1** Proportions of indicated and unindicated preoperative tests, drawn to scale. Numbers in parentheses represent sample sizes used. *CBC,* Complete blood cell; automated multiple analysis is the sixth factor; *PT/PTT,* prothrombin time/partial thromboplastin time. (From Kaplan EB, Scheiner LB, Boeckmann AJ, et al. The usefulness of preoperative laboratory screening. *JAMA.* 1985;253(24):3576-3581.)

coagulation studies are not cost effective and rarely provide useful clinical information unless indicated by history and physical examination, as the patient's menstrual history should identify women with bleeding disorders.

Other individualized preoperative laboratory testing should be determined based on the age of the woman, extent of the surgical procedure, and findings at the time of complete history and physical examination. It may be indicated to order limited blood screening tests for women older than 40 years or who have positive family histories or questionable histories of hepatic or renal disease. Determining the preoperative creatinine or blood urea nitrogen (BUN) level is especially important if the woman is going to be treated with antibiotics excreted by the kidneys. **A pregnancy test may be appropriate, depending on contraceptive and sexual history, but a preprocedure pregnancy risk questionnaire may also be used as an effective history-based screen on the day of surgery for women 18 years and older** (Fig. 24.2) (Wyatt, 2018). However, a preprocedure pregnancy test should almost always be performed if the patient is a teenager, as menstrual history is at best an imperfect indication of an early pregnancy. Serum electrolyte levels are ordered for women taking diuretics or those with a history of renal disease or heart disease. Also, serum electrolyte levels should be evaluated in women with vomiting, diarrhea, ileus, bowel obstruction, or any condition that affects electrolyte balance. Ideally, abnormal results from any laboratory test ordered preoperatively should result in some change in perioperative management.

Routine chest radiographs on all patients often do not affect perioperative management in elective gynecologic surgery. A history and physical examination are sufficient for screening, and

MAYO CLINIC

***Pre-Procedure Pregnancy Reasonably Excluded Guide (PREG)***

Page1 retained in medical record **Discard after electronic entry.** Page 2 instruction only, discard after use.

**Instructions:** To determine if we need to do a pregnancy test today, review each. Check any and that apply.

| **Mayo Clinic Number** | **Patient Name *(first, middle, last)*** | **Birth Date *(Month, DD, YYYY)*** |
|---|---|---|
| | | |

| | |
|---|---|
| A | ☐ I am pregnant.<br>☐ I have had a bilateral tubal ligation (ie, "tubes tied", Essure® with confirmatory testing).<br>☐ I have had a hysterectome or bilateral salpingo-oophorectomy (both ovaries removed), or both.<br>☐ I am menopausal and more than 45 year old. I have not had a period spontaneously for the past 12 months.<br>☐ I have a current IUD (eg, Mirena®, Skyla™, Paragard®, Liletta™) in place.<br>☐ I have a current contraceptive implant (eg, Nexplanon®, Implanon®) in place. |
| B | ☐ I have not had sexual intercourse with a man since the start of my last normal menstrual period.<br>☐ My partner has had a vasectomy and he has had a negative post-surgery semen analysis.<br>☐ I started bleeding from a normal period within the last seven days.<br>☐ I raliably use hormonal contraception (eg, "the pill", Depo-Provera® Shots, patch, ring). |
| C | ☐ I think I may be pregnant or would like a pregnancy test.<br>☐ None of the above in sections A–C apply. |

**Fig. 24.2** Pre-Procedure Pregnancy Reasonably Excluded Guide (PREG). This guide is an effective history-based pregnancy screen that can be used on the day of surgery for women 18 years and older. *IUD,* Intrauterine device. (From Wyatt, MA, Ainsworth AJ, DeJong SR, Cope AG, Long ME. Implementation of the "Pregnancy Reasonably Excluded Guide" for pregnancy assessment: a quality initiative in outpatient gynecologic surgery. *Obstet Gynecol.* 2018;132(5):1222-1228.

chest radiographs should be obtained in patients with positive findings. **A meta-analysis of studies of routine preoperative chest radiographs demonstrated that false-positive results leading to invasive procedures and associated morbidity are more common than the discovery of new findings leading to a change in management.** However, chest films should be ordered for women who are current or former smokers, women with cardiac or pulmonary symptoms, immigrants who have not had a recent chest film, and women older than 70 years (Qaseem, 2006), although there appears to be institutional variability regarding the absolute age cutoff.

**A baseline preoperative electrocardiogram (ECG) has been found to be cost effective** in asymptomatic women 60 years and older without a history of cardiac disease or significant risk factors. An ECG may also be indicated in younger women with a history of smoking and those with diabetes or renal disease, depending on the severity.

Based on the complete history, physical examination, and preoperative testing, the gynecologic surgeon should determine whether consultation with other specialists is necessary. This decision should take into account the severity of comorbidities and the complexity of the proposed operation.

## PATIENT EDUCATION AND INFORMED CONSENT

One of the primary responsibilities of the gynecologic surgeon is to educate the patient and her support team about the anticipated surgical procedure, hospitalization, and recovery. Informed consent is an important principle to ensure that the patient's right to self-determination is respected. **The ethical concept of the process of informed consent includes two components, comprehension and free consent.** Throughout the educational process, questions from the patient or her support team should be welcomed. Educating the patient can also address anxiety. Written information, when available, can be helpful. Psychological preparation of the patient's support team is equally important, and arrangements for appropriate communication with the patient's family or support team during the operation should be made.

Few concepts bring more ambivalence and concern to the physician than the doctrine of informed consent. In the present medicolegal climate, the absence of informed consent is cited as a major problem in many lawsuits. Some of these issues are discussed further in Chapter 6. It is important to differentiate between the concepts of consent and informed consent. **Consent involves a simple yes-no decision, but informed consent is an educational process that also includes shared decision making between surgeon and patient.** To obtain informed consent, the surgeon must explain the following to the patient in understandable terms: the nature and extent of the disease process; the nature and extent of the contemplated operation; the anticipated benefits and results of the surgery, including a conservative estimate of successful outcome; the risks and potential complications of the operative procedure; alternative methods of therapy; and any potential changes in sexual, reproductive, and other functions. The surgeon should also discuss with the patient what the operation will not accomplish. Questions from the patient should be encouraged and addressed. Any details specific to the situation should be clarified in the consent note in addition to stating that the procedure, alternative treatments, and risks have been discussed and questions have been answered. The possibility of unanticipated pathologic conditions should be discussed with the woman and permission obtained on the written consent form for the most extensive operative procedure that may be necessary.

One of the greatest dilemmas in the doctrine of informed consent is the extent and depth of discussions concerning potential complications of an operation. Attorneys who specialize in defending gynecologic surgeons in medical malpractice litigation strongly advise discussing the risks of all major complications, including death from surgery and rare, serious complications, such as urinary tract fistulas after hysterectomy. Studies have shown that approximately 70% of patients do not read the consent form before signing it. Ideally, to protect the surgeon, another member of the health care delivery team should witness the final discussion of the informed consent process. The surgeon should document critical highlights of this discussion in the patient's medical record.

The gynecologic surgeon must not only educate his or her patient but must be prepared to discuss other information that the patient has received, including information from the lay press and Internet. During the preoperative educational process, so much information may be given that it causes confusion. Studies have noted that the more information given, the less information is actually retained, much less correctly retained. A study by Sandberg and colleagues has noted that during the preoperative evaluation, information given by anesthesiologists and other health care providers vastly exceeds the short-term capacity of patients (Sandberg, 2008). Thus it is extremely helpful to provide written preoperative instructions and important information.

**TABLE 24.1** American Society of Anesthesiologists (ASA) Physical Status Classification

| ASA Physical Status Class | Description |
|---|---|
| 1 | A normal healthy patient |
| 2 | A patient with mild systemic disease |
| 3 | A patient with severe systemic disease |
| 4 | A patient with severe systemic disease that is a constant threat to life |
| 5 | A moribund patient who is not expected to survive without the operation |

From Koo CY, Hyder JA, Wanderer JP, et al. A meta-analysis of the predictive accuracy of postoperative mortality using the American Society of Anesthesiologists' Physical Status Classification System. *World J Surg.* 2015;39(1):88-103.

## PREOPERATIVE PREPARATION

Most procedures and orders are accomplished on an outpatient basis because most patients undergo same-day admission before elective surgery. Preoperative orders should be standardized to avoid omissions, and electronic order sets are standard at most institutions. Orders individualized to a patient should be written in specific detail to avoid confusion by nursing and other hospital personnel.

Before presentation to the hospital, the patient should be provided with a list of specific instructions for the 24 hours before surgery. If an enhanced recovery pathway is being used, **the patient can usually eat solid food up until midnight and clear liquids until 30 minutes before presenting to the hospital.** To avoid hypoglycemia, most enhanced recovery after surgery protocols allow patients to eat solid food up to 6 hours before surgery. Clear liquids are emptied from the stomach within minutes; however, fatty foods delay gastric emptying. Incomplete preparation of the upper gastrointestinal (GI) tract increases the risk of aspiration. Studies have documented the safety of allowing inpatients and outpatients to ingest clear liquids up until 2 hours before elective surgery, and this is reflected in current ASA guidelines (ASA Practice Guidelines, 2017). The extent of preoperative anxiety does not influence gastric fluid volume or acidity.

## CONSULTATION WITH ANESTHESIOLOGIST

Among patients with no or limited comorbidities, the consultation with their anesthesiologist may occur in the preoperative area on the day of surgery. During this time, the anesthesiologist reviews and obtains any additional medical information, evaluates the patient's airway, determines the ASA risk score for the patient, and writes any preoperative medication orders. Among patients with complex medical histories or comorbidities, prior complications with anesthesia, family history of anesthesia complications, or planned high complexity surgery, a preoperative evaluation with an anesthesiologist in an outpatient clinic a day or more before surgery is warranted. The goal for this evaluation is to ensure all preoperative assessments needed to optimize anesthesia safety have been performed.

Surgeons and anesthesiologists often have to determine whether to continue or interrupt medications during the perioperative period. If the medication is prescribed for a chronic medical illness, it is likely best to continue the drug throughout the perioperative period. However, it is essential to determine whether the drug will adversely affect the course of the anesthesia or surgery and whether it will interact with other drugs to be given during the procedure. **It is acceptable for the patient to take oral medications the morning of surgery.** The 30 to 60 mL of water needed to swallow the oral medication is negligible compared with gastric fluid volumes.

Anesthesiologists classify surgical procedures according to the patient's risk of mortality. In 1961, Dripps first published guidelines to determine the risk of death related to major operative procedures. This physical status scale (Table 24.1) has been adopted by the ASA and has been revalidated many times over the years. With minor modifications, these anesthetic risk classes are still widely used. An emergency operation doubles the mortality risks for classes 1, 2, and 3; produces a slightly increased risk in class 4; and does not change the risk in class 5 (Koo, 2015).

## PERIOPERATIVE MANAGEMENT

### Enhanced Recovery

***Enhanced recovery* refers to a bundled process with the aim of attenuating pathophysiologic changes and the stress response occurring with surgery.** These processes replace traditional but untested practices of perioperative care with the primary goal of hastening recovery. This challenge to traditional surgical paradigms—such as mechanical bowel preparation, the overnight fasting rule, delayed postoperative feeding, hypervolemia, and intravenous opioids—was first described in Europe in the 1990s (Kehlet, 1997). There has been widespread uptake of formalized evidence-based enhanced recovery after surgery (ERAS) protocols internationally, particularly in colorectal surgery. **Adoption of ERAS has resulted in an average reduction in length of stay of 2.5 days (Chambers, 2014; Varadhan, 2010) and a decrease in complications by as much as 50%.** Similarities between gynecologic oncology procedures and those performed in surgical specialties such as colorectal surgery suggest that patients with gynecologic cancer may obtain comparable benefits. Data also suggest women undergoing benign gynecologic surgery, including minimally invasive surgery (MIS), benefit from perioperative management on an ERAS pathway.

In one investigation of patients undergoing gynecologic surgery, 241 patients (81 complex cytoreductive, 84 staging, and 76 vaginal surgery cases) were managed with an ERAS protocol and compared with 235 historical controls matched by procedure (Kalogera, 2013). The protocol included omission of preoperative fasting (Brady, 2003), use of carbohydrate loading (Mathur, 2010; Nygren, 1995), omission of mechanical bowel preparation (Güenaga, 2011), use of preemptive analgesia, nausea and vomiting prophylaxis, and maintenance of perioperative euvolemia

(Brandstrup, 2003). Laparotomy wounds were injected with bupivacaine because epidural analgesia was not used for patients undergoing laparotomy in this series (Kalogera, 2013). Intrathecal analgesia was used in more than 40% of vaginal cases in this series. Nasogastric tubes (Nelson, 2007), surgical drains (Kalogera, 2012), and intravenous patient-controlled analgesia was avoided or omitted, whereas early feeding (Charoenkwan, 2007; Cutillo, 1999; Minig, 2009), laxative use, and early mobilization were encouraged (Table 24.2). The ERAS pathway achieved the greatest benefit in patients undergoing complex cytoreduction for ovarian cancer, of whom 57% underwent colonic or small bowel resection. Patient-controlled anesthesia use decreased from 99% to

**TABLE 24.2** Evidence-Based Enhanced Recovery after Surgery (ERAS) Protocol for Gynecologic Surgery Patients

| | |
|---|---|
| **PREOPERATIVE** | |
| Diet | Evening before surgery: carbohydrate-loading drink; may eat until midnight<br>May ingest fluids up to 4 hours before procedure<br>Eliminate use of mechanical bowel preparation; rectal enemas still performed |
| **INTRAOPERATIVE** | |
| Analgesia before OR entry | Celecoxib 400 mg PO once<br>Acetaminophen 1000 mg PO once<br>Gabapentin 600 mg PO once |
| Postoperative nausea and vomiting prophylaxis | Before incision (± 30 min): dexamethasone 4 mg IV once + droperidol 0.625 mg IV once<br>Before incision closure (± 30 min): granisetron 0.1 mg IV once |
| Fluid balance | Goal: maintain intraoperative euvolemia<br>Decrease crystalloid administration<br>Increase colloid administration if needed |
| Analgesia | Opioids IV at discretion of anesthesiologist supplemented with ketamine or ketorolac<br>After incision closure: injection of bupivacaine at incision site |
| Anesthesia in complex vaginal surgery | Subarachnoid block containing bupivacaine and hydromorphone (40-100 μg)<br>Sedation versus "light" general anesthetic at the discretion of the anesthesiologist<br>Ketorolac 15 mg at the end of the procedure for patients able to tolerate it<br>No wound infiltration with bupivacaine in this cohort |
| **POSTOPERATIVE** | |
| Activity | Evening of surgery: out of bed greater than 2 hours, including 1 or more walks and sitting in chair<br>Day after surgery and until discharge: out of bed greater than 8 hours, including 4 or more walks and sitting in chair<br>Patient up in chair for all meals |
| Diet | No nasogastric tube (NGT); if NGT used intraoperatively, remove at extubation<br>Patient encouraged to start low-residue diet 4 hours after procedure<br>Day of surgery: 1 box of liquid nutritional supplement. Encourage oral intake of at least 800 mL of fluid, but no more than 2000 mL by midnight.<br>Day after surgery until discharge: 2 boxes of liquid nutritional supplement. Encourage daily oral intake of 1500-2500 mL of fluids.<br>Osmotic diarrhetics: Senna and docusate sodium; magnesium oxide; magnesium hydroxide prn |
| Analgesia | Goal: no IV patient-controlled analgesia (PCA)<br>Oral opioids<br>Oxycodone 5-10 mg PO every 4 hours as needed for pain rated 4 or greater or greater than patient stated comfort goal (5 mg for pain rated 4-6 or 10 mg for pain rated 7-10). For patients who received intrathecal analgesia start 24 hours after intrathecal dose given.<br>Scheduled acetaminophen*<br>Acetaminophen 1000 mg PO every 6 hours for patients with no or mild hepatic disease; acetaminophen 1000 mg PO twice daily for patients with moderate hepatic disease; maximum acetaminophen should not exceed 4000 mg per 24 hours from all sources.<br>Scheduled NSAIDs<br>Ketorolac 15 mg IV every 6 hours for 4 doses (start no sooner than 6 hours after last intraoperative dose); then, ibuprofen 800 mg PO every 6 hours (start 6 hours after last Ketorolac dose administered)<br>If patient unable to take NSAIDs<br>Tramadol 100 mg PO four times a day (start at 6 a.m. day after surgery) for patients less than 65 years of age and no history of renal impairment or hepatic disease; tramadol 100 mg PO twice daily (start at 6 a.m. day after surgery) for patients 65 years of age or older or creatinine clearance less than 30 mL/min or history of hepatic disease.<br>Breakthrough pain (pain greater than 7 more than 1 hour after receiving oxycodone)<br>Hydromorphone 0.4 mg IV once if patient did not receive intrathecal medications; may repeat once after 20 minutes if first dose ineffective.<br>IV PCA<br>Hydromorphone PCA started only if continued pain despite two doses of IV hydromorphone |
| Fluid balance | Operating room fluids discontinued upon arrival to floor<br>Fluids at 40 mL/hour until 8:00 a.m. on day after surgery, then discontinued<br>Peripheral lock IV when patient had 600 mL PO intake or at 8:00 a.m. on day after surgery, whichever came first. |

From Kalogera E, Bakkum-Gamez JN, Jankowski CJ, et al. Enhanced recovery in gynecologic surgery. *Obstet Gynecol.* 2013;122(2 Pt 1):319-328.
*Doses for patients greater than 80 kg and less than 65 years of age; doses adjusted as appropriate for patients less than 80 kg and/or 65 years of age or older.
*IV,* Intravenous; *NSAID,* nonsteroidal antiinflammatory drug; *OR,* operating room; *PO,* administered orally.

33%, and total opioid use decreased by 80% in the first 48 hours with no increase in pain scores. Hospital stay was reduced by 4 days with 30-day cost savings of more than $7600 per patient (18.8% reduction). In benign vaginal cases, mean pain scores significantly improved and hospital stay was significantly reduced by 1 day with the use of intrathecal analgesia. Ninety-five percent of patients rated satisfaction with perioperative care as excellent or very good. Other investigations in patients undergoing gynecologic surgery have shown that **ERAS is safe and confers significant benefits in hospital length of stay, pain control, and overall recovery** (Carter, 2012; Chase, 2008; Eberhart, 2008; Gerardi, 2008; Kalogera, 2013; Marx, 2006; Wijk, 2014).

The popularity of thoracic epidural anesthesia (TEA) after major open gynecologic surgery is due to its effectiveness in controlling pain and the quicker return of bowel function seen in patients with epidural anesthetics (Ferguson, 2009). However, the role of TEA in an ERAS care plan is less clear because it can compete at times with some of the ERAS goals such as early ambulation and voiding. The use of TEA has been associated with more interventions to treat hypotension, longer length of hospital stay, and more complications in one series of early-stage endometrial cancer patients (Belavy, 2013). The estimated length of stay in most ERAS pathways for abdominal hysterectomy is approximately 1 to 2 days, and MIS hysterectomies are most often performed as outpatient procedures. TEA in these settings not only represents poor use of resources but also will likely interfere with the expected expedient discharge from the hospital. Further study is needed to determine whether TEA or other local or regional analgesic approaches in radical abdominal procedures such as ovarian cancer debulking improve the return of bowel function or shorten hospital stays.

### Gastrointestinal Tract Considerations

If GI symptoms are present before gynecologic surgery, preoperative endoscopy or imaging studies of the GI tract should be considered to better understand the cause of these symptoms. The effect of nausea, vomiting, or diarrhea on serum electrolyte levels and on the nutritional status of the patient also needs to be evaluated. The evaluation should be individualized to determine whether a primary gynecologic process is causing the GI symptoms.

If a bowel preparation is necessary, a single day of an oral solution can be used. Magnesium citrate, sodium phosphate (Fleet phospho-soda), and polyethylene glycol (PEG; GoLYTELY) are the three most commonly used agents. Oliveria and colleagues reported a large randomized trial comparing sodium phosphate and PEG-based oral lavage solutions. The efficacy of the two preparations was similar. However, there was superior subjective patient tolerance to the 90-mL dose of sodium phosphate (Oliveira, 1997). Care must be taken in selecting patients who are to receive oral sodium phosphate as a bowel preparation because it may lead to hypokalemia, has been associated with acute phosphate nephropathy, and is contraindicated in women with hepatic, renal, or heart disease. As a result, the U.S. Food and Drug Administration (FDA) issued a warning in late 2008 regarding the use of all oral sodium phosphate preparations when used as a bowel cleanser. Special care must be taken in patients older than 55 or younger than 18, patients taking medications that can affect kidney function, and patients who are dehydrated.

## REDUCING POSTOPERATIVE COMPLICATIONS

### Site Marking and Universal Protocol

Depending on the surgical procedure being performed, operative site marking may be required. Most institutions mandate site marking to be performed in the setting of surgical procedures that involve or remove one or both organs or structures that are paired. This is controversial in gynecologic surgery because the preoperative determination of adnexal laterality is not always reliable. **If site marking is done, it should performed in the preoperative area while the patient is awake and nonsedated. The patient should participate in Universal Protocol and confirm which organ(s) will undergo surgery**. Universal Protocol and site marking reduce the risks of wrong site, wrong procedure, and wrong person operations (Knight, 2010).

### Preoperative Briefing

It is now common practice to perform a preoperative briefing, or "huddle," before bringing the patient to the operating room. Usually performed in the preoperative area, **the entire surgical team should be briefed on the patient's diagnosis, surgical plan, positioning, relevant comorbidities, intraoperative orders, and perioperative considerations**. Medications to be administered, including antibiotics, prophylactic dose heparin, local analgesics, and specialty medications such as local or systemic dye injections or vasoactive medications should be discussed. The anesthesia plans and estimated blood loss for the procedure should be reviewed. Special equipment needed for the procedure should be noted so that it is immediately available when needed. The anticipated wound classification should be noted so that it is accurately documented in the patient's medical record. Ideally the entire operating room team should be present for the briefing, including the surgeon, resident/fellow, nurse, surgical assistant and technician, and anesthesia team. All team members' questions should be answered before bringing the patient to the operating room. **Once the patient is in the operating room and positioned and before the start of the operation a surgical "time-out" is performed**. The time-out involves the immediate members of the procedure team: the individual performing the procedure, anesthesia providers, circulating nurse, operating room technician, and any others who will be participating in the procedure. The patient is identified once again using two separate identifiers, usually name and medical record number, and the surgical site and planned procedure are also verified. Patient allergies, medications on the surgical table, and any special needs are reviewed. Finally, performing a fire risk assessment is considered a "best practice" as it increases awareness of the potential for fire, enhances communication among team members, and makes staff active participants in fire prevention when confirmed by all present.

### Positioning for Surgery

After anesthesia has taken effect and the abdominal wall is relaxed, a preoperative pelvic examination may be indicated depending on the planned surgical procedure; if so, it should have been part of the initial surgical consultation and informed consent process. The findings may influence the choice of incision or operative approach. Additionally, the surgeon should supervise the positioning of the patient to ensure that she is properly positioned for the procedure being performed. Pressure points should be avoided to protect against neuromuscular and skin injury, especially over bony prominences (Irvin, 2004).

### Surgical Site Infection Prevention

Surgical site infection (SSI) is one of the most common complications after surgery. SSIs dissatisfy patients and providers, but they also increase the cost of surgical care, increase morbidity, and can increase mortality (Bakkum-Gamez, 2013; Tran, 2015). Additionally, SSIs associated with hysterectomies performed through abdominal incisions (laparotomy, laparoscopy, or robotic) are reported to the Centers for Medicare and Medicaid Services (CMS) and are used to compare hospitals to the national benchmark for surgical quality. The occurrence of an SSI after

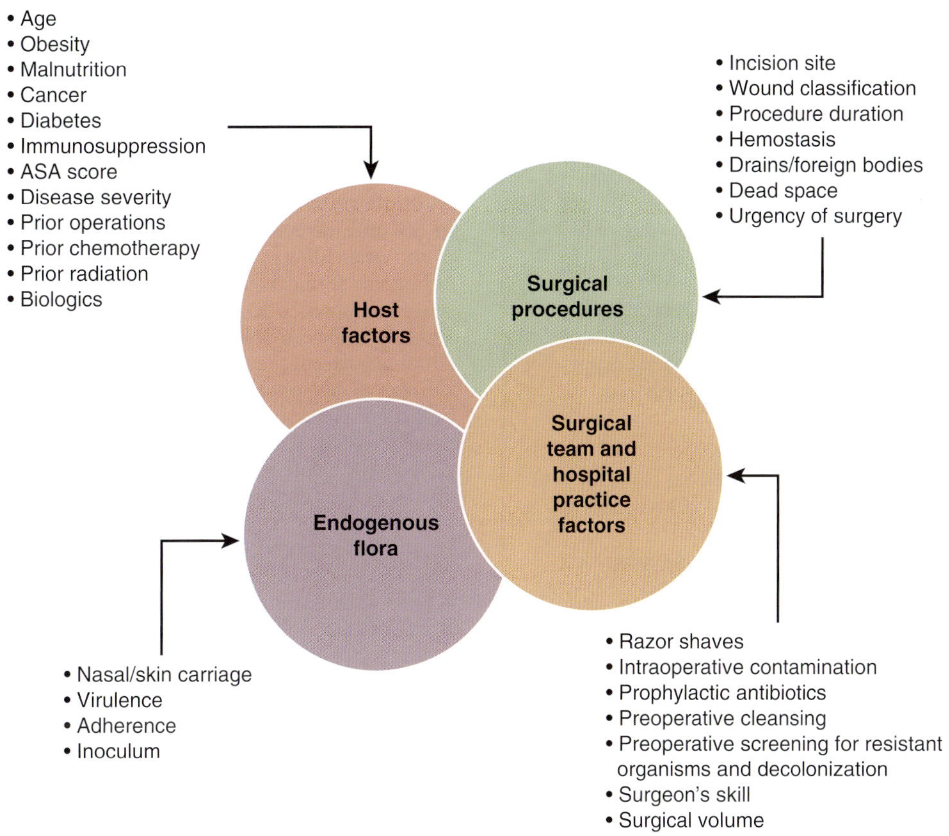


**Fig. 24.3** The causes of surgical site infections are multifactorial. *ASA,* American Society of Anesthesiologists.

hysterectomy may also influence third-party reimbursement. As such, there are multiple reasons to reduce SSI occurrences.

The causes of SSIs are multifactorial. There are host and endogenous flora factors that may or may not be modifiable. Additionally, surgical procedures, the surgical team, hospital practice factors, and prophylactic interventions influence the risk of SSI (Fig. 24.3). There are three categories of SSIs according to the Centers for Disease Control and Prevention (CDC) and the American College of Surgeons National Surgical Quality Improvement Program (ACS NSQIP): (1) superficial incisional, (2) deep incisional, and (3) organ/space (ACS NSQIP, 2011) (Box 24.1); each has different risk factors (Bakkum-Gamez, 2013). Given the implications of an SSI diagnosis, it is important to ensure that if a wound complication occurs, the surgeon classifies it appropriately. Additionally, if a wound is opened intentionally to evacuate a symptomatic hematoma or seroma, it should be cultured because a wound opened by the surgeon meets the definition of an SSI unless it is proven to be culture negative.

## Surgical Site Infection Reduction Bundles

**The combining of evidence-based medicine with consensus best practices into "bundles" of interventions has been shown to have some of the greatest impact in reducing SSIs.** The term *bundle* has been defined by the Institute for Healthcare Improvement (IHI) as a structured way of improving the processes of care and patient outcomes or a small, straightforward set of evidence-based practices that, when performed collectively and reliably, have been proved to improve patient outcomes. Elements shown to decrease SSI that are often included in reduction bundles include preoperative nicotine cessation (Sørensen, 2012), preoperative antiseptic showering (Webster, 2007) and chlorhexidine preparation (Darouiche, 2010), using hair clippers instead of a razor (Cruse, 1980; Kjønniksen, 2002), appropriate preoperative antibiotic selection (Bratzler, 2013), normothermia (Rajagopalan, 2008; Scott, 2006; Warttig, 2014), and glycemic control (Kwon, 2013). **SSI reduction bundles that include various combinations of these elements as well as additional evidence-based and best practices have been shown to decrease SSI after hysterectomy by 40% to 80%** (Revolus, 2014) and by more than 50% in general surgery and colorectal surgery (Cima, 2013; Johnson, 2016; van der Slegt, 2013; Waits, 2014). The colorectal surgery SSI reduction bundle at the Mayo Clinic (Fig. 24.4) has been validated in the gynecologic surgery practice as well (Cima, 2013) and yielded an 82% reduction in SSIs (Johnson, 2016). Additionally, at least one study of patients undergoing colorectal surgery reported an inverse association with SSI and the number of bundle elements used (Waits, 2014), suggesting it is the combination of interventions, rather than one element alone, that yields the impact.

## Prophylactic Antibiotics

The use of prophylactic antibiotics in gynecologic surgical procedures has become standard practice. Rigidly defined, prophylactic antibiotic use involves the administration of antibiotics to patients without evidence of current infection to prevent postoperative morbidity related to infection. The goal of antibiotic therapy is to prevent SSI by the endogenous flora of the lower female reproductive tract. **There is abundant literature supporting the use of prophylactic antibiotics in gynecologic surgery. The incidence of febrile morbidity may be reduced from 40% to 15% and the incidence of pelvic infection decreased from 25% to 3%** (Mahdi, 2014). The current guidelines for antimicrobial prophylaxis for any mode of hysterectomy include the first- and second-generation cephalosporins cefazolin, cefotetan, cefoxitin, and ampicillin-sulbactam. Among women

**BOX 24.1** Classification of Surgical Site Infections (SSI) by the Centers for Disease Control and Prevention (CDC) and American College of Surgeons National Surgical Quality Improvement Program (ACS NSQIP)

**SUPERFICIAL INCISIONAL SSI***

1. Purulent incisional drainage from above the fascia
2. Organisms isolated from an aseptically obtained culture of fluid or tissue from the superficial incision
3. Pain/tenderness, wound swelling, redness, or heat and the superficial incision is deliberately opened by the surgeon (unless it is culture negative)

**DEEP INCISIONAL SSI (INVOLVES DEEP SOFT TISSUES, SUCH AS THE FASCIA OR MUSCLE LAYERS OF THE INCISION)**

1. Purulent drainage from the deep incision
2. Spontaneous dehiscence or deliberate opening of the fascia in the setting of fever or localized pain/tenderness (unless it is culture negative)
3. An abscess is found involving the deep incision via physical examination, reoperation, or radiologic examination

**ORGAN/SPACE SSI**

1. Purulent drainage from an intraperitoneal drain
2. Presence of organisms in culture of fluid obtained aseptically from an organ or space
3. Abscess or other infection involving an organ or space on physical examination, reoperation, histopathologic or radiologic examination

From ACS NSQIP. Classic, essential, small-rural, targeted, and Florida variables & definitions. *American College of Surgeons National Surgical Quality Improvement Program Operations Manual.* Chicago: ACS; 2011:24-26.

*Surgeon diagnosis of any of the three types of SSI also meets NSQIP criteria.

with a beta-lactam allergy, the recommended combinations are (1) clindamycin or vancomycin plus an aminoglycoside; or (2) aztreonam; or (3) a fluoroquinolone, metronidazole, and aminoglycoside; or (4) a fluoroquinolone alone (Bratzler, 2013).

Emphasis has focused on short duration of therapy for prophylactic antibiotics. **Comparative studies have documented that single-dose therapy is as effective as 24 hours of antibiotics.** No advantage exists to continuing prophylactic antibiotics beyond the immediate operative period. This short duration of administration also reduces cost and complications. The incidence of serious complications, such as drug allergy and resistant bacteria, is directly related to the length of administration of the antibiotic.

The Surgical Care Improvement Project (SCIP) implemented by CMS focused on appropriate antibiotic selection and timing of administration with the goal of reducing SSI rates by 25% between 2006 and 2010. Despite high compliance to SCIP measures, which later included normothermia, glucose control, and hair removal guidelines, SSI rates do not correlate with SCIP compliance (Hawn, 2011). **Although antibiotic prophylaxis is an important element in SSI reduction, antibiotics alone cannot mitigate the SSI risk.**

## Minimally Invasive Surgery

With the introduction of laparoscopy and robotic surgery, the armamentarium of minimally invasive gynecologic surgery approaches changed dramatically. Vaginal surgery continues to carry the lowest risks of SSI (Lake, 2013) and should remain the preferred surgical approach when feasible. However, **when minimally invasive approaches to hysterectomy replace laparotomy, the risk of SSI can be reduced by up to 16-fold** (Bakkum-Gamez, 2013; Colling, 2015). As such, the use of minimally invasive surgery is a critical modifiable factor in the SSI prevention bundle.

## Hair Removal

**Multiple studies have documented a two- to threefold increase in SSI rate directly related to perioperative shaving.** Cruse and Foord studied approximately 63,000 operations over a 10-year period and found a 0.9% incidence of SSI when patients were not shaved as opposed to 2.5% when they were shaved (Cruse, 1980). Razors produce macroscopic and microscopic nicks and cuts that allow a protective environment for colonization by skin bacteria. Depilatory agents often produce intense burning if used on the perineum. A systematic review by Kjønniksen and associates has concluded that if the hair is mechanically in the way, it should be clipped just before the operation (Kjønniksen, 2002). Patients should also be advised not to shave themselves before surgery for this reason.

## Chlorhexidine/Alcohol Skin Preparation

A randomized trial comparing chlorhexidine gluconate with 70% isopropyl alcohol versus an aqueous solution of 10% povidone-iodine for skin preparation in the operating room showed a 40% reduction in SSIs in clean contaminated (type II) wound types (Darouiche, 2010). The solution is highly flammable, and care must be taken to ensure adequate drying time to avoid a fire when electrocautery is used.

## Smoking

The risk of an SSI is significantly increased in the setting of smoking (van Walraven, 2013). Ideally, patients should stop smoking for at least 8 weeks before surgery. However, abstinence from cigarettes for 2 to 4 weeks preoperatively is still beneficial. Providing nicotine replacement is helpful in alleviating the symptoms of acute nicotine withdrawal. Referral to preoperative smoking cessation programs not only decreases smoking around the time of surgery and related perioperative complications but also leads to an increased incidence of long-term smoking cessation. In one multicenter study, Lindström and associates noted that the patients in a smoking cessation program had perioperative complication rates of 21% versus 41% in controls (Lindström, 2008).

## Normothermia

Hypothermia, often defined as a core body temperature less than 36° C, has been shown to increase the incidence of SSI and postoperative myocardial events, increase perioperative blood loss, impair drug metabolism, and prolong postoperative recovery (Rajagopalan, 2008; Scott, 2006; Warttig, 2014). Patients undergoing laparotomy are at high risk of hypothermia as a result of prolonged periods with an open abdomen. Furthermore, general anesthesia induces peripheral vasodilation, leading to accelerated heat loss. Esophageal probes are often used to monitor temperature, and methods to maintain normothermia include the use of forced air devices (Galvão, 2010), underbody warming mattresses (Perez-Protto, 2010), and warmed intravenous fluids (Campbell, 2015). Whichever method is used, it is important to understand that preventing intraoperative hypothermia improves surgical outcomes.

## Glucose Control in Patients with and without Diabetes

The prevalence of diabetes is approximately 10% in women older than 65, and the incidence increases rapidly as women get older. The stress of surgery often produces changes in glucose tolerance and insulin resistance. Because pancreatic reserve is a continuum, even

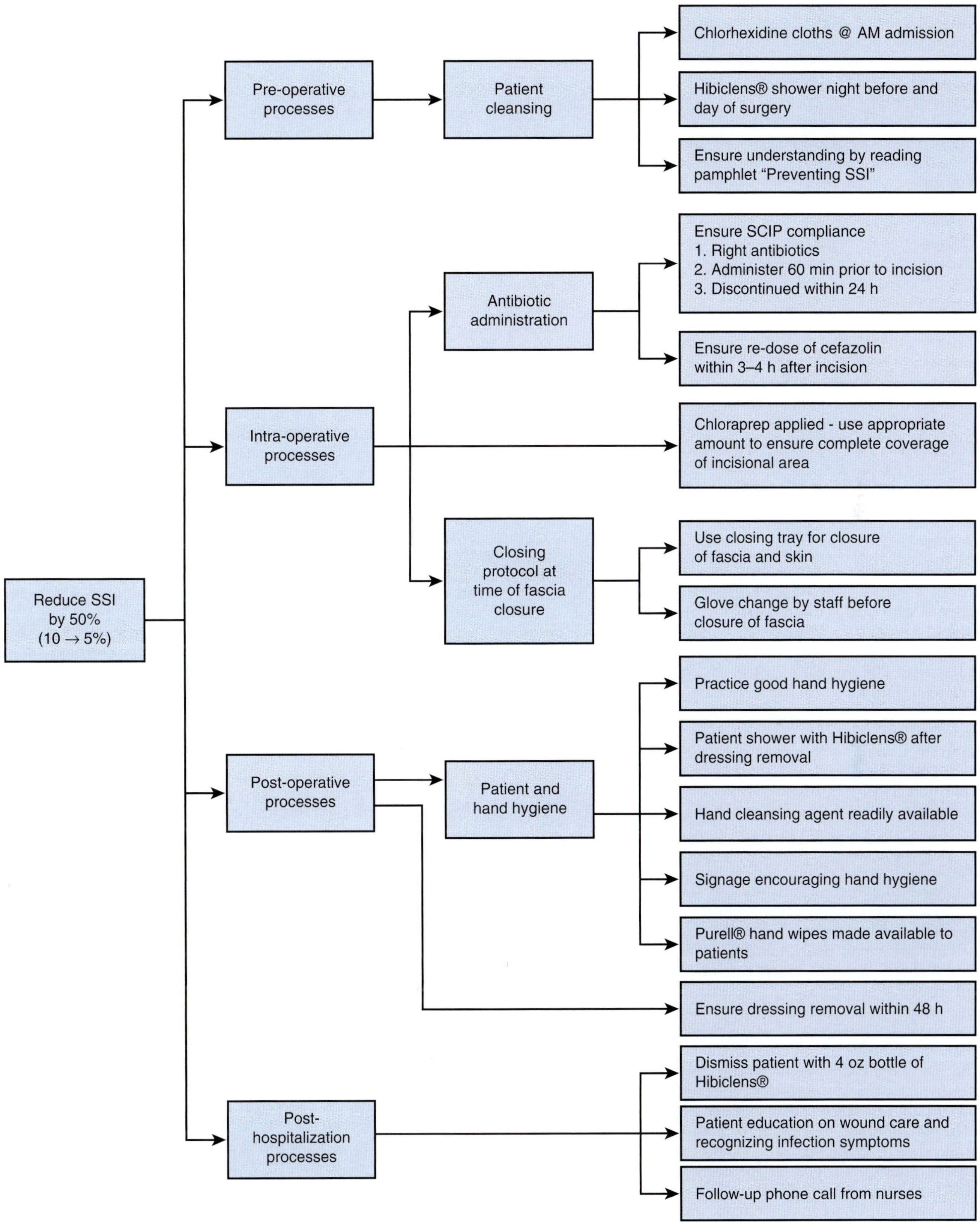


**Fig. 24.4** Surgical site infection (SSI) reduction bundle in colorectal surgery at Mayo Clinic. SSIs were reduced by more than 50% with the implementation of this full bundle. (From Cima R, Dankbar E, Lovely J, et al. Colorectal surgery surgical site infection reduction program: a national surgical quality improvement program–driven multidisciplinary single-institution experience. *J Am Coll Surg.* 2013;216(1):23-33.)

**BOX 24.2** Mechanisms Causing Adverse Outcomes From Poorly Controlled Diabetes

- Hyperglycemia
- Dehydration
- Academia from keto acids and lactate
- Nonenzymatic glycosylation of proteins central to immune function: complement, impaired IgG, inhibited neutrophil activity
- Fatigue and muscle wasting from lipolysis and protein catabolism
- Increased circulating fatty acids
- Increased skeletal muscle breakdown
- Cell membrane instability
- Decline in myocardial contractility and increased cardiac arrhythmias
- Inhibited endothelial function
- Insulin resistance
- Increased lipolysis
- Presence of insulin inhibits inflammatory factors
- Decreased endothelial-derived relaxing factor—nitric oxide
- Insulin and glucose inhibit proinflammatory cytokines

Modified from the American College of Endocrinology. Position statement on inpatient diabetes and metabolic control. *Endocr Pract.* 2004;10(1):77-82.

women who do not have diabetes by standard blood glucose criteria may develop detrimental hyperglycemia secondary to the physiologic stresses of surgery. **Glucose levels greater than 180 mg/dL among patients with and without diabetes increase the risk of SSI twofold** (Kwon, 2013). **Perioperative blood glucose levels among both patients with and without diabetes should be maintained at less than 200 mg/dL.** Category 1A evidence has demonstrated that strict glucose control (80 to 130 mg/dL) in patients with and without diabetes does not improve SSI rates compared with glucose levels less than 200 mg/dL (Chan, 2009), and strict control may have detrimental effects on postoperative outcomes (Gandhi, 2007).

In 2004, the American College of Endocrinology published a position paper, "Inpatient Diabetes and Metabolic Control," emphasizing not only the effects of elevated blood glucose levels but the beneficial effects of adequate insulin (Box 24.2). Insulin decreases lipolysis. Elevated free fatty acid levels are associated with arrhythmias. Insulin inhibits several inflammatory mediators, especially the proinflammatory cytokines, and adequate insulin also leads to an increase in nitric oxide levels in the endovasculature, inducing vasodilation.

**The principal postoperative complications in women with diabetes are increased risk of cardiac morbidity, SSI, and wound disruptions.** The increase in SSI rate is believed to be secondary to a decrease in cellular and humoral responses to bacteria. Women with diabetes have approximately a fivefold increase in incidence of SSI compared with age-matched controls. The increased incidence of wound disruptions is caused by a decreased tensile strength during healing, which is associated with insulin resistance and an elevated blood sugar level.

Important questions during the preoperative evaluation focus on the severity of the diabetes, types of medications, and recent diabetic control. Recent blood glucose and hemoglobin A1c (HbA1c) levels may be helpful predictors of perioperative morbidity, even if they are not modifiable. At the very least, their severity should be documented in the medical record to ensure accurate accounting of perioperative morbidity.

## Screening for *Staphylococcus aureus*

Approximately 25% of all SSIs are caused by *Staphylococcus aureus*. Patients at high risk for *S. aureus* SSI (those with previous *S. aureus* infection or colonization, obesity, or diabetes) likely benefit from preoperative *S. aureus* screening by nasal culture. If positive cultures are documented, eradication of colonization with chlorhexidine baths and twice-daily intranasal mupirocin has been shown to decrease the rate of SSI. Bode and colleagues demonstrated a decrease in SSI from 7.7% to 3.4% when *S. aureus* was detected and decolonization performed (Bode, 2010).

## Venous Thromboembolism Prevention

Venous thromboembolism (VTE) of the pelvic or leg veins is a common complication of gynecologic surgery. Studies using $^{125}$I-fibrinogen scanning techniques have documented that approximately 15% of women having gynecologic surgery for a benign disease and approximately 22% of women having surgery for malignant disease develop VTE (Bonnar, 1985). Most of these women will be asymptomatic. **Several aspects of pelvic surgery predispose women to VTE, including venous stasis, surgical injury to the walls of large veins, associated anaerobic infection, and hormonal status. Gynecologic malignancy also increases the risk of VTE.**

**Approximately 40% of deaths after gynecologic surgery are related to pulmonary emboli.** Although the initial venous injury most often occurs at the time of the operation, approximately 15% of symptomatic emboli cases do not present until the first week after discharge from the hospital. Because of the significant morbidity and mortality associated with a postoperative pulmonary embolus, every effort should be made to reduce the incidence of thrombophlebitis.

One method commonly used to determine the VTE risk for an individual patient is to calculate the Caprini score, which takes into consideration risk factors such as a history of previous VTE and personal or family history of hypercoagulability. The presence of such a history should also prompt an evaluation for a thrombophilia. Other risk factors for VTE include active malignancy, previous radiation therapy, congestive heart failure, chronic pulmonary disease, nephrotic syndrome, morbid obesity, venous disease, edema of the legs, active pelvic infection, age older than 40 years, current use of oral contraceptives or hormone replacement therapy up to the time of the operation, length of immobilization or preoperative hospitalization, and the length of the planned surgical procedure (Table 24.3). A Caprini score of 0 is very low risk for VTE, 1 to 2 is low risk, 3 to 4 is moderate risk, and 5 or more is considered high risk for VTE. Women in the very low-risk group have less than a 3% risk of VTE, women in the moderate group have a 10% to 30% risk, and women in the high-risk groups have a more than 30% risk of a VTE. The American College of Chest Physicians have published evidence-based clinical practice guidelines aimed at mitigating VTE risk in the setting of abdominopelvic surgery that vary by risk stratification (Table 24.4) (Gould, 2012). The use of an inferior vena cava (IVC) filter for primary VTE prevention is not recommended, in part because of the risk of long-term complications and also because that they are often not removed. Additionally, surveillance with lower extremity Doppler ultrasound for asymptomatic VTE is not recommended (Gould, 2012). These guidelines are widely accepted for VTE prevention.

The main complication from heparin prophylaxis is bleeding. Some women are transiently anticoagulated by the heparin and may experience excessive bleeding during or after the operative procedure. This complication is rare and experienced by approximately 2% of women. The risk of bleeding is significantly lower with low-molecular-weight heparin (LMWH). Women who are obese or extremely thin should have their dosage of heparin adjusted accordingly.

LMWH is superior to standard unfractionated heparin because it has a longer half-life, almost 100% bioavailability, dose-independent clearance, and a more consistent anticoagulation effect from dose to dose. Most studies have reported significantly fewer

**TABLE 24.3** Caprini Score Risk Assessment Model for Venous Thromboembolism

| 1 Point | 2 Points | 3 Points | 5 Points |
|---|---|---|---|
| Age 41-60 | Age 61-74 | Age ≥75 | Stroke (<1 mo) |
| Minor surgery | Arthroscopic surgery | History of VTE | Elective arthroplasty |
| BMI >25 kg/m² | Major open surgery (>45 min) | Family history of VTE | Hip, pelvis, or leg fracture |
| Swollen legs | Laparoscopic surgery (>45 min) | Factor V Leiden | Acute spinal cord injury (<1 mo) |
| Varicose veins | Malignancy | *Prothrombin 20210A* mutation | |
| Pregnancy or postpartum | Confined to bed (>72 h) | Lupus anticoagulant | |
| History of unexplained or recurrent spontaneous abortion | Immobilizing plaster cast | Anticardiolipin antibodies | |
| Oral contraceptives or hormone replacement | Central venous access | Elevated serum homocysteine | |
| Sepsis (<1 mo) | | Heparin-induced thrombocytopenia | |
| Serious lung disease, including pneumonia (<1 mo) | | Other congenital or acquired thrombophilia | |
| Abnormal pulmonary function | | | |
| Acute myocardial infarction | | | |
| Congestive heart failure (<1 mo) | | | |
| History of inflammatory bowel disease | | | |
| Medical patient at bed rest | | | |

From Gould MK, Garcia DA, Wren SM, et al. Prevention of VTE in nonorthopedic surgical patients: *Antithrombotic Therapy and Prevention of Thrombosis,* 9th ed. American College of Chest Physicians Evidence-Based Clinical Practice Guidelines. *Chest.* 2012;141(2 Suppl):e227S-e277S.
*BMI,* Body mass index; *VTE,* venous thromboembolism.

**TABLE 24.4** Venous Thromboembolism Prophylaxis Recommendations for Abdominal-Pelvic Surgery

| Risk Stratification | Prophylaxis Measures |
|---|---|
| Very low risk (Caprini score 0) | Early ambulation |
| Low risk (Caprini score 1-2) | Mechanical prophylaxis with SCDs |
| Moderate risk (Caprini score 3-4)<br>Not at high risk for bleeding | Daily prophylactic dose LMWH or thrice-daily prophylactic dose LDUH or SCDs |
| Moderate risk (Caprini score 3-4)<br>High risk for bleeding or consequences of bleeding severe | Mechanical prophylaxis with SCDs |
| High risk (Caprini score ≥5)<br>Not at high risk for bleeding | Daily prophylactic dose LMWH or thrice-daily prophylactic dose LDUH + elastic stockings or SCDs |
| High risk (Caprini score ≥5)<br>Undergoing surgery for cancer | Daily prophylactic dose LMWH or thrice-daily prophylactic dose LDUH + elastic stockings or SCDs<br>Extended duration (4 weeks) daily prophylactic dose LMWH |
| High risk (Caprini score ≥5)<br>LMWH and LDUH contraindicated | Low-dose aspirin or fondaparinux or SCDs |

Data from Gould MK, Garcia DA, Wren SM, et al. Prevention of VTE in nonorthopedic surgical patients: *Chest.* 2012;141(2):e227S-e277S.
*LDUH,* Low-dose unfractionated heparin; *LMWH,* low-molecular-weight heparin; *SCDs,* sequential compression devices.

hemorrhagic complications with LMWH than with unfractionated heparin. Also, the incidence of heparin-induced thrombocytopenia is significantly lower in women given LMWH than in those receiving unfractionated heparin. In the gynecologic surgical community there are two main approaches to the timing of pharmacologic prophylaxis. One approach includes a dose 1 to 2 hours before surgery and continuation postoperatively, and the other begins the pharmacologic prophylaxis between 6 and 12 hours after surgery. A meta-analysis of studies summarizing 1600 surgeries for elective hip repair, which is as high risk as gynecologic procedures, has found perioperative and postoperative LMWH initiation to be equally effective. The rates of deep vein thrombosis were 12.4% and 14.4%, respectively. The risks of bleeding were higher in the perioperative protocol groups, 6.3% versus 2.5% for postoperative dosing. It was concluded that dosing may begin 12 hours after the procedure in most cases and no less than 6 hours after the procedure (Raskob, 2003).

## CHRONIC ANTICOAGULATION AND BLEEDING DISORDERS

In women who are currently taking full anticoagulation because of an active VTE or cardiac indication, short-term interruption of blood thinning is indicated for surgical procedures that pose a greater risk of bleeding than a dilation and curettage (D&C). Bridging with LMWH preoperatively and postoperatively may be indicated, and oral anticoagulants should be restarted shortly after surgery. There are no randomized comparative effectiveness trials evaluating the benefits of anticoagulation bridging, and thus the decision to bridge should be individualized, include the physician managing the patient's anticoagulation, and address the benefits and risks of thrombosis and bleeding. In general, **warfarin should be held for at least 5 days before surgery, and the international normalized ratio (INR) should be less than 1.5 before incision.** Therapeutic-dose aspirin should be held for 7 days before surgery. Once-daily dosing of baby aspirin (81 mg/day) can usually be continued. The novel oral anticoagulants (NOACs), including factor Xa inhibitors (apixaban, rivaroxaban) and direct thrombin inhibitors such as fondaparinux, which inactivates factor Xa by binding antithrombin, have become more commonly prescribed than warfarin. **Factor Xa inhibitors should be held for 2 to 3 days** before surgery, depending on the individual drug's half-life. **Direct thrombin inhibitors should be held for 2 to 4 days before surgery**, depending on renal function. Depending on the indication for full anticoagulation, bridging with LMWH may be required, and this should be guided by the patient's primary prescribing physician as described earlier. Factor Xa inhibitors and direct thrombin inhibitors should be resumed when the surgeon feels the patient is stable and at low risk for postoperative bleeding from full anticoagulation; these oral anticoagulants have a short half-life and effectively fully anticoagulate within a matter of hours (Robertson, 2015). Patients with an acute VTE who cannot have their surgery delayed may require placement of a temporary IVC filter.

Bleeding disorders usually cause symptomatic issues in most patients earlier in their lives, and it is estimated that approximately 1% to 2% of patients in the United States have some type of bleeding diathesis. The most common is von Willebrand disease. Patients who have had symptoms of easy bruising, frequent nosebleeds, anemia, menorrhagia, and excessive bleeding with surgical procedures should be considered for a hematologic assessment. Any positive test result should be followed by consultation with a hematologist because supplementation with coagulation factors in the perioperative period may be required. Women with already confirmed bleeding problems should have a consultation for appropriate prophylaxis, and a hematologist should guide perioperative factor replacement.

## Stress-Dose Steroids

Glucocorticoids are prescribed for a variety of illnesses. **Exogenous glucocorticoid use may blunt the natural response of the hypothalamic-pituitary-adrenal (HPA) axis to stress depending on dose and duration of therapy.** In an attempt to prevent adrenal insufficiency, widespread use of stress-dose steroids was commonly administered perioperatively without high-level evidence to support or refute this practice. Any patient who received the equivalent dose of 20 mg of daily prednisone for more than 5 days was "at risk" for HPA suppression (Axelrod, 2003). The routine use of perioperative stress-dose steroids has been challenged, and more individualized treatment strategies assessing the risk of adrenal insufficiency have been created (Liu, 2017). Patients at high risk of HPA axis suppression (patients who have been treated with a glucocorticoid in doses equivalent to at least 20 mg/day of prednisone for more than 3 weeks or patients with clinical features of Cushing syndrome) would benefit from stress-dose steroid administration during the perioperative period. Table 24.5 summarizes a risk-based strategy for the administration of periprocedural steroids. Patients on chronic steroid therapy should receive their usual preoperative dose of steroids on the day of surgery. However, if HPA axis suppression is a clinical concern, perioperative stress-dose steroid administration appears to carry minimal risk compared with the risk of adrenal crisis.

**TABLE 24.5** Surgical Stress by Procedure and Recommended Steroid Dosing

| Surgery Type | Endogenous Cortisol Secretion Rate | Examples | Recommended Steroid Dosing |
|---|---|---|---|
| **Superficial** | 8-10 mg per day (baseline) | Dental surgery<br>Biopsy | Usual daily dose |
| **Minor** | 50 mg per day | Inguinal hernia repair Colonoscopy<br>Uterine curettage<br>Hand surgery | Usual daily dose<br>plus<br>Hydrocortisone 50 mg IV before incision Hydrocortisone 25 mg IV every 8 h × 24 h<br>Then usual daily dose |
| **Moderate** | 75-150 mg per day | Lower extremity revascularization<br>Total joint replacement Cholecystectomy<br>Colon resection<br>Abdominal hysterectomy | Usual daily dose<br>plus<br>Hydrocortisone 50 mg IV before incision Hydrocortisone 25 mg IV every 8 h × 24 h<br>Then usual daily dose |
| **Major** | 75-150 mg per day | Esophagectomy,<br>Total proctocolectomy Major cardiac/vascular Hepaticojejunostomy Delivery<br>Trauma | Usual daily dose<br>plus<br>Hydrocortisone 100 mg IV before incision<br>Followed by continuous IV infusion of 200 mg of hydrocortisone more than 24 h<br>or<br>Hydrocortisone 50 mg IV every 8 h × 24 h<br>Taper dose by half per day until usual daily dose reached plus<br>Continuous IV fluids with 5% dextrose and 0.2-0.45% NaCl (based on degree of hypoglycemia) |

From Liu MM, Reidy AB, Saatee S, Collard CD. Perioperative steroid management approaches based on current evidence. *Anesthesiology.* 2017;127:166-72.
*IV,* Intravenous.

## Assessment of Cardiopulmonary Comorbidities

Most healthy patients planning gynecologic surgery will not require extensive preoperative testing beyond a complete history, physical examination, and the basic preoperative testing described earlier. However, a patient with significant medical comorbidities will likely require more extensive testing and consultation with other specialties to optimize the patient's perioperative outcome. It is beyond the scope of this book to cover the full evaluation of the various medical comorbidities one will encounter in clinical practice, but a basic understanding of what the consulting physician will consider in his or her evaluation of the patient is important to help counsel the patient and set proper expectations.

### Pulmonary Disease

Pulmonary complications are a common form of postoperative morbidity experienced by approximately 5% of women after gynecologic surgery. The goals of the preoperative assessment of the respiratory system are to identify women at risk for developing postoperative pulmonary complications and prescribe appropriate preoperative therapy to reduce these risks. Similar to the evaluation of other organ systems, the history and physical examination are the most important parts of the pulmonary evaluation. Pulmonary function tests of lung volumes and flow rates are only indicated to evaluate women with a history or physical findings suggestive of restrictive or obstructive pulmonary disease. Pulmonary function tests help assess the pulmonary reserve and identify the extent to which the dysfunction is reversible by measuring lung volumes, forced vital capacity (FVC) and flow rates, and forced expiratory volume in 1 second ($FEV_1$) to help distinguish restrictive defects from obstructive defects. **Women who have compromised preoperative pulmonary function are especially susceptible to developing clinically significant postoperative atelectasis, which occurs after approximately 10% of gynecologic operations**. Predisposing factors that increase the incidence of atelectasis include morbid obesity, smoking, pulmonary disease, and advanced age. Increased pain, the supine position, abdominal distention, impaired function of the diaphragm, and sedation also contribute to decreased lung volumes and reduced dynamic measurements of pulmonary function postoperatively. Women with chronic lung disease often have shunting of blood in the lungs and arterial hypoxemia. A preoperative arterial blood gas may be able to demonstrate if the patient is hypoxic or hypercapneic, a serious sign, because the patient's respiratory drive may be refractory to hypercapnia. Hence, oxygen therapy for women with morbid obesity or symptoms of sleep apnea should be done with care because these conditions may further suppress respiratory drive.

**Asthma increases the incidence of perioperative respiratory problems approximately fourfold.** Women with asthma are susceptible to perioperative respiratory complications secondary to bronchial hyperresponsiveness, airflow obstruction, and hypersecretion of mucus. Ideally, a woman with asthma should have elective surgery when she is free of wheezing and her pulmonary function is optimal.

### Cardiovascular Disease

**Cardiac complications are the leading cause of postoperative deaths. Approximately 1.5% of adults who undergo inpatient noncardiac surgery die during the first 30 postoperative days**. (Devereaux, 2015). Unstable angina of less than 3 months' duration is a strong contraindication to an elective operation. After a myocardial infarction, it is important to delay an elective operation for approximately 6 months. **The excessive mortality rate associated with a noncardiac operative procedure within 3 months of an acute myocardial infarct is 27% to 37%.** After a 6-month interval, the chance of a reinfarction is 4% to 6% with elective operations.

The accurate assessment of cardiac risk is important for several reasons. First, it permits the patient to make an informed decision when weighing the risks and benefits of the proposed surgery. Second, the accurate estimation of cardiac risk can also guide preoperative interventions and postoperative care, including the intensity of monitoring. Finally, it allows for more accurate reporting of outcomes that are linked to the intensity of comorbid conditions. Two cardiac risk indexes are commonly used: the Revised Cardiac Risk Index (RCRI) is the most validated, and the National Surgical Quality Improvement Program risk index for Myocardial Infarction and Cardiac Arrest (NSQIP MICA) has the best predictive performance (http://www.surgicalriskcalculator.com/miorcardiacarrest). Both models assign points based on risk factors, but each defines a cardiac event a little differently, making direct comparisons difficult. For example, the RCRI assigns 1 point for each of the following: high-risk surgery; prior congestive heart failure, stroke, or transient ischemic attack; ischemic heart disease; use of insulin therapy; and creatinine level greater than 2 mg/dL. The risk of a myocardial infarction is 0.5% with 0 points, 1.3% with 1 point, 3.6% with 2 points, and 9.1% with 3 or more points. Unfortunately, clinical risk indexes tend to underestimate risk in patients who are immobile before surgery because they may lack some of the symptoms of cardiac disease simply because they are immobile. It is in this setting that noninvasive cardiac testing, such as stress nuclear scintigraphy, is used. However, it has been associated with up to a 30% false negative rate in postoperative patients.

One of the more common practices used to limit cardiac complications was the routine use of beta-blockers perioperatively as an attempt to blunt the sympathetic stress response. Unfortunately, **the use of beta-blockers perioperatively reduced the risk of nonfatal myocardial infarction but increased the risk of death, nonfatal stroke, hypotension, and bradycardia.** As a result, the common practice of perioperative beta-blockade has given way to its selective use to treat ischemia and tachycardia that can be safely and accurately identified by means of noninvasive cardiac monitoring.

## Prophylaxis Against Infective Endocarditis

The indications for prophylactic antibiotic use for the prevention of infective endocarditis (IE) have changed considerably since the American Heart Association guidelines were first published in 1955. In the current version of the guidelines, the indications for prophylaxis are very limited compared with prior guidelines (Wilson, 2007). The impetus behind the change is that **the risk of IE is greater from random spontaneous bacteremias associated with daily activities than from invasive GI, genitourinary (GU), or even dental procedures**. There are a lack of published data convincingly demonstrating that prophylaxis actually prevents IE. In addition, the use of prophylactic antibiotics may prevent a very small number of IEs, at the expense of more adverse antibiotic-associated events, tilting the risk-benefit scale in the wrong direction. As a result, the guidelines no longer recommend IE prophylaxis based solely on an increased lifetime risk of acquisition of IE. They restrict the use of prophylactic antibiotics to patients who are planning invasive, higher-risk procedures (Wilson, 2007). They do not recommend any prophylaxis to prevent IE for elective, invasive GU or GI procedures in noninfective patients. They acknowledge that there may be a very small number of instances of IE, if any, that could be prevented with prophylactic antibiotics use in this patient population. However, with no proved benefit, **the administration of prophylactic antibiotics solely**

**to prevent endocarditis is not recommended for patients who undergo GU or GI tract procedures.**

## SUMMARY

It is the gynecologic surgeon's responsibility to ensure his or her patient is adequately informed of the risks, benefits, and alternative treatments for each recommended surgical procedure. Caring for the patient as a team by involving the primary care provider or other long-term specialty physicians to guide management of medical conditions and long-term medications that may affect the surgical procedure or anesthesia is essential. Early consultation with an anesthesiologist is important when caring for patients with multiple comorbidities, those with prior anesthesia complications, and patients undergoing complex gynecologic operations to improve the preparation for and safety of the procedure. Universal Protocols, guidelines to prevent VTE, pathways to enhance postoperative recovery, and SSI prevention bundles improve the quality of gynecologic surgical care and should be used routinely.

### KEY REFERENCES


American College of Surgeons National Surgical Quality Improvement Program (ACS NSQIP). Classic, essential, small-rural, targeted, and Florida variables & definitions. In: *American College of Surgeons National Surgical Quality Improvement Program Operations Manual.* Chicago, IL: American College of Surgeons; 2011:24-26.

American Society of Anesthesiologists (ASA) practice guidelines for preoperative fasting and the use of pharmacologic agents to reduce the risk of pulmonary aspiration: application to healthy patients undergoing elective procedures: an updated report by the American Society of Anesthesiologists Task Force on preoperative fasting and the use of pharmacologic agents to reduce the risk of pulmonary aspiration. *Anesthesiology.* 2017; 126(3):376-393.

Axelrod L. Perioperative management of patients treated with glucocorticoids. *Endocrinol Metab Clin North Am.* 2003;32(2):367-383.

Bakkum-Gamez JN, Dowdy SC, Borah BJ, et al. Predictors and costs of surgical site infections in patients with endometrial cancer. *Gynecol Oncol.* 2013;130(1):100-106.

Belavy D, Janda M, Baker J, et al. Epidural analgesia is associated with an increased incidence of postoperative complications in patients requiring an abdominal hysterectomy for early stage endometrial cancer. *Gynecol Oncol.* 2013;131(2):423-429.

Bode LG, Kluytmans JA, Wertheim HF, et al. Preventing surgical-site infections in nasal carriers of Staphylococcus aureus. *N Engl J Med.* 2010;362(1):9-17.

Bonnar J. Venous thromboembolism and gynecologic surgery. *Clin Obstet Gynecol.* 1985;28(2):432-446.

Brady M, Kinn S, Stuart P. Preoperative fasting for adults to prevent perioperative complications. *Cochrane Database Syst Rev.* 2003;(4): CD004423.

Brandstrup B, Tønnesen H, Beier-Holgersen R, et al. Effects of intravenous fluid restriction on postoperative complications: comparison of two perioperative fluid regimens: a randomized assessor-blinded multicenter trial. *Ann Surg.* 2003;238(5):641-648.

Bratzler DW, Dellinger EP, Olsen KM, et al. Clinical practice guidelines for antimicrobial prophylaxis in surgery. *Am J Health Syst Pharm.* 2013; 70(3):195-283.

Campbell G, Alderson P, Smith AF, et al. Warming of intravenous and irrigation fluids for preventing inadvertent perioperative hypothermia. *Cochrane Database Syst Rev.* 2015;4:CD009891.

Carter J. Fast-track surgery in gynaecology and gynaecologic oncology: a review of a rolling clinical audit. *ISRN Surg.* 2012;2012:368014.

Chambers D, Paton F, Wilson P, et al. An overview and methodological assessment of systematic reviews and meta-analyses of enhanced recovery programmes in colorectal surgery. *BMJ Open.* 2014;4(5):e005014.

Chan RP, Galas FR, Hajjar LA, et al. Intensive perioperative glucose control does not improve outcomes of patients submitted to open-heart surgery: a randomized controlled trial. *Clinics (Sao Paulo).* 2009; 64(1):51-60.

Charoenkwan K, Phillipson G, Vutyavanich T. Early versus delayed (traditional) oral fluids and food for reducing complications after major abdominal gynaecologic surgery. *Cochrane Database Syst Rev.* 2007;(4): CD004508.

Chase DM, Lopez S, Nguyen C, et al. A clinical pathway for postoperative management and early patient discharge: does it work in gynecologic oncology? *Am J Obstet Gynecol.* 2008;199(5):541.e1-541.e7.

Cima R, Dankbar E, Lovely J, et al. Colorectal surgery surgical site infection reduction program: a national surgical quality improvement program-driven multidisciplinary single-institution experience. *J Am Coll Surg.* 2013;216(1):23-33.

Colling K, Glover J, et al. Abdominal hysterectomy: reduced risk of surgical site infection associated with robotic and laparoscopic technique. *Surg Infect (Larchmt).* 2015;16(5):498-503.

Committee on Standards and Practice Parameters, Apfelbaum JL, Connis RT, et al. Practice advisory for preanesthesia evaluation: an updated report by the American Society of Anesthesiologists Task Force on Preanesthesia Evaluation. *Anesthesiology.* 2012;116(3):522-538. (Reaffirmed 2018)

Cruse P, Foord R. The epidemiology of wound infection. A 10-year prospective study of 62,939 wounds. *Surg Clin North Am.* 1980;60(1):27-40.

Cutillo G, Maneschi F, Franchi M, et al. Early feeding compared with nasogastric decompression after major oncologic gynecologic surgery: a randomized study. *Obstet Gynecol.* 1999;93(1):41-45.

Darouiche RO, Wall Jr MJ, Itani KM, et al. Chlorhexidine-alcohol versus povidone-iodine for surgical-site antisepsis. *N Engl J Med.* 2010; 362(1):18-26.

Devereaux PJ, Sessler DI. Cardiac complications in patients undergoing major noncardiac surgery. *N Engl J Med.* 2015;373(23):2258-2269.

Eberhart LK, Koch T, Ploger B, et al. Enhanced recovery after major gynaecological surgery for ovarian cancer—an objective and patient-based assessment of a traditional versus a multimodal 'fast track' rehabilitation programme. *Anasthesiol Intensivmed.* 2008;49:180-194.

Ferguson SE, Malhotra T, Seshan VE, et al. A prospective randomized trial comparing patient-controlled epidural analgesia to patient-controlled intravenous analgesia on postoperative pain control and recovery after major open gynecologic cancer surgery. *Gynecol Oncol.* 2009;114(1):111-116.

Galvão CM, Liang Y, Clark AM. Effectiveness of cutaneous warming systems on temperature control: meta-analysis. *J Adv Nurs.* 2010;66(6): 1196-1206.

Gandhi GY, Nuttall GA, Abel MD, et al. Intensive intraoperative insulin therapy versus conventional glucose management during cardiac surgery: a randomized trial. *Ann Intern Med.* 2007;146(4):233-243.

Gerardi MA, Santillan A, Meisner B, et al. A clinical pathway for patients undergoing primary cytoreductive surgery with rectosigmoid colectomy for advanced ovarian and primary peritoneal cancers. *Gynecol Oncol.* 2008;108(2):282-286.

Gould MK, Garcia DA, Wren SM, et al. Prevention of VTE in nonorthopedic surgical patients: Antithrombotic Therapy and Prevention of Thrombosis, 9th ed: American College of Chest Physicians Evidence-Based Clinical Practice Guidelines. *Chest.* 2012;141(Suppl 2): e227S-e277S.

Güenaga K, Matos D, Wille-Jørgensen P. Mechanical bowel preparation for elective colorectal surgery. *Cochrane Database Syst Rev.* 2011; (9):CD001544.


**Full references for this chapter can be found on ExpertConsult.com.**

# 25 Perioperative Management of Complications

## Fever, Respiratory, Cardiovascular, Thromboembolic, Urinary Tract, Gastrointestinal, Wound, and Operative Site Complications; Neurologic Injury; Psychological Sequelae

*Leslie H. Clark, Paola Alvarez Gehrig, Fidel A. Valea*

### KEY POINTS

- Postoperative febrile morbidity is related to infection in approximately 20% of cases and noninfectious causes in 80% of cases.
- Infection in older adults will not always present with classic findings. The amount of temperature elevation may not reflect the severity of the infection. Not uncommonly, the first signs of infection in older adults will be mental status changes. Also, the degree of leukocytosis may not reflect infection, being blunted or absent.
- Minimum urine output is approximately 0.5 mL/kg per hour. The use of a 20-mL/hour benchmark for all women is only an approximation and should be adjusted for the patient's weight.
- Because of the shifts in water balance, the postoperative hemoglobin at 72 hours is a more accurate measurement of operative and postoperative blood loss than a hemoglobin at 24 hours.
- After subtracting the effects of the operative blood loss from the preoperative hemoglobin, a further reduction in hemoglobin of 1 to 2 points reflects a postoperative hemorrhage of approximately 500 mL.
- Women should be transfused when their hemoglobin falls to less than 7 or sooner if they are symptomatic or have significant cardiac or pulmonary comorbidities.
- Microatelectasis is a common occurrence developing during almost all pelvic surgeries and is persistent 24 hours postoperatively in approximately 50% of women. Studies have demonstrated that there is no association between fever and the amount of atelectasis diagnosed radiologically.
- Radiographic diagnoses are approximately 60% accurate for bacterial or viral pneumonia in women with laboratory-proved pneumonia.
- Rapid loss of 20% of a woman's blood volume produces mild shock, and a loss of greater than 40% of blood volume results in severe shock.
- Approximately 15% to 45% of surgical blood loss is absorbed onto drapes, pads, and other areas. Thus blood levels in the suction bottle are inaccurate markers of total operative blood loss.
- Massive blood loss has been defined as hemorrhage that results in replacement of 50% of circulating blood volume in less than 3 hours.
- Returning to the operating room to control hemorrhage is often a difficult decision. However, when indicated, this decision should be carried as soon as possible in conjunction with volume replacement.
- The extent of wound or pelvic hematomas is determined by the potential size of the compartment into which the bleeding occurs. Retroperitoneal or broad ligament hematomas may contain several units of blood.
- Superficial phlebitis is the leading cause of an enigmatic postoperative fever during the third, fourth, or fifth postoperative day.
- The clinical management of mild superficial thrombophlebitis includes rest, elevation, and local heat. Moderate to severe superficial thrombophlebitis may be treated with nonsteroidal antiinflammatory agents.
- Venous thrombosis and pulmonary embolism are the direct causes of approximately 40% of deaths after gynecologic surgery.
- Signs and symptoms of pulmonary emboli are nonspecific; however, the most common symptoms are chest pain, dyspnea, apprehension, tachypnea, rales, and an increase in the second heart sound over the pulmonic area.
- Intermittent in-and-out catheterization is preferable to continuous drainage with a Foley catheter for women with intermediate-term voiding dysfunction.
- Although symptoms of urinary incontinence may present within a few hours of the operative procedure, most fistulas present 8 to 12 days after operation and occasionally as late as 25 to 30 days after the operation.
- If there is a suspicion that trauma to the bladder has occurred during an operative procedure, continuous catheter drainage for 3 to 5 days usually results in spontaneous healing.
- Approximately 25% of adult women experience postoperative nausea and vomiting.
- Normal return of bowel function after abdominal surgery can take 3 to 7 days. The left colon takes the longest to resume function, approximately 72 hours after surgery. If return of bowel function does not occur by 7 days, a diagnosis of mechanical bowel obstruction or another cause for the ileus should be considered.
- Postoperative oral feeding is safe and efficacious. This practice is preferred because it facilitates recovery and shortens hospital stay.
- The difference between small bowel obstruction and adynamic ileus is subtle because adynamic ileus can be associated with partial obstruction of the small intestine. The use of diatrizoate (Gastrografin) contrast can be both diagnostic and therapeutic.
- Second- and third-generation cephalosporins are the antibiotics associated with the highest risk of developing *Clostridium difficile* diarrhea.
- The incidence of postoperative wound infection is increased eightfold when the woman's preoperative weight exceeds 200 pounds. The thickness of subcutaneous tissue is the greatest risk factor for wound infection in women undergoing abdominal hysterectomy.

*Continued*

KEY POINTS—cont'd

- Necrotizing fasciitis involves the subcutaneous tissue and superficial fascia. It rapidly expands in the subcutaneous spaces. This condition is a surgical emergency and patients should have operative debridement as soon as possible.
- The incidence of wound dehiscence is approximately 1 in 200 gynecologic operations. Wound infection is found in approximately 50% of women with wound disruption.
- The classic feature of an impending wound disruption is the spontaneous passage of copious serosanguineous fluid from the abdominal incision.
- Most postoperative pelvic infections are polymicrobial, usually from endogenous vaginal flora, and approximately 60% to 80% involve anaerobic organisms.
- Common causes of femoral neuropathy are continuous pressure from self-retaining retractors, particularly in thin women, or exaggerated hip flexion or abduction in the dorsal lithotomy position.
- Discharge instructions should be given in verbal and written forms, and the gynecologist should anticipate the most common questions.

**Appendixes A, B, and C are available at ExpertConsult.com.**

The goal of postoperative care is the restoration of a woman's normal physiologic and psychological health. The postoperative period includes the time from the end of the procedure in the operating room until the woman has resumed her normal routine and lifestyle.

**Postoperative complications may occur at any time; however, early recognition and management will often preclude larger problems.** Thus attention to postoperative details cannot be overemphasized. Complications increase the duration of the postoperative stay in the hospital and increase the risk of hospital readmission. Because many procedures are now performed using minimally invasive techniques, patients will usually leave less than or close to 24 hours after surgery, which is often before the signs and symptoms of a complication present. Before discharge, it is important that the patient receive education regarding expectations, signs and symptoms of infection and other complications, and appropriate contact information.

Significant risk factors in any surgical population include underlying cardiac and pulmonary disease, smoking, obesity, prior or current abdominal/thoracic surgery, and type of anesthesia. General caveats of postoperative management emphasize attention to the particular needs of each woman. Studies conflict on whether age alone is an independent risk factor for perioperative morbidity and mortality. Older patients tend to have more underlying disease, placing them at higher risk for perioperative complications. Unfortunately, this alone does not completely account for their worse outcomes. In one large population-based study, even *healthy* elderly patients continued to have higher morbidity and mortality (Deiner & Silverstein, 2012). It is likely that elderly patients respond differently to perioperative physiologic stressors and pharmacologic interventions. Individualization is especially important in the postoperative care of geriatric women. Special nursing attention and minimal doses of narcotics help prevent confusion and disorientation. Ongoing verbal communications with the nursing staff help eliminate misunderstandings that might result in less than ideal postoperative care.

Surgical stress invokes several physiologic responses meant as the body's defenses. Many of these responses may be more problematic than the actual surgery. For example, some women will respond to the insulin resistance from surgical trauma with severe hyperglycemia, which is detrimental to healing. Peri- and postoperative management strategies are aimed at minimizing or preventing these adverse effects, such as prevention of thromboembolism, or selective use of beta blockade in older patients to prevent cardiac complications (Fig. 25.1) (Kehlet, 2003).

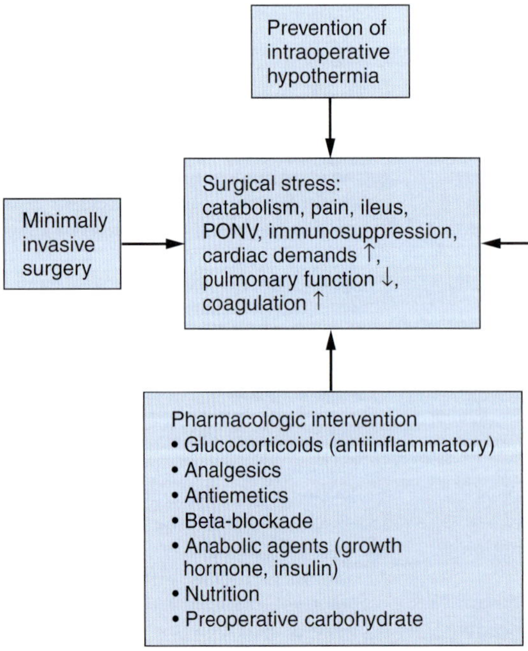

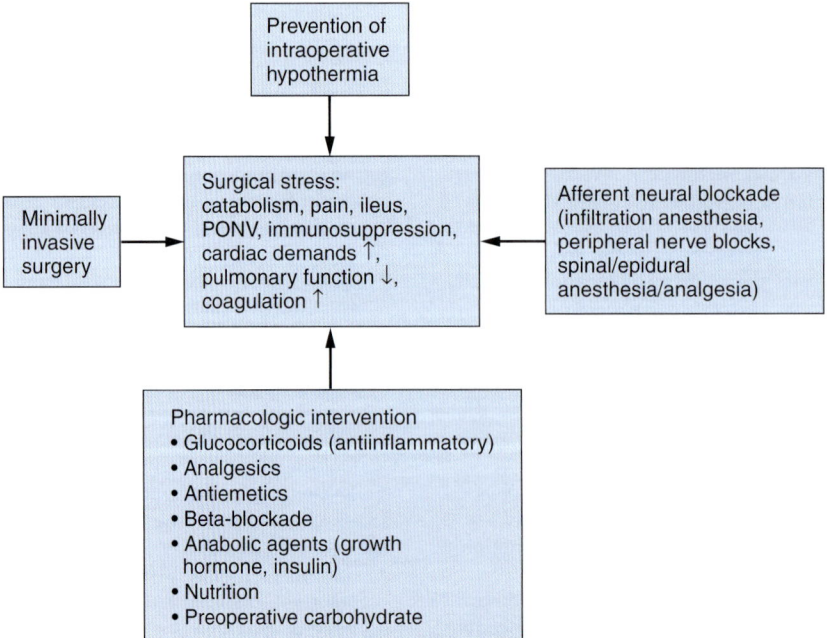

**Fig. 25.1** Stresses of surgery and interventions to counteract adverse responses. *PONV,* Postoperative nausea and vomiting. (Modified from Kehlet H, Dahl JB. Anesthesia, surgery, and challenges in postoperative recovery. *Lancet.* 2003;362:1921-1928.)

This chapter discusses major issues of management during the period from the end of surgery until the return to normal physiologic and psychological function. However, much of the data regarding postoperative complications only involve the period up through postoperative day 30. Problems and complications arise over the whole spectrum of the postoperative time frame and are interrelated. Thus the clinician must be aware at all times of a woman's changing status during recovery. For simplicity, this chapter is organized around organ systems and their potential complications.

## POSTOPERATIVE FEVER

The exact definition of postoperative febrile morbidity varies greatly among authors. Diurnal fluctuations are characteristic of the normal daily body temperature patterns of humans. Most definitions use a temperature greater than 38° C a day after surgery as the indicator of febrile morbidity. It is not unusual for gynecologic patients to have a mild temperature elevation during the first 72 hours of the postoperative period, especially during the late afternoon or evening. **Up to 75% of patients develop a temperature greater than 37° C, which is usually not associated with an infectious process.** The incidence of postoperative febrile morbidity after benign hysterectomy ranges from 14% to 16% with as few as 3% having a documented infectious source (Kendrick, 2008; Peipert, 2004).

**Fever is the most common morbidity in the postoperative patient. Common causes of a fever include atelectasis, pneumonia, urinary tract infection (UTI), nonseptic phlebitis, wound infection, and operative site infection.** Two intraoperative factors that dramatically increase the risk of postoperative fever are an operative time longer than 2 hours and the necessity for intraoperative transfusion. Increased intraoperative blood loss is associated with a 3.5-fold relative risk (RR; 95% confidence interval [CI], 1.8 to 6.8) of developing a postoperative fever (Peipert, 2004).

The physician's primary goal in examining the postoperative patient with fever is to determine the cause. Approximately 20% of postoperative fevers are directly related to infection and 80% are related to noninfectious causes (Schey, 2005). Some conditions necessitate active intervention, whereas others are self-limiting. Thus it is imperative not to treat a postoperatively febrile patient empirically with broad-spectrum antibiotics. Protocols limiting antibiotic use to high-risk patients (bowel operation, preoperative infection, immunodeficiency, indwelling vascular access, mechanical heart valves, or intensive care unit [ICU] admission) or those with persistent fevers greater than 101° F for more than 48 hours have been shown to be safe (Kendrick, 2008).

The pathophysiology of postoperative fever is primarily related to the release of cytokines. The cause of a postoperative fever may be simple and common, such as atelectasis or dehydration, or unusual, such as malignant hyperthermia or septicemia. The temporal relationship of the onset of a woman's febrile response to common postoperative complications is depicted in Table 25.1.

**TABLE 25.1** Onset of Fever for Various Postoperative Complications

| Causes | Day 1 | 2 | 3 | 4 | 5 | 6 | 1 Week or Longer |
|---|---|---|---|---|---|---|---|
| Atelectasis | — | — | → | | | | |
| Pneumonia | | | — | — | — | — | → |
| Wound infection | | | | | | | |
| Streptococcal or clostridial | — | → | | | | | |
| Other bacterial | | | | | — | — | → |
| Ovarian abscess | | | | | | | → |
| Cuff cellulitis | | | | — | — | → | |
| Phlebitis | | | | | | | |
| Superficial | | | | — | — | → | |
| Deep | | | — | — | — | — | → |
| Urinary tract infection | | | — | — | — | — | → |
| Ureteral or bladder injury | | | | | | | → |
| Bowel injury | — | — | — | — | — | — | → |

## Workup for Fever

The initial workup for a postoperative fever should focus on the most common problems. Medical students memorize the "five Ws" in the differential diagnosis of a postoperative fever: *wind* (atelectasis), *water* (UTI), *wound* (infection or hematoma), *walking* (superficial or deep vein phlebitis), and *wonder drugs* (drug-induced fever). The proper workup of a postoperative fever, similar to that of any problem in medicine, involves the three classic steps of history, physical examination, and laboratory evaluations, with major emphasis placed on the physical examination. The physical examination emphasizes the following: examination of the lungs for atelectasis and pneumonia; the wound and operative site for infection or hematoma formation; the costovertebral angles for tenderness, which may suggest pyelonephritis; and superficial veins in the arms for superficial phlebitis and deep veins in the legs for deep vein phlebitis.

The findings of the history and especially the physical examination influence the extent of laboratory tests ordered. The three most commonly ordered laboratory tests are complete blood cell count (CBC), chest radiography, and urinalysis, although a study by Schwandt and colleagues emphasized that chest radiography and urine cultures are best ordered only for specific clinical signs, not as reflex orders (Schwandt, 2001). Other common tests include culture and Gram stains of body fluids, including sputum, urine, and blood. One study of more than 300 women who were febrile after hysterectomy did not identify a single positive blood culture, whereas another study found a 9.7% positive blood culture rate in more than 500 patients, suggesting a role for judicious use of blood cultures (Kendrick, 2008; Schey, 2005). Women with persistent and undiagnosed fevers may need imaging studies, such as pelvic ultrasound or computed tomography (CT) to detect problems such as compromised ureters, abscesses, or foreign bodies, but routine imaging is likely low yield and may result in indeterminate results because of postoperative changes.

Each major complication will be discussed in detail later in the chapter; however, several specific generalizations concerning the type and characteristics of fever patterns should be emphasized. Fever is a common postoperative finding and rarely is the cause of the fever a serious infection. **Atelectasis is thought to be the cause of approximately 90% of fevers occurring in the first 48 hours after operation.** Patients who develop fever as a result of an indwelling catheter, such as intravenous (IV) lines or Foley catheters, are afebrile for several days and then experience an abrupt temperature spike. In contrast, wound or pelvic infections, which are usually clinically diagnosed from the fourth to seventh postoperative days, usually are associated with a low-grade fever that begins early in the postoperative period. An empiric trial of IV heparin for 72 hours is often a diagnostic and therapeutic trial for pelvic thrombophlebitis in refractory cases of postoperative fever of unknown origin.

Importantly, infection in the older woman will not always present with classic findings. The amount of temperature elevation may not reflect the severity of the infection. **Not uncommonly, the first signs of infection in older adults will be mental status changes.** Additionally, the degree of leukocytosis, being blunted or absent may not reflect infection.

A woman with a drug-induced fever feels better and does not look as ill as her temperature course indicates. The tachycardia associated with the elevated temperature is usually much less than usually anticipated with a similar temperature elevation secondary to inflammation or infection. The presence of eosinophilia suggests a drug-induced fever. However, drug fever is rare and is usually a diagnosis of exclusion. Presumptive evidence of a drug-induced fever is established when the fever disappears after discontinuation of the drug. The most commonly implicated drugs include allopurinol, carbamazepine, lamotrigine, phenytoin, sulfasalazine, vancomycin, minocycline, dapsone, and sulfamethoxazole. The risk of developing a drug-induced fever is higher in elderly and patients with human immunodeficiency virus (HIV).

Superficial thrombophlebitis often produces an enigmatic fever. Often there is tenderness at the IV site. IV catheters should be removed at the first sign of tenderness or erythema, but routine replacement (exchange) to prevent thrombophlebitis is not indicated (Webster, 2013). Transfusion reactions can also cause febrile events. Leukocyte or platelet antibodies usually cause these reactions. As long as a major blood type incompatibility is not found, treatment is usually conservative.

It is common practice to repeat the basic fever workup at regular intervals until the diagnosis is established. The woman should be reexamined and selective laboratory tests reordered. Rare causes of postoperative fever include pulmonary embolism (PE), thyroid storm, and malignant neoplasms. These diagnoses usually present with other signs and symptoms as well as temperature elevation. It is important to consider that fever is a potentially beneficial physiologic response of the patient. Therefore unless the woman is symptomatic secondary to the elevated temperature, it is not necessary to order antipyretic medications. Cellular damage usually occurs when the core temperature exceeds 41° C. Active cutaneous cooling does not reduce core temperature effectively and may have undesirable effects, such as increasing the metabolic rate and activating the autonomic nervous system.

## MANAGEMENT OF FALLING HEMOGLOBIN

Bleeding is one of the most worrisome postoperative complications. Significant arterial bleeding in the first 24 hours often necessitates reoperation. This complication is discussed later in the chapter, along with the management of shock and pelvic hematoma.

Vital signs should be ordered at frequent intervals during the first 24 hours because changes in vitals are often the first manifestation of hypovolemia. A 4-hour interval for vitals is appropriate for most floor patients. **Most women will have sufficient intravascular volume to compensate (during the early phases of hemorrhage) through the redistribution of blood flow from less vital to more vital organs, and as a result, low urine output may be the earliest sign of a decrease in intravascular volume.** Thus after an operation, sizable amounts of unrecognized intraperitoneal or retroperitoneal bleeding are sometimes present without the woman having subjective symptoms or appreciable changes in her vital signs. This may be the case particularly in young, healthy women. Typical teaching for appropriate postoperative urine output is at least 0.5 mL/kg per hour; however, many enhanced recovery protocols allow for permissive oliguria to help reduce overuse of IV fluids. **There should remain a low threshold to check a CBC or evaluate a patient if oliguria is seen in the postoperative period.** A consistent orthostatic decrease in blood pressure of more than 10 mm Hg can indicate a decrease of 20% of the blood volume, and therefore orthostatic vitals can be considered as part of the evaluation for postoperative hypovolemia caused by blood loss. Measuring the hemoglobin at two intervals during the postoperative course is helpful to allow for observation of change over time. It should be noted that a hemoglobin drawn within 24 hours after an operation may not truly reflect postoperative blood loss and a repeat hemoglobin evaluation 48 to 72 hours postoperatively will more accurately reflect the hemoglobin nadir from blood loss.

The normal physiologic response to the stress of the operation and tissue destruction is a release of aldosterone, cortisol, and antidiuretic hormone (ADH). The higher levels of aldosterone seen as a result of surgical stress produce an increase in sodium and water retention, whereas increased levels of ADH promote free water retention. This has been called the *ebb phase* of postoperative physiology. It is common for women to have notable lower extremity edema for the first few postoperative days as a result of these hormonal shifts and the use of perioperative IV fluids. Depending on the type and amount of intraoperative and postoperative IV fluids, the hemoglobin on the first postoperative day may be misleading and reflect fluid changes rather than intraoperative or postoperative hemorrhage. The hemoglobin from the third postoperative day is a more accurate measurement of postoperative change. If the patient is doing well, stress hormone levels decline, and water retention stops, the patient will begin to experience a brisk diuresis beginning around the third postoperative day. After the effects of the operative blood loss are subtracted from the preoperative hemoglobin, each further reduction in hemoglobin of 1 to 2 points reflects a postoperative hemorrhage of approximately 250 to 500 mL. Historically, patients were transfused to maintain a hemoglobin greater than 10, but mounting evidence supports the practice of more restrictive transfusion parameters with individualized consideration for transfusion. In hemodynamically stable patients who are asymptomatic from anemia, a hemoglobin level less than 7 is usually an indication for transfusion; however, a patient with cardiovascular disease and a hemoglobin level less than 8 should be considered for transfusion. In a patient with a hemoglobin of 8 to 10, transfusion is not indicated unless the patient is symptomatic, there is ongoing bleeding, or there is concern for acute coronary syndrome (Klein, 2007). The morbidity and mortality associated with a surgical procedure are directly related to the amount of intraoperative and postoperative blood loss and not the corresponding level of preoperative anemia.

## RESPIRATORY COMPLICATIONS

Alterations of pulmonary function are an expected physiologic change in women having general anesthesia and operations that enter the peritoneal cavity. Respiratory complications can occur in up to 10% to 30% of patients undergoing major abdominal surgery and can contribute significantly to the morbidity and mortality of surgery. The use of minimally invasive surgery for hysterectomy has resulted in fewer postoperative respiratory complications (~2%), which is attributed to less acute pain from the operative incision (Burks, 2017). Although postoperative respiratory status is improved, intraoperative ventilation is more challenging for anesthesia providers to manage with insufflation and Trendelenburg positioning.

### Atelectasis

The term *atelectasis* is derived from two Greek words that mean "imperfect expansion." The severity of atelectasis ranges from lack of expansion of a small group of terminal bronchioles and alveoli to complete collapse of a lung. In most patients, atelectasis is the failure to maintain patency of the small pulmonary airways and alveoli. **Atelectasis is the most common cause of postoperative temperature elevations.** Studies have demonstrated that there is no association between fever and the amount of atelectasis seen radiographically. The incidence of atelectasis depends on the number of predisposing risk factors and the vigor with which the clinical diagnosis is established.

Of all postoperative respiratory complications, 90% are related to atelectasis. The immediate postoperative period is characterized by a decrease in functional residual capacity and lung compliance (Fig. 25.2). Thus the work of breathing is increased. Microatelectasis

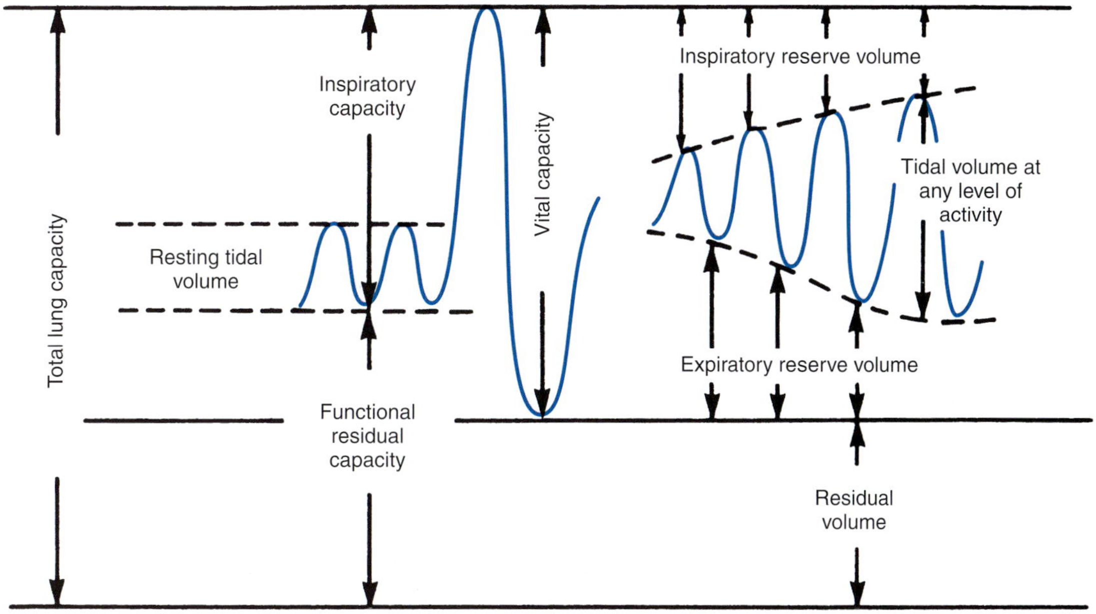


**Fig. 25.2** Graphic illustration of lung volumes and capacities. (From Wellman JJ. Respiratory care in the surgical patient. In: Lubin MF, Walker HD, Smith RB, eds. *Medical Management of the Surgical Patient.* Stoneham, MA: Butterworth; 1982.)

is most common when small airways (<1 mm in diameter) become blocked by secretions. When small airways remain closed by a combination of mucous plugs and bronchospasm, the gas distal to the obstruction is absorbed. This process results in atelectasis. These changes occur during the first 72 hours after an operation. When atelectasis becomes progressive and involves a large area of lung tissue, there is an associated decrease in oxygen saturation and a decrease in arterial oxygen pressure ($Po_2$). This is associated with a normal to low arterial carbon dioxide pressure ($Pco_2$).

Pulmonary and nonpulmonary factors that favor premature airway closure and development of atelectasis are listed in Box 25.1. **The supine position decreases the functional residual capacity by approximately 20% compared with the erect position; thus early ambulation should be encouraged.** Obesity, smoking, age older than 60 years, prolonged operative time, presence of a nasogastric tube, and coexisting medical conditions, such as cardiac or lung disease and pulmonary infection, all predispose women to atelectasis. **Insufflation of the abdomen for laparoscopic and robotic surgery also contributes to postoperative atelectasis by collapsing the dependent portion of the lung bases if adequate ventilation pressures are not used.**

In normal breathing, periodic, involuntary, deep inspirations help expand all areas of the lung. Incisional pain, the supine position, narcotics, and abdominal distention contribute to a pattern of monotonous shallow breathing without spontaneous deep sighs in the postoperative period. As a result of the incisional pain, chest wall breathing dominates over abdominal breathing. The resultant decrease in the movement of the diaphragm contributes to the development of atelectasis. A further decrease in functional residual capacity, a decrease in surfactant, and a depression of mucociliary transport, all contribute to ventilation-perfusion ($\dot{V}/\dot{Q}$) mismatches and reduced ($\dot{V}/\dot{Q}$) ratios. The results are gas trapping, atelectasis, and vascular shunting. In most individuals, microatelectasis is patchy and localized to small areas. However, the severity of atelectasis varies and may involve a complete lung. Distribution of pulmonary blood flow is influenced by gravity. A greater proportion of pulmonary blood flows to dependent areas of the lungs in the supine patient. Increased blood flow to dependent areas in combination with atelectasis in dependent areas results in impaired oxygenation and decreased elimination of carbon dioxide. **Elevation of the head of the bed in patients with obesity may help improve vital capacity and ventilation, thus decreasing atelectasis.**

**BOX 25.1** Nonpulmonary and Pulmonary Factors Favoring Premature Airway Closure and Atelectasis

**NONPULMONARY FACTORS**

- Supine position
- Obesity
- Increased abdominal girth (ileus, pneumoperitoneum)
- Breathing at low lung volumes
  - Bindings around the chest and abdomen
  - Incisional pain
  - Sedative narcotic drugs
  - Prolonged effect of paralyzing drugs
  - Immobility
  - Excessively high concentrations of oxygen for prolonged periods

**PULMONARY FACTORS**

- Interstitial edema
- Loss of surfactant with air space instability
- Airway obstruction
  - Inflammatory with swelling of bronchial and interbronchial tissue
  - Constriction of bronchial smooth muscle
  - Retained secretions

From Wellman JJ. Respiratory care in the surgical patient. In: Lubin MF, Walker HK, Smith RB, eds. *Medical Management of the Surgical Patient.* Stoneham, MA: Butterworth; 1982.

**Atelectasis may present as the classic triad of fever, tachypnea, and tachycardia developing within the first 72 hours after an operation.** On physical examination, decreased breath sounds and inspiratory rales may be heard. These findings are most prominent over the lung bases. If the atelectasis is not reversed with incentive spirometry and deep breathing, there will be an increase in productive cough and leukocytosis. Chest radiographs may demonstrate a patchy infiltrate with elevations of the diaphragm.

Atelectasis usually resolves spontaneously by the third to fifth postoperative day. Nevertheless, major efforts are made to prevent atelectasis, especially in high-risk individuals. Atelectasis prevention is based on the encouragement of uneven ventilation and the production of episodes of prolonged inspiration to increase functional residual capacity. Thus the patient is encouraged to walk, take deep breaths, cough, turn from side to side, remain semierect rather than supine, and use an incentive spirometer regularly. **Early mobilization and ambulation have been documented to be as effective as chest physical therapy in the prevention of pulmonary complications.** Keeping pain relief to a level at which the woman will be able to cooperate and not have monotonous shallow breathing is also helpful; however, excessive narcotic use can result in respiratory depression. Although neither the use of postoperative continuous positive airway pressure (CPAP) or incentive spirometry has been shown to reduce postoperative pulmonary morbidity, simple bedside incentive spirometry can be used to prevent and reverse atelectasis (do Nascimento, 2014; Ireland, 2014). **The primary risk of atelectasis is progression to pneumonia.**

## Pneumonia

Postoperative pneumonia is commonly associated with atelectasis because bacterial infections often begin in collapsed areas of the lungs. Predisposing factors to the development of pneumonia include chronic pulmonary disease, heavy cigarette smoking, alcohol abuse, obesity, advanced age, nasogastric tubes, long operative procedures, gram-negative bacterial infections, postoperative peritonitis, and debilitating illnesses.

**The symptoms and signs of pneumonia are fever, cough, dyspnea, tachypnea, and purulent sputum.** When pain occurs, it may be felt in the back or chest. **The classic physical finding of pneumonia is coarse rales over the infected area.** The patient usually has a higher temperature and more systemic toxicity than a woman with atelectasis. Leukocytosis is pronounced in most patients, although it may be delayed or attenuated in older women. Chest radiographs often demonstrate diffuse patchy infiltrates of the lung. **Radiographic diagnoses are approximately 60% accurate for bacterial or viral pneumonia in women with laboratory-proven pneumonia.** Gram staining of the sputum helps differentiate between bacterial colonization and infection. In cases of pneumonia the smear contains a large number of inflammatory cells with both intracellular and extracellular bacteria.

The management of pneumonia is similar to the management of atelectasis, with the addition of parenteral antibiotics. **Antibiotic choice is based on the type of pneumonia diagnosed.** Most postoperative patients will fall into one of the following categories: hospital-acquired pneumonia (HAP) occurring 48 hours or more after hospital admission or ventilator-acquired pneumonia (VAP) developing 48 to 72 hours after endotracheal intubation. The concept of health care–associated pneumonia (HCAP) occurring in a nonhospitalized patient with extensive health care contact was added as a category in 2005 and removed in 2016 in favor of a more stringent individual risk assessment and the use of hospital "antibiograms" to help guide treatment in each individual facility (Kalil, 2016). **Risk factors for multidrug-resistant pathogens are listed in Box 25.2.** Most patients with HAP and VAP who do not have significant risk factors for multidrug resistance and can be treated with empiric antibiotics using one of the following regimens: (1) cefepime 1–2 g intravenously every 8 hours, (2) piperacillin-tazobactam 4.5 g intravenously every 6 hours, (3) levofloxacin 750 mg intravenously daily, (4) imipenem 500 mg intravenously every 6 hours, (5) meropenem 1 g intravenously every 8 hours, or (6) aztreonam 2 g intravenously every 8 hours. However, in the setting of risk factors for multidrug resistance (see Box 25.2), one should choose one of the following: (1) an antipseudomonal cephalosporin (such as cefepime 2 g intravenously every 8 hours or ceftazidime 2 g intravenously every 8 hours), (2) an antipseudomonal carbapenem (such as meropenem 1 g intravenously every 8 hours or imipenem 500 to 1000 mg every 6 hours), or (3) piperacillin-tazobactam 4.5 g intravenously every 6 hours. In patients with severe penicillin allergies who cannot have these regimens, aztreonam 2 g intravenously every 6 to 8 hours should be used. In addition, the provider should add either an antipseudomonal fluoroquinolone (ciprofloxacin or levofloxacin), an aminoglycoside (gentamycin, tobramycin, or amikacin) or one of the polymyxins (Colistin or Polymyxin B). Finally, methicillin-resistant *Staphylococcus aureus* (MRSA) coverage should be provided with vancomycin (15 to 20 mg/kg intravenously every 8 to 12 hours) or linezolid (600 mg every 12 hours).

**BOX 25.2** Risk Factors for Multidrug-Resistant Pathogens

**RISK FACTORS FOR MDR VAP**

Prior intravenous antibiotic use within 90 days
Septic shock at time of VAP
ARDS preceding VAP
Five or more days of hospitalization prior to the occurrence of VAP
Acute renal replacement therapy prior to VAP onset

**RISK FACTORS FOR MDR HAP**

Prior intravenous antibiotic use within 90 days

**RISK FACTORS FOR MRSA VAP/HAP**

Prior intravenous antibiotic use within 90 days

**RISK FACTORS FOR MDR PSEUDOMONAS VAP/HAP**

Prior intravenous antibiotic use within 90 days

From Kalil AC, Metersky ML, Klompas M, et al. Management of adults with hospital-acquired and ventilator-associated pneumonia: 2016 Clinical Practice Guidelines by the Infectious Diseases Society of America and the American Thoracic Society. *Clin Infect Dis.* 2016;63(5):e61-e111.

*ARDS,* Acute respiratory distress syndrome; *HAP,* hospital-acquired pneumonia; *MDR,* multidrug resistant; *MRSA,* methicillin-resistant *Staphylococcus aureus; VAP,* ventilator-associated pneumonia.

Postoperative patients can also develop aspiration pneumonia as a result of loss of protective airway reflexes during intubation and extubation, or related to postoperative nausea and vomiting. **The most common pathogens in aspiration pneumonia are upper airway pathogens such as *Streptococcus pneumoniae*, *Haemophilus influenza*, *Staphylococcus aureus*, and gram-negative rods. The Infectious Disease Society of America and the American Thoracic Society in 2019 recommended that aspiration pneumonia is best treated with amoxicillin or doxycycline for outpatients with no comorbidities or risk factors for resistant bacteria.** Previously, macrolides were recommended as first-line antibiotics, but the new guideline lists macrolides as alternative options as a result of therapy failures in patients with macrolide-resistant *S. pneumoniae* and increasing macrolide resistance in United States; therefore, in that setting, azithromycin and clarithromycin are still options but erythromycin has been removed because of resistance (Metlay, 2019). For outpatients with comorbidities or risk factors, combination therapy is recommended with amoxicillin/clavulanate or cephalosporin plus a macrolide or doxycycline. One can also consider monotherapy with levofloxacin or moxifloxacin in this setting. For inpatients, combination therapy with a beta-lactam (ampicillin plus sulbactam 1.5 to 3 g every 6 hours, cefotaxime 1 to 2 g every 8 hours, ceftriaxone 1 to 2 g daily, or ceftaroline 600 mg every 12 hours) and a macrolide (azithromycin 500 mg daily or clarithromycin 500 mg twice daily) is recommended. Monotherapy with a respiratory fluoroquinolone (levofloxacin 750 mg daily, moxifloxacin 400 mg daily) can also be used in low-risk patients but should be used in combination with a beta-lactam for high-risk patients. Additional anaerobic coverage in patients with aspiration pneumonia is not recommended.

**Approximately 1 in 3000 surgical procedures are complicated by aspiration pneumonitis produced by the aspiration of gastric fluid (sterile and highly acidic).** The aspiration produces a severe chemical pneumonitis. Aspiration and its complications are a cause of approximately 30% of anesthetic mortalities. Risk factors for aspiration pneumonia include older age, obesity, hiatal hernia, or emergency surgery associated with a full stomach. The morbidity from aspiration is secondary to both particulate matter entering into the lungs and the caustic nature of gastric acid. The combination of these insults leads to a destructive inflammatory response. When aspiration is significant and severe, adult respiratory distress syndrome often develops. **Secondary infection usually complicates aspiration pneumonitis, and broad-spectrum antibiotics should be given when this diagnosis is entertained.** Preventive measures include avoiding the routine use of nasogastric suction, perioperative antacid ingestion, and the administration of H2 blockers, as well as judicious use of narcotics and sedatives.

## Sleep Apnea

**Sleep apnea has become a significant concern because of the rising incidence of obesity and morbid obesity in the United States.** The increased soft tissues of the head and neck can lead to airway compromise that leads to intermittent apnea and hypoventilation while a woman sleeps. The increased weight of the extra adipose tissue on the neck, chest, and abdominal wall lead to a decrease in pulmonary compliance. As a result, the relative hypoxia may induce systemic and pulmonary hypertension. Patients may also develop chronic hypercapnia as the respiratory drive shifts from a $CO_2$-driven response to a hypoxia-driven response in patients with sleep apnea. **It is important to note that when patients with morbid obesity are given higher levels of oxygen or narcotics, they are at increased risk for apnea.** These patients develop an increased sensitivity to narcotics that shuts down the respiratory drive. Patients with chronic hypoxia from any cause will often have an increased sensitivity to narcotics, but it is particularly problematic in the patient with obesity who is dependent on low levels of oxygen for respiratory stimulation. **These patients should be given oxygen as needed; however, during the postoperative period, when narcotics are given, the goal should be to keep the oxygen saturation in the 94% range.** At saturation levels of 96% to 99% these patients may lose respiratory drive and become hypercarbic and acidotic (Ahmad, 2008).

**Preoperatively patients who are thought to be at risk for sleep apnea may be queried by asking them the "STOP-BANG" questions.** These eight questions can predict sleep apnea with a high degree of sensitivity. The questions include the following: Do you *s*nore? Do you often feel *t*ired? Has anyone *o*bserved you stop breathing? Are you being treated for high blood *p*ressure? Is your *b*ody mass index >35? Are you older than *a*ge 50? Is your *n*eck size greater than 16 inches? Is your *g*ender male? A "yes" answer to zero to two questions implies that one is low risk for obstructive sleep apnea (OSA); three to four "yes" answers places one at intermediate risk for OSA; five to eight "yes" answers places one at high risk for OSA (Chung, 2008).

# CARDIOVASCULAR PROBLEMS

## Hemorrhagic Shock

***Shock* is defined as a condition in which circulatory insufficiency prevents adequate vascular perfusion of vital organs.** Systemic hypotension results in poor tissue perfusion and reduced capillary filling. Prolonged hypotension can result in oliguria, progressive metabolic acidosis, and multiple organ failure. Shock may be produced by hemorrhage, cardiac failure, sepsis, and anaphylactic reactions. **Hypovolemic shock is the most common cause of acute circulatory failure in gynecologic patients.** Cardiogenic shock and septic shock are less common. Shock from postoperative hemorrhage is usually seen in the first several hours after surgery. In the perioperative period, hypovolemia may be secondary to several factors, including preoperative volume deficiency, underreplaced blood loss during surgery, extracellular fluid loss during surgery, inadequate fluid replacement, and, most commonly, continued blood loss after the surgical procedure. **Tachycardia is the classic cardiovascular physiologic response to hypotension.** Progressive hypovolemia results in diminished urine output.

**The majority of perioperative cases of shock are related to hemorrhage secondary to inadequate hemostasis.** The development of shock from acute blood loss depends on the rate of bleeding; for example, slow venous oozing may produce a large amount of blood loss but not produce shock. Rapid loss of 20% of a woman's blood volume produces mild shock, whereas a loss of greater than 40% of blood volume results in severe shock. Even with the extensive use of suction equipment, the actual measurement of intraoperative blood loss is imprecise. Massive blood loss has been defined as hemorrhage that results in replacement of 50% of the circulating blood volume in less than 3 hours. The most common cause of postoperative bleeding is a less than ideal ligature or hemorrhage from a vessel that has retracted during the operation. Bleeding may come from an isolated artery or vein or may be more generalized when the bleeding is secondary to a clotting abnormality.

In addition to hemorrhage, hypotension in the immediate postoperative period may be secondary to the residual effects of anesthesia or oversedation. For example, older patients often experience prolonged vasodilation secondary to the sympathetic blockade produced by epidural or spinal anesthesia. The differential diagnosis of postoperative hypotension and tachycardia should include conditions such as pneumothorax, PE, aspiration, myocardial infarction, and acute gastric dilation. However, in the postoperative period the index of suspicion should be highest for bleeding.

In patients in whom ineffective coagulation is noted, the differential diagnosis includes medication-induced anticoagulation, sepsis, fibrinolysis, diffuse intravascular coagulation, and a previously unrecognized coagulation defect, such as von Willebrand disease. Coagulopathies can also develop from excessive transfusion and dilution of fibrinogen and other clotting factors. Blood product replacement for massive hemorrhage should incorporate adequate use of coagulation factors via fresh-frozen plasma (FFP) or cryoprecipitate and platelets because thrombocytopenia, impaired platelet function, and a decrease in factors V, VIII, and XI commonly occur with massive transfusions as a result of dilution of these factors with use of packed red cells alone. Further, **hemorrhagic shock results in progressive acidosis, which interferes with assembly of coagulation factor complexes, and hypothermia, which causes platelet dysfunction and decreased activity of thromboxanes.** Hypofibrinogenemia is the first to develop, followed by deficiencies of other coagulation factors. Thrombocytopenia is often the last defect to be recognized in the coagulopathy cascade, but the timing of its development varies among individuals. **Thus most hospitals have a massive transfusion protocol, which includes replacing packed red cells, plasma, and platelets in a 1:1:1 ratio.** In cases of submassive hemorrhage, transfusion of platelets should be determined by serial platelet counts (Box 25.3). Similarly, the transfusion of FFP can be performed as needed to match a clotting deficiency as measured by the prothrombin time (PT) and activated partial thromboplastin

**BOX 25.3** Suggested Transfusion Guidelines for Platelets

Recent (within 24 hr) platelet count <10,000/mm$^3$ (for prophylaxis)
Recent (within 24 hr) platelet count <50,000/mm$^3$ with demonstrated microvascular bleeding (oozing) or a planned surgical/invasive procedure
Demonstrated microvascular bleeding and a precipitous fall in platelet count
Adult patients in the operating room who have had complicated procedures or have required more than 10 units of blood *and* have microvascular bleeding. Giving platelets assumes that adequate surgical hemostasis has been achieved.
Documented platelet dysfunction (e.g., prolonged bleeding time >15 min, abnormal platelet function tests) with petechiae, purpura, microvascular bleeding (oozing), or surgical or invasive procedure
Unwarranted indications:
- Empirical use with massive transfusion when patient is not having clinically evident microvascular bleeding (oozing)
- Prophylaxis in thrombotic thrombocytopenic purpura, hemolytic-uremic syndrome, or idiopathic thrombocytopenic purpura
- Extrinsic platelet dysfunction (e.g., renal failure, von Willebrand disease)

From Rutherford EJ, Skeet DA, Schooler WG. Hematologic principles in surgery. In: Townsend CM, Beauchamp RD, Evers BM, eds. *Sabiston Textbook of Surgery.* 17th ed. Philadelphia, Saunders; 2004.

time (aPTT). Each unit of FFP can be expected to raise increase clotting protein levels by 2.5% to 10%.

**Two early signs of hypovolemia caused by hidden internal bleeding include tachycardia and decreased urine output.** The body's adrenergic response to hemorrhage includes perspiration, tachycardia, and peripheral vasoconstriction. Urine output decreases to less than 0.5 mL/kg per hour (20 to 25 mL/hr) as a result of poor perfusion of the kidneys. With further loss of blood, agitation, weakness, and skin pallor can appear; the extremities may feel cold and clammy; and, ultimately, systolic blood pressure drops to less than 80 mm Hg. Again, because of adaptive cardiovascular changes, **it takes a rapid loss of approximately one-third of the blood volume to produce significant hypotension.**

**Postoperatively, occult intraperitoneal and retroperitoneal bleeding often occurs without significant local symptoms.** Extraperitoneal bleeding may present as bleeding from the vaginal cuff. Abdominal distention, muscle rigidity, and shoulder pain are late signs of intraperitoneal hemorrhage. The diagnosis of clinically significant postoperative bleeding may be confirmed by serial changes in hemoglobin levels; however, it is important to caution that marked changes in hematocrit and hemoglobin levels require time to develop. Imaging studies may demonstrate hematomas or increased intraperitoneal free fluid.

The management goals of postoperative shock are to replace, restore, and maintain the effective circulating blood volume and establish normal cellular perfusion and oxygenation (Box 25.4). To accomplish this goal, an adequate cardiac output and appropriate peripheral vascular resistance must be maintained. The first priority is to provide adequate ventilation because poor respiratory gas exchange is the most common cause of death in these patients. The second, almost simultaneous priority is rapid fluid replacement with adequate amounts of blood and crystalloid solution (normal saline or lactated Ringer solution). The 3:1 rule suggests a ratio of 3 mL of crystalloid solution for every 1 mL of blood loss. The optimal fluid replacement is a fluid evenly distributed throughout multiple body compartments. **Randomized trials of crystalloid and colloid resuscitation solutions have shown no clear survival benefit to the use of colloids (albumin, gelatin, dextran, and hydroxyethyl starch), but a reduced rate of tissue edema, abdominal compartment syndrome, and hyperchloremic metabolic acidosis is demonstrated. The substantial cost of these agents should be weighed against potential benefits** (Bougle, 2013). Crystalloids should be considered the initial resuscitation fluid of choice in hemorrhagic shock; colloids are appropriate for resuscitation in conjunction with crystalloids when blood products are not immediately available. Guidelines for transfusion of packed red blood cells (PRBCs) are listed in Box 25.5.

The goals of fluid replacement are to maintain a systolic blood pressure that is similar to preoperative readings and a urine output greater than 0.5 mL/kg per hour (usually >30 mL/hr). Table 25.2 lists types of blood components used for replacement

**BOX 25.4** Management Priorities in Massive Transfusion*

Restore circulating blood volume.
Maintain oxygenation.
Correct coagulopathy.
Maintain body temperature.
Correct biochemical abnormalities.
Prevent pulmonary and other organ dysfunction.
Treat underlying cause of hemorrhage.

From Donaldson MDJ, Seaman MJ, Park GR. Massive blood transfusion. *Br J Anaesth.* 1992;69(6):621-630.
*The exact priority depends on the circumstances.

**BOX 25.5** Suggested Transfusion Guidelines for Red Blood Cells

Hemoglobin <8 g/dL or acute blood loss in an otherwise healthy patient with signs and symptoms of decreased oxygen delivery with two or more of the following:
- Estimated or anticipated acute blood loss of >15% of total blood volume (750 mL in 70-kg man)
- Diastolic blood pressure <60 mm Hg
- Systolic blood pressure drop >30 mm Hg from baseline
- Tachycardia (>100 beats/min)
- Oliguria, anuria
- Mental status changes

Hemoglobin <10 g/dL in patients with known increased risk of coronary artery disease or pulmonary insufficiency who have sustained or are expected to sustain significant blood loss
Symptomatic anemia with any of the following:
- Tachycardia (>100 beats/min)
- Mental status changes
- Evidence of myocardial ischemia, including angina
- Shortness of breath or dizziness with mild exertion
- Orthostatic hypotension

Unfounded or questionable indications:
- To increase wound healing
- To improve the patient's sense of well-being
- 7 g/dL < hemoglobin < 10 g/dL (or 21% < hematocrit < 30%) in otherwise stable, asymptomatic patient
- Mere availability of predesignated autologous blood without medical indication

From Rutherford EJ, Skeet DA, Schooler WG. Hematologic principles in surgery. In: Townsend CM, Beauchamp RD, Evers BM, eds. *Sabiston Textbook of Surgery.* 17th ed. Philadelphia: Saunders; 2004.

TABLE 25.2 Indications for Administration of Various Blood Products

| Product | Content | Indication: Acceptable | Indication: Unacceptable |
|---|---|---|---|
| Red blood cells | Red cells | To increase oxygen-carrying capacity in anemic women; for orthostatic hypotension secondary to blood loss | For volume expansion; to enhance wound healing; to improve general well-being |
| Platelet concentrates | Platelets | To control or prevent bleeding associated with deficiencies in platelet number or function | In patients with immune thrombocytopenic purpura (unless bleeding is life-threatening) |
| Fresh-frozen plasma | Plasma, clotting factors | To increase the level of clotting factors in patients with demonstrated deficiency | For volume expansion; as a nutritional supplement; prophylactically with massive blood transfusion |
| Cryoprecipitate | Factors I, V, VIII, XIII, von Willebrand factor, fibronectin | To increase the level of clotting factors in patients with demonstrated deficiency of fibrinogen, factor VIII, factor XIII, fibronectin, or von Willebrand factor | Prophylactically with massive blood transfusion |

From American Congress of Obstetricians and Gynecologists. *ACOG Tech Bull.* 1994;199:1.

therapy. Traditionally in patients with massive hemorrhage, replacement a ratio of 2 units of packed red blood cells to 1 unit of FFP has been the desirable ratio, but more recent literature in trauma surgery and massive hemorrhage suggests that a ratio of 1:1:1 for packed red cells, plasma, and platelets is superior (Holcomb, 2015). For every 6 units of packed red blood cells, a 6-pack of platelets will be required, as well as 6 units of FFP to maintain these ratios (Holcombe, 2015). Each unit or pack of platelets will raise the platelet level by 15,000/mm$^3$. The platelet count should be maintained at greater than 50,000/mm$^3$ in a woman who is bleeding (Stroncek, 2007). The importance of adequate transfusion is not only support of intravascular volume but also supply of oxygen.

Coagulation studies, PT, and activated PT should be obtained regularly during the bleeding episode to help guide resuscitation. The term *washout* is used to describe the loss of clotting factors as a woman uses up her blood volume and it is replaced with PRBCs and crystalloid. Disseminated intravascular coagulation (DIC) is an intravascular consumption and is different than washout. However, both conditions require replacement and ongoing evaluation. Although some consider off-label use of recombinant factor VIIa (70 to 90 μg/kg) in episodes of persistent severe bleeding, meta-analyses suggest there is no mortality benefit to its use and potential increased risk of thromboembolism. This combined with cost limits the utility of this product (Bougle, 2013, Yank, 2011).

**The decision to return to the operating room to control hemorrhage is often difficult to make because the offending artery or vein is often unable to be identified at the time or reoperation.** Additionally, friable inflamed postoperative tissues can result in further bleeding. If ongoing postoperative bleeding requires reoperation, this decision should not be postponed. It should be performed expediently after volume replacement and sometimes concomitantly. During this second operation, excellent anesthesia, a full selection of surgical instruments, and the value of good assistance cannot be overemphasized. Proper exposure is paramount for the success of this operation. Initially the old clots are removed and further bleeding is reduced by direct pressure over the presumed bleeding vessels while a systematic search is conducted in an effort to identify the individual vessels that are bleeding.

**Bilateral ligation of the anterior divisions of the hypogastric arteries distal to the posterior parietal branch is an effective operation to control persistent postoperative pelvic hemorrhage.** This procedure results in a reduction of pulse pressure, which allows a stable clot to form at the site where the pelvic vessels are injured. Classically, two ligatures are placed and tied around each hypogastric artery (Fig. 25.3). **The major potential complication of this procedure is injury to the hypogastric vein.** If there is generalized oozing, thrombocytopenia, DIC, or factor VIII deficiency should be suspected. If these conditions are excluded, venous oozing from small vessels in the pelvis may be controlled by the local application of topical hemostatic agents such as microfibrillar collagen compounds, gelatin compounds, or topical thrombin compounds (e.g., Avitene, Gelfoam, Floseal).

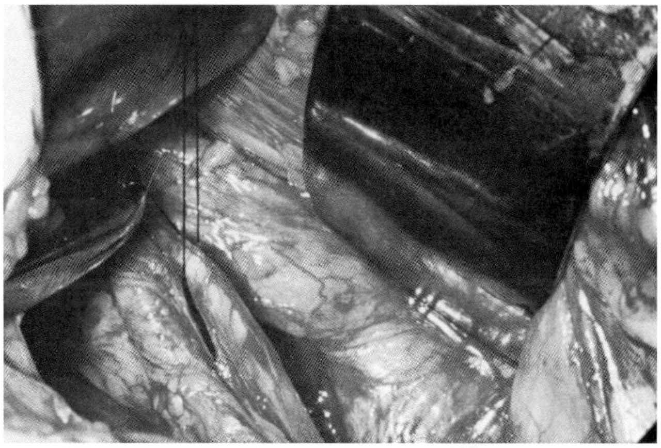

**Fig. 25.3** Ligation of internal iliac artery. Double loop is being directed toward bifurcation of common iliac artery. (From Breen JL, Gregori CA, Kindzierski JA. Hemorrhage in gynecologic surgery. In: Shaefer G, Graber EA, eds. *Complications in Obstetric and Gynecologic Surgery.* Hagerstown, MD: Harper & Row, 1981.)

Intraoperative rapid autologous blood transfusion is used extensively in cardiovascular and trauma surgery, but this technology is not often used by gynecologists. The major complication of rapid autologous transfusion is a 10% hemolysis rate. The risks of air embolism or infusion of particulate matter are minimal. Autologous blood does not contain platelets or clotting factors, so platelets and FFP have to be given concurrently for severe hemorrhage. **Rapid autologous transfusion is contraindicated in advanced pelvic infection or malignancy.**

**In many cases, angiographic embolization, instead of exploratory laparotomy, may be preferable for control of postoperative hemorrhage from an identifiable vessel** (Fig. 25.4). CT angiography has improved the rapid identification of bleeding vessels. Similarly, treatment of recurrent postoperative hemorrhage or

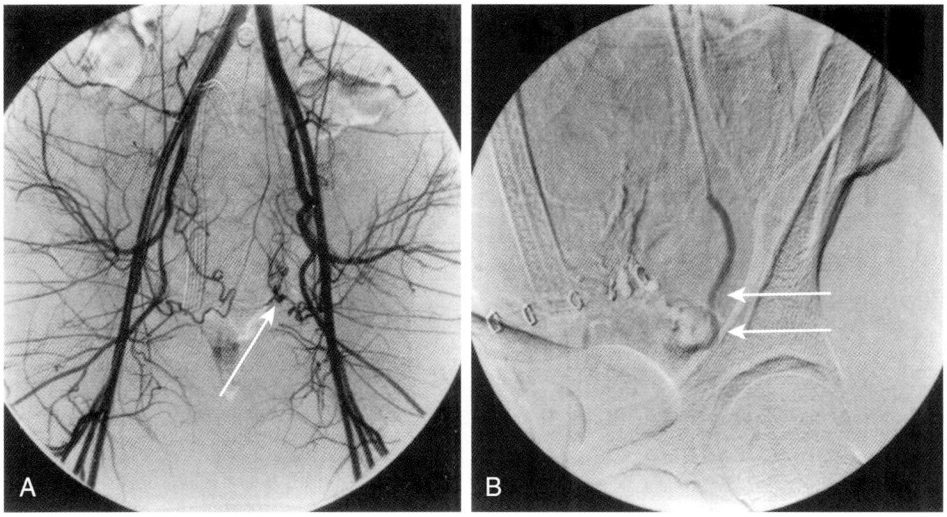


**Fig. 25.4 A,** Anteroposterior digital subtraction pelvic angiogram in 37-year-old woman with persistent pelvic bleeding after surgical myomectomy for uterine leiomyomas demonstrates contrast pooling *(arrows)* from branches of left uterine artery, consistent with active hemorrhage. **B,** Postembolization left uterine arteriogram shows occluded left uterine artery *(long arrows)* with no evidence of active bleeding. (From Vedantham S, Goodwin SC, McLucas B, et al. Uterine artery embolization: an underused method of controlling pelvic hemorrhage. *Am J Obstet Gynecol.* 1997;176:938-948.)

hemorrhage late in the postoperative course (7 to 14 days) may be performed with angiographic arterial embolization. Absorbable gelatin sponges are used to produce vascular occlusion for 10 to 30 days. For permanent occlusion metal coils, polyvinyl alcohol particles, microspheres or various "glues" are used.

## Hematomas

Management of delayed postoperative hematomas is challenging and controversial. The incidence of hematomas is inversely related to the extent to which meticulous hemostasis is obtained intraoperatively. Women who are given low-dose heparin or who take aspirin chronically are at a slightly higher risk of hematoma formation. Women on antiplatelet medication or anticoagulation are also at risk. **Hematomas result from intermittent or slow, continuous venous bleeding and are almost always self-limiting.** Eventually, the pressure of the expanding hematoma will exceed the venous pressure and a stable clot will form.

The extent of the hematoma is determined partially by the potential size of the compartment into which the bleeding occurs. Retroperitoneal or broad ligament hematomas may contain several hundred milliliters or even liters of blood. **A wound or pelvic hematoma should be suspected when the patient's hemoglobin continues to decline beyond the usual nadir on postoperative day 3.** Clinical examinations may reveal mild to moderate tenderness over the affected area. Generally by postoperative day 5, the hematoma will liquefy and may be easier to outline during bimanual examination. Distinguishing between an uninfected hematoma and a hematoma that has become secondarily infected is difficult before incision and drainage. Both clinical situations produce tenderness and fever secondary to the inflammation surrounding the hematoma. The diagnosis of a retroperitoneal hematoma may be made by physical examination; most helpful is a careful rectovaginal examination. However, radiologic imaging studies are indicated when a hematoma is suspected and cannot be palpated. Imaging is commonly used to make the diagnosis of a postoperative hematoma.

**Hematomas smaller than 5 cm in diameter may be treated conservatively.** Larger hematomas may be drained transcutaneously with CT or ultrasound guidance. If not treated, most large hematomas will become secondarily infected, even if treated with parenteral antibiotics. **Effective drainage of most pelvic and broad ligament hematomas usually can be accomplished vaginally or radiographically.** Small subcutaneous hematomas or fascial hematomas usually resolve spontaneously; however, they are associated with an increased incidence of wound infection and pain.

## Retained Foreign Body

With any operation there is the potential risk of an unrecognized retained foreign body, sponge, or laparotomy pad. **The exact incidence of this complication is difficult to establish but is estimated to be from 1 in 1200 to 1500 laparotomies, typically with correct sponge counts at the time of surgery.** When this complication is discovered during the first postoperative week, the woman usually has a tender pelvic mass that is infected. When this mass is discovered after the immediate postoperative course, patients are often asymptomatic or may exhibit minimal tenderness. The possibility of a retained foreign body should be considered in the differential diagnosis of pelvic hematomas and abscesses. A retrospective study of retained sponges by Gawande and associates noted that retained foreign bodies are more commonly associated with a higher body mass index (BMI), emergency surgeries, and an intraoperative change in the type of procedure to be performed (Gawande, 2003).

## Thrombophlebitis and Pulmonary Embolus

**Surgery is a time of hypercoagulability secondary to the stress response.** As such, the surgeon must be aware of the potential complications of thromboembolism throughout the postoperative course. Prophylaxis against **deep vein thrombosis (DVT)** is discussed in Chapter 24. However, prophylaxis must be continued throughout the hospital stay and, in certain high-risk cases, even after discharge. For example, patients with malignancy who undergo laparotomy, patients with previous blood clot or personal history of thrombophilia, and those who will have decreased ambulation may benefit from up to 4 weeks of **low-molecular-weight heparin (LMWH)** after leaving the hospital per guidelines from the American College of CHEST Physicians

(Kearon, 2016). Studies in patients with hip replacements and with abdominal pelvic malignancies have shown significant reductions (50% to 66%) in the incidence of DVT with prolonged anticoagulation, up to 4 weeks postoperatively. There is insufficient evidence to make recommendations for prolonged thromboprophylaxis in patients with routine gynecologic concerns, except in high-risk situations such as gynecologic cancer surgery (Guyatt, 2012). **There is a reduced risk of venous thromboembolism (VTE) with minimally invasive hysterectomy compared with abdominal hysterectomy.** Without specific guidelines, the length of time for thromboprophylaxis should be individualized and based on risk and bleeding assessment. Prophylaxis will not prevent all DVTs; thus part of daily rounds includes assessments for this complication.

## Superficial Thrombophlebitis

**Superficial thrombophlebitis is one of the most commonly occurring postoperative complications and is most often associated with IV catheters.** Superficial thrombophlebitis is often overlooked or disregarded as a cause of postoperative fever. Physical examination will reveal superficial tenderness and erythema over the course of the superficial veins. Women with established superficial varicosities in the lower extremities are especially susceptible because of localized stasis or pressure during the operative procedure and inactivity during the first 24 hours after operation. Superficial thrombophlebitis is a benign process; however, it is associated with deep vein thrombophlebitis in approximately 5% of cases. Thus the finding of superficial thrombophlebitis does not eliminate the necessity to consider DVT as well. Some series have documented the association of inherited thrombophilias with superficial phlebitis, increasing the risk by 4- to 13-fold. Recurrent superficial phlebitis, in varying anatomic sites, may be a sign of occult malignant disease. Detailed basic investigations have identified fibrin sheaths surrounding IV catheters in 60% to 100% of patients studied. The exact fate of the several inches of clot and fibrin sheath after the removal of the IV catheter is uncertain. Venography studies have found that these clots and fibrin sheaths do not break up on catheter removal but initially remain in situ.

IV catheters are also an important source of nosocomial infections. **Approximately 30% of all hospital-acquired bacteremias are secondary to IV lines.** The most serious complication of IV catheter use is infection of the thrombus, producing suppurative phlebitis or catheter sepsis. It was previously recommended that the IV catheters be removed and replaced in intervals ranging from 72 to 96 hours, regardless of whether signs or symptoms of superficial phlebitis are present, but a 2013 Cochrane review found no evidence to support routine catheter exchange without evidence of inflammation, infiltration, or blockage (Webster, 2013). **Although routine exchange is not indicated, venous catheters should be removed at the first sign of induration, erythema, or edema.**

**The clinical management of mild superficial thrombophlebitis includes rest, elevation, and local heat.** Moderate to severe superficial thrombophlebitis may be treated with a nonsteroidal antiinflammatory drug (NSAID), such as ibuprofen, or with low-dose heparin if refractory to supportive care. In the rare case of proximal progression of the inflammatory process, treatment with IV heparin and antibiotics is warranted.

## Deep Vein Thrombosis

Fifty percent of thromboembolic complications occur within the first 24 hours and 75% occur within 72 hours. Approximately 15% occur after the seventh postoperative day. **Diagnosis of DVT by physical examination alone is insensitive, and thus imaging studies are essential for establishing the correct diagnosis.** Venous thrombosis and PE are the direct causes of approximately 40% of deaths after gynecologic surgery. The incidence of fatal PE after gynecologic operations is approximately 0.2%. **Because women often die within a few hours of the appearance of initial symptoms, emphasis must be placed on prevention rather than treatment of this complication.** PE is not the only major consequence of deep venous thrombosis. Many women develop chronic venous insufficiency or postphlebitic syndrome of the legs as a major sequela. The resulting damage to valves of the deep veins produces shunting of blood to superficial veins, chronic edema, pain on exercise, and skin ulceration.

Historic incidence of DVT with gynecologic operations without prophylaxis varied from 7% to 45%, with an average of approximately 15% (Walsh, 1974). **Since the institution of universal mechanical prophylaxis, VTE rates as low as 0.6% for open hysterectomies and 0.2% for minimally invasive hysterectomies have been reported** (Barber, 2015). The incidence of thrombosis is directly dependent on risk factors such as the type and duration of operation; age of the woman; history of thrombophilia or DVT; peripheral edema; surgical blood loss; restrictions in perioperative ambulation or immobility; and history or presence of obesity, malignancy, sepsis, diabetes, current oral contraceptive or hormone use, and conditions that produce venous stasis, such as ascites and heart failure (Box 25.6)

**BOX 25.6** Conditions Associated With Increased Risk for Deep Vein Thrombosis

- Active cancer
- Acute medical illness (e.g., acute myocardial infarction, heart failure, respiratory failure, infection)
- Advancing age
- Antiphospholipid syndrome
- Behçet syndrome
- Central venous catheter
- Chronic care facility stay
- Congenital venous malformation
- Dyslipoproteinemia
- Heparin-induced thrombocytopenia
- Hormone replacement therapy
- Immobilization
- Inflammatory bowel disease
- Intravenous drug abuse
- Limb paresis
- Long-distance travel
- Myeloproliferative diseases
- Nephrotic syndrome
- Obesity
- Oral contraceptives
- Other drugs
  - Antipsychotics
  - Chemotherapeutic agents
  - Tamoxifen
  - Thalidomide
- Paroxysmal nocturnal hemoglobinuria
- Pregnancy, puerperium
- Previous venous thromboembolism
- Prolonged bed rest
- Superficial vein thrombosis
- Surgery
- Trauma
- Varicose veins
- Vena cava filter

From Kyrle PA, Eichinger S. Deep vein thrombosis. *Lancet.* 2005;365(9465):1163-1174.

**TABLE 25.3** Risk Categories of Thromboembolism in Gynecologic Operations

| | Risk Level | | |
|---|---|---|---|
| **Risk Category** | **Low** | **Medium** | **High** |
| Age (yr) | 40 | 40 | 50 |
| **Contributing Factors** | | | |
| Operation | Uncomplicated or minor | Major abdominal or pelvic | Major, extensive |
| Weight | | Moderately obese: 75-90 kg or >20% above ideal weight | Morbidly obese: >115 kg or >30% above ideal weight |
| Previous venous thrombosis | | | |
| Varicose veins | | | |
| Cardiac disease | | | |
| Diabetes (insulin-dependent) | | | |
| Calf vein thrombosis (%) | 2 | 10-35 | 30-60 |
| Iliofemoral vein thrombosis (%) | 0.4 | 2-8 | 5-10 |
| Fatal pulmonary emboli (%) | 0.2 | 0.1-0.5 | 1 |
| Recommended prophylaxis | Early ambulation | Low-dose heparin or intermittent pneumatic compression | Low-dose heparin or intermittent pneumatic compression |

From Mattingly RF, Thompson JD, eds. *Te Linde's Operative Gynecology.* 6th ed. Philadelphia: JB Lippincott; 1985.

(Kyrle, 2005). Older women and women with obesity have an increased incidence of thrombosis because of dilation of their deep venous system. **There is a two- to fourfold increased risk for venous thrombosis in women taking postmenopausal estrogen therapy.** The length of the surgical procedure also has an important influence on the development of thrombosis (Table 25.3).

The process of thrombosis usually begins in the deep veins of the calf. **It is estimated that 75% of pulmonary emboli originate from a thrombus in the leg.** If one leg is involved, the contralateral leg will have a thrombus in approximately 33% of women. Usually the thrombus remains localized, it lyses spontaneously, and the local symptoms resolve. In approximately 1 in 20 cases the process extends centrally to the veins of the upper leg and pelvis. Involvement of the femoral vein often results in lower extremity swelling. Pulmonary emboli from calf veins alone are rare, with only 4% to 10% of pulmonary emboli originating from this area. In contrast, there is a 50% risk of a PE if thrombosis of the femoral vein is not treated.

In 1854, Virchow described the three key predisposing or precipitating factors in the production of thrombi: an increase in coagulation factors, damage to the vessel wall, and venous stasis. Subsequent studies have documented that all three events occur with gynecologic operations. Blood flow in the iliac vein decreases by approximately 55% during an operation. During an operation, there are several normal physiologic changes that produce hypercoagulability, including increases in factors VIII, IX, and X, number of platelets, platelet aggregation and adherence, fibrinogen, and, lastly, thromboplastin-like substance from tissue necrosis.

The site of initial formation of the thrombus is most often near the base of a valve cusp in the calf of the leg (Fig. 25.5). The thrombus propagates and grows by repetitive layers of platelet aggregation and deposition of fibrin from fibrinogen. The most recently formed portion of the propagating thrombi are free floating (not attached to the vein) and are most likely to become pulmonary emboli. The body attempts to repair the area of thrombosis through an invasion of fibroblasts from the vein wall to encompass the base of the thrombus. Eventually the thrombus is attached to the vein wall, the area is reepithelialized, organization occurs, and symptoms resolve.

The signs and symptoms of DVT depend directly on the severity and extent of the process. Many localized cases of DVT in

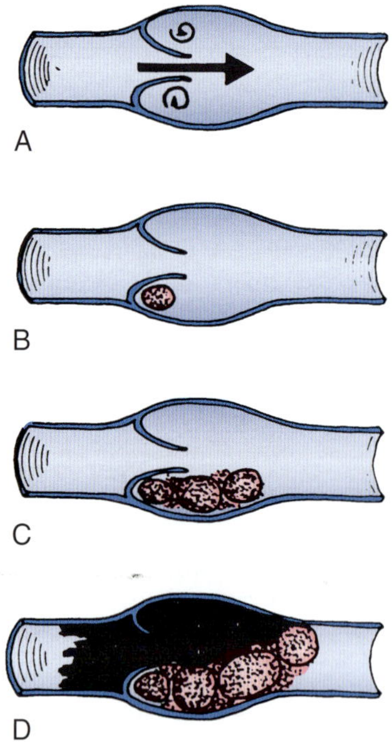


**Fig. 25.5** Stages in development of thrombus in valve pocket of deep veins of leg. **A,** Stasis in valve pocket results in thrombin generation. **B,** Platelet aggregation and fibrin formation. **C,** Propagation of platelet-fibrin nidus. **D,** Blockage of venous flow with resultant retrograde extension. (From Bloom AL, Thomas DP, eds. *Haemostases and Thrombosis.* Edinburgh: Churchill Livingstone; 1981:684.)

the calf are asymptomatic and are only recognized by a screening procedure such as duplex ultrasonography; however, even extensive areas of DVT may be asymptomatic and the first sign may be the development of a PE. In a woman who is asymptomatic, the pathophysiologic process may not totally obstruct the individual vein and drainage is obtained via associated competent collateral circulation.

Studies using $^{125}$I-labeled fibrinogen to screen the legs have documented that approximately half of women who develop DVT after gynecologic surgery is totally free of symptoms (Walsh, 1974). Among women who develop signs and symptoms, approximately 68% have induration of the calf muscles, 52% have minimal edema, 25% have calf tenderness, and 11% develop a difference of more than 1 cm in diameter of the leg. The Homan sign is present in 10%, and differential pain over the calf with a blood pressure cuff is present in approximately 40%. The clinical diagnosis of iliofemoral thrombosis is much easier—the woman usually develops severe symptoms caused by obstruction of venous return. Usually there is an acute onset of severe pain and swelling.

**The clinician must maintain a high degree of suspicion to begin the diagnostic workup for DVT.** The clinical symptoms and signs of DVT are nonspecific. Common clinical findings may include persistent low-grade fever or unexplained tachycardia. The tachycardia is often more rapid than one would expect with a low-grade fever. The finding of a definite difference in leg circumference is supportive evidence of DVT but not a sensitive test; further, physical examination of the legs produces false-positive findings in approximately 50% of cases. **Based on clinical examination, if the likelihood of DVT were low, the next step in nonsurgical patients, would be a D-dimer level; however, in the postoperative patient, D-dimer is not as reliable and should not be ordered.** D-Dimer is a protein from cross-linked fibrin after it has been degraded by plasmin in the fibrinolytic process; thus D-dimer may be elevated because of trauma, surgery, intravascular hemolysis, pregnancy, and other inflammatory states. If the signs and symptoms are suggestive or the woman is at high risk, the next step should be imaging.

**Imaging options for DVT include contrast venography (phlebography) and duplex ultrasound.** Most clinicians obtain a duplex lower extremity ultrasound when suspicious for DVT. Duplex ultrasound is a combination of color Doppler and real-time B-mode ultrasound. It has a high sensitivity and specificity in symptomatic women. Real-time ultrasound imaging provides visualization of the larger veins, and sensitive Doppler ultrasound is focused simultaneously on the suspicious vessel. The technology depends on changes in venous flow for a positive diagnosis. The documented sensitivity of duplex ultrasonography in detecting proximal thrombi is 95% (95% CI, 92% to 98%) and the specificity is 99% (95% CI, 98% to 100%) (Wells, 1995). The advantages of this method are that it is noninvasive, easy to use, highly accurate, objective, simple, and reproducible. Duplex ultrasonography may improve the diagnostic accuracy in larger veins. The main disadvantage of duplex ultrasound is its limited accuracy when investigating small vessels in the calf and vessels proximal to the inguinal canal. The inability to compress the deep vein by moderate pressure with the ultrasound probe is the most widely used criterion for the positive diagnosis of DVT.

The objectives of the clinical management of DVT associated with gynecologic surgery are early detection and early therapy. In reality, antithrombotic therapy is preventive medicine because the therapeutic agent interrupts progression of the disease (thrombus formation) but does not actively resolve the disease process. Anticoagulation with heparin (unfractionated or LMWH) is the initial treatment of choice for the diagnosis of DVT or PE (Table 25.4). **LMWH is as effective and has several advantages over unfractionated heparin, despite its increased cost.** Ease of dosing, lower risk of bleeding complications, and reduced risk of heparin-induced thrombocytopenia are among the most notable. LMWH has effectively replaced unfractionated heparin as the gold standard for treatment of DVT. **LMWH may be given subcutaneously with once or twice daily weight-based dosing; for example, for enoxaparin, the dosage would be 1.5 mg/kg daily or 1 mg/kg twice daily** (Guyatt, 2012). LMWH does not require monitoring in women with normal and stable renal function, LMWH has more stable pharmacokinetics, and there is actually a lower incidence of complications noted in some studies in terms of progression from DVT to pulmonary emboli. Additionally, studies comparing LMWH with unfractionated heparin have shown a greater effect with thrombus regression within the veins themselves. Testing of levels of LMWH is based not on the aPTT but on the anti–factor Xa activity level. Levels are calculated specifically for each LMWH. An aPTT of 1.5 times normal corresponds approximately to an anti–factor Xa activity level of 0.2. **Therapeutic levels are between 0.4 and 0.8.** Bleeding usually occurs when levels of the anti–factor Xa activity level rise more than 1.0 to 1.2. **If needed in patients with unstable renal status, levels may be checked approximately 4 hours after dosing.**

If unfractionated heparin is desired as an IV infusion, weight-adjusted or fixed-dose infusions are acceptable. The weight-adjusted

**TABLE 25.4** Options for Initial Anticoagulant Treatment of Deep Vein Thrombosis

| | | | Reported Risks (no./total no. [%]) | |
|---|---|---|---|---|
| **Drug** | **Method of Administration** | **Dosage*** | **Heparin-Induced Thrombocytopenia†** | **Major Bleeding** |
| Unfractionated heparin | IV | Loading dose, 5000 U or 80 U/kg of body weight with infusion adjusted to maintain aPTT within therapeutic range | 9/332 (2.7) | 35/1853 (1.9) |
| LMW heparin | | | 0/333 (0) | 20/1821 (1.1) |
| Dalteparin | Subcutaneous | 100 U/kg every 12 hr or 200 U/kg daily; maximum, 18,000 U/day | | |
| Enoxaparin | Subcutaneous | 1 mg/kg every 12 hr or 1.5 mg/kg daily; maximum, 180 mg/day | | |
| Tinzaparin | Subcutaneous | 175 U/kg daily; maximum, 18,000 U/day | | |
| Nadroparin | Subcutaneous | 86 U/kg every 12 hr or 171 U/kg daily; maximum, 17,100 U/day | | |

From Bates SM, Ginsberg JS. Treatment of deep-vein thrombosis. *N Engl J Med.* 2004;351(3):268-277.

*Doses vary in patients who are obese or who have renal dysfunction. Monitoring of anti–factor Xa levels has been suggested for these patients, with dose adjustment to a target range of 0.6 to 1.0 U/mL 4 hr after injection for twice-daily administration or 1.0 to 2.0 U/mL for once-daily administration. Even though there are few supporting data, most manufacturers recommend capping the dose for patients with obesity at the same dose as that for a 90-kg patient.

†The therapeutic range of activated partial thromboplastin time corresponds to heparin levels of 0.3 to 0.7 U/mL, as determined by anti–factor Xa assay. High levels of heparin-binding proteins and factor VIII may result in so-called heparin resistance. In patients requiring more than 40,000 U/day to attain a therapeutic aPTT, the dosage can be adjusted on the basis of plasma heparin levels.

*aPTT,* Activated partial thromboplastin time; *IV,* intravenous; *LMW,* low-molecular-weight.

dose is 80 IU/kg per hour bolus followed by 18 IU/kg per hour. The fixed dose uses an initial loading dose of 5000 IU, followed by a continuous infusion of 1000 IU/hr (Guyatt, 2012). The dosage of unfractionated IV heparin should be adjusted to prolong an aPTT to 2.5 times control values. Continuous heparin infusion is preferred over periodic bolus injections because there are fewer hemorrhagic complications (6% vs. 14%). The average half-life of heparin is 1 to 2 hours after IV injection. Failure to achieve adequate anticoagulation in the first 24 hours of therapy increases the risk of recurrent VTE 15-fold.

For women who are pregnant or have a malignancy, LMWH is the treatment of choice for long-term anticoagulation. Other women can be treated with oral warfarin or a direct oral anticoagulant (DOAC) such as dabigatran, rivaroxaban, apixaban, or edoxaban.

Standard dosing for warfarin is based on serial international normalized ratio (INR) laboratory values with a goal of 2.5 (range, 2 to 3). In general, a loading dose of warfarin is given with 5 to 10 mg nightly for two doses followed by INR-guided doses. Heparin or LMWH should be continued until the INR is greater than 2. The biologic half-life of warfarin is 2 to 3 days.

**DOAC medications are a new class of anticoagulant that work directly on the coagulation cascade via inhibition of either factor Xa (apixaban, edoxaban, and rivaroxaban) or thrombin (dabigatran).** They provide more consistent and reliable dosing than warfarin without laboratory monitoring and are widely used for DVT and PE in patients without malignancy. Their role in patients with malignancy is still an area of active research (Kearon, 2016), although they are commonly used in this setting.

**In general, anticoagulation is continued for 3 to 6 months for adequate treatment and secondary prophylaxis of a provoked thrombus, but individualized treatment for continuation beyond this period is considered.** For example, a provoked clot after an abdominal hysterectomy without other risk factors should be managed with 3 months of therapy (Guyatt, 2012). Patients with large DVT, antiphospholipid antibody syndrome, or malignancy may require extended therapy, which may be performed indefinitely while the risk factor is present and in conjunction with a hematologist.

**The primary risk of chronic anticoagulation therapy is the potential for major bleeding complications.** Major bleeding occurs in approximately 4% of woman-years of therapy. Approximately 1% of patients on full-dose heparin develop thrombocytopenia (platelet count <100,000/mm$^3$). If thrombocytopenia develops, heparin should be discontinued because of the potential risk of **paradoxical thrombosis.**

Inferior vena cava filters may be used to protect against pulmonary emboli in patients who cannot receive anticoagulation. However, this practice is becoming less popular because many of the fluoroscopically placed temporary vena cava filters are just not removed, leading to more risk of complications. **Routine perioperative use of vena cava filters has been shown to be of no benefit.**

**Routine screening for thrombophilia in all patients with VTE is not indicated.** The presence of a hereditary thrombophilia does not alter therapeutic or prophylactic management of a patient and has not been associated with improved outcomes. Patients who may benefit from testing include those with recurrent thrombosis, patients with a family history of thrombosis, patients with thrombosis in unusual locations (hepatic vein, portal vein, mesenteric vein, or arterial), and possibly patients younger than age 45 years. Patients with a provoked thrombosis from cancer, hormonal therapy, and surgery do not require testing for thrombophilias.

There is no evidence that bed rest is helpful for patients with DVT or that immobilization will prevent PE. Patients with confirmed DVT may receive NSAIDs because coagulation factors will be monitored. Patients should also be prescribed support stockings, which should be worn for several months and for up to 2 years. **The use of support stockings decreases the risks of postthrombotic syndrome.** In a systematic review, women who used stockings up to 2 years after DVT had up to a 50% reduction in the incidence of postthrombotic syndrome (Segal, 2007).

## Pulmonary Embolism

The accurate diagnosis of PE is essential for the prevention of morbidity from lack of treatment or unnecessary anticoagulation therapy. Autopsy studies have documented that pulmonary emboli are undiagnosed clinically in approximately 50% of women who experience this complication. Approximately 10% of women with a PE die within the first hour. **The mortality of women with correctly diagnosed and treated pulmonary emboli is 8%, in contrast to approximately 30% if the disease is not treated.** Most pulmonary emboli in gynecologic patients originate from thrombi in the pelvic and femoral veins. Predisposing risk factors are found in most women with PE.

No combination of symptoms or signs is pathognomonic for PE. They are nonspecific and similar to symptoms caused by other forms of cardiorespiratory disease. Many patients with PE will be asymptomatic. Common conditions considered in the differential diagnosis of PE include pneumonia, cardiac failure, atelectasis, aspiration, acute respiratory distress syndrome, and sepsis. Although the differential diagnosis is broad in scope, the symptoms should alert the physician to the possibility of a PE, thus allowing a proper diagnostic workup to establish or rule out the disease. **Chest pain, dyspnea, and apprehension are the most common symptoms.** The dyspnea is often of abrupt onset. The classic triad of shortness of breath, chest pain, and hemoptysis is seen in less than 20% of women with proved PE. Tachycardia, tachypnea, rales, and an increase in the second heart sound over the pulmonic area are the most commonly found signs of pulmonary emboli (Table 25.5). Approximately 15% of women with pulmonary emboli have an unexplained low-grade fever associated with a PE. A high fever is rarely associated with a PE but may occur. The clinical manifestations of PE are produced primarily by occlusion of the large branches of the pulmonary arteries by embolic material with subsequent associated reflex bronchial constriction and vasoconstriction that intensify symptoms.

**TABLE 25.5** Symptoms and Signs of Pulmonary Embolism

| Symptoms | Patients with Finding (%) |
|---|---|
| Predisposing factors* | 94 |
| Dyspnea | 84 |
| Pleuritic chest pain | 74 |
| Apprehension | 59 |
| Cough | 53 |
| Hemoptysis | 30 |
| Syncope | 14 |
| **Signs** | |
| Tachypnea | 92 |
| Rales | 58 |
| Accentuation of pulmonic valve closure | 53 |
| Tachycardia | 44 |
| Cyanosis | 20 |

From Blinder RA, Coleman RE. Evaluation of pulmonary embolism. *Radiol Clin North Am.* 1985;23(3):391-405.

*Prolonged immobilization, postoperative state, congestive heart failure, carcinomatosis.

More than 50% of clinically recognized pulmonary emboli are multiple. The most common location of pulmonary emboli is in the lower lobes of the right lung. Shock and syncope are associated with massive pulmonary emboli.

Although imaging techniques are the gold standard for establishing the diagnosis of pulmonary emboli, several studies have found that clinical assessment is almost as accurate (Goldhaber, 2003a, 2003b). Laboratory studies that may help in diagnosis and management include electrocardiograms (ECGs), chest radiographs, blood gas analyses, assessment of troponin, d-dimer (not reliable in postoperative patients), and brain natriuretic peptide (BNP). Less than 15% of ECGs demonstrate significant changes of right ventricular strain, with T-wave inversion in $V_1$ to $V_4$ with a PE. Most women with pulmonary emboli demonstrate hypoxemia on blood gas determinations, but as with other routine tests, these findings do not occur invariably. Diminished pulmonary vascular markings may be a suggestive finding on a chest film, but they are fairly nonspecific. The chest radiograph may be helpful in the differential diagnosis by demonstrating other pulmonary processes. **The most common findings on chest film examination in patients with a PE are infiltrate, pleural effusion, atelectasis, and enlargement of the heart or descending pulmonary artery.**

In women who are in mild to moderate distress, fractionated or unfractionated heparin should be started while imaging studies are being ordered. If there is any question of severe distress or hemodynamic instability, thrombolytic therapy may be indicated for the appropriate patient. In stable patients, a stepwise approach is useful. Many clinicians will order Doppler studies of the lower extremities. If the Doppler studies are positive, the woman will be anticoagulated and no further workup for a thrombotic source is necessary. If the tests are negative, further imaging is still necessary, because in the postoperative patient, pelvic clots may be the origin of the pulmonary embolus, not lower extremity clots. The next two options are a ventilation-perfusion ($\dot{V}/\dot{Q}$) scan or CT pulmonary angiography (CTPA). CTPA has largely replaced $\dot{V}/\dot{Q}$ scanning as the most common imaging technique to establish or exclude the diagnosis of PE (Fig. 25.6). CTPA uses IV contrast media to aid in the imaging of the pulmonary vessels. The procedure is minimally invasive and provides a volumetric image of the lung by rotating the detector at a constant rate around the woman. **A cost-effective analysis from Doyle and colleagues found that CTPA was the most cost-effective first-line test to diagnose pulmonary embolus.** A limitation of CTPA is a sixfold increase in radiation exposure

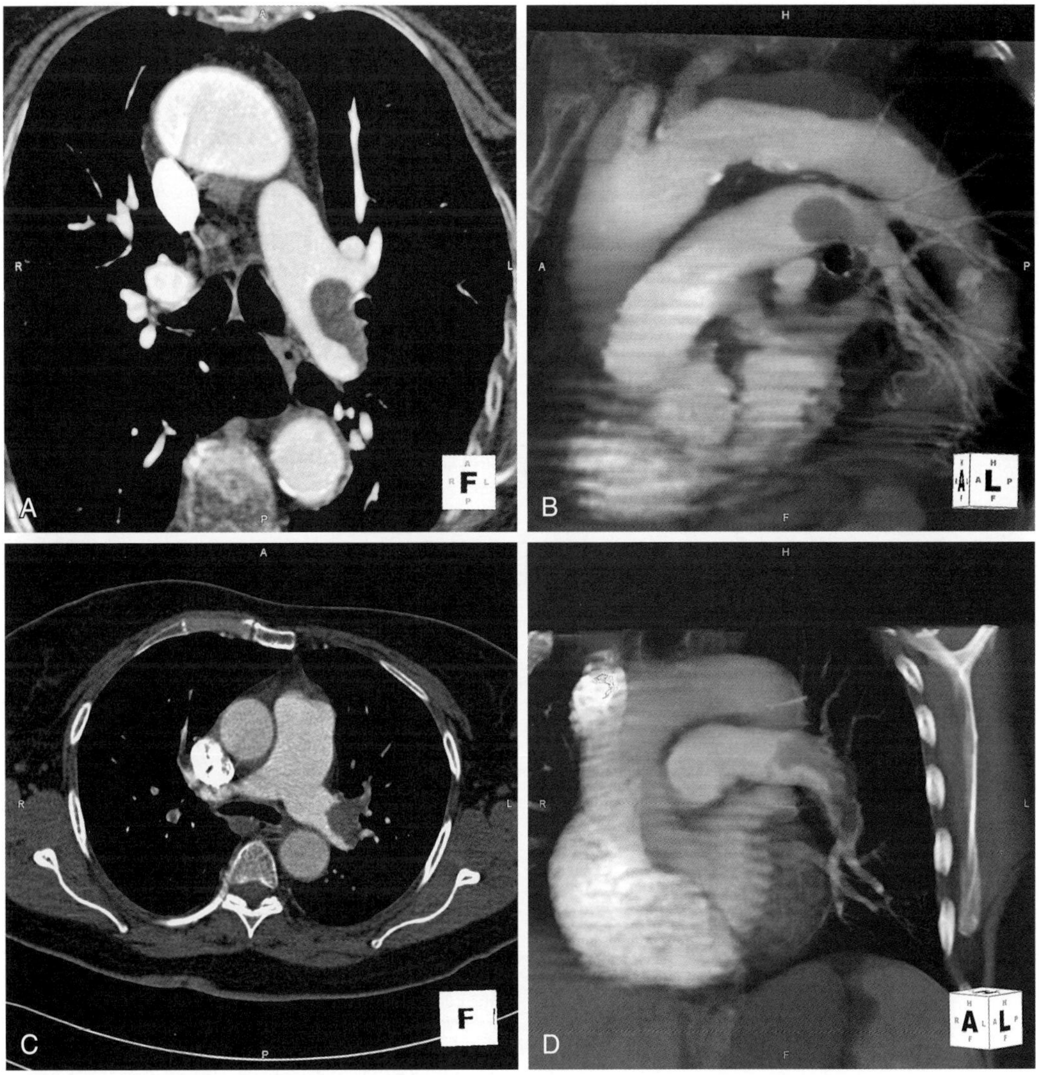


**Fig. 25.6 A** to **D,** Helical CT of pulmonary embolism. The letters on the cube help orient the viewer as the three-dimensional image is rotated. *A,* Anterior; *F,* foot; *H,* head; *L,* left. (Courtesy Dr. Charles McGlade, Sacred Heart Medical Center, Eugene, OR.)

compared with the $\dot{V}/\dot{Q}$ scan. This leads to a slightly increased risk of breast cancer (<1%). Before $\dot{V}/\dot{Q}$ scanning, a chest radiograph should be obtained. If the radiograph shows other findings, such as atelectasis, the $\dot{V}/\dot{Q}$ scan has a much higher chance of being nondiagnostic and CTPA should be ordered instead.

The $\dot{V}/\dot{Q}$ scan is a safe and relatively easy-to-perform test. The scan involves the injection of small radiocolloid particles into the circulation. They are trapped in small vessels; their distribution depends on regional pulmonary blood flow. Ventilation scintigraphy uses radionuclides of technetium aerosol or xenon gas. The combination of lack of symmetry and a mismatch in the ventilation scan is the abnormality that leads to the diagnosis. Whereas a normal result effectively rules out the diagnosis of PE, 40% of patients with a suspected PE will have a normal scan. The multicenter **Prospective Investigation of Pulmonary Embolism Diagnosis (PIOPED)** found that 4% of patients with normal or near-normal perfusion lung scans subsequently were discovered to have pulmonary emboli. This study emphasized a high sensitivity of 98% but a low specificity of 10% for $\dot{V}/\dot{Q}$ scans in the diagnosis of PE. The authors noted that almost all patients with acute PE had abnormal scans, but so did most patients without emboli. $\dot{V}/\dot{Q}$ scans have a high sensitivity but a variable specificity for the diagnosis of PE. For example, other cardiorespiratory diseases such as asthma may result in regional areas of decreased perfusion. If the scan documents multiple segments or lobar perfusion defects with a ventilation mismatch, the probability of pulmonary emboli is more than 85%. $\dot{V}/\dot{Q}$ scans with less extensive perfusion abnormalities or matching ventilation defects do not reliably exclude the diagnosis of PE.

The management of the majority of pulmonary emboli is with anticoagulation with IV unfractionated heparin or full-dose LMWH, similar to the management of DVT (Fig. 25.7). Prompt and early therapy with heparin provides anticoagulation and inhibits the release of serotonin from platelets, which potentially results in a decrease in the associated bronchoconstriction. Some women are candidates for thrombolytic therapy. The time window for effective use of thrombolysis is up to 14 days after the initial symptoms or signs of a PE, although it is rarely used beyond 48 to 72 hours. Thrombolytic therapy works by transforming plasminogen to plasmin. Use of thrombolytic therapy during the early postoperative period is contraindicated because of the increased risk of serious hemorrhage, except in very unique circumstances. Recombinant human tissue-type plasminogen activator (TPA) has been shown to be more rapid in onset and safer than urokinase for thrombolytic therapy. Thrombolytic therapy is the method of choice in patients with massive pulmonary emboli (angiographically, >50% obstruction of the pulmonary arterial bed) with associated moderate to severe hemodynamic instability, lobular obstruction, or multiple segmental profusion defects. Random trials of heparin versus thrombolytic therapy have shown that emboli clear more rapidly with initial thrombolytic therapy.

**The Management Strategies and Prognosis of Pulmonary Embolus–3 trial (MAPPET-3) found that in severely affected patients (but not those in shock), thrombolytic therapy was superior to heparin.** However, for all patients, particularly those with small emboli, the increased risks of intracranial bleeding may outweigh the benefits (1% to 3% of patients). Trials have evaluated thrombolytic therapy with heparin and found the combination superior to heparin alone. A thrombolytic agent is infused IV for the first 12 to 24 hours, and heparin therapy is continued for 7 to 10 days. The clinical assumption is that approximately 7 days are needed for the intravascular venous thrombus to become firmly attached to the vein's sidewall. In patients who have heparin allergies or develop heparin-induced thrombocytopenia (HIT), thrombin inhibitors are an alternative therapy.

One additional potential adjunct for treatment is vena cava filters. **The most widely accepted indication for vena cava filters is failure of medical management or a contraindication to heparin therapy.** Approximately 35% of vena cava filters are placed for prophylactic indications. A randomized trial reported by Decousos and colleagues compared vena cava filters with LMWH or unfractionated heparin. They concluded that the initial beneficial effect of vena cava filters for the prevention of PE is counterbalanced by an excess of recurrent DVT, without any difference in mortality rates. Treatment of a massive PE in an unstable woman involves a choice of thrombolytic therapy, pulmonary artery embolectomy, transvenous catheter embolectomy, or filter placement in the inferior vena cava.

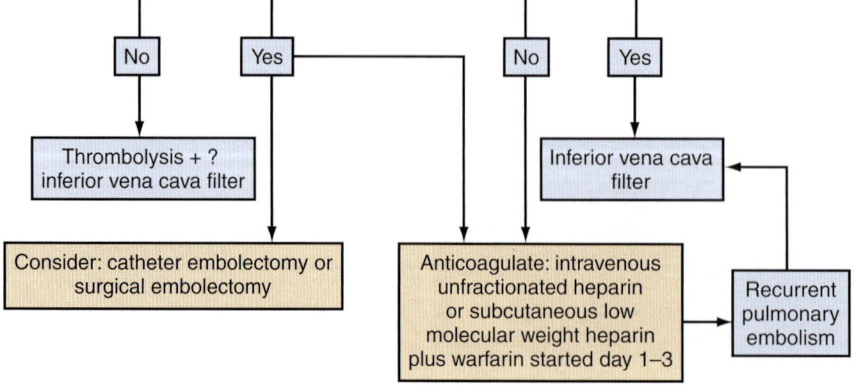

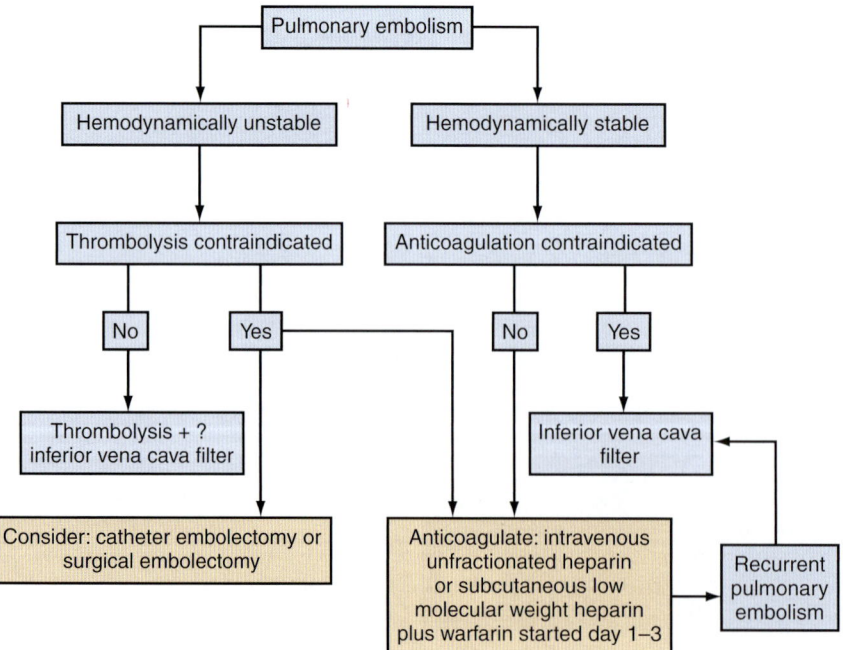


**Fig. 25.7** Algorithm for treatment of pulmonary embolism. (From Taj MR, Atwal AS, Hamilton G. Modern management of pulmonary embolism. *Br J Surg.* 1999;86:853-868.)

All patients with pulmonary emboli should have anticoagulation maintenance therapy for 3 or more months after assessment of the patient's bleeding risk (Guyatt, 2012). Options for treatment range from LMWH to warfarin or DOACs as discussed earlier. **The risk of a woman developing a subsequent fatal PE during the 3 months of anticoagulation therapy is approximately 1 in 70 to 100.**

## URINARY TRACT PROBLEMS

### Inability to Void

Many women experience an inability to void or an incomplete emptying of the bladder during the immediate postoperative period. The major pathophysiologic change is the direct trauma and edema produced by the surgical procedure to the perivesical tissues. Other factors that contribute include the potential of overdistention from excessive hydration and dyssynchronous contractions from the bladder neck. The differential diagnosis includes anxiety, mechanical interference, obstruction by swelling and edema, neurologic imbalance, and drug-associated detrusor hypotonia.

Most voiding dysfunction resolves without medication and with time. **If a mechanical obstruction is not suspected, intermittent straight catheterization is indicated to manage postoperative voiding dysfunction.** This will result in a lower incidence of UTI and facilitate a more rapid return to normal bladder function compared with prolonged catheterization. Overdistention of the bladder produces a temporary paralysis of the detrusor activity that may take several days to resolve and should be avoided. Rarely, medications may be given to patients who experience prolonged periods of inability to void. Reflex urethral spasm is common after surgery to repair an enterocele or rectocele. Urethral spasm may be diminished by an alpha-adrenergic receptor blocking agent such as phenoxybenzamine; however, hypotension is a potential side effect of this drug. Bladder hypotonia may occur as a result of overdistention, prolonged inactivity, or use of medications such as beta-blockers; it may be treated with bethanechol, 10 to 50 mg orally every 6 to 8 hours.

### Urinary Tract Infection

**The most commonly acquired infection in the hospital and the most common cause of gram-negative bacteremia in hospitalized patients is catheter-associated UTI.** Approximately 40% of nosocomial infections are UTIs, and 60% of these are directly related to an indwelling catheter. Of patients with infections from bladder catheters, 1% will develop bacteremia. **Therefore indwelling catheters should only be used when absolutely necessary and for as short a period as possible.**

The normal urothelium inhibits adherence of surface bacteria to the walls of the urethra and bladder. A bladder catheter disrupts this property and surface bacteria are able to colonize the lower urinary tract. Additionally, bacteria form a sheet or biofilm of microorganisms and bacterial bioproducts that adheres to the catheter. These biofilms protect bacteria from antibiotics. This characteristic of biofilms explains why antibiotic suppression is ineffective for patients with chronic catheterization and why replacement of a catheter is necessary in the treatment of systemic infection secondary to a colonized urinary tract. The incidence of a positive culture increases dramatically with time. After a Foley catheter has been in place for 36 hours, approximately 20% of women have bacterial colonization; after 72 hours, more than 75% have positive cultures. If the catheter drains into an open system for longer than 96 hours, 100% develop bacteriuria. **Women with an indwelling catheter in place with a closed drainage system develop UTIs at the rate of approximately 5% per 24 hours; this increases to 50% after 7 days of continuous catheterization.**

Catheter-related UTIs are related to the patient's age. In one study, 30% of women older than 50 years developed an infection compared with 16% of postoperative women younger than age 50 (Platt et al., 1986). Diabetes increased the incidence of catheter-related UTIs threefold. **The incidence of infection is directly related to how long the catheter is in place.** The incidence of a positive urine culture after a single in-and-out catheterization is approximately 1%. Sterile technique used during insertion, strict aseptic catheter care, and maintenance of a closed drainage system are all important steps for reducing the incidence of infection through reduced colonization. Bacteria ascend from the exterior to the bladder via the lumen of the catheter or around the outside of the catheter. A sterile, closed drainage system is another prophylactic measure to reduce the incidence of UTIs. In one study, strict closed drainage reduced the rate of infection from 80% to 23% (Kunin et al., 1966). Studies have documented a lower risk of infection with a suprapubic, transabdominal urinary catheter. The latter technique also decreases patient discomfort and permits earlier spontaneous voiding. Systemic prophylactic antibiotics exert a short-term effect, decreasing the initial incidence of infection. However, prophylactic antibiotics also have resulted in an increased emergence of antibiotic-resistant bacteria, and therefore prophylactic antibiotics should not be routinely used but determined on a case by case basis (e.g., in immunocompromised patients). With catheterization for longer than 3 weeks, all patients have bacterial colonization, regardless of the use of prophylactic antibiotics and a closed system.

The symptoms of UTI usually develop 24 to 48 hours after the Foley catheter is removed. Patients with lower UTIs usually do not have fever but experience urinary frequency and mild dysuria, which are difficult to distinguish from normal postoperative discomfort. Older women may manifest mental status changes as the first sign of problems. Women with upper UTIs usually have a high fever, chills, and flank pain. **If urinary tract symptoms persist after appropriate antibiotic therapy, one should obtain imaging studies to evaluate the possibility of obstruction in the urinary tract or renal abscess.** Obstruction of the ureter without associated infection may be asymptomatic or produce only mild flank tenderness. No appreciable change may be noted in urinary output or serum creatinine with an isolated unilateral ureteral obstruction.

The diagnosis of UTI is established by urinalysis and urine culture. **Women with high-volume urine output may demonstrate minimal findings on urinalysis but have a positive urine culture.** In a catheterized specimen, a bacterial concentration of $10^2$ organisms/mL is significant. More than 95% of patients with $10^2$ colony-forming units (CFU)/mL subsequently developed the standard criterion of infection, which is 100,000 CFU/mL for a midstream culture (Stark, 1984).

**A minimum of 3 days of antibiotic therapy for a woman who has developed cystitis after catheter use is the recommended treatment.** One-day, single-dose antibiotic treatment is not an effective treatment for catheter-associated UTI.

### Ureteral Injury and Urinary Fistula

Vesicovaginal and ureterovaginal fistulas are infrequent yet significant complications of operations for benign gynecologic conditions. In the United States gynecologic operations are found to be the cause of approximately 75% of urinary tract fistulas. Surprisingly, it is not the difficult cancer operation but rather the simple total abdominal hysterectomy for benign disease, such as myomas or abnormal bleeding, that is most often associated with this complication. Although initial concerns arose regarding increased urinary injury rates with minimally invasive gynecologic surgery, later reviews showed an **incidence of 0.3% of hysterectomies being complicated by urinary injury** (Wong, 2018). The role of universal cystoscopy has been evaluated for intraoperative detection of urinary injuries. Although some support its routine use, there are no high-quality data to support routine use of cystoscopy in preventing 30-day morbidity. Given the overall low rate of urinary injuries and increasing use of minimally invasive surgery with associated thermal injuries that often have a delayed presentation unlikely to be detected at the time of routine cystoscopy, surgeons should determine the role of cystoscopy on a case by case basis and rely on meticulous dissection in the retroperitoneum with ureteral identification to avoid injury. **The most common sites of ureteral injury are near the uterine artery, at the pelvic brim near the infundibulopelvic ligament, and at the lateral cuff closure.** Injuries may include transection, sutures that constrict or devascularize the ureter, and thermal injuries from cautery.

**The classic clinical symptom of a urinary tract fistula is the painless and almost continuous loss of urine, usually from the vagina.** On occasion, the uncontrolled loss of urine may be related to change in position or posture. Urinary incontinence that presents within a few hours of the operative procedure is usually secondary to a direct surgical injury to the bladder or ureter that was not appreciated during the surgery. **Most fistulas become symptomatic in 8 to 12 days and occasionally as late as 25 to 30 days after the operation, depending on the mechanism of injury.** Pelvic examination often reveals a small erythematous area of granulation tissue at the site of the fistula (Fig. 25.8).

A small vesicovaginal fistula may be clinically identified by placing a tampon in the vagina and instilling a dilute solution of methylene blue dye into the urinary bladder. This will also help differentiate between a vesicovaginal fistula and ureterovaginal fistula. If the blue coloring is discovered on the tampon, the defect is most likely in the bladder. If the tampon is not colored, administration of oral phenazopyridine can evaluate for ureterovaginal fistula. The subsequent finding of orange coloring on the tampon is presumptive evidence of an ureterovaginal fistula. **An IV pyelogram or CT urogram should be obtained in either case to detect obstruction of the ureter and diagnose compound (ureter and bladder) fistulas.**

As with most other postoperative complications, preventive medicine is paramount. The bladder should be adequately drained and the physician should obtain adequate exposure with meticulous dissection along tissue planes to mobilize the bladder and ureter away from the operative field. When operating near the bladder or ureter, bleeding vessels should be secured individually. If possible, the ureter should not be completely detached from the overlying peritoneum. With extensive dissection of the periureteral tissue, care should be taken to avoid interference with the longitudinal vascular supply of the ureter in the Waldeyer sheath. In the most difficult cases, in which anatomic landmarks are obscure, opening of the dome of the bladder and palpation with the index finger and thumb may help identify the proper surgical plane. The urinary system, especially the bladder, is very forgiving if given a short period of rest to recover. If trauma to the bladder is suspected, continuous catheter drainage for 3 to 5 days usually results in spontaneous healing.

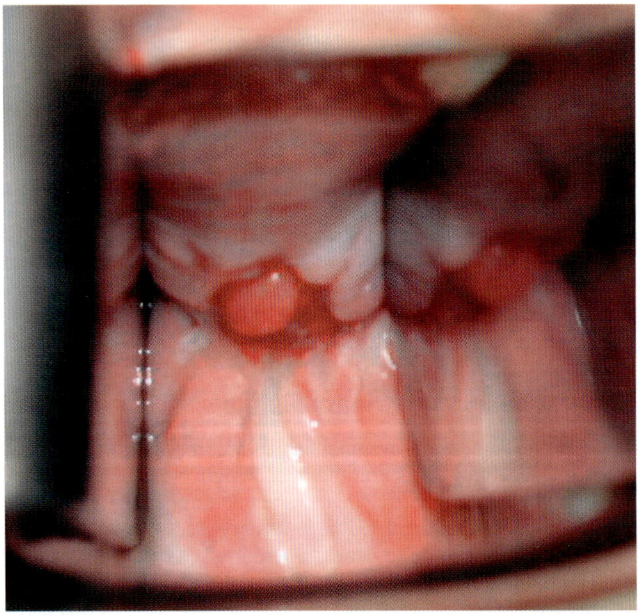

**Fig. 25.8** Vesicovaginal fistula with the classic "rosette" of inflammatory tissue denoting the opening to the fistulous track. (From Badlani GH, De Ridder D, Mettu JR, et al. Urinary tract fistulae. In: Wein AJ, Kavoussi LR, Partin AW, et al, eds. *Campbell-Walsh Urology.* 11th ed. Philadelphia: Elsevier; 2016.)

When leakage from the urinary tract is first discovered, the bladder should be drained with a Foley catheter. Ureteral injuries should be evaluated for treatment with retrograde ureteral catheters versus urinary diversion or primary repair. **Approximately 20% of bladder injuries and 30% of ureteral injuries that are drained and stented will heal spontaneously without further surgery, so conservative measures are often an appropriate first step.** Ureteral injuries that occur secondary to cauterization or coagulation may present several days to a few weeks after surgery. Symptoms may vary from pain, bloating, ileus, leukocytosis, and urinary ascites. Serum creatinine levels may be normal or elevated with intraabdominal leaking of urine. If levels are elevated in the presence of fever or ileus, imaging studies should be considered. With the increase in laparoscopic and robotic surgery, the incidence of thermal injury to the urinary tract has significantly increased. **Although initial series suggested a fourfold increase in urinary tract injury in laparoscopic total hysterectomies, later series did not confirm this and emphasized the importance of surgical technique** (Harmanli, 2009).

In cases in which the injury is seen at or around the time of surgery, immediate treatment facilitates healing of the defect before epithelialization of the aberrant tract occurs. Spontaneous healing usually occurs within the first 4 weeks. With a ureteral fistula, follow-up imaging should be considered to detect delayed ureteral strictures.

Operative repair of a vesicovaginal fistula is usually accomplished via a multilayered closure performed by the vaginal route. The principles for a successful operation include the following: adequate exposure, dissection, and mobilization of each tissue layer; excision of the fistulous tract; closure of each layer without tension on the suture line; and excellent hemostasis with closure of the dead space. Reliable bladder drainage is provided to avoid tension on the suture line for approximately 10 days. The Latzko operation is the simplest means of repairing a fistula at the vaginal apex. This technique of partial colpocleisis involves denudation of the vaginal mucosa surrounding the fistula and subsequent multilayer closure. The primary disadvantage of the procedure may be postoperative shortening of the vagina.

**Many ureteral injuries discovered during the immediate postoperative period will heal when treated by percutaneous nephrostomy and ureteral stents.** Ureterovaginal fistulas that do not heal spontaneously are usually repaired 2 to 3 months after the original operation. Reimplantation of the ureter into the bladder is the preferred repair for an injury involving the lower third of the ureter.

## GASTROINTESTINAL COMPLICATIONS

### Postoperative Diet

Most patients may be given a regular diet as soon as tolerated after elective gynecologic surgery, including patients who undergo bowel resection. This section discusses nausea and postoperative gastrointestinal (GI) complications, as well as glycemic control as it relates to postoperative nutrition. Part of the physiologic stress response to surgery is a drive for gluconeogenesis. This process is enhanced by a hormonally mediated insulin resistance. The resultant hyperglycemia is advantageous in the teleologic sense of the fight-or-flight response, but it is detrimental for wound healing, cardiovascular function, and inflammatory processes. Several studies have correlated clinical outcomes with glucose levels. **The American Association of Endocrinology has noted an 18-fold increase in hospital mortality in general medicine and general surgery patients with glucose levels greater than 200 mg/dL** (Garber, 2004).

Patients who are given insulin infusions during surgery should have their infusions continued until they are tolerating regular meals. At this point, they may be given subcutaneous insulin if necessary. Metformin is often avoided in the perioperative setting because of the potential risks of lactic acidosis. There is no clear consensus, but stopping metformin for 24 hours before surgery, with resumption when the patient resumes full oral intake, appears to adequately limit this risk. In women with a history of insulin resistance, women who are morbidly obese, and those older than 60 years, glucose levels should be checked at the bedside every 4 to 6 hours during the first postoperative day. **If a woman's glucose rises to more than 150 mg/dL, she should be treated; however, in multiples reviews there is not a significant benefit to strict perioperative glucose control to levels below 200 mg/dL.**

The American Diabetic Association recommendations suggest that critically ill patients have better outcomes with tighter glucose control—fasting levels less than 110 mg/dL and postprandial levels less than 140 mg/dL. Non–critically ill patients should have fasting levels less than 140 mg/dL and postprandial levels less than 180 mg/dL (Umpierrez, 2012). In a study of 6100 critically ill patients (NICE-SUGAR), tight control of fasting blood glucose levels (80 to 108 mg/dL) was associated with worse outcomes because of complications from iatrogenic hypoglycemia (Finfer, 2009). Studies of non–critically ill patients, in contrast, have found that hyperglycemia is associated with more wound infections. Ramos and associates have noted an increased incidence of infection by 30% for every increase in glucose of 40 mg/dL more than the recommended 110 mg/dL (Ramos, 2008).

Sliding-scale insulin treatments, though less effective than IV infusions in the first 24 hours, are easier to manage. Sliding-scale regular insulin is most appropriate for women without a previous history of diabetes and without risk factors and those with short surgeries who will resume normal activity and diet within 24 hours. **Infusions are preferable if glucose levels are elevated significantly, early in the postoperative course, and for women with longer surgeries who will not resume regular eating and activity for a few days.** Insulin infusions are begun with concomitant infusions of $D_5$ half-normal saline (5% dextrose in half-strength normal saline) with 10 mEq of KCl. The Portland Insulin Protocol allows for control of glucose levels and, with nursing support, can be effective (Appendix A).

When transitioning off insulin infusions, it is reasonable to use the rule of thumb of 80% of the previous 24-hour total insulin dose. This amount may be divided into split doses of NPH insulin or longer-acting glargine. Glargine is associated with less hypoglycemia. Initially a bolus of fast-acting insulin, lispro, may be added with meals. The bedside glucose level is measured every 4 hours. In patients who go home at 24 hours, oral medications or insulin may be restarted at the time of discharge with the same dose as that which was used before the operative period.

## Postoperative Nausea and Gastrointestinal Function

Minor disturbances in GI function are a normal consequence of anesthesia, perioperative medications, and surgical manipulation. Most women experience some nausea for approximately 12 to 24 hours, pass flatus some time during the first 48 hours, and have a spontaneous bowel movement by the third or fourth postoperative day after uncomplicated, benign gynecologic surgery. **The best practice for women after gynecologic surgery, including cancer and bowel resections, regardless of age, is early refeeding with quick advancement to a regular diet with cessation of nausea and as tolerated by the patient.** This principle is a staple of enhanced recovery protocols and is in direct opposition to traditional refeeding guidelines. Traditionally, patients were to have nothing by mouth until the passage of flatus and then were given a gradual resumption of diet from clear liquid to full liquid to soft to regular diet, commonly called *step-up diets.* Several studies have shown that delayed feeding such as this is unnecessary and, in some ways, detrimental. Steed and colleagues, in a study of major gynecologic surgeries, including oncologic cases, compared restricted oral intake with step-up diets to early full diet and found no adverse effects but did find shorter length of stay in the early feeding group (Steed, 2002). Similarly, a low-residual diet at 6 hours postoperative followed by a regular diet compared with a traditional delayed feeding and a step-up diet after return of bowel function lead to more nausea and emesis in the delayed feeding group, with a shorter length of stay in the early feeding group (Kalogera, 2013) (Table 25.6).

**TABLE 25.6** Gastrointestinal Information

| Category | Clear Liquid (N = 107) | Regular Diet (N = 138) |
|---|---|---|
| **MORBIDITY** | | |
| Nausea | 21 (19.6) | 26 (18.8) |
| Vomiting | 10 (9.3) | 19 (13.8) |
| Abdominal distention | 10 (9.3) | 18 (13.0) |
| Nasogastric tube use | 1 (0.9) | 8 (5.8) |
| **TOLERANCE** | | |
| Diet on first attempt | 101 (94.4) | 121 (87.7) |
| Regular diet on first attempt | 103 (96.3) | |
| If intolerant, time to tolerance (days) | 5.3 ± 1.5 | 3.6 ± 1.5 |
| Flatus before discharge | 55 (51.4) | 69 (50.0) |
| **INTERVALS (DAYS)** | | |
| Bowel sounds | 1.2 ± 0.5 | 1.2 ± 0.5 |
| Flatus | 2.8 ± 1.4 | 2.8 ± 1.0 |
| Regular diet* | 2.4 ± 2.5 | 1.1 ± 0.3 |
| Hospital stay | 3.6 ± 3.0 | 3.4 ± 1.7 |

From Pearl MI, Frandina M, Mahler L, et al. A randomized controlled trial of a regular diet as the first meal in gynecologic oncology patients undergoing intraabdominal surgery. *Obstet Gynecol.* 2002;100:232.
Data presented as mean ± standard deviation or N (%).
*$P < .05$; no other significant differences between groups.

**Approximately one-third of adult women experience postoperative nausea and vomiting (PONV).** Several factors affect the likelihood and severity of PONV, including preoperative anxiety, decreased threshold for nausea and vomiting, previous history of PONV, duration of surgery, drugs used for anesthesia, obesity, and postoperative pain medications. Gan and associates, in the 2014 Consensus Guidelines for the Management of Postoperative Nausea and Vomiting, have recommended certain preventive measures (Gan, 2014). These include avoiding general anesthesia with the use of more regional anesthesia, use of propofol for induction and maintenance, avoidance of nitrous oxide and other volatile anesthetics, adequate hydration, and minimizing the perioperative use of opioids. The list of recommended pharmacologic antiemetics for PONV prophylaxis can be seen in Table 25.7. Serotonin is the most

**TABLE 25.7** Antiemetics Used for Postoperative Nausea and Vomiting (PONV)

| Drugs | Dose | Evidence | Timing | Evidence |
|---|---|---|---|---|
| Aprepitant | 40 mg per os | A2[113,115] | At induction | A2[113] |
| Casopitant | 150 mg per os | A3[117,118] | At induction | |
| Dexamethasone | 4-5 mg IV | A1[121] | At induction | A1[326] |
| Dimenhydrinate | 1 mg/kg IV | A1[152_154] | | |
| Dolasetron | 12.5 mg IV | A2[84,85] | End of surgery; timing may not affect efficacy | A2[85] |
| Droperidol* | 0.625-1.25 mg IV | A1[138,139] | End of surgery | A1[140] |
| Ephedrine | 0.5 mg/kg IM | A2[223,224] | | |
| Granisetron | 0.35-3 mg IV | A1[91-93] | End of surgery | A1[108-110] |
| Haloperidol | 0.5-2 mg IM/IV | A1[146] | | |
| Methylprednisolone | 40 mg IV | A2[137] | | |
| Ondansetron | 4 mg IV, 8 mg ODT | A1[74,75] | End of surgery | A1[107] |
| Palonosetron | 0.075 mg IV | A2[105,106] | At induction | A2[105,106] |
| Perphenazine | 5 mg IV | A1[162] | | |
| Promethazine | 6.25-12.5 mg IV | A2[222,295] | | |
| Ramosetron | 0.3 mg IV | A2[102] | End of surgery | A2[102] |
| Rolapitant | 70-200 mg per os | A3[119] | At induction | |
| Scopolamine | Transdermal patch | A1[157,158] | Prior evening or 2 h before surgery | A1[157] |
| Tropisetron | 2 mg IV | A1[97] | End of surgery | Expert opinion |

From Gan TJ, Diemunsch P, Habib AS, et al. Consensus guidelines for the management of postoperative nausea and vomiting. *Anesth Analg.* 2014;118(1): 85-113.
All references are from the original source article.
These recommendations are evidence based, and not all the drugs have an Food and Drug Administration (FDA) indication for PONV. Drugs are listed alphabetically.
*See FDA black box warning.
*IM,* Intramuscularly; *IV,* intravenously; *ODT,* orally disintegrating tablet.

important neurotransmitter and intestinal hormone affecting nausea. Serotonin affects the GI nerves and also central nervous system (CNS) receptors, specifically through the 5-hydroxytryptamine (5-HT3) receptors. It should be no surprise that 5-HT3 receptor antagonists are effective and perhaps the most studied, specifically ondansetron. However, there are other 5-HT3 receptor antagonist medications, as well as neurokinin-1 (NK-1) receptor antagonists, corticosteroids, butyrophenones, antihistamines, and anticholinergics, that have activity and are currently used in clinical practice.

A randomized clinical trial of 5199 patients by Apfel and colleagues has examined several regimens for the prophylaxis of PONV. This multicenter trial documented several important principles for postoperative management. The antiemetic interventions of dexamethasone, ondansetron, and droperidol were found to be equally effective for treating nausea. Droperidol is associated with a rare but problematic side effect of prolonged QT intervals and has subsequently led to most pharmacies removing this medication from their formularies. Dexamethasone, 2.5 to 5 mg, should be given at the beginning of surgery to be most effective. The repeat use of medications for rescue effects is less efficacious if an agent has been given previously (Apfel, 2004). Previous studies have found that agents such as metoclopramide are ineffective for prophylaxis. Antiemetics in the phenothiazine class, such as promethazine and prochlorperazine, are effective but have some limitations because of side effects of sedation, dry mouth, and extrapyramidal effects, which may be worse for older women. Although ondansetron is the gold standard to which other antiemetics are compared, it is less effective than aprepitant for reducing emesis and palonosetron on PONV incidence.

Apfel and associates' study also looked at risk factors for PONV, and one of the strongest is female gender (RR, 3.13; 95% CI, 2.33 to 4.20). Thus prophylactic measures should be considered for all postoperative women. Other factors include 1.78 RR (95% CI, 1.35 to 2.95) for patients with hysterectomies, 1.57 RR (95% CI, 1.32 to 1.07) for nonsmokers, and 2.14 (95% CI: 1.75 to 2.61) for use of postoperative opioids (Apfel, 2004). The term *postdischarge nausea and vomiting* (PDNV) is used for patients going home within 24 hours of surgery. Several small randomized controlled trials (RCTs) have demonstrated efficacy in preventing PDNV with orally disintegrating ondansetron tablets, acupoint stimulation of P6, and transdermal scopolamine patches.

## Ileus

Ileus is a delay in the normal return of bowel function caused by an inhibition of the normal propulsive reflexes of the bowel that are regulated by the autonomic nervous system. Adynamic (paralytic) ileus is a misnomer because it is a normal event defined as delayed bowel function of minor to moderate degree in the absence of a mechanical obstruction. It may be expected to follow any intraperitoneal or pelvic operation. Brief declines in the motility of the GI tract are normal responses after surgery, and the stomach returns to full motility within 24 hours. However, some gastric secretions will continually pass into the duodenum. The stomach secretes 500 to 1000 mL of fluid/day, making the total output from the upper tract approximately 1 to 1.5 L daily. The pancreas secretes an additional liter. (Table 25.10 summarizes GI tract secretions.) The small intestine resumes peristalsis within 6 hours after surgery. The right colon resumes full motility in about 24 hours, but the left colon may take up to 72 hours. The incidence and duration of adynamic ileus are less after vaginal or laparoscopic hysterectomy than abdominal hysterectomy.

If the delay in bowel function persists longer than 5 to 7 days, the patient has an ileus and one should also consider the possibility causes: either a mechanical cause such as a bowel obstruction or some other condition leading to an adynamic, or paralytic, ileus such as an infection or retained foreign body.

Ileus, or specifically adynamic ileus, is believed to result from a lack of coordinated motor activity of the intestine, which results in disorganized propulsive activity. Electrical activity is present, but the pathophysiologic problem is continuous activity of the intrinsic inhibitor neurons in the wall of the small intestine. Usually the process is generalized but occasionally may be localized, involving only an isolated loop of bowel. The cause of prolonged postoperative ileus is a subject of continued debate. Generally the mechanisms include an increased neurologic inhibition of intestinal motility caused by sympathetic nerve activity, as well as edema and inflammation within the intestinal wall. Bauer and Boeckxstaens have described leukocytic infiltration secondary to cytokine production from manipulation of the bowel during surgery. The inflammation inhibits the appropriate neuromuscular reactions, which then decrease motility (Bauer, 2004). Postoperative narcotics also contribute to the problem by stimulating the mu-opioid receptors increasing the dyssynchronous contractions that are the hallmark of an ileus, further decreasing motility and increasing pain.

**The classic symptoms of a prolonged ileus include absence of flatus, abdominal distention, and obstipation.** Often these symptoms are associated with nausea and vomiting, and bowel sounds may be hypoactive or absent. This condition may be associated with abdominal tenderness, and the abdomen is usually tympanic to percussion. Nausea and vomiting that persist more than 24 hours after surgery are a cause for concern. Diagnostic films of the abdomen (supine, erect, lateral) may help establish the correct diagnosis but are often overused (Table 25.8). CT scanning has also been found to be a useful test for differentiating adynamic ileus from complete obstruction (Mattei, 2006).

Oral administration of radiocontrast material may be both therapeutic and diagnostic. The osmolality of the radiocontrast material is approximately six times greater than that of normal saline. Thus a large amount of fluid enters the small bowel and acts as a direct stimulant of peristalsis. In one study, after preliminary abdominal films were obtained, a dose of 120 mL 66% diatrizoate meglumine/10% diatrizoate sodium (Gastrografin) was administered orally or via nasogastric tube (Loftus, 2015). Passage of liquid stool occurred within a few hours in patients with adynamic ileus. Gastrografin, unlike barium, is nontoxic if it accidentally contaminates the peritoneal cavity during an operation for bowel obstruction.

**TABLE 25.8** Differential Radiography Findings in Ileus and Mechanical Obstruction

| Adynamic Ileus | Mechanical Obstruction |
|---|---|
| Small and large bowel distended in proportion to each other | In small bowel obstruction, there is dilated small bowel proximal to site of obstruction; in colonic obstruction, the colon is distended and small bowel distention is present with an incompetent ileocecal valve |
| Air-fluid levels in small bowel infrequent; when present, they at the same levels | Air-fluid levels are common and at different levels in the bowel |
| Quantitative difference in small bowel distention | Greater small bowel distention than with ileus |
| Small bowel distention in central part of abdomen with colon in periphery | Small bowel distention present in central part of abdomen; no peripheral large bowel distention |

From Buchsbaum HJ, Mazer J. The gastrointestinal tract. In: Buchsbaum HJ, Walton LA, eds. *Strategies in Gynecologic Surgery.* New York: Springer-Verlag; 1986.

**Early carbohydrate intake and also postoperative gum chewing have demonstrated some efficacy in decreasing the rates of postoperative ileus and promoting the return of normal bowel function;** a carbohydrate-loading drink the night before surgery and allowing fluids up to 4 hours before surgery may assist with postoperative recovery as well (Kalogera, 2013). **It is also known that early feeding decreases the incidence of postoperative ileus, most likely through stimulation of intestinal reflexes.** The workup of postoperative ileus should include evaluation of serum electrolyte and magnesium levels because hypokalemia and abnormal magnesium levels may contribute to the ileus. Narcotics, intraabdominal infection, urinary ascites, and retroperitoneal hematomas may all affect GI motility. The management of a postoperative ileus is controversial, with numerous remedies that are unproved but have demonstrated isolated, anecdotal success (Table 25.9).

Severe adynamic ileus is a self-limiting condition that responds to GI rest, IV fluids, and time. During the period of watchful expectancy, adequate fluid and electrolyte replacement is necessary. Patients experience mild cramping and passage of flatus and regain their appetite with the return of normal peristalsis. If adequate bowel sounds are present, a rectal tube, a Fleet enema, or a rectal suppository may facilitate the initial passage of flatus. Some advocate the routine postoperative administration of a "wetting agent," such as simethicone, to reduce surface tension of intestinal mucus and liberate entrapped gas. Opinions are mixed as to whether such an agent reduces the incidence or intensity of adynamic ileus. Randomized trials of the prokinetic agents erythromycin and metoclopramide have shown these agents to be ineffective in relieving ileus. Importantly, prophylactic nasogastric suctioning will not prevent ileus. In many studies, prophylactic nasogastric suctioning is associated with an increased risk of aspiration and an increased rate of ileus—the very symptom the treatment is supposed to prevent (Nelson, 2007). However, **if a severe ileus does not resolve, nasogastric suctioning is necessary because it prevents progression of the intestinal distention.** During periods when nasogastric suctioning is used, special attention should be given to correct replacement of fluid and electrolytes (Tables 25.10 and 25.11). A rare but worrisome complication of prolonged ileus is massive dilation of the cecum. Massive dilation of the colon related to a pseudo-obstruction produced by severe adynamic ileus in the absence of mechanical obstruction is known as Ogilvie syndrome. This condition may be treated medically by evacuating the air with colonoscopy or rectal tube, and in severe cases, cecostomy may be necessary. An alternative method of treating this condition is IV neostigmine.

## Intestinal Obstruction and Adhesions

**Adhesions are the most common cause of postoperative intestinal obstruction.** During subsequent operations, up to 90% of women are found to have some adhesions after abdominal laparotomy, although most are filmy. In a large retrospective cohort study after laparotomy for gynecologic conditions, approximately one in three women had adhesion-related readmissions to the hospital (Ellis, 1999). Less common causes of intestinal obstruction are hernias, mesenteric defects, intussusception, volvulus, and neoplasm. Large raw areas of the pelvis with hypoxic tissue facilitate the attachment of small intestine after pelvic surgery. Previous gynecologic surgeries are the most common cause of small bowel obstruction in women. The incidence of operation for obstruction of the small intestine after an abdominal hysterectomy is estimated to be approximately 2%. Interestingly, in one series, adhesions involving the pelvic peritoneum were responsible for the intestinal obstruction in 85% of cases, and adhesions

TABLE 25.9 Treatment Options for Postoperative Ileus

| Treatment | Potential Mechanism | Comments |
|---|---|---|
| **NONPHARMACOLOGIC OPTIONS** | | |
| Nasogastric tube | Gastric, small bowel decompression | No evidence nasogastric tubes reduce duration of POI<br>May increase pulmonary postoperative complications pulmonary postoperative complications |
| Early enteral nutrition | Stimulates gastrointestinal motility by eliciting reflex response and stimulating release of several hormonal factors | Appears safe, well tolerated<br>Some, but not all, studies suggest decrease in POI |
| Sham feeding | Cephalic-vagal reflex | Small clinical trials suggest some benefit |
| Early mobilization | Possible mechanical stimulation | No significant change in duration of POI but may decrease other postoperative complications |
| Laparoscopic surgery | Decreased opiate requirements, decreased pain, less abdominal wall trauma | Most studies find decreased duration of POI with laparoscopy |
| Psychological preoperative preparation | Improves bowel motility through visceral learning | One study found positive benefit in decreasing time to flatus and hospital discharge |
| **PHARMACOLOGIC TREATMENT OPTIONS** | | |
| Metoclopramide | Dopamine antagonist, cholinergic agent | |
| Cisapride | Dopamine antagonist, cholinergic agonist, serotonin receptor agonist | Possibly effective, withdrawn from U.S. market due to cardiovascular side effects |
| Erythromycin | Motilin agonist | Two RCTs suggest no benefit |
| Opiate antagonists | Block peripheral opiate receptors | One RCT shows ADL8-2698 decreases time to flatus, bowel movement, and hospital discharge, but not currently available outside of clinical trials<br>Other agents have not been evaluated in POI movement, and hospital discharge, but not currently available outside of clinical trials<br>Other agents have not been evaluated in POI |
| Epidural anesthesia | Inhibits sympathetic reflex at cord level, opioid-sparing analgesia | Several RCTs suggest benefit in decreasing POI, most effective when inserted at thoracic level |
| NSAIDs | Opiate-sparing analgesia, inhibits COX-mediated prostaglandin synthesis | Probable benefit. COX-2 selective medications need further evaluation |
| Laxatives | Stimulant, prokinetic effects | No RCTs<br>One nonrandomized, unblinded study suggests possible benefit |
| Antiadrenergic agents | Blocks sympathetic neural reflex | Little practical benefit in POI drugs often limited by cardiovascular side effects |
| Cholinergic agents | Acetylcholine modulation | Frequent systemic side effects<br>Neostigmine has possible benefit |
| Multimodality therapy | Combination therapy may work via multiple mechanisms | Possible benefit in reducing POI<br>No RCTs have been reported |

From Behm B, Stollman N. Postoperative ileus: etiologies and interventions. *Clin Gastroenterol Hepatol.* 2003;1(2):71-80.
*COX,* Cyclooxygenase; *NSAIDs,* nonsteroidal antiinflammatory drugs; *POI,* postoperative ileus; *RCTs,* randomized controlled trials.

TABLE 25.10 Average Daily Volume and Electrolyte Concentrations of Gastrointestinal Secretions

| | | Electrolyte Concentration (mEq/L) | | |
|---|---|---|---|---|
| **Secretion** | **Volume (mL/day)** | **$Na^+$** | **$K^+$** | **$Cl^-$** |
| Saliva | 1000-1500 | 10-40 | 10-20 | 6-30 |
| Gastric juice | 2000-2500 | 60-120 | 10-20 | 10-30 |
| Hepatic bile | 600-800 | 130-155 | 2-12 | 80-100 |
| Pancreatic juice | 700-1000 | 150-155 | 5-10 | 30-50 |
| Duodenal secretions | 300-800 | 90-140 | 2-10 | 70-120 |
| Jejunal and ileal secretions | 2000-3000 | 125-140 | 5-10 | 100-130 |
| Colonic mucosal secretions | 200-500 | 140-148 | 5-10 | 60-90 |
| Total: | 8000-10,000 | | | |

to the closure of the anterior abdominal wall accounted for the other 15%. Fortunately the fibrous adhesions that form during the first 2 to 3 weeks after an operation are soft and filmy, and thus intestinal strangulation during the postoperative period is extremely rare. Dense adhesions may develop several months after surgery. Adhesion formation after surgical procedures appears to be related to irritation of the peritoneum. The reaction of injured peritoneum involves a reepithelialization by peritoneal cells to cover raw intraabdominal surfaces. The process begins within 24 hours of surgery. Fibrin-rich exudates cover areas of denuded viscera and abdominal wall. Factors that increase adhesion formation include inflammation, infection, and trauma; thus suturing of peritoneum should be kept to a minimum. The greatest risk noted by Dubuisson and colleagues in a series of 1000 consecutive laparoscopies was in previous midline incisions, with more than 50% having adhesions, compared with less than 3% after a previous laparoscopy (Dubuisson, 2010). The incidence of intestinal obstruction depends on the type of gynecologic surgery performed. Approximately 2 in 1000 women develop an obstruction after a

**TABLE 25.11** Composition of Intravenous Solutions

| | | Component (mEq/L) | | | | | | | |
|---|---|---|---|---|---|---|---|---|---|
| **Solution** | **Glucose (g/L)** | **Na⁺** | **Cl⁻** | **$HCO_3^-$** | **$K^+$** | **$Ca^{2+}$** | **$Mg^{2+}$** | **$HPO_4^-$** | **$NH_4^-$** |
| Extracellular fluid | 1000 | 140 | 102 | 27 | 4.2 | 5 | 3 | 0.3 | |
| 5% Dextrose and water | 50 | | | | | | | | |
| 10% Dextrose and water | 100 | | | | | | | | |
| 0.9% Sodium chloride (normal saline) | | | 154 | 154 | | | | | |
| 0.45% Sodium chloride (half normal saline) | | | 77 | 77 | | | | | |
| 0.21% Sodium chloride (¼ normal saline) | | | 34 | 34 | | | | | |
| 3% Sodium chloride (hypertonic saline) | | | 513 | 513 | | | | | |
| Lactated Ringer's solution | | | 130 | 109 | 28* | 4 | 2.7 | | |
| 0.9% Ammonium chloride | | | 168 | | | | | | 168 |

From Miller TA, Duke JH. Fluid and electrolyte management. In: Dudrick SJ, Baue AE, Eiseman B, et al, eds, *Manual of Preoperative and Postoperative Care,* 3rd ed. Philadelphia: WB Saunders; 1983.
*Present in solution as lactate but is metabolized to bicarbonate.

**TABLE 25.12** Differential Diagnosis between Postoperative Ileus and Postoperative Obstruction

| Clinical Features | Postoperative Ileus | Postoperative Obstruction |
|---|---|---|
| Abdominal pain | Discomfort from distention but not cramping pains | Cramping, progressively severe |
| Relationship to previous operation | Usually within 48-72 hours of operation | Usually delayed; may be 5-7 days for remote onset |
| Nausea and vomiting | Present | Present |
| Distention | Present | Present |
| Bowel sounds | Absent or hypoactive | Borborygmi with peristaltic rushes and high-pitched tinkles |
| Fever | Only if related to associated peritonitis | Rarely present unless bowel becomes gangrenous |
| Abdominal radiograph | Distended loops of small and large bowels; gas usually present in colon | Single or multiple loops of distended bowel, usually small bowel with air-fluid levels |
| Treatment | Conservative with nasogastric suction, enemas, cholinergic stimulation | Partial—conservative with nasogastric decompression, *or* Complete—surgical |

benign gynecologic operation, whereas approximately 8% develop intestinal obstruction after radical cancer surgery. Intestinal obstruction occurs in the small intestine in approximately 80% of cases and in the colon in the remaining 20%. As noted, differentiating between bowel obstruction and ileus can be difficult in the postoperative period (Table 25.12).

The acute symptoms of intestinal obstruction usually present between the fifth and seventh postoperative days. Most patients have a short period of normal intestinal function before the onset of symptoms. Women with bowel obstruction appear to have more acute distress than women with an ileus. The abdominal pain is intermittent, colicky, and may be sharp in nature. Episodes of colicky pain usually last from 1 to 3 minutes. Associated symptoms include vomiting, abdominal distention, and constipation. Bowel sounds are loud, high-pitched, and rushing. Nasogastric drainage is usually more profuse than in patients with severe adynamic ileus.

Abdominal radiographs demonstrate a stepladder appearance, multiple air-fluid levels throughout the small intestine, with a paucity of gas in the colon and rectum. Pneumoperitoneum from an exploratory celiotomy usually persists for up to 7 days. Thus in the early postoperative period, free air under the diaphragm is not diagnostic of perforation of a hollow viscus. Obstruction of the colon may be diagnosed by retrograde infusion of contrast material or by flexible endoscopy.

**The foundation of early treatment of postoperative intestinal obstruction is decompression of the small intestine and adequate replacement of fluids and electrolytes.** Decompression may be accomplished by means of a nasogastric tube. Serial monitoring of white blood cell counts may be helpful in identifying patients who need further intervention. Repeat physical examinations and abdominal radiography are used to assess the degree of intestinal distention, and expectant management is successful in the majority of patients. Historically, less than 40% of patients with small bowel obstruction caused by adhesions will require surgery. Some advocate for immediate administration of Gastrografin on presentation for adhesive obstruction, with conservative management of patients in whom the Gastrografin does not reach the colon in 24 hours. **Patients in whom contrast reached the colon in 5 hours or less had a 90% success rate of conservative management** (Gowen, 2003).

**The major cause of morbidity and death with bowel obstruction is delay in diagnosis, with resultant strangulation, perforation, and secondary sepsis.** Women who develop strangulation experience a dramatic increase in the intensity of abdominal pain, and the pain becomes continuous. Strangulation of the small bowel is associated with localized peritoneal irritation, increase in temperature, and marked leukocytosis. Bowel obstruction may also lead to translocation of intestinal bacteria across the bowel wall, promoting sepsis. It has been shown that the more distal the obstruction, the greater the incidence of anaerobic septicemia.

Fecal impaction is most often seen in older patients. It results from loss of peristalsis in the colon, with an impaired perception of rectal fullness. This may result in diarrhea as intestinal contents pass around the impaction or obstipation. Treatment involves obtaining partial analgesia with lidocaine jelly and, subsequently, manually fragmenting and extracting the fecal mass.

## Rectovaginal Fistula

Rectovaginal fistulas and fecal incontinence secondary to perineal tears are usually obstetric complications and are only rarely associated with gynecologic surgery. In general, rectovaginal fistulas after hysterectomy or repair of an enterocele are usually located in the upper third of the vagina, whereas those secondary to a posterior colporrhaphy are in the lower third of the vagina. Other causes of rectovaginal fistula are carcinoma, radiation therapy, perirectal abscess, inflammatory bowel disease, lymphogranuloma venereum, and trauma.

The initial signs and symptoms associated with potential fistulous tracts between the rectum and vagina usually present 7 to 14 days after an operation. The first warning may be the rectal passage of several blood clots, indicating that a hematoma has ruptured into the rectum. Distressing symptoms include passage of gas from the vagina and, depending on the size of the opening, the passage of fecal material from the vagina. Associated with these classic symptoms and signs are a chronic, foul-smelling vaginal discharge and subsequent dyspareunia. Aside from the physical symptoms of the anatomic defect, fistulas cause severe emotional distress because they affect almost every aspect of the woman's daily life.

The diagnosis is not difficult to establish, and only very small openings present a diagnostic problem. What appears to be granulation tissue in the posterior aspect of the vagina is the dark red rectal mucosa, which stands out in contrast to the lighter vaginal mucosa. Usually the defect may be successfully defined with a small, malleable metal probe. If this is not successful, a Foley catheter should be placed in the rectum. Methylene blue dye or milk may then be instilled into the rectum with a tampon in the vagina, similar to the procedure for establishing the diagnosis of a vesicovaginal fistula. **Contrast enemas and colonoscopy may also be used in cases where there is a high degree of suspicion and the fistula cannot be identified by other means.**

**For initial treatment the woman should be obstipated with a low-residue diet and diphenoxylate hydrochloride (Lomotil).** Approximately one in four anatomic defects heal spontaneously before epithelialization of the tract. A low-residue diet or hyperalimentation may be helpful in facilitating spontaneous closure of some anatomic defects. Timing of the operative repair is important. The area surrounding the fistula should be free of edema, induration, and infection. Preoperative evaluation includes visualization of the entire vagina and sigmoidoscopy of the rectal mucosa in an attempt to discover more than one opening. Imaging studies and endoscopy are important diagnostic tools if there is any suspicion of coexistence of Crohn disease.

The operative technique used depends on the size and location of the fistula. Standard operative principles include removal of the entire fistulous tract and closure of tissue layers without tension on the suture line. In the repair of large rectovaginal fistulas in the lower part of the vagina, it is usually easier to convert the rectovaginal fistula into a fourth-degree laceration. Diverting colostomy should be used for all radiation-induced fistulas, most fistulas associated with inflammatory bowel disease, and some large postoperative fistulas at the apex of the vagina. The stool should be kept soft with low-residue diets and stool softeners such as mineral oil for the first 2 weeks after the operative repair.

## Antibiotic-Associated Diarrhea

Patients may develop diarrhea in the postoperative period after exposure to antibiotics. Oral and parenteral antibiotics produce similar rates of diarrhea, with some studies noting that up to one-third of patients receiving antibiotics will develop diarrhea. Antibiotic therapy, for prophylaxis or treatment, can disrupt the normal intestinal flora. The result is a disturbed breakdown of bile acids and carbohydrates that induce loose stools. Diarrhea may develop secondary to medications other than antibiotics, including oral contrast media, diabetic foods that contain artificial sweeteners, and many cardiac medications. If the woman is afebrile, the diarrhea is mild, and the abdominal examination is unremarkable, stopping or changing antibiotics and providing supportive care are all that is necessary. **If the woman has a temperature higher than 38°C, a leukocytosis, abdominal tenderness, severe abdominal distention, bloody diarrhea, or persistent diarrhea, evaluation for *Clostridioides difficile* infection is indicated** (Table 25.13).

**TABLE 25.13** Differences Between Antibiotic-Associated Diarrhea From *Clostridium difficile* and Diarrhea From Other Causes

| | Cause | |
|---|---|---|
| **Characteristic** | ***C. difficile* Infection** | **Other Causes** |
| Most commonly implicated antibiotics | Clindamycin, cephalosporins, penicillins | Clindamycin, cephalosporins, or amoxicillin-clavulanate |
| History | Usually no relevant history of antibiotic intolerance | History of diarrhea with antibiotic therapy common |
| **Clinical Features** | | |
| Diarrhea | May be florid; evidence of colitis with cramps, fever, and fecal leukocytes common | Usually moderate in severity (i.e., nuisance diarrhea) without evidence of colitis |
| Findings from CT or endoscopy | Evidence of colitis (not enteritis) common | Usually normal |
| Complications | Hypoalbuminemia, anasarca, toxic megacolon, relapses with treatment with metronidazole or vancomycin | Usually none except occasional cases of dehydration |
| Results of assay for *C. difficile* toxin | Positive | Negative |
| Epidemiologic pattern | May be epidemic for endemic in hospitals or long-term care facilities | Sporadic |
| **Treatment** | | |
| Withdrawal of implicated antibiotic | May resolve but often persists or progresses | Usually resolves |
| Antiperistaltic agents | Contraindicated | Often useful |
| Oral metronidazole or vancomycin | Prompt response | Not indicated |

From Bartlett JG. Antibiotic-associated diarrhea. *N Engl J Med.* 2002;346(5):334-339.
*CT,* Computed tomography.

*C. difficile* is a species of spore-forming, gram-positive anaerobic bacteria found normally in 5% of healthy adults. However, after antibiotic treatment and disruption of normal enteric flora, up to 25% of hospitalized adults will become colonized with *C. difficile*. The organism is spread by nosocomial oral-fecal contamination. Persistence of the spores of *C. difficile* and contamination of the environment are primary factors in cross infection. After colonizing the intestine, the organism may secrete toxins, which produce a spectrum of clinical disease. Symptoms from the infection are varied and range from a mild diarrhea to colitis to a pseudomembranous colitis that in rare cases may be fatal (McDonald, 2018). Almost any antibiotic has been associated with the development of *C. difficile* diarrhea, but **second- and third-generation cephalosporins are the antibiotics associated with the highest risk of developing *C. difficile* diarrhea.** Symptoms usually appear 5 to 10 days after the initiation of antibiotic therapy; however, they may appear from a few days to a few weeks after antibiotic exposure. Enzyme-linked immunosorbent assay (ELISA) testing for *C. difficile* cell cytotoxin B in the stool is the gold standard for diagnosis because it is the most sensitive and specific and is also relatively inexpensive. The results are usually available within 24 hours.

Use of drugs that slow intestinal transit time, such as diphenoxylate atropine (Lomotil) or narcotics, are generally felt to be contraindicated in the management of *C. difficile* colitis because the toxins of *C. difficile* remain in the GI tract for a longer period, but there is no high-quality evidence to support this hypothesis. **The preferred first-line treatment is vancomycin PO 125 mg four times daily for 10 days or fidaxomicin 200 mg twice a day for 10 days.** Alternatively, metronidazole with 500 mg three times daily for 10 days can be used, but this is no longer preferred. GI symptoms usually improve within the first 72 hours of therapy, and complete resolution of symptoms occurs within 10 days. Host factors are involved in the pathogenesis of the disease; older and more chronically ill patients usually develop more severe symptoms. Up to 25% of women may develop a recurrence or relapse. Studies have confirmed that more than 50% of recurrences of symptoms after initial response to treatment are caused by reinfection rather by a relapse. Recurrences usually can be successfully treated with oral antibiotics using longer courses (McDonald, 2018). In rare cases, fecal transplant has been used to treat recalcitrant disease.

## WOUND COMPLICATIONS

### Infection

A major wound infection prolongs the hospital stay by approximately 2 to 6 days. In a historic review of 23,649 operations, the incidence of abdominal wound infection after abdominal hysterectomy was approximately 5%. **Contemporary studies show rates of surgical site infection after hysterectomy of 3.9% for abdominal surgery and 1.8% for minimally invasive approaches ($P < .001$), with an odds ratio of 0.44 (CI 0.37 to 0.53)** (Gandaglia, 2014). Hysterectomy is classified as a clean-contaminated operative procedure because the bacterial flora of the vagina is in continuity with the operative site during the surgery. The Centers for Disease Control and Prevention have revised their nomenclature describing incisional infection. They subdivide incisional infections into superficial infections that involve only the skin and subcutaneous tissue and deep infections that involve the deep soft tissues, including fascia and muscles. **Although some infections are generally associated with specific organisms such as *Streptococcus* or clostridia, most gynecologic infections are polymicrobial.** Thus antibiotic treatments are aimed at providing broad-spectrum coverage for aerobic, anaerobic, and gram-negative organisms. A list of common antibiotics is found in Appendix B.

The pathophysiology of wound infection depends on an interaction between the number and virulence of bacterial contamination and the resistance of the woman. Inoculation of bacteria into the wound occurs in the operating room during the surgical procedure. A wide spectrum of common endogenous bacteria produce wound infections, including most gram-positive cocci and aerobic and anaerobic rods. Small numbers of bacteria are present in all surgical wounds; however, bacterial growth is facilitated by decreased tissue oxygen and excessive amounts of necrotic tissue. It takes from 100,000 to 1,000,000 bacteria per gram of tissue to produce infection in a surgical wound of the skin and subcutaneous tissue. The incidence of superficial skin infection is directly related to the length of the operative procedure, and each additional hour of surgery results in a doubling of the incidence of superficial skin infections. The primary source of bacterial contamination of an abdominal wound may be exogenous to the woman (e.g., a break in sterile technique) or endogenous (e.g., purulent material from a pelvic abscess).

Local and systemic factors contribute to the level of host resistance and thus to the incidence of wound infections. Local factors are more significant and include the presence of hematomas, necrotic tissue, foreign bodies, or dead space; use of cautery; and decreased local tissue perfusion. **Systemic factors include obesity, diabetes, liver disease, malnutrition, immunosuppression, defects in the reticuloendothelial system, age, and duration of preoperative hospitalization** (Box 25.7). The incidence of postoperative wound infection is increased eightfold when the woman's preoperative weight exceeds 200 pounds. In a series of women undergoing abdominal hysterectomy, the thickness of subcutaneous tissue was the greatest risk factor for wound infection (Soper, 1995). **If an abdominal incision is more than 4 cm in depth, the risk of a superficial skin infection is increased approximately threefold.** Multiple regimens and protocols have been studied to decrease rates of wound infection. Skin warming to improve circulation, supplemental oxygen, and antibiotics given before incision time have all been emphasized as techniques for infection prevention. The role of wound lavage is less clear.

**The first symptom of most wound infections usually appears between the fifth and tenth postoperative days.** Wound infection may occur as late as several months after surgery, but more than 90% of cases present within the first 2 weeks of the postoperative period. The first sign is usually fever, followed by tachycardia and varying degrees of increased incisional erythema, induration, tenderness, and pain. As the infection progresses,

**BOX 25.7 Factors Associated With Wound Infections**

- Preexisting skin and operative site infection
- Tissue with poor oxygenation
- Hematoma
- Necrotic tissue
- Foreign bodies
- Cauterized tissue
- Poor circulation from vascular disease
- Dead space within the wound
- Anemia
- Decreased perfusion from tension
- Obesity
- Long preoperative hospitalization
- Poor nutrition
  - Vitamin deficiencies
  - Mineral deficiencies (e.g., zinc)
- Glucocorticoids, other immunosuppressive medications
- Diabetes
- Liver disease
- Ionizing radiation
- Advanced age

many wounds develop areas that are fluctuant or firm, and some develop crepitus. There may be associated spontaneous purulent drainage from the wound later in the course of the infection.

Fever during the first 24 to 48 hours is usually secondary to atelectasis. However, two rare types of wound infections are so virulent that they produce toxicity within the first 48 hours. Typically these early infections are those produced by *Clostridium* spp. and acute beta-hemolytic streptococcal infection. Clinically, wound infections secondary to beta-hemolytic streptococci appear swollen and red and have an odorless discharge. In contrast, infections secondary to *Clostridium* are boggy and edematous and the discharge has a sweet odor.

**Initial treatment of any wound infection consists of opening and draining the wound.** Purulent material exhibits a wide range of consistency from the thin watery discharge typical of a streptococcal infection to the thick purulence associated with staphylococcal subcutaneous infections. **Gram staining with aerobic and anaerobic cultures of the wound should be performed.** These cultures are valuable in guiding treatment if the woman does not respond to initial management. In such cases the differential diagnosis would be between infections involving deeper tissue planes and infection for which host resistance has failed, even after drainage of the wound. Once a wound infection has been opened and drained, care is directed toward initial packing of the wound with gauze to effect debridement and periodic irrigation. If necrotic tissue is seen, the tissue should be resected back to the point where vital tissue can be identified. If there is a distinct zone of diffuse erythema surrounding a wound infection, the most likely organism is a streptococcal infection, and IV antibiotics are indicated. If methicillin-resistant *Staphylococcus aureus* (MRSA) is cultured, the great majority of women will respond solely to debridement. If the woman does not respond or responds slowly, antibiotics specific for MRSA should be used, such as clindamycin, sulfamethoxazole-trimethoprim, or vancomycin. Systemic antibiotics are always indicated for women with immunosuppression or concomitant disease with impaired defense mechanisms.

Most women with a wound infection will become afebrile within 48 to 72 hours after the wound has been opened and debrided. **When the woman becomes afebrile and granulation tissue begins to form, consideration may be given to delayed secondary closure. If the incision is large and debridement has been extensive, closure may be facilitated with the use of vacuum-assisted devices, which promote granulation, reduce edema in the subcutaneous tissue, and greatly speed healing.** The vacuum should be changed every 48 to 72 hours for wound evaluation, but it may be used on an outpatient basis (Fig. 25.9).

Prevention is the foundation of any approach to the treatment of wound infections. Prevention involves consideration of local and systemic factors, which, if unattended, predispose to infection. Prophylactic antibiotics, which are discussed in Chapter 24, decrease the incidence of wound infection. If the wound is grossly contaminated, it should be left open after surgery with wet to dry dressings or with negative pressure wound vacuum application. Delayed primary closure on the third or fourth postoperative day may be appropriate if healthy tissue is noted. Women who should be considered as candidates for delayed primary closure include those who are immunosuppressed or malnourished, have advanced malignancies, have a contaminated wound, or have morbid obesity. Delayed primary closure reduces the incidence of wound infection from 23% in a control group to 2%. When delayed primary closure is planned, sutures may be placed at the time of surgery and secured, but not tied. The incision should be packed loosely with gauze. If the wound is dry and without evidence of infection on postoperative day 3, the edges may be approximated with the preplaced sutures.

Delayed secondary closure may be accomplished in previously infected wounds after several days of drainage and debridement, once the wound exhibits nice healthy granulation tissue. Delayed secondary closure markedly reduces the time necessary for eventual closure of the skin defect by secondary intention. The woman's satisfaction is dramatically increased with delayed secondary closure. If delayed closure does not appear to be a likely option, such as in women who have more than 3 cm of subcutaneous tissue, application of a closed vacuum system should be initiated.

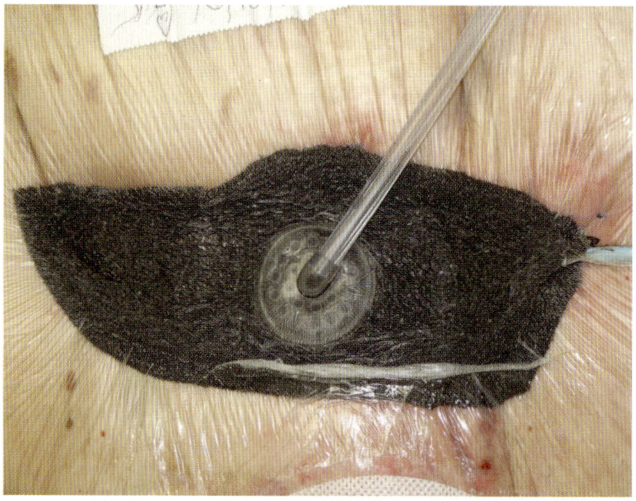

**Fig. 25.9** Wound-Vac device on an abdominal wound. The *black area* is the sponge within the incision. (From Heridge RT, Leong M, Phillips L: Wound healing. In: Townsend CM, Beauchamp RD, Evers BM, Mattox KL, eds. *Sabiston Textbook of Surgery.* 18th ed. Philadelphia: Saunders; 2008:191-216.)

**A virulent, rapidly progressing form of soft tissue wound infection is necrotizing fasciitis.** Often the diagnosis is not suspected during the early part of the infection because of the relative minor changes in the skin overlying the deeper infection. The early symptoms are local pain with systemic symptoms of tachycardia and fever, which are higher than would be expected with an uncomplicated wound infection. The woman may experience marked tenderness when the infected area is palpated. Conversely, necrotic tissue may become hypoesthetic, or completely numb. An appearance of an area that appears infected but is anesthetic should heighten the suspicion for the diagnosis of necrotizing fasciitis. As the disease progresses, the wound edges usually darken, with crepitus and bullae formation and anesthetic areas developing. Necrotizing fasciitis involves the subcutaneous tissue and superficial fascia. The infection rapidly expands in the subcutaneous spaces and often tracks far beyond the superficial margins of the involved skin.

**This condition is a life-threatening surgical emergency and patients should have debridement as soon as possible.** It is important for the gynecologist to have a high degree of suspicion for this condition because even with adequate surgical debridement the mortality rate is 30% to 50%. Only 35% of patients with necrotizing fasciitis will display evidence of subcutaneous gas on radiographs. If the diagnosis is questionable, a full-thickness core biopsy and frozen section of the tissue should be performed. This rare but potentially fatal condition necessitates wide debridement of all necrotic tissue, high levels of broad-spectrum antibiotics, and sometimes hyperbaric oxygen. Debridement to freely bleeding tissue helps determine the surgical margin. It is not unusual for the woman to need repetitive debridement. **Women with diabetes, malnutrition, immunosuppression, malignancy, obesity, and poor tissue perfusion are most susceptible to this complication.**

## Dehiscence and Evisceration

Dehiscence is a failure of normal healing and refers to a disruption of any of the layers of a surgical incision. The physiologic,

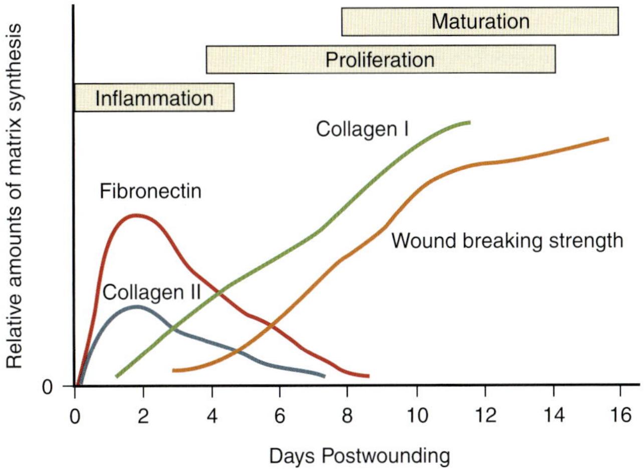


**Fig. 25.10** Wound healing over time. (From Heridge RT, Leong M, Phillips L. Wound healing. In: Townsend CM, Beauchamp RD, Evers BM, Mattox KL, eds. *Sabiston Textbook of Surgery.* 18th ed. Philadelphia: Saunders; 2008:191-216.)

biochemical, and structural changes that characterize normal wound healing are complex and, at best, imperfectly understood. However, the most important fact for the clinician is that the strength of the wound increases over time (Fig. 25.10). The strength of a skin incision increases at a rapid and almost constant rate for the first 4 months and at a much slower rate for the first year. Clinically, ***wound dehiscence*** refers to the separation of the skin, subcutaneous tissue, and fascia but not the peritoneum. This complication usually occurs during the first several days after an operation. **Wound evisceration** is a complete breakdown of the healing process through all levels of the abdominal incision, with omentum or bowel presenting through the fascia.

The incidence of wound dehiscence is approximately 1 in 200 gynecologic operations. The major short-term result of wound dehiscence is the prolongation of hospital stay; over the long term, dehiscence predisposes to incisional hernias. **Wound infection is present in approximately 50% of women with wound disruption.** As with wound infections, preventive management is the most important therapeutic consideration. The incidence of dehiscence has decreased with the use of longer-lasting and stronger sutures. Many clinicians prefer to use polydioxanone suture (PDS), a treated Vicryl, or a permanent suture such as polypropylene (Prolene) for greater strength and prolonged presence in the tissue. The rule of thumb is that the suture should remain strong in the tissue until the tissue can resume its original strength. In patients with a propensity for poor or prolonged healing, such as women with malignancy, diabetes, or immune suppression, the use of a permanent suture is reasonable. When infection is present, a monofilament suture is preferable to a braided or polyfilament suture (Tables 25.14 and 25.15).

The consensus regarding fascial disruption is that local factors are much more important in the pathophysiology of wound disruption than systemic factors, although both should be considered. Important mechanical factors predisposing to disruption are conditions that increase the tension on the incision line, such as abdominal distention and chronic lung disease, or a technically inadequate closure of the wound. Other factors include obesity, advanced age, malignancy, uremia, liver failure, diabetes, hypoproteinemia, hematoma formation, sepsis, corticosteroid use or chemotherapy, prior radiation therapy, and whether the incision is made through an area of a previous incision. Whether an incision is horizontal or vertical has little effect on the incidence of wound disruption. The pathophysiology of fascial dehiscence involves exaggerated collagen lysis in the wound. Clinically the sutures tear through the fascia rather than dissolving or becoming untied. For example, approximating and tying sutures too vigorously, especially with a figure-of-eight suture, may lead to strangulation and necrosis of the tissue and subsequent wound dehiscence. Primary mass closure with a continuous monofilament, delayed absorbable suture, helps avoid this problem in high-risk patients.

**The classic symptom and sign of wound disruption is the spontaneous passage of copious serosanguineous fluid from the abdominal incision.** This usually occurs between the fifth and eighth postoperative days. Patients with uninfected wounds generally have been asymptomatic but often report a "pop" after an episode of coughing or emesis. Patients who develop wound defects often lack the normal healing ridge of tissue that can be palpated in normal healing wounds.

Proper closure of the incision is imperative for prevention of wound dehiscence in a woman at high risk for less than optimum healing. Although there are many regional preferences for the choice of suture and method of closure, the most popular technique is some modification of the Smead-Jones closure with a monofilament suture (Fig. 25.11). **Closure with the Smead-Jones technique results in a dehiscence rate of approximately 1 in 1000 operations.** With this technique, it is important to place individual sutures at least 1 to 1.5 cm away from the adjacent sutures and include at least 2 cm of fascia on either side of the incision. **The alternative technique is the more common running mass closure using a monofilament suture material such as Prolene or PDS.**

**TABLE 25.14** Comparison of Absorbable Sutures

| Suture Reaction | Types | Raw Material | Tensile Strength Retention in Vivo | Tissue |
|---|---|---|---|---|
| Surgical gut suture | Chromic | Collagen derived from healthy beef and sheep | Individual patient characteristics can affect rate of tensile strength loss. | Moderate reaction |
| Monocryl suture (poliglecaprone 25) | Monofilament | Copolymer of glycolide and epsilon-caprolactone | ~50%-60% (violet, 60%-70%) remains at 1 wk; ~20%-30% (violet, 30%-40%) remains at 2 wk; lost within 3 wk (violet, 4 wk) | Minimal acute inflammatory reaction |
| Coated Vicryl (polyglactin 910) | Braided | Copolymer of lactide and glycolide coated with 370 and calcium stearate | ~75% remains at 2 wk | Minimal acute inflammatory reaction |
| Suture | Monofilament | | ~50% remains at 3 wk, 25% at 4 wk | |
| PDS II suture (polydioxanone) | Monofilament | Polyester polymer | ~70% remains at 2 wk; ~50% remains at 4 wk; ~25% remains at 6 wk | Slight |

Modified from Neumayer L, Vargo D. Principles of perioperative and operative surgery. In: Townsend CM, Beauchamp RD, Evers BM, Mattox KL, eds. *Sabiston Textbook of Surgery.* 18th ed. Philadelphia: Saunders; 2008:251-279.

**TABLE 25.15** Comparison of Nonabsorbable Sutures

| Suture | Types | Raw Material | Tensile Strength Retention in Vivo | Tissue Reaction |
|---|---|---|---|---|
| Perma-Hand—silk suture | Braided | Organic protein called *fibroin* | Progressive degradation of fiber may result in gradual loss of tensile strength over time | Acute inflammatory reaction |
| Ethilon—nylon suture | Monofilament | Long-chain aliphatic polymers nylon 6 or nylon 6,6 | Progressive hydrolysis may result in gradual loss of tensile strength over time | Minimal acute inflammatory reaction |
| Nurolon—nylon suture | Braided | Long-chain aliphatic polymers nylon 6 or nylon 6,6 | Progressive hydrolysis may result in gradual loss of tensile strength over time | Minimal acute inflammatory reaction |
| Mersilene—polyester fiber suture | Braided<br>Monofilament | Polyethylene terephthalate | No significant change known to occur in vivo | Minimal acute inflammatory reaction |
| Ethibond *Excel*—polyester fiber suture | Braided | Polyethylene terephthalate coated with polybutilate | No significant change known to occur in vivo | Minimal acute inflammatory reaction |
| Prolene—polypropylene suture | Monofilament | Isotactic crystalline stereoisomer of polypropylene | Not subject to degradation or weakening by action of tissue enzymes | Minimal acute inflammatory reaction |
| Pronova—polyvinylidene fluoride suture | Monofilament | Polymer blend of poly (vinylidene fluoride) and poly (vinylidene fluoride-cohexafluoropropylene) | Not subject to degradation or weakening by action of tissue enzymes | Minimal acute inflammatory reaction |

Modified from Neumayer L, Vargo D. Principles of perioperative and operative surgery. In: Townsend CM, Beauchamp RD, Evers BM, Mattox KL, eds. *Sabiston Textbook of Surgery.* 18th ed. Philadelphia: Saunders; 2008:251-279.

Rarely the vaginal cuff may separate, producing a dehiscence and possibly vaginal evisceration of abdominal contents. This complication often presents with sudden vaginal drainage, bleeding, and pain. **The incidence of vaginal cuff dehiscence varies by mode of surgery and is lowest in vaginal hysterectomy (0.11%), followed by abdominal hysterectomy (0.38%), and highest in laparoscopic hysterectomy (range, 0.75% to 4.93%)** (Hurr, 2011). Risk factors for vaginal cuff dehiscence are summarized in Table 25.16. If there is no evidence of infection at the time of repair, the vaginal cuff may be closed primarily without opening the abdomen. If there is any concern about an intraabdominal complication, an abdominal approach allows for a better intraabdominal evaluation, although reports of laparoscopic evaluation of the abdomen, even in the setting of evisceration with vaginal closure of the cuff, have been successful. Most would also consider antibiotic treatment with broad-spectrum coverage because of the association of vaginal dehiscence with vaginal cuff cellulitis. Vaginal evisceration is uncommon, but when it occurs it is usually several weeks after surgery and may follow intercourse. Reports have noted an increase in vaginal cuff disruption and evisceration with robotic surgery. This is postulated to be secondary to increased use of cauterization, leading to poor wound healing (Hurr, 2011). **This complication may present up to 8 weeks or more after surgery.** As a result, many gynecologists ask patients to refrain from intercourse for up to 12 weeks after surgery to allow time for the sutures to dissolve completely and for the tissue to heal.

The treatment of vaginal dehiscence is prompt reclosure in the operating room. Once the diagnosis is recognized, the wound and viscera should be covered with moist gauze and transported to the operating room supine and possibly in slight Trendelenburg position to help keep abdominal contents from eviscerating. Broad-spectrum antibiotics are usually begun, although there is no proof of their efficacy in this circumstance. Once the woman is anesthetized, the wound should be evaluated so that the full extent of the problem can be evaluated. The wound edges may have to be debrided and the wound closed with a wide mass closure, making sure not to incorporate the bladder or rectum in the closure.

### Wound Care for Patients With Obesity

**Obesity is one of the most significant risk factors for wound infection and disruption.** As noted, hyperglycemia is an associated risk factor in this population of patients. Optimal healing, collagen synthesis, and reepithelialization require good oxygenation. Adipose tissue is poorly vascularized and thus has suboptimal oxygenation. Poor ventilation after surgery in women with obesity further exacerbates this problem. Techniques to improve wound healing in patients with obesity have been summarized by Walsh and associates; these include maintaining normothermia in the operating suite, which decreases vasoconstriction; supplemental oxygen; and closure of the subcutaneous space if it is larger than 2 cm (Walsh, 2009). Subcutaneous drains do not decrease the infection or wound disruption rate. When patients weigh more than 120 kg, prophylactic antibiotic dose should be increased (e.g., from 2 g of cefazolin to 3 g). However, extending the dosing beyond surgery is not helpful. Maintaining euglycemia is essential, as previously discussed (Box 25.8).

## OPERATIVE SITE COMPLICATIONS

### Pelvic Cellulitis and Abscess

Infections of the contiguous retroperitoneal space immediately above the vaginal apex are common complications after abdominal or vaginal hysterectomy; however, the frequency of this postoperative complication has dramatically decreased in direct relation to the use of prophylactic antibiotics and minimally invasive surgery. These soft tissue infections range in severity from localized minor cellulitis to large pelvic abscesses and have many names, from cuff cellulitis to infected hematoma. Nevertheless, they are similar to soft tissue infections in other parts of the body. These infections prolong hospital stay and increase the cost of patient care. The bacterial spectrum that produces these infections includes aerobic and anaerobic bacteria from exogenous and endogenous sources. Most postoperative pelvic infections are polymicrobial, usually from endogenous vaginal flora, and approximately 60% to 80% involve anaerobic organisms.

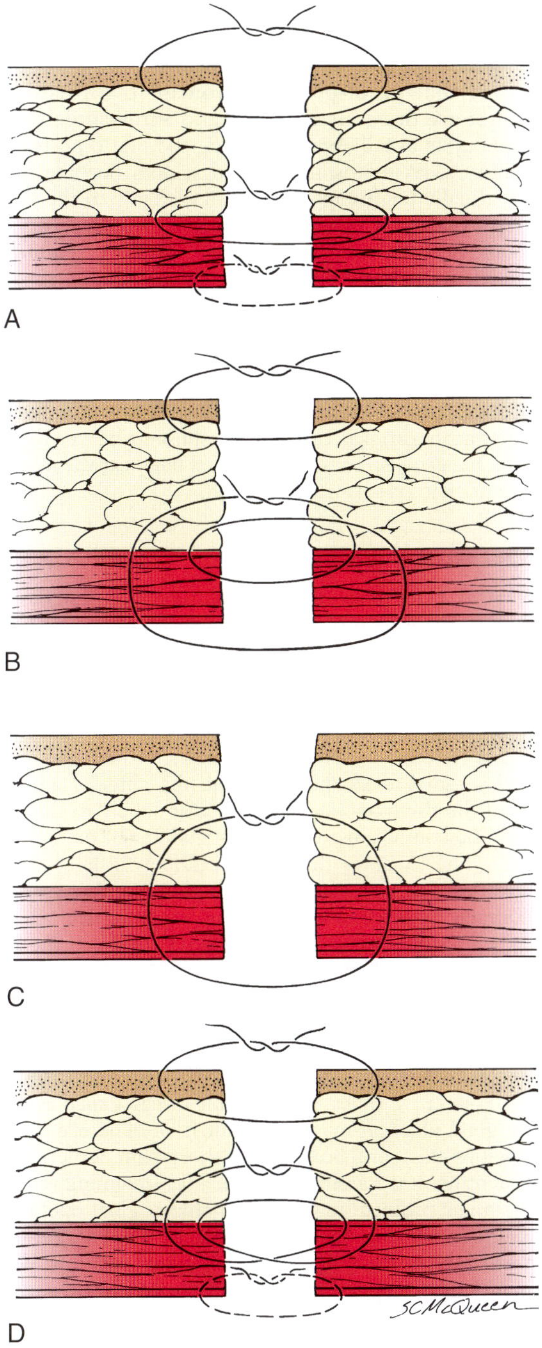


**Fig. 25.11** Types of abdominal incision closures. **A,** Layered. **B,** Smead-Jones. **C,** Through and through. **D,** Far near. (From Braun TE. Wound dehiscence. In: Schaefer G, Graber EA, eds. *Complications in Obstetric and Gynecological Surgery.* Hagerstown, MD: Harper & Row; 1981.)

The pathophysiology of the development of retroperitoneal infection is straightforward. The classic "clamp, crush, cut, and tie technique" used in pelvic surgery produces an abundance of hypoxic and anoxic tissue that helps establish an optimal environment for infection. In addition to this anoxic tissue, the retroperitoneal tissue produces an average of 40 mL of serosanguineous fluid daily during the first 72 postoperative hours. When the endogenous flora of the upper vagina colonize and multiply in this retroperitoneal serosanguineous fluid or pelvic hematoma, pelvic cellulitis and possibly a pelvic abscess can form.

**TABLE 25.16** Predisposing Factors to Evisceration*

| Predisposition | Clinical No./No. with Data Reported (%) |
|---|---|
| Postmenopausal (age >51 yr) | 9/12 (75) |
| Prior pelvic surgery | 10/12 (83) |
| Postmenopausal with surgery | 9/12 (75) |
| Enterocele and vaginal vault | 10/12 (83) |
| Posterior enterocele | 6/12 (50) |
| Vaginal cuff defect | 4/12 (33) |
| Coital trauma | 1/12 (8) |
| Spontaneous | 7/12 (58) |
| Trauma | 1/12 (8) |

From Croak AJ, Gelshart JB, Kingele CJ, et al. Characteristics of patients with vaginal vault rupture and evisceration. *Obstet Gynecol.* 2004; 103:573.

*Total numbers reported for each predisposition were limited by availability of data. Some patients had more than one predisposition.

**BOX 25.8** Techniques to Decrease Wound Disruption and Infection in Obese Surgical Patients

1. Chlorhexidine bath or shower the night before surgery
2. Women with BMI > 35—double the dosage of prophylactic antibiotics
3. Maintain core normothermia during the operation
4. Close subcutaneous tissue if >2 cm in depth
5. Sterile dressing for 24-48 hours
6. Maintain euglycemia
7. Subcutaneous drains do not improve outcomes

The major symptoms of an operative site infection are fever associated with lower quadrant abdominal and pelvic pain. The fever usually becomes prominent between the third and fifth postoperative days. As the infection becomes more severe, the fever spikes, the pain intensifies, and the patient develops moderate leukocytosis.

The diagnosis of cuff cellulitis is confirmed by pelvic examination. Pelvic tenderness and induration are prominent during the bimanual examination. A subtle difference exists between normal postoperative pelvic tenderness and induration and the tenderness and induration produced by an infection. Postoperative infection is accompanied by an increase in suprapubic pain and lateral parametrial tenderness. Cuff cellulitis sometimes responds to drainage by opening the vaginal cuff. Persistent cellulitis, one encompassing a large area, or a pelvic abscess necessitates parenteral antibiotic therapy. Large or complex fluid collections may be present without adverse clinical consequences. CT-directed drainage and culture may aid in diagnosis.

**Because of their polymicrobial origin, infections are usually treated with an aminoglycoside (gentamicin) and an antibiotic specific for anaerobic infection (clindamycin).** Metronidazole (Flagyl) may be substituted for clindamycin. An alternative therapy is substitution of a third-generation cephalosporin or the monobactam agent aztreonam (Azactam) for the aminoglycoside. IV antibiotics should be continued until the patient is afebrile for 24 hours. Once afebrile, the patient can be transitioned to a 10- to 14-day course of oral antibiotics, although some authors question the utility of this practice. Alternatives to the aminoglycoside-clindamycin regimen include broad-spectrum antibiotics combined with beta-lactamase inhibitors such as ampicillin-sulbactam, amoxicillin-clavulanate, piperacillin-tazobactam, or ticarcillin-clavulanate. These drugs have better coverage of *Enterobacteriaceae* spp. and *Enterococcus*. Ertapenem can also be used in this patient population.

**Drainage of an abscess through surgical intervention or interventional radiology is a key component of treatment.** The success rates seen with antibiotic therapy alone (without drainage) range from 34% to 87%, depending on the abscess size and location (Jaiyeoba, 2012). **Abscesses over 5 cm are more likely to benefit from drainage.** Appropriate cultures should be obtained from the center of an abscess cavity when the abscess is operatively incised. If a woman does not become afebrile within 48 hours of adequate drainage of a retroperitoneal abscess, a concomitant complication of pelvic thrombophlebitis should be suspected. If pelvic thrombophlebitis is suspected, a 72-hour trial of therapeutic heparin therapy with concurrent antibiotics should be considered.

## Granulation Tissue

Granulation tissue at the apex of the vaginal vault is a common complication after hysterectomy. **Small areas of friable, red granulation tissue are seen at the 6-week postoperative pelvic examination in more than 50% of women.** Granulation tissue is more common after abdominal than vaginal hysterectomy. In women undergoing total abdominal hysterectomy, polyglactin (Vicryl) has a reduced risk of developing granulation tissue compared with chromic catgut for closure of the cuff, 32% versus 68%.

Excessive granulation tissue is the result of an exaggerated healing response of the vascular-rich pelvic tissues. One of the causes is believed to be inversion of the vaginal epithelium between the margins of the edges of the incision at the apex of the vaginal vault. Some patients are asymptomatic, but many women experience spotting or a bloody discharge after intercourse. On speculum examination, the granulation tissue appears as a polypoid projection hanging from the vaginal suture line. The differential diagnosis includes a prolapsed fallopian tube and recurrent carcinoma in a woman with a pelvic malignancy. The polypoid mass is easily removed from the vaginal apex, and the remaining area of granulation tissue should be treated with a chemical cautery (e.g., silver nitrate, Monsel solution) in the office or by focal cryo- or electrocauterization if proper anesthesia is available.

## Incisional Hernia

**Vertical midline incisions produce the highest rate of abdominal wall hernias, 10% to 15%.** Most will present within 1 year of surgery. Diabetes, poor nutrition, and obesity are all predisposing factors for postoperative hernia. Transverse and Pfannenstiel incisions have a lower rate, followed by laparoscopic incisions, with the lowest rate of hernia formation. In patients with obesity and diabetes, it is prudent to close the fascia if the laparoscopic incision extends beyond 1 cm. Studies have noted a 2% to 3% hernia rate in laparoscopic sites of 12 mm or larger, although hernias can occur in smaller incisions. Studies performed since the institution of modern trocars have noted even lower rates of trocar site hernias (1%).

## Lymphocyst

A lymphocyst is a local collection of lymphatic fluid within the retroperitoneal spaces of the pelvis resulting from retrograde drainage of lymph. It is a rare complication, discovered most often after pelvic node dissections. In the past this complication occurred in approximately 20% of patients having undergone radical surgery; however, with meticulous attention to ligation of distal lymphatic channels, the widespread use of electrosurgery and abandonment of the practice of reperitonealization, this complication is reported in less than 5% of these cases. The incidence is lower in series in which palpation alone is used to identify the cysts. If ultrasound examination is used postoperatively to screen for lymphocysts, the incidence is 10-fold greater. **Conditions that predispose the woman to formation of a lymphocyst are previous radiation and anticoagulation.**

Lymphocysts usually present during the first 6 postoperative weeks. They vary greatly in size and seldom become infected. The cyst usually begins anteriorly and medially to the iliac vessels. As it expands, it may produce pelvic pain, leg pain, fever, obstruction or angulation of the ureter, pressure symptoms on the bladder, or partial venous obstruction. Small lymphocysts (<4 cm in diameter) are usually asymptomatic and regress spontaneously within 8 weeks. Larger cysts may necessitate treatment by intermittent aspiration or marsupialization that can be performed using minimally invasive surgery to create a peritoneal opening, or peritoneal window, that allows flow of the lymphatic fluid into the peritoneal cavity, with subsequent peritoneal resorption. One can also create an omental flap near the opening to further assist with resorption of lymph.

## Postoperative Neuropathy

Postoperative neuropathy is an uncommon but significant and sometimes debilitating problem. The most common causes of neuropathy in gynecologic surgery are improper patient positioning, the incorrect placement of surgical retractors, and direct surgical trauma.

The **femoral nerve** is the largest branch of the lumbar plexus and arises from the primary dorsal rami of L2, L3, and L4. It provides motor function to several leg muscles, including the quadriceps, and sensory fibers that innervate the anterior and medial surfaces of the thigh and leg. The vascular supply to the femoral nerve may be compromised during an abdominal or vaginal hysterectomy. The cause of this complication is usually related to continuous pressure, typically by a self-retaining retractor during an abdominal hysterectomy producing ischemic necrosis of the nerve. The vascular circulation of the nerve itself is compromised by diminished blood flow in the vasa nervorum. **The most common site of nerve compression is 4 to 6 cm above the inguinal ligament where the nerve pierces the psoas muscle.**

Factors that contribute to the development of this complication are abdominal wall thickness/BMI, long retractor blades, prolonged operative times, and systemic diseases such as diabetes mellitus, gout, alcoholism, and malnutrition. The classic patient who develops this complication is a short, thin, athletic woman who has a transverse incision in which a self-retaining retractor is used. A similar problem may develop after vaginal operations or laparoscopy in thin women who are placed into exaggerated hip flexion or abduction in the dorsal lithotomy position. **Femoral neuropathy after vaginal surgery is believed to be secondary to compromise of the nerve by prolonged severe angulation and not secondary to pressure injury from retractors.** Bohrer and associates found peripheral nerve injury in 1.8% of 616 patients with elective gynecologic procedures, with almost all related to positioning. Most of these could be related to exaggerated flexion for laparoscopic and vaginal surgeries. Two patients had motor and sensory losses. In this series, all but one woman had resolution of neuropathy with medical treatment (Bohrer, 2009).

Patients with femoral neuropathy may experience numbness, paresthesias, and difficulty with their gait. **Patients may have difficulty lifting the affected knee because of the involvement of the quadriceps.** Symptoms may present with a spectrum of severity, and usually the neurologic symptoms develop within the first 24 to 72 hours after surgery. Because of the inability to lift the leg, climbing stairs is a particular problem. Muscle and sensory function recover spontaneously over several weeks to several months. The patient should be seen by a physical therapist to facilitate ambulation and prevent muscle atrophy.

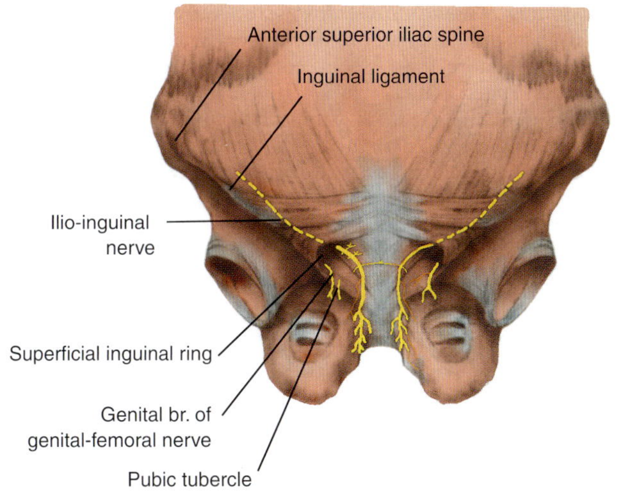


**Fig. 25.12** Ilioinguinal nerve entrapment during needle suspension for stress incontinence. (From Miyazaki F, Shook G. Ilioinguinal nerve entrapment during needle suspension for stress incontinence. *Obstet Gynecol.* 1992;80:246-248.)

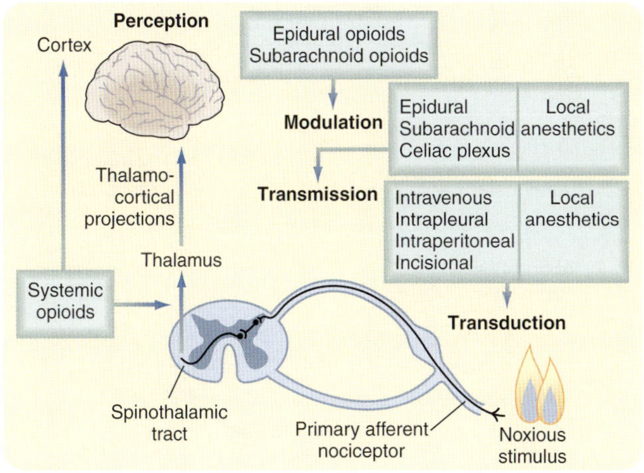


**Fig. 25.13** Schematic drawing of the pathways for transmission of painful stimuli. (From Sherwood E, Williams CG, Prough DS. Anaesthesiology principles, pain management, and conscious sedation. In: Townsend CM, Beauchamp RD, Evers BM, et al, eds. *Sabiston Textbook of Surgery.* 17th ed. Philadelphia: Saunders; 2004.)

To prevent this complication, it is important to avoid excess hip flexion and palpate the lateral pelvic wall after placement of a self-retaining retractor during a laparotomy. In a thin woman, placing folded towels between the skin surface and self-retaining retractor may help prevent this complication by decreasing the depth of penetration of the lateral retractor blades if short blades are not available.

The **ilioinguinal and iliohypogastric nerves** pass in a transverse and diagonal course through the anterior lower abdominal musculature medial to the inguinal ligament and through the inguinal canal. The nerves supply sensory fibers to the labia, mons pubis, and medial thigh. The nerves may become injured during surgery with a Pfannenstiel incision or during a urinary incontinence procedure (Fig. 25.12). These nerves are also potentially injured with lateral laparoscopic trocar placement and incision closure because they can be transected or entrapped by suture or scar formation. Sharp or burning pain may develop immediately postoperatively or usually within a few days. The pain may radiate to the groin or vulva. Most symptoms will resolve spontaneously. Severe pain may necessitate nerve block, suture removal, or segmented removal of the involved nerve. **To avoid injury, lateral sutures for Pfannenstiel incisions and trocar sites should remain two fingerbreadths medial to the anterior superior iliac spine and avoid excessive incorporation of tissue.**

Several specific postoperative neuropathies are related to specific procedures. Uterosacral ligament suspension may affect the sacral plexus (S2 to S4) and produce pain and numbness in the posterior thigh and buttocks. Genitofemoral neuropathy and injury to the obturator nerve can be seen after pelvic lymphadenectomy. If the nerve was not cut, most will resolve in time, although physical therapy is very helpful. Pudendal neuropathy has been reported with cystocele repairs and graft placement producing pain and numbness in the vulva and perineum. If symptoms are not relieved with analgesics and other medications, such as gabapentin, surgical removal of the sutures may be necessary. Peroneal neuropathy can occur from excessive pressure on the lateral knee compressing the peroneal nerve against the head of the fibula when a patient is placed in dorsal lithotomy position.

## PSYCHOLOGICAL SEQUELAE

### Pain Relief

The proper management of pain during the postoperative period should be an essential task and goal of all gynecologists; however, optimal pain control should be multimodal and opioid sparing while ensuring adequate pain control. Most women experience moderate to severe pain during the first 36 to 48 hours after a gynecologic operation. Pain is initiated at the local level through the trauma of the surgery. Systemic and neurologic pathways are then activated (Fig. 25.13). The most effective pain management strategies involve inhibiting the initiation and activation of these broader pain reflexes. Such inhibition is also associated with the fewest side effects. Factors that predict postoperative pain and the use of pain medications include preoperative pain, mental state, and type of surgery. Age is inversely correlated with pain and pain medication usage (Vivian, 2009). Studies comparing types of hysterectomy, abdominal, vaginal, and laparoscopic have found a descending order of postoperative pain, as may be anticipated.

The literature documents that pain relief is often treated inadequately in postoperative patients. Inadequate pain relief prolongs hospital stay and has adverse psychological consequences. Also, several investigators have noted that inadequately treated pain increases secondary morbidities, including atelectasis from decreased mobility, increased inflammatory response, and elevated glucose levels, with higher catecholamine levels. Syndromes of chronic pain are presumed to begin with inadequate pain relief in the postoperative period.

A schematic representation of the pain cycle and the potential delays in pain relief with traditional "as-needed" analgesic regimens is shown in Fig. 25.14. Thus optimal pain control incorporates scheduled pain medications with nonnarcotic medications and local and regional anesthetics, particularly for the first 36 to 48 hours after surgery. Narcotic pain medications should predominantly be used for breakthrough pain. IV patient-controlled analgesia (PCA) systems, popular in years past, lead to a great deal of postoperative bowel dysfunction and, as a result, are often deemphasized in postoperative enhanced recovery after surgery (ERAS) protocols, as discussed in Chapter 24. **The recommendation for postoperative pain relief is for multimodality therapy with NSAIDs, acetaminophen, and regional blocks with injection of long-acting local anesthetics such as bupivacaine with supplementary use of oral narcotics.** In general, patients use PCA much less frequently in this setting, but if PCA is used, the patient should be given instructions about its use. Additionally, families need instruction in not pushing the medication for the patient to help alleviate pain. Sample dosing for PCA is listed in Appendix C.

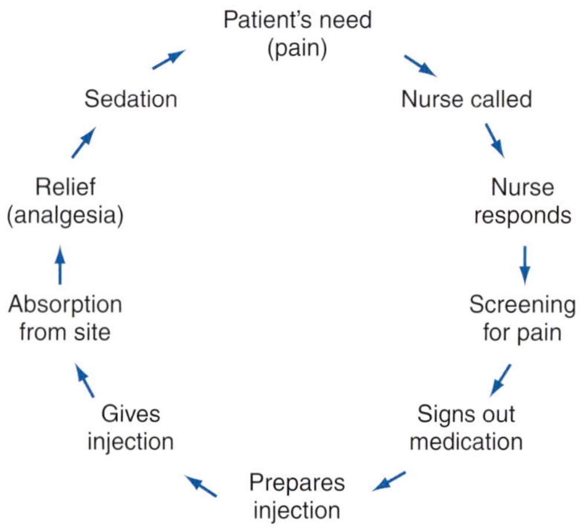


**Fig. 25.14** Pain cycle. (From White PF. Pain management [special report]. *Postgrad Med.* 1986;80:8.)

Some patients can also benefit from the use of continuous postoperative epidural anesthesia, especially patients who are undergoing planned extensive laparotomy with a more prolonged recovery. Perioperative intrathecal or epidural injections of opioids effectively relieve postoperative pelvic pain in most situations. Side effects are primarily itching and a risk of hypotension. Continuous PCA epidurals may also be used. The advantages and disadvantages of PCA and epidural anesthesia are presented in Table 25.17.

In addition to narcotics, NSAIDs are valuable as adjunctive agents. **NSAIDs are most effective when given as scheduled medications and as early as possible in the postoperative period.** Their mechanism of action is the inhibition of prostaglandin production. Through inhibition of prostaglandins, pain is prevented rather than blocked centrally.

NSAIDs have three potential side effects. The first is increased gastric acid, best treated by H2 blockers or proton pump inhibitors. The second is renal toxicity, which may be prevented by using set doses and prescribing only for women with normal renal function and adequate intravascular volume. The third is inhibition of platelet function with higher doses of NSAIDs. Some clinicians will wait 1 to 2 hours after surgery before giving these agents to avoid excessive bleeding, but there are no data to support this practice. Advantages of prostaglandin synthetase inhibitors are a lack of effect on GI motility and a much smaller effect on sensorium than narcotic agents.

Commonly used NSAIDs for postoperative pain include ibuprofen, naproxen, and ketorolac (Toradol); ketorolac should not be used for more than 4 consecutive days because of GI side effects. In older adults, changes in GI function may limit the usefulness of these agents. Stomach colonization with *Helicobacter pylori* increases with increasing age: Approximately 80% of women older than 80 years are colonized. These bacteria increase sensitivity to GI irritation. **Prophylactic H2 blockers or proton pump inhibitors should be considered when administering NSAID to older patients.** Further NSAID use should be limited in patients with prior gastric bypass surgery because of the risk of marginal ulcer development. There is also concern about the association of perioperative NSAID use and anastomotic leaks after colorectal surgery (Jamjittrong, 2019). This meta-analysis demonstrated a significant association between NSAID use and anastomotic leakage after colon resections (OR, 1.73; 95% CI, 1.31 to 2.29; $P < .0001$). Subgroup analyses suggest that nonselective NSAIDs, but not selective cyclooxygenase-2 inhibitors, were significantly associated with anastomotic leakage.

It is believed that giving preemptive analgesics in the perioperative period before the patient's sensation of pain leads to better pain control. Many studies have noted that the beneficial effects are significant when infiltration is given before the surgical incision. Because much pain arises from peritoneal irritation and fascial trauma, incisional infiltration is most effective with minimally invasive procedures such as laparoscopy. Infiltration is most commonly used with a local anesthetic, such as lidocaine 1% or bupivacaine 0.25%. Temporary indwelling infusion catheters that use local anesthetics have been shown in multiple studies and systematic reviews to benefit patients through decreased opioid use, earlier ambulation, and decreased PONV. Catheters are placed above and below the fascia and removed on day 3. **In patients who are expected to require large amounts of opioid, such as those already on chronic narcotics for pain, the addition of gabapentin decreases narcotic use, perceived pain levels, and PONV. A meta-analysis has found a 35% reduction in pain** (95% CI, 0.59 to 0.72). Most studies used 1200 mg/day.

**Patients with persistent incisional pain longer than 4 to 6 months should be evaluated for incisional neuromas.** Neuromas are thought to arise from damaged and transected peripheral nerves that develop a fibrous capsule. If a superficial small trigger area can be identified, an injection of 1% hydrocortisone with 2 to 3 mL of 0.25% bupivacaine may be attempted and is diagnostic if it helps. If this is unsuccessful, referral to a surgeon with expertise in peripheral nerves and chronic pain should be considered.

**TABLE 25.17** Advantages and Disadvantages of Epidural Analgesia and Patient-Controlled Analgesia

| Epidural Analgesia | Patient-Controlled Analgesia | Comments |
|---|---|---|
| Advantages | Immediate pain relief | Requires no special nursing or anesthesia support postoperatively |
| | May improve colon motility | Gives the patient personal control over administration of pain medication |
| | May improve postoperative pulmonary function after lower abdominal and pelvic surgery | |
| | Less sedating than patient-controlled analgesia | |
| Disadvantages | Requires a skilled anesthesiologist for correct placement | Patient may experience pain in the recovery room until an adequate serum level of medication is achieved |
| | May interfere with ambulation | |
| | May delay removal of Foley catheter | |

From Baker VV. Principles of postoperative care. In: Baker VV, Deppe G, eds. *Management of Perioperative Complications in Gynecology.* Philadelphia: WB Saunders; 1997.

## Postoperative Concerns in Older Surgical Patients

Patients older than 70 years, particularly those older than 80 years, need special consideration in the perioperative period. Studies of older women undergoing gynecologic surgery have found that for elective procedures, the complication rates are no different from those of younger women after adjusting for comorbidities. Box 25.9 summarizes physical changes that should be kept in mind when caring for older surgical patients. The cardiovascular system is affected with increased systemic vascular resistance and a poorer response to systemic catecholamines. Many anesthetic agents decrease cardiac contractility. Atrial fibrillation and cardiac failure are the two most common cardiac complications, and attention to intravascular volume is important to maintain cardiac output. Many older women have decreased appetites and poor nutrition; this should be addressed before elective surgery. The nursing staff often is hesitant to give enough pain medications for fear of oversedation; however, inadequate pain relief can lead to worse sequelae related to minimal early ambulation, including atelectasis, DVT, and ileus. Epidural PCA is an option for postoperative pain relief in this patient population to limit narcotic use.

**Postoperative delirium and postoperative cognitive dysfunction (POCD) are examples of altered levels of mental function occurring after surgery.** These conditions are more common in older adults. Prolonged and delayed mental status changes may be caused by decreased oxygen, decreased cardiac output, medications, and drug-drug interactions. In general, postoperative delirium occurs 24 to 72 hours after surgery. Disorientation, sleep deprivation, polypharmacy, and pain may all be contributing factors. **The condition occurs in 5% to 15% of older patients and increases the risk of patient falls.** POCD may occur for a few months after surgery and has been noted to some degree in up to 5% of older surgical patients. Further, postoperative disorientation and agitation are associated with higher risk of patient falls because patients attempt to get out of bed without assistance.

**BOX 25.9** Physiologic Changes in Older Adults That May Affect Surgery

**CARDIOVASCULAR**

Approximate 1% decrease in cardiac output per year after age 30
Decreased vascular compliance and increased systemic vascular resistance
Increased cardiovascular disease
Decreased cardiac output in response to stress
Increased susceptibility to conduction abnormalities

**PULMONARY**

Decreased pulmonary reserve
Decreased mucus-producing cells, with increased susceptibility to infection
Decreased elasticity in the lungs
Decreased forced expiratory volume in 1 second
Decreased functional residual capacity, exacerbated with postoperative pain, and atelectasis

**RENAL**

Decreased glomerular filtration rate—approximately 1% decrease per year after age 20
Serum creatinine level not effective measure of renal function in this situation

**SKELETAL**

Increased osteoporosis, with increase in injury from falls
Decreased rib expansion, so poorer response to need for postoperative lung expansion

**NUTRITIONAL**

Poorer nutrition
Greater incidence of vitamin deficiencies, including vitamin $B_{12}$

## Psychosexual Problems and Depression

The time immediately before and after a surgical procedure is a stressful period for all women and their families. Anxiety and fear are normal responses and should be anticipated by health care providers. Any surgery on the female reproductive organs stimulates questions and conflicts concerning body image, feminine identity, sexuality, and possibly future childbearing. The period after a gynecologic operation is one of transition and is a unique psychological challenge to the woman. After gynecologic surgery, every woman needs support to deal with this challenge, and it is important to emphasize that it may take many months to complete the process.

Personal issues that relate to a woman's body image and sexuality are particularly affected by hysterectomy. Open discussions with the woman that allow her to discuss issues regarding sexuality are important during preoperative and postoperative visits. Psychological studies have confirmed that sexual function after a hysterectomy is related to a number of factors. **Poor knowledge of reproductive anatomy, a negative expectation of sexual recovery after the operation, preoperative psychiatric morbidity, and a history of unsatisfactory sexual relationships are all associated with a poor outcome.** The effect of hysterectomy on sexual function is an exceedingly complex topic, with both physical and psychological factors known to have varying and almost unquantifiable influences.

## Mental Status Changes

Anxiety and mental status changes are not uncommon in the postoperative period. Medications, hemodynamic changes, fever, and altered sleep patterns contribute to changes in sensorium. These changes are most pronounced in older adults. Multivariate analyses have correlated pain levels, hematocrit less than 30%, smoking, and a history of psychiatric disorders with postoperative mental status changes. Other than hematocrit levels, these factors are difficult to control. Mental status change does require evaluation (Box 25.10). Changes in oxygenation, electrolyte imbalance, sepsis, medication interactions, and acute anemia need to be excluded.

**BOX 25.10** Causes of Acute Delirium

Drug intoxication (alcohol, antihistamines, sedatives)
Drug withdrawal (alcohol, narcotics, anxiolytics)
Acute cerebral disorders (edema, transient ischemic attack stroke, neoplasm)
Metabolic disturbances (electrolyte, imbalance, hypoglycemia)
Hemodynamic disturbances (hypovolemia, myocardial infarction, congestive heart failure)
Infections (septicemia, urinary tract infection, pneumonia)
Respiratory disorders (respiratory failure, pulmonary embolism)
Trauma (head injury, burns)

From Dayton MT. Surgical complications. In: Townsend CM, Beauchamp RD, Evers BM, et al, eds. *Sabiston Textbook of Surgery.* 17th ed. Philadelphia: Saunders; 2004.

A syndrome of nausea, sweating, tachycardia, tremors, delirium, and even grand mal seizures postoperatively is often misdiagnosed as a drug or anesthetic reaction. This constellation of signs and symptoms is usually caused by alcohol withdrawal, and the presence of a tremor should alert health care providers to the correct diagnosis. Benzodiazepines are the drug of choice in the treatment of post–alcohol withdrawal symptoms. In older women, especially after emergency surgery, postoperative confusion, anxiety, changes in personality, and memory impairment are common findings, and a large differential diagnosis must be considered.

## DISCHARGE INSTRUCTIONS AND POSTOPERATIVE VISITS

Simple but complete discharge instructions are an important component of postoperative care. The physician should anticipate the most common questions and give the woman explicit instructions. Particular attention should be given to limitations in physical activity, such as heavy lifting and resumption of sexual relations. Information should be given about vaginal spotting as sutures dissolve. Appropriate contact information should be provided in case of unanticipated complications and to schedule return appointments. Discharge instructions should not be given on the morning of discharge; rather, patients should receive these instructions before the day of discharge to ensure that, on the morning of discharge, instructions can be reviewed and questions answered to verify patient understanding. Instructions should be given in verbal and written format.

Because an increasing number of procedures are performed as outpatient surgeries or short stays, the physician must modify instructions to accommodate the gradual resumption of activity. The 24- to 48-hour postdischarge phone call to the recovering woman provides an excellent forum for answering questions and providing reassurance. Studies of outpatient surgeries have found this contact to be important. Additionally, it is difficult for the woman and her significant others to remember instructions received during the first 24 hours after surgery. Written guidelines are extremely valuable for outpatient procedures. Careful training of nursing and triage staff in regard to postoperative questions cannot be overemphasized. **Patients will usually be home when the first signs of complications occur.** These signs and symptoms may in themselves be minor, but they may presage a more serious complication that could evolve. Thus a much higher index of suspicion should be used with these patients.

Most clinicians will see patients one or more times in the postoperative period as patients are transitioning back to routine activities. Questions about appropriate levels of activity can be answered in person or via a postdischarge phone call. Discussions of reestablishing sexual relations and physical activity are important to review at several time points. Unless there is a problem or a specific issue, a pelvic examination may be deferred until 5 to 6 weeks after the procedure.

The discussion of surgical findings occurs at several points during the postoperative period. Initially, patients are drowsy after waking up from anesthesia or IV analgesics. Families may want to know the results before the patient hearing them. Preoperatively, it is important to clarify with the woman who in the family can know what information, and during the early postoperative period the gynecologist must judge how much information to provide. This should be tailored to what the patient can understand, depending on her level of awareness. By the end of the first few days, the discussion may move to details of surgical findings, treatment options, sequelae, and prognosis if a long-term problem has been found.

## KEY REFERENCES


Ahmad S, Nagle A, McCarthy RJ, et al. Postoperative hypoxemia in morbidly obese patients with and without obstructive sleep apnea undergoing laparoscopic bariatric surgery. *Anesth Analg.* 2008;107(1):138-143.

Apfel CC, Korttila K, Abdalla M, et al. A factorial trial of six interventions for the prevention of postoperative nausea and vomiting. *N Engl J Med.* 2004;350(24):2441-2451.

Barber EL, Neubauer NL, Gossett DR. Risk of venous thromboembolism in abdominal versus minimally invasive hysterectomy for benign conditions. *Am J Obstet Gynecol.* 2015;212(5):609.e1-609.e7.

Bauer AJ, Boeckxstaens GE. Mechanisms of postoperative ileus. *Neurogastroenterol Motil.* 2004;16(Suppl 2):54-60.

Bohrer JC, Walters MD, Park A, et al. Pelvic nerve injury following gynecologic surgery: a prospective cohort study. *Am J Obstet Gynecol.* 2009;201(5):531.e1-531.e7.

Bougle A, Harrois A, Duranteau J. Resuscitative strategies in traumatic hemorrhagic shock. *Ann Intensive Care.* 2013;3(1):1.

Burks C, Nelson L, Kumar D, et al. Evaluation of pulmonary complications in robotic-assisted gynecologic surgery. *J Minim Invasive Gynecol.* 2017;24(2):280-285.

Chung F, Yegneswaran B, Liao P, et al. Validation of the Berlin questionnaire and American Society of Anesthesiologists checklists and screening tools for obstructive sleep apnea in surgical patients. *Anesthesiology.* 2008;108(5):822-830.

do Nascimento Junior P, Módolo NS, Andrade S, et al. Incentive spirometry for prevention of postoperative pulmonary complications in upper abdominal surgery. *Cochrane Database Syst Rev.* 2014;2:CD006058.

Dubuisson J, Botchorishvili R, Perrette S, et al. Incidence of intraabdominal adhesions in a continuous series of 1000 laparoscopic procedures. *Am J Obstet Gynecol.* 2010;203(2):111.e1-111.e3.

Ellis H, Niran BJ, Thompson JN, et al. Adhesion-related hospital readmissions after abdominal and pelvic surgery: a retrospective cohort study. *Lancet.* 1999;353(9163):1476-1480.

Finfer S, Chittock DR, Su SY, et al. Intensive versus conventional glucose control in critically ill patients. *N Engl J Med.* 2009;360(13):1283-1297.

Gan TJ, Diemunsch P, Habib AS, et al. Consensus guidelines for the management of postoperative nausea and vomiting. *Anesth Analg.* 2014;118(1):85-113.

Gandaglia G, Ghani KR, Sood A, et al. Effect of minimally invasive surgery on the risk for surgical site infections: results from the National Surgical Quality Improvement (NSQIP) Database. *JAMA Surg.* 2014;149(10):1039-1044.

Garber AJ, Moghissi ES, Bransome Jr ED, et al. American College of Endocrinology Task Force on Inpatient Diabetes Metabolic Control: Position statement on inpatient diabetes and metabolic control. *Endocr Pract.* 2004;10(1):77-82.

Gawande AA, Studdert DM, Orav EJ, et al. Risk factors for retained instruments and sponges after surgery. *N Engl J Med.* 2003;348(3):229-235.

Goldhaber SZ, Elliot CG. Acute pulmonary embolism: part I. *Circulation.* 2003a;108(22):2726-2729.

Goldhaber SZ, Elliot CG. Acute pulmonary embolism: part II. *Circulation.* 2003a;108(23):2834-2838.

Gowen GF. Long tube decompression is successful in 90% of patients with adhesive small bowel obstruction. *Am J Surg.* 2003;185(6):512-515.

Guyatt GH, Akl EA, Crowther M, et al. Executive summary: Antithrombotic Therapy and Prevention of Thrombosis, 9th ed: American College of Chest Physicians Evidence-Based Clinical Practice Guidelines. *Chest.* 2012;141(Suppl 2):7S-47S.

Harmanli OH, Tunitsky E, Esin S, et al. A comparison of short-term outcomes between laparoscopic supracervical and total hysterectomy. *Am J Obstet Gynecol.* 2009;201(5):536.e1-536.e7.

Holcomb JB, Tilley BC, Baraniuk S, et al. Transfusion of plasma, platelets, and red blood cells in a 1:1:1 vs a 1:1:2 ratio and mortality in patients with severe trauma: the PROPPR randomized clinical trial. *JAMA.* 2015;313(5):471-482.

Hurr HC, Donnellan N, Mansuria S, et al. Vaginal cuff dehiscence after different modes of hysterectomy. *Obstet Gynecol.* 2011;118(4):749-801.

Ireland CJ, Chapman TM, Mathew SF, et al. Continuous positive airway pressure (CPAP) during the postoperative period for prevention of postoperative morbidity and mortality following major abdominal surgery. *Cochrane Database Syst Rev.* 2014;8:CD008930.

Jaiyeoba O. Postoperative infections in obstetrics and gynecology. *Clin Obstet Gynecol.* 2012;55(4):904-913.

Jamjittrong S, Matsuda A, Matsumoto S et al. Postoperative non-steroidal anti-inflammatory drugs and anastomotic leakage after gastrointestinal

anastomoses: systematic review and meta-analysis. *Ann Gastroenterol Surg.* 2019;4(1):64-75.
Kalil AC, Metersky ML, Klompas M, et al. Management of adults with hospital-acquired and ventilator-associated pneumonia: 2016 clinical practice guidelines by the Infectious Diseases Society of America and the American Thoracic Society. *Clin Infect Dis.* 2016;63(5):e61-e111.
Kalogera E, Bakkum-Gamez JN, Jankowski, et al. Enhanced recovery in gynecologic surgery. *Obstet Gynecol.* 2013;122(2 Pt 1):319-328.
Kearon C, Akl EA, Ornelas J, et al. Antithrombotic therapy for VTE Disease: CHEST Guideline and Expert Panel Report. *Chest.* 2016; 149(2):315-352.
Kehlet H, Dahl JB. Anaesthesia, surgery, and challenges in postoperative recovery. *Lancet.* 2003;362(9399):1921-1928.



**Full references and Suggested readings for this chapter can be found on ExpertConsult.com.**

# 26 Abnormal Uterine Bleeding

## Etiology and Management of Acute and Chronic Excessive Bleeding

*Timothy Ryntz, Roger A. Lobo*

### KEY POINTS

- The mean amount of menstrual blood loss in one cycle is approximately 35 mL but may be as much as 60 mL, with an average loss of 13 mg of iron. Heavy menstrual bleeding occurs in 9% to 14% of healthy women.
- Diagnostic tests in women with menorrhagia include measurement of hemoglobin, serum iron, serum ferritin, beta human chorionic gonadotropin, thyroid-stimulating hormone, and prolactin levels; endometrial biopsy and hysteroscopy; sonohysterography; and hysterosalpingography. Magnetic resonance imaging may be helpful in the diagnosis of adenomyosis or surgical planning for leiomyoma but is not part of the initial evaluation.
- High doses of oral or intravenous estrogen usually stops acute bleeding episodes in most cases of abnormal bleeding. An alternative regimen is high-dose oral progestogen for a week, with tapering of the dosage thereafter. Tranexamic acid (TXA) stops acute bleeding most rapidly and has particular efficacy for more chronic use in women with abnormal bleeding who ovulate.
- Patients who are being treated for abnormal uterine bleeding as a result of endometrial causes (and who are ovulatory) may be given oral contraceptives, nonsteroidal antiinflammatory drugs (antiprostaglandins), TXA or a prolonged course of progestogens, or levonorgestrel released locally from an intrauterine system (LNG-IUS). Those treated with the LNG-IUS have similar outcomes at 1 year to those treated by surgery, and the LNG-IUS is preferred in women with inherited bleeding disorders.
- Various endometrial ablation techniques achieve a 22% to 55% amenorrhea success rate at 1 year but an 86% to 99% satisfaction rate with regard to normalizing menstruation. Within 4 years after endometrial ablation, approximately 25% of women treated will have a hysterectomy.

**Abnormal uterine bleeding (AUB)** can present in many ways, from infrequent episodes, to excessive flow or prolonged duration of menses and intermenstrual bleeding. Alterations in the pattern or volume of blood flow of menses are among the most common health concerns of women. Infrequent uterine bleeding is called **oligomenorrhea** if the intervals between bleeding episodes vary from 35 days to 6 months, and **amenorrhea** is defined by no menses for at least 6 months. These are discussed in Chapter 38. Excessive or prolonged bleeding is discussed in this chapter, and an overview of several therapeutic modalities being used to treat excessive uterine bleeding is also provided.

To define excessive AUB, it is necessary to define normal menstrual flow. The mean interval between menses is 28 days (±7 days). Thus if bleeding occurs at intervals of 21 days or less or 35 days or more, it is abnormal. The mean duration of menstrual flow is 4 days. Few women with normal menses bleed more than 7 days, so bleeding for longer than 7 days is considered to be abnormally prolonged. It is useful to document the duration and frequency of menstrual flow with the use of menstrual diary cards; however, it is difficult to determine the amount of menstrual blood loss (MBL) by subjective means. Several studies have shown that there is poor correlation between subjective judgment and objective measurement of MBL (Chimbira, 1980).

Although subjective methods are used in predicting blood loss, and some investigators have used a pictorial bleeding assessment chart, a more accurate system is the alkaline hematic method, which measures hematin. Average MBL is 35 mL. Total volume, however, is twice this amount, being made up of endometrial tissue exudate. In the absence of disease, the amount of MBL increases with parity but not age. An MBL of 80 mL or greater is defined as heavy menstrual bleeding, which occurs in 9% to 14% of women (Shapley, 2004).

Although mortality and serious complications of AUB are uncommon, their effect on health-related quality of life is significant. Direct costs are calculated at more than $1 billion annually in the United States, and indirect costs as a result of lost work, social function, and vitality have been estimated at more than $12 billion annually (Liu, 2007).

## CAUSES OF ABNORMAL UTERINE BLEEDING

The causes of AUB can be described by a universally accepted systematic nomenclature. This system was reported by the International Federation of Gynecology and Obstetrics (FIGO) in 2011. It subdivides causes of AUB into nine main categories, which are arranged according to the acronym **PALM-COEIN**: polyp, adenomyosis, leiomyoma, malignancy and hyperplasia, coagulopathy, ovulatory dysfunction, endometrial, iatrogenic, and not yet classified. The causes that constitute the first group (**PALM**) are structural or histologic and are diagnosed through imaging or biopsy. Those that compose the second group (**COEIN**) are nonstructural (Fig. 26.1). The term *dysfunctional uterine bleeding (DUB)* is no longer favored and should be discarded. In the past this term represented causes of abnormal bleeding when structural causes and other specific defects, such as coagulation defects, had been excluded. Cases that previously would have been described as DUB are now referred to as AUB as a result of ovulatory dysfunction or endometrial causes.

According to FIGO, this classification system should be notated in a consistent and systematic manner. The acronym AUB is followed by the letters PALM-COEIN and a subscript

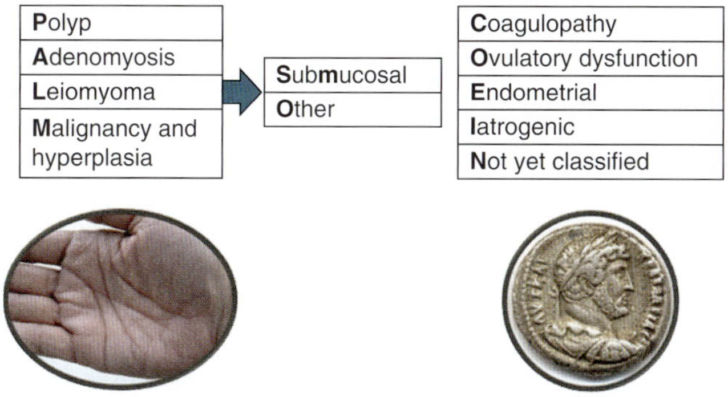


**Fig. 26.1** PALM-COEIN Classification System for Abnormal Uterine Bleeding. The basic system comprises four categories that are defined by visually objective structural criteria (PALM), four that are unrelated to structural anomalies (COEI), and one reserved for entities that are not yet classified (N). The leiomyoma category is subdivided into patients with at least one submucosal myoma ($L_{SM}$) and those with myomas that do not affect the endometrial cavity ($L_O$). *PALM-COEIN,* polyp, adenomyosis, leiomyoma, malignancy and hyperplasia, coagulopathy, ovulatory dysfunction, endometrial, iatrogenic, and not yet classified. (From Munro MG, Critchley HOD, Broder MS, Fraser IS. FIGO classification system [PALM-COEIN] for causes of abnormal uterine bleeding in nongravid women of reproductive age. *Int J Gynecol Obstet.* 2011;113(1):3-13.)

0 or 1 associated with each letter to indicate the absence or presence, respectively, of the abnormality. For example, a patient with abnormal bleeding caused by a polyp would be described as $AUB\text{-}P_1A_0L_0M_0\text{-}C_0O_0E_0I_0N_0$. Because patients may have abnormal bleeding as a result of more than one condition, this notation allows for description of simultaneous factors. For example, a patient with abnormal bleeding that is both irregular and heavy may have endometrial hyperplasia as a result of anovulation. As such, this patient's bleeding would be described as $AUB\text{-}P_0A_0L_0M_1\text{-}C_0O_1E_0I_0N_0$.

What follows is an introduction to each of the pathologic conditions described by the PALM-COEIN system. After this discussion, a diagnostic approach for women with AUB will be outlined. Treatments for acute and chronic bleeding as a result of these conditions conclude this chapter.

## Endometrial Polyps

Endometrial polyps (AUB-P) are localized overgrowths of endometrial tissue, containing glands, stroma, and blood vessels, covered with epithelium (Peterson, 1956). Endometrial polyps are most commonly found in reproductive-age women, and estrogen stimulation is thought to play a key role in their development. As such, polyps are rarely found before menarche. Molecular mechanisms involving overexpression of endometrial aromatase and gene mutations in *HMGIC* and *HMGI[Y]* have also been proposed (Maia, 2006; Tallini, 2000).

The majority of endometrial polyps are benign. A systematic review of the oncogenic potential of endometrial polyps demonstrated that symptomatic vaginal bleeding and postmenopausal status are associated with an increased risk of malignancy. Among symptomatic postmenopausal women with endometrial polyps, 4.5% had a malignant polyp compared with 1.5% in asymptomatic women (Lee, 2010). A strong correlation exists for both tamoxifen use and obesity and the development of malignancy in endometrial polyps. Diabetes mellitus and hypertension have not been reliably shown to increase the risk for malignancy in an endometrial polyp.

The importance of small and asymptomatic endometrial polyps is less clear. Transvaginal ultrasound detected asymptomatic polyps in up to 12% of women undergoing routine gynecologic examination; small endometrial polyps smaller than 1 cm appear to regress spontaneously (Hamani, 2013). Endometrial polyps were discovered in 32% of 1000 patients on office hysteroscopy about to undergo in vitro fertilization, suggesting a possible association between endometrial polyps and infertility (Hinckley, 2004). Women with symptomatic polyps can be treated safely and effectively with operative hysteroscopy.

## Adenomyosis

Adenomyosis (AUB-A) is defined by the presence of endometrial glands and stroma in the uterine myometrium. The presence of ectopic endometrial tissue leads to hypertrophy of the surrounding myometrium. Adenomyosis can occur as focal (adenomyoma) or diffuse, with a peak incidence in the fifth decade of life. Multiparity is considered the most significant risk factor for developing adenomyosis, but any process that allows for penetration of endometrial glands and stroma past the basalis layer (e.g., dilation and curettage, cesarean delivery, spontaneous abortion) is thought to contribute. There also appears to be a positive correlation between overexpression of immunoproteins interleukin-6, interleukin-18, and cyclooxygenase-2 and the presence of ectopic endometrial tissue, though these may not be causative (Leyendecker, 2004; Huang, 2010). Adenomyosis is a histologic diagnosis, but findings of an enlarged, asymmetric uterus on ultrasound and magnetic resonance imaging (MRI) are indicative. Anechoic avascular cysts scattered throughout the myometrium on sonography are considered pathognomonic for adenomyosis on ultrasound. MRI, which is both more sensitive and more specific than ultrasound, will demonstrate thickening of the junctional zone, the area between the endometrium and the myometrium, equal to or greater than 12 mm (Figs. 26.2 and 26.3) (Dueholm, 2007). Abnormal bleeding caused by adenomyosis is thought to be a result of altered uterine contractility and is commonly associated with profound dysmenorrhea.

## Leiomyoma

Leiomyoma (AUB-L), or fibroids, are benign tumors of the uterine myometrium with a complex and heterogeneous clinical presentation as varied as their biologic origins. Various genetic mutations

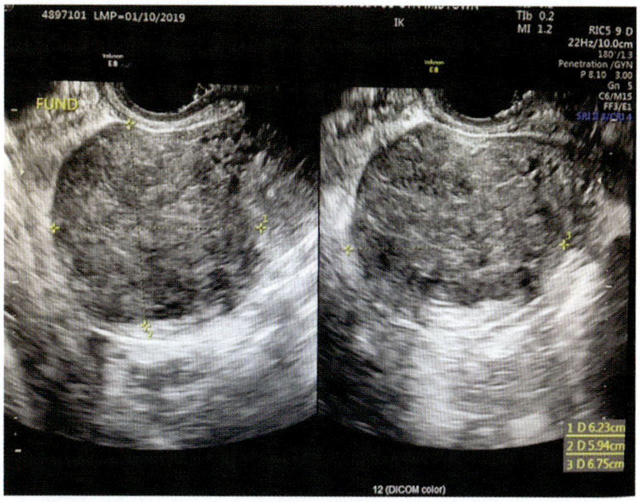


**Fig. 26.2** Transvaginal sonography of uterus with adenomyosis: heterogeneous and hypoechogenic, area in the fundal myometrium with characteristic anechoic lacunae, and ill-defined borders, sagittal view (**A**) and coronal and axial views (**B**). (Courtesy Dr. J. Lerner, Columbia University Medical Center, New York.)

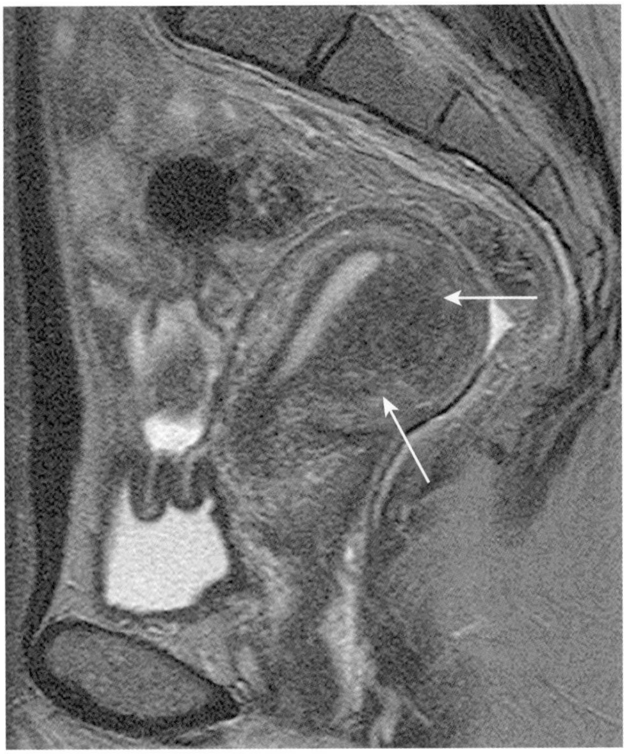

**Fig. 26.3** Magnetic resonance image of asymmetric adenomyosis, as indicated by *arrows*. (From Tamai K, Koyama T, Umeoka S, et al. Spectrum of MR features in adenomyosis. *Best Pract Res Clin Obstet Gynaecol.* 2006;20(4):583-602.)

are described in leiomyoma, but the pathogenesis is thought to initiate from myometrial injury leading to cellular proliferation, decreased apoptosis, and increased production of extracellular matrix. Critical in this pathway is the overexpression of transforming growth factor beta that leads to fibrosis of these tumors (Laughlin, 2011). Transforming growth factor beta also contributes to implantation failure in women with fibroids who are subfertile.

Although the prevalence of fibroids among women is approximately 70%, as many as 50% of these will be symptomatic (Gupta, 2008). Mechanisms by which fibroids cause abnormal bleeding are varied and depend on size, location, and number. Subclassification of leiomyomas describes their location throughout the myometrium (Fig. 26.4). Intracavitary fibroids (type 0) and submucosal fibroids, where more than 50% are intracavitary (type 1) or less than 50% are intracavitary (type 2), as well as intramural fibroids, which are large, may increase the overall surface area of the endometrial cavity or alter uterine contractility. These effects in turn lead to abnormal and excessive uterine bleeding. Whereas hysterectomy for fibroids remains among the leading indications for the procedure in the United States, treatments are diverse and include hormonal or surgical ablation of the endometrium, uterine artery embolization, radiofrequency ablation, and myomectomy through a variety of surgical approaches.

According to the FIGO system, leiomyomas can be notated in the PALM-COEIN system with a subscript 0 in their absence or by the number 1 when present. Additionally, the letters *SM* can be inserted to indicate a fibroid's location as submucosal.

## Malignancy

Malignancies (AUB-M) associated with the female reproductive tract include vulvar, vaginal, cervical, endometrial, uterine, and adnexal (ovarian or fallopian tube) cancers. Although vaginal cancers can cause abnormal bleeding, there are only approximately 3000 new cases reported annually in the United States. Bleeding from cervical malignancy classically presents as coital bleeding or intermenstrual bleeding; thus a thorough cervical evaluation is an important part of the workup of any woman with these symptoms. In a series of 73 women with coital bleeding referred for evaluation, squamous cell carcinoma of the cervix was present in 1.4% of patients, and 15% had cervical intraepithelial neoplasia.

AUB is the most common presenting symptom of endometrial cancer. Although endometrial cancer presents most often in the seventh decade, 15% of cases are diagnosed in premenopausal women, and 3% to 5% present in women younger than age 40 (Haidopoulos, 2010). Conditions that lead to increased circulating levels of estrogen are risk factors, for example, obesity is associated with increased estrone levels as a result of peripheral conversion by aromatase in adipose tissue, but the primary source of estrogen in premenopausal women remains the ovary. Impaired ovulation and the absence of progesterone withdrawal can result in sustained exposure of the endometrium to estrogen. This hyperestrogenic state can lead to the pathologic progression from normal endometrium to hyperplasia and ultimately to adenocarcinoma.

Lynch syndrome, or hereditary nonpolyposis colorectal cancer, is an autosomal dominant disease caused by a disruption in the mismatch repair *(MMR)* genes. Lynch syndrome also carries a 40% to 50% lifetime risk of endometrial cancer, with a significant proportion of endometrial cancers occurring before age 45. In addition, estrogen-producing ovarian tumors may manifest in AUB. Granulosa theca cell tumors are the most common tumors to have this presentation, although many ovarian tumors can produce estrogen.

## Coagulopathy

Systemic diseases, particularly disorders of blood coagulation (AUB-C) such as von Willebrand disease and prothrombin deficiency, may initially present as AUB (Minjarez, 2008). Routine screening for coagulation defects is mainly indicated for adolescents with prolonged heavy menses beginning at menarche. In adults, screening for these disorders is of little value unless otherwise indicated by clinical signs such as bleeding gums, epistaxis, or ecchymosis. Research has indicated that 20% of adolescent girls who require hospitalization for AUB have coagulation disorders (Claessens, 1981). Coagulation defects are present in approximately 25% of those whose hemoglobin levels fall to less than 10 g/100 mL, in one-third of those who require transfusions, and in 50% of those whose severe menorrhagia occurred at the time of the first menstrual period. Others report that a coagulation disorder is found in only 5% of adolescents hospitalized for heavy bleeding (Falcone, 1994).

Both studies indicated that the likelihood of a blood disorder in adolescents with heavy menses is sufficiently high that all adolescents should be evaluated to determine whether a coagulopathy is present.

Disorders of platelets are most often quantitative, but defects in platelet membrane or storage granules can result in normal circulating levels with altered function. Hemophilias A and B are X-linked recessive deficiencies of factor VIII and factor IX, respectively. Women who are carriers for these disorders can have reduced levels of factors VIII and IX, some less than 30% of normal and enough to be considered to have mild hemophilia. Rare inherited coagulopathies of the other clotting factors (V, VII, X, XI, XIII) include menorrhagia as a potential symptom. Other disorders that produce platelet deficiency, such as leukemia, severe sepsis, idiopathic thrombocytopenic purpura, and hypersplenism, can also cause excessive bleeding.

Chronic anticoagulation as a result of heparin, low-molecular-weight heparin, direct thrombin inhibitors, and direct factor Xa

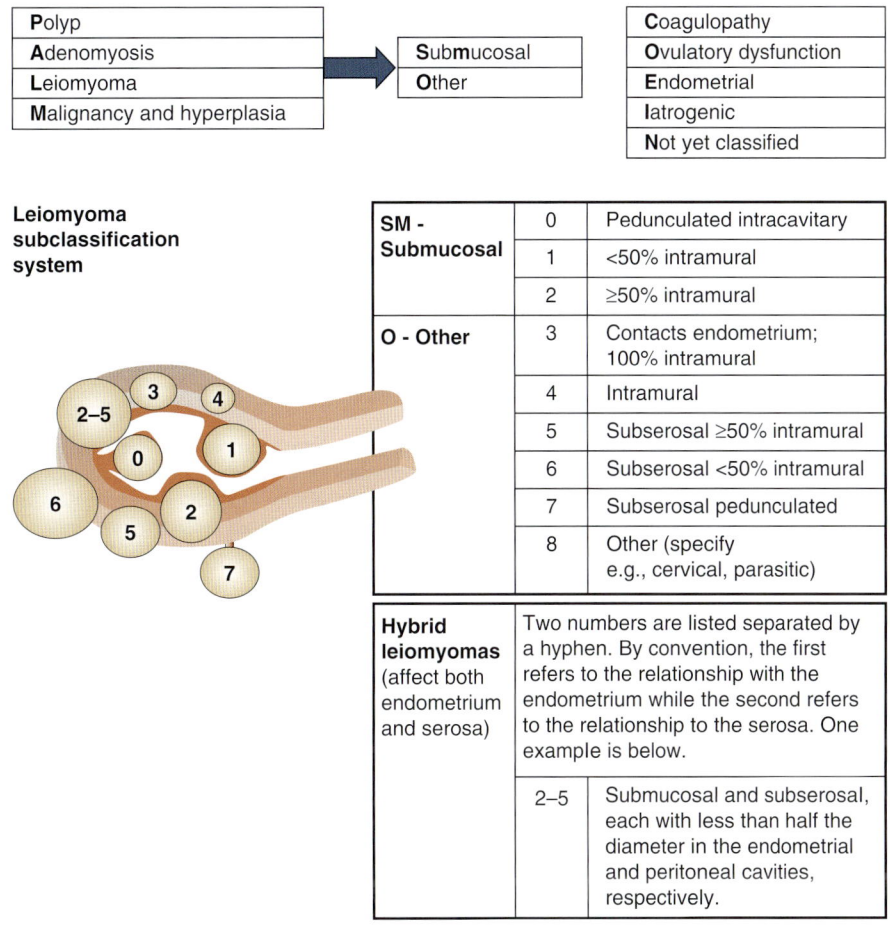

| PALM | |
|---|---|
| **P**olyp | |
| **A**denomyosis | **S**ub**m**ucosal |
| **L**eiomyoma | **O**ther |
| **M**alignancy and hyperplasia | |

| COEIN |
|---|
| **C**oagulopathy |
| **O**vulatory dysfunction |
| **E**ndometrial |
| **I**atrogenic |
| **N**ot yet classified |

**Leiomyoma subclassification system**

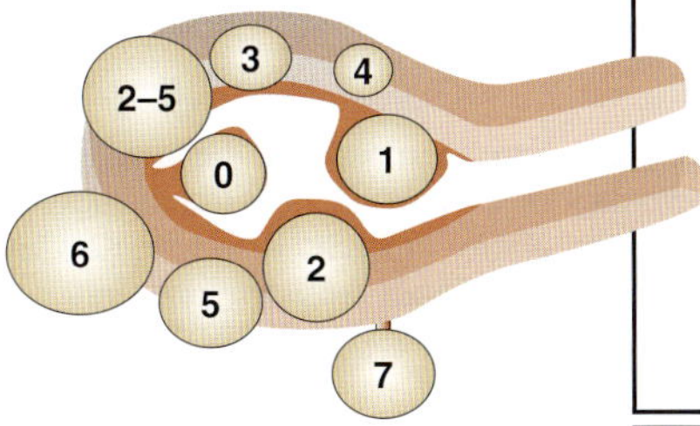


| | | |
|---|---|---|
| **SM - Submucosal** | 0 | Pedunculated intracavitary |
| | 1 | <50% intramural |
| | 2 | ≥50% intramural |
| **O - Other** | 3 | Contacts endometrium; 100% intramural |
| | 4 | Intramural |
| | 5 | Subserosal ≥50% intramural |
| | 6 | Subserosal <50% intramural |
| | 7 | Subserosal pedunculated |
| | 8 | Other (specify e.g., cervical, parasitic) |
| **Hybrid leiomyomas** (affect both endometrium and serosa) | Two numbers are listed separated by a hyphen. By convention, the first refers to the relationship with the endometrium while the second refers to the relationship to the serosa. One example is below. | |
| | 2–5 | Submucosal and subserosal, each with less than half the diameter in the endometrial and peritoneal cavities, respectively. |

**Fig. 26.4** Tertiary classification system of fibroids including submucosal, intramural, and subserosal fibroids. (From Munro MG, Critchley HOD, Broder MS, Fraser IS. FIGO classification system [PALM-COEIN] for causes of abnormal uterine bleeding in nongravid women of reproductive age. *Int J Gynecol Obstet.* 2011;113(1):3-13.)

inhibitors is necessary for prevention of thrombosis in women with inherited thrombophilias, those with mechanical heart valves, and those with rare anatomic disorders such as May-Thurner syndrome. In the absence of other gynecologic pathologic conditions, these patients present most often with heavy menstrual bleeding. Although it may seem that these patients could be considered to have iatrogenic abnormal bleeding as a result of prescribed medications, the heavy bleeding actually is a result of a derangement in the coagulation cascade and is thus categorized here.

## Ovulatory Dysfunction

The predominant cause of ovulatory dysfunction (AUB-O) in postmenarchal and premenopausal women is secondary to alterations in neuroendocrine function. In women with AUB-O, there is continuous estradiol production without corpus luteum formation and progesterone production. The steady state of estrogen stimulation leads to a continuously proliferating endometrium, which may outgrow its blood supply or lose nutrients with varying degrees of necrosis. In contrast to normal menstruation, uniform slough to the basalis layer does not occur, which produces excessive uterine bleeding.

Anovulatory bleeding occurs most commonly during the extremes of reproductive life—in the first few years after menarche and during perimenopause. In adolescents the cause of anovulation is an immaturity of the hypothalamic-pituitary-ovarian (HPO) axis and failure of positive feedback of estradiol to cause a luteinizing hormone (LH) surge. In perimenopausal women a lack of synchronization between the components of the HPO axis occurs as the woman approaches ovarian decline at menopause.

The pattern of anovulatory bleeding may be oligomenorrhea, intermenstrual bleeding, or heavy menstrual bleeding. Why different patterns of bleeding occur within a distinct entity of anovulatory bleeding is unclear but is probably related to variations in the integrity of the endometrium and its support structure. Up to 20% of women reporting normal menses may also be anovulatory.

What are the causes of anovulation? Apart from the extremes of reproductive life, as noted, women in their reproductive years often have a cause for anovulatory bleeding. This is most commonly because of polycystic ovary syndrome (PCOS), which may be suggested by other symptoms and signs, such as acne, hirsutism, and increased body weight (see Chapter 41). If not PCOS, anovulation can result from hypothalamic dysfunction, which could have no known cause or be related to weight loss, severe exercise, stress, or drug use. In addition, abnormalities of other nonreproductive hormones can lead to anovulation. The most common hormones involved are thyroid hormone, prolactin (PRL), and cortisol.

Hypothyroidism, evidenced by an elevated thyroid-stimulating hormone (TSH) level, can lead to anovulatory bleeding. Unexplained causes of endometrial problems in the face of normal ovulation (discussed later) may also be explained by subtle hypothyroidism. Hyperprolactinemia (PRL level >20 ng/mL) can also lead to anovulatory bleeding, as can hypercortisolism; however, Cushing syndrome is rare and may be considered only if other signs are present (e.g., obesity, moon facies, buffalo hump, striae, weakness). Accordingly, TSH and PRL assays should be part of the normal workup of anovulatory women.

## Iatrogenic

Iatrogenic bleeding (AUB-I) is abnormal bleeding resulting from medications. The most common of these are hormonal preparations, including selective estrogen receptor modulators, and gonadotropin-releasing hormone (GnRH) agonists and antagonists. All hormonal long-acting reversible contraceptives result in some degree of anovulation and irregular or intermenstrual bleeding; however, with time, most patients become amenorrheic. The prevalence of amenorrhea with depomedroxyprogesterone acetate users at 90, 180, 270, and 360 days are 12%, 25%, 37%, and 46%, respectively, as determined by a systematic review (Hubacher, 2009). In addition, chronic progestogen therapy of various types can lead to irregular spotting and bleeding. Similarly, irregular bleeding is an expected consequence of levonorgestrel intrauterine devices initially, but 20% of users are amenorrheic by 1 year. Implantable progestin devices have similar amenorrhea rates, but more than 40% of patients have irregular or prolonged bleeding. This pattern of bleeding is the most common reason for discontinuation of the subdermal implants within the first year (Mark, 2013).

Hyperprolactinemia can result from central nervous system dopamine antagonism of certain antipsychotic drugs. The prevalence of hyperprolactinemia among women taking risperidone was 88%, and among women taking conventional antipsychotics it was 47% in one study. As previously described, elevations in prolactin are disruptive to the HPO axis and can contribute to anovulation, with 48% of those women on risperidone experiencing AUB (Kinon, 2003).

It is well known that common combined and progestin-only oral contraceptives (OCs) may result in breakthrough bleeding (BTB). BTB most likely reflects alterations in the structural integrity, vascular density, and vascular morphology of the endometrial vasculature as a result of alterations in the expression of steroid receptors and the integrity of the endometrial epithelial layer (Smith, 2005). Compliance issues and interactions between OCs and other medications, such as antibiotics and anticonvulsants, may alter circulating levels of steroids, allowing follicular recruitment and increased endogenous levels of estrogen. These variations are a common cause of irregular bleeding in contraceptive users.

## Endometrial

Women who present with heavy menstrual bleeding in the absence of other abnormalities are thought to have underlying disorders of the endometrium (AUB-E) or are otherwise unclassified. In the past this category was called "ovulatory dysfunctional uterine bleeding."

The primary line of defense for excessive bleeding during normal menses is the formation of the platelet plug. This is followed by uterine contractility, largely mediated by prostaglandin F2 alpha (PGF2α). Thus prolonged and heavy bleeding can occur with abnormalities of the platelet plug or inadequate uterine levels of PGF2α. It has been shown that in some women with heavy menstrual bleeding, there is excessive uterine production of prostacyclin, a vasodilatory prostaglandin that opposes platelet adhesion and may also interfere with uterine contractility. Deficiency of uterine PGF2α or excessive production of prostaglandin E (PGE; another vasodilatory prostaglandin) may also explain ovulatory DUB (Smith, 1982). The ratio of PGF2α/PGE correlates inversely with MBL (Fig. 26.5). In addition to these, other uterine factors affecting blood flow, such as the endothelins and vascular endothelial growth factor, which controls blood vessel formation, may be abnormal in some women with heavy menstrual bleeding. Unfortunately, no commercially available assays exist, and endometrial causes of AUB remain a diagnosis of exclusion in most cases.

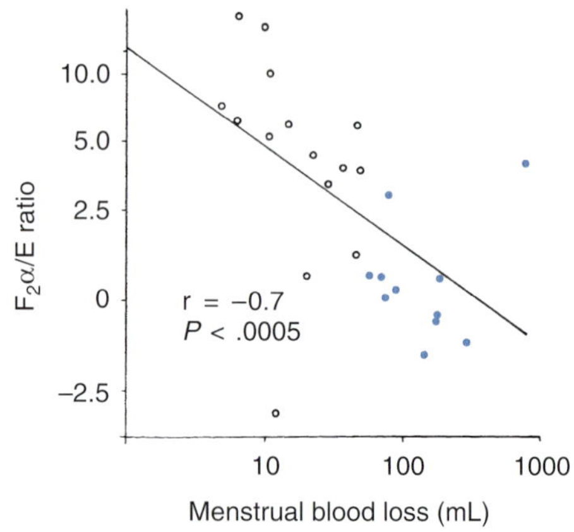


**Fig. 26.5** Correlation between the ratio of endogenous concentrations of prostaglandin F2 alpha (F2α) to prostaglandin E (E) and menstrual blood loss. (From Smith SK, Abel MH, Kelly RW, et al. The synthesis of prostaglandins from persistent proliferative endometrium. *J Clin Endocrinol Metab.* 1982;55(2):284-289.)

Chronic inflammatory changes of the endometrium as evidenced by plasma cell infiltration indicate endometritis; however, the causal relationship between inflammatory changes and abnormal bleeding is unclear, resulting from a variety of factors including infection, vascular endothelial damage, or alterations in vasculogenesis. Subclinical infection with *Chlamydia trachomatis* has also been associated with AUB.

## Not Otherwise Specified

Abnormal bleeding not classified in the previous categories is considered AUB-N. Examples of such conditions may include foreign bodies or trauma. Intermenstrual bleeding is associated with cesarean section scar dehiscence or niches, and can results in ectopic pregnancies in these defects as shown in the figure (Fig. 26.6). Heavy AUB may also be due to arteriovenous malformations. Treatment is tailored to the specific cause.

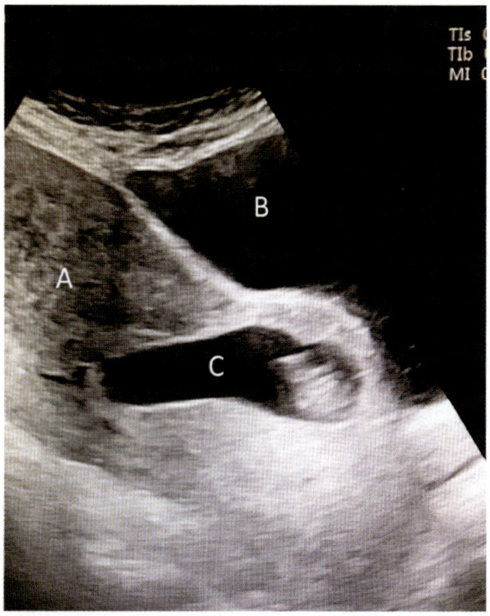


**Fig. 26.6** Transabdominal ultrasound of cesarean scar ectopic pregnancy: *A,* Uterus; *B,* bladder; *C,* gestational sac. (Courtesy Dr. J. Lerner, Columbia University Medical Center, New York.)

## DIAGNOSTIC APPROACH

When a woman presents with a complaint of abnormal bleeding, it is essential to take a thorough history regarding the frequency, duration, and amount of bleeding, as well as to inquire whether and when the menstrual pattern changed. This history is important for describing the menstrual abnormality as oligomenorrhea, polymenorrhea, heavy menstrual bleeding, or intermenstrual bleeding. History and physical examination provide clues about the diagnosis of ovulatory disorders and other systemic illnesses. Providing the woman with a calendar to record her bleeding episodes is a helpful way to characterize definitively the bleeding episodes. A number of commercially available smartphone applications exist to conveniently track abnormal bleeding, although none of these have been validated. Symptoms present for the majority of the preceding 6 months are considered chronic, but symptoms lasting 3 months sufficiently indicate the need for investigation.

Because there is a poor correlation between a woman's estimate of the amount of blood flow and the measured loss, as well as great variation in the amount of blood and fluid absorbed by different types of sanitary napkins and tampons (and by the same type in different women), objective criteria should be used to determine whether menorrhagia (blood loss > 80 mL) is present.

Because direct measurement of MBL is not generally possible, indirect assessment by measurement of hemoglobin concentration, serum iron levels, and serum ferritin levels are useful. The serum ferritin level provides a valid indirect assessment of iron stores in the bone marrow. Additional useful laboratory tests include a sensitive beta human chorionic gonadotropin (β-HCG) level determination and a sensitive TSH assay, as well as PRL. If PCOS is suspected, androgen level measurements may be considered but are not necessary.

For adolescent girls with heavy menstrual bleeding and older women with the constellation of systemic disease, easy bruising, and petechiae, a coagulation profile including platelet count, prothrombin time, von Willebrand factor, and ristocetin cofactor should be obtained to rule out a coagulation defect. Once thought to be extremely rare as a cause for abnormal bleeding, studies have found a fairly high prevalence of coagulation disorders in women presenting with heavy menstrual bleeding. Most abnormalities are platelet related. The single most common abnormality is a form of von Willebrand disease. It has been estimated that the prevalence of von Willebrand disease, the most common of these bleeding disorders, is 11% in women with heavy menstrual bleeding (Dilley, 2001). von Willebrand factor is responsible for proper platelet adhesion and protects against coagulant factor degradation. History is essential before a comprehensive hematologic workup is undertaken. This includes a history of menorrhagia, family history of bleeding, epistaxis, bruising, gum bleeding, postpartum hemorrhage, and surgical bleeding. In the absence of these clues, a comprehensive workup is probably unnecessary at the outset but should be considered in cases refractory to treatment. A hematologist should be consulted to assist in confirming the diagnosis and to suggest possible treatment (Fig. 26.7).

If the woman has regular cycles, it is helpful to determine whether she is ovulating; however, if bleeding is very irregular, it may be difficult to determine the phase of the cycle to document ovulatory function by means of serum progesterone level. Patients with chronic anovulation are at increased risk for endometrial hyperplasia and malignancy. If there is an enhanced risk for endometrial disease on the basis of history, endometrial sampling is indicated. Endometrial sampling is also recommended in patients with heavy menstrual bleeding older than age 45. Sampling is most often performed with a 3-mm Pipelle in the office, with little or no anesthesia. Sampling should include a measurement of the uterine length and subjective assessment of the quantity of tissue. When office endometrial biopsy is not

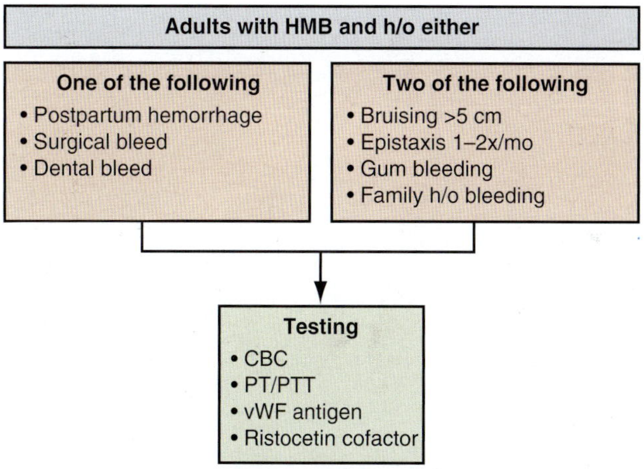


**Fig. 26.7** Diagnostic approach to adults with abnormal uterine bleeding as a result of coagulopathy. *CBC,* complete blood cell count; *HMB,* heavy menstrual bleeding; *h/o,* history of; *PT,* prothrombin time; *PTT,* partial thromboplastin time; *vWF,* von Willebrand factor. (Data from Kouides PA, Conard J, Peyvandi F, et al. Hemostasis and menstruation: appropriate investigation for underlying disorders of hemostasis in women with excessive menstrual bleeding. *Fertil Steril.* 2005;84(5):1345-1351.)

possible or if the tissue sample is insufficient, dilation and curettage (D&C) should be performed under anesthesia. The sensitivity of endometrial biopsy was 68% compared with hysterectomy specimens and was 78% compared with D&C in one meta-analysis, which concluded that a sampling error occurred in 0% to 54% of cases (Rodriguez, 1993). It thus works best in cases where pathologic change is global. In cases of regular heavy menstrual bleeding, a biopsy at the time of bleeding can also help determine whether the bleeding is caused by ovulatory function if it reveals a secretory endometrium.

Apart from performing a physical examination and obtaining a careful history, blood testing (as noted earlier), ultrasound, and endometrial biopsy (if indicated), it is often valuable to assess the uterine cavity through sonohysterogram (SHG) or flexible hysteroscopy. This is to rule out an intracavitary lesion before ascribing the diagnosis to endometrial disorders or ovulatory dysfunction.

For SHG, 10 to 15 mL of saline or sterile water is usually introduced through the cervix with an insemination catheter or with a special catheter that has a balloon for inflation in the cervical canal, allowing continuous infusion. Office-based flexible hysteroscopy is an excellent diagnostic technique that provides direct visualization of the endometrium and has the potential advantage of being able to treat the abnormality at the same time, for example, as removal of a polyp. The sensitivity and specificity of SHG and hysteroscopy are equivalent in diagnosing intracavitary lesions, but both are superior to transvaginal pelvic ultrasound alone (Kelekci, 2005). Studies show that both studies are well accepted by patients (Van Dongen, 2008) (Fig. 26.8).

Evaluation of the myometrium includes imaging modalities capable of detecting leiomyomas and adenomyosis. Ultrasonography is a sensitive screening tool and performs similarly to MRI in the detection of uterine fibroids with a sensitivity of 99% (Dueholm, 2002); however, with a wide array of treatment modalities available, assessment of the myometrium requires an exact understanding of fibroid position, size, and number. In most instances, MRI performs superiorly. Compared with findings at the time of hysterectomy, MRI, ultrasound and hysteroscopy perform equally well in the detection of submucous fibroids, but MRI performs superiorly in the evaluation of the extent of myoma invasion (Dueholm, 2001). In large uteri (>375 mL) or when fibroids

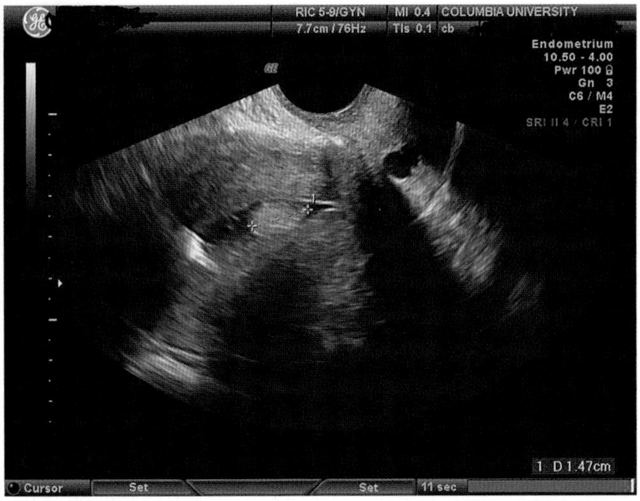


**Fig. 26.8** Saline sonography demonstrating a 1.4-cm diameter endometrial polyp in a woman with heavy menstrual bleeding. (Courtesy Dr. J. Lerner, Columbia University Medical Center, New York.)

number more than four, MRI is also superior to ultrasound in detecting and mapping fibroid location; however, hysteroscopy and sonohysterography continue to offer less expensive alternatives to MRI for adequate determination of endometrial distortion.

## TREATMENT OF ABNORMAL UTERINE BLEEDING

Treatment of abnormal bleeding requires an accurate diagnosis. Endometrial polyps that cause abnormal bleeding require surgical removal via hysteroscopy. The management of malignancy and hyperplasia is discussed elsewhere. Many of the following medical managements may be applied to leiomyoma, but large and complicated uteri or submucosal fibroids often require surgery. In the absence of an organic cause for excessive uterine bleeding, it is preferable to use medical instead of surgical treatment, especially if the woman desires to retain her uterus for future childbearing or will be undergoing natural menopause within a short time. There are several effective medical methods for the treatment of ovulatory or endometrial bleeding. These include estrogens, progestogen (systemic or local), nonsteroidal antiinflammatory drugs (NSAIDs), antifibrinolytic agents, and GnRH agonists. The type of treatment depends on whether it is used to stop an acute heavy bleeding episode or is given to reduce the amount of MBL in subsequent menstrual cycles. A definitive diagnosis is required before instituting long-term treatment and should be made on the basis of hysteroscopy, sonohysterography, or directed endometrial biopsies, if indicated.

This section is organized into treatment options for chronic conditions followed by management of severe acute bleeding. Whereas these medical options treat the underlying pathologic condition and manage the symptoms in patients with ovulatory dysfunction and endometrial causes, medical treatment options may be initiated in patients with adenomyosis or leiomyoma not severe enough to require surgery. Last, a brief overview of surgical options is presented.

### Abnormal Uterine Bleeding: Ovulatory Dysfunction

In adolescents, after ruling out coagulation disorders, the main direction of therapy is to temporize because with time and maturity of the HPO axis the problem will be corrected. A cyclic progestogen—for example, medroxyprogesterone acetate (MPA), 10 mg for 10 days each month for a few months—is all that is needed to produce reliable and controlled menstrual cycles. This may be continued for up to 6 months with the situation reevaluated thereafter. Alternatively, some clinicians prefer to use an OC, although this may not be necessary and does not allow the HPO to mature on its own. If the problem persists beyond 6 months, OCs become an option in that the condition may be more chronic.

In the perimenopausal woman who has dysregulation of the HPO axis, there is much variability and unpredictability of cycles because the HPO axis is in flux, moving toward ovarian failure. Although most of the bleeding in this setting is caused by anovulation, occasional ovulation can occur, with or without a normal luteal phase, which is highly variable and erratic. In this case it is more efficient to use a low-dose (20-μg) OC in a woman who does not smoke. Although they help the endometrium by preventing endometrial tissue from building up because of anovulation, when used cyclically progestogens do not control bleeding reliably because of the unpredictability of the hormonal situation.

During reproductive life, chronic anovulatory bleeding is primarily caused by hypothalamic dysfunction or PCOS. OCs work well in this setting, although an alternative is cyclic progestogens, as noted previously. Some of these women may also wish to conceive, in which case ovulation induction is indicated.

### Abnormal Uterine Bleeding: Endometrial

For women with heavy menstrual bleeding with no known cause and in whom anatomic lesions have been ruled out, the aim of therapy is to reduce the amount of excessive bleeding. As noted, some women with AUB-E have abnormal prostaglandin production and some have alterations of endometrial blood flow.

Options for treatment to reduce blood loss include a more prolonged regimen of progestogens (3 weeks each month); shorter cyclic therapy does not work in this situation. Doses in excess of 10 mg daily of MPA have been used, but large doses can cause side effects and weight gain when used for several months and may not be necessary. OCs reduce blood loss by at least 35% in women with AUB-E (Shabaan, 2011). Another beneficial option is the use of the levonorgestrel-releasing intrauterine system (LNG-IUS), whereby menorrhagia can be substantially reduced (discussed later). It should be noted that in ovulatory heavy menstrual bleeding, even if all obvious lesions have been ruled out, some anatomic abnormalities cannot be easily diagnosed. These include endometriosis and, in particular, adenomyosis, although the chance of diagnosis may be improved with MRI. Thus other options also have to be considered for reducing blood loss.

#### Local Progestogen Exposure

The LNG-IUS has an effective duration of action of more than 5 years. Research on the use of this IUS as treatment for heavy menstrual bleeding found that at the end of 3 months, it caused an average 80% reduction in MBL, which increased to 100% at the end of 1 year. This reduction in MBL was significantly greater than that achieved with an antifibrinolytic agent or a prostaglandin synthetase inhibitor in studies by the same investigators (Fig. 26.9) (Milsom, 1991). Other studies have shown that the LNG-IUS reduces MBL by 74% to 97% and is effective in increasing hemoglobin levels, decreasing dysmenorrhea, and reducing blood loss caused by fibroids and adenomyosis.

Although endometrial ablation achieves a more rapid return to normal flow, studies comparing the LNG-IUS to endometrial ablation show similar bleeding profiles after 1 year, with similar patient satisfaction scores (Kaunitz, 2009). In addition, the LNG-IUS has also been compared with hysterectomy for menorrhagia and has been considered to be a viable alternative.

Patients with AUB caused by coagulopathy, especially secondary to anticoagulation therapy, also can be managed successfully

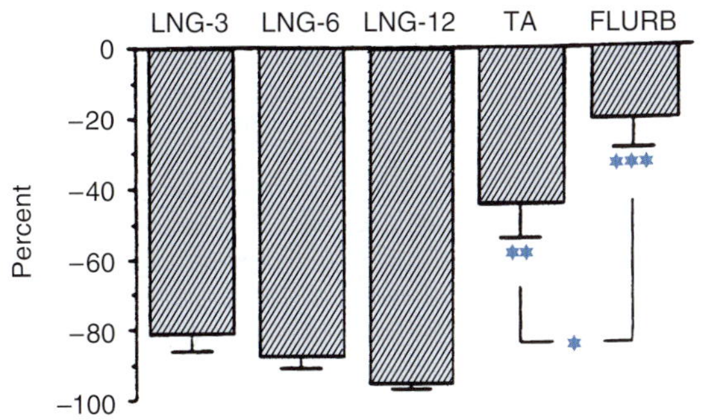


**Fig. 26.9** Reduction in menstrual blood loss expressed as a percentage of the mean of two control cycles for each form of treatment. Significance of difference between treatment with levonorgestrel (LNG)–releasing intrauterine device and tranexamic acid (TA) and flurbiprofen (FLURB), indicated by double asterisks ($P < .01$) and triple asterisks ($P < .001$), and between treatment with TA and FLURB indicated by a single asterisk ($P < .05$). (From Milson I, Andersson K, Andersch B, et al. A comparison of flurbiprofen, tranexamic acid, and a levonorgestrel-releasing intrauterine contraceptive device in the treatment of idiopathic menorrhagia. *Am J Obstet Gynecol.* 1991;164:879.)

with the LNG-IUS. In one series of 23 patients, MBL was reduced in 59% of LNG-IUS users on oral anticoagulation (Pisoni, 2006). Similar results have been demonstrated in patients with von Willebrand disease (Kingman, 2004). Importantly, a systematic review failed to answer whether the risk of thrombosis is decreased in hormonal contraceptive users while taking oral anticoagulation (Culwell, 2009). The World Health Organization states that combined OCs should not be used in patients with active deep venous thrombosis (DVT), but the benefits of progesterone-only methods outweigh the risks (Mohllajee, 2005). As such, the LNG-IUS has become an appropriate initial therapy in patients with heavy menstrual bleeding as a result of anticoagulation therapy.

## Nonsteroidal Antiinflammatory Drugs

NSAIDs are prostaglandin synthetase inhibitors that inhibit the biosynthesis of the cyclic endoperoxides, which convert arachidonic acid to prostaglandins. In addition, these agents block the action of prostaglandins by interfering directly at their receptor sites. To decrease bleeding of the endometrium, it would be ideal to block selectively the synthesis of prostacyclin alone, without decreasing thromboxane formation, because the latter increases platelet aggregation. Presently there are no NSAIDs that possess this ability. All NSAIDs are cyclooxygenase inhibitors and thus block the formation of both thromboxane and the prostacyclin pathway. Nevertheless, NSAIDs have been shown to reduce MBL, primarily in women who ovulate, although the mechanisms whereby prostaglandin inhibitors reduce MBL are not yet completely understood and their therapeutic action may take place through some as yet undiscovered mechanism. Several NSAIDs have been administered during menses to groups of women with menorrhagia and ovulatory AUB and have been found to reduce the mean MBL by approximately 20% to 50% (Vargyas, 1987). Drugs used in various studies have included mefenamic acid (500 mg three times daily), ibuprofen (400 mg three times daily), meclofenamate sodium (100 mg three times daily), and naproxen sodium (275 mg every 6 hours after a loading dose of 550 mg), as well as other NSAIDs. These drugs are usually given for the first 3 days of menses or throughout the bleeding episode. All appear to have similar levels of effectiveness.

Not all women treated with these agents have reduction in blood flow, but those without a decrease usually did not have excessive bleeding to begin with. The greatest amount of MBL reduction occurs in women with the greatest pretreatment blood loss. The treatment of heavy menstrual bleeding with mefenamic acid in 36 women for longer than 1 year resulted in a significantly sustained reduction in the amount of MBL and in a significant increase in serum ferritin levels (Fraser, 1983). Thus this approach can be used for long-term treatment because the side effects, mainly gastrointestinal (GI), are mild.

Although NSAIDs have been studied as the sole therapy to treat women with MBL who ovulate, they can also be given in combination with OCs or progestogens. With this combined approach, a reduction in MBL can be achieved more effectively than with the use of any of these agents alone.

### Antifibrinolytic Agents

ϵ-Aminocaproic acid (EACA), tranexamic acid (AMCA), and para-aminomethylbenzoic acid (PAMBA) are potent inhibitors of fibrinolysis and therefore have been used in the treatment of various hemorrhagic conditions. These lysine analogs act as reversible inhibitors of plasminogen activator, thereby inhibiting the breakdown of clots. Nilsson and Rybo compared the effect on blood loss of EACA, AMCA, and OCs in 215 women with menorrhagia. EACA was given in a dose of 18 g/day for 3 days and then 12, 9, 6, and 3 g daily on successive days. The total dosage was always at least 48 g. AMCA was administered at a dosage of 6 g/day for 3 days, followed by 4, 3, 2, and 1 g/day on successive days. The total dosage of AMCA was at least 22 g. There was a significant reduction in blood loss after treatment with EACA, AMCA, and OCs, and use of each of these agents resulted in approximately a 50% reduction in MBL (Nilsson, 1971) (Table 26.1). Of interest was the finding that the greatest reduction in blood loss with antifibrinolytic therapy occurred in women who exhibited the greatest pretreatment MBL. Preston and colleagues compared the effects of 4 g of AMCA daily for 4 days each cycle with 10 mg of norethindrone for 7 days each cycle in a group of women with ovulatory menorrhagia with a mean MBL of 175 mL. AMCA reduced MBL by 45%, but there was a 20% increase with norethindrone. The side effects of this class of drugs, in decreasing order of frequency, are nausea, dizziness, diarrhea, headaches, abdominal pain, and allergic manifestations. These side effects are much more common with EACA than with AMCA. Other investigators have compared the use of AMCA with placebo in double-blind studies and have found no significant differences in the occurrence of side effects. Renal failure, pregnancy, and history of thrombosis are contraindications to the use of antifibrinolytic agents.

Antifibrinolytic agents clearly produce a reduction in blood loss and may be used as therapy for women with heavy menstrual

**TABLE 26.1** Reduction of Menstrual Blood Loss with Treatment

| Agent Used | Decrease in Menstrual Blood Loss (%) |
|---|---|
| EACA | 47 |
| AMCA | 44-54 |
| NSAID | 21-50 |
| Oral contraceptives | 52 |
| Levonorgestrel IUD at 3, 6, and 12 months | 82, 88, 96 |
| Endometrial ablation | Up to 100; 68%-78% of patients achieve normal menses |
| Hysterectomy | 100 |

*AMCA,* Tranexamic acid; *EACA,* ϵ-aminocaproic acid; *IUD,* intrauterine device; *NSAID,* nonsteroidal antiinflammatory drug.

bleeding who ovulate. Side effects and can be minimized by reducing the dose and limiting therapy to the first 3 to 5 days of bleeding. Antifibrinolytics may have value in treating bleeding as a result of structural causes as well. AMCA administered in doses of 3.9 g/day demonstrated a statistically significant reduction of MBL in women with fibroids, with greatest reductions on days 2 and 3 (Eder, 2013). Thus AMCA has a role in decreasing acute blood loss from any cause. In this regard, its rapid onset of action, with a decrease in blood loss occurring in approximately 3 hours, is more rapid than other approaches such as the use of high-dose estrogen. Because of the increased risks of thrombosis and myocardial infarction, antifibrinolytic agents should not be combined with OCs. Combined treatment with AMCA and the OC pill has been implicated in coronary ulcerated plaque and acute myocardial infarction (Iacobellis, 2004).

### GnRH Agonists

GnRH agonists may be used to inhibit ovarian steroid production because estrogen production is necessary for endometrial proliferation. In a study of four women, daily administration of a GnRH agonist for 3 months markedly reduced MBL from 100 to 200 mL per cycle to 0 to 30 mL per cycle. Unfortunately, after therapy was discontinued, blood loss returned to pretreatment levels (Shaw, 1984). Two other observational studies, one using sequential add-back in 20 women and another using goserelin in 60 women, also showed some benefit (Cheung, 2005). Because of the expense and side effects of these agents, their use for heavy menstrual bleeding is limited to women with severe MBL who fail to respond to other methods of medical management and wish to retain their childbearing capacity. More commonly, GnRH agonists are an effective means of bridging patients to surgical treatment, allowing for correction of anemia. Use of an estrogen or progestogen (add-back therapy) together with the agonist helps prevent bone loss.

## MANAGEMENT OF ACUTE BLEEDING

In women who are bleeding heavily and are hemodynamically unstable, the quickest way to stop acute bleeding is with curettage. This should also be the preferred approach for older women and those with medical risk factors for whom high-dose hormonal therapy may pose a great risk.

## Pharmacologic Agents for Acute Bleeding

To stop acute bleeding that does not require curettage the most effective regimen involves high-dose estrogen. This treatment, aimed at stopping acute bleeding, is diagnosis-independent and is merely a temporary measure.

There has also been some experience with using high-dose progestogens alone for the management of acute bleeding (discussed later).

### Estrogens

The rationale for the therapeutic use of estrogen for the treatment of AUB is based on the fact that estrogen in pharmacologic doses causes rapid growth of the endometrium. This strategy is for the acute management of abnormal bleeding. The bleeding that results from most causes of abnormal bleeding will respond to this therapy because a rapid growth of endometrial tissue occurs over the denuded and raw epithelial surfaces. This effect is independent of the cause of abnormal bleeding. To control an acute bleeding episode, oral conjugated equine estrogen (CEE), 10 mg/day in four divided doses, has been found to be a clinically useful therapeutic regimen. It is possible that in addition to the rapid growth mechanism of action, these large doses of CEE may alter platelet activity, thus promoting platelet adhesiveness. Six hours after infusion of an average dose of 30 mg of CEE to individuals with a prolonged bleeding time caused by renal failure, the bleeding time was significantly shortened. In this study, measurements of various clotting factors were unchanged after CEE infusion. Acute bleeding from most causes is usually controlled, but if bleeding does not decrease within the first 24 hours, consideration must be given to an organic cause and curettage should be considered.

Intravenous (IV) administration of estrogen is also effective in the acute treatment of menorrhagia. Compared with women given a placebo, a significantly greater percentage of women had cessation of bleeding 2 hours after the second of two 25-mg doses of CEE was administered intravenously 3 hours apart. There was no significant difference in cessation of bleeding between women administered estrogen and those given a placebo 3 hours after the first infusion (DeVore, 1982). This study indicated that at least several hours are required to induce mitotic activity and growth of the endometrium, whether the estrogen is administered orally or parenterally. Thus IV estrogen therapy with its rapid metabolic clearance does not appear to offer a significant advantage compared with a comparable dose of estrogen given orally as long as the oral dosing can be tolerated in terms of symptoms such as nausea. From a practical standpoint, if IV therapy is chosen, it usually requires that women remain in the office or clinical setting for 4 to 6 hours to receive at least a second dose.

Estrogen therapy usually reduces the amount of uterine bleeding within the first 24 hours after treatment is initiated; however, because most women with an acute heavy bleeding episode bleed because of anovulation, progestogen treatment is also required. Therefore after bleeding has ceased, oral estrogen therapy is continued at the same dosage and a progestogen, such as MPA 10 mg once daily, is added. Both hormones are administered for another 7 to 10 days (or longer if desired and tolerated by the woman), after which treatment is stopped to allow withdrawal bleeding, which may have an increased flow but is rarely prolonged. After the withdrawal bleeding episode, one of several other treatment modalities should be used. Before instituting long-term treatment, a definitive diagnosis should be made after reviewing the endometrial histologic report. Definitive treatment should be based on these findings. OCs are usually the best long-term treatment in the absence of contraindications.

A more convenient method to stop acute bleeding than the sequential high-dose estrogen-progestin regimen is the use of a combination OC containing both estrogen and progestin. Four tablets of an OC containing 30 to 35 μg of estrogen taken every 24 hours in divided doses usually provides sufficient estrogen to stop acute bleeding and simultaneously provides progestin. Treatment is continued for at least 1 week after the bleeding stops. This regimen is successful and convenient and is thus the preferred method of some clinicians. The expectation that the IV regimen is more effective than using OCs is not well documented. A theoretic reason for this suggestion may be that the combined use of estrogen and progestin does not cause the rapid endometrial growth that estrogen alone produces, because the progestin decreases the synthesis of estrogen receptors and increases estradiol dehydrogenase in the endometrial cell, thus inhibiting the growth-promoting action of estrogen.

It must be noted that high-dose estrogen, even for a short course, may be contraindicated for some women (e.g., those with prior thrombosis, certain rheumatologic diseases, or estrogen-responsive cancer). In these cases the options are therapy with progestogen alone given continuously or intermittently. Although invasive, curettage remains the fastest way to stop acute bleeding and should be used in women who are volume depleted and severely anemic (hemodynamically unstable).

When ultrasound is available, it is more logical to use estrogen therapy if there is prolonged heavy bleeding in the setting of a thin endometrium (<5-mm stripe). Conversely, if the endometrium is thick (>10 to 12 mm) or if an anatomic finding is suspected, curettage should be considered. Unless bleeding is extremely heavy (in which case estrogen therapy is preferred), progestogens may be used initially and help by organizing the endometrium. In the setting of a thickened irregular endometrium, if curettage is not performed, an endometrial biopsy should be obtained.

Although the World Health Organization recommends against the use of OCs in patients on anticoagulation with a history of thrombosis, there is evidence suggesting their safety. In a secondary analysis of 1866 women on rivaroxaban or warfarin for treatment of DVT, the incidence of recurrent DVT was 3.8% per year on estrogen/progesterone and 4.7% off hormones. There was also a reduced incidence of transfusion for heavy menstrual bleeding in those on hormone therapy compared with those off hormones (Martinelli et al., 2016).

### Progestogens

Progestogens not only stop endometrial growth but also support and organize the endometrium so that an organized slough occurs after their withdrawal. In the absence of progesterone, erratic, unorganized breakdown of the endometrium occurs. With progestogen treatment, an organized slough to the basalis layer allows a rapid cessation of bleeding. In addition, progestogens stimulate arachidonic acid formation in the endometrium, increasing the PGF2α/PGE ratio. Some studies support the efficacy of progestogens alone in the management of acute bleeding.

In one randomized trial, MPA at a dose of 60 mg daily (20 mg three times daily) for 7 days followed by 20 mg/day for 3 weeks stopped bleeding in 76% of women in 3 days and had equal efficacy to an OC given as three tablets a day for 7 days, followed by one tablet a day for 3 weeks. In another uncontrolled short-term study, depo-MPA 150 mg intramuscularly followed by oral MPA 60 mg (20 mg three times daily) for 3 days stopped bleeding in all 48 women within 5 days (Ammerman, 2013).

High-dose progestogens in this setting may be expected to exert direct stabilizing effects on the endometrium in a rapid sequence. Similarly, large doses of norethindrone acetate (30 mg/day) may be expected to perform equally well. In addition, higher doses of norethindrone may be efficacious on the basis of some conversion to ethinyl estradiol (thus mimicking the use of a low-dose OC) (Chu, 2007). For longer-term management of abnormal bleeding, the mainstay of progestogen therapy is opposing the effects of estrogen in anovulatory women. For women with a history of bothersome intermenstrual bleeding, it is advisable to use intermittent progestogens for several months or to use an OC.

MPA 10 mg/day for 10 days each month is a successful therapeutic regimen that produces regular withdrawal bleeding in women with adequate amounts of endogenous estrogen to cause endometrial growth; 19-norprogestogens, such as norethindrone or norethindrone acetate (2.5 to 5 mg) may be used in the same regimen. Although more androgenic progestogens are less favorable for metabolic parameters (e.g., high-density lipoprotein [HDL] cholesterol, carbohydrate tolerance), when used as prolonged therapy, short-term cyclic therapy is not harmful.

In summary, if a curettage is not required, which is often the case, high-dose estrogen is the typical first-line approach for management of acute bleeding; however, the onset of reduction in bleeding occurs in approximately 5 hours with IV CEEs and in 10 hours with oral estrogen. This compares with a rapid onset of action of approximately 3 hours for TXA as discussed earlier. Other agents require more time for action: approximately 36 hours for OCs, 72 hours for oral progestogens, and up to a week for GnRH agonists.

## OTHER APPROACHES FOR ABNORMAL BLEEDING

### Androgens

Danazol is a synthetic androgen used in doses of 200 mg daily for the treatment of heavy menstrual bleeding and appears to be more effective than placebo, oral progestogens, OCs, and NSAIDs; however, a Cochrane review noted that although nine randomized controlled trials (RCTs) were identified that examined treatment with danazol, the studies have been generally underpowered. In addition, compared with NSAIDs, danazol's side effects of weight gain and skin problems were sevenfold and fourfold greater, respectively, compared with progestogens (Beaumont, 2002). Consequently, its use is limited.

### Selective Progesterone Receptor Modulators

Ulipristal acetate is a selective progesterone receptor modulator (SPRM) with antiproliferative effects on fibroid cells. Amenorrhea is achieved within 2 to 4 days in 73% and 82% of women taking ulipristal 5 mg and 10 mg, respectively, for 13 weeks for management of AUB-L. Repeated courses of ulipristal appear to be safe and to reduce fibroid volume by more than 50% (Donnez, 2015). Menstruation usually returns in 4 to 5 weeks after cessation. Common side effects include headache and breast tenderness. SPRMs have been associated with benign, nonproliferative changes in the endometrium termed P receptor modulator–associated endometrial changes and characterized by cystic glandular dilation, apoptosis, glandular crowding, and low mitotic activity in the glands and stroma. These changes are reversible with discontinuation of ulipristal.

While the SPRMs appear to be very effective therapy for fibroids and probably have a role in management of abnormal bleeding from other causes as well, there have been some safety concerns limiting their use. Recently clinical trails have been terminated because of some safety issues.

### Surgical Therapy: Dilation and Curettage

The performance of a D&C can be diagnostic and is also therapeutic for the immediate management of severe bleeding. For women with markedly excessive uterine bleeding who may be hypovolemic, a D&C is the quickest way to stop acute bleeding, and thus it is the treatment of choice in women who suffer from hypovolemia. A D&C may be preferred as an approach to stop an acute bleeding episode in women older than 35, when the incidence of pathologic findings increases.

The use of D&C for the treatment of anovulatory bleeding has been reported to be curative only rarely. Temporary cure of the problem may occur in some women with chronic anovulation because the curettage removes much of the hyperplastic endometrium; however, the underlying pathophysiologic cause is unchanged. D&C has not proved useful for the treatment of women who ovulate and have heavy menstrual bleeding. More than 1 month after D&C, there is no change in MBL in women with menorrhagia who ovulate (Nilsson, 1971). Therefore D&C is only indicated for women with acute bleeding resulting in hypovolemia and for older women who are at higher risk of having endometrial neoplasia. All other women, after having an endometrial biopsy, sonohysterography, or diagnostic hysteroscopy to rule out organic disease, are best treated with medical therapy, as outlined earlier, without D&C.

### Surgical Therapy: Endometrial Ablation

Abnormal bleeding may be treated by endometrial ablation (EA) if medical therapy is not effective or is contraindicated. Exceptions are women who have very large uteri caused by fibroids or abnormal pathologic conditions, such as endometrial hyperplasia or cancer. Various EA methods are available as alternatives to hysterectomy or to the use of the LNG-IUS, which is also highly effective (discussed earlier).

Although the concept of EA was developed in 1937, the hysteroscopic technique was first used in 1981 with the introduction of the neodymium:yttrium-aluminum-garnet (Nd:YAG) laser. Laser-based approaches were largely replaced with resectoscopic techniques to resect, vaporize, or electrodesiccate the endometrium. Most commonly, various global EA (GEA) devices have been approved by the U.S. Food and Drug Administration (FDA) for this type of treatment.

Endometrial resection is usually carried out with a loop electrode, roller ball, or grooved or spiked electrode to vaporize the endometrium. Hysteroscopic surgical techniques have the advantage of dealing definitively with associated pathologic conditions (e.g., polyps, submucous fibroids), although they require greater surgical skill, have longer procedure times, and have higher complication rates compared with nonresectoscopic methods.

Most systems, except the Hydro ThermAblator (Boston Scientific, Marlborough, MA), are used without hysteroscopic monitoring. The Hydro ThermAblator uses heated normal saline delivered through a 7.8-mm sheath. The uterus is distended and causes a closed circuit process, heating the saline to 90° C and maintaining this temperature for 10 minutes, followed by a 1-minute cooling process. The closed system is automated to shut down if there is 10 mL or more leakage of fluid via the cervix or fallopian tubes.

The NovaSure radiofrequency electricity system (Hologic, Bedford, MA) uses a 7.2-mm probe with a bipolar gold mesh electrode that opens to conform to the shape of the uterus. A fixed volume of $CO_2$ is injected and monitored to confirm the integrity of the endometrial cavity. Suction is carried out during the application of radiofrequency energy to remove debris stream. The vaporization and desiccation are carried out until a current resistance of 50 ohms is met or until 90 seconds have passed.

Before any EA techniques, endometrial sampling is required as part of the workup evaluation of the woman with abnormal bleeding. The uterine cavity should be evaluated for size and for the presence of pathologic conditions that may limit some of the techniques. With the possible exception of the use of the NovaSure system, a review by Sowter confirmed the benefit of pretreatment with danazol or a GnRH agonist before an ablation. GEA is more successful when a thin endometrial lining is present. Most systems typically treat to a depth of 4 to 6 mm. In the evaluation it is important to note that there is no thinning of the myometrium from some other cause, such as prior surgery, particularly with the microwave method. It is suggested that the myometrium should be no less than 10 mm anywhere in the uterus. Most methods of GEA may be beneficial in treating submucous fibroids up to 2 cm in size.

Complications are infrequent with GEA if adherence to the manufacturer's guidelines is maintained. Cervical lacerations and perforations occur more commonly with endometrial resection. Lower genital tract burns may occur, as well as endometritis (1%), and there is a syndrome of tubal pain after EA, which is caused by trapping of endometria at the cornual recesses and is more likely in women with a tubal ligation. If pregnancy occurs unexpectedly, there is a high incidence of poor outcomes, including prematurity and placenta accreta. Contraception is recommended for all sexually active patients after GEA.

Use of GEA in patents with AUB-O should be judicious. Women with ovulatory dysfunction often have numerous risk factors for endometrial cancer. The length of time between ablation procedure and diagnosis of endometrial cancer was 6 months to 10 years in a systematic review (AlHilli, 2011). Although the length of time did not affect the ability to diagnose endometrial cancer and all cancers were stage 1, the issue remains that destruction of the uterine cavity may prevent early presentation of symptoms or impede accurate sampling of the lining for prompt diagnosis.

GEA procedures can be safely performed in an office setting with paracervical block and conscious sedation. Although amenorrhea may not always occur (only up to 55% of the time), bleeding is significantly improved for most women. Of note, the success rate is slightly worse in women with a retroverted uterus. Up to 20% of patients will pursue hysterectomy after EA, with the most common reasons being persistent bleeding and pain. A history of dysmenorrhea, cesarean delivery and structural abnormalities and having the procedure performed in an office increased the risk of subsequent hysterectomy (AlHilli, 2011).

### Surgical Therapy: Hysterectomy

The decision to remove the uterus should be made on an individual basis and should usually be reserved for women with other indications for hysterectomy, such as leiomyoma or uterine prolapse. Hysterectomy should only be used to treat persistent AUB after all medical therapy has failed, medical therapy is contraindicated, the amount of MBL has been documented to be excessive by direct measurement, or bleeding causes significant disruption to a woman's daily activities. Although the number of hysterectomies performed for the treatment of fibroids, endometriosis, and other benign causes has declined from 1998 to 2010, the number of hysterectomies performed for the treatment of benign AUB has remained stable at 200,000 cases per year. AUB is now the leading cause of hysterectomy in the United States and elsewhere (Wright, 2013). A Cochrane review on the treatment found that medical and conservative surgical treatments had similar efficacy at 1 year, with more side effects in hormone users. Although hysterectomy can reliably provide complete cessation of bleeding and improved mental health at 6 months compared with conservative treatments, it is associated with a greater number of serious complications (Marjoribanks, 2006).

Uterine artery embolization is not particularly effective unless fibroids are the cause of excessive bleeding.

If hysterectomy is chosen, many options are available, including vaginal hysterectomy, laparoscopic-assisted vaginal hysterectomy (LAVH), laparoscopic or supracervical hysterectomy, laparoscopic total hysterectomy, robotic hysterectomy, and abdominal supracervical hysterectomy. Compared with abdominal hysterectomy, minimally invasive approaches result in shorter hospital stays, less pain, and a better quality of life, with equivalent complication rates.

## Summary of Approaches to Treatment

Having reviewed the various options, an important perspective is to approach the woman with AUB according to her acute and chronic needs or short-term and long-term therapy. Acute bleeding, which necessitates immediate cessation of bleeding, requires the use of pharmacologic doses of estrogen or curettage; the latter is used more liberally in older women with risk factors or in those who are hemodynamically compromised. This approach is not dependent on whether the woman is anovulatory or ovulatory. Although estrogen is temporarily helpful, even if there are abnormal anatomic findings such as fibroids, it is preferable to perform curettage if a pathologic condition is suspected.

In our view there is less experience with large doses of progestogens used acutely to stop bleeding; however, this is an option and may be preferable for some women who could be sensitive to or have contraindications to the use of estrogens.

After the acute episode, it is imperative to determine the exact cause or causes of a woman's abnormal bleeding. Causes most commonly are structural, hormonal, or both. Less common causes are coagulopathies, idiopathic, endometrial, or unclassified. In adolescents, 10 mg MPA 10 days each month for at least 3 months should be prescribed and patients observed carefully thereafter. In this group, additional diagnostic studies should be performed to detect possible defects in the coagulation process, particularly if bleeding is severe. For women of reproductive age, long-term therapy depends on whether they require contraception, induction of ovulation, or treatment of anovulatory bleeding alone. In the latter case, oral OCs or MPA can be administered monthly for at least 6 months, whereas OCs and clomiphene citrate are used for the other indications. For perimenopausal women who characteristically have fluctuating amounts of circulating estrogen, use of cyclic progestogen alone often is not curative. In these women, abnormal bleeding is best treated with low-dose OCs.

The most difficult type of abnormal bleeding to treat is chronic ovulatory heavy menstrual bleeding caused by an endometrial defect. If anatomic abnormalities are absent, long-term treatment is necessary to reduce MBL. For these women, NSAIDs, progestins, OCs, antifibrinolytics, and GnRH analogs are all useful therapeutic modalities. A combination of two or more of these agents is often required to obviate the need for EA or hysterectomy. The LNG-IUS has become one of the most successful options and is the first-line therapy in patients with bleeding caused by anticoagulation.

## KEY REFERENCES


Ammerman SR, Nelson AL. A new progestogens-only medical therapy for outpatient management of acute, abnormal uterine bleeding: a pilot study. *Am J Obstet Gynecol.* 2013;208(6):499.e1-499.e5.

Beaumont HY, Augood C, Duckitt K, et al. Danazol for heavy menstrual bleeding. *Cochrane Database Syst Rev.* 2002;(2):CD001017.

Cheung TH, Lo KW, Yim SF, et al. Dose effects of progesterone in add-back therapy during GnRHa treatment. *J Reprod Med.* 2005;50(1):35-40.

Chu MC, Zhang X, Gentzschein E, et al. Formation of ethinyl estradiol in women during treatment with norethindrone acetate. *J Clin Endocrinol Metab.* 2007;92(6):2205-2207.

Culwell KR, Curtis KM. Use of contraceptive methods by women with current venous thrombosis on anticoagulant therapy: a systematic review. *Contraception.* 2009;80(4):337-345.

Dilley A, Drews C, Miller C, et al. von Willebrand disease and other inherited bleeding disorders in women diagnosed with menorrhagia. *Obstet Gynecol.* 2001;97(4):630-636.

Donnez J, Hudecek R, Donnez O, et al. Efficacy and safety of repeated use of ulipristal acetate in uterine fibroids. *Fertility and Sterility.* 2015; 103(2), 519-527.e3.

Dueholm E, Lundorf E. Transvaginal ultrasound or MRI for diagnosis of adenomyosis. *Curr Opin Obstet Gynecol.* 2007;19(6):505-512.

Dueholm M, Lundorf E, Hansen ES, et al. Accuracy of magnetic resonance imaging and transvaginal ultrasound in the diagnosis, mapping, and measurement of uterine myomas. *Am J Obstet Gynecol.* 2002;186(3):409-415.

Dueholm M, Lundorf E, Hansen ES, et al. Evaluation of the uterine cavity with magnetic resonance imaging, transvaginal ultrasound, sonohysterogram examination, and diagnostic hysteroscopy. *Fertil Steril.* 2001; 76(2):350-357.

Eder S, Baker J, Gersten J, et al. Efficacy and safety of oral tranexamic acid in women with heavy menstrual bleeding and fibroids. *Womens Health (Lond).* 2013;9(4):397-403.

Haidopoulos D, Simou M, Akrivos N, et al. Risk factors in women 40 years of age and younger with endometrial cancer. *Acta Obstet Gynecol Scand.* 2010;89(10):1326-1230.

Hamani Y, Eldar I, Sela H, et al. The clinical significance of small endometrial polyps. *Eur J Obstet Gynecol Reprod Biol.* 2013;170(2):497-500.

Hinckley MD, Milki AA. 1000 office-based hysteroscopies prior to in vitro fertilization: feasibility and findings. *JSLS.* 2004;8(2):103-197.

Hubacher D, Lopez L, Steiner MJ, et al. Menstrual pattern changes from levonorgestrel subdermal implants and DMPA: systematic review and evidence-based comparisons. *Contraception.* 2009;80(2):113-118.

Kaunitz AM, Meredith S, Inki P, et al. Levonorgestrel-releasing intrauterine system and endometrial ablation in heavy menstrual bleeding: a systematic review and meta-analysis. *Obstet Gynecol.* 2009;113(5):1014-1016.

Kelekci S, Kaya E, Alan M, et al. Comparison of transvaginal sonography, saline infusion sonography, and office hysteroscopy in reproductive-aged women with or without abnormal uterine bleeding. *Fertil Steril.* 2005;84(3):682-686.

Kingman CE, Kadir RA, Lee CA, Economides DL. The use of levonorgestrel-releasing intrauterine system for treatment of menorrhagia in women with inherited bleeding disorders. *BJOG.* 2004;111:1425-1428.

Leyendecker G, Wildt L, Mall G. The pathophysiology of endometriosis and adenomyosis: tissue injury and repair. *Arch Gynecol Obstet.* 2004; 280(4):529-538.

Liu Z, Doan QV, Blumentahl P, et al. A systematic review evaluating health-related quality of life, work impairment, and health-care costs and utilization in abnormal uterine bleeding. *Value Health.* 2007;10(3):183-194.

Maia Jr H, Pimentel K, Silva TM, et al. Aromatase and cyclooxygenase-2 expression in endometrial polyps during the menstrual cycle. *Gynecol Endocrinol.* 2006;22(4):219-224.

Marjoribanks J, Lethaby A, Farquhar C. Surgery versus medical therapy for heavy menstrual bleeding. *Cochrane Database Syst Rev.* 2006;19(2):CD003855.

Mark A, Sonalkar S, Borgatta L. One-year continuation of the etonogestrel contraceptive implant in women with portabortion or interval placement. *Contraception.* 2013;88(5):619-623.

Martinelli I, Lansing AWA, Middeldorp S et al. Recurrent venous thromboembolism and abnormal uterine bleeding with anticoagulant and hormone therapy. *Blood* 2016 127:1417-1425.

Minjarez DA, Bradshaw KD. Abnormal uterine bleeding in adolescents. *Obstet Gynecol Clin North Am.* 2008;27(1):63-78.

Okolo S. Incidence, aetiology and epidemiology of uterine fibroids. *Best Pract Res Clin Obstet Gynaecol.* 2008;22(4):571-588.

Pisoni C, Cuadrado MJ, Khamashta MA, et al. Treatment of menorrhagia associated with oral anticoagulation: efficacy and safety of the levonorgestrel releasing intrauterine device (Mirena coil). *Lupus.* 2006;15(12):877-880.

Rodriguez GC, Yaqub N, King ME. A comparison of the Pipelle device and the Vabra aspirator as measured by endometrial denudation in hysterectomy specimens: the Pipelle device samples significantly less of the endometrial surface than the Vabra aspirator. *Am J Obstet Gynecol.* 1993; 168: 55–59.

Shabaan MM, Zakherah MS, El-Nashar SA, et al. Levonorgestrel-releasing intrauterine system compared to low dose combined oral contraceptive pills for idiopathic menorrhagia: a randomized clinical trial. *Contraception.* 2011;83(1):48-54.

Sheppard BL, Dockeray CJ, Bonnar J. An ultrastructural study of menstrual blood in normal menstruation and dysfunctional uterine bleeding. *Br J Obstet Gynaecol.* 1983;90:259.

Tamai K, Koyama T, Umeoka S, et al. Spectrum of MR features in adenomyosis. *Best Pract Res Clin Obstet Gynaecol.* 2006;20(4):583-602.


**Full references and Suggested readings for this chapter can be found on ExpertConsult.com.**

# PART IV Gynecologic Oncology

# 27 Molecular Oncology in Gynecologic Cancer

## Immunologic Response, Cytokines, Oncogenes, and Tumor Suppressor Genes

*Premal H. Thaker, Anil K. Sood*

### KEY POINTS

- The immune system consists of the innate and adaptive immune systems. The innate system is present at birth and consists of natural barriers, natural killer (NK) cells, macrophages, and the complement system. The adaptive immune system adapts to infection and consists of T and B cells.
- The cellular immune response occurs as a result of T lymphocytes reacting via a surface **T-cell receptor** (TCR) that processes antigens presented to it by an antigen-presenting cell (APC) in conjunction with human leukocyte (HLA) (major histocompatibility complex; MHC) molecules.
- T-cell activation can result in activation of helper or inducer (Th) cells, cytotoxic or **suppressor T cells**, or cytokine production.
- Th cells recruit macrophages and cytotoxic or suppressor cells.
- Cytotoxic T cells have the ability to lyse infected cells or signal B cells to produce antibody.
- Humoral immunity results from antigenic stimulation of a B lymphocyte, which differentiates into a plasma cell and secretes antibody (immunoglobulin).
- The complement cascade provides a basis for the inflammatory response and can also mediate cytotoxicity.
- Cytokines **(lymphokines)** are regulatory substances of the immune system produced as a result of T-cell activation caused by cell damage as a result of a virus or other cells, such as macrophages and monocytes, involved in the immune response.
- Passive therapy transfers components of the acquired immune system to the recipient with cancer (e.g., monoclonal antibodies directed toward tumor-specific antigens).
- Active immunotherapy uses a patient's own immune system for protection against infection (e.g., vaccines).
- Three types of genes are associated with malignant development—oncogenes, tumor suppressor genes, and DNA mismatch repair genes.
- Malignant change is seen with point mutations, chromosomal aberration, gene amplification (increase in number of copies), or chromosomal translocation.
- *Ras* oncogenes are part of a group of signal transducer oncogenes that relay messages from the membrane to the cell nucleus. Generally they are activated by point mutations.
- Growth factor genes include *C-erb-B2 (Her-2/neu)*, which can be overexpressed and act as a tumor-specific target for monoclonal antibody therapy; these are especially useful in breast cancer therapy.
- Nuclear oncogenes include *myc* and *fos* and can activate other genes as well as stimulate DNA replication.
- Angiogenesis is the formation of new blood vessels, allowing tumors to grow.
- Tumor suppressor genes such as *Rb* and *p53* restrain cell growth. They have two copies and, in general, alteration of both copies leads to a mutant expression, which allows tumorigenesis to occur.
- *BRCA1* and *BRCA2* mutations confer a high lifetime risk of breast and/or ovarian cancer. Mutation screening may be appropriate for women with family histories suggesting a hereditary predisposition to breast or ovarian cancer. All epithelial nonmucinous ovarian cancer patients and the majority of breast cancer patients should be offered genetic testing.
- DNA mismatch repair genes act by recognizing and fixing errors in the DNA helix resulting from incorrect pairings of nucleotides. They prevent the accumulation of genetically damaged material in the cell.

Cancer develops because of the accumulation of successive and multiple molecular lesions that result in an altered cellular phenotype that is self-sufficient in growth signaling; insensitive to antigrowth signals; and capable of tissue invasion and metastasis, limitless replicative potential, sustained **angiogenesis**, evading **apoptosis**, deregulating cellular energetics, genome instability, and avoiding immune destruction (Hanahan, 2011). These molecular changes can include **overexpression**, **amplification**, or **mutation** of **oncogenes**; the failure of **tumor suppressor gene** function because of a mutation, copy number loss, deletion, or viral infection; and the inappropriate expression of **cytokines**, growth factors, or cellular receptors. Also, natural or induced immune responses may play a role in the modulation of cancer growth because immune cells such as tumor-associated **macrophages** may actually cause tumors to grow. Based on a growing understanding of the immune response, biologic pathways, and cancer development, new immunotherapy and targeted therapies for gynecologic malignancies are being developed and are reviewed and summarized in this chapter.

## THE IMMUNOLOGIC RESPONSE

The immune system has adapted to fight off bacterial or viral infections, but it also plays an important role in the surveillance and control of cancer cell growth. The immune system has two types of responses, innate and adaptive. Innate responses are non–antigen specific, rapid, and do not increase with repetitive exposure to a given **antigen**. Components of the innate immune system include physical barriers such as epithelial surfaces, macrophages, **natural killer** (NK) cells, neutrophils, dendritic cells, and components of the **complement** system. Dendritic cells and macrophages are phagocytic cells that act as **antigen-presenting cells** (APCs). Macrophages also play an important role in the production of cytokines. Innate immune system forms the initial immune response to invading pathogens and contributes to adaptive immunity, which is composed of **T lymphocytes** (T cells) and **B lymphocytes** (B cells) that are involved in cell-mediated immunity and **humoral immunity**, respectively.

## Innate Immunity

In contrast to the adaptive immune system, which can recognize a variety of foreign substances, including tumor antigens, the innate immune system can only recognize microbial substances. For the most part, neutrophils, macrophages, NK cells, and dendritic cells are involved in the innate immune response and depend on the recognition of pattern recognition receptors (PRRs), which are encoded in the germline and identically expressed by effector cells. These receptors recognize pathogen-associated molecular patterns (PAMPs), which are expressed by microbes and trigger intracellular signaling cascades that result in inflammation and microbial death. PRRs are expressed constitutively in the host and are not dependent on immunologic memory (Fig. 27.1). Toll-like receptors (TLRs) are PRRs that stimulate type 1 **interferon** (IFN) production, which has antimicrobial, antiviral, and anticancer activity (Takeuchi, 2009). TLR agonists are being evaluated for use as vaccine adjuvants in immunotherapy trials for ovarian cancer. NK cells are a subset of the lymphocyte population, can directly kill infected cells, and recognize cells that lack **major histocompatibility complex** (MHC) class I molecules, such as bacteria (Di Vito, 2019). Moretta and colleagues have reported that NK cells are cytotoxic to tumor cells, probably because of a similar lack of MHC class I molecules (Moretta, 2005).

The complement system plays an important role in the innate immune system and is a complex system consisting of a large group of interacting plasma proteins. Activation by binding to antigen-complexed **antibody** molecules activates what is termed the *classical pathway*. In contrast, the alternative pathway is activated by recognition of microbial surface structures in the absence of antibody. Activation of these pathways leads to cleavage of C3 protein into a larger C3b fragment that is deposited on the microbial surface, leading to complement activation of C3a, which serves as a chemoattractant for neutrophils. Complexing of downstream complement proteins C6, C7, C8, and C9 produces a membrane pore in tagged cells that ultimately results in cell lysis. Unfortunately, tumor cells are often resistant to complement-dependent cytotoxicity. The innate immune system is intricately linked to the adaptive immune system by activated macrophages that enhance T-cell activation and complement fragments that can activate B cells and antibody production.

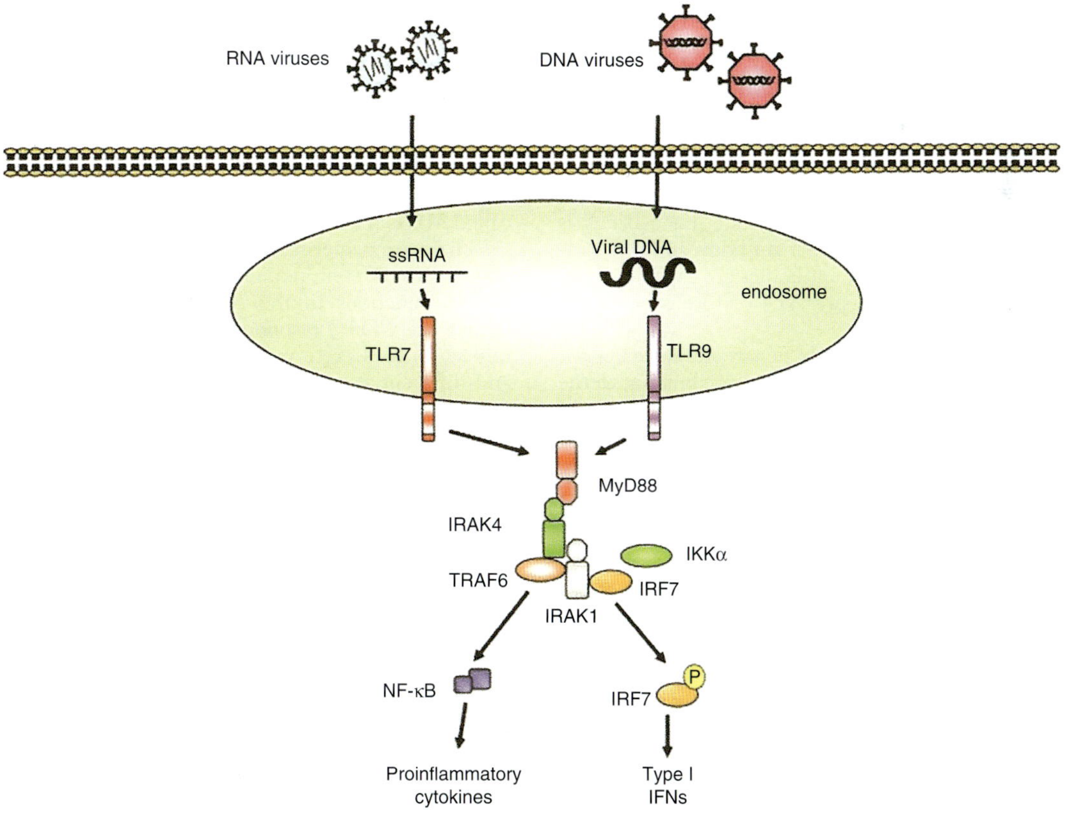


**Fig. 27.1** Toll-like receptors (TLRs). TLRs are pattern recognition receptors that recognize microbes, viruses, and cancer cells. TLRs recruit MyD88, which is an adaptor protein that ultimately activates interferon and proinflammatory cytokines. *IKK,* Inhibitor of nuclear factor kappa B (IκB) kinase; *IRAK-4,* interleukin-1R–associated kinase-4; *IRF-3,* interferon regulatory factor-3; *IRF-7,* interferon regulatory factor-7; *TNF,* tumor necrosis factor; *TRAF6,* TNF receptor–associated factor 6. (From Takeuchi O, Akira S. Recognition of viruses by innate immunity. *Immunol Rev.* 2007;220:214-224.)

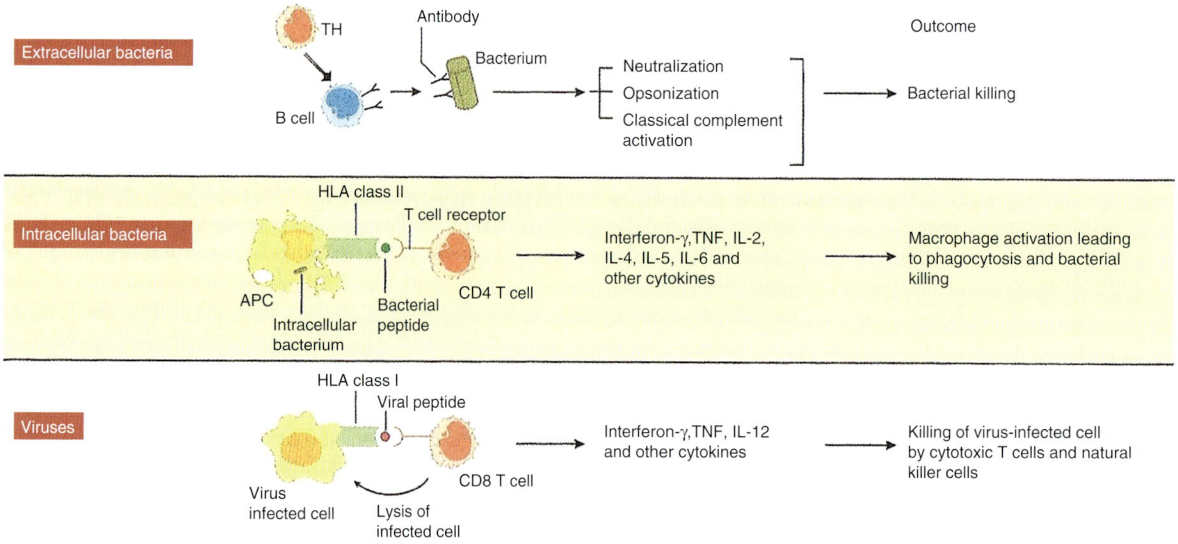


**Fig. 27.2** Overview of specific immune responses. *Top row,* Humoral immunity. B lymphocytes eliminate microbes by secreting antibodies. *Middle and lower rows,* Cell-mediated immunity. Helper T lymphocytes activate macrophages or dendritic cells that kill phagocytosed molecules or cytotoxic T lymphocytes that eliminate infected cells. (*APC,* Antigen presenting cell; *IL,* interleukin; *TH,* helper T cell; *TNF-a,* tumor necrosis factor alpha. From Chapel H, Haeney M, Misbah S, Snowden N. *Essentials of Clinical Immunology.* 5th ed. Malden, MA: Blackwell; 2006:35.)

## Adaptive Immunity

### Humoral Immunity: B Cells and Immunoglobulins

In humans, B cells are derived from hematopoietic stem cells and aggregate in the lymph nodes, gastrointestinal tract, or spleen. B lymphocytes synthesize antibodies in response to an activated $CD8^+$ cell or **helper T cell** (Th2). B lymphocytes then differentiate into **plasma cells** that secrete large quantities of antibody (**immunoglobulin**) in response to an antigen. Unlike T cells, B cells recognize antigens in an unprocessed state. Each B cell is programmed to secrete a specific type of antibody, and it is estimated that more than $10^7$ different antibodies are capable of being produced in response to the presence of foreign antigens (Fig. 27.2).

Overall, antibodies have the same basic structure, except for extensive variability in the portion of the structure binding to the specific antigen. Two identical heavy and light chains comprise the basic immunoglobulin (Ig) structure. Each pair is connected by a disulfide bond. Both the heavy and light chains have a variable (V) region at the amino terminus and a constant region (C) at the carboxy terminus. The V region participates in antigen recognition and confers specificity, and the C region enables the antibody to bind to the phagocyte. Five Ig molecules (IgG, IgM, IgA, IgD, and IgE) exist and serve different effector functions. Early in the antibody response, IgM and IgD production occurs and the membrane-bound forms of IgM and IgD bind antigen and activate naïve B cells, leading to B-cell proliferation and clonal selection. IgM is also involved in the activation of the classical pathway of the complement system. Later in the antibody response, the IgG response develops. IgG has a higher specificity for particular antigens and is also responsible for neonatal immunity in the transfer of maternal antibodies across the placenta and gut. Also, IgG causes **opsonization** of the antigen for phagocytosis by macrophages and neutrophils, as well as activation of the classical pathway of the complement system. NK cells and other leukocytes can bind to IgG- and IgE-coated cells to facilitate antibody-dependent cytotoxicity. IgE mediates hypersensitivity reactions, and IgA is responsible for mucosal immunity.

### Cellular Immunity: T Cells

T cells originate in the bone marrow, differentiate in the thymus, and then circulate in the blood or are harbored in the lymph nodes, spleen, or Peyer patches of the intestine. In contrast to the humoral response, the cellular immune response (**cellular immunity**) depends on direct cell-cell contact. Although antibodies and B-cell receptors may recognize multiple types of antigens, T cells are restricted to peptide antigens and only recognize peptide sequences in the context of membrane-bound host proteins called MHC molecules (Fig. 27.3).

There are two classes of MHC molecules. Each class presents antigens to different populations of T cells and is responsible for various functions in the cellular immune response. Th cells (which are $CD4^+$) respond to antigens bound to class II MHC molecules to secrete cytokines that stimulate the proliferation and differentiation of T cells, other B cells, and macrophages. Class II MHC molecules are expressed primarily by professional APCs, which present phagocytosed and processed extracellular peptides to Th cells.

There are two subsets of Th cells, which differ in their cytokine profiles and elicit different responses. Th1 cells secrete **interleukin** (IL)–2 and IFN-gamma (IFN-γ) to elicit a cell-mediated inflammatory response. Th2 cells secrete IL-4, IL-5, IL-6, and IL-10 to promote antibody secretion and the humoral response. Although both types are involved in most immune responses, they regulate the magnitude of each through mutual inhibition of cytokine production such that Th2 cell cytokines suppress production of Th1 cell cytokines and vice versa.

Unlike class II MHC molecules, class I MHC molecules are expressed by all nucleated cells in the body and are used to present intracellular peptides for surveillance to circulating **cytotoxic T lymphocytes** (CTLs). CTLs are also known as $CD8^+$ T cells and directly destroy cells that express foreign antigens that arise after a viral infection or are expressed as a result of tumorigenesis. Therefore CTLs are considered to be primarily responsible for the antitumor immune response. Zhang and colleagues reported that the presence of intratumoral T cells was associated with improved progression-free and overall survival in ovarian cancer

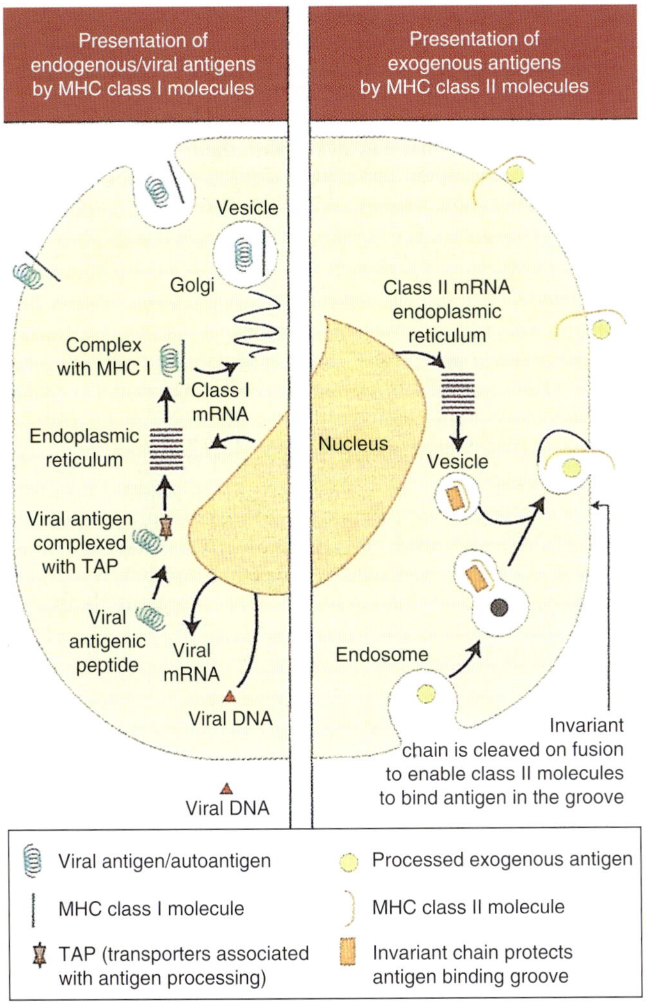


**Fig. 27.3** Different routes of antigen presentation. After the antigen is processed into smaller fragments, the major histocompatability complex class (I or II) and these fragments interact with the receptor on the surface of the T cell to activate cytotoxic or helper T cells. (From Chapel H, Haeney M, Misbah S, Snowden N. *Essentials of Clinical Immunology.* 5th ed. Malden, MA: Blackwell; 2006:7.)

patients (Zhang, 2003). This association was confirmed by Sato and colleagues, who documented a survival advantage in patients with a higher $CD8^+/CD4^+$ ratio of intratumoral cells in ovarian cancer patients (Sato, 2005). Pedersen and associates have successfully treated six platinum-resistant ovarian cancer patients with an infusion of tumor-infiltrating lymphocytes preceded by lymphodepleting chemotherapy and followed by decrescendo IL-2 (Pedersen, 2018). Another adoptive immunotherapy strategy is the adoptive transfer of genetically modified T cells, such as chimeric antigen receptor (CAR)–expressing T cells. There are ongoing phase I trials using CAR-T targeting mesothelin (NCT03608618), MUC16 (NCT02498912), and NY-ESO-1 (NCT01567891).

A third class of T cells, regulatory T cells (Tregs), are $CD4^+$ T cells that are present in the peripheral circulation, inhibit immune responses, and prevent autoimmunity. Because most tumor-associated antigens are self-antigens, recognition by immune effector cells is regulated by Tregs through peripheral tolerance. High numbers of Tregs have been found in the peripheral blood of patients with epithelial ovarian cancer, and Tregs preferentially accumulate in the tumor environment, such as ascites and ovarian tumor islets. Curiel and associates have shown that high levels of Tregs are found to be predictive of poor overall survival in a cohort of 70 patients with ovarian cancer (Curiel, 2004). Based on these data, a goal of immunotherapy is to eliminate Tregs with the aim of enhancing innate antitumor immunity, which may be achieved with the use of low-dose cyclophosphamide (Ghiringhelli, 2004).

## Cytokines

Cytokines are proteins secreted by immune cells that are produced in different phases of the immune response to control its duration and extent. During the activation phase of the immune response, cytokines stimulate growth and differentiation of lymphocytes, whereas in the effector phase of the immune response, they activate other effector cells to help eliminate antigens and microbes. The major classes of cytokines include those that regulate innate immunity, regulate adaptive immunity, and stimulate hematopoiesis.

### Cytokines That Mediate Innate Immunity

#### Interleukins

Interleukins are potent cytokines produced by some leukocytes to affect other leukocytes. IL-1 is released in response to cell damage by macrophages, endothelial cells, and some epithelial cells. Although IL-1 has actions similar to those of **tumor necrosis factor** (TNF), it lacks the ability to cause septic shock symptoms. Macrophages can secrete a variety of ILs. M1 macrophages secrete IL-12, IL-18, IL-23, IFN-γ, and TNF-alpha (TNF-α) and promote immune responses against tumors and intracellular microbes. IL-12 plays an important role in the transition between cell-mediated immunity and adaptive immunity. IL-12 stimulates NK cells and T cells to produce IFN-γ, which activates macrophages to kill phagocytosed foreign substances; IL-12 also increases cytolytic activity by stimulating $CD8^+$ cells. M2 macrophages produce vascular endothelial growth factor (VEGF), IL-6, IL-10, and prostaglandin E2, all of which have immunosuppressive functions and are found selectively in established tumors. The other ILs stimulate NK and T-cell activation and proliferation and IFN-γ synthesis.

#### Chemokines

Chemokines are small secreted proteins that are part of the largest known cytokine family. There are approximately 47 peptides and 19 G protein–coupled receptors in humans. Functionally, chemokines released in response to stimuli that cause leukocyte recruitment are considered to be inflammatory, whereas chemokines that cause migration of leukocytes to lymphoid organs are considered to be homeostatic. Chemokines affect tumor establishment in the following ways: determining the extent and type of leukocyte infiltration, promoting angiogenesis, controlling site-specific metastasis, and affecting tumor cell proliferation. Chemokines have been classified into four main subfamilies: CXC, CC, CX3C, and XC. The CXC chemokines (CXCL9, CXCL10, and CXCL11) are induced by IFN-γ and are typical chemoattractants of NK cells (Ben-Baruch, 2008; Tokunaga, 2018). In ovarian cancer patients, the expression of CXCR4/CXCL12 correlates with decreased progression-free and overall survival (Barbieri, 2010; Jiang, 2006; Righi, 2011). Because of the importance of chemokines in gynecologic and other malignancies, CXCR4 inhibitors such as peptide antagonists and neutralizing antibodies have been tested in phase I trials (NCT02179970).

#### Interferons

Type 1 IFNs, IFN-α and IFN-β, are stimulated by intracellular TLRs and mediate the early innate immune response to viral infections. These cytokines inhibit viral replication, increase expression of class I MHC molecules, and promote a Th1 cell–mediated immune response by promoting T-cell proliferation and NK cell cytolytic activity. IFN-γ, a type II IFN, is principally responsible for macrophage activation and the effector functions of innate and adaptive immune responses.

## Cytokines That Mediate Adaptive Immunity

In addition to IFN-γ and transforming growth factor beta (TGF-β), IL-2, IL-4, IL-5, and IL-13 are all involved in the regulation of adaptive immunity. After antigen recognition, the T cells produce IL-2, which causes clonal expansion of activated T cells and additional production of cytokines such as IFN-γ and IL-4. IL-2 stimulates antibody synthesis and B cells by acting as a growth factor. IL-4 not only promotes IgE production from B cells but also stimulates the development of Th2 cells from naïve T cells. IFN-γ is produced by T cells in response to antigen recognition or by NK cells in response to microbes or IL-12. IFN-γ activates the microbicidal function of macrophages, stimulates the expression of class I and II MHC and costimulatory molecules by APCs, promotes the maturation of cells expressing CD4 into Th1 cells, and inhibits the Th2 cell pathway, thereby effectively promoting a cellular immune response. TGF-β inhibits the proliferation of and differentiation of T cells and contributes to immune evasion of tumor cells by inhibiting antitumor host immune responses.

## Cytokines That Mediate Hematopoiesis

**Colony-Stimulating Factors**

IL-3 is a multilineage **colony-stimulating factor** that allows for the differentiation of cells into myeloid progenitor cells, granulocytes, monocytes, and dendritic cells. Granulocyte colony-stimulating factor (G-CSF) is a cytokine produced by macrophages, fibroblasts, and endothelial cells and promotes the mobilization of neutrophils from the bone marrow. Granulocyte-macrophage colony-stimulating factor (GM-CSF) is produced by T cells, macrophages, endothelial cells, and fibroblasts. GM-CSF stimulates the maturation of bone marrow cells into dendritic cells and monocytes. G-CSF and GM-CSF are available pharmacologically and are used in patients undergoing chemotherapy and bone marrow transplantation.

# Tumor Cell Killing and Immunotherapy

Immunotherapy has been developed to recognize and destroy tumor cells (Fridman, 2017). Immune modulation, passive therapy, and active therapy are the three major classes of immunotherapy. Immune modulation relies on nonspecific means such as the administration of IL-2, IFNs, checkpoint inhibitors, or bacille Calmette-GueÅÅrin to elicit an immune response. Passive therapy transfers components of the acquired immune system to the cancer patient (**passive immunity**). An example of passive therapy is the use of monoclonal antibodies directed toward **tumor-specific antigens**. Active therapy uses the woman's immune system to elicit a response; examples include vaccines composed of peptides, proteins, DNA, or RNA.

Immune modulation has been used in ovarian cancer in the form of adjuvant IFN treatment after surgery and as consolidation therapy after surgery and standard chemotherapy. A phase III trial randomly assigned patients with advanced ovarian cancer to intravenous (IV) cisplatin and cyclophosphamide chemotherapy versus the same regimen with intraperitoneal IFN-γ. Windbichler and colleagues have shown an improvement in progression-free but not overall survival in the IFN arm, with acceptable toxicity (Windbichler, 2000). Possible explanations for the improvement in the chemotherapy plus IFN include induction of CTLs, stimulation of NK cells and macrophages, an antiangiogenic effect on tumor vasculature, and the direct inhibition of oncogene expression by high IFN-γ levels in the tumor microenvironment. This study was redone with the standard chemotherapy of carboplatin and paclitaxel with IFN-γ versus chemotherapy alone and showed a survival disadvantage in patients receiving IFN-γ but no difference in progression-free survival (PFS) (Alberts, 2008).

Tumor cells have specific tumor-associated antigens or receptors on their surface that may distinguish them from normal cells. The antigen most often targeted in ovarian cancer is CA-125, a glycoprotein present at elevated levels in the serum of more than 80% of patients with epithelial ovarian cancer. A murine monoclonal antibody (MAb) to CA-125 (oregovomab) was investigated for its therapeutic usefulness as a consolidation treatment in ovarian cancer patients but did not demonstrate an overall survival advantage over control (Berek, 2008). However, a subset of patients who had evidence of a robust antiantibody immune response in the form of antimurine antibodies had evidence of tumor protection after treatment. Trials of oregovomab, with or without chemotherapy, have also been conducted in patients with recurrent or upfront disease (NCT01616303), and induction of anti–CA-125 T-cell responses correlated with improved survival times (Fernandina, 2017). Bevacizumab (Avastin) is a monoclonal antibody directed against VEGF. In two large phase III trials (GOG [Gynecologic Oncology Group] 218 and ICON7 [International Collaborative Group for Ovarian Neoplasm 7]), the incorporation of bevacizumab to primary treatment of ovarian cancer patients produced a clinical benefit (Burger, 2011; Perren, 2011). In GOG 218 the median PFS was 10.3 months in the control chemotherapy group, 11.2 months in the upfront chemotherapy and bevacizumab and placebo maintenance group, and 14.1 months in the upfront chemotherapy and bevacizumab-throughout group. Additionally, bevacizumab combined with chemotherapy has been approved to be used in recurrent platinum-resistant ovarian cancer because there is a 3.3-month improvement in PFS (Pujade-Lauraine, 2014). Bevacizumab-based therapy is also approved for use in platinum-sensitive ovarian cancer based on an average of 3.4- to 4-month improvement in PFS, as demonstrated in the OCEANS (Ovarian Cancer Study Comparing Efficacy and Safety of Chemotherapy and Anti-Angiogenic Therapy in Platinum-Sensitive Recurrent Disease) and GOG 213 clinical trials (Aghajanian, 2012; Coleman, 2017).

Adoptive T-cell immunotherapy uses the transfer of T cells expanded ex vivo in large numbers because of their ability to kill tumor cells specifically and to proliferate and persist for long periods after transfer. A strong rationale exists for the development of adoptive T-cell therapies in the treatment of ovarian cancer. First, tumor-specific T cells can be found in the peripheral circulation or in tumors in up to 50% of ovarian cancer patients. Second, the fact that intratumoral T cells are associated with improved survival suggests that administering adoptive immunotherapy could produce clinical results (Lanitis, 2015). T cells used for adoptive immunotherapy can be derived from peripheral blood lymphocytes (PBLs) or tumor-infiltrating lymphocytes (TILs); however, because TILs are labor intensive and only successful in a subset of patients, investigators are focusing on genetic modification of PBLs to exhibit tumor antigen specificity. T cells can be genetically modified to express either a tumor antigen–specific T-cell receptor (TCR) encoding α and β chains with specificity for tumor-restricted peptide expressed on a given human leukocyte antigen (HLA) molecule or a CAR encoding a transmembrane protein comprising the tumor antigen–binding domain of an Ig linked to one or more T-cell costimulatory molecules (Gajewski, 2006).

Another promising immunotherapy in gynecology has been the human papillomavirus (HPV) vaccine for the prevention of vulvar, vaginal, or cervical dysplasia and the corresponding cancers. A study conducted by Munoz and workers has shown that the quadrivalent vaccine against HPV-6, -11, -16, and -18 was up to 100% effective in reducing the risk of HPV-16 and HPV-18–related high-grade cervical, vulvar, and vaginal dysplasias, which may lead to reduction in rates of cervical, vulvar, and vaginal cancers (Munoz, 2010). *Listeria monocytogenes*, which secretes the antigen HPV-16 E7 and is fused to a nonhemolytic listeriolysin O protein, has been used as a therapeutic vaccine for patients with advanced cervical cancer (Basu, 2018). HPV vaccine therapy is efficacious and has tremendous implications for the prevention and treatment of gynecologic HPV-related dysplasias and cancers.

## MOLECULAR ONCOLOGY

Cancer development can be sporadic if it is caused by acquired mutations or can be hereditary if caused by inheritance of a mutated gene followed by acquisition of an acquired mutation in the other **allele**. Genetic alterations occur in three major categories of genes—oncogenes, tumor suppressor genes, and DNA **mismatch repair** (MMR) **genes**. Knowledge of how these genes function is a rapidly expanding field and well beyond the scope of this text, but a general overview is provided here.

### Oncogenes

An oncogene is a set of genes that when altered are associated with the development of a malignant cell. Functionally, oncogenes are involved in cell proliferation, signal transduction, and transcriptional alteration. Mechanisms of alteration in oncogene function include gene amplification (an increase in the number of copies of the genes in the cell), **translocation**, or overexpression, which refers to excessive and abnormal protein production. Several classes of oncogenes, such as peptide growth factors, cytoplasmic factors, and nuclear factors, exist. Examples are described in the following section (Table 27.1).

#### Peptide Growth Factors

**Epidermal Growth Factor Receptor Family**

There are four types of *Erb*B receptors: *Erb*B1 (commonly known as epidermal growth factor receptor [EGFR], human epidermal growth factor receptor [HER]1), *Erb*B2 (also known as HER2/neu), *Erb*B3 (also known as HER3), and *Erb*B4 (also known as HER4). All *Erb*B receptors share an extracellular domain that binds ligand, a transmembrane domain, and an intracellular tyrosine kinase domain. In the *Erb*B pathway, homodimers and heterodimers are formed from the various classes of receptors, resulting in activation of the Ras–Raf–mitogen-activated protein kinase (MAPK) pathway and the phosphoinositide 3-kinase (PI3K)–activated AKT pathway. Although *Erb*B3 lacks intrinsic kinase activity and *Erb*B2 has no specific ligand, the formation of heterodimers leads to activation of these classes of receptors.

The Ras-Raf-MAPK pathway is a major downstream target of the *Erb*B family of receptors and leads to the activation of Ras, causing the activation of MAPKs to regulate transcription of molecules linked to cell proliferation, survival, and transformation (Tebbutt, 2013). Also, the PI3K-activated AKT pathway serves as another downstream target of the *Erb*B pathway; it drives tumor progression via increased cell growth, proliferation, survival, and motility. A number of mechanisms such as receptor gene amplification and overexpression, receptor mutations, and autocrine ligand production cause *Erb*B pathway disruption, leading to tumor formation. *EGFR* gene mutations have been found in glioblastomas, non–small cell lung cancer, and ovarian cancer. Although, Slamon and colleagues have reported that Her2/neu amplification is found in 20% to 30% of breast cancers and 10% of ovarian cancers, uterine papillary serous cancer have higher Her2/neu expression and *HER2* gene amplification than ovarian cancer (Slamon, 1989). Because of the multitude of cancers with genetic alterations or changes in the *Erb*B family, several potential strategies exist for targeting EGFR, including monoclonal antibodies, low-molecular-weight tyrosine kinase inhibitors (TKIs, many of which are in advanced clinical development), antisense oligonucleotides, and intracellular single-chain Fv fragments of antibodies. A 2018 randomized phase II trial demonstrated an improved progression-free benefit of 4.6 months by adding trastuzumab (a humanized monoclonal antibody targeting Her2/neu) to carboplatin and paclitaxel in patients with advanced or recurrent uterine serous cancer that overexpress Her2/neu (Fader, 2018).

**TABLE 27.1 Classes of Genes Involved in Growth Stimulatory Pathways**

| Peptide Growth Factors | Corresponding Receptors |
|---|---|
| Epidermal growth factor (EGF) and transforming growth factor alpha (TGF-α) | EGF receptor (*erb*-B1), *erb*-B2 (Her-2/Neu), *erb*-B3, *erb*-B4 |
| Heregulin | |
| Vascular endothelial growth factor (VEGF) A, VEGF-B, VEGF-C, VEGF-D, VEGF-E, placental growth factor (PlGF) 1, PlGF2 | VEGFR-1, VEGFR-2, VEGFR-3, neuropilins |
| Insulin-like growth factors (IGF-I, IGF-II) | IGF-I and IGF-II receptors |
| Platelet-derived growth factor (PDGF) | PDGF receptor |
| Fibroblast growth factor (FGF) | FGF receptors |
| Macrophage colony-stimulating factor (M-CSF) | M-CSF receptor (FMS) |
| Cytoplasmic Factors | Examples |
| Tyrosine kinases | Eph family |
| G proteins | K-Ras, H-Ras, N-Ras, RAF |
| Serine-threonine kinases | AKT |
| Nonreceptor tyrosine kinases | Focal adhesion kinase (FAK), src |
| Nuclear Factors | Examples |
| Transcription factors | C-myc, C-jun, C-fos, ARID1A, MYC |
| Cell cycle progression factors | Cyclins, E2F |

Adapted from Boyd J, Berchuck A. Oncogenes and tumor suppressor genes. In Hoskins WJ, Young RC, Markman M, et al., eds. *Principles and Practice of Gynecologic Oncology.* Philadelphia: Lippincott Williams & Wilkins; 2005:93-122.

### Angiogenesis and VEGF

Cancer growth requires a sufficient blood supply to extend beyond 1 $mm^3$ in size. Angiogenesis occurs by sprouting (branching of new blood vessels from preexisting blood vessels) or by nonsprouting (requires the enlargement and splitting of preexisting blood vessels). The tumor vascular environment is characterized by vessels that are irregularly shaped, dilated, tortuous, and disorganized. Angiogenesis is dependent on the relative increase of proangiogenic factors such as VEGF, platelet-derived growth factor (PDGF), and ephrins and their receptors. Also, endothelial cells are genetically stable, unlike tumor cells, thereby potentially increasing the therapeutic value of targeting angiogenesis for cancer therapy (Baeriswyl, 2009).

VEGF is critical to endothelial cell survival, vascular permeability, cell fenestration, and vasodilation. There are seven proteins in this family: VEGF-A, VEGF-B, VEGF-C, VEGF-D, VEGF-E, placental growth factor (PlGF) 1, and PlGF2. Most human tumors, including those of the lung, thyroid, breast, gastrointestinal, female reproductive tract, and urinary tract, have marked expression of VEGF. There are three VEGF receptors: VEGFR-1, VEGFR-2, and VEGFR-3. VEGFR-3 is expressed on the vascular and lymphatic endothelium, unlike the other two receptors, which are expressed on the vascular endothelium. Also, a second class of VEGFRs known as the neuropilins (NRPs) potentiate VEGF-A– and VEGFR-2–mediated actions. Similar to the EGFR family, there are many ligands to receptors in the VEGF family. Ultimately, activation of the VEGF receptors can lead to downstream effects on the MAPK pathway, v-src sarcoma viral oncogene homologue (SRC), PI3K-AKT, focal adhesion kinase (FAK), and Ras-Raf-MAPK superfamily (Apte, 2019; Carmeliet, 2000; Dvorak, 2002). Because of the clinical significance of the VEGF pathway in many cancers, anti-VEGF antibodies such as bevacizumab, VEGFR TKIs, and vascular targeting agents have been developed to target this critical pathway (Choi, 2015; Montor, 2018).

Cediranib is a receptor TKI against VEGFR-1 to -3, platelet-derived growth factor alpha (PDFR-α), and c-kit. In the ICON6 trial, patients with platinum-sensitive recurrent ovarian cancer who received chemotherapy plus cediranib followed by 18 months of cediranib maintenance had a median PFS of 11.0 versus 8.7 months (hazard ratio [HR], 0.57; 95% confidence interval [CI], 0.45 to 0.74) (Lederman, 2016). Cediranib is being combined with the poly(adenosine diphosphate [ADP]–ribose) polymerase (PARP) inhibitor olaparib in both patients with platinum-sensitive and platinum-resistant ovarian cancer. Liu and colleagues reported an improved PFS of 23.7 versus 5.7 months ($P$ =.002) and overall survival benefit of 37.8 versus 23.0 months ($P$ = .047) in patients with platinum-sensitive germline *BRCA* wild-type/unknown cancer receiving the combination of cediranib and olaparib compared with olaparib (Liu, 2019b).

### Ephrin Family of Ligands and Receptors

Tyrosine kinases provide a transfer of a phosphate from adenosine triphosphate (ATP) to tyrosine residues on specific cellular proteins; however, they can also play a role in the development of cancer and tumor progression. Attention has been given to elucidating the role of the ephrin receptor A2 (EphA2) in tumorigenesis and therapeutic targeting. EphA2 belongs to the largest known family of protein tyrosine kinase receptors, the Eph family, and two Eph receptors, A and B, have corresponding ligands. The normal cellular function of EphA2 in epithelial tissue is not completely understood, but in cancer, EphA2 modulates cell growth, survival, migration, and angiogenesis (Pasquale, 2008). EphA2 overexpression has been correlated with disease severity and is predictive of a poor outcome in patients with ovarian cancer. Several therapeutic approaches exist for targeting EphA2, including agonist monoclonal antibody, immunotherapy, soluble EphA receptors, and neutral liposomal **small interfering RNA** (siRNA), some of which are already in clinical trials (Carles-Kinch, 2002; Thaker, 2004).

### Phosphoinositide 3-Kinase Pathway

The PI3K family is composed of lipid and serine-threonine kinases that control second messengers through phosphorylation. AKT is the predominant downstream target of PI3K and has many targets, including mammalian target of rapamycin (mTOR), signal transducer and activation of transcription (STAT), MAPK, nuclear factor–kappa βÔÄ¨ and protein kinase C. The activation of the PI3K-AKT pathway controls cell survival with inhibition of apoptosis, cell growth, cell metabolism, RNA translation, and cell proliferation. Also, this pathway has been implicated in chemotherapy resistance (Fruman, 2014).

RAS, another cytoplasmic factor, is a G protein involved in the transmission of growth stimulatory signals from the cell membrane to the nucleus. The RAS family of G proteins is positioned downstream of cell surface receptor tyrosine kinases and upstream of the cytoplasmic cascade of kinases, such as mitogen-activated protein (MAP) kinases. MAP kinases in turn activate nuclear transcription factors such as c-myc, c-jun, and c-fos. It is estimated that about one-third of cancers have point mutations in RAS genes, such as *KRAS*, *HRAS*, and *NRAS* (Mammas, 2004). Because RAS requires the posttranslational modification of the addition of a farnesyl group to the C-terminus to move from the cytoplasm to the inner plasma membrane, inhibitors to farnesylation had been developed but with disappointing results; however, research is ongoing regarding work to use switch II pocket (SII-P) inhibitors to target a pocket in the SW2 region of RAS and inhibitors to target nucleotide exchange (O'Bryan, 2019).

### Tumor Suppressor Genes

Tumor suppressor genes control cell growth cellular proliferation, and aberrations in tumor suppressor genes can cause malignancy. The retinoblastoma *(Rb)* gene was the first tumor suppressor gene to be identified and encodes a nuclear protein that regulates G1 phase cell cycle arrest. Knudson and colleagues have proposed the "two-hit" theory to explain the action of tumor suppressor genes. The first hit is the inheritance of the *Rb* mutated gene and the second hit is the somatic mutation that occurs later and leads to cancer.

In gynecologic malignancies, the most common deregulated tumor suppressor gene is *p53*, which is located on the short arm of chromosome 17. *p53* has key roles as a transcription factor and regulator of the cell cycle and apoptosis. Normal *p53* binds to transcriptional regulatory elements in the DNA and acts as a gatekeeper of the genome by responding to DNA damage with the activation of apoptotic effectors such as BAX, FAS, and bcl-2. Missense mutations that change a single amino acid in the encoded protein in exons 5 to 8 are the most common mutations of *p53*. The resultant mutant proteins can no longer bind to DNA but can bind to and inactivate any normal *p53* in a cell. Cells with mutant *p53* do not experience cell cycle arrest at the $G_1$-S checkpoint before DNA replication and at the $G_2$-M checkpoint before mitosis, nor do they undergo apoptosis (Baretk, 1997; Hollstein, 1991; Li, 2019).

Tumor suppressor genes such as *p53* are found in approximately 10% to 20% of endometrioid cancers, predominantly grade 3, and in many late and sporadic ovarian cancers. In cervical carcinogenesis, the E6 oncoprotein of HPV types 16 and 18 associates with *p53* and targets it for degradation, and the E7 oncoprotein of HPV type 16 binds to *Rb* in infected cells to upregulate proliferation (Scheffner, 1990; Werness, 1990). Although *p53* mutations are one of the most common mutations in cancer, therapeutic targeting of *p53* has met with less than optimal results in several disease sites.

Phosphatase and tensin homologue (PTEN) is the regulatory counterpart of PI3K as a result of dephosphorylating proteins phosphorylated by PI3K. *PTEN* is a tumor suppressor gene and is found in approximately 20% of endometrial hyperplasia and 50% of endometrioid cancers. Mutations of *PTEN* occur in exons 3, 4, 5, 7, and 8 targeting the phosphatase domain and regions that control protein stability and localization. Decreased or absent expression of *PTEN* results in many of the mutations found in endometrioid cancers. Also, **epigenetic** mechanisms such as promoter hypermethylation and subcellular localization can affect *PTEN* function in the absence of intragenic mutations.

### BRCA1 and BRCA2

Approximately 5% to 10% of breast and 15% of ovarian cancers arise in the setting of a genetic predisposition. Genetic testing for mutations has clinical implications for the patient and patient's family. The vast majority of these cases are associated with germline mutations in the BRCA1 gene located on chromosome 17q21 and the BRCA2 gene located on chromosome 13q12.3 (Antoniou, 2005). Other important pathogenic germline mutations predisposing to ovarian cancer are *PALB2, BARD1, BRIP1, RAD51C,* and *RAD51D.* The pattern of inheritance is autosomal dominant, and the prevalence of the mutated gene occurs more often in women of Ashkenazi Jewish descent and in certain French Canadian women. The following women should be tested for a *BRCA* or other mutations (Karlan, 2007; NCCN, 2019; Norquist, 2015):

- A woman with a family history of two or more women with breast cancer or ovarian cancer at any age

or

- A woman with breast cancer before age 50 years, triple negative breast cancer before age 60, two breast cancer primaries, or breast cancer at any age with a family history of other cancers (breast cancer at age younger than 50, ovarian cancer, male breast cancer, pancreatic cancer, or high-grade/metastatic prostate cancer)

or

- A woman at any age with epithelial nonmucinous histology ovarian, fallopian tube, or primary peritoneal cancers

The cumulative risk of developing ovarian cancer by age 70 years is 40% to 50% for *BRCA1* mutation and 20% to 25% for *BRCA2* mutation carriers, but there is equal breast cancer penetrance in *BRCA1* or *BRCA2* mutation carriers. The *BRCA2* mutation is also associated with male breast cancer and pancreatic, urinary tract, and biliary tract cancers. Unfortunately, a woman with this mutation develops breast or ovarian cancer at a younger age than those who develop sporadic cancers.

*BRCA1* and *BRCA2* are tumor suppressor genes that encode for large proteins. Similar to other hereditary cancer syndromes, inheritance of a *BRCA* mutation confers an increased susceptibility to cancer but not an absolute guarantee of developing cancer unless a second inactivation of the allele occurs. Both *BRCA1* and *BRCA2* encode proteins that are involved in the repair of DNA strand breaks. Most detected mutations are nonsense or frameshift alterations that lead to truncated proteins. BRCA1 and BRCA2 proteins are involved in the pathway mediated by RAD51, which is a protein important in repairing double DNA strand breaks. BRCA1 is also involved in tumor suppression by transcriptional regulation of gene expression, such as being a *p53*-independent transactivator of cyclin kinase inhibitor p21. *BRCA2* has been identified as a FANCD1 gene, a member of the Fanconi anemia complex. Cells with deficient *BRCA1* or *BRCA2* are incapable of repairing DNA strand breaks, which leads to genetic instability and tumorigenesis. In *BRCA*-deficient cells, the defective maintenance of genomic integrity may not only accelerate cancer initiation and progression but also render the cancer more susceptible to therapeutic agents whose cytotoxic potential is mediated through the induction of a specific type of DNA damage that *BRCA* normally functions to repair. For example, cisplatin and radiation cause DNA interstrand cross-links.

PARPs are a family of multifunctional enzymes that repair DNA single-strand breaks through the repair of base excisions. The inhibition of PARPs leads to the accumulation of DNA double-strand breaks, which are normally repaired by BRCA proteins and thereby provide selectivity of treatment in this *BRCA* mutation population. Approximately 7% of ovarian cancers will have somatic mutations in *BRCA* and even more will have a homologous recombination signature, increasing the number of patients who can benefit from PARP inhibitors. Currently there are three commercially available PARP inhibitors: olaparib, rucaparib, and niraparib. PARP inhibitors can be used as first-line maintenance in patients with a germline or somatic *BRCA* mutation, as second-line maintenance after platinum-sensitive recurrence, and as treatment for patients with germline *BRCA* mutations (Mullen, 2019). In a large randomized phase III clinical trial (SOLO-1), Moore and colleagues found that patients with ovarian cancer with a germline or somatic *BRCA1/2* mutation who had achieved a partial or complete response after initial chemotherapy and had olaparib maintenance had a 70% decrease in the risk of disease progression or death at a median follow-up of 41 months compared with the placebo maintenance group (Moore, 2018). There are ongoing trials with combinations of PARP inhibitors with antivascular agents and checkpoint inhibitors in gynecologic malignancies.

### DNA Mismatch Repair Genes

Hereditary nonpolyposis colorectal cancer (HNPCC), also known as Lynch syndrome, is an autosomal dominant cancer syndrome that predisposes an individual to colorectal, endometrial, gastric, biliary tract, urinary tract, or ovarian cancer. This syndrome is thought to account for all cases of hereditary endometrial cancer and up to 5% of hereditary ovarian cancers. The estimated lifetime risk for endometrial cancer in *HNPCC* gene carriers is 40% to 60%, corresponding to a relative risk of 13 to 20, whereas that of ovarian cancer is 6% to 20%, corresponding to a relative risk of 4 to 8. Linkage analysis of high-risk families led to the discovery of Lynch syndrome. It was found to be caused by germline mutations in genes responsible for recognizing and fixing errors in the DNA helix, resulting from incorrect pairings of nucleotides during replication or the formation of abnormal loops of DNA. *MSH2* (MutS homologue 2) and *MLH1* (MutL homologue 1) are the most commonly mutated MMR genes and are located on chromosomes 2p16 and 3p21, respectively. Other MMR genes are *MSH6, PMS1,* and *PMS2,* but these occur at a lower frequency. Cells with a defective MMR system exhibit **microsatellite instability** (MSI). MSI occurs as DNA mismatches cause a shortening or lengthening of repetitive DNA sequences and these mismatches go unchecked. This results in the cancer containing a greater or lesser number of repeats than are present in the normal cells of the individual (Adar, 2018). A consensus panel of five microsatellite markers (D2S123, D5S346, D17S250, Bat 25, and Bat 26) can be used to identify HNPCC-related cancers compared with sporadic cancers (Boland, 1998; Karlan, 2007; Sood, 2001). In endometrial cancer, MSI can occur from promoter methylation and must be distinguished from MSI caused by an inherited MMR defect.

Taking a family history is the first step in identifying patients with HNPCC. The Bethesda criteria (Box 27.1) seem to be the most sensitive for predicting MMR gene mutations, but the Amsterdam II criteria are more specific. Amsterdam II criteria include the following: colorectal carcinoma and/or endometrial cancer or transitional cell of the ureter or renal pelvis or carcinoma of the small bowel in at least three individuals; one of the patients is a first-degree relative of two other patients; disease occurs in at least two other family members; one of the diagnoses should be made before age 50 years; there is histologic confirmation of the

**BOX 27.1 Bethesda and Amsterdam II Criteria for Hereditary Nonpolyposis Colorectal Cancer**

Any one of the following meet Bethesda Criteria:

- Colorectal cancer in person younger than 50 years
- Presence of synchronous or metachronous HNPCC-related carcinomas regardless of age (colorectal, endometrial, stomach, ovarian, pancreas, ureter, renal pelvis, biliary tract, sebaceous gland, and small bowel)
- Colorectal cancer with specific histologic features in individuals younger than age 6o years
- Colorectal cancer diagnosed in one or more first-colorectal degree relatives with colorectal cancer or other HNPCC-related tumors. One of the cancers must have been diagnosed before age 50 years (this includes adenomas, which must have been diagnosed before age 40 years)
- Colorectal cancer in two or more first- or second-degree relatives with a HNPCC-related tumor, regardless of age

or

All of the following meet Amsterdam II Criteria:

- Colorectal and/or endometrial cancer or transitional cancer of the ureter or renal pelvis or cancer of the small bowel in at least three individuals in the same family
- One of the patients is a first-degree relative of the other patients
- Disease occurs in at least two other family members
- At least one of the diagnoses was made before age 50
- The diagnoses must be histologically confirmed
- Familial adenomatous polyposis is excluded

Vasen HF, Mecklin JP, Khan PM, Lynch HT. The International Collaborative Group on Hereditary Non-Polyposis Colorectal Cancer (ICG-HNPCC). *Dis Colon Rectum*. 1991;34:424–425; Vasen HF, Watson P, Mecklin JP, Lynch HT. New clinical criteria for hereditary nonpolyposis colorectal cancer (HNPCC, Lynch syndrome) proposed by the International Collaborative Group on HNPCC. *Gastroenterology*. 1999;116:1453–1456; Rodriguez-Bigas MA, Boland CR, Hamilton SR, et al. A National Cancer Institute workshop on hereditary nonpolyposis colorectalcancer syndrome: meeting highlights and Bethesda guidelines. *J Natl Cancer Inst* 1997;89:1758–1762; Umar A, Risinger JI, Hawk ET, Barrett JC. Testing guidelines for hereditary non-polyposiscolorectal cancer. *Nat Rev Cancer*. 2004;4:153–158.
*HNPCC*, Hereditary nonpolyposis colorectal cancer.

diagnosis; and familial adenomatous polyposis has been excluded. Immunohistochemistry-based universal screening for all colon and endometrial cancer patients will identify 50% more patients with Lynch syndrome than using Amsterdam II or Bethesda criteria.

## Future Directions

With the continued improved understanding of molecular oncogenesis and tumor progression, promising biologically targeted therapies such as antibody-drug conjugates, and oncolytic viruses, innovative immune approaches continue to emerge (described in later sections) (Sterman, 2006). One such therapy is siRNA, which can be designed to target and silence oncogenes involved in all steps of cancer initiation, proliferation, and metastasis. Unlike small molecule inhibitors or fully humanized antibodies, siRNAs can target multiple downstream pathways or targets specifically and effectively based on direct, homology-dependent, posttranscriptional gene silencing. The major challenges to the development of siRNA as a therapeutic tool have been its degradation by serum nucleases, poor cellular uptake, and rapid renal clearance after administration. However, the development of nuclease-resistant chemically modified siRNAs and neutral nanoliposomes such as 1,2-dioleoyl-*sn*-glycero-3-phosphatidylcholine (DOPC) for improved delivery should overcome these obstacles (Barata, 2016; Chen, 2018). Preclinically, neutral nanoliposomal EphA2 siRNA injection every 4 days decreased tumor growth in two ovarian cancer cell lines compared with control siRNA, and when EphA2-targeted siRNA was combined with paclitaxel, there was a statistically significant decrease in tumor growth in both cell lines (Landen, 2005). An ongoing phase I clinical trial (NCT01591356) is recruiting women with advanced recurrent ovarian cancer who have biopsy results demonstrating EphA2 overexpression to receive twice weekly IV infusions of siRNA-EphA2-DOPC.

Another potential therapeutic target is noncoding RNA (ncRNA). This includes a broad range of regulatory RNA molecules, such as ribozymes, antisense, siRNA, micro-RNA, and aptamers (Van Roosbroeck, 2017). Small ncRNAs elicit at least four types of responses that trigger specific gene inactivation, which are important in a variety of cancers—destruction of homologous messenger RNA, inhibition of translation, de novo methylation of genomic regions that block transcription of target genes, and chromosomal rearrangement. These flexible molecules have proven to have enormous potential as diagnostic and therapeutic tools in cancer medicine.

# GYNECOLOGIC MALIGNANCIES

Cancer is a complex multistep process that requires self-sufficient growth signals, insensitivity to antigrowth signals, tissue invasion and metastasis, limitless replicative potential, sustained angiogenesis, evasion of apoptosis deregulating cellular energetics, genome instability, and immune destruction avoidance. The clinical diversity of gynecologic cancers such as histologic type, stage, and outcome is probably attributable to molecular differences among cancers. The role of oncogenes and tumor suppressor genes vary not only among cancers but also within a given type of cancer. Our understanding of the molecular pathogenesis of gynecologic cancers is in its infancy, but with new molecular profiling technologies, this understanding is expanding rapidly. With this improved characterization, new insights into the origin, prevention, and treatment of gynecologic cancers should follow. In the following sections we describe the role of oncogenes and tumor suppressor genes that lead to the development of gynecologic cancers.

## Endometrial Cancer

### Endometrial Cancer and Tumor Suppressor Genes

Endometrial cancer is divided into two types—type 1, which is thought to be caused by unopposed estrogen and develops in a background of endometrial hyperplasia, and type 2, which is composed of nonendometrioid and more aggressive cancers. Inactivation of tumor suppressor gene *p53* is among the most common genetic events in endometrial cancer. Also, overexpression of *p53* occurs more often in advanced endometrial cancer and has been associated with worse survival after controlling for stage, suggesting that loss of *p53* tumor suppressor function leads to a more aggressive phenotype. Endometrial glandular dysplasia has been proposed as a precursor for type 2 serous carcinomas, and both the precursor and serous carcinoma have demonstrated overexpression of *p53* (Jia, 2008). In uterine sarcomas, overexpression of mutant *p53* occurs in malignant mixed mesodermal tumors (MMMTs), leiomyosarcomas, and undifferentiated endometrial sarcomas (Han, 2018).

The *PTEN* gene is on chromosome 10q and encodes a phosphatase that functions by opposing the activity of PI3K (Cancer Genome Atlas Research Network, 2013). Mutations in this gene are usually deletions, insertions, or nonsense mutations that lead to truncated protein products and are associated with endometrioid histology, early stage, and favorable clinical behavior (Risinger, 1998). Dellas and coworkers found that loss of *PTEN* and p27 protein expression in patients with obesity and endometrial cancer is associated with a significantly better prognosis (Dellas, 2009). Sometimes, *PTEN* mutation status can be used to differentiate an ovarian metastasis from an endometrial cancer versus synchronous primary cancers. *PTEN* mutations are common according to The Cancer Genome Atlas (TCGA) analysis. Because tumor cells lacking PTEN contain high levels of activated AKT, PTEN is necessary for the appropriate regulation of the PI3K/AKT pathway (Mahdi, 2015). Studies have identified the AKT kinase as a potential mediator of tumorigenesis in endometrial cancer cell lines. The finding of PTEN mutations in the majority of endometrial cancer suggests that the loss of PTEN function may be one mechanism by which AKT activity is increased in this disease. Because PTEN-deficient cancer cells may have upregulated activity of mTOR, which is downstream of AKT, these cells may be sensitive to mTOR inhibition (Slomovitz, 2015). PI3K inhibitors have shown a clinical benefit rate of 21% to 52% in recurrent disease. Because estrogen receptor (ER) signaling is important in type 1 endometrial cancers and there is cross regulation between ER and PI3K/AKT/mTOR pathways, the GOG ran a study using the combination of everolimus (an mTOR inhibitor) with letrozole (an aromatase inhibitor) versus tamoxifen and medroxyprogesterone (standard-of-care arm) in patients with recurrent endometrial cancer. The results demonstrated that the everolimus and letrozole combination was an active regimen in terms of PFS (6.3 months vs. 3.8 months in control arm), especially in chemotherapy-naïve patients (Yang et al., 2019; Slomovitz, 2018).

Germline mutations in DNA MMR genes are essential to HNPCC. Endometrial cancer is the second most common malignancy in women with HNPCC after colon cancer. Unlike colon cancer, loss of MMR function in endometrial cancer has not been consistently associated with improved survival (Cohn, 2006) (see earlier section on HNPCC for further details); however, immunotherapy is beneficial in the recurrent setting for these patients (Yamashita, 2018).

### Endometrial Cancer and Oncogenes

Unlike inactivation of tumor suppressor genes, fewer alterations in oncogenes have been found in endometrial cancer. *Her2/neu* has been found to be expressed in approximately 20% of endometrioid and serous carcinomas and was associated with aggressive phenotype and poor survival in a population-based series (Engelsen, 2008). Racial differences in the expression of *Her2/neu* have been found as well (Santin, 2005). Regardless, the levels of *Her2/neu* overexpression are much lower than in breast cancer, but nonetheless there is benefit in using trastuzumab (an anti-*Her2/neu* antibody) for the treatment of recurrent serous endometrial cancer (Fader, 2018; Fleming, 2010).

KRAS mutations occur most often in type 1 endometrial cancers and in hyperplasia, suggesting that *KRAS* mutation is an early event in the development of type 1 endometrial cancers. The *BRAF* mutations were found in endometrial cancers with MMR deficiency and have different frequencies in various populations (Feng, 2005).

The beta-catenin (β-catenin) gene maps to chromosome 3p21 and is important for cell differentiation, maintenance of normal tissue architecture, and signal transduction. Mutations in exon 3 of β-catenin result in stabilization of the protein, cytoplasmic and nuclear accumulation, and participation in signal transduction and transcriptional activation through the formation of complexes with DNA-binding proteins. These mutations occur in approximately 14% to 44% of endometrial cancers and are independent of the presence of MSI and the mutational status of *PTEN* and *KRAS*. Data regarding the prognostic significance of these mutations are unclear but they are thought to be associated with good prognoses (Arend, 2018; Coenegrachts, 2015).

### Immunotherapy and Endometrial Cancer

Although endometrial cancer is the most common gynecologic cancer and the fourth most common cancer in women, investigations have revealed that endometrial cancer is immunogenic and immunotherapy can be beneficial. TCGA classification of high-grade endometrial cancers has demonstrated that polymerase ϵ exonuclease (POLE) mutated and microsatellite unstable tumors show higher mutation rates and a higher rate of TILs compared with the high copy number/serous-like or low copy number tumors (Howeitt, 2015). Pembrolizumab is a monoclonal antibody targeting the anti–programmed death-1 (anti-PD1) protein found on T cells that has efficacy in a variety of tumors that are mismatch deficient or MSI high, and this was the Food and Drug Administration's (FDA's) first accelerated approval for a tissue site–agnostic therapeutic. The approval was based on a pooled analysis of five trials showing an objective response rate of 39.6% that lasted greater than 6 months. In the KEYNOTE-28 (Phase IB Study of Pembrolizumab [MK-3475] in Subjects With Select Advanced Solid Tumors) trial, the endometrial cancer cohort had a favorable safety profile; however, the objective response rate was 13% in patients with recurrent microsatellite-stable endometrial cancer (Ott, 2017). Makker and colleagues found that adding lenvatinib, a multikinase inhibitor of VEGFR-3, fibroblast growth factor receptor 1 to 4, PDGF-alpha, and the oncogenes *RET* and *KIT* to pembrolizumab in biomarker-unselected patients with recurrent endometrial cancer had an objective response rate of 39.6% at 6 months in a phase II trial; a randomized phase III trial is ongoing (Makker, 2019). Because indoleamine 2,3 dioxygenase (IDO) is prevalent in endometrial cancer and MMR-deficient cancers, combinations of anti-IDO and anti-PD1/PD-L1 are being investigated (Mills, 2018).

## Ovarian Cancer

### Ovarian Cancer and Tumor Suppressor Genes

To date, alteration of the *p53* tumor suppressor gene is the most common genetic event in ovarian cancers. Advanced-stage and serous cancers have a higher rate of *p53* mutations than early-stage and nonserous cancers. Overall, 70% of advanced ovarian cancers have missense or truncation mutations in *p53*. Evidence suggests that inactivation of *Rb* greatly enhances tumor formation in ovarian cells with *p53* mutations (Flesken-Nikitin, 2003). Various *p53* mutations exist and can lead to aberrations in the amino-terminal area, oligodimerization domain, or DNA-binding domain of the gene. Hence, targeting this gene has been elusive and toxic, but there are ongoing trials with pharmacologic rescue of mutant *p53* conformation and function by using a small-molecule oral drug such as COTI-2 (NCT02433626) (Sabapathy, 2018).

Cyclin-dependent kinase inhibitors (CDKIs) also act as tumor suppressors because they inhibit cell cycle progression from the $G_1$ to S phases. The *p16* gene *(CDKN2A)* undergoes homozygous deletion in approximately 15% of ovarian cancers. *BRCA1* and *p16* may be inactivated by transcriptional silencing because of promoter methylation rather than mutation and/or deletion (Somasundaram, 1997).

### Oncogenes and Ovarian Cancer

Unlike in breast cancer, in which 30% of cases express increased levels of *Her2/neu*, a minority of ovarian cancers have increased *Her2/neu* expression. The GOG has conducted a trial to evaluate the response rate of patients with ovarian cancer to single-agent anti-*Her2/neu* antibody therapy and found the rate of response to be approximately 7% (Bookman, 2003). *KRAS* mutations are commonly found in borderline tumors of the ovary and mucinous ovarian cancers but not in serous ovarian tumors. PI3K, ARID1A, and β-catenin are rarer mutations but are more likely to be found in endometrioid and clear cell tumors of the ovary (Sarrio, 2006).

### Immunotherapy and Ovarian Cancer

Because the clinical history of ovarian cancer entails periods of remission and relapse of sequentially shortened duration as chemotherapy resistance develops, immune-based strategies should be contemplated in women with minimal disease burden. The immune system protects the host against the development of cancer but also creates tumor immunogenicity. Immunotherapy trials are generally focused on the effector phase of the immune response to elicit primarily an antibody response, produce humoral and cellular responses, or cause the activation or generation of antigen-specific CTLs and Th cells. The cancer-testis antigen New York esophageal squamous cell carcinoma 1 (NY-ESO-1) vaccines have been developed and used in a clinical trial of high-risk patients with ovarian cancer in first clinical remission. Overall these vaccines were found to have a low side effect profile and induced specific T-cell immunity but did not delay PFS (Verheijen, 2006; Diefenbach, 2008). Also, antiidiotype vaccines, which try to increase the immunogenicity of tumor-associated antigens by presenting the desired **epitope** to the host in a different molecular environment, have been used to increase antibody production. The Arbeitsgemeinschaft Gynakologische Oncologie group performed a phase III trial using abagovomab vaccination as maintenance therapy and found that it was safe but did not prolong relapse-free or overall survival in patients with ovarian cancer in first remission (Sabbatini, 2013).

A major barrier to the success of the implementation of immunotherapy for ovarian cancer patients is the immunosuppressive tumor microenvironment. Evidence in several cancer types has shown that T-cell expression of inhibitory immune checkpoint receptors is one mechanism by which tumors evade or dampen the host immunity. These receptors negatively regulate T-cell function and include cytotoxic T-lymphocyte-associated protein 4 (CTLA-4), PD-1, lymphocyte-activation gene 3 (LAG-3), and others. To date, there has been limited single-agent activity of using CTLA-4 or PD-1/PD-L1 inhibitors in ovarian cancer therapy. Hence, there are ongoing clinical trials to evaluate these inhibitors in combination with chemotherapy and/or bevacizumab or PARP inhibitors or as maintenance therapy (Chodon, 2018; Odunsi, 2017; Pakish, 2017).

IL-12 is a pleiotropic cytokine and is one of the most potent inducers of antitumor immunity, with multiple mechanisms, including activation of NK cells, maturation and activation of cytotoxic $CD8^+$ T cells, potentiation of antibody-dependent cell-mediated cytotoxicity, and interference with Treg differentiation (Robertson, 1996; Tugues, 2015). Additionally, it has antiangiogenic effects through IFN-γ–inducible protein. GEN-1 is a novel plasmid vector that encodes the p35 and p40 subunits of the human *IL12* gene, and because of its synthetic lipopolymer delivery system it does not have the side effect profile of previous IL-12 drugs (Thaker, 2019). In a phase I trial with escalating doses of intraperitoneal weekly GEN-1 and intravenous weekly paclitaxel and every-3-week carboplatin for patients with neoadjuvant ovarian cancer, there was a PFS of 21 months (Thaker, 2019). The translational data demonstrate a less immunosuppressive environment with the administration of GEN-1. OVATION II (NCT03393884) is a randomized phase I/II trial to further study GEN-1 in a neoadjuvant setting.

## Cervical Cancer: Oncogenes, Tumor Suppressor Genes, and Immunotherapy

Because only a small proportion of women with HPV develop cervical cancer, additional genetic alterations must occur. However, compared with other gynecologic cancers, the roles of oncogenes and tumor suppressor genes are not as well elucidated. The allelic loss of possible tumor suppressor genes at loci on chromosomes 3p, 11p, and others has been noted, but specific tumor suppressor genes remain unidentified (Choi, 2007). Also, Mammas and colleagues have found that the oncogenes *Hi* and *NRAS* are upregulated in cervical cancer independently of HPV infection (Mammas, 2004). Because cervical cancers have mutations in *PIK3CA* and *KRAS*, a single-arm phase II trial evaluated trametinib (a MEK inhibitor) and GSK2141795 (an AKT inhibitor) in patients with recurrent cervical cancer demonstrated minimal activity even in patients with PI3K or RAS pathway alterations (Liu, 2019a). Similar to endometrial and ovarian cancers, gene silencing caused by promoter hypermethylation may also be involved in cervical cancer development. The methylation status of the oncogene human telomerase reverse transcriptase and the tumor suppressor genes death-associated protein kinase (DAPK) and O6-methylguanine-DNA methyltransferase (MGMT) could be used to distinguish the progression from normal to cervical dysplasia to invasive cancer (Iliopoulos, 2009).

There has been substantial progress in immunotherapy options for cervical cancer patients. Stevanovic and colleagues used adoptive T-cell therapy by administering HPV TIL cell product to patients with HPV-positive recurrent cervical cancer. Objective tumor responses occurred in 5 of 18 (28%) of the cervical cancer patients with two complete responses ongoing at 67 and 53 months posttreatment (Stevanovic, 2019). In June 2018 the FDA approved pembrolizumab for PD-L1–positive cervical cancer, defined as combined positive score of 1 or higher; this was based on response rates of 14.3% to 17% in the KEYNOTE-28 and KEYNOTE-158 trials (Chung, 2018; Frenel, 2017). Based on these encouraging results, KEYNOTE-826 was launched, which is a randomized phase III trial evaluating platinum and taxane chemotherapy with or without bevacizumab per physician choice with randomization to the addition of pembrolizumab (NCT03635567).

## CONCLUSION

Cancer pathogenesis is a complex process, but with the advent of high-throughput molecular technologies, a new understanding is rapidly advancing. This understanding of the biology and immunology of the disease offers hope for better means for prevention, early detection, and treatment.

### Acknowledgments

Portions of this chapter were supported by grants from the National Institutes of Health (CA016672, UH3TR000943, P50 CA217685, P50 CA098258, R35 CA209904, U01 CA213759, CA177909), Ovarian Cancer Research Fund, Inc. (Program Project Development Grant), The Blanton-Davis Ovarian Cancer Research Program, the American Cancer Society Research Professor Award, and the Frank McGraw Memorial Chair in Cancer Research.

## KEY REFERENCES

Alberts DS, Marth C, Alvarez RD, et al. Randomized phase 3 trial of interferon g-1b plus standard carboplatin/paclitaxel versus carboplatin/paclitaxel alone for first-line treatment of advanced ovarian and primary peritoneal carcinomas: Results from a prospectively designed analysis of progression-free survival. *Gynecol Oncol.* 2008;109:174-181.

Apte RS, Chen DS, Ferrara N. VEGF in signaling and disease: beyond discovery and development. *Cell.* 2019;176:1248-1264.

Baeriswyl V, Christofori G. The angiogenic switch in carcinogenesis. *Semin Cancer Biol.* 2009;19:329-337.

Boland CR, Thibodeau SN, Hamilton SR, et al. A National Cancer Institute workshop on microsatellite instability for cancer detection and familial predisposition: development of international criteria for the determination of microsatellite instability in colorectal cancer. *Cancer Res.* 1998;58:5248-5257.

Burger RA, Brady MF, Bookman MA, et al. Incorporation of bevacizumab in the primary treatment of ovarian cancer. *N Engl J Med.* 2011;365: 2473-2483.

Carmeliet P. Mechanisms of angiogenesis and arteriogenesis. *Nat Med.* 2000;6:389-395.

Chodon T, Lugade AA, Battaglia S, Odunsi K. Emerging role and future directions of immunotherapy in advanced ovarian cancer. *Hematol Oncol Clin North Am.* 2018;32:1025-1039.

Di Vito C, Mikulak J, Zaghi E, et al. NK cells to cure cancer. *Semin Immunol.* 2019;41:101272.

Fridman WH, Zitvogel L, Sautes-Fridman C, Kroemer G. The immune contexture in cancer prognosis and treatment. *Nat Rev Clin Oncol.* 2017;14:717-734.

Fruman DA, Rommel C. PI3K and cancer: lessons, challenges and opportunities. *Nat Rev Drug Discov.* 2014;13:140-156.

Hanahan D, Weinberg RA. Hallmarks of cancer: the next generation. *Cell.* 2011;144:646-674.

Hollstein M, Sidransky D, Vogelstein B, et al. p53 mutations in human cancers. *Science.* 1991;253:49-53.

Karlan BY, Berchuck A, Mutch D. The role of genetic testing for cancer susceptibility in gynecologic practice. *Obstet Gynecol.* 2007;110: 155-167.

Moore K, Colombo N, Scambia G, et al. Maintenance olaparib in patients with newly diagnosed advanced ovarian cancer. *N Engl J Med.* 2018;379:2495-2505.

Montor WR. Salas AROSE, Melo FHM. Receptor tyrosine kinases and downstream pathways as druggable targets for cancer treatment: the current arsenal of inhibitors. *Mol Cancer.* 2018;17:55.

Munoz N, Kjaer SK, Sigurdsson K, et al. Impact of human papillomavirus (HPV)-6/11/16/18 vaccine on all HPV-associated genital diseases in young women. *J Natl Cancer Inst.* 2010;102:325-339.

Pakish JB, Jazaeri AA. Immunotherapy in Gynecologic Cancers: Are We There Yet? *Curr Treat Options Oncol.* 2017;18:59.

Pasquale EB. Eph-ephrin bidirectional signaling in physiology and disease. *Cell.* 2008;133:38-52.

Sabapathy K, Lane DP. Therapeutic targeting of p53: all mutants are equal, but some mutants are more equal than others. *Nat Rev Clin Oncol.* 2018;15:13-30.

Takeuchi O, Akira S. Innate immunity to virus infection. *Immunol Rev.* 2009;227:75-86.

Tebbutt N, Pedersen MW, Johns TG. Targeting the ERBB family in cancer: couples therapy. *Nat Rev Cancer.* 2013;13:669-673.

Zhang L, Conejo-Garcia JR, Katsaros D, et al. Intratumoral T cells, recurrence, and survival in epithelial ovarian cancer. *N Engl J Med.* 2003;348:203-213.

**Full references for this chapter can be found on ExpertConsult.com.**

# 28 Principles of Radiation Therapy and Chemotherapy in Gynecologic Cancer

## Basic Principles, Uses, and Complications

*Judith A. Smith, Anuja Jhingran*

### KEY POINTS

- Electromagnetic radiation is a form of energy that has no mass or charge and travels at the speed of light.
- The inverse square law states that the energy measured from a radiation source is inversely proportional to the square of the distance from the radiation source.
- Each delivered radiation dose kills a constant fraction of tumor cells irradiated. Oxygen can render radiation-induced DNA damage permanent.
- The effect of photon radiation (low linear energy transfer [LET]) on tissues is altered by tissue oxygenation, whereas neutron radiation (high LET) is independent of oxygenation.
- The cell replication cycle consists of M (mitosis), $G_1$ (Gap1 = RNA and protein synthesis), S (DNA synthesis), and $G_2$ (Gap2 = RNA and protein synthesis). When the cell is not in the replication cycle, it is in the $G_0$ phase.
- The dose of radiation delivered to a tumor depends on the energy of the source, the size of the treatment field, and the depth of the tumor beneath the surface. Increasing the dose increases the depth of maximum dose beneath the skin surface.
- Radiation acts on cells primarily in the M phase, making rapidly proliferating cells the most radiosensitive.
- Normal tissues repair the radiobiologic effects of radiation more effectively than tumor tissue.
- Uncommon side effects include lowering of the circulating blood cells, dysuria and urinary frequency, diarrhea, bowel injury, and fistula formation.
- Cytotoxic chemotherapeutic agents act on various phases of the cell cycle, primarily affecting rapidly proliferating cells, and at a given dose destroy a constant fraction of tumor cells.
- Growth factors or granulocyte colony-stimulating factor [G-CSF] are used to limit the hematologic toxicity of chemotherapy.
- After the completion of the staging and primary surgical treatment, the current standard of care is six cycles of a taxane–platinum-containing chemotherapy regimen. After completion of adjuvant chemotherapy, consider consolidation with bevacizumab or poly(adenosine diphosphate [ADP]-ribose) polymerase (PARP) inhibitor.
- If recurrence is less than 6 months after completion of chemotherapy, the tumor is defined to be platinum or taxane resistant.
- The antitumor activity of second-line chemotherapy regimens is similar; the choice of treatment for recurrent disease depends on residual toxicities, physician preference, and patient convenience. Participation in a clinical trial is also a reasonable option for these patients.
- Often in the recurrent setting, in patients not tolerating adverse effects or schedule, switch maintenance chemotherapy regimen such as a PARP inhibitor.

**This chapter describes the underlying concepts and principles of radiation therapy and chemotherapy as they pertain to the treatment of gynecologic malignancies. The rationale and logistics of individual cancer treatments are detailed separately in other chapters specifically dedicated to each gynecologic malignancy.**

Included with the basic concepts of radiation physics are discussions of atomic and nuclear structure, particles, and nomenclature; radiation production; interactions of radiation with body tissues; the biologic effects of radiation on cells; and the factors that modify these effects. Common radiation sources and their properties are illustrated as they relate to the treatment of specific gynecologic malignancies. Basic principles of normal tissue tolerance and the complication risks of radiation therapy as they relate to gynecologic malignancies are also presented.

Cell growth, division, and metabolism are modified by cancer-related changes in gene expression and protein regulation and by chemotherapeutic alteration of cellular metabolism. Treating physicians must recognize the various classes of chemotherapeutic agents, their actions in gynecologic malignancies, and their treatment-related toxicities. General approaches are to be followed in administering chemotherapy, specifically including the monitoring of patients receiving these agents. This chapter reviews all these factors.

## RADIATION THERAPY

### Radiation Therapy Principles

Radiation therapy is the safe clinical application of radiation for the local treatment of abnormally proliferating benign or malignant tumors. The principles of radiation physics and radiobiology underlying treatment are discussed, but several key therapeutic goals deserve mentioning first. **The dose response of tumor cells after radiation treatment follows a sigmoid curve, with increasingly effective tumor cell kill or arrest of division associated with increasing dose (Fig. 28.1). A similar treatment response exists for normal tissues, and the ability of radiation therapy to control malignancy depends on the greater tolerance of normal tissues to radiation exposure and a diminished capacity of cancer cells to recover from radiation-induced damage.** Thus if one were to treat up to the total radiation dose that causes no normal tissue damage, only a small proportion of a tumor would be controlled by radiation-induced damage. Conversely, if one were to treat to a total dose that could eradicate almost the entire tumor, irreparable damage to normal tissue would often occur. This would lead to an unacceptable series of complications or even patient death after radiation treatment. The therapeutic goal of radiation therapy is to balance attempts at maximum local tumor control while

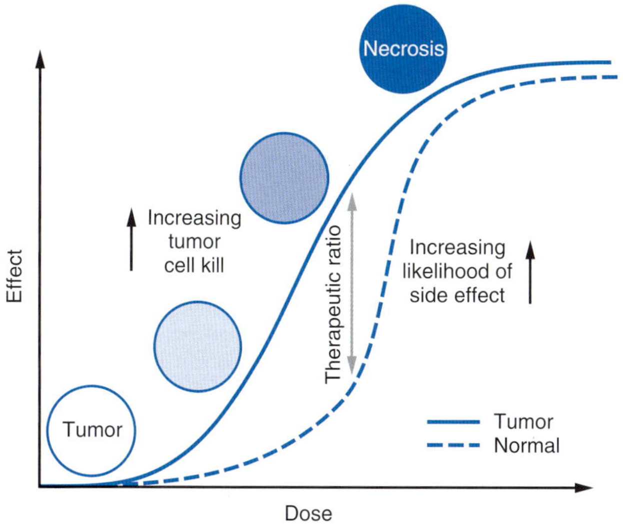


**Fig. 28.1** Therapeutic ratio. The concept of the therapeutic ratio for radiation therapy compares the radiation dose–response curves for tumor control and normal tissue side effect rate. Optimally, the tumor control curve lies to the left of the normal tissue curve. For every incremental increase in total dose needed to control tumor, there is a corresponding increase in the likelihood of normal tissue side effects from treatment. The magnitude of the difference between effective tumor cell kill and the likelihood of treatment-related side effects corresponds to the therapeutic ratio *(gray arrow).* Improved tumor-directed, image-guided radiotherapy planning, use of radiation sensitizers, and use of chemotherapeutic agents (which push the tumor control curve to the left) or the use of radioprotectors (which push the normal tissue curve to the right) can widen the therapeutic ratio.

minimizing adverse symptoms of treatment and normal tissue damage. Basic radiation therapy principles are detailed throughout the chapter but briefly include the following (Hall, 2000):

- ***Fractional cell kill:*** Each radiation dose kills a constant fraction of the tumor cell population. Tumor cell kill follows a linear-quadratic relationship with the potential for cell-mediated repair of radiation-induced damage between radiation dose fractions.
- ***Radiation dose rate:*** Large radiation doses per fraction produce the greatest number of tumor cell kills; these same large radiation doses also produce the greatest damage burden on normal tissues, leading to early and late adverse complications.
- ***Radiation resistance:*** Although all tumor cells are sensitive to the effects of radiation, select malignant tumor cells show reduced radiosensitivity, resulting in slow tumor regression or renewed tumor repopulation during or after radiation treatment. Radiation resistance is associated with (1) enhanced cell-mediated repair of radiation-induced damage, (2) active concentration of chemical radioprotectors, or (3) cellular hypoxia or nutritional deficiency.
- ***Cell cycle dependency of cell kill:*** Actively proliferating tumor cells are most often killed by radiation therapy. Ionizing radiation imparts its greatest cell kill effect during the mitotic phase (M phase) and, to a lesser extent, during the late Gap1 phase and early DNA synthesis phase ($G_1$/S). Radiation has little effect during the late synthetic phase (S phase). Before each phase of the cell cycle, genomic integrity is monitored; if found intact, a cell then progresses through the next phase. If, however, genomic damage is detected, a cell arrests the cell cycle so that the damage may be repaired. If the normal monitors of genomic integrity are faulty, as in the case of most cancers, then a cell traverses the cell cycle with radiation-induced damage, leading to mitotic cell death or loss of critical genomic information vital to future cell survival.

With these basic fundamental principles of radiation therapy discussed, it is important to examine in depth the effects of electromagnetic radiation on biologic systems as they pertain to the treatment of gynecologic malignancies.

## Basic Radiation Physics

Matter is made up of subatomic particles bound together by energy to form atoms. The simplest representation of the atom consists of a central core of one or more positively charged protons (+1; 933 MeV [mega electron volt]) and zero or more uncharged neutrons (±0; 933 MeV) surrounded by a cloud of negatively charged orbital electrons (−1; 0.511 MeV). As Bowland described, four fundamental forces hold these subatomic particles together: the strong force ($10^1$ N), electromagnetic or coulomb force ($10^{-2}$ N), weak force ($10^{-13}$ N), and gravitational force ($10^{-42}$ N). The strong nuclear force acts over a short range ($10^{-14}$ m), keeping an atom's protons from repelling one another because of the similar electrostatic charge. The coulomb force of attraction binds orbital electrons to the nucleus so that the closer an electron is to the nucleus, the higher the binding energy of the electron. As described later, the strength of the binding energy of orbital electrons relates to the interaction of radiation on matter and its subsequent biologic effects. The chemical identity of an atom relates to its number of protons, and this number identifies the atom's atomic number (Z). The neutron number (N) varies among atoms and increases as the atomic number increases to stabilize the nucleus. An atom's atomic mass number (A) is approximately the sum of the proton number and the neutron number (A = Z + N). Radionuclides are represented by the following notation: $^{A}X$.

When an atom is neutral, it has no electric charge, meaning that the number of protons equals the number of electrons. If incident energy is transferred to an atom, an ionization event can occur whereby the atom acquires a positive or negative charge. When a charge is acquired, an atom is said to be ionized. Removal of an orbital electron results in an atom with a positive charge; the energy required to strip an electron off an atom must exceed the binding energy of that particular electron. Addition of an orbital electron results in an atom with a negative charge. This can occur when an electron passes close enough to an atom to experience a strong attractive force from the nucleus. Atoms can also undergo excitation, a process whereby an incident particle's energy is not sufficient to eject an atom's orbital electron but rather raises one or more electrons to a higher orbital energy state. It is through these types of interactions in atoms that radiation therapy elicits biologic consequences within tissues.

Radiation itself can be defined as the emission and propagation of energy through space or a physical medium. Radiation can be particulate, meaning that units of matter with discrete mass and momentum propagate energy (e.g., alpha particles, protons, neutrons, electrons), or it can be electromagnetic (photons), meaning that energy travels in oscillating electric and magnetic fields that have no mass and no charge, with a velocity of the speed of light ($c = 3.8 \times 10^8$ m/sec). Both particulate radiation and electromagnetic radiation can ionize atoms, events that occur randomly throughout the medium.

**In the treatment of gynecologic malignancies, the most common source of radiation is electromagnetic (photon) radiation.** Photons are generally referred to as *x-rays* (extranuclear or from the atom) or *gamma rays* (from the nucleus) based on their origin. Important properties of a photon include its wavelength ($\lambda$), frequency ($\nu$), speed c = ($\lambda\nu$), and energy E = ($h\nu$), where *h* is Planck's constant. A photon's energy (E) is proportional to its frequency—that is, higher energies are transmitted at a higher frequency. Because the frequency of a photon is inversely proportional to the wavelength, electromagnetic radiation with a shorter wavelength has a higher frequency and thus a higher energy. As Kahn described in his textbook on the physics of radiation therapy, the energy that is produced is measured in electron volts, 1 eV = 1.6 × $10^{-19}$ J, and it takes approximately 34 eV to generate one ion pair in water. The photons used to treat gynecologic malignancies can be generated externally at a distance from the woman's tumor (teletherapy) or internally, close to the woman's tumor (brachytherapy). Teletherapy x-ray radiotherapy units can deliver a range of photon energies from 50,000 eV (50 keV) to more than 30 MeV, depending on their radiation source or linear accelerator design. Nuclear decay of radioactive isotopes generates the gamma ray photons used in brachytherapy; such decay or disintegration was measured historically in a unit called a *curie (Ci)*. One Ci is defined as 3.7 × $10^{10}$ disintegrations/sec, which is equivalent to the rate of disintegration of 1 g of radium. The modern standard unit for activity is the becquerel (Bq), which is 1 disintegration/sec, or 2.7 × $10^{-11}$ Ci.

Regardless of the source of electromagnetic or photon radiation, the transmitted energy diverges as the distance it travels from the source increases. This divergence causes a decrease in energy, a relationship described by the inverse square law. The inverse square law states that the energy dose of radiation per unit area decreases proportionately to the square of the distance from the site to the source ($1/r^2$). For example, the dose of radiation 3 cm from a point source is only one ninth of the value of the dose at 1 cm (Fig. 28.2) (Bowland, 2000; Kahn, 2003).

## Therapeutic Radiation Production

**In general, two techniques are used in radiation therapy treatment: teletherapy (external) and brachytherapy (internal).** Teletherapy in the form of external beam radiation treatment produces ionizing radiation through radioactive decay of unstable radionuclides such as cobalt ($^{60}Co$) or, more commonly, through acceleration of electrons. In a typical linear accelerator teletherapy unit, electrons are "boiled" off a filament and accelerated under vacuum along an accelerating waveguide using alternating microwave fields. These accelerated electrons can be used to treat the patients themselves or can hit a high Z material transmission target to produce photons of various energies by an interaction known as *bremsstrahlung*, which means braking radiation. Most treatment machines generate photon energies of 4 to 20 MeV and, similar to $^{60}Co$ teletherapy units, have 360-degree gantry rotation around a patient. Typical linear accelerator dose rates are 3 Gy/min at 100 cm from the source. Alternate forms of teletherapy treatment are available, but they are rarely used to treat gynecologic malignancies. A teletherapy radiation dose can be delivered using alpha particles (helium nucleus), neutrons, or protons. Alpha particles produce a large number of ionizations over a short distance, but they have limited use as a mode of therapy because of their short range in tissue. Neutrons are highly penetrating into tissue because of their lack of charge; they cause high-energy collisions with atomic nuclei, principally of hydrogen, to produce recoil protons that then lose energy in surrounding tissues by ionization. Accelerated protons, as positively charged particles, used as therapy deposit a radiation dose sparingly along their path until near the end of their range, where the peak dose is delivered, the so-called *Bragg peak*. Neutron and proton therapies are used to treat cancer but are not used routinely in the treatment of gynecologic malignancies.

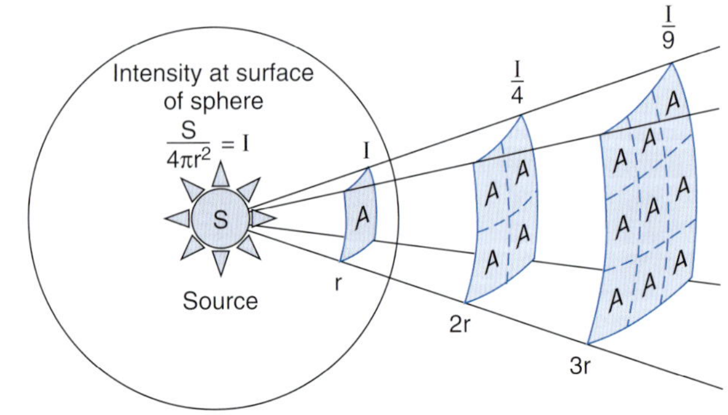


**Fig. 28.2** Inverse square law. Radiation intensity decreases with the square of the distance away from a point source of radiation. The intensity *(I)* of radiation at any given radius *(r)* is the source strength *(S)* divided by the area *(A)* of the sphere. For example, the energy intensity three times as far from a point source is spread over nine times the area—hence, one-ninth the intensity.

To produce a consequential radiobiologic effect in tissues or tumor, incident photons or other forms of radiation must interact with matter. Kahn has noted that there are five possible electromagnetic (photon) interactions with matter (Kahn, 2003):

1. ***Coherent scattering*** (<10 keV) occurs when an incident photon scatters off an atom's outer orbital electron without losing energy. This produces no radiobiologic effect.
2. ***Photoelectric effect*** (10 to 60 keV) occurs when an incident photon interacts with an inner orbital electron and the photon's energy is completely absorbed by that electron. If enough energy is transferred to the orbital electron to exceed the binding energy of the inner orbital electron, it is ejected, leaving a vacancy that an outer orbital electron fills. When an outer orbital electron fills the vacancy, a characteristic x-ray is produced with energy equal to the difference in binding energy between the two electron orbitals. The probability of a photoelectric effect event happening is proportional to $Z^3/E^3$. Diagnostic radiographic or computed tomography (CT) images that are acquired at relatively low photon energies have high tissue–bone contrast detail because the $Z^3/E^3$ ratio is maximized.
3. ***Compton effect*** (60 keV to 10 MeV) occurs when an incident photon (Eγ) loses some or all of its energy to an outer orbital electron. The photon, if it remains, is scattered at some angle away from the atom. An electron that has acquired energy exceeding its binding energy ($E_{BE}$) leaves the atom with sufficient kinetic energy ($E_{KE} = E\gamma - E_{BE}$) to penetrate tissue and produce molecular damage through downstream ionizations. For simplicity, at common therapeutic photon energies (4 to 18 MeV), the Compton effect is biologically most important in that incident photons interact predominantly with cellular water. Human and mammalian tissues are principally composed of water (90%) and functional biomolecules such as proteins and DNA (Fig. 28.3). Incident photons ionize water to produce an ion radical ($H_2O^+$) and a free electron ($e^-$). The ion radical is highly reactive (half-life of $10^{-10}$ second) and can interact with another molecule of water to form a hydroxyl radical (ċOH). Hydroxyl radicals are also highly reactive (half-life of $10^{-9}$ second) and can break chemical bonds in target molecules such as proteins and DNA (ċR). Breaks in the chemical bonds of DNA can lead to DNA base damage, DNA cross-links, DNA single-strand breaks, and DNA double-strand breaks. As discussed later, DNA strand breaks can result in the loss of vital genomic material during subsequent cell divisions, potentially leading to mitotic death of the damaged cell. In this way, therapeutic radiation leads to significant radiobiologic effects by functionally modifying cellular proteins and damaging DNA.
4. ***Pair production*** (>10 MeV) occurs when an incident photon has an energy greater than 1.022 MeV. This threshold is required because the photon disappears to form an electron-positron pair,

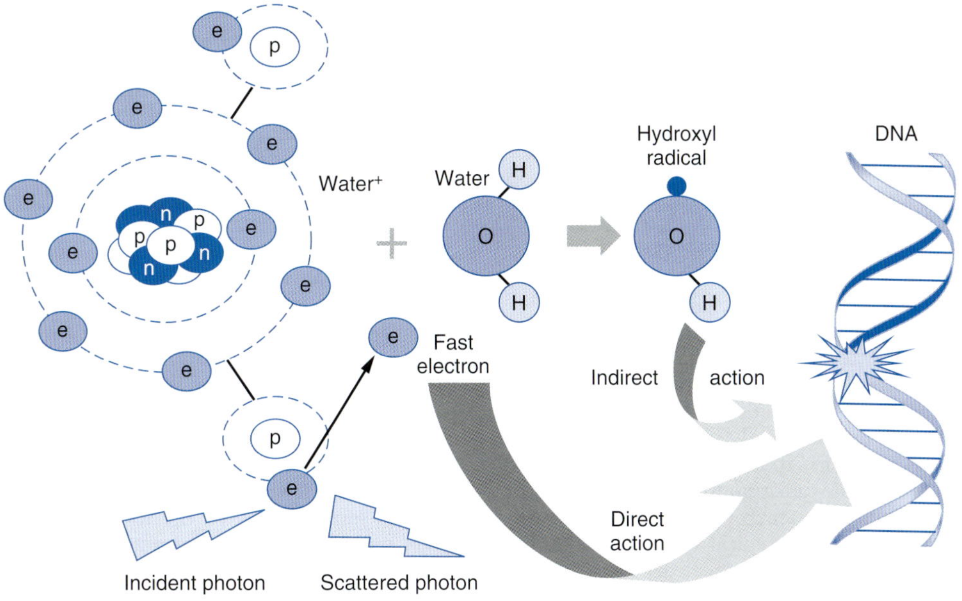


**Fig. 28.3** Compton effect. Cells are composed of biomolecules dissolved in an aqueous solution (≈90% water by weight). Incident photons (p) randomly ionize *(left)* cellular water to produce an ion radical (water$^+$) and a free fast electron (e$^-$) that can damage biomolecules such as DNA. The water ion radical interacts with another molecule of water to form a hydroxyl radical (ċOH). Most often (≈66%), formed hydroxyl radicals diffuse throughout the cell, breaking chemical bonds in target molecules such as proteins and DNA *(right)*. Breaks in the chemical bonds of DNA can lead to DNA base damage, DNA cross-links, DNA single-strand breaks, and DNA double-strand breaks, contributing to the loss of vital genomic material during subsequent cell divisions and possibly mitotic death of the damaged cell. *n,* Neutron.

with each particle having an energy of 0.511 MeV. Once formed, free electrons slow by nuclear attraction and are quickly stopped in tissue; however, the formed positron is highly reactive and short lived in that it is annihilated with surrounding electrons to create two photons of 0.511 MeV, each traveling 180 degrees apart from one another. Positron emission tomography (PET) scanners build images based on the coincident detection of photons formed by this process.

5. ***Photodisintegration*** (>10 MeV) occurs when an energetic photon penetrates the nucleus of an atom and dislodges a neutron. Emitted neutrons cannot ionize tissue themselves because they have no charge; rather they collide with surrounding atomic nuclei to produce recoil, positively charged protons that elicit radiobiologic effects through subsequent ionizations.

## Radiation Biology

Munro has shown that nuclear DNA is unquestionably one essential target of therapeutic radiation (Munro, 1970). **In his textbook on radiobiology, Hall reported that one-third of radiation-induced DNA damage is from the direct interaction of incident photons ionizing atoms within DNA itself (Hall, 2000). Two-thirds of radiation-induced DNA damage is a consequence of the indirect damage done by freely diffusing hydroxyl radicals (ċOH); however, Hall and Hei described a bystander effect whereby lethal damage to cellular proteins, organelles, or the cell membrane in an irradiated cell can lead to neighboring cell death in cells that would not have died on their own (Hall, 2003).** The bystander effect suggests that damage to cellular proteins or organelles in one cell may also result in cell lethality. **Note that not all radiation damage is lethal to the cell; some damage to DNA can undergo repair—namely, sublethal DNA damage repair. Sublethal DNA damage repair occurs in normal cells and malignant cells, but it occurs much less so in malignant cells because these often have abnormal DNA repair mechanisms.** A variety of complex and redundant repair mechanisms have been identified, including base excision repair and nucleotide excision repair for damage to the DNA base and deoxyribose backbone, homologous recombination repair for DNA single-strand breaks, and nonhomologous end-joining repair for DNA double-strand breaks. As the time interval between radiation doses lengthens, cell survival increases because of the prompt repair of radiation-induced damage. The repair process is usually complete within 1 to 2 hours, although this period may be longer in some slowly renewing cellular tissues. Before discussing the consequences of DNA damage, it is important to understand key factors that can modify the rate at which DNA damage accumulates.

**Intracellular molecular oxygen importantly modifies radiation-induced DNA damage as it fixes damage done by free hydroxyl radicals.** Palcic and Skarsgard reported that molecular oxygen, when present during or within microseconds of photon-induced ionization events, reacts with the altered chemical bonds of ionized molecules (ċR) to produce organic peroxides ($RO_2$), a nonrepairable form of the target molecule (Palcic, 1984). Molecules fixed in this manner are permanently altered and may function abnormally. Thus tumor and tissue oxygenation have practical implications in radiation therapy insofar as a rapidly proliferating gynecologic malignancy may have a poor blood supply, which decreases tumor cell oxygenation, particularly at the center of large tumors. Tumor tissue hypoxia leads to radiation resistance, as reflected by increased cell survival after radiation treatment (Dunst, 2003). Laboratory experiments have shown that the radiation dose necessary to kill the same proportion of hypoxic cells compared with aerated cells approaches 3:1 (Siemann, 2003). This ratio is commonly referred to the *oxygen enhancement ratio.* For oxygen to have its maximal effect, the dissolved oxygen concentration in a tumor must be approximately 3 mm Hg (venous blood is 30 to 40 mm Hg), according to Hall

(2000). In the treatment of gynecologic malignancies, Dunst and coworkers found that cervical cancer patients undergoing radiation therapy with a serum hemoglobin level greater than 10 mg/dL have improved tumor oxygenation, resulting in superior local control and superior clinical outcomes compared with patients whose hemoglobin level is less than 10 mg/dL (Dunst, 2003). Also, hypoxic cell sensitizers such as the nitroimidazoles, as studied by Adams and colleagues, and the bioreductive drug tirapazamine, as reported by Goldberg and coworkers, improve the radiosensitivity of hypoxic cells within tumors (Adams, 1991; Goldberg, 2001). The potential benefit of these agents in the treatment of gynecologic cancers has been explored in clinical trials.

The rate at which energy is lost per unit path length of medium, or linear energy transfer (LET), also has an effect on the accumulation of radiation-induced DNA damage. For photons, energy loss is infrequent along its path length, typical of low-LET radiation. Sparsely ionizing, low-LET radiation produces one or more sublethal events, and thus multiple hits are needed to kill the cell. Heavy particulate radiation from alpha particles or protons is densely ionizing because energy is deposited more diffusely along its path length. This is typical of high-LET radiation. Because the probability of producing a lethal event in a cell is much higher with high- LET radiation, cell death in this case is independent of tumor oxygenation. Thus research efforts have been directed toward the development of heavy particle generators that can overcome the limitation of poor oxygenation of cancer cells.

Within the cell, molecules that have sulfhydryl moieties at one end and a strong base such as an amine at the other end are capable of scavenging free radicals produced by radiation-induced ionization events. These molecules can also donate hydrogen atoms to ionized molecules before molecular oxygen can fix the damage done by radiation-induced hydroxyl radicals. As Utley and associates reported, amifostine is a nonreactive phosphorothioate that accumulates (1) readily in normal tissues by active transport to be metabolized into an active compound to scavenge free radicals and (2) slowly in tumors by passive diffusion, with limited or no conversion to the active compound (Utley, 1976). It is reasonable to conclude that the presence of a radioprotector such as amifostine would decrease radiation-induced DNA damage and limit normal tissue radiation-related side effects. Clinical trials have been investigating the radioprotective effect of amifostine in gynecologic malignancies but, at present, amifostine has shown the most promise as a chemoprotectant and has been approved to reduce the renal toxicity associated with repeated administration of cisplatin chemotherapy in women with advanced ovarian cancer.

What constitutes cell death in the traditional sense—cessation of cellular respiration and vital function—is not the same in radiation biology. Death in radiation biology is the loss of reproductive integrity or the inability to maintain uninterrupted cellular proliferation with high fidelity. Thus radiation kills without the actual physical disappearance of malignant cells, although body macrophages often remove the dead cells, causing tumors to shrink in size. Malignant cells may remain a part of a tumor but have discontinued cellular metabolism and proliferation. Most cells, when exposed to radiation, die a mitotic death, meaning that cells die at the next or a subsequent cell division, with all progeny also dying. Inflammation can accompany mitotic cell death, potentially resulting in local adverse side effects. Jonathan and associates noted that alternative forms of loss in reproductive capacity caused by radiation include terminal differentiation, senescence, and apoptosis (Jonathan, 1999). In apoptosis, cells undergo a complex process of programmed cellular involution and phagocytosis by neighboring cells. There is no inflammatory response resulting from apoptosis. One remarkable example of apoptosis is the formation of the spaces between the digits of the hand during human fetal development.

Returning to radiation-induced DNA damage, electromagnetic radiation (x-ray or gamma) deposits energy in cells, which may damage DNA directly or indirectly through hydroxyl radicals (OH). In relative terms, more than 1000 DNA base-damaging events, 1000 DNA single-strand breaks, and 40 DNA double-strand breaks occur with each typical radiation dose fraction. Although base and DNA single-strand breaks must be repaired so that mutations are not propagated, DNA double-strand breaks are believed to be the most crucial radiobiologic effect of radiation therapy. There is an increased statistical probability that a cell will be unable to repair a DNA double-strand break, resulting in the loss of genetic material at cell division. Also, attempts by cells to repair the DNA double-strand breaks often result in bizarre chromosome arrangements that interfere with the normal division of the cell. Cell death ensues through loss of critical genes or impaired cell division.

**Cell death after radiation therapy is modeled by a linear-quadratic relationship (Fig. 28.4). The initial slope of the cell survival curve is shallow and curvilinear, whereas the terminal slope is more linear. In the low-dose region of the survival curve typical of daily dose fractions used in radiation therapy, the fraction of cells surviving is high because of the repair of single-event sublethal damage (e.g., multiple base damage or DNA single-strand breaks). In the high-dose region of the survival curve, the fraction of cells surviving is low because of multiple event damage in the form of DNA double-strand breaks or the accumulation of too many sublethal events that can be repaired before the next cell division. Capacity to repair sublethal damage depends on radiation quality (LET), tissue oxygenation, and cell cycle time.**

As shown in Fig. 28.5 and as described by Deshpande and associates and Pawlik and Keyomarsi, there are four highly regulated phases of the cell cycle (Deshpande, 2005; Pawlik, 2004). After completing mitosis, cells enter a gap phase ($G_1$), variable in time span, in which the cell performs protein synthesis and other

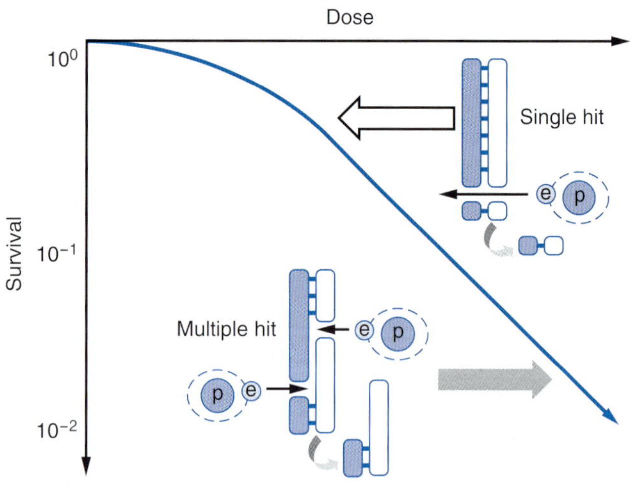


**Fig. 28.4** Cell survival curves. A radiation survival curve plots cell survival on a logarithmic scale against radiation dose on a linear scale. Survival represents the number of cells retaining reproductive capacity to form approximately 50 cell colonies (i.e., approximately five to six cell divisions) after a specified radiation dose. The initial slope is shallow, forming a shoulder in the low-dose region (1 to 3 Gy/fraction) caused by repair of sublethal damage. Occasionally a single hit will produce a DNA double-strand break, resulting in the loss of genetic material *(open arrow)*. In the high-dose region (>3 Gy/fraction), the slope steepens because of multiple damaging events leading to DNA double-strand breaks. If not repaired, significant vital genetic material may be lost at a subsequent cell division and the cell may die. *e,* Electron; *p,* photon.

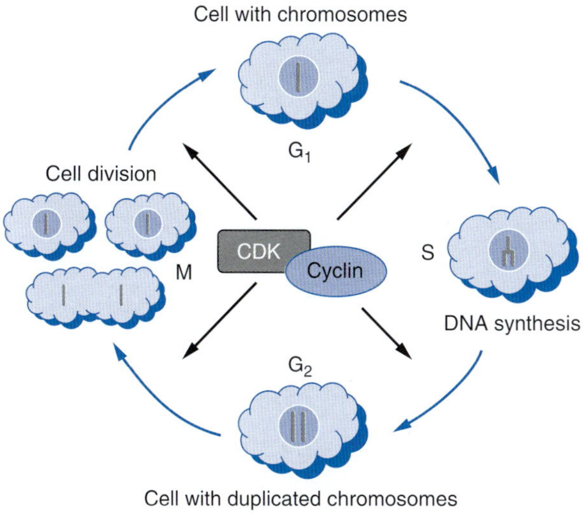


**Fig. 28.5** Phases of the cell. After mitosis (M), there is an interval of variable duration during which there is RNA and protein synthesis and a diploid DNA content ($G_1$ [Gap1]). The cell may also enter a prolonged or resting phase ($G_0$) and then reenter the cycle during DNA synthesis, the S phase, in which DNA is duplicated. During the $G_2$ (Gap2) phase, there again is protein and RNA synthesis. During the M phase, the cell divides into two cells, each of which receives diploid DNA content. *CDK*, Cyclin-dependent kinase.

functional metabolic and biologic processes. Under the influence of complex, finely regulated intercellular and intracellular signaling, cells then enter the DNA replication phase (S phase) in which the cell must exactly replicate its DNA to produce an identical set of chromosomes. Entry into the S phase is controlled by sequentially activated, highly regulated cyclin-dependent kinases (CDKs) responsible for differentially recruiting and amplifying specific gene products necessary for DNA replication. Moreover, there are corresponding cell cycle inhibitory proteins (cyclin-dependent kinase inhibitor proteins [CDKIs]) that negatively regulate cell cycle progression. After DNA replication, the cell enters a second gap phase ($G_2$), in part to ensure high DNA replication fidelity in the newly formed chromosomes. At the completion of the $G_2$ phase, cells undergo mitosis, whereby two identical daughter cells are produced.

To maintain genetic integrity through the cell cycle, the cell has multiple checkpoints through which it must pass, notably at the $G_1$-S and $G_2$-M transitions, as described by Pawlik and Keyomarsi (Pawlik, 2004). The $G_1$-S checkpoint prevents the replication of damaged DNA, as in the case of radiation therapy. Malumbres and Barbacid have reported that proteins critical to the $G_1$-S checkpoint include p53, p21, and the retinoblastoma protein (Rb), all of which modulate the activity of CDKs responsible for the transition to S phase (Malumbres, 2001). Briefly, Rb lacks phosphorylated subunits in its active form, binding to the E2F transcription factors and preventing E2F translocation to the nucleus to recruit genes needed for the S phase. Sequential phosphorylation of RB by CDK 4/6–cyclin D and CDK2–cyclin E complexes releases the E2F transcription factors. Radiation-induced DNA damage results in the accumulation of the $G_1$ checkpoint regulatory protein p53, which in turn activates the CDKI p21; p21 inhibits the phosphorylation of RB, delaying the $G_1$-S transition. The G2/M checkpoint prevents the segregation of aberrant chromosomes at mitosis. Two molecularly distinct checkpoints have been identified, one that is regulated by the ataxia-telangiectasia mutated gene product (ATM) and one that is ATM independent. ATM has multiple phosphorylation products that modulate CDKs at the $G_2$-M transition (Chk1 and Chk2) and p3 expression through modification of its degradation pathway. According to Xu and associates, phosphorylation of Chk1 and Chk2 inhibits the cdc2 protein kinase, blocking cells at the $G_2$-M transition (Xu, 2002). ATM's essential role in DNA damage recognition is highlighted by the extreme radiosensitivity of patients with mutated ATM. Malignant cells that often have mutated cell cycle checkpoint proteins have an impaired ability to repair damage done to nuclear DNA and thus accumulate lethal DNA-damaging events that lead to cell kill in a few cell cycles.

**Cells show different radiosensitivities during the cell cycle. M-phase cells are particularly radiosensitive because the DNA is packaged tightly into chromosomes, so ionization events have a high likelihood of causing lethal DNA double-strand breaks. S-phase cells are particularly radioresistant because enzymes responsible for ensuring high-fidelity DNA replication are relatively overexpressed and recognize altered DNA bases or inappropriate strand breaks. Cells in the $G_1$ or $G_2$ phase of the cell cycle are relatively radiosensitive compared with the S phase. Chemotherapies that inhibit cell cycle–dependent pathways or impede DNA repair enhance the radiobiologic effect of radiation (Amorino, 1999; Lawrence, 2003).**

## Radiation Treatment: Brachytherapy and Teletherapy

In general, two techniques are used in radiation treatment: brachytherapy (internal) and teletherapy (external). **Brachytherapy involves the placement of radioactive sources within an existing body cavity (e.g., the vagina) in close proximity to the tumor.** In the treatment of gynecologic malignant tumors, radioactive sources can be placed within hollow needles that are implanted directly into the tissue to be irradiated (interstitial implant) or within a hollow cylinder, or they can be inserted in tandem into the uterus through the cervical os, respectively. For the treatment of cervical cancer, two vaginal ovoids are positioned in the vaginal fornices (intracavitary therapy). One of the most widely used intracavitary applicator is the Fletcher-Suit applicator, which is useful for the treatment of a cervical tumor or a tumor located near the cervix (Fig. 28.6). **For interstitial and intracavitary brachytherapy, the radiation dose delivery to the tumor and surrounding tissues follows the inverse square law as modified by source and tissue photon attenuation.** With the increased use of high-dose rate brachytherapy, a tandem and ring may be used where the ring replaces the ovoids (see Fig. 28.6). In the past, interstitial or intracavitary brachytherapy needles or applicators without radioactive sources are placed first in the operating room with the patient under anesthesia. After postanesthesia patient recovery, the position of the needles or applicators is confirmed by radiographic imaging. These radiographic images help guide radiotherapy planning. With the increased use of high-dose brachytherapy described later, the majority of patients are just sedated or spinal anesthesia is used during the procedure. The instruments are placed and then the patient undergoes imaging, usually a CT or magnetic resonance imaging (MRI) scans, and planning is done on these images instead of plain films. Once the plan is completed, the patient is treated in the radiation oncology department and then released to go home. The approximately time for the entire procedure varies from 3 to 5 hours. The entire procedure is done on an outpatient basis and is usually repeated three to six times, usually twice a week.

Several radioisotopes with various photon energies and half-lives are used in gynecologic brachytherapy. Although uncommon, radioisotopes with a short half-life (e.g., $^{198}$Au [gold]) may be placed within the woman and left permanently. Radioisotopes with a long half-life (e.g., $^{137}$Cs [cesium]) are placed temporarily within interstitial or intracavitary needles or applicators and are removed after a prescribed radiation dose has been administered.

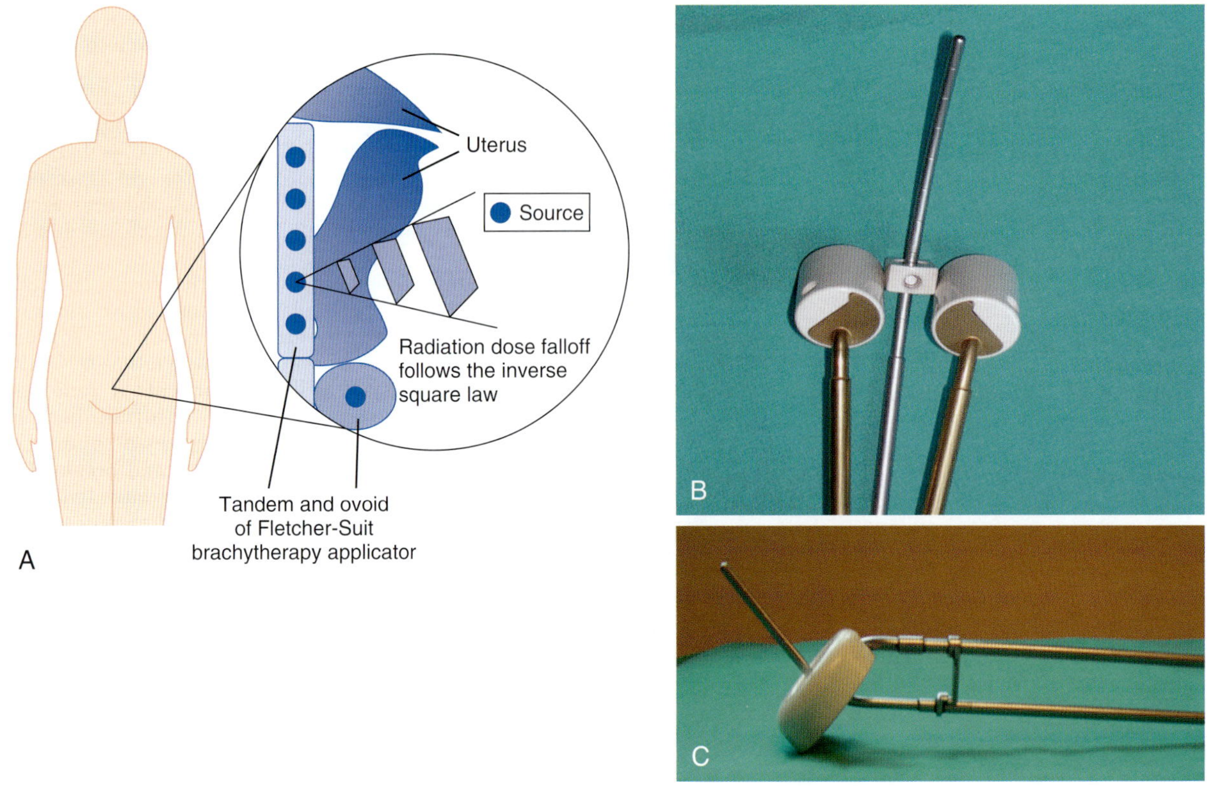


**Fig. 28.6** Brachytherapy. For the treatment of gynecologic malignancies, brachytherapy usually consists of the placement of radiation sources *(dark circles)* in close proximity to the tumor **(A).** This can be accomplished by the intracavitary placement of hollow applicators such as the Fletcher-Suit applicator *(inset)* **(B)** or tandem and ring **(C)** placed within the uterine cavity and vaginal vault or by the interstitial placement of hollow needles through the tissues themselves. The radiation dose decreases as the square of the distance away from the radiation source.

Historically, brachytherapy for most gynecologic malignancies consisted of temporary low-dose rate (40 to 70 centigray [cGy]/hr) sources in place for 1 to 3 days. A low-dose rate requires that the woman be in a shielded hospital room with medical personnel supervision, on bed rest, with prolonged analgesia and prophylactic anticoagulation, and limited family contact during radiation dose administration. High-dose rate, catheter-based brachytherapy has become popular because the procedure can be performed in 1 day on an outpatient basis. The high-dose rate uses a thin wire tipped with iridium ($^{192}$Ir) to deliver radiation doses at rates exceeding 200 cGy/min. Unlike low-dose rate therapy, high-dose rate therapy is performed in a shielded treatment room requiring patient immobilization for a short period and minimal patient analgesia and anesthesia. Table 28.1 indicates the half-lives of some of the isotopes commonly used in treating gynecologic cancers. It is also important that a uniform distribution of radiation be achieved in the adjacent tissues to avoid hot spots, which can damage normal tissue, as well as cold spots, which can lead to reduced dose delivery to the tumor.

**Teletherapy in the form of external beam radiotherapy means that the source of radiation is at a distance from the woman, sometimes located at a distance 5 to 10 times more than the depth of the tumor being irradiated. This distance is referred to as the *source-to-surface distance (SSD)* and is used to calculate dose using the inverse square law.** When using an SSD patient treatment setup, the SSD is used along with tumor depth, radiation beam energy, depth of the point of maximum dose, and output parameters for a given treatment field size to determine the daily radiation dose. Alternatively, with the use of different angles and ports of treatment, the concept of source-axis distance has been introduced; it denotes the distance from the radiation source to the central axis of machine rotation. The woman is positioned so that this axis passes through the center of the tumor, and treatment ports are arranged around this axis to optimize tumor dose. When using a source-axis distance patient treatment setup, the daily radiation dose is calculated using machine output and beam attenuation at the depth for a given treatment field size.

**TABLE 28.1** Half-Lives of Commonly Used Radioisotopes for Gynecologic Malignancies

| Radionuclide | Half-Life |
|---|---|
| Gold ($^{198}$Au) | 2.7 days |
| Phosphorus ($^{32}$P) | 14.3 days |
| Iridium ($^{192}$Ir) | 73.8 days |
| Cobalt ($^{60}$Co) | 5.26 years |
| Cesium ($^{137}$Cs) | 30 years |
| Radium ($^{226}$Ra) | 1620 years |

Conventional external beam radiation is delivered with beams of uniform intensity. **Advances in computer-guided planning and treatment have made the use of beams of varying intensity more commonplace. This approach of planned dose intensification allows the high-dose region to be conformed precisely to the shape of the planned treatment volume, a technique called *intensity-modulated radiotherapy (IMRT)*. The advantage of this technique is that there may be more sparing of normal tissue, especially small bowel, and therefore hopefully decrease**

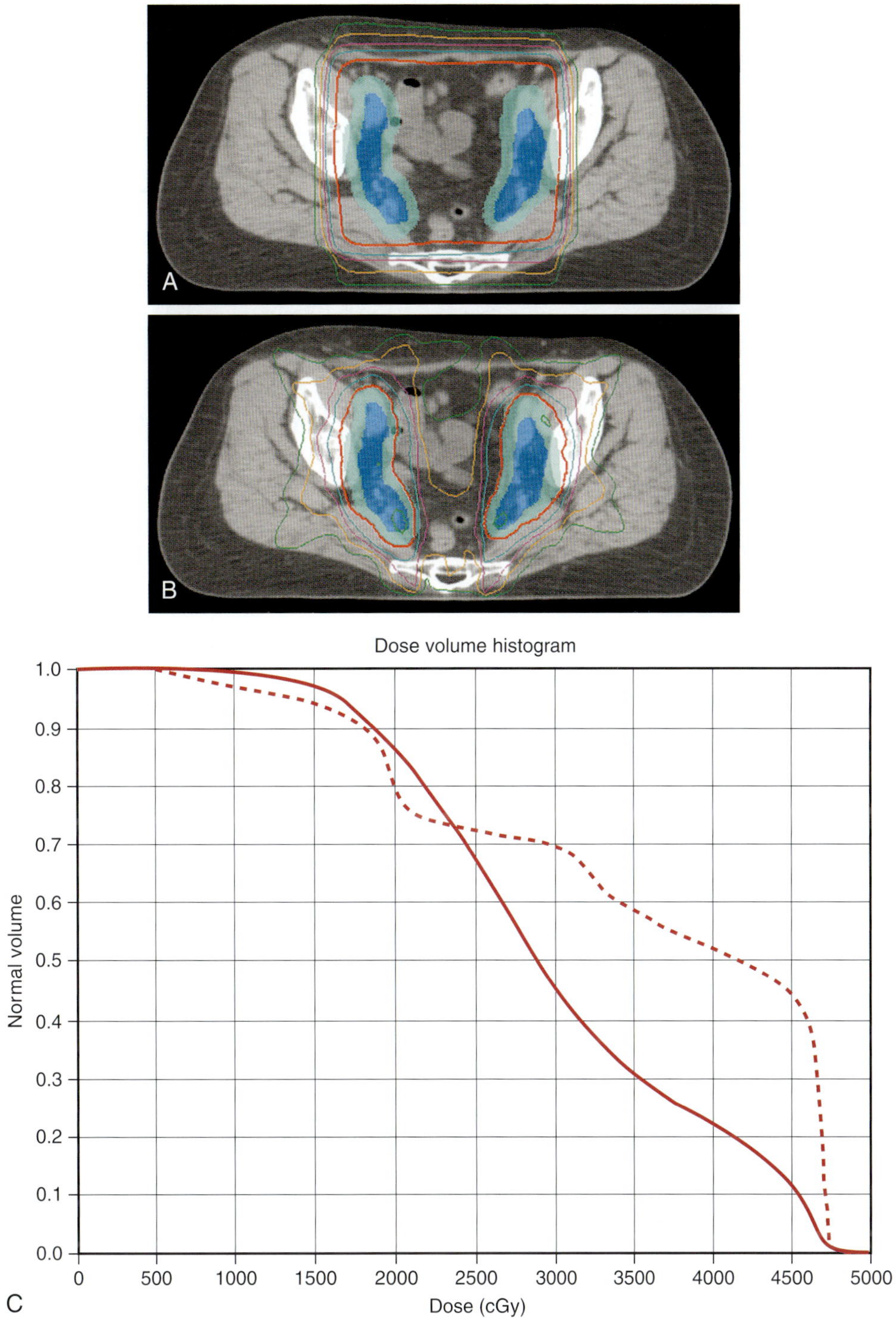


**Fig. 28.7** Treatment plan. **A,** The distribution of dose with a standard three-dimensional (3D) plan. The red line is the 45 Gy isodose line and, as shown, everything within the red line gets 45 Gy, including all the bowel. **B,** The distribution of dose using intensity-modulated radiotherapy (IMRT). Again, the red line is the 45 Gy isodose line, and what can clearly be seen is the sparing of bowel using IMRT. **C,** The dose to bowel—the *dotted line* is the bowel dose using the 3D plan and the *solid line* is the bowel dose using the IMRT plan. As shown, with IMRT, the bowel gets a less high dose compared with the 3D plan.

**both short-term and long-term toxicity (Fig. 28.7).** Advances in radiotherapy delivery systems have allowed linear accelerators to be coupled with helical CT scanners. Image-guided radiation therapy using this type of device is called *helical tomotherapy*. In conventional therapy, and in IMRT and helical tomotherapy, beams from the external radiation source can be sculpted using high electron-dense material collimators. Collimators limit scatter radiation and block portions of the treatment beam from delivering an intolerant radiation dose to critical tissues (Fig. 28.8). In general, the higher the energy source of the radiation, the deeper the beam can penetrate into tissue. Thus high-energy radiation has its predominant effect in deeper tissues and spares the surface of the skin of a radiation effect.

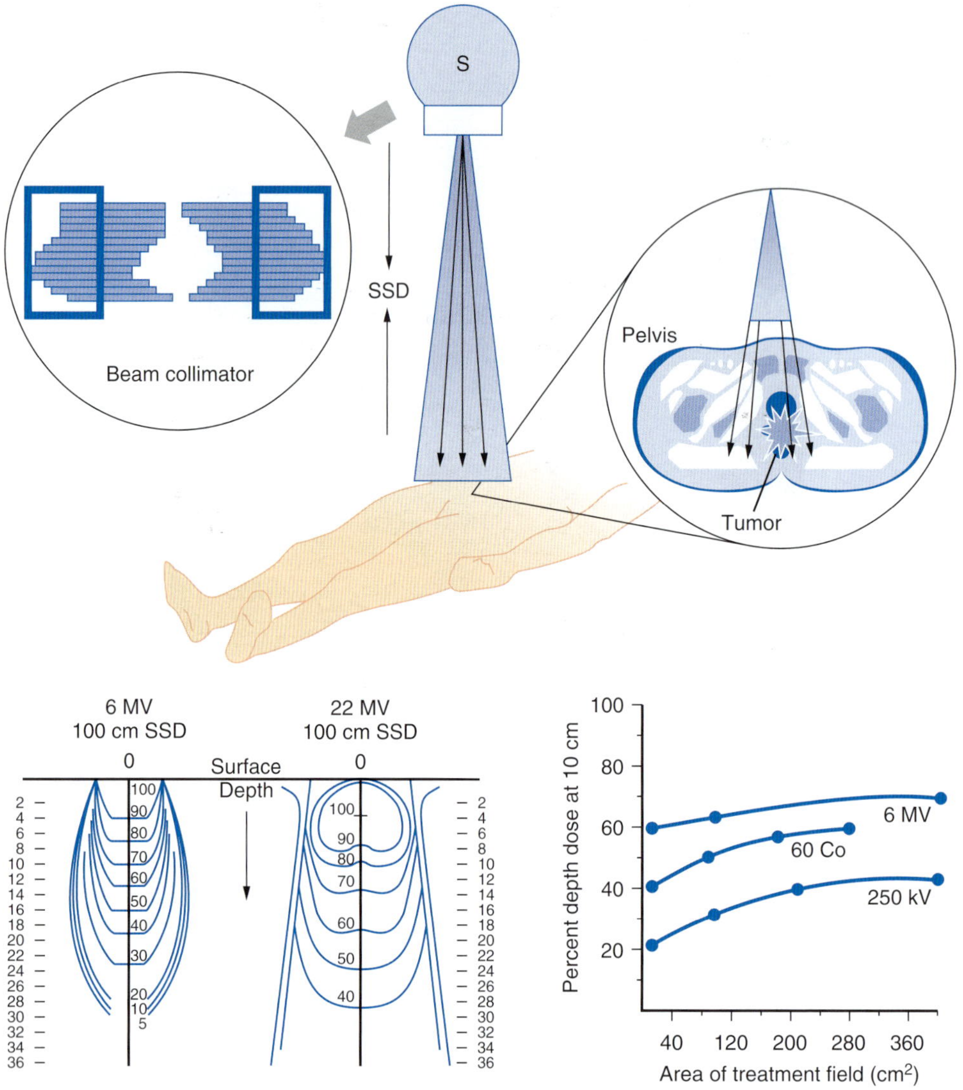


**Fig. 28.8** Teletherapy. Conventional external beam radiotherapy is the delivery of radiation dose to tissues at a distance (SSD) away from the radiation source (S). As the beam emerges from the treatment machine, the beam diverges and can be shaped by high-Z material leaflets of a beam collimator *(top)* or custom blocks. As the treatment beam hits the patient, photon interactions occur, producing ionization events *(inset)*. Energy deposition within tissue creates isodose curves. Isodose curves and depth-dose distributions for 6- and 22-MV photons are shown *(bottom left)*. Note that the higher-energy machine delivers radiation to a greater depth for the same surface dose, resulting in skin sparing. As treatment field size varies, the dose delivered at a specified depth varies *(bottom right)*.

An isodose curve is a line that connects points in the tissue that receive equivalent doses of irradiation. Fig. 28.8 contrasts the isodose curves for 6- and 22-MeV machines. For the 6-MeV machine, the maximum dose is near the surface, with a more rapid falloff in the deeper tissues. For the 22-MeV machine, the maximum dose is deep to the surface, sparing the effects of radiation on the overlying skin. In addition to the energy of the beam, the energy of radiation absorbed at various depths is affected by the size of the field being treated. Larger fields contain more scattered radiation, which leads to a greater dose at a given depth. Fig. 28.8 shows the effect of increasing the size of the field with an increasing dose at a given depth for three different types of energy sources.

Thus the radiation dose delivered to the tumor is affected by the energy of the source, depth of the tumor beneath the surface, and size of the field undergoing irradiation. With external therapy, usually 180 to 200 cGy/day is given five times per week.

## Tissue Tolerance and Radiation Complications

**Adverse radiation effects are commonly divided into two broad categories, early and late, which demonstrate markedly different patterns of response to radiation dose fractionation. It is important for the treating physician to understand critical tissues and organ systems at risk of radiation damage. Table 28.2 presents the approximate tolerance of tissues to radiation therapy.**

Early or acute effects manifest as the result of death in a large population of cells and can occur within days to weeks after the initiation of radiation therapy. **For early effects, the total dose of radiation and, to a lesser extent, the dose per fraction determine the severity of the side effect. Radiation acutely affects tissues undergoing rapid cell division to replace lost normal functioning cells. This is most pronounced in areas such as the skin, intestinal mucosa, mucosa of the vagina and bladder, and hematopoietic system, in which precursor stem cells are renewing**

**TABLE 28.2** Normal Tissue Tolerance to Radiation Therapy

| Tissue | Tolerance (Gy) |
|---|---|
| Kidney | 20-23 |
| Liver | 25-35 |
| Small bowel | 45-50 |
| Rectum | 60-70 |
| Bladder | 60-70 |
| Vaginal mucosa | 70-75 |
| Cervix | >120 |

**functional mature cells. The radiation dose given in multiple small fractions reduces the untoward adverse effects of cell damage on normal tissue and allows normal healing to occur between treatment fractions through sublethal DNA damage repair (the shallow curvilinear portion of the cell survival curve).** During the treatment of gynecologic malignancies, most adverse early treatment-related toxicities can be managed with medication. It is preferred practice that radiation treatment not be interrupted for treatment-related toxicities caused by radiation-induced tumor accelerated repopulation. Only rarely does a treatment program have to be temporarily discontinued for treatment-related toxicities.

**Late effects occur after a delay of months or years after radiation therapy.** Late effects are often the product of parenchymal connective tissue cell loss and vascular damage. **Late effects may be seen in slowly renewing tissues such as the lung, kidney, heart, and liver and in the central nervous system. In the treatment of gynecologic malignancies, late adverse effects include tissue necrosis and fibrosis, as well as fistula formation and ulceration.** In contrast to early effects, late effects depend primarily on the dose per fraction. Fractionated radiation therapy using a daily radiation dose of 180 to 200 cGy minimizes the risk of late effects. Second cancers (mostly sarcomas) induced after radiation are rare (1 in 500 to 1000 cases) and do not usually appear until 15 to 20 years after radiation exposure. Arai and associates noted an excess of rectal cancer, bladder cancer, and leukemia in women with carcinoma of the cervix treated by radiation compared with those treated by surgery (Arai, 1991).

The skin overlying the tumor being treated visibly reveals the effects of radiation-induced normal tissue damage. Skin effects are manifest by reddening of the skin and loss of hair where the radiation treatment beam enters the body. Erythema may progress to dry or moist skin breakdown or desquamation caused by loss of the actively proliferating basal layer of the epidermis that renews the overlying epithelium. This is less common now than in prior years because higher-energy radiation beams, which spare the surface, are used; however, during the treatment of vulvar malignancies, the skin surface and superficial groin nodes are the radiotherapeutic target, so desquamation is more commonly observed. Medical treatments consisting of non–metal-containing creams and emollients during therapy reduce discomfort and allow healing within 2 to 4 weeks after completion of radiation therapy. Late skin fibrosis may produce a rough, leathery texture to the skin in the irradiated field. Chiao and Lee as well as Gothard and coworkers have reported on the use of pentoxifylline and vitamin E to promote healing of late subcutaneous and deep tissue fibrosis after radiation (Chiao, 2005; Gothard, 2005).

**In the treatment of gynecologic malignancies, other sites at risk of radiation-induced normal tissue damage are the bladder, rectum, and large and small bowel. Risk factors for late complications include a history of smoking and body habitus.** The bladder epithelium consists of a basal layer of small diploid cells covered by large transitional cells. Radiation damage to the diploid cells results in slow renewal of the overlying transitional cells that are periodically sloughed off during urination. Radiation cystitis manifested as dysuria and urinary frequency results in bladder irritation. Treatment with analgesics such as phenazopyridine (Pyridium) can alleviate symptoms. Hematuria may also occur. Therapy with sclerosing solutions or fulguration through a cystoscope may be necessary. McIntyre and colleagues noted that ureteral stricture after radiation for stage I carcinoma of the cervix is 1% at 5 years and 2.5% at 20 years, a rare but important complication (McIntyre, 1995). In rare cases, urinary diversion may be required. Bladder fibrosis and reduced bladder capacity are late effects of pelvic radiation therapy.

In the intestine, the renewing stem cells are found at the bottom of the crypts of Lieberkuhn. Within 2 to 4 days after the start of radiation, these cells can become depleted, leading to atrophy of intestinal mucosa. Damage to the bowel usually occurs in the form of inflammation (sigmoiditis or enteritis), which commonly results in increased bowel motility or diarrhea but also, rarely, may be associated with severe bleeding and cramping pain. Less severe cases can often be controlled with a low-roughage diet and antispasmodic medications. Although uncommon, severe cases may require bowel resection or permanent bowel diversion through a colostomy. Covens and coworkers noted that those who require operation for radiation damage to the bowel have an approximately 25% risk of dying in 2 years, with ileal damage being the most risky (Covens, 1991). Those with complications not requiring surgery often have decreased vitamin $B_{12}$ and bile acid absorption. Late bowel toxicities include radiation proctitis caused by small vessel vascular damage in the epithelium, which may progress to intermittent rectal bleeding. Bowel stenosis or obstructions resulting from fibrosis and adhesion formation may occur, especially in patients who have had previous pelvic or abdominal surgery. Occasionally, enteric fistulas can develop, and bowel perforation may occur. In the latter case, surgical therapy is required, usually to bypass the affected area of the intestine. As a rule, extensive dissection of irradiated tissue is avoided. Montana and Fowler have shown that the risks of proctitis and cystitis are dose related (Montana, 1989). For example, they found severe proctitis and cystitis at doses of 6750 and 6900 cGy, respectively, whereas such complications were not observed in patients whose median dose was 6300 and 6500 cGy. Extensive work looking at dose response and late toxicity is presently being done through a large multiinstitutional study (EMBRACE).

**A lowering of circulating lymphocytes, granulocytes, platelets, and red blood cells can be seen with pelvic radiation therapy for gynecologic malignancies.** The stem cells of the bone marrow in an adult reside in the axial skeleton (vertebrae, ribs, and pelvis). Usual external beam radiation therapy treatment fields for gynecologic malignancies encompass the sacrum and lower vertebrae and pelvis, thereby reducing precursor stem cells for circulating blood cells. This is an important consideration if the woman is to receive concurrent radiosensitizing chemotherapy or subsequent cytotoxic chemotherapy. Growth factor support with synthetic erythropoietin or granulocyte colony-stimulating factor (G-CSF) is often required for patients receiving multiagent chemotherapy after treatment with pelvic radiation therapy.

**Finally, fistulas between the vagina and bladder or between the vagina and rectum may develop when there has been extensive radiation damage to the intervening tissues. As a rule, such complications generally occur 6 to 24 months after treatment, although they may develop many years after primary therapy.** Diverting surgery or resection of the fistulas is often needed to correct these serious complications.

## CHEMOTHERAPY

Although many patients with gynecologic cancers present initially with a clinically appreciable mass or tumor, only a minority of patients have localized disease, curable with surgery or radiation treatment alone. More often, the cancer has spread to regional lymph nodes or disseminated to other organs, even though these sites may not be clinically appreciated at the time of initial diagnosis.

Chemotherapy regimens for gynecologic cancers have evolved since the 1940s. Initially, Li and colleagues demonstrated the first successful effort in gynecologic cancer using the antimetabolite methotrexate, which could cause permanent remission of metastatic trophoblastic disease. Shortly thereafter, treatment regimens emerged with single-agent melphalan followed by single-agent cyclophosphamide. When cisplatin was introduced into clinical practice, it added significantly improved activity to cyclophosphamide; this combination then became the standard of care. In the 1980s, clinical studies to evaluate paclitaxel for treatment of ovarian cancer were undertaken. Paclitaxel soon replaced cyclophosphamide, and paclitaxel plus cisplatin became the standard of care for ovarian cancer; since then, it has become a popular treatment option for all gynecologic malignancies (McGuire, 1996; Piccart, 2003). Because of toxicity associated with cisplatin, numerous studies were conducted to justify substitution with carboplatin for cisplatin because of its improved toxicity profile, but controversy remains over which taxane or platinum agent is preferred (Ozols, 2003). Overall, the consensus is that primary chemotherapy should include a taxane and a platinum agent (Ozols, 2006).

Historically, there has been no clear difference or advantage in regard to which taxane or platinum agent was used or which dose intensity was selected until the clinical trial by Katsumata and colleagues. This study suggested that there is an advantage with a weekly schedule or dose density compared with the standard platinum-taxane, every 3-week regimen (Katsumata, 2009); however, there are concerns about the toxicity associated with the dose-dense regimen; questions about the feasibility of this regimen have arisen with the typical older women seen in clinical practice, so a confirmatory Gynecologic Oncology Group (GOG 262) phase III study is ongoing.

In addition to dosing schedule, the route of chemotherapy administration has also been an area of research interest. For decades, many researchers have conducted numerous clinical trials of intraperitoneal (IP) chemotherapy. In 2006, Armstrong and colleagues published the first IP therapy clinical trial to demonstrate a survival advantage over the standard intravenous (IV) regimen (Box 28.1) (Armstrong, 2006); however, these advances in chemotherapy for the treatment of advanced ovarian cancer have not translated into major changes in overall 5-year survival, which remains less than 30%.

A number of general principles have been developed during the study of chemotherapeutic agents. These provide guidelines for their recommended use and administration (see Box 28.1).

**BOX 28.1** Clinical Pearls

- The use of intraperitoneal (IP) chemotherapy as first-line treatment of advanced ovarian cancer has been recommended by the National Comprehensive Cancer Network guidelines. The key lesson learned from the study by Armstrong and colleagues is that patient selection is critical for tolerability of this regimen. Those who are younger, with optimal tumor debulking, no significant bowel resection, and good organ function, will tolerate IP therapy better.
- Patient assessment before each regimen of chemotherapy is essential to minimize toxicity. This includes evaluation of complete blood cell count, liver function tests, and calculation of renal function. Consider the use of growth factors or dose adjustments as appropriate.

## Chemotherapy Principles and Guidelines

Some of the concepts used in antibiotic therapy for infections have been applied to the chemotherapeutic approach to cancer management; however, major differences exist. Infections are often caused by a single virus or even multiple types of bacteria with specific growth patterns and sensitivities to antibiotics. Although it is believed that a cancer can originate from a single cell, clinically evident disease is composed of a heterogeneous population of cells with different cell cycle durations, varying growth fractions, and diverse expression of genes, potential mutations, and proteins responsible for cell proliferation and metastasis. Intrinsic and acquired drug resistance remains one of the daunting challenges in the treatment of gynecologic cancers.

Basic principles for cancer chemotherapy arose from experiments in murine tumor models, notably mice leukemias, conducted by Skipper and colleagues at the Southern Research Institute (Skipper, 1965). These principles include the following:

- *Fractional cell kill:* Each dose of chemotherapy kills a constant fraction of the tumor cell population. Tumor cell kill usually correlates in a linear relationship with the pharmacokinetic parameter of the area under the curve (AUC) for drug concentration.
- *Dose intensity:* High chemotherapy doses interspersed with short rest periods produce the greatest tumor cell kill in rapidly proliferating malignancies.
- *Drug resistance:* Single-agent chemotherapy administration selectively isolates drug-resistant tumor cells, leading to an outgrowth of hardy, resistant malignant cells. Chemotherapy drug resistance has been associated with the following: (1) cell-mediated modification of drug targets, (2) active drug transport out of the cell, and (3) alteration of drug activation or targeting.
- *Cell cycle dependency of cell kill:* Actively proliferating tumor cells are most often killed by chemotherapy agents; drugs inhibiting DNA processing act during the S phase and those impairing cell division act during the M phase. If the normal monitors of genomic integrity are intact, a cell may suspend the cell cycle to repair any detected damage. If, however, these monitors are abnormal, a cell may continue progression through the cell cycle, which may lead to unrecoverable cell cycle arrest or irreparable damage to critical genes vital for future cell survival. Malignant cancer cells often demonstrate abnormal monitors of genomic integrity, in part permitting their rapid proliferation but also increasing their sensitivity to chemotherapies.

## Approaches to Treatment

Chemotherapy is employed in four settings in gynecologic oncology. First, chemotherapy is often given before primary surgical treatment or neoadjuvant in attempts to reduce tumor size and extent of disease before surgery. In some cases, ***neoadjuvant* chemotherapy helps reduce tumor burden before surgery so that optimal debulking can be achieved.** Most commonly chemotherapy after primary surgery is an ***adjuvant* treatment intended to resolve or eliminate any residual disease.** After completing adjuvant chemotherapy in those patients that achieve a clinical complete response, there is an option to continue chemotherapy as *consolidation* treatment in an attempt to eliminate any microscopic or undetectable disease or decrease the risk of recurrence. Chemotherapy is the primary treatment modality used in the setting of recurrent disease. Over the past few decades, with the introduction and optimization of numerous chemotherapy regimens, patients can often achieve stable disease for extended intervals on what is commonly described as *maintenance* chemotherapy. Over time, patients may develop cumulative toxicity during maintenance chemotherapy or just prefer difference schedule or route of administration; thus ***switch maintenance* chemotherapy is common and defined as changing between effective agents in presence of stable disease because of toxicity or patient preference.**

The dose of an anticancer chemotherapy agent is usually calculated as a function of body surface area (square meters), which provides a better measure of potential toxicity than body weight. This is partly because of the observation that body surface area more closely reflects cardiac output and blood flow than body weight alone. Chemotherapeutic agents have varying toxicities (discussed later). A major problem with most agents is bone marrow toxicity, requiring careful monitoring of mature cell and stem cell turnover in the hematopoietic system. Most gynecologic cancer chemotherapy agents are administered intravenously in cycles varying from weekly to 3- or 4-week intervals between each cycle. If mature white blood cells (i.e., absolute neutrophil count) and platelets have not recovered adequately by the time the next cycle is due, treatment delay or a dose reduction is often considered. In patients with a history of prolonged myelosuppression or with regimens associated with significant myelosuppression, the proactive use of growth factor support is often helpful in allowing chemotherapy treatments to continue at full dose and on time, as scheduled.

Additional considerations about the toxicity of chemotherapeutic agents relate to hepatic metabolism or renal excretion. It may be necessary to modify the dose of the drug administered when renal or hepatic function is compromised. For example, consider the following:

- Doxorubicin (Adriamycin) and paclitaxel are metabolized in the liver, and dose reductions must be made if the drug is administered to a woman with hepatic dysfunction.
- Methotrexate and cisplatin effects are increased in patients with renal damage, necessitating a dose reduction in these patients.
- Cisplatin not only has its effects intensified in patients with renal insufficiency but also is toxic to the kidney, requiring particular caution if administered to those with compromised renal function or those undergoing therapy with other renal toxic medications.

Plasma protein binding (PPB) can also alter the toxicity profile. For example, paclitaxel and topotecan both are associated with PPB greater than 80%. When PPB drugs are displaced, the unbound or free fraction of drug increases, which may increase toxicity or the effects of chemotherapy. Furthermore, a low serum albumin level leads to an increase in the free fraction of the chemotherapeutic agent, which is one reason why malnourished patients have a heightened toxicity to chemotherapy.

Various chemotherapeutic agents can be differentially toxic to other organ systems of the body, including the gastrointestinal, nervous, pulmonary, and reproductive systems. The primary toxicities affecting gynecologic cancer patients are nausea and vomiting, prolonged myelosuppression, and neuropathies. Acute nausea and vomiting can usually be prevented with the combination of a serotonin antagonist with a steroid. Despite the introduction of newer agents such as aprepitant and palonosetron, delayed nausea and vomiting continue to constitute therapeutic challenges. Unfortunately there are limited options for the prevention and management of chemotherapy-induced neuropathy other than dose reduction or switching chemotherapy agents.

Myelosuppression is a manageable toxicity with most chemotherapy regimens. Prevention of myelosuppression with the use of a myeloid growth factor (e.g., G-CSF) has better efficacy than waiting until prolonged neutropenia develops. Although not often relevant for patients with gynecologic cancer, loss of ovarian function and fertility is often an important consideration when selecting adjuvant treatments for younger women with other cancers. The goal of treatment is to provide as high a dose of the chemotherapeutic agent at a planned frequency, as defined by clinical trial data to produce maximum chemotherapeutic effectiveness without causing unacceptable toxicity or side effects.

**TABLE 28.3** Response Evaluation Criteria in Solid Tumors (RECIST) Criteria to Assess Clinical Response to Therapy

| Criterion | Features |
|---|---|
| CR (complete response) | Disappearance of all target lesions |
| PR (partial response) | 30% decrease in sum of greatest diameters of target lesions |
| PD (progressive disease) | 20% increase in sum of greatest diameters of target lesions |
| SD (stable disease) | Small changes that do not meet the above criteria |

In assessment of the effect of chemotherapeutic agents, a number of definitions are used to describe the response of the tumor being treated. Clinical response should be assessed on an individual basis, with tumors in some patients monitored by physical examination and in some patients through imaging, typically with CT or MRI. Other means of assessing response to therapy include serial assessment of specific tumor markers (e.g., CA-125 for ovarian cancer or beta human chorionic gonadotropin [β-HCG] for gestational trophoblastic disease) or identification of changes in hypermetabolic foci by PET.

In 2000, an international committee endorsed a technique for measuring tumors by CT and MRI that is easy and highly reproducible. This is known as RECIST (*r*esponse *e*valuation *c*riteria *i*n *s*olid *t*umors) and is applicable for patients with at least one measurable target lesion. The greatest diameters of all target lesions are summed, and changes in this sum during treatment are used to assign a response (Table 28.3).

## Chemotherapeutic Agents

A large number of chemotherapeutic drugs have been used in the treatment of gynecologic cancers (Fig. 28.9). In general these agents can be classified into platinum compounds, taxanes, antitumor antibiotics, topoisomerase I inhibitors, alkylating agents, antimetabolites, vinca alkaloids, biologic and targeted therapy, and anticancer hormones. Agents currently used alone or in combination for the treatment of gynecologic cancer are discussed here.

### Platinum Analogs

Cisplatin and carboplatin are two of the most active and widely used chemotherapeutic agents in the treatment of gynecologic malignancies and are used in the primary treatment of ovarian, tubal, peritoneal, endometrial, cervical, and vulvar cancers, as well as some cases of metastatic gestational trophoblastic disease.

Platinum (PLT) analogs form PLT-DNA adducts that intercalate the DNA, interrupting DNA synthesis. Although its cell cycle specificity has not been clearly defined, cisplatin's radiosensitizing mechanisms include the formation of toxic intermediates in the presence of radiation-induced free radicals, radiation-induced increased cellular platinum uptake, inhibition of radiation-induced DNA repair, and cell cycle arrest at the $G_2$-M transition. For the treatment of most gynecologic malignancies, cisplatin is given by an IV or IP infusion. Cisplatin is emetogenic but can be appropriately managed with serotonin antagonists. Hypomagnesemia is a problem in patients receiving cisplatin, often requiring frequent magnesium replacement. Because cisplatin is nephrotoxic, copious hydration and mannitol infusion usually accompany cisplatin administration to prevent renal tubular necrosis because the drug is excreted in the urine in its active form. Cisplatin also induces myelosuppression and high-frequency ototoxicity. Audiograms may be obtained before and

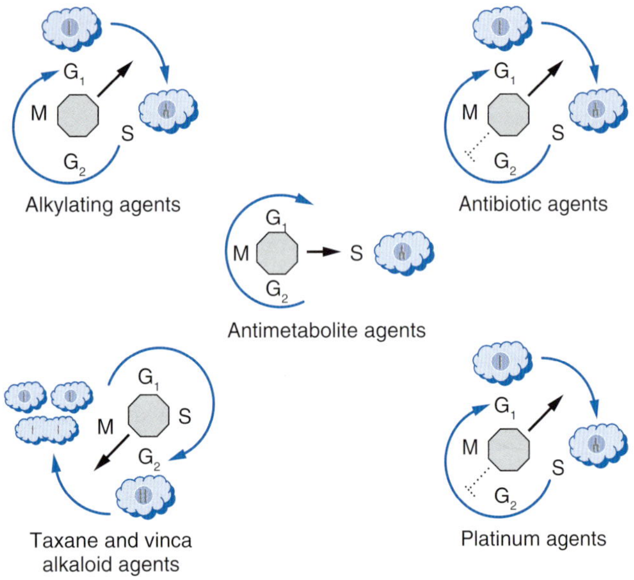


**Fig. 28.9** Chemotherapy cell cycle activity. Chemotherapeutic agents demonstrate variable antitumor cytotoxic and radiosensitizing activities, depending on their mechanism of action during the cell cycle. Alkylating agents facilitate the transfer of alkyl groups to DNA, disrupting the $G_1$/S transition *(top left).* Agents derived from bacteria deregulate normal DNA and RNA processing, slowing progression through the $G_1$/S and $G_2$/M transitions *(top right).* Antimetabolites result in faulty base insertion into replicated DNA or specifically inhibit rate-limiting enzymes such as ribonucleotide reductase that are needed to produce deoxyribonucleotides for DNA replication during the S phase *(center).* Taxane and vinca alkaloid agents alter the mitotic spindle during mitosis, preventing cell division *(bottom left).* Platinum agents show activity throughout the cell cycle and form DNA structural adducts, limiting progression at various cell cycle checkpoints. Chemotherapeutic agents themselves are cytotoxic but also increase tumor cell sensitivity to ionizing radiation during critical periods of the cell cycle in which radiation has a maximal effect. The safe combination of these various classes of chemotherapeutic agents and radiation is an area of active clinical research.

during treatment to assess ototoxicity. Cisplatin induces severe peripheral neuropathy, which may improve somewhat after cessation of therapy but tends to be long lasting.

Carboplatin is an analog of cisplatin; a study conducted by Ozols and colleagues has reported that it has activity in ovarian epithelial carcinoma comparable with that of cisplatin (Ozols, 2003). Its mechanism of action and antitumor activity throughout the cell cycle are similar to those of cisplatin, but carboplatin is less potent in producing DNA interstrand cross-links compared with cisplatin. Yang and coworkers found that the cellular uptake of carboplatin increases after ionizing radiation treatment with a concomitant increase in drug–DNA binding (Yang, 1995).

Carboplatin is dosed based on the woman's specific renal function. Often, the calculated creatinine clearance is used in place of the measured **glomerular filtration rate (GFR) to estimate renal function. Carboplatin is dosed based on a target AUC from 5 to 7 mg/mL × min; the dose is calculated using the Calvert formula:**

$$\textbf{Dose (mg)} = \textbf{Target AUC} \times (\textbf{GFR} + 25)$$

Although carboplatin is renally eliminated because of this dose algorithm, it is not associated with the degree of nephrotoxicity as cisplatin; thus rigorous prehydration is not required, allowing for it to be administered on an outpatient basis. The adverse drug effects associated with carboplatin include neurotoxicity, nausea, and vomiting, but to a lesser extent compared with cisplatin. Myelosuppression, primarily thrombocytopenia, is the dose-limiting toxicity (DLT) associated with carboplatin.

The DLT of carboplatin is myelosuppression, primarily thrombocytopenia, although neutropenia and anemia also occur. Typically, after dosing single-agent carboplatin, the nadir occurs between 15 and 20 days. Because carboplatin's typical dose is individualized based on the woman's specific renal function, it appears to have an improved toxicity profile. It is important to keep in mind that appropriate parameters must be used to estimate renal function to minimize toxicity. Less common toxicities include alopecia, hepatotoxicity, neurotoxicity, and ototoxicity.

Both platinum analogs can be associated with delayed hypersensitivity reactions. Because carboplatin is used more often in a recurrent setting, there are more hypersensitivity reactions reported with carboplatin. There is a high cross-sensitivity, so patients who react to one platinum agent will be at significant risk for another reaction if exposed to another platinum analog. Desensitization protocols with complete histamine blockade (H1 and H2) and steroids have been successful and allow continuation of treatment with the platinum agent.

## Taxanes

Paclitaxel is a taxane that is naturally derived from the bark of the Pacific or Western yew *(Taxus brevifolia).* Docetaxel are derived from the bark of the English yew *(Taxus baccata).* Both chemotherapeutic agents promote microtubule assembly, stabilizing microtubules to prevent and inhibit depolymerization of tubulin during mitosis (M phase). By arresting cell division through a functional block of the M phase, paclitaxel and docetaxel are potent chemotherapeutic agents, with activity in most solid tumors. Although administration of both taxanes can be accompanied by severe hypersensitivity reactions and hypotension, these responses are more commonly observed with paclitaxel because of its diluent, polyethoxylated castor oil (Cremophor EL) and ethanol. Thus premedication with antihistamines and steroids are recommended to minimize infusion-related hypersensitivity reactions. Neutropenia is the major toxic side effect, but sensory peripheral neuropathy is also a serious problem. Bradycardia and severe cardiac problems have been reported with the administration of paclitaxel, but they are rare. A rare complication has been the report of bowel perforation in a few individuals while on paclitaxel therapy, as noted by Rose and Piver (Rose, 1995). In addition to its use in the treatment of ovarian cancer, paclitaxel or docetaxel is being used in the treatment of other cervical cancers, endometrial cancer, and uterine sarcomas.

## Antitumor Antibiotics

Antitumor antibiotics are derived from products of bacterial or fungal cultures. The chemotherapeutic agents generally used for gynecologic malignancies are actinomycin D (dactinomycin), doxorubicin, and bleomycin (Blenoxane).

Actinomycin D is derived from the bacteria *Streptomyces parvulus* and is used primarily in the treatment of gestational trophoblastic disease. It lodges between adjacent purine-pyrimidine (guanine-cytosine) base pairs, blocking DNA-dependent ribosomal RNA synthesis by RNA polymerase. Actinomycin D is maximally effective in the G1 phase of the cell cycle, but data suggest that this drug may act throughout the entire cell cycle. Because bound actinomycin D dissociates slowly from DNA, cells actively progressing through the cell cycle are stopped from doing so at the $G_1$-S checkpoint for genomic integrity, leading to cell death. If radiation is delivered in the presence of the drug, treated cells show a radiosensitizing effect. The drug causes severe myelosuppression, often leading to leukopenia and thrombocytopenia (nadir, 7 to 10 days). Toxicity to the gastrointestinal mucosa is associated with vomiting within 20 hours, stomatitis, and nonbloody diarrhea. Reversible alopecia may also occur. Dermatitis resulting from radiation recall has also been noted, meaning that skin erythema and inflammation arise in skin areas previously irradiated.

Doxorubicin and its liposomal formulation are anthracyclines derived from the bacteria *Streptomyces peucetius*, var. *caesius*. Within the cell nucleus, doxorubicin wedges between stacked nucleotide pairs in the DNA helix and, because of its bulk, inhibits binding of enzymes needed for DNA-directed RNA and DNA transcription, as well as DNA replication. Doxorubicin therefore has maximal activity in the $G_1$ and S phases of the cell cycle. A second mechanism of action noted for doxorubicin includes the inhibition of topoisomerase II in the $G_2$ phase of the cell cycle. Topoisomerase II assists in the coiling and supercoiling of DNA before mitosis by facilitating enzymatic DNA double-strand breaks. Doxorubicin has been shown to stabilize the double-strand break generated by topoisomerase II, thereby promoting loss of genetic material during mitotic division. Doxorubicin must be administered carefully by IV injection because extravasation leads to soft tissue and skin necrosis and ulceration. Doxorubicin is metabolized by the liver, and dosages must be reduced in patients with compromised hepatic function. Myelosuppression occurs regularly with therapeutic doses. Complete but reversible alopecia is a side effect (Table 28.4). Because the doxorubicin metabolism creates free radicals that bind to cardiac myocytes, it can cause significant cardiac toxicity, leading to irreversible congestive heart failure. Therefore cardiac function is assessed routinely before administration, and cumulative doses are kept to less than 450 mg/m$^2$. Liposomal doxorubicin has a synthetic lipidlike membrane around the doxorubicin molecule that is proposed to promote tumor uptake and protect against cardiotoxicity. Cardiomyopathy is less common with liposome-encapsulated doxorubicin, but skin toxicity, notably palmar-plantar erythrodysesthesia (PPE), is more common.

Bleomycin is derived from the bacteria *Streptomyces verticillus* and, when complexed with ferrous iron, is a potent oxidase, producing single-strand DNA breaks by hydroxyl radical formation. Bleomycin may be administered intravenously, intramuscularly, or subcutaneously. It is excreted via the kidney, and some dose reduction is made if renal function is compromised. The drug does not produce significant myelosuppression, in contrast to most of the other cytotoxic agents. It is, however, highly toxic to the lungs in that pneumonitis and pulmonary fibrosis occurs in 10% of patients. Thus particular care must be used in persons with compromised lung function. To prevent this complication, cumulative doses of less than 400 units are given. If pneumonitis develops, as evidenced by symptoms of low-grade fever and nonproductive cough, treatment is a tapered course of oral corticosteroid therapy. Bleomycin is also toxic to skin and can produce erythema, peeling, and pigmentation. It has been used as part of combination therapy, with particular effectiveness against ovarian germ cell tumors, and has been tried for a variety of other gynecologic malignancies, particularly carcinoma of the cervix.

**TABLE 28.4** Side Effects of Drugs Often Used or Being Tested in Gynecologic Oncology

| Agent | Common Toxicities |
|---|---|
| Altretamine | Nausea and vomiting, diarrhea, abdominal cramping, myelosuppression |
| Bevacizumab | Hypertension (DLT), proteinuria, congestive heart failure, increase risk of bleeding, thromboembolism, GI perforation |
| Bleomycin | Interstitial pneumonitis, pulmonary fibrosis (DLT), mucocutaneous toxicity, fever |
| Capecitabine | Diarrhea (DLT), paresthesias, palmar-plantar erythrodysesthesia (PPE), dermatitis, hyperbilirubinemia, fatigue, anorexia |
| Carboplatin | Nausea and vomiting, myelosuppression (DLT), nephrotoxicity, electrolyte wasting, diarrhea, stomatitis, hypersensitivity reactions |
| Cyclophosphamide | Hemorrhagic cystitis, SIADH, alopecia, myelosuppression (DLT) |
| Dactinomycin | Myelosuppression (DLT), hepatotoxicity, alopecia, fatigue, myalgia, pneumonitis, malaise, lethargy |
| Docetaxel | Myelosuppression, fluid retention, hyperlacrimation, nail disorders |
| Etoposide | Myelosuppression, nausea and vomiting, hypotension, anorexia, alopecia, headache, fever |
| 5-Flurouracil | Nausea and vomiting, diarrhea, anorexia, myelosuppression, PPE, cardiotoxicity |
| Gemcitabine | Myelosuppression (DLT), flulike symptoms, headache, somnolence, nausea and vomiting, stomatitis, diarrhea, constipation, rash |
| Letrozole | Nausea and vomiting, bone pain, arthralgias, hot flashes |
| Leuprolide acetate | Peripheral edema, gynecomastia, hot flashes, hyperphosphatemia, nausea and vomiting, weight gain |
| Liposomal doxorubicin | Myelosuppression, stomatitis, mucositis, alopecia, flushing, shortness of breath, hypotension, headaches, cardiotoxicity, hand-foot syndrome |
| Methotrexate | Stomatitis, nausea and vomiting, myelosuppression, nephrotoxicity, elevation in hepatic enzymes, interstitial pneumonitis |
| Paclitaxel | Hypersensitivity reactions, peripheral neuropathy (DLT), nausea and vomiting, alopecia |
| Tamoxifen | Thromboembolism, hot flashes, decreased libido, nausea and vomiting, thrombocytopenia, anemia |
| Topotecan | Myelosuppression (DLT), nausea and vomiting, diarrhea, stomatitis, abdominal pain, alopecia, SGOT and SGPT elevation |
| Vincristine | Neurotoxicity, constipation (DLT), alopecia |
| Vinorelbine | Myelosuppression (DLT), neurotoxicity, constipation, asthenia, fatigue |

*DLT,* Dose-limiting toxicity; *GI,* gastrointestinal; *SGOT,* serum glutamic pyruvic transaminase; *SGPT,* serum glutamic pyruvic transaminase; *SIADH,* syndrome of inappropriate antidiuretic hormone secretion.

## Topoisomerase I and II Inhibitors

As noted, topoisomerases are DNA enzymes that control the topology of DNA double-helix cellular functions during transcription and replication of genetic material. There are two classes of topoisomerases, I and II. Drugs that prevent these functions are referred to as *topoisomerase inhibitors*.

### *Topotecan*

Topotecan is in the class of camptothecins and is used for the treatment of cervical and epithelial ovarian cancers. Camptothecins inhibit topoisomerase I, causing stabilization of the cleavable complex and resulting in an accumulation of single-strand and double-strand DNA breaks, and ultimately cell death. It has been approved by the U.S. Food and Drug Administration (FDA) to be used in combination with cisplatin for the treatment of platinum-sensitive recurrent cervical cancer.

Topotecan is a semisynthetic analog of camptothecin, a chemical derived from the *Camptotheca acuminata* tree native to China.

This drug stabilizes single-strand breaks made by topoisomerase I, an enzyme that relaxes DNA structural tension by facilitating single-strand breaks and subsequent relegation. Topotecan has the greatest activity during the $G_1$-S phases of the cell cycle. Toxicities include bone marrow suppression, nausea and vomiting, alopecia, mucositis, and diarrhea.

***Etoposide***

Etoposide is an epipodophyllotoxin derived from the root of the mayapple or mandrake plant that stabilizes DNA strand breaks made by topoisomerase II during coiling and supercoiling of DNA during mitosis. The primary toxicity of etoposide is myelosuppression, leading to depression of leukocytes and platelets. Other common toxicities include anorexia, nausea and vomiting, stomatitis, and severe hypotension if infused in less than 30 minutes. Uncommon toxicities include cardiotoxicity, bronchospasm, and somnolence. It is important to recognize that oral etoposide has an erratic absorption, with significant interpatient variability, from 0% to 100% bioavailability. Oral etoposide is typically used in the recurrent setting after failure of other second-line agents. Oral etoposide should never be used in place of the IV formulation when there is a curative intent—that is, a BEP regimen (bleomycin sulfate, etoposide phosphate, and cisplatin) for germ cell tumors.

## Alkylating Agents

Alkylating agents are chemical compounds that facilitate the replacement of hydrogen for an alkyl group, potentially disrupting normal function of the altered molecule. As chemotherapeutic agents, alkylating agents interact directly with DNA by transferring positively charged alkyl groups to negatively charged chemical groups intrinsic to the DNA molecule. Examples of this class include cyclophosphamide and ifosfamide. In general, the effectiveness of these agents appears to be similar, but there are some variations in toxicity. As a drug class, alkylating agents affect rapidly dividing cells and are particularly toxic to bone marrow, leading to severe myelosuppression.

Cyclophosphamide and its structural analog ifosfamide are bifunctional cyclic phosphamide esters of nitrogen mustard. Both drugs interact with the N7 position of guanine in the DNA helix to form cross-link bridges between the same strand of DNA (intrastrand), opposite strands of DNA (interstrand), and DNA and cellular proteins. By forming intrastrand and interstrand DNA bridges, cyclophosphamide and ifosfamide impair the functional binding of enzymes used to process and replicate DNA, disrupting the $G_1$-S phase transition of the cell cycle. These drugs are inactivated in the liver and exclusively excreted by the kidney. Their urinary metabolite acrolein may accumulate within the urinary system, causing severe urothelial damage that may result in hemorrhagic cystitis within 24 hours or weeks after administration. Prophylactic hydration (3 L/day) to increase dilute urinary output and administration of 2-mercaptoethane sulfonate (mesna), a compound that binds to acrolein and prevents urotoxicity, can be used to prevent this complication. Administration of these agents also leads to leukopenia (nadir, 8 to 14 days) and thrombocytopenia (nadir, 18 to 21 days), alopecia, nausea and vomiting, and amenorrhea. Therapy with alkylating agents has been associated with a subsequent risk of developing acute leukemia. This risk may range from 2% to 10% and appears to be related to the dose and duration of alkylating agent treatment. They may be administered intravenously or orally but are only rarely used in the primary treatment of gynecologic malignancies.

## Antimetabolites

Antimetabolites interfere with cell metabolism by competing with naturally occurring purines or pyrimidines, whose chemical structure they resemble. In this way they interfere with or prevent vital biochemical reactions.

The antimetabolite 5-fluorouracil (5-FU) is a fluorinated pyrimidine analog resembling the DNA nucleoside thymine; it differs from the RNA nucleoside uracil by a fluorinated carbon in the fifth position in the nucleoside ring, as described by Grem. Conversion of 5-FU into fluorodeoxyuridine monophosphate blocks DNA synthesis by covalently binding to thymidylate synthase. This inhibits the formation of de novo thymidylate, a necessary precursor of thymidine triphosphate essential for DNA synthesis and cell division. The conversion of 5-FU into fluorouridine triphosphate results in the erroneous incorporation of fluorouridine triphosphate into RNA strands, which interferes with RNA processing and protein synthesis. By these actions, 5-FU perturbs normal progression through the $G_1$-S transition, bringing about impaired cell division caused by altered nucleotide pools and DNA repair. As such, 5-FU is a potent radiosensitizer. One advantage of the drug is that 5-FU can be administered as a bolus or continuous IV infusion or orally as a prodrug (e.g., capecitabine) that is metabolized to 5-FU. Common toxicities associated with 5-FU have been reported and include myelosuppression, stomatitis, diarrhea, alopecia, nail changes, dermatitis, acute cerebellar syndrome, cardiac toxicity, hyperpigmentation over the vein used for infusion, and PPE (see Table 28.4). The 5-FU given intravenously is normally used in conjunction with cisplatin as a radiation sensitizer in the treatment of advanced cervical and vulvar cancers. Oral 5-FU (capecitabine) is often used in the treatment of recurrent ovarian and endometrial cancers.

Methotrexate is a folic acid analog that binds tightly to dihydrofolate reductase, which plays a critical role in intracellular folate metabolism. This prevents the metabolic transfer of one carbon unit within the cell and thereby arrests DNA, RNA, and protein synthesis. Cells exhibit sensitivity to this drug predominantly in the S-phase portion of the cell cycle. The effects of methotrexate can be overcome by the administration of folinic acid (citrovorum factor) 24 hours after methotrexate, which replenishes the tetrahydrofolate. Some chemotherapeutic protocols have used very high doses of methotrexate to treat the tumor, followed by citrovorum rescue to avoid severe toxic side effects (see Table 28.4). Methotrexate is administered intravenously, intramuscularly, or orally using a variety of dose regimens. It is excreted in the urine, and dose adjustments must be made if there is decreased renal function. Methotrexate results in severe myelosuppression (nadir, 6 to 13 days). Stomatitis, nausea, and vomiting are reported. Hepatotoxicity resulting in liver enzyme elevation may be seen within 12 hours after high-dose treatment. Therapeutic serum methotrexate levels are evident long after treatment in patients with ascites or pleural effusion because these act as a reservoir for the drug. The predominant use of the drug for gynecologic malignancies has resulted in the effective treatment of trophoblastic disease.

Gemcitabine, a synthetic deoxycytidine nucleoside analog, targets ribonucleotide reductase (RR), the rate-limiting enzyme in deoxyribonucleotide metabolism during the S phase. Gemcitabine is triphosphorylated in tumor cells by the enzyme deoxycytidine kinase, inhibiting DNA polymerase activity and interrupting DNA replication. As a nucleoside analog, gemcitabine is incorporated as a fraudulent base pair in DNA; as a diphosphate, it inhibits the regulatory subunit of the RR enzyme, which leads to the depletion of deoxyribonucleotide pools needed for DNA synthesis in the S phase of the cell cycle. Reported treatment toxicities include myelosuppression, transient elevation of liver enzyme levels, nausea, vomiting, flulike symptoms, and fatigue (see Table 28.4). Gemcitabine is used in the treatment of recurrent ovarian cancer, endometrial cancer, and uterine sarcomas.

## Vinca Alkaloids

The vinca alkaloids bind to the beta-tubulin subunits of the mitotic spindles, blocking polymerization of the microtubules in mitosis. For gynecologic malignancies, the vinca alkaloids used most often include vinorelbine and vincristine. Vincristine is derived from the periwinkle plant *(Vinca rosea)* and acts in a cell cycle–dependent manner, blocking the assembly of tubulin and causing toxic destruction of the mitotic spindle, which arrests cellular mitosis. Vinorelbine is a semisynthetic vinca alkaloid derived from vinblastine. By affecting the late $G_2$ and M phases of the cell cycle, these drugs are potent cytotoxins and increase cell radiosensitivity by slowing the $G_2$-M transition in which radiation effects are maximal. Vincristine is severely neurotoxic and can produce numbness, motor weakness, and constipation as a result of its autonomic effects. The DLT of vinorelbine is myelosuppression (see Table 28.4).

## Altretamine

Altretamine has been used for a number of years but in more recent years it has been replaced with more active agents. The exact mechanism of action of altretamine is not known. It does not act as an alkylating agent in vitro but is possibly activated to one in vivo. Altretamine is metabolized by cytochrome P450 (CYP450) and the reduced form of nicotinamide adenine dinucleotide phosphate (NADPH) to N-hydroxymethyl pentamethylmelamine, which has been shown to bind covalently to DNA. Additional N-methylmelamines formed may also mediate some of the cytotoxicity of this agent.

It is an oral agent that is usually given in four divided doses. Altretamine therapy may be associated with some nausea, vomiting, diarrhea, abdominal cramping, and myelosuppression (see Table 28.4). In addition, a pharmacist should monitor for potential CYP450 drug interactions in patients on multiple prescriptions and alternative medications.

## Biologic and Targeted Agents

Since the early 2000s, there have been major efforts toward the incorporation of monoclonal antibodies such as bevacizumab and cetuximab and small-molecule tyrosine inhibitors such as sunitinib, gefitinib, and sorafenib into first-line and recurrent treatment regimens for gynecologic cancers. Although as single-agent therapy the biologic agents have not demonstrated significant activity against gynecologic cancers, there are mounting clinical data to support the implementation of agents such as bevacizumab into first-line adjuvant, consolidation, recurrent, and maintenance regimens to improve progression-free survival, specifically for ovarian cancer.

### Bevacizumab

Bevacizumab is a recombinant humanized monoclonal antibody that targets and inactivates vascular endothelial growth factor (VEGF) to inhibit the angiogenesis pathway. As a single agent in the recurrent ovarian cancer setting, bevacizumab has had only a moderate response ranging from 16% to 21% (Cannistra, 2007; Monk, 2006); however, in combination with chemotherapy, bevacizumab has had promising response rates, ranging from 15% to 80% (Micha, 2007; Penson, 2009). There are significant limitations to incorporating bevacizumab with chemotherapy regimens because of the high risk of bowel perforation in ovarian cancer patients that was first observed in phase II studies; hence, the current recommendation is that patients should not have had recent bowel surgery or a history of significant bowel resections.

Bevacizumab has been evaluated in combination with oral cyclophosphamide, paclitaxel, and gemcitabine for the treatment of recurrent ovarian cancer. The integration of bevacizumab into a first-line treatment regimen has focused on the benefits with paclitaxel plus carboplatin followed by maintenance with bevacizumab alone. Based on the encouraging results of the ICON7 trial that incorporated bevacizumab into front-line therapy, the GOG initiated a confirmatory phase III study comparing six cycles of standard paclitaxel plus carboplatin to six cycles of the same regimen with bevacizumab to determine whether bevacizumab improves efficacy of front-line treatment (Oza, 2015); however, the duration of consolidation with bevacizumab remains an area of therapeutic and pharmacoeconomic controversy. Bevacizumab is approved as both single agent and in combination with chemotherapy (Fig. 28.10).

### Targeted Agents

Tyrosine kinase inhibitors (TKIs) such as sorafenib, sunitinib, pazopanib, and cediranib also target the VEGF angiogenesis

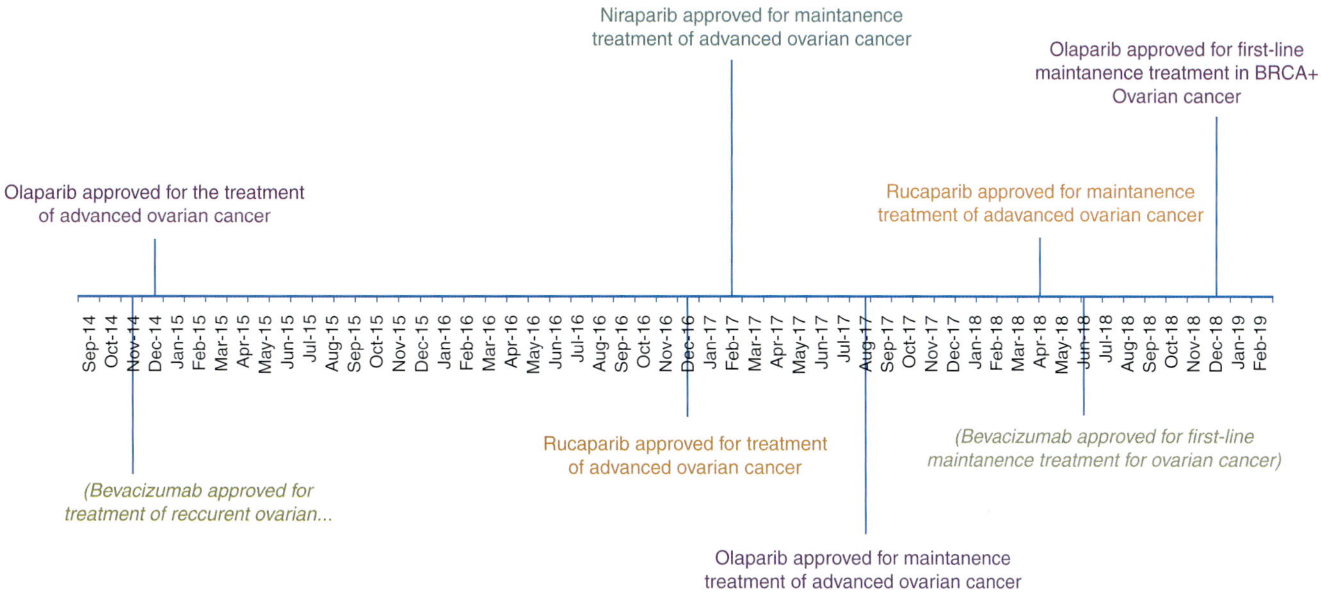


**Fig. 28.10** In the past 5 years there have been multiple approvals for treatment options for consolidation, treatment, and maintenance chemotherapy for ovarian cancer. This timeline summarized the sequential and expedited time of each these approvals.

pathway via inhibition of the VEGF receptor (VEGFR). Research efforts have been focused on combination regimens of these TKIs with cytotoxic agents for first-line treatment and also for the treatment of recurrent ovarian cancer. Another agent of interest is aflibercept (VEGF-Trap), which is a fusion protein that targets VEGF-A. Initial studies have demonstrated that it is beneficial in the treatment of malignant ascites. Unfortunately, the popular epidermal growth factor receptor (EGFR) agents such as erlotinib, which have had so much benefit in the treatment of other cancers, have not demonstrated activity alone or in combination with chemotherapy or with bevacizumab for the treatment of gynecologic cancers. Finally, the newer classes of targeted therapies, such as platelet-derived growth factor (PDGF) inhibitors, are being incorporated into numerous clinical studies in an attempt to improve progression-free and overall survival.

***PARP Inhibitors***

A major breakthrough for targeted therapy in 2014 was the first approval of a poly(adenosine diphosphate [ADP]-ribose) polymerase (PARP) inhibitor for treatment of ovarian cancer. PARP plays a critical role in the repair of single-strand DNA (ssDNA) breaks and double-strand DNA (dsDNA) breaks via the base-excision repair pathway. Three proposed mechanisms contribute to the toxicity of the PARP inhibitors: inhibition of PARP, PARP trapping, and synthetic lethality. More specifically, PARP promotes the functioning of the low-fidelity nonhomologous end-joining DNA repair machinery mechanisms. PARP inhibition results in dsDNA breaks that cannot be repaired in cancer cells with homologous recombinant deficiency such as those with *BRCA1/2* mutations. The activity of the new class of the PARP inhibitors may depend on *BCRA* status or the "*BRCA*ness" of the tumor. Three oral PARP inhibitors are commercially available—olaparib, rucaparib, and niraparib—with drug-specific FDA-labeled approvals as maintenance therapy in the recurrent setting. Both olaparib and rucaparib also have FDA-approved indications for treatment of recurrent platinum-sensitive ovarian cancers.

In 2015, olaparib, the first PARP inhibitor, was approved for treatment of recurrent, platinum-sensitive, *BRCA1/2*-positive ovarian cancer after failure of at least three prior treatments (Kaufman, 2015). The second agent to gain approval in the treatment of recurrent disease was rucaparib. Progression-free survival was increased in patients with *BRCA* mutations in a recent phase II trial (ARIEL2) assessing rucaparib as recurrence therapy for patients with platinum-sensitive ovarian cancer after failure of two or more lines of chemotherapy (Coleman, 2017). Patients with platinum-sensitive disease have a higher response rate to PARP inhibitors compared with those with platinum-resistant disease (66% vs. 20% to 30%) (Kristeleit, 2017); however, PARP inhibitors are considered a preferred option in this setting because of the lack of active agents in platinum-resistant disease (NCCN, 2018).

All three PARP inhibitors have FDA-labeled indications as maintenance therapy options in patients with recurrent disease. Niraparib was specifically approved for maintenance treatment regardless platinum sensitivity and *BRCA* status. The approval for these agents was based on improvements in progression-free survival ranging from 9 to 14 months (Mirza, 2016; Pujade-Lauraine, 2017).

The common adverse effects associated with PARP inhibitors include nausea and vomiting requiring management with antiemetics and significant anemia with associated fatigue often requiring transfusion support. Additional serious but infrequent toxicities include thrombocytopenia, neutropenia, and, rarely, progression of malignant neoplasms. The challenge of combining PARP inhibitors with chemotherapy has been the fatigue, nausea, and significant hematologic toxicity, primarily anemia, thrombocytopenia, and neutropenia. Currently four FDA-approved PARP inhibitors are available—three with specific indications in ovarian cancer. Although initially approvals were focused on treatment indications or switch maintenance therapy in the recurrent setting, in 2018, olaparib was approved to be used as consolidation chemotherapy after the completion of adjuvant chemotherapy in patients with *BRCA* mutations. Almost a year later, preliminary results from the niraparib first-line adjuvant consolidation therapy suggested benefits of PARP inhibitors regardless of *BRCA* status.

### Anticancer Hormone Therapy

Hormone therapy has been effectively developed for the treatment of breast cancer. Estrogen and progesterone receptors have been clearly identified in endometrial carcinomas and have been found in other types of gynecologic cancers, particularly ovarian epithelial carcinomas. Progestins such as megestrol (Megace), depot medroxyprogesterone acetate (Depo-Provera), and 17-hydroxyprogesterone caproate (Delalutin), as well as antiestrogens such as tamoxifen and raloxifene, have been used in the treatment of endometrial carcinomas and seem to have their best effects against well-differentiated tumors.

## Drug Resistance

A daunting challenge is overcoming drug resistance, which occurs fairly often in the recurrent setting of all gynecologic malignancies. Platinum sensitivity is defined by a disease-free interval longer than 6 months after treatment with a platinum agent. If they are platinum sensitive, patients can be retreated with a platinum agent, which usually will be single-agent carboplatin because it is tolerated better. **Platinum resistance is present when there is tumor progression while receiving a platinum agent or disease relapse within less than 6 months after the completion of chemotherapy, and alternative agents must be considered.** Taxane resistance follows the same parameters.

The optimal chemotherapeutic agent or regimen in the treatment of platinum-resistant disease is currently unknown. Ideally the agent should be active in gynecologic cancer and should be non–cross resistant with taxanes or platinum agents. Overall, regardless of the agent, the response rate is low for all the agents in platinum-refractory (resistant) cancer. Typically it is recommended to give three cycles before evaluation for response to the new agent unless there is a more than 50% doubling of CA-125. Because tumor regression is so rare in the recurrent setting, even achieving stable disease is considered a treatment success. **If no response is observed after three cycles, an alternative chemotherapy regimen may be selected.**

## Evaluation of New Agents

In the development of new oncology drugs, serial evaluations are necessary to assess the effectiveness of the drug and ascertain its toxicity. A number of trials are necessary to move a new agent from the point of evaluation to allow it to be used in regular medical practice. Unlike other areas of drug development, clinical trials for cytotoxic agents can only be conducted in those with active cancer, often those who have already failed current standard therapy treatment options.

A standard method commonly used to measure a patient's general functional condition before enrollment in clinical chemotherapy trials of new agents is the Karnofsky Performance Status Scale (Table 28.5). In general, patients are poor candidates from clinical trials if their score is 50 or less. Cooperative research groups, such as the GOG, have modified the Karnofsky scoring system to reflect a five-point graded classification.

After extensive preclinical evaluation, investigational new drug (IND) applications are filed to move new drugs into human studies. The human clinical trial process is a fairly rigorous and

TABLE 28.5 Assessment of Performance Status

| Score | Karnofsky Performance Status Scale |
|---|---|
| 100 | Normal, no complaints; no evidence of disease |
| 90 | Able to carry on normal activity; minor signs or symptoms of disease |
| 80 | Normal activity with effort; some signs or symptoms of disease |
| 70 | Cares for self but unable to carry on normal activity or do active work |
| 60 | Requires occasional assistance but is able to care for most personal needs |
| 50 | Requires considerable assistance and frequent medical care |
| 40 | Disabled; requires special care and assistance |
| 30 | Severely disabled; hospitalization indicated, although death not imminent |
| 20 | Very sick; hospitalization necessary; active support treatment necessary |
| 10 | Moribund; fatal process progressing rapidly |
| 0 | Dead |
| **Grade** | **Gynecologic Oncology Group Performance Status Scale** |
| 1 | Fully active, able to carry on all predisease performance without restriction |
| 2 | Restricted in physically strenuous activity but ambulatory and able to carry out work of a light or sedentary nature (e.g., light housework, office work) |
| 3 | Capable of only limited self-care, confined to bed or chair >50% of waking hours |
| 4 | Completely disabled; cannot carry on any self-care; totally confined to bed or chair |
| 5 | Dead |

costly process to determine not only safety and efficacy but also improvement over the current standard of care for each new agent proposed, sometimes alone or in various combination regimens. A general outline of phase trials is as follows:

- *Phase I trial:* A phase I trial tests new drugs at various doses to evaluate toxicity and determine tolerance to the drug. At the various doses tested, some therapeutic effects may be observed, although this is not the primary aim of the trial.
- *Phase II trial:* A phase II trial tests the therapeutic effectiveness and extent of toxicity of the drug at doses expected to be effective against a specific tumor type.
- *Phase III trial:* A phase III trial compares new treatment therapies against the current treatment standard of care. For example, this trial design assesses whether a new drug therapy is superior, equivalent, or inferior to the chemotherapeutic agent currently used.

Numerous programs have been implemented to facilitate drug approval and access to investigational drugs, such as the Fast Track Drug Approval Program and Orphan Drug Approval. Special consideration for either program requires preapplication and approval by the FDA. Often, in the gynecologic oncology setting, FDA approval for new gynecologic indications is not sought because of small patient populations and the inability to conduct phase III studies in a timely fashion. Compendia listings are often granted based on peer-reviewed published literature, which expands reimbursement for treatment recommendations.

Progress has been slow and unsuccessful in finding a cure for ovarian cancer and recurrent endometrial or cervical cancers. In the absence of a curative treatment for recurrent disease, selecting an investigational trial treatment still remains the best option for ovarian cancer patients. Research is needed to identify and develop new approaches for preventing recurrence and new options for treating advanced primary and recurrent disease. Efforts should especially focus on agents to modulate or overcome drug resistance or new molecular targets to optimize chemotherapy outcomes.

## REFERENCES


Amorino GP, Freeman ML, Carbone DP, et al. Radiopotentiation by the oral platinum agent, JM216: role of repair inhibition. *Int J Radiat Oncol Biol Phys.* 1999;44:399–405.

Armstrong DK, Bundy B, Wenzel L, et al. Intraperitoneal cisplatin and paclitaxel in ovarian cancer. *N Engl J Med.* 2006;354:34–43.

Cannistra SA, Matulonis UA, Penson RT, et al. Phase II study of bevacizumab in patients with platinum-resistant ovarian cancer or peritoneal serous cancer. *J Clin Oncol.* 2007;25:5180–5186.

Coleman RL, Oza AM, Lorusso D, et al. Rucaparib in relapsed, platinum-sensitive high-grade ovarian carcinoma (ARIEL2 Part 1): an international, multicentre, open-label, phase 2 trial. *Lancet Oncol.* 2017;18:75–87.

Covens A, Thomas G, DePetrillo A, et al. The prognostic importance of site and type of radiation-induced bowel injury in patients requiring surgical management. *Gynecol Oncol.* 1991;43:270–274.

Dunst J, Kuhnt T, Strauss HG, et al. Anemia in cervical cancers: impact on survival, patterns of relapse, and association with hypoxia and angiogenesis. *Int J Radiat Oncol Biol Phys.* 2003;56:778–787.

Hall EJ, Hei TK. Genomic instability and bystander effects induced by high-LET radiation. *Oncogene.* 2003;22:7034–7042.

Jonathan EC, Bernhard EJ, McKenna WG. How does radiation kill cells? *Curr Opin Chem Biol.* 1999;3:77–83.

Katsumata N, Yasuda M, Takahashi F, et al. Dose-dense paclitaxel once a week in combination with carboplatin every 3 weeks for advanced ovarian cancer: a phase 3, open-label, randomized controlled trial. *Lancet.* 2009;374:1331–1338.

Kaufman B, Shapira-Frommer R, Schmutzler RK, et al. Olaparib monotherapy in patients with advanced cancer and a germline BRCA1/2 mutation. *J Clin Oncol.* 2015;33:244–250.

Lawrence TS, Blackstock AW, McGinn C. The mechanism of action of radiosensitization of conventional chemotherapeutic agents. *Semin Radiat Oncol.* 2003;13:13–21.

McIntyre JF, Eifel PJ, Levenback C, et al. Ureteral stricture as a late complication of radiotherapy for stage IB carcinoma of the uterine cervix. *Cancer.* 1995;75:836–843.

Micha JP, Goldstein BH, Rettenmaier MA, et al. A phase II study of outpatient first-line paclitaxel, carboplatin, and bevacizumab for advanced-stage epithelial ovarian, peritoneal, and fallopian tube cancer. *Int J Gynecol Cancer.* 2007;17:771–776.

Mirza MR, Monk BJ, Herrstedt J, et al. Niraparib maintenance therapy in platinum-sensitive, recurrent ovarian cancer. *N Engl J Med.* 2016; 375:2154–2164.

Monk BJ, Han E, Josephs-Cowan CA, et al. Salvage bevacizumab (rhuMAB VEGF)-based therapy after multiple prior cytotoxic regimens in advanced refractory epithelial ovarian cancer. *Gynecol Oncol.* 2006;102:140–144.

Montana GS, Fowler WC. Carcinoma of the cervix: analysis of bladder and rectal radiation dose and complications. *Int J Radiat Oncol Biol Phys.* 1989;16:95–100.

National Comprehensive Cancer Network (NCCN). *Practice Guidelines in Oncology—Ovarian Cancer, V2.* 2018. Available at http://www.nccn.org. Accessed February 18, 2018.

Oza AM, Cook AD, Pfisterer J, et al. Standard chemotherapy with or without bevacizumab for women with newly diagnosed ovarian cancer (ICON7): overall survival results of a phase 3 randomised trial. *Lancet Oncol.* 2015;16:928–936.

Ozols RF, Bundy BN, Greer BE, et al. Phase III trial of carboplatin and paclitaxel compared with cisplatin and paclitaxel in patients with optimally resected stage III ovarian cancer: a Gynecologic Oncology Group study. *J Clin Oncol.* 2003;21:3194–3200.

Pawlik TM, Keyomarsi K. Role of cell cycle in mediating sensitivity to radiotherapy. *Int J Radiat Oncol Biol Phys.* 2004;59:928–942.

Penson RT, Dizon DS, Cannistra SA, et al. Phase II study of carboplatin, paclitaxel, and bevacizumab with maintenance bevacizumab as

first-line chemotherapy for advanced mullerian tumors. *J Clin Oncol.* 2009;28:154–159.
Pujade-Lauraine E, Ledermann JA, Selle F, et al. Olaparib tablets as maintenance therapy in patients with platinum-sensitive, relapsed ovarian cancer and a BRCA1/2 mutation (SOLO2/ENGOT-Ov21): a double-blind, randomised, placebo-controlled, phase 3 trial. *Lancet Oncol.* 2017;18:1274–1284.
Siemann DW, Shi W. Targeting the tumor blood vessel network to enhance the efficacy of radiation therapy. *Semin Radiat Oncol.* 2003;13:53–61.
Xu B, Kim ST, Lim DS, et al. Two molecularly distinct G(2)/M checkpoints are induced by ionizing irradiation. *Mol Cell Biol.* 2002;22:1049–1059.

**Suggested readings for this chapter can be found on ExpertConsult.com.**

# 29 Intraepithelial Neoplasia of the Lower Genital Tract (Cervix, Vagina, Vulva)

## Etiology, Screening, Diagnosis, Management

*Mila Pontremoli Salcedo, Natacha Phoolcharoen, Kathleen M. Schmeler*

### KEY POINTS

- Human papillomavirus (HPV) infection is the cause of virtually all cases of cervical dysplasia/cancer and many cases of vaginal and vulvar dysplasia/cancer.
- The majority of HPV infections regress spontaneously, but if the infection persists, dysplasia and cancer may develop.
- Smoking increases the likelihood that an HPV infection will persist or progress.
- Preventive vaccines are available that prevent HPV infection and the development of dysplasia and cancer.
- When Papanicolaou (Pap) testing is used widely, it decreases the incidence of cervical cancer by approximately 50% to 70%.
- The Bethesda System terminology is used for the reporting of cervical cytologic specimens.
- Colposcopy is used to evaluate women with abnormal Pap tests and/or positive HPV tests.
- In some cases an HPV infection can lead to a precancerous lesions of the cervix, called cervical intraepithelial neoplasia (CIN) or squamous intraepithelial lesion (SIL). CIN is graded as 1, 2, or 3 depending on the depth of the epithelial thickness involved.
- CIN 1 should be observed rather than treated because it usually regresses spontaneously.
- Excisional treatment is preferred for histologic HSIL (CIN 2 or CIN 3) in the United States and is recommended for adenocarcinoma in situ (AIS).

## INTRODUCTION

Cervical cancer is one of the leading causes of cancer and cancer-related deaths among women worldwide, with an estimated 570,000 new cases and 311,000 deaths annually (IARC GLOBOCAN, 2018). In May 2018, the director-general of the World Health Organization (WHO) announced a global call to action toward the elimination of cervical cancer (WHO, 2018). The focus of this initiative is on low- and middle-income countries (LMICs), where more than 85% of cervical cancer cases and deaths occur primarily because of a lack of organized screening programs (Bray, 2018). Cervical cancer was previously the leading cause of cancer-related death among women in the United States; however, the incidence and mortality has decreased by approximately 70% over the past 40 years. This decline largely is due to the introduction in 1941 of the Papanicolaou (Pap) test, which led to a systemic effort to detect early cervical cancer and precancerous lesions (Papanicolaou, 1941); however, cervical cancer continues to be the first or second leading cause of cancer and cancer-related death among women in LMICs and many underserved parts of the United States because of the lack of organized screening and early detection programs. Cervical cancer is a preventable disease, with excellent tools for prevention (vaccination) and screening (Pap and **human papillomavirus [HPV]** testing). Furthermore, there is a treatable preinvasive phase that lasts several years before progressing to invasive cancer.

## ETIOLOGY: HUMAN PAPILLOMAVIRUS

Virtually all cases of cervical cancer are caused by **persistent infection with high-risk types of the HPV** (Walboomers, 1999). HPV is the most common sexually transmitted infection, and it is estimated that approximately 80% of women will be infected with HPV at some point in their lifetime. The initial infection usually occurs during adolescence or early adulthood, with the majority of women clearing the infection within 18 to 24 months (Chesson, 2014; Moscicki, 1998, 2004, 2008; Wheeler, 1996); however, in 3% to 5% of women the HPV infection persists and they develop significant preinvasive disease, and in less than 1% of all women invasive cancer develops. HPV infection is therefore necessary but not sufficient for cervical cancer development. HPV infection is also the causative agent of other malignancies, including cancer of the oropharynx, anus, penis, vulva, and vagina.

HPV is a double-stranded DNA virus that replicates within epithelial cells (Chang, 1990; Wolf, 2001). To date more than 120 HPV types have been identified, and approximately 40 HPV types are known to infect the genital tracts of men and women. Of these, approximately a dozen are considered high-risk types, with HPV-16 and -18 being responsible for more than 70% of cervical cancers. High-risk HPV causes neoplastic cellular changes when viral DNA becomes integrated into the host cell genome. When this happens, certain repressor areas of the viral genome are lost. Consistently, the loss of these control mechanisms allows for the expression of the viral E6 and E7 genes. The production of oncoproteins results in the inactivation of the p53 and retinoblastoma tumor suppressors (Munger, 2004). These changes are believed to lead to cell immortalization and rapid cell proliferation; however, in most cases the transformed cells are managed by the individual's immune system and the infection clears or intraepithelial neoplasia regresses. In some women the transformed cells replicate, and if left untreated, a cancer can develop after a period of several years.

## RISK FACTORS

In the United States, cervical cancer is most commonly diagnosed between ages 35 and 44 years (American Cancer Society,

2019). The lifetime risk of developing cervical cancer by age 74 is 0.9% in high-income countries (HICs) compared with 1.6% in LMICs. Similarly, the lifetime risk of death from cervical cancer is 0.3% in HICs compared with 0.9% in LMICs (Torre, 2015). Despite widespread infection with HPV, most women do not develop cervical cancer (Fig. 29.1). The search for a predictive measure to distinguish between women who are infected and will clear the virus and those in whom the infection will persist and who will develop cancer has been difficult. Although it is clear that women who have a compromised immune system from any cause (e.g., genetic, iatrogenic, infectious) have a greater risk of developing a persistent HPV infection (Ahdieh, 2001), there is no way to predict which healthy women are unable to clear the virus spontaneously. The risk factors associated with cervical cancer include HPV infection, immunosuppression, smoking, parity, increased number of sexual partners, and oral contraceptive use (CDC, 2017).

## PRIMARY PREVENTION: HPV VACCINATION

Three preventive vaccines are commercially available. The bivalent vaccine (Cervarix) targets two high-risk HPV types (16 and 18) that account for 70% of the cervical cancer cases worldwide and is no longer available in the United States. The quadrivalent vaccine (Gardasil) targets high-risk HPV types 16 and 18, as well as two low-risk HPV types (6 and 11) that cause genital warts. The nonavalent vaccine (Gadasil-9) targets the same HPV types as the quadrivalent vaccine (6, 11, 16, and 18) and also types 31, 33, 45, 52, and 58 (FUTURE II Study Group, 2007; Joura, 2015; Paavonen, 2009). In randomized clinical trials all three vaccines have been shown to have 93% to 98% efficacy in the prevention of cervical dysplasia (and presumably cervical cancer) in women not previously infected with HPV-16 and -18. In addition, several studies have shown the vaccines to be safe, with no scientific evidence that HPV vaccination increases the risk of serious adverse events. The vaccines are most effective if given before sexual debut and exposure to HPV (FUTURE II Study Group, 2007; Joura, 2015; Paavonen, 2009). Only Gardasil-9 is available in the United States.

The Centers for Disease Control and Prevention (CDC) recommends that the **HPV vaccine** be given to both boys and girls between the ages of 11 and 12 years, but it can be administered as early as 9 years (CDC, 2019). If given before age 15 years, only two doses are now required (0 and 6 to 12 months). If given at age 15 years or older, or in immunocompromised individual, three doses are required (0, 1 to 2 months, and 6 months). Catch-up vaccination should be offered for females and males aged 13 to 26 years who have not been previously vaccinated (Meites, 2016). In 2018, the U.S. Food and Drug Administration (FDA) approved the use of Gardasil-9 up to the age of 45 years for both men and women (FDA, 2018); however, the Advisory Committee on Immunization Practices (ACIP) and the CDC stated that vaccination of men and women between ages 27 and 45 is not recommended for all individuals but should be considered on a case-by-case basis through shared clinical decision making between patient and doctor (CDC, 2019).

Unfortunately, the uptake of HPV vaccination in the United States has been poor, with only 50% of eligible children receiving all the recommended doses (CDC, 2018). The uptake in other HICs (Canada, Australia, the United Kingdom) has been much higher, approximately 70%, likely because of government-supported, school-based programs. Several LMICs have instituted HPV vaccination programs because the Global Alliance for Vaccination and Immunization (GAVI) has made the HPV vaccine available to low-income countries for $4 to $5 per dose (compared with approximately $150 per dose in the United States); however, economic, political and logistical barriers in many LMICs have limited universal mass vaccination programs. It is not yet known whether vaccination protection is lifelong or whether a booster dose will be required. Because the vaccines available do not provide protection against all cancer-associated HPV types, and because the duration of immunity is not yet known, routine cervical screening is still recommended in vaccinated women.

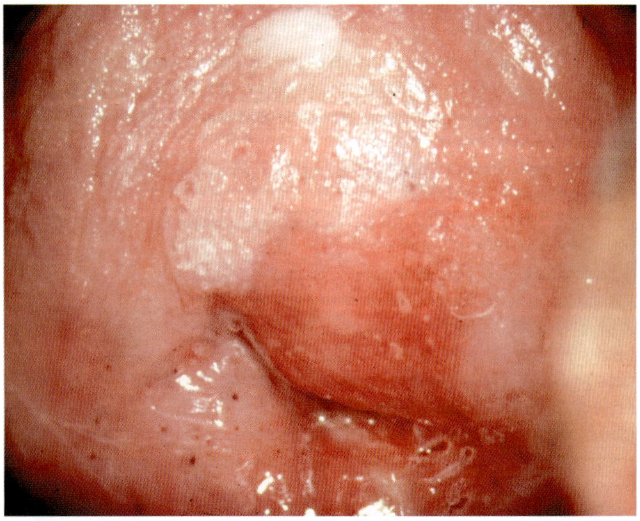

**Fig. 29.1** Colpophotograph of a cervix with an active human papillomavirus infection. The patient had a cytologic sample reported as a low-grade squamous intraepithelial lesion. She was followed without treatment, and the lesions regressed over the next year.

## SECONDARY PREVENTION

### Cervical Cytology Testing

**Cervical cytologic testing** (Pap test) became available in the 1950s after the studies of Dr. Papanicolaou demonstrated that cancer and its precursors could be identified by examining a properly prepared and stained cellular sample scraped from the uterine cervix. The 1941 monograph by Papanicolaou and Traut remains one of the sentinel breakthroughs in the history of preventive medicine. Their work led to the demonstration that local therapy of precancerous lesions can prevent the development of cancer. Despite the fact that it has a low sensitivity, widespread Pap testing has reduced the incidence of cervical cancer by 50% to 70%. In part, the success of this screening technique relies on the fact that it takes many years for invasive cancer to develop after a persistent HPV infection and development of dysplasia and that most women are tested repeatedly (Papanicolaou, 1941). Generally, in the United States, women who develop invasive cervical cancer have never been tested, have not been tested for many years, or had an abnormal Pap test but were unable to return for diagnostic or treatment services.

The Pap test (conventional Pap smear) is performed by scraping cervical cells using a spatula and endocervical brush (Figs. 29.2 and 29.3). Cells are sampled from the transformation zone (TZ), which is the area of the cervix where cervical cancer develops. The TZ includes the squamocolumnar junction, which is the area where the squamous epithelium of the ectocervix meets the columnar epithelium of the endocervix, and is dynamic throughout a woman's lifetime; the squamocolumnar junction migrates from the ectocervix into the endocervical canal as women age and reach menopause. In the past the collected sample was placed on a glass slide and fixed with alcohol. In recent years in the United States and some HICs, this method has been replaced by a liquid-based approach, where the sample is placed in a liquid medium that also can be used for HPV DNA testing.

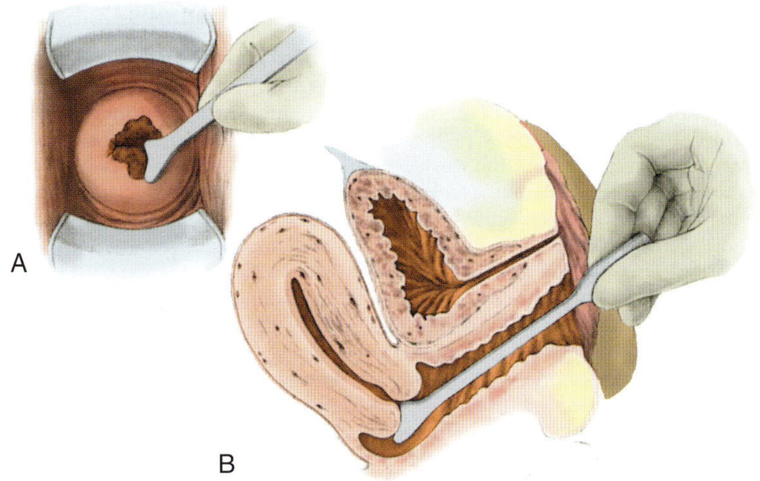


**Fig. 29.2** Conventional Papanicolaou test. A spatula is often used to obtain a specimen from the exocervix. It must be used with an instrument that samples the endocervix. **A,** Cervix as seen through a speculum, with the spatula being used to obtain a cell sample. **B,** Longitudinal view at the same point in the procedure.

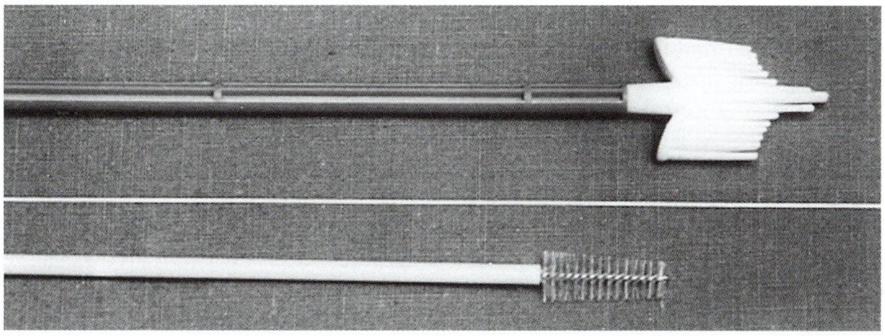

**Fig. 29.3** Both these instruments can be used to obtain a cytologic sample from the endocervix: cervical broom (Unimar) (*top*); cytobrush (Medscand, Cooper Surgical, Trumbull, CT) (*bottom*).

## Primary HPV Testing

There is increasing evidence that **HPV testing** is effective for cervical cancer screening. A number of studies have demonstrated that HPV testing is more sensitive than Pap testing, with only a small loss in positive predictive value (Castle, 2011; Dillner, 2008; Huh, 2015; Monsonego, 2015). Although the Pap test is still the most widely used screening test in developed countries, cotesting with HPV is now also recommended. The HPV DNA testing has been recommended in countries or regions of the world with any level of available resources (Jeronimo, 2017; WHO, 2015). Ogilvie and colleagues conducted a large randomized study in Canada that included 19,009 women screened for cervical cancer with HPV testing versus liquid-based cytologic examination. They concluded that HPV primary testing had a significantly lower likelihood of identifying CIN 3+ at 48 months than liquid-based cytologic examination (Ogilvie, 2018).

## Cervical Cancer Screening Guidelines

The American Society of Colposcopy and Cervical Pathology (ASCCP) guidelines in the United States recommend screening women for cervical cancer between ages 21 and 65 (Saslow, 2012). Cervical cancer screening should not be performed in women younger than 21 years, regardless of age of onset of sexual activity. The screening guidelines are as follows:

- 21 to 29 years: Pap testing every 3 years; no HPV testing.
- 30 to 65 years: Cotesting with Pap and HPV every 5 years (preferred) or Pap testing alone every 3 years.
- Screening is NOT recommended for women older than 65 years who have had three consecutive negative Pap tests or two consecutive negative HPV tests, provided they have no history of **high-grade dysplasia (cervical intraepithelial neoplasia [CIN]** 2/3) or cancer (CIN 2+) in the past 20 years; however, women presenting at age 65 years or older who have not had previous screening should undergo Pap and HPV testing.
- Screening with a Pap test and/or HPV testing is NOT recommended for women who have had a hysterectomy with removal of the cervix and who do not have a history of CIN 2+.

Of note, these guidelines do not apply to those special populations with additional risk factors and other complicating history.

Primary high-risk HPV screening test has been recommended by the U.S. Preventive Services Task Force (USPSTF) as an alternative screening method in the United States, starting at the age of 30 years. The USPSTF recommends that this group of women could be screened with cervical cytologic testing alone every 3 years, high-risk HPV testing alone every 5 years, or cotesting (cervical cytologic and high-risk HPV testing) every 5 years (USPSTF, 2018).

## Cervical Cytology Reporting: The Bethesda System

In 1988, the National Cancer Institute convened a conference in Bethesda, Maryland to develop a uniform terminology for the reporting of Pap test results; the result is known as the Bethesda System (TBS) (Solomon, 2002). Almost all laboratories in the United States and those in many countries throughout the world use this terminology. Fig. 29.4 shows how TBS, CIN, and dysplasia categories correspond to tissue changes.

The first part of a TBS report states whether the sample is satisfactory or unsatisfactory. A sample may be unsatisfactory if there is lack of a label, loss of transport medium, scant cellularity, or contamination by foreign material. Few samples are reported as unsatisfactory if a liquid-based technique is used. The report next indicates whether the cellular material is normal. If other than normal, the abnormalities are further divided into squamous and glandular. The cytologist may also comment on whether there is evidence of infection, such as yeast, or changes consistent with a diagnosis of bacterial vaginosis.

## Management of Abnormal Cervical Screening Tests

In the current guidelines from the American Society of Colposcopy and Cervical Pathology (ASCCP), the recommendations are based on risk of CIN 3+ (CIN 3, adenocarcinoma in situ, or cancer) determined by current tests results combined with patient's past history. If primary HPV screening is used and the results show positive HPV, it is recommended to perform both a reflex HPV genotyping test, if this is not previously done, and a reflex cytology test. If this is not feasible, referral for colposcopy is acceptable. If positive HPV 16 or 18 and negative cytology (negative for intraepithelial lesion or malignancy, NILM) is documented, a colposcopy is recommended. If minimally abnormal screening results (HPV positive and negative cytology, HPV negative and LSIL with unknown previous screening history) are found, the recommendation is for surveillance with close follow-up at 1 year (Perkins, 2020; Egemen 2020).

## Atypical Squamous Cells

The most common squamous abnormality is **atypical squamous cell (ASC) of undetermined significance (ASC-US)**. This finding indicates that there are few cellular abnormalities or changes that are not consistent with a more precise diagnosis of CIN. ASC-US changes are reported in approximately 3% to 5% of all Pap samples. The management of ASC-US and other cytological abnormalities is based on the recommendations of the ASCCP management guidelines (Perkins 2020; Egemen 2020; Solomon, 2001). Women with HPV positive ASC-US cytology in their initial screening should undergo colposcopy, as their immediate risk of CIN 3+ is approximately 4.5%. Women with HPV negative ASC-US cytology screening in the setting of an unknown history can be re-evaluated at 3 years (estimated 5-year CIN 3+ risk 0.40%) (Perkins, 2020).

The second ASC abnormality is **ASC-H (atypical squamous cells, cannot exclude a higher-grade lesion)**. Approximately 5% to 10% of ASC cases are classified at ASC-H. Women with this diagnosis should be evaluated with colposcopy regardless of HPV result (Massad, 2013; Perkins, 2020).

## Low-Grade Squamous Intraepithelial Lesion

**Low-grade squamous intraepithelial lesion (LSIL)** is often found to be consistent with histologic reports of low-grade dysplasia or **CIN 1** (Fig. 29.5). LSIL may resolve spontaneously or progress to more severe dysplasia and should be managed according to the ASCCP guidelines (Perkins, 2020). One-year follow-up is recommended in HPV-negative LSIL with unknown previous screening history. Colposcopy is recommended after an HPV-positive LSIL screening results in the general population with unknown previous screening history. A 1-year follow-up is also recommended in a patient with a new positive HPV test and LSIL cytology after a documented negative HPV test or co-test within an appropriate screening interval or colposcopic examination less than CIN 2 within the past year. Surveillance is recommended

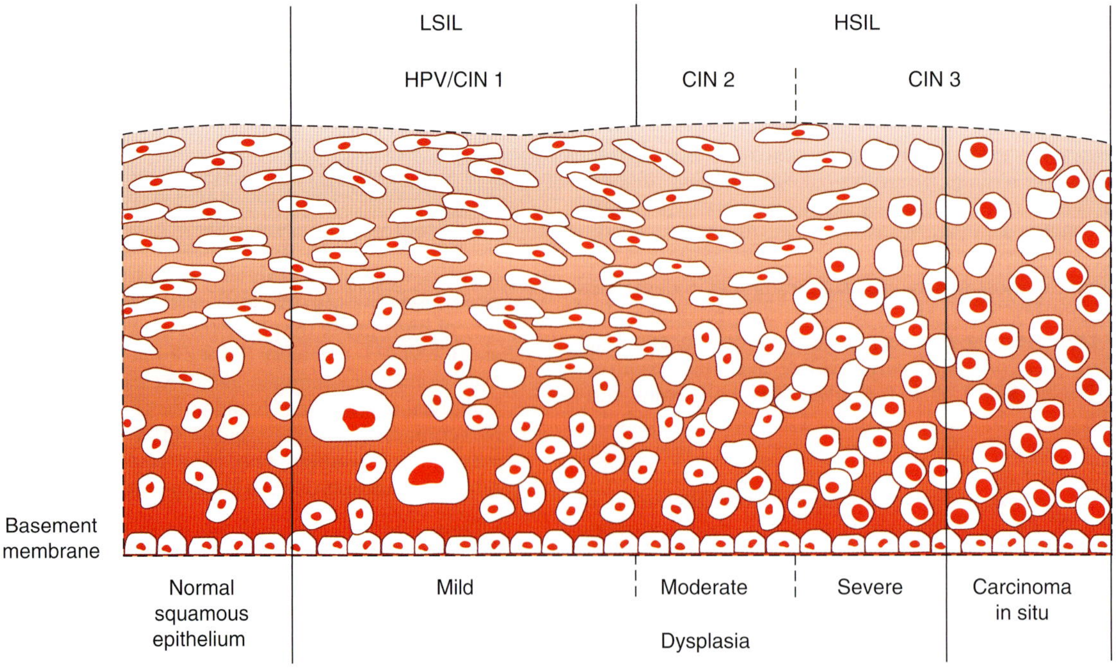


**Fig. 29.4** Diagram of cervical epithelium showing various terminologies used to characterize progressive degrees of cervical neoplasia. *CIN,* Cervical intraepithelial neoplasia; *HPV,* human papillomavirus; *HSIL,* high-grade squamous intraepithelial lesion; *LSIL,* low-grade squamous intraepithelial lesion.

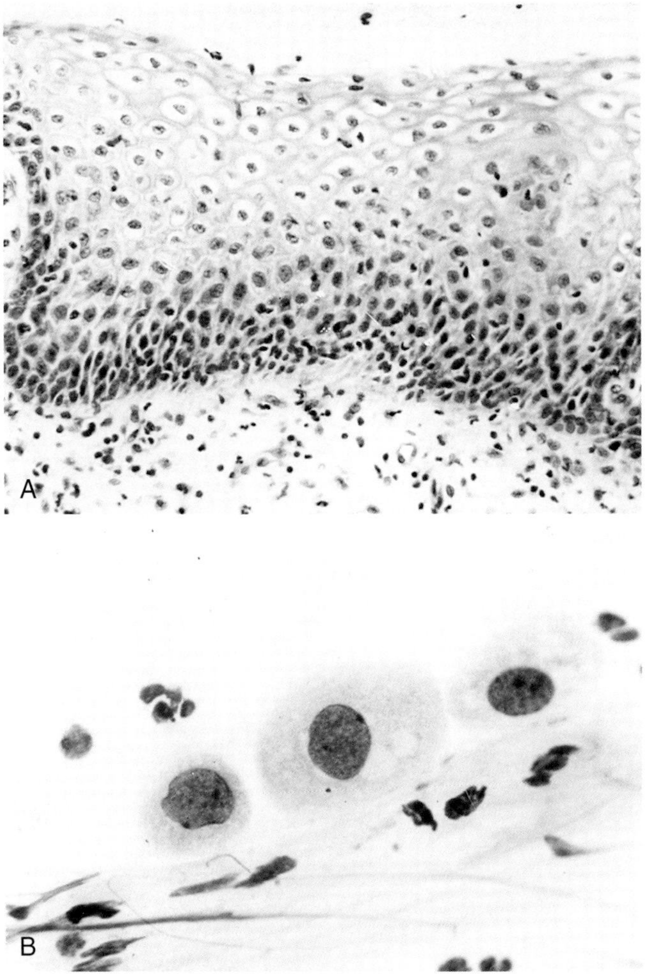


**Fig. 29.5 A,** Cervical intraepithelial neoplasia 1 (mild dysplasia). Atypical cells are present in the lower one-third of the epithelium (hematoxylin-eosin stain, original magnification ×250). **B,** Low-grade squamous intraepithelial lesion cytologic view. These cells show an altered nuclear-to-cytoplasmic ratio with enlargement and have granular chromatin (Papanicolaou stain, original magnification ×800).

rather than immediate colposcopy for low-grade abnormalities (HPV-positive ASC-US or LSIL), if a patient has at least one previous negative HPV-based test. After a low-grade cytology (HPV positive and negative for intraepithelial lesion or malignancy cytology, ASC-US or LSIL) without evidence of cytologic or histologic HSIL, continued surveillance according to risk estimation using available data is recommended (Perkins, 2020).

## High-Grade Squamous Intraepithelial Lesion

A diagnosis of **high-grade squamous intraepithelial lesion (HSIL)** indicates more severe dysplasia or **CIN 2/3** (Figs. 29.6 and 29.7). If untreated, approximately 15% of patients with HSIL will progress to cervical cancer (ACOG, 2013; Massad, 2013). In non-pregnant patients 25 years or older, expedited treatment (excisional procedure without preceding histologic confirmation) is preferred, but colposcopy with biopsy is acceptable, when the risk of CIN 3+ is 60% or higher. If HSIL cytology and HPV 16 positive are presented, the immediate CIN 3+ risk is 60% and cancer risk is 8.1%, thus expedited treatment is preferred. If an estimated immediate risk of CIN 3+ is 25% or greater and less than 60%, treatment with excisional procedure without

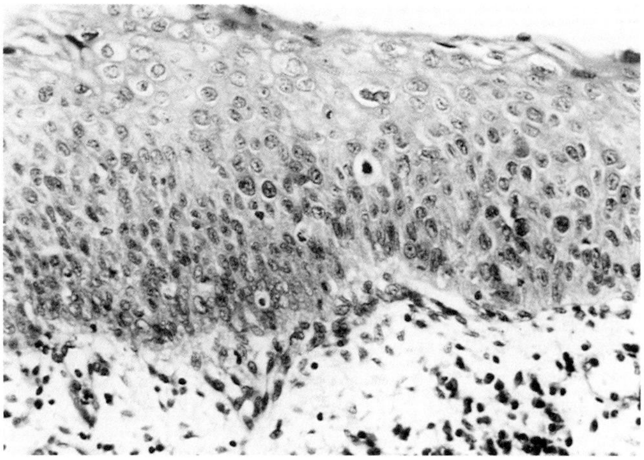

**Fig. 29.6** Cervical intraepithelial neoplasia 2 (moderate dysplasia). The atypical cells extend approximately halfway through to the epithelium (hematoxylin-eosin stain, original magnification ×300).

preceding histologic confirmation or histologic evaluation with colposcopy and biopsy are both acceptable (Perkins, 2020).

## Atypical Glandular Cells

**Atypical glandular cells (AGCs)** have an incidence of approximately 0.05% to 2.1%. The risk of underlying CIN 3+ is approximately 9% and invasive cancer is 3% in women with AGC cytologic results (ACOG, 2013; Marques, 2011; Massad, 2013). Per the ASCCP guidelines, the recommendation is for colposcopy with endocervical sampling, except in pregnancy. Endometrial sampling should also be performed in non-pregnant women who are older than 35 years or at risk for endometrial cancer (abnormal uterine bleeding, obesity, conditions suggesting chronic anovulation). For women presenting atypical endometrial cells specified, initial evaluation with endometrial and endocervical sampling is preferred, with colposcopy acceptable at the same time at the initial evaluation (Perkins, 2020).

# COLPOSCOPY

**Colposcopy** is often the first step in the evaluation of women with abnormal cytologic results. The colposcope is a low-power binocular microscope with a powerful light source that is used to carefully examine the cervix for the presence of lesions. Dilute acetic acid (3% to 5%) is applied to the cervix and after 30 to 60 seconds the cervix is again examined. Acetic acid dehydrates the epithelial cells, and dysplastic cells with large nuclei will reflect light and appear white. An experienced colposcopist can identify those tissue patterns associated with cervical dysplasia and determine or the appropriate site to perform a biopsy (Fig. 29.8).

For a thorough and complete examination, the entire TZ must be assessed and the colposcopy must therefore be satisfactory or adequate. Eventually some portions of the TZ cannot be visualized as they extend into the endocervical canal or for other reasons, and the examiner is unable to determine the presence or extent of abnormal tissue (unsatisfactory/inadequate) (Bornstein, 2012). In the case of abnormal cytologic results and an unsatisfactory or inadequate colposcopy, it is recommended that an endocervical curettage (ECC) should be performed. Cervical biopsies should be performed of acetowhite lesions noted (Fig. 29.9). It is common for a small amount of bleeding to occur after biopsy, and this can be controlled with ferric subsulfate (Monsel solution) or silver nitrate sticks. Cervical biopsy

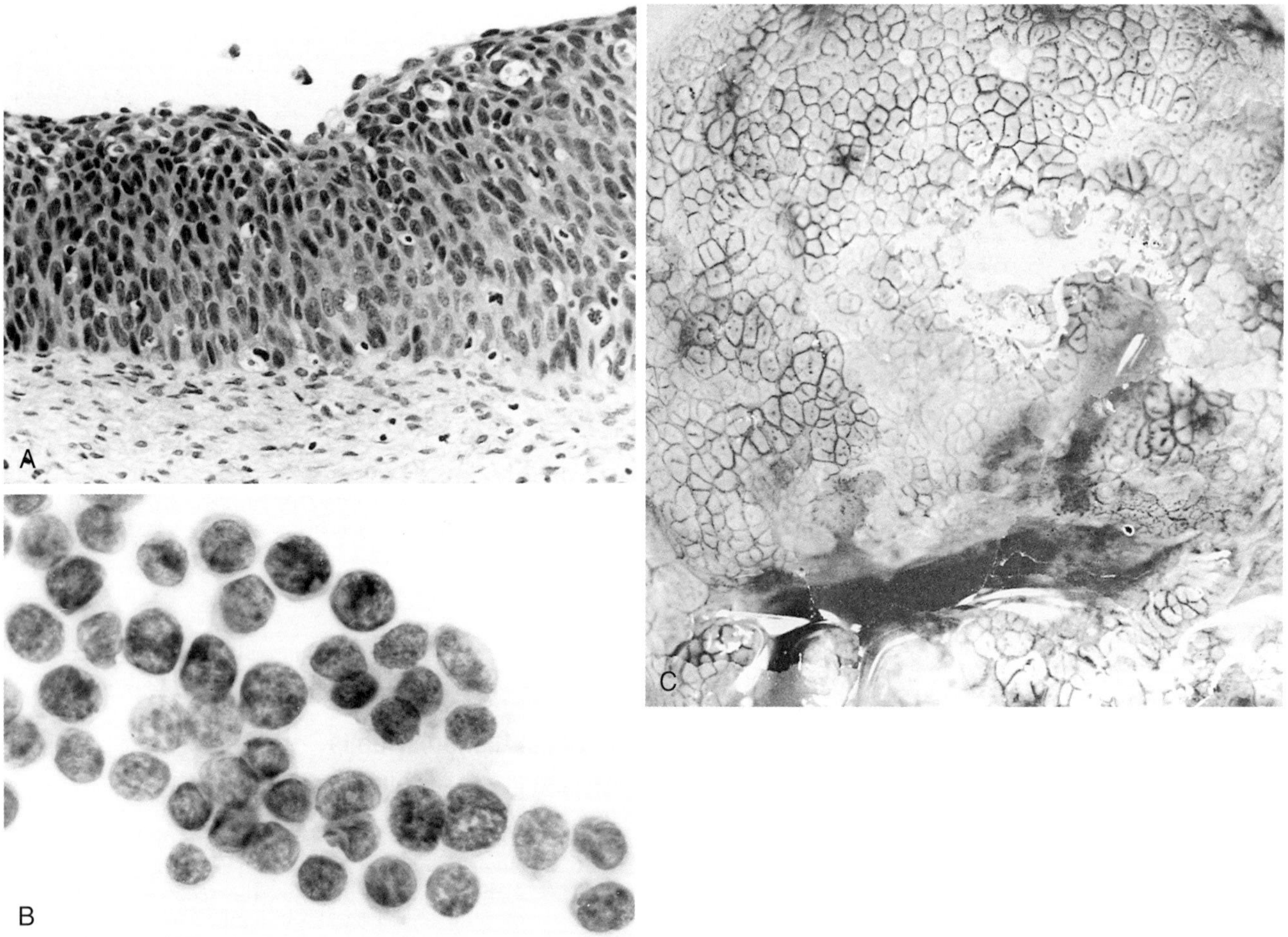


**Fig. 29.7 A,** Cervical intraepithelial neoplasia 3 (severe dysplasia, carcinoma in situ). There is a lack of squamous maturation throughout the thickness of the epithelium. Almost all the cells have enlarged nuclei with granular chromatin. Note that the basement membrane is intact, showing that this process is confined to the epithelial layer only. **B,** High-grade squamous intraepithelial lesion. These cells exhibit large nuclei with granular chromatin. Very little cytoplasm can be seen (Papanicolaou stain, original magnification ×800). **C,** Extensive cervical intraepithelial neoplasia 3 (CIN 3) lesion covering most of the epithelium visible in this colpophotograph. The predominant feature is a mosaic pattern. There is umbilication of many of the tiles with a punctate vessel, a common feature of CIN 3. Although this large lesion needs to be examined carefully for evidence of atypical vessels, a hallmark of invasive cancer, none are seen in this view (colpophotograph, original magnification ×8). (From Kolstad P, Stafl A. *Atlas of Colposcopy*. Baltimore, MD: University Park Press; 1972.)

specimens are very small, and the biopsy site usually heals within a few days (Fig. 29.10).

## Cervical Dysplasia in Pregnancy

During pregnancy the cervix becomes larger, the blood supply is increased, and decidual changes in the epithelium can be confused with CIN. The ASCCP provides guidelines for the management of abnormal cytologic testing in pregnancy (Perkins, 2020). Colposcopy is safe in pregnancy; however, biopsies should only be performed if there is a suspicion of invasive disease. It is highly unlikely that dysplasia will progress significantly during pregnancy, and for most patients further evaluation can be postponed until at least 4 weeks after delivery. If invasive cancer is suspected, a cervical biopsy is indicated and can be performed safely during pregnancy; however, ECC, endometrial biopsy, and treatment without biopsy are unacceptable during pregnancy should never be performed during pregnancy. If CIN 2/3 is diagnosed, examination during pregnancy, surveillance colposcopy and testing (cytology and/or HPV Test depending on age) is preferred every 12 to 24 weeks, but further colposcopy is acceptable to be delayed until the postpartum period. Treatment of CIN 2 or CIN 3 during pregnancy is not recommended

## Natural History of Cervical Intraepithelial Neoplasia

CIN, the precancerous lesion of the squamous epithelium of the cervix, is a histologic diagnosis based on tissue examination of a cervical biopsy specimen. The current 2019 ASCCP Risk-Based Management Consensus Guidelines for Abnormal Cervical Cancer Screening Tests and Cancer Precursors recommended histopathology reports based on Lower Anogenital Squamous Terminology (LAST)/World Health Organization (WHO). The recommendations are for reporting histologic HSIL with CIN 2 or CIN 3 qualifiers, i.e., HSIL (CIN 2) and HSIL (CIN 3) (Perkins, 2020). CIN is graded as 1, 2, or 3 depending on the how much of the epithelial layer contains atypical cells. CIN 1, or mild dysplasia, often spontaneously regresses, usually within 6 to

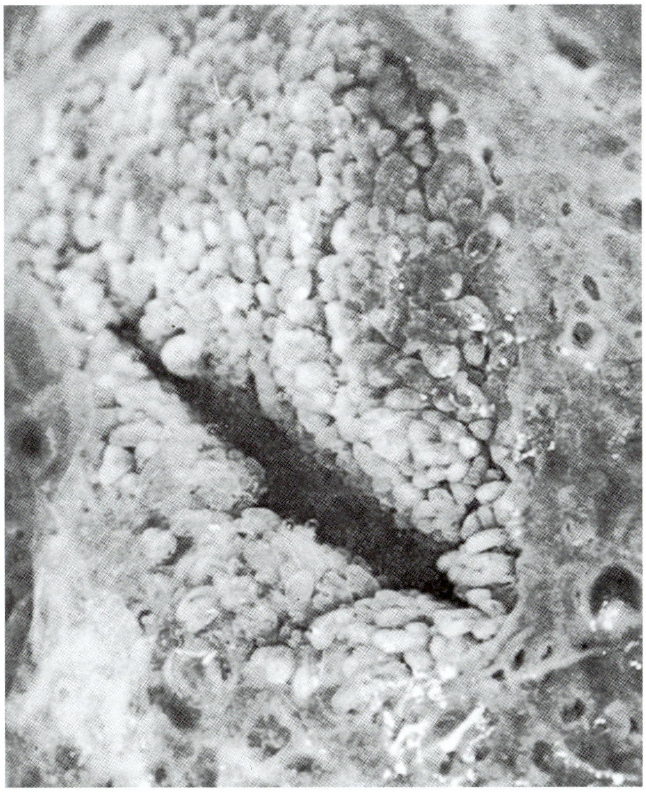

**Fig. 29.8** Normal cervix as seen through a colposcope at approximately 6× magnification. The central grapelike structures are covered with columnar epithelium. The tissue outside this area represents squamous metaplasia. There are multiple gland openings in this area, indicating that columnar epithelium is being replaced by squamous epithelium. This area between the columnar and squamous epithelia is known as the transformation zone. (From Coppleson M, Pixley E, Reid B. *Colposcopy—A Scientific and Practical Approach to the Cervix in Health and Disease*. Springfield, IL: Charles C Thomas; 1971.)

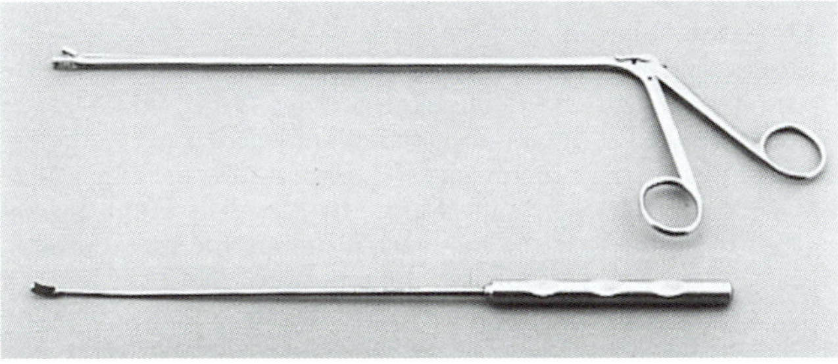

**Fig. 29.9** Cervical biopsy instruments: cervical biopsy forceps (*top*); endocervical curette (*bottom*).

12 months (Bansal, 2008). When cellular atypia involves two-thirds of the thickness of the epithelium, it is designated as CIN 2. The process remains reversible at this stage, with approximately 40% regressing spontaneously without treatment (Castle, 2009). When the cellular atypia involves more than two-thirds of the epithelium, it is designated as CIN 3. This term encompasses what was once called severe dysplasia and carcinoma in situ (CIS). CIN 3 is a precursor to invasive cancer; however, approximately one-third of these lesions may spontaneously regress (Ostör, 1993).

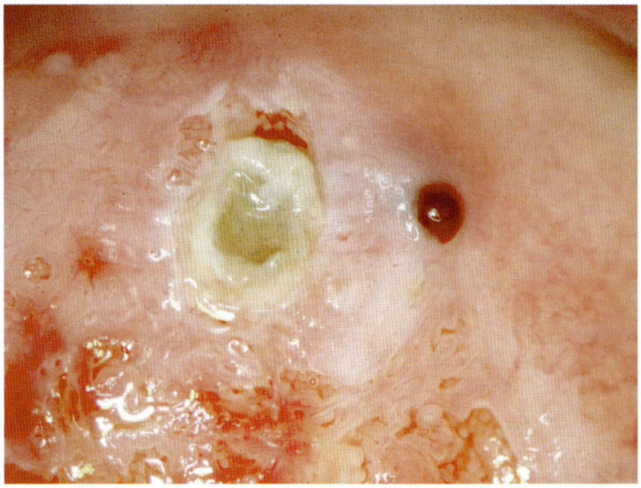

**Fig. 29.10** Colpophotograph (≈ ×12) of a cervical biopsy site 72 hours after the procedure. The eschar is already beginning to separate from the cervix.

## TREATMENT OF CERVICAL DYSPLASIA

The approach to treatment of CIN lesions over the past 40 years has changed and continues to evolve. Many early lesions disappear spontaneously, and treatment is indicated for those lesions that have demonstrated a potential for further progression. The ASCCP provides regularly updated guidelines for the management of cervical dysplasia (Perkins, 2020).

### CIN 1

Almost all CIN 1 is a manifestation of a transient HPV infection, and the regression rates are high. Patients with CIN 1 usually do not require treatment but do require follow-up to ensure that the lesion regresses. Observation is preferred to treatment for CIN 1.

## CIN 1

Given the high rates of spontaneous regression, CIN 1 with LSIL cytologic characteristics is usually managed with observation. Histologic LSIL (CIN 1) and cytologic ASC-US/HPV positive and cytology showing LSIL are biologically the same and should be managed similarly. A small percentage of CIN 1 lesions progress to CIN 2 or 3, but it is not possible to determine which lesions have this potential, so continued follow-up is recommended. When CIN 1 or no lesion are found on histology (colposcopy with biopsy) after HPV positive and cytology with ASC-US or LSIL, there is a 5-year risk of CIN 3+ of approximately 2%. One-year surveillance is recommended after colposcopy with biopsies of histologic LSIL (CIN 1) or less, preceded by a low-grade cotest result (HPV positive and LSIL cytology, HPV-positive and ASC-US cytology, or repeated HPV positive and negative for intraepithelial lesion or malignancy cytology) (Perkins, 2020).

For women 25 years or older, if histologic LSIL (CIN 1) persists for more than 2 years, observation is preferred but treatment is acceptable. If the decision is in favor of treatment and the entire squamocolumnar junction and all lesions are fully visualized on colposcopy, either excision or ablation treatments are acceptable. Treatment of CIN 1 in less than 2-year follow-up is an acceptable option based on patient preference, after shared decision making, but it is considered a special situation, as the immediate estimated CIN3+ risk is less than 25% (Perkins, 2020). If the diagnosis of CIN 1 is preceded by cytologic testing showing HSIL, there is a higher chance of underlying CIN 2/3. When CIN1 is preceded by ASC-H, observation in 1 year with

HPV-based testing is recommended, if the colposcopic examination can visualize the entire squamocolumnar junction and the upper limit of lesions, and the endocervical sampling, if collected, is negative. When CIN1 is preceded by HSIL, it is acceptable to review the cytologic, histologic, and colposcopic findings. If the review changes the diagnosis, the guidelines should be followed for management. If cytology shows HSIL and biopsy shows histology CIN 1 or less, either a diagnostic excisional procedure or observation with HPV-based testing and colposcopy in 1 year is acceptable (only if colposcopy visualized the entire squamocolumnar junction and upper limit of lesions and endocervical sampling is less than CIN 2) (Perkins, 2020). It is acceptable to review the cytologic, histologic, and colposcopic findings for CIN 1 histology after an ASC-H or HSIL cytology result. If the review demonstrate a revised findings or interpretation, management should follow guidelines for the revised diagnosis.

## CIN 2/3

It is difficult to distinguish CIN 2 from CIN 3 pathologically, so the two diagnoses are often managed similarly. Approximately 40% of CIN 2 lesions and 30% of CIN 3 lesions regress spontaneously (Castle, 2009); however, 22% of CIN 2 progress to CIN 3 and 5% progress to cancer. Furthermore, approximately 15% of CIN 3 progress to cancer. Treatment is recommended in non-pregnant women presenting with HSIL (CIN 3), and observation is unacceptable. Treatment is recommended in nonpregnant women presenting with HSIL (CIN 2), unless the patient's concerns about the effect of treatment on future pregnancy outweigh concerns about cancer, then either treatment or observation is acceptable (Perkins, 2020). If observation is the option, it may include careful observation, including colposcopy and HPV-based testing every 6-month for up to two years. Observation is unacceptable if the entire squamocolumnar junction or the upper limit of lesions are not visualized or when the results of an endocervical sampling, if performed, is CIN 2+ or higher. If treatment is the option for HSIL histology (CIN 2 or CIN 3), the excisional treatment is preferred to ablative (Perkins, 2020). Pregnant women with CIN 2/3 and no evidence of invasion may be observed during the pregnancy, with evaluation delayed until 4 weeks postpartum. Women with a history of CIN 2/3 are more likely to develop another lesion in the future. Therefore **long-term follow-up for at least 25 years is recommended**, even if this extends screening past age 65 (ACOG, 2013; Perkins, 2020). These recommendations do not apply for rare abnormalities or special populations. For recommendations for women younger than 25 years, pregnant, with additional risk factors and/or other complicating history, ASCCP guidelines should be consulted. After immediate treatment, surveillance and the next steps in the management should follow ASCCP guidelines.

## Treatment of Cervical Dysplasia

Treatment of CIN can be accomplished by ablation or excision, and these methods have first-treatment success rates of greater than 90% in properly selected patients (Martin-Hirsch, 2013; Massad, 2013; Mitchell, 1998; Ostör, 1993; Soutter, 1997). Ablative methods include cryotherapy, $CO_2$ laser ablation, and thermal ablation. Excisional procedures include **loop electrosurgical excision procedure (LEEP)**, cold knife conization (CKC), and $CO_2$ laser conization. The choice of treatment modality depends on the availability of equipment and experience and expertise of the clinician. Hysterectomy is unacceptable as primary therapy solely for the treatment of histologic HSIL (Perkins, 2020). Furthermore, if high-grade dysplasia is present, conization must first be performed to rule out underlying invasive cancer, which may require more extensive procedures such as radical hysterectomy, radical trachelectomy, and lymph node dissection.

### Ablative Methods

Ablative procedures treat CIN but do not provide further diagnostic information. To qualify for ablative therapy, there should be no suspicion of invasive cancer and the lesion and the TZ should be entirely visualized. Specific criteria for ablative therapies include the following:

- A satisfactory colposcopy has been performed with visualization of the entire cervical squamocolumnar junction.
- The lesion and TZ should be entire visualized on colposcopy or visual inspection with acetic acid (VIA) and/or negative ECC (if available).

#### Cryotherapy

Cryotherapy is a commonly used treatment for CIN lesions that is safe, effective, and relatively simple to perform; however, it does not provide a specimen for pathology review and in many high-resource settings has been replaced by LEEP. Contraindications to cryotherapy include large lesions (covering >75% of the cervix and/or cannot be covered by the cryoprobe) and lesions that extend into the endocervical canal or lesions suspicious for cancer. In addition, if the patient had an endocervical curettage performed and it shows evidence of high-grade dysplasia, cryotherapy is contraindicated.

The procedure includes performing VIA or colposcopy to confirm that the lesion is confined to the exocervix. A probe is selected that will cover the entire lesion. $N_2O$ or $CO_2$ is used as the refrigerant. The cervix will freeze quickly, but the probe must remain in place until the ice ball extends to at least 5 mm beyond the edge of the instrument. In most cases this takes 3 minutes. The refrigerant is then turned off, and the probe is allowed to thaw and separate from the cervix. It is recommended that a 3-5-3 double freeze–thaw cycle is performed with 3 minutes of freezing, followed by 5 minutes of thawing, and another 3 minutes of freezing. Most patients experience minimal discomfort during the procedure. Because the tissue that was destroyed remains on the cervix, the patient will experience vaginal discharge within a few hours. It may take as long as 3 weeks for the discharge to stop. The patient should be cautioned to place nothing in the vagina for at least 3 weeks after the procedure to avoid dislodgment of the eschar.

#### $CO_2$ Laser Ablation

$CO_2$ laser ablation became available in the 1980s but has largely been replaced by LEEP in the United States. A focused $CO_2$ laser beam is directed at the cervical epithelium where water in the tissue absorbs the laser energy and the tissue is destroyed by vaporization. The lesion is typically ablated to a depth of 5 mm. Several safety procedures must be followed, including the use of protective eyewear by all personnel in the procedure room, the use of a blackened or brushed speculum to avoid damage to surrounding tissues by misdirected laser beams, and the use of wet towels and cloth drapes to prevent fire. Because little devitalized tissue is left after the procedure, there is no prolonged vaginal discharge as there is with cryotherapy. The success rate is similar to cryotherapy and excisional procedures. The advantages of this technique are that the area of tissue destruction can be minimized and there is no prolonged vaginal discharge. Similar to cryotherapy, there is no specimen for pathologic evaluation. Treatment success depends on the correct choice of laser energy delivered and achieving the proper depth and extent of treatment.

#### Thermal Ablation

**Thermal ablation** (TA) was developed in 1966 and can be used to treat all grades of CIN (Dolman, 2014; Haddad, 1988; Semm, 1966). This process uses heat generated by electricity to thermally ablate cervical lesions at temperatures of 100° to 120° C. TA treatment results are comparable to other current ablative methods such as cryotherapy (Dolman, 2014; Vink, 2013). In a study with 4569 women, Dolman and colleagues found that TA is 96% effective at treating CIN grade 1 and 95% effective at treating grades 2 and 3 (Dolman, 2014). A 2019 meta-analysis revealed the overall response rate for TA treatment of biopsy proven CIN 2+ was 93.8% (Randall, 2019).

The TA device is an FDA-approved, portable, handheld, and battery-operated device designed to treat CIN lesions in less than 1 minute (Langell, 2019). It was developed for global use, avoiding limitations imposed by limited resource availability, especially in LMICs. Additionally, its short duration of treatment and simplicity of use deliver compatibility with the WHO-recommended screen-and-treat approach, which is designed to reduce patient loss to follow-up, especially in remote areas. In 2019, the WHO recommended TA for the treatment of confirmed CIN 2+ and for use in those who have been screened positive by a screen-and-treat approach. The eligibility criteria for ablation include women who screened positive by colposcopy or VIA, in whom the whole lesion/TZ was visualized and able to be covered by the probe tip, and in whom there is no suspicion of invasion or glandular disease (WHO, 2019).

## Excisional Methods

Excisional procedures have the advantage compared with ablative procedures because they provide a pathologic specimen for further diagnostic information. The specific indications for an excisional procedure compared with an ablative procedure include the following (WHO, 2014):

- Suspected microinvasion
- Adenocarcinoma in situ or other glandular abnormalities
- Unsatisfactory/inadequate colposcopy where the TZ is not fully visualized
- Lack of correlation between cytologic testing and colposcopy/biopsy results
- Unable to rule out invasive disease
- Lesion extending into the endocervical canal
- Endocervical curettage indicating CIN or a glandular abnormality
- Recurrence after an ablative or previous excisional procedure

### Loop Electrosurgical Excision Procedure

**LEEP, also called large loop excision of the transformation zone (LLETZ)**, is the most common method of treatment for CIN 2/3 in the United States. It involves the removal of the TZ of the cervix under local anesthesia and can be performed safely in the office. The cervix is infiltrated with an anesthetic/vasoconstrictor solution (1% to 2% lidocaine with epinephrine), and a cone-shaped piece of the cervix inclusive of the TZ is removed (Martin-Hirsch, 2013). The LEEP procedure uses a thin wire in the shape of a loop and an electrosurgical generator, providing a cutting current to remove the tissue. The loops are available in a variety of shapes and sizes, allowing selection of a loop best fitted to the patient's lesion (Fig. 29.11). Bleeding areas can be cauterized with a ball electrode attached to the current generator set to cautery.

The removed tissue is examined histologically for diagnosis and evaluation of margin status. Management guidelines for positive margins are provided by the ASCCP and include reexcision versus follow-up cytologic testing, colposcopy, and endocervical sampling in 4 to 6 months depending on pathology results and patient age and desire for future fertility (Massad, 2013). Hysterectomy is rarely indicated for the treatment of CIN unless a repeat diagnostic procedure is recommended but not feasible because of minimal remaining cervix.

### Cold Knife Conization

CKC is an excisional procedure similar to LEEP but is performed with a scalpel under anesthesia in the operating room.

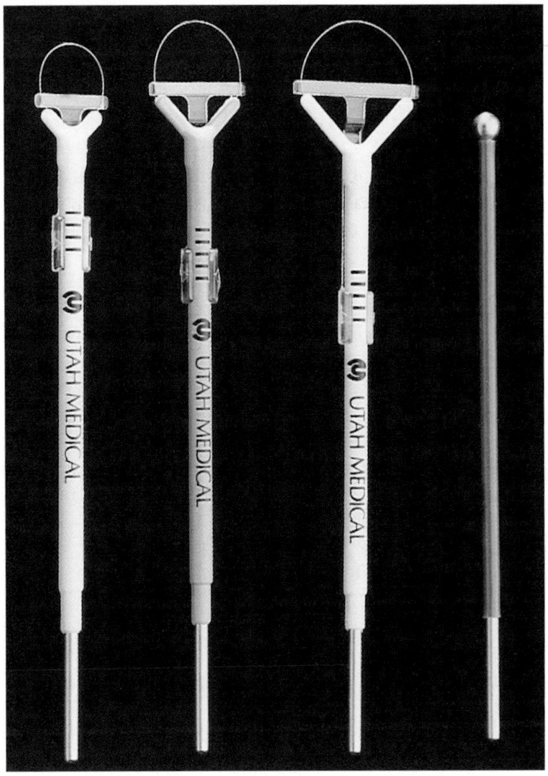


**Fig. 29.11** Electrodes (Utah Medical, Midvale, UT) used for a loop electroexcision procedure. The width of the excised tissue specimens can vary, and the specimen depth can be adjusted by sliding the guard attached to the electrode shaft. After excision, the base of the cervix is often gently cauterized with a ball electrode. (Courtesy Dr. Steven E. Waggoner, University of Chicago, Chicago, IL.)

For the evaluation of squamous lesions, CKC offers little advantage over LEEP; however, CKC is advantageous in patients with glandular abnormalities or suspicion of invasive cancer because CKC uses a scalpel and avoids the thermal artifact sometimes seen at the margins of specimens obtained by LEEP. Once the specimen is removed, bleeding can be controlled with cauterization and the application of ferric subsulfate (Monsel solution). Sutures to control bleeding are rarely necessary.

## Follow-up After Treatment of Cervical Dysplasia

The rate of recurrent or persistent disease after excisional or ablative treatment for CIN 2/3 is 5% to 17%, with no significant differences in outcomes among the different treatment modalities. (Martin-Hirsch, 2013). Factors associated with recurrent or persistent disease include the following (Demopoulos, 1991; Ghaem-Maghami, 2007; Manchanda, 2008; Mitchell, 1998):

- Large lesion size
- Endocervical gland involvement
- Positive margins

The current ASCCP recommendations for surveillance after excision of CIN 2/3 consists of HPV-based testing at 6 months (preferred). If HPV-based tests are positive, colposcopy and appropriate biopsies should be performed. Follow-up at 6 months with colposcopy and endocervical curettage is acceptable. After this, annual HPV or co-testing is preferred until three consecutive negative tests have been obtained for at least 25 years as long as the patient is in a good health (Perkins, 2020).

## Cervical Cancer Prevention in LMICs

Although the screening and diagnosis algorithms described earlier are effective, they are expensive and require high-level infrastructure and well-trained personnel. In addition, they require three separate patient visits with communication of test results between visits. Therefore there is a significant need for alternative solutions, particularly in low-resource settings in the United States and in LMICs, where there is often lack of trained personnel, infrastructure, and pathology services.

One commonly used approach in low-resource settings is VIA, in which acetic acid is applied to the cervix, and if there is whitening of the epithelium indicating a precancerous lesion, immediate ablation treatment is performed (screen-and-treat). VIA and ablation therapy (cryotherapy or TA) can be performed by nonphysicians, such as community health workers (CHWs) or promotoras (Jeronimo, 2017; WHO, 2015). Such a program using VIA has been shown to decrease cervical cancer mortality by more than 30% in unscreened communities in India (Adsul, 2017; Shastri, 2014). HPV DNA testing has also been recommended as a primary cervical screening option in LMICs (Jeronimo, 2017; WHO, 2015).

## Vaginal Intraepithelial Neoplasia

**Vaginal intraepithelial neoplasia (VaIN)** is similar to CIN and is defined as squamous atypia without invasion. The true incidence of VaIN is unknown, but it is estimated to be approximately 0.1 in 100,000 in the United States (Watson, 2009). It is most commonly diagnosed in women aged 50 to 60 years (Boonlikit, 2010; Kim, 2018). Classification is similar to CIN and reflects the depth of involvement of the epithelial layer (VaIN 1, 2, and 3). Risk factors for VaIN include current or previous neoplasia elsewhere in lower genital tract (cervix, vulva) and persistent HPV infection. Previous studies have shown 50% to 90% of patients with VaIN had prior or concurrent intraepithelial neoplasia or carcinoma of the cervix or vulva (Aho, 1991; Cheng, 1999; Gunderson, 2013; Sillman, 1997).

Most cases of VaIN are discovered incidentally during colposcopy because of abnormal cytologic results. Presenting symptoms of postcoital discharge or spotting are rare. Suspicious lesions should be biopsied to confirm the diagnosis. The most common site of VaIN (87% to 97%) is the upper third of the vagina (Boonlikit, 2010; Kim, 2018).

Patients with VaIN 1 are followed with surveillance similar to patients with CIN 1 because of the low risk of progression to invasive cancer; however, it is recommended that patients with VaIN 2 or VaIN 3 undergo treatment because the risk of progression to vaginal cancer is estimated to be 2% to 5%. Treatment options include excision, ablation, and topical therapy with 5-fluorouracil or imiquimod (Audet-Lapointe, 1990; Cardosi, 2001; Sopracordevole, 2016; Tranoulis, 2018). There is a high recurrence rate of 20% to 30% regardless of the treatment modality used, and these patients should be carefully followed long term. There are no standard guidelines for the follow-up of patients with VaIN 2/3, but it is reasonable to perform cytologic testing and colposcopy every 6 to 12 months (Zeligs, 2013). The role of HPV testing in patients with VaIN is still unknown. In a study of 44 women with VaIN, posttreatment HPV testing had a sensitivity of 90% and a specificity of 78% (Frega, 2007).

## VULVAR INTRAEPITHELIAL NEOPLASIA

**Vulvar intraepithelial neoplasia (VIN)** is defined as squamous atypia of the vulva (Fig. 29.12). The incidence of VIN 3 is approximately 2.86 per 100,000 women in the United States (Judson, 2006). VIN was traditionally classified as (1) VIN, usual type, or (2) VIN, differentiated type (ACOG, 2016; Sideri, 2005); however, the International Society for the Study of Vulvovaginal Disease (ISSVD) recommends the terms (1) *LSIL of the vulva* or *vulvar LSIL*, encompassing flat condyloma or HPV effects; (2) *vulvar HSIL* (formerly termed usual type VIN); and (3) *differentiated type* (ACOG, 2016; Bornstein, 2016).

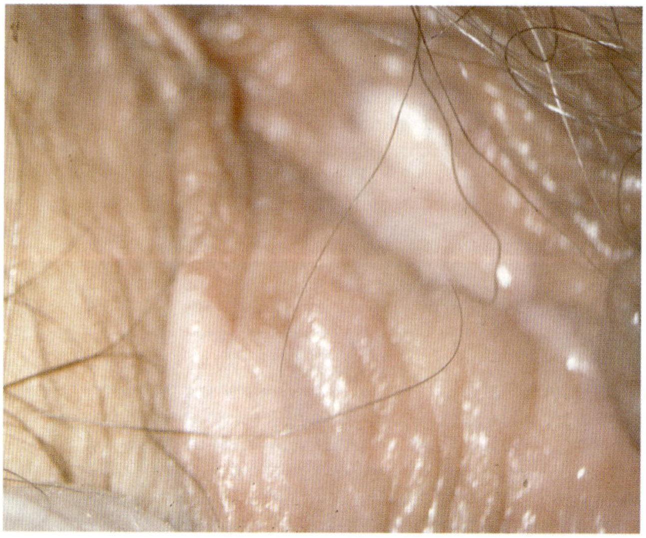

**Fig. 29.12** Vulvar intraepithelial neoplasia (VIN) 3 lesion as seen through a colposcope after the application of acetic acid. A second lesion is out of focus but can be seen in the background. VIN is often multifocal.

VIN, usual type, or vulvar HSIL, is the most common form of VIN and is an HPV-associated condition. It occurs in younger women, may be multifocal, and is associated with cervical and vaginal dysplasia. VIN, differentiated type, is less common and is unrelated to HPV infection but is associated with chronic inflammatory conditions such as lichen sclerosus and lichen planus. Symptoms of VIN include pruritus, pain, and burning; however, many patients are asymptomatic and VIN is incidentally discovered during a thorough pelvic examination. Punch biopsies should be performed of any lesions noted on the vulva, particularly those that persist or are not responsive to therapy for other conditions. Furthermore, colposcopy of the vulva with biopsies of any lesions should be performed in all patients with CIN or VaIN because of the association with these other HPV-related conditions.

VIN 1 is a benign entity, and treatment for asymptomatic disease is not necessary; however, patients with VIN 2/3 should undergo treatment because of the risks of underlying cancer and progression of disease. Treatment modalities include excision, ablation, and topical therapies (ACOG, 2016; Jones, 2005; Ribeiro, 2012). All modalities have similar effectiveness (Wallbillich, 2012). The modality used depends on the risk of invasive disease, location of the lesion, and extent of disease and symptoms. If underlying invasive disease is suspected, patients with VIN 2/3 should undergo wide local excision. Other options for diffuse disease include $CO_2$ laser ablation and topical therapies. The most commonly used topical therapy is imiquimod, a topical immune response modifier that is applied to vulvar lesions three times per week for 16 weeks. Small studies have shown imiquimod to be very effective with a complete response rate of 51%, a partial response rate of 25%, and a recurrence rate of 16% (Mahto, 2010; van Seters, 2008). Similar to VaIN, VIN recurrence rates are high. There are no standard guidelines for the follow-up of patients with VIN 2/3, but it is reasonable to perform colposcopy of the vulva every 6 to 12 months for 2 years. The role of HPV testing in patients with VIN is unknown.

## KEY REFERENCES

American College of Obstetricians and Gynecologists (ACOG). Practice Bulletin No. 140: management of abnormal cervical cancer screening test results and cervical cancer precursors. *Obstet Gynecol.* 2013; 122(6):1338-1367. doi: 10.1097/01.AOG.0000438960.31355.9e.

American College of Obstetricians and Gynecologists (ACOG). Committee Opinion No.675: Management of vulvar intraepithelial neoplasia. *Obstet Gynecol.* 2016;128(4):e178-e182. doi: 10.1097/aog.0000000000001713.

Bornstein J, Bentley J, Bosze P, et al. 2011 colposcopic terminology of the International Federation for Cervical Pathology and Colposcopy. *Obstet Gynecol.* 2012;120(1):166-172. doi: 10.1097/AOG.0b013e318254f90c.

Bornstein J, Bogliatto F, Haefner HK, et al. The 2015 International Society for the Study of Vulvovaginal Disease (ISSVD) Terminology of Vulvar Squamous Intraepithelial Lesions. *J Low Genit Tract Dis.* 2016;20(1):11-14. doi: 10.1097/LGT.0000000000000169.

Bray F, Ferlay J, Soerjomataram I, et al. Global cancer statistics 2018: GLOBOCAN estimates of incidence and mortality worldwide for 36 cancers in 185 countries. *CA Cancer J Clin.* 2018;68(6):394-424. doi: 10.3322/caac.21492.

Cardosi RJ, Bomalaski JJ, Hoffman MS. Diagnosis and management of vulvar and vaginal intraepithelial neoplasia. *Obstet Gynecol Clin North Am.* 2001;28(4):685-702.

Castle PE, Schiffman M, Wheeler CM, et al. Evidence for frequent regression of cervical intraepithelial neoplasia-grade 2. *Obstet Gynecol.* 2009;113(1):18-25. doi: 10.1097/AOG.0b013e31818f5008.

Centers for Disease Control and Prevention (CDC). *More US Adolescents Up To Date on HPV vaccination.* Division of Cancer Prevention and Control, Centers for Disease Control and Prevention; August 23, 2018. Available at: https://www.cdc.gov/media/releases/2018/p0823-HPV-vaccination.html. Accessed May 30, 2019.

Chang F. Role of papillomaviruses. *J Clin Pathol.* 1990;43(4):269-276. doi: 10.1136/jcp.43.4.269.

Dolman L, Sauvaget C, Muwonge R, et al. Meta-analysis of the efficacy of cold coagulation as a treatment method for cervical intraepithelial neoplasia: a systematic review. *BJOG.* 2014;121(8):929-942. doi: 10.1111/1471-0528.12655.

FUTURE II Study Group. Quadrivalent vaccine against human papillomavirus to prevent high-grade cervical lesions. *N Engl J Med.* 2007;356(19):1915-1927. doi: 10.1056/NEJMoa061741.

Ghaem-Maghami S, Sagi S, Majeed G, et al. Incomplete excision of cervical intraepithelial neoplasia and risk of treatment failure: a meta-analysis. *Lancet Oncol.* 2007;8(11):985-993. doi: 10.1016/S1470-2045(07)70283-8.

International Agency for Research on Cancer (IARC). Cervix uteri. GLOBOCAN; 2018. Available at http://gco.iarc.fr. Accessed May 5, 2019.

Jeronimo J, Castle PE, Temin S, et al. Secondary prevention of cervical cancer: ASCO resource-stratified clinical practice guideline. *J Glob Oncol.* 2017;3(5):635-657. doi: 10.1200/JGO.2016.006577.

Martin-Hirsch PP, Paraskevaidis E, Bryant A, et al. Surgery for cervical intraepithelial neoplasia. *Cochrane Database Syst Rev.* 2013(12): CD001318. doi: 10.1002/14651858.CD001318.pub3.

Massad LS, Einstein MH, Huh WK, et al. 2012 updated consensus guidelines for the management of abnormal cervical cancer screening tests and cancer precursors. *J Low Genit Tract Dis.* 2013;17(5 Suppl 1): S1-S27. doi: 10.1097/LGT.0b013e318287d329.

Mitchell MF, Tortolero-Luna G, Cook E, et al. A randomized clinical trial of cryotherapy, laser vaporization, and loop electrosurgical excision for treatment of squamous intraepithelial lesions of the cervix. *Obstet Gynecol.* 1998;92(5):737-744.

Monsonego J, Cox JT, Behrens C, et al. Prevalence of high-risk human papilloma virus genotypes and associated risk of cervical precancerous lesions in a large U.S. screening population: data from the ATHENA trial. *Gynecol Oncol.* 2015;137(1):47-54. doi: 10.1016/j.ygyno.2015.01.551.

Moscicki AB, Shiboski S, Hills NK, et al. Regression of low-grade squamous intra-epithelial lesions in young women. *Lancet.* 2004; 364(9446):1678-1683. doi: 10.1016/S0140-6736(04)17354-6.

Ogilvie GS, van Niekerk D, Krajden M, et al. Effect of screening with primary cervical HPV testing vs cytology testing on high-grade cervical intraepithelial neoplasia at 48 months: The HPV FOCAL Randomized Clinical Trial. *JAMA* 2018;320(1):43-52. doi: 10.1001/jama.2018.7464.

Ostör AG. Natural history of cervical intraepithelial neoplasia: a critical review. *Int J Gynecol Pathol.* 1993;12(2):186-192.

Paavonen J, Naud P, Salmeron J, et al. Efficacy of human papillomavirus (HPV)-16/18 AS04-adjuvanted vaccine against cervical infection and precancer caused by oncogenic HPV types (PATRICIA): final analysis of a double-blind, randomised study in young women. *Lancet.* 2009;374(9686):301-314. doi: 10.1016/S0140-6736(09)61248-4.

Papanicolaou GN, Traut HF. The diagnostic value of vaginal smears in carcinoma of the uterus. *Am J Obstet Gynecol.* 1941;42:193-206.

Randall TC, Sauvaget C, Muwonge R, et al. Worthy of further consideration: an updated meta-analysis to address the feasibility, acceptability, safety and efficacy of thermal ablation in the treatment of cervical cancer precursor lesions. *Prev Med.* 2019;118:81-91. doi: 10.1016/j.ypmed.2018.10.006.

Saslow D, Solomon D, Lawson HW, et al. American Cancer Society, American Society for Colposcopy and Cervical Pathology, and American Society for Clinical Pathology screening guidelines for the prevention and early detection of cervical cancer. *J Low Genit Tract Dis.* 2012;16(3):175-204. doi: 10.1097/LGT.0b013e31824ca9d5.

Semm K. New apparatus for the "cold-coagulation" of benign cervical lesions. *Am J Obstet Gynecol.* 1966;95(7):963-966.

Solomon D, Davey D, Kurman R, et al. The 2001 Bethesda System: terminology for reporting results of cervical cytology. *JAMA.* 2002; 287(16):2114-2119.

Torre LA, Bray F, Siegel RL, et al. Global cancer statistics, 2012. *CA Cancer J Clin.* 2015;65(2):87-108. doi: 10.3322/caac.21262.

World Health Organization (WHO). *WHO guidelines for treatment of cervical intraepithelial neoplasia 2-3 and adenocarcinoma* in situ*: cryotherapy, large loop excision of the transformation zone, and cold knife conization;* 2014. Available at https://www.who.int/reproductivehealth/publications/cancers/treatment_CIN_2-3/en/. Accessed May 15, 2019.

World Health Organization (WHO). WHO Guidelines for the Use of Thermal Ablation for Cervical Pre-Cancer Lesions; May 28, 2019. https://apps.who.int/iris/handle/10665/329299

**Full references for this chapter can be found on ExpertConsult.com.**

# 30 Neoplastic Diseases of the Vulva and Vagina

Michael Frumovitz

## KEY POINTS

### VULVAR PREMALIGNANT AND MALIGNANT DISEASE

- Squamous cell carcinomas constitute 90% of primary vulvar malignancies. More than 80% of patients are older than 50 years at the time of diagnosis.
- Cancer of the vulva accounts for approximately 4% of malignancies of the lower female genital tract and occurs less often than uterine, ovarian, and cervical cancers.
- Paget disease generally occurs in postmenopausal women and is usually treated by wide excision. Invasive carcinomas at other sites should be ruled out.
- Prolonged use of fluorinated corticosteroids to treat itching accompanying vulvar dystrophy can lead to vulvar contraction.
- Topical testosterone is sometimes beneficial to treat lichen sclerosus but is absorbed systemically and occasionally can produce masculinizing symptoms.
- Studies have indicated that symptomatic lichen sclerosus is a premalignant condition preceding carcinoma by a mean of 4 years. The tumors that develop tend to be clitoral in location and identified in patients older than age 40 years.
- Human papillomavirus (HPV) vulvar infection is common. Intraepithelial neoplasia occurs much less often.
- HPV-positive tumors tend to occur in younger patients, and these tumors tend to have a better prognosis than HPV-negative tumors.
- A clear progression of dysplasia–carcinoma in situ (vulvar intraepithelial neoplasia [VIN] I, II, and III) to invasive carcinoma in the vulva has not been clearly established. VIN may spontaneously regress. VIN III has an approximately 3.4% risk of progression to invasive carcinoma.
- Intraepithelial neoplasia of the vulva is usually treated by local excision. Laser therapy of the atypical area may be used for younger patients who do not have raised lesions.
- Vulvar carcinomas less than 2 cm in diameter and depth of invasion less than 1 mm rarely metastasize to regional nodes.
- Unilateral vulvar tumors (>2 cm from midline) usually metastasize to ipsilateral inguinofemoral nodes only.
- Prognosis in vulvar cancer is primarily related to lesion size, lymph node status, and stage.
- The risk of lymph node groin metastases is related to tumor differentiation, lesion thickness, lymphovascular space involvement, patient age, and tumor size.
- The deep pelvic nodes do not become involved with metastatic vulvar cancer unless the inguinofemoral nodes are affected.
- The 5-year survival rate of vulvar carcinoma with negative nodes is more than 95%. With one positive node, the 5-year survival is approximately the same, 94%; with two nodes, it decreases to 80% and with three or more to 12%.
- Advanced vulvar tumors encroaching on the urethra or anus may be treated by radiation followed by wide radical excision rather than exenteration. Enhanced results have also been reported with the combined use of chemotherapy and radiation.
- Verrucous carcinomas are a variant of squamous cancer that do not metastasize to regional nodes. Radiation therapy is contraindicated, and local surgical excision is the treatment of choice.
- Melanomas constitute 5% of vulvar cancers and are the most common non–squamous cell malignancies.
- The overall 5-year survival of patients with vulvar melanoma is approximately 50%.
- Superficial spreading melanomas tend to occur in younger patients and have a better prognosis than nodular melanomas.
- Prognosis of vulvar melanoma is related to tumor invasion (Clark level) and to tumor thickness.
- Basal cell carcinoma of the vulva is treated by wide local excision.

### VAGINAL PREMALIGNANT AND MALIGNANT DISEASE

- Predisposing factors associated with the development of vaginal intraepithelial neoplasia include infection with HPV, previous radiation therapy to the vagina, immunosuppressive therapy, and human immunodeficiency virus (HIV) infection.
- The tendency of intraepithelial squamous neoplasia to develop anywhere in the lower female genital tract is termed a *field defect* and describes the increased risk of premalignant changes occurring in the cervix, vagina, or vulva.
- Most cases of vaginal intraepithelial neoplasia (VAIN) occur in the upper third of the vagina.
- VAIN can be treated by excision, laser, 5-fluoroucacil (5-FU), or imiquimod. Excision is often used for VAIN-3. Laser treatment is generally used for discrete lesions once invasion has been ruled out, and 5-FU and imiquimod cream are used to treat diffuse, multicentric, low-grade disease.
- The most common primary vaginal malignancy is squamous cell carcinoma (90%).
- Most cancers occurring in the vagina are metastatic.
- Vaginal cancers constitute less than 2% of gynecologic malignancies.
- Tumors of the upper vagina have a lymphatic drainage to the pelvis similar to cervical tumors. Tumors of the lower third of the vagina drain to the pelvic nodes and also to the inguinal nodes, similar to vulvar tumors.
- Radical surgery may be used to treat low-stage tumors, primarily of the upper vagina, in younger patients.
- Radiation therapy is the most commonly used modality for the treatment of squamous cell carcinoma of the vagina. Ideally at least 7000 to 7500 cGy is administered in less than 9 weeks. Concurrent chemoradiation should strongly be considered.
- The overall 5-year survival rate of patients treated for squamous cell carcinoma of the vagina is approximately 45%.
- Clear cell adenocarcinoma is often associated with prenatal diethylstilbestrol (DES) exposure. Prognosis is improved if the patient is older than 19 years, the tumor has a predominant tubulocystic tumor pattern, and the disease is low stage. Those with a maternal history of DES exposure have a better prognosis.
- Local therapy for small, stage I clear cell adenocarcinoma of the vagina is best considered if the tumor is smaller than 2 cm in diameter, invades less than 3 mm, and is predominantly of the tubulocystic histologic type. Pelvic nodes should be sampled and be free of tumor.

KEY POINTS—cont'd

- The overall 5-year survival rate of patients treated for clear cell adenocarcinoma is approximately 80%, partially because of the high proportion of low-stage cases.
- Vaginal melanomas are usually fatal. They occur primarily in patients older than 50 years.
- Endometrioid adenocarcinomas of the vagina may occur through the malignant transformation of endometriosis, often associated with the use of unopposed estrogen or tamoxifen.
- Endodermal sinus tumors occur in children younger than 2 years. They secrete alpha-fetoprotein and are usually treated by multiagent chemotherapy, followed by surgical excision.
- Sarcoma botryoides occurs primarily in children younger than 8 years. It is treated by a multimodality approach using multiagent chemotherapy with surgical removal and occasionally irradiation.

This chapter reviews the clinical and pathologic aspects of premalignant vulvar lesions and vulvar atypias (Box 30.1). This is followed by consideration of the diagnosis, natural history, and management of invasive cancers of the vulva, which includes not only the squamous cell carcinomas but also the rarer melanomas and sarcomas. The second part of the chapter reviews the diagnosis and treatment of premalignant and malignant diseases of the vagina.

## PREMALIGNANT AND MALIGNANT LESIONS OF THE VULVA

Cancer of the vulva accounts for approximately 5% of malignancies of the lower female genital tract, ranking it fourth in frequency after cancers of the endometrium, ovary, and cervix. Well-defined predisposing factors for the development of vulvar carcinoma have not been identified. In general, premalignant and malignant changes often arise at multifocal points on the vulva. Human papillomavirus (HPV) has been noted in almost 70% of patients with carcinoma of the vulva (Saraiya, 2015), and invasive carcinoma may arise from areas of carcinoma in situ, similar to the mechanism in cervical squamous cell carcinoma (see Chapter 29); however, some cases of squamous cell carcinoma of the vulva appear to develop in the absence of HPV or premalignant changes in the vulvar epithelium. Other factors, such as granulomatous disease of the vulva, diabetes, hypertension, smoking, and obesity, have been suggested as causative factors, but data do not provide consistent evidence regarding their association with vulvar carcinoma. Carcinoma of the vulva occurs with increasing frequency in those who have been treated for squamous cell carcinoma of the cervix or vagina, presumably as a result of the increased risk of carcinogenesis in the squamous epithelium of the lower genital tract in these patients. It appears that HPV DNA is involved in the development of a subset of vulvar carcinomas that tend to occur in younger patients, as noted by Crum (Crum, 1987). **Monk and colleagues demonstrated that not only were the HPV DNA–associated carcinomas found in younger patients but also that patients who are HPV negative appear to have had a poorer prognosis with tumors that were more likely to recur and lead to patient death (Monk, 1995).** As demonstrated by Hording and coworkers, HPV-positive tumors tend to have a warty or basaloid appearance, whereas HPV-negative tumors tend to be keratinized (Hørding, 1994). The former tend to be associated with premalignant vulvar changes (vulvar intraepithelial neoplasia [VIN]). The incidence of vulvar carcinoma in situ has increased by more than 400% since the 1980s, with most of the increase in new cases occurring in women younger than 50 years (Judson, 2006).

Most vulvar malignancies are squamous cell carcinomas and most occur in women older than 50 years. In fact, although more than 80% of patients with vulvar carcinoma in situ are younger than 50, less than 20% of women with invasive carcinoma are younger than 50. The age-specific incidence of vulvar cancer increases with each decade of life but overall has remained relatively stable since the 1980s (Fig. 30.1). Although most patients with carcinoma of the vulva are older than 60, those with carcinoma in situ of the vulva are usually 10 to 15 years younger—that is, aged 40 to 55. Premalignant changes of the vulva have been seen with increasing frequency among younger patients, often in their 20s and 30s, possibly as a result of an increasing rate of multiple sexual contacts and increased exposure to venereal infections, particularly HPV, in this population. Carter and colleagues reported a link between immunosuppression and invasive squamous cell carcinoma of the vulva in women younger than 40 years (Carter, 1993). Similar to cervical cancer, HPV-related infections would presumably progress through dysplasia to invasive cancer in these immunocompromised women.

**BOX 30.1** Classification of Vulvar Atypias

Squamous cell hyperplasia (formerly hyperplastic dystrophy)
Lichen sclerosus
Intraepithelial neoplasia
VIN I: Mild dysplasia
VIN II: Moderate dysplasia
VIN III: Severe dysplasia–carcinoma in situ
Others
  Paget disease
  Melanoma in situ (level 1)

*VIN,* Vulvar intraepithelial neoplasia.

## VULVAR ATYPIAS

### Specific Conditions

#### Vulvar Atypias: Intraepithelial Neoplasia

Lichen sclerosus (Fig. 30.2) is a change in the vulvar skin that often appears whitish; microscopically the epithelium becomes markedly thinned, with a loss or blunting of the rete ridges. **In some cases there is also a thickening or hyperkeratosis of the surface layers (Fig. 30.3), and inflammation is usually present. In a study of 3038 women in the Netherlands, Bleeker and associates found that the cumulative incidence of squamous cell carcinoma of the vulva for women with a prior diagnosis of lichen sclerosis was 6.7% (Bleeker, 2016).** The latency period between diagnosis of lichen sclerosis and subsequent vulvar cancer in those who developed the malignancy was 3.3 years. Concurrent VIN and age 70 or older at the time of the diagnosis of lichen sclerosis were independent risk factor for subsequent development of vulvar cancer. For women with lichen sclerosis, the standard incidence ratio (SIR) for developing vulvar

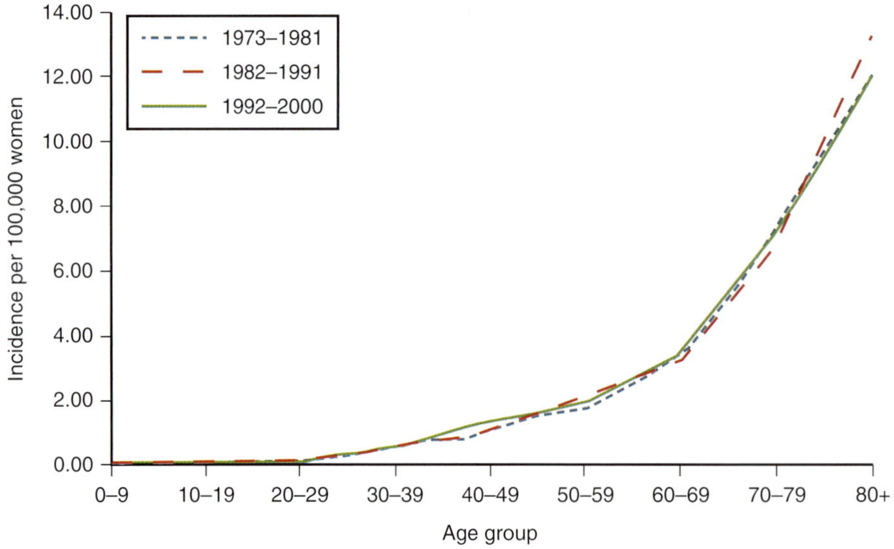


**Fig. 30.1** Incidence of invasive vulvar cancer by age and diagnosis year. (Modified from Judson PL, Habermann EB, Baxter NN, et al. Trends in the incidence of invasive and in situ vulvar carcinoma. *Obstet Gynecol.* 2006;107:1018-1022.)

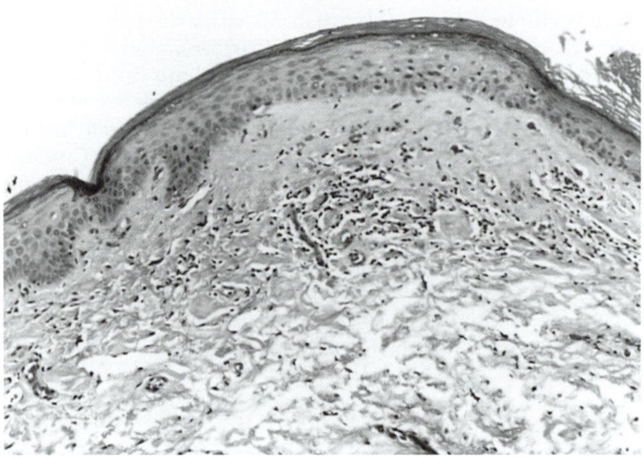

**Fig. 30.2** Lichen sclerosus et atrophicus. Homogeneous collagen in the papillary dermis is accompanied by a scattered lymphocytic infiltrate and atrophy of the epithelium (hematoxylin and eosin stain, ×80). (Courtesy Dr. Anthony Montag, Department of Pathology, University of Chicago, Chicago.)

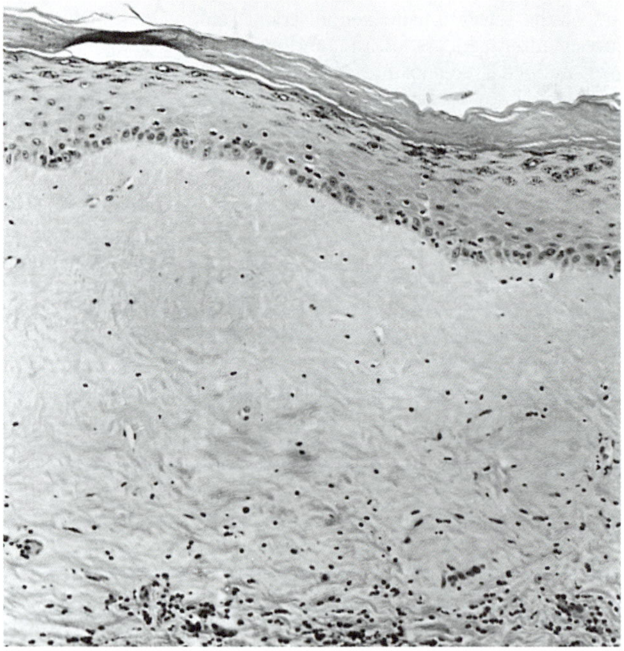

**Fig. 30.3** Lichen sclerosus. Hyperkeratosis is occasionally present. (From Friedrich EG, Wilkinson EJ. The vulva. In: Blaustein A, ed. *Pathology of the Female Genital Tract.* New York: Springer-Verlag; 1982.)

cancer is 33.6 and 3.69 for developing vaginal cancer (Halonen, 2017). For women who are compliant with topical corticosteroid therapy, the risk of developing vulvar dysplasia or carcinoma approaches 0% compared with noncompliant women, whose risk is 4.7% (Lee, 2015). Squamous hyperplasia (formerly called hyperplastic dystrophy) involves the elongation and widening of the rete ridges, which may be confluent (Fig. 30.4). There may also be hyperkeratotic surface layers, and the tissue grossly is often whitish or reddish.

Atypical changes may appear in the vulvar epithelium. These are often marked by a loss of the maturation process usually seen in squamous epithelium, as well as an increase in mitotic activity and nuclear/cytoplasmic ratio (Fig. 30.5). Mild dysplasia (atypia) is diagnosed if these changes involve the lower third of the epithelium, moderate dysplasia (atypia) if half to two-thirds of the epithelium is involved, and severe dysplasia (atypia) if more than two-thirds of the epithelium is affected. Carcinoma in situ involves the full thickness of the epithelium. The term *VIN I* is used for mild atypia, *VIN II* for moderate atypia, and *VIN III* for severe atypia and carcinoma in situ. It is sometimes difficult to distinguish between squamous hyperplasia and intraepithelial neoplasia. Crum has suggested that VIN usually contains nuclei that are fourfold or greater different in size, whereas differences in the size of nuclei in condyloma or nonneoplastic epithelia are threefold or less (Crum, 1987). Furthermore, abnormal mitoses are usually observed in VIN.

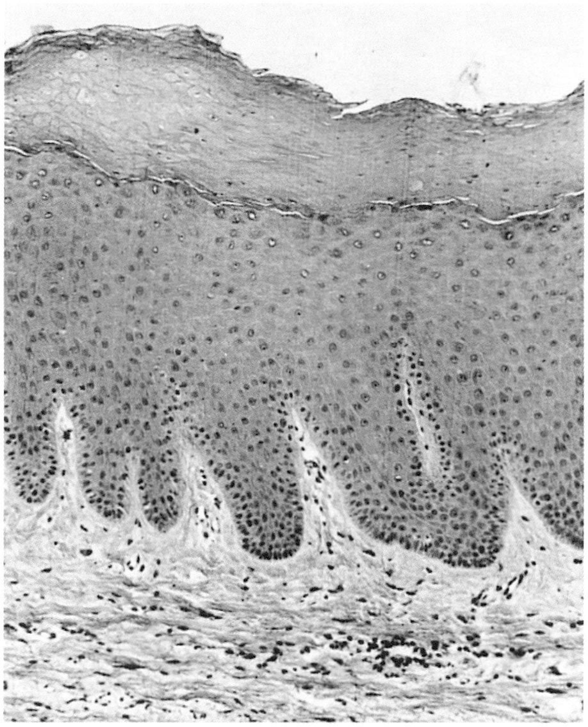

**Fig. 30.4** Squamous hyperplasia (formerly hyperplastic dystrophy), benign. Hyperkeratosis, acanthosis, and mild inflammation are present. (From Friedrich EG, Wilkinson EJ. The vulva. In: Blaustein A, ed. *Pathology of the Female Genital Tract.* New York: Springer-Verlag; 1982.)

### Carcinoma in Situ (VIN III)

Carcinoma in situ is diagnosed if the full thickness of the epithelium is abnormal (Fig. 30.6). Occasionally the process may histologically resemble carcinoma in situ of the cervix, and in many lesions there are multinucleated cells, abnormal mitoses, an increased density in cells, and an increase in the nuclear-to-cytoplasmic ratio.

### Paget Disease

Paget disease is a rare intraepithelial disorder that occurs in the vulvar skin and histologically resembles Paget disease in the breast. Paget cells are large pale cells (Fig. 30.7). The cells often occur in nests and infiltrate upward through the epithelium. Histologic abnormalities of the apocrine glands of the skin often may be noted in these lesions. **There has been an increased association of Paget disease of the vulva with underlying invasive adenocarcinoma of the vulva, vagina, and anus, as well as distant sites, including the bladder, cervix, colon, stomach, and breast.** Paget disease of the vulva tends to spread, often in an occult fashion, and recurrences are common after treatment.

## Diagnosis

### Clinical Presentation

Atypias of the vulva present with a variety of symptoms and signs. Irritation or itching is common, although some patients do not report these symptoms. The vulva often has a whitish change because of a thickened keratin layer. In the past, the term *leukoplakia* was used. This term has been discarded, in part because

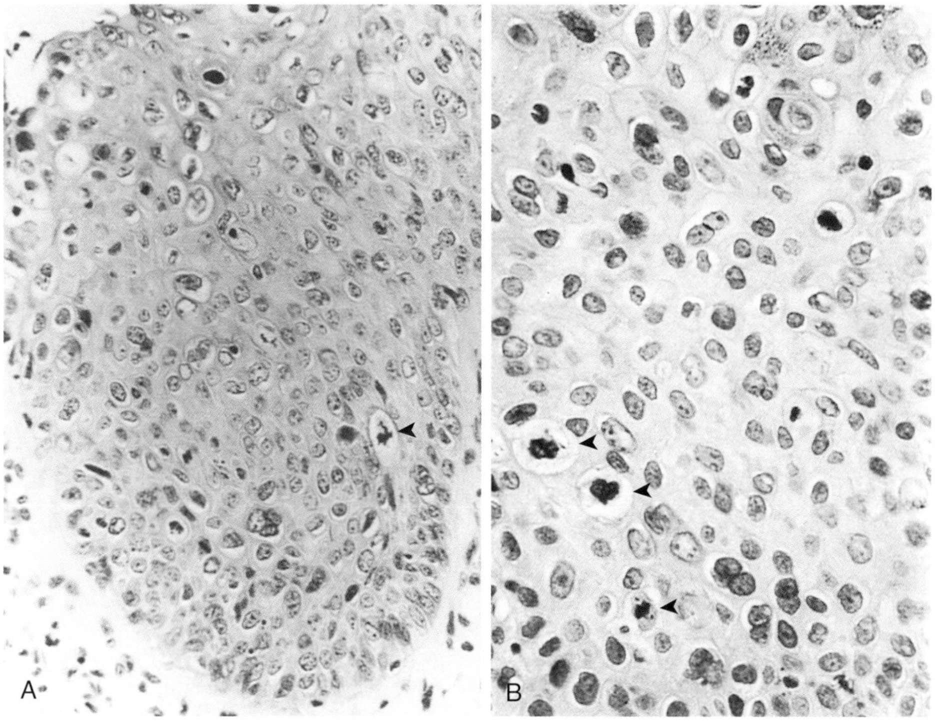


**Fig. 30.5 A,** Vulvar intraepithelial neoplasia from which human papillomavirus type 16 was isolated. Characteristic features displayed here include abnormal mitoses (a two-group metaphase is denoted by the *arrowhead*), a full-thickness population of abnormal cells, and abnormal differentiation. Superficial cells contain perinuclear halos, which in contrast to condylomata are small and concentric. **B,** The higher-power photomicrograph of vulvar intraepithelial neoplasia illustrates the marked variability in nuclear size and staining, with both enlarged nuclei and multinucleated cells. Coarsely clumped mitoses *(small arrowheads)* and a three-group metaphase *(large arrowhead)* are present. (From Crum CP. *Pathology of the Vulva and Vagina.* New York: Churchill Livingstone; 1987.)

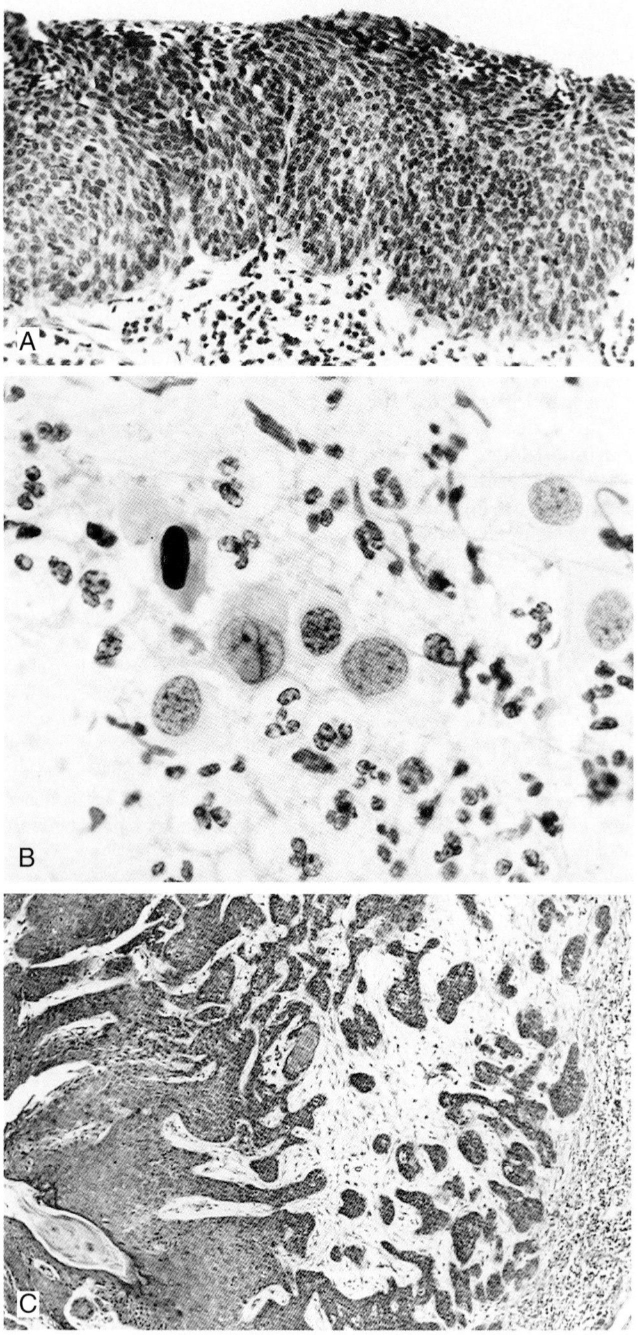

Fig. 30.6 **A,** Carcinoma in situ, histology. The full thickness of the epithelium is replaced by hyperchromatic cells with poorly defined cellular borders (×80). **B,** Carcinoma in situ, cytology. Cells derived from carcinoma in situ of the vulva may exhibit varying sizes and shapes, as depicted in this photomicrograph. Note variation in nuclear pattern from one nucleus to another. Degenerated polymorphonuclear leukocytes are present in the background (×800). **C,** Invasive squamous carcinoma, histology. Tumor nests and cords infiltrate stroma. The squamous nature of the tumor is more apparent on surface *(left),* where cells have abundant dense cytoplasm. Keratin is also seen (×80).

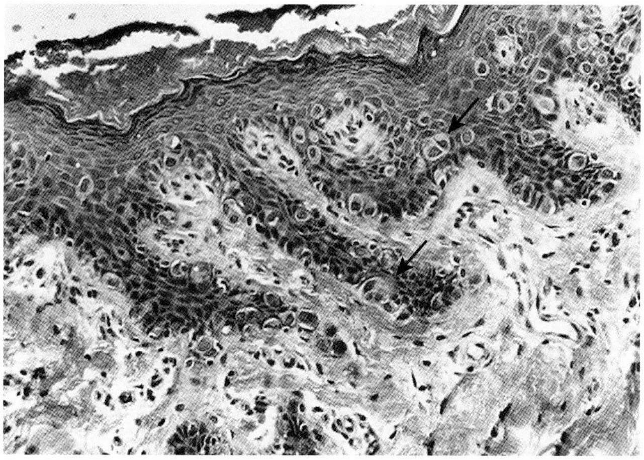

**Fig. 30.7** Vulvar epidermis with Paget disease. Malignant cells *(arrows)* are seen infiltrating the epidermis and spreading along the dermal-epidermal junction (hematoxylin and eosin stain, ×160). (Courtesy Anthony Montag, MD, Department of Pathology, The University of Chicago.)

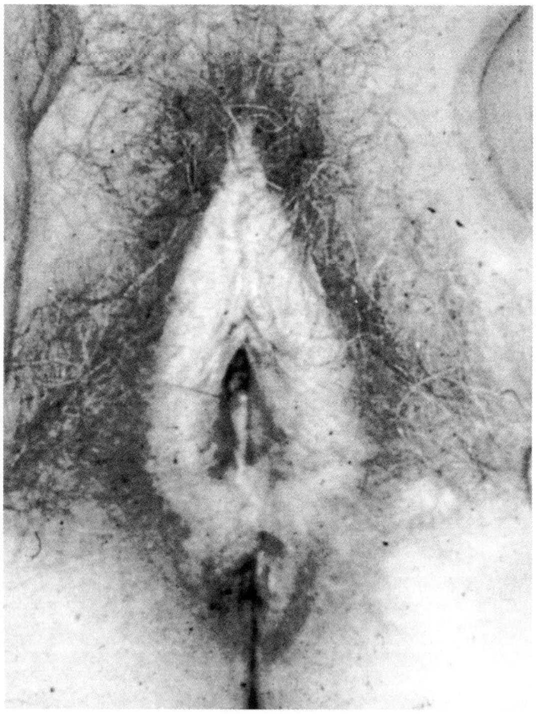

**Fig. 30.8** Vulva, lichen sclerosus. The tissue of the labia minora and perineum have a white, brittle, cigarette paper appearance. (From Kaufman RH, Gardner HL, Merrill JA. Diseases of the vulva and vagina. In: Romney SL, Gray MJ, Little AB, et al, eds. *Gynecology and Obstetrics.* New York: McGraw-Hill; 1980.)

abnormal lesions of the vulva require biopsy to establish a correct diagnosis. When lichen sclerosus is present, there is usually a diffuse whitish change to the vulvar skin (Fig. 30.8). The vulvar skin often appears thin and there may be scarring and contracture. In addition, fissuring of the skin is often present, accompanied by excoriation secondary to itching. Areas of squamous hyperplasias (formerly called *hyperplastic dystrophy without atypia*) also appear as whitish lesions in general, but the tissues of the vulva usually appear thickened and the process tends to be more focal or multifocal than diffuse (Fig. 30.9).

Abnormal areas of vulvar atypia or VIN may also appear as white, red, or pigmented areas on the vulva, although the clinical appearance of VIN is variable. Friedrich and colleagues estimated that approximately one-third of patients with carcinoma in situ present with pigmented lesions, emphasizing the importance of a biopsy to establish the diagnosis (Friedrich, 1980). The lesions

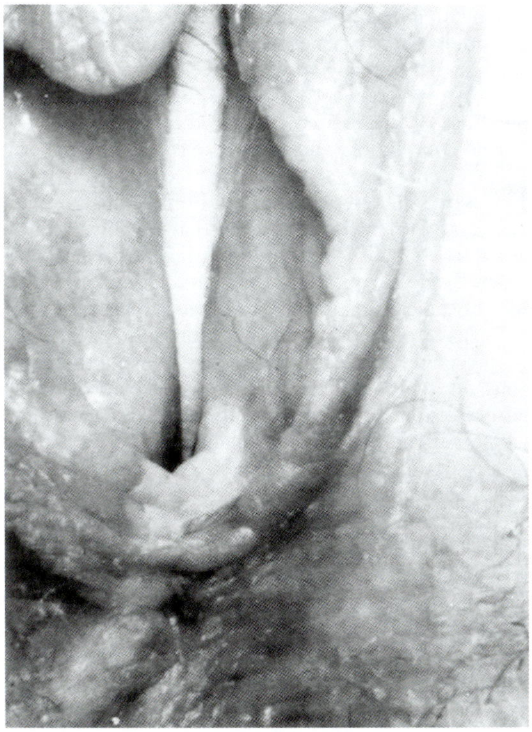

Fig. 30.9 Vulva, hyperplastic dystrophy. A sharply demarcated, raised, white area is noted at lower tip of white pointer. (From Kaufman RH, Gardner HL, Merrill JA. Diseases of the vulva and vagina. In: Romney SL, Gray MJ, Little AB, et al, eds. *Gynecology and Obstetrics.* New York: McGraw-Hill; 1980.)

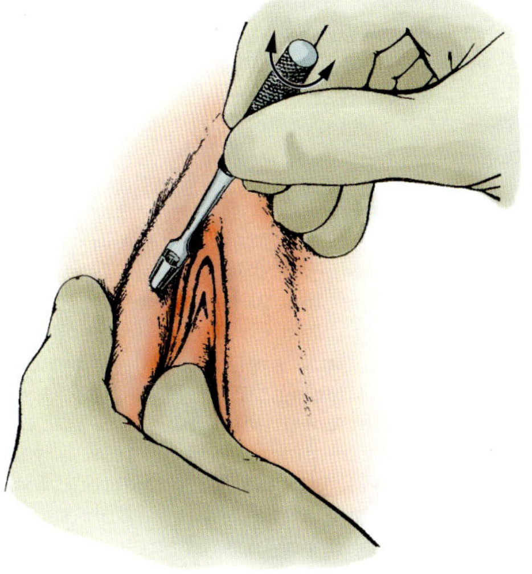

**Fig. 30.10** Diagnostic Keyes punch biopsy. (From Friedrich EG. *Vulvar Disease.* 2nd ed. Philadelphia: WB Saunders; 1983.)

tend to be discrete and multifocal and occur more commonly in those who have had squamous cell neoplasia of the cervix. In addition, reddish nodules may be foci of Paget disease as well as of carcinoma in situ, and Paget disease often has a reddish eczematoid appearance. **However, it should be reemphasized that these conditions cannot be accurately diagnosed from their clinical appearance, and biopsies are needed.**

### Diagnostic Methods

In general, cytologic evaluation (Papanicolaou [Pap] smear) of the vulva has not proved helpful, in part because the vulvar skin is thick and keratinized and does not shed cells as readily as the epithelium of the vagina and cervix; however, in some cases, particularly if there is ulceration of the vulva, a cytologic smear can be helpful diagnostically (see Fig. 32.6, *B*). A tongue depressor moistened with normal saline or tap water is scraped over the surface portion of the vulva to be sampled, and the specimen is placed on a glass slide and then fixed.

The toluidine blue test (1% toluidine blue applied for 1 minute, followed by 1% acetic acid) with biopsy of the retained blue-staining areas has generally been discarded because it appears to be very nonspecific.

Colposcopy of the vulva is difficult because the characteristic changes in vascular appearance and tissue patterns that are seen in the cervix are not present (see Chapter 28). Nevertheless, the magnification of the colposcope may be used to help follow patients with VIN and to identify the discrete whitish or pigmented areas that warrant biopsy. The colposcope is not used for routine vulvar examination but is primarily used for those who are being evaluated or followed for vulvar atypia or VIN. The addition of 3% acetic acid highlights whitish areas for biopsy.

Biopsy of the vulva can be conveniently accomplished with a Keyes dermal punch biopsy (Fig. 30.10). Usually, a 3- to 5-mm diameter punch is used. Each area in which a biopsy sample is to be obtained is usually infiltrated with local anesthesia using a fine 25-gauge needle. The punch is then rotated and downward pressure applied so that a disk of tissue is circumscribed. When the entire thickness of the skin has been incised, the specimen is elevated with forceps and removed with a sharp scissors. Occasionally, a larger biopsy is needed, in which case a larger field is anesthetized and a small scalpel or cervical punch biopsy (see Fig. 30.14 later in the chapter) is used to obtain the specimen. Little bleeding typically is encountered, and generally can be controlled by applying silver nitrate or ferrous subsulfate (Monsel solution). Depending on the size of the atypical area and the variety of atypical-appearing areas, one or multiple biopsy specimens may be needed.

## Treatment

### Vulvar Atypias

Most vulvar atypias have pruritus as the major symptom, so the relief of itching is often the woman's main concern. Once the correct diagnosis has been established by biopsy, appropriate therapy can be undertaken. Most whitish lesions will be benign because lichen sclerosus is the most common condition encountered.

Topical steroids can be used for atrophic conditions of the vulva, particularly lichen sclerosus. **The most commonly used option for the treatment of lichen sclerosus is 0.05% clobetasol propionate ointment. This can be used anywhere from nightly to twice weekly for up to 12 weeks and then used to retreat as necessary.** Although lichen sclerosus can be associated with the development of squamous cell carcinoma as described previously, use of a potent steroid cream may offer protection from malignant evolution.

A newer class of drug, topical calcineurin inhibitors (TCIs), has been evaluated as a nonsteroidal treatment of lichen sclerosis. Both the TCIs, pimecrolimus and tacrolimus, have been compared with clobetasol. In one study, twice daily usage of pimecrolimus 1% cream was compared with once daily application of clobetasol 0.05% cream in 38 women with biopsy-proven vulvar lichen sclerosis (Goldstein, 2011). Although clobetasol was superior in improving inflammation, patients who used pimecrolimus did have some reduction in inflammation and showed equivalent improvement in pruritus and burning/pain. Another study compared nightly tacrolimus 0.1% ointment with nightly clobetasol 0.05% cream in 55 women with lichen sclerosis (Funaro, 2014). Both groups had significant improvement in disease-related symptoms, although the clobetasol group had a larger improvement. Most would agree that clobetasol should still be used as first-line therapy in the treatment of lichen sclerosis, with consideration of TCIs in women who fail clobetasol or have other contraindications to topical steroid therapy.

When clobetasol and TCIs are ineffective, some advocate the use of hormonal creams, although results from small clinical trials using testosterone and progesterone creams have been mixed. A preparation of 2% testosterone propionate in petrolatum can be used twice daily, with once-daily maintenance after the first week. Often, reducing the dosage of testosterone cream to twice weekly is a sufficient maintenance dose. Side effects, such as clitoral hypertrophy and increased hair growth, can occur. If there are undesirable side effects with testosterone, local progesterone cream is sometimes tried, with variable success. Those who have a beneficial response to testosterone should be continued on the medication indefinitely.

The control of local irritation of the vulva is discussed in Chapter 18 (Benign Gynecologic Lesions). In addition to local measures to diminish irritation (e.g., cotton underclothes, avoidance of strong soaps and detergents, avoidance of synthetic undergarments), topical fluorinated corticosteroids are helpful to control itching. Commonly used preparations are 0.025% or 0.1% triamcinolone acetonide (Aristocort, Kenalog), fluocinolone acetonide (Synalar), and 0.01% or 0.1% betamethasone valerate. These are usually applied twice daily to control the itching, which is often relieved in 1 to 2 weeks. Unfortunately, the prolonged use of fluorinated topical steroids can lead to vulvar atrophy and contraction, and thus once the symptoms of itching are controlled, the dose of topical corticosteroids is tapered off or, if long-term therapy is needed, a nonfluorinated compound such as 1.0% hydrocortisone is used to avoid vulvar contraction. Occasionally, 1% hydrocortisone is sufficient for initial therapy. In some cases the corticosteroids are not successful, and numerous types of topical therapy must be tried to control symptoms. Gentle soaps are helpful. Burow's solution (5% solution of aluminum acetate) is often used as a wet dressing to help control irritation and itching. Doak tar, 3%, in petrolatum (USP) or in 1% hydrocortisone ointment is useful for severe cases.

In some patients with lichen sclerosus, severe contracture of the vulva, particularly in the area of the posterior fourchette, occurs with concomitant scarring and tenderness. Intercourse may then become painful for these patients. Woodruff and coworkers described a useful surgical technique to treat these vaginal outlet disorders by repair of the perineum (Woodruff, 1981). The contractured and fissured area in the posterior fourchette is excised, which results in an elliptic defect. This is then closed by undermining the distal 3 to 4 cm of the posterior vaginal mucosa and suturing the freed mucosa to the perineal skin (Fig. 30.11).

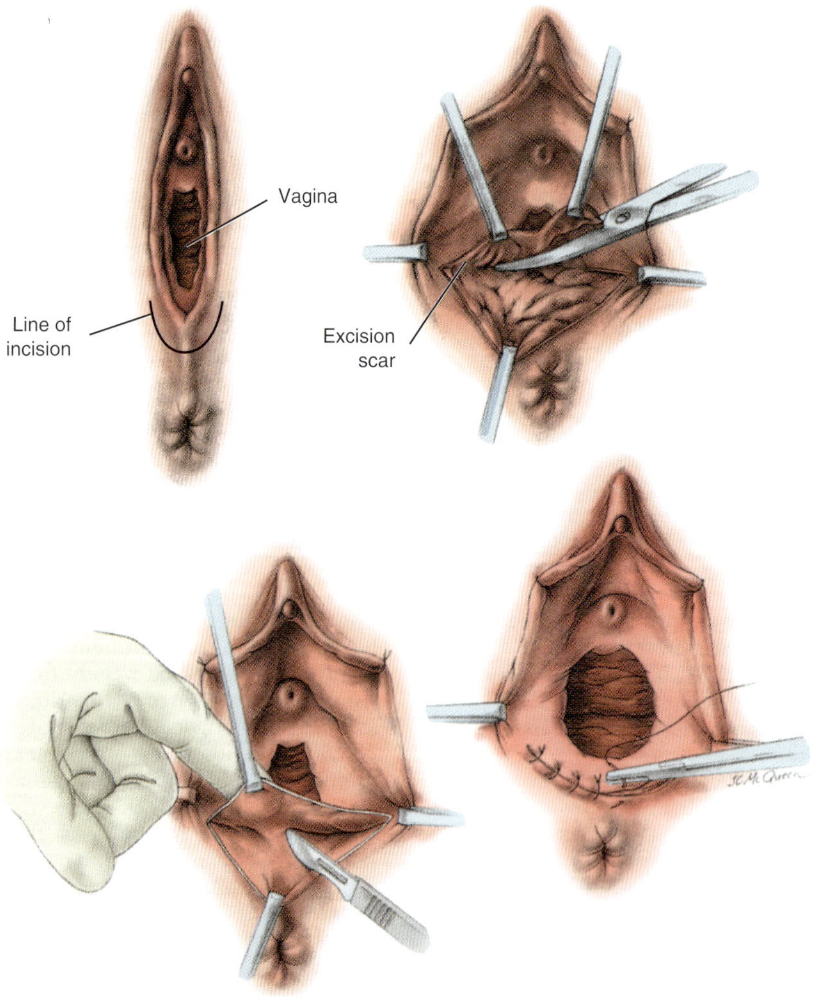


**Fig. 30.11** Surgical correction of perineal scars. (From Woodruff JD, Julian C. Surgery of the vulva. In: Ridley JH, ed. *Gynecologic Surgery: Errors, Safeguards, Salvage.* Baltimore: Williams & Wilkins; 1974.)

## Vulvar Intraepithelial Neoplasia

Once the diagnosis of VIN has been established by biopsy, therapy is performed to eradicate the area containing the neoplasia. The clinician must be aware that the progress of vulvar atypia (mild dysplasia [VIN I]) to moderate dysplasia (VIN II) to severe dysplasia and carcinoma in situ (VIN III) and then to invasive carcinoma is not as well documented for vulvar neoplasia as it is for squamous cell neoplasia of the cervix. Moreover, vulvar neoplasia is often multifocal, requiring treatment of several areas. An additional complication is that some cases originally diagnosed as intraepithelial neoplasia have been reported to regress spontaneously.

In 1972, Friedrich reported bowenoid atypia (histologically similar to carcinoma in situ) in a pregnant woman that regressed spontaneously postpartum (Friedrich, 1972). Others also reported spontaneous regression of this lesion. These spontaneously regressing lesions tend to be discrete elevations in young women. Some may be explained by studies of the nuclear DNA content of vulvar atypias that suggest that not all lesions with this designation are premalignant. Fu and colleagues noted that only four of eight cases of vulvar atypia had an aneuploid (neoplastic) distribution. A polyploid distribution was noted in four of the cases, which is consistent with a benign process, whereas aneuploidy is consistent with intraepithelial neoplasia (Fu, 1981).

**Although VIN has been diagnosed more commonly in younger women, the risk of progression to invasive cancer is higher for those who are older and for those who are immunosuppressed, such as women with acquired immunodeficiency syndrome (AIDS) or transplant recipients.** Chafe and associates studied 69 patients with a diagnosis of VIN treated by surgical excision (Chafe, 1988). Unsuspected invasion was found in 13 patients. The median age was 36 years for those without invasive carcinoma, whereas the median age was 58 years ($P = .003$) for those with invasion found in the excision specimen, emphasizing the increased risk of invasion in the older patients. Furthermore, the risk of invasion was higher in those who had raised lesions with irregular surface patterns. Thus patients who were older and those with irregular raised lesions had the greatest risk of unrecognized invasive carcinoma. A study by Modesitt and colleagues of 73 women, with a mean age of 45 years, found an invasive carcinoma in 22% of VIN III excision specimens (Modesitt, 1998). Not surprisingly, the risk of recurrence was almost 50% if the margins were positive and only 17% if they were negative. The risk of progression from intraepithelial disease to invasive carcinoma appears to be less for vulvar cases than for cervical disease (see Chapter 28).

Women with HIV and AIDS are also more likely to develop vulvar carcinoma in situ and invasive cancer than the general population. In a large population-based study, Chaturvedi and colleagues found a relative risk (RR) of 1.59 for developing VIN III in the 28 to 60 months after the onset of AIDS and an RR of 4.91 for developing invasive carcinoma in this group (Chaturvedi, 2009).

Studies have suggested that the potential of VIN to develop into invasive cancer is low. Buscema and coworkers followed 102 patients with vulvar carcinoma in situ for 1 to 15 years without treatment; 4 patients developed invasive disease, 2 of whom were immunosuppressed (Buscema,1980). Unfortunately, current techniques do not allow precise prediction of which lesions of VIN are at the greatest risk of progression to invasive disease. A population-based study from Norway has confirmed an increasing frequency of VIN III that nearly tripled from the mid-1970s to 1988 to 1991 but, during the same period, the age-adjusted frequency of invasive vulvar carcinomas remained almost constant (Iversen, 1998). Iversen and Tretli further noted an estimated conversion rate of VIN III to invasive carcinoma of approximately 3.4% for these in situ lesions (Iversen, 1998). **For women with a known diagnosis of VIN, risk factors for progression to invasive disease include immunosuppression (odds ratio [OR], 4.0), multifocal lesions (OR, 3.1), and smoking (OR, 3.0) (Fehr, 2013).**

HPV types 6 and 11 have generally been recognized as being found most often in benign vulvar warts, whereas primarily HPV types 16, 18, 31, 33, and 35 are more often associated with intraepithelial neoplasia or invasive carcinoma (see Chapter 28). The Centers for Disease Control and Prevention (CDC) has estimated that 80% of women aged 50 will have acquired a genital HPV infection at some point in their lives. Beutner and associates predicted that as many as 1 million new cases of perineal warts will occur annually in the United States (Beutner, 1998). An additional complication is that HPV type 16 infection is not always accompanied by histologic evidence of VIN. Moreover, HPV types 6, 11, and 16 can be recovered from a single site, including those that show only condyloma as well as those that show carcinoma. Thus a unique role for HPV types in VIN has not been elucidated. With current data, therapy should be based on histologic findings and not on the presence or absence of HPV infection or specific HPV types. Studies by Buscema and associates have suggested that HPV type 16 is often found in vulvar neoplasia and, as noted, HPV 16 has been commonly associated with some vulvar carcinomas (Buscema, 1980).

### HPV Therapy

The problem of the management of vulvar HPV infection is particularly complicated because it is extremely prevalent and the risk of progression from HPV infection to VIN is small. Planner and Hobbs evaluated 148 women with cytologic evidence of vulvar HPV infection and found that two-thirds of them had pruritus and dyspareunia (Planner, 1988). Results of the biopsy revealed that 11 of the 148 women had VIN. Follow-up identified spontaneous regression of HPV infection in 56 patients, whereas VIN III developed in 2 and invasive cancer eventually developed in 1. It appears that the best approach is to restrict therapy to those with clinically bothersome symptoms such as warts or to eradicate lesions with VIN, particularly VIN II and III. Cytologic or histologic evidence of an asymptomatic HPV infection, such as koilocytosis, is not an indication for therapy. Riva and colleagues treated lower genital tract HPV infection with laser to include the cervix, vagina, and vulva; 25 patients had proven subclinical HPV infection, and their male partners were also evaluated and treated (Riva, 1989). All 25 patients suffered severe pain, and many required hospitalization. At 3 months after therapy, 24 of 25 again had evidence of subclinical HPV infection and 22 had persistent histologic evidence of koilocytosis, indicating the futility of trying to eradicate HPV infection by this method.

Many VIN lesions tend to be posterior, predominantly in the perineal area. Surgical removal has been effectively used, but the type of operation has been changing. In the past, simple vulvectomy was widely performed to treat carcinoma in situ of the vulva, but this disfiguring operation is now uncommon, particularly because the disease is occurring in younger women. To improve the cosmetic result and sexual function, Rutledge and Sinclair introduced the method of skinning vulvectomy (Rutledge, 1968). This removes the superficial vulvar skin, preserving the clitoris, and replaces the removed skin with a split-thickness vulvar graft. In many cases, however, such extensive surgery is not needed. Often the abnormal area of the vulva can be removed only with wide local excision. Of the patients in the series reported by Buscema and coworkers, 62 were treated with local excision; 68% showed no recurrence (Buscema, 1980). For comparison, in 28 patients treated by vulvectomy, 70% showed no recurrence. The risk of recurrence is higher if neoplastic epithelium is found at the resection margin. Friedrich has noted a 10% risk of recurrence if the surgical margins are free of disease compared with a 50% risk if the surgical margins are involved with neoplasia (Friedrich, 1980). In addition to positive margins, other risk factors for recurrence of VIN include smoking and larger tumor size. (Wallbillich, 2012). Because recurrence may develop even if the resection margins are negative, long-term follow-up is mandatory.

**The carbon dioxide laser has been used to treat VIN, usually to a depth of 2 to 3 mm, with a deeper depth being used for areas that contain hair.** This results in eradication of the abnormal vulvar tissue and healing without scarring. Most patients require a single treatment but some require more, particularly those with large or multiple lesions. Usually, patients can be treated on an outpatient basis with local, regional, or general anesthesia. The laser is particularly useful for younger patients. **It is essential to be certain that the woman does not have invasive disease before using the laser, so a biopsy of any suspicious lesions should be performed before laser ablation.** The surgeon should be experienced in the diagnosis and treatment of vulvar disease before using laser ablation. Older patients and those with raised lesions should be treated by surgical excision.

Laser ablation treatment is usually carried out to a depth of 2 to 3 mm, and healing is usually complete within 2 to 3 weeks. Leuchter and associates treated 142 patients with carcinoma in situ of the vulva (Leuchter, 1984). Of the 42 treated by laser, 17% had recurrence; 4 of the 16 treated with vulvectomy (25%) and 15 of 45 treated by local excision (33%) also had recurrence. In view of the risk of unsuspected carcinoma in older patients, as noted by the studies of Chafe and colleagues (1988), those older than 45 years and those with raised or irregular lesions should have an excision performed and the entire tissue submitted for histologic evaluation. Posterior lesions near the anus require particular attention because the anal canal is often involved and this abnormal tissue also should be removed.

Treatment with 5-fluorouracil (5-FU) cream has been attempted for carcinoma in situ of the vulva, but it causes severe burning and is generally not used. Investigators have had promising results with 5% imiquimod cream as a primary treatment for VIN III. Van Seters and coworkers performed a randomized control study of 5% imiquimod topical cream versus placebo in 52 women with VIN II and III (van Seters, 2008). Most women included in the study (96%) were positive for HPV before initiation of therapy. In the treatment group, 81% had at least a reduction in the size of the primary lesion by more than 25% at 20 weeks and 35% had a complete response. In the placebo group there were no patients with partial or complete responses. At 12 months after enrollment, however, 3 patients (6%) had progressed to microinvasive vulvar carcinoma (1 in the treatment group, 2 in the placebo group).

Therapeutic vaccines using HPV peptides have also been explored for the treatment of VIN III. Kenter and colleagues combined long peptides from the E6 and E7 oncoproteins of HPV-16 into a vaccine and immunized 20 women with HPV-16–positive VIN III (Kenter, 2009). At 12 months after last vaccination, 79% had a clinical response, with 47% achieving complete response. Of note, all the women who had a complete response by 12 months also remained disease free at 24 months.

## Paget Disease of the Vulva

Paget disease generally occurs in postmenopausal women with an average age of approximately 65 years and is more common in white women. The disease typically appears grossly as a diffuse erythematous eczematoid lesion that has usually been present for a prolonged time. Itching is a common problem. **The major importance of Paget disease of the vulva is the common association with other invasive carcinomas. Squamous cell carcinoma of the vulva or cervix, adenocarcinoma of the sweat glands of the vulva, or Bartholin gland carcinoma may be present. Cases of adenocarcinoma of the gastrointestinal (GI) tract and breast accompanying Paget disease have also been reported.** Once a diagnosis of Paget disease of the vulva is made, it is important for the gynecologist to rule out the presence of breast and GI malignancies. In a review by Fanning and associates, 20% of patients with vulvar Paget had nonvulvar malignancies, including cancers of the breast, uterus, pancreas, lung, stomach, thyroid, and skin. In addition, 12% had invasive Paget disease of the vulva and 4% had invasive adenocarcinoma of the vulva (Fanning, 1999).

If no local or distant primary malignancy is uncovered, a wide excision of the affected area can be performed. It is important to remove the full thickness of the skin to the subcutaneous fat to ensure that all the skin adnexal structures are excised because they may have a subclinical malignancy. Bergen and coworkers evaluated 14 patients with Paget disease of the vulva treated by surgery, usually vulvectomy, skinning vulvectomy with graft, or hemivulvectomy (Bergen, 1989). With a median follow-up of 50 months, all patients were free of disease, although 2 with positive margins and 1 with negative margins required treatment for recurrence. Fishman and colleagues studied 14 patients with Paget disease treated by various surgical procedures (Fishman, 1995). Frozen-section or gross visual inspection was used to judge the operative margins. In this series, visual estimation was as useful as frozen section insofar as the error rate for judging margins by the final pathology report was approximately 35%. In addition, 2 of 5 patients with positive margins had a recurrence after the initial operation compared with 3 of 9 with negative margins. This small series therefore suggests that gross visual inspection may be as useful as frozen section when judging the extent of surgical operation. Other small series evaluating Mohs micrographic surgery for treating vulvar extramammary disease have failed to reduce recurrence significantly. A conservative approach involving removal of gross Paget disease with approximately a 1-cm margin appears to be the most appropriate, with the understanding that reexcision may be required for recurrence in the future. The full thickness of the vulvar skin to the adipose layer should be removed.

Even if resection margins are free of Paget disease at the time of surgical excision, local recurrence remains a risk. Women who have been treated for Paget disease of the vulva should have as part of their routine follow-up an annual examination of the breast, cytologic evaluation of the cervix and vulva, and screening for GI disease, at least by testing for occult blood in the stool. Progression of Paget disease of the vulva to invasive adenocarcinoma has been rarely reported.

Investigators have also explored using topical imiquimod cream as a nonsurgical therapy for extramammary Paget disease of the vulva. In one retrospective study, 21 women with Paget disease were treated with imiquimod cream and 11 (52%) had a complete response to therapy, whereas an additional 6 (29%) had a partial response with no cases of progressive disease (Luyten, 2014). In another small study, 6 of 8 patients with vulvar Paget disease (75%) treated with imiquimod cream had a complete pathologic response at 12 weeks; however, 4 of the 6 patients who had a complete response (67%) eventually did have recurrent disease (Cowan, 2016). Because treatment of Paget disease not associated with underlying malignancies is largely for symptom control, a trial of imiquimod may be a reasonable approach for patients who do not desire surgery or are not surgical candidates. In addition, because achieving negative margins with surgical resection is rare, some may consider using a course of imiquimod adjuvantly after surgical resection in an effort to reduce recurrence.

## MALIGNANT CONDITIONS

### Squamous Cell Carcinoma

Squamous cell carcinomas comprise approximately 90% of primary vulvar malignancies, but a variety of other vulvar cancers are encountered; the major types are listed in Box 30.2. Melanomas account for approximately 4% to 5%, and the other types make up the remainder.

#### Morphology and Staging

Grossly, vulvar carcinomas usually appear as raised, flat, ulcerated, plaquelike, or polypoid masses on the vulva (Fig. 30.12). A biopsy sample of the lesion reveals the characteristic histologic appearance of squamous cell carcinoma (see Fig. 30.6, *C*).

**BOX 30.2** Primary Vulvar Malignancies

Squamous cell carcinoma
Adenocarcinoma (including Bartholin gland)
Verrucous carcinoma
Basal cell carcinoma
Melanoma
Sarcoma

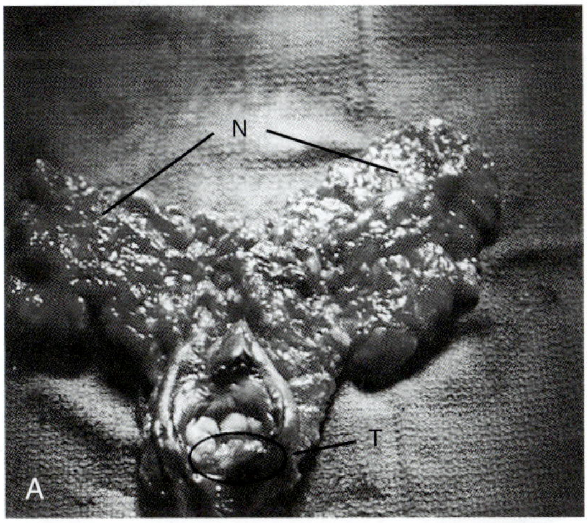


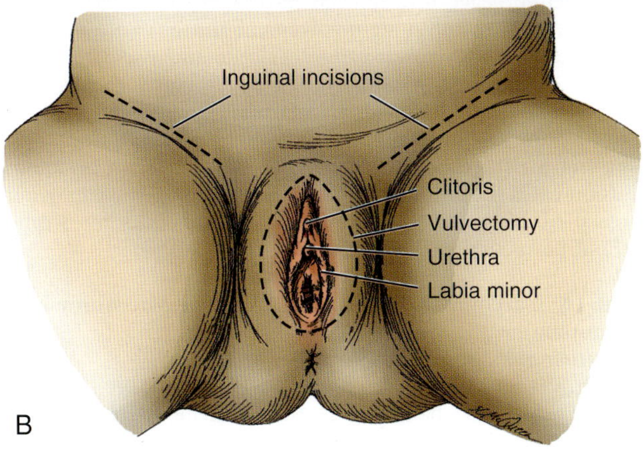


**Fig. 30.12 A,** Radical vulvectomy specimen. **B,** Vulvectomy with operative incision lines shown. Note groin incisions.

Four clinical stages are defined for carcinoma of the vulva according to the International Federation of Gynecology and Obstetrics (FIGO), similar to the system used for other gynecologic malignancies. In addition, many centers use the TNM system (tumor, nodes, metastases) for classification; *T* denotes the size and extent of the tumor, *N* the clinical status of the nodes, and *M* the presence or absence of metastatic disease.

In the clinical staging system, lymph node status was assessed clinically and incorporated into the stage. Enlarged or clinically suspicious lymph nodes were assigned a higher stage, regardless of disease status documented at surgery. Clinically negative nodes were assigned an earlier stage, which was upheld even if they were found to harbor metastasis after surgical removal and pathologic examination. Therefore in 1988 the FIGO staging was modified to a surgical staging system for vulvar cancer to reflect lymph node status more accurately. In addition, a location on the perineum is no longer assigned to stage III. This system, with the modifications introduced in 2009 by FIGO and in 2017 by the American Joint Committee on Cancer (AJCC) for new definitions of stages I to IV, is shown in Box 30.3.

#### Natural History, Spread, and Prognostic Factors

The vulvar area is rich in lymphatics, with numerous cross connections. The main lymphatic pathways are illustrated in Fig. 30.13. Tumors located in the middle of either labium tend to drain initially to the ipsilateral inguinofemoral nodes, whereas perineal tumors can spread to the left or right side. Tumors in the clitoral or urethral areas can also spread to either side. From the inguinofemoral nodes, the lymphatic spread of tumor is cephalad to the deep pelvic iliac and obturator nodes. **Although there has been concern in the past that tumors in the clitoral-urethral area would spread directly to the deep pelvic nodes, this rarely, if ever, occurs.** The characteristics of lymph drainage of the vulva have been evaluated by Iversen and Aas, who injected technetium-99m colloid subcutaneously into the anterior and posterior labia majora, anterior and posterior labia minora, clitoral area, and perineum (Iversen, 1983). They then measured the radioactivity in the pelvic lymph nodes, which were surgically removed 5 hours later. More than 98% of the radioactivity was found in the ipsilateral node and less than 2% on the contralateral side. The anterior labial injections resulted in a 92% concentration of radioactivity in the ipsilateral side, with 8% on the contralateral side. The clitoral and perineal injections developed a bilateral nodal distribution of radioactivity in all the patients. It is of interest that two-thirds of the patients with labial injections had a small amount of detectable radioactivity in the contralateral nodes. Thus anastomoses of the lymphatics do exist, but a direct connection from the clitoris to the deep nodes was not demonstrated.

**The prognosis of a woman with vulvar carcinoma is related to the stage of the disease (Fig. 30.14), lesion size, and the presence or absence of cancer in regional nodes.**

The status of the regional lymph nodes is the most important factor prognostically and therapeutically. Numerous studies, including a multicenter collaborative investigation from the Gynecologic Oncology Group (GOG), have indicated that tumor stage, location on the vulva, microscopic differentiation, presence or absence of vascular space involvement, and tumor thickness are all important prognostic factors. In a GOG study of 588 patients reported by Homesley and colleagues, the risk of lymph node metastases was related to lesion size (19% for $<2$ cm and 42% for $>2$ cm) (Homesley, 1991). Additional independent predictors of positive nodes were as follows: (1) tumor grade; (2) suspicious, fixed, or ulcerated lymph nodes; (3) lymphovascular space involvement; (4) older age of the woman; and (5) tumor thickness. Table 30.1 summarizes these factors.

**BOX 30.3** TNM and Staging Classifications of Carcinoma of the Vulva

**TNM**

T: Primary tumor
Tis: Preinvasive carcinoma (carcinoma in situ)
T1: Tumor confined to the vulva and/or perineum
 T1a: Tumor confined to the vulva or perineum, ≤2 cm in diameter and with stromal invasion <1 mm
 T1b: Tumor confined to the vulva or perineum, >2 cm in diameter or tumor any size with stromal invasion >1 mm
T2: Tumor of any size with adjacent spread to the urethra, vagina, anus, or all of these
T3: Tumor of any size infiltrating the bladder mucosa, rectal mucosa, or both, including the upper part of the urethral mucosa or fixed to the anus
N: Regional lymph nodes
NX: Regional lymph nodes cannot be assessed
N0: No regional lymph node metastasis
N1: Regional lymph node metastasis with one or two lymph node metastases each less than 5 mm, or one lymph node metastasis greater than or equal to 5 mm
 N1a: One or two lymph node metastases each less than 5 mm
 N1b: One lymph node metastasis greater than or equal to 5 mm
N2: Regional lymph node metastasis with three or more lymph node metastases each less than 5 mm, or two or more lymph node metastases greater than or equal to 5 mm, or lymph node(s) with extranodal extension
 N2a: Three or more lymph node metastases each less than 5 mm
 N2b: Two or more lymph node metastases greater than or equal to 5 mm
 N2c: Lymph node(s) with extranodal extension
N3: Fixed or ulcerated regional lymph node metastasis
 M: Distant metastases
 M0: No clinical metastases
 M1: Distant metastases (including pelvic lymph node metastases)

**STAGING (FIGO), MODIFIED 2009**

Stage I—T1, N0, M0: Tumor confined to vulva or perineum
 IA: Lesions ≤2 cm in size, confined to the vulva or perineum and with stromal invasion ≤1 mm; no nodal metastasis
 IB: Lesions >2 cm in size or with stromal invasion >1.0 mm, confined to the vulva or perineum, with negative nodes
Stage II—T2, N0, M0: Tumor of any size with extension to adjacent perineal structures (one-third lower urethra, one-third lower vagina, anus) with negative nodes
Stage III—T1-2, N1/2, M0: Tumor of any size with or without extension to adjacent perineal structures (one-third lower urethra, one-third lower vagina, anus), with positive inguinofemoral lymph nodes
 IIIA: (i) With one lymph node metastasis (≥5 mm) or (ii) one or two lymph node metastasis(es) (<5 mm)
 IIIB: (i) With two or more lymph node metastases (≥5 mm) or (ii) three or more lymph node metastases (<5 mm)
 IIIC: With positive nodes with extracapsular spread
Stage IV—T3 or any T, any N, M1: Tumor invades other regional (two-thirds upper urethra, two-thirds upper vagina) or distant structures
 IVA: Tumor invades any of the following: (i) upper urethral or vaginal mucosa, bladder mucosa, rectal mucosa, or fixed to pelvic bone; or (ii) fixed or ulcerated inguinofemoral lymph nodes
 IVB: Any distant metastasis including pelvic lymph nodes.

Modified from FIGO Committee on Gynecologic Oncology, European Institute of Oncology, Milan, Italy: Revised FIGO staging for carcinoma of the vulva, cervix, and endometrium. *Int J Gynecol Obstet.* 2009;105:103; and American College of Surgeons, Chicago, Illinois. The original source for this information is the American Joint Committee on Cancer's *Cancer Staging Manual, Eighth Edition* (2017) published by Springer International Publishing. Corrected at 4th printing, 2018.
*FIGO,* International Federation of Gynecology and Obstetrics; *TNM,* tumor-node-metastasis.

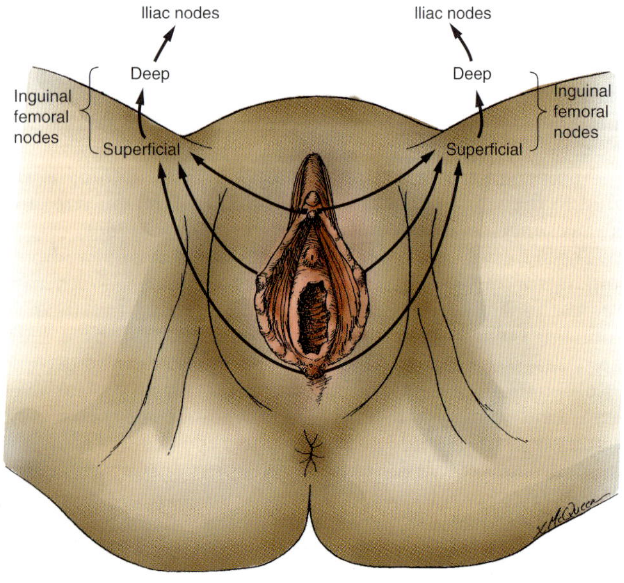


**Fig. 30.13** Vulvar lymph drainage is shown in this general schematic representation of major drainage channels of vulva.

Lymphovascular space invasion also appears to be a prognostic factor in vulvar tumors, as it is in cervical carcinoma (see Chapter 28). In a small study of 22 patients, Rowley and associates noted no metastases in 20 patients without lymphovascular space invasion and in 2 patients with lymphovascular space invasion (Rowley, 1988).

Perineural space invasion has also been shown to be a risk factor for both lymph node involvement and survival. In a study of 421 patients with vulvar cancer, Salcedo and associated found the rate of perineural invasion was 7.6%. Patients with perineural invasion had a 50% risk for lymph node metastases compared with 22% for those without. In addition, on multivariate analyses adjusting for stage, women with vulvar cancers with perineural invasion had a hazard ratio for death of 2.71 and a median overall survival of 26 months compared with 94 months for women without perineural invasion (Salcedo, 2019).

### Stage IA: Carcinoma of the Vulva (Early or Microinvasive Carcinoma)

#### *Definition and Clinicopathologic Relationships*

The term *microinvasive carcinoma of the vulva* typically refers to a lesion considered to be stage IA—that is, smaller than 2 cm, with less than 1 mm invasion—and is used to identify early tumors unlikely to spread to regional nodes. However, varying clinicopathologic results are reported when this definition is used.

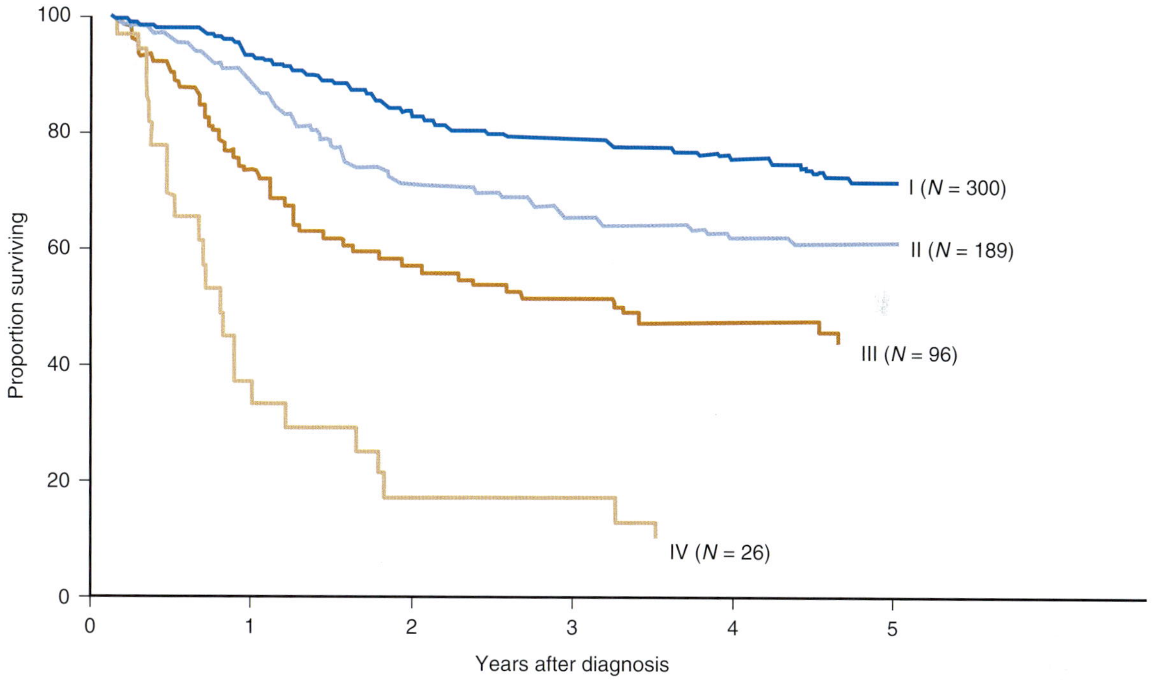


| Strata | Patients (N) | Mean age (years) | Overall survival at 1 year | 2 year | 3 year | 4 year | 5 year | Hazards ratio[a] (95% Confidence intervals) |
|---|---|---|---|---|---|---|---|---|
| I | 300 | 64.7 | 92.3% | 82.3% | 78.7% | 75.7% | 71.4% | Reference |
| II | 189 | 67.4 | 86.5% | 71.0% | 65.8% | 62.2% | 61.3% | 1.94 (1.36–2.75) |
| III | 96 | 69.4 | 72.0% | 57.2% | 51.3% | 47.5% | 43.8% | 3.84 (2.55–5.78) |
| IV | 26 | 72.8 | 33.3% | 16.7% | 16.7% | 8.3% | 8.3% | 12.2 (7.08–21.2) |

**Fig. 30.14** Carcinoma of the vulva, patients treated from 1990 to 1992; survival by International Federation of Gynecology and Obstetrics stage (epidermoid invasive cancer only; N = 611). [a]Hazards ratio and 95% confidence intervals obtained from a Cox model adjusted for country. (From Pecorelli S, Creasman WT, Pettersson F, et al. *FIGO Annual Report on the Results of Treatment in Gynaecological Cancer.* Vol. 23. Milan, Italy: International Federation of Gynecology and Obstetrics; 1998.)

**TABLE 30.1** Factors Related to Positive Inguinal Nodes (588 Cases)

| GOG Grade | % Positive Nodes | Tumor Thickness (mm) | % Positive Nodes | Age (yr) | % Positive Nodes | LVSI | % Positive Nodes |
|---|---|---|---|---|---|---|---|
| 1 | 2.8 | ≤1 | 2.6 | <55 | 25.2 | + | 75 |
| 2 | 15.1 | 2 | 8.9 | 55-64 | 25.4 | – | 27 |
| 3 | 41.2 | 3 | 18.6 | 65-74 | 36.4 | | |
| 4 | 59.7 | 4 | 30.9 | >75 | 46 | | |
| | | ≥5 | 43 | | | | |

Modified from Homesley H, Bundy BN, Sedlis A, et al. Prognostic factors for groin node metastasis in squamous cell carcinoma of the vulva (a Gynecologic Oncology Group study). *Gynecol Oncol.* 1993;49:279.
*GOG,* Gynecologic Oncology Group; *LVSI,* lymphovascular space invasion.

Part of the confusion is because of different reference points from which the depth of invasion is measured—that is, from the surface or basement membrane. Dvoretsky and coworkers carefully analyzed the microscopic aspects of 36 cases of superficial vulvar carcinoma (Dvoretsky, 1984) Tumor penetration into the stroma was measured from the surface of the squamous epithelium (neoplastic thickness; Fig. 30.15, *A*) and also from the tip of the adjacent epithelial ridge (stromal invasion; see Fig. 30.15, *B*). In 6 of the 36 cases, disease had spread to the regional nodes, and all had invaded more than 3 mm from the surface. Yoder and associates found that no women with squamous cell carcinoma of the vulva invading less than 1 mm had nodal disease. **For women with lesions invading 1 to 3 mm, the risk of nodal spread was 6% and for those with lesions invading 3 to 5 mm, the risk of nodal spread increased to 20%. Furthermore, none of the patients with tumors invading less than 1 mm had local recurrence at 258 months' follow-up (Yoder, 2008).**

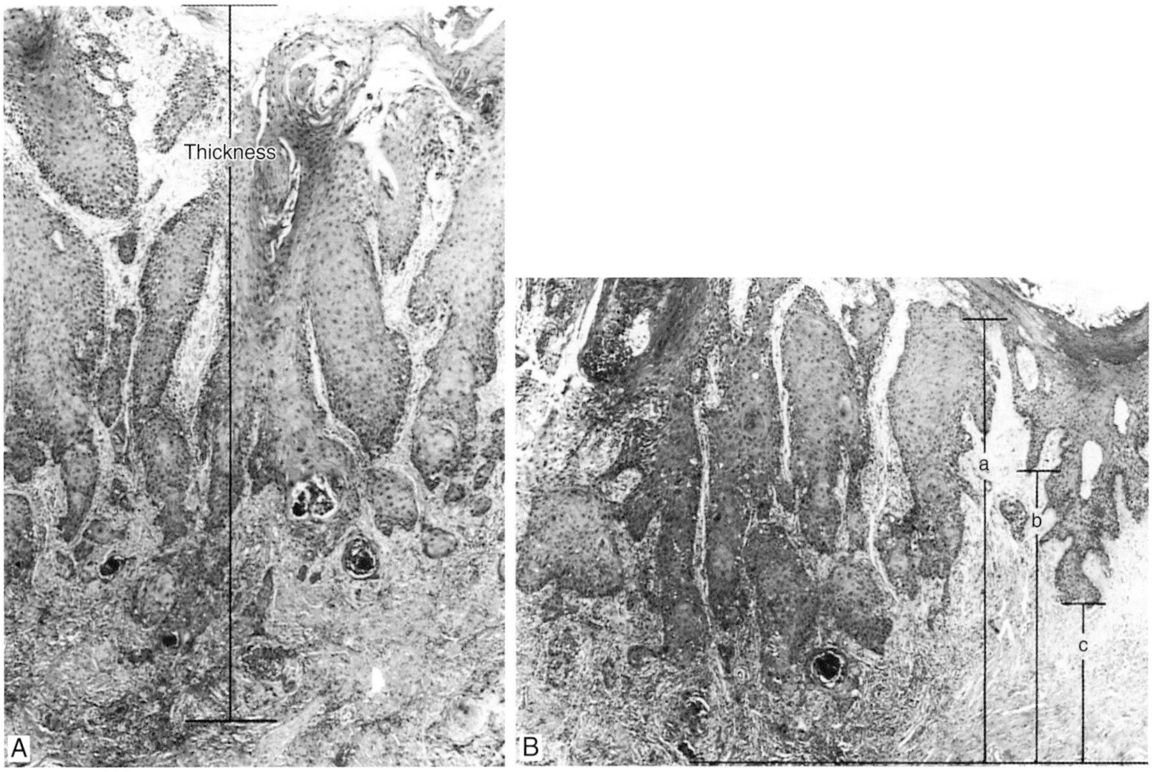


**Fig. 30.15 A,** Measurement of neoplastic thickness in squamous cell carcinoma (×35). **B,** Superficially invasive squamous cell carcinoma. The reference point used to measure the depth of stromal invasion is demonstrated by line b. Note the striking variation in the measurement of stromal invasion, depending on which reference point is chosen (line a, b, or c; ×35). (From Dvoretsky PM, Bonfiglio TA, Helkamp BF, et al. The pathology of superficially invasive thin vulva squamous cell carcinoma. *Int J Gynecol Pathol.* 1984;3:331.)

The presence of carcinoma in situ in the primary lesion decreases the risk of node involvement in these cases. Ross and Ehrman have noted that only 1 of 35 patients with adjacent carcinoma in situ had nodal metastases, and this tumor penetrated the stroma 1.7 mm (Ross, 1987). In contrast, 5 of 27 superficial stage I patients (2.1 to 5.0 mm penetration) without adjacent carcinoma in situ had positive nodes. Thus spread to regional lymph nodes in stage IA carcinoma of the vulva is unlikely, particularly if the tumor is well differentiated (grade 1), invades less than 3 mm measured from the surface, or has a depth of invasion measured from the adjacent rete pegs of less than 1 mm and is without vascular space involvement. The presence of carcinoma in situ is a favorable factor. Less well-differentiated tumors or those with vascular involvement or confluence and with greater depths of invasion have an increased risk of lymph node involvement by cancer.

*Treatment*

**Based on available evidence, it would appear prudent that most patients with stage IA carcinoma of the vulva based on the criteria described earlier should be treated at least with a wide excision to give a margin of 1 to 2 cm. Depending on the location of the tumor, a hemivulvectomy may be needed. The lymph node dissection may be omitted or deferred, depending on the final pathologic evaluation of the tumor in the surgical specimen.** For younger patients, especially with tumors that involve the labia or perineum at a distance from the clitoris, an operation that spares the clitoris should be used. Even if the criteria for stage IA are rigorously applied, a rare nodal metastasis may occur, as reported by Van der Velden and associates (Van der Velden, 1992). However, a report by Magrina and coworkers on 40 patients with T1 lesions (<2 cm in diameter and <1 mm invasion) indicated that they could be effectively treated with wide excision (Magrina, 2000). No nodal metastases were noted in this small group, and excision appeared to be as effective as a more radical operation in preventing recurrent disease.

## Invasive Carcinoma of the Vulva

Fig. 30.12, *A*, shows a typical carcinoma of the vulva, which usually appears as a polyploid mass. The woman often reports a sore that has not healed. She may also report bleeding, but this does not usually occur early in the course of the disease. Unfortunately, the delay in diagnosis is common because older patients often fail to seek prompt medical attention and, often when they do, a biopsy is not initially performed. For example, some patients with symptoms of irritation or itching are treated with various medications to eradicate the symptoms. It is vital that a biopsy sample be taken of any vulvar lesion before undertaking therapy, as was emphasized earlier. A biopsy of a tumor such as that shown in Fig. 30.12, *A*, can easily be obtained on an outpatient basis using local anesthesia and biopsy forceps such as a Kevorkian punch as illustrated in Chapter 28, Intraepithelial Neoplasia of the Lower Genital Tract.

Effective therapy of clinical stage I or II and early stage III vulvar carcinoma can be accomplished with a wide radical excision and inguinofemoral node dissection. Lesions located more than 2 cm from the midline typically need only an ipsilateral inguinofemoral lymphadenectomy, whereas midline lesions necessitate bilateral groin dissections or sentinel lymph node biopsies (see later). **Because the deep pelvic nodes are almost never involved unless the inguinal nodes are also involved, only the**

**inguinofemoral nodes are removed at the time of the primary operation and the deep pelvic nodes subsequently treated with external radiation if the superficial nodes are involved with tumor.** The inguinofemoral node dissection is performed through separate inguinal incisions followed by the vulvectomy portion. Fig. 30.12, *A*, shows the type of specimen that can be obtained through separate groin incisions. The operative incisions are shown in Fig. 30.12, *B*. It appears that an adequate surgical dissection with decreased wound complications can be accomplished by this technique. If a complete inguinofemoral lymphadenectomy is performed, it is advisable to use suction drainage in the inguinal area until all drainage is complete, which usually takes 7 to 10 days, and drains are also occasionally used in the vulvar area. If sentinel lymph node biopsy only is performed, drains are not necessary. It is important that an adequate margin, usually 1 to 2 cm, be obtained around the primary tumor at the time of surgery. Grimshaw and colleagues reported on 100 cases operated on through separate incisions and noted superb results with a corrected 5-year survival rate in stage I of 96.7% and stage II of 85% (Grimshaw, 1993). Similar excellent results for separate skin incisions were reported by Farias-Eisner and associates on 74 patients, with 5-year survival rates of 97% and 90% for stages I and II, respectively (Farias-Eisner, 1994). Tumor recurrence has occurred rarely in the skin bridge over the symphysis when separate groin incisions are used without an en bloc dissection of the vulva and intervening lymph tissue.

In treating clinical stage I and stage II tumors of the vulva, the results of histologic evaluation of the inguinofemoral nodes are important. Many initially treat the superficial nodes above the cribriform fascia (Fig. 30.16). If these nodes are negative, the deep nodes are spared. The procedure can usually be accomplished with preservation of the saphenous vein, which was traditionally sacrificed. These modifications reduce the risk of leg edema. If the lymph nodes, particularly the upper femoral group, are involved with tumor, the deep pelvic nodes require treatment. Homesley and coworkers reported improved survival for those who received radiation (4500 to 5000 rad) to the deep pelvic nodes compared with those who had a pelvic node dissection (Homesley, 1986).

The results of therapy in patients with clinical stages I and II disease relate not only to the stage of the disease but also to the status of the regional pelvic nodes. If the nodes do not contain metastatic tumor and the woman can be successfully treated by radical vulvectomy and bilateral node dissection, 5-year survival rates of approximately 95% have been reported. Iversen and associates, in a series of 424 patients, noted lymph node metastasis in 10.5% of clinical stage I cases, 30% of clinical stage II, 66% of clinical stage III, and 100% of clinical stage IV (Iversen, 1980). The number of positive nodes in the radical vulvectomy specimen correlates with the size of the primary tumor and also with the woman's survival. In a study of T1 and T2 tumors, Andrews and coworkers noted that only unilateral inguinal node metastases occurred and, furthermore, the deep nodes were involved only if the superficial nodes were positive (Andrews, 1994); however, there was a small (2% to 3%) risk of contralateral node involvement of the larger T2 lesions. In a study of 113 patients, Hacker and colleagues noted an actuarial 5-year survival rate of 96% for those with negative nodes, but there was a progressive decrease in the survival rate to 94% for those having one positive node, 80% for two positive nodes, and 12% for three or more positive nodes (Hacker, 1983). **In the various cases that have been studied, the deep pelvic nodes do not contain tumor unless the upper inguinofemoral nodes contain metastatic disease.** The number of nodes involved and the size of the metastasis are both important. Hoffman and associates noted that 14 of 15 patients with inguinal lymph node metastases smaller than 36 mm$^2$ survived free of disease at 5 years compared with 12 of 29 whose lymph node metastases measured more than 100 mm$^2$ (Hoffman, 1985). These results should be taken into consideration when planning additional therapy for patients with positive nodes.

If tumor spread to the regional inguinofemoral nodes is identified, further treatment should be considered. If only one node is microscopically involved with tumor and the woman has

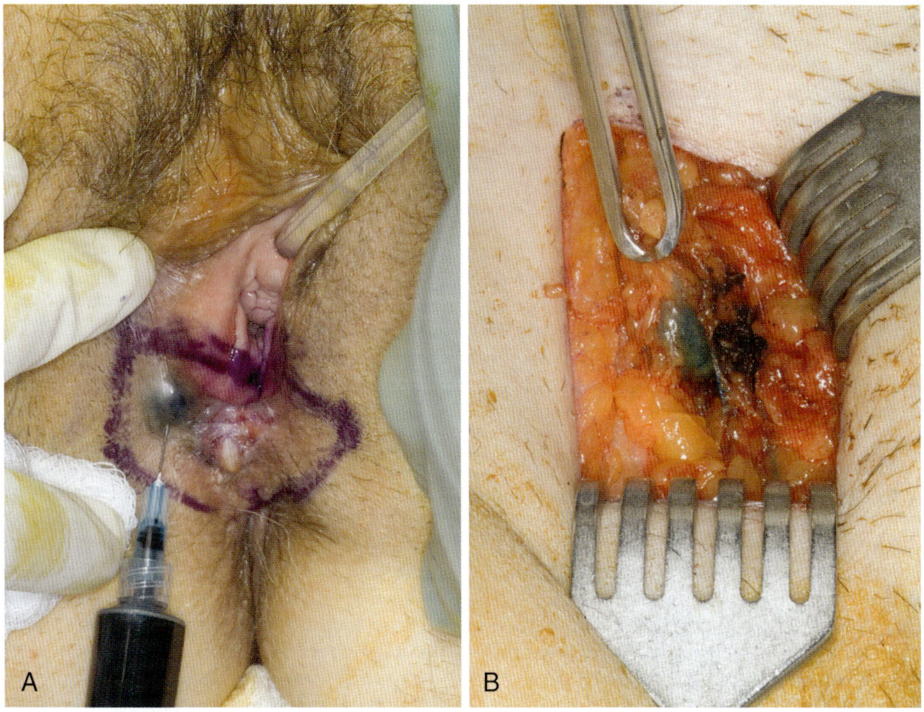


**Fig. 30.16 A** and **B,** Injection of blue dye into vulvar lesion and identification of sentinel node in inguinofemoral triangle.

undergone a complete lymph node dissection of the groin, no further therapy is usually needed, particularly if only a small volume is present; however, if one node is microscopically positive and the woman has undergone a superficial inguinofemoral lymph node dissection, many clinicians would be uncomfortable not treating the groin with adjuvant radiation therapy. If three or more nodes are involved, pelvic radiation as outlined is usually prescribed. For patients with only two nodes involved, the decision for further therapy will depend on the location of the nodes, extent of groin dissection performed, and size of the metastatic deposit of tumor, although most clinicians would opt for radiotherapy in such cases.

## Advanced Vulvar Tumors

Large tumors of the vulva, particularly those that encroach on the anal-rectal area or urethra, may require more extensive treatment than radical vulvectomy to achieve effective tumor control. In such cases it may be necessary to remove the anus or urethra as part of a primary operative procedure, in which case diversion of the urinary or fecal stream is required (see the discussion of exenterative surgery for carcinoma of the cervix in Chapter 29.

For tumors that encroach on the urethra or anus, making procurement of negative margins improbable, multidisciplinary organ-sparing approaches may be used in an effort to reduce the morbidity of exenterative procedures. **A useful therapeutic approach has been to treat large vulvar tumors with external radiation and then, after the tumor has been reduced in size, to remove the residual tumor surgically, usually by radical vulvectomy.** External radiation is used to deliver approximately 4000 cGy to the tumor and 4500 cGy to the pelvis and inguinal nodes. The operation is usually performed approximately 5 weeks after the completion of radiation therapy. Although a large series of patients have not been treated by this technique, a sufficient number have been treated to demonstrate that marked tumor regression does occur. The primary cancer can be eradicated by a procedure that does not require diversion of the urine or feces. Boronow and associates initially summarized the treatment of 26 patients with primary carcinoma of the vaginal vulvar area with this technique and noted a 5-year survival rate of 80% (Boronow, 1987). Rotmensch and colleagues reported on 16 patients, 13 with stage III disease and 3 stage IV, and achieved an overall 5-year survival rate of 45% with this technique, somewhat better than might be expected with stages III and IV (see Fig. 30.14) (Rotmensch, 1990). Recurrences are more likely if the resection margins were within 1 cm of the tumor.

Chemotherapy with radiation appears to offer a therapeutic advantage. Koh and coworkers studied 20 patients with stages III and IV disease and 3 with recurrence, using 5-FU with radiation (Koh, 1993). In addition, some patients also received cisplatin with concurrent radiotherapy. Actuarial 3- and 5-year survival rates in this small group were 59% and 49%, respectively. Similar results with 5-FU and radiation, occasionally with the addition of cisplatin, were also reported by Russell and associates in 25 patients (Russell, 1992). Moore and colleagues reported on a phase II GOG study and noted the need for a less extensive operation when chemotherapy with cisplatin and 5-FU were combined with preoperative radiation (Moore, 1998). Multiple chemoradiation programs are available, but a convenient outpatient regimen consists of weekly intravenous (IV) cisplatin with radiation, usually to 4500 cGy. Other complications reported include stenosis of the introitus, urethral stenosis, and rectovaginal fistula, but this technique is an effective alternative to primary exenteration for large vulvar vaginal carcinomas and is preferred in most treatment centers, although success with exenteration can occasionally be achieved.

### Radiation Therapy and Recurrences

In a few cases the medical condition of the woman precludes surgery, and radiation therapy may be used as the sole treatment. However, the vulvar skin is at risk for radiation dermatitis, fibrosis, and ulceration, making irradiation as the sole form of therapy a less desirable treatment, and therefore irradiation is seldom used as the sole treatment of carcinoma of the vulva. To manage recurrences, reoperation is often tried. Piura and colleagues analyzed 73 patients whose disease recurred only on the vulva (Piura, 1993). Salvage was achieved with wide radical local excision, which appeared to be successful in 30 patients in whom the recurrence was only on the vulva.

As may be expected, the risk of recurring carcinoma rises as the stage of the disease increases. In an analysis of 224 patients with vulvar carcinoma, Podratz and associates noted a recurrence rate of 14% in stage I and 71% in stage IV (Podratz, 1983). Local vulvar recurrences were the most common and were noted in 40 of 74 cases of recurrence (54%). The remaining recurrences were in the groin, pelvis, or distant sites. Radiation therapy or additional operations for local vulvar recurrences usually provide effective control and yield 5-year survival rates of approximately 50%. The risk of recurrence of the disease in the vulva requires careful attention to the surgical resection margins at the time of initial operation.

Combined chemotherapy and radiation has been used for primary treatment of late-stage advanced vulvar tumors, as noted. It has also been applied to recurrences, especially those near the anus or urethra. Radiation alone may also be used for vulvar recurrences, although chemoradiation would appear to be a more effective choice.

Treatment of patients with disseminated disease requires chemotherapy, but unfortunately no chemotherapeutic regimen has been successful for treatment of this disease. Squamous cell carcinomas of the female genital tract have generally not been responsive to cytotoxic chemotherapy; the protocols followed are similar to those described for recurrent squamous cell carcinomas of the cervix (see Chapter 29).

### Quality of Life and Vulvar Carcinoma

There have been few studies regarding quality of life in patients with vulvar cancer. Body image disturbance is significant and may account for decreased or absent sexual activity in women who have undergone vulvectomy. Interestingly, Green and colleagues noted that the extent of surgery or type of vulvectomy performed does not correlate well with the degree of sexual dysfunction (Green, 2000). They demonstrated a significant need to address sexual problems with all women undergoing any type of vulvectomy. The Functional Assessment of Cancer Therapy–Vulvar (FACT-V) is a valid and reliable instrument to assess quality of life in women with vulvar cancer. Perhaps this tool can be used to help assess quality of life and also facilitate vital communication about quality-of-life issues in women with this disease.

### Lymphatic Mapping and Sentinel Lymph Node Biopsy

As noted, regional lymph node dissections are routinely performed in the surgical treatment of vulvar cancer because the status of regional lymph nodes is essential for therapeutic planning and overall prognosis. More than 80% of women with clinical stages I and II disease, however, will have no metastatic disease found in the lymph nodes, therefore making an extensive lymphadenectomy unnecessary while increasing postoperative morbidities, such as lymphedema and lymphocyst formation. Lymphatic mapping and sentinel lymph node biopsy, as used for the treatment of patients with melanoma and breast cancer, are appealing techniques for patients with vulvar cancer. The sentinel nodes are those that directly drain the primary tumor and are thought to predict the metastatic status of the upper echelon or nonsentinel nodes in the groin. **If the sentinel node is negative, in theory all the other groin nodes would also be negative and surgeons could abandon full groin dissections, thereby greatly reducing the associated morbidities of lymphocyst, lymphedema, and wound separation** (see Fig. 30.16).

Van der Zee and colleagues performed a prospective observational study in 403 women with clinical stage I squamous cell carcinoma of the vulva smaller than 4 cm (GROningen INternational Study on Sentinel nodes in Vulvar cancer [GROINSS-V]) (Van der Zee, 2008). Women enrolled in this study underwent a sentinel node biopsy, with omission of complete inguinofemoral lymphadenectomy if no metastatic disease was found. Patients with negative sentinel nodes were triaged to no further therapy and observed for recurrence. With a median follow-up of 35 months, only six groin recurrences (2.3%) have been noted in patients without multifocal disease. In a validation study, Levenback and colleagues set out to determine the true sensitivity and negative predictive value of the sentinel node technique in 453 women with vulvar cancer (GOG 173) (Levenback, 2012). In contrast to GROINSS-V, all women in GOG 173 underwent a sentinel node biopsy followed by a complete inguinofemoral lymphadenectomy. They found a sensitivity of 90.1% and a negative predictive value of 95.7%. Therefore if the sentinel node was negative, there was only a 4.3% chance that disease was present in that groin (false-negative predictive value). In an accumulation of data from smaller studies on the subject, Frumovitz and colleagues reviewed the combined data on 279 patients with vulvar cancer who had undergone lymphatic mapping and sentinel lymph node identification (Frumovitz, 2008). They found the overall sensitivity of the sentinel node for detecting metastatic disease in patients with vulvar cancer to be 97.7% and the false-negative rate for the procedure to be 2.3%. The overall negative predictive value was 99.3%. Although these numbers are promising, lymphatic mapping and sentinel lymph node biopsy are still considered experimental, with the standard of care remaining full inguinofemoral node dissection.

## Other Vulvar Malignancies

### Bartholin Gland Carcinoma

Bartholin gland carcinomas are adenocarcinomas that constitute approximately 1% to 2% of vulvar carcinomas. An enlargement of Bartholin gland in a postmenopausal woman should raise suspicion for this malignancy. These tumors are treated similarly to primary squamous cell carcinoma of the vulva; radical vulvectomy with bilateral inguinofemoral lymphadenectomy is the treatment of choice. If the regional lymph nodes are free of tumor, the prognosis is good.

### Basal Cell Carcinoma

Basal cell carcinoma can arise in the vulva, as it can arise in the skin elsewhere in the body. It is rare and comprises approximately 2% of vulvar carcinomas. Therapy consists of wide local excision of the lesion, which is generally ulcerated. If the surgical resection margins are free of tumor, the disease is cured.

### Verrucous Carcinoma

Verrucous carcinomas of the vulva are a rare special variant of squamous cell cancer, with distinctive histologic features. Clinically they appear as a large condylomatous mass on the vulva; histologically they consist of mature squamous cells and extensive keratinization, with nests that invade the underlying vulvar tissue. It is often necessary to perform multiple biopsies of the condylomatous lesion to establish a diagnosis of malignancy. Radiation therapy is ineffective and can worsen the prognosis by causing anaplastic changes in the tumor and is therefore contraindicated. The treatment of an authentic verrucous carcinoma is wide excision.

In 24 cases of verrucous carcinoma, Japaze and coworkers noted no lymph node metastases (Japaze, 1982). Some of the primary tumors were as large as 10 cm in diameter. Recurrences developed in 9 patients, 5 of whom had previous radiation therapy. Wide local excision is effective therapy. Depending on the size and location of the tumor, simple vulvectomy may be needed, but a radical vulvectomy or inguinal node dissection is not indicated. The 17 patients treated surgically who were reported on by Japaze and colleagues had a 5-year survival rate of 94%.

It is important to take a large biopsy specimen to establish the diagnosis. This is particularly important when dealing with a malignant-appearing tumor from a biopsy specimen that has been reported as benign, which can lead to incorrect therapy for condyloma acuminata. Conversely, too shallow a biopsy may fail to show areas of squamous cell carcinoma that can coexist with verrucous carcinoma, but in the presence of areas of squamous cell carcinoma, local excision is inadequate therapy. Verrucous tumors with squamous cell carcinoma elements can metastasize to regional nodes; these tumors should not be treated as true verrucous carcinomas.

### Melanoma

**Melanoma is the most common non–squamous cell malignancy of the vulva. It comprises approximately 5% of primary cancers of this area.** As is true elsewhere in the body, melanomas arise from junctional or compound nevi. Pigmented lesions of the vulva are usually junctional nevi, and all such lesions should be removed by excision.

Patients with malignant melanoma of the vulva vary widely in age, from the late teens to women in their 80s. The average age is approximately 50 years. Clinically, melanomas appear as brown, black, or blue-black masses on the vulva. The lesion can be flat or ulcerated; occasionally, it is nodular, and small, darkly pigmented areas (satellite nodules) may surround the primary lesion. Some melanomas may be without pigment and can grossly resemble squamous cell carcinoma of the vulva. Most melanomas of the vulva occur on the labia minora or the clitoris (Fig. 30.17).

Vulvar melanomas should be staged using the AJCC TNM staging system for cutaneous melanoma and not the FIGO staging system for vulvar cancer. The AJCC TNM staging system has

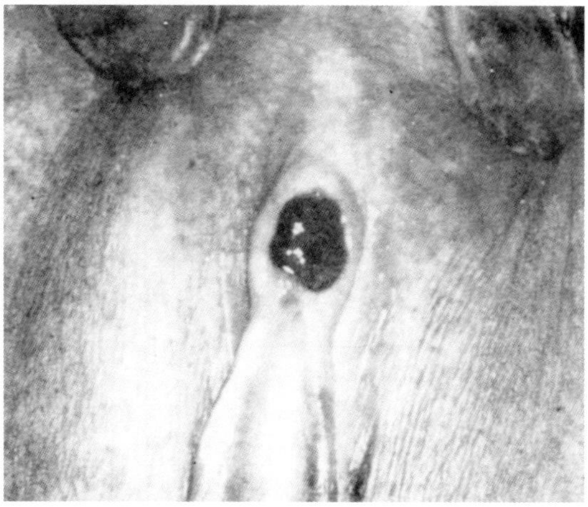

**Fig. 30.17** Nodular melanoma arising directly from glans clitoris. (Courtesy Dr. J.M. Morris [deceased], Yale University School of Medicine, New Haven, CT.)

been shown to be a better predictor of recurrence-free survival compared with the FIGO staging system. However, staging may not be as useful a prognostic indicator as is the depth of invasion. A staging system for vulvar melanoma analogous to that used by Clark for cutaneous melanomas has been adopted. Five levels (I to V) have been defined based on the Clark classification. Fig. 30.18 shows the depth of invasion for each level of superficial spreading melanoma and nodular melanoma, the two most common varieties of melanomas that occur on the vulva. Superficial spreading melanoma is more common and fortunately has a better prognosis, with a 5-year survival rate of 71% reported in the series by Podratz and associates (Podratz, 1983). The 5-year survival for nodular melanoma, which is more invasive, was only 38%. The level of invasion correlates with survival, which varies from 100% for level II, to 83% for level IV, to 28% for level V.

Tumor thickness is also useful to evaluate the tumor. Breslow has reported that overall prognosis is excellent, and spread to a regional node is not likely for melanomas whose thickness is less than 0.76 mm, measured from the surface epithelium to the deepest point of penetration (Breslow, 1970). Most of these lesions would correspond to level I or II penetration by the modified Clark system. Stefanon and coworkers, in a study of 28 patients, noted no lymph node metastasis if melanoma thickness was less than 3 mm; the 5-year survival rate in this group was 50% compared with 25% for those whose melanomas were more than 3 mm thick (Stefanon, 1987). In a comprehensive long-term study of 219 Swedish women, Ragnarsson-Olding and coworkers noted that tumor thickness and ulceration are prognostic factors (Ragnarsson-Olding, 1999). In addition, gross amelanosis and advanced age worsened the prognosis. They further noted that amelanotic tumors were seen in approximately 25% of patients and that overall the vulvar melanomas were approximately 2.5 times more common than cutaneous melanomas. A preexisting nevus was not necessary; de novo melanoma development does appear to occur on the vulva, particularly in the glabrous (hairless) skin.

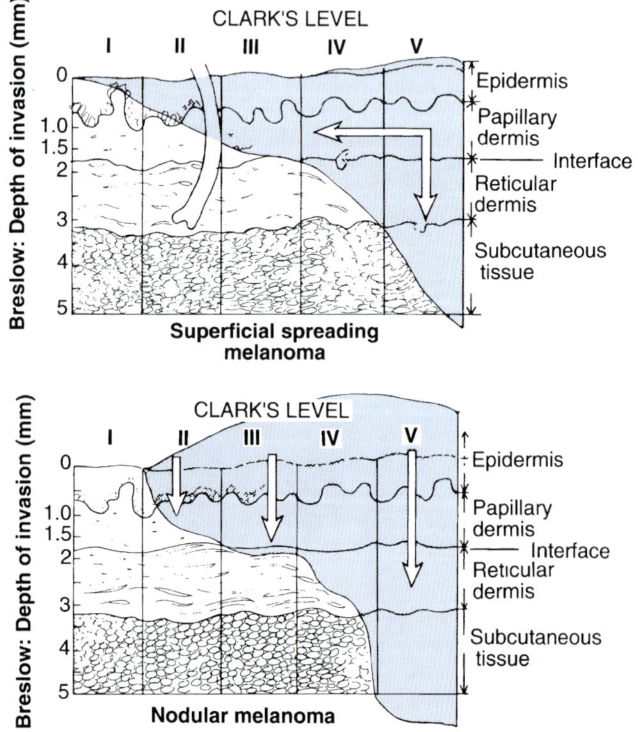


Fig. 30.18 Level of invasion for superficial spreading melanoma and nodular melanoma. (From Podratz KC, Gaffey TA, Symmonds RE, et al. Melanoma of the vulva: an update. *Gynecol Oncol.* 1983;16:153.)

The standard therapy for vulvar melanoma is a wide excision of the primary tumor and consideration for lymphatic mapping with sentinel lymph node biopsy. Detection of disease in the lymph nodes may only be prognostic because some studies shown no survival benefit with primary excision plus complete inguinofemoral lymphadenectomy compared with resection of primary lesion alone in these patients (Trimble, 1992). However, with the evolution of immunotherapy and targeted therapies as adjuvant therapy in patients with metastatic cutaneous melanoma at other sites, sentinel lymph node biopsy may make sense in these patients. Because the tumors are rare, a large clinical experience is not available. It was believed that melanoma of the vulva could metastasize to pelvic nodes, bypassing the inguinofemoral nodes, but it is now thought that there is no pelvic node involvement without previous inguinal node involvement. A further therapeutic consideration is that patients with melanoma whose pelvic nodes are involved with tumor usually do not survive the disease.

Excision margins have been extensively studied for cutaneous melanomas. Veronesi and colleagues found that cutaneous melanomas less than 2 mm thick could be adequately treated with a 1-cm margin, which was as effective as a 3-cm margin for these thin lesions (Veronesi, 1988). Although comparable data do not exist for vulvar melanomas, evidence from studies of cutaneous melanomas has suggested that a 1-cm margin may be used for very thin vulvar melanomas. In a report of 36 melanoma cases, Rose and associates noted that wide excision was as effective as radical vulvectomy (Rose, 1988). They found that the prognosis was improved in younger patients, presumably because most of them had superficial spreading (good prognosis) rather than nodular (poor prognosis) melanomas. Although firm recommendations from available data are not possible, a reasonable approach would be to excise a melanoma with a 2-cm margin without node dissection for tumors that are smaller than 0.76 mm thick. An excision with a 2- to 3-cm margin combined with node dissection would be carried out for more advanced melanomas.

For lesions that correspond to Clark level I or II—that is, less than 0.76 mm thick—a wide local excision results in 5-year survival rates of approximately 100%. The prognosis is poor for patients with melanomas more than 3 mm thick. If the regional nodes are negative, the survival rate is greater than 60% but decreases to less than 30% if the regional nodes are involved with tumor. Most series of malignant melanoma have reported overall survival rates of approximately 50%. Although metastases of melanoma to regional inguinal nodes are usually fatal, isolated cases of prolonged survival have been observed.

Distant metastases are commonly noted, and no effective program of chemotherapy has been described. Regressions (but not cures) have been reported with various multiagent cytotoxic programs. Research efforts now are devoted to developing an effective program of bioimmunotherapy.

## Sarcoma

Sarcomas of the vulva are extremely rare, accounting for less than 3% of vulvar cancers. Leiomyosarcomas are the most common histologic subtype found, followed by liposarcomas, neurofibrosarcomas, angiosarcomas, and epithelioid sarcomas. Surgical removal of the primary tumor is the treatment of choice. Chemotherapeutic considerations are the same as those for sarcomas of other sites in the female genital tract.

## Granular Cell Myoblastoma

Granular cell myoblastoma is also an extremely rare tumor that is almost invariably benign but morphologically shows pleomorphism. Local excision is generally sufficient therapy. The tumor appears as a solitary, firm, nontender, slowly growing nodule in the subcutaneous tissue of the vulva.

## PREMALIGNANT AND MALIGNANT LESIONS OF THE VAGINA

Premalignant changes in the vagina occur less often than comparable lesions in the cervix and vulva, although the histologic appearance of intraepithelial neoplasia of the vagina is similar to that described for the cervix (see Chapter 28). These changes are also similarly designated as dysplasia (mild, moderate, or severe) and carcinoma in situ. The term *VAIN* (vaginal intraepithelial neoplasia) has been used to describe these histologic changes; the comparable categories are VAIN-1 (mild dysplasia), VAIN-2 (moderate dysplasia), and VAIN-3 (severe dysplasia to carcinoma in situ). VAIN-1 is classified as a low-grade squamous intraepithelial lesion, whereas VAIN-2 and VAIN-3 are grouped as high-grade squamous intraepithelial lesions (Audet-Lapointe, 1990). The cytologic and histologic features of these changes are illustrated in Fig. 30.19.

VAIN occurs more commonly in patients previously treated for cervical intraepithelial neoplasia. The frequency of vaginal premalignancy in these patients is approximately 1% to 3%. Similarly, there is an increased risk of VAIN in those previously treated for squamous cell neoplasia of the vulva. The tendency to develop premalignant changes in the lower genital tract is known as a *field defect* and denotes the increased risk of squamous cell neoplasia arising anywhere in the lower genital tract in such individuals. Most VAIN cases are related to infection with HPV. Additional risk factors include HIV infection, cigarette smoking, previous radiation therapy of the genital tract,

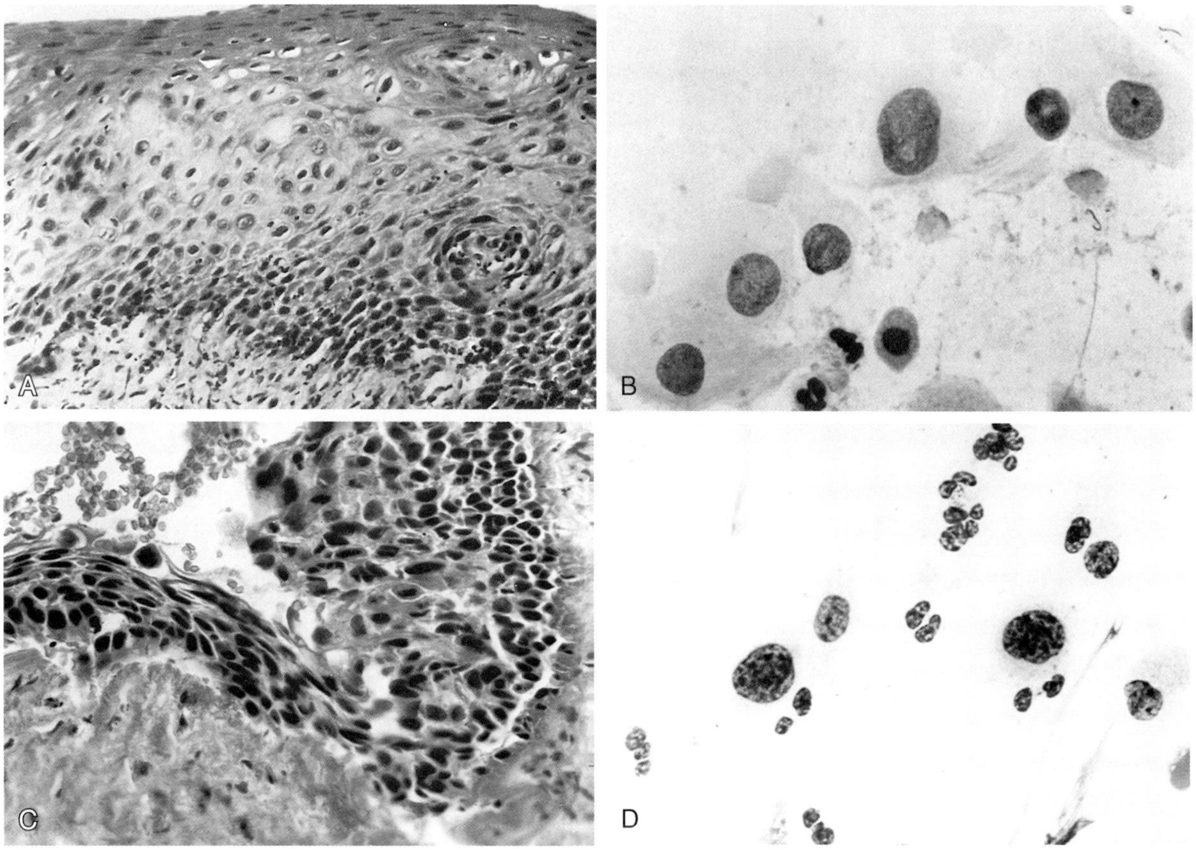


**Fig. 30.19 A,** Section of a vagina showing dysplasia. The epithelium appears thickened and shows abnormal maturation. Immature hyperchromatic cells occupy the lower two to four layers. The middle and upper thirds of mucosa show evidence of cytoplasmic differentiation with well-defined cellular borders. Nuclei in these areas are enlarged and pleomorphic. Parakeratosis is apparent on the surface. Because immature cells are confined to the lower third of the mucosa, dysplasia is classified as mild (hematoxylin and eosin [H&E] stain, ×250). **B,** Cytologic specimen showing mild dysplasia. Note the sheet of dysplastic cells. Cells show well-defined cytoplasmic borders. Nuclei are enlarged, and the nuclear contour is smooth. Chromatin is uniformly and finely granular. Focal condensations of chromatin (chromocenters) are present in some nuclei. Nucleoli are not present (Papanicolaou [Pap] stain, ×1000). **C,** Section showing severe dysplasia to carcinoma in situ. The entire epithelial thickness is occupied by hyperchromatic dysplastic cells. Marked nuclear variation and mitoses are seen. Because of occasional cells with squamous differentiation (spindle-shaped cells, cells with well-defined cytoplasmic borders) in superficial layers, this lesion is sometimes classified as severe dysplasia. In carcinoma in situ, immature cells replace the full thickness, and there is no evidence of squamous differentiation on the surface (H&E stain, ×400). **D,** Cytologic specimen showing carcinoma in situ. Several isolated immature cells with a high nuclei-to-cytoplasm ratio and poorly defined cytoplasmic borders can be seen. Chromatin is coarsely granular, and no nucleoli are present. In the background are several polymorphonuclear leukocytes and strings of mucus (Pap stain, ×1000).

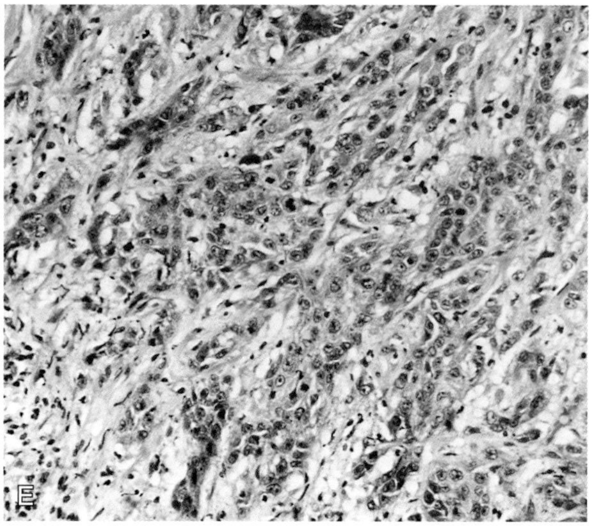


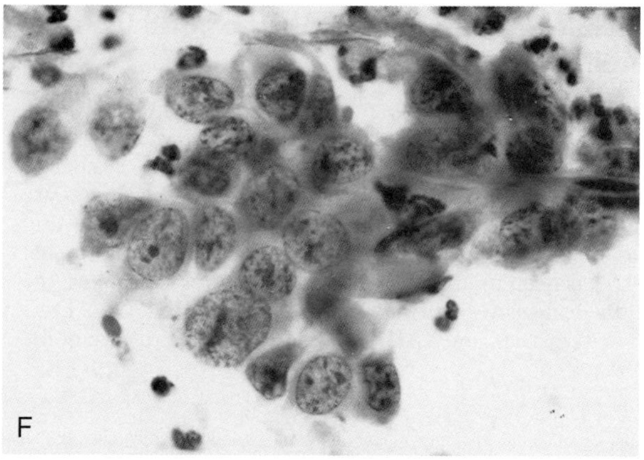


**Fig. 30.19 cont'd E,** Section showing invasive squamous carcinoma. Cords and sheets of poorly differentiated tumor cells infiltrate the stroma. Nuclei are pleomorphic and nucleoli are distinct. The mitotic rate is high. Squamous differentiation (keratin pearl formation, single-cell keratinization) was present in other areas of tumor (H&E stain, ×200). **F,** Cytologic specimen showing invasive squamous cell carcinoma. Note aggregate of tumor cells. Cellular boundaries are poorly defined, and nuclear orientation is lacking. Chromatin is irregularly distributed and has areas of clumping and clearing. Note nucleoli in some cells, which were absent in cells of patients with dysplasia and carcinoma in situ (Pap stain, ×800).

**TABLE 30.2** Common Primary Vaginal Cancers

| Tumor Type | Predominant Age (Years) | Clinical Correlations |
|---|---|---|
| Endodermal sinus tumor (adenocarcinoma) | <2 | Extremely rare, alpha-fetoprotein secretion, often fatal, multimodality therapy |
| Sarcoma botryoides | <8 | Aggressive malignancy, multimodality therapy |
| Clear cell adenocarcinoma | >14 | Associated with intrauterine exposure to diethylstilbestrol |
| Melanoma | >50 | Very rare, poor survival |
| Squamous cell carcinoma | >50 | Most common primary vaginal cancer |

and immunosuppressive therapy. In situ and invasive vaginal neoplasias have many of the same risk factors as cervical cancer, including a strong association with HPV infection. Women who have previously been treated for anogenital cancer, particularly for cervical cancer, have a high relative risk of being diagnosed with vaginal cancer (Shrivastava, 2015).

Primary cancer of the vagina is rare and constitutes less than **2% of gynecologic malignancies. Most vaginal malignancies are metastatic, primarily from the cervix and endometrium. Less commonly, ovarian and rectosigmoid carcinomas, as well as choriocarcinoma, metastasize to the vagina.** The most common histologic type of primary vaginal cancer is squamous cell carcinoma, which is usually seen in women older than 60 years. Other types of carcinoma, including melanomas and adenocarcinomas, occur less commonly. Malignant transformation of endometriosis has been described in the vagina and rectovaginal septum. Clear cell adenocarcinoma, historically associated with young women exposed in utero to diethylstilbestrol (DES), may also occur in unexposed women. Primary vaginal sarcoma is rare and usually a disease of children. Table 30.2 summarizes the major primary malignancies of the vagina arranged according to age at occurrence.

## PREMALIGNANT DISEASE OF THE VAGINA

### Detection and Diagnosis

Because premalignant disease of the vagina is generally asymptomatic, detection depends primarily on cytologic screening (see Fig. 30.19, *B* and *D*). Usually the changes will be observed in patients who have undergone previous therapy for intraepithelial disease of the cervix. This fact underscores the importance of continued examinations and Pap smears for women, even after hysterectomy for dysplastic conditions. VAIN usually occurs in the upper half of the vagina or along the vaginal cuff suture line. Once an abnormal smear from vaginal epithelium is identified, a biopsy is required for histologic identification (see Fig. 30.19, *A* and *C*). A colposcopic examination is usually performed to identify the areas requiring biopsy. As in the case of cervical neoplasia, a repeat Pap smear is often taken before the colposcopic examination. Vaginal colposcopic techniques are similar to those described for the cervix. A large speculum is used to aid in visualizing the entire vaginal wall. Although the abnormal colposcopic findings resemble those of the cervix (see Chapter 28), full visualization of the entire vaginal wall is often difficult and time consuming. A useful adjunct to colposcopy for identifying an area in which to perform a biopsy is to stain the vaginal epithelium with Lugol solution and to take a biopsy sample from the nonstaining areas. The vaginal epithelium must be adequately estrogenized so that sufficient epithelial glycogen is present for the normal tissue to stain dark brown. The more rapidly dividing dysplastic epithelium uses up its glycogen and thus does not pick up the iodine stain. Vaginal estrogen cream used for 1 to 2 weeks before examination is helpful for evaluating postmenopausal women and those with atrophic vaginitis who present with cytologic atypia. The estrogen cream will not only increase epithelial glycogen but also helps mature the squamous epithelium, reducing the number of parabasal cells at the surface. Parabasal cells, with their large nuclei, are a common cause of false-positive Pap tests in this age group.

A biopsy is performed with small instruments, such as the Kevorkian or Eppendorf punch biopsy forceps (Fig. 30.20) or

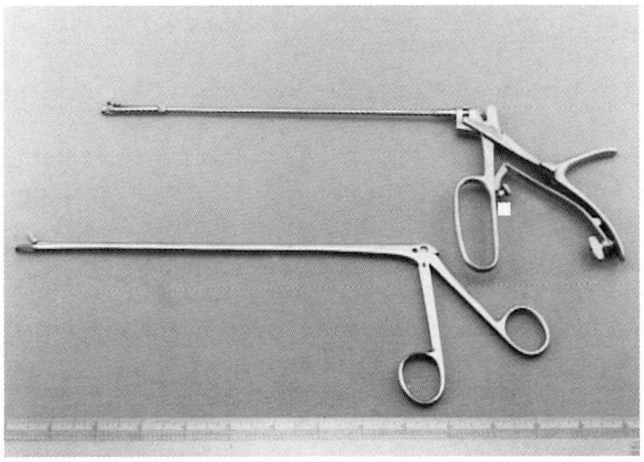

**Fig. 30.20** Eppendorf *(upper)* and Kevorkian *(lower)* punch biopsy instruments.

similar instruments that are also used for the cervix. Occasionally it is necessary to use a fine instrument, such as a nerve hook, to provide traction on the vaginal epithelium to obtain a biopsy sample. Most patients experience some discomfort during the biopsy. Local anesthesia is often helpful, although injection of the anesthetic may be as uncomfortable as the biopsy itself. Vaginal neoplasia is often multifocal. Although the process is most often located in the vaginal apex, it can occur anywhere along the vaginal canal, necessitating examination of the vagina in its entirety (Jentschke, 2015).

## Treatment

There is limited information regarding the natural history of VAIN. The risk of progression to invasive cancer is thought to be low, approximately 9%. Those at highest risk of progression are women with high-risk strains of HPV, those with VAIN-3, cigarette smokers, and women who are immunocompromised (Gadducci, 2015). Significantly, Aho and colleagues have found that 28% of women undergoing evaluation for VAIN-3 have an underlying invasive carcinoma (Aho, 1991). This has led many to recommend surgical excision rather than destructive procedures for the treatment of VAIN-3.

The principles of managing VAIN are to rule out and prevent invasive disease and preserve vaginal function. As is true for cervical dysplasia, biopsy-proven VAIN-1, particularly those lesions associated with low-risk strains of HPV, can be observed, provided that the woman is compliant with follow-up. VAIN-2 and VAIN-3 are generally treated. Treatment options include $CO_2$ laser vaporization, topical 5-FU cream, and wide local excision. The choice of treatment depends largely on the number of lesions, their location, and the level of concern for possible invasion. Radiation therapy, previously used to treat VAIN-2 and VAIN-3, often leads to scarring and fibrosis and is generally not recommended for the treatment of noninvasive disease. Because of the proximity of the bladder and rectum, cryotherapy is generally not used.

The main advantage of the $CO_2$ laser is that it vaporizes the abnormal tissue without shortening or narrowing the vagina, thereby preserving vaginal function. Criteria for $CO_2$ laser vaporization include a lesion that is discrete and easily visible and proof that invasive cancer has been ruled out. The beam is directed colposcopically. Iodine staining of the vagina can help outline those areas requiring therapy. Treatment is occasionally performed on an outpatient basis with a local anesthetic and an analgesic. More often, general or regional anesthesia is required. The intensity of therapy is regulated by adjusting the wattage of the laser, most commonly 15 to 20 W carried to a depth of 1.5 to 2 mm. Care must be taken not to apply the laser too deeply because of the proximity of the bladder and bowel, particularly in older women whose vaginal epithelium may be quite thin. The woman will experience a discharge for 1 to 2 weeks after therapy. Healing usually requires a few weeks. The success rates of laser in treating VAIN vary in the literature but are generally in the range of 60% to 85% (Petrilli, 1980). Regular follow-up every 4 months, including a Pap smear and colposcopy, is required during the first year and usually 6 to 12 months thereafter. The primary disadvantages of laser treatment are the lack of a pathologic specimen for evaluation of the adequacy of margins and the fact that the procedure can be tedious and difficult because of the many folds and crevices at the vaginal apex. It is often difficult to obtain a uniform depth of destruction in these areas (Piovano, 2015).

Topical chemotherapy, 5% 5-FU cream, can be self-administered to cover the entire area at risk. It is most often used for widespread multifocal lesions of HPV-associated VAIN-1 or VAIN-2. Half of a vaginal applicator (approximately 5 g) is inserted into the vagina at bedtime for 7 days. Because the cream is irritating, protective ointment such as zinc oxide should be applied to the vulva. If excess leakage occurs, less than half of an applicator should be used. In addition, the treatment should be discontinued before the 7-day course is completed if the woman notes excessive irritation. A cycle of therapy should be repeated in 3 to 4 weeks if intraepithelial neoplasia persists. In some cases, the application of 5-FU is continued for 10 to 14 days, in which case the nontherapy interval is increased to 2 or 3 months. In contrast, many postmenopausal women tolerate only small doses of 5-FU, presumably because of relatively thin vaginal epithelium. In one study, patients used one-third of an applicator of 5% 5-FU weekly for 10 weeks, and 17 of 20 patients with vaginal condyloma were free of disease at 3 months. Three patients received a second cycle, and 16 of 18 were free of disease at 10 to 20 months. Success rates of 80% to 90% for patients with VAIN after multiple treatment cycles have been reported. The disadvantage of topical therapy with 5-FU cream is related to the high level of motivation required to complete therapy. The 5-FU cream causes exfoliation and erosion of the vaginal mucosa and can be extremely painful. Only a small percentage of patients are able to complete a full course; thus use of this topical therapy is limited. Imiquimod has been evaluated for the treatment of vaginal intraepithelial neoplasia. Complete regression of neoplasia has been reported in 26% to 100% of patients, whereas 0% to 60% have partial regression. Recurrence of neoplasia was identified in 0% to 37% of the patients. The most commonly reported side effects were local burning and tenderness, although not severe enough to discontinue treatment. Because patients who experience disease partial regression will require less extensive excision, this treatment may prove to be a promising option (de Witte, 2015).

Wide local excision (upper vaginectomy) is the treatment of choice for VAIN-3, especially for lesions occurring at the cuff after hysterectomy. Excision gives the surgeon the ability to excise the specimen to rule out invasion and ascertain margin adequacy and also has a high success rate (84%). Upper vaginectomy, however, can result in vaginal shortening, which can be ameliorated by the use of topical estrogen cream and a vaginal dilator (or frequent intercourse) once healing is complete (Ait Menguellet, 2007).

## MALIGNANT DISEASE OF THE VAGINA

### Symptoms and Diagnosis

Primary vaginal cancers usually occur as squamous cell carcinomas in women older than 60 years. To be considered a primary vaginal tumor, the malignancy must arise in the vagina and not involve the external os of the cervix superiorly or the vulva inferiorly. If this occurs, the tumor is classified as cervical or vulvar. To rule out primary carcinoma of the cervix, biopsy is mandatory if the cervix is intact. This is also an important therapeutic consideration, insofar as the same management techniques apply to small tumors of the upper third of the vagina and cervical carcinomas. Tumors of the lower third of the vagina are treated similarly to vulvar cancers. Table 30.3 lists the staging criteria for vaginal cancers according to FIGO, which are illustrated in Fig. 30.21 (Rajaram, 2015).

Delay in the diagnosis of these cancers is common, in part because of their rarity. Lack of recognition that abnormal symptoms may be caused by malignancy can also contribute to a delay.

**TABLE 30.3** International Federation of Gynecology and Obstetrics Staging Classification for Vaginal Cancer

| Stage | Characteristics |
|---|---|
| I | Carcinoma limited to vaginal wall |
| II | Carcinoma involves subvaginal tissue but has not extended to pelvic wall |
| III | Carcinoma extends to pelvic wall or to pelvic lymph nodes and/or causing hydronephrosis or nonfunctioning kidney |
| IV | Carcinoma extends to the bladder, rectum, or beyond the pelvis (IVA) or to a distant part of the body (IVB) (bullous edema as such does not assign a patient to stage IV) |

The most common symptom of vaginal cancer is abnormal bleeding or discharge. Pain is usually a symptom of an advanced tumor. Urinary frequency is also reported occasionally, particularly in the case of anterior wall tumors, whereas constipation or tenesmus may be reported when the tumors involve the posterior vaginal wall. In general, the longer the delay in diagnosis, the poorer the prognosis and the more difficult the therapy. Vaginal cancer is usually diagnosed by direct biopsy of the tumor mass (see Fig. 30.19, *E*). Abnormal cytologic findings (see Fig. 30.19, *F*) may prompt a thorough pelvic examination that will lead to diagnosis of vaginal cancer. It is important during the course of the pelvic examination to inspect and palpate the entire vagina and to rotate the speculum carefully to visualize the entire vagina because a small tumor may occupy the anterior or posterior vaginal wall.

## TUMORS OF THE ADULT VAGINA

### Squamous Cell Carcinoma

Squamous cell carcinoma is the most common vaginal malignancy and accounts for 90% of primary vaginal cancers. Although reported in women in their 30s, the disease occurs primarily in women older than 60, and 20% are older than 80 years. Most squamous cell carcinomas occur in the upper third of the vagina, but primary tumors in the middle and lower thirds

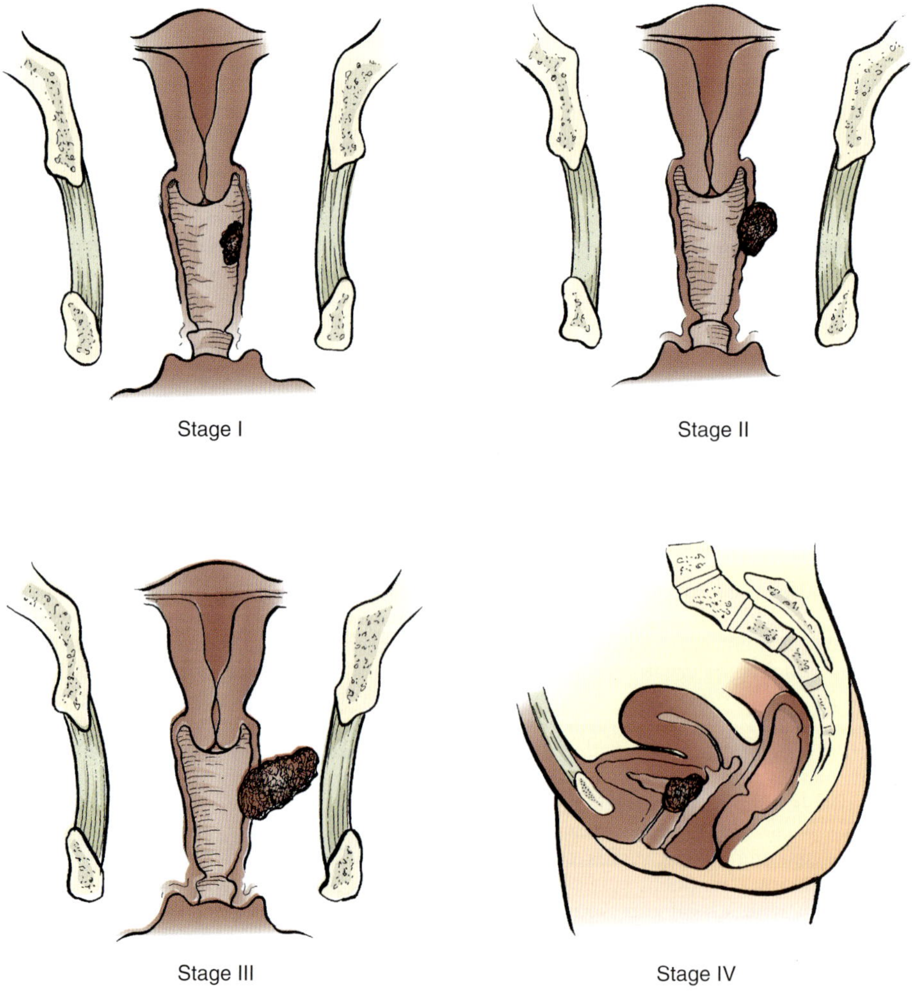


**Fig. 30.21** Staging of vaginal cancer.

may also occur. Grossly the tumor appears as a fungating, polypoid, or ulcerating mass, often accompanied by a foul smell and discharge related to secondary infection. Microscopically (see Fig. 30.19, *E*) the tumor demonstrates the classic findings of an invasive squamous cell carcinoma infiltrating the vaginal epithelium.

**Treatment of these tumors is based on the size, vaginal tumor stage, and location of the lesion.** Therapy is limited by the proximity of the bladder anteriorly and the rectum posteriorly. It is also influenced by the location of the tumor in the vagina, which determines the area of lymphatic spread (Fig. 30.22).

The lymphatics of the vagina envelop the mucosa and anastomose with lymphatic vessels in the muscularis. Those of the mid- to upper vagina communicate superiorly with the lymphatics of the cervix and drain into the pelvic nodes of the obturator and internal and external iliac chains. In contrast, the lymphatics of the distal third of the vagina drain to the inguinal nodes and pelvic nodes, similar to the drainage of the vulva. The posterior wall lymphatics anastomose with the rectal lymphatic system and then to the nodes that drain the rectum, such as the inferior gluteal, sacral, and rectal nodes.

## Treatment

Once the diagnosis of vaginal malignancy is established, a thorough bimanual and visual examination documenting the size and location of the tumor and assessment of spread to adjacent structures (submucosa, vaginal sidewall, bladder, rectum) should be performed to determine the clinical stage. Cystoscopy or proctoscopy may be helpful, depending on clinical concern, to rule out bladder or rectal invasion. Distant spread may be evaluated by computed tomography (CT) of the chest, abdomen, and pelvis or by positron emission tomography (PET).

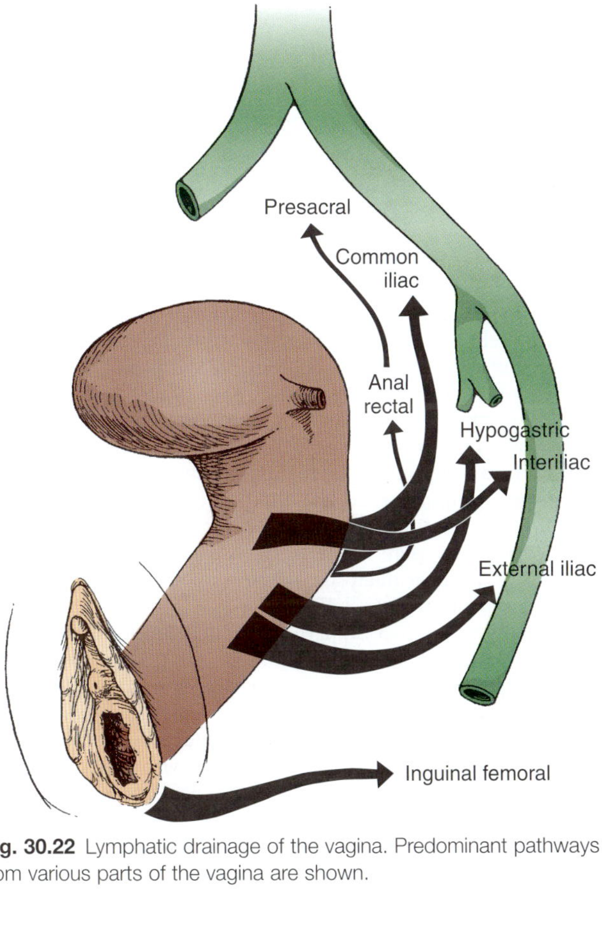


**Fig. 30.22** Lymphatic drainage of the vagina. Predominant pathways from various parts of the vagina are shown.

Similar to cervical carcinoma, early-stage vaginal carcinoma, without lymph node involvement (stage I or II), may be treated with surgery or radiation. Young patients with early-stage disease and upper vaginal lesions may be treated with radical upper vaginectomy, parametrectomy, and pelvic lymphadenectomy (Davis, 1991). **Radiation therapy is the most common mode of treatment because most women with vaginal carcinoma are older and have a poorer surgical risk and radiation is highly effective and can be used for early and advanced disease.** Pelvic exenteration can be used primarily to treat advanced disease in the absence of lymph node metastasis, but it is usually reserved for patients with localized recurrence after radiation. Cisplatin-based chemotherapy administered concurrently with radiation has been used with increasing frequency for squamous cell carcinomas of the vagina because of the well-documented improvements in outcomes for patients with squamous lesions of the cervix treated in this fashion. Although there have been no randomized prospective trials proving its effectiveness in this disease, the numerous similarities in pathophysiology between squamous lesions of the cervix and vagina would lead to the logical conclusion that concurrent chemotherapy with radiation will have increased efficacy over radiation alone in the treatment of vaginal carcinoma.

Stage I vaginal carcinoma may be treated with brachytherapy alone, without external beam therapy. Grigsby has recommended vaginal brachytherapy using vaginal cylinders, in one or two applications, delivering a dose of 65 to 80 Gy to the entire length of the vagina (Grigsby, 2002). For more advanced lesions, a combination of external beam and brachytherapy is used. External radiation therapy with megavoltage equipment is initially used to shrink the tumor. The size and extent of the radiation field will be determined by the presence or absence of nodal disease, as determined by the pretreatment PET or CT scan. The whole pelvis is generally treated to a dose of approximately 5040 cGy. This is followed by a local cesium or radium implant placed interstitially with needles or by intracavitary radiation using a vaginal cylinder or tandem and ovoids if the cervix is still present. The brachytherapy will bring the total dose to between 7000 and 8500 cGy. The prognosis appears to improve if the interval from the end of external therapy to the initiation of brachytherapy is less than 28 days (Gadducci, 2015).

DiSaia and coworkers have reported using a fixed perineal template (Syed-Neblett applicator) to achieve reproducible isodose delivery to a large vaginal tumor volume (DiSaia, 1990). For lesions of the upper vagina after hysterectomy, a laparoscopy may be performed to remove any bowel loops from the vaginal apex. The omentum may be used to provide additional layer of separation of the bowel from the vaginal apex. Paley and associates have reported using a retropubic approach in a small series of six patients to achieve direct visualization of needle placement (Paley, 1998). Treatment is individualized, depending on tumor size and stage. For larger lesions, the dose of the external component of radiation therapy is increased, with a concomitant reduction in the local vaginal component of treatment of the primary tumor. Usually a total tumor dosage of approximately 7500 cGy is administered. Implants cannot be used in some patients with stage III or IV carcinoma; in such cases, only external therapy can be used, and a central boost is given after an initial 5000-cGy whole-pelvis treatment. Severe complications have been noted if the vaginal dose exceeds 9800 cGy. Kucera and Vavra, in a series of 434 patients treated with irradiation, noted that results were best for low-stage tumors, those in the upper third of the vagina, and when the tumor was well differentiated (Kucera, 1991). Kirkbride and colleagues have reported that stage, tumor size, and tumor grade are prognostic and that the tumor dose must reach at least 7000 cGy, consistent with other studies (Kirkbride, 1995). Treatment time is also important; as noted by Lee and colleagues, it is preferable to complete the radiation therapy within 9 weeks (Lee, 1994).

## Survival

Overall 5-year survival rates for patients with primary carcinoma of the vagina have been reported to be approximately 45%. The stage of the tumor is the most important predictor of prognosis. In one series of 89 patients treated with surgery or irradiation, 5-year survival rates were 82% and 53%, respectively, for stage I and stage II disease. The use of concomitant chemotherapy with radiation can be expected to produce improved survival rates (Creasman, 1998).

# Clear Cell Adenocarcinoma

Clear cell adenocarcinomas in young women have been more common since 1970 as a result of the association of many of these cancers with intrauterine exposure to DES (Herbst, 1971). Therapeutic considerations are similar to those for squamous cell carcinoma, taking into account the young age of the patients undergoing therapy. Cervical clear cell adenocarcinomas are treated in the same manner as primary cervical carcinomas. The results of therapy for vaginal and cervical clear cell adenocarcinoma in young women are discussed together in this section. These tumors are also staged according to FIGO classification (see Table 30.3). Most tumors (80%) have been diagnosed as stage I or II. The overall results of therapy, based on the stage of the tumor at the time of treatment, are shown in Table 30.4. The survival rate is related directly to the stage of the tumor, similar to other gynecologic malignancies at these sites.

In general, surgery is the primary treatment modality because of the young age of the patients. For stage I and early stage II tumors, radical hysterectomy with partial or complete vaginectomy, pelvic lymphadenectomy, and reconstruction of the vagina with split-thickness skin grafts has been the most common approach. In most cases, ovarian function is preserved. In addition, efforts have been made to preserve fertility in patients who have small tumors of the vagina by the use of local irradiation of the primary tumor and immediate adjacent tissues to spare the ovaries. Because metastases to regional pelvic nodes can occur, even with small stage I tumors, retroperitoneal lymph node dissections are usually performed before local therapy.

Local excision of the tumor can be performed before irradiation to facilitate local application. Senekjian and associates have noted that the survival of patients with small vaginal tumors treated by local excision and then local irradiation is comparable with that obtained with conventional extensive therapy (Senekjian, 1989). The best candidates are those with tumors smaller than 2 cm in diameter, a predominant tubulocystic pattern (Fig. 30.23), and depth of invasion less than 3 mm. After wide local excision, the pelvic nodes are sampled to rule out tumor spread. If these are negative, local irradiation can then be given. Patients treated in this manner have become pregnant. Patients with larger tumors, however, receive full pelvic irradiation, in addition to an intracavitary implant. In a few cases, exenterative surgery has been successfully performed. This procedure is preferably applied to central recurrences that develop after primary irradiation. Local vaginal excision as the sole therapy is not usually adequate for small tumors because the tumor often recurs.

Three predominant histologic patterns are found in patients with clear cell adenocarcinoma (see Fig. 30.23). In addition, a number of prognostic factors have been identified. Older patients (older than 19 years) have been found to have a more favorable prognosis compared with younger patients (younger than 15 years). This difference is associated with a more favorable outcome for those with the tubulocystic pattern of clear cell adenocarcinoma, the most common histologic pattern found in older patients. In addition, smaller tumor diameter and superficial depth of invasion correlate with improved patient survival. Waggoner and coworkers have shown that patients with clear cell adenocarcinoma and a maternal history of DES use survive longer than those without a maternal history of DES use (Waggoner, 1994). If the regional pelvic nodes are free of tumor, the prognosis is also more favorable. It is more likely that the regional pelvic lymph nodes will be free of tumor if other factors are favorable.

Clear cell adenocarcinomas can spread locally and via lymphatics and blood vessels. Metastases to regional pelvic nodes are found in approximately one sixth of patients with stage I disease. Spread to regional pelvic nodes becomes more common in higher-stage tumors. Depending on the location of the tumor recurrence, therapy has consisted of additional radical surgery or extensive radiation in localized pelvic disease and systemic chemotherapy in cases of metastatic disease. Unfortunately, no single agent or combination of chemotherapeutic agents has emerged as an effective therapy. Prolonged follow-up is necessary for these patients because recurrences have been reported as long as 20 years after primary therapy, particularly in the lungs and supraclavicular areas. Data from the Registry on Hormonal Transplacental Carcinogenesis (Herbst, 1990) indicate that ovarian preservation with concomitant estrogen stimulation does not adversely affect survival in patients with clear cell adenocarcinoma of the vagina.

**TABLE 30.4** The 5- and 10-Year Survival Rates for 588 Patients With Clear Cell Adenocarcinoma of the Vagina and Cervix

| Stage | 5-Year Survival (%) | 10-Year Survival (%) |
|---|---|---|
| I | 91 | 85 |
| IIA | 80 | 67 |
| IIB | 56 | 47 |
| II (vagina) | 82 | 67 |
| III | 37 | 25 |
| IV | 0 | 0 |

Modified from Registry Data, University of Chicago; Herbst A, Anderson D. Clear cell adenocarcinoma of the vagina and cervix secondary to intrauterine exposure to diethylstilbestrol. *Semin Surg Oncol.* 1990;6(6):343-346.

# Malignant Melanoma

Vaginal melanomas are rare and highly malignant. Only approximately 2% to 3% of primary vaginal cancers are melanomas. The most common presenting symptoms are vaginal discharge, bleeding, and a palpable mass. These lesions appear as darkly pigmented, irregular areas and may be flat, polypoid, or nodular. The average age of affected women is 57 years. Vaginal melanomas tend to metastasize early, via the bloodstream and lymphatics, to the iliac or inguinal nodes, lungs, liver, brain, and bones. Patients with vaginal melanoma have a poorer prognosis than those with vulvar melanoma, in part probably because of delay in diagnosis compared with vulvar carcinomas and in part because of their mucosal location, which seems to predispose patients to developing early metastasis (Kirschner, 2013).

Treatment usually consists of surgery with wide excision of the vagina and dissection of the regional nodes (pelvic, inguinal-femoral, or both), depending on the location of the lesion; improved outcomes have been associated with the removal of all gross disease (Buchanan, 1998). Therapy is usually tailored to the extent of disease. Surgery, radiation, chemotherapy, and immunotherapy have all been described, but no single therapy or combination treatment is uniformly successful.

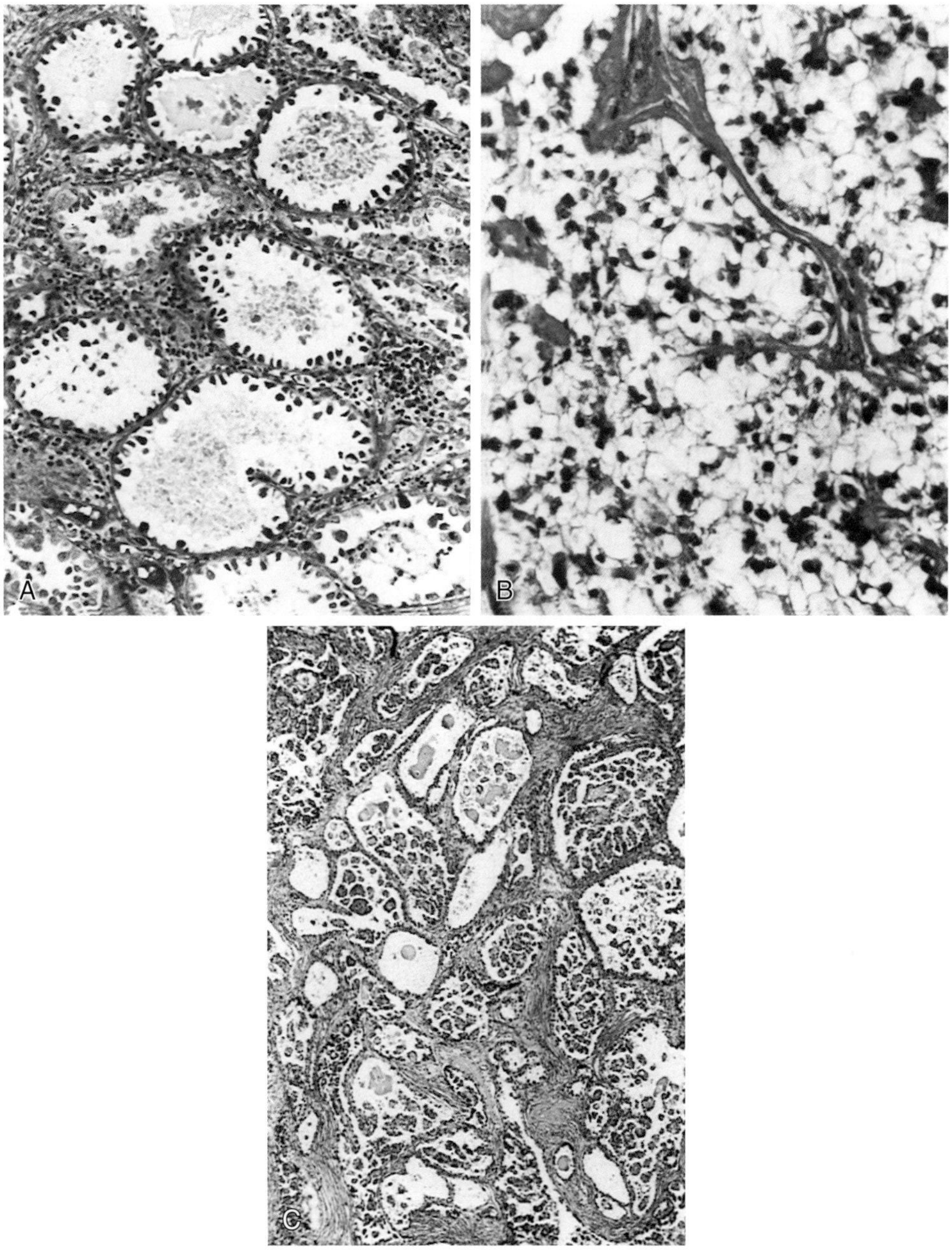


**Fig. 30.23** Clear cell adenocarcinoma. **A,** Tubulocystic cell pattern. Note hobnail cells extruding into the lumina of tubular structures (hematoxylin and eosin [H&E] stain, ×180). **B,** Solid pattern (H&E stain, ×300). **C,** Papillary pattern (H&E stain, ×50). (**A** and **B,** From Scully RE, Robboy SJ, Herbst AL. Vaginal and cervical abnormalities, including clear cell adenocarcinoma, related to prenatal exposure to stilbestrol. *Ann Clin Lab Sci.* 1974;4(4):222-233. **C,** From Scully RE, Robboy SJ, Welch WR. Pathology and pathogenesis of diethylstilbestrol-related disorders of the female genital tract. In: Herbst AL, ed. *Intrauterine Exposure to Diethylstilbestrol in the Human.* Washington, DC: American College of Obstetricians and Gynecologists; 1978.)

Local and distant recurrences are common, and the disease is usually fatal. Even with local control, distant failure is common in patients with melanoma. The overall 5-year survival rate is 8.4%, with an overall median survival of 20 months. Prognostic indicators include tumor size, mitotic index, and Breslow tumor thickness. Improved survival has been noted for patients whose tumors had fewer than six mitoses per 10 high-power fields (HPFs). Van Nostrand and associates have reported a 2-year survival for three of four patients with tumors smaller than 10 $cm^2$—that is, approximately 3 cm in diameter (Van Nostrand, 1994). However, Neven and coworkers have noted that among nine patients, all those with melanomas more than 2 mm thick died or had a recurrence regardless of type of therapy, emphasizing the importance of tumor thickness in melanoma prognosis (Neven, 1994).

## Vaginal Adenocarcinomas Arising in Endometriosis

The malignant transformation of extraovarian endometriosis is rare but has been reported with increasing frequency. The reason for this increase is not known. The rectovaginal septum is the most common extragonadal location (Yazbeck, 2005). When these tumors occur in the vagina or rectovaginal septum, the typical clinical presentation is pain, vaginal bleeding, or the presence of a vaginal mass in a woman who has previously undergone extirpative surgery for endometriosis. Risk factors include use of unopposed estrogen and tamoxifen use. The most common histologic type is endometrioid adenocarcinoma, followed by sarcomas (25%) and other tumors of müllerian differentiation. Treatment usually includes surgery plus radiation or chemotherapy. Leiserowitz and colleagues have reported a relatively favorable prognosis for women with endometriosis-related malignancies, with 70% alive at a mean follow-up of 31 months (2003).

## VAGINAL TUMORS OF INFANTS AND CHILDREN

### Endodermal Sinus Tumor (Yolk Sac Tumor)

Endodermal sinus tumor, a type of adenocarcinoma, is a rare germ cell tumor that usually occurs in the ovary. This tumor secretes alpha-fetoprotein, which provides a useful tumor marker to monitor patients treated for these neoplasms. Approximately 69 cases of this unusual malignancy originated in the vagina of infants, predominantly those younger than age 2 years. This tumor is aggressive, and most patients have died (Anderson, 1985). Young and Scully reported on six patients who were free of disease 2 to 9 years after surgery, irradiation, or both, who also received vincristine, *actinomycin* D, and cyclophosphamide (VAC) chemotherapy (Young, 1984). Copeland and colleagues have reported similar good results with combination chemotherapy and excision (Copeland, 1985). The combination of bleomycin, etoposide, and cisplatin (BEP) has also been used to treat this disease (Tao, 2012).

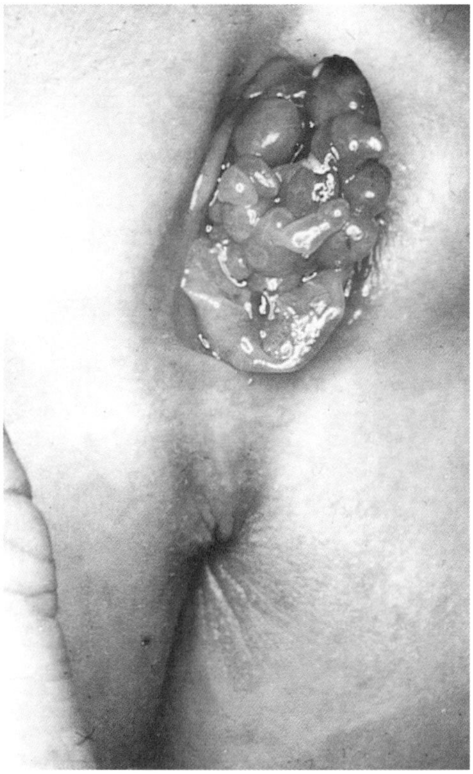

**Fig. 30.24** Sarcoma botryoides protruding through the vaginal introitus. (From Herbst AL. Cancer of the vagina. In: Gusberg SB, Frick HC, eds. *Gynecologic Cancer.* 5th ed. Baltimore: Williams & Wilkins; 1978.)

### Sarcoma Botryoides (Embryonal Rhabdomyosarcoma)

Sarcoma botryoides is an uncommon vaginal sarcoma usually diagnosed in young girls. Rarely does it occur in a young child older than 8 years, although cases in adolescents have been reported. The most common symptom is abnormal vaginal bleeding, with an occasional mass present at the introitus (Fig. 30.24). The tumor grossly resembles a cluster of grapes forming multiple polypoid masses (Copeland, 1985).

These tumors are believed to begin in the subepithelial layers of the vagina and expand rapidly to fill the vagina. They are often multicentric. Histologically they have a loose myxomatous stroma with malignant pleomorphic cells and occasional eosinophilic rhabdomyoblasts that often contain characteristic cross-striations (strap cells; Fig. 30.25).

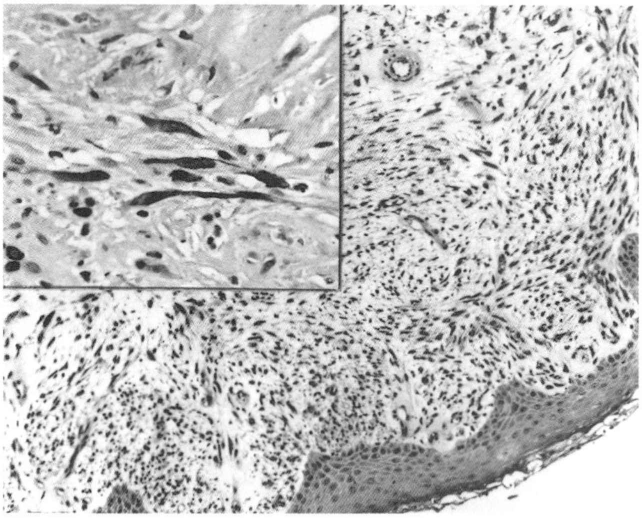

**Fig. 30.25** Vaginal mucosa with sarcoma botryoides showing condensation of malignant cells under the epithelium (hematoxylin and eosin stain, ×100). *Insert,* Immunohistochemical stain for desmin illustrating strap cells (×240). (Courtesy Dr. A. Montag, University of Chicago.)

In the past, sarcoma botryoides lesions were treated by radical surgery, such as pelvic exenteration; however, effective control with less radical surgery has been achieved with a multimodality approach consisting of multiagent chemotherapy (VAC) combined with surgery. Radiation therapy has also been used. Andrassy and associates reported on 21 patients with vaginal rhabdomyosarcomas who received chemotherapy (Andrassy, 1995); 7 relapsed, 5 of whom had residual disease after incomplete resection. One had disseminated disease. In 17 patients who received chemotherapy for 8 to 48 weeks, a delayed excision could be performed. Long-term survival data for a large number of patients are not available, but such a combined approach appears to result in effective treatment with less mutilating surgery (Piver, 1988).

A multimodal approach, including chemotherapy, was used by Flamant and coworkers in 17 women with rhabdomyosarcoma of the vagina or vulva (Flamant, 1990). At the time of their report, 15 appeared cured; 11 of 12 pubescent patients had experienced menses, and 2 had successfully conceived and delivered healthy children. This was emphasized in a report from the Intergroup Rhabdomyosarcoma Study by Andrassy and colleagues (Andrassy, 1995). They found VAC chemotherapy to be effective for disease confined to the vagina without nodal spread. This therapy was effective without irradiation for disease that was locally resected, suggesting that for these patients, chemotherapy plus surgery can be effective therapy.

## Pseudosarcoma Botryoides

*Pseudosarcoma botryoides* refers to a rare, benign vaginal polyp that resembles sarcoma botryoides and is found in the vagina of infants and pregnant women. Although large atypical cells may be present microscopically, strap cells are absent. Grossly these polyps resemble the grapelike appearance of sarcoma botryoides. Treatment by local excision is effective (Lin, 1995).

### KEY REFERENCES


Andrews SJ, Williams BT, DePriest PD, et al. Therapeutic implications of lymph nodal spread in lateral T1 and T2 squamous cell carcinoma of the vulva. *Gynecol Oncol.* 1994;55:41.

Bergen S, DiSaia PJ, Liao SY, et al. Conservative management of extramammary Paget's disease of the vulva. *Gynecol Oncol.* 1989;33:151.

Beutner KR, Reitano MV, Richwald GA, et al. External genital warts: report of the American Medical Association consensus conference. *Clin Infect Dis.* 1998;27:796.

Bleeker MC, Visser PJ, Overbeek LI, van Beurden M, Berkhof J. Lichen sclerosus: incidence and risk of vulvar squamous cell carcinoma. *Cancer Epidemiol Biomarkers Prev.* 2016;25(8):1224-1230. doi: 10.1158/1055-9965.EPI-16-0019.

Boronow RC, Hickman BT, Reagan MT, et al. Combined therapy as an alternative to exenteration for locally advanced vulvovaginal cancer. II. Results, complications, and dosimetric and surgical considerations. *Am J Clin Oncol.* 1987;10:171-181.

Breslow A. Thickness, cross-sectional areas, and depth of invasion in the prognosis of cutaneous melanoma. *Ann Surg.* 1970;172:908.

Buscema J, Woodruff JD, Parmley TH, et al. Carcinoma in situ of the vulva. *Obstet Gynecol.* 1980;55:225.

Carter J, Carlson J, Fowler J, et al. Invasive vulvar tumors in young women—a disease of the immunosuppressed? *Gynecol Oncol.* 1993;51:307.

Chafe W, Richards A, Morgan L, et al. Unrecognized invasive carcinoma in vulvar intraepithelial neoplasia (VIN). *Gynecol Oncol.* 1988;31:154.

Chaturvedi AK, Madeleine MM, Biggar RJ, et al. Risk of human papillomavirus-associated cancers among persons with AIDS. *J Natl Cancer Inst.* 2009;101:1120.

Cowan RA, Black DR, Hoang LN, et al. A pilot study of topical imiquimod therapy for the treatment of recurrent extramammary Paget's disease. *Gynecol Oncol.* 2016;142(1):139-143.

Crum CP. Vulvar intraepithelial neoplasia: histology and associated viral changes. In: Wilkinson EJ, ed. *Pathology of the Vulva and Vagina.* New York: Churchill Livingstone; 1987.

Dvoretsky PM, Bonfiglio TA, Helkamp BF, et al. The pathology of superficially invasive thin vulva squamous cell carcinoma. *Int J Gynecol Pathol.* 1984;3:331.

Fanning J, Lambert HC, Hale TM, Morris PC, Schuerch C. Paget's disease of the vulva: prevalence of associated vulvar adenocarcinoma, invasive Paget's disease, and recurrence after surgical excision. *Am J Obstet Gynecol.* 1999;180(1 Pt 1):24-27.

Farias-Eisner R, Cirisano FD, Grouse D, et al. Conservative and individualized surgery for early squamous carcinoma of the vulva: the treatment of choice for stage I and II (T1-2 N0-1 M0) disease. *Gynecol Oncol.* 1994;53:55.

Fehr MK, Baumann M, Mueller M, et al. Disease progression and recurrence in women treated for vulvovaginal intraepithelial neoplasia. *J Gynecol Oncol.* 2013;24(3):236-241.

Fishman DA, Chambers SK, Schwartz PE, et al. Extramammary Paget's disease of the vulva. *Gynecol Oncol.* 1995;56:266.

Friedrich Jr EG. Reversible vulvar atypia: a case report. *Obstet Gynecol.* 1972;39:173.

Friedrich EG, Wilkinson EJ, Fu YS. Carcinoma in situ of the vulva: a continuing challenge. *Am J Obstet Gynecol.* 1980;136:830.

Frumovitz M, Levenback CF. Lymphatic mapping and sentinel node biopsy in vulvar, vaginal, and cervical cancers. *Oncology (Williston Park).* 2008;22(5):529-536.

Fu YS, Reagan JW, Townsend DE, et al. Nuclear DNA study of vulvar intraepithetial and invasive squamous neoplasms. *Obstet Gynecol.* 1981; 57:643.

Funaro D, Lovett A, Leroux N, Powell J. A double-blind, randomized prospective study evaluating topical clobetasol propionate 0.05% versus topical tacrolimus 0.1% in patients with vulvar lichen sclerosus. *J Am Acad Dermatol.* 2014;71(1):84-91.

Goldstein AT, Creasey A, Pfau R, Phillips D, Burrows LJ. A double-blind, randomized controlled trial of clobetasol versus pimecrolimus in patients with vulvar lichen sclerosus. *J Am Acad Dermatol.* 2011; 64(6):e99-e104.

Green MS, Naumann RW, Elliot M, et al. Sexual dysfunction following vulvectomy. *Gynecol Oncol.* 2000;77:73.

Grimshaw RN, Murdoch JB, Monaghan JM. Radical vulvectomy and bilateral inguinal-femoral lymphadenectomy through separate incisions: experience with 100 cases. *Int J Gynecol Cancer.* 1993;3:18.

Hacker NF, Berek JS, Lagasse LD, et al. Management of regional lymph nodes and their prognostic influence in vulvar cancer. *Obstet Gynecol.* 1983;61:408.

Halonen P, Jakobsson M, Heikinheimo O, Riska A, Gissler M, Pukkala E. Lichen sclerosus and risk of cancer. *Int J Cancer.* 2017;140(9): 1998-2002. doi: 10.1002/ijc.30621.

Hoffman JS, Kumar NB, Morley GW. Prognostic significance of groin lymph node metastases of squamous carcin

Kenter GG, Welters MJ, Valentijn AR, et al. Vaccination against HPV-16 oncoproteins for vulvar intraepithelial neoplasia. *N Engl J Med.* 2009;361(19):1838-1847.

Rotmensch J, Rubin SJ, Sutton HG, et al. Preoperative radiotherapy followed by radical vulvectomy with inguinal lymphadenectomy for advanced vulvar cancer. *Gynecol Oncol.* 1990;36:181.


**Full references and Suggested readings for this chapter can be found on ExpertConsult.com.**

# 31 Malignant Diseases of the Cervix

## Microinvasive and Invasive Carcinoma: Diagnosis and Management

*Anuja Jhingran, Larissa A. Meyer*

### KEY POINTS

- Carcinomas of the cervix are predominantly squamous cell carcinomas (85% to 90%), and approximately 10% to 15% are adenocarcinomas.
- Squamous cell carcinomas are strongly associated with human papillomavirus (HPV) infection.
- Cervical carcinoma is the third most common malignancy of the lower female genital tract, after endometrial and ovarian cancer, and the second most common cause of death, after ovarian cancer.
- Definitive diagnosis of microinvasive carcinoma is established only by means of cervical conization, not biopsy. The margins of the cone should be free of neoplastic epithelium before conservative therapy is undertaken.
- Microinvasive carcinoma of the cervix can be effectively treated by total hysterectomy, with a 5-year survival rate of almost 100%, but recurrent neoplasia can develop after 5 years; however, a precise and reliable definition of microinvasion is controversial.
- Prognosis in squamous cell cancer of the cervix is related to tumor stage and lesion size, depth of invasion, and spread to lymph nodes.
- Cervical carcinomas are locally invasive tumors that spread primarily to the pelvic tissues and then to the pelvic and paraaortic lymph nodes. Less commonly, hematogenous spread to the liver, lung, and bone occurs.
- The risk of the spread of cervical carcinoma to pelvic nodes is approximately 15% for stage I, 29% for stage II, and 47% for stage III. For the paraaortic nodes, the figures are 6% for stage I, 19% for stage II, and 33% for stage III.
- Surgery is often used to treat stage IB and early stage IIA carcinomas of the cervix, particularly for smaller tumors and in younger patients to preserve their ovarian function. Surgery produces less scarring and vaginal fibrosis than radiation and is preferred for women with a pelvic infection or a history of conditions such as inflammatory bowel disease, which increase the risk for radiation complications.
- Minimally invasive radical hysterectomies are associated with increased rates of recurrence and decreased survival rates compared with an open abdominal surgical approach.
- High-stage tumors are treated by chemoradiation. Programs usually use cisplatin, 40 mg/m$^2$ weekly, during external treatment and with brachytherapy.
- Most cancers of the cervix are treated by radiation therapy (teletherapy and brachytherapy). Radiation doses vary with tumor size and stage but are approximately 50 to 65 Gy at point B and 80 to 85 Gy at point A. Brachytherapy should be used whenever feasible because data indicate that use of brachytherapy improves survival compared with any other type of modality.
- Complications after radiation are related to dose and volume of tissue treated; these include radiation inflammation of the bladder or bowel, which may lead to pain, bleeding, or, infrequently, fistula formation. The normal cervix is resistant to radiation, and the dose can be as high as 200 to 250 Gy over 2 months. The rectum should be limited to doses of 70 Gy or less and the bladder to doses of 80 Gy or less. Overall, the rate of moderate to severe radiation complications for treatment of all stages is approximately 10%.
- Worldwide 5-year survival rates reported for patients with carcinomas of the cervix are as follows: stage IA, 95%; stage IB, 80%; stage II, 70%; stage III, 50%; and stage IV, 20% with radiation therapy alone.
- Pregnancy does not adversely affect the survival rate for women with carcinoma of the cervix, stage for stage.
- Approximately one-third of patients treated for cervical carcinoma develop tumor recurrence, and approximately 50% of these recurrences are located in the pelvis; most occur within 2 years.
- Patients whose recurrences occur more than 3 years after primary therapy have a better prognosis than those with earlier recurrence.
- Pelvic exenteration in carefully selected patients with central pelvic recurrence can lead to a 5-year survival rate of 50% or better.
- Chemotherapy of recurrent squamous cell carcinoma of the cervix does not produce long-term cures, but results suggest that cisplatin-paclitaxel-bevacizumab should be considered the standard treatment for patients with stage IVB recurrent or metastatic cervix cancer.

The majority of cervical malignancies are carcinomas; a summary of the more common histologic types is shown in Box 31.1. Approximately 80% to 85% of these tumors are squamous cell carcinomas, and 15% to 20% are adenocarcinomas. The incidence of adenocarcinomas has increased in most developing countries, particularly among younger women. Carcinoma of the cervix is closely associated with early and frequent sexual contact and cervical viral infection, particularly human papillomavirus (HPV), as detailed in Chapter 29. According to the American Cancer Society, the frequency of cervical cancer has been steadily decreasing, in part because of the effect of widespread screening for premalignant cervical changes by cervical cytologic testing (Papanicolaou [Pap] smear). In the United States there will be an estimated 13,240 new cases of invasive cervical cancer diagnosed in 2018, with 4170 related deaths (Siegel, 2018). Racial and ethnic disparities continue in the United States in both the incidence and mortality from cervical cancer. The incidence of cervical carcinoma in the United States is higher among the Hispanic

**BOX 31.1 Summary of Major Categories of Cervical Carcinoma**

**SQUAMOUS CELL CARCINOMAS**

Large cell (keratinizing or nonkeratinizing)
Small cell
Verrucous

**ADENOCARCINOMAS**

Typical (endocervical)
Endometrioid
Clear cell
Adenoid cystic (basaloid cylindroma)
Adenoma malignum (minimal deviation adenocarcinoma)

**MIXED CARCINOMAS**

Adenosquamous
Glassy cell carcinoma

population (9.7 per 100,000) compared with white (7 per 100,000) and African American populations (9.5 per 100,000) (Siegel, 2018); however, the mortality rate from cervical cancer is the highest among African Americans compared with other races and ethnicities, partly because African Americans tend to be diagnosed at a later stage. Invasive cervical cancers are diagnosed at a localized stage in 47% of white women and 37% of African American women. This chapter details the various types of cervical carcinoma and considers the natural history, methods of diagnosis and evaluation, and details of therapy. Primary sarcomas and melanomas of the cervix are extremely rare and are not considered separately.

## HISTOLOGIC TYPES

Varieties of squamous cell carcinoma of the cervix are illustrated in Fig. 31.1. An early form, microinvasive carcinoma, is considered separately in the next section. Most squamous cell

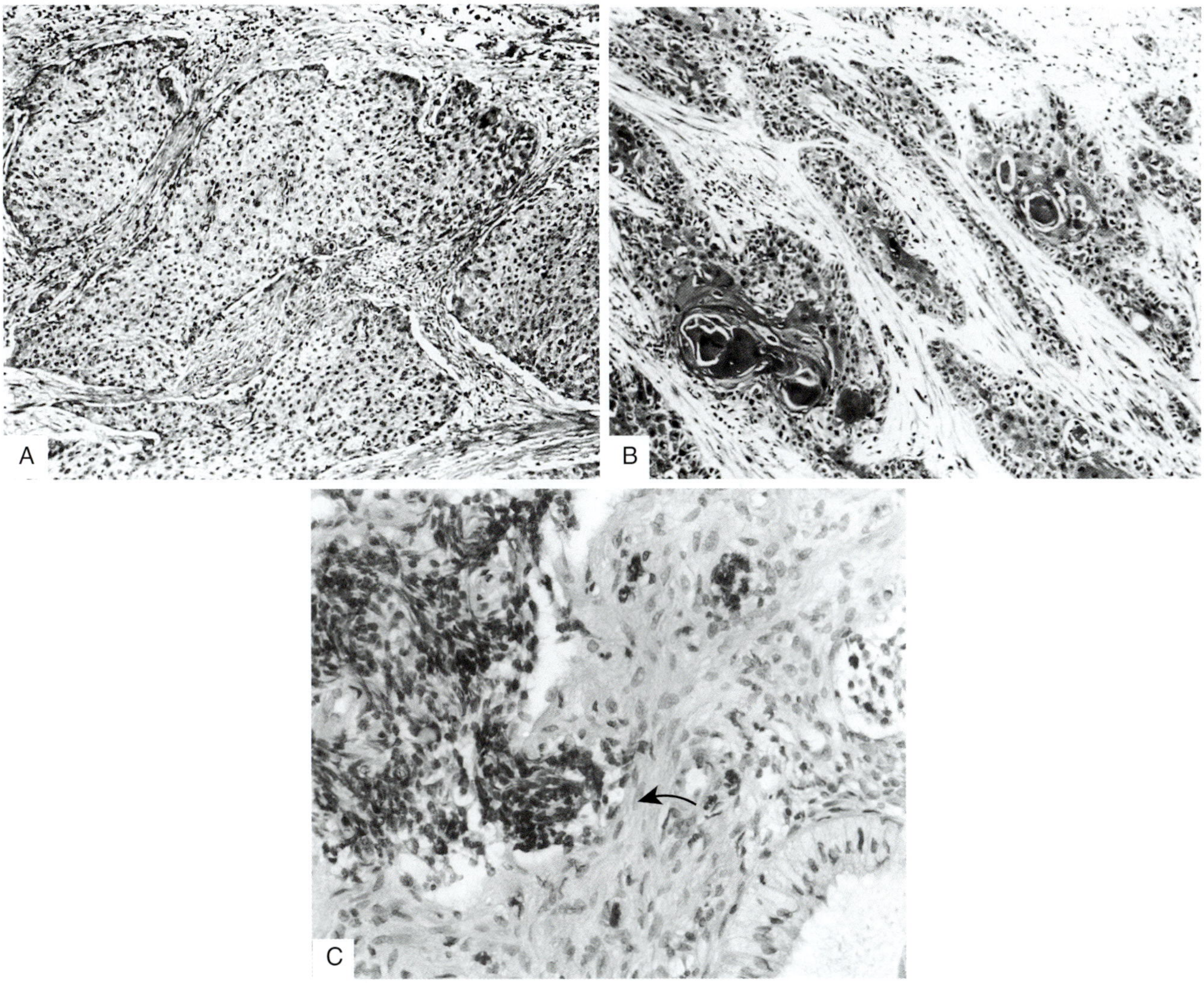


**Fig. 31.1** **A,** Large-cell, nonkeratinizing squamous cell carcinoma. Discrete islands of uniform, large cells with abundant cytoplasm are separated by fibrous stroma (original magnification ×160). **B,** Keratinizing squamous cell carcinoma. Irregular nests of squamous cells forming several pearls are separated by fibrous stroma. The nests have pointed projections (original magnification ×160). **C,** Small cell neuroendocrine carcinoma of the cervix *(arrow)* infiltrating between normal endocervical glands (hematoxylin-eosin, original magnification ×240). (**A** and **B,** From Clement PB, Scully RE. Carcinoma of the cervix: histologic types. *Semin Oncol.* 1982;9: 251-264; **C,** Courtesy Dr. Anthony Montag, Department of Pathology, University of Chicago, Chicago.)

carcinomas of the cervix are reported to be of the large cell, nonkeratinizing type, but some are keratinized, and squamous pearls may be seen. The degree of differentiation of the tumors is usually designated by three grades: G1, well differentiated; G2, intermediate; and G3, undifferentiated; however, there is no consensus on the value of tumor grade as a major prognostic factor for squamous cell carcinoma of the cervix.

A rare variety of squamous cell carcinoma is the so-called verrucous carcinoma, which is morphologically similar to that found in the vulva (see Chapter 30). These warty tumors appear as large bulbous masses (Fig. 31.2). They rarely metastasize but unfortunately may be admixed with the more virulent, typical squamous cell carcinomas, in which case metastatic spread is more likely.

Adenocarcinomas may have a number of histologic varieties. The typical variant often contains intracytoplasmic mucin and is related to the mucinous cells of the endocervix (endocervical pattern; Fig. 31.3); however, on occasion the cells contain little or no mucin, and then the tumor may resemble an endometrial carcinoma (endometrioid pattern). It may be difficult histologically to ascertain whether these carcinomas arise in the cervix or endometrium. Although not independently diagnostic, the immunohistochemical panel that is recommended to assist in differentiating endocervical from endometrial primary malignancies includes estrogen receptor (ER), vimentin, monoclonal carcinoembryonic antigen (CEA), and p16. Typically an endocervical carcinoma stains diffusely positive for p16 and CEA and is negative for ER and vimentin.

A rare but important virulent variety of adenocarcinoma is adenoma malignum. These microscopically innocuous-appearing tumors consist of well-differentiated mucinous glands (Fig. 31.4) that vary in size and shape and infiltrate the stroma. Despite their bland histologic appearance, they tend to be deeply invasive and metastasize early. The term *minimal deviation adenocarcinoma* is applied to these tumors.

Clear cell adenocarcinomas of the cervix are histologically identical to those of the ovary (see Chapter 33) and vagina (see Chapter 30). They are uncommon in the cervix and can be associated with intrauterine diethylstilbestrol exposure, although they also may develop spontaneously in the absence of diethylstilbestrol exposure.

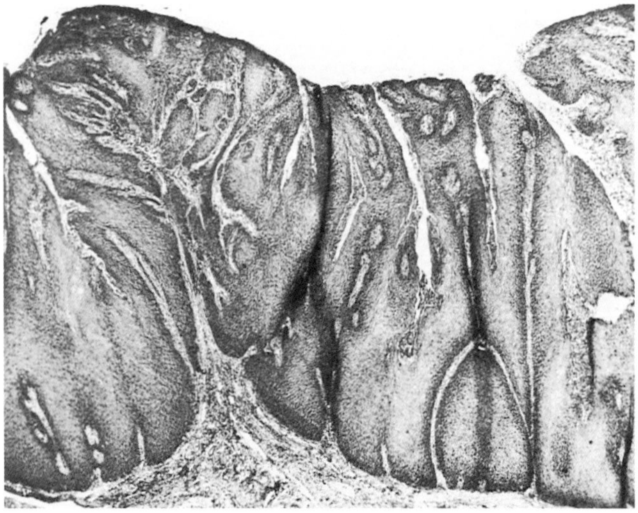

**Fig. 31.2** Verrucous carcinoma. Downgrowths of papillae have broad bases. Tumor cells are well differentiated (original magnification ×34). (From Clement PB, Scully RE. Carcinoma of the cervix: histologic types. *Semin Oncol.* 1982;9:251-264.)

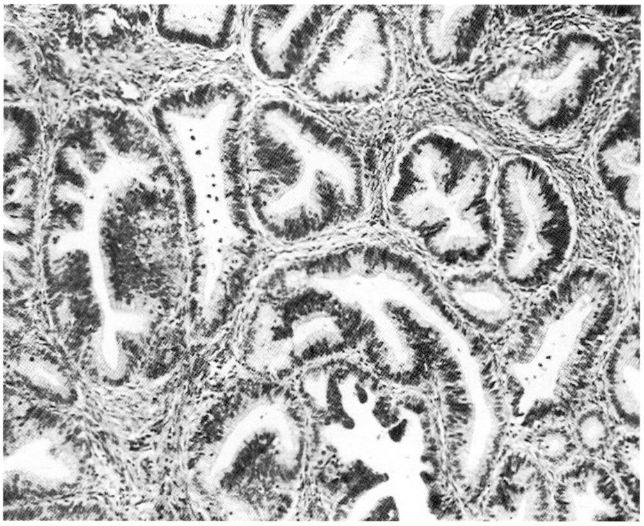

**Fig. 31.3** Typical adenocarcinoma. Irregular glands are lined by stratified mucin-containing epithelium. Mitotic figures are numerous (original magnification ×160). (From Clement PB, Scully RE. Carcinoma of the cervix: histologic types. *Semin Oncol.* 1982;9:251-264.)

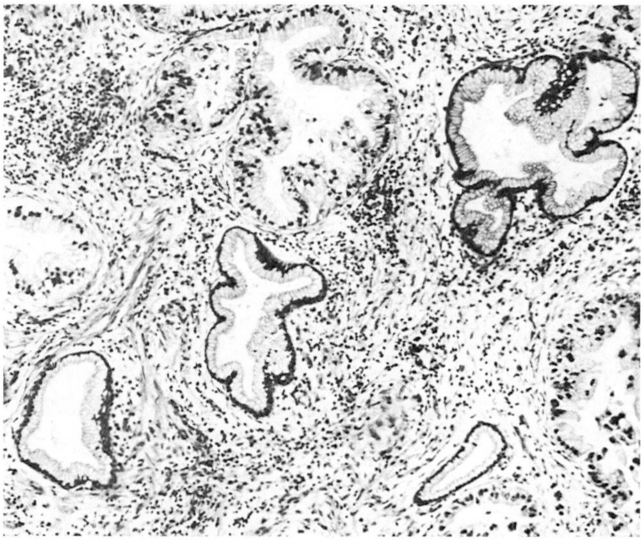

**Fig. 31.4** Adenoma malignum. Glands are mostly well differentiated, appearing normal except for their irregular shapes. A few obviously malignant glands are also present (original magnification ×160). (From Clement PB, Scully RE. Carcinoma of the cervix: histologic types. *Semin Oncol.* 1982;9:251-264.)

Adenoid cystic carcinomas are rare. Berchuk and Mullin summarized 88 cases reported in the literature (Berchuk, 1985). These tumors are aggressive and may resemble cylindromas of salivary gland or breast origin and histologically may resemble basal cell carcinomas of the skin (adenoid basal, or basaloid, carcinomas). Most patients with these tumors are older than 60 years. The basaloid variety appears to be less aggressive.

Adenosquamous carcinomas, as the name implies, consist of squamous carcinoma and adenocarcinoma elements in varying proportions (Fig. 31.5). They occur often in pregnant women. A particularly virulent variety is termed *glassy cell carcinoma* (Fig. 31.6). This is an undifferentiated tumor consisting of large

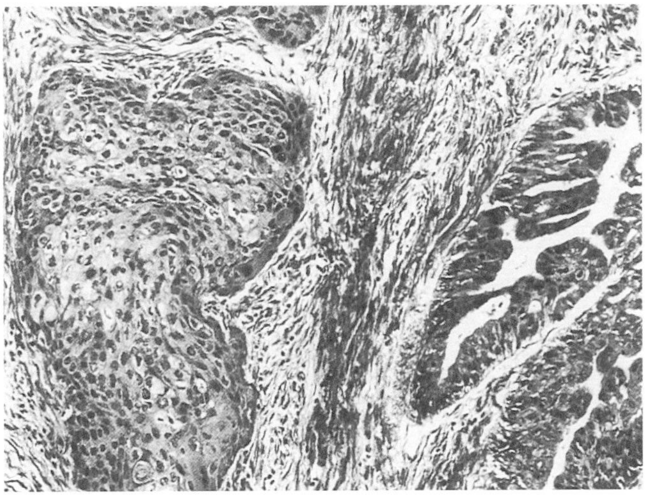

**Fig. 31.5** Well-differentiated adenosquamous carcinoma. Glandular structure lies adjacent to a nest of nonkeratinizing large squamous cells (original magnification ×400). (From Clement PB, Scully RE. Carcinoma of the cervix: histologic types. *Semin Oncol.* 1982;9:251-264.)

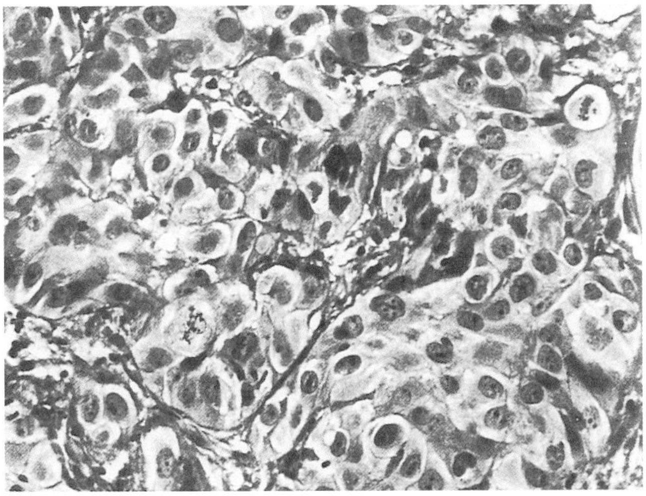

**Fig. 31.6** Glassy cell carcinoma. Cells have sharp borders, ground-glass–type cytoplasm, and nuclei containing prominent nucleoli (original magnification ×1000). (From Clement PB, Scully RE. Carcinoma of the cervix: histologic types. *Semin Oncol.* 1982;9:251-264.)

cells containing cytoplasm, with a ground-glass appearance. Glassy cell carcinomas tend to metastasize early to lymph nodes and to distant sites and usually have a fatal outcome.

Small cell carcinoma of the cervix is rare, comprising less than 5% of all carcinomas of the cervix. Women with small cell carcinoma are likely to be 10 years younger than those with squamous cell carcinoma. Cervical small cell carcinoma is composed of small anaplastic cells with scant cytoplasm that behave aggressively and are often associated with widespread metastasis to multiple sites, including bone, liver, skin, and brain. Efforts to treat these cancers with approaches typically used for small cell carcinoma of the lung have had mixed results.

Another variant that is not in the World Health Organization (WHO) classification is non–small cell neuroendocrine tumors. These tumors contain intermediate to large cells, high-grade nuclei, and eosinophilic cytoplasmic granules of the type seen in neuroendocrine cells. Reported survival rates for patients with these aggressive carcinomas are similar to those of patients with small cell tumors, and an optimal therapy has yet to be established.

# CARCINOMA OF THE CERVIX

## Clinical Considerations

Patients with carcinoma of the cervix characteristically present with abnormal bleeding or brownish discharge, often noted after douching or intercourse and also occurring spontaneously between menstrual periods. These patients often have a history of not having had a cytologic (Pap) smear for many years. Other symptoms, such as back pain, loss of appetite, and weight loss, are late manifestations and occur when there is extensive spread of cervical carcinoma. The patients tend to be in their 40s to 60s, with a median age of 52 years. Preinvasive intraepithelial carcinoma of the cervix (see Chapter 29) occurs primarily in women in their 20s and 30s and has become more common in those in their 20s, leading to a gradual increase in the incidence of invasive carcinoma in younger patients.

The diagnosis is established by biopsy of the tumor; a specimen can easily be obtained during an office examination. A Kevorkian, Eppendorf, Tischler, or similar punch biopsy instrument is convenient to use. Occasionally it is necessary to biopsy nodularity or indurations in the vagina near the cervix to ascertain the limit of tumor spread and define a correct tumor stage. If the woman's cytologic smear suggests invasive carcinoma, with no gross lesion visible, and endocervical curettage does not demonstrate carcinoma, or if an adequate biopsy specimen to establish carcinoma cannot be obtained, cervical conization should be performed.

## Staging

Historically the staging of carcinoma of the cervix depended primarily on the pelvic examination, with no changes to staging based on operative findings. **In 2018, the staging system underwent revisions that allow imaging and pathologic findings from surgery, where available, to assign the stage. Table 31.1** describes the four stages of cervical carcinoma according to the International Federation of Gynecology and Obstetrics (FIGO; revised in 2018) (Bhatla, 2018). The types of tumor distributions that may be observed in the various stages are illustrated in Fig. 31.7.

## Natural History and Spread

Carcinoma of the cervix is initially a locally infiltrating cancer that spreads from the cervix to the vagina and paracervical and parametrial areas. Grossly the tumors may be ulcerated (Fig. 31.8), similar to carcinomas occurring elsewhere in the female genital tract, and may have an exophytic growth pattern or cauliflower-like appearance extruding from the cervix. Alternatively, they may be endophytic, in which case they are asymptomatic, particularly in the early stage of development, and tend to be deeply invasive when diagnosed. These usually start initially from an endocervical location and often fill the cervix and lower uterine segment, resulting in a barrel-shaped cervix. The latter tumors tend to metastasize to regional pelvic nodes and, because of the tendency of late diagnosis, are often more advanced than the exophytic variety. The primary path for distant spread is through lymphatics to the regional pelvic nodes. Bloodborne metastases from cervical carcinomas do occur but are less common and are usually seen late in the course of the disease.

**Initially, cervical carcinoma spreads to the primary pelvic nodes, which include the pericervical node; presacral, hypogastric (internal iliac), and external iliac nodes; and nodes in the obturator fossa near the vessels and nerve. From this**

TABLE 31.1 Clinical Stages of Carcinoma of the Cervix Uteri

| Stage | Characteristics |
|---|---|
| I | Carcinoma is strictly confined to the cervix (extension to the corpus should be disregarded) |
| IA | Invasive cancer that can be diagnosed only by microscopy, with deepest invasion <5 mm* |
| IA1 | Measured stromal invasion <3 mm in depth |
| IA2 | Measured stromal invasion of ≥3 mm and <5 mm in depth |
| IB | Invasive carcinoma with measured deepest invasion ≥5 mm (greater than stage IA), lesion limited to the cervix uteri† |
| IB1 | Invasive carcinoma >5 mm depth of stromal invasion, and ≤2 cm in greatest dimension |
| IB2 | Invasive carcinoma >2 cm and ≤4 cm in greatest dimension |
| IB3 | Invasive carcinoma lesion >4 cm in greatest dimension |
| II | The carcinoma invades beyond the uterus, but has not extended onto the lower third of the vagina or to the pelvic wall |
| IIA | Involvement limited to the upper two-thirds of the vagina without parametrial involvement |
| IIA1 | Invasive carcinoma <4 cm in greatest dimension |
| IIA2 | Invasive carcinoma mensionn greatest dimension |
| IIB | With parametrial involvement but not up to the pelvic wall |
| III | The carcinoma involves the lower third of the vagina and/or extends to the pelvic wall and/or causes hydronephrosis or nonfunctioning kidney and/or involves pelvic and/or paraaortic lymph nodes‡ |
| IIIA | The carcinoma involves the lower third of the vagina, with no extension to the pelvic wall |
| IIIB | Extension to the pelvic wall and/or hydronephrosis or nonfunctioning kidney (unless known to be due to another cause) |
| IIIC | Involvement of pelvic and/or paraaortic lymph nodes, irrespective of tumor size and extent (with r and p notations)‡ |
| IIIC1 | Pelvic lymph node metastasis only |
| IIIC2 | Paraaortic lymph node metastasis |
| IV | The carcinoma has extended beyond the true pelvis or has involved (biopsy-proven) mucosa of the bladder or rectum; a bullous edema, as such, does not permit a case to be allotted to stage IV |
| IVA | Spread to adjacent pelvic organs |
| IVB | Spread to distant organs |

When in doubt, the lower staging should be assigned.

*Imaging and pathologic examination can be used, where available, to supplement clinical findings with respect to tumor size and extent, in all stages.

†The involvement of vascular/lymphatic spaces does not change the staging. The lateral extent of the lesion is no longer considered.

‡Adding notation of r (imaging) and p (pathology) to indicate the findings that are used to allocate the case to stage IIIC. Example: If imaging indicates pelvic lymph node metastasis, the stage allocation would be stage IIIC1r, and if confirmed by pathologic findings, it would be stage IIIC1p. The type of imaging modality or pathology technique used should always be documented.

(From: Bhatla N, Aoki D, Sharma DN, Sankaranarayanan R. Cancer of the cervix uteri. *Intl J Gynaecol Obstet* 2018; 143 S2:22. Available at: https://obgyn.onlinelibrary.wiley.com/doi/full/10.1002/ijgo.12611. Updated with information from: Corrigendum to revised FIGO staging for carcinoma of the cervix uteri. *Intl J Gynaecol Obstet* 2019; 147:279.)

**primary group, tumor spread proceeds secondarily to the common iliac and paraaortic nodes.** Rarely the inguinal nodes are involved; however, if the lower third of the vagina is involved, the median inguinal nodes should be considered primary. The distribution of lymph node involvement in 26 cases of untreated carcinoma of the cervix was studied in detail by Henriksen (Fig. 31.9) (Henriksen, 1949). A series studying the incidence and distribution pattern of retroperitoneal lymph node metastases in 208 patients with stages IB, IIA, and IIB cervical carcinomas who underwent radical hysterectomy and systemic pelvic node dissection reported that 53 patients (25%) had node metastasis (Sakuragi et al., 1999). The obturator lymph nodes were the most commonly involved, with a rate of 19% (39 of 208), and the authors proposed them as sentinel nodes for cervical cancers. An important distal node that becomes involved after the paraaortic group is the left scalene node—that is, the left supraclavicular node. A biopsy of this node may be performed in the assessment of advanced cervical carcinoma to clarify whether the tumor has spread outside the abdomen. In addition to nodal spread, hematogenous spread of cervical carcinoma occurs primarily to the lung, liver, and, less often, bone (see Recurrence later in the chapter).

## Prognostic Factors

**FIGO stage is the most important determinant of prognosis for carcinoma of the cervix (Table 31.2); however, there are other factors, including tumor and patient characteristics, that are prognostic. One of the most important predictors is tumor size for local recurrence and death for patients treated with surgery or radiation therapy (Eifel, 1994).** The 2018 FIGO staging classification for stage IB disease was further modified based on tumor diameter (i.e., IB1, <2 cm; IB2, ≥2 cm and <4 cm; and IB3, ≥4 cm). **Another important prognostic factor is involvement of lymph nodes, which is now included in the staging system as stage IIIC disease.** In several surgical series, after a radical hysterectomy, patients with positive pelvic lymph nodes had a 35% to 40% lower 5-year survival rate than patients with negative nodes. Patients with positive paraaortic nodes have a survival rate that is approximately 50% that of patients with similar stage disease and negative paraaortic nodes. With extended-field radiation therapy, patients with positive paraaortic nodes have approximately a 40% to 50% 5-year survival rate. **There is a strong correlation between positive nodes and positive lymph–vascular space**

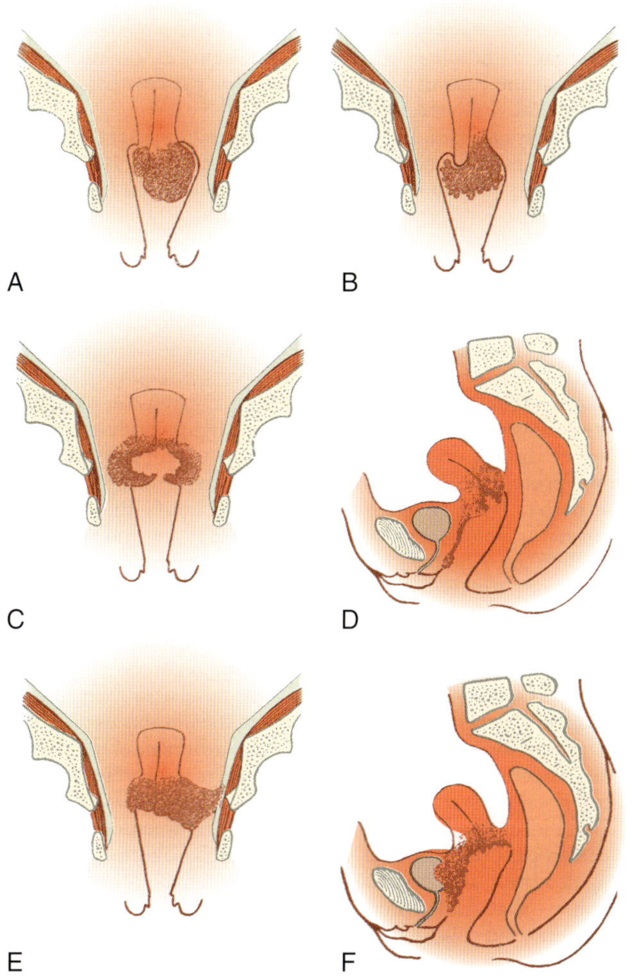


**Fig. 31.7** Staging of cervical carcinoma. **A,** Stage IB, nodular cervix. **B,** Stage IIA, carcinoma extending into left vault. **C,** Stage IIB, parametrium involved on both sides, but carcinoma has not invaded pelvic wall; endocervical crater. **D,** Stage IIIA, submucosal involvement of anterior vaginal wall and small papillomatous nodule in its lower third. **E,** Stage IIIB, parametrium involved on both sides; at left, carcinoma has invaded pelvic wall. **F,** Stage IVA, involvement of bladder. (From Pettersson F, Bjorkholm E. Staging and reporting of cervical carcinoma. *Semin Oncol.* 1982;9:287-298.)

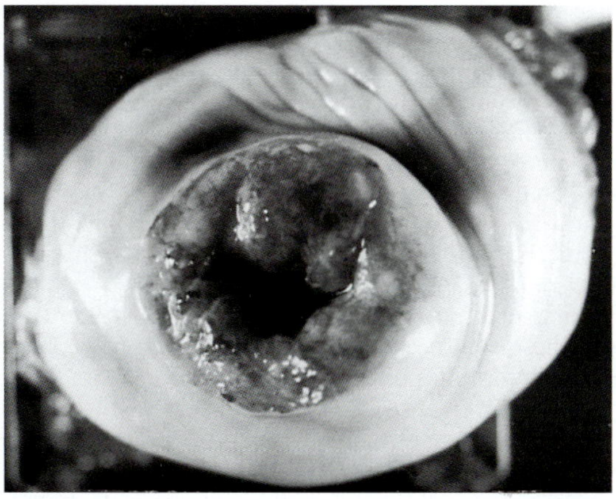

**Fig. 31.8** Carcinoma of the cervix (gross specimen).

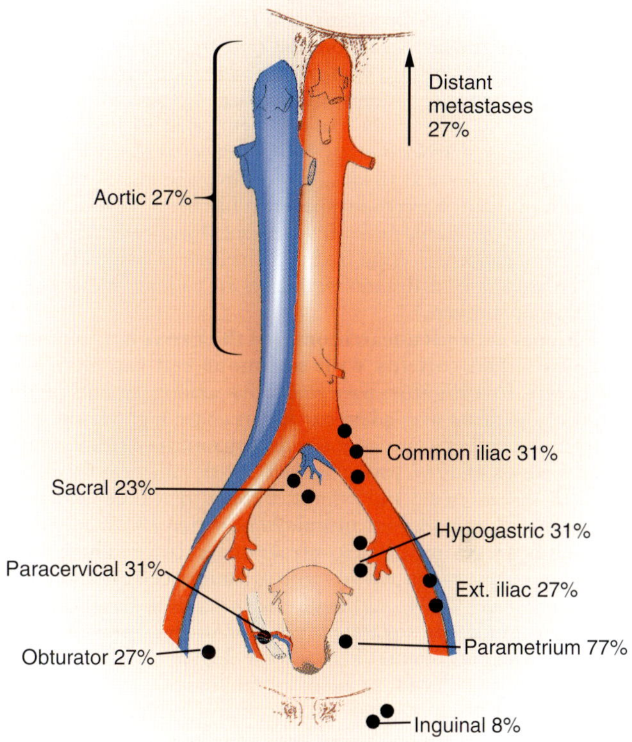


**Fig. 31.9** Frequency of lymph node metastases in cervical carcinoma. Shown is the incidence of node group involvement in 26 nontreated cases of cervical carcinoma. *Ext,* External. (From Henriksen E. The lymphatic spread of carcinoma of the cervix and of the body of the uterus. *Am J Obstet Gynecol.* 1949;58:924-942.)

**TABLE 31.2** Carcinoma of the Uterine Cervix: Distribution by Stage and 5-Year Survival Rates for Patients Treated in 1990-1992 (n = 11,945)

| Stage | No. of Patients (n) | 5-Year Survival |
|---|---|---|
| IA | 902 | 95.01% |
| IB | 4657 | 80.1% |
| II | 3364 | 64.2% |
| III | 2530 | 38.31% |
| IV | 492 | 14% |

Modified from Pecorelli S, Creasman WT, Pettersson F, et al. *FIGO Annual Report on the Results of Treatment in Gynaecological Cancer.* Vol. 23. Milan, Italy: International Federation of Gynecology and Obstetrics; 1998.

**invasion (LVSI) in the tumor specimen in patients with cervical carcinoma; however, LVSI may be an independent predictor of prognosis, as shown in a number of larger surgical series.**

**In patients who have had a radical hysterectomy, histologic evidence of extracervical spread (≥10 mm), deep stromal invasion (>70% invasion), and LVSI are associated with a poorer prognosis. A** randomized trial from the Gynecologic Oncology Group (GOG) compared observation versus adjuvant radiation therapy in patients after radical hysterectomy with a combination of two of the factors mentioned earlier; patients who received radiation therapy had better local control and improved overall survival (Sedlis, 1999). Involvement of the parametrium in the hysterectomy specimen has been correlated with higher rates of lymph node involvement, local recurrence, and death from cancer. Uterine body involvement is associated with an increased rate of distant metastases in patients treated with radiation or surgery.

**Patients with adenocarcinomas of the cervix have a poorer prognosis than patients with squamous cell carcinomas of the cervix. Investigators** have found that among patients treated surgically, patients with adenocarcinomas have high relapse rates compared with rates in patients with squamous cell carcinomas. In an analysis of 1767 patients treated with radiation for FIGO stage IB disease, Eifel and associates found that independent of age, tumor size, and tumor morphology, patients with adenocarcinomas had the same pelvic control rate but twice as high a rate of distant metastasis as patients with squamous cell carcinomas of the cervix (Eifel, 1994). Although the prognostic significance of histologic grade for squamous carcinomas has been disputed, there is a clear correlation between the degree of differentiation and the clinical behavior of adenocarcinomas.

There has been a great interest in molecular markers for prognosis and treatment in carcinoma of the cervix. One of the most studied markers is the serum squamous cell carcinoma antigen. Studies have shown that pretreatment levels of this antigen correlate well with stage of disease, tumor histologic characteristics, grade, type of tumor (exophytic vs. infiltrative), microscopic depth of invasion, and risk of lymph node metastases in patients with early-stage disease. Possible clinical applications of this antigen may be to predict clinical outcome and as a marker for monitoring the course of disease and response to treatment in patients with cervical cancer. Several investigators have reported significantly lower survival rates in patients with elevated values compared with patients with normal baseline levels, independent of stage. For detection of tumor recurrence, serial squamous cell carcinoma antigen testing has proved to be more specific than sensitive, with specificities ranging from 90% to 100% and sensitivities ranging from 60% to 90%. Further investigation is needed in these areas. Some investigators have found a higher rate of recurrence in patients with HPV-positive nodes (although negative for malignancies) and poor prognosis with the presence of HPV messenger RNA (mRNA) in the peripheral blood of cervical cancer patients. Other markers that have been investigated include epidermal growth factor receptor, cyclooxygenase-2, DNA-ploidy, tumor vascularity, and S-phase fraction. Programmed death ligand 1 (PDL1) expression may be useful for treatment decisions in the recurrent setting (Frenel, 2017).

## Treatment

### Pretherapy Evaluation

Once a woman has been diagnosed as having an invasive carcinoma, a pretreatment evaluation is conducted to determine the extent of disease, arrive at an accurate clinical staging, and plan the program of therapy. The usual evaluation consists of a thorough history and physical examination, routine blood studies, intravenous pyelogram (IVP) or computed tomography (CT), and chest radiography. Demonstration of an obstructed ureter or nonfunctioning kidney caused by tumor automatically assigns the case at least to stage III (see Table 31.1). A barium enema test or flexible sigmoidoscopy, as well as a cystoscopy, is sometimes performed in the case of large tumors or for patients who will be receiving radiation treatment.

The best radiographic imaging technique for detecting lymph node metastases is unclear. CT and magnetic resonance imaging (MRI) are good for identifying enlarged nodes; however, the accuracy of these techniques in the detection of positive nodes is compromised by their failure to detect small metastases, and many enlarged nodes are caused not by metastases but by inflammation associated with advanced disease. The accuracy of MRI in the detection of lymph node metastases (72% to 93%) is similar to that of CT but better than CT and physical examination for the evaluation of tumor location, tumor size, depth of stromal invasion, vaginal extension, and parametrial extension of cervical cancer; however, with regard to detecting lymph node metastases or other distant disease, positron emission tomography (PET) shows promise. Several studies from a single institution have shown that $^{18}$F-fluorodeoxyglucose PET (FDG-PET) detects abnormal lymph nodes more often than CT, and those findings with PET are a better predictor of survival than those with CT or MRI in patients with carcinoma of the cervix. Medicare has approved PET/CT as part of the initial staging evaluation for patients with cervical carcinoma, and most insurance companies approve PET/CT for a 3-month follow-up.

Surgical sampling of lymph nodes is the most sensitive method of evaluating whether regional lymph nodes contain metastases; however, it is invasive, expensive, and may delay treatment of the primary lesion. Laparoscopic lymph node dissection may decrease the time between surgery and the start of treatment and may be associated with less late radiation-related morbidity than open transperitoneal staging. Laparoscopic extraperitoneal paraaortic lymphadenectomy has also been described and may further decrease radiation-related bowel morbidity by avoiding entrance into the peritoneal cavity. In a study by Ramirez and colleagues, 22% of patients who had positive pelvic but negative paraaortic nodes on PET/CT had histopathologically positive paraaortic nodes (Ramirez, 2011).

### Treatment for Stage I

#### Stage IA

The term *microinvasion* has been used for years to describe patients with minimally invasive cervical cancer, but this term is not part of the FIGO staging system. Microinvasion was used to describe patients with 3-mm invasion or less and essentially no risk of metastatic spread. There is ample evidence that patients with small-volume tumors measured only by depth of invasion have a low risk of relapse and death with radical surgery or more conservative surgical approaches.

The diagnosis of microinvasive tumor cannot be made based on a biopsy specimen alone; a cervical conization must be performed. If the margin of the cervical cone specimen contains neoplastic epithelium, the risk of invasive tumor in the remaining uterus is increased. Decisions on treatment should be based on an adequate cone biopsy specimen. If a woman has positive margins, the cone can be repeated. Sometimes, deeper invasion will be uncovered and more radical treatment will be required. In some patients, conization alone is adequate.

The measured stromal invasion of stage IA1 tumors is 3 mm or less. These measurements are determined on a cone biopsy, which also determines other prognostic factors (e.g., lymph vascular space involvement, histologic subtype, grade). These factors do not alter the stage assignment, in spite of their adverse prognostic significance. In the absence of LVSI or high-risk histologic subtypes, the risk of lymph node metastases is remote and nonradical surgery is adequate. This may include cone biopsy, simple trachelectomy, or simple hysterectomy, depending on the circumstances and patient preference.

Patients with stage IA2 tumors have a measured stromal invasion of 5 mm or less. Patients in this category, even without LVSI, are at a low risk of nodal involvement. Thus radical or modified radical approaches are usually recommended, which include modified radical hysterectomy or trachelectomy and pelvic lymphadenectomy. Stage IA1 patients who have LVSI are treated in the same manner as stage IA2 patients.

There continues to be interest in determining the necessity of treating the parametrium in patients with low-stage cervical cancer. Several investigators have noted that the risk of parametrial involvement is 1% or less in patients undergoing radical hysterectomy in low-risk situations. Parametrial resection contributes significant short-term and long-term morbidity to surgery. Lymphatic mapping techniques suggest that parametrial sentinel lymph nodes can be identified and resected without a radical dissection. In the future, as cervical cancer surgery trials mature, the indications for surgery that omits the parametrial resection may grow.

### Stage IB

Stage IB encompasses tumors that are larger than stage IA, meaning 5 mm or larger in measured stromal invasion.

**Patients with stage IB1 and IB2 disease have tumor limited to the cervix that is 4 cm or less in diameter. These patients have equally good outcomes with radical surgery or radiotherapy. A major factor in favor of radical surgery is younger age, especially premenopausal patients for whom ovarian preservation is an option.** In addition, there is now increasing availability of ovum transfer and pregnancy surrogates. Other factors favoring radical surgery are smaller size, desire to preserve fertility, and absence of other comorbidities that escalate the risk of surgery. Factors that favor radiotherapy are the presence of indicators that would result in postoperative radiotherapy if surgery were the primary therapy. These include larger size, extensive LVSI, suspicious findings on preoperative imaging, high-risk histologic subtypes, and deep stromal invasion on imaging or examination that increases the risk of close margins.

The decision regarding radical surgery or radiotherapy should be made with the active involvement of the woman, the gynecologic oncologist, and the radiation oncologist. Both modalities are associated with the potential for significant short- and long-term complications. Some complications, such as bladder atony, food intolerance, and loss of sexual function, are not easy to measure and can persist for years after treatment. Long-term survival data are similar for well-selected patient populations. Some data suggest more long-term patient satisfaction with outcomes related to surgery than radiotherapy.

**Most gynecologic oncologists and radiation oncologists recommend concurrent chemoradiation for patients with stage IB3 cervical cancer. Reports demonstrate that up to 80% of patients with tumor size greater than 4 cm who have undergone a radical hysterectomy have clear indications for postoperative radiotherapy.** Our experience is that postoperative radiotherapy results in greater toxicity than treatment with the cervix intact. The counterargument is that radical hysterectomy obviates the need for high-dose brachytherapy, which is associated with the most severe and difficult to manage complications, notably pelvic fistulas. A number of innovations in treatment targeting techniques appear to be having a beneficial impact on reduction of posttreatment fistulas. Concurrent chemoradiation is our primary recommendation for stage IB3 patients and is discussed later in this chapter.

## Operative Therapy: Radical Hysterectomy and Pelvic Node Dissection

Radical hysterectomy and bilateral pelvic lymphadenectomy are effective for the treatment of stage IB1 to IB2 and some early stage IIA1 cancers. It is important that the surgery removes the same volume of tissue that has received tumoricidal doses of radiation in patients for whom radiation is the sole therapy. The amount of tissue removed, particularly in the paracervical and parametrial areas near the ureter, depends on the extent and location of the tumor. Piver and colleagues defined five classes to describe the extent of the operation (Piver, 1974). Class I guarantees the removal of the entire cervix and uterus. The ureter is not disturbed from its bed. In many cases this is described as an extrafascial hysterectomy, the type used after preoperative radiation for treatment of a barrel-shaped cervix (discussed later). A class II operation (Fig. 31.10) removes more paracervical tissue than class I; the ureters are retracted laterally but are not dissected from their attachments distal to the uterine artery, and the uterosacral ligaments are ligated approximately halfway between the uterus and rectum. The operation, which is usually performed with pelvic lymphadenectomy and is often termed a *modified radical hysterectomy*, is useful to treat small microscopic carcinomas of the cervix. Magrina and colleagues used modified radical hysterectomy primarily for tumors smaller than 2 cm (median, 1.1 cm), with a 5-year survival of 96% (Magrina, 1999). This procedure may occasionally be used to treat small, central cervical recurrences of carcinoma that are diagnosed after radiation therapy of the primary tumor. For a class III operation, the uterine artery is ligated at its origin from the anterior division of the hypogastric artery and the uterosacral ligaments are ligated deep in the pelvis near the rectum (see Fig. 31.10). This operation is usually termed a *radical hysterectomy* (Meigs-Wertheim hysterectomy) and is performed for stage IB2 and, rarely, for stage IIA carcinomas of the cervix.

Class IV and V operations are infrequently performed. A class IV procedure involves a complete dissection of the ureter from its bed and sacrifice of the superior vesical artery. A class V operation involves resection of the distal ureter, bladder, or both, with reimplantation of the ureter into the bladder (ureteroneocystostomy). Both are designed to remove small, central recurrent disease and would be attempted to avoid an anterior exenteration (see later). Extensive data are not available, but the latter two procedures appear to have high complication rates.

Other classification systems for radical hysterectomy exist. Querleu and Morrow described a classification that is principally based on the lateral extent of resection (four types, A through D) with subtypes that address nerve preservation and paracervical lymphadenectomy (Querleu, 2008). Within this classification, four levels of lymph node dissection (1 to 4) are also defined according to arterial anatomy and overall radicality of the procedure.

Preoperative preparation for a woman who is to undergo a radical hysterectomy includes the same basic considerations for anyone undergoing a major operative procedure. Graduated compression, below-the-knee leg stockings, and perioperative prophylactic doses of heparin or other low-molecular-weight heparin formulations are used to reduce the risk of thromboembolism. Prophylactic antibiotics prior to incision are also recommended. During the course of the operation, care is taken not to grasp the ureters with instruments such as forceps to avoid damaging the periureteral capillary blood supply.

An important complication of pelvic lymphadenectomy is lymphocyst formation. Most gynecologic oncologists have abandoned the use of closed suction drains in patients undergoing radical hysterectomy, instead leaving the pelvic peritoneum open to allow lymph fluid to drain internally in the peritoneal cavity. Sentinel lymph node mapping and biopsies increasingly are replacing full lymphadenectomy.

Ovarian function may be preserved in younger patients if there is little likelihood of postoperative radiation. If intraoperative findings suggest that radiotherapy will be given postoperatively, the ovaries may be transposed superior and lateral to preserve their function. This technique has some liabilities, including early loss of ovarian function and abdominal pain from ovarian cysts.

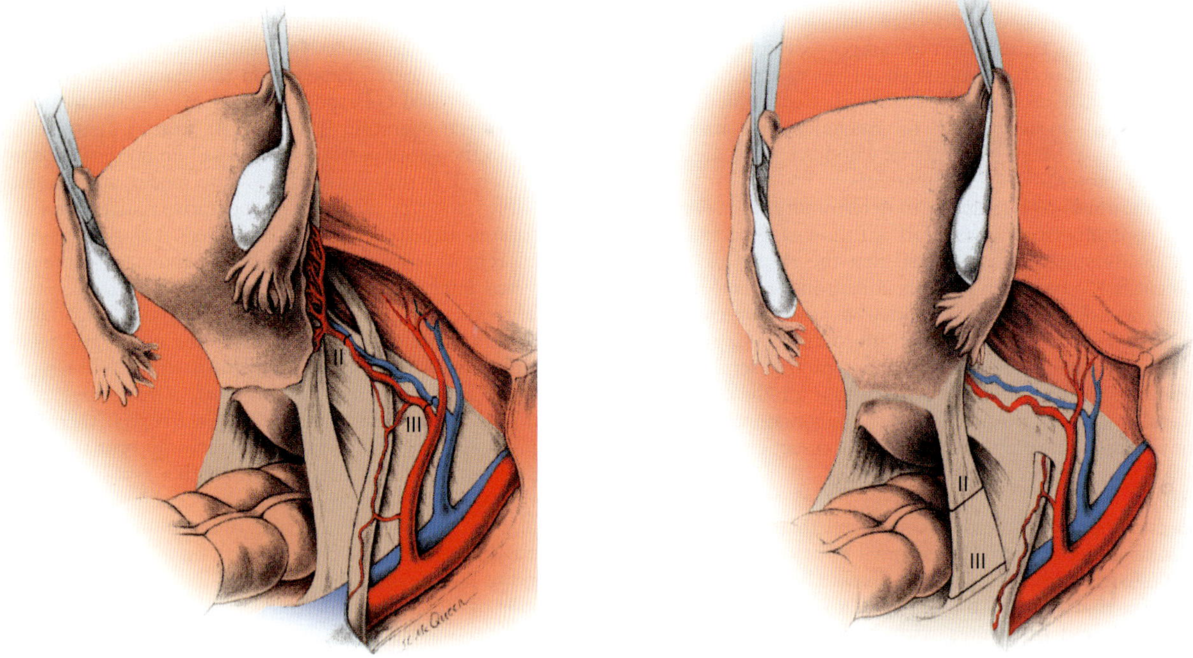


**Fig. 31.10** Classes I and II radical hysterectomy with points of dissection shown (see text).

In clinical patients with stage I disease treated by radical hysterectomy and node dissection, the results obtained are related primarily to the status of the pelvic nodes and the surgical resection margins around the primary tumor (ideally, >1 cm). If the pelvic nodes are free of tumor, the 5-year survival rate can be expected to exceed 90%, whereas if the nodes are found to contain tumor (surgical stage IIIC), the 5-year survival rate drops to 45% to 50%. If the woman is found to have extensive spread of gross disease to the pelvic nodes, the studies of Potter and coworkers (Potter, 1990) have suggested that it is preferable to cease the operation and complete radiation therapy to improve pelvic control of tumor; however, Hacker and associates reported an estimated 5-year survival of 80% for 34 patients whose tumor-positive pelvic or paraaortic nodes were resected and the areas subsequently radiated (Hacker, 1995). In a GOG study, Sedlis and coworkers evaluated disease-free survival for patients treated with radical hysterectomy who had negative lymph nodes and surgical margins but with intermediate risk factors, including more than one-third stromal invasion, capillary lymphatic space involvement, adenocarcinoma, and large tumor diameter by randomly allocating patients to pelvic radiotherapy or observation (Sedlis, 1999). Survival was improved in those who received postoperative pelvic radiation; however, there were radiation complications, including bowel obstruction and death.

Nerve-sparing radical hysterectomy is an innovation described by Hockel and others (Hockel, 2003). Bladder atony is a difficult-to-study outcome of radical hysterectomy. The incidence of complete bladder atony requiring self-catheterization or nerve stimulators is low, but milder forms are common. The severity of bladder atony is directly related to the trauma inflicted on the hypogastric nerves, which may be traumatized during radical hysterectomy. The impact of the nerve-sparing approach on sexual function is not known.

### Fertility-Sparing Surgery

Dargent developed a combined laparoscopic and vaginal technique for removal of the pelvic lymph nodes, cervix, parametrium, and upper vagina (Dargent, 1995). Dargent trained gynecologic oncologists from around the world to perform radical vaginal trachelectomy and laparoscopic pelvic lymphadenectomy (Dargent, 1995). Long-term outcomes reported by Plante, Diaz, and others have confirmed that in well-selected patients, oncologic outcomes are identical to radical hysterectomy outcomes (Plante, 2005; Diaz, 2008). First-trimester pregnancy loss rates are approximately the same for radical trachelectomy patients as for the general population. Second-trimester pregnancy loss is approximately doubled in trachelectomy patients compared with the general population, presumably because of the loss of cervical stroma. Typically a permanent cerclage is placed at the time of radical trachelectomy. Approximately two-thirds of patients have a successful pregnancy after radical trachelectomy.

When fertility-sparing surgery was first described, the assumption was that it would be offered to only a small proportion of patients. From a cohort of more than 400 patients who underwent radical hysterectomy, Sonoda and colleagues determined that approximately 50% of those younger than 40 years had low-risk histologic types and tumor size smaller than 2 cm, making them candidates for radical trachelectomy (Sonoda, 2004).

In spite of the contribution of radical vaginal surgery to fertility preservation, the technique has been difficult for gynecologic oncologists in the United States to master. Vaginal surgical skills are diminishing and there are no other indications for radical vaginal surgery. American gynecologic oncologists, unlike their counterparts in Canada and Europe, appear to have been discouraged by the long learning curve and have not invested the time to master the approach. Gynecologic oncologists in the United States have described abdominal radical trachelectomy as an alternative to the vaginal approach. Although smaller numbers have been published, it is anticipated that oncologic and fertility outcomes will be similar to the laparoscopic-vaginal approach.

Patient selection is important when considering fertility-sparing surgery. Preoperative pelvic MRI is recommended for all patients with a visible lesion. Patients should have a desire to preserve fertility, no evidence of metastatic disease to lymph nodes or distant metastases, age younger than 45, and stage IAI with LVSI, IA2, or IB1 disease (lesion size ≤2 cm) with limited endocervical extension assessed by colposcopy and MRI.

### Minimally Invasive Surgery

Minimally invasive techniques for treatment of cervical cancer are attractive for several reasons. Minimally invasive surgery (MIS) is associated with shorter length of stay, less pain, few postoperative infections, fewer thromboembolic complications, and reduced blood loss compared with abdominal procedures.

Minimally invasive radical surgery has become more popular over time, with minimally invasive radial hysterectomies increasing from 2% in 2006 to 33% in 2010 (Wright, 2012). For gynecologic oncologists in practice, the long learning curve associated with laparoscopy has been an impediment to advancement. **The most recent minimally invasive technique, robotic laparoscopic surgery, offers new advantages and increased the use of MIS for radical hysterectomies; however, data have demonstrated that patients who had a radical hysterectomy by a minimally invasive approach (laparoscopic or radical) have a higher risk of recurrence and death compared with those who had an open abdominal radical hysterectomy (Melamed, 2018; Ramirez, 2018).** An international randomized trial reported that disease-free survival at 4.5 years was 86% in the MIS arm compared with 96.5% with open surgery. The 3-year overall survival rates were also lower in the minimally invasive group (93.8% vs. 99.0%) (Ramirez, 2018).

### Sentinel Node Biopsy

Cervical cancer, like most solid tumors, spreads primarily lymphatically. Surgical management of solid tumors, as pioneered more than 100 years ago by Halsted, is based on the resection of all regional lymph nodes and lymphatic channels connecting the lymph nodes to the primary tumor. Implicit in this approach is that all regional lymph nodes have the same risk of containing metastatic disease. Morton, working in patients with cutaneous melanoma, demonstrated that there are sentinel lymph nodes that are the first nodes to receive lymphatic drainage from the primary tumor and are therefore the first site of metastasis (Morton, 2001). Experience with thousands of patients with melanoma and breast cancer has validated this concept, which has been successfully extended to other disease sites, notably vulvar cancer.

**Cervical cancer is an excellent target for the sentinel lymph node concept because the tumor is easy to inject and the regional lymph nodes can be reached through an incision.** Lymphatic drainage of the cervix is complex; however, most sentinel lymph nodes of the cervix are found along the external iliac artery or vein, obturator space, or parametrium. A number of investigators have reported their experience with sentinel lymph node biopsy in patients undergoing radical hysterectomy. In one series of 188 patients, the sensitivity of sentinel lymph node mapping in cervical cancer was calculated to be 96.4%, with a negative predictive value of 99.3% and a 3.6% false-negative rate (Salvo, 2017). Various protocols have been used to perform sentinel lymph node mapping in cervical cancer. Common mapping strategies use technetium-99m, blue dyes (methylene blue, isosulfan blue, patent blue), and, more recently, indocyanine green (ICG).

### Surgical Complications

After radical hysterectomy, many patients experience long-term complications. Montz and associates noted a 5% frequency of small bowel obstruction, which increases to 20% if radiation is used postoperatively (Montz, 1994). Fistulas from the urinary tract, particularly ureterovaginal fistulas, have been reported to occur in approximately 1% of cases. The low rate appears to result from the administration of antibiotics, prevention of retroperitoneal serosanguineous collections, and avoidance of direct manipulation of the ureter to avoid injury to the periureteral blood supply. Most gynecologic oncologists do not reperitonealize the pelvis, which allows direct drainage of lymphatic fluid to the peritoneal cavity, where it is reabsorbed.

Many women suffer postoperative bladder dysfunction. In part, this appears to be caused by disruption of the sympathetic nerve supply to the bladder; however, the dysfunction may be temporary. Low and associates noted an increase in bladder pressure with a decrease in urethral pressure after radical hysterectomy (Low, 1981). There was reduced bladder compliance with detrusor instability. The bladder can develop hypotonicity, and overdistention can then become a problem. If overdistention of the bladder and infection are avoided, progressive improvement of bladder function usually occurs. Forney correlated the degree of bladder dysfunction after radical hysterectomy with the extent of resection of the cardinal ligament (Forney, 1980). Those who had a complete resection of cardinal ligaments could void satisfactorily at an average of 51 days compared with 20 days for those with only partial resection of the ligaments. All patients experienced a decrease in bladder sensation. In a few patients the decrease in bladder sensation can be permanent. For patients in whom it is temporary, recovery usually occurs after continuous drainage of the bladder with an indwelling catheter. Westby and Asmussen observed that by 1 year after surgery a slight decrease in urethral pressure persists but that the decrease is not as great as that noted immediately after the operation (Westby, 1985). After 1 year, the postoperative changes and bladder function usually recover. Newer nerve-sparing surgical techniques where the uterosacral ligament is transected after separation of the hypogastric nerve and preservation of the bladder branches of the pelvic plexus have been associated with improved bladder function without compromising oncologic outcomes and survival.

In a 1999 study from Sweden, Bergmark and coworkers noted compromised sexual activity, decreased lubrication, and shortened vaginas in women treated for cervical cancer by surgery or radiation (Bergmark, 1999). During the consent process, patients should be informed regarding the potential impact of radical hysterectomy on their sexual function.

Lymphedema is another complication of radical pelvic surgery that can affect quality of life. The areas most affected are the mons, lower abdomen, and upper thighs. Lymphedema massage may help reduce this problem, but treatment options are limited and of only modest effectiveness.

### Outcomes After Surgical Treatment

Reported 5-year survival rates for women with stage IB cervical cancer treated with radical hysterectomy and pelvic lymphadenectomy are approximately 80% to 90%. **Patients with positive or close margins or positive lymph nodes have the highest risk of recurrence and poor outcome.** In large prospective studies, 3-year disease-specific survival rates of 85.6% in patients with negative nodes and 50% to 74% in patients with positive nodes were reported. A randomized study found that postoperative chemoradiation improves survival in patients with positive lymph nodes and positive surgical margins (Peters, 1999).

## Radiation Treatment

Most patients with carcinoma of the cervix are treated by radiation. The principles of external megavoltage treatment (teletherapy) and local implants (brachytherapy) are reviewed in Chapter 28. External beam radiation is administered in fractions, usually 180 cGy/day, 5 days a week, to destroy the tumor without causing permanent damage to normal tissues. This delivers uniform doses to the entire pelvis, including the regional pelvic nodes. The local implant delivers its highest energy locally to the cervix, surface of the vagina, and paravaginal and paracervical tissues. The radiation from the implant diminishes according to the inverse square law. The uterus and cervix serve as receptacles for arranging and holding the intracavitary applicator stem (tandem) and accompanying vaginal applicators (ovoids or ring) in a fixed and optimal position for delivering the desired radiation dosimetry. Usually the tandem and ovoids or a tandem and ring are inserted and a pack is placed into the vagina to stabilize the apparatus and increase the distance from the mucosa of the bladder and rectum. After the position of the applicator has been confirmed to be satisfactory by imaging, the radioactive source, such as cesium-137 or iridium-192, is inserted (afterloading technique). Other types of applicators are available, but the principle of delivering intense radiation to the cervix and paracervical areas is the same. The goal is to increase the total dose of radiation to the maximum allowable to achieve tumor control without introducing a major risk of complications and injury to adjacent normal tissue. The specific protocols followed in various treatment centers differ; individualization for specific patients is often needed depending on the stage and size of the cervical tumor as well as the patient's local anatomy. In general, external therapy is given first to treat the regional pelvic nodes and shrink the central tumor mass, which then is more amenable for a local implant. In some patients, external therapy can lead to excessive shrinkage of the vaginal apex, making safe, effective implantation of local radiation sources difficult. This can be a problem, particularly in older or postmenopausal patients. Occasionally, in those patients, the implantation is done first, especially for smaller stage I tumors. Intraoperative ultrasounds may be helpful especially in difficult cases for optimal implant positioning. In some cases the central pelvis is shielded during external radiation therapy to allow for subsequent higher doses from the implant. Occasionally, interstitial therapy in the form of needles implanted into the area of the tumor is needed to achieve effective local tumor control. Although criteria differ, patients with stage III disease or poor vaginal anatomy are most often considered candidates for interstitial brachytherapy.

Intracavitary radiation therapy may be delivered at either a low-dose rate or a high-dose rate. The advantage of high-dose-rate brachytherapy is that it is given on an outpatient basis and can be done with 3 to 4 hours. High-dose-rate brachytherapy and low-dose-rate brachytherapy have similar survival and toxicity and high-dose-rate brachytherapy has become the most common type of brachytherapy available throughout the world. The number of fractions varies from two to five; the most common one in the United States is 5.5 Gy to 6 Gy to point A in five fractions. Brachytherapy in combination with external beam should be used in the treatment of locally advance cervical cancer whenever feasible because data reveal that there is an increase in survival with the use of brachytherapy compared with any other modality (Gill, 2014; Han, 2013).

In calculating the doses of radiation, two reference points, A and B, are used (Fig. 31.11). Point A is 2 cm above the external os and 2 cm lateral to the cervical canal. Point B is 5 cm lateral to the cervical canal and 3 cm lateral to point A, which places point B in the vicinity of the lateral pelvic wall (see Fig. 31.11). The total dose administered depends on tumor stage but, in general, at the pelvic wall, it is in the range of 50 to 65 Gy, with the higher doses used for high-stage disease. At point A, it varies, but approximately 80 Gy is given for small IB1 lesions and doses higher than 85 Gy for larger lesions. The normal cervix is particularly resistant to radiation and can tolerate doses as high as 200 to 250 Gy over 2 months, whereas the adjacent bladder and, in particular, the rectum are much more sensitive, and their exposure in general should be limited at the point of maximal radiation to 80 Gy to the bladder and 70 Gy to the rectum, with overall average doses in the range of 65 to 70 Gy. The small bowel can be damaged at doses greater than 45 to 50 Gy, especially if adhesions limit intestinal mobility and a large volume is treated.

There has been increased interest in the use of image-based three-dimensional treatment planning for intracavitary and interstitial brachytherapy. Among the many potential advantages of image-based planning are its ability to provide a better sense of the actual doses delivered to critical structures and possibly a more solid basis for comparisons among institutions. Studies have used CT- and MRI-based images; at present, a large multi-institutional study of image-based brachytherapy is ongoing in Europe and worldwide.

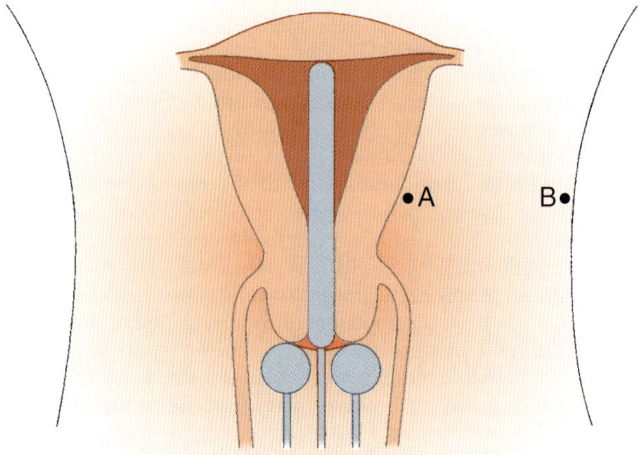

**Fig. 31.11** Points A and B with central stem (tandem) and two ovoids in place.

### Outcomes

Radical radiation therapy achieves excellent survival and pelvic disease control rates in patients with stage IB or IIA cervical cancer. Eifel and associates reported 5-year disease-specific survival of 90%, 86%, and 67% in patients with stage IB tumors with cervical diameters less than 4 cm, 4 to 4.9 cm, and larger than 5 cm, respectively (Eifel, 1994). In 1961, a report suggested that adjuvant hysterectomy improved local control in patients with stage IB disease with tumors larger than 6 cm; however, several studies since then have shown no improvement in local control but an increase in toxicity. One of these studies was a large GOG study in which patients were randomly allocated to a trial of radiation, with or without extrafascial hysterectomy; results showed no difference in survival or local control but a higher complication rate (Keys, 1999). Therefore there is no clear evidence that adjuvant hysterectomy improves outcome in patients with early-stage disease and large tumor size. The 5-year survival for patients with stage IIA disease is similar to that for patients with stage IB disease. For patients with more advanced disease, 5-year survival rates of 65% to 75%, 35% to 50%, and 15% to 20% have been reported for stages IIB, IIIB, and IV tumors, respectively. The addition of chemotherapy has further improved local control and survival for stage IB2 and higher (discussed later).

### Chemoradiation

**In 1999, prospective randomized trials involving concurrent cisplatin-containing chemotherapy to standard radiotherapy showed such improved survival that the trials were preliminarily halted to release the results, which changed clinical practice. In** one of the studies by GOG, Rose and colleagues treated patients with advanced squamous cell, adenosquamous, or adenocarcinoma of the cervix (stages IIB, III, or IVA) (Rose, 1999). The patients received external radiation therapy (40.8 to 51 Gy) followed by one or two brachytherapy implants. The patients were randomly assigned to receive one of three concomitant chemotherapy regimens: hydroxyurea; cisplatin, 5-fluorouracil, and hydroxyurea; or cisplatin alone. The best results were obtained with the cisplatin-containing regimens, with the least complications seen with weekly cisplatin (40 $mg/m^2$) alone. Progression-free survival at 24 months was an impressive 67% for this very high-risk group of patients.

In another collaborative trial, Keys and associates studied 369 women with bulky stage IB carcinoma (>4 cm) in diameter (Keys, 1999). They were randomly assigned to receive radiation alone or with concomitant weekly cisplatin (40 $mg/m^2$). Adjuvant extrafascial hysterectomy was performed 3 to 6 weeks after conclusion of the chemoradiation treatments. The therapeutic results were markedly better in the chemoradiation group, with a 3-year 83% disease-free survival compared with 74% in the radiation group alone ($P$ = .008), and they noted no added benefit with the addition of extrafascial hysterectomy. At the same time, the Radiation Therapy Oncology Group also conducted a trial comparing paraaortic–pelvic radiation therapy with concurrent chemotherapy and pelvic radiation in patients with stages IB to IVA tumors and also found a significant improvement in outcome for all stages of disease with concurrent chemotherapy compared with radiation therapy alone (Eifel, 2004). Another trial studied concurrent chemotherapy with radiation therapy in patients who had undergone a radical hysterectomy for cervical cancer and were found to have pelvic lymph node metastases, positive margins, or parametrial involvement. In this trial, patients who received chemoradiation had a better disease-free survival rate than patients who received radiation therapy alone (Peters, 1999).

Only one large randomized trial has failed to demonstrate a significant advantage from concurrent cisplatin-based chemotherapy in cervical cancer patients. This trial, in Canada, was the smallest of six trials of concurrent cisplatin and radiation therapy (Pearcey, 2002).

In North America, the primary focus has been on cisplatin-based chemotherapy regimens, but international trials have evaluated others. In a large trial from Thailand, patients were randomly allocated to one of four arms: radiation therapy alone, radiation therapy with concurrent mitomycin and oral fluorouracil, radiation therapy with adjuvant fluorouracil, or radiation with concurrent and adjuvant chemotherapy (Lorvidhaya, 2003). Patients in the two treatment groups that included concurrent chemotherapy had higher disease-free survival rates and lower rates of local recurrence than patients in the other two groups. More recently, Dueños-Gonzales published a trial comparing cisplatin–radiation therapy to cisplatin–gemcitabine–radiation therapy followed by two courses of cisplatin-gemcitabine (Dueñas-Gonzales, 2011). Patients who received gemcitabine had better overall survival and disease-free survival compared with patients who did not.

**A meta-analysis of trials that included a comparison of chemotherapy plus radiation to radiation therapy alone found a 6% improvement in 5-year survival with chemoradiotherapy (Chemoradiotherapy for Cervical Cancer Meta-Analysis Collaboration, 2008).** A larger survival benefit was seen for the two trials in which chemotherapy was administered after chemoradiotherapy. There was a significant survival benefit for patients in the group of trials that used platinum-based and non–platinum-based chemoradiotherapy, but no evidence of a difference in the size of the benefit by radiotherapy or chemotherapy dose or scheduling was seen. Chemoradiotherapy also reduced local and distant recurrence and progression and improved disease-free survival.

### Neoadjuvant Chemotherapy

Neoadjuvant chemotherapy may be given before surgery or before radical radiation therapy. Advantages of chemotherapy before surgery include the potential for reducing tumor volume, increasing resectability, and helping to control micrometastatic disease. Neoadjuvant chemotherapy may also have the potential to provide a viable alternative when access to radiotherapy is poor or if there are unavoidable delays in delivering radiotherapeutic treatment. In one study by Sardi and coworkers, 205 patients with stage IB1 were randomly allocated to neoadjuvant chemotherapy plus radical hysterectomy or to radical hysterectomy alone (Sardi, 1993). They reported that the patients who received neoadjuvant chemotherapy had more resectable tumors and better overall survival than patients who did not receive neoadjuvant chemotherapy. In the United States, the GOG closed a trial with 258 patients with stage IB2 cervical tumors who were randomly assigned to neoadjuvant chemotherapy plus radical hysterectomy or to radical hysterectomy alone. They found no difference in the two arms in the rate of surgery performed (79% chemotherapy plus surgery vs. 54% surgery) or in the surgical-pathologic findings, specifically in progression-free survival (56% chemotherapy plus surgery vs. 54% surgery) and overall survival (63% chemotherapy plus surgery vs. 61% surgery) at 5 years. A meta-analysis of six randomized trials of neoadjuvant chemotherapy plus surgery compared with surgery alone found that although progression-free survival was improved with neoadjuvant chemotherapy, there was no significant survival benefit, and distant recurrence and rates of resection only tended to favor the neoadjuvant chemotherapy (Rydzewska, 2010). The authors observed heterogeneity in the trials but concluded that it remains unclear whether neoadjuvant chemotherapy consistently offers a benefit over surgery alone for women with early stage or locally advanced cervical cancer. In the United States, neoadjuvant chemotherapy is rarely used; however, internationally there is much interest in using neoadjuvant chemotherapy, especially in countries in which radiotherapy is not easily accessible.

The other use of neoadjuvant chemotherapy is before radiation therapy. Seven randomized trials have studied neoadjuvant chemotherapy plus radiation therapy compared with radical radiation therapy alone. Other randomized trials have studied neoadjuvant chemotherapy plus surgery compared with radical radiation therapy in locally advanced cervical cancer. A meta-analysis published in 2004 evaluated 21 of these trials (NACCCMA Collaboration, 2004); however, all the trials that were included in this analysis were carried out before 1999, when the concurrent chemotherapies were all published. Much heterogeneity was found in the trials, which made them difficult to analyze; however, it was concluded that the timing and dose intensity of cisplatin-based neoadjuvant chemotherapy appeared to have an important impact on whether it benefited women with locally advanced cervical cancer; further exploration was recommended.

Data from two newer studies have been presented and may help with the question of neoadjuvant chemotherapy. The EORTC study was presented at the 2019 meeting of the American Society of Clinical Oncology (ASCO); in this study, patients with stage IB2-IIB cervical cancer were randomly allocated to neoadjuvant chemotherapy followed by surgery or definitive chemotherapy and radiation therapy. Forty percent of the patients in the surgery arm received postoperative radiation therapy. There was no statistical difference between the two arms, with a 5-year overall survival of 72% in the surgery arm and 75% in the chemotherapy and radiation arm (Kenter et al., 2019). The second study, from India (Gupta, 2018), also randomly allocated patients with stage IB2-IIB cervical cancer to neoadjuvant chemotherapy followed by surgery or definitive chemotherapy and radiation therapy. A total of 639 patients were included; researchers reported was a 7% improvement in disease-free survival with definitive chemotherapy and radiation therapy compared with neoadjuvant chemotherapy and surgery.

**Paraaortic Node Involvement**

Numerous small series of patients having documented paraaortic node involvement have demonstrated that some patients have long-term disease-free survival. Patients with microscopic involvement have a better survival duration than those with gross involvement; however, even patients with gross involvement have a 15% to 20% survival rate with aggressive management. Laparoscopy and laparotomy using the extraperitoneal approach allow the removal of positive nodes and sampling of other paraaortic nodes, which may enhance control with radiation therapy and help design the treatment field.

Patients with paraaortic lymph node involvement can be treated effectively with extended-field radiation. The superior boundary of the extended field is usually placed at the T12 vertebral body to cover the paraaortic nodes. Patients are treated with a combination of external beam radiation therapy and brachytherapy. The 5-year survival rates range from 25% to 50%. At present, the standard treatment for patients with positive paraaortic nodes is extended-field radiation therapy with concurrent weekly cisplatin.

**Radiation Complications**

**Complications after radiation therapy are related to dose, volume treated, and sensitivity of the various tissues receiving radiation.** The patient's habitus and presence of diseases that affect circulation, such as diabetes and high blood pressure, increase the risk, as does previous intraabdominal surgery. Acute minor complications, such as diarrhea and nausea, subside after radiation therapy is completed. Complications usually develop in 1 to 2 years but can occur as early as 6 months or as late as many years after radiation therapy has been completed. Scarring of normal tissues can lead to severe radiation fibrosis. The rare development of a second primary cancer after radiation for cervical cancer was reported by Kleinerman and associates from 13 population-based European registries (Kleinerman, 1995). With 30 years of survival, there was approximately a doubling of the risk of a new primary in an irradiated pelvic organ, including the ovaries and bladder, as well as the vagina and vulva.

The treatment of radiation complications depends on the symptoms and location of the complication. Vaginal or cervical ulcerations occasionally occur, and local treatment with topical antibiotics and estrogen creams is usually satisfactory. Postradiation cystitis may manifest itself as urinary frequency or dysuria. After infection has been ruled out, symptomatic treatment is undertaken with drugs such as antispasmodics or urinary analgesics (e.g., phenazopyridine, oxybutynin, tolterodine, solifenacin); these are prescribed until the symptoms clear. Occasionally, hemorrhagic cystitis develops, which may require hospitalization for continuous bladder irrigation or instillation of agents to control bleeding, such as silver nitrate or possibly fulguration of the bleeding points. In cases of hematuria, recurrent tumor should first be ruled out. Periureteral fibrosis can lead to ureteral obstruction and loss of kidney function. McIntyre and coworkers studied 1784 patients with stage IB carcinomas who were treated by radiation therapy and found 29 cases of ureteral stenoses, which increased from a frequency of 1% at 5 years to 2.5% at 20 years (McIntyre, 1995). Although tumor recurrence was the most common cause of early ureteral obstruction, radiation fibrosis can be a rare but occasionally fatal late complication.

Bowel complications tend to be more common than urinary complications. Proctosigmoiditis can lead to diarrhea, severe pain on defecation, or gastrointestinal bleeding. Conservative therapy with stool softeners and a low-roughage diet may suffice; occasionally, local corticosteroids (e.g., cortisone enema) are of assistance. Fistulas or rectal ulcerations occasionally occur in the area adjacent to the tip of the cervix, which is also the area maximally radiated during local vaginocervical implantation. If a fistula, ulceration, or severe bleeding and pain develops, a diverting colostomy is required. Serious small bowel complications may occur, leading to obstruction, fistula formation, or necrosis. The use of parenteral nutrition and intravenous hyperalimentation are excellent measures to help deal with these problems. Follow-up studies by Klee and colleagues have shown that bladder and bowel symptoms tend to be chronic in some patients, but long-term fatigue is also reported. In most patients it regresses in a few months (Klee, 2000).

Compromise of sexual function because of inelastic vaginal walls and decreased use was noted in studies by Bergmark and associates (Bergmark, 1999). In a randomized trial of experimental psychoeducational intervention involving regular vaginal dilation, Robinson and coworkers noted a reduced fear of sexual activity posttreatment in the experimental group (Robinson, 1999).

## Special Considerations

### Cervical Stump Tumors

Some patients undergo supracervical hysterectomy for nonmalignant disease. Carcinomas that subsequently develop in the cervical stump pose special problems because of the shortness of the cervical canal and absence of the uterus, both of which curtail the effective use of brachytherapy, especially insertion of an intracervical tandem. There is also the risk that bowel adhesions to the apex of the vagina and cervix will increase the chances of radiation complications; a pretherapy barium study of the small and large bowel may be helpful to identify loops that adhere to the cervical apex. For patients with small stage IB tumors, an operative approach similar to radical hysterectomy can be considered; however, most patients are treated with radiation. External treatment is emphasized because of the difficulty of an optimal intracavitary implant. A transvaginal cone may also be used to supplement external pelvic therapy. Effective treatment of cervical stump carcinoma can be achieved, resulting in overall 5-year survival rates ranging from 45% to 60%; however, because of the previous supracervical hysterectomy, there is an increased risk of complications compared with patients treated with a supracervical hysterectomy. Results of chemoradiation studies of these tumors are not available but, based on data already presented, radiation, combined with weekly cisplatin, appears to be optimal.

### Carcinoma of the Cervix Inadvertently Removed at Simple Hysterectomy

Unfortunately, the situation occasionally arises in which a woman undergoes a simple total hysterectomy and an invasive carcinoma of the cervix is found after operation. Patients with unsuspected invasive cervical carcinoma detected after simple hysterectomy have been classified into five groups according to the amount of disease and presentation: (1) microinvasive cancer, (2) tumor confined to the cervix with negative surgical margins, (3) positive surgical margins but no gross residual tumor, (4) gross residual tumor by clinical examination documented by biopsy, and (5) patients referred for treatment more than 6 months after hysterectomy (usually for recurrent disease).

The treatment plan is based on the amount of residual disease. Sometimes the surgeon can subsequently perform a radical operation, removing the tissues that would normally be removed at radical hysterectomy, including the regional pelvic nodes, and this approach particularly has been used in younger patients, especially those with small tumors; however, most women are usually treated with some sort of radiation therapy. Patients with minimal or no known residual disease at most require brachytherapy to the vaginal apex; patients with gross disease at the specimen margin require full-intensity therapy. Patients with minimal or no gross residual disease (groups 1 to 3) have excellent 5-year survival rates (59% to 79%), whereas rates for patients with gross residual disease (groups 4 and 5) are poorer (in the range of only 41%).

### Carcinoma of the Cervix in Pregnancy

Rarely an invasive carcinoma of the cervix is discovered in a pregnant woman. Within each stage, survival statistics are similar in pregnant and nonpregnant women. A concern has been that the delivery of a fetus through a cervix replaced by carcinoma might worsen the prognosis because of tumor dissemination, but there is no clear evidence to indicate that the birth process causes tumor dissemination; however, tumor recurrence in episiotomy sites after vaginal delivery has been reported in some studies. The major risk to the patient of delivery through a cervix containing invasive carcinoma is that of hemorrhage as a result of tearing of the tumor during cervical dilation and delivery.

A problem arising in pregnancy is whether a woman with an abnormal cytologic smear has intraepithelial neoplasia or invasive cancer. In general, if the cytologic and histologic findings of colposcopically directed biopsies are comparable and suggest intraepithelial neoplasia or carcinoma in situ, the woman is observed and delivered, with final evaluation and therapy completed approximately 6 weeks after delivery. Even if there is a question of microinvasion, a woman so diagnosed in the last trimester of pregnancy is usually followed and evaluated further after delivery. Cervical conization during pregnancy can lead to severe complications, particularly hemorrhage and loss of the fetus. If it is necessary to perform a conization or preferably a wedge resection of the cervix during pregnancy, it is probably best to perform this procedure during the second trimester, when the risks of fetal loss and hemorrhage are minimal. For patients in whom invasive cancer is diagnosed, a therapeutic plan must be developed to deliver appropriate care, with regard also for the outcome of the pregnancy.

The therapy of carcinoma during pregnancy is influenced by the stage of the disease, time in pregnancy when the cancer is diagnosed, and beliefs and desires of the woman in terms of initiating therapy that can terminate the pregnancy, as opposed to postponing therapy until fetal viability is achieved. If carcinoma is diagnosed in the first trimester or early in the second trimester (before 20 weeks), treatment may be undertaken immediately because of the concern that a delay could lead to tumor progression or spread. If the woman has a resectable tumor (stage IB or early IIA), effective treatment consists of radical hysterectomy and node dissection (class III). This procedure usually can be carried out without difficulty on a pregnant woman. Increased uterine motility and edema of the pelvic tissue planes help simplify the procedure for the experienced surgeon, but pregnancy does increase the risk of blood loss. For higher-stage tumors, therapy begins with external beam radiation (teletherapy), and, usually in 4 to 6 weeks, this leads to spontaneous abortion. The dose of external therapy prescribed varies depending on the stage of the tumor, but approximately 40 to 50 Gy is given. Although the results of a published series are not available, it would appear preferable to augment the radiation with weekly cisplatin because the pregnancy in this case would be terminated. After abortion, the uterus involutes and an implant (brachytherapy) is placed. If the pregnancy does not spontaneously abort, dilation and curettage, prostaglandin-assisted delivery, or, rarely, hysterotomy may be necessary to empty the uterus before brachytherapy. Alternatively, if the initial tumor was small and has completely regressed, an extrafascial hysterectomy or modified radical hysterectomy may be performed.

For patients beyond the 20th week of gestation, therapy is often delayed until fetal viability. The health and maturity of the fetus are determined by appropriate ultrasound studies and amniotic fluid analysis to ensure fetal lung maturity. Delivery is usually accomplished by cesarean section; after this, therapy is completed by surgery or radiation with the usual considerations of tumor stage and size. Overall, treatment results in pregnant patients are similar to those in nonpregnant patients, stage for stage. It should be noted that many published studies dealing with carcinoma of the cervix in pregnancy include cases treated as long as 1 year postpartum, which assumes that the carcinoma was present during pregnancy. Hacker and coworkers summarized the results of 1249 cases reported in various series in the literature (Hacker, 1982). Overall, a 5-year survival rate of 49.2% was recorded for pregnant patients compared with 51% for nonpregnant patients treated during the same period. Their statistics included not only patients treated during pregnancy but also those treated up to 6 months after delivery, and the postpartum group had the poorest survival statistics. Survival was most closely related to stage, as expected, and those diagnosed during the first trimester had a better prognosis than those diagnosed during the third trimester.

## RECURRENCE

Approximately one-third of patients treated for cancer of the cervix will experience tumor recurrence, which is defined as the reappearance of tumor 6 months or more after therapy. Metastases can occur anywhere, but most are in the pelvis—centrally in the vagina or cervix or laterally near the pelvic walls—or, less commonly, distally in the periaortic nodes, lung, liver, or bone. It should be noted that liver, lung, and distal bone metastases outside the pelvis likely result from hematogenous tumor spread.

The symptoms caused by recurrence depend on the site and extent of metastatic disease. Vaginal discharge and abnormal bleeding are often symptoms of an early central pelvic recurrence. Malaise, loss of appetite, and general symptoms associated with widespread metastatic disease are late manifestations of recurrence. Lateral pelvic recurrences often have a retroperitoneal component, which can lead to sciatic nerve irritation and cause severe pain around the distribution of the sciatic nerve in back of the leg, as well as loss of muscle strength, causing the woman to walk with a limp. Unilateral leg edema often accompanies such metastases, or leg swelling may occur from fibrosis of lymphatics after surgery or radiation. In addition, tumor recurrence can also cause ureteral obstruction, leading to unilateral or bilateral compromise of kidney function. Low back pain commonly occurs.

Patients treated for carcinoma of the cervix are examined according to the same schedule as patients with other malignancies—every 3 months the first 2 years, every 6 months from years 3 to 5, and yearly thereafter. More frequent examinations are done if abnormal symptoms or signs develop. Examination consists of physical and pelvic examination at every visit and a Pap smear annually unless an abnormality is detected on the Pap smear. Generally a PET/CT is repeated 3 to 6 months after chemoradiation therapy and chest radiographs are done annually. Other imaging tests are only ordered if the patient has symptoms or there are other indications. Renal function tests may be indicated because ureteral fibrosis can occur more than 5 years after the completion of radiation therapy. Once recurrent disease is suspected, verification is usually obtained by biopsy of an accessible mass or CT-directed thin-needle aspiration, depending on the location of the tumor recurrence.

### Pelvic Recurrence

Approximately 50% of recurrences develop in the pelvis. In addition to clinical assessment and CT, a vaginal ultrasound scan is often useful to document pelvic recurrence. Recurrences of adenocarcinoma are less common in the pelvis and are more likely to be at distant sites, such as the lung or supraclavicular areas. For patients who were initially treated by surgery, radiation is usually prescribed for pelvic recurrences; approximately 45- to 50-Gy whole-pelvis irradiation is given. Supplemental interstitial or intracavitary radiation is also prescribed, depending on the size and location of recurrence in the pelvis. As noted, chemoradiation is preferable. Patients who have isolated central recurrences without pelvic wall fixation or regional metastasis can be cured in as many as 60% to 70% of cases. The prognosis is much poorer when the pelvic wall is involved; usually, 10% to 20% of patients survive 5 years after radiation therapy. For patients who were initially treated with radiation who have developed a localized pelvic recurrence, surgical eradication of the tumor should be considered because further effective radiation is not possible and limited surgical resection of the pelvic recurrence may not lead to a cure but will often cause severe complications of wound healing and intestinal and urinary fistulas; however, in rare, carefully selected patients initially treated with primary radiation therapy, radical hysterectomy may be a feasible alternative to exenterative surgery. Coleman and associates reported on 50 patients who underwent a radical hysterectomy for persistent or recurrent disease and found 5- and 10-year survival rates of 72% and 60%, respectively, with complication rates of 64% for severe complications and 42% for permanent complications (Coleman, 1994). The authors concluded that a radical hysterectomy was an alternative to exenteration in patients with small, centrally recurrent cervical cancer, but that it should be used only in carefully selected patients. If neither surgery nor radiation is a feasible alternative, palliative chemotherapy is considered.

### Pelvic Exenteration

Exenterative therapy for central pelvic tumor recurrence is an extensive operative procedure used only if the preoperative evaluation suggests that the patient's condition has the potential be cured by this procedure. Exenteration is not performed for palliation. Three types of procedures may be used. Anterior pelvic exenteration is removal of the bladder, uterus, cervix, and all or part of the vagina. Posterior pelvic exenteration is removal of the anus and rectum and resection of the uterus, cervix, and all or part of the vagina. Total exenteration removes all the pelvic contents. Shepherd and coworkers noted that patients older than 69 years, those who had a recurrence within 3 years, or those who had persistent disease or positive resection margins had a poorer prognosis for the procedure (Shepherd, 1994). Rarely, select patients with recurrence involving the sidewall that would not be standard candidates for total pelvic exenteration secondary to concern for a positive surgical margin may be considered for an extended pelvic resection, or the laterally extended endopelvic resection (LEER procedure) (Hockel, 2003, 2008). This procedure requires multidisciplinary advanced surgical support and carries high risk of surgical morbidity, but it may be contemplated as a possible curative option for very select patients.

Before an exenterative operation is undertaken, the patient is thoroughly evaluated for any evidence of disease spread outside the pelvis. At operation, abdominal exploration is carried out to ensure that the tumor is resectable. Biopsy specimens of any enlarged lymph nodes or suspicious areas outside the pelvis are taken, and frozen-section studies are performed, including evaluation of the operative margins. Usually, total exenteration is performed.

Several surgical innovations have expanded the reconstruction options. The introduction of continent urinary diversion provides an alternative incontinent urinary conduit. Generally the urinary stoma is located in the abdomen on the right side and the intestinal stoma on the left side. The use of intestinal stapling devices sometimes allows preservation of the rectal sphincter and anal function and avoids a permanent colostomy. Long-term complications are usually ureteral stricture or difficulty catheterizing the intestinal reservoir.

Continent conduits require the woman to catheterize the pouch every 4 hours, but no external appliance is required. Goldberg and colleagues reported long-term dissatisfaction among women with continent conduits, and in our practice we have done an increasing number of incontinent diversions (Goldberg, 2006).

Transverse rectus abdominis myocutaneous (TRAM) flaps have provided a welcomed alternative to gracilis flaps. TRAM flaps, even small ones, as described by Sood and associates, are reliable and provide patients with the option of intercourse (Sood, 2005).

Severe postoperative and intraoperative complications can occur with this extensive procedure, and perioperative mortalities as high as 10% to 20% were reported in the past. Infection and bowel obstruction are the major risks; however, current surgical techniques of preoperative bowel preparation, use of antibiotics, careful intraoperative fluid and volume monitoring, and use of parenteral nutrition have reduced the immediate postoperative mortality to less than 5%. The use of a peritoneal graft or an omental flap, created from the right or left side of the omentum and placed in the pelvis to protect the denuded pelvic floor, can help avoid bowel obstruction and reduce postoperative morbidity. Occasionally, gracilis myocutaneous grafts are used to create a new vagina and bring a new blood supply to the previously irradiated pelvis, which aids in wound healing. No patients with positive nodes in the operative specimen survived (Morley et al., 1989).

## Nonpelvic Recurrence

Recurrences outside of the pelvis can be treated with radiation, surgery, or chemotherapy. Localized recurrences in areas not previously irradiated are occasionally treated by radiation. Resection of the metastasis is rarely done; it is usually restricted to a localized lesion that occurs 3 to 4 years after primary therapy on the assumption that such a solitary metastasis can be effectively treated with local resection; however, in general, distant metastases are usually manifestations of systemic disease and are not cured with local therapy.

## Chemotherapy as Treatment for Recurrence

Patients with advanced, recurrent, or persistent cervical cancer are the most difficult to treat, and chemotherapy offers the best hope for this patient population. Cisplatin is the single most active drug in the treatment of cervical cancer. Several phase II studies have evaluated novel single agents or the combination of cisplatin with other agents, including mitolactol, ifosfamide, gemcitabine, topotecan, paclitaxel, and vinorelbine, and all have shown promising results. This has led to several phase III studies evaluating chemotherapy in patients with recurrent, advanced, or persistent cervical cancer.

The GOG has published results from four randomized phase III trials (protocols 110, 149, 169, and 179) trying to find the optimal platinum doublet to treat women with metastatic disease. The first of these trials to be published was GOG protocol 110, which compared single-agent cisplatin with cisplatin-mitolactol and cisplatin-ifosfamide (Omura, 1997). Despite the fact that overall response rates were 17.8% in the cisplatin-only arm, 21.1% in the cisplatin-mitolactol, and 31.1% in the cisplatin-ifosfamide arm ($P$ = .004), there was no significant difference in overall survival and greater toxicity with the cisplatin-ifosfamide regimen. GOG protocol 149 demonstrated that the addition of bleomycin did not enhance the activity of the cisplatin-ifosfamide doublet (Bloss, 2002), and GOG protocol 169 showed that the addition of paclitaxel to cisplatin or increasing the dose of cisplatin only improved response rate and prolonged progression-free survival but not overall survival (Moore, 2004).

GOG protocol 179 was a notable trial that demonstrated a significant improvement in overall survival (Long, 2005). In this trial, patients were randomly assigned to single-agent cisplatin or cisplatin and topotecan. There was a 2.9-month improvement in median survival in patients receiving the combination of cisplatin-topotecan versus cisplatin alone with no increase in toxicity. The result of this trial led to GOG protocol 204, which compared cisplatin-paclitaxel with cisplatin-topotecan, cisplatin-gemcitabine, and cisplatin-vinorelbine in patients with advanced, recurrent, or persistent disease in an attempt to find the optimal platinum doublet (Monk, 2009). The trial was closed early because of futility; however, in 513 patients there was no difference in overall survival among the four arms but there was a trend in response rate, progression-free survival, and overall survival that favored the cisplatin-paclitaxel arm, and the conclusion of the study was that cisplatin-paclitaxel should be considered the standard treatment for patients with stage IVB or metastatic cervical cancer.

There has been a major step forward in the treatment of patients with recurrent or metastatic cervix with the addition of targeted therapy. In GOG 240, patients were randomly assigned to treatment with one of two chemotherapy regimens (cisplatin plus paclitaxel vs. paclitaxel plus topotecan) and to bevacizumab versus no bevacizumab (Tewari, 2014). There was no difference in outcomes between the two chemotherapy regimens; however, the addition of bevacizumab significantly improved overall survival (17 months vs. 13.3), progression-free survival (8.2 months vs. 5.9 months), and response rate (48% vs. 36%) compared with chemotherapy alone. The cisplatin-paclitaxel-bevacizumab triplet has been listed as category 2A in the National Comprehensive Cancer Network (NCCN) Clinical Practice Guidelines for cervical cancer (NCCN, 2014).

Despite the results of GOG 240, the prognosis of patients with stage IVB or recurrent cervical cancer remains poor and represents an urgent unmet need worldwide. In addition to more robust prevention and screening strategies, better therapeutic strategies must be explored, including determining prognostic factors, the administration of novel agents that may improve the therapeutic index of definitive chemoradiation, and various immunotherapeutic approaches.

Immunotherapy options continue to evolve. There are trials investigating therapeutic vaccines, immune checkpoint inhibitors, and adoptive immunotherapy with adoptive transfer of in vitro tumor-infiltrating lymphocytes (TILs). In patients who have cervical cancer that has recurred or progressed after chemotherapy and whose tumors express PDL1, a 17% response rated was noted to treatment with pembrolizumab (Frenel, 2017). These results from the KEYNOTE 158 trial (NCT02628067) led to approval by the Food and Drug Administration (FDA) for patients with recurrent or metastatic cervical cancer with disease progression on or after chemotherapy whose tumors express programmed death-ligand 1 (PDL-1) (combined positive score [CPS] $\geq$ 1) as determined by the FDA-approved test. Participation in ongoing clinical trials is necessary to determine the most effective strategies for treating advanced and recurrent cervical cancer.

## REFERENCES


Bhatla N, Aoki D, Sharma D, Sankaranarayanan R. Cancer of the cervix uteri. *Int J Gynaecol Obstet.* 2018;143(Suppl 2):22-36.

Bloss JD, Blessing J, Behrens R, et al. Randomized phase III trial of cisplatin and ifosfamide with or without bleomycin in squamous carcinoma of the cervix: a Gynecology Oncology Group study. *J Clin Oncol.* 2002;20:1832.

Chemoradiotherapy for Cervical Cancer Meta-Analysis Collaboration. Reducing uncertainties about the effects of chemoradiotherapy for cervical cancer: a systematic review and meta-analysis of individual patient data from 18 randomized trials. *J Clin Oncol.* 2008;26:5802-5812.

Coleman RL, Keeney ED, Freedman RA, et al. Radical hysterectomy after radiotherapy for recurrent carcinoma of the uterine cervix. *Gynecol Oncol.* 1994;55:29-35.

Dargent D, Mathevet P. Schauta's vaginal hysterectomy combined with laparoscopic lymphadenectomy. *Baillieres Clin Obstet Gynaecol.* 1995;9:691.

Diaz JP, Sonoda Y, Leitas MM, et al. Oncologic outcome of fertility-sparing radical trachelectomy versus radical hysterectomy for stage IB1 cervical carcinoma. *Gynecol Oncol.* 2008;111:255.

Eifel PJ, Morris M, Wharton JT, et al. The influence of tumor size and morphology on the outcome of patients with FIGO stage IB squamous cell carcinoma of the uterine cervix. *Int J Radiat Oncol Biol Phys.* 1994;29:9.

Frenel JS, Le Tourneau C, O'Neil B, et al. Safety and efficacy of pembrolizumab in advanced, programmed death ligand 1-positive cervical cancer: results from the phase Ib KEYNOTE-028 Trial. *J Clin Oncol.* 2017;35(36):4035.

Goldberg GL, Sukumvanich P, Einstein MH, et al. Total pelvic exenteration: the Albert Einstein College of Medicine/Montelior Medical Experience (1987 to 2003). *Gynecol Oncol.* 2006;101(2):261-268.

Gupta S, Maheshwari A, Mahantshetty U, et al. Neoadjuvant chemotherapy followed by radical surgery versus concomitant chemotherapy and radiotherapy in patients with stage IB2, IIA or IIB Squamous cervical cancer: a randomized controlled trial. *J Clin Oncol.* 2018; 36(16):1548-1555.

Hacker NF, Wain GV, Nicklin JL. Resection of bulky positive lymph nodes in patients with cervical carcinoma. *Int J Gynecol Cancer.* 1995;5:250-256.

Hockel M. Laterally extended endopelvic resection (LEER)-principles and practice. *Gynecol Oncol.* 2008;111(Suppl 2):S13-S17.

Hockel M, Horn LC, Hentschel B, et al. Total mesometrial resection: high resolution nerve-sparing radical hysterectomy based on developmentally defined surgical anatomy. *Int J Gynecol Cancer.* 2003;13(6): 791-803.

Kenter G, Greffi S, Vergote S, et al. Results from neoadjuvant chemotherapy followed by surgery compared to chemoradiation for stage Ib2-IIb cervical cancer, EORTC 55994. *J Clin Oncol.* 2019;37(15 suppl), abstract 5503.

Long III HJ, Bundy B, Grendys EC, et al. Randomized phase III trial of cisplatin with or without topotecan in carcinoma of the uterine cervix. A Gynecologic Oncology Group study. *J Clin Oncol.* 2005;23: 4626-4633.

Magrina JF, Goodrich MA, Lidner TK, et al. Modified radical hysterectomy in the treatment of early squamous cervical cancer. *Gynecol Oncol.* 1999;72:183-186.

Monk BJ, Sill MW, McMeekin DS, et al. Phase III trial of four cisplatin-containing doublet combinations in stage IVB, recurrent or persistent cervical carcinoma: a Gynecology Oncology Group study. *J Clin Oncol.* 2009;27:4649-4655.

Moore D, Blessing J, McQuellon R, et al. Phase III study of cisplatin with or without paclitaxel in stage IVB, recurrent or persistent squamous cell carcinoma of the cervix: a Gynecologic Oncology Group study. *J Clin Oncol.* 2004;22:3113-3119.

Morley G, Hopkins M, Lindenauer JR. Pelvic exenteration, University of Michigan: 100 patients at 5 years. *Obstet Gynecol.* 1989;74(6):934-943.

Omura G, Blessing J, Vaccarello L, et al. Randomized trial of cisplatin versus cisplatin plus mitolactol versus cisplatin plus ifosfamide in advanced squamous carcinoma of the cervix: a Gynecologic Oncology Group study. *J Clin Oncol.* 1997;15:165-171.

Pearcey R, Brundage M, Drouin P, et al. Phase III trial comparing radical radiotherapy with and without cisplatin chemotherapy in patients with advanced squamous cell cancer of the cervix. *J Clin Oncol.* 2002;20: 966-972.

Peters WAI, Liu PY, Barrett R, et al. Cisplatin, 5-fluorouracil plus radiation therapy are superior to radiation therapy as adjunctive therapy in high-risk, early-stage carcinoma of the cervix after radical hysterectomy and pelvic lymphadenectomy. Report of a Phase III Intergroup Study. *Gynecol Oncol.* 1999;72:443.

Piver MS, Rutledge F, Smith JR. Five classes of extended hysterectomy for women with cervical cancer. *Obstet Gynecol.* 1974;44: 265-272.

Plante M, Renaud MC, Roy M. Radical vaginal trachelectomy: a fertility-preserving option for young women with early stage cervical cancer. *Gynecol Oncol.* 2005;99(Suppl 1):S143-S146.

Querleu D, Morrow CP. Classification of radical hysterectomy. *Lancet Oncol.* 2008;9(3):297-303.

Ramirez PT, Jhingran A, Macapinlac HA, et al. Laparoscopic extraperitoneal para-aortic lymphadenectomy in locally advanced cervical cancer: a prospective correlation of surgical findings with positron emission tomography/computed tomography findings. *Cancer.* 2011;117(9):1928-1934.

Ramirez PT, Frumovitz M, Pareja R, et al. Minimally invasive versus abdominal radical hysterectomy for cervical cancer. *N Engl J Med.* 2018;379(20):1895-1904.

Sakuragi N, Satoh C, Takeda N, Hareyama H, Takeda M, Yamamoto, R, et al. Incidence and distribution pattern of pelvic and paraaortic lymph node metastasis in patients with Stages IB, IIA, and IIB cervical carcinoma treated with radical hysterectomy. *Cancer.* 1999;85(7):1547-1554.

Salvo G, Ramirez PT, Levenback CF, et al. Sensitivity and negative predictive value for sentinel lymph node biopsy in women with early-stage cervical cancer. *Gynecol Oncol.* 2017;145(1):96-101.

Sedlis A, Bundy BN, Rotman MZ, et al. A randomized trial of pelvic radiation therapy versus no further therapy in selected patients with stage IB carcinoma of the cervix after radical hysterectomy and pelvic lymphadenectomy: a Gynecologic Oncology Group study. *Gynecol Oncol.* 1999;73:177-183.

Siegel RL, Miller KD, Jemal A. Cancer statistics, 2018. *CA Cancer J Clin.* 2018;68(1):7-30.

Tewari KS, Sill MW, Long III HJ, et al. Improved survival with bevacizumab in advanced cervical cancer. *N Engl J Med.* 2014;370:734-743.

**Suggested readings for this chapter can be found on ExpertConsult.com.**

# 32 Malignant Diseases of the Uterus

## Endometrial Hyperplasia, Endometrial Carcinoma, Sarcoma: Diagnosis and Management

*Pamela T. Soliman, Karen H. Lu*

### KEY POINTS

- Endometrial carcinoma is the most common malignancy of the female genital tract. In the United States the lifetime risk of endometrial cancer is 3%.
- Most women who develop endometrial cancer are aged 50 to 65 years.
- Women with Lynch syndrome (hereditary nonpolyposis colorectal cancer syndrome) have a 40% to 60% lifetime risk of endometrial cancer, which is similar to their lifetime risk of colon cancer.
- Chronic unopposed estrogen stimulation of the endometrium leads to endometrial hyperplasia and in some cases adenocarcinoma. Other important predisposing factors include obesity, nulliparity, late menopause, and diabetes.
- The risk of a woman developing endometrial carcinoma is three times higher if her body mass index is greater than 30 $kg/m^2$.
- Tamoxifen use increases the risk of endometrial neoplasia two- to threefold.
- The primary symptom of endometrial carcinoma is postmenopausal bleeding. Women with abnormal bleeding should undergo endometrial sampling to rule out endometrial pathologic conditions.
- Cytologic atypia in endometrial hyperplasia is the most important factor in determining malignant potential.
- Studies have found that there is a 40% concurrent rate of endometrial cancer in patients with a preoperative diagnosis of complex atypical hyperplasia.
- Prognosis in endometrial carcinoma is related to tumor grade, tumor stage, histologic type, and degree of myometrial invasion.
- Older patients with atypical hyperplasia are at increased risk of malignant progression compared with younger patients.
- A key determinant of the risk of nodal spread of endometrial carcinoma is depth of myometrial invasion, which is often related to tumor grade.
- Well-differentiated (grade 1) endometrial carcinomas usually express steroid hormone receptors, whereas poorly differentiated (grade 3) tumors usually do not express receptors.
- Uterine serous carcinoma is an aggressive histologic subtype associated with metastatic disease even in the absence of myometrial invasion.
- Ninety percent of recurrences of adenocarcinoma of the endometrium occur within 5 years.
- Overall survival rates for patients with adenocarcinoma of the endometrium by stage are as follows: stage I, 86%; stage II, 66%; stage III, 44%; stage IV, 16% (overall 72.7% 5-year survival rate combining clinical and operative staging systems).
- Histologic variants of endometrial carcinoma with a poor prognosis include uterine serous carcinoma and clear cell carcinoma.
- The most common sites of distant metastasis of adenocarcinoma of the endometrium are the lung, retroperitoneal nodes, and abdomen.
- Primary treatment of endometrial cancer includes hysterectomy, bilateral salpingo-oophorectomy, lymph node assessment, and resection of all disease. The exceptions include young premenopausal women with stage I and grade 1 endometrial carcinoma associated with endometrial hyperplasia and women with increased risk of mortality secondary to medical comorbidities.
- Postoperative adjuvant radiation has not been shown to improve overall survival.
- Patients with high-stage or recurrent disease should be treated with a multimodal approach including chemotherapy, radiation, and/or hormone therapy.
- Uterine sarcomas comprise less than 5% of uterine malignancies.
- Uterine sarcomas are treated primarily by operation including removal of the uterus, tubes, and ovaries.
- Endometrial stromal sarcomas are low-grade sarcomas with an indolent course.
- Multiagent chemotherapeutic regimens are usually prescribed for metastatic sarcomas; complete responses are rare and usually temporary.

Endometrial carcinoma is the most common malignancy of the lower female genital tract in the United States. Lifetime risk for endometrial cancer is 3%, and approximately 61,880 new cases develop in the United States each year, according to 2019 figures from the American Cancer Society. The rising rates of obesity in the United States correlate with rising rates of endometrial cancer. Approximately 12,000 deaths occurred annually in women with uterine cancer, more than for cervical cancer (4250) and fewer than the estimated 14,000 for ovarian cancer.

This chapter reviews the clinical and pathologic features of endometrial hyperplasias and carcinomas, the factors that contribute to the development of these diseases, and the appropriate methods of management. Sarcomas of the uterus and their clinical behavior and therapy are also presented.

## EPIDEMIOLOGY

Adenocarcinoma of the endometrium affects women primarily in the perimenopausal and postmenopausal years and is most often diagnosed in those between ages 50 and 65; however, these cancers can also develop in young women during their reproductive years. Approximately 5% of the cases are diagnosed in women younger than 40 and approximately 10% to 15% in women younger than age 50. Women diagnosed before age 50 years are also at risk for synchronous ovarian cancer (Soliman, 2004). Fig. 32.1 plots a typical age–incidence curve for cancers of the endometrium. The curve rises sharply after age 45 and peaks between 55 and 60; then there is a gradual decrease.

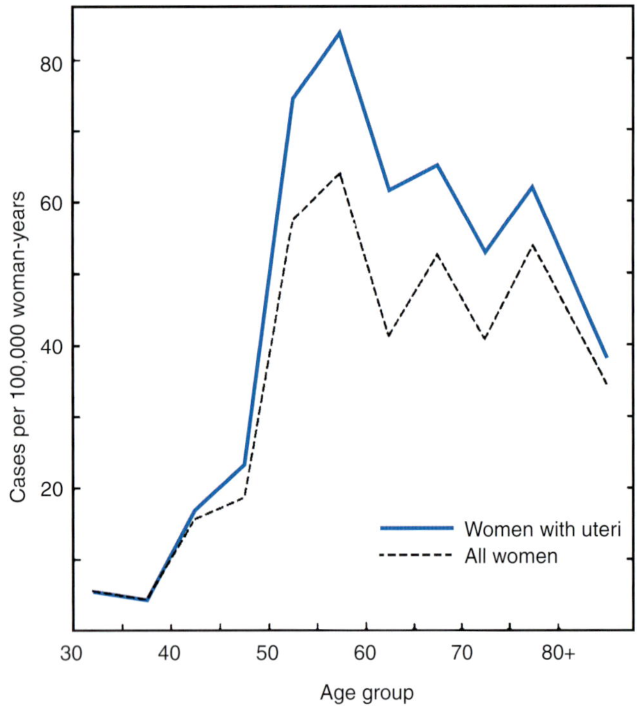


**Fig. 32.1** Incidence curve for carcinoma of the endometrium by age. (From Elwood JM, Cole P, Rothman KJ, Kaplan SD: Epidemiology of endometrial cancer. *J Natl Cancer Inst.* 1977;59:1055.)

Complex atypical hyperplasia, also referred to as endometrial intraepithelial neoplasia (EIN), is a precursor to endometrioid endometrial cancer. Some endometrial cancers develop without previous hyperplasia. These non–estrogen-related carcinomas with serous histology tend to be poorly differentiated and clinically more aggressive.

Multiple factors increase the risk of developing endometrial carcinoma (Box 32.1). Obesity is a strong risk factor for endometrial cancer. **Women who are obese (body mass index > 30) have a two- to threefold increased risk, and this risk increases with increasing weight.** The association is believed to be due in part to increased circulating estrogen levels that result from conversion of androstenedione to estrone in the adipose tissue, decreased sex hormone-binding globulin, and other factors, including insulin resistance. Although more historical than clinically relevant, unopposed estrogen stimulation is strongly associated with endometrial cancer, increasing the risk four to eight times for a woman using estrogen alone for menopausal replacement therapy. The risk increases with higher doses of estrogen (>0.625 mg conjugated estrogens) and more prolonged use but can be markedly reduced with the use of progestin (see Chapter 42, Menopause). Similarly, combination (progestin-containing) oral contraceptives decrease the risk, as noted by Grimes and Economy, with most studies showing a relative risk reduction to approximately 0.5 (Grimes 1995). The protection begins after 1 year of use and lasts approximately 15 years after discontinuation. Other conditions leading to long-term estrogen stimulation of the endometrium, including the polycystic ovary syndrome (Stein-Leventhal syndrome) and the much more rare feminizing ovarian tumors, are also associated with increased risk of endometrial carcinoma.

### BOX 32.1 Endometrial Carcinoma Risk Factors

**INCREASES THE RISK**

Obesity (2-5 times)
Nulliparity (2-3 times)
Diabetes (2.8 times)
Lynch syndrome
Insulin resistance
Estrogen-secreting ovarian tumors
Polycystic ovary syndrome
Tamoxifen therapy for breast cancer
Unopposed estrogen stimulation
Unopposed menopausal estrogen (4-8 times) replacement therapy

**DIMINISHES THE RISK**

Ovulation
Progestin therapy
Combination oral contraceptives
Menopause before 49 years
Multiparity

Patients who receive the selective estrogen receptor modulator (SERM) tamoxifen are also at increased risk of developing endometrial carcinoma. **In the National Surgical Adjuvant Bowel and Breast P-1 trial examining tamoxifen as a chemopreventive agent, risk of endometrial cancer was elevated 2.5-fold.** Risk increased with duration of use. The majority of endometrial cancers that developed in tamoxifen users had endometrioid histology and were of low grade and stage; however, high-grade endometrial cancers and sarcomas have also been reported in women taking tamoxifen. There is a high false-positive rate with transvaginal ultrasonography as a screening technique because tamoxifen causes subendometrial cyst formation, which makes the endometrial stripe appear abnormally thick. Women taking tamoxifen should be counseled about the increased risk of endometrial cancer, and all women on tamoxifen who have irregular vaginal bleeding (if premenopausal) or any vaginal bleeding (if postmenopausal) should undergo endometrial sampling or dilation and curettage (D&C).

Various other factors increase the risk of endometrial cancer. Nulliparity is associated with a twofold increased risk in endometrial cancer. Diabetes increases the risk by 2.8-fold and has been found to be an independent risk factor. Hypertension is often related to obesity and diabetes but is not considered an independent risk factor. Insulin resistance or metabolic syndrome has also been recognized as a risk factor for endometrial cancer. Regarding racial factors, the incidence of endometrial cancer among white women is approximately twice the rate in black women; however, studies of Hill and coworkers demonstrated that black women tend to develop a much higher percentage of poorly differentiated tumors. The National Cancer Database report by Partridge and colleagues confirmed that patients who are black and have a low income do present at an advanced stage and have a poor survival compared with non-Hispanic white patients. The difference in survival between black and non-Hispanic white women does not appear to be solely based on access to care issues, and there are likely biologic differences that account for the disparity in survival.

Lynch syndrome, or hereditary nonpolyposis colorectal cancer (HNPCC) syndrome, is an autosomal dominant hereditary cancer susceptibility syndrome caused by a germline defect in a DNA mismatch repair gene (*MLH1*, *MSH2*, *MSH6*, or *PMS2*). Women with *MLH1* or *MSH2* mutations have a 40% to 60% lifetime risk for developing endometrial cancer, a 40% to 60% lifetime risk of developing colon cancer, and a 12% lifetime risk of developing ovarian cancer. This contrasts sharply with the general population risk of 3% for endometrial cancer, 5% for colon cancer, and 1.7% risk of ovarian cancer. Women with *MSH6* mutations have a high rate of endometrial cancer, but the occurrence is often at a later age. Endometrial cancers in Lynch syndrome can be of any histology and grade. **Broaddus and Lu reported that although most endometrial cancers in women with Lynch syndrome were early stage, approximately one-fourth were high grade, high stage, or of a poor histologic type (Broaddus, 2006).** Given that there are few longitudinal cohort studies, screening recommendations for gynecologic cancers are based on expert opinion and can include endometrial biopsy every 1 to 2 years. Schmeler reported on the efficacy of prophylactic hysterectomy and salpingo-oophorectomy to decrease endometrial and ovarian cancer risk (Schmeler, 2006). Women with Lynch syndrome should be offered this option after childbearing is complete. Lynch syndrome is likely to account for approximately 2% of all endometrial cancers. Women with endometrial cancer and a family history of colon, endometrial, or ovarian cancer should be referred for genetic evaluation and colonoscopy. In addition, women who have a personal history of both endometrial and colon cancer have a significant risk for Lynch syndrome and should be referred. Although synchronous endometrial and ovarian cancers are fairly common, Soliman and colleagues estimated the risk of Lynch syndrome in this cohort to be less than 10% (Soliman, 2005).

In 2013 the Cancer Genome Atlas Program published a comprehensive genomic analysis on more than 300 endometrial cancers (Levine, 2013). Four molecular subtypes emerged: polymerase-epsilon *(POLE)* ultramutated, microsatellite instability high (MSI-H), copy number low, and copy number high. Copy number–low tumors include most low-grade, estrogen receptor–positive endometrial cancers, which contain defects in the PTEN and KRAS pathways. Copy number–high tumors include endometrial cancers of serous histologic type, which contain p53 mutations, and high-grade endometrioid cancers. MSI-H tumors can occur in women with Lynch syndrome; more commonly, they result from somatic hypermethylation of the MLH1 promoter. Finally, a small subset of endometrial cancers with mutations in *POLE* are associated with a large number of mutations and have an improved clinical outcome.

## ENDOMETRIAL HYPERPLASIA

The normal morphologic changes that occur in the endometrium during the menstrual cycle are reviewed in Chapter 4, Reproductive Endocrinology. Endometrial hyperplasia is believed to result from an excess of estrogen or an excess of estrogen relative to progestin, such as occurs with anovulation. In 2014 the World Health Organization changed its categorization of endometrial hyperplasias. There are two important separate categories: hyperplasia without atypia and hyperplasia with atypia, often referred to as complex atypical hyperplasia or EIN.

### Hyperplasia without atypia

*Hyperplasia without atypia* encompasses the older terms *simple hyperplasia* and *complex hyperplasia without atypia*. The endometrium may have dilated glands with some outpouching and abundant endometrial stroma (Fig. 32.2). Alternatively, the glands may demonstrate crowding with very little endometrial stroma, a very complex gland pattern, and outpouching formations but no cytologic atypia (Fig. 32.3).

### Hyperplasia with atypia

*Hyperplasia with atypia* refers to hyperplasias that contain glands with cytologic atypia and are considered premalignant. There is an increase in the nuclear/cytoplasmic ratio with irregularity in the size and shape of the nuclei (Fig. 32.4). The term *complex atypical hyperplasia* can also be used, as well as the term *endometrial intraepithelial neoplasia (EIN)*.

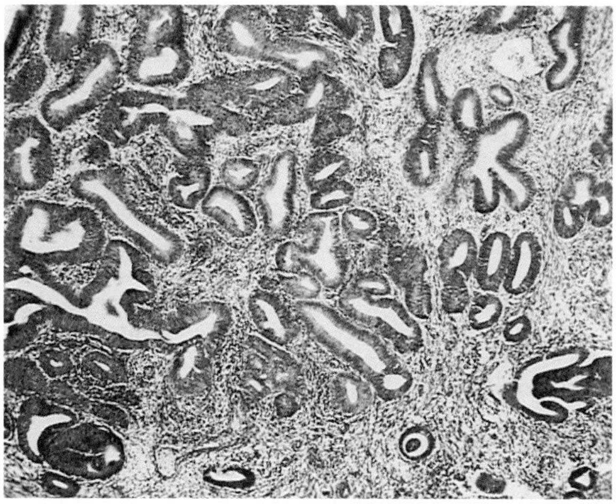

**Fig. 32.2** Benign simple hyperplasia. (From Kurman RJ, Kaminski PF, Norris HJ. Behavior of endometrial hyperplasia: a long-term study of "untreated" hyperplasias in 170 patients. *Cancer.* 1985;56:403.)

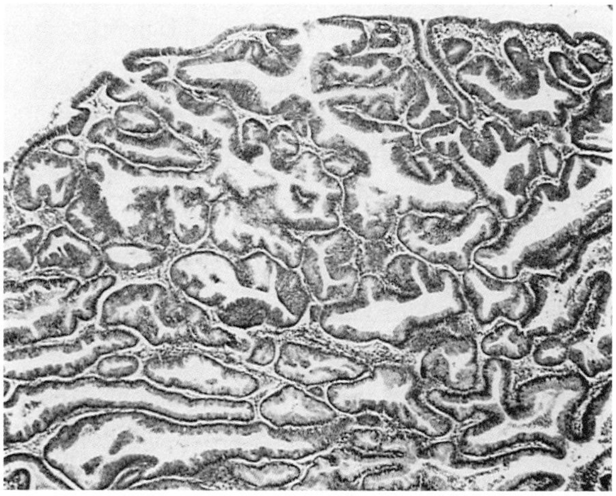

**Fig. 32.3** Complex hyperplasia characterized by crowded back-to-back glands with complex outlines. (From Kurman RJ, Kaminski PF, Norris HJ. Behavior of endometrial hyperplasia: a long-term study of "untreated" hyperplasias in 170 patients. *Cancer.* 1985;56:403.)

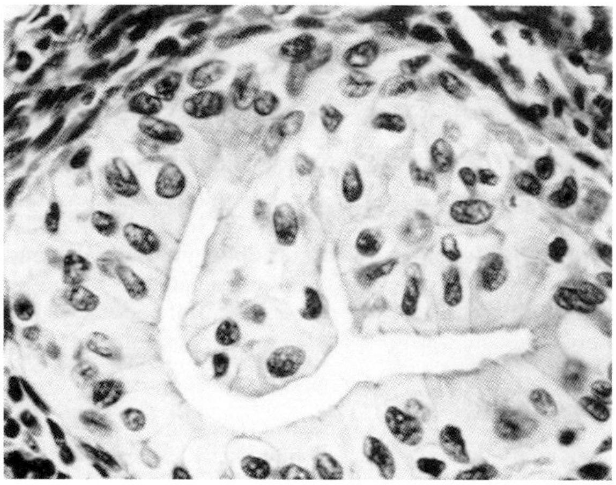

**Fig. 32.4** Severely atypical hyperplasia (complex) of the endometrium with marked irregularity of nuclei (original magnification ×720). (From Welch WR, Scully RE: *Hum Pathol.* 1977;8:503, 1977.)

## Natural History

The rate at which endometrial hyperplasia progresses to endometrial carcinoma has not been accurately determined because many of the studies have been retrospective and were based on the 1994 classification of endometrial hyperplasia. Kurman and associates studied 170 patients with endometrial hyperplasia diagnosed by D&C at least 1 year before hysterectomy. Overall, complex atypical hyperplasias had the highest risk of progression to carcinoma. Simple hyperplasia had a 1% rate of progression to cancer, complex hyperplasia without atypia had a 3% rate of progression to cancer, and complex atypical hyperplasia had a 29% rate of progression to cancer. **Lacey found up to 27.5% cumulative risk of endometrial cancer in women with atypical hyperplasia, compared with a 4.6% cumulative risk of endometrial cancer in women with nonatypical hyperplasia** (Lacey, 2010). In addition to possible progression to cancer, 42% of women who undergo hysterectomy for complex atypical hyperplasia have a concurrent endometrial cancer in their hysterectomy specimen. This high rate of cancer suggests that complex atypical hyperplasia often may be present with low-grade endometrial cancer and that endometrial sampling may not identify an endometrial cancer when admixed with a complex atypical hyperplasia. Clearly there is a spectrum of histologic types that make a definitive diagnosis of atypical hyperplasia/EIN difficult, and the clinician must be aware of this fact when planning management strategies.

## Diagnosis and Endometrial Sampling

Abnormal vaginal bleeding is the most common symptom of endometrial hyperplasia. In younger patients, hyperplasia may develop during anovulatory cycles and may be detected after prolonged periods of oligomenorrhea or amenorrhea. It can occur at any time during the reproductive years but is most common with abnormal bleeding in the perimenopausal period. Premenopausal women with irregular vaginal bleeding and postmenopausal women with any vaginal bleeding should be evaluated with an office endometrial sampling or a D&C. The office sampling instruments, such as a thin plastic Pipelle, are introduced through the cervical os into the endometrial cavity and can provide sufficient tissue for accurate histologic diagnoses. Studies have had conflicting results regarding whether a D&C provides more sensitivity in detecting cancer compared with an office Pipelle procedure. Importantly, both modalities still miss a significant number of cancers. Suh-Bergmann reported that preoperative D&C lowered the risk of an unrecognized cancer in women with complex atypical hyperplasia from 45% to 30%.

Transvaginal ultrasonography has been evaluated as an adjunct for the diagnosis of endometrial hyperplasia and cancer. In postmenopausal women with any vaginal bleeding, Gull and colleagues found that an endometrial stripe of less than 4 mm had a 100% negative predictive value. **A finding of endometrial thickness less than 4 mm is a reasonable predictor of lack of endometrial pathologic changes, even in a postmenopausal patient with bleeding; however, persistent vaginal bleeding should lead to endometrial sampling regardless of the ultrasound findings.** In addition, measurement of endometrial stripe in a premenopausal woman is not clinically useful.

## Management

The therapy employed for endometrial hyperplasia depends on the patient's age, desire for future childbearing, comorbidities, and the type of hyperplasia. For younger women with benign endometrial hyperplasia, the risk of developing endometrial cancer is extremely low and patients can be treated with progestins or combination oral contraceptive agents. **For patients with hyperplasia with atypia/EIN, the risk of developing endometrial cancer may be close to 30%.**

For patients who do not desire future childbearing, hysterectomy is the definitive treatment. Oophorectomy can be considered, but long-term risks and benefits should be discussed with the patient. Because of the 40% risk of a concomitant cancer, many surgeons send the uterus for frozen section evaluation intraoperatively, with staging as needed.

Women who desire preservation of childbearing function or who are poor surgical candidates are treated with progestin therapy, usually megestrol acetate 40 mg four times a day. A common alternative is the use of a progestin-eluting intrauterine device (IUD), which has the benefit of local delivery to the endometrium with minimal systemic side effects and which has an overall response rate for women with complex atypical hyperplasia of 80% (Pal, 2018). One study found a higher rate of regression in patients treated with a progestin-eluting IUD compared with those treated with oral progestins (Gallos, 2013). Patients require long-term follow-up and periodic sampling. In these patients the risk factors that led to the development of hyperplasia with atypia/EIN are likely to remain. In those for whom progestin therapy is ineffective, hysterectomy should be considered.

# ENDOMETRIAL CARCINOMA

## Symptoms, Signs, and Diagnosis

Postmenopausal bleeding, abnormal premenopausal bleeding, and perimenopausal bleeding are the primary symptoms of endometrial carcinoma.

The diagnosis of endometrial carcinoma is established by histologic examination of the endometrium. Initial diagnosis often can be made on an outpatient basis, with an office endometrial biopsy. A routine cytologic examination (Papanicolaou [Pap] smear) from the exocervix, which screens for cervical neoplasia, detects endometrial carcinoma in only approximately 50% of the cases.

If adequate outpatient evaluation cannot be obtained or if the diagnosis or cause of the abnormal bleeding is not clear from the tissue obtained, a hysteroscopy and D&C should be performed. If cervical involvement is suspected, the endocervix should be sampled first, followed by hysteroscopy to visualize the endometrial cavity and then a complete uterine curettage.

## Histologic Types

The various types are listed in Box 32.2. Fig. 32.5 illustrates typical adenocarcinomas of the endometrium and demonstrates varying degrees of differentiation (G1, well differentiated; G2, intermediate differentiation; G3, poorly differentiated). Grading is determined by the percentage of solid components found in the tumor: Grade 1 has less than 5% solid components, grade 2

**BOX 32.2 Endometrial Primary Adenocarcinomas**

Typical endometrioid adenocarcinoma
Adenocarcinoma with squamous elements*
Clear cell carcinoma
Serous carcinoma
Secretory carcinoma
Mucinous carcinoma
Squamous carcinoma

*Previously termed adenoacanthoma or adenosquamous carcinoma.

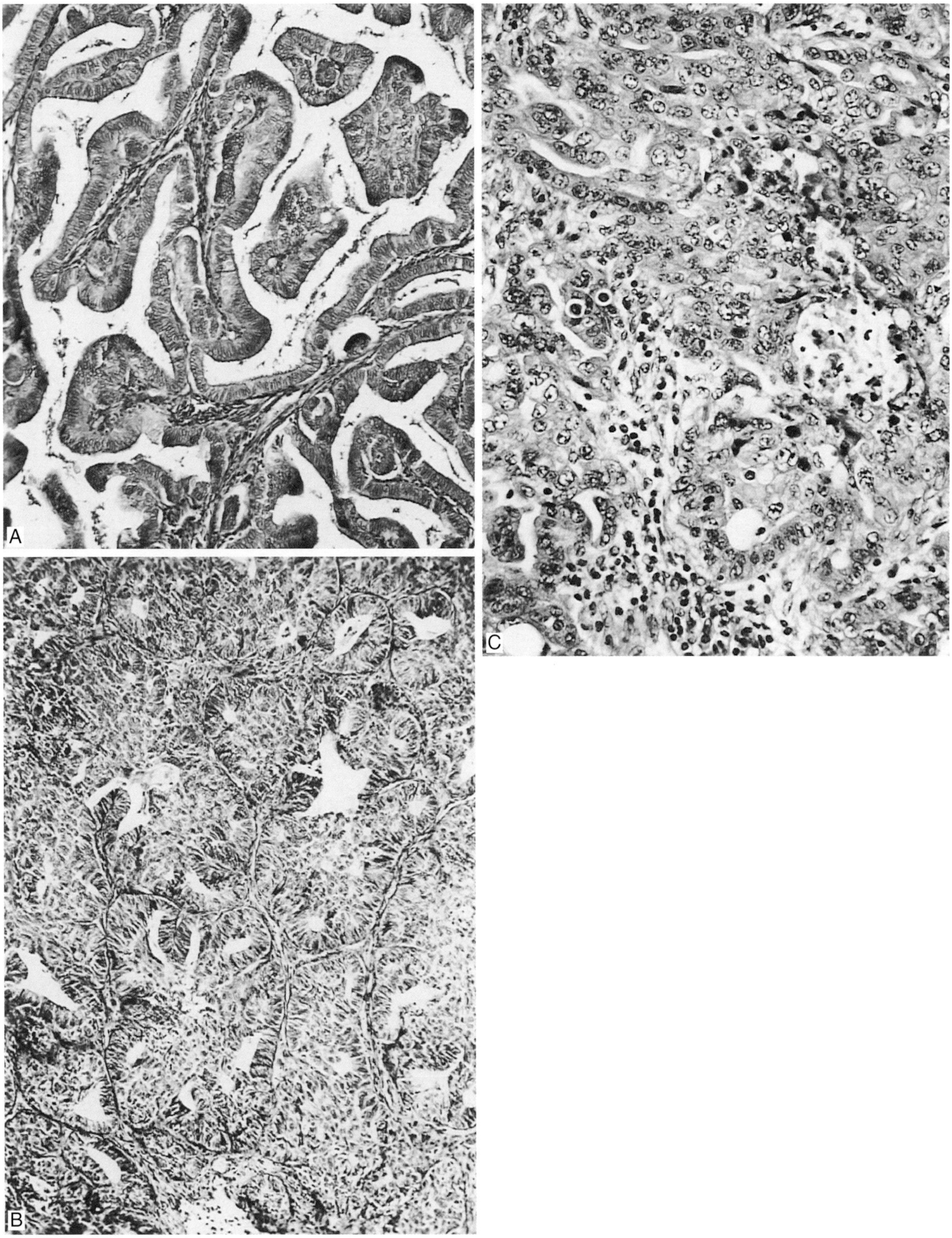

Fig. 32.5 **A,** Well-differentiated adenocarcinoma of the endometrium. The glands are confluent. (Original magnification ×130.) **B,** Moderately differentiated adenocarcinoma of the endometrium. The glands are more solid, but some lumens remain. (Original magnification ×100.) **C,** Poorly differentiated adenocarcinoma of the endometrium. The epithelium shows solid proliferation with only a rare lumen. (Original magnification ×100.) (From Kurman RJ, Norris HJ. Endometrial neoplasia: hyperplasia and carcinoma. In Blaustein A, ed. *Pathology of the Female Genital Tract.* 2nd ed. New York: Springer-Verlag; 1982.)

has 6% to 50% solid components, and grade 3 has more than 50% solid components.

Squamous epithelium commonly coexists with the glandular elements of endometrial carcinoma. Previously the term *adenoacanthoma* was used to describe a well-differentiated tumor and *adenosquamous carcinoma* to describe a poorly differentiated carcinoma with squamous elements. More recently, the term *adenocarcinoma with squamous elements* has been used with a description of the degree of differentiation of both the glandular and squamous components. Zaino and colleagues, in a Gynecologic Oncology Group (GOG) study of 456 cases with squamous elements, showed that prognosis was related to the grade of the glandular component and the degree of myometrial invasion. They suggested the term *adenocarcinoma with squamous differentiation*, and this has been generally adopted.

Uterine serous carcinomas are a highly virulent and a less common histologic subtype of endometrial carcinomas (5% to 10%). These tumors histologically resemble papillary serous carcinomas of the ovary (Fig. 32.6). Slomovitz and associates evaluated 129 patients with uterine serous carcinoma (USC) and found a high rate of extrauterine disease even in cases without myometrial invasion. They recommend a thorough operative staging (see the next section) with all cases of these tumors because of the high risk of extrauterine disease even in cases where the tumor is admixed with other histologic types (endometrial and/or clear cell).

Clear cell carcinomas of the endometrium are less common (<5%). Histologically they resemble clear cell adenocarcinomas of the ovary, cervix, and vagina; they tend to develop in postmenopausal women and carry a prognosis much worse than typical endometrial adenocarcinomas. Survival rates of 39% to 55% have been reported, much less than the 65% or better usually recorded for endometrial carcinoma. When diagnosed at an early stage, however, prognosis can be favorable. Armbruster and colleagues reviewed 112 cases of clinical early stage clear cell cancer of the uterus. Patient with pure clear cell or mixed tumors with more than 50% clear cell type had an overall survival approaching 10 years. Women older than 70 years had the worst prognosis

## Staging

In 2009, a revised International Federation of Gynecology and Obstetrics (FIGO) surgical staging classification was introduced in which the staging was modified to better define clinically relevant risk strata based on the FIGO Annual Report and other supporting publication (Table 32.1).

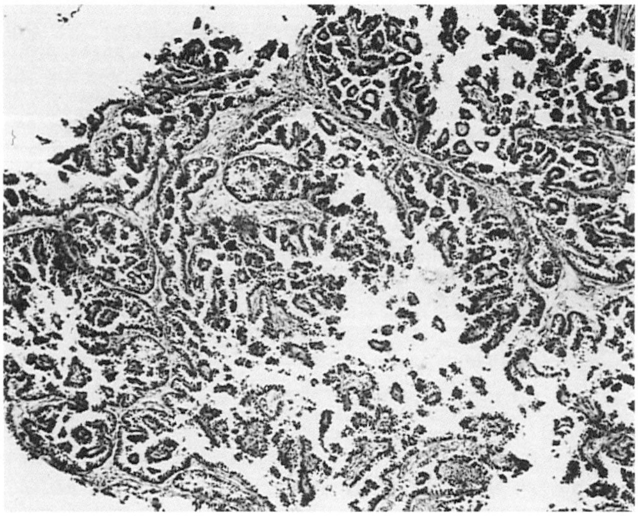

**Fig. 32.6** Serous carcinoma characterized by a complex papillary architecture resembling serous carcinoma of the ovary. (From Kurman RJ. *Blaustein's Pathology of the Female Genital Tract.* 3rd ed. New York: Springer-Verlag; 1987.)

**TABLE 32.1 Revised FIGO Staging for Endometrial Cancer (adopted 2009)**

| Stages | Characteristic |
|---|---|
| I* | Tumor confined to the corpus uteri |
| IA* | No or less than half myometrial invasion |
| IB* | Invasion equal to or more than half of the myometrium |
| II* | Tumor invades cervical stroma but does not extend beyond the uterus† |
| III* | Local and/or regional spread of the tumor |
| IIIA* | Tumor invades serosa of the corpus uteri and/or the adnexae‡ |
| IIIB* | Vaginal and/or parametrial involvement‡ |
| IIIC* | Metastases to pelvic and/or paraaortic lymph nodes‡ |
| IIIC1* | Positive pelvic nodes |
| IIIC2* | Positive paraaortic lymph nodes with or without positive pelvic lymph nodes |
| IV* | Tumor invades bladder and/or bowel mucosa and/or distant metastasis |
| IVA* | Tumor invades bladder and/or bowel mucosa |
| IVB* | Distant metastases, including intraabdominal and/or inguinal lymph nodes |

*Either G1, G2, or G3.
†Endocervical glandular involvement only should be considered stage I and no longer stage II.
‡Positive cytologic testing has to be reported separately without changing the stage.
*FIGO,* International Federation of Gynecology and Obstetrics.

## Prognostic Factors

Many variables affect the behavior of endometrial adenocarcinomas. These variables can be divided into clinical and pathologic factors. The clinical determinants are patient age at diagnosis, race, and clinical tumor stage. The pathologic determinants are tumor grade, histologic type, tumor size, depth of myometrial invasion, microscopic involvement of vascular spaces in the uterus by tumor, and spread of tumor outside the uterus to the retroperitoneal lymph nodes, peritoneal cavity, or uterine adnexa.

### Clinical Factors

Older patients have tumors of a higher stage and grade compared with younger patients. White patients have a higher survival rate than black patients, a finding partially explained by higher-stage and higher-grade tumors among black women. In addition, black women are more likely to develop USCs. In the series reported by Aziz and coworkers, the 10-year survival of 136 black patients was 40% compared with 72% for 135 white patients.

### Pathologic Factors

Tumor stage is a well-recognized prognostic factor for endometrial carcinoma (Table 32.2). Fortunately, most cases are diagnosed in stage I, which provides a favorable prognosis.

The histologic grade of the tumor is a major determinant of prognosis. Endometrial carcinomas are divided into three grades: grade 1, well differentiated; grade 2, intermediate differentiation;

**TABLE 32.2 Carcinoma of the Corpus Uteri: Patients Treated in 1990-1992: Survival by 1988 FIGO Surgical Stage, N = 5562**

| Stage | 5-Year Survival Rate |
|---|---|
| IA | 90.9% |
| IB | 88.2% |
| IC | 81.0% |
| II | 71.6% |
| III | 51.4% |
| IV | 8.9% |

Modified from Pecorelli S, Creasman WT, Pettersson F, et al. FIGO annual report on the results of treatment in gynaecological cancer. Vol 23. Milano, Italy. *J Epidemiol Biostat.* 1998.
*FIGO,* International Federation of Gynecology and Obstetrics.

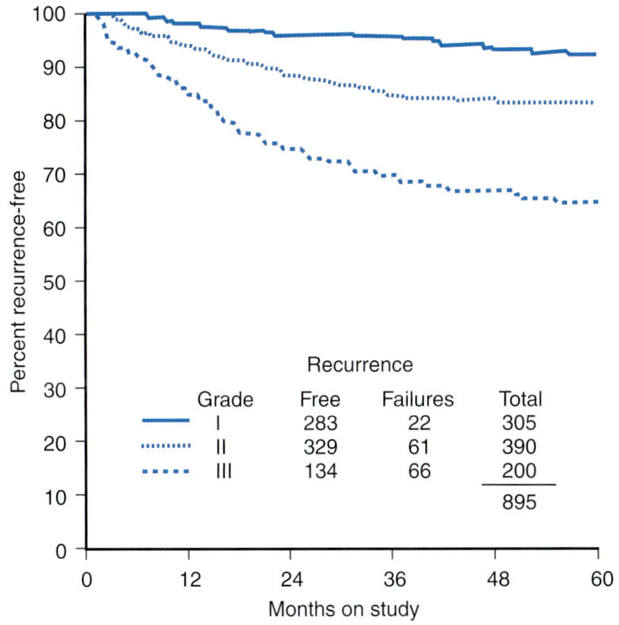


**Fig. 32.7** Recurrence-free interval by histologic grade. (Redrawn from Morrow CP, Bundy BN, Kurman RJ, et al. Relationship between surgical-pathologic risk factors and outcome in clinical stage I and II carcinoma of the endometrium: a Gynecologic Oncology Group study. *Gynecol Oncol.* 1991;40:55.)

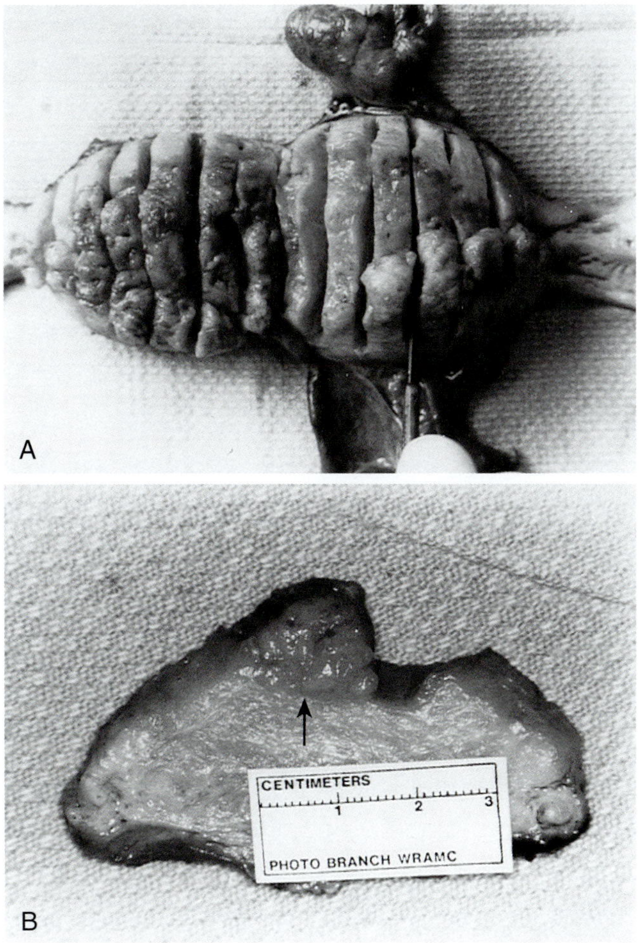


**Fig. 32.8 A,** Technique for intraoperative assessment of the depth of myometrial invasion. **B,** Cross section of uterine wall demonstrating superficial myometrial invasion. *Arrow* shows the tumor–myometrial junction. (From Doering DL, Barnhill DR, Weiser EB, et al. Intraoperative evaluation of depth of myometrial invasion in stage I endometrial adenocarcinoma. *Obstet Gynecol.* 1989;74:930.)

and grade 3, poorly differentiated. Fig. 32.7 shows the survival of 895 patients studied by the GOG that relates endometrial carcinoma survival to tumor grade and demonstrates the worsening of prognosis with advancing grade.

The histologic type of the endometrial carcinoma is also related to prognosis, with the best prognosis associated with endometrioid adenocarcinomas, in particular well-differentiated tumors. Approximately 80% of all endometrial carcinomas fall into the favorable category. Histologic types that carry poor prognoses are serous carcinoma, clear cell carcinoma, carcinosarcoma, and poorly differentiated carcinoma with or without squamous elements.

**The degree of myometrial invasion correlates with the risk of tumor spread outside the uterus, but the higher-grade and higher-stage tumors in general are more likely to have deep myometrial penetration (Fig. 32.8).** In a study by Schink and colleagues, tumor size greater than 2 cm was also found to be prognostic. Only 4% of those with tumors 2 cm or less had lymph node metastases. The rate increased to 15% for those with tumors greater than 2 cm and to 35% when the entire endometrial cavity was involved. Table 32.3 summarizes the clinical and pathologic factors affecting outcomes in patients with early-stage tumors. Peritoneal cytologic characteristics have been studied as a prognostic factor, and the results are conflicting. In a study of 567 surgical stage I cases, Turner and associates found that positive peritoneal cytologic evaluation was an independent prognostic factor. In contrast, Grimshaw and coworkers evaluated 322 clinical stage I cases and found that positive peritoneal cytology was an adverse prognostic factor, but they did not find it to be an independent risk factor when other variables were considered. In 2018 Seagle and colleagues evaluated 16,851 women though the National Cancer Database and found that positive washings were associated with decreased survival among women with stage I/II endometrial cancer, including those with low-grade tumors. In addition, treatment of women with positive cytology with adjuvant chemotherapy was associated with increased survival. Although these large database studies have limitations, this is something to consider. In the 2009 revised FIGO surgical staging, positive cytology is no longer classified as stage IIIA.

**TABLE 32.3 Surgical Stage I and II Tumors: The Proportional Hazards Modeling of Relative Survival Time**

| Variable | Regression Coefficient | Relative Risk | Significance Test* (*P* value) |
|---|---|---|---|
| **ENDOMETRIOID** | | | |
| Grade 1 | — | 1.0 | — |
| Grade 2 | 0.28 | 1.3 | 2.7 (.1) |
| Grade 3 | 0.56 | 1.8 | |
| Endometrioid with squamous differentiation | | | 0.1 (.7) |
| Grade 1 | 0.20 | 1.2 | |
| Grade 2 | –0.01 | 1.0 | 0.3 (.6) |
| Grade 3 | 0.22 | 0.8 | |
| Villoglandular | | | 2.2 (.1) |
| Grade 1 | –4.91 | 0.01 | |
| Grade 2 | –0.59 | 0.5 | 10.4 (.001) |
| Grade 3 | 3.73 | 41.9 | |
| **MYOMETRIAL INVASION** | | | |
| Endometrium only | — | 1.0 | |
| Superficial | 0.39 | 0.5 | |
| Middle | 1.20 | 3.3 | 19.6 (.0002) |
| Deep | 1.53 | 4.6 | |
| Age | 0.17 | — | |
| Age | –0.000837 | — | 20.7 (.0001) |
| 45 (arbitrary reference) | — | 1.0 | |
| 55 | 0.85 | 2.3 | |
| 65 | 1.52 | 4.6 | |
| 75 | 2.03 | 7.6 | |
| Vascular space involvement | 0.32 | 1.4 | 1.2 (.3) |

Modified from Zaino RJ, Kurman RJ, Diana KL, Morrow CP. Pathologic models to predict outcome for women with endometrial adenocarcinoma. *Cancer.* 1996;77:1115.

*P* value for grading is for overall grade within cell type.

*Wald $x^2$ test.

**Patterns of Spread of Endometrial Carcinoma.** Plentl and Friedman noted four major channels of lymphatic drainage from the uterus that serve as sites for extrauterine spread of tumor: (1) a small lymphatic branch along the round ligament that runs to the inguinal femoral nodes; (2) branches from the tubal and (3) ovarian pedicles (infundibulopelvic ligaments), which are large lymphatics that drain into the paraaortic nodes; and (4) the broad ligament lymphatics that drain directly to the pelvic nodes. The pelvic and paraaortic node drainage sites (2, 3, and 4) are the most important clinically. In addition, direct peritoneal spread of tumor can occur through the uterine wall or via the lumen of the fallopian tube. Therefore the clinician must assess the retroperitoneal nodes, the peritoneal cavity, and the uterine adnexa for the spread of endometrial carcinoma (Fig. 32.9).

Extensive studies by the GOG have elucidated both the frequency of lymph node metastases in endometrial carcinoma and the pathologic factors that modify this risk in stage I disease. Tumor grade, size of the uterus, and degree of myometrial invasion were studied. Table 32.4 illustrates the frequency of lymph node metastases according to tumor grade and depth of myometrial invasion. **The frequency of nodal involvement becomes much greater with high-grade tumors and with greater depth of myometrial invasion.** The risk of lymph node involvement appears to be negligible for endometrial carcinoma involving only the endometrium. With invasion of the inner third of the myometrium, there is minimal risk of node involvement for grade 1 and 2 cases. If the outer third of the myometrium is involved, the risk of nodal metastases is greatly increased. These data emphasize the importance of myometrial invasion and tumor spread, providing the basis for the FIGO Surgical Staging System. Tables 32.5 and 32.6 summarize the risk of nodal metastases based on the GOG studies published by Creasman and colleagues. Mariani and colleagues at the Mayo Clinic found that tumor size could also be incorporated into a staging paradigm to identify patients at highest risk for nodal spread. **They found that in grade 1 and 2 tumors with less than 50% invasion and tumor size less than 2 cm, the risk of lymph node involvement was virtually zero (Mariani, 2000).**

## Evaluation

In addition to the usual routine preoperative evaluation, the patient should have a chest radiographic examination. For high-risk histologic types, preoperative imaging in the form of a computed tomography (CT) scan is often done; however, a study by Connor and associates noted that preoperative computed tomography scan had only a 50% positive predictive value for nodal disease. A 2019 study by Stewart and colleagues examined preoperative positron emission tomography (PET)/CT in women with high-risk endometrial cancer. They found that PET/CT was not reliable in detecting extrauterine disease, either nodal or peritoneal.

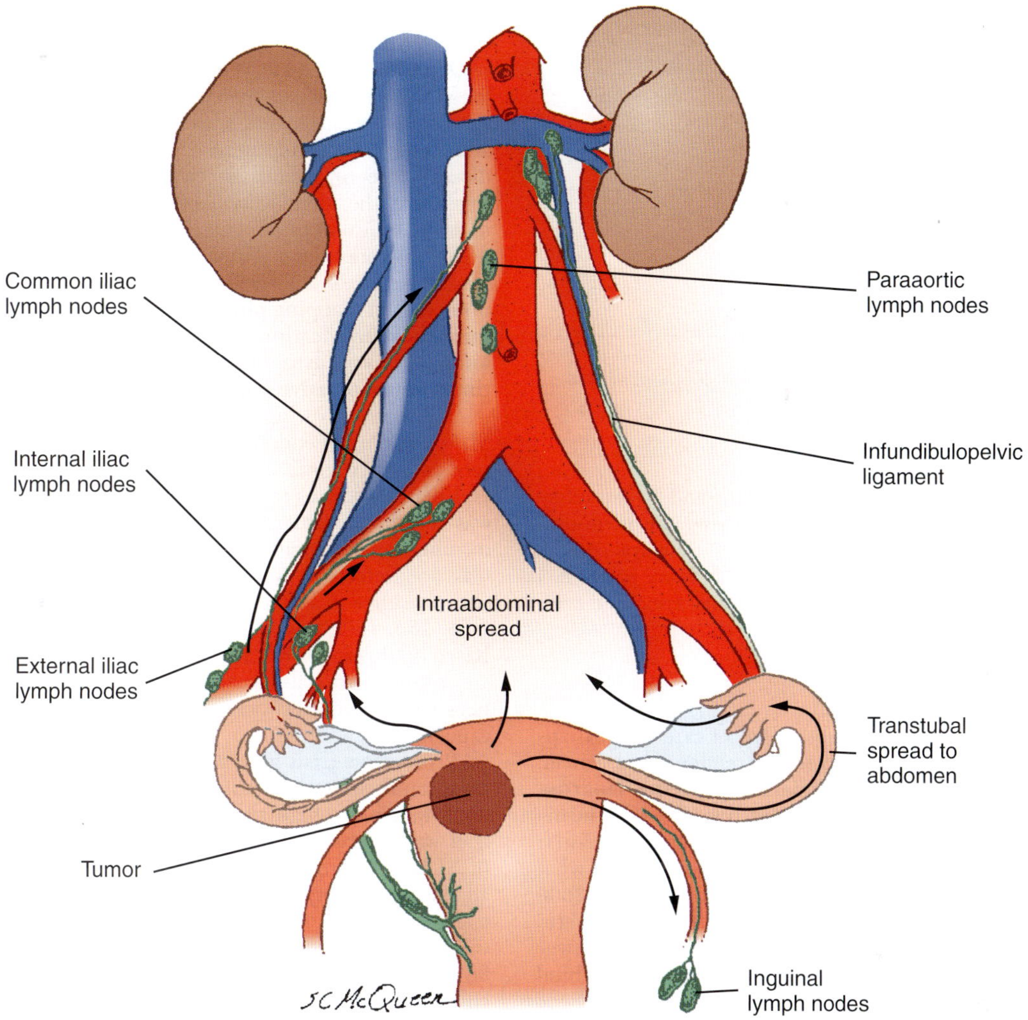


**Fig. 32.9** Spread of endometrial carcinoma. The major pathways of tumor spread are illustrated (see text).

**TABLE 32.4 Grade, Depth of Myometrial Invasion, and Node Metastasis—Stage I**

| Depth of Invasion | G1 n = 180 | G2 n = 288 | G3 n = 153 |
|---|---|---|---|
| **Pelvic** | | | |
| Endometrium only (n = 86) | 0 (0%) | 1 (3%) | 0 (0%) |
| Inner (n = 281) | 3 (3%) | 7 (5%) | 5 (9%) |
| Middle (n = 115) | 0 (0%) | 6 (9%) | 1 (4%) |
| Deep (n = 139) | 2 (11%) | 11 (19%) | 23 (34%) |
| Aortic | | | |
| Endometrium only (n = 86) | 0 (0%) | 1 (3%) | 0 (0%) |
| Inner (n = 281) | 1 (1%) | 5 (4%) | 2 (4%) |
| Middle (n = 115) | 1 (5%) | 0 (0%) | 0 (0%) |
| Deep (n = 139) | 1 (6%) | 8 (14%) | 15 (23%) |

Adapted from Creasman WT, Morrow CP, Bundy BN, et al. Surgical pathologic spread patterns of endometrial cancer. *Cancer* 1987;60:2035.
*G*, grade.

**TABLE 32.5 FIGO Staging and Nodal Metastasis**

| Staging | Metastasis: Pelvic | Metastasis: Aortic |
|---|---|---|
| IA G1 (n = 101) | 2 (2%) | 0 (0%) |
| G2 (n = 169) | 13 (8%) | 6 (4%) |
| G3 (n = 76) | 8 (11%) | 5 (7%) |
| IB G1 (n = 79) | 3 (4%) | 3 (4%) |
| G2 (n = 119) | 12 (10%) | 8 (7%) |
| G3 (n = 77) | 20 (26%) | 12 (16%) |

From Creasman WT, Morrow CP, Bundy BN, et al. Surgical pathologic spread patterns of endometrial cancer. *Cancer.* 1987;60:2035.
*FIGO,* International Federation of Gynecology and Oncology; *G,* grade.

## Management

Surgery is the primary treatment modality for patients with endometrial carcinoma. Complete surgical staging includes hysterectomy, with or without bilateral salpingo-oophorectomy, and lymph node assessment. Surgical staging allows accurate surgical and histologic assessment of (1) tumor spread within the uterus,

**TABLE 32.6 Risk Factors for Nodal Metastases—Stage I**

| Factor | Pelvic | Aortic |
|---|---|---|
| Low risk<br>Grade 1<br>Endometrium only<br>No intraperitoneal spread | 0/44 (0%) | 0/44 (0%) |
| Moderate risk<br>Grade 2 or 3<br>Invasion to middle third | 15/268 (6%) | 6/268 (2%) |
| High risk<br>Invasion to outer third | 21/116 (18) | 17/118 (15%) |

Adapted from Creasman WT, Morrow CP, Bundy BN, et al. Surgical pathologic spread patterns of endometrial cancer. *Cancer.* 1987;60: 2035.

(2) degree of penetration into the myometrium, and (3) extrauterine spread to retroperitoneal nodes, adnexa, and the peritoneal cavity. Exceptions include women with significant medical comorbidities and young, premenopausal women who desire future fertility with grade 1 endometrial adenocarcinoma associated with endometrial hyperplasia.

## Stage I

Minimally invasive surgery is the standard of care surgical approach for women with newly diagnosed endometrial cancer. **Several randomized controlled trials comparing laparoscopy with laparotomy have shown the benefits of a minimally invasive approach.** The GOG LAP2 study was the first reported randomized trial comparing laparoscopy with what was then the standard of care, laparotomy, with more than 2600 women enrolled (Walker, 2009). Although the conversion rates were high at 25.8%, laparoscopy was associated with fewer postoperative adverse events and shorter length of hospital stay. In a similar trial (Laparoscopic Approach to Cancer of the Endometrium [LACE] trial) conducted in Australia, New Zealand, and Hong Kong, laparoscopy was associated lower rates of postoperative complications and serious adverse events (Janda, 2010). Both studies reported improved short-term quality of life after laparoscopy.

Long-term outcomes from both trials have also been published. In 2012, the follow-up data on GOG LAP2 reported a small difference in recurrence rate between the two groups (11.4% after laparoscopy and 10.2% after laparotomy); however, the 5-year overall survival was almost identical in both arms at 89.8%. The authors concluded that laparoscopic hysterectomy in endometrial cancer was a safe alternative to traditional laparotomy. More recently, the long-term outcomes of the LACE trial were reported. **In this study the disease-free and overall survival rates were equivalent between laparoscopy and abdominal hysterectomy, confirming that minimally invasive surgery should be considered for all patients with clinical stage I endometrial cancer.**

## Lymphadenectomy

Surgical management of endometrial cancer historically included exploratory laparotomy, pelvic washings, hysterectomy, bilateral salpingo-oophorectomy, selective biopsies of suspicious areas, and lymph node sampling in patients at risk for extrauterine disease. Complete surgical staging is not only prognostic but also facilitates targeted therapy to maximize survival while minimizing morbidity by reducing both under- and overtreatment. Unfortunately, patients with endometrial cancer can be poor surgical candidates because of obesity, diabetes, and hypertension, which are common risk factors for this disease. As a result, different strategies have been used to determine which patients need more extensive evaluation based on their risk for distant spread.

A complete staging procedure, including lymphadenectomy, for all women with endometrial cancer continues to remain controversial. **Two randomized studies evaluating the role of lymphadenectomy in endometrial cancer showed no benefit in disease-free or overall survival.** Despite these findings, many agree that the identification of metastatic disease in the lymph nodes is critical in the diagnosis and treatment of women with endometrial cancer and lymph node metastases are an important prognostic factor in overall survival. **The use of sentinel lymph node (SLN) mapping plus ultrastaging could potentially maximize the identification of positive nodes, while minimizing the known risks of lymphadenectomy, including longer surgical times, intraoperative injury, blood loss, and lymphedema.**

There is a growing body of evidence supporting the role of SLN mapping in endometrial cancer. Published studies have described SLN detection rates as high as 85% to 100% with bilateral detection rates of 60% to 97%. Memorial Sloan Kettering was the first to describe an SLN algorithm that included performing a side-specific pelvic lymphadenectomy when an SLN was not detected. Retrospective implementation of this algorithm resulted in a significant decrease in their false-negative rate from 15% to 2% in women with low-risk endometrial cancer. Based on this and other studies, SLN mapping was recognized as an option for nodal assessment in the 2014 National Comprehensive Cancer Network (NCCN) guidelines for endometrial cancer.

Prospective trials have shown that sentinel lymph node mapping can accurately identify women with positive nodes in both the low-risk and high-risk populations. The Rossi (2017) FIRES trial was a prospective, multicenter trial evaluating the efficacy of SLN mapping using the robotic platform in patients with all histologic subtypes with required completion pelvic lymphadenectomy with or without paraaortic lymphadenectomy to validate the SLN algorithm. SLN mapping was successful in 86% of patients with a false negative rate of 2.8%. Soliman and colleagues confirmed the accuracy of SLN mapping in high-risk patients with an 89% successful mapping rate and a false-negative rate of 4.3%. These studies further validated the sentinel lymph node algorithm in both low-risk and high-risk women, leading to its adoption in a majority of clinical practices.

## Nonsurgical Options

For patients with significant medical comorbidities, radiation therapy alone can be used. Radiation as the sole method of therapy, however, yields inferior results, as Bickenbach and colleagues noted, with an 87% 5-year survival rate for patients with stage I carcinoma treated by surgery alone, compared with a 69% survival rate for those treated with radiation therapy alone. For those who cannot tolerate surgery or external beam therapy, treatment by intracavitary radiation alone offers some benefit. Lehoczky and associates reported on 170 elderly patients treated with brachytherapy alone with uncorrected 5-year survival rates for stages IA and IB of 46% and 30%, respectively. For patients with grade 1 cancers, progesterone therapy can be considered if patients are not medically fit for surgery. **Success rates of progesterone therapy for the treatment of grade 1 endometrial cancer have been as high as 90%.** See the later section on hormonal therapy for further details.

# Stage II

Three therapeutic options have been employed for the treatment of stage II carcinoma of the endometrium that also involves the endocervix: (1) primary operation (radical hysterectomy and lymph node assessment), (2) primary radiation (intrauterine and vaginal implant and external irradiation) followed by an extrafascial hysterectomy, and (3) simple hysterectomy followed by external beam irradiation. Radical hysterectomy and pelvic dissection have been used as effective therapy. Mariani and colleagues reported on 57 patients with endocervical involvement at the time of diagnosis. Of these, 61% underwent radical hysterectomy and staging. There were no recurrences in the radical hysterectomy group if their nodes were negative at the time of surgery. Five-year disease-related survival and recurrence-free survival in the radical hysterectomy patients was 76% and 71%.

Another option for patients with stage II carcinoma of the endometrium is treatment with a combination of radiation and extrafascial hysterectomy. A protocol includes external radiation (45 Gy) and a single brachytherapy implant usually followed by extrafascial total abdominal hysterectomy, bilateral salpingo-oophorectomy, and paraaortic node sampling. Podczaski and coworkers noted that those with gross cervical tumor had a poor prognosis and were likely to have extrauterine disease at operation. For patients with cervical involvement on biopsy but no gross tumor, Trimble and Jones found radiation treatment by a single implant alone followed by a hysterectomy to be effective, and they added external therapy depending on the nodal findings and myometrial invasion. Andersen reported on 54 patients with stage II tumors and found a 70.6% survival rate in patients treated by abdominal hysterectomy followed by radiation.

### Adjuvant Radiation Therapy for Early-Stage Disease

A number of phase III randomized trials evaluating the use of adjuvant radiotherapy in patients with high-risk stage I endometrial cancer have shown no improvement in overall survival (Table 32.7). In a Norwegian study comparing brachytherapy versus brachytherapy and pelvic radiation, local recurrences were decreased in the group of patients receiving pelvic radiation. In the PORTEC trial from The Netherlands, Creutzberg and colleagues reported on 714 patients with presumed stage I disease (Creutzberg, 2000). Patients received full pelvic radiotherapy or observation. Although locoregional control was better in the treatment arm, there was no difference in overall survival. In a GOG trial, Keys and associates randomly assigned almost 400 patients who underwent complete surgical staging to pelvic radiation versus observation. Similar to the PORTEC trial, there was a decrease in local recurrences in the radiation arm with no difference in overall survival (Keys, 2004). In PORTEC-2 researchers compared pelvic external beam radiation versus vaginal brachytherapy and found no difference in local recurrence or overall survival. They concluded that vaginal cuff radiation should be standard for this group of patients, with similar benefit from pelvic radiation.

## Adjuvant Systemic Therapy for Early-Stage Endometrial Cancer

In addition to radiation therapy, adjuvant chemotherapy has been explored for patients with endometrial cancer and high-risk features. Although the addition of postoperative radiation to high-risk, early-stage patients does reduce the local recurrence rate, distant metastasis continues to be problematic. In approximately 25% of patients with low-stage, grade 3 lesions, the disease recurs at a distant site. In addition, 20% of clinical stage II patients and at least 30% of patients who present with extrauterine disease have recurrences at distant sites even after patients have received adjuvant pelvic radiation.

A 2019 study, GOG-249, compared adjuvant pelvic radiation with vaginal brachytherapy plus paclitaxel/carboplatin in high intermediate and high-risk, early-stage endometrial cancer. In this phase III, randomized trial of patients with stage I/II disease, there was no difference in overall survival between the two groups. The vaginal brachytherapy with chemotherapy arm had higher acute toxicity, and similar long-term toxicity was found in the two groups.

## Stage I or II Uterine Serous Carcinoma

The best treatment for early-stage USCs is still unknown because of the rarity of this disease and lack of prospective trials. Recommendations for adjuvant therapy have developed through a better understanding of patterns of recurrence and retrospective data reviews. **Several studies have consistently shown that patients who have undergone a complete surgical staging and are found to have no residual disease in the uterus have a low risk of recurrence and therefore do not require adjuvant therapy.** Patients with residual disease in the uterus, even if minimal, are at higher risk for recurrent disease. Fader and colleagues (2013) found that patients with noninvasive USC had a recurrence risk of 0% to 30% and those with any myometrial invasion had a 29% to 80% recurrence risk with observation alone. As a result, adjuvant chemotherapy with or without volume-directed radiation is often considered. Hamilton and colleagues (2006) in a retrospective series of stage I patients found that treatment with paclitaxel and carboplatin with or without vaginal brachytherapy resulted in a recurrence rate of 9.2% versus 24% among those who did not receive adjuvant therapy ($P =$ .016). They also found a significant difference in 5-year progression-free survival (PFS) among those who received adjuvant chemotherapy (81.5%) compared with those observed (64.7%) or treated with radiation alone (64.1%). In a multiinstitutional retrospective study of early-stage USC, The combination of carboplatin and paclitaxel in the adjuvant setting was effective in improving survival and limiting recurrences. Based on these data and other studies, adjuvant therapy is considered an acceptable treatment options in the NCCN guidelines. Prospective studies, however, could help us further determine which subset of patients really benefit from adjuvant therapy and those who may not require additional treatment.

## Stage III

In stage III carcinoma the disease has spread outside the uterus but remains confined to the pelvis or the retroperitoneal nodes. Patients with stage IIIA disease include those with disease spread to the adnexa and/or the serosa of the uterus. Stage IIIB involves

**TABLE 32.7 Summary of Randomized Trials of Adjuvant Radiotherapy in Stage I Endometrial Carcinoma**

| Trial | Surgery | Randomization | Locoregional Recurrences | Survival |
|---|---|---|---|---|
| Norwegian 1968-1974 | TAH-BSO | Brachytherapy vs. brachy and pelvic RT | 7% vs. 2% at 5 years ($P < .01$) | 89% vs. 91% at 5 years ($P =$ NS) |
| PORTEC | TAH-BSO | Obs vs. pelvic RT | 14% vs. 4% at 5 years ($P < .001$) | 85% vs. 81% at 5 years ($P = .31$) |
| GOG | TAH-BSO, nodes | Obs vs. pelvic RT | 12% vs. 3% at 2 years ($P < .01$) | 86% vs. 92% at 4 years ($P = .56$) |

*GOG*, Gynecologic Oncology Group; *NS*, nonsignificant; *RT*, radiotherapy.

the vagina. Stage IIIC includes spread to the retroperitoneal lymph nodes. In the revised FIGO staging, stage IIIC was further divided into those with positive pelvic nodes only (stage IIIC1) and those with positive paraaortic nodes (stage IIIC2). Stage III accounts for approximately 7% of all endometrial carcinomas. Adjuvant treatment is often a combination of tumor-directed radiation and systemic chemotherapy; however, there continues to be controversy regarding the role of radiation in this patient population.

Both PORTEC-3 and GOG-258 trials evaluated the role of adjuvant therapy in patients with advanced endometrial cancer after surgical staging. PORTEC-3 was a prospective randomized trial, which included patients with stage III disease and compared pelvic radiation alone with cisplatin with radiation followed by paclitaxel and carboplatin. The addition of chemotherapy did not improve overall survival but did improve failure-free survival by 11% in patients with stage III disease. **Although the toxicity was higher in the combination arm, the authors concluded the addition of chemotherapy may be warranted in the higher-risk patients, including those with stage III disease.**

GOG-258 was a prospective randomized trial comparing cisplatin with tumor-directed radiation followed by paclitaxel and carboplatin (similar to PORTEC-3 regimen) versus paclitaxel and carboplatin alone in women with locally advanced endometrial cancer (stage IIIA to IVA) or stage I/II serous or clear cell carcinoma with positive cytologic results. Risk for locoregional and nodal recurrence was higher in the chemotherapy-only arm, but there was no difference in overall survival. **Although data consistently show that radiation can decrease local recurrence, there does not appear to be an improvement in overall survival.**

## Stage IV

Extrauterine disease is found in approximately 10% to 15% of new endometrial cancer cases. These cases account for more than 50% of all uterine cancer-related deaths, with survival rates as low as 5% to 15%. For patients with peritoneal disease treatment often consists of radical surgery followed by any combination of radiation, chemotherapy, and novel therapeutic agents. Support for initial maximal cytoreductive effort is provided by data showing that the extent of residual disease among advanced-stage endometrial cancer appears to have a direct influence on survival. In a retrospective comparative study of women with advanced endometrial cancer, patients with optimal cytoreduction had improved median overall survival compared with those with residual disease (29 vs. 17 months; $P = .02$) (Rajkumar, 2019). In older reports, patients in whom the tumor was determined to be unresectable had median survivals of 2 to 8 months, regardless of adjuvant treatment with radiation and/or chemotherapy (Goff, 1994; Shih, 2011). In contrast, when patients underwent optimal cytoreductive surgery, survival was twice that of those who underwent a suboptimal cytoreduction. In a study by Bristow and colleagues, the median survival for patients who had less than 1 cm residual disease was 15 months, compared with 40 months among those who had microscopic disease (Bristow, 2000). A similar study by Shih and colleagues reported median survival for patients with no residual disease of 40 months compared with 19 months for those who had any residual disease (Shih, 2011). **Although the data come from small studies and single-institution reviews, the findings are consistent that patients benefit from a maximal surgical effort when feasible.**

### Treatment in Advanced or Recurrent Disease

Several chemotherapeutic agents or combinations have demonstrated activity in patients with endometrial cancer. Combination therapy is more effective than single-agent therapy in treating this disease. In a GOG randomized phase III study, cisplatin and doxorubicin in combination had a higher response rate compared with single-agent doxorubicin (45% vs. 27%), but there was no difference in overall survival. The European Organisation for Research and Treatment of Cancer (EORTC) performed a similar trial comparing the same two regimens with a modest survival advantage found in those patients who received the combination regimen. The median overall survival in cisplatin- and doxorubicin-treated patients was 9 months compared with 7 months in the patients who received doxorubicin alone ($P = .065$).

Single-agent paclitaxel has shown significant activity in chemotherapy-naive patients with recurrent endometrial cancer with a response rate of 36%. The antitumor effect of single-agent paclitaxel led to the incorporation of paclitaxel into combination therapy regimens. In a phase II study the combination of cisplatin and paclitaxel demonstrated a 67% response rate. In a phase III study, the GOG found similar activity between the combination of cisplatin and doxorubicin versus doxorubicin and paclitaxel. After this study, the GOG performed a phase III trial evaluating doxorubicin and cisplatin compared with paclitaxel (Taxol), doxorubicin (Adriamycin), and cisplatin (Platinol) with granulocyte colony-stimulating factor (Miller, 2012). The TAP regimen yielded a superior response rate (57% vs. 34%; $P < .001$), longer PFS (8.3 vs. 5.3 months; $P < .001$), and longer overall survival (15.3 vs. 12.3 months; $P = .037$).

In a phase II study the combination of paclitaxel and carboplatin was evaluated in patients with advanced and recurrent disease. In patients with advanced endometrioid endometrial cancer, there was a 78% response rate to this combination. The median failure-free survival time was 23 months and the 3-year overall survival rate was 62%. In patients with recurrent disease, the response rate was 56% and the median failure-free interval was 6 months.

The combination of carboplatin and paclitaxel has a more favorable toxicity profile than TAP. GOG-209 was a phase III randomized, noninferiority study comparing TAP with carboplatin and paclitaxel. The preliminary results showed that paclitaxel and carboplatin were not inferior to TAP in terms of progression-free and overall survival. **As a result, paclitaxel and carboplatin are now considered first-line standard of care for advanced and recurrent endometrial cancer.**

Prognosis is very poor for patients for whom first-line chemotherapy is ineffective. A number of studies done through the GOG in women with recurrent endometrial cancer have shown poor responses to salvage chemotherapy. Paclitaxel was the only active single-agent chemotherapeutic with a response rate (RR) of 27.3% in women with advanced or recurrent endometrial cancer. These data, however, were in women without prior treatment with taxane-based chemotherapy (Lincoln, 2003). Now that the combination of paclitaxel and carboplatin is often used at first-line treatment in advanced or recurrent endometrial cancer, the focus of second-line therapy has been on nontaxane treatment. Other agents studied, including etoposide, liposomal doxorubicin, and topotecan, have shown less than promising results, with RRs between 4% and 13%. Bevacizumab was approved in the recurrent setting based on a 6-month PFS of 40% and an overall RR of 13.5% (Aghajanian et al., 2011). A major focus of clinical research studies has included alternative treatment strategies.

For patients with an isolated recurrence in the pelvis, radiotherapy can be useful. Ackerman and coworkers treated 21 patients with pelvic relapse and found radiation achieved pelvic control of disease in 14 (67%). The best results were with recurrences in the vaginal mucosa. Similarly, Sears and colleagues treated 45 patients with vaginal recurrence of endometrial cancer with radiation and achieved a 44% 5-year survival rate. As noted previously, Carey and associates salvaged 15 of 17 patients with vaginal recurrence initially treated by operation alone. The addition of chemotherapy at the time of radiation is being evaluated. In patients who have had previous irradiation, pelvic exenteration can be considered for those with an isolated central recurrence.

## Chemotherapy for Advanced and Recurrent Uterine Serous Carcinoma

For a majority of the trials, USCs were included among all patients with advanced or recurrent endometrial cancer except for a trial by Fader and colleagues (2018) for advanced of recurrent, chemotherapy-naive patients with uterine serous cancer. This trial evaluated the addition of trastuzumab to carboplatin/paclitaxel compared with paclitaxel and carboplatin alone. **The addition of trastuzumab significantly improved PFS. The greatest benefit was seen in the 41 patients with stage III or IV HER2/neu-positive USC undergoing primary treatment (9.3 vs. 17.9 months; *P* = .013; hazard ratio [HR], 0.40; 90% confidence interval [CI], 0.20 to 0.80).** A smaller benefit was seen in patients with recurrent USC who had received one or two prior lines of treatment (n = 17; 83% 9.2 vs. 6.0 months; HR, 0.14; 90% CI, 0.05 to 0.54; *P* = .003), although overall survival data are still immature.

## Hormone Therapy

### Progestins for Advanced or Recurrent Disease

For the past 50 years, progestational agents have been valuable in the armamentarium against endometrial cancer, particularly in patients with recurrent disease. Progestins are well tolerated; side effects are usually minor and include weight gain, edema, thrombophlebitis, headache, and occasionally hypertension. In patients with medical comorbidities, use of hormonal agents may be preferable to cytotoxic chemotherapy. Initial clinical trials in patients with advanced or recurrent endometrial cancer demonstrated response rates of 30% to 50%. Larger studies with more specific response criteria reported more modest response rates, usually between 11% and 24%. Podratz and colleagues treated 155 patients with advanced or recurrent endometrial cancer with progesterone. The objective response rate was 11%. Overall, survival after initiation of hormone therapy was 40% at 1 year, 19% at 2 years, and 8% at 5 years. In a GOG phase II study, patients who had no previous exposure to chemotherapy or hormonal agents were treated with megestrol acetate (800 mg/day). The overall response rate was 24%. The PFS and overall survival were 2.5 months and 7.6 months, respectively.

Recommendations for progestin therapy include oral medroxyprogesterone acetate (Provera), intramuscular medroxyprogesterone acetate (Depo-Provera), and megestrol acetate (Megace). Although no randomized studies have directly compared different formulations of progestins, response rates are similar. In addition, although a dose-response effect of progestin therapy has been reported in patients with breast cancer, there is no evidence of this effect in patients with endometrial cancer. In a randomized trial of oral medroxyprogesterone acetate, patients receiving the low-dose regimen (200 mg/day) had a higher response to therapy than those receiving the high-dose regimen (1000 mg/day).

A number of tumor characteristics increase the likelihood of response to hormone therapy. These include low-grade tumors, the presence of steroid hormone receptors (i.e., tumors that are progesterone receptor [PR] and estrogen receptor [ER] positive), and a longer disease-free interval. The GOG demonstrated a response rate of 8% in women whose tumors were PR negative and 37% for women whose tumors were PR positive. In addition, there was a 7% response rate in women with ER-negative tumors compared with a 26% response rate in women with ER-positive tumors. Patients with poorly differentiated tumors or hormone receptor–negative tumors have significantly lower response rates to progestin therapy.

Because of the low toxicity profile and modest efficacy, progestins should be considered in patients with recurrent endometrial cancer. In particular, all patients not eligible for clinical trials with well-differentiated hormone receptor–positive recurrent or advanced disease can be given a trial of progestin therapy. If the patient has an objective response, the progestin may be continued indefinitely until there is disease progression.



#### Selective Estrogen Receptor Modulators and Aromatase Inhibitors

SERMs with antiestrogenic effects in the uterus have been used to treat women with recurrent endometrial cancer. First-generation SERMs such as tamoxifen have mixed estrogenic agonist and antagonist activity. Early response rates for tamoxifen in advanced or recurrent endometrial cancer were between 20% and 36%; however, in a GOG phase II study of tamoxifen given at a dose of 20 mg twice daily, only 10% of patients demonstrated an objective response. Grade 1 and 2 tumors were more likely to respond to tamoxifen than grade 3 tumors.

Short-term administration of tamoxifen can cause an increase in the progesterone receptor levels in postmenopausal women with endometrial cancer. Studies with alternating tamoxifen and progestins have been performed to determine whether this upregulation increases the response to progestin therapy. **Phase II trials of tamoxifen plus alternating cycles of progestin demonstrated a 27% to 33% response rate.** The Eastern Cooperative Oncology Group found no difference in response rates between patients treated with progestin alone and those treated with progestin in combination with tamoxifen.

Anastrozole, an oral nonsteroidal aromatase inhibitor, is approved by the U.S. Food and Drug Administration for postmenopausal women with progressive breast cancer after tamoxifen therapy. Aromatase is elevated in the stroma of endometrial cancer. In a phase II trial by the GOG, anastrozole was found to have minimal activity (9% response rate) in an unselected population of patients with advanced or recurrent endometrial cancer. More than 25% of the patients in this study had nonendometrioid histologic subtypes, and only 22% of the patients had ER- and PR-positive tumors or demonstrated a response to previous therapy. In the subset of women with FIGO grade 1 and 2 tumors with endometrioid histologic type, the response rate was 30%.

## Targeted Therapy

Several molecular aberrations are commonly seen in endometrioid adenocarcinomas, the most common being abnormalities in the PTEN/AKT pathway, and a number of clinical trials exploiting this pathway have shown promising results in women with recurrent endometrial cancer. Several studies have found efficacy for mTOR inhibitors, including temsirolimus, everolimus, and ridaforolimus, in endometrial cancer recurrence. In the first-line setting, response rates have been 9% to 24%, with clinical benefit rates up to 90%. **Combining agents such as everolimus and letrozole produced a reported response rate of 31% with a median duration of response of 12.5 months (Slomovitz, 2015).** The GOG has an ongoing study comparing this combination with tamoxifen alternating with megestrol acetate, which is considered the standard hormonal regimen.

## Immunotherapy

There has been an increasing interest in the role of immunotherapy across cancer types, and responses rates and duration of responses have been remarkable in nongynecologic cancers. **Approximately 20% of endometrial cancers are thought to have mismatch repair deficiency or MSI.** In 2017 the U.S. Food and Drug Administration (FDA) granted accelerated approval to pembrolizumab (anti–PD-1) for mismatch repair (MMR)–deficient solid tumors that progressed after prior treatment. In a single-arm, phase II trial of MMR–deficient noncolorectal cancer, the response rate to pembrolizumab was 71%, with an immune-related PFR rate of 67% at 20 weeks. In a separate study, 3 out of 8 patients with MMR-deficient endometrial cancers (37%) demonstrated an objective response to single-agent avelumab (Konstantinopolous, 2019). The KEYNOTE-028 phase IB trial reported a 13% partial response rate in 24 patients with pretreated PD-L1–positive endometrial cancer, with the median duration of response not reached, and an additional 13% with prolonged stable disease, with a median duration of response of 25 weeks (Ott, 2017).

**In September 2019 the FDA approved combination pembrolizumab and lenvatinib for the treatment of recurrent endometrial cancer without MSI-H or mismatch repair deficiency (dMMR) (Makkar, 2019). Objective response rates were nearly 40% at 24 weeks in patients who had received up to two prior therapies for recurrence.** Numerous ongoing studies are evaluating the role of immunotherapy in combination with chemotherapy and in the maintenance setting after front-line therapy in advanced or recurrent disease.

## SARCOMAS

Sarcomas comprise less than 5% of uterine malignancies and are much less common than endometrial carcinomas, particularly in Western countries. Numerous terms have been used to describe the many histologic types. One useful classification is based on determination of the resemblance of the sarcomatous elements to mesenchymal tissue normally found in the uterus (homologous sarcomas) in contrast to tissues foreign to the uterus (heterologous sarcomas). Homologous types include leiomyosarcoma, endometrial stromal sarcoma (ESS), and, rarely, angiosarcoma. Heterologous types include rhabdomyosarcoma, chondrosarcoma, osteosarcoma, and liposarcoma. These sarcomas may exist exclusively or may be admixed with epithelial adenocarcinoma, in which case the term *carcinosarcoma* (malignant mixed müllerian tumor) is applied. Box 32.3 shows a morphologic classification for uterine sarcomas. A study by Zelmanowicz and colleagues suggested that risk factors for these tumors are similar to those of endometrial carcinoma—that is, estrogens and obesity increase the risk, and oral contraceptive use decreases the risk. No uniformly defined staging criteria exist for these tumors, and the most widely used definitions are similar to those for endometrial carcinoma: stage I, confined to the corpus; stage II, corpus and cervix involved; stage III, spread outside the uterus but confined to the pelvis or retroperitoneal lymph nodes; and stage IV, spread outside the true pelvis or into the mucosa of the bladder or rectum. **Similar to endometrial adenocarcinoma, operative stage is the most important predictor of survival.**

### BOX 32.3 Modified Classification of Uterine Sarcomas

I. Pure sarcoma
  A. Homologous
    1. Smooth muscle tumors
      a. Leiomyosarcoma
      b. Leiomyoblastoma
      c. Metastasizing tumors with benign histologic appearance
        i. Intravenous leiomyomatosis
        ii. Metastasizing uterine leiomyoma
        iii. Leiomyomatosis peritonealis disseminata
    2. Endometrial stromal sarcomas
      a. Low grade: endolymphatic stromal myosis
      b. High grade: endometrial stromal sarcoma
  B. Heterologous
    1. Rhabdomyosarcoma
    2. Chondrosarcoma
    3. Osteosarcoma
    4. Liposarcoma
  C. Other sarcomas
II. Carcinosarcoma—malignant mixed müllerian tumors
  A. Homologous (carcinosarcoma): carcinoma + homologous sarcoma
  B. Heterologous: carcinoma + heterologous sarcoma
III. Müllerian adenosarcoma
IV. Lymphoma

Modified from Clemet P, Scully RE. Pathology of uterine sarcomas. In Coppleson M, ed. *Gynecologic Oncology.* New York: Churchill Livingstone; 1981:591. Reprinted with permission.

## Leiomyosarcoma

Leiomyosarcomas represent 1% to 2% of uterine malignancies and approximately one-third of uterine sarcomas (Fig. 32.10). Although the exact cause is unknown, leiomyosarcomas are not thought to arise from benign leiomyomas. Leibsohn and coworkers noted that among 1423 patients who had hysterectomies for presumed leiomyomas with a uterine size comparable to a 12-week pregnancy or larger, the risk of sarcoma increased with age, from 0.4% for those in their 30s to 1.4% for those in their 50s. The determination of malignancy is made in part by ascertaining the number of mitoses in 10 high-power fields (HPF) and by the presence of cytologic atypia, abnormal mitotic figures, and nuclear pleomorphism (see Fig. 32.10). Vascular invasion and extrauterine spread of tumor are associated with worse prognoses. A finding of more than 5 mitoses per 10 HPF with cytologic atypia leads to a diagnosis of leiomyosarcoma; when there are four or fewer mitoses per 10 HPF, the tumors usually have a more benign clinical course. The prognosis worsens for tumors with more than 10 mitoses per 10 HPF. The presence of bizarre cells may not necessarily establish the diagnosis because they can occasionally be seen in benign leiomyomas and in patients receiving progestational agents. Furthermore, it is important to note that an increase in mitotic count in leiomyomas occurs in pregnancy and during oral contraceptive use. This can occasionally cause confusion in the histologic diagnosis.

Usually the patient has an enlarged pelvic mass, occasionally accompanied by pain or vaginal bleeding. Approximately 85% of

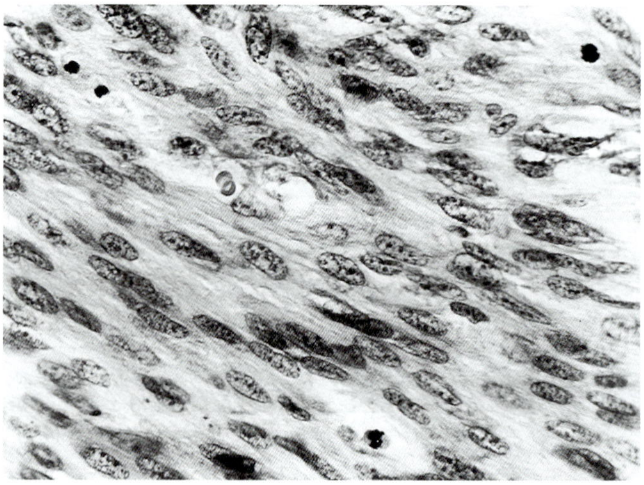

**Fig. 32.10** Leiomyosarcoma. Nuclear hyperchromatism and mitotic figures are present. (Original magnification ×660.) (From Clement PB, Scully RE. Pathology of uterine sarcomas. In Coppleson M, ed. *Gynecologic Oncology.* Edinburgh: Churchill Livingstone; 1981. Reprinted with permission.)

women diagnosed with a leiomyosarcoma have clinical stage I or II disease (i.e., disease that is limited to the uterus and cervix). The risk of lymph node involvement is very low. Primary treatment includes total hysterectomy, bilateral salpingo-oophorectomy, and staging. **Despite the low incidence of high-stage disease, approximately 50% of patients have a recurrence within 2 years.** The recurrence in most of these patients is outside the pelvis.

The GOG evaluated the role of adjuvant radiation therapy in patients (N = 48) with clinical stage I and II disease. There was no difference in the progression-free interval, absolute 2-year survival rate, or site of first recurrence between patients who received pelvic radiation (N = 11) and those who did not (N = 37). This is not surprising because most recurrences were outside the pelvis (83%). There was recurrence in 48% of the patients, and most of these patients had a recurrence within 17 months of diagnosis. In the adjuvant chemotherapy trial by the GOG, patients treated with doxorubicin had fewer recurrences than those in the observation arm (44% vs. 61%); however, this difference was not statistically significant. There is no known benefit to adjuvant radiation or chemotherapy in women with leiomyosarcoma limited to the uterus.

Several studies have evaluated treatment of advanced or recurrent leiomyosarcoma. Hannigan and colleagues used vincristine, actinomycin D, and cyclophosphamide (Cytoxan) (VAC) and noted a 13% complete response rate and 16% partial response rate in 74 patients with advanced metastatic uterine sarcomas. A large collaborative trial was conducted by the GOG and reported by Omura and associates. The best responses were obtained for patients with lung metastases who received doxorubicin and dacarbazine (DTIC). Evidence suggests that a multidrug program offers the greatest response for these patients. Cisplatin, doxorubicin, paclitaxel, ifosfamide, and etoposide (VP-16) all appear to have some effectiveness. Gemcitabine and docetaxel have been evaluated in a phase II study for patients with recurrent leiomyosarcoma. In this study, 34 patients with leiomyosarcoma were treated. The overall response rate was 53%; however, the duration of response was only 5.6 months. This regimen is used commonly for advanced and recurrent disease. A phase III study completed by the GOG failed to show any benefit to the addition of bevacizumab to gemcitabine and docetaxel in the treatment of this disease.

## Endometrial Stromal Sarcoma

Overall, stromal tumors comprise approximately 10% of uterine sarcomas. Their behavior correlates primarily with mitotic rate. These tumors are divided into low grade and high grade. Prognosis depends on the extent of disease and ability to remove the entire tumor at the time of surgery. A large National Cancer Database Study suggested that women with low-grade tumors have a significantly better prognosis than those with high-grade tumors Seagle, 207. In addition, a subset of women with high endometrial stromal sarcomas may benefit from adjuvant therapy after surgery, even in disease confined to the uterus.

Low-grade ESS tends to recur locally in the pelvis or peritoneal cavity and often spreads to the lungs. In treating metastatic disease, it should be remembered that these tumors can contain estrogen and progestin steroid hormone receptors and may be sensitive to hormone therapy. Complete resolution has been reported with megestrol acetate, medroxyprogesterone (Provera), letrozole (Femara), tamoxifen, and 17α-hydroxyprogesterone caproate (Delalutin).

## Carcinosarcoma (Malignant Mixed Müllerian Tumors)

As shown in Box 32.3, carcinosarcomas consist of both carcinoma and sarcoma elements native to the uterus and may resemble the endometrial stroma of smooth muscle (homologous) or of sarcomatous tissues foreign to the uterus (heterologous). Spanos and colleagues reviewed 188 patients with mixed mesodermal tumor and found both the prognosis and the pattern of survival similar for both homologous and heterologous tumors. The study of George and coworkers showed that patients with these tumors had a markedly worse prognosis than patients with high-grade endometrial carcinomas. Unlike patients with endometrial stromal sarcoma or leiomyosarcoma, those with carcinosarcoma tend to be older and primarily postmenopausal, usually older than age 62 years. Previous pelvic irradiation has been identified as an occasional predisposing factor and was experienced by 17 of the 136 patients reviewed by Norris and Taylor. The heterologous and homologous tumors occur with approximately equivalent frequency. These tumors can spread locally into the myometrium and pelvis or distally to the abdominal cavity, lungs and pleura, a pattern similar to the spread of endometrial carcinoma.

A common symptom is postmenopausal bleeding, often accompanied by an enlarged uterus. Occasionally the diagnosis is made using tissue removed by D&C, and the tumor may appear to be a polypoid mass protruding through the cervix.

As is true for other sarcomas, the primary treatment is surgical removal of the uterus. The extent of the tumor and the depth of myometrial invasion are important prognostic factors. Those with deep myometrial invasion are more likely to have spread to pelvic or paraaortic nodes. Patients with tumors confined to the uterus and little or no myometrial spread have the best prognosis. A comprehensive surgical staging procedure is recommended for all patients with this diagnosis. Nielsen and coworkers reported a 5-year survival rate of 58% for these when the disease was confined to the uterus.

In a phase I/II study of ifosfamide and cisplatin as adjuvant therapy in patients with high-stage carcinosarcoma, the GOG found this combination to be tolerable. Progression-free and overall survival rates at 2 years were 69% and 82%, respectively. For patients with advanced or recurrent disease, the GOG evaluated ifosfamide versus ifosfamide and cisplatin in a phase III randomized study. The response rate to the combination therapy was superior (54% vs. 36%); however, the toxicity was significantly higher. In addition, no significant difference in overall survival was seen. A follow-up study compared ifosfamide with ifosfamide and paclitaxel in a phase III randomized study. Response rates in the combination arm were superior (45% vs. 29%), but more importantly there was a significant difference in overall survival (13 months vs. 8 months). Finally, a phase II study showed efficacy of paclitaxel and carboplatin in women with advanced or recurrent carcinosarcoma with an overall response rate of 54% using this well-tolerated regimen (Powell, 2010). Paclitaxel and carboplatin is the standard treatment for women with carcinosarcoma.

## Müllerian Adenosarcoma

Müllerian adenosarcoma is a rare low-grade malignancy composed of both a sarcomatous stroma (homologous) and a proliferation of benign glandular elements that are intimately associated. It occurs predominantly in women older than 60 years. Total abdominal hysterectomy with bilateral salpingo-oophorectomy is the treatment of choice. Mitotic index and sarcomatous overgrowth are related to prognosis.

### REFERENCES

Aghajanian C, Sill MW, Darcy KM, et al. Phase II trial of bevacizumab in recurrent or persistent endometrial cancer: a Gynecologic Oncology Group study. *J Clin Oncol.* 2011;29:2259-2265.

Broaddus RR, Lu KH. Women with HNPCC: a target population for the chemoprevention of gynecologic cancers. *Front Biosci.* 2006;11:207-280.

Creutzberg CL, van Putten WLJ, Kiper PCM, et al. Surgery and postoperative radiotherapy versus surgery alone for patients with stage-1 endometrial carcinoma: Multicentre randomised trial. *Lancet.* 2000; 355:1404.

de Boer SM, Powell ME, Mileshkin L, et al. Adjuvant chemoradiotherapy versus radiotherapy alone in women with high-risk endometrial cancer (PORTEC-3): patterns of recurrence and post-hoc survival analysis of a randomised phase 3 trial. *Lancet Oncol.* 2019;20:1273-1285.

Dowdy SC, Borah BJ, Bakkum-Gamez JN, et al. Prospective assessment of survival, morbidity, and cost associated with lymphadenectomy in low-risk endometrial cancer. *Gynecol Oncol.* 2012;127:5-10.

Fader AN, Santin AD, Gehrig PA. Early stage uterine serous carcinoma: management updates and genomic advances. *Gynecol Oncol.* 2013;129: 244-250.

Fader AN, Roque DM, Siegel E, et al. Randomized phase II trial of carboplatin-paclitaxel versus carboplatin-paclitaxel-trastuzumab in uterine serous carcinomas that overexpress human epidermal growth factor receptor 2/neu. *J Clin Oncol.* 2018;36:2044-2051.

Hamilton CA, Cheung MK, Osann K, Chen L, Teng NN, et al. Uterine papillary serous and clear cell carcinomas predict for poorer survival compared to grade 3 endometroid corpus cancers. *Br J Cancer*. 2006 Mar 13;94(5):642-646. doi: 10.1038/sj.bjc.6603012. PMID: 16495918.

Janda M, Gebski V, Davies LC, et al. Effect of total laparoscopic hysterectomy vs total abdominal hysterectomy on disease-free survival among women with stage I endometrial cancer: a randomized clinical trial. *JAMA.* 2017;317:1224-1233.

Keys HM, Roberts JA, Brunetto VL, et al. A phase III trial of surgery with or without adjunctive external pelvic radiation therapy in intermediate risk endometrial adenocarcinoma: a Gynecologic Oncology Group study. *Gynecol Oncol.* 2004;92:744-751.

Konstantinopoulos PA, Luo W, Liu JF, Gulhan DC, Krasner C, et al. Phase II study of Avelumab in patients with mismatch repair deficient and mismatch repair proficient recurrent/persistent endometrial cancer. *J Clin Oncol.* 2019 Oct 20;37(30):2786-2794. doi: 10.1200/JCO.19.01021. Epub 2019 Aug 28. PMID: 31461377.

Lacey Jr JV, Sherman ME, Rush BB, et al. Absolute risk of endometrial carcinoma during 20-year follow-up among women with endometrial hyperplasia. *J Clin Oncol.* 2010;28(5):788-792.

Levine D, Getz G, Gabriel S. et al. Integrated genomic characterization of endometrial carcinoma. *Nature.* 2013;497:67-73.

Lincoln S, Blessing JA, Lee RB, Rocereto TF. Activity of paclitaxel as second-line chemotherapy in endometrial carcinoma: a Gynecologic Oncology Group study. *Gynecol Oncol.* 2003;88:277-281.

Makker V, Rasco D, Vogelzang NJ, et al. Lenvatinib plus pembrolizumab in patients with advanced endometrial cancer: an interim analysis of a multicentre, open-label, single-arm, phase 2 trial. *Lancet Oncol.* 2019;20:711-718.

Miller D, Filiaci V, Fleming G, et al. Randomized phase III noninferiority trial of first line chemotherapy for metastatic or recurrent endometrial carcinoma: a Gynecologic Oncology Group study. *Gynecol Oncol.* 2012;125:771-773.

Ott PA, Bang YJ, Berton-Rigaud D, et al. Safety and antitumor activity of pembrolizumab in advanced programmed death ligand 1-positive endometrial cancer: results from the KEYNOTE-028 study. *J Clin Oncol.* 2017;35:2535-2541.

Pal N, Broaddus RR, Urbauer DL, et al. Treatment of low-risk endometrial cancer and complex atypical hyperplasia with the levonorgestrel-releasing intrauterine device. *Obstet Gynecol.* 2018;131(1):109-116.

Powell MA, Filiaci VL, Rose PG, et al. Phase II evaluation of paclitaxel and carboplatin in the treatment of carcinosarcoma of the uterus: a Gynecologic Oncology Group study. *J Clin Oncol.* 2010;28(16):2727-2731.

Rajkumar S, Nath R, Lane G, Mehra G, Begum S, Sayasneh A. Advanced state (IIIC/IV) endometrial cancer: role of cytoreduction and determinants of survival. *Eur J Obstet Gynecol Reprod Biol.* 2019 Mar;234:26-31. doi: 10.1016/j.ejogrb.2018.11.029. Epub 2018 Dec 21. PMID: 30639953.

Rossi EC, Kowalski LD, Scalici J, et al. A comparison of sentinel lymph node biopsy to lymphadenectomy for endometrial cancer staging (FIRES trial): a multicentre, prospective, cohort study. *Lancet Oncol.* 2017;18:384-392.

Schmeler KM, Lynch HT, Chen LM, et al. Prophylactic surgery to reduce the risk of gynecologic cancers in the Lynch syndrome. *N Engl J Med.* 2006;354:261-269.

Seagle BL, Shilpi A, Buchanan S, Goodman C, Shahabi S. Low-grade and high-grade endometrial stromal sarcoma: A National Cancer Database study. *Gynecol Oncol.* 2017;146:254-262.

Shih KK, Yun E, Gardner GJ, Barakat RR, Chi DS, Leitao MM Jr. Surgical cytoreduction in stage IV endometrioid endometrial carcinoma. *Gynecol Oncol.* 2011 Sep;122(3):608-611. doi: 10.1016/j.ygyno.2011.05.020. Epub 2011 Jun 12. PMID: 21664663.

Slomovitz BM, Jiang Y, Yates MS, et al. Phase II study of everolimus and letrozole in patients with recurrent endometrial carcinoma. *J Clin Oncol.* 2015;33(8):930-936.

Soliman PT, Westin SN, Dioun S, et al. A prospective validation study of sentinel lymph node mapping for high-risk endometrial cancer. *Gynecol Oncol.* 2017;146:234-239.

Stewart KI, Chasen B, Erwin W, et al. Preoperative PET/CT does not accurately detect extrauterine disease in patients with newly diagnosed high-risk endometrial cancer: a prospective study. *Cancer.* 2019;125(19): 3347-3353.

Walker, JL, Piedmonte MR, Spirtos NM, et al. Laparoscopy compared with laparotomy for comprehensive surgical staging of uterine cancer: Gynecologic Oncology Group Study LAP2. *J Clin Oncol.* 2009;27(32): 5331-5336.

**Suggested readings for this chapter can be found on ExpertConsult.com**

# 33 Malignant Diseases of the Ovary, Fallopian Tube, and Peritoneum

*Robert L. Coleman, Shannon N. Westin, Pedro T. Ramirez, Gloria Salvo, David M. Gershenson*

## KEY POINTS

- Ovarian cancer is the leading cause of death from gynecologic cancer, but it occurs less often than endometrial cancers.
- Ovarian cancers in women older than 50 years are diagnosed at a more advanced stage, leading to a worse prognosis than for younger women.
- The risk of ovarian cancer is decreased by oral contraceptive use. Tubal ligation and hysterectomy also appear to decrease the risk.
- The normal postmenopausal ovary is approximately 1.5 to 2 cm in diameter.
- A cystic adnexal mass smaller than 8 cm in diameter in a menstruating female is most commonly functional.
- A vaginal ultrasound finding of a unilocular cyst of 5 cm or smaller in a perimenopausal woman can usually be followed without surgical intervention.
- Ovarian cancer risk rises from approximately 1.4% in general to 5% to 7% if the woman has one or two first- or second-degree relatives with ovarian cancer.
- There is no known effective screening for ovarian cancer.
- Risk-reducing surgery is an option for women at high risk for ovarian cancer.
- Patients with ovarian cancer are at increased risk of developing breast cancer and endometrial cancer.
- Genetic testing and tissue-based testing are recommended for all patients diagnosed with epithelial ovarian cancer. Approximately 15% to 18% of patients with high-grade serous carcinoma will have a germline *BRCA* mutation. In addition, of those who test negative for a germline *BRCA* mutation, 5% to 7% will be positive for a somatic *BRCA* mutation on tissue-based testing.
- It is important that the follow-up of ovarian cancer patients includes monitoring for breast cancer.
- Epithelial tumors are the most common ovarian neoplasm. They account for two-thirds of all ovarian neoplasms and 85% of ovarian cancers.
- The major ovarian epithelial ovarian cancer subtypes are high-grade serous (the most common), mucinous, clear cell, endometrioid, and low-grade serous.
- The risk of an ovarian tumor being malignant is approximately 33% in a woman older than 45, whereas it is less than 1 in 15 for those aged 20 to 45. More than 50% of ovarian cancers occur in women older than 50.
- Most ovarian carcinomas start from small microscopic foci and spread throughout the peritoneum before becoming clinically evident (de novo origin), especially serous and poorly differentiated tumors.
- Ovarian carcinomas having a cystic origin are primary mucinous or endometrioid and are more likely to be discovered at an early stage.
- Most ovarian carcinomas are diagnosed in stage III or IV.
- The primary distribution spread of epithelial carcinoma is transcoelomic to the visceral and parietal peritoneum, diaphragm, and retroperitoneal nodes.
- The risk of retroperitoneal node spread of epithelial carcinoma in apparent stage I cases is greatest for poorly differentiated tumors, for which the risk can reach 10% to 20%. The risk of retroperitoneal node spread increases in higher-stage cases.
- The prognosis of a patient with ovarian epithelial carcinoma is related primarily to tumor stage and tumor grade and to the amount of residual tumor remaining after primary resection.
- Laparoscopic or robotic staging of early ovarian cancers appears to be feasible without compromising survival, based on retrospective data.
- For women with apparent metastatic ovarian cancer, diagnostic laparoscopy can be used to determine those patients who benefit most from primary cytoreductive surgery versus neoadjuvant chemotherapy followed by interval cytoreductive surgery.
- Optimal surgical debulking (R0-microscopic residual) appears to confer a survival advantage in cases of stages III and IV ovarian carcinoma.
- Systematic pelvic and paraaortic lymph node dissection in advanced ovarian cancer is not beneficial based on randomized clinical trials.
- Interval cytoreduction has little additional effect on overall survival if a maximal attempt is made at primary surgery.
- Neoadjuvant chemotherapy can reduce surgical morbidity; randomized trials have indicated that this strategy may be equivalent to standard treatment for advanced-stage patients with surgery followed by chemotherapy.
- Minimally invasive surgery for interval cytoreductive surgery should not be performed outside a clinical trial.
- Hyperthermic intraperitoneal chemotherapy (HIPEC) should not be recommended outside a clinical trial for primary or recurrence treatment.
- The addition of HIPEC to interval debulking surgery is associated with longer recurrence-free and overall survival compared with surgery plus conventional chemotherapy.
- Assessing the ovarian CA-125 level is useful to help monitor patients with ovarian carcinoma. Reaction to the antigen is positive in approximately 80% of cases.
- A rapid decrease in CA-125 values after treatment indicates a more favorable prognosis.
- More than 80% of patients with epithelial ovarian cancer will be disease free at the completion of primary chemotherapy. Initial treatment usually includes a combination of platinum and taxane agents.
- PARP inhibitors have demonstrated efficacy in epithelial ovarian cancer patients in both the treatment and maintenance settings.
- Recurrent ovarian cancer is difficult to cure.
- Factors determining response to recurrent chemotherapy regimens include time to treatment progression, distribution and volume of disease, and performance status.
- Bevacizumab tends to augment the activity of platinum-based chemotherapy in the frontline and recurrent (both platinum-sensitive and platinum-resistant) settings.
- Secondary cytoreductive surgery may be of benefit only in select patients with prolonged disease-free interval, single site of disease, no evidence of carcinomatosis, and optimal cytoreduction at initial primary surgery.
- The 5-year survival rate for patients with borderline epithelial ovarian carcinoma (grade 0) is close to 100% for stage I and more than 90% for all stages.

*Continued*

## KEY POINTS—cont'd

- Germ cell tumors are the second most common type of ovarian neoplasms and account for approximately 20% to 25% of all ovarian tumors.
- In women younger than 30 years, the most common ovarian neoplasm is a germ cell tumor; approximately one-third of these germ cell tumors are malignant in those younger than 21. For women younger than 30 years, the most common ovarian neoplasm is the dermoid.
- The most common germ cell tumor is the benign cystic teratoma (dermoid). It is bilateral in 10% to 15% of the cases. Approximately 30% are calcified.
- Malignant germ cell tumors are usually unilateral except dysgerminomas, which are bilateral in approximately 10% to 15% of patients.
- Dysgerminomas are the most common malignant germ cell tumors and account for 1% to 2% of ovarian cancers.
- The prognosis for a patient with an immature teratoma is related to tumor grade and tumor stage. These tumors are the second most common type of malignant germ cell tumor.
- The 5-year survival rate of stage IA pure dysgerminoma treated by unilateral salpingo-oophorectomy is more than 90%.
- Pure dysgerminomas are radiocurable; however, multiagent chemotherapy, particularly with etoposide and platinum, with or without bleomycin, will often result in complete remission. Approximately two-thirds of cases present as stage IA.
- Most patients with malignant ovarian germ cell tumors can be treated successfully with fertility-sparing surgery followed by bleomycin, etoposide, and cisplatin (BEP) chemotherapy. Patients who do not require postoperative chemotherapy include those with stage IA dysgerminoma and stage IA, grade 1, immature teratoma; however, there has been a trend toward surveillance rather than chemotherapy for patients with stage I tumors of any histologic subtype.
- Multiagent chemotherapy has improved survival in patients with malignant germ cell tumors, preserving childbearing function in most cases. Standard chemotherapy consists of the BEP regimen.
- Gonadoblastomas are sex cord–stromal germ cell tumors that usually arise in dysgenetic gonads in patients with a Y chromosome; these are cured by removal.
- Granulosa cell tumors and Sertoli-Leydig tumors usually behave as low-grade malignancies, but there may be late recurrences.
- For patients with primary metastatic or recurrent sex cord–stromal tumors of the ovary, platinum-based chemotherapy is the treatment of choice. Commonly used regimens include BEP and paclitaxel-carboplatin.
- Some metastatic granulosa cell tumors may respond to hormone therapy, such as leuprolide acetate, tamoxifen, or aromatase inhibitors.
- Fibroma is the most common benign solid ovarian tumor.
- The most common sites of origin of tumors metastatic to the ovary are the lower reproductive tract, gastrointestinal tract, and breast.
- There is increasing evidence that many cases of ovarian and peritoneal carcinoma may actually arise from the fallopian tube, thereby underestimating the incidence of fallopian tube carcinoma.
- Fallopian tube and peritoneal cancers have similar clinical characteristics, patterns of spread, and response to treatment compared with ovarian cancer.
- The primary risk factor for fallopian tube and peritoneal cancer is an inherited mutation in the *BRCA1* or *BRCA2* tumor suppressor gene.
- The most common histologic subtype of fallopian tube and peritoneal carcinoma is high-grade serous carcinoma.
- The treatment of fallopian tube and peritoneal cancer is identical to that for ovarian cancer and typically includes a combination of surgery and chemotherapy.

Ovarian cancer is the second most common malignancy of the lower part of the female genital tract, occurring less often than cancers of the endometrium but more often than cancers of the cervix; however, it is the most common cause of death from gynecologic neoplasms in the United States. Cancer Statistics 2019 has reported that approximately 22,530 new cases of ovarian cancer will be diagnosed yearly in the United States, and there will be 13,980 deaths (Siegel, 2019). A major contributing factor to the high death rate from the relatively few cases stems from the frequent detection of the disease after metastatic spread, when symptoms direct clinical investigation or raise clinical concern. Surprisingly, most women diagnosed with ovarian cancer do report symptoms for months before diagnosis. As detailed later, only the severity and duration of symptoms differentially segregate cancer patients from noncancer patients. The incidence of ovarian cancer (Fig. 33.1) increases with age, becoming most marked beyond 50 years, with a gradual increase continuing to age 70 years followed by a decrease for those older than 80. Previous studies have noted that those older than 65 are more likely to have their cancers diagnosed at an advanced stage, leading to a worse prognosis and poorer survival compared with those younger than 65 years. Although much of the demographic information regarding this disease has been static over the past several decades, a remarkable trend of increasing prevalence has been noted. Surveillance, Epidemiology, and End Results (SEER) estimates of disease prevalence for 2015 suggest more than 225,000 women are currently alive with ovarian cancer in the United States (Howlader, 2019). Successful incorporation of new treatment and specialized care are believed to be driving this metric.

Despite numerous epidemiologic investigations, a clear-cut cause of ovarian cancer has not been defined. A number of theories, particularly those associated with ovulation (e.g., parity, breastfeeding, hormonal contraception, infertility), have been previously supported. Because certain forms of hormonal manipulation of ovulation have been associated with a substantially reduced lifetime risk of ovarian cancer, even among those carrying a germline mutation in *BRCA1* or *BRCA2*, an ovarian epithelial origin has been suggested; however, salpingectomy and tubal ligation are also associated with a reduced risk of ovarian cancer, and direct transitions from benign to malignant states have been difficult to demonstrate in ovarian surface epithelia and inclusion cysts. More recently, focus has been placed on transitional states in the fallopian tube, particularly for the most common histologic type, high-grade serous ovarian cancer (HGSOC). Next-generation sequencing of primary HGSOCs reported in the Cancer Genome Atlas (TCGA) demonstrate that nearly all these tumors have a mutation in *TP53*. Similar findings were reported in detailed analyses of serous tubal intraepithelial carcinomas (STICs) found in the normal-appearing fallopian tubes of unaffected women undergoing risk-reducing salpingo-oophorectomy. In these studies microinvasive tubal lesions were also identified, providing a serial link of an acquired p53 signature in normal noninvasive tissue to transformed cells migrating to the ovarian

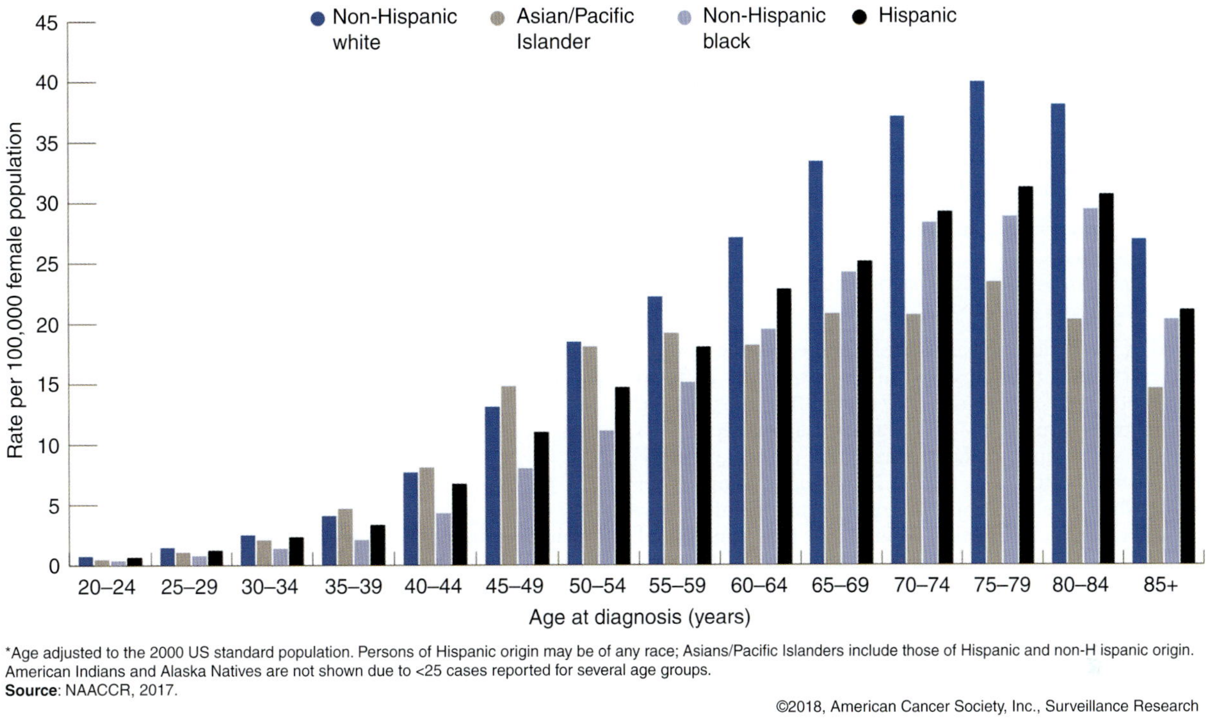


**Fig. 33.1** Epithelial ovarian cancer incidence rates by age and race, United States, 2010 to 2014. (From *Cancer Facts and Figures, 2018: Special Section: Ovarian Cancer.* Atlanta: American Cancer Society; 2018:33.)

surface and peritoneal cavity with invasion. In further investigation from Labidi-Galy and colleagues, they performed whole-exome sequencing and copy number analyses of laser-captured microdissected STICs, invasive fallopian tube and ovarian cancers, and metastases from nine patients. Interestingly, tumor-specific alterations in *TP53*, *PTEN*, and *BRCA1/2* were present in most of the samples, and functional evaluation of the sample supported the precursor status of these lesions and the development of invasive disease. It was estimated from this work that an evolutionary window of about 7 years separated the events. Even more recently, though, primary ovarian epithelial cells were found to produce STIC-like lesions in the ovary primarily under controlled gene expression (Zhang, 2019). This field continues to evolve as multiomics investigations continue to describe ovarian carcinogenesis. Other traditional risk factors, including smoking, benign ovarian diseases such as polycystic ovarian syndrome, pelvic inflammatory disease, and endometriosis, continue to provide clues to carcinogenesis, including the most strongly linked, family or personal history of ovarian/breast cancer or known germline mutation of *BRCA1/2*. Table 33.1 lists the various epidemiologic factors that are thought to alter ovarian cancer risk.

**TABLE 33.1** Putative Associations of Increasing and Decreasing Risks of Ovarian Epithelial Carcinoma

| Increases | Decreases |
|---|---|
| Age | Breast-feeding |
| Diet | Oral contraceptives |
| Family history | Pregnancy |
| Industrialized country | Tubal ligation and hysterectomy, with ovarian conservation |
| Infertility | |
| Nulliparity | |
| Ovulation | |
| Ovulatory drugs | |
| Talc (?) | |

From Herbst AL. The epidemiology of ovarian carcinoma and the current status of tumor markers to detect disease. *Am J Obstet Gynecol.* 1994;170(4):1099-1105.

## FAMILIAL OVARIAN CANCER

In a case-control study, Hartge and colleagues showed that a familial history of breast cancer and a personal history of breast cancer are ovarian cancer risk factors. Lynch and associates reported on families with these hereditary ovarian cancers and noted that they tend to occur at a younger age than in the general population. It appears that germline mutations of the *BRCA* tumor suppressor gene on chromosome 17q are responsible for a large proportion of hereditary cancers (discussed later); however, these are a small proportion of all ovarian carcinomas. Risk alteration in these patients through oral contraceptive use is of uncertain impact. Narod and coworkers suggested that it might be possible to reduce incident risk by their administration; however, Modan and colleagues conducted a case-control study of Jewish women in whom *BRCA* founder mutational analysis was performed; they evaluated the risk of cancer development based by parity and oral contraceptive use. They were able to establish a protective effect by oral contraceptive use in the cohort, but subanalysis by carrier status demonstrated no effect in those harboring a *BRCA* founder mutation (odds ratio [OR], 1.07; 95% confidence interval [CI], 0.63 to 1.83). Further studies are needed.

**Hereditary ovarian cancers are uncommon, accounting for approximately 10% to 15% of all incident cases; however,**

**identification of affected or unaffected women with significant familial risk is important, given their accelerated risk of ovarian and other cancers.** In addition, these patients are commonly diagnosed at a younger age (median, 50 years), and unaffected individuals are able to consider prophylactic procedures that can affect their lifetime risk. The term *familial ovarian cancer* denotes an inherited trait that predisposes to ovarian cancer development. It has been widely studied, and two definitions are important:

1. A *first-degree relative* is a mother, sister, or daughter of an affected individual.
2. A *second-degree relative* is a maternal or paternal aunt or grandmother.

As noted in the review by Kerlikowske and colleagues, previous studies suggested an increase from approximately 1.5% to 5% in the lifetime risk of ovarian cancer with one first-degree relative; with two or more, the risk reaches may exceed 7% to 12%. Because contemporary family size may preclude disease penetrance, careful attention to *BRCA*-associated cancers in either gender should be performed in a multigenerational history. Furthermore, the high association of fallopian tube cancer and underlying *BRCA* mutation has prompted some to call for routine *BRCA* testing in all such cases.

Most ovarian cancers develop sporadically. For the woman with a familial history of ovarian cancer (not the dominant genetic hereditary type), periodic surveillance with transvaginal ultrasonography 6 months after the age of 35 years has been suggested (see the ultrasonography discussion presented later in this chapter). Unfortunately, such a strategy has not been shown to be worthwhile or cost effective in disease prevention and may, on occasion, lead to additional tests or unnecessary procedures when a questionable ultrasound result is. The use of prophylactic oophorectomy in patients whose mothers had ovarian cancer has been a controversial topic. Kerlikowske and colleagues and Herbst have provided reasons opposing the widespread use of this practice; however, there is a clear benefit to the use of risk-reducing salpingo-oophorectomy in the population with mutations in *BRCA1/2*. **In a meta-analysis performed by Rebbeck and colleagues, this surgery was found to yield a 79% reduction in the risk of ovarian or fallopian tube cancer among patients with *BRCA1* or *BRCA2* mutations (hazard ratio [HR], 0.21; 95% CI, 0.12 to 0.39). Importantly, there was also a significant reduction in the risk of breast cancer with this procedure (HR, 0.49; 95% CI, 0.37 to 0.65).** The utility of risk-reducing surgery has been validated in several prospective studies, confirming the reduction in breast and ovarian cancer risk, as well as all-cause mortality, breast cancer–specific mortality, and ovarian cancer–specific mortality (Domchek, 2010; Finch, 2014). For patients with a significant family history in whom an operation such as hysterectomy is required, consideration of removal of both tubes and ovaries at the time of operation is appropriate. Similarly, mutation carriers who have finished childbearing may reduce their subsequent cancer risk by undergoing salpingo-oophorectomy. The recommendation for hysterectomy at this time is controversial but has been advocated by some to ensure complete removal of the fallopian tube (cornual segment). The woman must be aware that peritoneal carcinomatosis, a process resembling serous carcinoma of the ovary, can develop (rarely) despite the removal of both ovaries.

Because evidence has suggested a significant proportion of ovarian carcinomas arise from preinvasive intraepithelial carcinomas in the fallopian tube, interest in a two-step approach to removal of the adnexa has arisen. Preserving ovarian function in high-risk women while mitigating risk via removal of the fallopian tubes has appeal for maintaining quality of life and avoidance of the risks from premature castration. Nevertheless, much is unknown regarding the efficacy and safety of this approach, including the strength of the risk mitigation and the degree to which retaining the ovary increases the risk of breast cancer in these at-risk women. Finally, the timing for oophorectomy is unknown. Fortunately, several prospective clinical trials are under way to address this novel approach to risk reduction surgery.

**TABLE 33.2** World Health Organization Classification: Frequency of Ovarian Neoplasms

| Class | Approximate Frequency (%) |
|---|---|
| Epithelial stromal (common epithelial) tumors | 65 |
| Germ cell tumors | 20-25 |
| Sex cord–stromal tumors | 6 |
| Lipid (lipoid) cell tumors | <0.1 |
| Gonadoblastoma | <0.1 |
| Soft tissue tumors (not specific to ovary) | |
| Unclassified tumors | |
| Secondary (metastatic) tumors | |
| Tumorlike conditions (not true neoplasm) | |

The following section describes the classification and histologic characteristics of the major ovarian neoplasms. Pertinent microscopic findings, clinical behavior, and appropriate therapy are presented.

## CLASSIFICATION OF OVARIAN NEOPLASMS

The most widely used classification of ovarian neoplasms is that of the World Health Organization (WHO), which was last updated in 2014 (Kurman, 2014). This modified classification is shown in Table 33.2.

Epithelial tumors (common epithelial tumors) are the most common ovarian neoplasms. They are believed to arise from the surface (coelomic) epithelium. Germ cell tumors are the second most common and are the most common among young women. Histologically they may be composed of extraembryonic elements or may have features that resemble any or all of the three embryonic layers (ectoderm, mesoderm, or endoderm). Germ cell tumors are the main cause of ovarian malignancy in young women, particularly those in their teens and early 20s. Sex cord–stromal tumors are the third most common and contain elements that recapitulate the constituents of the ovary or testis. These tumors may secrete sex steroid hormones or may be hormonally inactive.

## EPITHELIAL OVARIAN NEOPLASMS

According to Scully (1953, 1994, 1998, 2000), two-thirds of ovarian neoplasms are epithelial tumors; malignant epithelial tumors account for approximately 85% of ovarian cancers. Table 33.3 summarizes the five cell types that most commonly constitute epithelial ovarian tumors, indicating their relative frequency.

Epithelial tumors can be categorized as benign (adenoma), malignant (adenocarcinoma), or of an intermediate form, known as borderline tumor or tumor of low malignant potential. The thinking regarding their origin has undergone considerable modification and debate (Chan, 2012; Howitt, 2015; Karnezis, 2017; Prat, 2018).

Serous tumors are the most common ovarian epithelial tumors. There are two types of serous borderline tumors—atypical proliferative serous tumor and the micropapillary variant (noninvasive low-grade serous carcinoma) (Fig. 33.2, *A* and *B*). The current classification for invasive serous carcinoma divides them into low-grade serous and high-grade serous subtypes

**TABLE 33.3** Epithelial Ovarian Tumor Cell Subtypes

| Sub Type | Mutations | Clinical Prognosis | Frequency |
|---|---|---|---|
| High-grade serous | *TP53, BRCA1, BRCA2, CDK12* | Often diagnosed at late stage and chromosomally unstable. | ~65% |
| Low-grade serous | *BRAF, KRAS, NRAS, ERBB2* | Often diagnosed in younger patients, less aggressive, gnomically stable. | ~5% |
| Endometrioid | *PTEN, CTNNB1, PPP2R1a, MMR* deficient | Favorable prognosis and response to chemotherapy. | ~20% |
| Clear cell carcinoma | *PIK3CA, KRAS, PTEN, ARID1A* | Low response to chemotherapy and intermediate prognosis. | ~5% |
| Mucinous | *KRAS, HER-2* amplification | Low response to chemotherapy. | ~5% |

From Hirst et al. Ovarian cancer genetics: subtypes and risk factors. In Devaja O, ed. *Ovarian Cancer: From Pathogenesis to Treatment.* London: IntechOpen; 2018.

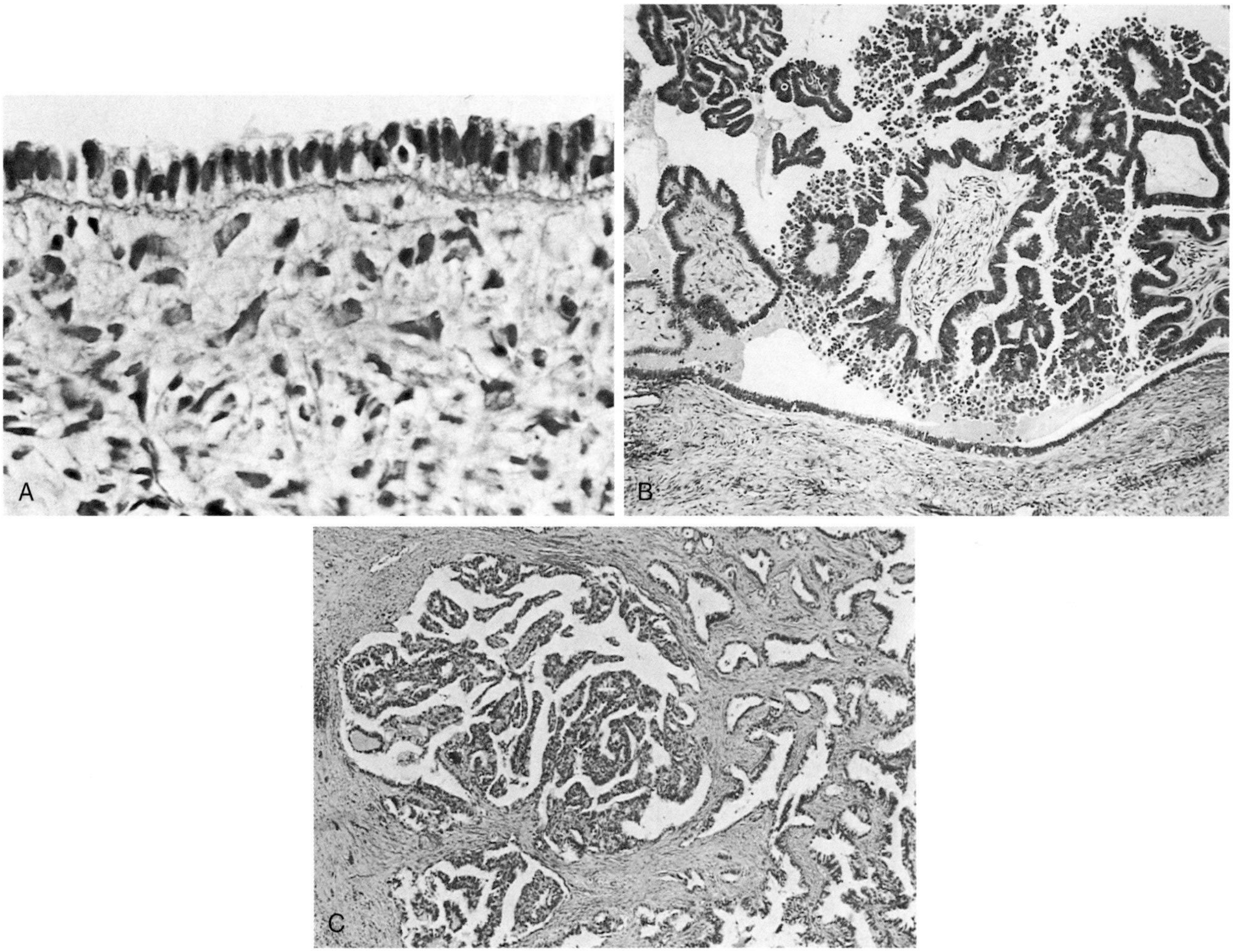


**Fig. 33.2 A,** Ciliated epithelium of a well-differentiated serous tumor (original magnification ×800). **B,** Serous papillary cystadenoma of borderline malignancy. The epithelium resembles that of the fallopian tube, and a well-developed papillary pattern is present (original magnification ×80). **C,** Serous papillary adenocarcinoma (original magnification ×50). The neoplastic epithelium invades the stroma. (**A** and **C,** From Serov SF, Scully RE, Sobin LH. *Histologic Typing of Ovarian Tumors.* Geneva: World Health Organization; 1973. **B,** Courtesy Dr. R. E. Scully.)

based on microscopic criteria (nuclear atypia and mitotic count) and molecular signatures (Fig. 33.2, *C* and *D*). Although the origin of low-grade serous carcinoma is unclear, various theories suggest that they may arise from serous borderline tumors, ovarian surface epithelium, or endometriosis. The mitogen-activated protein (MAP) kinase pathway appears to play a prominent role in their pathogenesis. On the other hand, high-grade serous carcinomas have a p53 signature, and an undetermined proportion are thought to arise from the fimbriated end of the fallopian tube.

Mucinous tumors (Fig. 33.3, *A* and *B*) consist of epithelial cells filled with mucin; most are benign. These cells resemble cells of the endocervix or may mimic intestinal cells, which can pose a problem in the differential diagnosis of tumors that appear to originate from the ovary or intestine. Benign mucinous tumors

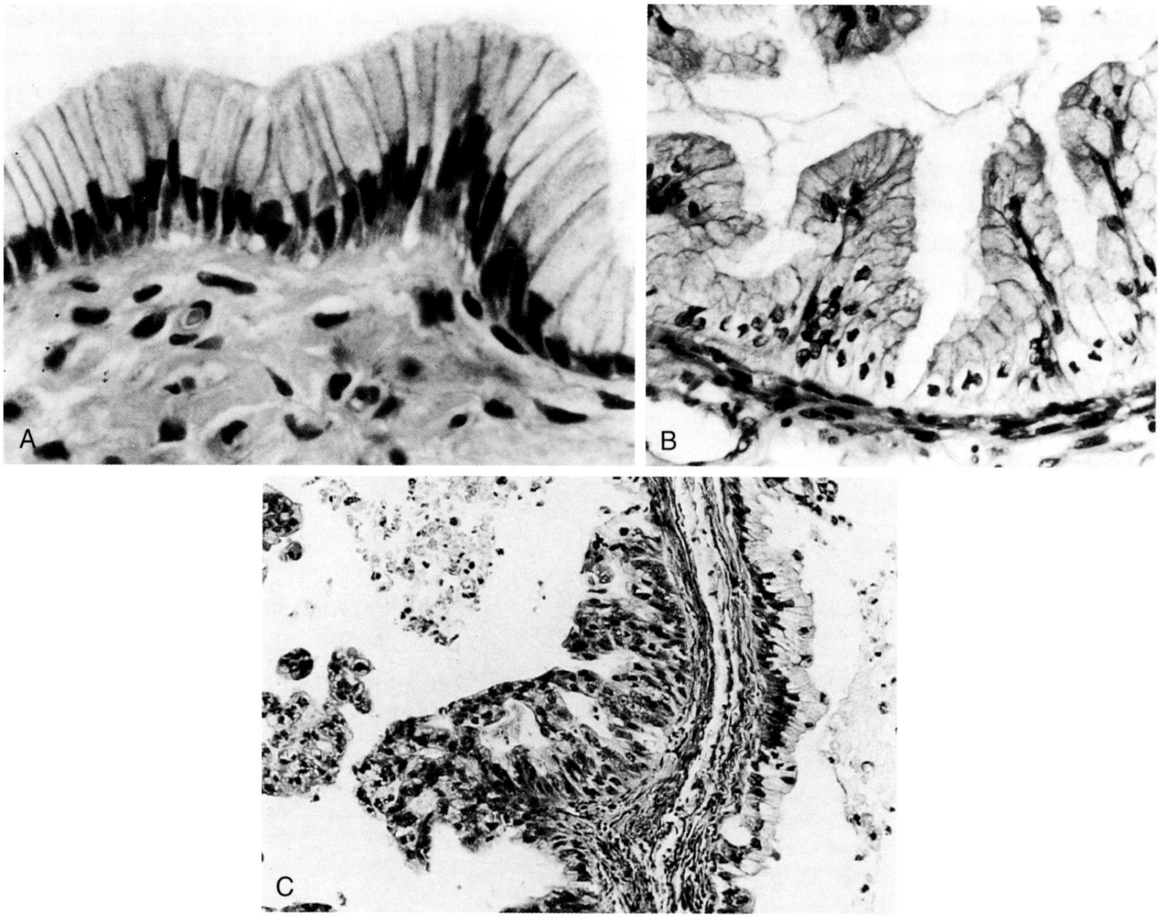


**Fig. 33.3** **A,** Mucinous cystadenoma (original magnification ×800). **B,** Mucinous borderline tumor. Epithelium resembles that of the endocervix. **C,** Mucinous carcinoma (original magnification ×120). Incomplete stratification of cells, and atypicality is present. (**A** and **C,** From Serov SF, Scully RE, Sobin LH. *Histologic Typing of Ovarian Tumors.* Geneva: World Health Organization; 1973. **B,** Courtesy Dr. R. E. Scully.)

are found primarily during the reproductive years, and mucinous carcinomas (Fig. 33.3, *C*) usually occur in those in the 30- to 60-year age range. Overall they can account for approximately 25% of ovarian tumors and as many as 10% of ovarian cancers. Molecular studies have revealed *KRAS* mutations in approximately 30% to 40% of mucinous carcinomas and HER-2 amplification in 18% to 20%.

Endometrioid tumors (Fig. 33.4), as the name implies, consist of epithelial cells resembling those of the endometrium. In the ovary these neoplasms are less common (approximately 5% to 10%) than serous or mucinous tumors, but the malignant variety accounts for approximately 20% of ovarian carcinomas. Endometrioid carcinomas usually occur in women in their 40s and 50s. They may be seen in conjunction with endometriosis and ovarian endometriomas and are most commonly diagnosed in the early stages. ARID1A mutations occur in 30%, and *PTEN* mutations are also common.

Clear cell tumors contain cells with abundant glycogen (Fig. 33.5, *A*) and so-called *hobnail cells* (Fig. 33.5, *B*), in which the nuclei of the cells protrude into the glandular lumen. Tumors with identical histologic features are found in the endometrium, cervix, and vagina, the latter two often associated with intrauterine diethylstilbestrol (DES) exposure. Molecular evaluation of these tumors suggests a homology to similar pathologic changes occurring in the kidney, which may have therapeutic implications. Clear cell ovarian tumors account for approximately 5% of ovarian cancers, and most are unilateral and early stage. They occur primarily in women aged 40 to 70 years and are highly aggressive. *ARID1A* mutations occur in 50%, and hepatocyte nuclear factor 1beta is upregulated.

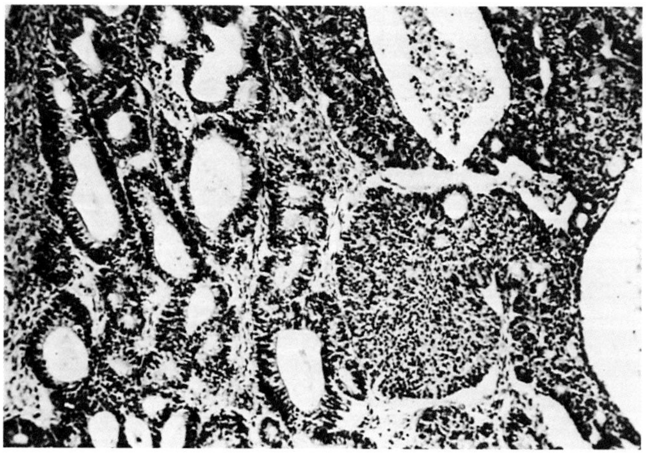

**Fig. 33.4** Endometrioid carcinoma. Tubular glands are lined by stratified endometrium (original magnification ×80). (Courtesy Dr. R. E. Scully.)

The major cell types of ovarian epithelial tumors recapitulate the müllerian duct–derived epithelium of the female reproductive system (serous-endosalpinx, mucinous-endocervix,

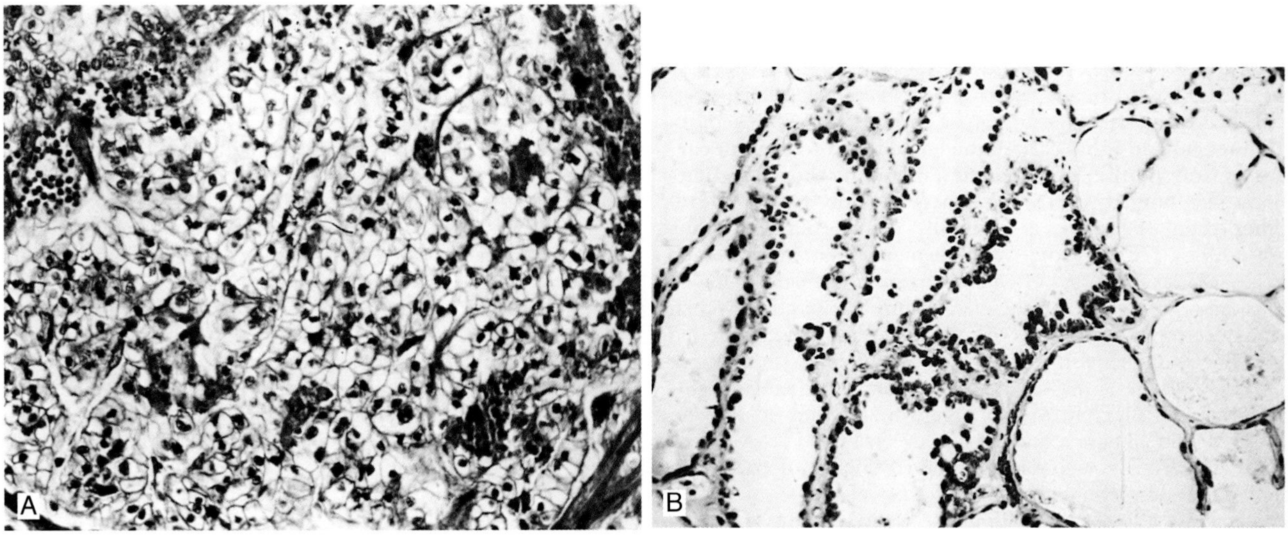


**Fig. 33.5 A,** Clear cell adenocarcinoma (original magnification ×200). A solid pattern of abundant polyhedral tumor cells containing abundant clear cytoplasm is present. **B,** Clear cell adenocarcinoma (original magnification ×200). *Left:* Hobnail cells with scant cytoplasm; protruding nuclei line shows tubules. *Right:* Cysts lined by flattened tumor cells. (**A,** From Barlow JF, Scully RE. "Mesonephroma" of ovary: tumor of müllerian nature related to the endometrioid carcinoma. *Cancer.* 1967;20(9):1405-1417. **B,** Courtesy Dr. R.E. Scully.)

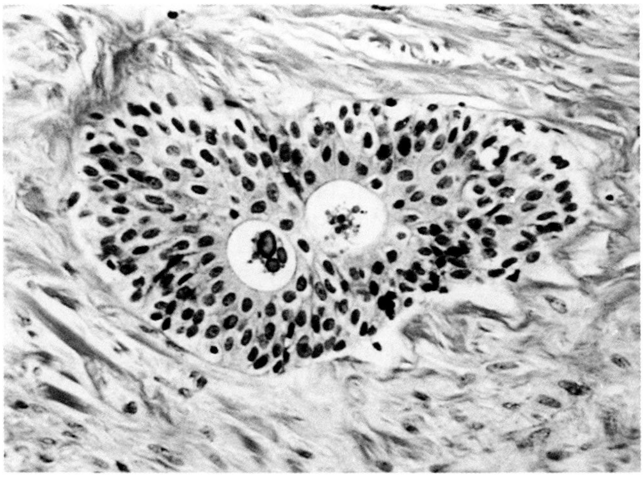

**Fig. 33.6** Brenner tumor (original magnification ×350). Note the nest of transition-like epithelium containing spaces with eosinophilic material. (From Scully RE. *Atlas of Tumor Pathology,* fascicle 16, series 2. Washington, DC: Armed Forces Institute of Pathology; 1979.)

**TABLE 33.4** Bilaterality of Ovarian Tumors

| Type of Tumor | Occurrence (%) |
|---|---|
| **Epithelial Tumors** | |
| Serous cystadenoma | 10 |
| Serous cystadenocarcinoma | 33-66 |
| Mucinous cystadenoma | 5 |
| Mucinous cystadenocarcinoma | 10-20 |
| Endometrioid carcinoma | 13-30 |
| Benign Brenner tumor | 6 |
| **Germ Cell Tumors** | |
| Benign cystic teratoma (dermoid) | 12 |
| Immature teratoma (malignant) | 2-5 |
| Dysgerminoma | 5-10 |
| Other malignant germ cell tumors | Rare |
| **Sex Cord–Stromal Tumors** | |
| Thecoma | Rare |
| Sertoli–Leydig cell tumor | Rare |
| Granulosa-theca cell tumor | Rare |

endometrioid-endometrium). This differentiation occurs even though the ovary is not derived directly from the müllerian ducts (see Chapter 2). The clear cell tumors also mimic this müllerian tendency, commonly being admixed with endometrioid carcinomas and with ovarian endometriomas.

Brenner tumors (Fig. 33.6) consist of cells that resemble the transitional epithelium of the bladder and Walthard nests of the ovary. There is abundant stroma. These tumors constitute only 2% to 3% of all ovarian tumors.

In addition to the cell types shown in Table 33.3, epithelial tumors may be classified as undifferentiated if the tumor consists of poorly differentiated epithelial cells that are not characteristic of any particular cell type. They may be considered unclassifiable if they cannot be placed in any of the categories shown in this table.

Many epithelial ovarian tumors can be bilateral, and the risk of bilaterality is an important consideration in therapy, particularly when an ovarian tumor is discovered in a young woman of reproductive age. Widely varying percentages have been reported for bilaterality in ovarian tumors; the most widely quoted are summarized in Table 33.4. Compared with benign epithelial tumors, malignant epithelial tumors more often tend to involve both ovaries. Serous tumors also tend to be bilateral more commonly than mucinous tumors.

## ADNEXAL MASS AND OVARIAN CANCER

CA-125 was described by Bast and colleagues in the 1980s. It is expressed by approximately 80% of ovarian epithelial carcinomas but less often by mucinous tumors. **The marker is increased in endometrial and tubal carcinoma, in addition to ovarian carcinoma, and in other malignancies, including those originating in the lung, breast, and pancreas (Box 33.1). A level higher than 35 U/mL is generally considered to be increased.** Box 33.2 lists some of the benign conditions for which the CA-125 level also has often been found to be increased.

As can be seen, many of these are commonly found in women of childbearing age. This lack of specificity must be remembered when one is interpreting increased CA-125 levels in younger women with adnexal masses or when screening is being considered (discussed later). In addition, there are rare individuals who have no disease but are found to have levels of CA-125 as high as 200 to 300 U/mL as a consequence of developing idiopathic antibodies to mouse immunoglobulin (Ig) G.

One must also be cautious in the interpretation of an increased CA-125 level, particularly in a premenopausal woman with an adnexal mass. The specificity appears to be better for increased values in the postmenopausal woman. In a study of 3511 patients, Van Calster and colleagues noted that among patients with benign masses, CA-125 level was increased in a higher proportion of premenopausal patients compared with postmenopausal patients (Van Calster, 2011). Conversely, in the setting of malignancy, postmenopausal patients had higher levels of CA-125. Similar findings have been observed in a number of different prospective studies best described in the meta-analysis by Myers and colleagues (2006).

**BOX 33.1** Cancer Antigen 125 Associations

**CANCER**

Ovarian, primary peritoneal, fallopian tube
Uterine
Colon
Breast
Stomach
Liver

**DISEASE**

Leiomyomata
Endometriosis
Pelvic infection
Liver, heart, kidney failure
Alcoholism
Peritonitis
Pancreatitis

**CONDITION**

Pregnancy
Mild menstrual cycle

**BOX 33.2** Benign Conditions in Which CA-125 Level Is Elevated

Endometriosis
Peritoneal inflammation, including pelvic inflammatory disease
Leiomyoma
Pregnancy
Hemorrhagic ovarian cysts
Liver disease

In addition to CA-125 and transvaginal ultrasound (TVUS), other biomarkers have been evaluated for their ability to preoperatively discriminate between benign disease and cancer. One test, OVA1, has been approved to aid this decision by providing a probability estimate of cancer based on a proprietary mathematical algorithm of five independent biomarkers: CA-125, beta$_2$-microglobulin, transferrin, apolipoprotein A1, and transthyretin. OVA1 was the first blood test cleared by the U.S. Food and Drug Administration (FDA) to help evaluate the likelihood that a woman's ovarian mass is malignant or benign before a planned surgery. The OVA1 test, when performed in 516 women with adnexal masses deemed appropriate for surgical excision, improved the sensitivity of cancer versus noncancer discrimination in a double-blind clinical study from 72% to 92% when using the biomarker panel. When administered by gynecologic oncologists, the sensitivity increased from 86% to 99%. Although not approved for surveillance or diagnosis, the test may complement clinical decision making, particularly if a gynecologic oncologist is not available to perform appropriate staging should cancer be identified.

### Evaluation of the Adnexal Mass

Ultrasound has helped define criteria to allow conservative follow-up and the risk of malignancy of some adnexal masses. Goldstein and associates studied 42 postmenopausal patients whose ultrasound scans showed unilocular cysts smaller than 5 cm in diameter; 28 were explored, none had malignancy, and 14 were followed for as long as 6 years with no change in ultrasound appearance. Finkler and colleagues noted that the addition of a CA-125 serum assay to their ultrasound criteria in postmenopausal women increases the accuracy of preoperative evaluation. In a study to evaluate the performance of the Society of Radiologists in Ultrasound consensus guidelines for risk stratification of adnexal masses, Maturen and colleagues evaluated adnexal cysts in 500 women. Of 219 with simple unilocular cysts, only one was malignant. In contrast, malignancy rates were 12.5% (12 of 84) for complex cysts and all four predominantly solid masses were malignant. Among the 132 cysts in postmenopausal women, 14 (10.6%) were malignant. Conversely, among 438 cysts in premenopausal women, 4 (0.9%) were malignant. In an ultrasound study of cystic ovarian masses in women older than 50 years, Bailey and coworkers noted that unilocular cysts smaller than 10 cm in diameter are rarely malignant, whereas complex cysts or those with solid areas are at high risk of malignancy.

Several scoring systems have been proposed to try to determine the risk of an ovarian mass being malignant. They usually include the following:

1. Is the finding a simple (unilocular) or complex (multicystic or multilocular with solid components) cyst?
2. Are there papillary projections?
3. Are the cystic walls or septa regular and smooth?
4. What is the echogenicity (tissue characterization)?

These terms, definitions, and measurements have been standardized under a consensus opinion from the International Ovarian Tumor Analysis (IOTA) group and help refine the likelihood of malignancy. Shalev and coworkers combined transvaginal ultrasonography and normal CA-125 values in 55 postmenopausal women with simple cystic or septate cystic ovarian masses; all 55 had benign disease. Although this was a small study, it suggests the potential of applying stringent ultrasound criteria with CA-125 evaluation of ovarian masses in postmenopausal women.

Others have advocated using transvaginal pulsed Doppler color-enhanced flow studies to differentiate benign from malignant masses. The resistance index, which measures resistance to flow in the vessels, has been used and presumably is low in the presence of the neovascularization that is seen with malignant tumors. The vessels of neoangiogenesis are abnormal in their distribution, with disorganized branching and a loss of the muscularis layer, all of which contribute to the decreased resistance to flow. A resistance of 0.40 or less was found useful by Kurjak and coworkers in a study of 254 women. In contrast, Bromley and colleagues, in a study of 33 postmenopausal women, used a cutoff of 0.6, which did not greatly add to their specificities; they relied on morphologic criteria (e.g., solid elements, papillary projections) to diagnose malignancy.

Valentin and associates evaluated the characteristics of 1066 adnexal masses; 266 were malignant (55 borderline ovarian tumors, 144 primary invasive epithelial cancers, 25 nonepithelial ovarian cancers, 42 metastatic cancers). A scoring system was used as well as information from color Doppler studies. They reported that borderline and stage I ovarian cancers shared similar morphology but had different characteristics from more advanced-stage tumors. They were larger, contained more papillary projections, and were more often multilocular, without solid components, but were less often purely solid and less likely to be associated with ascites. Significant variation was noted, however. Similarly, Twickler and colleagues described a scoring model to create an ovarian tumor index for women with adnexal disease. Of 244 women with follow-up, 214 had nonmalignant findings and 30 had cancer. In addition to age, TVUS variables, including ovarian volume, the Sassone morphology scale, and Doppler determination of angle-corrected systole, diastole, and time-averaged velocity, were evaluated. An ovarian tumor index was created from discriminant variables (continuous and weighted) correctly classifying the two cohorts. The area under the receiver operator characteristic curve (AUC) was highly significant (AUC, 0.91). Unfortunately, scoring systems such as these, developed from data produced by highly skilled and proficient sonographers, are difficult to generalize and, although promising, are highly operator dependent. The IOTA group has temporally and externally validated the diagnostic performance of two logistic regression models containing clinical and ultrasound variables for malignancy identification. In this study the prevalence of invasive cancer was 3%. The likelihood of cancer from a positive screen exceeded 6 for both models; a negative likelihood ratio was less than 0.1, suggesting that the criteria may be of use for evaluating women with an adnexal masses.

It should be noted that there is a difference in using ultrasonography to screen for ovarian cancer compared with using different modalities of ultrasonography to characterize an ovarian mass as benign or malignant. For example, the addition of color Doppler sonography, which measures blood flow and direction of flow, and power Doppler sonography, which can detect slow flow in small vessels, can add useful information. These permit visualization of flow location (peripheral, central, or within a septum). Most malignant tumors have a central flow (75% to 100%) compared with only 5% to 40% of benign ovarian tumors. Schelling and colleagues studied transvaginal B-mode and color Doppler sonography for the diagnosis of malignancy in 257 adnexal masses with unclear malignant status. They achieved 92% sensitivity and 94% specificity. The development of three-dimensional (3D) ultrasonography may allow more accurate volume assessments. In addition, color Doppler with 3D ultrasonography may permit better detection of vessel irregularity, coiling, and branching. Another possibility is the use of contrast media to quantify and permit earlier detection of abnormal angiogenesis, as noted by Abramowicz. Contrast-enhanced (microbubble) power 3D Doppler sonography has been investigated to evaluate the efficacy of antiangiogenic biologic agents in serial scanning.

## Ovarian Cancer Screening

Although ovarian cancer is characterized by advanced-stage disease at diagnosis and high mortality, early-stage disease is often curable. The greatest impact on these statistics, other than prevention, would be screening to identify early-stage disease. Four modalities, used individually or in combination, have been the common theme of this effort: physical examination, biomarkers (e.g., CA-125), proteomics-genomics (experimental), and sonography. For a disease to be amenable to screening, it should be sufficiently severe (high mortality); it should have a natural history that is well characterized from latency to overt disease; and there should be a successful outcome if early disease is treated. The screening modality should have high positive and negative predictive values; have high sensitivity and specificity; and be acceptable to the population, cost-effective, and widely available. The screening population should be identifiable, and effective therapy should be available for those in whom early disease is identified. Although ovarian cancer satisfies many of these mandates, it is rare in the general population (1/2500 postmenopausal women) and not readily characterized by an identifiable precursor, thus producing a high bar for any modality.

Of the three most commonly used modalities, the least sensitive and specific is physical examination. It is estimated that just one early ovarian cancer will be identified in 10,000 physical examinations. Although the easiest to implement, poor sensitivity limits this intervention as an effective strategy.

Biomarkers such as CA-125 are of great interest because they are easy to obtain and serial evaluation can be tracked. CA-125 has been used most consistently since being discovered as a reliable biomarker to monitor epithelial nonmucinous ovarian cancer, particularly during treatment; however, large, population-based studies highlighted its limitation as a sole strategy for ovarian cancer screening. Einhorn and associates screened 5550 women and in 1992 reported that only two stage I cancers in 175 women with elevated CA-125 values were identified. As noted, a differential effect would be expected between pre- and postmenopausal women. Using the modality in women with a pelvic mass (in whom prevalence is increased) has substantial effects on assay performance but overlooks the obvious need for cancer identification before gross ovarian enlargement. This has led to the development of combined evaluation (sonography) as described here.

Ultrasonography as an isolated modality has also been advocated for screening. Although more expensive and less amenable to population-wide screening, it has become increasingly accurate in identifying early changes within the ovary, as noted. Campbell and coworkers screened 5479 patients and obtained 338 abnormal scans. Five early-stage ovarian cancers were identified. The positive predictive value was only 1.5%. Similarly, van Nagell screened 1300 patients and obtained 33 abnormal scans. Two early-stage ovarian cancers were identified. As with single-modality testing, sonography is too insensitive to be widely used for screening.

Population-based ovarian cancer screening programs have been difficult to recommend and implement because poor sensitivity and positive predictive value characteristics accompany expensive and inefficient testing methodology and triage algorithms. Menon and colleagues approached this problem by evaluating a prospectively based algorithm in a population-based screening program in the United Kingdom. The population cohort used to evaluate this screening strategy involved 13,582 menopausal women 50 years or older with at least one ovary, of whom 6532 randomly allocated women completed a first screen; the remainder served as controls. The screening strategy was a staged process in which each CA-125 sample drawn underwent a calculation using the Risk of Ovarian Cancer Algorithm (ROCA) based on the woman's age and CA-125 value relative to her personal baseline. In this trial an estimated risk of less than 1 in 2000 was considered normal, whereas a risk of more than 1 in 500 was considered increased; those in between were considered intermediate and required repeat testing. Those not considered normal were referred for a second stage of screening that incorporated a TVUS scan and repeat CA-125 testing. A TVUS scan was considered normal, abnormal, or equivocal based on ovarian volume and morphology. From the combination of CA-125 risk estimation and transvaginal ultrasound scan, a follow-up recommendation was made that could be a gynecologic oncology referral, repeat CA-125 testing, or TVUS scan or annual screening. In the screened group, almost 80% continued with annual screening; 91 (1.4%) were considered at increased risk. Among the intermediate group, repeat testing was normal in 92%, leaving 188 (2.9% of the initial population) to undergo second-stage evaluation. Of the 144 who stayed in the program, 95 were returned to annual screening based on CA-125 and TVUS scan findings; 6 were found to have nongynecologic malignancies; and 43 were referred to a gynecologic oncologist, of whom 27 women were returned to annual screening and 16 underwent surgery. From this group, 5 cases of ovarian cancer were identified (4 malignant epithelial and 1 borderline); the 11 remaining women had benign ovarian neoplasms. Compared with the authors' previous algorithm based on flat CA-125 values (normal = 30 U/mL), the new process referred less than 50% to secondary screening. It was concluded that this algorithm increased screening precision.

Two other prospective trials of general population screening deserve mention: the Prostate, Lung, Colorectal and Ovarian (PLCO) study and the UK Collaborative Trial of Ovarian Cancer Screening (UKCTOCS) (Buys, 2011; Jacobs, 2016). The primary objective of the PLCO study is to evaluate the impact of annual screening with TVUS and CA-125 on ovarian cancer mortality. The study is prospectively following a cohort of more than 78,000 largely postmenopausal women with intact ovaries using an algorithm indicating that an abnormal CA-125 level (≥35 U/mL) or an abnormality on TVUS is considered a positive screen. Follow-up procedures for a positive screen are not prespecified but have been tracked, along with any surgical interventions resulting from these findings. Depending on when patients joined the study, between four and six rounds of screening could be experienced. Compliance of screening decreased slightly over the 6 years of postbaseline evaluation but remained greater than 75%; in years 5 and 6 TVUS was not administered. CA-125 screen positives ranged from 1.4% to 1.8% during six screening rounds and from 2.9% to 4.6% during the four screening rounds with TVUS. Ovarian cancer was diagnosed in 212 women in the intervention group and 176 in the usual care, control group. The relative risk (RR) for incident disease was 1.21 (95% CI, 0.99 to 1.48). Accordingly, 118 and 100 deaths were recorded in the intervention and usual care groups, respectively, over a median follow-up of 12.4 years. The RR for ovarian cancer mortality was 1.18 (95% CI, 0.82 to 1.71). In addition, of the cases diagnosed, no stage migration was experienced. Collectively, this suggests that annual screening with combined CA-125 and TVUS is insufficiently sensitive to affect ovarian cancer natural history.

The UKCTOCS was designed to definitively assess the effect of ovarian cancer screening on mortality, as well as comprehensively address the cost, acceptance, physical and psychosocial morbidity, and performance characteristics of multimodal screening and ultrasound-based screening. Between 2001 and 2005, a total of 202,638 postmenopausal women 50 to 74 years of age were randomly assigned to control (no screening), annual CA-125 screening (based on the ROCA), and second-line ultrasound testing (multimodal screening [MMS]) or annual TVUS screening (USS) alone in a 2:1:1 ratio. In the prevalence screen, 50,078 women (98.9%) underwent MMS and 48,230 (95.2%) underwent USS. Overall, 9% of the MMS cohort and 12% of the USS cohort required repeat testing. Surgery was undertaken in a small proportion of both cohorts but was significantly more likely after USS. Ovarian neoplasms, benign and malignant, were identified in both screening cohorts. The proportion of stage I and II cases

**TABLE 33.5** Screening Performance of Multimodal and Transvaginal Ultrasound in the United Kingdom Collaborative Trial of Ovarian Cancer Screening Prevalence Study

| | Screening Modality | |
|---|---|---|
| **Parameter** | **Multimodal Screening** | **Transvaginal Ultrasound** |
| Repeat testing | 9% | 12% |
| Clinical evaluation | 0.3% | 3.9% |
| Surgery | 0.2% | 1.8% |
| Number of ovarian cancers | 42 | 45 |
| Borderline cancers | 8 | 20 |
| Stage I and II cancers (48.3% of cancers identified) | 16 | 12 |
| Sensitivity | 89.5% | 75% |
| Specificity | 99.8% | 98.2% |
| Positive predictive value | 35.1% | 2.8% |

was 48.3% and was balanced between the two screening algorithms; however, specificity was significantly higher for the MMS cohort (99.8%) relative to USS (98.2%). The primary endpoint was reported in 2016 with 50,639 patients randomly allocated to USS and 50,640 patients to MMS (with 101,359 controls). Over a median follow-up of 11 years, 1282 women were diagnosed with ovarian cancer: 338 in the MMS group, 314 in the USS group, and 630 in the control group. The percentage of screened patients dying from ovarian cancer was 0.29%, 0.30%, and 0.34% for the MMS, USS, and control groups, respectively. The reduction in mortality relative to control over years 0 to 14 was 15% (95% CI, −3 to 30; $P$ = .10) with MMS and 11% (−7 to 27; $P$ = .21) with USS. In detailed analysis of time-dependent risk reduction, the strongest effect was late in the screening interval (years 7 to 14). In a sensitivity analysis, removing the prevalent cases of ovarian cancer (those diagnosed in the first year of screening) raised the hypothesis that MMS could, in fact, reduce mortality (averaging 20% over 14 years of screening). These two studies establish the feasibility of screening; determining efficacy will required further work to firmly establish a change in clinical practice (Table 33.5).

One strategy to improve the predictive index is to address a population in which prevalence is increased. A number of studies have been undertaken using transvaginal ultrasonography to screen for ovarian malignancy in higher-risk women. Bourne and colleagues screened 775 women who had at least one first-degree (n = 677) or second-degree (n = 98) relative with ovarian cancer. Overall, 43 women were referred for surgery with abnormal-appearing ovaries and 39 underwent surgery, with three stage IA ovarian carcinomas discovered (3.9 of 1000 screened); one of these was a borderline tumor. One screened patient was found to have peritoneal carcinomatosis 11 months after a normal screening study. The remainder had nonmalignant findings. The UK Familial Ovarian Cancer Screening Study (UKCTOCS) evaluated the Bayesian ROCA every 4 months with annual TVUS, if normal; if ROCA values were elevated, TVUS was to be performed within 2 months. A total of 4348 women were enrolled and followed for a median 4.8 years; 19 cases of ovarian or fallopian tube cancer were diagnosed, with 10 (52.6%) at stage I/II. Mortality data are immature. Similarly, Skates and colleagues evaluated ROCA screening with every 3 months of CA-125 testing in 3692 high-risk women. At the time of the report approximately half of incident cancers were stage I/II.

Given the potential value of an effective screening algorithm, investigation into more sensitive modalities continue. For instance, based on a deeper understanding of tissue and blood-borne factors associated with ovarian cancer, molecular-based and enhanced standard imaging are entering the clinical domain. In addition, multiomic assays, such as proteomics, microRNAs, circulating tumor DNA, exosomes, and TP53 autoantibodies, are under investigation (Nebgen, 2019).

## Diagnosis, Staging, Spread, Preoperative Evaluation, and Prognostic Factors

Ovarian carcinomas are usually diagnosed by detection of an adnexal mass on pelvic or abdominal examination. Occasionally the diagnosis is made from a radiographic survey carried out for the evaluation of nonspecific gastrointestinal symptoms. Unfortunately, the diagnosis is commonly made only after the disease has spread beyond the ovary, as noted earlier when we described the de novo origin of these tumors. Scully has estimated that the risk of malignancy in a primary ovarian tumor increases to approximately 33% in a woman older than 45, whereas it is less than 1 in 15 for women aged 20 to 45. In general, more than 50% of ovarian carcinomas occur in women older than 50. In a hospital-based study of ovarian neoplasms in 861 women, Koonings and associates noted that the risk of malignancy was 13% in premenopausal women but rose to 45% in postmenopausal women. More than 90% of women diagnosed with ovarian cancer report symptoms before diagnosis. Unfortunately, these symptoms are vague and not specific for early-stage disease or even ovarian cancer. Goff and colleagues conducted a prospective survey of women seeking medical care. The case patients were those about to undergo surgery for a known or suspected pelvic or ovarian mass; the controls were women presenting to one of two primary care clinics, in which approximately two-thirds were being seen for a specific problem. The voluntary questionnaire instrument administered to both cohorts asked the respondents to score the severity, frequency, and duration of 20 symptoms generally reported by ovarian cancer patients. In both groups, recurring symptoms were common and nonspecific. Symptoms in control patients were related to the purpose of their visit (general checkup vs. specific complaint), underlying disease comorbidities, and menopausal status. Not surprisingly, women with the final diagnosis of ovarian cancer generally reported numerically more symptoms and symptoms of greater severity but of shorter duration of onset compared with the clinic controls and patients with benign ovarian tumors. Patients with ovarian cancer were also statistically more likely to report increased abdominal size, bloating, urinary urgency, and pelvic pain. Because the combination of increased abdominal size, bloating, and urinary urgency was reported five times more often and had greater severity in cancer patients than in controls, the authors recommended further clinical investigation when identified. The diagnosis is established by histologic examination of tumor tissue removed at operation, although occasionally the initial diagnosis is suggested by malignant cells found in ascitic or pleural fluid obtained at paracentesis or thoracentesis, respectively.

On abdominal pelvic examination, patients may present with a suspicious or palpable pelvic mass, ascites, abdominal distention, and/or other symptoms that may not indicate an obvious source of malignancy. These may include bloating, pelvic or abdominal pain, difficulty eating or feeling full quickly, and urinary symptoms such as urgency or frequency. The initial workup for such patients, as suggested by the 2019 National Comprehensive Cancer Network (NCCN) guidelines, should include an abdominal/pelvic examination, an ultrasound, and/or abdominal/pelvic computed tomography (CT) or magnetic resonance imaging (MRI) as indicated. A chest CT is generally obtained when an ovarian malignancy is suspected. Tumor markers such as CA-125 should be obtained; other tumor markers may include inhibin, beta human chorionic gonadotropin (β-HCG), alpha-fetoprotein (α-fetoprotein), lactate dehydrogenase (LDH), carcinoembryonic antigen (CEA), and CA-19-9. A thorough family history assessment should be performed; if the patient is not being evaluated by a gynecologic oncologist, when findings are indicative of a primary ovarian malignancy, a referral to a gynecologic oncologist should be made (NCCN Ovarian Cancer Guidelines, 2019).

**TABLE 33.6** Staging of Ovarian Carcinomas*

| Stage | Characteristics |
|---|---|
| I | Tumor confined to the ovaries |
| IA | Growth limited to one ovary (capsule intact); no tumor on ovarian surface; no malignant cells in the ascites or peritoneal washings |
| IB | Tumor limited to both ovaries (capsule intact); no tumor on ovarian surface; no malignant cells in the ascites or peritoneal washings |
| IC | Tumor limited to one or both ovaries |
| 1C1 | Surgical spill |
| 1C2 | Capsule ruptured before surgery or tumor on ovarian surface |
| 1C3 | Malignant cells in the ascites or peritoneal washings |
| II | Tumor involves one or both ovaries with pelvic extension |
| IIA | Extension or metastases to the uterus or fallopian tubes |
| IIB | Extension to other pelvic intraperitoneal tissues |
| III | Tumor involving one or both ovaries with cytologically or histologically confirmed spread to the peritoneum outside the pelvis or metastasis to the retroperitoneal lymph nodes |
| IIIA1 | Positive retroperitoneal lymph nodes only (cytologically or histologically proved) |
| IIIA1 (i) | Metastasis up to 10 mm in greatest dimension |
| IIIA1 (ii) | Metastasis more than 10 mm in greatest dimension |
| IIIA2 | Microscopic extrapelvic (above the pelvic brim) peritoneal involvement with or without positive retroperitoneal lymph nodes |
| IIIB | Macroscopic peritoneal metastasis beyond the pelvis up to 2 cm in greatest dimension, with or without metastasis to the retroperitoneal lymph nodes |
| IIIC | Macroscopic peritoneal metastasis beyond the pelvis more than 2 cm in greatest dimension, with or without metastasis to the retroperitoneal lymph nodes (includes extension of tumor to capsule of liver and spleen without parenchymal involvement of either organ) |
| IV | Distant metastases excluding peritoneal metastases |
| IVA | Pleural effusion with positive cytology |
| IVB | Parenchymal metastases and metastases to extraabdominal organs (including inguinal lymph nodes and lymph nodes outside of the abdominal cavity) |

*According to the International Federation of Gynecology and Obstetrics (FIGO), 2014.

The staging of ovarian cancer (Table 33.6) is designed according to the criteria of the International Federation of Gynecology and Obstetrics (FIGO), which are based on the results of operative exploration. Involvement of certain sites in the abdominal or pelvic cavity would lead to disease being considered inoperable to achieve an optimal cytoreduction (no gross residual disease). These include retroperitoneal suprarenal lymph node enlargement, mesenteric disease, portal hepatis disease, and bilateral parenchymal liver metastases.

Radiologic imaging has an important role in the management of ovarian cancer. Ultrasonography may be used to confirm the presence of an ovarian mass and to help distinguish between a benign or malignant lesion. CT is more commonly used to determine extent of disease and treatment response, although one of the limitations of such imaging is that it may not detect small tumor implants (<2 cm). $^{18}$F-2-fluoro-2-deoxy-D-glucose positron emission tomography/CT (FDG-PET/CT) is a hybrid metabolic and anatomic imaging technique. In the setting of ovarian cancer, it is not routinely performed in the initial evaluation but rather more so in patients with suspected recurrence based on elevated serum CA-125 or when findings on traditional CT scans are nonspecific (Khiewvan, 2017).

Occasionally, a diatrizoate (Gastrografin) enema or colonoscopy is performed to evaluate pelvic or gastrointestinal symptoms. Consideration of gastrointestinal pathologic changes is of importance for the potential of a primary colon carcinoma, which may present initially as an adnexal mass in the older woman. Approximately 4% of colon cancers have metastatic involvement of the ovary at diagnosis. Determination of the serum CEA level may be useful in this setting and is recommended as part of the preoperative evaluation of a pelvic mass when there is suspicion of metastatic disease to the ovary. An endoscopic or gastrointestinal radiographic examination is performed if there is evidence of gastrointestinal bleeding or the suggestion of any gastrointestinal pathologic condition.

Preoperatively the use of routine bowel preparation before major abdominal surgery for advanced ovarian cancer is no longer considered the standard of care. In a Cochrane review of 260 trials including 43,451 participants with colorectal cancer, the authors aimed to determine whether rates of postoperative surgical wound infection were affected by prophylactic antibiotics compared with no treatment. The main findings from that study were that antibiotics delivered orally or intravenously before elective colorectal surgery reduced the risk of surgical wound infection. The risk of postoperative surgical wound infection was reduced by as much as 75%. (Nelson, 2014). In another study by Koller et al., the investigators aimed to determine the relationship between bowel preparation and surgical site infection. The analysis included 32,359 patients who underwent elective colorectal resections in the American College of Surgeons National Surgery Quality Improvement Program. Mechanical bowel preparation was not associated with decreased risk of surgical site infection compared with no bowel preparation. In contrast, both oral antibiotics or oral antibiotics and mechanical bowel preparation were associated with decreased risk of any surgical site infection compared with no bowel preparation. Venous thromboembolism prophylaxis is of particular importance in patients with ovarian cancer because a large tumor burden is associated with venous stasis and prolonged operation times. Treatment with variable-compression leg support stockings and heparin (fractionated and unfractionated) appears to reduce the risk of thromboembolism in gynecologic oncology patients undergoing surgical tumor extirpation.

Ovarian carcinomas infiltrate the peritoneal surfaces of the parietal and intestinal areas, as well as the undersurface of the diaphragm, particularly on the right side (Fig. 33.7). This is particularly important because tumors that at operation appear to be confined to the ovary may have small areas of diaphragmatic involvement as the sole site of extraovarian spread. As noted earlier, most ovarian carcinomas, particularly the serous type, appear to arise from microscopic ovarian sites and do not become clinically evident until there is widespread metastatic disease. Lymphatic dissemination is also a prominent part of disease spread (Fig. 33.8), and it is particularly important to note that the paraaortic nodes are at risk through lymphatics that run parallel to the ovarian

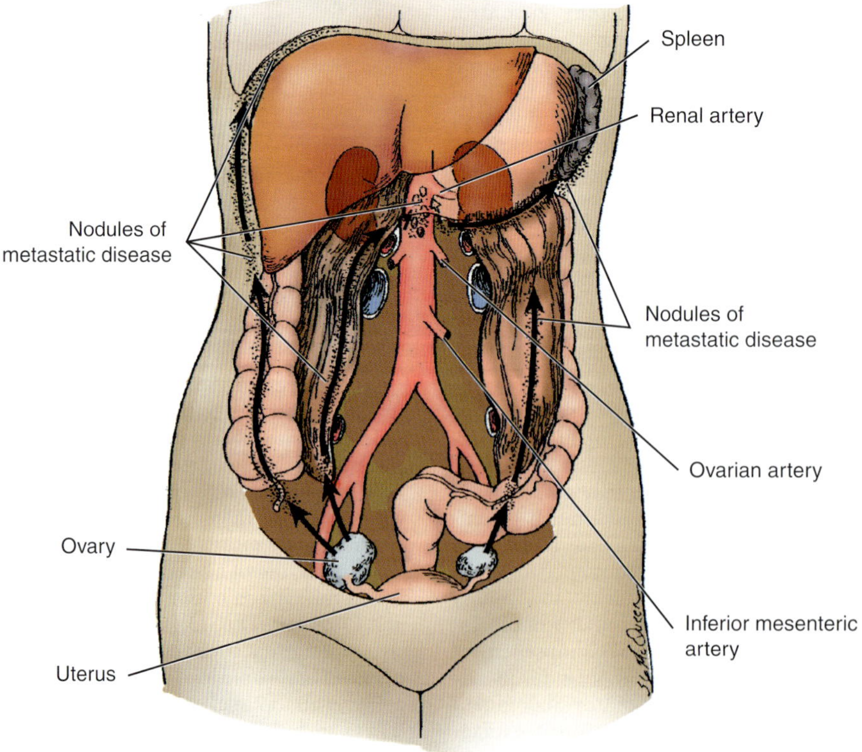


**Fig. 33.7** Peritoneal spread of ovarian cancer. Portions of the omentum, small intestine, and transverse colon have been resected. (From Knapp RC, Berkowitz RS, Leavitt T Jr. Natural history and detection of ovarian cancer. In: *Gynecology and Obstetrics*. Vol. 4. Philadelphia: JB Lippincott; 1986.)

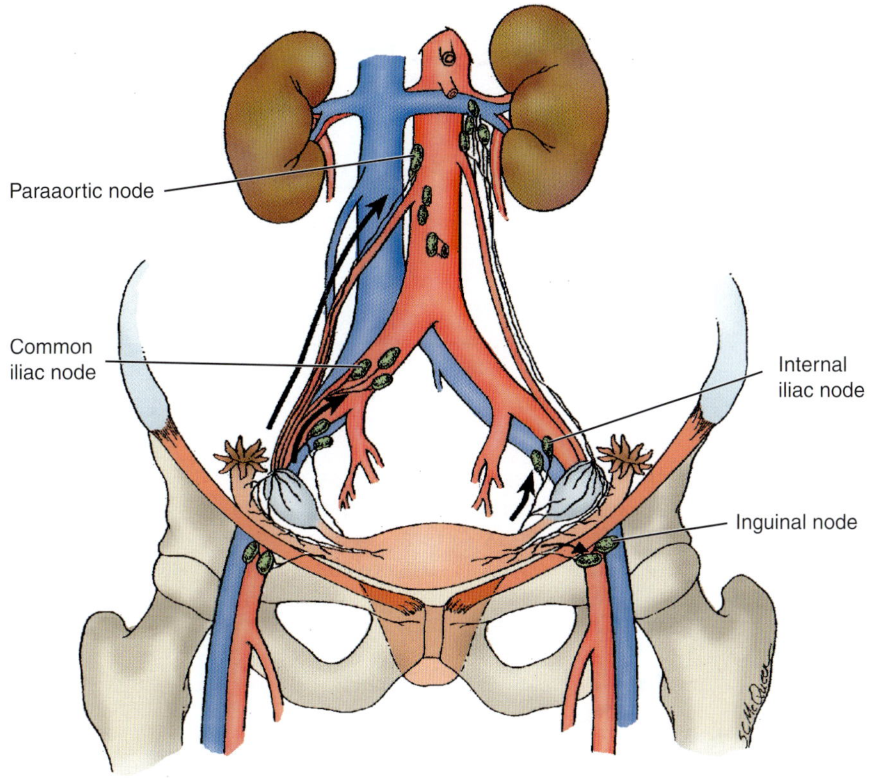


**Fig. 33.8** Lymph nodes draining ovaries. Primary routes of spread to the pelvic and paraaortic nodes are illustrated. (Modified from Musumeci R, Banfi A, Bolis G, et al. Lymphangiography in patients with ovarian epithelial cancer: an evaluation of 289 consecutive cases. *Cancer.* 1977;40:1444-1449.)

vessels. In a study of 180 patients, Burghardt and coworkers observed that the proportion of positive nodes increases with higher-stage tumors: 24% in stage I, 50% in stage II, and 73.5% in stages III and IV. A study conducted by Schmeler and colleagues has evaluated the prevalence of lymph node involvement in women with primary mucinous ovarian carcinomas. A total of 107 patients were identified. Of the patients with tumor grossly confined to the ovary at surgical exploration who underwent lymphadenectomy, none had metastatic disease to the pelvic or paraaortic lymph nodes. In addition, the authors found no significant differences in progression-free survival or overall survival between patients who underwent lymphadenectomy and those who did not.

The prognosis for patients with ovarian carcinoma is related to tumor stage, tumor grade, cell type, and amount of residual tumor after resection. Information from the SEER database is presented in Table 33.7.

Cell type has been reported to be an important factor in prognosis, as shown in Fig. 33.9, which summarizes the 10-year survival rate of a group of patients. The most common invasive epithelial cancers, serous carcinomas, have the worst prognosis; prognosis may be better for mucinous and endometrioid tumors. A variant of papillary serous carcinoma termed *transitional cell carcinoma* is thought by some to be a rare but more chemosensitive tumor; however, this has not been established in multiinstitutional studies. Endometrioid carcinoma may be associated with endometriosis; such cases more commonly occur in younger women and have a better prognosis than typical endometrioid carcinomas of the ovary. Clear cell cancers have a worse prognosis, but Kennedy and associates noted that mitotic activity and tumor stage are important prognostic features of this tumor in their series. Serous tumors tend to be more poorly differentiated and discovered at a higher stage than mucinous tumors.

**TABLE 33.7** Carcinoma of the Ovary: Survival by International Federation of Gynecology and Obstetrics (FIGO) Stage*

| Stage | 5-Year Survival (%) |
|---|---|
| IA | 94% |
| IB | 92% |
| IC | 85% |
| IIA | 78% |
| IIB | 73% |
| IIIA | 59% |
| IIIB | 52% |
| IIIC | 39% |
| IV | 17% |

*Data from the American Cancer Society. Information is based on patients diagnosed from 2004 to 2010 and obtained from the National Cancer Institute and the Surveillance, Epidemiology, and End Results (SEER) Database.

In addition to stage, the grade of the tumor is a major determinant of patient prognosis. Fig. 33.10 demonstrates the survival of 442 patients with ovarian carcinoma by grade, with a markedly worse prognosis for poorly differentiated tumors (grade 3). The relationship between grade and survival also exists when the results are examined separately for each stage of disease.

The development of gene expression profiling has enabled a more precise evaluation of clinical behavior in some tumors. Bonome and coworkers studied the gene expression of low malignant

A

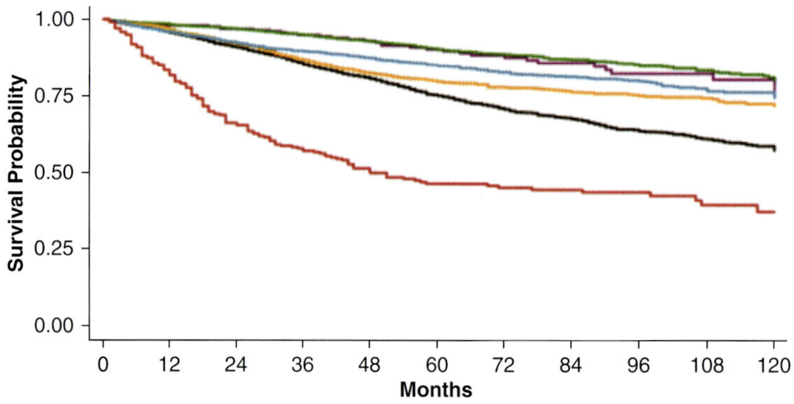


**Number at risk**

| | | | | | | | | | | | |
|---|---|---|---|---|---|---|---|---|---|---|---|
| High-grade serous | 3939 | 3378 | 2892 | 2395 | 1942 | 1525 | 1177 | 901 | 661 | 418 | 206 |
| Low- grade serous | 330 | 291 | 262 | 226 | 182 | 150 | 110 | 82 | 59 | 42 | 14 |
| Endometrioid | 2452 | 2151 | 1867 | 1615 | 1378 | 1122 | 910 | 702 | 520 | 337 | 163 |
| Clear cell | 1950 | 1674 | 1419 | 1161 | 932 | 768 | 614 | 469 | 350 | 237 | 113 |
| Mucinous | 1935 | 1618 | 1391 | 1176 | 1000 | 835 | 661 | 536 | 403 | 253 | 134 |
| Carcinosarcoma | 342 | 244 | 173 | 140 | 109 | 87 | 71 | 59 | 43 | 25 | 9 |

B

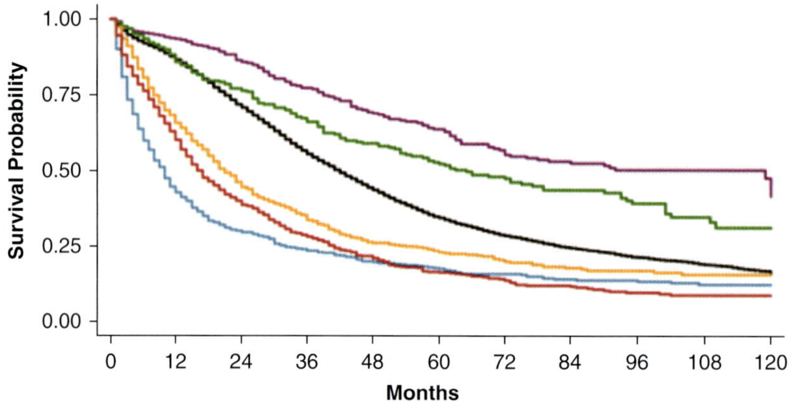


**Number at risk**

| | | | | | | | | | | | |
|---|---|---|---|---|---|---|---|---|---|---|---|
| High-grade serous | 13898 | 11098 | 8173 | 5622 | 3824 | 2526 | 1710 | 1150 | 726 | 424 | 179 |
| Low- grade serous | 378 | 320 | 277 | 222 | 181 | 147 | 109 | 87 | 62 | 34 | 16 |
| Endometrioid | 330 | 262 | 211 | 166 | 131 | 105 | 80 | 57 | 42 | 21 | 9 |
| Clear cell | 745 | 464 | 279 | 189 | 117 | 93 | 68 | 45 | 31 | 19 | 10 |
| Mucinous | 706 | 285 | 181 | 134 | 102 | 76 | 60 | 42 | 34 | 22 | 12 |
| Carcinosarcoma | 1039 | 560 | 319 | 201 | 130 | 84 | 60 | 42 | 26 | 17 | 6 |

High-grade serous — Low-grade serous — Endometrioid
Clear cell — Mucinous — Carcinosarcoma

**Fig. 33.9** Epithelial ovarian cancer survival by stage and histotype. **A,** Local and regional-stage disease. **B,** Distant-stage disease. (From Peres LC, et al. *J Natl Cancer Inst.* 2019;111(1):60-68.)

potential (LMP) serous neoplasms and invasive low-grade and high-grade serous tumors. A distinct and separate clustering was observed between LMP tumors and high-grade cancers. Low-grade serous tumors generally clustered with LMP neoplasms. High-grade tumors differentially expressed genes linked to cell proliferation, chromosomal instability, and epigenetic silencing. Based on these findings, high-grade epithelial cancers appear to have a distinct profile relative to LMP neoplasms. Low-grade serous tumors are remarkably similar to LMP serous neoplasms. These observations have ushered in the reclassifying invasive malignant cancers into two categories, low grade and high grade.

## Treatment

### Borderline Ovarian Tumors: Ovarian Carcinomas of Low Malignant Potential

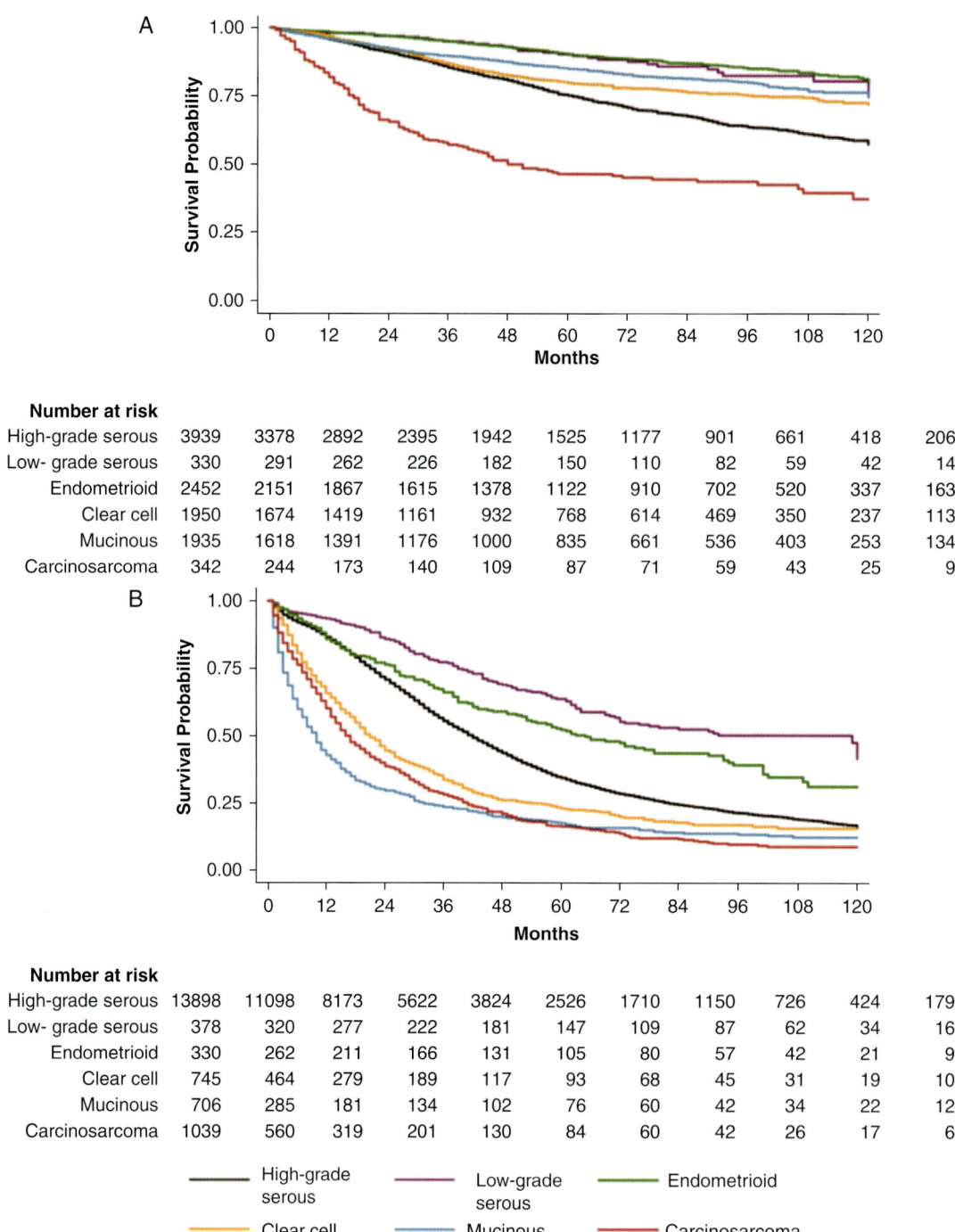

**Approximately 20% of ovarian epithelial cancers are tumors of LMP and usually have an excellent prognosis, regardless of stage.** Most studies have been confined to borderline tumors of the serous (see Fig. 33.2, *B*) and mucinous (see Fig. 33.3, *B*) varieties, which are the most common histologic types; however, other epithelial types (see Table 33.3) can occur. **Serous borderline**

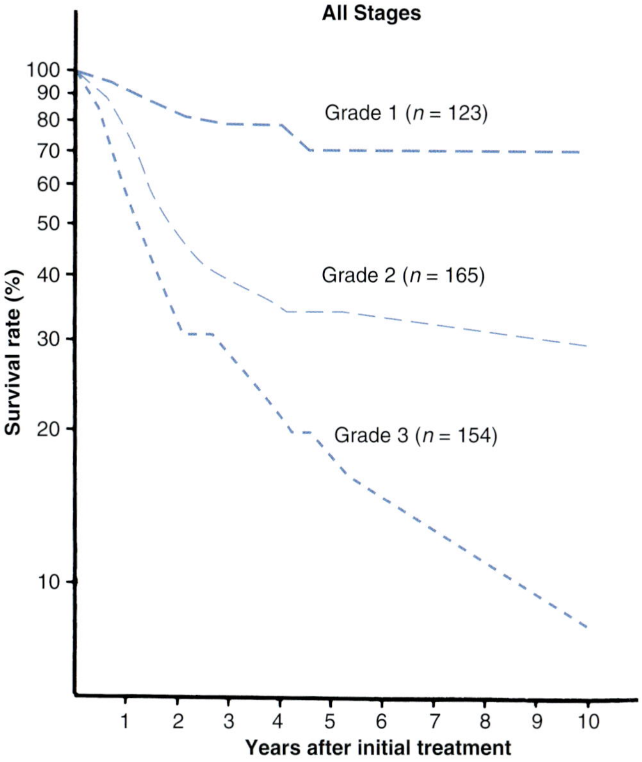


**Fig. 33.10** Survival rates for patients with ovarian cancer by tumor grade. Survival curves for the complete series according to the histologic degree of differentiation. All differences between curves are highly significant. (From Kosary CL. Ovarian carcinoma clinical trial. *Semin Surg Oncol.* 1994;10(1):31-46.)

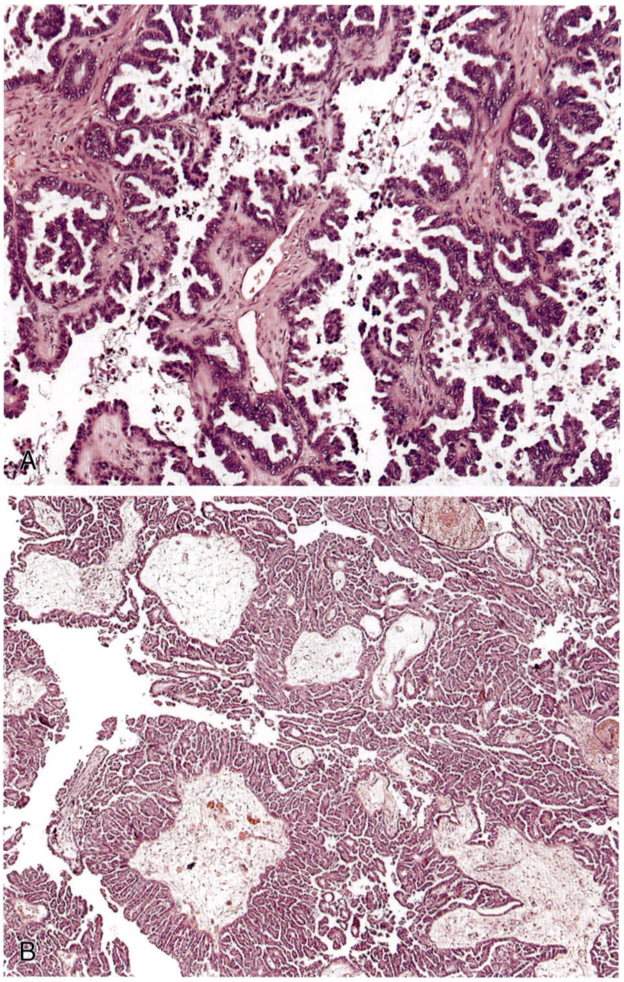


**Fig. 33.11** Serous borderline ovarian tumor histologic examination. **A,** Atypical proliferating tumor. **B,** Micropapillary/cribriform (noninvasive low-grade serous carcinoma) pattern.

**tumors include two patterns—atypical proliferating tumor and micropapillary/cribriform (also known as noninvasive low-grade serous carcinoma) (Fig. 33.11).** The cells of these epithelial tumors do not invade the stroma of the ovary. It is extremely important that the ovarian tumor be thoroughly sampled by the pathologist to ensure that a borderline tumor is not mixed with invasive elements. Numerous studies have confirmed that borderline tumors have a slower growth rate than invasive ovarian carcinomas, manifested by prolonged survival

**Surgery is the primary treatment for women with borderline ovarian tumors. The principal objectives of surgery are as follows: (1) diagnosis, (2) fertility-sparing surgery for patients who have not completed childbearing or who are young and have only unilateral ovarian involvement, (3) surgical staging for apparent early-stage disease, and (4) cytoreductive surgery for the minority of patients who have obvious advanced-stage disease.**

The typical scenario is surgery for an adnexal mass of unknown type. One of the initial considerations in planning surgery for a pelvic mass is the surgical approach—minimally invasive or open technique. Factors to be considered in the selection of minimally invasive surgery (laparoscopic or robotic) include size of the ovarian mass(es), extent of tumor metastasis, number and type of previous operations, and body habitus. Several reports have documented the feasibility and safety of the minimally invasive approach when appropriately used (Romagnolo, 2006; Song, 2017).

Once the mass is excised, frozen-section examination is a key element in ensuring appropriate decision making. If the frozen section suggests a borderline ovarian tumor, considerations for fertility-sparing surgery include the woman's age, her desire for future childbearing, and the degree of involvement of the ovaries—unilateral versus bilateral disease. Options for fertility-sparing surgery include ovarian cystectomy and unilateral adnexectomy. Even with bilateral borderline ovarian tumors, bilateral ovarian cystectomies or ovarian cystectomy plus unilateral adnexectomy may be performed, depending on the extent of ovarian disease. Lim-Tan and associates reported on 33 cases of stage I serous borderline tumors initially treated by cystectomy. Only 3 of 33 patients undergoing cystectomy had recurrence or persistence of borderline tumor, and these patients had positive resection margins or multiple cysts present in the ovary, emphasizing the effectiveness of conservative operation; however, for most stage IA cases, unilateral adnexectomy is performed and, if the opposite ovary looks normal, no biopsy or wedge resection is done.

Surgical staging for borderline ovarian tumors remains somewhat controversial. **The most compelling reason for surgical staging in a woman with borderline tumor on frozen-section examination is the risk of invasive carcinoma on final pathologic diagnosis.** For women with pathologically confirmed borderline tumors, the incidence of lymph node involvement is only approximately 5%. Therefore most investigators have recommended against routine pelvic and paraaortic lymphadenectomy; however, omental and peritoneal biopsies are recommended because peritoneal implants are usually small or microscopic (Harter, 2014).

As noted earlier, there are two types of serous borderline tumors: atypical proliferating tumor and micropapillary pattern. The former is more common, and the latter is more often associated with relapse. For stage I serous borderline tumors, surgery alone is the standard of care because the cure rate associated with this treatment approaches 100%. On the other hand, approximately 30% of women will have peritoneal implants, which are classified as noninvasive (see Fig. 33.11) or invasive (now classified as invasive low-grade serous carcinoma based on the 2014 WHO classification) (Fig. 33.12). For these women, the recurrence rate associated with noninvasive implants is 20% to 50% and the recurrence rate with invasive implants (Fig. 33.13) (invasive low-grade serous carcinoma) is 50% to 70%. **No studies to date have convincingly demonstrated any benefit to postoperative therapy for women with stages II to IV disease with noninvasive implants; however, for women with invasive implants (invasive low-grade serous carcinoma), postoperative treatment—paclitaxel-carboplatin chemotherapy or hormonal therapy—is recommended.**

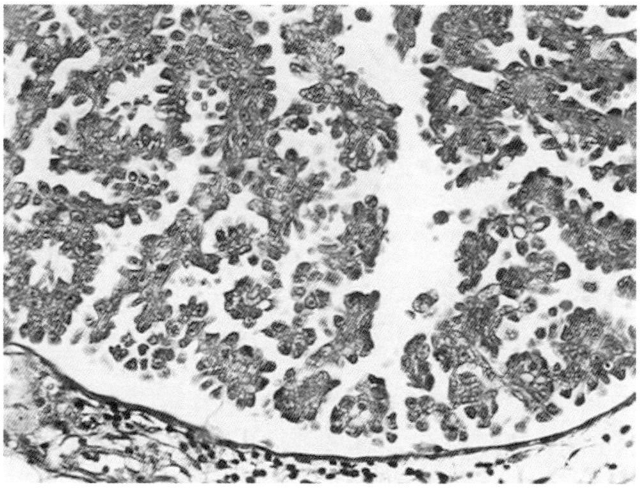

**Fig. 33.12** Noninvasive implant, epithelial type. Branching papillae and detached clusters of polygonal cells showing moderate cytologic atypicality are present (hematoxylin-eosin stain, original magnification ×313). (From Bell DA, Weinstock MA, Scully RE. Peritoneal implants of ovarian serous borderline tumors: histologic features and prognosis. *Cancer.* 1988;62(10):2212-2222.)

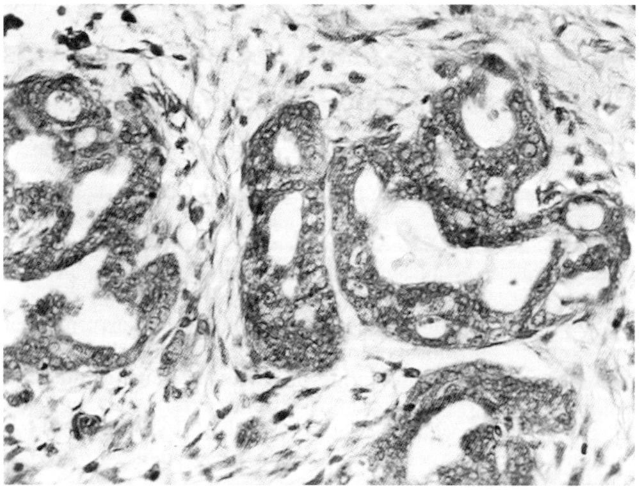

**Fig. 33.13** Invasive implant. Glands with an irregular contour lined by severely atypical epithelial cells with extensive intraglandular bridging are present (hematoxylin-eosin stain, original magnification ×313). (From Bell DA, Weinstock MA, Scully RE. Peritoneal implants of ovarian serous borderline tumors: histologic features and prognosis. *Cancer.* 1988;62(10):2212-2222.)

Outcomes are influenced by pathologic, clinical, and other factors. Pathologic factors that may be associated with an increased risk of relapse include the presence of the micropapillary/cribriform pattern or microinvasion in the primary ovarian serous LMP tumor and the presence of peritoneal implants (Longacre, 2005). Clinical factors include age at diagnosis, baseline serum CA-125, conservative surgery, and residual disease.

Mucinous borderline tumors also are associated with an excellent prognosis. Hart and Norris reviewed 97 patients aged 9 to 70 years (median, 35 years) with stage I tumors. More than 10% of the tumors were discovered during pregnancy or in the immediate postpartum period. Follow-up data were available on 87 of the patients, and there were only three tumor-related deaths during the 5- to 10-year follow-up. The actuarial survival was 98% at 5 years and 96% at 10 years. This was also noted by Bostwick and colleagues, who reported on 109 borderline tumors, 33 of which were mucinous and all of which were stage I, contributing to the good prognosis.

Mucinous borderline tumors include two distinct subtypes, gastrointestinal and seromucinous or endocervical. In the seromucinous type, the association of endometriosis is high (40%). They also may have associated microinvasion and lymph node involvement. The prognosis associated with the seromucinous type is excellent. Conversely, the gastrointestinal type may rarely be associated with the condition known as *pseudomyxoma peritonei*, consisting of widespread growth of mucin-producing cells in the peritoneum. The result may be the accumulation of large amounts of mucinous material, which is sometimes associated with recurrent episodes of bowel obstruction. Studies by Young and coworkers suggested that pseudomyxoma peritonei usually arises in the appendix. The review of Ronnett and coworkers supports a primary appendiceal origin for these tumors and suggest that therefore appendectomy may be indicated for women with an intraoperative diagnosis of a mucinous ovarian tumor. On the other hand, more recent studies have recommended appendectomy only if the appendix appears abnormal (Kleppe, 2014). The disease tends to recur and is commonly characterized by repeated laparotomy to relieve bowel obstruction. Chemotherapy and mucolytic agents have been tried but are usually not successful.

## Invasive Epithelial Carcinomas

The primary treatment of ovarian epithelial carcinoma is removal of all resectable gross disease. The woman's abdomen is explored through a vertical incision. If ascitic fluid is present, it is sent for cytologic evaluation; if ascites is not present, 200 to 400 mL of normal saline solution is used to obtain cytologic samples from the peritoneum by irrigating at least the pelvis, upper abdomen, and right and left paracolic gutters before any resection is done. The diaphragm can be cytologically sampled by scraping the undersurface with a sterile tongue depressor and the sample placed on a glass slide and sprayed with a fixative. Biopsy or, preferably, excision of any suspicious nodules is performed. A total abdominal hysterectomy, bilateral salpingo-oophorectomy, and infracolic omentectomy are performed if technically possible. When there is no gross disease outside the pelvis, in the setting of early-stage disease, paraaortic and pelvic lymph node sampling is recommended. Evidence suggests that if all gross disease can be resected, the duration of patient survival is enhanced. Although randomized clinical trials have not been performed to document this effect, a meta-analysis of 6885 patients gathered from 81 cohorts has suggested a linear relationship between the degree of cytoreduction and overall survival. In this report, Bristow and colleagues noted that for each 10% increase in cytoreduction, a 5.5% increase in survival was observed. The surgical procedures required to achieve maximal cytoreduction may be extensive and involve splenectomy, diaphragmatic stripping resection, and posterior exenteration. It may occasionally be necessary to resect bowel to relieve impending obstruction or remove a tumor nodule, thereby eliminating all gross disease from the peritoneal cavity. Heintz and coworkers noted that prognosis is improved in patients younger than 50 years, those with good initial performance status (Karnofsky score > 80), and those whose disease could be cytoreduced to less than 1.5 cm. In a small collaborative Gynecologic Oncology Group (GOG) study, Hoskins and colleagues found that those who started with large-volume disease did worse than those who initially had small-volume disease; no survival advantage could be demonstrated for the debulking operation in the large-volume disease group. Chi and associates noted that those with advanced disease and a preoperative CA-125 level greater than 500 U/mL had less than a 20% chance of an optimal surgical debulking (discussed later).

One exception to the required removal of the uterus and opposite ovary occurs in the case of well-differentiated (grade 1) ovarian tumors confined to one ovary (stage IA). DiSaia and coworkers outlined criteria for preserving childbearing function in a young woman with stage IA, grade 1 ovarian epithelial carcinoma, as follows:

1. Tumor confined to one ovary
2. Tumor well differentiated (grade 1), with no invasion of capsule, lymphatics, or mesovarium
3. Peritoneal washings negative
4. Omental biopsy specimen negative
5. Young woman of childbearing years with a strong desire to preserve reproductive function

These criteria can be applied to all types of epithelial ovarian tumors but are more likely to be satisfied in the case of mucinous tumors, which are more commonly well differentiated and unilateral than serous carcinomas. Wedge resection of a normal-appearing contralateral ovary is unlikely to uncover an occult tumor. In these cases it is reasonable to follow the woman closely with vaginal ultrasonography for any evidence of future ovarian enlargement.

**Mutations in *BRCA1/2* are clearly associated with increased risk of development of ovarian cancer (Norquist, 2016; Pal, 2005). Thus genetic testing with or without genetic counseling is recommended during the workup of any patient with high-grade, nonmucinous, epithelial ovarian cancer (NCCN Ovarian Cancer Guidelines, 2019).** This has been clearly supported by a number of national organizations, including the NCCN, the American Society of Clinical Oncology, and the Society of Gynecologic Oncology. Genetic testing should be performed even in the absence of traditional risk factors for hereditary breast and ovarian cancer syndromes. Testing can be focused on the *BRCA1/2* genes alone or can be accomplished with panel testing, which may include more than 20 genes from the homologous recombination pathway that are relevant to ovarian cancer risk (LaDuca, 2014). Results are not only important for patient and family risk of cancer but may also affect choice of therapy (discussed later). In addition to germline testing for *BRCA*, the use of next-generation sequencing to test for tumor tissue–based (somatic) *BRCA1/2* mutations is also indicated in ovarian cancer. As detailed later, PARP (poly [ADP-ribose] polymerase) inhibitors have equivalent activity in patients with germline or somatic mutations in *BRCA*, and thus the performance of somatic testing is critical to guide treatment decisions.

## Early-Stage Ovarian Carcinomas

### Stage I

The standard therapy for all patients with early-stage ovarian cancer (EOC) includes hysterectomy (usually performed via celiotomy) with bilateral salpingo-oophorectomy. In patients interested in preserving fertility, unilateral salpingo-oophorectomy with preservation of the contralateral ovary and uterus is often feasible. In addition, all patients with early-stage disease should undergo pelvic washings, omental biopsy, cytologic sampling of the surface of the diaphragm, complete bilateral pelvic and paraaortic lymphadenectomy or lymph node sampling, and bilateral biopsies of the paracolic gutters and pelvic peritoneal surfaces. It is important to emphasize that careful assessment of the subdiaphragmatic areas and inspection of the entire peritoneum and the retroperitoneal paraaortic and pelvic nodes are important, particularly in view of the risk of diaphragmatic and nodal spread in higher-grade tumors that initially appear to be at stage I, especially those on frozen section that appear to be less well differentiated than grade 1.

Le and colleagues compared a group of patients who underwent minimal staging performed by a general gynecologist with a group of patients who underwent comprehensive staging performed by a gynecologic oncologist. They found the risk of recurrence to be increased for patients operated on by the general gynecologist. Another study by Mayer and associates showed that patients operated on by a gynecologic oncologist had a 24% improvement in 5-year overall survival.

### Rupture of Ovary

Occasionally, during removal, a stage I ovarian carcinoma is inadvertently ruptured (stage IC; see Table 33.6). There are conflicting opinions as to the potential adverse effects on prognosis. In an analysis of 394 patients, Sjövall and associates found that rupture during surgery did not affect survival, whereas there was marked reduction in survival in that study among those whose ovarian rupture occurred *before* the operation. In general, the spilled fluid and all residual tumor should be removed promptly from the operative field after a rupture (discussed later). Presumably, higher-grade and larger tumors are most at risk for rupture.

A study by Dembo and colleagues of 519 stage I patients found that adverse factors were grade of tumor, dense pelvic adherence (no invasion but adhesion), or more than 250 mL of ascites. Patients without these features had a 98% 5-year survival rate. It appears that patients with stage I, grade 3 tumors should have postoperative therapy, but data are unclear for stage I, grade 2 patients.

### Minimally Invasive Surgical Staging

An estimated 15% of women with EOC have early-stage disease at diagnosis. In these patients, comprehensive surgical staging is required to provide accurate prognostic information and plan treatment options. Commonly the diagnosis of EOC is made incidentally during adnexal surgery for other indications. Because minimally invasive surgical procedures are becoming more common in gynecology and more in demand by the public at large, determining the feasibility and safety of these procedures for the staging of presumed early-stage EOC has become a necessity.

Laparoscopy often leads to a shorter hospital stay, less intraoperative blood loss, and a shorter recovery period than laparotomy; however, surgical staging for EOC requires meticulous inspection of the peritoneal cavity and careful dissection of lymph nodes, vessels, and other abdominal and pelvic structures. Thus to assess the feasibility of minimally invasive surgical staging, several issues must be considered, such as the frequency of complications, frequency of conversion to laparotomy, and recurrence rate after laparoscopic staging.

In a study by Gallota and colleagues, the authors evaluated the safety and perioperative outcomes of laparoscopic staging of patients with apparent EOC (Gallota, 2014). A total of 300 patients were selected: 150 had been submitted to immediate laparoscopic staging (group 1), and 150 had undergone delayed laparoscopic staging (group 2). No significant differences in postoperative complications were observed between the two groups. Histologic data revealed more serous tumors (0.06), grade 3 ($P$ = .0007), and final upstaging ($P$ = .001) in group 1. **Recurrence and death of disease were documented in 25 patients (8.3%) and 10 patients (3.3%), respectively. The 3-year disease-free survival (DFS) and overall survival (OS) rates were 85.1%, and 93.6%, respectively, in the whole series. There was no difference between group 1 and group 2 in terms of DFS ($P$ = .39) and OS ($P$ = .27). The authors concluded that laparoscopic management of early ovarian cancer is safe and feasible.**

In summary, it appears that minimally invasive surgical staging of presumed EOC is safe and effective when performed by a trained gynecologic oncologist.

### Adequacy of Minimally Invasive Surgery Compared with Laparotomy for Staging of Ovarian Neoplasms

Important concerns have been raised about laparoscopic staging for ovarian neoplasms, including concerns about the adequacy of the lymph node dissection, differences between laparoscopy and laparotomy in operative time, postoperative complications, and postoperative recovery. In one meta-analysis of laparoscopic staging surgery in patients with presumed EOC, Park and colleagues identified 11 observational studies (Park, 2013). The combined results of three retrospective studies showed that the estimated blood loss in laparoscopy was significantly lower than that for laparotomy ($P < .001$). The overall upstaging rate after laparoscopic surgery was 22.6% (95% CI, 18.1 to 27.9) without significant heterogeneity among all study results. The overall incidence of conversion from laparoscopy to laparotomy was 3.7% (95% CI, 2.0 to 6.9). The overall rate of recurrence in studies with a median follow-up period of 19 months or more was 9.9% (95% CI, 6.7 to 14.4). The authors concluded that the operative outcomes of a laparoscopic approach in patients with EOC could be compatible with those of laparotomy.

Data on the application of robotic surgery for ovarian cancer staging are scant. In a study by Brown and associates, the authors evaluated the safety and feasibility of robotic-assisted systematic lymph node staging in the management of EOC. A total of 26 patients with EOC were identified. The mean operating time was 2.90 hours, and the estimated blood loss was 63 mL; there were no intraoperative complications, although one patient's surgery was significantly prolonged because of pelvic adhesions. The mean number of pelvic and paraaortic lymph nodes removed was 14.6 (2.3% incidence of pelvic lymph node metastases) and 5.8 (3.3% incidence of paraaortic lymph node metastases), respectively. The patients' mean duration of hospital stay was 18.4 hours, and 2 patients were readmitted for either a postoperative wound infection or vaginal dehiscence. The authors concluded that robotic-assisted surgical staging was feasible and safe; however, there was a low incidence of lymph node metastasis (2.3%), and the authors stressed the value of a systematic lymph node dissection.

### Stage II

Stage II ovarian cancer is initially treated by removal of all gross disease, in addition to removal of the uterus, tubes, ovaries, and omentum. The pelvic and paraaortic nodes are sampled.

### Postoperative Management for Stages I and II

Recommendations for postoperative or adjuvant therapy generally have evolved around the identification of patients in whom a sufficient risk of recurrence is observed. The precision to make this assessment is low and has been based on morphologic features such as grade, histology, and presence of rupture and residuum. Historically, several modalities have been evaluated alone and in combination by prospective studies of unselected patients, including chemotherapy, radiation therapy, and immunotherapy. Guthrie and coworkers evaluated 656 patients treated for epithelial ovarian carcinomas that had been totally excised. Most carcinomas were stage I or II, and patients were randomly assigned to receive postoperative treatment of radiation therapy alone, chemotherapy alone, radiation therapy and chemotherapy, or no postoperative therapy. Perhaps surprisingly, the lowest frequency of death or recurrence was noted in the group receiving no postoperative therapy (2%), whereas in the other groups, the death or recurrence incidence was 14% to 17%. Thus this study found no benefit for adjuvant therapy and highlights the need for careful case selection and pathologic review. In addition, because survivorship of low-stage cancer is better, long-term follow-up is necessary to tease out the merits of intervention.

Two large multicenter trials have been conducted and were combined for analytic purposes to address this issue. The International Collaborative Ovarian Neoplasm 1 (ICON1) and Adjuvant ChemoTherapy in Ovarian Neoplasm (ACTION) trials compared platinum-based chemotherapy with observation in patients after surgery with EOC. The two trials differed somewhat in patient eligibility, with ICON1 predominantly enrolling postoperative stages I and II patients with limited staging and ACTION enrolling patients who were postoperative stage IA and IB, grades 2 and 3, stages IC to IIA, all grades, and clear cell tumor. Overall, 925 patients were collectively enrolled (477 in ICON1 and 448 in ACTION) and followed for a median 4 years. **The OS rate at 5 years was 82% in the chemotherapy arm and 74% in the observation arm (HR, 0.67; 95% CI, 0.5 to 0.9; $P$ = .001). Recurrence-free survival at 5 years was also significantly higher in the chemotherapy arm compared with observation (HR, 0.64; 95% CI, 0.5 to 0.82).** In select patients, platinum-based therapy appears to improve survival and lower recurrence at 5 years compared with observation. In all, three randomized clinical trials have addressed platinum-based chemotherapy versus observation in EOC. These three trials were evaluated via meta-analysis to assess the role of adjuvant chemotherapy. As expected, the combined data mirror the results of the two larger studies with regard to the impact of adjuvant chemotherapy (HR, 0.71; 95% CI, 0.53 to 0.93) on 5-year survival; however, when subcategorized by surgical staging, this benefit retained significance only in the group in whom nonoptimal staging was performed. **These data highlight the importance of accurate surgical staging information when devising an appropriate postoperative treatment plan.**

The ideal regimen and number of courses of chemotherapy needed for EOC are still debated. Bell and associates reported the results of a randomized study comparing three and six cycles of adjuvant paclitaxel and carboplatin for women with stages IA and IB, grade 3, all stage IC, clear cell tumor, and completely resected stage II epithelial ovarian cancer. A total of 457 patients were recruited; 344 were alive a median of 6.8 years since entry. **The overall treatment effect was a nonsignificant 24% reduction in recurrence for the six-cycle arm (HR, 0.76; 95% CI, 0.51 to 1.13; $P$ = .18).** The improved impact on estimated recurrence at 5 years was 5%, and there was no difference in OS between the arms. A post hoc analysis of the survival results by histologic type raises the hypothesis that six cycles of therapy may benefit patients with serous histologic type to a different degree than the others included in the trial.

A follow-up study, GOG-175, addressed the role of maintenance therapy in this setting. Women with the same eligibility as GOG-157 were randomly allocated to three cycles of paclitaxel and carboplatin followed by normal surveillance or 24 infusions of low-dose (40 mg/m$^2$) weekly paclitaxel (Mannel, 2011). Eighty percent of patients randomly allocated to the maintenance arm received all assigned therapy. Toxicity was similar between the two arms. The HRs for progression-free survival (PFS) and OS were 0.81 (95% CI, 0.56 to 1.15) and 0.78 (95% CI, 0.52 to 1.17), respectively. Subgroup analysis demonstrated no effect by stage, histologic type, or grade. There was remarkable consistency between the two GOG studies in the 5-year survival recorded by the three-cycle cohort. Although the optimal treatment is still not known, high-risk, early-stage patients clearly benefit from therapy.

## Advanced-Stage Ovarian Cancer

### Role of Imaging Studies and Serum Markers in Determining Ideal Surgical Candidate

To determine which patients would be less likely to benefit from primary surgery, a number of attempts have been made to predict outcomes of primary cytoreductive surgery by using imaging modalities, tumor markers, and laparoscopic scores. The use of preoperative CT scan imaging has shown inconsistent results. The same issue has been encountered when exploring the use of serum CA-125. One should note that studies attempting to identify preoperative predictors have been limited by their retrospective design, sample size, broad inclusion criteria, and heterogeneous rates of optimal cytoreduction.

Suidan and colleagues reported on a prospective, nonrandomized, multicenter trial of patients who underwent primary cytoreduction for stage III-IV ovarian, fallopian tube, and peritoneal cancer. A CT scan of the abdomen and pelvis and a serum CA-125 level were obtained within 35 and 14 days before surgery; respectively. Four clinical and 20 radiologic criteria were assessed. A total of 669 patients were enrolled and 350 patients met eligibility criteria. The optimal (<1 cm) debulking rate was 75%. On multivariate analysis, three clinical and six radiologic criteria were associated with suboptimal debulking: age 60 years or older; serum CA-125 more than 500 U/mL; American Society of Anesthesiology (ASA) 3 to 4; suprarenal retroperitoneal lymph nodes greater than 1 cm; diffuse small bowel adhesions or thickening; and lesions greater than 1 cm in the small bowel mesentery, root of the superior mesenteric artery, perisplenic area, and lesser sac. The authors identified nine criteria associated with suboptimal cytoreduction and developed a predictive model in which the suboptimal rate was directly proportional to a predictive value score.

### Role of Laparoscopy in Assessing Resectability to R0 in Advanced Ovarian Cancer

Laparoscopy has been proposed as a reliable predictor of R0 resection. Here we review the existing literature on the proposed criteria to predict the outcome of cytoreductive surgery and the role of laparoscopy-based scores in the management of advanced ovarian cancer. This principle was initially introduced by Fagotti and colleagues. In a study evaluating the prognostic impact of routinely using laparoscopy in patients with advanced ovarian cancer, the authors submitted all patients to laparoscopy before undergoing either primary debulking surgery or neoadjuvant chemotherapy. Among 300 consecutive patients, there were no complications related to the surgery and the laparoscopic evaluation showed that almost half of the patients (46.3%) had a high tumor load. A total of 148 patients (49.3%) were considered suitable for primary debulking surgery and the remaining 152 (50.7%) were treated with neoadjuvant chemotherapy. The authors concluded from that study that **the inclusion of laparoscopy in this setting did not appear to have a negative impact on survival and that it might be helpful to individualize treatment by avoiding unnecessary laparotomies** and surgical complications. The same group of investigators subsequently demonstrated that the laparoscopic assessment of peritoneal spread was a concept that could be reproduced among different institutions in a multicentric trial (Multicentre Italian Trials in Ovarian Cancer [MITO]-13) (Fagotti, 2013).

Gómez-Hidalgo and colleagues published a comprehensive review of the evolution of laparoscopy as a tool to help identify ideal patients with advanced ovarian cancer for optimal cytoreduction (R0). The authors concluded that existing studies point to a highly valuable role for laparoscopy for objectively assessing the feasibility of optimal primary and interval cytoreductive surgery for patients with advanced-stage ovarian cancer (FIGO stages III and IV). They went on to suggest that the Fagotti laparoscopy-based score is a useful predictor of optimal cytoreduction.

Nick and colleagues published an algorithm that identifies patients in whom complete gross resection at primary surgery is likely to be achieved. Such an algorithm is currently being used to ensure that the rate of optimal cytoreduction (R0) increases and the rate of patients unnecessarily undergoing neoadjuvant chemotherapy decreases. In addition, the algorithm allows surgeon to obtain tissue before the initiation of therapy, thus targeting molecular pathways in a much more precise and personalized strategy.

In a 2018 study by Fleming and colleagues, the authors evaluated the impact of the laparoscopic scoring algorithm to triage patients with advanced ovarian cancer to immediate or delayed debulking to improve complete gross surgical resection rates and evaluate clinical outcomes. A total of 488 patients met inclusion criteria; 215 patients underwent laparoscopic scoring. The patients were stratified according to scoring of less than 8 (58.1%) or 8 or more (39%). The authors also evaluated the concordance between two surgeons in predicting the laparoscopic score. This resulted in a bivariate concordance of 98%. **The implementation of this laparoscopic algorithm lead to no gross residual disease (R0) in 88% of patients in the primary surgery group and 74% in the neoadjuvant chemotherapy group.**

Lastly, a 2017 multicenter, prospective randomized trial was performed within eight gynecologic cancer centers in the Netherlands (Rutten, 2017). The goal of the study was to investigate whether diagnostic laparoscopy can prevent futile primary cytoreduction by identifying patients with advanced-stage ovarian cancer in whom more than 1 cm of residual disease will be left after primary surgery. A total of 201 participants were included, of whom 102 were assigned to diagnostic laparoscopy and 99 to primary surgery. **Results showed that futile laparotomy occurred in 10% in the laparoscopy group versus 39% of patients in the primary surgery group. These data suggested that diagnostic laparoscopy may help avoid futile laparotomy when considering primary surgery.**

## Primary Cytoreductive Surgery

Most patients with ovarian cancer present with disease that has spread beyond the pelvis and into the upper abdomen. The routine recommendation for patients with advanced disease who are surgical candidates is to perform a total abdominal hysterectomy, bilateral salpingo-oophorectomy, complete omentectomy, and resection of all visible tumor. Bristow and colleagues performed a retrospective population-based study of consecutive patients diagnosed with epithelial ovarian cancer (Bristow, 2015). A total of 9933 patients were identified (stage I, 22.8%; stage II, 7.9%; stage III, 45.1%; stage IV, 24.2%), and 8.1% of patients were treated at comprehensive cancer centers (National Cancer Institute Comprehensive Cancer Center [NCI-CCC]). Overall, 35.7% of patients received NCCN guideline–adherent care, and NCI-CCC status (OR, 1.00) was an independent predictor of adherence to treatment guidelines compared with high-volume hospitals (HVHs) (OR, 0.83; 95% CI, 0.70 to 0.99) and low-volume hospitals (LVHs) (OR, 0.56; 95% CI, 0.47 to 0.67). The median ovarian cancer–specific survivals according to hospital type were NCI-CCC 77.9 months (95% CI, 61.4 to 92.9), HVH 51.9 months (95% CI, 49.2 to 55.7), and LVH 43.4 months (95% CI, 39.9 to 47.2) ($P < .0001$). NCI-CCC status (HR, 1.00) was a statistically significant and independent predictor of improved survival compared with HVH (HR, 1.18; 95% CI, 1.04 to 1.33) and LVH (HR, 1.30; 95% CI, 1.15 to 1.47).

Aletti and associates sought to estimate the effect of aggressive surgical resection on the survival of epithelial ovarian cancer patients. They found that the 5-year disease-specific survival rate was markedly better for patients operated on by surgeons who were most likely to use radical procedures than for patients operated on by surgeons who were least likely to use radical procedures (44% vs. 17%; $P < .001$). Also, the rate of optimal resection was 84% for the surgeons most likely to use radical procedures compared with 51% for the surgeons least likely to use radical procedures, highlighting the value of extensive surgical effort.

Zivanovic and colleagues evaluated the impact of upper abdominal disease (UAD) cephalad to the greater omentum on surgical outcomes for 490 patients with stage IIIC ovarian, fallopian tube, and primary peritoneal cancers. Patients were divided into three groups according to the amount of disease in the upper abdomen. Group 1 was defined as no disease in the upper abdomen, group 2 as having tumors smaller than 1 cm, and group 3 as having bulky disease, larger than 1 cm. The authors found that optimal cytoreduction was achieved in 81%, 63%, and 39% of patients in groups 1, 2, and 3, respectively. In the largest study of postoperative tumor residuum and outcome, resection to no visible intraperitoneal disease was substantially related to PFS and OS. The study population (n = 3126) was generated from three randomized phase III trials assessing primary chemotherapy regimens in patients with advanced-stage disease. Median OS was 99.1 months for patients with no postoperative tumor residua compared with 36.2 months for those with visible disease 1 cm or smaller and 29.6 months in those with more than 1 cm of tumor residua.

Chang and associates sought to quantify the impact of complete cytoreduction to no gross residual disease on OS among patients with advanced-stage ovarian cancer treated during the platinum-taxane era (Chang, 2013). A total of 18 relevant studies (13,257 patients) were identified for analysis. After controlling for other factors on multiple linear regression analysis, each 10% increase in the proportion of patients undergoing complete cytoreduction to no gross residual disease was associated with a significant and independent 2.3-month increase (95% CI, 0.6 to 4.0, $P = .011$) in cohort median survival compared with a 1.8-month increase (95% CI, 0.6 to 3.0, $P = .004$) in cohort median survival for optimal cytoreduction (residual disease ≤1 cm). Each 10% increase in the proportion of patients receiving intraperitoneal chemotherapy was associated with a significant and independent 3.9-month increase (95% CI, 1.1 to 6.8, $P = .008$) in median cohort survival time. The authors found that the proportions of patients left with no gross residual disease and receiving intraperitoneal chemotherapy are independently significant factors associated with the most favorable cohort survival time.

**The role of surgery in the upfront setting in patients with advanced ovarian cancer remains a topic of controversy and debate.** There are many who argue that rather than residual disease as the primary determinant of oncologic outcomes, it may be other elements such as tumor biology that impart the most influence on such outcomes. Two ancillary data analyses have explored this question. The first was a subanalysis of the SCOTROC-1 (Scottish Randomized Trial in Ovarian Cancer 1) trial data by Crawford and colleagues. The authors reviewed the data on 889 patients with FIGO stage IC to IV ovarian cancer. A prognostic scoring system that reflected each patient's preoperative biologic characteristics based on FIGO stage, tumor histologic type, preoperative CA-125 levels, and omental cake was established using a multivariate Cox model. In that study **the authors concluded that the survival benefit associated with optimal surgery was limited to patients with less aggressive disease and that tumor biology was the primary survival determinant.**

A subsequent study by Horowitz and colleagues retrospectively reviewed the GOG-182 trial data on 2655 patients with FIGO stage III or IV ovarian cancer. PFS and OS were analyzed based on three indices: preoperative disease score, surgical complexity score, and residual disease. Disease score was defined as low, with pelvic and retroperitoneal spread; moderate, with additional spread to the abdomen but sparing the upper abdomen; or high, with the presence of UAD affecting the diaphragm, spleen, liver, or pancreas. In that study **the authors found that PFS and OS decreased with increasing disease score, and patients with high disease score had the worst PFS and OS.** Interestingly, in patients with no gross residual disease, the high disease score still had a worse influence on PFS and OS compared with those with low-moderate disease scores. **The authors concluded that although complete cytoreduction to no gross residual disease may be achieved, initial tumor burden is a primary determinant in survival and aggressive surgery alone does not seem to have a strong impact on outcomes.** Both these studies have drawn some criticism for including patients with less advanced disease, having a nonobjective definition of surgical aggressiveness, defining optimal cytoreduction in the SCOTROC trial analysis as less than 2 cm, and use of complexity score as a surrogate of aggressive surgery in the GOG-182 subanalysis.

Most retrospective evidence suggests that **patients with advanced ovarian cancer treated at HVHs by high-volume surgeons have better outcomes than those treated at the JVHs and by low-volume surgeons** (Bristow, 2015).

### Utility of Video-Assisted Thoracoscopy

Unfortunately, no tools are available that allow surgeons to predict with high confidence whether there is disease in the pleural cavity. Video-assisted thoracoscopic surgery (VATS) allows surgeons, through a minimally invasive approach, to not only drain the pleural cavity of fluid but also evaluate whether pleural disease is present.

In a review by Di Guilmi and colleagues the authors summarized the literature on VATS and its applicability in patients with advanced ovarian cancer. A total of 187 patients with suspected ovarian cancer who underwent VATS procedure were identified for the analysis. The median patient age was 59.4 years (range, 20.3 to 83) and the median operative time was 32 minutes (range, 5 to 65). In 89 patients (48%), VATS revealed macroscopic disease in the pleural cavity. After VATS, 44 patients underwent neoadjuvant chemotherapy, and the remaining 143 patients underwent primary cytoreductive surgery. VATS led to a change in disease stage or management in 76 patients (41%). Among patients with pleural effusion, VATS revealed pleural disease in 57% of patients, and 73% of patients with positive pleural cytologic results had evidence of pleural disease. Interestingly, 23.5% of patients with negative pleural cytologic results had evidence of pleural disease. Whether VATS should be routinely performed in the setting of advanced ovarian cancer remains a topic of debate.

### Diaphragmatic Stripping or Resection

At initial surgical exploration, diaphragmatic disease may be the largest-volume metastatic disease. Unfortunately, the presence of diaphragmatic disease is one of the most common factors precluding optimal tumor reduction surgery. Aletti and coworkers evaluated the therapeutic value of diaphragmatic surgery in patients with advanced ovarian cancer and found that patients who underwent diaphragmatic surgery (stripping of the diaphragm peritoneum, full- or partial-thickness diaphragm resection, or excision of nodules) had an improved 5-year OS rate relative to patients who did not undergo diaphragmatic surgery (53% vs. 15%, $P < .0001$).

A study by Pathiraja and colleagues compared the surgical morbidity of diaphragmatic peritonectomy versus full-thickness diaphragmatic resection with pleurectomy at radical debulking. A total of 42 patients were eligible for the study; 21 underwent diaphragmatic peritonectomy (DP, group 1) and 21 underwent diaphragmatic full-thickness resection (DR, group 2). Forty patients out of 42 (93%) had complete tumor resection with no residual disease. Histologic examination confirmed the presence of cancer in the diaphragmatic peritoneum of 19 patients out of 21 in group 1 and all 21 patients of group 2. The overall complications rate was 19% in group 1 versus 33% in group 2. The pleural effusion rate was 9.5% versus 14.5%, and the pneumothorax rate was 14.5% only in group 2. Two patients in each group required postoperative chest drains (9.5%). The authors concluded that patients in the pleurectomy group experienced pneumothorax and a higher rate of pleural effusion, but none had long-term morbidity or additional surgical interventions.

In a 2016 study by Muallem and colleagues, the authors reported on 268 patients who underwent diaphragmatic interventions. The comparison group was another 268 patients who did not undergo any diaphragmatic procedure. The surgical interventions varied between diaphragmatic partial resection (44.8%), stripping (53%), and only infrared coagulation (2.2%). The postoperative complication rate was higher in the diaphragm-intervention group compared with the group without any diaphragmatic intervention (49.6% vs. 38.8%); however, the authors recognized that most of the postoperative complications were not directly related to the diaphragmatic intervention itself. Pleural effusion was the only increased complication with a direct correlation with diaphragmatic surgery (25.4% vs. 14.2%).

Given the high risk for potential complications after diaphragmatic surgery, it would be of value to the surgeon to predict which patients would require a diaphragmatic resection to achieve optimal cytoreduction. A 2018 study evaluated the positive predictive value of preoperative imaging and the proportion of CT scans with false-negative results in patients who underwent cytoreductive surgery (Pounds, 2018). A total of 536 patients were analyzed in the study; diaphragmatic disease was found intraoperatively in 40.1%, and 16% underwent a diaphragmatic procedure. The positive predictive value for preoperative radiologic identification of diaphragmatic disease was 78.6%. CT imaging failed to detect diaphragmatic involvement despite obvious diaphragm disease during surgery in 29.4% of cases, thus leading to a low negative predictive value of 64.8%. The sensitivity and specificity for CT imaging in detecting diaphragm disease was 44.3% and 93.8%, respectively. The authors concluded that preoperative assessment with CT imaging is not reliable in accurately detecting diaphragmatic involvement.

### Splenectomy

For optimal cytoreductive surgery, a splenectomy may be required if there is disease involving the hilum, capsule, or parenchyma of the spleen. Magtibay and colleagues evaluated 112 patients who underwent splenectomy as part of primary or secondary cytoreductive surgery. They found that the most common indications for splenectomy were direct metastatic involvement (46%), facilitation of an en bloc resection of perisplenic disease (41%), and intraoperative trauma (13%). In that same study, the authors found that 65% of patients had hilar involvement, 52% capsular involvement, and 16% parenchymal metastases. Interestingly, patients with disease directly involving the splenic parenchyma did not have a worse prognosis than patients with disease involving the splenic hilum or capsule.

A 2018 large study by Sun and colleagues evaluated 2882 patients who underwent ovarian cancer cytoreductive surgery. Of these, a total of 38 patients (1.3%) underwent spleen resection. One patient underwent splenectomy because of trauma, but the remaining 37 patients had splenic metastases. Of these, 27 patients underwent splenectomy because of direct tumor spread in the spleen and 10 patients underwent resection because of hematogenous metastases. The authors concluded that splenectomy should be attempted, when feasible, to achieve optimal cytoreduction.

### Hepatic Resection

The clinical significance of hepatic parenchymal metastasis on survival in patients with advanced ovarian cancer has been studied. Lim and coworkers reported on a series of patients with hepatic parenchymal metastases. In this series, patients underwent wedge resection, segmentectomy, or hemihepatectomy as part of their tumor-reductive surgery. The 5-year PFS and OS rates for patients with stage IIIC disease and patients with stage IV disease and hepatic parenchymal metastasis from peritoneal seeding were 25% and 23% and 55% and 51%, respectively. The authors advocated that complete hepatic resection should be attempted for patients with hepatic parenchymal metastasis.

### Bowel Resection

Because ovarian cancer often presents with confluent tumor in the cul de sac, rectosigmoid resection—along with or en bloc with hysterectomy and bilateral salpingo-oophorectomy—is often necessary to achieve complete tumor resection in the pelvis. This results in high rates of optimal cytoreduction, with acceptable morbidity. An average of 26% of women with ovarian cancer undergo colon resection as part of their primary cytoreductive operation according to a study by Aletti and colleagues. Peiretti and associates aimed to determine the impact of rectosigmoid resection, at the time of primary cytoreductive surgery, on morbidity and survival of patients with advanced ovarian cancer. A total of 238 patients were identified; 180 (75%) had stages IIC to IIIC and 58 (25%) had stage IV. Complete cytoreduction was achieved in 41% of the cases. Stapled coloproctostomy was performed in 98%, whereas hand-sewn coloproctostomy was performed in only 2%; a protective ileostomy and colostomy were necessary (constructed) in 2 (0.8%) and 5 (2%) cases, respectively. The complications associated to rectosigmoid resection were anastomotic leakage in 7 patients (3%) and pelvic abscess in 9 patients (3.7%) . Fifty percent of patients recurred during the study period, but only 5% of them showed a relapse at the level of the pelvis, whereas 8% presented with abdominal recurrence associated with pelvic disease as well. The median OS time among patients with complete cytoreduction was 72 months compared with 42 months among the rest of patients ($P = .002$). The authors concluded that rectosigmoid colectomy may significantly contribute to a complete primary cytoreduction for advanced stage ovarian, tubal, and peritoneal cancers and that pelvic complete debulking accomplished by rectosigmoid resection could be associated with a lower rate of pelvic recurrence as well.

One of the main concerns after bowel resection is the risk of anastomotic leak, and this is particularly important in patients who have undergone multiple bowel resections. In a study by Grimm and colleagues, the authors aimed to identify risk factors for anastomotic leakage in patients undergoing primary surgery for advanced ovarian cancer. In that study, 30.1% of patients had multiple bowel resections. In a multivariate model after correcting for comorbidities, duration of surgery, patient age, and blood loss during pregnancy, the authors were not able to identify an independent predictor of anastomotic leak. The authors concluded that rate of anastomotic leak was mainly influenced by rectosigmoid resection and only marginally increased by additional bowel resections.

### Retroperitoneal Lymphadenectomy

Whether systematic removal of retroperitoneal lymph nodes should be part of optimal cytoreductive surgery had been a topic of debate for many years. We now have evidence that systematic lymphadenectomy in patients with grossly uninvolved lymph nodes provides no benefit to the woman. A prospective randomized trial by Benedetti-Panici and colleagues showed that systematic lymphadenectomy improves PFS but not OS in women with optimally debulked advanced ovarian cancer. In addition, the median operating time was longer (300 vs. 210 minutes; $P < .001$) and the percentage of patients requiring blood transfusions was higher (72% vs. 59%; $P = .006$) in the systematic lymphadenectomy arm. A 2019 prospective randomized trial (LIONS [Lymphadenectomy in Ovarian Neoplasms]) assigned patients with newly diagnosed advanced ovarian cancer (FIGO stage IIB to IV) who underwent macroscopically complete resection and had normal lymph nodes both before and during surgery to either undergo or not undergo lymphadenectomy. A total of 647 patients underwent randomization; the results showed that systematic pelvic and paraaortic lymphadenectomy in patients with advanced ovarian cancer was not associated with longer overall or PFS compared with no lymphadenectomy and was associated with a higher incidence of postoperative complications (Harter, 2019).

## Postoperative Therapy for Advanced Epithelial Carcinomas (Stages III and IV)

For historical interest, early adjuvant therapy attempts in advanced disease included single-agent and combination chemotherapy regimens based on the alkylating agents. A limited number of responses were observed, and treatment often continued for 1 to 3 years. With the discovery of cisplatin (and carboplatin, subsequently), several randomized trials were conducted comparing platinum and platinum combinations with nonplatinum regimens. These pivotal trials secured platinum as the agent of choice in primary adjuvant therapy, which continues to this day. In addition, several clinical trials have established that little additional benefit to treatment is observed beyond four cycles of therapy. Most recently, the development of the taxanes has documented the importance of this agent (discussed later). By convention, six to eight cycles of combination platinum- and taxane-based therapy are now recommended as adjuvant therapy for most patients with advanced disease.

The pivotal trial establishing the importance of paclitaxel in primary ovarian cancer management was reported by McGuire and associates on behalf of the GOG. They conducted a randomized trial comparing cisplatin, 75 mg/m$^2$, with cyclophosphamide, 750 mg/m$^2$, or paclitaxel, 135 mg/m$^2$, over 24 hours and demonstrated a survival advantage in the paclitaxel arm. All patients had residual tumors larger than 1 cm after the primary operation. Response rates improved with paclitaxel relative to control in patients with measurable disease (73% vs. 60%). The median PFS was 18 months in the paclitaxel arm compared with 13 months in the platinum arm ($P < .001$). OS was similarly improved (38 vs. 24 months; HR = 0.6; 95% CI, 0.5 to 0.8; $P < .001$).

The results of this study were confirmed in similar randomized clinical trials conducted worldwide. The taxane-platinum combination was generally considered to be the recommended first-line therapy for ovarian cancer. The platinum analog carboplatin was found to be less nephrotoxic and neurotoxic and easily administered without prehydration, thus shortening the time of infusion. After several randomized clinical studies demonstrating the equivalence of this agent to cisplatin in ovarian cancer, carboplatin was substituted for cisplatin in taxane-based regimens. In addition, paclitaxel infused over 3 hours was found likely to be equivalent to paclitaxel infused over 24 hours and, in combination with carboplatin, enabled the combination to be given on an outpatient basis. Phase III studies by Ozols and coworkers showed that paclitaxel-carboplatin is a feasible outpatient regimen with less toxicity than paclitaxel-cisplatin and is associated with equivalent survival.

It should be noted that carboplatin is quantitatively excreted by the kidney and its effective serum concentration can be calculated from a formula based on the woman's glomerular filtration rate (GFR). This can be determined by various methods but is generally estimated by calculating the creatinine clearance. The Calvert formula is most commonly used and determines a total dose by this formula:

AUC-based dosing is preferred for carboplatin because the AUC most accurately reflects observed dose-specific toxicity and is more reliable across patients than dosing based on the body mass index. A usual dose for carboplatin is calculated for AUC values of 5 to 7.5. Both paclitaxel and platinum compounds are neurotoxic, as noted by Warner, and this is often the dose-limiting toxicity. The taxane, docetaxel, was found to be potentially less neurotoxic than paclitaxel. Vasey and colleagues reported on a large phase III study comparing docetaxel and carboplatin with paclitaxel and carboplatin in patients with stages IC to IV ovarian cancer. Almost identical survival parameters were observed between the two agents. The docetaxel arm was significantly less neurotoxic; however, it was associated with more myelosuppression. Neurotoxicity, as evaluated by several objective measures, returned to parity several months after treatment. Granulocyte colony-stimulating factor is occasionally needed to reduce the duration of significant neutropenia in these regimens. A commonly used regimen is paclitaxel, 175 mg/m$^2$ over 3 hours, or docetaxel, 75 mg/m$^2$ over 1 hour, and carboplatin (AUC, 5 to 6) given as a 1-hour infusion every 3 weeks. Premedication is required for both taxanes to combat hypersensitivity reactions, which have been attributed to the taxane itself and the carrier vehicle required to make these agents water soluble. In addition, steroid administration is necessary after treatment for docetaxel to combat fluid retention and effusion, a complication that may occur in as many as 25% of patients without prophylaxis.

## Alterations in Frontline Treatment Strategies

Although the preferred sequence in primary advanced ovarian cancer management is surgery followed by chemotherapy, several authors have attempted to take advantage of the disease's intrinsic chemosensitivity to improve outcomes in patients with extensive disease. Two avenues have been pursued:

- Neoadjuvant chemotherapy, in which, after biopsy or limited surgery, chemotherapy is administered for a reduced number of cycles (usually three to four) and an operation is planned for removal of the primary tumor (if present) and residual metastases
- Interval cytoreduction, when an unsuccessful maximal attempt at cytoreduction is followed by a reduced number of chemotherapy cycles (usually three to four), followed by a second cytoreduction attempt

Both strategies are followed by three to four cycles of chemotherapy after surgery. This latter strategy has been evaluated in randomized clinical trials with conflicting results; the former was evaluated in a randomized evaluation.

### Neoadjuvant Chemotherapy

Neoadjuvant chemotherapy is practiced as an alternative for patients thought to have substantial operative risk or preoperative disease distribution that could preclude optimal cytoreduction. Several authors have noted the potential benefits to this strategy, including the opportunity to allow for an improvement in performance status, decreasing operative morbidity through less extensive surgery, and increasing the opportunity to achieve an optimal result. Each of these goals has been demonstrated in several single-institution retrospective and prospective trials. In this approach, selected patients are given three to four cycles of combination chemotherapy before a planned surgical attempt. Adjuvant therapy to complete six to eight cycles is commonly administered. Because primary cytoreduction is deferred, concerns have been raised against a potential trade-off in survival benefit among patients who were not too infirm or harboring unresectable disease. Given these concerns, calls were made for prospective randomized controlled trials to examine the safety and efficacy. To date, three trials have been conducted with remarkably similar outcomes.

The first trial reported was the European Organization for Research and Treatment of Cancer (EORTC) 55971, a 670-patient randomized, noninferiority designed clinical trial; OS was the primary endpoint (Vergote, 2010). Of these patients, 632 (94.3%) were eligible and started the treatment. The majority had extensive stage IIIC or IV disease at primary debulking surgery (metastatic lesions that were larger than 5 cm in diameter in 74.5% of patients and larger than 10 cm in 61.6%). The largest residual tumor was 1 cm or less in diameter in 41.6% of patients after primary debulking and in 80.6% of patients after interval debulking. Postoperative rates of adverse effects and mortality tended to be higher after primary debulking than after interval debulking. The HR for death (intention/treat analysis) in the group assigned to neoadjuvant chemotherapy followed by interval debulking, compared with the group assigned to primary debulking surgery followed by chemotherapy, was 0.98 (90% CI, 0.84 to 1.13, $P$ = .01 for noninferiority), and the HR for disease progression was 1.01 (90% CI, 0.89 to 1.15). Complete resection of all macroscopic disease (at primary or interval surgery) was the strongest independent variable in predicting OS.

In the second trial, Chemotherapy or Upfront Surgery (CHORUS), Kehoe and colleagues randomized 552 evaluable patients to primary cytoreduction followed by six cycles of platinum-taxane chemotherapy or three cycles of neoadjuvant platinum-based therapy followed by interval cytoreduction and three additional cycles of therapy (Kehoe, 2015). The trial was designed to follow the eligibility and testing procedures of the EORTC trial with the intent of combining the databases for a future meta-analysis. In this trial 552 women with stage III or IV ovarian cancer were randomly allocated 1:1 to either primary surgery followed by six 3-week cycles of a carboplatin regimen (usually in combination with paclitaxel) or to three induction cycles of chemotherapy followed by surgery followed by three adjuvant cycles of chemotherapy. The primary endpoint was OS, which was similar (primary debulking surgery [PDS] 22.6 months vs. neoadjuvant chemotherapy (NACT) 24.1 months, upper bound of the one-sided 90% CI, 0.98), favored the NACT arm, unable to reject the noninferiority null hypothesis. High-grade adverse events related to surgery, including mortality, were higher in the PDS arm; however, like the EORTC trial, OS in the trial (both cohorts) was much lower than expected, reflecting low rates of complete cytoreduction (PDS, 17%; NACT, 39%) and heterogeneity in treatment care (76% of both arms receiving paclitaxel and carboplatin). Criticisms for both trials lie in patient selection and surgical effort potentially confounding the interpretation of contemporary management.

The third trial was conducted by the Japanese Clinical Oncology Group (JCOG-0602; Onda, 2018). Similar to the EORTC and CHORUS trials, this trial was designed to assess OS in a noninferiority design. In all, 301 patients were randomly allocated; unlike the previous two trials, patients who had a suboptimal cytoreduction at initial tumor reduction were allowed to undergo a second attempt. Of interest, this strategy was the focus of another randomized phase III trial conducted by the GOG (GOG-152), which failed to demonstrate any benefit on PFS or OS with a second surgical attempt in such patients (Rose, 2004). Nevertheless, median OS was 44.3 months versus 49.0 months for chemotherapy versus PDS, respectively, corresponding to a HR for survival of 1.05 (90.8% CI, 0.83 to 1.33; $P$ = .24 for noninferiority) favoring the latter. Heterogeneity in outcomes was seen in low-volume centers and patients with poor medical or performance characteristics. Compared with the EORTC and CHORUS trials, the absolute OS values are substantially longer in the JCOG trial, which is not completely clear from patient or operative characteristics among the three trials. Because the absolute PFS values are more aligned, the differential improvement in OS may reflect the recency of the latter trial and the availability of newer therapeutic agents.

### Interval Cytoreduction

Cytoreductive surgery performed after an initial failed attempt or in patients who were initially not considered candidates for cytoreductive surgery is referred to as interval cytoreductive surgery. This approach is interictally linked to the neoadjuvant chemotherapy approach described earlier, which has been largely the result of celiotomy. More recently, there has been an increased interest in the implementation of minimally invasive surgery when performing interval debulking surgery. In a study by Aletti and colleagues, the authors assessed the feasibility and early complication rates of minimally invasive surgery in 52 patients with stage III/IV ovarian cancer after undergoing neoadjuvant chemotherapy. The authors found that the median operative time was 285 minutes (range, 124 to 418) and the median estimated blood loss was 100 mL (range, 50 to 200). A microscopic residual was obtained in 96.6% of patients. No early postoperative complications were registered. Median time to restart of chemotherapy was 20 days (range, 10 to 30). **The authors concluded that minimally invasive interval debulking surgery after neoadjuvant chemotherapy was safe and feasible.** Subsequently, Fagotti and colleagues evaluated the role of minimally invasive surgery at the time of interval debulking surgery in different gynecologic cancer centers. A total of 127 patients were included. Among them, 96.1% of patients had no residual tumor. The rate of intraoperative complications was 4.7%, and 4.7% of patients experienced a postoperative short-term complication. The conversion rate to laparotomy was 3.9%. **The authors concluded that minimally invasive surgery may be considered for the management of patients with advanced ovarian cancer when surgery is limited to low-complexity procedures.**

One critical element when introducing a novel surgical modality or approach is ensuring that it does not compromise cancer-related outcomes. Although minimally invasive surgery has been shown to be safe and feasible, there is a paucity of prospective randomized data showing equivalence or noninferiority of minimally invasive interval debulking compared with open surgery. A study by Melamed and colleagues used the National Cancer Database to identify a cohort of patients diagnosed with stage IIIC and IV epithelial ovarian cancer who underwent neoadjuvant chemotherapy and interval debulking surgery by laparoscopy or open surgery and determined the 3-year survival rates, length of hospitalization, perioperative mortality, risk of readmission, and residual disease. The authors identified 3071 patients, of whom 450 (15%) underwent surgery initiated by laparoscopy. **The authors found no difference in 3-year survival between patients undergoing laparoscopy (47.5%) and laparotomy (52.6%), $P$ = .12).** Postoperative hospitalization was shorter in the laparoscopy group (median 4 compared with 5 days, $P < .001$). Readmission (5.3% vs. 3.7%; $P$ = .26), death within 90 days of surgery (2.8% vs. 2.9%, $P$ = .93), and suboptimal debulking (20.6% vs. 22.6%, $P$ = .29), did not differ between patients undergoing laparoscopy versus laparotomy.

### Hyperthermic Intraperitoneal Chemotherapy

**The value of hyperthermic intraperitoneal chemotherapy (HIPEC) in epithelial ovarian cancer appears to be inconclusive, as evidenced by contradictory and inconsistent results.** Although it has been used routinely in the setting of metastasizing appendiceal cancer and later in colon cancer, the integration of HIPEC in the management of patients with ovarian cancer, particularly after upfront cytoreductive surgery, should remain experimental; however, there is evidence from prospective

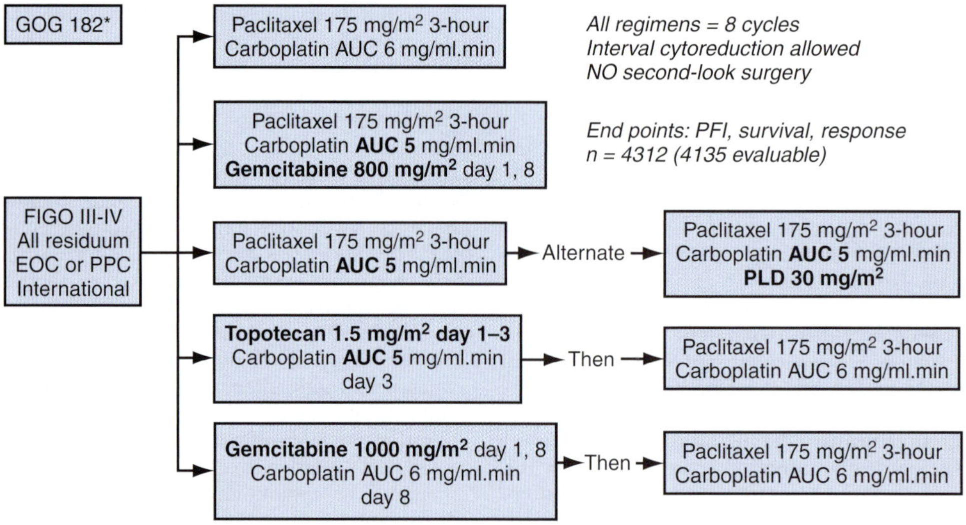


**Fig. 33.14** The GOG-182 trial that randomized 4312 patients to one of four experimental arms against paclitaxel and carboplatin. (Modified from Bookman MA, Brady MF, McGuire WP, et al. Evaluation of new platinum-based treatment regimens in advanced-stage ovarian cancer: a phase III trial of the Gynecologic Cancer Intergroup. *J Clin Oncol.* 2009;27:1419-1425.)

randomized data that HIPEC may have a role in treating patients undergoing interval cytoreductive surgery. In a 2018 multicenter, phase III randomized trial, van Driel and colleagues evaluated whether the addition of HIPEC to interval cytoreductive surgery would improve outcomes among patients who had undergone neoadjuvant chemotherapy for stage III epithelial ovarian cancer. A total of 245 patients with at least stable disease after neoadjuvant chemotherapy were randomly assigned to undergo interval cytoreductive surgery either with or without HIPEC. The authors found that the median survival was 33.9 months in the surgery group and 45.7 months in the surgery-plus-HIPEC group. Interestingly, they found that the percentage of patients who had adverse events was similar in the two groups (25% in the surgery group and 27% in the surgery-plus-HIPEC group). **The authors concluded that the addition of HIPEC to interval cytoreductive surgery resulted in longer recurrence-free survival and OS than surgery alone and that it did not result in higher rates of side effects.**

### Additions to the Paclitaxel and Carboplatin Backbone

It has been postulated that agents with nonoverlapping cross-resistance mechanisms or alternative mechanisms of action may be complementary opportunities in primary ovarian cancer patients to improve the therapeutic index. Several trials have been completed, with mixed results. The prevalent strategy has been to add to platinum and taxane therapy or substitute another agent for paclitaxel. The largest trial reported to date is GOG-182, which randomly allocated 4312 patients to one of four experimental arms against paclitaxel and carboplatin (Bookman, 2009). Two of the experimental arms involved a three-drug strategy (adding gemcitabine or pegylated liposomal doxorubicin to paclitaxel and carboplatin, with the latter triplet given every other course) and two others substituted topotecan or gemcitabine for paclitaxel for four of the eight planned cycles in a sequential administration design (Fig. 33.14).

Although considered a highly successful trial in terms of global participation and recruitment, the trial failed to improve outcomes by any parameter (response, PFS, or OS); however, as anticipated, the three-drug regimens were more toxic. Two other trials, the MITO-2, which randomized patients to an experimental regimen with carboplatin and pegylated liposomal doxorubicin, and OVAR9, which randomly assigned patients to an experimental arm of paclitaxel, carboplatin, and gemcitabine, also failed to demonstrate superiority to this strategy (du Bois, 2010; Pignata, 2011). It is unclear whether the addition or substitution of available cytotoxic agents in this setting will improve outcomes in primary disease, given the probability for overlapping toxicities.

Based on efficacy data regarding angiogenesis inhibition on ovarian cancer response and prevention of progression, several trials were launched with the agent bevacizumab. GOG-0218 included two experimental arms with chemotherapy in combination with bevacizumab—one arm also administered bevacizumab as a maintenance agent for sixteen 21-day cycles after primary therapy and the other experimental arm administered only placebo in maintenance (Burger, 2011). ICON7 was a two-armed trial in which bevacizumab was administered with chemotherapy at half the dose of GOG-0218 (7.5 mg/kg) but for 12 cycles in maintenance after administration with paclitaxel and carboplatin for five or six cycles (Perren, 2011). The trials have important differences (Table 33.8). **Both met their primary endpoint, PFS, but yielded no difference in OS data. In GOG-218 the improvement in PFS over paclitaxel and carboplatin was seen only for arm 3, in which bevacizumab was administered with chemotherapy and in the maintenance setting (HR, 0.717; 95% CI, 0.625 to 0.824). Similarly, there was a significant PFS benefit in the ICON7 trial favoring bevacizumab in combination with chemotherapy followed by bevacizumab maintenance (HR, 0.81; 95% CI, 0.70 to 0.94).** Both studies reported post hoc analyses indicating the greatest benefit for bevacizumab combination therapy in patients at high risk for recurrence. In ICON7, this was defined as patients with suboptimal stage III or stage IV disease. In GOG-0218, *high risk* was defined as those patients with stage IV disease. Importantly, there was an OS benefit for patients with stage IV disease treated with the bevacizumab combination in GOG-0218 (HR, 0.75; 95% CI, 0.59 to 0.95) (Tewari, 2019).

Additional studies of other molecules targeting one or more processes of angiogenesis and novel targets, such as the folate receptor and DNA damage repair (discussed later), are being pursued in this setting.

### Intraperitoneal Therapy

One promising but relatively old strategy that has been investigated is chemotherapy given by the intraperitoneal (IP) route. Ovarian cancer appears to be IP friendly because the distribution of disease is largely confined to this space, the pharmacokinetics

**TABLE 33.8** Comparison of GOG-0218 and ICON7 Study Characteristics

| | Trial | |
|---|---|---|
| **Parameter** | **GOG-0218** | **ICON7** |
| Setting and design | Double blinded, placebo controlled<br>Three-arm study<br>Bevacizumab for 16 cycles (maintenance)<br>Bevacizumab dose, 15 mg/kg every 3 weeks | Open label<br>Two-arm study<br>Bevacizumab for 12 cycles<br>Bevacizumab dose, 7.5 mg/kg every 3 weeks |
| Patient population | Stage III (suboptimal)<br>Stage III (optimal, visual or palpable)<br>Stage IV | Stage I or IIA (grade 3/clear cell histologic type)<br>Stages IIB-IV (all) |
| Additional endpoint | OS analysis (formal testing at time of PFS)<br>IRC | Defined final OS analysis (end, 2012)<br>No IRC |

*GOG*, Gynecologic Oncology Group; *ICON*, International Collaborative Ovarian Neoplasm; *IRC*, independent radiology review; *OS*, overall survival; *PFS*, progression-free survival.

of drug delivery are favorable, and the tumor is considered chemosensitive. Pharmacologic studies in the 1970s and 1980s demonstrated favorable profiles of relatively high direct drug exposure (high $C_{max}$ and AUC) for a number of agents subsequently identified to be important for ovarian cancer treatment. In this regard, platinum (cisplatin and carboplatin) and taxanes (paclitaxel and docetaxel) have been shown to have superior pharmacokinetic profiles when delivered into the peritoneum directly compared with intravenous (IV) administration.

**Administration is done principally via an implantable vascular access device placed during surgery.** More than eight randomized clinical studies formally evaluating the efficacy of IP-based chemotherapy compared with IV-based chemotherapy in patients with advanced-stage ovarian cancer have been reported. **A meta-analysis of these studies has been published and concluded that the route of administration "has the potential to improve cure rates from ovarian cancer" (Jaaback et al., 2016). Similarly, the NCI issued a clinical announcement accompanying the publication of a large GOG study stating that the IV and IP regimen "conveys a significant survival benefit among women with optimally debulked epithelial ovarian cancer, compared with intravenous administration alone"** (NCI, 2006). In this latter study, patients with stage III epithelial ovarian cancer rendered optimal (defined as postoperative residual disease <1 cm) were eligible for random allocation to standard IV cisplatin and paclitaxel (24-hour infusion) or to IV paclitaxel (135 mg/m$^2$ on day 1), IP cisplatin (100 mg/m$^2$ on day 2), and IP paclitaxel (60 mg/m$^2$ on day 8) (Armstrong, 2006). Both cohorts were to undergo repeat cycles every 21 days for six total infusions. The primary endpoints were PFS and OS, and reassessment operations, if planned, were indicated at random allocation.

Overall, 415 eligible patients made up the study population. Both PFS and OS were significantly improved in the intent to treat the IP cohort ($HR_{PFS}$, 0.80; 95% CI, 0.64 to 1.00; $HR_{Death}$, 0.75; 95% CI, 0.58 to 0.97, respectively). The recorded median OS of 65.6 months is among the longest ever observed in an adjuvant therapy phase III ovarian cancer study. The results are even more impressive given that most (58%) randomly allocated IP patients did not complete all six cycles of their assigned therapy via IP administration. This was largely because of significant differences in hematologic and nonhematologic toxicities associated with the IP regimen. In a reflection of these observed adverse events, health-related quality-of-life assessments were significantly lower throughout the trial but returned to parity 12 months after therapy. It was concluded that the IP regimen provides superior survival efficacy and is associated with significant but manageable toxicity. The authors encouraged the use of IP therapy in clinical practice.

Lesnock and colleagues reported on the impact of somatic or germline *BRCA* mutation status relative to IP (vs. IV) therapy (Lesnock, 2013). In this trial just less than half (48%) of the population had aberrant *BRCA* expression in the tumor. Patients with tumors harboring aberrant *BRCA* expression who received IP therapy had substantially longer PFS and OS relative to patients with aberrant *BRCA* expression receiving IV chemotherapy. This highlights the important role *BRCA* alterations have on outcomes, particularly in those receiving IP therapy. Toxicity concerns and a number of unanswered fundamental questions regarding efficacy (e.g., optimal agent, schedule, future trial designs) and the impact of alternative agents such as biologic therapies (e.g., vascular endothelial growth factor and epidermal growth factor targeting) limited the general acceptance of this strategy in the clinical community. Subsequent randomized controlled trials have again called the utility of IP therapy into question. **In GOG-252, 1560 patients were randomly allocated between dose-dense IV paclitaxel with IV carboplatin versus dose-dense IV paclitaxel with IP carboplatin versus every-3-weeks IV paclitaxel with IP cisplatin and IP paclitaxel. Bevacizumab was included in all arms. There was no difference in PFS or OS between the three arms** (Walker, 2019).

### Dose-Dense Chemotherapy

One additional strategy, dose-dense and dose-intense chemotherapy, has received attention based on positive results reported in patients with primary ovarian cancer (Katsumata, 2009). The trial, conducted by the Japanese Gynecologic Oncology Group (JGOG) and published in 2009, randomly assigned 631 patients to standard paclitaxel (180 mg/m$^2$) and carboplatin (AUC 6) or weekly paclitaxel (80 mg/m$^2$ per week) and carboplatin (AUC 6) for six to nine cycles. The dose density (measured in mg/m$^2$ per week) was 33% greater in the experimental arm. **Despite just 62% of patients receiving six or more cycles of the dose-dense strategy (vs. 73% in the control arm), the median PFS was 28 versus 17.2 months (HR, 0.714; $P$ = .0015). OS, although early, also demonstrated a significant difference, with 3-year OS in the experimental arm at 72.1% versus 65.1% in the control arm (HR, 0.75; $P$ = .03).** The remarkable results of JGOG-3026 prompted reevaluation of this strategy in different patient populations. In MITO-7, 810 patients were randomly assigned to paclitaxel (175 mg/m$^2$) plus carboplatin (AUC 6) on a 3-week schedule or weekly paclitaxel (60 mg/m$^2$) plus carboplatin (AUC 2) on days 1, 8, and 15 of a 21-day cycles. PFS and OS were coprimary endpoints (Pignata, 2014). Approximately half the patients in both arms had an optimal cytoreduction (≤1 cm residual disease), and both regimens were well tolerated, although more dose interruptions or delays and lower dose intensity was seen with the weekly arm. **Nevertheless, after a median follow-up of 22.3 months the median PFS was 17.3 months for the 3-week arm versus 18.3 months for the weekly arm (HR, 0.96; 95% CI, 0.80 to 1.16; *P* = .66); for OS, the estimated probability of survival at 24 months was 78.9% in the 3-week arm versus 77.3% in the weekly arm (HR, 1.20; 95% CI, 0.90 to 1.61; *P* = .22).**

The 2019 ICON8 trial reported on the evaluation of a 3-week infusion schedule (paclitaxel 175 mg/m$^2$ plus carboplatin AUC 5 or 6) to two weekly schedules: one with paclitaxel 80 mg/m$^2$ plus 3-week carboplatin AUC 5 or 6, and one with paclitaxel 80 mg/m$^2$ with carboplatin AUC 2 administered weekly (Clamp, 2019). All arms were followed a planned 21-day cycle, with day 15 infusions dropped on day 15 of cycle 3 for tolerance. Overall, 1565 patients were randomly allocated 1:1:1; both primary debulking and neoadjuvant therapy could be used. **In the intent-to-treat population, the median PFS was 17.9 months for the 3-week arm and 20.6 months and 21.1 months for the weekly paclitaxel/3-week carboplatin and weekly paclitaxel/weekly carboplatin arms, respectively. These were not statistically different.** As expected, patients undergoing neoadjuvant therapy as a group fared worse than those undergoing primary surgery, but there was no difference among these cohorts by chemotherapy type. Adverse events were similar between arms in the initial presentation. Data on OS were immature.

Another trial evaluating dose-dense strategy was GOG-262, which was conducted in women with suboptimal (defined as postoperative tumor residuum of greater than 1 cm) cytoreduction or undergoing NACT (Chan, 2016). In this phase III trial, 692 women were randomly allocated 1:1 to dose-dense paclitaxel (80 mg/m$^2$, weekly) plus carboplatin AUC 6 or standard 3-week paclitaxel/carboplatin. Bevacizumab could be added at the discretion of the physician and, if chosen, was to be administered in maintenance until progression. Overall, 84% of patients received bevacizumab and more than 87% underwent a primary debulking attempt. **In contrast to the JGOG trial, no significant difference was observed between the arms for PFS or OS; however, looking at just the cohort who opted not to receive bevacizumab, the dose-dense strategy was more effective on PFS.** When bevacizumab was added, this effect was lost. This strategy is the subject of ongoing phase III studies with similar designs, addressing intraperitoneal infusion, and with the addition of bevacizumab (e.g., IPocc, GOG-252). In all, it is unclear that dose-dense chemotherapy offers an advantage across all patient cohorts. The outlier is the JGOG3026 trial, which may indicate differential cytotoxicity of this dosing administration in Asian–Pacific Islander populations. More work will be needed to establish optimal therapy.

### Evaluation of Chemotherapy Results

Chemotherapy is usually administered every 3 weeks. The patient is monitored with careful physical examination; blood tests to measure hematologic, liver, and kidney function; and radiographic studies, such as chest radiography, ultrasound, or, usually, CT of the abdomen and pelvis. Granulocyte colony-stimulating factor is added as needed to combat neutropenia. Mild neutropenia after chemotherapy can be managed expectantly, but for the patient who develops severe neutropenia with fever and an absolute neutrophil count of less than 500 cells/mL, antibiotics are prescribed to prevent septic complications.

After completion of chemotherapy, imaging is typically obtained to assess response. If tumor is suspected on CT scan, biopsy may be used to document the presence of persistent or recurrent disease. A negative CT scan, however, does not guarantee complete clinical response. Goldhirsch and coworkers noted that 5 of 26 patients with tumor nodules larger than 1 cm have negative CT scans. In 1989 Reuter and colleagues reported improved results of 8% false negatives using newer equipment, with CT slices at 10- to 15-mm intervals. Patsner has reported that 24 of 60 patients with negative CT scans have a positive second-look operation, calling into question the value of this imaging study. CA-125 levels are used to monitor the course of the woman with carcinoma. As noted, Buller and colleagues calculated that the CA-125 level follows an exponential regression curve in successfully treated patients. This provides the possibility of mathematically estimating the patient's response to chemotherapy early in treatment. Bridgewater and associates reported that a greater than 50% decrease in the CA-125 level is a good sign of clinical response.

### Maintenance Therapy

Unfortunately, many patients develop recurrent disease, even after evidence of clinical complete response. Rubin and associates noted a high rate of recurrence (45%) in patients with a negative second-look laparotomy. Those who initially have higher-stage and higher-grade tumors are more likely to have a recurrence; however, those who were disease free at 5 years are likely to remain disease free by the subsequent follow-up period. Nonetheless, this high recurrence risk has prompted the evaluation of additional treatment at the identification of a complete response to primary treatment. This is often termed *maintenance* or *consolidation therapy*, although the former term is favored, given that the decision for treatment is based on the effect of primary therapy. Several randomized and nonrandomized clinical trials have been conducted in this arena, including hormones, vitamins, radiation therapy, chemotherapy, radioimmunoconjugates, immunotherapy, vaccines, gene therapy, biologic therapy, complementary medicines, and holistic approaches. Unfortunately, the majority have been negative in regard to improving OS. A randomized study of two regimens of paclitaxel did show an improvement in PFS. Markman and coworkers studied whether 3 or 12 additional months of paclitaxel could influence the time until progression in women who had achieved a complete clinical remission after primary treatment. The trial was designed to accrue 450 patients; however, at a planned interim analysis (after 277 patients were randomly allocated), a statistically significant benefit for the longer treatment was demonstrated, which closed the trial to further accrual. **The initial report demonstrated a 7-month improvement in median PFS (28 vs. 21 months; *P* = .0035); a later report with a long follow-up confirmed these earlier results (median PFS, 21 vs. 14 months; *P* = .006). No effect on survival was demonstrated, however.** As noted, the addition of a maintenance biologic agent such as bevacizumab improved PFS relative to placebo, but there was no impact on OS.

Several additional biologic agents have entered phase III in this setting with mixed results. Pazopanib, an oral tyrosine kinase inhibitor (TKI) of vascular endothelial growth factor receptor (VEGFR), platelet-derived growth factor receptor (PDGFR) c-Kit, and fibroblast growth factor receptor (FGFR), was studied in women without evidence of progression on primary chemotherapy (du Bois, 2014). In all, 940 women were randomly assigned to either placebo or pazopanib for up to 24 months. The primary endpoint was PFS, which was extended by 5.6 months on the median (HR, 0.77; 95% CI, 0.64 to 0.91; *P* = .0021). Unfortunately, no difference was seen in OS, and the regimen was associated higher rates of hepatotoxicity, hypertension, and gastrointestinal adverse events.

Another TKI targeting the epidermal growth factor receptor (EGFR) pathway, erlotinib, was studied as a primary maintenance intervention in a phase III randomized trial (Vergote, 2014). In this trial, 835 patients achieving complete clinical response (CR) to six to nine cycles of platinum-based chemotherapy were randomly allocated to either erlotinib (150 mg/day) for 24 months or observation. The primary endpoint was PFS, which was similar between the two arms (erlotinib, 12.7 months; observation, 12.4 months; *P* = .91). Similarly, OS was no different between the arms. Of interest, PFS was not associated with aberrations in EGFR, Ras, Raf, and phophatidylinositol-3-kinase (PI3K).

Another strategy that has been tried and continues to be of great interest is immunotherapy (discussed in detail later). Acting against the ability of a tumor to evade the immune system holds great promise in the maintenance setting, and a number of ongoing trials have incorporated immunotherapy, alone and in combination with PARP inhibitors, antiangiogenics, and other targeted therapies, to leverage this potential.

### CA-125 Surveillance After Primary Therapy

Because patients with advanced ovarian cancer commonly have CA-125 values that pace tumor response and progression during therapy, a common practice for monitoring patients after therapy involves serial CA-125 level determinations. The supposition is that earlier identification of recurrent disease can be better controlled by earlier initiation of therapy. To formally address this hypothesis, the EORTC conducted a randomized phase III trial in which women in complete clinical remission after primary surgery and chemotherapy were enrolled into a blinded surveillance program (Rustin, 1996). Follow-up visits were scheduled every 3 months, when an examination was performed and blood was taken for CA-125 level assessment. All registrants were blinded to their CA-125 values during this time; however, when an individual's CA-125 level rose to twice the upper limit of normal, the patient was randomly allocated 1:1 to unblinding of the result (early) or continued blinded surveillance (delayed). In this latter group, intervention was determined by the development of clinical or symptomatic relapse. Postprogression therapy was determined by local standard of care. The primary endpoint of the study was OS. In all, 1442 patients were registered, of whom 529 were randomly assigned to the treatment groups. Patients unblinded and made aware of their rising CA-125 values generally started treatment immediately, 4.8 months (median) before those in the delayed group. After a median follow-up of almost 57 months from random allocation and 370 deaths, there was no difference in OS between the arms (HR, 0.98; 95% CI, 0.8 to 1.2). Median survival in the early treatment group was 25.7 months compared with 27.1 months in the delayed group. For patients receiving third-line therapy, the time differential to initiation was almost the same as the time differential to initiation of second-line therapy (median 4.6 months). Interestingly, a first deterioration in Global Health score occurred significantly sooner in the early treatment group. The authors concluded that no benefit in survival was gained by treatment dictated solely by an asymptomatic rise in CA-125 level and challenged the practice of routine biomarker surveillance in this setting. Of note, this study was completed before the availability of targeted therapies such as antiangiogenic and DNA-damaging agents. The utility of early identification of recurrence in the setting of potential targeted therapy is unknown.

**The decision to follow CA-125 during disease surveillance remains an important conversation between a patient and her physician.** Although practice standards may have changed on the based on the trial just described, counseling patients to watchful waiting is a challenge in the setting of rising CA-125 level without measurable recurrent disease.

### Recurrent Ovarian Cancer Management

Unfortunately, as many as 70% of patients who present with advanced-stage disease will exhibit recurrent or persistent disease after primary treatment. These women may have prolonged survival despite developing recurrence; however, they are rarely cured. For this reason, treatment is generally considered palliative and must balance efficacy with toxicity. The choice of therapy is largely empirical; the treatment plan usually involves several agents in sequence, depending on treatment history, observed and expected toxicity, and performance status. Surgery, chemotherapy, immunotherapy, radiation therapy, biotherapy, and hormone therapy are options, alone and in combination, in this cohort of patients. It is not uncommon for a woman to undergo five or more different chemotherapy regimens, including cycles of retreatment with one or more agents. This characteristic reflects the increasing number of agents available for use, the short duration of response, and the general health of those receiving therapy.

Although there are few specific treatment guidelines addressing how recurrence should be approached, initial consideration is most often guided by the interval of time until recurrence is identified. Patients are categorized as potentially platinum sensitive, platinum resistant, or platinum refractory based on the time from the completion of primary therapy until recurrence is identified. By convention, patients exhibiting a treatment-free interval of 6 months or longer are considered as having potentially platinum-sensitive disease. Those who achieved a complete response and were identified with recurrence under this benchmark are considered platinum resistant, and those who did not achieve a complete response or had disease progression during frontline therapy are considered platinum refractory. In reality, the probability for subsequent chemotherapy response likely represents a continuum based on this interval of time; however, clinically the arbitrary division is used commonly to make treatment decisions.

## Platinum-Refractory Disease

Patients who fall into the designation of platinum refractory have a difficult disease to treat because their objective response to almost all available agents is low and the duration of any individual therapy is short. The choice of therapy depends on the woman's wishes and comorbidities. Because expectations for response to standard agents are low, these women are good candidates for investigative clinical studies, in which new agents with alternative mechanisms of action or targets are being evaluated. Under these expectations, some patients may opt to continue active treatment, whereas others may choose supportive care.

### Platinum-Resistant Disease

Patients demonstrating an abbreviated initial response to frontline therapy represent cohorts who are unlikely to respond well to platinum retreatment. This is not to imply that some of these patients would not respond to retreatment with a platinum compound, just that the probability of response would be no greater than with any other agent and potentially lower. A recommendation for most of these patients is to consider an alternative nonplatinum agent for the first treatment of recurrence. Table 33.9 lists the potential agents for treating these patients, their respective response rates, and significant common toxicities. Patients achieving stable disease or better are usually treated until the agent no longer demonstrates a clinical benefit or toxicity precludes further infusion.

Because expected OS is shorter in patients with this phenotype, a number of clinical trials with novel agents have been completed or are ongoing (see Targeted Therapy later in the chapter).

### Platinum-Sensitive Disease

Patients in whom disease recurrence is identified more than 6 months after the completion of frontline treatment are considered potentially platinum sensitive. These patients are good candidates for retreatment with platinum or a platinum-based combination regimen. In many cases this combination is similar to that received in frontline treatment, paclitaxel and carboplatin; however, other two-drug and three-drug combinations have been investigated. A limited number of phase III studies have been conducted in this setting, but only one has demonstrated an OS advantage for the use of a taxane- and platinum-based regimen. The ICON4-AGO-OVAR 2.2 study randomly assigned 802 women with recurrent ovarian cancer to paclitaxel and platinum

**TABLE 33.9** Clinical Efficacy of Cytotoxic Agents in Platinum-Resistant and Platinum-Sensitive Ovarian Cancer Toxicity

| | Response Rate (%) | | |
|---|---|---|---|
| **Agent** | **Platinum Resistant** | **Platinum Sensitive** | **Principal Toxicity** |
| PLD | 14-20 | 28 | PPE, mucositis |
| Topotecan | 14-18 | 33 | Myelosuppression |
| Hexamethylmelamine | 10-18 | 27 | Nausea, vomiting |
| Gemcitabine | 16 | | Myelosuppression |
| Etoposide | 27 | 35 | Myelosuppression, leukemia |
| Ifosfamide | 12 | | Hemorrhagic cystitis, CNS |
| Tamoxifen | 10-15 | 10-15 | Hot flashes, thromboembolic |
| Docetaxel | 22-25 | 38 | Myelosuppression |
| Paclitaxel | 12-33 | 20-41 | Myelosuppression |
| Vinorelbine | 21 | 29 | Myelosuppression |

*CNS,* Central nervous system neurotoxicity; *PLD,* pegylated liposomal doxorubicin; *PPE,* palmar-plantar erythrodysesthesia.

or a nontaxane platinum regimen. The objective response was 66% in the taxane arm compared with 54% in the non-taxane arm ($P$ = .06). PFS was significantly improved (12 vs. 9 months; HR, 0.76; 95% CI, 0.66 to 0.89), as was OS (29 vs. 24 months; HR, 0.82; 95% CI, 0.69 to 0.97). Approximately 75% of women in both groups had a treatment-free interval of at least 12 months, and 64% were taxane naïve at random allocation. These are important factors when considering the study's conclusions. In all, six phase III clinical trials in platinum-sensitive patients have been completed. They differ substantially by agents investigated, sample size, use of measurable patients, prior exposure to paclitaxel and platinum in frontline therapy, and median progress-free interval before registration. Each of these factors has important consequences in regard to the data reported, making cross-trial comparisons among experimental groups hazardous. Table 33.10 summarizes the key features of these trials. It is noteworthy that two of these efforts included the use of nonplatinum agents in potentially platinum-sensitive patients, according to the definition provided earlier. These are important trials to consider given the high rate of drug hypersensitivity (platinum or taxane), intolerance, and lack of a clear benefit between platinum-containing and nonplatinum-containing agents in patients with moderate platinum-sensitive disease, such as those recurring between 6 and 12 months after primary therapy.

Novel targeted therapies, including antiangiogenesis agents and PARP inhibitors, have been used to enhance the efficacy of platinum-based treatment in potentially platinum-sensitive disease (These are outlined later in the section on Targeted Therapy; their efficacy has led to new FDA approvals.) To better characterize the heterogeneity of patients with recurrent disease, new descriptive criteria have been suggested, including treatment-free interval (<3 months, 3 to 12 months, >12 months), *BRCA1/2* status (mutation, BRCA-like [homologous recombination deficiency (HRD)], other), histologic type (high-grade serous or endometrioid, other), and number of prior regimens (three or fewer, more than three) (Alvarez, 2016). Understanding individual patient and tumor characteristics in the setting of recurrent disease has become vital to optimizing both strategy and care for these women, who are expected to endure a significant time in postprogression survivorship.

## Secondary Cytoreduction

The recurrence rate in patients with advanced epithelial ovarian cancer ranges from 50% to 90%. Therefore secondary cytoreductive surgery might be a viable treatment option for a select group of patients. Although there is some inconsistency in the definition of secondary cytoreduction procedures, the specific intent in this setting is resection of disease at recurrence, with the intent of debulking. The treatment of recurrent epithelial ovarian cancer is variable and dependent on a number of important criteria, which are evaluated at the time the recurrence is diagnosed. These include but are not limited to the time from completion of initial adjuvant therapy, site of disease, number of disease sites, and the woman's performance status. Most studies in the literature suggest that patients with platinum-resistant disease (recurrent disease within 6 months of completing platinum-based treatment) do not benefit from secondary cytoreductive surgery; however, others have argued for a role of surgery in this patient population.

In observational studies, secondary cytoreductive surgery has been associated with improved survival; however, its implementation has drawn significant controversy since the improved outcomes of surgery may reflect selection bias rather than the superiority of secondary surgery over systemic therapy. A 2018 study by Gockley and colleagues compared the OS of women with platinum-sensitive recurrent ovarian cancer treated at NCI–designated cancer centers who underwent secondary surgery versus chemotherapy. The study had the primary outcome of OS. Propensity-score matching was used to compare similar women who received secondary surgery versus chemotherapy. Data on a total of 626 women were analyzed; 146 women (23%) received secondary surgery, and 480 (77%) received chemotherapy. In adjusted analyses, patients who received secondary surgery were younger ($P$ = .001), had earlier-stage disease at diagnosis ($P$ = .002), and had longer disease-free intervals ($P$ < .001) compared with those receiving chemotherapy. The median survival was 54 months in patients who received secondary surgery and 33 months in those treated with chemotherapy ($P$ < .001). Among patients who received secondary surgery, 102 (70%) achieved optimal secondary cytoreduction. The authors concluded that patients who underwent secondary surgery had a superior median OS compared with patients who underwent chemotherapy (Gockley, 2018).

In a study by Zang and colleagues, the authors aimed to identify prognostic factors and to develop a risk model predicting survival in patients undergoing secondary cytoreductive surgery (SCR) for recurrent epithelial ovarian cancer (Zang, 2011). Individual data for 1100 patients with recurrent ovarian cancer of a progression-free interval at least 6 months who underwent SCR were pooled and analyzed. Complete SCR was strongly associated with the improvement of survival, with a median survival of

**TABLE 33.10** Phase III Trials in Patients with Platinum-Sensitive Recurrent Disease

| Control | Experimental | No. of Patients | TTP/PFS (wk) | *P* | OS (wk) | *P* | Comments |
|---|---|---|---|---|---|---|---|
| Carboplatin* | Carboplatin Epirubicin | 190 | 65 vs. 78 | NS | 109 vs. 122 | NS | TFI 17 mo; grade 4 ANC, 45%; T RBC, 30%, Plt, 25% |
| Platinum† | Platinum Paclitaxel | 802 | 43 vs. 52; HR, 0.76 | <.001 | 104 vs. 130 HR, 0.82 | .023 | TFI 75% >12 mo; neuro 1% vs. 20%; infection, 17%; hematologic, 46% vs. 29% |
| Carboplatin‡ | Carboplatin Gemcitabine | 356 | 23 vs. 35 HR, 0.72 | <.001 | 75 vs. 78 | NS .0016 | TFI 60% >12 mo; RR 31% vs. 47% ANC, Plt more common in combination |
| Carboplatin, Paclitaxel§ | Carboplatin PLD | 976 | 41 vs. 49 HR, 0.82 | .001 (noninferiority) .005 (superiority) | 30.7 vs. 33.0 | .94 | TFI nonhematologic, 37% vs. 29%; HSR, 19% vs. 6%; grade 2-3 PPE, 2% vs. 12% |
| Topotecan‖ | Topotecan/etoposide Topotecan/gemcitabine | 502 | HR, 0.84 HR, 0.84 | NS NS | HR, 1.13 HR, 1.07 | NS NS | TFI 64% >12 mo More hematologic toxicity, less alopecia in topotecan-gemcitabine arm |
| PLD¶ | PLD Trabectedin | 672 | 25 vs. 32 HR, 0.79 | 0.019 | 82 vs. 97 HR, 0.86 (*P* = .08) | PLD | TFI (32% >12 mo); effect seen only in PS cohort; PPE less in combination; ANC, LFTs |

*Bolis G, et al. Carboplatin alone vs carboplatin plus epidoxorubicin as second-line therapy for cisplatin- or carboplatin-sensitive ovarian cancer. *Gynecol Oncol.* 2001;81:3-9.

†Parmar MK, et al. Paclitaxel plus platinum-based chemotherapy versus conventional platinum-based chemotherapy in women with relapsed ovarian cancer: the ICON4/AGO-OVAR-2.2 trial. *Lancet.* 2003;361:2099-2106. This arm was mostly single agent platinum; however, platinum combinations were also allowed.

‡Pfisterer J, et al. Gemcitabine plus carboplatin compared with carboplatin in patients with platinum-sensitive recurrent ovarian cancer: an intergroup trial of the AGO-OVAR, the NCIC CTG, and the EORTC GCG. *J Clin Oncol.* 2006;24:4699-4707.

§Pujade-Lauraine E, et al. Pegylated liposomal doxorubicin and carboplatin compared with paclitaxel and carboplatin for patients with platinum-sensitive ovarian cancer in late relapse. *J Clin Oncol.* 2010;28:3323-3329. Wagner U, Marth C, Largillier R, et al. Final overall survival results of phase III GCIG CALYPSO trial of pegylated liposomal doxorubicin and carboplatin vs paclitaxel and carboplatin in platinumsensitive ovarian cancer patients. *Br J Cancer.* 2012;107(4):588-91.

‖Sehouli J, et al. Nonplatinum topotecan combinations versus topotecan alone for recurrent ovarian cancer: results of a phase III study of the North-Eastern German Society of Gynecological Oncology Ovarian Cancer Study Group. *J Clin Oncol.* 2008;26:3176-3182.

¶Monk BJ, et al. Trabectedin plus pegylated liposomal doxorubicin (PLD) versus PLD in recurrent ovarian cancer: overall survival analysis. *Euro J Cancer.* 2012;48:2361-2368.

*ANC,* Absolute neutrophil count; *HR,* hazard ratio; *HSR,* hypersensitivity reaction; *LFTs,* liver function tests; *NA,* not available; *NS,* not significant; *OS,* overall survival; *PFS,* progression-free survival; *PLD,* pegylated liposomal doxorubicin; *Plt,* platelet count; *PPE,* palmar-plantar erythrodysesthesia; *RR,* response rate; *TFI,* treatment-free interval; *T RBC,* blood transfusion; *TTP,* time to treatment progression.

57.7 months, compared with 27 months in those with residual disease of 0.1 to 1 cm and 15.6 months in those with residual disease greater than 1 cm, respectively ($P < .0001$). Progression-free interval (≤23.1 months vs. >23.1 months; HR, 1.72; score, 2), ascites at recurrence (present vs. absent; HR, 1.27; score, 1), extent of recurrence (multiple vs. localized disease; HR, 1.38; score, 1), and residual disease after SCR (R1 vs. R0: HR, 1.90, score, 2; R2 vs. R0: HR, 3.0, score, 4) entered into the risk model.

In the AGO study, researchers also reported their efforts in establishing (DESKTOP OVAR I [Descriptive Evaluation of Preoperative Selection Criteria for Operability in Recurrent Ovarian Cancer] trial) and validating (DESKTOP OVAR II trial) a panel of features that would reliably predict optimal (no visible disease) secondary surgical outcomes in women with platinum-sensitive disease (Harter, 2006, 2011). The researchers found, as did others, that **only complete surgical cytoreduction was associated with an improved OS and that this could be reliably achieved (>67% of the time)** in patients who had a performance status of 0 or 1, were in the early stage, or had no visible tumor residuum after initial surgical cytoreduction and the absence of ascites.

GOG protocol 213 evaluated the role of SCR in patients with recurrent, platinum-sensitive ovarian cancer and the merit of adding an antiangiogenic agent (bevacizumab) to a combination of carboplatin and paclitaxel. In addition, this study evaluated the usefulness of maintenance bevacizumab until progression relative to control (Coleman, 2019). **The authors found that secondary cytoreduction can be safely performed in women with platinum-sensitive recurrent ovarian cancer. Complete gross resection was achieved in 68% of the per protocol population and was significantly higher (79%) among women with preoperative oligometastatic disease.** Women with oligometastatic disease undergoing surgery had longer PFS and OS than those with greater preoperative tumor burden; however, neither patients with oligometastatic disease nor those with a long preoperative platinum-free interval had superior OS compared with chemotherapy alone.

### Targeted Therapy

The processes that govern cell transformation and immortalization, tumor growth, and metastases for ovarian cancer are complex and nonuniform. Nonetheless, several critical targets have been identified that appear to be differentially expressed in tumors cells relative to normal cells. Novel agents that target disruption or inhibition of these specific processes have been incorporated into the care of ovarian cancer patients. The most developed of these are agents that disrupt the signals to engender

**TABLE 33.11** Randomized Phase III Trials of Combination Chemotherapy in Platinum-Resistant Ovarian Cancer Patients

| Control | Experimental | N | PFS (mo) | *P* | OS (mo) | *P* | Comment |
|---|---|---|---|---|---|---|---|
| PLD* | PLD + trabectedin | 228 | 3.7 vs. 4 | NS | 14.2 vs. 12.4 | NS | RR: 16% vs. 23% |
| Paclitaxel weekly† | Paclitaxel + trebananib | 480 | 5.6 vs. 3.8 | HR, .65 | NA | NA | OS: effect in ascites |
| Chemotherapy (paclitaxel weekly, gemcitabine, topotecan)‡ | Chemotherapy + bevacizumab | 361 | 3.4 vs. 6.7 | <.001 | 16.6 vs. 13.3 | NS | RR: 12% vs. 27% (RECIST) |
| Chemotherapy + placebo (paclitaxel weekly, gemcitabine, topotecan)§ | Chemotherapy + pertuzumab | 156 | 4.3 vs. 2.6 | NS | 10.3 vs. 7.9 | NS | Similar to AURELIA except all low Her3 (64%) Placebo controlled |

*Monk BJ, et al. Trabectedin plus pegylated liposomal doxorubicin in recurrent ovarian cancer. *J Clin Oncol.* 2010;28:3107-3114.
†Monk BJ, et al. Anti-angiopoietin therapy with trebananib for recurrent ovarian cancer (TRINOVA-1): a randomised, multicentre, double-blind, placebo-controlled phase 3 trial. *Lancet Oncol.* 2014;15:799-808.
‡Pujade-Lauraine E, et al. Bevacizumab combined with chemotherapy for platinum-resistant recurrent ovarian cancer: the AURELIA open-label randomized phase III trial. *J Clin Oncol.* 2014;32:1302-1308.
§Kurzeder C, et al. Efficacy and safety of chemotherapy (CT) ± pertuzumab (P) for platinum-resistant ovarian cancer (PROC): AGO-OVAR 2.20/ ENGOT-ov14/ PENELOPE double-blind placebo-controlled randomized phase III trial. *J Clin Oncol.* 2015;33.
*HR,* Hazard ratio; *NA,* not available; *NS,* not significant; *OS,* overall survival; *PFS,* progression-free survival; *PLD,* pegylated liposomal doxorubicin; *RR,* response rate.

new vessel growth and development or angiogenesis. This process appears critical for a tumor to continue its growth beyond 8 mm$^3$. A number of cytokines have been described that tip the balance to sustained angiogenesis, but the most potent is vascular endothelial growth factor (VEGF). Prognostically, VEGF expression has been documented in all stages of ovarian cancer and has been correlated with impaired survival. VEGF overexpression has also been directly associated with ascites formation. This clinical feature is the result VEGF-induced endothelial hyperpermeability. The compound furthest in development for the treatment for ovarian cancer is bevacizumab, which has been investigated for primary and recurrent ovarian cancers (discussed earlier); however, a number of agents targeting VEGF, its receptors, angiopoietin, the EGFR family, the PI3K/Akt/mTor pathway, and other cellular signaling pathways are also under investigation. In addition, new cytotoxics with alternative mechanisms of action, such as the tubulin poisons, and new topoisomerase inhibitors, agents that bind the minor groove of DNA (trabectedin), have been under phase III investigation. A summary of the outcomes of these trials is provided in Table 33.11. A detailed discussion of these trials is beyond the scope of this chapter; however, one trial deserves mention as it provided the background for the first approval of a biologically targeted agent in platinum-resistant disease. The AURELIA trial was a phase III open-label randomized trial comparing standard chemotherapy (weekly paclitaxel, pegylated liposomal doxorubicin, topotecan) to standard chemotherapy with bevacizumab (Pujade-Lauraine, 2014). The designation of chemotherapy was left to physician's choice, but each cohort was capped to provide equal representation in the randomization strata. The trial's primary endpoint was PFS. In the overall population, the addition of bevacizumab to chemotherapy significantly improved PFS (median 6.7 months vs. 3.4 months; HR, 0.48; 95% CI, 0.38 to 0.60; $P < .001$). The observation was consistent in each chemotherapy stratum; in addition, objective response was significantly improved, both of which may have contributed to the increased frequency of adverse events; however, quality-of-life indicators demonstrated improvement in global symptoms despite these observations. No difference was seen in OS. These data, along with a substantial database of bevacizumab use in ovarian and other cancers, led to the approval of bevacizumab in combination with chemotherapy for patients with recurrent platinum-resistant disease who have received one or two prior regimens.

Similarly, investigative efforts continue with novel therapies in patients with platinum-sensitive disease. A summary of the outcomes from these trials (newly diagnosed, platinum sensitive, and platinum resistant) is presented in Table 33.12. Each of these trials has demonstrated a significant effect in improving PFS, but the impact on OS has been less robust and may directly relate to the opportunities for treatment crossover and factors associated with long posttreatment survival. Only GOG-213 has demonstrated a significant improvement in both PFS and OS in women with platinum-sensitive recurrent disease (Coleman, 2017). This trial was unique in that it explored two primary objectives, both with the OS as the primary endpoint. The first objective was to evaluating the addition of bevacizumab to paclitaxel and carboplatin in women with first recurrent ovarian cancer with a minimum 6-month platinum-free interval. Patients were first considered for surgical candidacy (see earlier); if not, they were randomly allocated 1:1 to paclitaxel 175 mg/m$^2$ and carboplatin AUC 5 or the same chemotherapy plus bevacizumab 15 mg/kg every 21 days for up to 8 total cycles. Patients on the experimental arm went on to continue bevacizumab maintenance until disease progression or unacceptable toxicity if they had not progressed before maintenance. If surgical candidacy was met, eligible patients underwent random allocation 1:1 to surgery or no surgery before chemotherapy random allocation. In all, 674 women were enrolled and randomly assigned to a treatment arm; 107 of these women also underwent surgical random allocation. After a median follow-up of 49.6 months, the median OS for chemotherapy was 37.3 months compared with 42.2 months in the chemotherapy plus bevacizumab cohort (HR, 0.829; 95% CI, 0.683 to 1.005; $P = .056$). After a correction in the platinum-free interval stratification factor, the adjusted HR for OS was 0.823 (95% CI, 0.680 to 0.996; $P = .0447$). A similar significant improvement in PFS was seen. Median PFS in the control arm was 10.4 months versus 13.3 months, corresponding to an HR of 0.628 (95% CI, 0.534 to 0.739; $P < .001$). The results of these along with the favorable PFS seen with bevacizumab combined with gemcitabine/carboplatin in the Ovarian Cancer Study Comparing Efficacy and Safety of Chemotherapy and Anti-Angiogenic Therapy in Platinum-Sensitive Recurrent Disease (OCEANS) trial led to FDA approval of bevacizumab in combination with chemotherapy (Aghajanian, 2012). A third trial, reported in 2018, comparing pegylated liposomal doxorubicin, carboplatin, and bevacizumab to gemcitabine, carboplatin, and bevacizumab confirmed that this

**TABLE 33.12** Summary of Phase III Trials Evaluating the Addition of Antiangiogenesis Targeted Agents in Patients with Ovarian Cancer

| Study | Agent | Target | HR-PFS (95% CI) | HR-OS (95% CI) |
|---|---|---|---|---|
| GOG-0218* | Bevacizumab | VEGF ligand | 0.72 (0.63-0.82) | 0.89 (0.75-1.04) |
| ICON7† | Bevacizumab | | 0.81 (0.70-0.94) | 0.99 (0.85-1.14) |
| AURELIA‡ | Bevacizumab | | 0.48 (0.38-0.60) | 0.85 (0.66-1.08) |
| OCEANS§ | Bevacizumab | | 0.53 (0.41-0.70) | 0.96 (0.76-1.21) |
| GOG-0213‖ | Bevacizumab | | 0.628 (0.53-0.74) | 0.83 (0.68-1.005)<br>Adjusted: 0.823 (0.686-0.996) |
| ENGOT-Ov17¶ | Bevacizumab | | 0.51 (0.41-0.65) | NR |
| AGO-OVAR 2.21# | Bevacizumab | | 0.81 (0.68-0.96) | NR |
| AGO-OVAR12** | Nintedanib | VEGFR, FGFR, PDGFR | 0.84 (0.72-0.98) | NR |
| AGO-OVAR16†† | Pazopanib | | 0.77 (0.64-0.91) | 0.99 (0.75-1.32) |
| ICON6‡‡ | Cediranib | VEGFR | 0.56 (0.44-0.72) | 0.77 (0.51-1.07) |
| TRINOVA-1§§ | Trebananib | Ang ligand | 0.66 (0.57-0.77) | 0.86 (0.69-1.08) |

*Burger R, et al. Incorporation of bevacizumab in the primary treatment of ovarian cancer. *N Engl J Med.* 2011;365(26): 2473-2483.
†Perren T, et al. A phase 3 trial of bevacizumab in ovarian cancer. *N Engl J Med.* 2011;365(26):2484-2496.
‡Pujade-Lauraine E, et al. Bevacizumab combined with chemotherapy for platinum-resistant ovarian cancer: the AURELIA open-label randomized phase III trial. *J Clin Oncol.* 2014;32:1302-1308.
§Aghajanian C, et al. OCEANS: a randomized, double-blind, placebo-controlled phase III trial of chemotherapy with or without bevacizumab in patients with platinum-sensitive recurrent epithelial ovarian, primary peritoneal, or fallopian tube cancer. *J Clin Oncol.* 2012;30(17):2039-2045.
‖Coleman RL, et al. Bevacizumab and paclitaxel-carboplatin chemotherapy and secondary cytoreduction in recurrent, platinum-sensitive ovarian cancer (NRG Oncology/Gynecologic Oncology Group study GOG-0213): a multicenter, open-label, randomized, phase 3 trial. *Lancet Oncol.* 2017;18: 779-791.
¶Pignata S, et al. Chemotherapy plus or minus bevacizumab for platinum-sensitive ovarian cancer patients recurring after a bevacizumab containing first line treatment: the randomized phase 3 trial MITO16B-MaNGO OV2B-ENGOT OV17. *J Clin Oncol.* 2018;36(15 suppl):5506.
#Pfisterer J, et al. Carboplatin/pegylated liposomal doxorubicin/bevacizumab (CD-BEV) vs. carboplatin/gemcitabine/bevacizumab (CG-BEV) in patients with recurrent ovarian cancer: a prospective randomized phase III ENGOT/GCIG-Intergroup study. *Ann Oncol* 2018;29:vii332-vii358.
**du Bois A, et al. Standard first-line chemotherapy with or without nintedanib for advanced ovarian cancer (AGO-OVAR 12): a randomized, double-blind, placebo-controlled phase 3 trial. *Lancet Oncol.* 2016;17:78-89.
††Vergote I, et al. AGO-OVAR 16: a phase III study to evaluate the efficacy and safety of pazopanib monotherapy versus placebo in women who have not progressed after first line chemotherapy for epithelial ovarian, fallopian tube, or primary peritoneal cancer—overall survival (OS) results. *J Clin Oncol.* 2018;36(15 suppl):5518.
‡‡Ledermann JA, et al. Overall survival results of ICON6: a trial of chemotherapy and cediranib in relapsed ovarian cancer. *J Clin Oncol.* 2017;35 (15 suppl):5506.
§§Monk BJ, et al. Anti-angiopoietin therapy with trebananib for recurrent ovarian cancer (TRINOVA-1): a randomized, multicenter, double-blind, placebo-controlled phase 3 trial. *Lancet Oncol.* 2014;15(8):799-808.
*Ang,* Angiopoietin; *FGFR,* fibroblast growth factor receptor; *HR,* hazard ratio; *OS,* overall survival; *PDGFR,* platelet derived growth factor receptor; *PFS,* progression-free survival; *VEGF,* vascular endothelial growth factor; *VEGFR,* vascular endothelial growth factor receptor.

third platinum-based triplet is efficacious in patients with platinum-sensitive recurrent ovarian cancer (Pfisterer, 2018).

### PARP Inhibitors

Preclinical data demonstrated the extreme sensitivity of *BRCA*-deficient cells to inhibition of the single-strand DNA repair enzyme PARP. Inhibition of PARP leads to an accumulation of single-strand DNA breaks, which can lead to double-strand breaks at replication forks. Normally these breaks are repaired through homologous recombination, in which the *BRCA* genes play a major role; however, synthetic lethality occurs when these genes themselves function improperly because of mutation or silencing. This prompted the clinical development of PARP inhibitors, which theoretically hold promise for patients whose tumors rely on PARP for continued cell growth. Early clinical studies confirmed this theory, and additional mechanisms for PARP inhibitor activity have been discovered, including PARP trapping and enhancement of error prone DNA repair mechanisms such as nonhomologous end joining and alternative end joining. Thus PARP inhibitors may have activity outside of BRCA mutant tumors across a number of tumor types (Patel, 2011).

In early studies, clear activity by PARP inhibitors was identified in patients with *BRCA* germline mutations. A phase II study in *BRCA* carriers enrolled patients into two consecutive dosing cohorts of the PARP inhibitor olaparib. Overall, response rates were notable (>25%) in patients with platinum-resistant disease (Fong, 2009). This promising degree of clinical activity was confirmed in a larger study of patients with multiple solid tumors including ovarian cancer (n = 60) (Kaufman, 2015). **Objective responses to single-agent olaparib (capsule formation) 400 mg twice daily, orally, continuously were observed in 31% (95% CI, 25% to 38%). This is favorably referenced to expected responses from chemotherapy in a similar setting. These data along an extensive safety database led to an accelerated regulatory approval of olaparib in *BRCA*-mutation carriers with three or more lines of prior therapy.** A subsequent randomized phase III study of olaparib (tablet formation) versus physician-choice standard chemotherapy in recurrent platinum-sensitive ovarian cancer was performed (Penson, 2019). This study demonstrated superior response rates and PFS for olaparib, confirming the earlier studies.

**Rucaparib is a highly potent PARP inhibitor that also has an FDA indication in recurrent *BRCA* mutant ovarian**

**cancer. Importantly, this includes patients with germline or somatic mutations.** This indication was based on data from two studies, Study 10 in *BRCA* mutant tumors and the ARIEL 2 study in recurrent platinum-sensitive ovarian cancer. Across both studies, BRCA-mutant tumors had an overall response rate of 53.8% and median response duration of 9.2 months (Oza, 2017). Another objective of the ARIEL2 trial was to evaluate the ability of HRD testing to predict response to PARP inhibition (Swisher, 2017). This study demonstrated a difference in PFS based on genomic status. Patients with *BRCA* mutant tumors had a median PFS of 9.4 months. *BRCA*-like tumors, including those without *BRCA* mutation that displayed evidence of genome-wide loss of heterozygosity, had a median PFS of 7.1 months. *BRCA*-negative tumors had the lowest evidence of activity, with a median PFS of 3.7 months. These data are undergoing confirmation in a randomized controlled trial comparing rucaparib with standard chemotherapy in a recurrent setting (ARIEL4).

Interesting clinical activity has also been seen in the maintenance setting for ovarian cancer. **Three PARP inhibitors are FDA approved as maintenance therapies for platinum-sensitive recurrent ovarian cancer: olaparib, niraparib, and rucaparib. All three are indicated as maintenance treatment for recurrent epithelial ovarian cancer after complete or partial response to platinum-based chemotherapy, regardless of *BRCA* mutation status.** These indications are based on four trials in patients with recurrent platinum-sensitive ovarian cancer who had received two or more lines of platinum-based chemotherapy and had response to the most recent regimen (Coleman, 2017; Mirza, 2016; Pujade-Lauraine, 2017).

Study 19 was a randomized phase II trial of olaparib compared with placebo in the maintenance setting. In this study, patients taking olaparib had a median time to treatment progression of 8.4 months versus 4.8 months in patients taking placebo (HR, 0.35; 95% CI, 0.25 to 0.49). A post hoc analysis of patients with *BRCA1/2* mutation demonstrated an even greater effect (Ledermann, 2012). The follow-up study, SOLO2, was a randomized phase III trial of olaparib versus placebo in *BRCA* mutant recurrent platinum-sensitive ovarian cancer (Pujade-Lauraine, 2017). Patients in SOLO2 also experienced significantly improved PFS with olaparib versus placebo (HR, 0.30; 95% CI, 0.22 to 0.41).

Niraparib was evaluated as a maintenance therapy in any patient with platinum-sensitive recurrent ovarian cancer in the NOVA study (Mirza, 2016). This study demonstrated significant improvement in PFS for patients on niraparib compared with placebo, regardless of the presence of a *BRCA* mutation (HR, 0.27; 95% CI, 0.17 to 0.41). The greatest PFS benefit was observed in the *BRCA* mutant and homologous recombination–deficient cohorts, but there was still modest PFS benefit in the biomarker-negative cohort.

ARIEL3 compared rucaparib maintenance with placebo in all comers with platinum-sensitive recurrent ovarian cancer (Coleman, 2017). The trial included two nested cohorts; one included patients with *BRCA* mutations (germline or somatic), and one included HRD tumors defined by high loss of heterozygosity. In a hierarchical testing analysis, ARIEL3 found significant improvement in *BRCA*-mutated subgroup (HR, 0.23; 95% CI, 0.16 to 0.34), the HRR-deficient subgroup (HR, 0.32; 95% CI, 0.24 to 0.42), and the overall population (HR, 0.36; 95% CI 0.30 to 0.45).

OS data for SOLO2, NOVA, and ARIEL3 are immature; however, there was a trend toward OS benefit for patients treated with olaparib in Study 19. Of note, this study was not powered for the OS endpoint (Coleman, 2017; Friedlander, 2018; Mirza, 2016; Pujade-Lauraine, 2017).

Activity in the recurrent setting led to exploration of PARP inhibitor maintenance in earlier lines of therapy. SOLO1 was a phase III randomized control trial of olaparib as maintenance compared with placebo in patients with *BRCA* mutant (germline or somatic) ovarian cancer after completion of primary therapy (Moore, 2018). All patients had complete or partial response after upfront treatment with surgery and chemotherapy. **Olaparib provided a statistically significant improvement in PFS compared with placebo (HR, 0.30; 95% CI, 0.23 to 0.41). This agent is FDA approved for this indication.**

Niraparib was also found to be active in this setting. The PRIMA study evaluated niraparib maintenance after completion of primary therapy in women with epithelial ovarian cancer. Of note, this trial was performed in a high-risk group of women with residual disease after surgery or a stage IV diagnosis. **Niraparib demonstrated significant benefit in PFS in all comers (HR, 0.62; 95% CI, 0.50 to 0.76) with the greatest benefits in tumors with HRD (HR, 0.43; 95% CI, 0.31 to 0.59)** (Gonzalez-Martin, 2019).

Overall, PARP inhibitors have been difficult to combine with chemotherapy because of overlapping myelosuppressive toxicities; however, the PARP inhibitor veliparib has lower PARP trapping, which may allow successful combination. The VELIA study combined veliparib with standard paclitaxel and carboplatin chemotherapy in patients with untreated advanced epithelial ovarian cancer (Coleman, 2019). This was a three-arm study that included one arm with veliparib during chemotherapy only and another arm that followed the veliparib and chemotherapy combination with a veliparib maintenance phase. **Compared with the control arm, the combination arm including maintenance veliparib demonstrated a statistically significant improvement in PFS (HR, 0.68; 95% CI, 0.56 to 0.83) in the intention-to-treat population. Additional exploratory analyses revealed maximum benefit in the population with BRCA mutations.**

An active area of contemporary research is the exploration of PARP inhibitor combinations, particularly with other biologic agents such as angiogenesis inhibitors, immune checkpoint inhibitors, cell cycle checkpoint inhibitors, cyclin-dependent kinases, MAPK pathway inhibitors, and PI3K pathway inhibitors (Dalton, 2015; Liu, 2014). These combinations will have special relevance given the movement of PARP inhibition into the frontline treatment of ovarian cancer. Earlier exposure to PARP inhibition has the potential to lead to resistance to these agents. A goal of combination therapy is to overcome the development of therapy resistance in addition to potentially increase efficacy in the biomarker negative group. The bulk of these combination studies are being explored in platinum-sensitive and platinum-resistant recurrent disease. Additional studies are moving these combinations into the upfront setting as well. Major recent PARP inhibitor studies are shown in Table 33.13.

#### Immunotherapy

Work from TCGA demonstrated that ovarian cancers have a moderate mutational load and thus the possibility for a high degree of expressed neoantigens, making them a prime target for immune-targeted therapy (Bell, 2011); however, early attempts at immune therapy in ovarian cancer were not successful. For example, IP immunotherapy approaches with agents such as interferon, lymphokine-activated killer cells, interleukin-2, and tumor necrosis factor were only minimally successful. Berek and coworkers conducted a phase I and II trial of IP cisplatin (60 mg/m$^2$) and interferon-alpha (25 $\times$ 10$^6$ IV) given every 4 weeks. Among 18 patients, there were three complete and four partial responses. Unfortunately, a randomized trial comparing interferon-alpha with no further treatment in women achieving complete response after primary chemotherapy has shown no benefit. A frontline phase III study adding interferon-gamma to paclitaxel and carboplatin was terminated early when an interim analysis of OS demonstrated a detrimental effect from the intervention. Additional studies of vaccination strategies including oregovomab, abagovomab, and agents targeting Mucin-1 (Muc-1) and Mucin-16 (Muc-16) were also disappointing (Berek, 2004).

**TABLE 33.13** PARP Inhibitor Trials

| Study | Agent | BRCA | N | BRCA mt HR-PFS (95% CI) | Non-BRCA mt/ HRD+HR-PFS (95% CI) | Non-BRCA mt HR-PFS (95% CI) |
|---|---|---|---|---|---|---|
| **UPFRONT MAINTENANCE STUDIES** | | | | | | |
| SOLO1* | Olaparib | BRCA mutant | 391 | 0.30 (0.23-0.41) | Not tested | Not tested |
| PRIMA† | Niraparib | All comers | 733 | 0.43 (0.31-0.59) | 0.50 (0.31-0.83) | 0.68 (0.49-0.94) |
| PAOLA‡ | Olaparib + bevacizumab | All comers | 537 | 0.33 (0.25-0.45) | 0.43 (0.28-0.66) | 0.92 (0.72-1.17) |
| VELIA§ | Veliparib + chemotherapy | All comers | 1140 | 0.44 (0.28-0.68) | 0.74 (0.52-1.06) | 0.81 (0.60-1.09) |
| **RECURRENT PLATINUM-SENSITIVE MAINTENANCE STUDIES** | | | | | | |
| SOLO2‖ | Olaparib | BRCA mutant | 295 | 0.30 (0.22-0.41) | Not tested | Not tested |
| NOVA¶ | Niraparib | All comers | 553 | 0.27 (0.17-0.41) | 0.38 (0.24-0.59) | 0.58 (0.36-0.92) |
| ARIEL3# | Rucaparib | All comers | 564 | 0.23 (0.16-0.34) | 0.44 (0.29-0.66) | 0.58 (0.40-0.85) |

*Moore K, et al. Maintenance olaparib in patients with newly diagnosed advanced ovarian cancer. *N Engl J Med. 2018*;379(26):2495-2505.
†Gonzalez-Martin A, et al. Niraparib in patients with newly diagnosed advanced ovarian cancer. *N Engl J Med.* 2019;381:2391-2402.
‡Ray-Coquard I, et al. Olaparib plus bevacizumab as first-line maintenance in ovarian cancer. *N Engl J Med.* 2019;381:2416-2428.
§Coleman RL, et al. Veliparib with first-line chemotherapy and as maintenance therapy in ovarian cancer. *N Engl J Med.* 2019;381:2403-2415.
‖Pujade-Lauraine E, et al. Olaparib tablets as maintenance therapy in patients with platinum-sensitive, relapsed ovarian cancer and a BRCA1/2 mutation (SOLO2/ENGOT-Ov21): a double-blind, randomized, placebo-controlled, phase 3 trial. *Lancet Oncol.* 2017;18(9):1274-1284.
¶Mirza MR, et al. Niraparib maintenance therapy in platinum-sensitive, recurrent ovarian cancer. *N Engl J Med.* 2016;375:2154-2164.
#Coleman RL, et al. Rucaparib maintenance treatment for recurrent ovarian carcinoma after response to platinum therapy (ARIEL3): a randomized, double-blind, placebo-controlled, phase 3 trial. *Lancet.* 2017;390:1949-1961.
*CI,* Confidence interval; *HR,* hazard ratio; *HRD,* homologous recombination deficiency; *mt,* mutation; *OS,* overall survival; *PFS,* progression-free survival.

**TABLE 33.14** Immunotherapy of Ovarian Cancer

| Study (PD1/PDL1) | n | RR | Disease Control Rate | Prior Treatment |
|---|---|---|---|---|
| Nivolumab*<br>Cohort 1: 1 mg/kg every 2 wk<br>Cohort 2: 3 mg/kg every 2 wk | 10<br>10 | 1 (PR)/10 (10%)<br>2 (CR)/10 (20%) | 5/10 (50%)<br>4/10 (40%) | ≥2 prior regimens<br>Platinum resistant |
| Avelumab†<br>10 mg every 2 wk | 125 | 12 (1 CR 11 PR)/125 (9.6%)<br>2/2 clear cell | 65/125 (52%) | No limit on priors (median, 3; range, 0-10)<br>Platinum resistant |
| Pembrolizumab‡<br>10 mg/kg every 2 wk | 26 | 3 (1 CR, 2PR)/26 (12%) | 9/26 (35%) | No limit on priors (>80% ≥4 priors)<br>PDL1 IHC positive (49/96, 51%) |
| Atezolizumab§<br>0.3 mg–15 mg/kg every 3 wk | 12 | 2 (CR)/9 (22%) | 2/9 (22%) | ≥2 lines of therapy<br>Platinum resistant |
| Ipilumumab‖<br>3 mg/kg every 2-3 mo | 9 | 11% (1/10) | 3/9 (33%) | Previously treated with GVAX vaccine |

*Hamanishi J, et al. Safety and antitumor activity of anti-PD-1 antibody, aivolumab, in patients with platinum-resistant ovarian cancer *J Clin Oncol.* 2015;33:4015-4022.
†Disis ML, et al. Efficacy and safety of avelumab for patients with recurrent or refractory ovarian cancer: phase 1b results from the JAVELIN solid tumor trial. *JAMA Oncol.* 2019;5(3):393-401.
‡Varga A, et al. Pembrolizumab in patients with programmed death ligand 1-positive advanced ovarian cancer: analysis of KEYNOTE-028. *J Clin Oncol.* 2015;33(15 suppl):5510.
§Infante JR, et al. Immunologic and clinical effects of antibody blockade of cytotoxic T lymphocyte-associated antigen 4 in previously vaccinated cancer patients. *Ann Oncol.* 2016;27(6):296-312. Abstract 871P.
‖Hodi FS, et al. *Proc Natl Acad Sci U S A.* 2008;105:3005-3010.
*CR,* complete response; *GVAX,* autologous tumor cells engineered to secrete GM-CSF; *IHC,* immunohistochemistry; *PR,* partial response; *RR,* response rate.

Despite early setbacks of immune therapy in ovarian cancer, the field is in a renaissance with the discovery of mechanisms providing immune escape. The development of various immune checkpoint inhibitors has been explored in ovarian cancer and is summarized in Table 33.14. **Single-agent studies of agents targeting programmed cell death protein 1 (PD1) and programmed death ligand 1 (PDL1), including avelumab, atezolizumab, nivolumab, ipilimumab, and pembrolizumab, have been only modestly successful in ovarian cancer.** In general, response rates range between 10% to 25% in the unselected platinum-resistant setting (Disis, 2019; Hamanishi, 2015; Hodi, 2008; Infante, 2016; Varga, 2019). The lack of universal benefit in ovarian cancer has led to exploration of a number of combination therapies, including checkpoint inhibition with PARP inhibitors, antiangiogenic agents, and other immune therapy techniques.

In addition to these trials, the use of tumor-directed T cells (adoptive T-cell therapy) is also under exploration in ovarian cancer.

### Gene Therapy

The therapeutic impact of gene therapy in ovarian cancer has yet to be totally explored. Although the IP nature of this disease makes it well suited for this approach, various gene- or virus-based gene therapy programs have yielded mixed results at best. Several therapeutic models have been used in early investigations, including replacement of a tumor suppressor gene (e.g., *BRCA* and *P53*), suicide gene therapy, and inhibition of growth factor suppressors and regulators. As noted by Berchuck and Bast, there are a number of obstacles to developing this type of therapy to clinical usefulness; however, intensive investigation has been underway in a few centers to develop efficient and efficacious therapeutic programs.

### Radiation Therapy

Radiation has a limited role in ovarian cancer. At least one report has suggested ovarian clear cell cancer may be responsive to radiotherapy, providing a potential treatment option for patients with this chemoresistant disease (Hoskins, 2012). The modality has also been used to treat recurrent disease. Cmelak and Kapp treated 41 patients with platinum-refractory ovarian cancer who had undergone secondary cytoreduction. They treated the whole abdomen with 28 Gy and a pelvic boost to 48 Gy. For 28 patients with residual disease smaller than 1.5 cm, the 5-year survival rate was 53%, which is better than would be expected with chemotherapy; however, no large-scale trial data are available for this technique. Because of the risk of complications and lack of extensive data regarding its effectiveness, whole abdominal radiation has generally not been used in these cases; however, localized radiation can be of use in select patients with isolated recurrences or persistent disease after chemotherapy or to manage localized symptomatic disease, such as bone metastases.

## Complications and Other Considerations

### Malignant Effusions

Pleural effusions are a common and devastating complication of advanced malignancies. Women with ovarian cancer commonly develop ascites, hydrothorax, or both, requiring repeated drainage by paracentesis or thoracentesis. In the majority of cases, malignant pleural effusion is associated with an incurable disease, with high morbidity and mortality. For the same reason, several studies have argued in favor of a palliative approach, rather than a conventional curative approach for treatment of this condition. Occasionally, sclerosing solutions are used in the thoracic cavity to prevent the reaccumulation of fluid, with resultant adherence of the pleural surfaces. New modalities, such as pleuroscopy and long-term indwelling pleural catheters, offer cost-effective outpatient or minimal hospital stay and less discomfort.

In a review by Musani and associates, it was reported that several mechanisms have been proposed to explain the development of malignant effusion. The inability of the parietal pleura to reabsorb pleural fluid because of the involvement of mediastinal lymph nodes by tumor is likely the most common cause of malignant pleural effusion. Therefore, tumors that involve the mediastinal lymph nodes, such as lung cancer, breast cancer, and lymphoma, are responsible for most malignant pleural effusions. Other possible mechanisms include direct tumor invasion, as is sometimes seen in lung cancer, chest wall neoplasms, breast cancer, and ovarian cancer, as well as hematogenous spread to the parietal pleura.

There are several options for therapy, such as thoracentesis, chemical pleurodesis with chest tubes, VATS, pleuroperitoneal shunts, and chronic indwelling pleural catheters. The advantage of a thoracentesis largely relies on the rapid relief of symptoms; however, it is unfortunately often associated with reaccumulation of fluid, multiple procedures and hospital visits, and associated complications, such as pneumothorax or reexpansion pulmonary edema. The option of chemical pleurodesis offers the advantage that it is highly effective; however, this treatment may be associated with required hospitalization and high cost. The VATS procedure is also highly effective and can be diagnostic in addition to therapeutic. The disadvantages are its cost, its invasiveness, and its contraindication for patients who cannot tolerate single-lung ventilation. A pleuroperitoneal shunt may be considered in patients who have recurrent reaccumulation of fluid and those who have failed pleurodesis; however, this approach is not practical for patients with advanced or recurrent ovarian cancer because disease in these patients often also causes significant ascites. The option of a chronic indwelling catheter is ideal for patients who have recurrent episodes of reaccumulation of the pleural effusion. This approach is minimally invasive, cost effective, and successful. One of the major disadvantages is the risk for infection and the fact that the woman must be motivated to learn how to drain; otherwise, a family member or visiting nurse is required for home drainage.

A number of strategies have been studied in prospective trials. Most efficacious for problematic pleural effusion is pleurodesis with a sclerotic agent (e.g., talc slurry, antibiotic), decortication, or placement of an infusion catheter that can be operated by the woman. Tan and coworkers conducted a systematic review. Symptomatic ascites can also be problematic because few sclerodesis or surgical decortication-type procedures are available for long-term care. It is also not uncommon for patients to develop implants of tumor in the subcutaneous tissues after aspiration. Numnum and colleagues reported some success using bevacizumab as an adjuvant for this problem.

### Malignant Bowel Obstruction

Intestinal obstruction is a common complication in patients with advanced epithelial ovarian cancer and is estimated to occur in 25% to 50% of patients. The onset of bowel obstruction is rarely an acute event. In cancer patients, compression of the bowel lumen develops slowly and often remains partial. Obstruction can result from partial or total occlusion of the bowel lumen or from alteration of the normal peristaltic motion. The initial symptoms are often abdominal cramps, nausea, vomiting, and abdominal distention that present periodically and resolve spontaneously.

Contrast radiography may help in defining the site and extent of the obstruction. Although barium may provide excellent radiographic definition, it is not absorbed well and may cause severe impaction. Diatrizoate meglumine and diatrizoate sodium solution is ideal for this type of contrast radiography because it offers similar radiographic definition and, in certain cases, may restore the intestinal transit. Abdominal CT is usually recommended because it can provide information about the location of the obstruction and the extent of disease. Surgical options may be offered to the woman, depending on a number of factors that dictate the success of surgical management. These include the site of obstruction, number of obstructions along the small or large bowel, number of prior chemotherapy regimens, and prior episodes of bowel obstruction; the nutritional status of the woman; and her overall functional status.

Pothuri and colleagues reviewed a series of patients undergoing surgery for intestinal obstruction caused by recurrent epithelial ovarian cancer and found that the mean time from original diagnosis of epithelial ovarian cancer to obstruction was 2.8 years. Surgical correction (intestinal surgery performed to relieve the obstruction) was achieved in 84% of cases, and successful palliation (the ability to tolerate a regular or low-residue diet by 60 days after surgery) was achieved in 71% of cases. The median survival in patients with successful palliation was 11.6 versus 3.9 months for all other patients. Major surgical morbidity was documented in 22% of patients. Interestingly, postoperative chemotherapy was administered to 79% of patients for whom surgical correction was possible. The authors noted that with respect to quality of life, it is important to consider that 56% of patients undergoing surgery for bowel obstruction had a colostomy or permanent gastrostomy tube. They also recommended that patients are not ideal surgical candidates if they have bulky carcinomatosis, rapidly progressive disease, multiple sites of obstruction, poor performance status, or heavy pretreatment with chemotherapy and radiation.

In patients who refuse palliative surgery or are considered poor surgical candidates, a percutaneous endoscopic gastrostomy (PEG) tube may offer symptomatic relief without the discomfort or complications of a nasogastric tube. The study by Pothuri and associates has shown that symptomatic relief (defined as the absence of nausea or vomiting) is achieved in 91% of patients with advanced epithelial ovarian cancer and bowel obstruction within 7 days of placement of a PEG tube. Only 13% of patients had resolution of obstruction and removal of the PEG tube after chemotherapy was administered. The median survival from the date of PEG tube placement was 8 weeks. The complication rate was 18%, and the most common complication was leakage. This study also demonstrated that the administration of total parenteral nutrition after PEG tube placement was not associated with a survival benefit. It is important to note that PEG tube placement is feasible for patients with a tumor encasing the stomach, diffuse carcinomatosis, or ascites.

Another potential nonsurgical option for the management of bowel obstruction is the use of metallic stents. These stents are flexible and self-expanding and can be inserted using radiologic or endoscopic techniques. The most important reported complications include local pain, gastric ulceration, gastroesophageal reflux, bleeding, and bowel perforation. Metallic stents are contraindicated in patients with multiple obstructions and peritoneal carcinomatosis. The literature on the usefulness of metallic stents for bowel obstruction in patients with gynecologic cancers is limited.

### Summary

Therapy for epithelial ovarian carcinoma is based on the removal of all gross disease and sampling of areas at high risk of spread in the peritoneal cavity and retroperitoneal nodes. Postoperative therapy is used according to the stage and grade of the primary tumor. Multiagent platinum- and taxane-based chemotherapy is commonly used as adjunctive treatment for poorly differentiated tumors, such as stage I or grade 3, or for stage II cases without residual tumor.

For high-stage tumors and for patients with residual disease after initial operation, multiagent chemotherapy, usually paclitaxel and carboplatin, is used. It is accompanied by a number of short- and long-term toxic side effects, but initial response rates in stage III cases may exceed 90%. Five-year survival rates decrease to 30% or less. Long-term randomized trials and the development of new agents will be needed to improve rates of salvage and optimize therapy for epithelial ovarian carcinomas. Second-line chemotherapy offers remission to some patients, but the best response rates are achieved with initial chemotherapy.

## RARE EPITHELIAL OVARIAN CANCER SUBTYPES

### Clear Cell Carcinoma

Clear cell carcinoma is an aggressive subtype and accounts for approximately 5% to 10% of all epithelial ovarian cancers. It appears to be more prevalent in Japan. More than 50% are diagnosed in the stage I-II category, and outcomes are similar to those of women with high-grade serous carcinoma (Okamoto, 2014). For women with stage III or IV disease, however, the outcomes are worse than those associated with high-grade serous carcinoma (Mackay, 2010). A proportion of clear cell carcinomas appear to arise from endometriosis. The prevailing thought is that clear cell carcinomas are relatively resistant to conventional platinum/taxane chemotherapy. The most common alterations include mutations in *ARID1A* and the *PI3K/AKT/mTOR* pathway (Kuo, 2009; Wiegand, 2010). The angiogenesis pathway and *MET* amplification appear to be good potential targets as well (Mabuchi, 2010; Yamashita, 2013). There has been increasing interest in targeted therapies for this subtype, and several clinical trials have been completed or are ongoing (Chan, 2018; Konstantinopoulos, 2018; Tan, 2013). In addition, immune checkpoint inhibitors hold promise in the treatment of clear cell carcinoma (Hamanishi, 2015).

**Current NCNN guidelines include the following: (1) stage IA, IV platinum-based therapy or observe; (2) stage IB to IC, IV platinum-based therapy; (3) stage II to IV, chemotherapy as per epithelial ovarian cancer.**

### Low-Grade Serous Carcinoma

**Low-grade serous carcinoma is a rare subtype constituting approximately 10% of all serous carcinomas.** The stage distribution is very similar to that of high-grade serous carcinoma, with more than 70% of cases in the stage III or IV category. **Compared with high-grade serous carcinoma, low-grade serous carcinoma is characterized by young age at diagnosis, relative chemoresistance, and prolonged survival (Gershenson, 2015).** Hormonal therapy has excellent activity for some patients (Gershenson, 2012). Likewise, antiangiogenic therapy appears to be active as well (Dalton, 2017; Grisham, 2014). Translational research investigations have indicated that *KRAS* mutations occur in these tumors with a frequency of 20% to 40%, and *BRAF* mutations occur with a frequency of approximately 5%. MEK (mitogen-activated protein kinase kinase enzyme) inhibitor therapy has demonstrated promising activity in the recurrent setting; second-generation, phase II/III clinical trials—MEK inhibitor in Low-Grade Serous Ovarian Cancer (MILO/ENGOT) and GOG-0281—have completed accrual, and results have been published (MILO/ENGOT ov11) or presented (GOG-0281). In the MILO/ENGOT ov11 trial, the MEK inhibitor, binimetinib (45 mg orally twice daily), was compared against physician's choice chemotherapy, which included pegylated liposomal doxorubicin (40 $mg/m^2$) intravenously on day 1 of every 28 days, paclitaxel (80 $mg/m^2$ IV on days 1, 8, and 15) of a 28-day cycle, or topotecan (1.25 $mg/m^2$ IV on days 1-5) every 21-days. Treatment continued until locally determined progressive disease, unacceptable toxicity, or inability to continue on protocol-directed therapy. A total of 303 patients were randomly assigned 2:1 to binimetinib or physician's choice chemotherapy. The primary endpoint was PFS as assessed by a blinded independent central radiology (BICR) review. Median PFS (at interim futility assessment) was 9.1 months (95% CI, 7.3 to 11.3) for binimetinib and 10.6 months (95% CI, 9.2 to 14.5) for chemotherapy (HR:1.21; 95%CI, 0.79 to 1.86), resulting in study termination. Objective response rate (ORR) was 16% with a median duration of repsonse of 8.1 months for binimetinib versus an overall ORR of 13% and a median duration of response of 6.7 months for physician's choice chemotherapy. Safety results were consistent with the known safety profile of the administered agents (Monk et al., 2020). In contrast, GOG-0281 randomized 260 women with low-grade serous ovarian cancer 1:1 to the MEK inhibitor, trametinib (2 mg daily) or one of five standard of care treatment options (pegylated liposomal doxorubicin [40 $mg/m^2$] intravenously on day 1 of every 28 days, paclitaxel [80 $mg/m^2$ IV on days 1, 8, and 15] of a 28-day cycle, topotecan [1.25 $mg/m^2$ IV on days 1-5] every 21 days, or letrozole 2.5 mg orally once daily or tamoxifen 20 mg orally twice daily). Patients who progressed on the control arm could cross over to trametinib. The primary endpoint, investigator-assessed PFS, was significantly improved PFS versus control (median, 13.0 vs. 7.2 months; hazard ratio 0.48; 95% confidence interval [CI], 0.36-0.64; p <0.0001). Objective response was 26.2% for trametinib versus 6.2% for control (odds ratio 5.4; 95% CI, 2.39-12.21; p <0.0001). Similarly, toxicity was consistent with the known adverse effects of the individual agents. Median OS was 37.0 months for trametinib versus 29.2 months for control therapy (hazard ratio 0.75 [95% CI, 0.51-1.11; p = 0.054]) (Gershenson et al., 2019). Interestingly, despite the association of this histology with aberrations in the MAPK pathway, the presence of KRAS, BRAF, or NRAS mutations was not predictive of response or PFS for either MEK inhibitor.

**NCCN guidelines include the following: (1) stage IA/IB, observe; (2) stage IC or higher, observe or platinum-based therapy or hormonal therapy; (3) stage II to IV, chemotherapy followed by observation or maintenance hormonal therapy or primary adjuvant hormonal therapy.**

### Mucinous Carcinoma

Mucinous carcinoma accounts for approximately 5% of epithelial ovarian cancers and is commonly confused histologically with mucinous tumors of the gastrointestinal tract. It is usually unilateral and is diagnosed in the stage I category in more than 50% of cases. Stage I is associated with an excellent prognosis. Women with advanced-stage mucinous carcinoma have a worse outcome than those with advanced-stage serous carcinoma, and standard platinum/taxane chemotherapy does not appear to be active in this subtype. Consequently, colorectal cancer–type regimens have been recommended by some. An international, phase III randomized trial, mEOC/GOG-0241 (mucinous epithelial ovarian cancer/GOG-0241), randomly allocated women with stage II to IV mucinous carcinoma or recurrent stage I to paclitaxel/carboplatin or capecitabine/oxaliplatin, each for six cycles, with a secondary random allocation to bevacizumab or no bevacizumab. Unfortunately, the trial was stopped after 50 patients were accrued because of slow accrual, and thus no definite conclusions could be made regarding optimal adjuvant chemotherapy (Gore, 2019).

**Current NCCN guidelines include the following: (1) stage IA/IB, observe; (2) stage IC, observe or IV platinum-based therapy for three to six cycles or 5-fluorouracil (5-FU) plus leucovorin plus oxaliplatin or capecitabine plus oxaliplatin; (3) stage II to IV, primary chemotherapy regimens for stage II to IV disease or 5-FU plus leucovorin plus oxaliplatin with or without bevacizumab or capecitabine plus oxaliplatin with or without bevacizumab.**

Although information on the biology of mucinous carcinoma is somewhat limited, potential genes or pathways for therapeutic targeting include *HER2*/neu amplification, *KRAS*, *src*, and the angiogenesis pathway.

### Endometrioid Carcinoma

Endometrioid carcinoma accounts for approximately 5% to 10% of all epithelial ovarian cancers. They are thought to arise from endometriosis in most cases. A higher proportion of endometrioid carcinomas are diagnosed in stage I compared with serous carcinomas. They are graded as well differentiated (grade 1), moderately differentiated (grade 2), or poorly differentiated (grade 3). Grade 3 endometrioid carcinomas appear to behave similar to high-grade serous carcinomas and are treated the same. Grade 1 and 2 tumors are more likely to express the estrogen and progesterone receptors and are more likely to respond to endocrine therapy. **NCCN guidelines for grade 1 endometroid carcinoma include the following: (1) stage IA/IB, observe; (2) stage IC, observe, or IV platinum-based therapy for three to six cycles or hormonal therapy; (3) stage II to IV, chemotherapy followed by observation or maintenance hormonal therapy or primary hormonal therapy.**

## SMALL CELL CARCINOMA

Dickersin and colleagues described a virulent type of ovarian malignancy that occurs in young women, usually between ages 15 and 30 years. Because of its histologic appearance, it has been designated a small cell carcinoma. The tumor is often but not always accompanied by hypercalcemia, as noted by Young and associates in an analysis of 150 cases.

Small cell carcinoma of the ovary, hypercalcemic type (SCCOHT), is rare, with fewer than 300 cases reported. It primarily affects young women and children, with a mean age at diagnosis of 24 years (Benrubi, 1993; Callegaro-Filho, 2016; Estel, 2011; Harrison, 2006; Reed, 1995; Young, 1994). Regardless of stage, the disease recurs, and most patients die of the disease within a short period, with a 1-year survival of 50% and a 5-year survival of 10% (Dykgraaf, 2009).

Primary treatment of SCCOHT consists of surgery followed by adjuvant, multiagent, platinum-based chemotherapy (Callegaro-Filho, 2016; Senekjian, 1989); however, there is no standard regimen. The most common regimens are etoposide/cisplatin; bleomycin, etoposide, and cisplatin (BEP); and the combination of vinblastine, cisplatin, cyclophosphamide, bleomycin, doxorubicin (Adriamycin), and etoposide (VPCBAE). Although the role of radiotherapy is unknown, several studies have reported long-term survival in patients who received this modality in addition to chemotherapy (Callegaro-Filho, 2014; Dickersin, 2006; Young, 1994). Jelinic (2018) reported PDL1 expression in 8 of 11 cases of SCCOHT and reported responses in 4 patients treated with anti-PD1 immune checkpoint inhibitor therapy.

The molecular biology of SCCOHT has been elucidated. Germline and somatic *SMARCA4* mutations have been identified in a high proportion of these patients, and this information coupled with recent pathology reviews have led to the conclusion that these neoplasms are actually malignant rhabdoid tumors (Jelinic, 2014; Ramos, 2014; Witkowski, 2014).

### Carcinosarcoma

Carcinosarcomas are extremely rare ovarian malignancies that histologically resemble comparable tumors in the uterus. Treatment involves operation for cytoreduction, as noted by Muntz and associates, with added therapy, usually in the form of multiagent chemotherapy. Stage is a prognostic factor, and advanced stages are associated with poor survival.

As noted by Hellstrom and coworkers, approximately 500 of these rare tumors have been reported. In their series of 36 of these cases over 20 years, the median survival was 16.6 months, with a 5-year actuarial survival rate of 18%. Per NCCN guidelines, recommended regimens for stage I to IV disease include paclitaxel/carboplatin, cisplatin/ifosfamide, carboplatin/ifosfamide, or paclitaxel/ifosfamide. Although some reports indicate the carcinosarcomas have outcomes equivalent to high-grade serous carcinomas, other reports conclude that they have a worse prognosis.

## GERM CELL TUMORS

These tumors are derived from the germ cells of the ovary. As a group, they are the second most frequent type of ovarian neoplasms and account for approximately 20% to 25% of all ovarian tumors. The classification of germ cell tumors, according to the WHO designation, is shown in Box 33.3.

The most common germ cell tumor is the benign cystic teratoma (dermoid); overall, 2% to 3% of germ cell tumors are

**BOX 33.3** World Health Organization Classification of Germ Cell Tumors

Dysgerminoma
- Endodermal sinus tumor
- Embryonal carcinoma
- Polyembryoma
- Choriocarcinoma
- Teratomas
- Immature
- Mature
    - Solid
    - Cystic

Dermoid cyst (mature cystic teratoma)
Dermoid cyst with malignant transformation
- Monodermal and highly specialized
    - Struma ovarii
    - Carcinoid
    - Struma ovarii and carcinoid
    - Others
- Mixed forms

malignant. Of the malignant germ cell tumors, the most common is the dysgerminoma, which accounts for approximately 45% of malignant germ cell tumors. Next in frequency are immature teratomas and then yolk sac tumors (endodermal sinus tumors). In women younger than 30 years, germ cell tumors are the most common ovarian neoplasm, and approximately one-third of the germ cell tumors found in those younger than 21 years are malignant.

The histogenesis of germ cell tumors has been extensively studied and summarized by Talerman. Fig. 33.15 shows the theoretical histogenesis of these tumors. They are thought to originate from the primitive germ cell and gradually differentiate to mimic the developmental tissues of embryonic origin (ectoderm, mesoderm, or endoderm) and extraembryonic tissues (yolk sac and trophoblast). Germ cell tumors that originate in the ovary have homologous counterparts in the testes (e.g., dysgerminoma and seminoma). Germ cell tumors are usually unilateral, except for benign cystic teratomas and dysgerminomas (see Table 33.4). The morphologic and clinical aspects of each of the various types of germ cell tumors are considered separately.

## Teratoma

Teratomas consist of tissues that recapitulate the three layers of the developing embryo (ectoderm, mesoderm, and endoderm). One or more of the layers may be represented, and the tissues can be mature (benign) or immature (malignant). Chromosomal studies indicate that teratomas appear to arise from a single germ and have an XX karyotype. In the older literature, terms such as *malignant teratoma* and *teratocarcinoma* were used to denote the malignant variety of these tumors, but these terms have been replaced by the nomenclature shown in Box 33.3.

### Benign Cystic Teratoma (Dermoid)

**Benign cystic teratomas are the most common germ cell tumors and account for 25% of all ovarian neoplasms.** They primarily occur during the reproductive years but may occur in postmenopausal women and in children. The risk of malignant transformation (discussed later) is markedly increased if these tumors are found in postmenopausal women. One of the interesting facets of teratomas is their ability to produce adult tissue, including skin, bone, teeth, hair, and dermal tissue. The presence of calcified bone or teeth allows the tumor to be diagnosed preoperatively by ultrasonography or radiography (Fig. 33.16).

Dermoids are usually unilateral, but 10% to 15% are bilateral. The outside wall of the tumor tends to be smooth, with a yellowish appearance caused by the sebaceous fatty material that fills the tumor. Hair is also a prominent feature once the cyst is opened (Fig. 33.17). Usually the tumors are asymptomatic but can cause severe pain if there is torsion or if the sebaceous material perforates the cyst wall, leading to a reactive peritonitis. This rare complication is severe and can occur during pregnancy. Microscopically a number of adult tissues are seen (Fig. 33.18).

Treatment of the reproductive-age woman or child consists of ovarian cystectomy or unilateral oophorectomy. In most cases it should be possible to remove only the cyst and preserve normal ovarian tissue. The opposite ovary should be inspected. If it is grossly normal, nothing further needs to be done. Treatment involves preservation of the contralateral ovary without any biopsy if it grossly appears normal. In women beyond childbearing years, therapy for a dermoid usually consists of removal of the uterus, both tubes, and the ovaries.

Occasionally teratomas may be solid and may consist only of adult tissues, leading to the diagnosis of a solid mature teratoma. These benign germ cell tumors are rare.

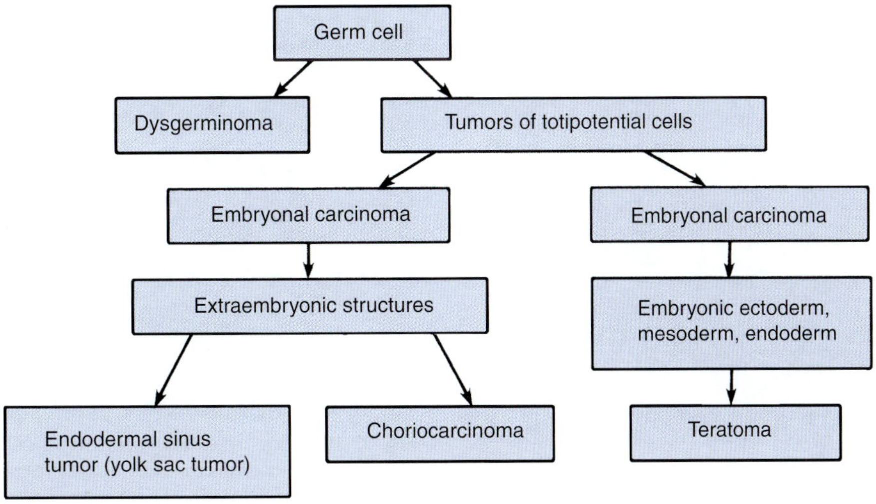


**Fig. 33.15** Histogenesis of germ cell tumors. (Modified from Talerman A. Germ cell tumors of the ovary. In: Blaustein A, eds. *Pathology of the Female Genital Tract—New York: Springer Verlag; 1982.*

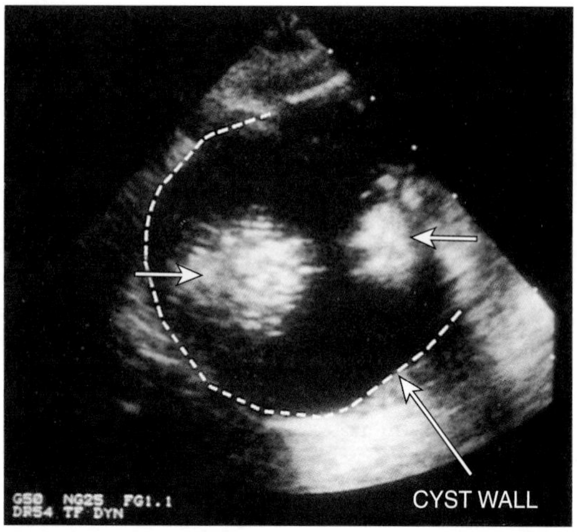


**Fig. 33.16** Transvaginal ultrasound image of an ovarian dermoid cyst. *Arrows* indicate balls of hair. (Courtesy Dr. Zubie Sheikh, Department of Obstetrics and Gynecology, University of Chicago, Chicago.)

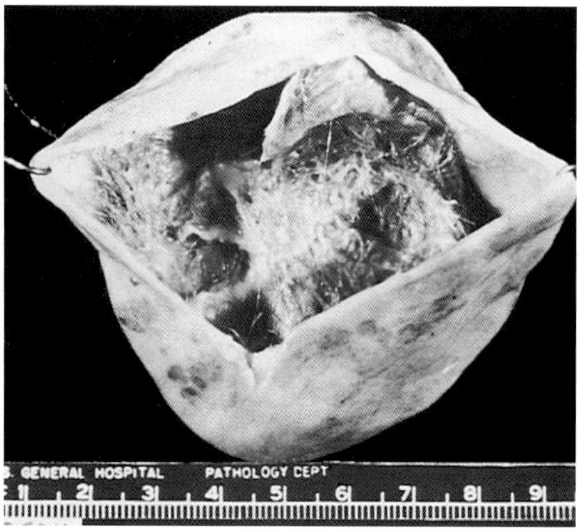


**Fig. 33.17** Gross specimen of a dermoid cyst that was filled with sebaceous material and hair. (Courtesy Dr. R. E. Scully.)

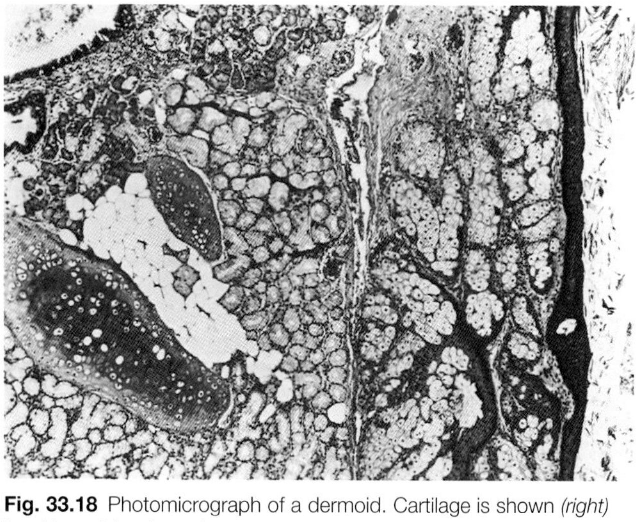

**Fig. 33.18** Photomicrograph of a dermoid. Cartilage is shown *(right)* lined by epidermis and accompanying appendages *(left)* (original magnification ×50). (From Serov SF, Scully RE, Sobin LH. *Histologic Typing of Ovarian Tumors.* Geneva: World Health Organization; 1973.)

A cystic teratoma can undergo malignant degeneration, usually after menopause. Generally it occurs in the squamous epithelial elements of the dermoid, producing a squamous cell carcinoma. It is a rare complication, estimated to occur in less than 2% of these tumors. If the malignant tissue has spread beyond the confines of the ovary, the prognosis is poor. In such cases, additional therapy for squamous cell carcinoma with radiation therapy, chemotherapy, or both is used.

## Immature Teratoma

Immature teratomas are malignant and account for as many as 20% of the malignant ovarian tumors found in women younger than 20 years, but less than 1% of all ovarian cancers. They rarely occur in women after menopause. They consist of immature embryonic structures that can be admixed with mature elements. Approximately one-third of immature teratomas express serum α-fetoprotein.

The prognosis for patients with immature teratomas is related to the stage (FIGO) and grade of the tumor. The grade of the tumor is based on the degree of immaturity of the various tissues. Grade 3 tumors consist of the most immature tissues and often have a high proportion of immature neuroepithelium. Kurman and Norris reported that patients with stage IA immature teratoma have a 10-year actuarial survival rate of 70% after unilateral salpingo-oophorectomy; this rate is comparable with that recorded after bilateral salpingo-oophorectomy.

In a database study of 179 patients (98 children and 81 adults) with pure immature teratoma, **Pashankar reported that 90 children were treated with surgery alone, and all adults received adjuvant chemotherapy (Pashankar, 2016).** Relapse occurred in none of the grade 1 patients, regardless of stage, in only one adult with grade 2, and in 8 of 38 patients with grade 3 tumors (21%). The authors concluded that grade was the most important risk factor for relapse.

## Dysgerminoma

Dysgerminomas are the most common type of malignant germ cell tumors. They consist of primitive germ cells with stroma infiltrated by lymphocytes (Fig. 33.19), are analogous to

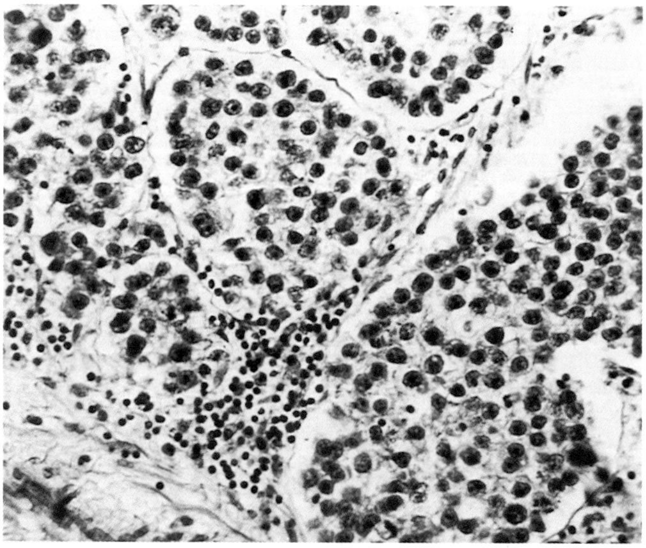

**Fig. 33.19** Dysgerminoma (original magnification ×300). Dysgerminoma cells are demonstrated as well as infiltration of stroma by lymphocytes. (From Scully RE: Germ cell tumors of the ovary and fallopian tube. In: Meigs JV, Sturgis SH, eds. *Progress in Gynecology.* Vol 4. New York: Grune & Stratton; 1963.)

seminoma in the male testis, and constitute approximately 1% of ovarian malignancies. Dysgerminomas occur primarily in women younger than 30 years. The tumor can be discovered during pregnancy. Some arise in dysgenetic gonads (discussed later). Unlike other malignant germ cell tumors, dysgerminomas are bilateral in approximately 10% of cases (see Table 33.4). Approximately 15% of dysgerminomas produce HCG related to areas of syncytiotrophoblast tissue.

### Yolk Sac Tumor (Endodermal Sinus Tumors)

Yolk sac tumors, which comprises 10% of malignant germ cell tumors, in part resemble the yolk sac of the rodent placenta, thus recapitulating extraembryonic tissues (see Fig. 33.15). One typical histologic pattern is shown in Fig. 33.20. The tumor secretes α-fetoprotein, which is a specific marker useful for identifying and following these tumors clinically. These rapidly growing tumors occur in females between ages 13 months and 45 years. Kurman and Norris noted a median age of 19 years at diagnosis.

### Choriocarcinoma

Nongestational choriocarcinoma is a highly malignant rare germ cell tumor resembling extraembryonic tissues. Like gestational choriocarcinoma (see Chapter 35), it consists of malignant cytotrophoblasts and syncytiotrophoblast; HCG is a useful tumor marker. This tumor mostly develops in women younger than 20 years, primarily in the ovary.

### Embryonal Carcinoma

Embryonal carcinoma is a rare malignant germ cell tumor composed of primitive embryonal cells. It occurs in young females between the ages of 4 and 28 years. Kurman and Norris summarized 15 cases. Trophoblastic elements may be present; both HCG and α-fetoprotein have also been reported to be present.

### Polyembryoma

Polyembryomas are exceedingly rare tumors that are usually found in the testes. They can occur in the ovary and consist of embryonal bodies that resemble early embryos. Trophoblastic elements with HCG and placental lactogen secretion have been reported.

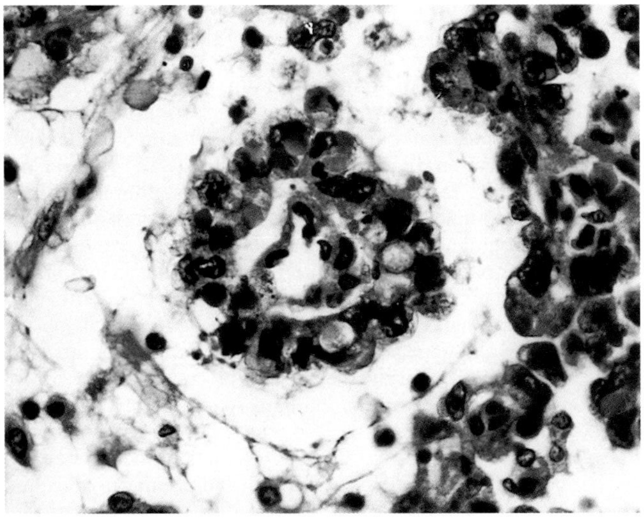

**Fig. 33.20** Schiller-Duvall body associated with numerous hyaline droplets in an endodermal sinus tumor (original magnification ×350). (From Kurman RJ, Norris HJ. Malignant germ cells of the ovary. *Hum Pathol.* 1977;8(5):551-564.)

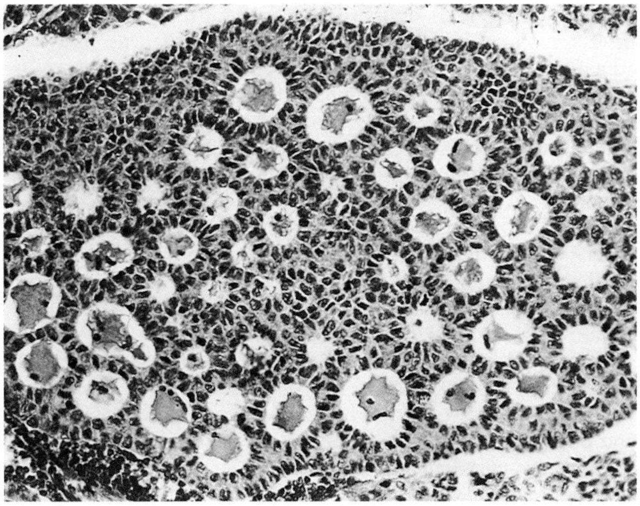

**Fig. 33.21** Granulosa cell tumor (original magnification ×460). (From Scully RE, Morris J. Functioning ovarian tumors. In: Meigs JV, Sturgis SH, eds. *Progress in Gynecology.* Vol. 3. New York: Grune & Stratton; 1957.)

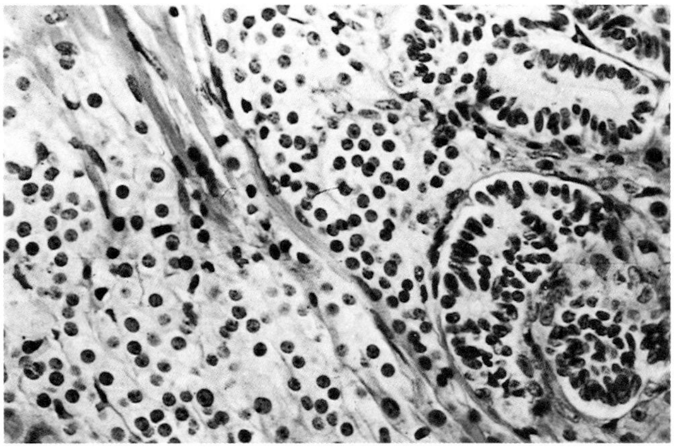

**Fig. 33.22** Sertoli–Leydig cell tumor. Tubules of Sertoli cells *(right)* and Leydig cells *(left)* are shown (original magnification ×250). (Courtesy Dr. R.E. Scully.)

### Mixed Germ Cell Tumor

Mixed germ cell tumors are combinations of any of the germ cell tumors of the ovary described earlier. They can be bilateral if dysgerminoma elements are involved; otherwise, they are unilateral.

## Treatment of Malignant Germ Cell Tumors

**Current treatment modalities result in cure rates approaching 100% for patients with stage I malignant germ cell tumors and more than 75% for patients with advanced-stage disease (stages III and IV).** Because most patients are young and most of these tumors are unilateral, fertility-sparing surgery consisting of unilateral salpingo-oophorectomy with preservation of the contralateral ovary and the uterus is appropriate. After unilateral adnexal excision, frozen-section examination should be performed to confirm the diagnosis preliminarily. Once a malignant ovarian germ cell tumor is documented, routine biopsy of a normal contralateral ovary should be avoided because such an intervention could lead to future infertility related to peritoneal adhesions or ovarian failure. If bilateral ovarian masses are encountered at surgery, a unilateral salpingo-oophorectomy of the more suspicious side is appropriate. If the opposite ovary contains tumor or is dysgenetic, bilateral salpingo-oophorectomy is generally indicated. In the case of bilateral ovarian dysgerminomas in nondysgenetic ovaries, although not proved to be entirely safe, unilateral salpingo-oophorectomy and contralateral ovarian cystectomy may be considered in an effort to preserve fertility. Conversely, if a contralateral ovary contains a mature cystic teratoma, which is more likely because it is present in 10% to 15% of cases, ovarian cystectomy is indicated.

If the tumor appears to be grossly confined to the ovary, comprehensive surgical staging is recommended, with cytologic washings, omentectomy, peritoneal biopsies, and bilateral pelvic and paraaortic lymphadenectomy. If obvious extraovarian metastases are present, the guiding principle is maximum cytoreductive surgery. The philosophy regarding comprehensive surgical staging for patients with malignant ovarian germ cell tumors is based primarily on that for common epithelial ovarian cancers and may or may not apply. For example, a very different perspective prevails in the pediatric surgery community. Based on an intergroup study report in which deviations from standard surgical guidelines did not adversely influence survival, Billmire and colleagues proposed a different set of surgical guidelines: collection of ascites or cytologic washings, examination of peritoneal surfaces with biopsy or excision of any nodules, examination and palpation of retroperitoneal lymph nodes and sampling of any firm or enlarged nodes, inspection and palpation of omentum with removal of any adherent or abnormal areas, biopsy or excision of any other abnormal areas, and complete resection of the tumor-containing ovary with sparing of the fallopian tube if not involved.

**Historically, for most patients with malignant ovarian germ cell tumors, postoperative chemotherapy has been recommended. Notable exceptions include patients with stage IA pure dysgerminoma and patients with stage IA, grade 1, immature teratoma; these patients have a high cure rate with surgery alone.** In the 1970s the VAC regimen (vincristine, 1.5 mg/m$^2$ IV weekly for 8 to 12 weeks, and actinomycin D, 300 μg/m$^2$ per day for 5 days every 4 weeks, with cyclophosphamide [Cytoxan] 150 mg/m$^2$ per day for 5 days every 4 weeks) was the first effective combination chemotherapy regimen for patients with malignant germ cell tumors. VAC was the most widely used regimen during the 1970s and early 1980s and produced a relatively high proportion of cures in stage I disease (82%), but in patients with metastatic disease, the cure rate was less than 50%. By the mid-1980s, BEP, the combination of bleomycin, etoposide, and cisplatin, became the standard and remains so today. Most patients require three to four cycles of therapy. In 1990 Gershenson and colleagues reported that 25 of 26 patients treated with BEP for malignant germ cell tumors were in sustained remission. Subsequently, Williams and associates, reporting the GOG experience, noted that 89 of 93 patients (96%) with completely resected stage I, II, or III disease remained continuously disease free.

Special note should be made regarding dysgerminoma. Historically, for patients with metastatic dysgerminoma, the traditional postoperative treatment was radiotherapy. Although dysgerminoma is exquisitely radiosensitive and survival rates with this treatment were excellent, most patients suffered loss of fertility. With the advent of successful combination chemotherapy, such as BEP, chemotherapy has almost exclusively supplanted radiotherapy, with a high rate of fertility preservation. In a GOG report, adjuvant chemotherapy with etoposide and carboplatin for 39 patients with completely resected stage IC to III dysgerminoma resulted in no relapses (Williams, 2004).

**There has been a trend toward surveillance, with careful follow-up after surgery as an alternative to chemotherapy in select patients.** Bonazzi and colleagues treated 32 patients with operation alone for stage I or II, grade 1 or 2, tumors. All patients with grade 3 or stage III tumors, or those with tumor recurrence, received BEP. Most patients underwent fertility-sparing surgery, and 10 received chemotherapy. All patients were free of disease with a median follow-up of 47 months, and 5 had delivered healthy infants. A Pediatric Oncology Group study reported by Cushing and associates indicated that patients younger than 15 years with a pure immature teratoma could be followed without chemotherapy; however, more than 90% of the tumors in their series were grade 1 or 2. Patterson and associates reported on surveillance in patients with stage IA malignant ovarian germ cell tumor. Relapses were reported in 8 of 22 patients with nondysgerminomatous tumors (36%) and 2 of 9 patients with dysgerminomas (22%). All relapses occurred within 13 months of diagnosis, and 1 patient was not salvaged with chemotherapy. Mangili and colleagues reported 28 patients with stage I immature teratoma (9 grade 1, 12 grade 2, and 7 grade 3), 19 of whom were treated with surgery alone. A total of 24 patients underwent fertility-sparing surgery; 4 patients treated with surgery alone relapsed—2 with mature teratoma and 2 with immature teratoma. All were successfully given salvage secondary surgery, with the 2 patients with immature teratoma receiving chemotherapy as well.

The Children's Oncology Group (COG) conducted a clinical trial in the pediatric population that included surveillance of a low-risk cohort, consisting of all patients with apparent stage I disease with close follow-up of serum markers and initiation of chemotherapy only if relapse occurred (Billmire, 2014). Twenty-five girls were enrolled in the trial. After a median follow-up of 42 months, 12 patients had persistent or recurrent disease. Eleven of the 12 patients were successfully given salvage chemotherapy. **An ongoing international clinical trial sponsored by COG (AGCT1531) includes a cohort of patients with stage IA or IB ovarian yolk sac tumors, grade 2 or 3 immature teratomas, embryonal carcinomas, and nongestational choriocarcinomas who undergo surveillance after primary surgery. Chemotherapy is administered only if relapse occurs.**

There is no standard surveillance for patients with malignant ovarian germ cell tumors after completion of primary therapy. For patients who have completed standard surgery plus chemotherapy, we generally recommend evaluation of serum tumor marker every 1 to 2 months for up to 2 years, every 3 months for the third year, and then every 6 months until 5 years from diagnosis. Patients treated with fertility-sparing surgery should be closely followed with periodic TVUS. Office visits, with a physical examination, are generally recommended every 3 months for the first 2 years and less frequently thereafter.

With the success of cure in a high proportion of young patients with malignant ovarian germ cell tumors has come an increasing focus on the late effects of therapy, particularly fertility preservation. In a report of 40 patients, Gershenson and colleagues noted that 27 had normal menses after multiagent chemotherapy for germ cell tumors, and 11 of 16 patients who attempted pregnancy were successful in bearing 22 children. Most of these patients received nonplatinum-based chemotherapy. Peccatori and associates reported on 139 patients with malignant germ cell tumors, 108 of whom had fertility-sparing operations. Multiagent platinum-containing chemotherapy was used, with a 96% survival rate and a mean follow-up of 55 months. In a GOG study, Williams and associates reported on 93 patients treated with BEP for three cycles. Of 93 patients, 91 were free of disease 4 to 90 months after treatment, although leukemia developed in one patient and lymphoma in a second patient. Brewer and coworkers reported on 26 patients treated with BEP, with 25 alive and disease free at a median follow-up of 89 months. They reported that 71% resumed normal menstrual function and 6 patients conceived. Three additional large studies from Australia, Italy, and the United States have provided further support for the concept of preservation of fertility in most treated with fertility-sparing surgery and chemotherapy. In a GOG matched control study of 132 survivors (all of whom were treated with surgery and platinum-based chemotherapy) and 137 controls, 71 survivors (54%) underwent fertility-sparing surgery. Of the fertile survivors, 87% reported having normal menstrual function and 24 survivors had 37 offspring after cancer therapy; however, compared with controls, cancer survivors had significantly greater reproductive concerns and less sexual pleasure.

Options for fertility preservation in young patients with malignant ovarian germ cell tumors include prechemotherapy oocyte retrieval with oocyte or embryo cryopreservation or gonadotropin-releasing hormone agonist prophylaxis during chemotherapy; however, the latter strategy remains controversial (Blumenfeld, 1996; Demeestere, 2016; Lambertini, 2018).

### Specialized Germ Cell Tumors: Struma Ovarii and Carcinoid

Specialized ovarian germ cell tumors are rare; two types are commonly recognized (see Box 33.3): the struma ovarii and carcinoids. Struma ovarii are dermoids with thyroid tissue exclusively or with thyroid tissue as a major component. The thyroid tissue can be functional, leading to clinical hyperthyroidism. Most of these tumors are benign, but malignant changes are possible. Metastatic disease, if present, has been reported to be effectively treated with iodine-131 ($^{131}I$), as for primary thyroid carcinoma.

Carcinoids are ovarian teratomas that histologically resemble similar tumors in the gastrointestinal tract. Carcinoids are rare and are unilateral in the ovary. In approximately 30% of cases, a true carcinoid syndrome will develop, and 5-hydroxyindoleacetic acid can be detected and used to monitor the tumor postoperatively. These tumors occur primarily in older women and tend to grow slowly; the prognosis after hysterectomy and bilateral salpingo-oophorectomy is excellent. For a young woman desiring preservation of childbearing function, a stage IA carcinoid can be treated by unilateral salpingo-oophorectomy.

## GONADOBLASTOMA (GERM CELL SEX CORD–STROMAL TUMOR)

The term *gonadoblastoma* was introduced by Scully in 1953 to describe a tumor that consists of germ cell and sex cord–stromal elements. Approximately 100 cases have been reported. The germ cells usually resemble dysgerminoma, whereas the sex cord–stromal elements may consist of immature granulosa and Sertoli cells. Leydig cells and luteinized cells may be present. The tumor usually occurs in patients with abnormal (dysgenetic) gonads. Most patients have a female phenotype, but they may be virilized. These patients have a Y chromosome detected in their karyotype, and patients with gonadal dysgenesis and a Y chromosome are at risk for the development of gonadoblastoma or malignant germ cell tumors, predominantly dysgerminoma, which may occur in those as young as 6 months. Removal of these gonads is indicated when they are discovered. Both gonads should be removed; if the presence of pure gonadoblastoma is confirmed, the prognosis is excellent because these tumors have not been reported to metastasize.

## SEX CORD–STROMAL TUMORS

Sex cord–stromal tumors are derived from the sex cords of the ovary and the specialized stroma of the developing gonad. The elements can have a male or female differentiation, and some of these tumors are hormonally active. This group accounts for approximately 6% of ovarian neoplasms and most hormonally functioning ovarian tumors. For the female derivatives, the sex cord component is the granulosa cell and the stromal component is the theca cell or fibroblast. For the male counterpart, the similar components are the Sertoli cell and Leydig cell. Granulosa–theca cell tumors and Sertoli–Leydig cell tumors tend to behave as low-grade malignancies. Their clinical and morphologic aspects considered separately.

### Granulosa–Theca Cell Tumors

Granulosa cell tumors consist primarily of granulosa cells and a varying proportion of theca cells, fibroblasts, or both. One characteristic microscopic pattern is shown in Fig. 33.23, which demonstrates the so-called *Call-Exner bodies*, eosinophilic bodies surrounded by granulosa cells. Functional granulosa cell tumors are primarily estrogenic. Approximately 5% occur before puberty and they can be one cause of precocious puberty, but the tumors have been described in women of all ages. In postmenopausal women, these tumors can produce increased levels of blood estrogens, uterine bleeding, and occasionally endometrial carcinoma. It is estimated that approximately 25% to 50% of granulosa cell tumors are associated with endometrial hyperplasia and 5% to 10% are associated with endometrial carcinoma. In menstruating women the functional granulosa cell tumor can produce abnormal menstrual patterns, menorrhagia, and even amenorrhea.

These tumors can become large and may present as a ruptured mass, leading to laparotomy for an acute abdomen with hemoperitoneum. Because of the low-grade malignant character of these tumors, recurrences are commonly more than 5 years after primary therapy. In general, prognosis does not correlate with the histologic pattern of the tumor. **Approximately 90% of granulosa cell tumors present as stage I. Advanced clinical stage, the presence of tumor rupture, a large primary tumor (>15 cm), and a high mitotic rate have been associated with a poorer prognosis.** Overall 10-year survival rates of 90% have been reported. Studies by Klemi and colleagues and others have suggested that most granulosa cell tumors have a diploid pattern and a low S-phase fraction (<60%) when analyzed by flow cytometry. Those with an aneuploid pattern had a worse prognosis. A variant found predominantly in females younger than 20 years is known as *juvenile granulosa cell tumor*. It was described by Young

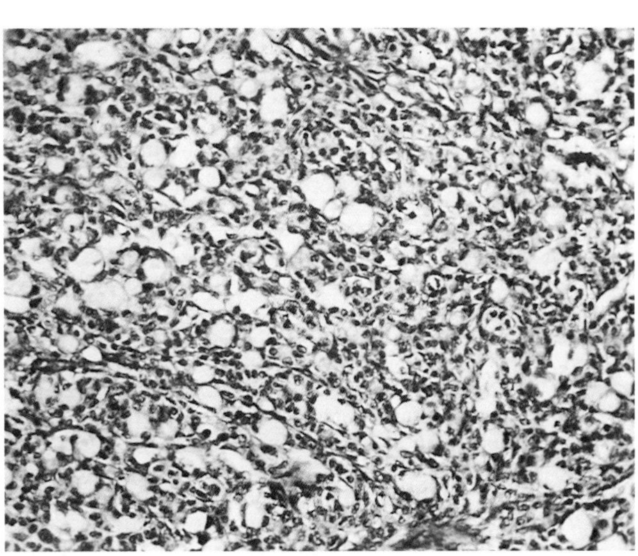

**Fig. 33.23** Krukenberg tumor (original magnification ×256). Mucin-filled signet ring cells are present. (Courtesy Dr. R.E. Scully.)

and coworkers and has an excellent prognosis, particularly if the tumor is confined to one ovary.

**Molecular profiling investigations have found that almost all granulosa cell tumors have a *FOXL2* mutation (Shah, 2009). *FOXL2* is a member of the forkhead-winged-helix family of transcription factors and one of the earliest markers of ovarian differentiation.**

The primary therapeutic approach is surgery. Because these tumors are rarely bilateral (<5%), young patients with stage IA tumors can be treated by unilateral adnexectomy. Lack and colleagues reported on 10 cases of granulosa cell tumors in premenarchal female patients, all of whom were treated by unilateral salpingo-oophorectomy. Two tumors were ruptured. All 10 of the patients were alive with no evidence of disease 2 to 33 years after therapy. Evans and associates noted a higher recurrence rate in women who were treated by unilateral salpingo-oophorectomy for stage IA cases compared with those treated with bilateral salpingo-oophorectomy. This finding has led to the recommendation that women of reproductive age treated for granulosa cell tumor by unilateral salpingo-oophorectomy have close follow-up. For women who have completed childbearing, abdominal hysterectomy and bilateral salpingo-oophorectomy are recommended. Regardless of the treatment of the pelvic organs, if a granulosa cell tumor is diagnosed on frozen-section examination, comprehensive surgical staging is recommended; however, routine pelvic and paraaortic lymphadenectomy not recommended related to information that the incidence of lymph node metastases associated with this tumor type is low. In a study of 262 patients with sex cord–stromal tumors reported by Brown and colleagues, 178 patients were diagnosed with granulosa cell tumors. None of the patients who underwent lymphadenectomy had evidence of lymph node metastasis.

Tumor markers may be helpful for monitoring the clinical course of granulosa cell tumors. Studies by Lappohn and colleagues have suggested that the peptide hormone inhibin is secreted by some granulosa cell tumors and serum measurements could serve as a tumor marker. In addition, serum CA-125, serum estradiol, or serum testosterone levels may occasionally serve as markers that should be followed serially, and one study of 123 women indicated that monitoring of both antimüllerian hormone (AMH) and inhibin levels was superior to inhibin alone in detection of macroscopic disease (Farkkila, 2015).

Historically, radiotherapy, the VAC regimen (discussed earlier), or the combination of cisplatin, doxorubicin, and cyclophosphamide have been used for the treatment of metastatic granulosa cell tumors, but none of these options are recommended for general application. Many questions remain regarding recommendations for postoperative treatment. For patients with stage IA granulosa cell tumors, surgery alone is recommended. The recommendation for those with stage IC disease remains controversial, but consideration can be given to adjuvant therapy based on the probable increased risk of relapse. Postoperative therapy is recommended for all patients with stages II to IV disease and for those patients with recurrent tumor.

Because of the rarity of granulosa cell tumors, no standard regimen exists. The GOG has reported the largest series of women treated with the BEP regimen. Homesley and associates reported on 57 eligible patients; 41 had recurrent disease and 16 had primary metastatic disease. Of these patients, 48 had granulosa cell tumors. Overall, 11 of 16 primary disease patients and 21 of 41 recurrent disease patients remained progression free at a median follow-up of 3 years; however, toxicity was fairly severe, with two bleomycin-related deaths reported.

Brown and coworkers reported the MD Anderson Cancer Center experience with taxane-based chemotherapy in a study of 44 patients with sex cord–stromal tumors of the ovary treated for primary metastatic or recurrent disease. The response rate for 30 patients treated with a taxane plus platinum for recurrent measurable disease was 42%. In a phase II trial of single-agent paclitaxel for recurrent ovarian stromal tumors, the objective response rate was 29% (Burton, 2016). The combination of paclitaxel and carboplatin is also an option for these patients. NRG Oncology (GOG) is conducting a randomized phase II study comparing BEP with the combination of paclitaxel and carboplatin for women with newly diagnosed or chemo-naïve recurrent sex cord–stromal ovarian tumors. In general, however, the value of chemotherapy for ovarian sex cord–stromal tumors has been questioned (Meisel, 2015; van Meurs, 2014a). The rarity of these tumors and the indolent nature of some subtypes are features that complicate the assessment of the efficacy of chemotherapy.

Hormonal therapy may also be considered for patients with metastatic granulosa cell tumors. Responses of these tumors to medroxyprogesterone acetate and gonadotropin-releasing hormone antagonists have been reported. Fishman and colleagues treated six patients with recurrent or persistent granulosa cell tumors with leuprolide acetate; of five patients with assessable disease, two had partial responses and three had stable disease. Van Meurs and associates reviewed the literature and made a case for hormonal therapy as a good treatment alternative for granulosa cell tumors (van Meurs, 2014b). In addition, a phase II trial of bevacizumab in patients with recurrent sex cord–stromal tumors showed an objective response rate of 16.7% (Brown, 2014).

For patients with recurrent granulosa cell tumors, SCR is a major option, depending on the extent and distribution of tumor implants. Options for systemic therapy include conventional chemotherapy, hormonal therapies, bevacizumab alone or in combination, and potential clinical trials.

**As with malignant ovarian germ cell tumors, fertility-sparing surgery may be an option for young patients, particularly those with stage IA disease.** Wang and colleagues reported fertility-sparing surgery in 61 of 113 patients with stage IA granulosa cell tumors. Of the 22 patients desiring pregnancy, 19 had 20 singleton pregnancies. The pregnancy rate was 86.4%, and the live birth rate was 95%.

## Thecoma and Fibroma

A thecoma is a benign tumor that consists entirely of stroma (theca) cells. It predominantly occurs in women in their perimenopausal and menopausal years. These tumors can be associated with estrogen production but not as often as granulosa cell tumors. Removal of the tumor alone is adequate treatment for women in their reproductive years. For older women, total abdominal hysterectomy and bilateral salpingo-oophorectomy are performed. Rarely, thecomas have been reported to be malignant, and these are most likely fibrosarcomas. A closely related tumor is the fibroma, which is the most common benign solid ovarian tumor and accounts for 4% of all ovarian tumors. Like the thecoma, it can occur at any age but is more common in older women; it does not secrete hormones. These tumors contain spindle cells and can grow large, but they are benign and excision is adequate treatment. They are associated with ascites in approximately 40% of cases if the tumor is larger than 10 cm, according to Samanth and Black. They can also be responsible for hydrothorax with a benign ascites (Meigs syndrome), which regresses after tumor removal.

## Sertoli–Leydig Cell Tumor (Androblastoma)

Sertoli–Leydig cell tumors are very rare. Sertoli (sex cord) and Leydig (stromal) cells are present in varying amounts, and the tumor may consist almost entirely of Sertoli or Leydig cells (Fig. 33.24). These tumors tend to occur in young women of reproductive age and often are the cause of masculinization and hirsutism related to production of testosterone. The symptoms of

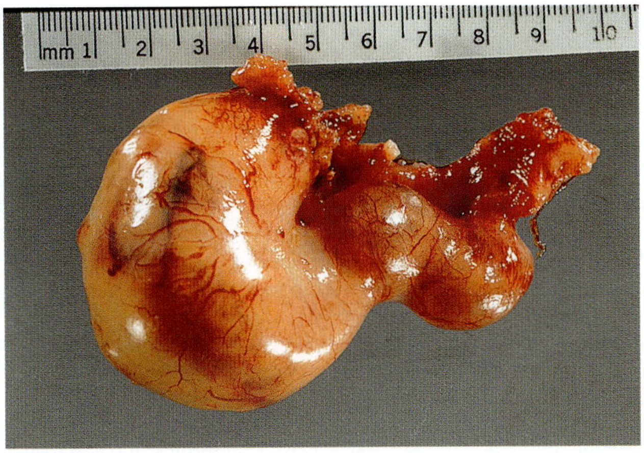

**Fig. 33.24** Adenocarcinoma of the fallopian tube revealing a dilated fallopian tube with an obstructed fimbriated end. (From Voet RL. *Color Atlas of Obstetric and Gynecologic Pathology.* St. Louis: Mosby-Wolfe; 1997.)

virilization usually regress after tumor removal, but temporal hair recession and a deeper voice tend to remain. Rarely, they have also been reported to have estrogenic activity, leading to the same symptoms and signs as those of granulosa cell tumors. The tumors tend to behave as low-grade malignancies, and the 5-year survival rate can vary from 70% to 90%; however, poorly differentiated types tend to have a poor prognosis, as do higher-stage tumors. Young and Scully reviewed 207 cases; 75% were in those aged 30 or younger and less than 10% were older than 50 years. One-third of patients had evidence of androgen excess. Both ovaries were involved in only three cases. The well-differentiated tumors behaved clinically as benign tumors, whereas recurrence or extrauterine spread was noted occasionally in women with intermediate differentiation (11%) and commonly in those with poor differentiation (59%). Of 164 patients available for follow-up, 18% had metastasis or recurrence.

**Studies have established that *DICER1* mutations are found in a relatively high percentage of patients with Sertoli–Leydig cell tumors (Heravi-Moussavi, 2012; Schultz, 2011). These mutations may be either germline or somatic and may be associated with familial pleuropulmonary blastoma.**

Treatment of metastatic Sertoli–Leydig cell tumors is similar to that for granulosa cell tumors. In addition, because the prognosis for patients with stage I poorly differentiated Sertoli–Leydig cell tumors is so poor, adjuvant chemotherapy is recommended (Gui, 2012; Sigismondi, 2012); however, it should be emphasized that there are no therapeutic data in this setting, and if treatment is recommended, the optimal regimen remains unclear. The BEP regimen or the combination of paclitaxel and carboplatin may be considered for these patients. For patients with stage IC to IV disease or relapse, platinum-based chemotherapy or other conventional chemotherapy regimens (if the patient is platinum-resistant) are recommended.

### Other Sex Cord–Stromal Tumors

#### Gynandroblastoma

Gynandroblastomas are rare sex cord–stromal tumors consisting of female (granulosa cells) and male (Sertoli cells) cell types. Theca or Leydig cells may also be present. Patients with this tumor typically present with androgenic manifestations, but stigmata associated with hyperestrogenism may also be observed. These tumors are usually unilateral and generally considered to be of LMP.

#### Sex Cord Tumors with Annular Tubules

Sex cord tumors with annular tubules are unusual. As suggested by the name, there is a prominent tubular pattern. Features of both Sertoli and granulosa cell tumors are present. Young and colleagues reviewed 74 cases; 27 were associated with mucocutaneous pigmentation and gastrointestinal tract polyposis (Peutz-Jeghers syndrome). The tumors may have estrogenic manifestations. Those associated with Peutz-Jeghers syndrome are benign and those not associated with this syndrome can be malignant. It is of interest that 4 of these 74 cases were associated with a virulent form of cervical adenocarcinoma (adenoma malignum).

#### Leydig Cell Tumor

Leydig cell tumors are rare. They are composed of Leydig cells or cells of the ovarian hilus. Their cytoplasm contains hyaline bodies known as *crystalloids of Reinke*. They usually cause virilization and are benign. They tend to be small (<6 cm) and develop primarily in perimenopausal women.

## LIPID (LIPOID) TUMOR

Lipid tumors are infrequently occurring ovarian tumors composed of large cells that resemble Leydig cells, luteinized cells, or cells that arise in the adrenal cortex. Approximately 100 tumors have been reported. These tumors usually cause virilization but have also been associated with excess cortisol production. There is not enough experience with them to delineate an effective form of treatment; however, metastases of lipid cell tumors have been reported.

## METASTATIC OVARIAN TUMORS

Tumors from distant primary sites can metastasize to the ovary. Commonly, metastases are from primary tumors that originate elsewhere in the female reproductive tract, particularly from the endometrium and fallopian tube. Distant sites of origin occur most commonly from the breast and gastrointestinal tract. Metastatic tumors from the gastrointestinal tract to the ovary can be associated with sex hormone production, which usually leads to estrogenic manifestations. One special type of metastatic ovarian tumor is known as a Krukenberg tumor, which histologically consists of nests of mucin-filled signet ring cells in a cellular stroma (Fig. 33.25). The most common

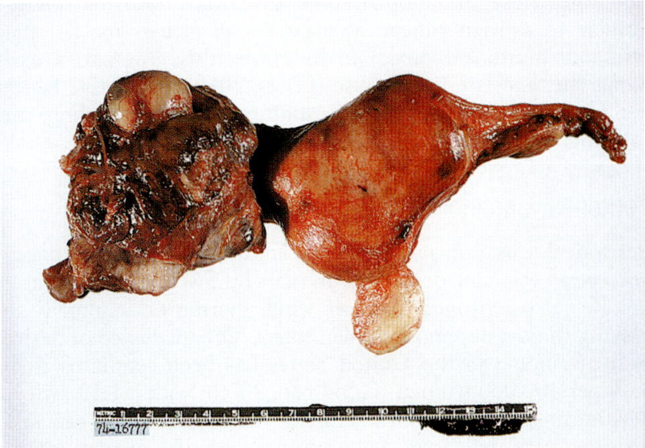

**Fig. 33.25** Adenocarcinoma of the fallopian tube. (From Anderson MC, Robboy SJ, Russell P. The fallopian tube. In: Robboy SJ, Anderson MC, Russell P, eds. *Pathology of the Female Reproductive Tract.* Edinburgh: Churchill Livingstone; 2002.)

gastrointestinal tract origin for these tumors is the stomach, and the next common is the large intestine; however, breast metastases to the ovary can on occasion reveal the same histologic picture. A few cases of Krukenberg tumors have been described, with no apparent distant primary malignancy, suggesting the rare possibility of a primary ovarian tumor with the histologic features of a Krukenberg tumor. A primary gastrointestinal tract malignancy should be considered in older women with an adnexal mass, particularly if it is bilateral and solid. A pretherapy evaluation to rule out a gastrointestinal tract or breast primary tumor is indicated. The tumor should be removed when discovered, and the primary site should be treated. The prognosis is poor; it is rare for a woman to survive for 5 years or longer after treatment.

## Fallopian Tube and Peritoneal Cancers

Fallopian tube and peritoneal cancers have similar clinical characteristics, patterns of spread, response to treatment, and survival rates compared with ovarian cancer. In addition, the most common histologic type for all three malignancies is high-grade serous carcinoma; however, fallopian tube and peritoneal cancers have several distinct clinical and pathologic findings.

### Fallopian Tube Cancer

Fallopian tube carcinoma is rare, accounting for approximately 0.2% of cancers among women. The estimated incidence of fallopian tube cancer in the United States is 0.41 per 100,000 women (Stewart, 2007); however, it has been suggested that many cases of ovarian carcinoma may actually arise from the epithelial lining of the fallopian tube fimbria, thereby grossly underestimating the incidence of primary fallopian tube carcinoma (Carlson, 2008a; Kindelberger, 2007).

Similar to ovarian cancer, the primary risk factor for fallopian tube cancer is an inherited mutation in the *BRCA1* and *BRCA2* tumor suppressor genes associated with hereditary breast and ovarian cancer syndromes. Women with *BRCA1* and *BRCA2* mutations have a 40% to 60% and 20% to 30% lifetime risk, respectively, for developing ovarian, fallopian tube, or peritoneal cancer (Chen, 2007; Mavaddat, 2013). Furthermore, previous reports have shown that approximately 15% to 45% of women with fallopian tube cancers have a *BRCA* mutation (Levine, 2003; Cass, 2005). Risk-reducing bilateral salpingo-oophorectomy (rrBSO) is therefore recommended for women with a *BRCA* mutation once they have completed childbearing (Domchek, 2010; Kauff, 2002; Rebbeck, 2002, 2009); however, in women without a *BRCA* mutation, the cause of fallopian tube carcinoma remains unclear. Similar to ovarian cancer, associated risk factors for fallopian tube and peritoneal cancer include infertility, low parity, early menarche, and late menopause (Gates, 2010). Protective factors include oral contraceptive use, multiparity, breastfeeding, and tubal ligation (Cibula, 2011; Tsilidis, 2011).

### Peritoneal Carcinoma

Peritoneal carcinoma (previously known as *primary peritoneal carcinoma*) was first described in 1959 by Swerdlow. It diffusely involves the peritoneal surfaces while sparing or minimally involving the ovaries and fallopian tubes. The incidence of peritoneal carcinoma in the United States has been estimated to be 0.46 per 100,000 women (Goodman, 2009); with a 1:10 ratio of peritoneal cancer to ovarian cancer cases. Peritoneal cancer is histologically indistinguishable from epithelial ovarian cancer and has similar clinical characteristics, patterns of spread, response to treatment, and survival rates (Fromm, 1990; Halperin, 2001). Risk factors for primary peritoneal carcinoma are similar to those for ovarian and fallopian tube cancer, including *BRCA* mutation and low parity; however, peritoneal cancer has also been associated with older age at diagnosis and increased rates of obesity compared with ovarian cancer (Barda, 2004; Jordan, 2008).

The pathogenesis of peritoneal carcinoma is not well characterized. The germinal epithelium of the ovary and mesothelium of the peritoneum arise from the same embryonic origin, and it was previously suggested that primary peritoneal cancer may develop from a malignant transformation of these cells (Lauchlan, 1972). Another proposed theory was a field effect, with the coelomic epithelium lining the abdominal cavity (peritoneum) and ovaries (germinal epithelium) manifesting a common response to an oncogenic stimulus (Parmley, 1974; Truong, 1990). Molecular studies have been inconclusive in determining whether the tumor arises from the ovarian surface epithelium and spreads throughout the peritoneum or if a multifocal malignant transformation process occurs. Peritoneal carcinoma has therefore become a diagnosis of exclusion when a primary ovarian or fallopian tube carcinoma cannot be identified.

### Serous Tubal Intraepithelial Carcinoma

There is increasing evidence that many cases of ovarian and peritoneal carcinoma may actually arise from the fallopian tube (Carlson, 2008a; Kindelberger, 2007). This hypothesis is supported by studies of women with *BRCA* mutations who have undergone risk-reducing bilateral salpingo-oophorectomy (rrBSO). Between 5% and 15% of women undergoing rrBSO have been reported to have occult serous cancers (Callahan, 2007; Finch, 2006; Leeper, 2002; Lu, 2000; Reitsma, 2013). A large number of these early cancers involve the fallopian tube as invasive fallopian tube carcinoma or as a precursor lesion known as serous tubal intraepithelial carcinoma (STIC). In most cases, the tumor involves the fimbriated end of the fallopian tube. These studies have suggested that the fallopian tube may be the primary source of ovarian and peritoneal serous carcinomas in women with *BRCA* mutations. It is therefore recommended that after rrBSO the ovarian and fallopian tube specimens undergo careful examination for neoplasm. This consists of serial sectioning and extensively examining the fimbrial end of the fallopian tube using the sectioning and extensively examining the fimbriated end (SEE-FIM) protocol (Mehrad, 2010; Powell, 2005).

Studies of unselected women with ovarian and peritoneal cancer have also shown a significant number of cases to coexist with a STIC. Kindelberger and colleagues reported that a STIC was present in 47% of 43 tumors classified as primary ovarian cancers (Kindelberger, 2007). Similarly, Carlson and coworkers found a STIC present in the fallopian tube of 47% of 19 women with serous peritoneal cancers (Carlson, 2008a). In addition, *P53* mutational analyses have shown the same mutations in STIC and distant tumors, providing a genetic link between the two (Kuhn, 2012).

### Diagnosis, Clinical Findings, and Staging

Similar to ovarian cancer, the diagnosis of fallopian tube or peritoneal cancer may be suspected based on imaging studies, CA-125 level, or symptoms, as well as physical examination findings; however, a definitive diagnosis is usually made at the time of surgery.

**Ultrasound**

The classic ultrasound findings for fallopian tube cancer include a fluid-filled, tubular or ovoid mass with internal papillary areas, mural nodules, or septations that is separate from the uterus and ovaries. In peritoneal and fallopian tube cancers, ascites or peritoneal implants may be present. With both malignancies, the ovaries are often normal in appearance.

### Other Imaging Modalities

CT, MRI, and PET scans may provide additional information in women with suspected fallopian tube or peritoneal cancer. These studies can provide information regarding the extent of disease and sites of metastatic spread, allowing the physician to plan appropriate intervention and treatment.

### CA-125 Level

The CA-125 level is elevated in more than 80% of women with fallopian tube and peritoneal cancer. CA-125 value is useful for monitoring response to treatment or evaluating a woman in whom the disease is suspected.

The mean age at diagnosis of fallopian tube carcinoma is 58 years, with a range of 26 to 85 years; however, in women with *BRCA*-associated fallopian tube carcinoma, the age at diagnosis is considerably younger. Cass and colleagues reported the median age at diagnosis to be 57 years in *BRCA* mutation carriers compared with 65 years in sporadic cases (Cass, 2005). Fallopian tube cancer is more common among white women (age-adjusted incidence rate, 0.41), compared with black (0.27), Hispanic (0.27), and Asian and Pacific Islander women (0.25) (Stewart, 2007).

The presenting symptoms of fallopian tube carcinoma are largely related to the degree of obstruction of the distal tube. Many women are asymptomatic; however, the most commonly reported signs and symptoms include abnormal vaginal bleeding or serosanguineous vaginal discharge (35% to 60%), a palpable adnexal mass (10% to 60%), and crampy lower abdominal pain caused by tubal distention and forced peristalsis (20% to 50%). *Hydrops tubae profluens* is the term used to describe intermittent expulsion of clear or serosanguineous fluid from the vagina caused by contraction of a distended, distally occluded fallopian tube (Sinha, 1959). The discharge may be followed by shrinkage or resolution of the adnexal mass. The triad of intermittent serosanguineous discharge, colicky pain, and a mass (Latzko triad) is considered to be pathognomonic of fallopian tube cancer but occurs in only approximately 15% of patients. In addition, approximately 10% to 40% of women with fallopian tube carcinoma have abnormal cervical cytologic test results, including adenocarcinoma or atypical glandular cells of undetermined significance (AGUS). Evaluation with a CA-125 level and TVUS to rule out ovarian and fallopian tube cancer should be considered in women with these cytologic findings who have a negative workup for endocervical and endometrial carcinoma.

Patients with peritoneal cancer tend to be older than women with ovarian or fallopian tube cancer, with the median age at diagnosis reported to range from 63 to 66 years. Similar to those with ovarian cancer, women with peritoneal cancer typically present with pain, abdominal distention, pressure, or gastrointestinal symptoms. A small proportion of patients are asymptomatic. Occasionally, primary peritoneal cancer is detected during exploratory surgery for other reasons.

The staging of fallopian tube and peritoneal carcinomas is combined in the FIGO classification system with ovarian carcinoma (Table 33.6); however, the staging does require that the site of origin be noted if known (ovary, fallopian tube, peritoneum) (Mutch, 2014).

## Pathologic Findings

### Fallopian Tube Carcinoma

Fallopian tube carcinomas arise in either tube with similar frequency and are bilateral in 3% to 8% of cases. The fimbriated end of the fallopian tube is grossly occluded in approximately 50% of patients, resulting in a dilated lumen filled with tumor or fluid (see Figs. 33.24 and 33.25). Histologically, 80% to 90% of fallopian tube carcinomas are adenocarcinomas (Fig. 33.26).

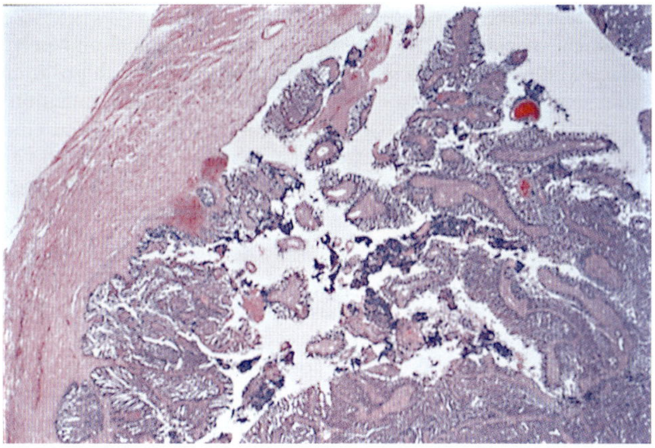

**Fig. 33.26** Microscopic appearance of an adenocarcinoma of fallopian tube confined to the endosalpinx, with minimal invasion into the muscular wall. (From Voet RL. *Color Atlas of Obstetric and Gynecologic Pathology.* St. Louis: Mosby-Wolfe; 1997.)

Most of these are serous carcinomas, followed by endometrioid and clear cell adenocarcinomas. Other rare histologic subtypes include sarcomas, carcinosarcomas, germ cell tumors, and gestational trophoblastic tumors.

Similar to ovarian cancer, most patients with fallopian tube cancer have grade 2 or 3 tumors, with less than 5% being grade 1 tumors. Previous reports have shown stage at diagnosis to be evenly distributed among localized disease, regional spread, and distant metastases; however, serous adenocarcinomas are more likely to be diagnosed at advanced stages and endometrioid adenocarcinomas at earlier stages (Stewart, 2007).

It can be challenging to distinguish primary fallopian tube carcinoma from ovarian or peritoneal carcinomas. Hu and colleagues (Hu, 1950) initially developed pathologic diagnostic criteria in 1950 for the diagnosis of primary fallopian tube carcinoma. These were subsequently modified by Sedlis and associates in 1978 (Sedlis, 1978), and included the following:

1. The main tumor lies in the tube and arises from the endosalpinx.
2. The histologic pattern reproduces the papillary epithelium of tubal mucosa.
3. A transition can be demonstrated between the malignant and nonmalignant tubal epithelium.
4. The ovaries and uterus are normal or contain less tumor than the fallopian tube.

Data also suggest that if a STIC is present and there is minimal involvement of the ovary, a primary fallopian tube origin should be assigned. In contrast, if the majority of the tumor is in the ovary and no STIC is present, then an ovarian origin is considered (Carlson, 2008b).

The patterns of spread of fallopian tube carcinoma are largely related to the degree of obstruction of the distal tube. If the fimbriated end of the tube is obstructed by tumor, previous injury, or infection, the by-products of tumor growth, such as blood and increased serous fluid, distend the tube and are discharged intermittently through the vagina. If the distal portion of the fallopian tube is patent, the malignancy spreads more easily out the distal end of the tube, resulting in tumor seeding of the peritoneal cavity, ascites, and omental caking. IP spread may also occur as the tumor grows through the muscular wall of the tube. The peritoneum is therefore the most common site of metastatic spread; however, lymphatic spread also occurs to the pelvic and paraaortic lymph nodes. Occult lymph node metastases may be present in patients with tumor that grossly appeared to be confined to the fallopian tube.

**Peritoneal Carcinoma**

Peritoneal carcinoma tends to involve the abdominal and pelvic surfaces diffusely. The most common histologic type is high-grade serous carcinoma, but cases of endometrioid, clear cell, mucinous, and carcinosarcoma have also been reported. Given the difficulty in distinguishing primary peritoneal carcinoma from ovarian carcinoma, the GOG previously developed the following pathologic criteria for the diagnosis of primary peritoneal carcinoma:

1. Both ovaries must be physiologically normal in size or enlarged by a benign process.
2. Involvement in the extraovarian sites must be greater than involvement on the surface of either ovary.
3. Microscopically, the ovarian component must be one of the following:
   a. Nonexistent
   b. Confined to the ovarian surface epithelium with no evidence of cortical invasion
   c. Involving ovarian surface epithelium and underlying cortical stroma but with any given tumor size smaller than 5 × 5 mm
   d. Tumor smaller than 5 × 5 mm within the ovarian substance, with or without surface disease
4. The histologic and cytologic characteristics of the tumor must be predominantly of the serous type that is similar or identical to ovarian serous papillary adenocarcinoma of any grade.

## Treatment And Prognosis

The treatment of fallopian tube and peritoneal cancers is identical to that of epithelial ovarian cancer. As with ovarian cancer, the prognosis for patients with fallopian tube cancer is strongly related to the stage of disease. The 5-year survival rates are 81% for stage I disease, 67% for stage II disease, 41% for stage III disease, and 33% for stage IV disease (Heintz, 2006). Other prognostic factors for early-stage disease include the degree of invasion of the fallopian tube wall and the location of the tumor within the tube (fimbrial versus nonfimbrial). Similar to ovarian cancer, improved survival has been seen if the tumor can be completely removed at the time of surgery. In addition, patients with a *BRCA* mutation have been shown to have higher survival rates. Most studies have reported a better survival for patients with advanced-stage fallopian tube cancer compared with primary ovarian cancer. In contrast, retrospective case-control studies have shown no difference in survival rates between patients with peritoneal cancer and patients with ovarian cancer. This favorable prognosis for patients with fallopian tube cancer may be the result of a higher rate of *BRCA* mutation carriers among women with fallopian tube cancer compared with ovarian and peritoneal cancers; however, if a subset of ovarian and peritoneal carcinomas actually arises from the fallopian tube, the prognosis for women with fallopian tube, peritoneal, and ovarian cancer may actually be similar.

## REFERENCES


Armstrong DK, Bundy B, Wenzel L, et al. Intraperitoneal cisplatin and paclitaxel in ovarian cancer. *N Engl J Med.* 2006;354(1):34-43.

Bell D, Berchuck A, Birrer M, et al. Integrated genomic analyses of ovarian carcinoma. *Nature.* 2011;474(7353):609-615.

Burger RA, Brady MF, Bookman MA, et al. Incorporation of bevacizumab in the primary treatment of ovarian cancer. *N Engl J Med.* 2011;365(26):2473-2483.

Chan JK, Brady MF, Penson RT, et al. Weekly vs. every-3-week paclitaxel and carboplatin for ovarian cancer. *N Engl J Med.* 2016;374(8): 738-748.

Clamp AR, James EC, McNeish IA, et al. Weekly dose-dense chemotherapy in first-line epithelial ovarian, fallopian tube, or primary peritoneal carcinoma treatment (ICON8): primary progression free survival analysis results from a GCIG phase 3 randomised controlled trial. *Lancet.* 2019;394(10214):2084-2095.

Coleman RL, Brady MF, Herzog TJ, et al. Bevacizumab and paclitaxel-carboplatin chemotherapy and secondary cytoreduction in recurrent platinum-sensitive ovarian cancer (NRG Oncology/Gynecologic Oncology Group study GOG-0213: a multicenter, open-label, randomized, phase 3 trial. *Lancet Oncol.* 2017;18(6):779-791.

Coleman RL, Fleming GF, Brady MF, et al. Veliparib with first-line chemotherapy and as maintenance therapy in ovarian cancer. *N Engl J Med.* 2019;381(25):2403-2415. doi: 10.1056/NEJMoa1909707.

Coleman RL, Oza AM, Lorusso D, et al. Rucaparib maintenance treatment for recurrent ovarian carcinoma after response to platinum therapy (ARIEL3): a randomized, double-blind, placebo-controlled, phase 3 trial. *Lancet.* 2017;390(10106):1949-1961.

Coleman RL, Spirtos NM, Enserro D, et al. Secondary surgical cytoreduction for recurrent ovarian cancer. *N Engl J Med.* 2019;381(20): 1929-1939.

Disis ML, Taylor MH, Kelly K, et al. Efficacy and safety of avelumab for patients with recurrent or refractory ovarian cancer: Phase Ib results from the JAVELIN solid tumor trial. *JAMA Oncol.* 2019;5(3)384-392.

Fader AN, Bergstrom J, Jernigan A, et al. Primary cytoreductive surgery and adjuvant hormonal monotherapy in women with advanced low-grade serous ovarian carcinoma: Reducing overtreatment without compromising survival? *Gynecol Oncol.* 2017;147:85-91.

Fagotti A, Vizzielli G, Fanfani F, et al. Introduction of staging laparoscopy in the management of advanced epithelial ovarian, tubal and peritoneal cancer: Impact on prognosis in a single institution experience. *Gynecol Oncol.* 2013;131:341-346.

Gershenson DM, Bodurka DC, Coleman RL, et al. Hormonal maintenance therapy for women with low-grade serous cancer of the ovary or peritoneum. *J Clin Oncol.* 2017:35:1103-1111.

Gershenson DM, Miller A, Brady W, et al., A randomized phase II/III study to assess the efficacy of trametinib in patients with recurrent or progressive low-grade serous ovarian or peritoneal cancer. *Ann Oncol.* 2019;30(suppl_5):v851-v934.

Gonzalez-Martin A, Pothuri B, Vergote I, et al. Niraparib in patients with newly diagnosed advanced ovarian cancer. *N Engl J Med.* 2019;381: 2391-2402. doi: 10.1056/NEJMoa1910962.

Hamanishi J, Mandai M, Ikeda T, et al. Safety and antitumor activity of anti-PD-1 antibody, nivolumab, in patients with platinum-resistant ovarian cancer. *J Clin Oncol.* 2015;33:4015-4022.

Harter P, Sehouli J, Reuss A, et al. Prospective validation study of a predictive score for operability of recurrent ovarian cancer: the Multicenter Intergroup Study DESKTOP II. A project of the AGO Kommission OVAR, AGO Study Group, NOGGO, AGO-Austria, and MITO. *Int J Gynecol Cancer.* 2011;21(2):289-295.

Jacobs IJ, Menon U, Ryan A, et al. Ovarian cancer screening and mortality in the UK Collaborative Trial of Ovarian Cancer Screening (UKCTOCS): a randomized controlled trial. *Lancet.* 2016;387(10022): 945-956.

Kehoe A, Hook J, Nankivell M, et al. Primary chemotherapy versus primary surgery for newly diagnosed advanced ovarian cancer (CHORUS): an open-label, randomised, controlled, non-inferiority trial. *Lancet.* 2015;386:249-257.

Kurman RJ, Carcangiu ML, Herrington CS, Young RH, eds. Chapter 1: Tumours of the ovary. In: *WHO Classification of Tumours of Female Reproductive Organs.* 4th ed. Lyon: IARC: 2014:11-40.

Mirza MR, Monk MD, Herrstedt J, et al. Niraparib maintenance therapy in platinum-sensitive, recurrent ovarian cancer. *N Engl J Med.* 2016;375:2154-2164.

Monk BJ, Grisham RN, BAnerjee S, et al., MILO/ENGOT ov11: Binimetinib versus physician's choice chemotherapy in recurrent or persistent ow-grade serous carcinomas of the ovary, fallopian tube or prrimary peritoneum. *J Clin Oncol.* (2020)38:3753-3762.

Moore K, Colombo N, Scambia G, et al. Maintenance olaparib in patients with newly diagnosed advanced ovarian cancer. *N Engl J Med.* 2018;379(26):2495-2505.

Mutch DG, Prat J. FIGO staging for ovarian, fallopian tube and peritoneal cancer. *Gynecol Oncol.* 2014;133(3):401-404.

NCI Clinical Announcement on Intraperitoneal Chemotherapy in Ovarian Cancer (January 5, 2006) https://ctep.cancer.gov/highlights/20060105_ovarian.htm. Accessed December 21, 2020.

NCCN Clinical Practice Guidelines in Oncology (NCCN Guidelines). *Ovarian Cancer Including Fallopian Tube Cancer and Primary peritoneal Cancer.* Version 3.2019 - November 26, 2019.

Pashankar F, Hale JP, Dang H, et al. Is adjuvant chemotherapy indicated in ovarian immature teratomas? A combined data analysis from the Malignant Germ Cell Tumor International Collaborative. *Cancer.* 2016;122(2):230-237.

Prat J, D'Angelo E, Espinosa I. Ovarian carcinomas: at least five different diseases with distinct histological features and molecular genetics. *Hum Pathol.* 2018;80:11-27.

Pujade-Lauraine E, Hilpert F, Weber B, et al. Bevacizumab combined with chemotherapy for platinum-resistant recurrent ovarian cancer: The AURELIA open-label randomized phase III trial. *J Clin Oncol.* 2014;32(13):1302-1308.

Siegel RL, Miller KD, Jemal A. Cancer statistics, 2019. *CA Cancer J Clin.* 2019;69(1):7-34.

Varga A, Piha-Paul S, Ott PA, et al. Pembrolizumab in patients with programmed death ligand 1-positive advanced ovarian cancer: analysis of KEYNOTE-028. *Gynecol Oncol.* 2019;152(2):243-250.

Vergote I, Trope CG, Amant F, et al. Neoadjuvant chemotherapy or primary surgery in stage IIIC or IV ovarian cancer. *N Engl J Med.* 2010;363:943-953.

Walker JL, Brady MF, Wenzel L, et al. Randomized trial of intravenous versus intraperitoneal chemotherapy plus bevacizumab in advanced ovarian carcinoma: an NRG Oncology/Gynecologic Oncology Group study. *J Clin Oncol.* 2019;37(16):1380-1390.

**Suggested readings for this chapter can be found on ExpertConsult.com.**

# 34 Gestational Trophoblastic Disease

## Hydatidiform Mole, Nonmetastatic and Metastatic Gestational Trophoblastic Tumor: Diagnosis and Management

*Andra Nica, Geneviève Bouchard-Fortier, Allan Covens*

### KEY POINTS

- Persistent abnormal bleeding after normal pregnancy, abortion, or ectopic pregnancy should lead to a consideration of the diagnosis of gestational trophoblastic disease (GTD). Pulmonary nodules present on chest radiographs after a normal pregnancy suggest GTD. Beta human chorionic gonadotropin ($\beta$-HCG) levels is elevated in these situations.
- Investigation of a young woman with metastatic disease of unknown primary should include a $\beta$-HCG level measurement.
- The risk of GTN after complete hydatidiform mole (HM) is 15% to 20% and is 1% to 5% after partial HM.
- Approximately 50% of cases of GTN occur after molar pregnancy, 25% occur after normal pregnancy, and 25% occur after abortion or ectopic pregnancy.
- The major risk factors for molar pregnancy include maternal age (older than 45 and younger than 15 years) and a history of prior HM.
- The risk of HM is approximately 1 in 1000 pregnancies in North America.
- The risk of a subsequent HM after a primary mole is 1 in 100.
- Complete moles are of paternal origin, are diploid, and carry a 15% to 20% risk of GTD sequelae.
- Partial moles are of maternal and paternal origin, are triploid, and are rarely (2% to 4%) followed by GTD. They nonetheless require follow-up for potential malignant sequelae, as done for a complete mole.
- The monitoring of trophoblastic disease and its follow-up is accomplished by measurement of the $\beta$-HCG level.
- The diagnosis of a molar pregnancy can be established with ultrasonography and may coexist with a normal pregnancy.
- Hydatidiform moles are effectively and safely evacuated from the uterus using suction dilation and curettage.
- Medical complications of HM are rare but may include anemia, gestational hypertension before 20 weeks, hyperthyroidism, hyperemesis gravidarum, cardiac failure, and, rarely, pulmonary insufficiency.
- Patients are classified into low- or high-risk categories. Low-risk patients are treated with single-agent methotrexate or actinomycin D; high-risk patients receive combination chemotherapy, usually with EMA/CO (etoposide, methotrexate, actinomycin D, cyclophosphamide, vincristine [Oncovin]).
- The cure rate for low-risk patients approaches 100%.
- Patients with high-risk metastatic GTN are successfully treated with chemotherapy in up to 80% of cases.
- Surgery plays an important role in the treatment of placental site trophoblastic tumor (PSTT) and epithelioid trophoblastic tumor (ETT).
- PSTT and ETT are both relatively chemoresistant.
- Patients treated for GTD should not become pregnant for approximately 6 months after treatment to allow accurate follow-up of $\beta$-HCG levels.
- Fertility rates and pregnancy outcomes are similar in patients treated for GTD compared with those in the general population.
- Patients treated with the EMA/CO regimen have an increased rate of secondary malignancies, particularly hematologic malignancies.

**Gestational trophoblastic disease (GTD)** is considered one of the most curable gynecologic malignancies. Early disease recognition, effective chemotherapy regimens, and sensitive beta human chorionic gonadotropin ($\beta$-HCG) assays have contributed to the excellent oncologic outcome of these patients. Understanding the disease process cannot be overstated to the general gynecologist, who is usually responsible for the initial diagnosis and management of GTD, as well as the timely referral to gynecologic oncology for further management of gestational trophoblastic neoplasia (GTN). A structured approach to diagnosis and management will result in cure for most patients, even in the setting of advanced disease, without adversely affecting future fertility.

GTD describes a heterogeneous spectrum of diseases of abnormal trophoblastic proliferation ranging from benign to premalignant and malignant, with varying predilections toward local invasion and distant metastasis. Benign trophoblastic lesions include placental site nodule and exaggerated placental reaction. Hydatidiform moles, which include **complete hydatidiform mole (CHM)** and **partial hydatidiform mole (PHM)**, are considered premalignant conditions given their potential for invasion. An intermediate lesion arising from chorionic-type intermediate trophoblast, termed atypical placental site nodule (APN), has been described (Kaur, 2015; McCarthy. 2019), but it is not yet part of the World Health Organization (WHO) classification. APN have been associated with a diagnosis of **placental site trophoblastic tumor (PSTT)** or **epithelioid trophoblastic tumor (ETT)** 14% of the time, either concurrently or within months of diagnosis (Kaur, 2015). Gestational trophoblastic neoplasia (GTN) includes four subtypes: invasive mole, choriocarcinoma, PSTT, and ETT (Box 34.1).

In 2000, the International Federation of Gynecology and Obstetrics (FIGO) released a new staging for GTD incorporating the modified WHO Prognostic Scoring System, which has standardized the method for reporting the disease (FIGO, 2009). GTD is classified according to histopathologic, cytogenetic, and clinical features, using the WHO classification of GTD. GTN is diagnosed based on clinical, laboratory, and histologic criteria, and those tumors have a tendency to invade and metastasize.

**BOX 34.1** World Health Organization Classification of Gestational Trophoblastic Disease

**BENIGN TROPHOBLASTIC LESIONS**

Placental site nodule
Exaggerated placental reaction

**HYDATIDIFORM MOLES**

Complete hydatidiform mole
Partial hydatidiform mole

**GESTATIONAL TROPHOBLASTIC NEOPLASIA**

Invasive mole
Choriocarcinoma
Placental site trophoblastic tumor
Epithelioid trophoblastic tumor

# HYDATIDIFORM MOLE

## Epidemiology

The incidence of GTD is as common as 1 in 1000 pregnancies, but there are marked regional variations worldwide (Altieri, 2003; Melamed, 2016). The precise estimate of the incidence of GTD is difficult to establish as a result of a number of factors, such as low prevalence of the disease, inconsistencies between hospital- and population-based data, and disparity in access to centralized pathology review (Lurain, 2010). Prior estimates based on hospital data overestimated the incidence because deliveries (as opposed to pregnancies) were used in the denominator. Nonetheless, with the introduction of census data, true denominators have added validity to reported incidence rates. Similarly, improvements in central reporting through tumor registries have increased the certainty of case ascertainment. Other factors leading to the improved accuracy of incidence estimations include standardized definitions of GTD variants, improvements in cytogenetics, and recognition of rare variants, such as PSTT and ETT.

The incidence of PHM in the United Kingdom, where all GTD cases are registered in a national database, is 3 in 1000 pregnancies, and that of CHM ranges from 1 to 3 in 1000 pregnancies (Seckl, 2010). A similar rate (2.2 in 1000 pregnancies) was reported in a population-based study from Nova Scotia, Canada. Population-based studies suggest that the incidence of HM is higher in Asia than in North America or Europe (Lurain, 2010; Seckl, 2010); however, the incidence of hydatidiform mole (HM) in Asian countries has been decreasing in recent decades, perhaps because of a combination of improved diet, decreased birth rates, and improved measurement of population incidence (Martin, 1998; Ngan, 2015). In a North American cohort, race and ethnicity were strongly associated with the risk of both CHM and PHM. After adjusting for age, Asian women were twice as likely to develop a CHM compared with white women, whereas black and Hispanic women had the lowest risk of CHM (Melamed, 2016).

The increased incidence of GTD in certain ethnic groups has not been explained by looking at genetic traits, cultural factors, or difference in reporting. More recent evidence suggests that women from lower socioeconomic status from various geographic and cultural backgrounds (East Asia, Middle East, North and South America) have an increased risk of HM compared with women from higher socioeconomic statuses in the same regions (Mangili, 2014; Soares, 2010).

## Risk Factors

### Age

Pregnancy occurring at extremes of maternal age (younger than 15 and older than 45 years) is a well-established risk factor for HM, with incidence rates following a J-shaped distribution curve (Altman, 2008; Sebire, 2002). Risk increases after age 35, and a 5- to 10-fold increase is seen in women conceiving after age 40, rising precipitously thereafter. This increase is accounted for by abnormal gametogenesis or abnormal fertilization with advanced maternal age; however, due to the decreased fecundity in this cohort, the overall effect on incidence rates is low.

### Reproductive History

A reproductive history including HM is another risk factor, increasing the risk in future pregnancies by 5- to 40-fold that of the general population. Subsequent pregnancies have an approximate 1% to 1.7% risk, increasing to 11% to 25% when the number of previous HM is two or more (Seckl, 2013; Vargas, 2014). The risk is not affected by changing partners. Patients with recurrent molar pregnancies are also at increased risk for the malignant sequelae of GTN. A history of infertility and of two or more miscarriages is associated with a modest increased risk of both CMH and PHM of 1.9 to 3.2 times the population baseline risk (Acaia, 1988; Berkowitz, 1995).

### Diet

Dietary risk factor analyses have shown conflicting results. Several case-control studies have shown an increased risk of CHM with decreasing consumption of animal fat and beta-carotene (precursor to vitamin A) (Berkowitz, 1985). Vitamin A deficiency is more prevalent in countries where the incidence of GTD is higher. Dietary factors may somewhat explain geographic variations in the incidence of CHM; however, other studies detailing food intake have failed to show a decreased incidence with increasing consumption of dietary protein or fat. To date, no association between diet and partial mole has been reported.

### Genetics

Recurrent HM, defined as the occurrence of two or more HMs in the same patient, may be sporadic or familial. A rare autosomal recessive disorder known as *familial recurrent HM* has been identified on chromosome 19q 13.3-13.4 (Murdoch, 2006; Wang, 2009); it affects 1.5% to 9% of women with a previous HM (Nguyen, 2018a). Affected women have a mutation of the *NLRP7* gene and, more rarely, the *KHDC3L* gene, and they are predisposed to abnormal pregnancies characterized by CHM. Approximately 60% of cases of recurrent HM occur in women who have a mutation in both alleles of the same gene (Nguyen, 2018a). HMs in women with biallelic mutations are all genetically normal, with chromosomes from each parent (diploid biparental CHM); HMs in women without mutations are heterogeneous, with only a small percentage constituted by diploid biparental CHM and the majority being PHMs and the more common, diploid androgenic CHM type (Nguyen, 2018b). The mechanism of recurrent HM is through disruption of normal genomic imprinting, with silencing of maternal imprinted genes and preferential expression of paternal imprinted genes (El-Maarri, 2003). These patients are unlikely going to achieve a normal pregnancy, and egg donation with in vitro fertilization is often necessary.

## Histopathology and Cytogenetic Features

During early embryonic differentiation, trophoblasts are derived from the outer blastocyst layer, with three distinct trophoblasts recognized: cytotrophoblasts, syncytiotrophoblasts, and intermediate trophoblasts. Cytotrophoblasts are the trophoblastic stem cells that differentiate along a villous and extravillous pathway. The villous trophoblast forms the interface between maternal

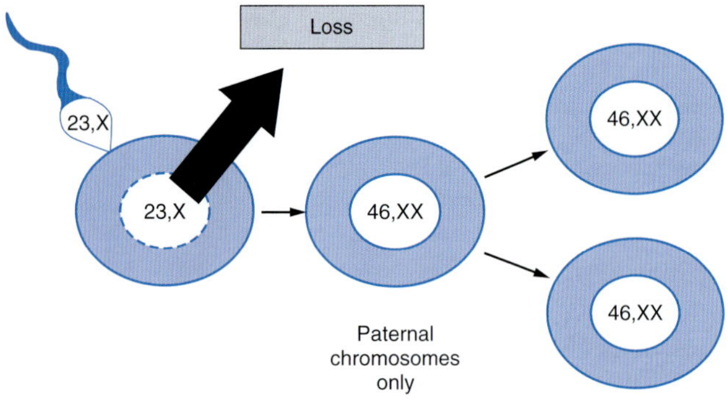


**Fig. 34.1** Paternal chromosomal origin of a complete classic mode (46,XX). *Left to right:* Entry of normal sperm with haploid set of 23,X into an egg whose 23,X haploid set is lost. The egg is taken over by paternal chromosomes, which duplicate (without cell division) to reach the requisite complement of 46. Observe that almost the same result can be obtained through fertilization by two sperm gaining entry into an empty egg (dispermy). (From Szulman AE, Surti UL. The syndromes of partial and complete molar gestation. *Clin Obstet Gynecol.* 1984;27:172-180.)

and fetal tissues (chorionic villi) and is composed of cytotrophoblasts and syncytiotrophoblasts. This layer is responsible for molecular exchange across compartments and, in the case of syncytiotrophoblasts, production of the pregnancy-associated hormones $\beta$-HCG and human placental lactogen (HPL). Along the extravillous pathway, they differentiate into intermediate trophoblasts in the placental bed at the implantation site. This layer is responsible for establishing the maternal-fetal circulation and infiltrating the decidua, myometrium, and spiral arteries.

In HM, chromosomal abnormalities differentiate the disease, with complete and partial moles having distinct chromosomal profiles (Figs. 34.1 and 34.2). CHMs are completely derived from paternal origin, with greater than 90% having a 46,XX genotype, produced by fertilization of an empty (anuclear) ovum by a single haploid (23,X) sperm, which then duplicates in the ovum. A small percentage of CHMs have a 46,XY or 46,XX genotype, produced by dispermy, in which a 23,X sperm and a 23,Y or 23,X sperm fertilize an empty ovum. Rarely, complete moles may be triploid or aneuploid. The mechanism for production of the empty ovum is unknown.

In contrast, PHMs are derived from paternal and maternal chromosomes, resulting in a triploid genotype. A haploid ovum is fertilized by two haploid spermatozoa, resulting in a triploid gestation 69,XXX, 69,XXY or 69,XYY. Although a triploid karyotype is usually seen in PHM, not all triploid pregnancies show histologic changes consistent with a partial mole. In addition, PHM may present in conjunction with a viable fetus, showing signs of triploidy such as multiple congenital anomalies or severe growth retardation. Conditions that may be confused pathologically with PHM include Beckwith-Wiedemann syndrome, placental angiomatous malformation, twin gestation with complete mole and an existing fetus, early complete mole, and hydropic complete mole.

The histopathologic differences between CHM and PHM are well defined. The gross appearance of CHM may be impressive, with a large volume of grapelike vesicles made up of edematous enlarged villi (Fig. 34.3). Histopathologic characteristics include the following: (1) lack of fetal or embryonic tissues, (2) hydropic (edematous) villi, (3) diffuse trophoblastic hyperplasia, (4) marked atypia of trophoblasts at the implantation site, and (5) absence of trophoblastic stromal inclusions. In comparison, the gross appearance of PHM may only show subtle abnormalities, with generally a smaller volume of hydropic villi and the possible presence of a fetus or fetal tissue. The histopathologic features are the following: (1) presence of fetal or embryonic tissues; (2) less diffuse, focal hydropic swelling of villi; (3) focal trophoblastic hyperplasia; (4) less pronounced trophoblastic atypia at the molar implantation site; and (5) presence of trophoblastic scalloping and stromal inclusions.

Differentiation between CHM and PHM in early first-trimester abortions can be difficult because of less pronounced trophoblastic proliferation and only subtle hydropic swelling of the villi. Absence of the immunohistochemical nuclear stain p57 gene product of *CDKN1C* (a paternally imprinted, maternally expressed gene) suggests paternal origin and can be used to differentiate between CHM from PHM or nonmolar pregnancies. Further studies such as flow cytometry, ploidy analysis by in

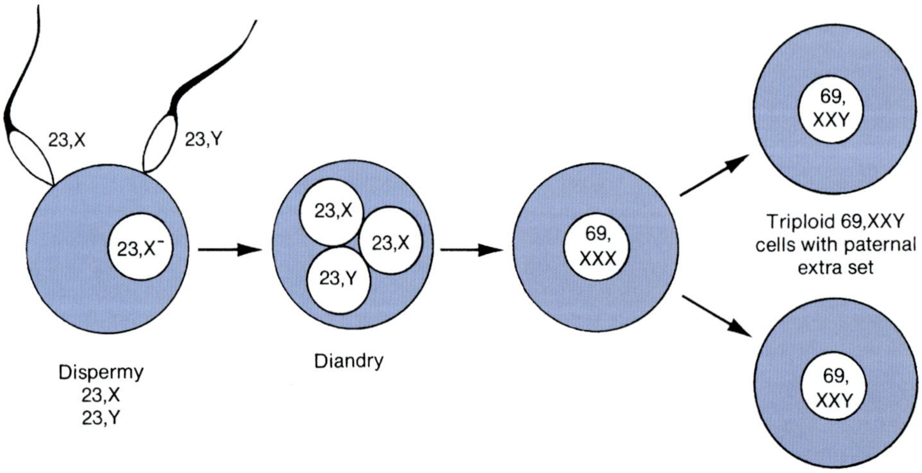


**Fig. 34.2** Triploid chromosomal origin of partial mole (69,XXY dispermy). Fertilization of an egg equipped with a normal 23,X complement by two independently produced sperm (dispermy) to give a total of 69 chromosomes. Observe that triploidy can also result through fertilization by sperm carrying father's total complement of 46,XY. (From Szulman AE, Surti UL. The syndromes of partial and complete molar gestation. *Clin Obstet Gynecol* 1984;27:172-180.)

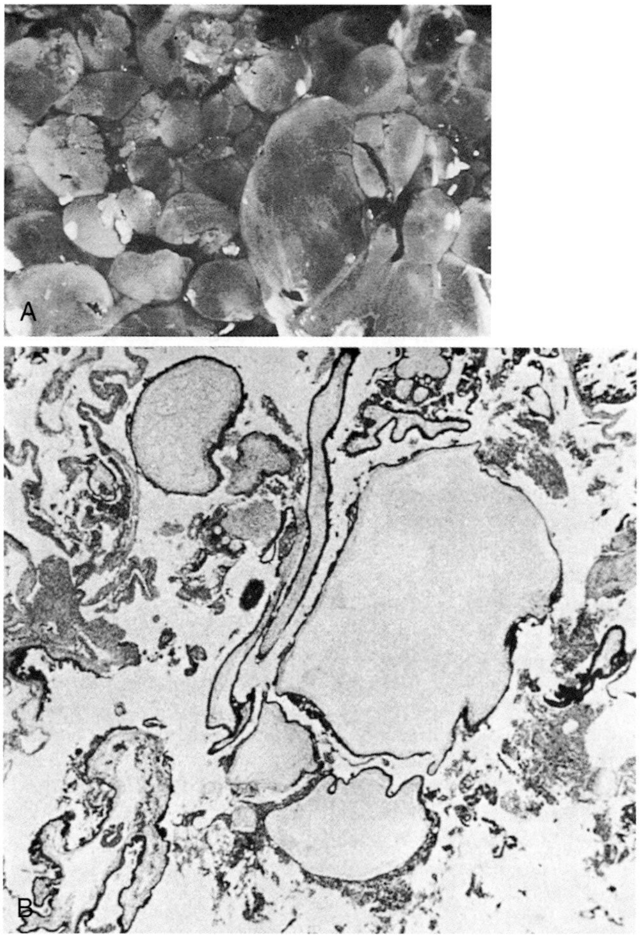


**Fig. 34.3 A,** Hydatidiform mole. A few vesicles approach 1 cm in diameter. The background is formed by smaller vesicles. **B,** Hydatidiform mole aborted by suction curettage. A large intact vesicle is near the center. Many vesicles, however, have been ruptured and have collapsed. (From Bigelow B. Gestational trophoblast disease. In: Blaustein A, ed. *Pathology of the Female Genital Tract.* 2nd ed. New York: Springer-Verlag; 1982.)

**TABLE 34.1** Features of Complete and Partial Hydatidiform Moles

| Feature | Complete Moles | Partial Moles |
|---|---|---|
| Fetal or embryonic tissue | Absent | Present |
| Hydatidiform swelling of chronic villi | Diffuse | Focal |
| Trophoblastic hyperplasia | Diffuse | Focal |
| Trophoblastic stromal inclusions | Absent | Present |
| Genetic parentage | Paternal | Bipaternal |
| Karyotype | 46,XX; 46,XY | 69,XXX, 69,XXY; 69,XYY |
| Persistent human chorionic gonadotropin | 15%-20% of cases | 1%-5% of cases |

From Eifel PJ, Gershenson DM, Kavanagh JJ, Silva EG. *Gynecologic Cancer.* New York: Springer-Verlag; 2006:230.

**TABLE 34.2** Changing Clinical Presentation of Complete Hydatidiform Mole at the New England Trophoblastic Disease Center (%)

| Symptom or Sign | 1988-1993 (N = 74) | 1965-1975 (N = 306) |
|---|---|---|
| Vaginal bleeding | 84 | 97 |
| Size greater than dates | 28 | 51 |
| Anemia | 5 | 54 |
| Preeclampsia | 1.3 | 27 |
| Hyperemesis | 8 | 26 |
| Hyperthyroidism | 0 | 7 |
| Respiratory distress | 0 | 2 |
| Asymptomatic | 9 | 0 |

From Valena S-W, Bernstein M, Goldstein DP, Berkowitz R. The changing clinical presentation of complete molar pregnancy. *Obstet Gynecol.* 1995;86:775-779.

situ hybridization, or molecular genotyping have been described to differentiate PHM (triploid) from CHM and nonmolar hydropic abortions. A summary of the genetic and histopathologic differences between CHM and PHM is presented in Table 34.1.

## Clinical Features

Dramatic presentations of advanced HMs have become less common in the developed world, largely because of the increased use of ultrasonography and improvements in the sensitivity of $\beta$-HCG assays, both leading to earlier detection. The average gestational age of diagnosis of CHM today is 9.6 weeks versus 17 weeks in the 1960s. After a delayed menses, CHM typically presents in the first trimester as vaginal bleeding, with or without the passage of molar vesicles. Other classic signs of CHM include a large-for-date uterus, absence of fetal movement, anemia secondary to occult hemorrhage, gestational hypertension before 20 weeks' gestation, presence of theca lutein cysts, hyperemesis, hyperthyroidism, and respiratory distress from trophoblastic emboli to the lungs.

When uterine enlargement is more than 14 to 16 weeks, 25% of patients will have medical complications related to the high levels of $\beta$-HCG commonly seen in CHM and proportional to the volume of trophoblastic hyperplasia. $\beta$-HCG is homologous to thyrotropin-releasing hormone, and the $\beta$-HCG isoforms seen in CHM may have a greater affinity for the thyrotropin-stimulating hormone receptor than normal $\beta$-HCG, causing excessive thyroid stimulation in some patients. Similarly, $\beta$-HCG is homologous to luteinizing hormone (LH), the purported mechanism whereby ovarian stimulation leads to the formation of theca lutein cysts in some patients.

Despite the possible medical complications associated with the disease, data from the New England Trophoblastic Disease Center have revealed the changing clinical presentation over time of HM (Table 34.2). This change in clinical presentation of HM was also demonstrated in China and Thailand, suggesting a worldwide phenomenon. Patients are now more likely to present with minimal symptoms; nonetheless, if medical complications are present, the woman should be stabilized, followed by evacuation of the HM as soon as possible.

PHM usually presents incidentally after histopathologic examination of the products of conception from uterine evacuation of a suspected missed or therapeutic abortion. Medical complications such as gestational hypertension, hyperthyroidism, theca

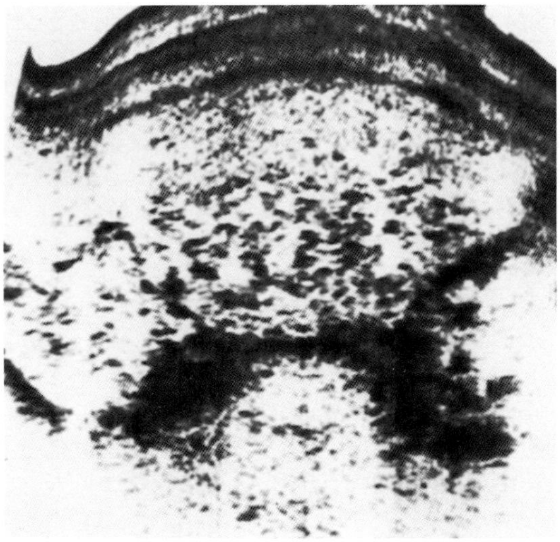

**Fig. 34.4** Ultrasound scan of uterus demonstrating snowstorm appearance of hydatidiform mole.

lutein cysts, and respiratory distress are rare with PHM. With a low clinical suspicion for PHM, missed diagnosis is a risk, reflecting the importance of a thorough histopathologic examination of curettage specimens to ensure quality care. It is recommended to measure serum or urine HCG level 4 to 6 weeks after uterine evacuation of a suspected missed or therapeutic abortion if symptoms of pregnancy persist (persistent vaginal bleeding or amenorrhea).

## Diagnosis

The various symptoms associated with HM, such as vaginal bleeding or a large-for-date uterus, often prompt an ultrasound (US) examination to determine whether a pregnancy is viable. US is the standard imaging modality for the diagnosis of a mole, although CHMs are easier to diagnose by US than PHMs, which are difficult to differentiate from incomplete or missed abortion. A CHM has the appearance on US of multiple hypoechoic foci accompanying an enlarged uterus, the so-called snowstorm appearance (Fig. 34.4). As the molar pregnancy progresses into the second trimester, the anechoic spaces of the molar vesicles become more evident. A transvaginal US may show the interface between molar tissue, endometrium, and dilated vesicles in the first trimester better, but it can worsen vaginal bleeding in the setting of metastatic disease to the vagina. Features suggestive of CHM on US are (1) absence of fetal or embryonic tissue, (2) absence of amniotic fluid, (3) enlarged placenta with multiple cysts, and (4) ovarian theca lutein cysts. Features suggestive of PHM on US are (1) presence of fetal or embryonic tissue, (2) presence of amniotic fluid, (3) abnormal placenta with multiple cysts or increased echogenicity of chorionic villi, (4) increased transverse diameter of gestational sac, and (5) absence of theca lutein cysts (Benson, 2000).

Although US may be the imaging modality of choice, Fowler and associates reviewed 859 cases of histologically proven HM and have shown that only 44% of cases had a preevacuation US suggesting HM, reinforcing the importance of histologic examination for diagnosis (Fowler, 2006). The accuracy was higher for CHM (79%) than for PHM (29%).

### Human Chorionic Gonadotropin

The anterior pituitary produces a series of glycoproteins that differ only in their beta subunits, including HCG, follicle-stimulating hormone (FSH), LH, and thyroid-stimulating hormone (TSH). Outside of pregnancy, an elevated $\beta$-HCG level signifies the following: (1) GTN, (2) nongestational tumors secreting HCG, (3) false positives, and (4) pituitary HCG (secondary to LH elevation and cross-reactivity of assays) (Cole, 2008).

An unexpectedly elevated $\beta$-HCG level during pregnancy may suggest the diagnosis of CHM. $\beta$-HCG typically plateaus in pregnancy at approximately 10 weeks' gestation, with levels peaking at 100,000 IU/L and then falling thereafter. Genest and coworkers found that 46% of patients with CHM managed over a 10-year period had pretreatment $\beta$-HCG levels higher than 100,000 IU/L (Genest, 1991). Conversely, Berkowitz and colleagues reported in one series that PHM presented with an elevated $\beta$-HCG greater than 100,000 IU/L in 2 of 30 cases (6%) (Berkowitz, 1985).

## Treatment

Preevacuation diagnosis of HM allows for optimal treatment planning, but the diagnosis of most patients will be made histologically after surgery. If HM is suspected preoperatively, a chest radiograph should be performed because evacuation may transiently shower the lungs with trophoblastic emboli, complicating the interpretation of a postevacuation chest radiograph. A complete blood cell count (CBC), blood typing with antibody screen, $\beta$-HCG level, TSH and creatinine levels, coagulation profile, and liver function testing should also be performed. As the RhD factor is expressed on the trophoblasts, patients who are Rh negative with an Rh positive or Rh unknown partner should be treated with Rho(D) immune globulin after evacuation. The anesthesia team should be made aware of the suspected diagnosis and be ready to manage potential complications such as severe hemorrhage, thyroid storm, and acute respiratory distress from trophoblastic emboli.

### Suction Dilation and Curettage

The preferred method of uterine evacuation of HM is suction dilation and curettage (D&C) under general anesthetic. The cervix is serially dilated and then a 12- to 14-mm suction curette is advanced just past the endocervix into the endometrial canal. After activating the suction device, a solution of crystalloid and oxytocin (20 U/L) is infused to increase uterine tone; this is continued for several hours postoperatively to promote uterine contractility and reduce bleeding. Because of the propensity for heavy bleeding, blood products should be available when the uterine size is greater than 16 weeks' gestation (Berkowitz, 2009). A gentle sharp curettage may be performed to complete the procedure. Care must be taken during D&C to avoid perforation of the enlarged soft uterus in HM. The D&C may be performed under intraoperative US guidance to decrease the risk of uterine perforation and to establish when evacuation of all products of conception is complete.

### Hysterectomy

For patients diagnosed with HM preoperatively for whom continued fertility is not an issue, hysterectomy with preservation of the ovaries is a treatment option. The risk of developing GTN is 53% in women older than 40 and up to 60% in women older than 50 (Elias, 2010, 2012), compared with 15% to 20% after CHM and 1% to 5% after PHM, which has been observed in the general population (Berkowitz, 2013). A meta-analysis showed that hysterectomy in women 40 years of age and older decreases the risk of postmolar GTN (odds ratio [OR], 0.21; confidence interval [CI], 0.11 0.38; $P < .00001$) and thus the need for chemotherapy. A hysterectomy eliminates the risk of local (myometrial) persistence (Zhao, 2019), but it does not eliminate the risk

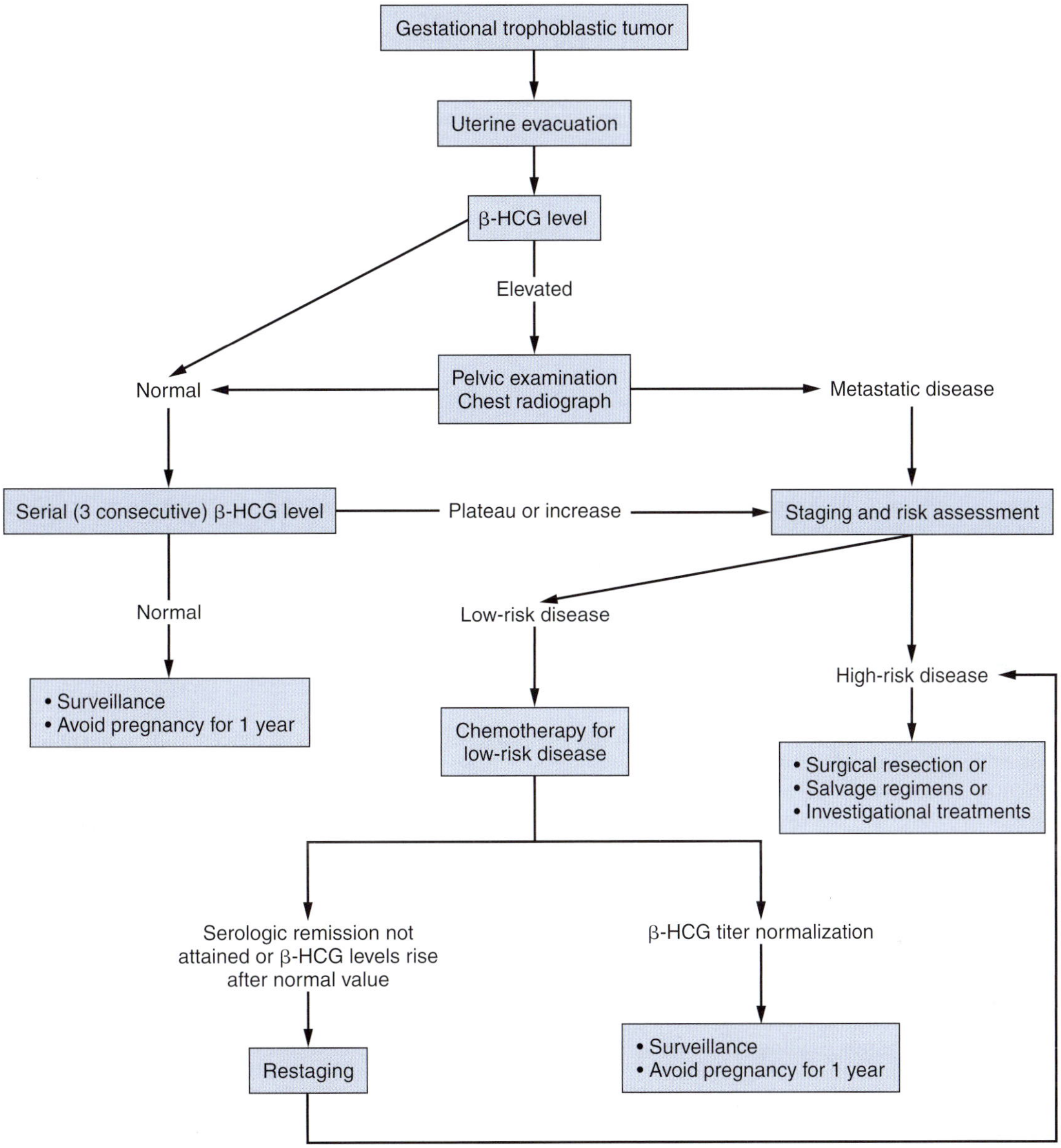


**Fig. 34.5** Treatment algorithm. This is a diagnostic and therapeutic approach to gestational trophoblastic disease as practiced at the University of Texas M.D. Anderson Cancer Center. *β-HCG*, Beta human chorionic gonadotropin. (Modified from Eifel PJ, Gershenson DM, Kavanagh JJ, Silva EG. *Gynecologic Cancer.* New York: Springer-Verlag; 2006:235.)

of distant metastases. Because of high rates of postmolar GTN (30% to 58%), two out of the six studies included in the meta-analysis were not in favor of hysterectomy, but the pooled analysis favored hysterectomy in this age group. As a result of the ongoing risk of postmolar GTN after hysterectomy, continued *β*-HCG monitoring is necessary (Berkowitz, 2013).

## Prophylactic Chemotherapy

After surgical evacuation, postmolar GTN, usually in the form of a locally invasive mole, occurs in 15% to 20% of CHM cases (>50% of cases in woman older than 40 years) and only rarely (<5%) after PHM (Curry, 1975). Fig. 34.5 outlines a treatment algorithm for GTD. If postevacuation follow-up is anticipated to be compromised, patients with high-risk CHM may be considered for treatment with prophylactic chemotherapy. High-risk HM is defined as the presence of one or more of the following: initial serum *β*-HCG greater than 100,000, uterine size larger than gestational age, theca lutein cysts larger than 6 cm, maternal age older than 40, previous GTD, or the presence of hyperthyroidism or trophoblastic embolization (Berkowitz, 1995).

A 2017 Cochrane review evaluated the evidence for the effectiveness and safety of prophylactic chemotherapy to prevent GTN after HM (Wang, 2017). After excluding nonrandomized studies and studies that enrolled patients who already had a GTN diagnosis, three studies were included in the data synthesis. Two of the three studies were found to have a high risk of bias, and overall the quality of the evidence was low to very low. The meta-analysis showed that prophylactic chemotherapy reduced the risk of GTN by approximately two-thirds in all patients with HM, including in the high-risk cohort; however, patients who received prophylactic chemotherapy had a delayed diagnosis of GTN and required more courses of chemotherapy than the average to treat subsequent GTN. Therefore prophylactic chemotherapy is an option in high-risk patients who have limited access to follow-up; however, its routine use is not recommended because of the morbidity associated with treatment, potential delays in diagnosis of invasive GTN and the development of drug resistance, the requirement for surveillance regardless, and the ultimate high cure rates eventually achieved in GTN.

**Surveillance After Hydatidiform Mole Evacuation**

After evacuation of a HM, surveillance with serial $\beta$-HCG serum measurements are required to ensure a timely diagnosis of postmolar malignant GTN (discussed later in the section Gestational Trophoblastic Neoplasia, Clinical Features). Within 48 hours of evacuation, a baseline $\beta$-HCG level should be obtained and repeated weekly until the level returns to normal (<5 mIU/mL). Most cases of postmolar GTN occur within 6 months of evacuation; a retrospective study of 6701 women with HM reported that only 3 were subsequently diagnosed with GTN at 13, 23 and 42 months after evacuation (Sebire, 2007). Therefore weekly $\beta$-HCG monitoring is recommended after normalization for 2 additional weeks (three normal weekly values), and then monthly for an additional 6 months (GTN, 2018). Prolonged follow-up is not recommended because of the low yield of diagnosis and the increased financial and emotional burden.

Although the minimum conventional period for observation is 6 months, such a long duration of follow-up has been questioned, particularly for women with a narrow window of fertility because of advanced age. Older small scale studies (Bagshawe, 1986; Schmitt, 2013; Wielsma, 2006) had suggested that the risk of persistent GTN is zero after a normal $\beta$-HCG in patients with PHM and in patients with CHM in whom the $\beta$-HCG normalized within 56 days and stated that prolonged surveillance was not necessary. A large population-based study from the United Kingdom (Coyle, 2018) reported the risk of GTN to be extremely low but not zero (1 in 3195, or <1%) after $\beta$-HCG normalization and lower still (1 in 9584) after 6 months of normal $\beta$-HCG. In contrast, after CHM, the risk of GTN is 1 in 420 after $\beta$-HCG normalization, falling to 1 in 839 after 4 months and 1 in 1677 after 12 months. Patients who had $\beta$-HCG normalization within 56 days from evacuation were almost 4 times less likely to develop GTN. The resulting recommendations are that for women who are eager to get pregnant after PHM, surveillance may stop after the first normal $\beta$-HCG. Further, after CHM, if the patient wishes to attempt another pregnancy sooner, surveillance may stop 6 months after evacuation when the $\beta$-HCG normalizes within 56 days but should continue for 6 months after normalization when the $\beta$-HCG is still positive at 56 days.

During this period of surveillance, use of reliable contraception is strongly recommended to ensure that a rise in $\beta$-HCG level represents postmolar GTN and not a new pregnancy. IUD use should be avoided until normalization of $\beta$-HCG because of the potential risk of uterine perforation. One randomized controlled trial (RCT) has shown that use of the oral contraceptive pill (OCP) results in 50% fewer pregnancies during the surveillance period when compared to barrier methods of contraception (Curry, 1989). In the past there was concern that OCP use increased the risk of GTN, but two RCTs have shown no association between OCP use during postmolar surveillance and the incidence of GTN (Costa, 2006).

Prognostic factors associated with the development of GTN have been identified in various reports. As noted, advanced maternal age (older than 40 years) increases the risk of invasive mole (Berkowitz, 2013), as does a history of HM (Seckl, 2013). Ultrasound findings of uterine invasion may also be predictive of the development of GTN. In a retrospective analysis, Garavaglia and coworkers have shown that the presence of hyperechoic lesions (nodules) within the myometrium or increased signal intensity suggesting hypervascularization at baseline US was associated with an OR of 17.57 for the development of GTN ($P < .001$) (Garavaglia, 2009).

***Phantom* β*-HCG***

Persistent low levels of $\beta$-HCG must be evaluated to rule out false-positive assay results or phantom HCG, a rare finding that is secondary to heterophilic antibodies or proteolytic enzymes that mimic HCG. The diagnosis is made when a serum $\beta$-HCG test is positive but a corresponding urine $\beta$-HCG test taken at the same time is negative. Alternatively, despite serial dilutions of serum, the test result will usually remain positive if heterophilic antibodies are the cause. Finally, physicians can test against multiple $\beta$-HCG assays, when available; heterophilic antibodies may cause a positive result in one test and a negative result in another. The reason for the negative urine $\beta$-HCG test is that heterophilic antibodies are large glycoproteins unable to cross the glomeruli and thus are not excreted in the urine. These antibodies—typically derived from exposure to mouse, rabbit, goat, or sheet antigens—are acquired through immunizations or time spent in agricultural settings, and they persist over time.

***Quiescent GTD***

After a hydatidiform mole, choriocarcinoma, or spontaneous abortion, the persistence of low levels (range, 1 to 212 IU/L) of $\beta$-HCG for 3 months or longer with no obvious increase or decrease in the $\beta$-HCG level trend along with the absence of clinical or radiologic evidence of GTN is termed *quiescent GTD*. This process is more common after a CHM but may occur after PHM, invasive mole, or choriocarcinoma and has been identified in patients treated with single-agent or multiagent chemotherapy. It is best described as a premalignant condition given that 25% of these cases progress to GTN-choriocarcinoma over a time frame ranging from 6 months to 10 years. Cole and colleagues have shown that the incorporation of hyperglycosylated HCG (HCG-H), a marker of invasive cytotrophoblasts, will detect 100% of quiescent GTD cases that require no further treatment and 96% of self-resolving HM cases that require ongoing surveillance, differentiating these from GTN-choriocarcinoma cases that require further treatment (Cole, 2006, 2010). This methodology, however, requires validation in a prospective fashion.

***Pituitary* β*-HCG***

In perimenopausal or postmenopausal women, persistent low levels (typically <10 mIU/mL) of $\beta$-HCG may be due to increased pituitary gland production, which naturally occurs in both older men and women (Snyder, 2005). The form of $\beta$-HCG produced by the pituitary is a sulfated variant, and it is detectable in the laboratory as such [(Cole, 2012). The diagnosis can also be made clinically after the administration of a combined OCP for 3 weeks, which inhibits gonadotropin-releasing hormone (GnRH) production and consequently also production of the $\beta$-HCG by the pituitary (Cole, 2008).

## GESTATIONAL TROPHOBLASTIC NEOPLASIA

GTN includes invasive mole/postmolar GTN, choriocarcinoma, PSTT, and ETT.

### Characteristics

#### Histopathology and Cytogenetic Features

**Invasive moles** are HMs characterized by syncytiotrophoblast or cytotrophoblast hyperplasia, with the presence of villi. The presence of these villi extending into the myometrium constitutes invasion, hence the name. Most of these tumors, as in HM, are diploid; anaplastic tumors are the exception.

The dominant histologic type in metastatic GTN is gestational choriocarcinoma after an HM or nonmolar pregnancy, which occurs in approximately 1 to 50,000 pregnancies (Smith, 2003). The characteristic appearance of choriocarcinoma is sheets of anaplastic trophoblastic tissue containing cytotrophoblast and syncytiotrophoblast cells without chorionic villi. These cells invade adjacent tissues, with a propensity for vascular infiltration, necrosis, and hemorrhage. Immunohistochemistry in trophoblast cells shows strong staining with markers for β-HCG, inhibin, and cytokeratin. Primary gonadal (nongestational) choriocarcinomas, a type of ovarian germ cell tumors, can develop without pregnancy, and the estimated incidence is 1 in 369,000,000. They are highly aggressive, secrete β-HCG, and share the same histologic appearance as gestational choriocarcinoma. Nongestational choriocarcinomas are derived from differentiation of malignant germ cells into trophoblastic structures. The absence of paternal DNA within the tumor using DNA analysis differentiates nongestational choriocarcinomas from gestational choriocarcinomas. Furthermore, metastatic GTN must be distinguished from extragonadal germ cell tumors. Those rare tumors originating from midline locations such as the anterior mediastinum and retroperitoneum have no primary tumor in the ovaries but do secrete β-HCG. The fluorescence in situ hybridization (FISH) method for identifying single-nucleotide variants in exons and introns on individual RNA transcripts is used to differentiate gestational choriocarcinoma from extragonadal germ cell tumors by quantifying allelic expression and differentiating maternal from paternal chromosomes.

PSTT is a rare tumor composed almost entirely of intermediate trophoblasts, lacking the syncytiotrophoblasts and cytotrophoblasts seen in other forms of GTD. PSTT has an infiltrative pattern, with nests or sheets of cells invading between myometrial cells and fibers. Compared with choriocarcinoma, PSTT is less at risk for vascular invasion, necrosis, and hemorrhage. Immunohistochemical staining is often positive for HPL, CD146, placental alkaline phosphatase, and, in less than 10% of cases, for β-HCG.

ETT was recognized by the WHO tumor classification in 2003. It is considered a rare variant of PSTT and is also derived from intermediate trophoblasts. Similar to PSTT, these cells are arranged in sheets or nests and form tumor nodules in the myometrium. Immunohistochemical staining is positive for multiple markers, such as cytokeratin and inhibin A.

## Clinical Features

After surgical evacuation of HM, β-HCG values decrease exponentially, with an expected initial steep decline followed by a slower decrease in β-HCG levels. Symptoms associated with invasive mole include irregular vaginal bleeding, uterine subinvolution, and theca lutein cysts. Most GTN is identified in patients undergoing surveillance after evacuation of HM on the basis of β-HCG criteria, as outlined by FIGO (Box 34.2). These include a plateau in β-HCG values (remaining within ±10% of the previous results) over a 3-week period (four values on days 1, 7, 14, and 21); a rising β-HCG value of 10% or more over a 2-week period (three values on days 1, 7, 14); and a histologic diagnosis of choriocarcinoma or evidence of metastases (clinically or radiologically). Experts in the United Kingdom also start chemotherapy to help with heavy vaginal bleeding requiring transfusion, even if the β-HCG is falling, and in any patients in whom the β-HCG is 20,000 or more 4 weeks after evacuation (Seckl, 2013). A persistently elevated β-HCG 6 months after evacuation is no longer an accepted criteria for treatment because evidence suggests that the β-HCG eventually normalizes in almost all patients left on surveillance (Braga, 2016).

**BOX 34.2** International Federation of Gynecology and Obstetrics Criteria for Diagnosis of Gestational Trophoblastic Neoplasia

The International Federation of Gynecologists and Obstetricians (FIGO) standardized criteria for diagnosing gestational trophoblastic neoplasia GTN after an HM are as follows:

1. Four β-HCG values plateauing (±10%) over a 3-week period (days 1, 7, 14, 21)
2. A rising β-HCG value of 10% or greater seen on three values measured over a 2-week period (days 1, 7, 14)
3. Histologic diagnosis of choriocarcinoma
4. Evidence of metastases (clinically or radiologically)

β-HCG, Beta human chorionic gonadotropin; *GTN,* gestational trophoblastic neoplasia; *HM,* hydatidiform mole.

### Malignant Gestational Trophoblastic Neoplasia

Most metastatic GTN results from choriocarcinoma. Nonetheless, PSTTs are associated with metastases at the time of initial diagnosis in 40% of cases, with the lung being the most common site, and 50% of ETT present with metastases at time of diagnosis. Choriocarcinomas, PSTT, and ETT may follow after any pregnancy event. A longer time interval from antecedent pregnancy is a negative prognostic factor (Frijstein, 2019; Powles, 2006; Schmid, 2009). The initial study by Schmid and colleagues described in a retrospective cohort that all 13 PSTT patients who presented 48 months or later from antecedent pregnancy died, whereas 1 out of 49 patients who presented before 48 months died (Schmid, 2009). A retrospective review of the international PSTT and ETT database (Frijstein, 2019) also found that a time from antecedent pregnancy of longer than 47 months was significantly associated with worse overall survival (hazard ratio [HR], 13.3; $P = .015$). Compared with choriocarcinoma, PSTT and ETT are slower growing, chemoresistant, and secrete low levels of β-HCG. Metastases result from hematogenous dissemination, with almost any site possible. These tumors tend to be hemorrhagic and necrotic. Local metastases may include the vagina, and distant metastasis to the lung, brain, liver, gastrointestinal (GI) tract, and kidney have been reported. The lungs usually represent the first organ involved, followed by dissemination via the systemic circulation. Metastatic lesions are highly vascularized with thin-walled fragile vessels. Symptoms of metastatic GTN, such as hemoptysis or headache, may be related to hemorrhage at involved sites. When metastases are suspected, image-guided biopsy is contraindicated because of the potential risk of uncontrollable hemorrhage.

## Classification and Staging

In 2000, a revised FIGO-WHO Prognostic Scoring System was adopted to attain uniformity in reporting, while indicating the extent of disease spread and risk factors important for predicting persistent disease and therefore appropriate chemotherapy treatment (Table 34.3). The stage of the disease relates to tumor spread, with stage I disease confined to the uterus, stage II disease including spread to the adnexa, vagina, and broad ligament, stage III disease defined by lung metastases, and stage IV disease including all other sites of metastases. Prognostic factors included in the WHO Prognostic Scoring System are age, antecedent pregnancy, interval months from index pregnancy, pretreatment serum β-HCG levels, largest tumor size (cm), site of metastases, number of metastases, and previous failed chemotherapy. A WHO score of 6 or lower is considered low risk and 7 or greater is considered high risk. Generally, stage relates to risk scoring, with stage I patients usually low risk and stage IV patients high risk.

**TABLE 34.3** International Federation of Gynecology and Obstetrics (FIGO) 2000 Classification for Gestational Trophoblastic Neoplasia

| Staging | | Features | | |
|---|---|---|---|---|
| Stage I | | Disease confined to uterus | | |
| Stage II | | GTN extends outside uterus but is limited to genital structures (adnexa, vagina, broad ligament) | | |
| Stage III | | GTN extends to lungs, with or without known genital tract involvement | | |
| Stage IV | | All other metastatic sites | | |
| | | | **Scoring** | |
| **Parameter** | **0** | **1** | **2** | **4** |
| Age (yr) | <40 | ≥40 | — | — |
| Antecedent pregnancy | Mole | Abortion | Term | — |
| Interval from index pregnancy (mo) | <4 | 4-6 | 7-12 | >12 |
| Pretreatment β-HCG (IU/mL) | $<10^3$ | $10^3$-$10^4$ | $10^4$-$10^5$ | $>10^5$ |
| Largest tumor size (cm; including uterus) | <3 | 3 to <5 cm | ≥5 cm | — |
| No. of metastases | 0 | 1-4 | 5-8 | >8 |
| Previous failed chemotherapy | — | — | Single drug | Two or more drugs |
| Site of metastasis | Lung | Spleen, kidney | GI tract | Brain, liver |

*β-HCG*, Beta human chorionic gonadotropin; *GI*, gastrointestinal; *GTN*, gestational trophoblastic neoplasia.

The WHO Prognostic Scoring System does not apply to patients with PSTT and ETT, but they are staged using FIGO stage I to stage IV. Therefore those tumors are not described as low or high risk.

## Diagnosis

Diagnosis of persistent disease via β-HCG monitoring should prompt a complete history and physical examination accompanied by quantitative β-HCG, CBC, and renal, liver, and thyroid function testing. Invasive mole and choriocarcinoma typically produce a high β-HCG level, ranging from 100 to 100,000 mIU/mL, whereas PSTT and ETT produce low levels of β-HCG (usually <1000 mIU/mL). As a diagnostic imaging test, US will rule out concurrent intrauterine pregnancy and provides superior visualization compared with computed tomography (CT) for discerning the interface between normal myometrium and trophoblastic tissue. Examination via Doppler US may show hypervascularity and areas of tumor necrosis.

Uterine artery pulsatility index (UAPI) is a noninvasive method that can be used as a surrogate marker of tumor vascularity. UAPI is inversely proportional to tumor vascularity, with low values representing high arteriovenous shunting and abnormal neoangiogenesis (Agarwal, 2012). Although not part of the WHO score, UAPI can be used to further risk stratify patients with low-risk GTN, for whom single-agent chemotherapy is ineffective up to one-third of the time. UAPI has been shown to be an independent predictor of methotrexate resistance, with patients who were found to have low UAPI almost three times as likely to require combination chemotherapy (Agarwal, 2012).

In addition, US will identify patients whose large-volume uterine disease is best treated surgically. After US of the pelvis, FIGO recommends a chest radiograph as the test of choice to rule out lung metastases. If the chest radiograph is negative, CT of the thorax may demonstrate small-volume metastases, but these findings have been shown to be of little to no clinical relevance. Although 40% of patients with a normal chest radiograph have evidence of micrometastases on CT, this does not appear to affect outcomes (Darby, 2009); however, if lung metastases are seen on chest radiographs and are greater than 1 cm, magnetic resonance imaging (MRI) of the brain and body CT are recommended to exclude metastatic disease of the brain or liver, which would change prognosis and alter management decisions (Seckl, 2013). In low-risk cases, a retrospective study found that the WHO score would have been changed in 79.2% of cases after a chest CT was obtained (Darby, 2009). Despite this, there was no significant difference in the odds of requiring second-line therapy between the group of patients who did and did not have a change in WHO risk score from low to high, and the cure rate was 100%.

Most patients with brain metastases do experience some neurologic symptoms. An assessment of central nervous system (CNS) involvement, typically found at the gray matter–white matter junction, can be assessed with CT or MRI. If brain imaging is unclear, or if it is negative and the patient is experiencing neurologic symptoms, a lumbar puncture can be considered. A cerebrospinal fluid β-HCG–to–plasma ratio lower than 1:60 is considered normal and can be used to rule out occult brain involvement (Bakri, 2000). For asymptomatic patients with a negative chest radiograph and CT scan of the abdomen, further investigation is not required to assign a risk score because high-risk sites of metastasis are rarely seen without evidence of pulmonary metastases (Savage, 2015).

Identification of lung metastases or the diagnosis of choriocarcinoma, PSTT, or ETT necessitates further imaging with CT of the chest, abdomen, and pelvis, as well as brain MRI. Use of intravenous (IV) contrast will identify metastases as round enhanced masses, which are usually multiple, heterogenous, and hypoechoic in appearance.

MRI is also the preferred imaging modality for assessment of vaginal or parametrial lesions. Extrauterine disease is more common in patients with a diagnosis of choriocarcinoma, PSTT, or ETT; therefore those patients should be screened with pelvic US, CT of the abdomen, and brain MRI. The role of $^{18}$F-fluorodeoxyglucose positron emission tomography (FDG-PET) in GTN is undefined, but its high sensitivity and specificity in other disease sites may make it a useful test when other modalities are equivocal; studies to date are limited to small case series.

## Treatment

### Low-Risk Gestational Trophoblastic Neoplasia

**Low-risk GTN** includes localized and metastatic disease and is defined by a WHO prognostic score of 6 or lower. The management of malignant GTN is based more on clinical presentation than histologic diagnosis. For these patients, clinicians can expect an excellent outcome with single-agent chemotherapy consisting of either methotrexate (MTX) or actinomycin D (ActD). While on chemotherapy, patients require monitoring of $\beta$-HCG level as well as hematologic and metabolic studies to gauge treatment toxicity. In addition, patients require reliable contraception, preferably with OCP, to prevent intercurrent pregnancies that would be adversely affected by the teratogenic chemotherapy and confuse the evaluation of $\beta$-HCG follow-up.

For patients with localized disease for whom fertility preservation is not an issue, hysterectomy may be undertaken. Bolze and colleagues (Bolze, 2018) reported a high rate of cure (82.4%) with hysterectomy alone in patients with nonmetastatic GTN and a low WHO score. Patients should be counseled that even after surgery, chemotherapy may still be required to treat occult disease. In this small retrospective study of 76 patients (Bolze, 2018), patients with choriocarcinoma and patients with uterine tumors larger than 5 cm were, respectively, 9 and 14 times more likely to require subsequent chemotherapy after hysterectomy. There have been no RCTs of combined hysterectomy and chemotherapy, but if chemotherapy has been given preoperatively, it should be continued postoperatively until $\beta$-HCG levels are normal.

Another surgical treatment option for patients with low-risk GTN is second curettage, as a means to "debulk" residual disease. A phase II single-arm prospective study from the Gynecologic Oncology Group (GOG) (Osborne, 2016) found that in a cohort of 64 women, 28 of them (47%) were able to avoid chemotherapy after second curettage as first-line treatment. In this study there was only one reported uterine perforation, and one patient suffered grade 3 hemorrhage; however, previous studies report uterine perforation rates up to 8%. Only 5 patients in this study had a WHO score of 5 or 6, and none of the 5 were cured with second curettage, compared with 24 out of 55 patients (44%) with WHO scores of 0 to 4, suggesting that second curettage is unlikely to be of benefit in patients with intermediate WHO scores of 5 to 6. Interestingly, three patients were found to have PSTT on second curettage central pathology review, and second curettage may allow earlier diagnosis of those patients. An analysis of predictors of surgical failure is under way. Nonetheless, the value of repeated D&C remains controversial given that chemotherapy achieves exceptional cure rates (nearly 100%) without the additional surgical risks.

A review of first-line therapies in low-risk GTN cases has identified 13 different treatment regimens. The most commonly used first-line treatments are MTX and ActD, with various dosing schedules used. MTX can be given on a 5-day schedule, once weekly, or every 2 weeks on an 8-day schedule, with or without folinic acid rescue; ActD can be given on a 5-day or 1-day schedule repeated every 2 weeks, the latter termed a *pulsed dose*. There is no consensus on the optimal regimen.

Worldwide the most common first-line regimen for low-risk disease is 8-day MTX alternating with folinic acid rescue because of factors such as established activity, low toxicity, and low cost. The described 8-day MTX regimen uses 1 mg/kg or a standard dose of MTX 50 mg intramuscularly (IM) on days 1, 3, 5, and 7 with folinic acid 15 mg orally (PO) on days 2, 4, 6, and 8. This regimen achieves complete remission in 67% to 88% of women (Maestá, 2018; McNeish, 2002). MTX use requires normal liver and renal function because of altered hepatic metabolism followed by renal excretion of the drug. Depending on the regimen used, patients may experience cutaneous side effects, mucositis, serositis, GI toxicities, alopecia, or hematologic suppression. ActD side effects increase with more dose-intense regimens. The 5-day regimen side effects include alopecia, nausea, and myelotoxicity. ActD is a vesicant, causing tissue necrosis if IV extravasation occurs. The effectiveness of pulse ActD versus the 5-day regimen appears to be equivalent, with decreased toxicity and cost and fewer patient visits with the pulsed regimen.

A Cochrane review (Lawrie, 2016) evaluated the evidence of various first-line chemotherapy regimens in low-risk GTN. Six RCTs were included (Lertkhachonsuk, 2009; Mousavi, 2012; Osborne, 2011; Shobeiri, 2014; Yarandi, 2008, 2016). Three of these studied weekly MTX with ActD every 2 weeks, and the other three randomly allocated patients to 5-day MTX or ActD every 2 weeks, 8-day MTX or 5-day ActD, and 8-day MTX or ActD every 2 weeks. Irrespective of the regimen used, ActD was more likely to lead to primary remission than MTX (relative risk [RR], 0.65; 95% CI, 0.57 to 0.75). Moreover, first-line chemotherapy was more likely to fail with MTX than with ActD (RR, 3.55; 95% CI, 1.81 to 6.95). The most commonly encountered adverse effects were nausea, fatigue, and anemia. There were no significant differences in the probability of women experiencing these symptoms with the two drugs. Alopecia was only described in three out of the six studies, and one study (Lertkhachonsuk, 2009) found an increase in alopecia with the 14-day ActD regimen, suggesting a dose response. This review was criticized because of substantial heterogeneity between studies and the relatively low total number of patients (667) among all six studies. A large, phase III GOG RCT of pulse ActD and multiday MTX for the treatment of low-risk GTN is closed because of issues with accrual (*Dactinomycin or Methotrexate in Treating Patients With Low-Risk Gestational Trophoblastic Neoplasia*, 2019).

Treatment continues until disease remission, defined as three consecutive weekly $\beta$-HCG levels less than 5 mIU/mL. Once complete remission is achieved, patients should continue to receive chemotherapy for a few consolidation cycles to prevent relapse. Data are scare with respect to the ideal number of consolidation cycles. A study from Netherlands and the United Kingdom showed that only receiving two consolidation cycles resulted in a higher probability of recurrence compared with three cycles (8.3% vs. 4%).

Although most women with low-risk GTN are cured with a first-line chemotherapy regimen, tumor resistance and relapse do occur. Chemotherapy resistance is defined as an increase or a plateau in $\beta$-HCG noted on two consecutive weekly measurements (Golfier, 2007) or when new metastases are detected (McNeish, 2002). In patients treated with single-agent MTX, resistance requiring a change to alternative first-line treatment can be expected in 10% to 31% of patients. The experience from the Charing Cross Hospital GTD database reveals that relapse after attaining a normal $\beta$-HCG level occurs in 4% of cases (Lybol, 2012).

Box 34.3 provides an overview of management for low-risk GTN. The conventional period of observation with monthly $\beta$-HCG measurements before attempting pregnancy is 12 months because most relapses occur during this period. Irrespective of which first-line agent is used, cure rates approaching 100% can be achieved with diligent follow-up and salvage therapy for failures. Some reports suggest that one WHO score of 5 to 6 is associated with a higher rate of resistance and a lower rate of remission of 30% with single-agent chemotherapy (Sita-Lumsden, 2012). Salvage therapy with pulsed ActD after failed MTX treatment in patients with low-risk GTN achieved complete response in 74% with a median of four cycles in a phase III trial (GOG-176) (Covens, 2006).

**BOX 34.3** Management of Low-Risk Gestational Trophoblastic Neoplasia

After metastatic evaluation and determination of low-risk disease:

1. Initiate single-agent methotrexate or actinomycin D; consider hysterectomy if fertility is not desired.
    1. Monitor hematologic, renal, and hepatic indices before each cycle of chemotherapy.
    2. Monitor β-HCG levels while on treatment.
    3. If severe toxicity or resistance develops, switch to the alternative single agent.

    If resistance to the alternative agent develops:
2. Repeat the metastatic evaluation.
3. If resistant or recurrent disease is present after second-line single-agent chemotherapy, treat with combination EMA/CO even if patient still meets low-risk criteria.
4. Consider hysterectomy if disease is confined to the uterus.
5. Treat with multiagent therapy with EMA/CO if patient meets criteria for high-risk disease regardless of initial treatment choice (see treatment of high-risk GTN, Box 34.4).

Remission is defined as three consecutive weekly β-HCG values in the normal range. After the first normal β-HCG, continue with three cycles of maintenance or consolidation chemotherapy. Monitor β-HCG levels for 12 months, with the patient counseled to use reliable contraception in this period.

β-HCG, Beta human chorionic gonadotropin; *EMA/CO,* etoposide, methotrexate, actinomycin D, cyclophosphamide, vincristine; *GTN,* gestational trophoblastic neoplasia.

**BOX 34.4** Management of High-Risk Gestational Trophoblastic Neoplasia (excluding PSTT/ETT)

After metastatic evaluation and determination of high-risk disease:

1. Initiate treatment with EMA/CO (see Table 34.4); monitor hematologic, renal, and hepatic indices before each cycle of chemotherapy.
    1. Monitor β-HCG levels while on treatment.
    2. Avoid extended intervals between courses because of myelosuppression.
    3. If severe myelosuppression develops, use granulocyte colony-stimulating factor (G-CSF) to maintain neutrophil count and treatment intensity.
    4. Consider omitting the day 2 dose of etoposide and actinomycin D occasionally if ongoing severe myelosuppression occurs.
2. If patients meet criteria for ultra-high-risk disease, start with low-dose induction etoposide and cisplatin (EP) treatment.
    1. Etoposide and cisplatin only on days 1 and 2.
    2. Repeat EP weekly for 1 to 2 cycles.
    3. Start EMA/CO or EMA/EP.
3. In patients with CND disease:
    1. Obtain neurosurgical consult.
    2. Consider using one dose of single-agent methotrexate or low-dose induction EP.
    3. Use modified EMA/CO with high-dose intravenous methotrexate (1000 mg/m$^2$ over 24 hours) for high CNS penetrance or with intrathecal methotrexate.
    4. Consider whole-brain radiation therapy to control bleeding and facilitate tumor shrinkage.
4. Surgery is reserved for recurrent or resistant foci of disease.

Remission is defined as three consecutive weekly β-HCG values in the normal range. After the first normal β-HCG, continue with four cycles of maintenance or consolidation chemotherapy. Monitor β-HCG levels for 24 months, with the patient counseled to use reliable contraception in this period.

*β-HCG,* Beta human chorionic gonadotropin; *CNS,* central nervous system; *EMA/CO,* etoposide, methotrexate, actinomycin D, cyclophosphamide, vincristine (Oncovin); *ETT,* epithelioid trophoblastic tumor *GTN,* gestational trophoblastic neoplasia; *PSTT,* placental site trophoblastic tumor.

## High-Risk Gestational Trophoblastic Neoplasia

In the developed world, **high-risk GTN** cases are uncommon. The timely involvement of specialist teams with experience in treating high-risk disease is key to achieving optimal outcomes. Patients with high-risk GTN, defined as a WHO prognostic score of 7 or higher, are at increased risk of treatment failure with single-agent therapy, hence the use of combination chemotherapy for this group (Lurain, 1995). Box 34.4 provides an overview of management for high-risk disease. As for low-risk disease, multiple treatment regimens exist but no quality RCTs have been conducted comparing regimens. A 2012 Cochrane review design to determine the efficacy and safety of combination chemotherapy in treating high-risk GTN found only one RCT (42 women) comparing MAC (MTX, ActD, and chlorambucil) or the modified CHAMOCA (cyclophosphamide, hydroxyurea, ActD, MTX with colonic acid rescue, vincristine (Oncovin), melphalan, and doxorubicin [Adriamycin]) (Curry et al., 1989; Deng, 2013). Direct comparison is further complicated by the various scoring systems used to classify the disease over time.

The greatest experience with combination treatment for high-risk GTN is with **EMA/CO (etoposide, MTX, ActD, cyclophosphamide, vincristine [Oncovin])**; however, no RCTs have been done (Table 34.4) (Lurain, 2006). This intensive regimen consists of etoposide, MTX, and ActD alternating with cyclophosphamide and vincristine. A number of case series, the largest being from the Charing Cross group, have reported complete response rates of 78% to 80% using primary treatment with EMA/CO (Newlands, 1991). In the Charing Cross cohort, 17% developed resistance to EMA/CO, but 70% of these were salvaged with the addition of platinum-based chemotherapy. Deaths from GTN occurred in 4% of patients, and two women developed acute myeloid leukemia after treatment with EMA/CO. Side effects include universal alopecia, stomatitis, and hematologic and gastrointestinal toxicities. Patients may require granulocyte colony-stimulating factor to prevent dose delays in the setting of neutropenia. The risk of secondary malignancies (e.g., acute myeloid leukemia, colon cancer, breast cancer), mainly related to cumulative etoposide dosing, is 50% greater than expected in a standardized nontreated cohort.

Although less than 5% of patients with low-risk disease relapse after apparent remission, this increases to 25% in patients with high-risk disease. Consolidation therapy with at least three additional course of chemotherapy after normalization of β-HCG level is warranted to reduce risk of relapse. The approach to these patients is multimodality treatment, including surgical resection of chemotherapy-resistant sites and salvage second-line (or third-line) chemotherapy. EMA/EP (substituting etoposide and cisplatin for cyclophosphamide and vincristine in EMA/CO) achieves complete response in 90% of patients with recurrent disease, but alternative regimens, including TE-TP (paclitaxel [Taxol], etoposide, cisplatin [Platinol]), BEP (bleomycin, etoposide, cisplatin), VIP (vinblastine, ifosfamide, cisplatin), and ICE (ifosfamide, carboplatin, etoposide), have also been used with success.

**TABLE 34.4** Chemotherapy Regimen for Intermediate- and High-Risk Gestational Trophoblastic Disease

| Drug Regimen | Administration |
|---|---|
| **EMA/CO (Preferred Regimen)—Course I (EMA)*** | |
| **Day 1** | |
| Etoposide | 100 mg/m² IV over 30 min |
| Methotrexate | 100 mg/m² IV bolus |
| Methotrexate | 200 mg/m² IV as 12-hr continuous infusion |
| Actinomycin D | 0.5 mg IV bolus |
| **Day 2** | |
| Etoposide | 100 mg/m² IV over 30 min |
| Folinic acid | 15 mg IV/IM/PO every 12 hr for four doses, to be started 24 hr after start of methotrexate |
| Actinomycin D | 0.5 mg IV bolus |
| Course II (CO) | |
| **Day 8** | |
| Cyclophosphamide | 600 mg/m² IV over 30 min |
| Vincristine | 1 mg/m² IV bolus |

Modified from Kantarjian HM, Wolf RA, Koller CA. *M.D. Anderson Manual of Medical Oncology.* New York: McGraw-Hill; 2006.
*Cytokine support may be used.
*EMA/CO,* Etoposide, methotrexate, actinomycin D, cyclophosphamide, vincristine (Oncovin)—EMA alternates with CO every week; *IV,* intravenous.

## Ultra-High-Risk Gestational Trophoblastic Neoplasia

Patients with WHO scores 13 or greater, those with major bleeding, and those with extensive disease in the chest, liver, or brain are considered to be at higher risk of early death and are treated with a low-dose induction EP (etoposide and cisplatin) chemotherapy on days 1 and 2, and repeated weekly for 1 to 2 cycles, before starting EMA/CO or EMA/EP (Alifrangis, 2013). In a retrospective study from Charing Cross (Alifrangis, 2013), 23% of high-risk patients received low-dose EP induction. These patients had a higher number of metastases, more brain metastases, and higher WHO score. EP induction was not associated with increased EMA/CO or EMA/EP resistance. These higher-risk patients did have higher but not statistically significant rates of recurrence and death. A longer consolidation period with four instead of three cycles can be considered (Ngan, 2015).

Moreover, frontline treatment with EMA/EP in patients who have brain or liver metastases was shown to have good results in this high-risk group and may be considered as a means to avoid the need for salvage chemotherapy (Cyriac, 2011).

### Central Nervous System Metastases

Brain metastases portend a poor prognosis. Favorable outcomes have been achieved using a combination chemotherapy, with select craniotomy in some cases; 30 of 39 patients in one series achieved remission (Newlands, 2002). Whole-brain radiotherapy to achieve hemostasis and tumor shrinkage has been used in conjunction with chemotherapy for patients with brain metastasis, but given the high success with chemotherapy and the deleterious long-term effects on overall function in survivors, including global intellectual impairment, chemotherapy is the preferred option. Many authors initiate steroid treatment and use one dose of single-agent MTX or low-dose EP induction, as described in the previous section, as a first regimen before EMA/CO to limit massive tumor necrosis, which may precipitate an intracranial bleed. Antiepileptic drugs are not routinely given. Others have used a modified EMA/CO regimen, including intrathecal MTX in the CO portion of scheduling; however, given the vascular nature of these tumors and the fact that they are not protected by the blood-brain barrier, intrathecal chemotherapy is probably unnecessary. Nonetheless, a study of 27 GTN patients with brain metastases used EMA/CO or EMA-EP with an enhanced CNS MTX dose combined with intrathecal MTX (Savage, 2015). Eighty-five percent (23 of 27) were long-term survivors, with only 4 deaths. All the patients who died had chemotherapy refractive disease.

### Pulmonary Metastases

Respiratory failure secondary to pulmonary metastases is a concern in patients with chest pain, cyanosis, anemia, and more than 50% lung field opacification. Cao and associates reported on 62 patients who underwent lobectomy for pulmonary metastasis, with complete response (CR) seen in 89% of patients with recurrent disease, 79% of patients with drug-resistant disease, and 100% of patients in whom a satisfactory response to chemotherapy was seen in the setting of residual pulmonary lesion (Cao, 2009). They recommended operative treatment of pulmonary metastases for recurrent drug-resistant disease in patients with adequate performance status to tolerate surgery, no evidence of active tumor elsewhere, and pulmonary metastases limited to one lung.

### Liver Metastases

Patients with liver metastases are at increased risk of hemorrhage with chemotherapy initiation. In addition to high-risk chemotherapy regimens, other treatment modalities described include radiation therapy, embolization, and surgical resection.

### Vaginal Metastases

Patients with vaginal metastases are at high risk for hemorrhage. Embolization or surgery may be used to control acute bleeding.

## Resistant or Recurrent Disease

Recurrences after remission relate to the initial stage of disease. Goldstein and coworkers reported recurrences in 3% for stage I disease, 8% for stage II, 4% for stage III, and 9% for stage IV (Goldstein, 2012). The mean time from the last detectable $\beta$-HCG to recurrence was 6 months. For all stage I, II, and III patients, remissions were achieved with additional chemotherapy, whereas all stage IV patients with recurrences died of their disease. Ngan and colleagues found no relationship between time to relapse and mortality, with an overall survival of 78% in patients with relapse (Ngan, 2007). In contrast, the reported recurrence rate of PSTT and ETT range from 20% to 30%, and despite salvage treatment (chemotherapy or surgery), only 30% will achieve long-term remission.

All patient who develop resistance to chemotherapy or recurrence require restaging. If patients still meet criteria for low-risk disease and have been treated with first-line single-agent MTX or ActD, treatment should be switched to the second-line single-agent alternative or to combination EMA/CO after second-line single agent treatment (Seckl, 2013). If after restaging patients meet the criteria for high-risk disease, they should be treated with EMA/CO as per high-risk treatment recommendations.

For patients with resistant or recurrent disease after EMA/CO and EMA/EP, a number of multiagent drug combinations have been described; however, none have yet been identified as the optimal treatment. These include paclitaxel and etoposide alternating weekly with paclitaxel and cisplatin (TE-TP) (Wang, 2008); BEP;

ICE; cisplatin, vinblastine, and bleomycin (PVB); and paclitaxel and carboplatin (PC) (Rathod, 2015). Single-agent treatment regimens also have been considered recurrent, advanced, or metastatic GTN with paclitaxel (Jones, 1996), pegylated liposomal doxorubicin, and capecitabine (Bianconi, 2007).

A novel promising treatment option is pembrolizumab, a programmed-death protein 1 receptor monoclonal antibody (anti-PD1). Signaling through this receptor pathway occurs through programmed cell death ligand 1 (PD-L1), which has been shown to be strongly expressed in GTN (Ghorani, 2017). A case series (Ghorani, 2017) of four patients treated with pembrolizumab included patients with recurrent or progressive disease, including choriocarcinoma (2), PSTT, and mixed PSTT/ETT histologic types. PD-L1 expression ranged from 90% to 100%. Three out of the four patients achieved remission with pembrolizumab (2 mg/kg every 3 weeks) after multiple previous lines of combination chemotherapy. The drug was well tolerated, with mild toxicities. Another PD-L1 antibody, avelumab, is under investigation, with recruiting for the study estimated to be complete in 2023 (*Avelumab in Chemo-resistant Gestational Trophoblastic Neoplasias*, 2019). Animal studies have not shown an increase in the risk of birth defects in survivors after treatment with anti-PD1/PD-L1 agents, but data in humans is lacking at this time (Johnson, 2017; Duma and Lambertini, 2020).

## Treatment of Placental Site Trophoblastic Tumor and Epithelioid Trophoblastic Tumor

PSTTs and ETTs are rare trophoblastic tumors occurring with a frequency of less than 1%, with clinical behavior ranging from relatively benign to highly malignant. The International Society for the Study of Trophoblastic Diseases (ISSTD) has established an international database of all the cases of PSTT and ETT to further inform on management of these rare tumors. Metastases are seen in approximately 30% of patients with PSTT and 50% of patients with ETT at the time of diagnosis and develop in a further 10% during posttreatment follow-up (Frijstein, 2019; Lan, 2010; Zhang, 2013). These types of GTN are relatively chemoresistant compared with invasive mole and choriocarcinoma. Therefore surgery is the cornerstone for the treatment of nonmetastatic PSTT and ETT, with hysterectomy being sufficient provided that the ovaries are normal (Baergen, 2006). Patients with metastatic PSTT and ETT have a poor prognosis. A retrospective study found that five out of six stage IV PSTT patients (83%) died despite multiagent chemotherapy (Hyman, 2013). The largest retrospective case series, which included 108 patients with PSTT, reported 94.4% survival for stage I disease (Zhao, 2016). Despite the lack of strong prospective evidence, surgery, followed by combination chemotherapy with EMA/EP or TP-TE (alternating weekly paclitaxel-cisplatin and paclitaxel-etoposide), has been recommended in patients with advanced disease. Zhao and colleagues (Zhao, 2016) reported initial response rates to chemotherapy of 92%, a relapse rate of 20.6%, and a mortality of 13.5% in patients with advanced (stage II to IV) disease. In this large case series of 108 patients, the most common treatment strategies were a sandwich pattern of chemotherapy, followed by surgery and chemotherapy. The most used chemotherapy regimens were FAV (floxuridine, ActD, vincristine), FAEV (FAV and etoposide), and EMA/CO.

Data for ETT are even more limited than for PSTT, but it appears to be even more chemoresistant (Davis, 2015). A series from the international database of ETT and PSTT (Frijstein, 2019) reported on 45 patients with ETT and 9 with PSTT/ETT; 43% of patients were diagnosed at an early stage and treated with surgery alone; 96% of them (22 out of 23) survived. The 17 patients with advanced (stage II to IV) disease were treated with surgery and chemotherapy or chemotherapy alone; 59% were alive after a median follow-up of 39 months. A total of 18 different chemotherapy regimens were used in this cohort, and no conclusions could be drawn regarding the optimal regimen.

## Surveillance After Gestational Trophoblastic Neoplasia

After $\beta$-HCG remission is achieved for three weekly cycles, patients with low-risk GTN require monthly testing for 12 months, whereas patients with high-risk GTN require repeat testing every 2 weeks for 3 weeks and then monthly for a minimum of 2 years. Patients with a history of PSTT or ETT may be considered for longer follow-up. Patients with stage IV disease are encouraged to maintain monthly testing for 24 months. The risk of relapse beyond the first year is less than 1% (Seckl, 2013).

Reliable contraception in the post-GTN period is required, and the OCP is the method of choice. Cross-reactivity of LH, and therefore false positives, may occur with some assays. Furthermore, patients treated with multiagent chemotherapy may develop ovarian dysfunction, either transient or eventually premature ovarian failure, particularly those in their 30s or 40s. OCP has been recommended for those patients with the thought that it may suppress the production of LH from the pituitary glands and therefore protect the ovaries, although it remains controversial because of a lack of high-quality studies.

## Pregnancy After Gestational Trophoblastic Neoplasia

After molar pregnancy or GTN, patients can expect normal reproductive outcomes. Garner and associates summarized pregnancy outcomes after GTD from multiple centers (Garner, 2002). In a total of 2657 pregnancies after treatment for persistent GTN, 77% had live births, with 72% term deliveries, 5% preterm births, 1% stillbirths, 14% spontaneous abortions, and 2% of children born with congenital anomalies—pregnancy outcomes similar to those of the general population.

After a molar pregnancy, however, there is an increased risk of subsequent molar pregnancy, increasing from roughly 1 to 3 in 1000 pregnancies to 1 to 2 in 100. After two molar pregnancies, the risk in a subsequent pregnancy may be as high as 20% (Seckl, 2013). Changing partners has not been proved to decrease this risk.

When a patient with a history of GTD or GTN becomes pregnant, an early US to confirm a normal pregnancy in the first trimester is recommended, after which patient care can be transferred to the obstetric provider. The $\beta$-HCG level should be checked at 6 and 10 weeks postpartum to rule out new or recurrent disease (Seckl, 2013).

## Psychosocial Considerations

Diagnosis and treatment for GTN may have long-lasting psychosocial sequelae for patients, including sadness with a sense of loss after pregnancy, low self-esteem, sexual dysfunction, and anxiety about future pregnancies. Petersen and coworkers used validated questionnaires to assess quality of life in patients after treatment for molar pregnancy and found that more than 50% showed psychological symptoms suggestive of an underlying psychiatric disorder (Petersen, 2005). They recommended a multidisciplinary approach to care to address the emotional and social aspects of a woman's well-being after treatment for GTN.

## Centralization of Care

Because of the rare incidence of GTN, care in GTN centers of excellence with a multidisciplinary approach has been proposed as a means to ensure consistency of care and progress in the field. Centralization of care would allow for central pathology review, the opportunity for a prospective patient registry, and systematic surveillance and treatment recommendations at a minimum. When feasible, patient referral and transfer of care would be ideal.

## REFERENCES


Alazzam M, Tidy J, Hancock BW. First-line chemotherapy in low-risk gestational trophoblastic neoplasia. *Cochrane Database Syst Rev.* 2012; 7:CD007102.

Alifrangis C, Agarwal R, Short D, et al. EMA/CO for high-risk gestational trophoblastic neoplasia: good outcomes with induction low-dose etoposide-cisplatin and genetic analysis. *J Clin Oncol.* 2013;31(2):280–286.

Altieri A, Franceschi S, Ferlay J, et al. Epidemiology and aetiology of gestational trophoblastic diseases. *Lancet Oncol.* 2003;4(11):670–678.

Berkowitz RS, Goldstein DP. Clinical practice. Molar pregnancy. *N Engl J Med.* 2009;360(16):1639–1645.

Berkowitz RS, Goldstein DP. Current advances in the management of gestational trophoblastic disease. *Gynecol Oncol.* 2013;128(1):3–5.

Braga A, Torres B, Burlá M, et al. Is chemotherapy necessary for patients with molar pregnancy and human chorionic gonadotropin serum levels raised but falling at 6months after uterine evacuation? *Gynecol Oncol.* 2016;143(3):558–564.

Cole LA, Muller CY. Hyperglycosylated hCG in the management of quiescent and chemorefractory gestational trophoblastic diseases. *Gynecol Oncol.* 2010;116:3–9.

Cole LA. hCG, the wonder of today's science. *Reprod Biol Endocrinol.* 2012;10:24.

Coyle C, Short D, Jackson L, et al. What is the optimal duration of human chorionic gonadotrophin surveillance following evacuation of a molar pregnancy? A retrospective analysis on over 20,000 consecutive patients. *Gynecol Oncol.* 2018;148(2):254–257.

Deng L, Zhang J, Wu T, Lawrie TA. Combination chemotherapy for primary treatment of high-risk gestational trophoblastic tumour. *Cochrane Database Syst Rev.* 2013;1:CD005196

Elias KM, Goldstein DP, Berkowitz RS. Complete hydatidiform mole in women older than age 50. *J Reprod Med.* 2010;55(5-6):208–212.

Elias KM, Shoni M, Bernstein M. Complete hydatidiform mole in women aged 40 to 49 years. *J Reprod Med.* 2012;57(5-6):254–258.

Frijstein MM, Lok CAR, van Trommel NE, et al. Management and prognostic factors of epithelioid trophoblastic tumors: results from the International Society for the Study of Trophoblastic Diseases database. *Gynecol Oncol.* 2019;152(2):361–367.

Fu J, Fang F, Xie L, et al. Prophylactic chemotherapy for hydatidiform mole to prevent gestational trophoblastic neoplasia. *Cochrane Database Syst Rev.* 2012;10:CD007289.

Ghorani E, Kaur B, Fisher RA, et al. Pembrolizumab is effective for drug-resistant gestational trophoblastic neoplasia. *Lancet.* 2017;390(10110): 2343–2345.

Lawrie TA, Alazzam M, Tidy J, et al. First-line chemotherapy in low-risk gestational trophoblastic neoplasia. *Cochrane Database Syst Rev.* 2016; (6):CD007102.

Maesta I, Nitecki R, Horowitz NS, et al. Effectiveness and toxicity of first-line methotrexate chemotherapy in low-risk postmolar gestational trophoblastic neoplasia: The New England Trophoblastic Disease Center experience. *Gynecol Oncol.* 2018;148(1):161–167.

Mangili G, Lorusso D, Brown J, et al. Trophoblastic disease review for diagnosis and management: a joint report from the International Society for the Study of Trophoblastic Disease, European Organisation for the Treatment of Trophoblastic Disease, and the Gynecologic Cancer InterGroup. *Int J Gynecol Cancer.* 2014;24(9 Suppl 3):S109–S116.

National Comprehensive Cancer Network. Gestational Trophoblastic Neoplasia. Version 3. October 29 2020. https://www.nccn.org/professionals/physician_gls/pdf/gtn_blocks.pdf. Accessed November 30 2020.

Ngan HY, Seckl MJ, Berkowitz RS, et al. Update on the diagnosis and management of gestational trophoblastic disease. *Int J Gynaecol Obstet.* 2015;131(Suppl 2):S123–S126.

Osborne RJ, Filiaci V, Schink JC, et al. Phase III trial of weekly methotrexate or pulsed dactinomycin for low-risk gestational trophoblastic neoplasia: a gynecologic oncology group study. *J Clin Oncol.* 2011;29(7): 825–831.

Osborne RJ, Filiaci VL, Schink JC, et al. Second curettage for low-risk nonmetastatic gestational trophoblastic neoplasia. *Obstet Gynecol.* 2016;128(3):535–542.

Savage P, Kelpanides I, Tuthill M, et al. Brain metastases in gestational trophoblast neoplasia: an update on incidence, management and outcome. *Gynecol Oncol.* 2015;137(1):73–76.

Sebire NJ, Foskett M, Short D, et al. Shortened duration of human chorionic gonadotrophin surveillance following complete or partial hydatidiform mole: evidence for revised protocol of a UK regional trophoblastic disease unit. *BJOG.* 2007;114(6):760–762.

Seckl MJ, Sebire NJ, Fisher RA, et al. Gestational trophoblastic disease: ESMO Clinical Practice Guidelines for diagnosis, treatment and follow-up. *Ann Oncol.* 2013;24(Suppl 6):vi39–vi50.

Vargas R, Barroilhet LM, Esselen K, et al. Subsequent pregnancy outcomes after complete and partial molar pregnancy, recurrent molar pregnancy, and gestational trophoblastic neoplasia: an update from the New England Trophoblastic Disease Center. *J Reprod Med.* 2014;59 (5-6):188–194.

Wang Q, Fu J, Hu L, et al. Prophylactic chemotherapy for hydatidiform mole to prevent gestational trophoblastic neoplasia. *Cochrane Database Syst Rev.* 2017;9:CD007289.

Zhang X, Lü W, Lü B. Epithelioid trophoblastic tumor: an outcome-based literature review of 78 reported cases. *Int J Gynecol Cancer.* 2013; 23(7):1334–1338.

Zhao J, Lv WG, Feng FZ, et al. Placental site trophoblastic tumor: a review of 108 cases and their implications for prognosis and treatment. *Gynecol Oncol.* 2016;142(1):102–108.

Zhao P, Lu Y, Huang W, et al. Total hysterectomy versus uterine evacuation for preventing post-molar gestational trophoblastic neoplasia in patients who are at least 40 years old: a systematic review and meta-analysis. *BMC Cancer.* 2019;19(1):13.


**Suggested readings for this chapter can be found on ExpertConsult.com.**

# 35 Primary and Secondary Dysmenorrhea, Premenstrual Syndrome, and Premenstrual Dysphoric Disorder

## Etiology, Diagnosis, Management

*Vicki Mendiratta, Gretchen M. Lentz*

### KEY POINTS

- Approximately 75% of all women complain of primary dysmenorrhea. Approximately 15% have severe symptoms.
- Education, supportive therapy, and nonsteroidal antiinflammatory drugs are the treatments of choice for primary dysmenorrhea. Combined oral contraceptives (COCs) reduce the prevalence and severity of dysmenorrhea. They can be used in extended cycles for better relief. This is also a reasonable first-line treatment, especially if contraception is desired.
- Secondary dysmenorrhea can be due to a variety of both gynecologic and nongynecologic causes. Extensive history with directed physical and imaging are key to determining the specific diagnosis.
- Approximately 3% to 8% of all women suffer from clinically relevant premenstrual syndrome (PMS), with 2% demonstrating premenstrual dysphoric disorder (PMDD). The most useful diagnostic tool in evaluating women with potential PMS or PMDD is a prospective symptom diary.
- Therapy with psychoactive drugs, particularly selective serotonin reuptake inhibitors (SSRIs), has been demonstrated in randomized controlled trials to relieve PMS and PMDD symptoms. These medications should be considered first-line therapy. Specific cautions for the use of these agents must be followed. For women who also desire contraception, COCs are a valid option that have produced demonstrated improvement in PMS/PMDD symptoms.

Dysmenorrhea, premenstrual syndrome, and premenstrual dysphoric disorder afflict a large percentage of women in their reproductive years. These conditions have a negative effect on the quality of these women's lives and the lives of their families, and they are also responsible for a huge economic loss as a result of the cost of medications, medical care, and decreased productivity. This chapter discusses current thinking with respect to the causes, pathophysiology, and management of these three conditions.

## DYSMENORRHEA

**Dysmenorrhea is defined as a cyclic, painful cramping sensation in the lower abdomen often accompanied by other biologic symptoms, including sweating, tachycardia, headaches, nausea, vomiting, diarrhea, and tremulousness, all occurring just before or during the menses. *Primary dysmenorrhea* refers to pain with no obvious pathologic pelvic disease.** It is currently recognized that these patients are suffering from the effects of endogenous prostaglandins. ***Secondary dysmenorrhea*, on the other hand, is due to pelvic pathologic conditions** (Smith, 2016). Primary dysmenorrhea almost always first occurs in women younger than 20. Indeed, the woman will report pain as soon as she establishes ovulatory cycles. Secondary dysmenorrhea may occur in adolescents and in women of any age.

## INCIDENCE AND EPIDEMIOLOGY

Several studies have attempted to determine the prevalence of dysmenorrhea; a wide range (16% to 90%) has been reported. These studies have been performed on students, teenagers, and their mothers, as well as individuals from various specific populations, such as industrial workers or college students. **The best estimate of the prevalence of primary dysmenorrhea is approximately 75%.** Andersch and Milsom (1982) surveyed all the 19-year-old women in the city of Gothenburg, Sweden. A total of 90.9% of these women responded to a randomly distributed questionnaire, and 72.4% of these stated that they suffered from dysmenorrhea. In addition, 34.3% of the total population reported mild menstrual symptoms, 22.7% cited moderate symptoms that required analgesia, and 15.4% stated that they had severe dysmenorrhea that clearly inhibited their working ability and that could not be adequately assuaged by general analgesia (Andersch, 1983) (Table 35.1). A 2005 Canadian study of 1546 menstruating women reported that 60% had primary dysmenorrhea and 60% of those affected reported their pain as moderate or severe (Burnett, 2005). Similarly, 17% missed school or work. Most women do not have any specific risk factors for this disorder; however, factors that may *reduce* the risk of developing dysmenorrhea include the following:

- Younger age at first childbirth
- Higher parity
- Physical exercise
- Oral contraceptive pill use

Risk factors that have been reported to *increase* the risk of dysmenorrhea include (Latthe, 2006) the following:

- Age younger than 30
- Body mass index less than 20 $kg/m^2$
- Prolonged duration of menses
- Irregular or heavy menses

**TABLE 35.1** Severity of Primary Dysmenorrhea*

| Severity | Number of Women | Percentage of Total |
|---|---|---|
| None | 162 | 27.6 |
| Mild† | 201 | 34.3 |
| Moderate‡ | 133 | 22.7 |
| Severe§ | 90 | 15.4 |

*In a population of 586 19-year-old Swedish women.
†No systemic symptoms, medication rarely required, work rarely affected.
‡Few systemic symptoms, medication required, work moderately affected.
§Multiple symptoms, poor medication response, work inhibited.
Data from Andersch B, Milsom I. An epidemiologic study of young women with dysmenorrhea. *Am J Obstet Gynecol.* 1982;144:655.

- Premenstrual syndrome
- Pelvic inflammatory disease
- Sterilization
- History of sexual assault
- Heavy smoking
- Family history (particularly if mother or sister has dysmenorrhea as well)

## Relationship to Menstruation and the Menstrual Cycle

Andersch and Milsom (1982) have demonstrated a significant positive correlation among the severity of dysmenorrhea and duration of menstrual flow, amount of menstrual flow, and early menarche. They showed no relationship with the actual duration of the menstrual cycle. In their series, 38.3% of patients reported that they had experienced dysmenorrhea for the first time during the first year after menarche, and only 20.8% reported that dysmenorrhea had not occurred until 4 years after menarche.

# PRIMARY DYSMENORRHEA

## Pathogenesis

**The pathogenesis of dysmenorrhea is that of elevated prostaglandin F2 alpha (PGF2α) and E2 (PGE2) levels in the secretory endometrium resulting in uterine hypercontractility, thus leading to the symptoms of severe cramping.** When menses begins, the simultaneous decreases in circulating progesterone and estradiol lead to increased transcription of endometrial collagenases, matrix metalloproteinases (MMPs), and inflammatory cytokines. Upregulated MMPs target and break down endometrial tissue, freeing phospholipids from the cellular membrane. Phospholipases convert uterine phospholipids to arachidonic acid. Arachidonic acid, the precursor to prostaglandin production, has been found in increased amounts in the endometrium during ovulatory cycles. Arachidonic acid is converted to PGF2α, PGE2, and leukotrienes, which are involved in increasing myometrial contractions.

**During menses, these contractions decrease uterine blood flow and cause ischemia and sensitization of pain fibers (Fig. 35.1).** Endometrial concentrations of PGF2α and PGE2 correlate with the severity of dysmenorrhea; cyclooxygenase inhibitors decrease menstrual fluid prostaglandin levels and decrease pain. In a small 2018 study, magnetic resonance imaging (MRI) correlated uterine cramping with myometrial changes of both uterine pressure and hemodynamic dysfunction with decreased blood flow (Fig. 35.2). PGF2α and PGE2 affect other

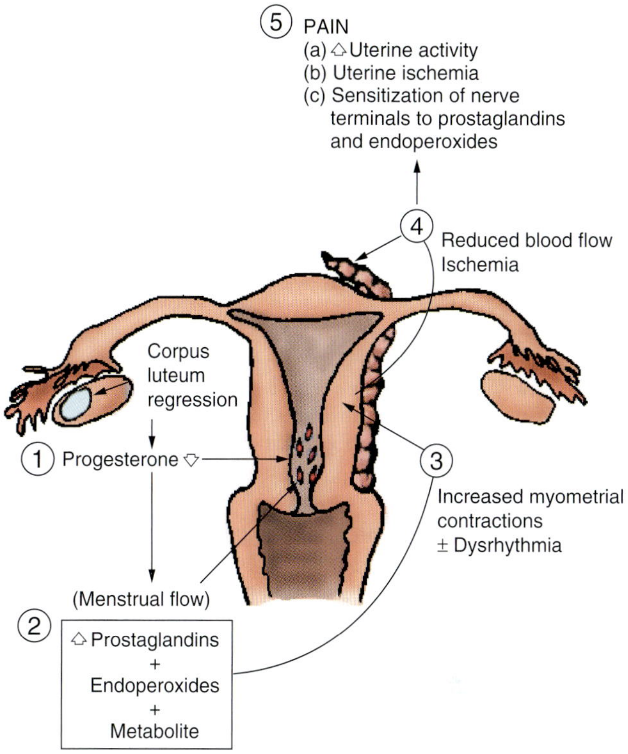


**Fig. 35.1** Mechanisms contributing to generation of pain in primary dysmenorrhea. (From Dawood MY. Nonsteroidal anti-inflammatory drugs and reproduction. *Am J Obstet Gynecol.* 1993;169:5.)

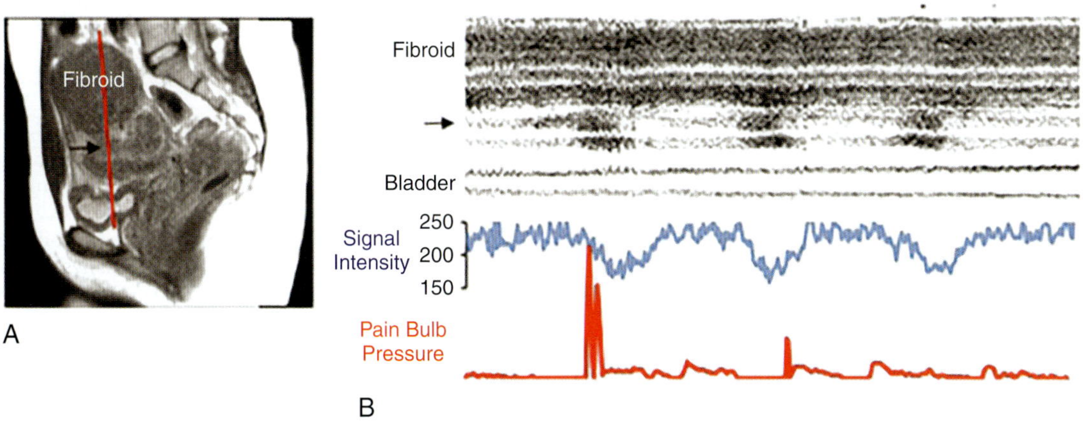


**Fig 35.2** Example of measurements of myometrial signal. (From Hellman KM, Kuhn CS, Tu FF, et al. Cine MRI during spontaneous cramps in women with menstrual pain. *Am J Obstet Gynecol.* 2018;218(5):506.e1-506.e8.)

organs such as the bowel and result in nausea, vomiting, and diarrhea.

## Diagnosis

**The diagnosis of primary dysmenorrhea is made largely by history and physical examination.** Patients typically complain of midline, crampy, lower abdominal or suprapubic pain, which begins with the onset of menstruation. The pain gradually resolves over 12 to 72 hours. Pain does not occur at times other than menses and only occurs in ovulatory cycles. Diarrhea, headache, fatigue, and malaise may be reported. Women with primary dysmenorrhea have a normal pelvic examination. Pelvic ultrasound should be considered in the evaluation of dysmenorrhea to evaluate for secondary causes. There are no laboratory or imaging abnormalities associated with primary dysmenorrhea.

Canadian 2017 consensus guidelines include a dysmenorrhea history checklist:

1. Menstrual history
2. Relationship between menarche and onset of dysmenorrhea
3. Timing of pain in relation to menses and amount of menstrual flow
4. Characterization, severity, chronology, and resulting disability
5. Sexual history, including inquiry about sexual abuse
6. Inquiry about chronic pain syndromes and medical conditions
7. Presence of symptoms of depression, anxiety, or other psychiatric disorders
8. Previous treatment, including dose, duration of use, side effects, and response

They also include a primary dysmenorrhea treatment algorithm (Fig. 35.3).

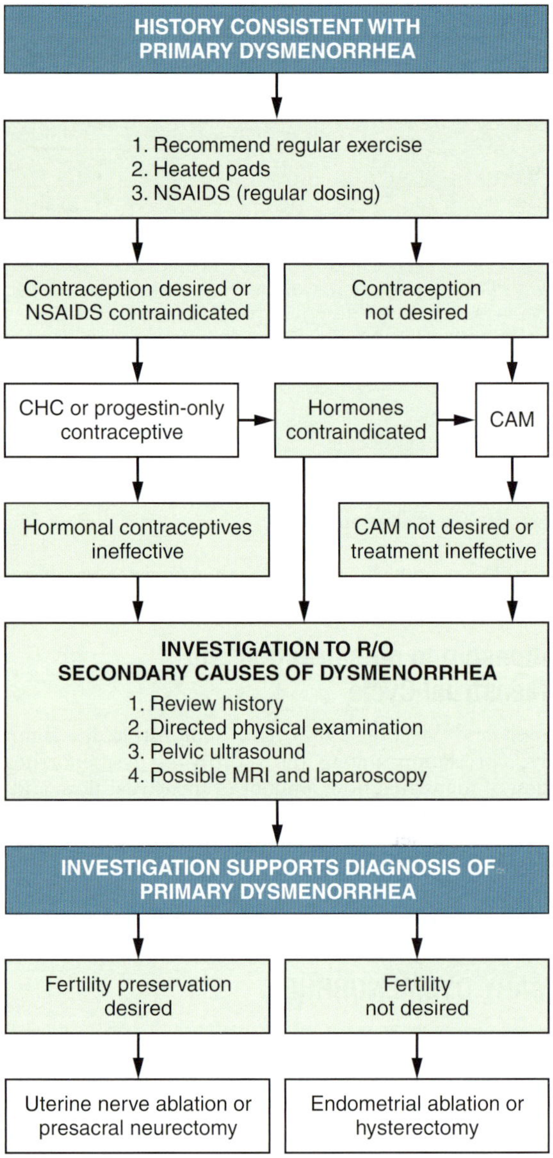


**Fig. 35.3** Primary dysmenorrhea treatment algorithm. (From Burnett M, Lemyre M. No. 345-primary dysmenorrhea consensus guideline. *J Obstet Gynaecol Can.* 2017;39(7):585-595.)

## Treatment

Treatment for primary dysmenorrhea begins with providing patient education and reassurance. Individualized, supportive therapy can then be tailored to the patient's specific symptoms, degree of disability from those symptoms, and other health care considerations, such as need for contraception (Smith, 2016).

## Nonpharmacologic Interventions

### Exercise

Cochrane conducted a systematic review of the literature in 2010. Only one randomized controlled trial (RCT) was included that demonstrated efficacy of aerobic exercise in reducing dysmenorrhea. In 2018, a more contemporary systematic review concluded that physical activity may be effective for mitigating primary dysmenorrhea. Although the included studies were of low to moderate quality (Matthewman, 2018), **the many other benefits from exercise warrant its recommendation as first-line therapy for women suffering from significant dysmenorrhea.**

### Heat

Two RCTs have shown that heat applied to the low abdomen, in the form of a patch or wrap, was effective in reducing dysmenorrhea. Unlike medications, this intervention has no side effects.

## Behavioral Interventions

In 2007, a Cochrane review revealed some evidence from five RCTs that a variety of behavioral interventions may help reduce cyclic menstrual pain; however, the authors cautioned that the data were of limited quality, with small sample sizes, and the included studies suffered from some methodologic limitations. Interventions that have been used and studied include relaxation training, biofeedback, Lamaze exercises, hypnotherapy, imagery, coping strategies, and desensitization procedures (Proctor, 2007).

## Vitamins and Diet

Dietary and vitamin therapies may be beneficial but to date have not been studied in a rigorous fashion. A low-fat vegetarian diet decreased menstrual pain in one study, and vitamin E was more effective than placebo in reducing dysmenorrhea in adolescents. Vitamins $B_1$ and $B_6$, fish oil supplements, fish oil plus $B_1$, ginger (750 to 2000 mg), valerian, zinc, and a Japanese herbal combination have been helpful in reducing pain compared with placebo in small trials.

## Medications

**Nonsteroidal antiinflammatory drugs (NSAIDs) are first-line therapies for primary dysmenorrhea.** NSAIDs are prostaglandin synthetase inhibitors (PGSIs). They are divided into two chemical groups: the arylcarboxylic acids, which include acetylsalicylic acid (aspirin) and fenamates (mefenamic acid); and the arylalkanoic acids, including the arylpropionic acids (ibuprofen, naproxen, and ketoprofen) and the indoleacetic acids (indomethacin). The more specific cyclooxygenase (COX-2) inhibitors such as celecoxib have similarly been shown to alleviate the primary dysmenorrheal symptoms. COX-2 expression in the uterine glandular epithelium was maximal during menstruation in one trial of ovulatory women, suggesting a possible association with the cause. The increased expression of COX-2 was eliminated with continuous use of oral contraceptives (OCs), which also offer an effective treatment (discussed later). The specific effect of these agents on the uterine musculature is reduction of contractility, as measured by reduction of intrauterine pressure. COX-2 inhibitors may be considered for women with gastrointestinal toxicity caused by NSAIDs; however, these agents carry a risk of serious adverse events and now contain a black box warning. These medications therefore should only be used with caution and full disclosure.

In 2015, Marjoribanks provided a review to the Cochrane Database of RCTs of NSAIDs in the treatment of dysmenorrhea. Eighty RCTs were included, including 20 different NSAIDs (both nonselective and COX-2–specific formulations). **NSAIDs were substantially more effective than placebo in pain reduction** (odds ratio [OR], 4.37; 95% confidence interval [CI], 3.76 to 5.09). There was no significant difference if efficacy among the variety of NSAIDs. Side effects involving the gastrointestinal track and neurologic systems occurred in 11% to 14% of women taking NSAIDs and should be considered when prescribing these medications (Marjoribanks, 2015).

**NSAIDs should be given the day before the expected menses or at the onset of menses. If one NSAID is ineffective, switching to a different class of NSAIDs may be helpful.** NSAIDs should not be given to patients who have shown previous hypersensitivity to such drugs. They are also contraindicated for women who have had nasal polyps, angioedema, and bronchospasm related to aspirin or NSAIDs. In addition, these agents are contraindicated for individuals with a history of chronic ulceration or inflammatory reaction of the upper or lower gastrointestinal (GI) tract and for those with preexisting chronic renal disease. During the use of these agents, autoimmune hemolytic anemia, rash, edema and fluid retention, and central nervous system (CNS) symptoms, such as dizziness, headache, nervousness, and blurred vision, can occur. In up to 15% of users, a slight elevation of hepatic enzyme levels may also be found. Table 35.2 lists some NSAIDs commonly used for the treatment of dysmenorrhea.

Roughly 18% of women have dysmenorrhea that is resistant to NSAIDs. Fig. 35.4 summarizes potential mechanisms that may be responsible lack of NSAID response.

**Combined contraceptives (CCs) containing estrogen and progesterone will relieve the symptoms of primary dysmenorrhea in approximately 90% of patients.** CCs suppress ovulation and endometrial proliferation, and the progestin component also blocks the production of the precursor to prostaglandin formation. The thinned endometrium from CCs then contains less arachidonic acid, which is the precursor to prostaglandins. As a result of these mechanisms, there is less uterine contractility and resultant pain with menses. If the woman also requires contraception, CC therapy may prove to be the treatment of choice.

In 2009, Wong and colleagues provided a review to the Cochrane Database of RCTs comparing combined oral contraceptives (COCs) with differing dosages of COCs, placebo, and NSAIDs. Six studies revealed that COCs were significantly more effective than placebo for the treatment of dysmenorrhea (OR, 2.99; 95% CI, 1.76 to 5.07) (Wong, 2009).

In small RCTs, low-dose oral contraceptives (OCs with 20 μg ethinyl estradiol) were effective in reducing dysmenorrhea in adolescents and adult women. **Continuous OC administration compared with traditional monthly cyclic dosing in systematic review seems to be more effective at reducing dysmenorrhea.** Breakthrough bleeding can be an undesirable side effect, although a review of RCTs reported bleeding and discontinuation rates to be similar. The extended-cycle OCs available are also associated with less dysmenorrhea than are monthly cyclic OCs.

The vaginal ring CC has also been shown to reduce dysmenorrhea in a similar fashion as COCs. Dysmenorrhea was not, however, as well controlled in women using the transdermal CC patch compared with COCs (Smith, 2016).

**TABLE 35.2** Commonly Used Nonsteroidal Antiinflammatory Drugs*

| Class | Brand Name | Generic Name | Usual Regimen (mg)* | Initial Dose | Subsequent Dose |
|---|---|---|---|---|---|
| Propionic acid | Motrin | Ibuprofen | 400 (qid)–800 (tid) | 500 | 250 tid-qid |
| | Naprosyn | Naproxen | 250 (qid)–500 (bid) | | |
| | Anaprox | Naproxen sodium | 275 (qid)–550 (bid) | | |
| | N/A | Ketoprofen | 25-75 (tid) | | |
| | Nalfon | Fenoprofen calcium | 200 (qid) | | |
| Fenamic acid | Ponstel | Mefenamic acid | 250 (qid) | 550 | 275 tid-qid |
| | N/A | Meclofenamate | 100 (qid) | | |
| Acetic acid | Indocin | Indomethacin | 25 (tid) | 50 | 25-50 tid-qid |
| | Voltaren | Diclofenac | 75 (bid) | | |
| | N/A | Tolmetin | 400 (tid) | | |
| | N/A | Diflunisal | 500 (bid) | | |
| | N/A | Etodolac | 400 (tid-qid) | | |
| | Toradol | Ketoralac | 10 (qid) | | |
| Oxicams | Feldene | Piroxicam | 20 (qd) | 500 | 250 qid |

*Maximum doses.
*bid,* Two times a day; *N/A,* not applicable; *qd,* once daily; *qid,* four times a day; *tid,* three times a day.

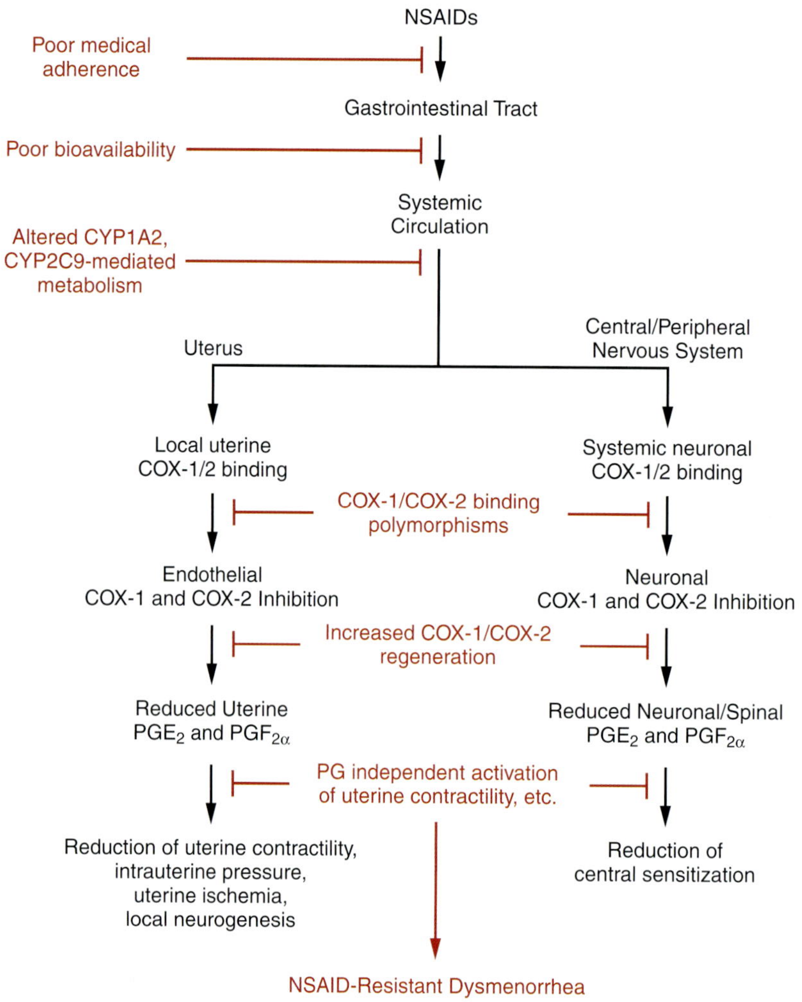


**Fig. 35.4** Nonsteroidal antiinflammatory drug–resistant dysmenorrhea. (From Oladosu FA, Tu FF, Hellman KM. Nonsteroidal antiinflammatory drug resistance in dysmenorrhea: epidemiology, causes, and treatment. *Am J Obstet Gynecol*. 2018;218(4):390-400.)

### Progestin-Only Formulations

Depot medroxyprogesterone (DMPA), a long-acting injectable contraceptive, has not been studied specifically for primary dysmenorrhea. Trials in contraceptive studies report a reduction in dysmenorrhea in adolescents. Systemic progestins result in thinned endometrium and can lead to infrequent menses or amenorrhea. **After 1 year of DMPA use, approximately 50% of women experience amenorrhea and resultant cessation of dysmenorrhea.**

**The 20 $\mu$g levonorgestrel-releasing intrauterine system (LNG-IUS) has been shown in RCTs to reduce menstrual pain.** Levonorgestrel is a 19-nortestosterone derivative affecting endometrial progesterone receptors, leading to an atrophic endometrial lining. In 2013 a smaller LNG-IUS containing only 14 $\mu$g of levonorgestrel was approved by the U.S. Food and Drug Administration (FDA) and may represent another option for the management of dysmenorrhea (Smith, 2016). Of note, by comparison, the copper T380A intrauterine device (IUD) often increases dysmenorrhea.

**The single-rod etonogestrel-releasing contraceptive (current version, Nexplanon)** has also been shown in clinical trials to reduce dysmenorrhea. This long-acting reversible contraceptive also offers excellent contraption for those women who need it.

### Tocolytics

Because of their ability to block uterine contractility, tocolytics may be beneficial in the treatment of dysmenorrhea. Studies using nifedipine at a dose of 20 to 40 mg orally have demonstrated pain relief. Moderate pain relief was noted in 36 of 40 women, but side effects of facial flushing, tachycardia, and headache can occur. Glyceryl trinitrate and magnesium have also been studied in limited fashion and have demonstrated effectiveness in reducing cyclic menstrual pain. Ongoing large-scale research is needed to assess safety and efficacy; therefore these medications are not often used for contemporary management of dysmenorrhea.

## Other Treatments

Narcotic analgesics are often used in treating patients with general chronic pain syndromes; however, because of the very real potential for dependency or abuse, they should not be used in dysmenorrhea management.

A meta-analysis of three trials has reported that transcutaneous electrical nerve stimulation (TENS) is more effective than placebo in relieving dysmenorrhea, although it is not as effective as analgesics. Milsom and colleagues in Sweden and Smith and

Heltzel in the United States have noted that TENS relieves menstrual pain without reducing intrauterine pressure, suggesting that its mode of action may be in the CNS. High-frequency TENS provides more dysmenorrheal pain relief compared with placebo or low-frequency TENS (Milsom, 1994; Smith, 1991).

Acupuncture and acupressure have been used for the management of dysmenorrhea. Several studies have evaluated the effectiveness of these complementary alternatives; however, they were of low quality. A 2018 randomized study used a smartphone application for self-acupressure in 221 women. Modest differences were notes with some reduction in mean pain scores. There is limited evidence that acupuncture may be of benefit.

A 2005 meta-analysis of eight RCTs of surgical interruption of nerve pathways concluded that there was insufficient evidence to advise laparoscopic uterine nerve ablation (LUNA) or laparoscopic presacral neurectomy (LPSN) for primary dysmenorrhea (Proctor, 2005).

## SECONDARY DYSMENORRHEA: CAUSES AND MANAGEMENT

Many other conditions cause or are associated with dysmenorrhea. **Pelvic disease should be considered in patients who do not respond to NSAIDs or CCs or a combination of these agents for presumed primary dysmenorrhea.** The diagnosis should also be considered when symptoms appear after many years of painless menses. Pelvic pathologic conditions may occur at any age, and in most cases the pain experienced is secondary to the pathologic process of the condition or a specific result of it. These constitute the secondary dysmenorrhea group of conditions as outlined in Box 35.1 (Howard, 2013).

### Cervical Stenosis

Severe narrowing of the cervical canal, particularly at the level of the internal os, may impede menstrual flow, causing an increase in intrauterine pressure at the time of menses. In addition, retrograde menstrual flow through the fallopian tubes into the peritoneal cavity may take place. Thus severe cervical stenosis may eventually be associated with pelvic endometriosis as well. The origin of cervical stenosis may be congenital or secondary to cervical injury, such as with electrocautery, cryocautery, or operative trauma (e.g., conization). The condition may also result from an inflammatory process caused by infection, the application of caustic substances, or hypoestrogenism. After any of these conditions, the cervical canal may narrow because of the contraction of scar tissue.

The possibility of cervical stenosis should be considered if there is a history of scant menstrual flow and if severe cramping continues throughout the menstrual period. Hematometra or pyometra may occur.

The diagnosis is suspected when the external os appears scarred or when it is impossible to pass a cervical brush or uterine sound through the internal os. Diagnosis can be verified via hysterosalpingogram or hysteroscopy. With complete stenosis, a probe will not be able to pass through the internal os. In other cases, passage through the internal os may be difficult but often can be accomplished with patience and/or ultrasound guidance. Self-administration of buccal or intravaginal misoprostol before the procedure may aid in the ease with which cervical dilation can be accomplished. Misoprostol is not FDA approved for this particular indication, but many studies have evaluated its effectiveness for procedures such as IUD insertion and hysteroscopy.

Treatment consists of dilating the cervix, which may be accomplished by dilation and curettage (D&C) with progressive dilators or by the use of progressive *Laminaria* tents. Unfortunately, cervical stenosis often recurs after therapy, necessitating repeat procedures. Pregnancy and vaginal delivery often afford a more lasting cure.

Often other problems obstructing the cervix can have a similar presentation. Fig. 35.5 shows anteroposterior and lateral views of a hysterogram in an 18-year-old nulliparous woman who had a 2-year history of severe disabling dysmenorrhea that usually required morphine therapy with each menstrual period. At hysteroscopy, she was found to have a tissue band across her internal os, at which site a large endocervical polyp had formed. Transecting the band and removing the polyp completely relieved the dysmenorrhea, and she had no further symptoms after 3 years.

**BOX 35.1** Causes of Secondary Dysmenorrhea

**GYNECOLOGIC PATHOLOGY**

- Cervical stenosis
- Endometriosis
- Adenomyosis
- Pelvic infection (pelvic inflammatory disease) and adhesions
- Uterine polyps or fibroids
- Ovarian cyst or mass
- Pelvic congestion
- Congenital obstructed müllerian malformations

**NONGYNECOLOGIC DISORDERS CAUSING PELVIC PAIN**

- Mental health issues/disorders
  - Somatization
  - Depression
  - Drug-seeking behavior and opioid dependency
  - History of physical or sexual abuse
- Bowel disease
  - Irritable bowel syndrome
  - Inflammatory bowel disease
  - Celiac sprue
  - Lactose intolerance
- Urinary tract disease
  - Ureteral obstruction
  - Interstitial cystitis
  - Nephrolithiasis

### Endometriosis

**The presence of endometrial glands and stroma outside the uterus defines endometriosis. Endometriosis is a chronic condition that may manifest in generalized pelvic pain, cyclic pain, dysmenorrhea, dyspareunia, infertility, and bowel or bladder dysfunction. This condition affects 6% to 10% of reproductive age women and is found in approximately 70% to 80% with chronic pelvic pain** (American College of Obstetricians and Gynecologists [ACOG], 2010). **Endometriosis is the most common cause of secondary dysmenorrhea among adolescents, in particular.** Approximately one-third of women undergoing diagnostic laparoscopy as a result of chronic pelvic pain (CPP) will have endometriosis confirmed visually or by biopsy. Endometriosis should be considered when there is a history of pain becoming more severe during menses. Pertinent physical findings may include uterosacral ligament nodules, evidence for endometriosis in the vagina or cervix, and lateral displacement of the cervix. Pelvic ultrasonography and diagnostic laparoscopy should be considered in the evaluation. Treatment options for endometriosis are discussed in Chapter 19.

### Adenomyosis

The presence of endometrial glands and stroma in the myometrium defines adenomyosis. This ectopic endometrial tissue may

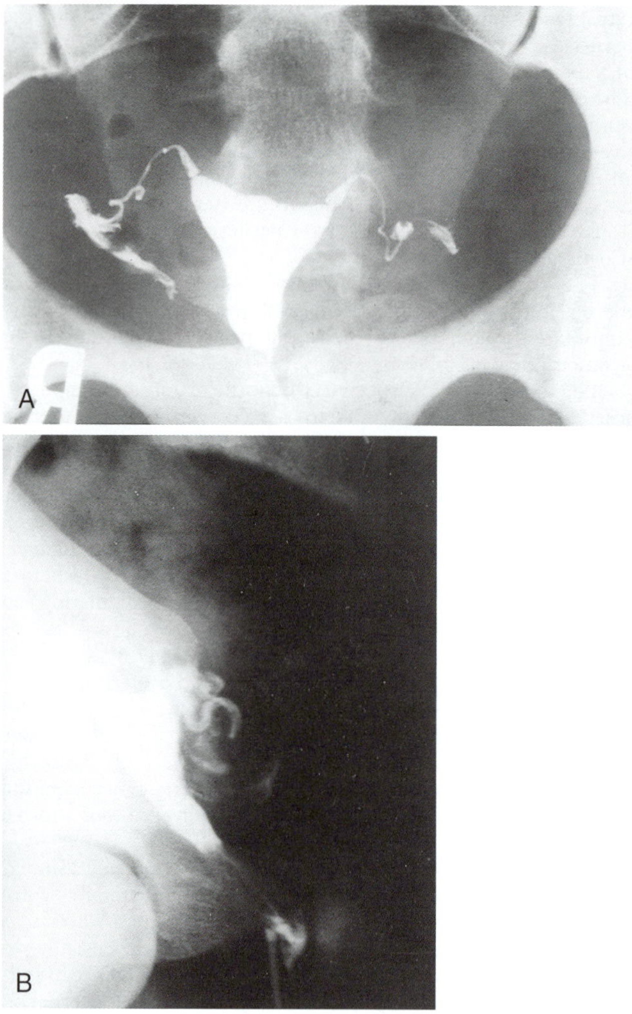


**Fig. 35.5** Hysterogram. Anteroposterior (**A**) and lateral (**B**) views of an 18-year-old patient with severe disabling dysmenorrhea. At hysteroscopy, she was found to have a tissue band across the internal os and an endocervical polyp at this site. Removal of the polyp and transection of the band completely relieved the dysmenorrhea.

induce hypertrophy and hyperplasia of the adjacent myometrium. It typically manifests in heavy, painful menses that tends to be progressive. Women may appreciate bulk symptoms as the uterus enlarges.

Koike and colleagues, in an in vitro experiment using tissue slices, found that the prostaglandin level in endometriosis implants is significantly higher than in normal endometrium, myometrium, leiomyomata, and normal ovarian tissue, and that adenomyosis implants produce larger amounts of 6-keto-PGF1 when the dysmenorrhea has been severe. They believe that prostaglandins in these conditions increase painful menstruation (Koike, 1994). Treatment options for adenomyosis are discussed in Chapter 18.

### Pelvic Inflammation

Pelvic infections secondary to gonorrhea, chlamydia, or other microbes may cause pelvic inflammation or pelvic abscess and, with healing, may be associated with pelvic adhesions and tubal damage that may cause pelvic pain. **Pelvic inflammatory disease (PID) can lead to CPP in up to 30% of women.** This may often be aggravated during menses, causing dysmenorrhea. Infections secondary to other conditions, such as appendicitis or IUD use, may create a similar response. The pain may be secondary to the congestion and edema that occur normally at menses, which may subsequently be aggravated by the healed inflammatory areas and adhesions. Pelvic infections are further discussed in Chapter 23.

## OTHER STRUCTURAL ABNORMALITIES OF THE REPRODUCTIVE TRACT

**Although most structural lesions of the uterus, such as fibroids or polyps, and structural lesions of the ovaries, such as cysts or masses, do not cause isolated dysmenorrhea, they should be considered in the differential diagnosis.** Pelvic examination and ultrasound are useful in the evaluation of anatomic abnormalities. Hysteroscopy or saline infusion sonography may reveal pathologic conditions that could contribute to dysmenorrhea (Fig. 35.6).

### Pelvic Congestion Syndrome

Pelvic congestion syndrome (PCS), which was first described by Taylor in 1949, results from the engorgement of pelvic vasculature. Controversy exists regarding whether this is an actual disorder because it has been difficult to prove. It is a poorly understood disorder of the pelvic venous circulation. PCS is defined by chronic pelvic discomfort (often burning or throbbing in nature) worsened by prolonged standing and intercourse in women who have periovarian varicosities on imaging studies. The cause of PCS is unclear and the optimum treatment is uncertain. Development of an evidence-based approach to managing these patients has been limited by the absence of definitive diagnostic criteria.

Physical examination of the vagina and cervix may reveal vasocongestion, uterine enlargement and global tenderness of the cervix, uterus, and adnexa on palpation. Diagnosis is made by history and physical imaging, such as pelvic ultrasound, venography, computed tomography (CT), or MRI, and by laparoscopy, which not only rules out other causes of pelvic pain but also demonstrates congestion of the uterus and engorgement or varicosities of the broad ligament and pelvic sidewall veins.

No standard therapeutic approach is available, so therapies range from ovarian hormone suppression, local sclerotherapy (for vulvar varices), and embolization of the hypogastric vein to resection of the gonadal vein to hysterectomy. A 2010 systematic review by Tu and coworkers has found 6 diagnostic and 22 treatment studies but no consensus on diagnostic studies or treatment, although progestins and gonadotropin-releasing hormone (GnRH) agonists were effective in decreasing pain symptoms (Tu, 2010).

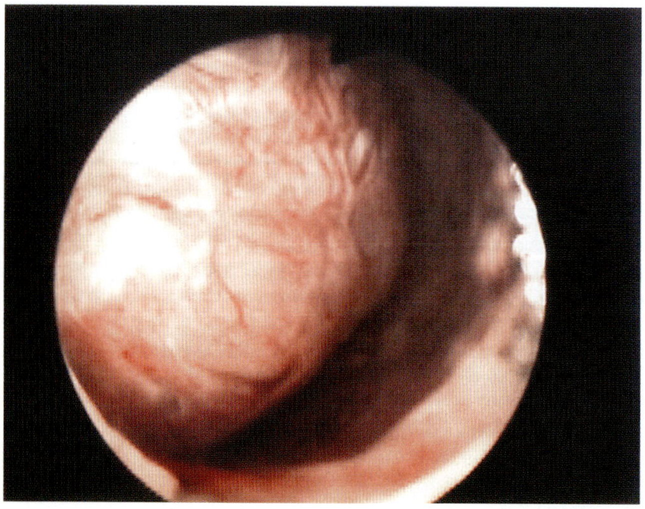

**Fig. 35.6** Submucous myoma blocking the internal os causing secondary dysmenorrhea.

## CONGENITAL OBSTRUCTIVE ANOMALIES

Obstructive anomalies of the reproductive tract, which include anomalies of the hymen and vagina and müllerian anomalies of the uterus, can result in secondary dysmenorrhea. It is estimated that these occur in up to 3.8% of young women (ACOG, 2018). Careful examination, sometime necessitating examination under anesthesia, and/or imaging are necessary to evaluate for this group of pathologic conditions. The goal of surgical correction is to create a patent outflow tract and relieve symptoms.

## NONGYNECOLOGIC CAUSES FOR PELVIC PAIN

### Mental Health Conditions

In individuals with strong family histories of dysmenorrhea, or when a careful history demonstrates a possibility for societal reward or control because of the symptoms of pain, a conditioned behavior should be considered. It is important to obtain a careful medical and social history and to rule out all other causes of acquired dysmenorrhea. Dysmenorrhea has been positively associated with the presence and severity of chronic pelvic pain and chronic nonpelvic pain any may be a general risk factor or chronic pain (Li, 2020). Conditions that may manifest in CPP including dysmenorrhea include somatization, opiate dependency, history of physical or sexual abuse, and depression. **Women with CPP often have psychological issues, so careful evaluation of the patient's past and present social situation, administering a depression screen, and performing a mental status examination may be revealing.** Referral to a mental health provider may be beneficial for further diagnostic testing, counseling, or medical therapy.

### Relation to Functional Bowel Disease

Crowell and coworkers studied 383 women aged 20 to 40 using a Neuroticism-Extraversion-Openness (NEO) Personality Inventory on entry into the program, a Moos' Menstrual Distress Questionnaire, and a bowel symptom inventory every 3 months for 12 months. Dysmenorrhea was diagnosed in 19.8% of these women. Functional bowel disorder, defined as abdominal pain with altered bowel function, occurred in 61% of the women with dysmenorrhea but in only 20% of the others ($P < .05$) (Crowell, 1994). Bowel symptoms were significantly correlated with dysmenorrhea, even after controlling for the effects of neuroticism. Prostaglandin levels in vaginal fluid were elevated in patients with dysmenorrhea but did not consistently differentiate the diagnostic groups. It was concluded that there was a strong covariance of menstrual and bowel symptoms, along with an overlap in their diagnosis, suggesting a common physiologic basis. Adolescents with irritable bowel syndrome (IBS) were found to have significantly higher rates of primary dysmenorrhea and premenstrual syndrome (Bahrami, 2019).

In a study of women with IBS and menstrual cycle symptoms, dysmenorrhea was twice as prevalent among women with IBS as in controls (21% vs. 10%; $P = .09$), although this was not statistically significant. Women with IBS who took OCs had significantly less dysmenorrhea than women in the control group who were not on OCs (11% vs. 28%, $P = .02$). One case report found an association of celiac sprue and dysmenorrhea, but little is known about this finding.

### Other Causes

There are nongynecologic causes for pain during menses that should be considered in the differential diagnosis. These include appendicitis, lactose intolerance, celiac sprue, abdominal mass, and a number of urinary tract conditions (e.g., urinary tract infection, painful bladder syndrome/interstitial cystitis, nephrolithiasis, and ureteral obstruction).

## PREMENSTRUAL SYNDROME AND PREMENSTRUAL DYSPHORIC DISORDER

**Premenstrual syndrome (PMS) is defined as a group of mild to moderate symptoms, physical and behavioral, that occur in the second half of the menstrual cycle and that may interfere with work and personal relationships.** Common physical complaints include breast tenderness, bloating, and headache. Common behavioral symptoms may include irritability, anxiety, and depression. These are followed by a period entirely free of symptoms. Frank first described the condition in 1931 and attempted to relate symptoms of the so-called *premenstrual tension* with hormonal changes of the menstrual cycle (Frank, 1931). The term *premenstrual syndrome* was first used by Dalton in 1953. The symptoms vary from woman to woman, and more than 150 symptoms have been linked with the disorder.

**Premenstrual dysphoric disorder (PMDD) represents a more severe disorder, with marked behavioral and emotional symptoms. This condition is included in the American Psychiatric Association *Diagnostic and Statistical Manual of Mental Disorders*, fifth edition (DSM-V) (APA, 2014). PMDD differs from PMS in the severity of symptoms and the fact that women with PMDD must have at least one severe affective symptom that occurs regularly during the last week of the luteal phase in most menstrual cycles.** A number of physical symptoms may also be present (Box 35.2). In contrast to PMS, women suffering from PMDD have substantial impairment in personal functioning. PMS and PMDD are similar in that the symptoms manifest in the luteal phase of the menstrual cycle and resolve during menses.

### Incidence and Epidemiology

**Premenstrual symptoms occur in 75% of women at some point in their reproductive lives. The incidence of clinically relevant PMS occurs in 3% to 8% of women.** Using DSM-V diagnostic criteria, 2% of reproductive-age women will suffer from PMDD (Yonkers, 2016). The average age of onset is 26 years. Risk factors for PMS include the following:

- Family history of PMS in the mother
- Personal past or current psychiatric illness involving mood or anxiety disorders
- History of alcohol abuse
- History of postpartum depression
- Nulliparity
- Earlier menarche
- High caffeine intake
- High levels of stress
- High body mass index

Some racial and ethnic differences have been reported, but PMS/PMDD appears consistently in all cultures studied. Data from a California PMS Severity Study of 1194 women found that women of Hispanic descent reported greater severity of symptoms than non-Hispanic white and black women, and Asian women reported less (Sternfeld, 2002). Similar to PMS, PMDD prevalence is noted in many countries studied, including Croatia, Italy, Iceland, and Japan. A Japanese study found a 1.2% prevalence of PMDD, suggesting a cultural difference in prevalence or reporting.

In the Harvard Study of Moods and Cycles by Cohen and colleagues, a population-based, cross-sectional sample of 4164 premenopausal women was studied retrospectively regarding PMDD prevalence. A PMDD diagnosis was made in 6.4% of the women, and PMDD was associated with lower education, a history of major depression, and current smoking (Cohen, 2002). This confirms the results of earlier studies reporting a significant lifetime comorbidity of PMDD and affective disorders. Past sexual abuse has been reported more often in women attending PMS clinics compared with women in the general population.

**BOX 35.2** Premenstrual Dysphoric Disorder, DSM-V

**DIAGNOSTIC CRITERIA**

**625.4 (N94.3)**

A. In the majority of menstrual cycles, at least five symptoms must be present in the final week before the onset of menses, start to *improve* within a few days after the onset of menses, and become *minimal* or absent in the week post menses.

B. One (or more) of the following symptoms must be present:
- Marked affective lability (e.g., mood swings; feeling suddenly sad or tearful, or increased sensitivity to rejection).
- Marked irritability or anger or increased interpersonal conflicts.
- Marked depressed mood, feelings of hopelessness, or self-deprecating thoughts.
- Marked anxiety, tension, and/or feelings of being keyed up or on edge.

C. One (or more) of the following symptoms must additionally be present, to reach a total of *five* symptoms when combined with symptoms from Criterion B above.
- Decreased interest in usual activities (e.g., work, school, friends, hobbies).
- Subjective difficulty in concentration.
- Lethargy, easy fatigability, or marked lack of energy.
- Marked change in appetite; overeating; or specific food cravings.
- Hypersomnia or insomnia.
- A sense of being overwhelmed or out of control.
- Physical symptoms such as breast tenderness or swelling, joint or muscle pain, a sensation of "bloating," or weight gain.

*Note:* The symptoms in Criteria A–C must have been met for most menstrual cycles that occurred in the preceding year.

D. The symptoms are associated with clinically significant distress or interference with work, school, usual social activities, or relationships with others (e.g., avoidance of social activities; decreased productivity and efficiency at work, school, or home).

E. The disturbance is not merely an exacerbation of the symptoms of another disorder, such as major depressive disorder, panic disorder, persistent depressive disorder (dysthymia), or a personality disorder (although it may co-occur with any of these disorders).

F. Criterion A should be confirmed by prospective daily ratings during at least two symptomatic cycles. (**Note:** The diagnosis may be made provisionally prior to this confirmation.)

G. The symptoms are not attributable to the physiologic effects of a substance (e.g., a drug of abuse, a medication, other treatment) or another medical condition (e.g., hyperthyroidism).

From American Psychiatric Association (APA). Premenstrual dysphoric disorder. In: *Diagnostic and Statistical Manual of Mental Disorders.* 5th ed (DSM-V). American Psychiatric Association: Arlington, VA; 2014.

## Symptoms

In a review by O'Brien, a number of common somatic and affective symptoms were enumerated (see Box 35.2). **The most common somatic symptoms relate to abdominal bloating, breast tenderness, and various pain constellations, such as headache. Psychological symptoms vary from fatigue, irritability, and tension to anxiety, labile mood, and depression** (O'Brien, 1982). In the California PMS Severity Study, consistency of symptoms was found over two consecutive cycles, especially for emotional symptoms (Sternfeld, 2002).

Depression is a common complaint in the population in general and also in PMS-PMDD sufferers during the luteal phase. Mortola and coworkers have shown that 16 PMS patients had marked worsening of scores on the Profile of Mood States and Beck Depression Inventory during the luteal phase compared with 16 controls; however, 6 patients suffering from endogenous depression had scores threefold higher on both indices than PMS patients who were in the luteal phase. Also, the amplitude of cortisol secretion pulses was higher in the depressed patients than in the PMS patients or control patients (Mortola, 1989). The data demonstrate that PMS patients have more episodes of depression during the luteal phase compared with controls, but these episodes are distinctly different from those suffered by patients with endogenous depression. The National Institute of Mental Health's Sequenced Treatment Alternatives to Relieve Depression (STAR-D) trial of clinically depressed women found that 64% of 433 participants not on OCs reported worsening of their depressive symptoms before menses (Kornstein, 2005). Therefore it can be challenging to differentiate women with PMS/PMDD from women with depression and premenstrual exacerbations of depressive symptoms.

## Causes

When Frank first described the syndrome, it was attributed to estrogen excess. Others have offered theories that the disorder is related to an imbalance of estrogen and progesterone, endogenous hormone allergy, hypoglycemia, vitamin $B_6$ deficiency, prolactin excess, fluid retention, inappropriate prostaglandin activity, elevated monoamine oxidase (MAO) levels, endorphin malfunction, and a number of psychological disturbances. In 1981, Reid and Yen reviewed the subject and concluded that **PMS was a multifactorial psychoendocrine disorder** (Reid, 1981). Fig. 35.7 shows a schematic of the proposed causes. **Studies indicate that cyclic gonadal hormonal alterations and serotonergic neuronal mechanisms in the CNS may interact and be major causative factors for PMS in susceptible women.** Evidence for this conclusion is indirect but includes successful clinical trials with selective serotonin reuptake inhibitors (SSRIs) and other neurotropic agents thought to affect the serotonin pump mechanism between CNS neurons. Other indirect evidence includes the fact that platelet tritium-labeled, imipramine-binding sites are thought to be reduced in patients suffering from depression and are believed to represent receptor sites that label for a presynaptic serotonin transporter on the presynaptic nerve terminal. In some studies, binding sites returned to normal several months after clinical remission of depression or during the response to psychotropic medications or electroconvulsive therapy. These platelet-binding sites therefore have been used as an indirect measure of the neuron receptor site. Steege and coworkers have demonstrated lower platelet tritium-labeled imipramine binding in women with late luteal phase dysphoric disorder (now called *PMDD*); they believe that this result supported the hypothesis that such patients suffer from alterations of the central serotonergic systems (Steege, 1992). **More recently, beta-endorphin and gamma-aminobutyric acid (GABA) neurotransmitters have been implicated. Estrogen has been found to modulate neurotransmitters such as GABA and dopamine, which may serve as inhibitory or excitatory agents in the brain.**

That fact that ovarian steroids are important in this syndrome has been known for some time. Studies related to the relationship of estrogen and progesterone in the circulation and the severity of the symptoms have not been fruitful. There are no consistent differences between estrogen and progesterone levels in PMS sufferers and those in controls. These women may have an abnormal response to normal cyclic ovarian steroid changes. Although symptom relief has been noted in several studies using GnRH agonists to block ovulation completely, no relief was found in a study by Chan and colleagues, who blocked progesterone receptors with the progesterone antagonist RU-486 (Chan, 1994).

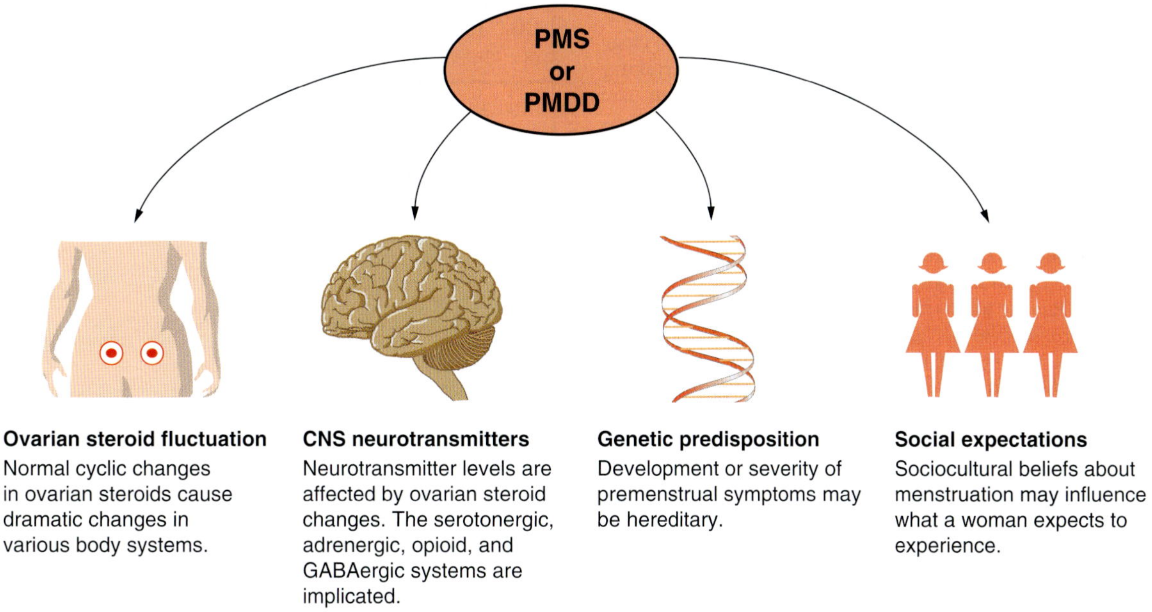


**Fig. 35.7** Proposed causes of premenstrual syndrome and premenstrual dysphoric disorder. *GABA,* γ-Aminobutyric acid. (From Ling F, Mortola J, Pariser S, et al. *Premenstrual Syndrome and Premenstrual Dysphoric Disorder: Scope, Diagnosis, and Treatment.* Crofton, MD: Association of Professors of Gynecology and Obstetrics; 1998.)

Rapkin and colleagues have evaluated the anxiolytic 3α, 5α reduced progesterone metabolite allopregnanediol during the luteal phase of 35 women with PMS and 36 controls (Rapkin, 1997). Serum progesterone and allopregnanediol levels were measured on days 19 and 26 of the cycles as determined by luteinizing hormone (LH) kits. Allopregnanediol levels were significantly lower in the PMS patients than controls on day 26, but there were no significant differences with respect to progesterone itself. They concluded that because PMS patients had lower levels of this anxiolytic metabolite during the luteal phase, they could be at greater susceptibility for various mood symptoms such as anxiety, tension, and depression. Allopregnanediol enhances GABA-A receptor function. Chuong and associates have demonstrated that beta-endorphin levels throughout the periovulatory phase are lower in PMS patients than in controls, especially in postovulatory days 0 to 4 (Chuong, 1994). Similarly, Halbreich and coworkers have demonstrated that PMS patients treated with 200 mg/day of danazol for 90 days have complete relief of symptoms in 23 anovulatory cycles, but relief of symptoms occurred in only 6 of 32 ovulatory cycles. They concluded that the beneficial effect of danazol in the treatment of PMS was achieved only when the anovulatory state eliminated the hormonal cyclicity of the normal cycle and not because of action of the drug per se (Halbreich, 1991). O'Brien and Abukhalil have advanced further evidence for this conclusion. They studied 100 women with PMS and premenstrual breast pain using a randomized, double-blind, placebo-controlled study of three menstrual cycles, using danazol 200 mg/day as the active drug. Treatment was given only during the luteal phase. Danazol did not effectively reduce the general symptoms of PMS, but it did relieve mastalgia (O'Brien, 1999). Severe PMS has been shown to be relieved by total abdominal hysterectomy and bilateral salpingo-oophorectomy, even with hormone replacement therapy using an estrogen, but some women on cyclic estrogen and progesterone therapy postmenopausally continue to complain of PMS symptoms. A 2003 study by Roca and colleagues has suggested that women with PMS may have an abnormal response to progesterone. Women with PMS failed to show a normal increased luteal phase hypothalamic-pituitary-adrenal axis response to exercise stress testing compared with controls (Roca, 2003). This response is distinctly different in PMS patients compared with women with major depression.

Another potential causative factor is a genetic contribution. Twin studies have demonstrated a high heritability of PMS symptoms; the concordance rate is twice as high in monozygotic twins as in dizygotic twins.

Concerning other possible causes, most dietary and vitamin deficiency theories have been difficult to prove and have not been found to be a major cause of this syndrome; however, data from Bertone-Johnson and associates' case-control study involving the Nurses' Health Study II cohort (2005) have suggested that a high intake of calcium and vitamin D may reduce the risk of PMS, so further research is needed. Several studies have looked for prolactin excess because some of the women complain of breast tenderness, but no positive findings have been found. Although some of the symptoms seems to relate to prostaglandin activity, and these symptoms are often reduced with treatment with NSAIDs, a direct cause and effect has not been established.

In summary, **the cause of PMS and PMDD is associated with ovarian steroids and ovulation, which seem to produce alterations in neurohormones and neurotransmitters that lead to a reduction of serotonergic function during the luteal phase.** The most effective evidence-based treatments for moderate to severe PMS and PMDD symptoms are SSRIs and agents that block ovulation. The temporal relationship between menstrual phase PMS and PMDD symptoms suggests a role of the reproductive hormones, not a direct linear role, but a more complex vulnerability to these cyclic hormonal shifts. Only 60% of women with PMDD respond to SSRI treatment, so serotonergic dysfunction may not be the only pathway involved. Beta-endorphin, GABA, the autonomic nervous system, and social expectations may all play a role in these complex disorders.

## Diagnosis

**The diagnosis of PMS and PMDD is made by the history of two consecutive menstrual cycles demonstrating luteal phase symptoms of PMS and PMDD.** The facts given by the woman may allow the physician to construct a specific, individualized treatment regimen. It is important that the physician have a clear understanding of the woman's symptoms before undertaking therapy. After a complete history and physical examination, the physician should rule out any medical problems that could be influencing the symptomatology. There is limited utility in blood tests; however, it is reasonable to screen for thyroid disease with a serum thyroid-stimulating hormone (TSH) test. The physician should then ask the woman to keep a diary of her symptoms throughout two menstrual cycles. Although she and her physician may focus on the second half of the menstrual cycle, the woman should be encouraged to keep track of all symptoms, regardless of the stage of the menstrual cycle. **A number of validated tools with diary sheets and symptom checklists are available. The Daily Record of Severity of Problems (DRSP) is most commonly used.** It is necessary to track symptoms for a full 2 months to compare follicular phase symptoms to luteal and menstrual phase data. At the end of two cycles, the physician should review the symptom diary. A change in the symptom severity score between 30% and 50% between the follicular and luteal phases suggests PMS and PMDD.

ACOG defines PMS as the presence of at least one symptom during the luteal phase of the cycle leading to significant impairment in functioning. It is important to differentiate PMS from other illnesses with similar symptoms. Women with depression and anxiety disorders may present believing that they have PMS. A differentiating aspect is that PMS patients suffer their symptoms only during the luteal phase. **Diagnosis can be difficult because women with depression and anxiety disorders can have premenstrual exacerbation of their symptoms, and PMS and PMDD can coexist with psychiatric disorders.**

Many women who do not actually have PMS may be self-referred to a facility that treats this condition. In one study, Plouffe and coworkers carefully analyzed 100 consecutive women prospectively entering the uniform diagnostic and treatment protocol for PMS and found that 38 women had PMS, 24 had premenstrual magnification syndrome (i.e., other conditions that were magnified during the luteal phase), and 13 had affective or other psychiatric disorders. Only 44% of the women previously given a diagnosis of PMS were found to have this syndrome. Overall, in this study, 84% of the women with PMS and premenstrual magnification syndrome responded to treatment (Plouffe, 1993). A variety of currently accepted therapies were used.

Other conditions to consider based on patient symptoms include anemia, diabetes, endometriosis, autoimmune disorders, chronic fatigue syndrome, collagen vascular disorders, and many psychiatric disorders (e.g., depression, anxiety, dysthymia, bipolar disorder).

The diagnosis of PMS is therefore made by symptom diary and by the elimination of other diagnoses.

**The diagnosis of PMDD is made after the DSM-V criteria, which require 5 of 11 symptoms of PMS, including one affective symptom (APA, 2014). These symptoms should be occurring for most of the preceding year. Affective symptoms include feeling sad or hopeless or having self-deprecating thoughts; anxiety or tension; mood lability and crying; and persistent irritability, anger, and increased interpersonal conflicts.** Prospective menstrual cycle charting is required for the diagnosis. Box 35.3 lists physical and psychiatric disorders that should be considered in the differential diagnosis of PMDD.

**BOX 35.3 Considerations in the Differential Diagnosis of Premenstrual Dysphoric Disorder**

Premenstrual syndrome
Endometriosis
Dysmenorrhea
Physical disorders with premenstrual exacerbations
Autoimmune disorders
Diabetes mellitus
Anemia
Hypothyroidism
Psychiatric disorders with luteal phase exacerbation
Depression
Anxiety
Dysthymic disorder
Bipolar disorder

## Treatment

### Diet, Supplements, Exercise, and Lifestyle Changes

Reassuring women with mild PMS without serious coexisting gynecologic disorders that this is a common problem should be part of the counseling. Thus the selection of medications and lifestyle changes should be tailored to the symptomatic needs of the patient. Lifestyle modifications can be recommended for 2 months while the woman completes the prospective diary for diagnosis.

Several dietary studies have been performed, but most were not rigorously controlled. Two trials have studied increasing complex carbohydrate intake, which reduced the severity of PMS mood symptoms. Complex carbohydrates may increase tryptophan availability and thereby increase serotonin. Because food cravings or increased appetite, mood changes, sleep disturbances and irritability, and fluid retention are listed among the key 17 symptoms, symptom severity may be affected by reducing or eliminating sugar, alcohol, caffeine, salty foods, and red meat.

A multicenter RCT of 466 women has shown that 1200 mg of calcium/day for three cycles reduces PMS symptoms significantly compared with placebo (48% versus 30%; $P < .001$) (Thys-Jacobs, 1998). This is a treatment to consider because some amount of calcium supplementation is helpful for bone health as well. Caution must be taken, however, because higher supplementation may be linked to heart disease.

Vitamin $B_6$ (pyridoxine) deficiency in PMS patients has been suggested because vitamin $B_6$ is a coenzyme involved in the biosynthesis of dopamine and serotonin, and neurotransmitters have been implicated in the cause of PMS. A review of nine RCTs of vitamin $B_6$ for the treatment PMS found no high-quality trials, although several suggested relief of PMS symptoms compared with placebo (Wyatt, 1999). A double-blind placebo-controlled trial of 94 women with PMDD found a greater decrease in psychiatric symptoms with 80 mg of vitamin $B_6$ (Kashanian, 2007). **Vitamin $B_6$ supplement at the rate of 50 mg/day can be tried for mild PMS symptoms.** Higher doses of pyridoxine should be administered with caution because neuropathy can occur in patients treated with as little as 200 mg/day. Other side effects, such as sensory deficit, paresthesia, numbness, ataxia, and muscle weakness, may occur.

There is inconclusive evidence from four RCTs that magnesium (200 to 400 mg/day) reduces PMS symptoms (Canning, 2006). A 2019 systematic review of 13 studies found no association with serum magnesium and PMS.

Patients should be encouraged to regularly exercise for general health reasons. A general recommendation is exercise for at least 30 minutes, on most days of the week, including during the luteal phase when symptoms are present. **Small trials have suggested aerobic exercise to be beneficial for PMS sufferers, and one trial found high-intensity aerobic exercise to be superior to low-intensity aerobic exercise for PMS treatment.**

Many other adjunct treatments as well as complementary and alternative medicines (CAMs) have been studied. These therapies include massage, biofeedback, yoga, acupuncture, chiropractic manipulation, evening primrose oil, and Chinese herbal medicines. A 2009 Cochrane review concluded that there is insufficient evidence to recommend the use of Chinese herbal therapies for this condition (Jing, 2009). A systematic review of several trials has suggested that of all the alternative therapies, bright light therapy, which may increase serotonin, may be a reasonable option for PMDD. Avoiding stressful activities in the luteal phase and having enough sleep may also alleviate PMS and PMDD symptoms.

## Cognitive Behavioral Therapy

Studies in the 1950s showed that 50% of patients improved with psychotherapy alone. More recently, Lustyk and coworkers reviewed seven studies, three of which were RCTs, and reported **efficacy of cognitive behavioral therapy for the management of PMS and PMDD** (Lustyk, 2009). Group psychoeducation in managing symptoms of PMS has been efficacious. Relaxation therapy may benefit patients with significant stress and anxiety components.

## Pharmacologic Agents

### Psychoactive Drugs

**SSRIs have been shown to be extremely effective for treating PMS and have become first-line treatment for PMDD.** In 2013 a Cochrane review included 31 RCTs studying 4372 women affected with PMS. Included studies compared paroxetine, sertraline, escitalopram, fluoxetine, or citalopram versus placebo. The authors concluded that both continuous and luteal phase SSRIs were effective for PMS (Marjoribanks, 2013). Medication dosages are generally lower than those used for depression. The onset of action can be rapid, within 1 to 2 days, unlike when SSRIs are used for depression (for dosing, see Table 35.3). Some patients may prefer a luteal phase regimen because it is less expensive and has fewer side effects. This is started on cycle day 14 and continues until the onset of menses or for a few more days thereafter. Even for PMDD, using the psychoactive drugs in only the luteal phase of the menstrual cycle can be effective; however, Shah and colleagues' 2008 meta-analysis of 20 RCTs and 2964 women found that although SSRIs are effective for treating PMS and PMDD (OR, 0.40; 95% CI, 0.31 to 0.51), intermittent dosing was less effective (OR, 0.55) than continuous dosing (OR, 0.28) (Shah, 2008). **If luteal phase treatment is not effective after 3 months, a trial of continuous SSRIs is warranted. No SSRI was demonstrably better than another.** If one SSRI is ineffective, other agents may still be effective. **SSRIs are effective in approximately 60% of PMS sufferers.** Venlafaxine, a serotonin and norepinephrine reuptake inhibitor, has also been found in RCTs to be more effective than placebo (Freeman, 2001). This medication may be helpful for patients who have side effects or no benefit on other SSRIs. After three cycles of SSRI treatment for PMDD, symptoms recurred with the first cycle after drug discontinuation, suggesting that prolonged therapy may be necessary.

**TABLE 35.3** SSRIs for Premenstrual Dysphoric Disorder

| SSRI | Effective Doses |
|---|---|
| Fluoxetine hydrochloride* | 20 mg/day |
| Sertraline hydrochloride | 50-150 mg/day |
| Paroxetine hydrochloride* | 20-30 mg/day |
| Paroxetine controlled release (CR) | 25 mg/day |
| Citalopram | 20-30 mg/day |
| Escitalopram | 10-20 mg/day |
| **SNRI** | **Effective Doses** |
| Venlafaxine | 37.5-112.5 mg/day |

*Only fluoxetine and paroxetine are approved for PMDD.
*PMDD,* Premenstrual dysphoric disorder; *SNRI,* selective norepinephrine reuptake inhibitor; *SSRI,* selective serotonin reuptake inhibitor.

Serious adverse effects from SSRIs can occur and must be weighed against the severity of the woman's symptoms. Approximately 15% of women on SSRIs have significant side effects, including sexual dysfunction (anorgasmia), sleep alterations, GI distress (including nausea), and CNS complaints such as headache and jitteriness. Some SSRIs can precipitate anxiety reactions, so caution should be used if anxiety symptoms predominate. Increased suicide rates have been observed with some SSRIs, so caution is needed if significant depressive symptoms are noted. This should be a low risk, given the low dose and intermittent luteal phase dosing.

In a carefully performed double-blind, placebo-controlled, crossover study of 19 patients suffering from PMS using alprazolam (Xanax), Smith and coworkers noted that the drug significantly relieved the severity of premenstrual nervous tension, mood swings, irritability, anxiety, depression, fatigue, forgetfulness, crying, cravings for sweets, abdominal bloating, cramps, and headaches compared with the placebo. They prescribed alprazolam, 0.25 mg three times per day on days 20 to 28 of each cycle and then tapering to 0.25 mg twice daily on day 1 and 0.25 mg on day 2 (Smith, 1987). Several RCTs have shown that doses higher than 0.75 mg/day are necessary to reduce PMS symptoms significantly. **Alprazolam may be more effective for depressive and anxiety symptoms than for other PMS complaints**; however, approximately 50% of women complain of drowsiness and sedation on these doses. Patients with a strong tendency to habituation should not be treated with this regimen. **Therefore alprazolam is considered second-line treatment.** Buspirone has less addictive potential than alprazolam and has been found in two RCTs to reduce symptoms. Continuous use of psychoactive drugs, such as tricyclics and lithium, has not yielded good PMS symptom relief.

Before using psychoactive drugs, it is extremely important to be sure of the diagnosis, because these drugs may not be effective and may actually be contraindicated in other psychiatric conditions that mimic PMS.

### Hormonal Suppression

#### *Progesterone*

Although a common treatment previously, many studies to date have shown progestogens to have mixed results in the treatment of PMS and PMDD. A 2012 Cochrane review concluded that progestin therapy did not show a significant improvement for patients with PMS (Ford, 2012).

#### *Oral Contraceptives*

Early RCTs and descriptive studies using cyclic OCs have shown mixed results for the treatment of PMS, but OCs are likely beneficial because they inhibit ovulation. OCs mainly help physical symptoms such as breast pain, bloating, acne, and appetite. If used, monophasic OCs appear to be better. In Sulak and associates' retrospective review of 220 patients using an extended OC regimen and shortened hormone-free interval (3 to 4 days), 45% of patients chose this regimen for control of PMS symptoms and 40% for dysmenorrhea and pelvic pain symptoms (Sulak, 2004). Continuous COCs should suppress ovulation and provide symptom relief. A 2005 review found that few studies have reported on premenstrual symptoms on continuous- or extended-use OCs, but relief was noted in headaches, tiredness, bloating, and menstrual pain (Edelman, 2005). Finally, a prospective 2006 study by Coffee and colleagues has shown that an extended regimen of 30 μg of ethinyl estradiol with 3 mg of drospirenone for 168 days significantly reduces PMS symptoms compared with typical 21-day cyclic OCs. The FDA has approved a 20-μg ethinyl estradiol and 3-mg drospirenone combination OC for the treatment of PMDD, although limiting use to women with PMDD who also need contraception was mentioned. Because of drospirenone's antimineralocorticoid and antiandrogenic properties, it has been hypothesized to be more effective (Coffee, 2006). A 2012 Cochrane systematic review supported its efficacy (Lopez, 2012). **For women with PMS/PMDD who also desire contraception, this OC is a reasonable first therapy.**

### Nonsteroidal Antiinflammatory Drugs

For patients who complain of cramping or other systemic symptoms such as aches, diarrhea, or heat intolerance, a trial with an NSAID may be useful. RCTs with mefenamic acid and naproxen have shown improvement in pain, mood, and somatic symptoms. It should be noted, however, that a toxic complication of NSAID use is nonoliguric renal failure. Because it is more likely to occur with NSAID use associated with severe dehydration, the agent should be discontinued if severe diarrhea is present and should not be used with diuretics.

### Diuretics

Historically, potassium-sparing diuretics were included in treatment consideration if the woman's complaints involve bloating, fluid retention, and a perceived change in body habitus during the luteal phase of the cycle. Study results on efficacy of this treatment, however, have been mixed. Spironolactone (100 mg/day) has been studied in four RCTs; three trials demonstrated moderate efficacy for breast tenderness and fluid retention, and two found reduced irritability symptoms. Diuretics should be avoided in patients with chronic renal disease or in those who are suffering from diarrhea or other fluid loss.

### Bromocriptine

Bromocriptine may be used for patients with cyclic mastalgia and may be helpful for some other symptoms of PMS, although its use in any individual case will need to be evaluated. A dose of 5 mg/day during the luteal phase is appropriate.

### Gonadotropin-Releasing Hormone Agonists

**At least 10 RCTs have shown GnRH agonists (leuprolide, 3.75 mg intramuscularly [IM] monthly) to be effective for ovulation suppression and treatment of PMS and the physical symptoms of PMDD.** GnRH agonists are less effective in treating the psychiatric symptoms of PMDD; however, they are expensive, can have marked side effects, and are limited in duration of use because of hypoestrogenism and osteoporosis. Using add-back estrogen and progesterone has been studied to offset the hypoestrogenic side effects without aggravating PMS and PMDD symptoms. The optimal add-back regimen is unclear from existing studies if GnRH agonists are to be used long term. Minimizing hormonal fluctuations with continuous estrogen and progesterone or minimizing the periods of exposure to progesterone seems prudent.

## Surgical Treatment: Bilateral Oophorectomy With or Without Hysterectomy

For women with severe, disabling symptoms who have been refractory to other medical therapies, surgical management may be considered. Three observational studies found bilateral oophorectomy, typically with hysterectomy, to be effective in this group of rare patients. **Although this approach is not offered as standard therapy for severe PMS, it may be a reasonable alternative for select patients for whom all other treatment regimens have failed.** The use of a GnRH analog for 3 to 6 months, with or without estrogen add-back, demonstrating efficacy is important before determining whether the patient may benefit from surgical treatment.

The physician should be cautious when determining a treatment regimen for any individual patient and should attempt to verify the patient's symptoms and add medications only when relief has not been achieved. Because of the myriad PMS symptoms, it is not surprising that individualization of treatment is essential. Many of the therapies mentioned, however, offer relief of most symptoms and hope for many sufferers.

## KEY REFERENCES


Andersch B. Bromocriptine and premenstrual symptoms: a survey of double-blind trials. *Obstet Gynecol Surv.* 1983;38:643.

American College of Obstetricians and Gynecologists (ACOG). ACOG Committee Opinion No. 760: Dysmenorrhea and Endometriosis in the Adolescent. *Obstet Gynecol.* 2018;116(1):e249–258.

American Psychiatric Association (APA). Premenstrual dysphoric disorder. In: *Diagnostic and Statistical Manual of Mental Disorders.* Arlington, VA: (DSM-V). American Psychiatric Association; 2014.

Andersch B, Milsom I. An epidemiologic study of young women with dysmenorrhea. *Am J Obstet Gynecol.* 1982;144:655.

Bahrami A, Gonoodi K, Khayyatzadeh SS, et al. The association of trace elements with premenstrual syndrome, dysmenorrhea and irritable bowel syndrome in adolescents. *Eur J Obstet Gynecol Reprod Biol.* 2019;233:114–119.

Burnett M, Lemyre M. No. 345-Primary Dysmenorrhea Consensus Guideline. *J Obstet Gynaecol Can.* 2017;39(7)585–595.

Burnett MA, Antao V, Black A, et al. Prevalence of primary dysmenorrhea in Canada. *J Obstet Gynaecol Can.* 2005;27(8):765.

Canning S, Waterman M, Dye L. Dietary supplements and herbal remedies for premenstrual syndrome (PMS): a systematic research review of the evidence for their efficacy. *J Reprod Infant Psyc.* 2006;24(4):363–378.

Li R, Li B, Kreher DA, Benjamin AR, Gubbels A, Smith SM. Association between dysmenorrhea and chronic pain: a systematic review and meta-analysis of population-based studies. *Am J Obstet Gynecol.* 2020 Sep;223(3):350–371. doi: 10.1016/j.ajog.2020.03.002. Epub 2020 Mar 7. PMID: 32151612.

O'Brien PM, Abukhalil IE. Randomized controlled trial of the management of premenstrual syndrome and premenstrual mastalgia using luteal phase-only danazol. *Am J Obstet Gynecol.* 1999 Jan;180(1 Pt 1):18–23. doi: 10.1016/s0002-9378(99)70142-0. PMID: 9914571.

Steege JF, Stout AL, Knight DL, Nemeroff CB. Reduced platelet tritium-labeled imipramine binding sites in women with premenstrual syndrome. *Am J Obstet Gynecol.* 1992 Jul;167(1):168–172. doi: 10.1016/s0002-9378(11)91653-6. PMID: 1442921.


**Full references and Suggested readings for this chapter can be found on ExpertConsult.com.**

# 36 Primary and Secondary Amenorrhea and Precocious Puberty

*Roger A. Lobo*

KEY POINTS

- Primary amenorrhea is diagnosed if no menstrual function has occurred by age 15, or 5 years after initial breast development.
- Menarche is delayed approximately 0.4 year for each year of premenarchal athletic training.
- Gonadal failure is the most common cause of primary amenorrhea, accounting for almost 50% of patients with this disorder.
- Individuals with gonadal failure should have a peripheral karyotype obtained to determine whether a Y chromosome is present. If it is present, or if there are signs of hyperandrogenism, the gonads should be removed to prevent the development of malignancy.
- Amenorrhea with low estrogen levels is associated with decreased bone density.
- If signs of pubertal progression (precocious puberty) are present in a girl, a workup is warranted by the age of 8 years.
- The two primary concerns of parents of children with precocious puberty are the social stigma associated with the child being physically different from her peers and the diminished ultimate height caused by the premature closure of epiphyseal centers.
- The exact cause of the majority of cases of GnRH-dependent (true or central) precocious puberty is unknown; however, approximately 30% of cases are secondary to central nervous system disease.
- The most common cause of gonadotropin-releasing hormone–independent precocious puberty is a functioning ovarian tumor. Granulosa cell tumors are the most common type accounting for 60% of neoplasms.

## PRIMARY AND SECONDAY AMENORRHEA

**Amenorrhea** is defined as the absence of menstrual bleeding and may be primary (never occurring) or secondary (cessation sometime after initiation).

**Primary amenorrhea** is defined as the absence of menses in a **woman who has never menstruated by the age of 15 years** (Practice Committee of the American Society for Reproductive Medicine, 2008.) Another definition includes girls who have not menstruated within 5 years of breast development, if occurring by age 10. **Breast development (thelarche) should occur by age 13** or otherwise requires evaluation as well. The incidence of primary amenorrhea is less than 0.1%. **Secondary amenorrhea** is defined as the absence of menses for an arbitrary period, usually longer than 6 to 12 months. The incidence of secondary amenorrhea of more than 6 months' duration in a survey of a general population of Swedish women of reproductive age was found to be 0.7% but has been cited to be as high as 3% (Practice Committee of the American Society for Reproductive Medicine, 2008). The incidence is significantly higher in women younger than 25 years and those with a history of menstrual irregularity.

Outside the United States, it is common to see women who have been categorized according to the World Health Organization (WHO) classification. ***WHO type I* usually refers to women with low estrogen levels and low follicle-stimulating hormone (FSH) and normal prolactin (PRL) levels without central nervous system (CNS) lesions; *type II* refers to a normal estrogen status with normal FSH and PRL levels; *WHO type III* refers to low estrogen levels and a high FSH level, denoting ovarian failure.**

## PHYSIOLOGY LEADING UP TO MENARCHE

Before the onset of menses, the normal female goes through a progressive series of morphologic changes produced by the pubertal increase in estrogen and androgen production. In 1969 Marshall and Tanner defined five stages of breast development and pubic hair development (Carel, 2008; Marshall, 1969) (Fig. 36.1; Table 36.1). These changes sometimes are combined and called ***Tanner*, or *pubertal*, stages 1 through 5**. The first sign of puberty is usually the appearance of breast budding, followed within a few months by the appearance of pubic hair.

Thereafter the breasts enlarge, the external pelvic contour becomes rounder, and the most rapid rate of growth occurs (peak height velocity). These changes precede menarche. Thus breast budding is the earliest sign of puberty and menarche the latest. The mean ages of occurrence of these events in American women are shown in Table 36.2 and the mean intervals (with standard deviation [SD]) between the initiation of breast budding and other pubertal events are shown in Table 36.3 (Frisch, 1971). The mean interval between breast budding and menarche is 2.3 years, with an SD of approximately 1 year. Some individuals can progress from breast budding to menarche in 18 months, and others may take 5 years. As stated previously, **if thelarche has not occurred by age 13, a diagnostic evaluation should be performed.**

The mean time of onset of menarche was previously thought to occur when a critical body weight of approximately 48 kg (106 lb) was reached; however, **it is now believed that body composition is more important than total body weight in determining the time of onset of puberty** and menstruation. Thus the ratio of fat to both total body weight and lean body weight is probably the most relevant factor that determines the time of onset of puberty and menstruation. Individuals who are moderately obese, between 20% and 30% more than the ideal body weight, have an earlier onset of menarche than women who are not obese. Malnutrition, such as occurs with **anorexia nervosa** or starvation, is known to delay the onset of puberty.

One of the major links between body composition and the hypothalamic-pituitary-ovarian (HPO) axis, and thus menstrual cyclicity, is the adipocyte hormone **leptin**. Leptin is produced by adipocytes and correlates well with body weight. **Leptin is also important for feedback involving gonadotropin-releasing hormone (GnRH) and luteinizing hormone (LH) pulsatility** and also binds to specific receptor sites on the ovary and

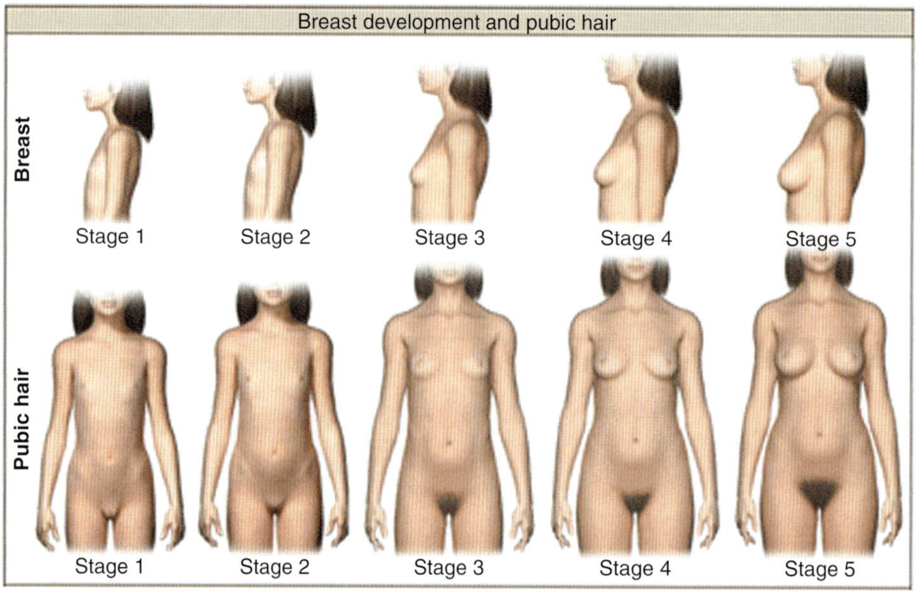


**Fig. 36.1** Pubertal rating according to Tanner stage. *Top row,* Breast development in girls is rated from 1 (prepubertal) to 5 (adult). Stage 2 breast development (appearance of the breast bud) marks the onset of gonadarche. *Bottom row,* For girls, pubic hair stages are rated from 1 (prepubertal) to 5 (adult). Stage 2 marks the onset of adrenarche. (From Herring JA. *Tachdjian's Pediatric Orthopedics: From the Texas Scottish Rite Hospital for Children.* 5th ed. Philadelphia: Elsevier; 2014.)

**TABLE 36.1** Classification of Breast Growth and Pubic Hair Growth

| Classification | Description |
|---|---|
| **Breast Growth** | |
| B1 | Prepubertal: elevation of papilla only |
| B2 | Breast budding |
| B3 | Enlargement of breasts with glandular tissue, without separation of breast contours |
| B4 | Secondary mound formed by areola |
| B5 | Single contour of breast and areola |
| **Pubic Hair Growth** | |
| PH1 | Prepubertal—no pubic hair |
| PH2 | Labial hair present |
| PH3 | Labial hair spreads over mons pubis |
| PH4 | Slight lateral spread |
| PH5 | Further lateral spread to form inverse triangle and reach medial thighs |

**TABLE 36.2** Mean Ages of Girls at the Onset of Pubertal Events (United States)

| Event | Mean Age ± SD (yr) |
|---|---|
| Initiation of breast development | 10.8 ± 1.10 |
| Appearance of pubic hair | 11.0 ± 1.21 |
| Menarche | 12.9 ± 1.20 |

Modified from Frisch RE, Revelle R. Height and weight in menarche and a hypothesis of menarche. *Arch Dis Child.* 1971;46:695.
*SD,* Standard deviation.

**TABLE 36.3** Pubertal Intervals

| Interval | Mean Age ± SD (yr) |
|---|---|
| B2—peak height velocity | 1.0 ± 0.77 |
| B2—menarche | 2.3 ± 1.03 |
| B2-PH2 | 3.1 ± 1.04 |
| B2-B5 (average duration of puberty) | 4.5 ± 2.04 |

Modified from Frisch RE, Revelle R. Height and weight in menarche and a hypothesis of menarche. *Arch Dis Child.* 1971;46:695.
*B2,* Initiation of breast development; *PH2,* appearance of pubic hair; *SD,* standard deviation.

endometrium. Leptin administration has been shown to affect LH pulsatile activity (Laughlin, 1997) and to restore cyclicity in women with amenorrhea. Another hormone, a gastric peptide, ghrelin, interacts with leptin in this regard particularly when menstrual function is perturbed (Schneider, 2006).

Body weight and body fat content have been shown to be important for menstruation; a fatness nomogram is depicted in Fig. 36.2 (Frisch, 1971). Well-nourished individuals with prepubertal strenuous exercise programs resulting in less total body fat have also been shown to have a delayed onset of puberty. Warren and colleagues have reported that ballet dancers, swimmers, and runners have menarche delayed to approximately age 15 if they began exercising strenuously before menarche (Warren, 1980) (Fig. 36.3). It is greater in those athletic activities requiring lower body weight and where success is more subjective (ballet, gymnastics) compared with swimming. It was also determined that stress per se is not the cause of the **delayed menarche** in these exercising girls, because girls of the same age with stressful musical careers did not have a delayed onset of menarche (Warren, 1980). Young women with strenuous exercise programs have sufficient

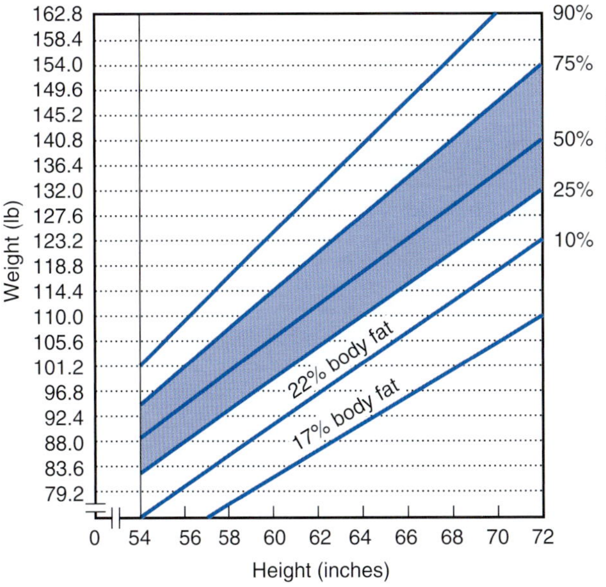


**Fig. 36.2** Fatness index nomogram. (Modified from Frisch RE, Revelle R. Height and weight in menarche and a hypothesis of menarche. *Arch Dis Child.* 1971;46:695.)

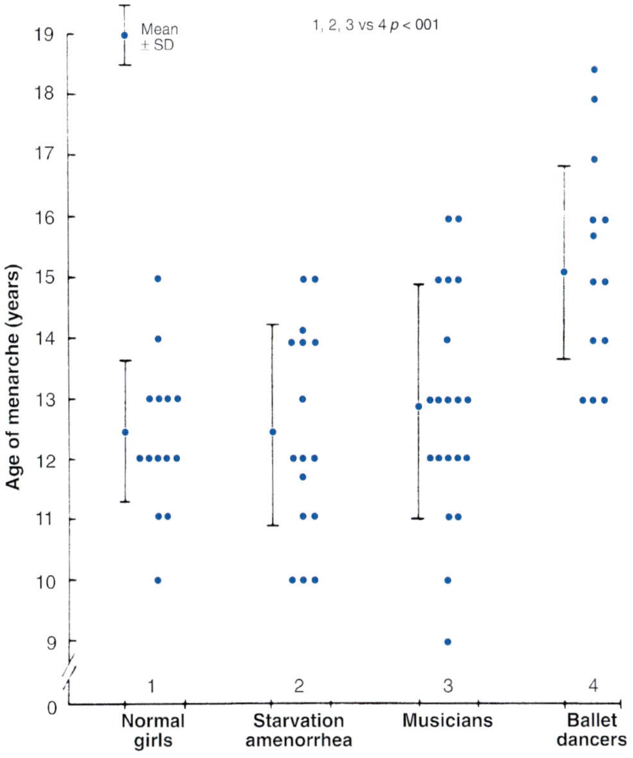


**Fig. 36.3** Ages of menarche in ballet dancers compared with those of three other groups. *SD,* Standard deviation. (From Warren MP. The effects of exercise on pubertal progression and reproductive function in girls. *J Clin Endocrinol Metab.* 1980;51:1150.)

estrogen to produce some breast development and thus do not need extensive endocrinologic evaluation if concern arises about the lack of onset of menses. Frisch and coworkers have reported that for girls engaged in premenarchal athletic training, menarche is delayed 0.4 year for each year of training. Individuals who exercise strenuously should be counseled that they will usually have a delayed onset of menses, but it is not a health problem. They should be told that they will most likely have regular ovulatory cycles when they stop exercising or become older.

The metabolic features of amenorrheic athletes, who are considered to be in a state of negative energy balance, are fairly characteristic. These include elevated serum FSH and insulin-like growth factor-binding protein 1 (IGFBP-1) and lowered insulin-like growth factor (IGF) levels.

**Emotional stress can lead to inhibition of the GnRH axis.** The mechanism involves an increased secretion of corticotropin-releasing hormone (CRH), releasing adrenocorticotropic hormone (ACTH), opioid peptides such as beta-endorphin, and cortisol. CRH itself is known to inhibit GnRH.

Before puberty, circulating levels of LH and FSH are low, with an FSH/LH ratio greater than 1. The CNS-hypothalamic axis is extremely sensitive to the negative feedback effects of low levels of circulating estrogen. As the critical weight or body composition is approached, the CNS-hypothalamic axis becomes less sensitive to the negative effect of estrogen and GnRH is secreted in greater amounts, causing an increase in LH and, to a lesser extent, FSH levels. This release from the prepubertal "brake" on GnRH secretion is depicted in Fig. 36.4, which also illustrates the integral role of **neuropeptides such as kisspeptin** (Terasawa, 2013). The initial endocrinologic change associated with the onset of puberty is the occurrence of episodic pulses of LH during sleep (Boyar, 1974) (Fig. 36.5). These pulses are absent before the onset of puberty. After menarche, the episodic secretions of LH occur during sleep and while awake. The last endocrinologic event of puberty is activation of the positive gonadotropin response to increasing levels of estradiol ($E_2$), which results in the midcycle gonadotropic surge and ovulation.

## PRIMARY AMENORRHEA

### Causes

Although numerous classifications have been used for the various causes of primary amenorrhea, it has been found useful to group causes on the basis of whether secondary sexual characteristics (breasts) and female internal genitalia (uterus) are present or absent (Box 36.1). Thus the findings on a physical examination can alert the clinician to possible causes and indicate which laboratory tests should be performed. In a series of 62 individuals reported by Mashchak, the largest subgroup with primary amenorrhea (29; 47%) were individuals in whom breasts were absent but where a uterus was present; the second largest subgroup (22; 35%) had both breasts and a uterus; lack of a uterus together with breast development accounted for the third largest category (9; 14.5%); and individuals without breasts or a uterus were the least common (2; <1%) (Mashchak, 1981). This breakdown of the various accompanying conditions of primary amenorrhea reflects the referral pattern to the center. In one study, a "physiologic delay" occurring in 14% and polycystic ovary syndrome (PCOS) in 7% (Reindollar, 1981).

#### Breasts Absent and Uterus Present

It would seem logical, because breast development is a biomarker of ovarian estrogen production, that individuals with no breast development and a uterus present have no estrogen production. This is either the result of a primary ovarian disorder or an abnormality of the CNS hypothalamic–pituitary axis, which provides the normal signal to the ovary. The phenotype of individuals with either of these causes of low estrogen status is similar.

**Gonadal Failure (Hypergonadotropic Hypogonadism)**

**Failure of gonadal development is the most common cause of primary amenorrhea,** occurring in almost 50% of those with this

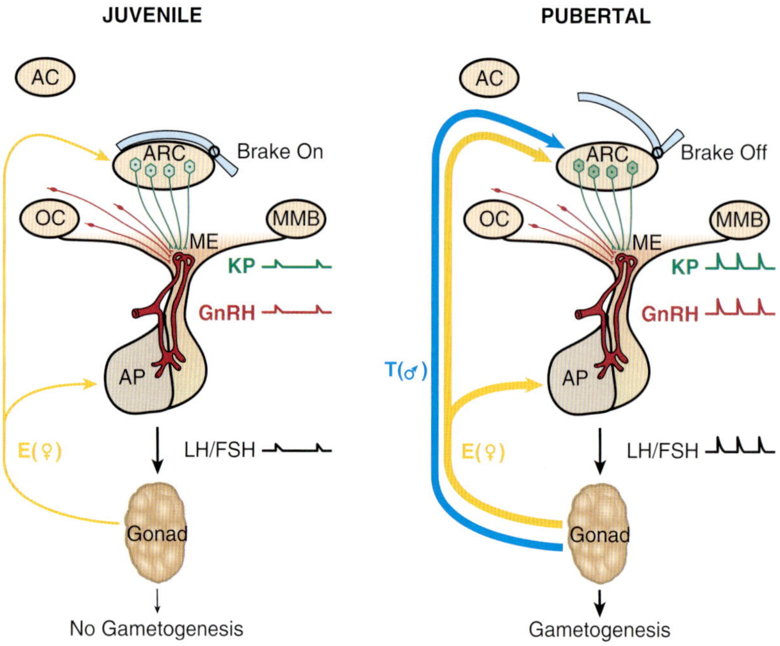


**Fig. 36.4** A model for the control of the timing of puberty. The figure depicts the key role of kisspeptin (KP) signaling in generating GnRH release. In the juvenile state *(left panel)* a physiologic "brake" is operational, and in the pubertal state *(right panel)* the "brake" is off, allowing for kisspeptin and GnRH release and a fully integrated negative feedback system for testosterone *(blue)* in the male or estradiol *(gold)* in the female. *AC,* anterior commissure; *AP,* anterior pituitary; *ARC,* arcuate nucleus; *E,* estradiol; *FSH,* follicle-stimulating hormone; *GnRH,* gonadotropin-releasing hormone; *LH,* luteinizing hormone; *ME,* median eminence; *MMB,* mammillary body; *OC,* optic chiasm; *T,* testosterone. (Modified from Terasawa E, Guerrier KA, Plant TM. Kisspeptin and puberty in mammals. In: Kauffman AS, Smith JT, eds. *Kisspeptin Signaling in Reproductive Biology.* New York: Springer; 2013:253.)

symptom. **Gonadal failure** is most commonly caused by a chromosomal disorder or deletion of all or part of an X chromosome, but it is sometimes caused by another chromosomal genetic defect and, rarely, defective CYP-17 leading to 17α-hydroxylase deficiency. The chromosomal disorders are usually caused by a random meiotic or mitotic abnormality (e.g., nondisjunction, anaphase lag) and thus are not inherited; however, if gonadal development is absent in the presence of a 46,XX (called **pure gonadal dysgenesis**), a gene disorder may be present, because it has been reported to occur in siblings. Reindollar reported that all individuals with gonadal failure and an X chromosome abnormality were shorter than 63 inches in height (Reindollar, 1981). Approximately one-third also had major cardiovascular or renal anomalies.

Deletion of the entire X chromosome (as occurs in Turner syndrome) or of the short arm (p) of the X chromosome results in short stature. Deletions of only the long arm (q) usually do not affect height. In place of the ovary a band of fibrous tissue called a **gonadal streak** is present (Federman, 1967) (Fig. 36.6). When ovarian follicles are absent, synthesis of ovarian steroids and inhibin does not occur. Breast development does not occur because of the low circulating $E_2$ levels. Because the negative hypothalamic-pituitary action of estrogen and inhibin is not present, gonadotropin levels are markedly elevated, with FSH levels being higher than LH. Estrogen is not necessary for müllerian duct development or wolffian duct regression, so the internal and external genitalia are phenotypically female.

An occasional individual with mosaicism, an abnormal X chromosome, pure gonadal dysgenesis (46,XX), or even Turner syndrome (45,X) may have a few follicles that develop under endogenous gonadotropin stimulation early in puberty and may synthesize enough estrogen to induce breast development and a few episodes of uterine bleeding, resulting early in **premature ovarian failure**, usually before age 25. Rarely, ovulation and pregnancy can occur.

Goldenberg reported that all individuals with primary amenorrhea and plasma FSH levels higher than 40 mIU/mL have no functioning ovarian follicles in the gonadal tissue. Thus in women with primary amenorrhea, the diagnosis of gonadal failure can be established if the FSH levels are consistently elevated, without requiring ovarian tissue evaluation.

### 45,X and Related Abnormalities

**Turner syndrome occurs in approximately 1 per 2000 to 3000 live births but is much more common in abortuses.** In addition to primary amenorrhea and absent breast development, these individuals have other somatic abnormalities, the most prevalent being short stature (<60 inches in height), webbing of the neck, a short fourth metacarpal, and cubitus valgus. Cardiac abnormality, renal abnormalities, and hypothyroidism are also more prevalent.

A wide variety of chromosomal mosaics are associated with primary amenorrhea and normal female external genitalia, the most common being X/XX. In addition, individuals with X/XXX and X/XX/XXX mosaicism have primary amenorrhea. These individuals are generally taller and have fewer anatomic abnormalities than individuals with a 45,X karyotype. In addition, some of them may have a few gonadal follicles and approximately 20% have sufficient estrogen production to menstruate. Occasionally, ovulation may occur, as stated earlier. Isolated phenotypic features of Turner syndrome (without gonadal failure) may also occur in males and is known as *Noonan syndrome.*

### Structurally Abnormal X Chromosome

Although individuals with this disorder have a 46,XX karyotype, part of one X chromosome is structurally abnormal. If there is deletion of the long arm of the X chromosome (Xq), normal height has been reported to occur, but, in Reindollar's series,

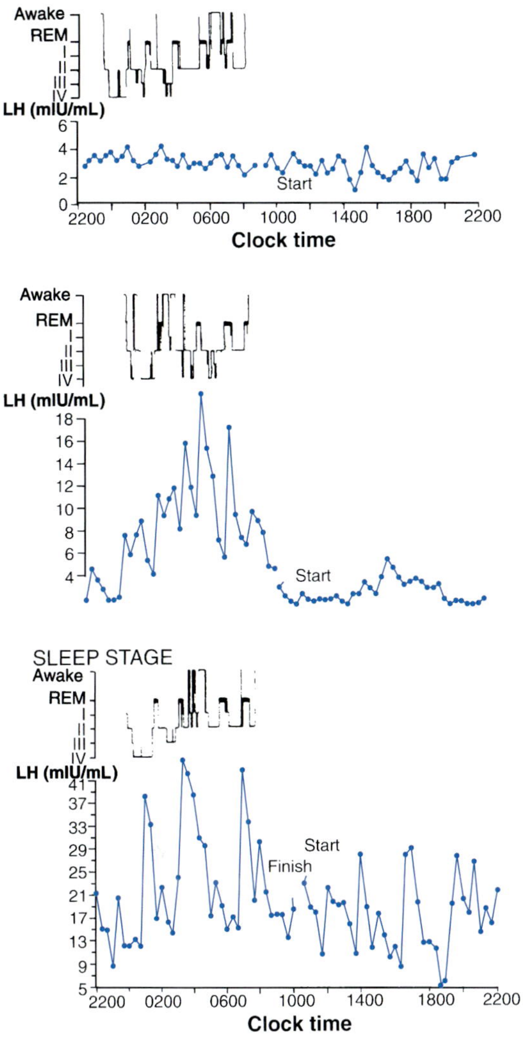


**Fig. 36.5** Plasma luteinizing hormone (LH) concentration measured every 20 minutes for 24 hours in normal prepubertal girl *(upper panel),* early pubertal girl *(center panel),* and normal late pubertal girl *(lower panel).* In top and center panels, sleep histogram is shown above period of nocturnal sleep. Sleep stages are awake, rapid eye movement (REM), and stages I to IV by depth of line graph. Plasma LH concentrations are expressed as mIU/mL. (Modified from Boyar RM, Katz J, Finkelstein JW, et al. Anorexia nervosa: immaturity of the 24-hour luteinizing hormone secretory pattern. *N Engl J Med.* 1974;291:861.)

these individuals were all relatively short (Reindollar, 1981). They have no somatic abnormalities; however, if there is deletion of the short arm of the X chromosome (Xp), the individual will be short. A similar phenotype occurs in those with isochromosome of the long arm of the X chromosome. Other X chromosome abnormalities include a ring X and minute fragmentation of the X chromosome.

### *Pure Gonadal Dysgenesis (46,XX and 46,XY With Gonadal Streaks)*

As noted, this abnormality may have a familial/genetic association and has been reported in siblings. Abnormalities in genes involved in gonadal development are expected to be involved. These individuals have normal stature and phenotype, absence of secondary sexual characteristics, and primary amenorrhea. Some of these women have a few ovarian follicles, develop breasts, and may even menstruate spontaneously for a few years.

**BOX 36.1** Classification of Disorders With Primary Amenorrhea and Normal Female Genitalia

**I ABSENT BREAST DEVELOPMENT; UTERUS PRESENT**

A. Gonadal failure
   1. 45,X (Turner syndrome)
   2. 46,X, abnormal X (e.g., short- or long-arm deletion)
   3. Mosaicism (e.g., X/XX, X/XX,XXX)
   4. 46,XX or 46,XY pure gonadal dysgenesis
   5. 17α-hydroxylase deficiency with 46,XX
B. Hypothalamic failure secondary to inadequate GnRH release
   1. Insufficient GnRH secretion because of neurotransmitter defect
   2. Inadequate GnRH synthesis (Kallmann syndrome)
   3. Congenital anatomic defect in central nervous system
   4. CNS neoplasm (craniopharyngioma)
C. Pituitary failure
   1. Isolated gonadotrophin insufficiency (thalassemia major, retinitis pigmentosa)
   2. Pituitary neoplasia (chromophobe adenoma)
   3. Mumps, encephalitis
   4. Newborn kernicterus
   5. Prepubertal hypothyroidism

**II BREAST DEVELOPMENT; UTERUS ABSENT**

A. Androgen resistance (testicular feminization)
B. Congenital absence of uterus (uterovaginal agenesis)

**III ABSENT BREAST DEVELOPMENT; UTERUS ABSENT**

A. 17,20-desmolase deficiency
B. Agonadism
C. 17α-hydroxylase deficiency with 46,XY karyotype

**IV BREAST DEVELOPMENT; UTERUS PRESENT**

A. Hypothalamic cause
B. Pituitary cause
C. Ovarian cause
D. Uterine cause

*CNS,* Central nervous system; *GnRH,* gonadotropin-releasing hormone.

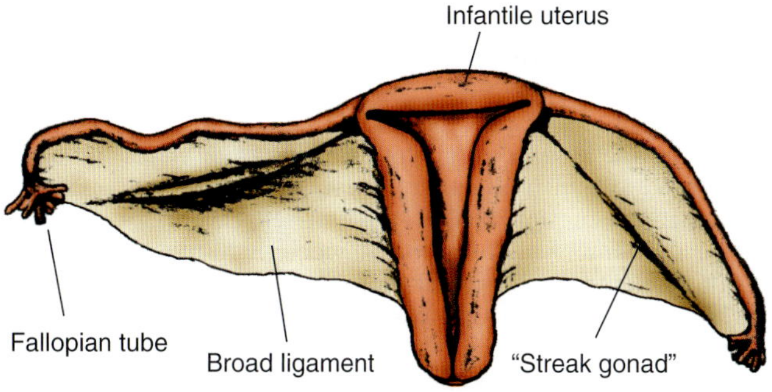


**Fig. 36.6** Internal genitalia of patient with gonadal dysgenesis (Turner syndrome), featuring normal but infantile uterus, normal fallopian tubes, and pale, glistening streak gonads in both broad ligaments. (From Federman DD. Disorders of gonadal development: gonadal dysgenesis [Turner syndrome]. In: Federman DD, ed. *Abnormal Sexual Development: A Genetic and Endocrine Approach to Differential Diagnosis.* Philadelphia: WB Saunders; 1967.)

**46,XY gonadal dysgenesis** is the result of an abnormal testis in utero. There can be incomplete forms with some degree of testicular tissue, but in this context the "pure" form as a dysgenetic streak as in other forms of ovarian dysgenesis and previously has been referred to as **Swyer syndrome.**

If a Y chromosome is present (as in 46,XY gonadal dysgenesis) or is found as part of a mosaic karyotype, with or without any clinical signs of androgenization, gonadectomy should be performed.

*17α-Hydroxylase Deficiency with 46,XX Karyotype*

A rare gonadal cause of primary amenorrhea without breast development and normal female internal genitalia is deficiency of the enzyme 17α-hydroxylase (P450 CYP-17) in an individual with a 46,XX karyotype (it can also occur in genetic males 46,XY), who may present in a similar fashion. Only a few such individuals have been described in the literature, but it is important for the clinician to be aware of this entity because, in contrast to those described earlier, these individuals have hypernatremia and hypokalemia. Because of decreased cortisol, ACTH levels are elevated. The mineralocorticoid levels are also elevated, because 17α-hydroxylase is not necessary for the conversion of progesterone to deoxycortisol or corticosterone. **Thus there is excessive sodium retention and potassium excretion, leading to hypertension and hypokalemia.** Serum progesterone levels are also elevated because progesterone is not converted to cortisol. In addition to sex steroid replacement, these individuals need cortisol administration. They usually have cystic ovaries and viable oocytes. Pregnancies have been documented after in vitro fertilization–embryo transfer (IVF-ET), despite low levels of endogenous sex steroids.

### Genetic Disorders with Hyperandrogenism

Hyperandrogenism occurs in approximately 10% of women with gonadal dysgenesis. Most have a Y chromosome or fragment of a Y chromosome, but some may only have a DNA fragment that contains the testes-determining gene (probably *SRY*) without a full Y chromosome. **Those with hypergonadotropic hypogonadism and a female phenotype who have any clinical manifestation of hyperandrogenism, such as hirsutism, should have a gonadectomy**, even if a Y chromosome is not present, because gonadal neoplasms are common.

### CNS-Hypothalamic-Pituitary Disorders

With CNS-hypothalamic-pituitary disorders, the low estrogen levels are caused by an abnormal or absent signal to the ovary, resulting in very low circulating gonadotropin levels. The cause of low gonadotropin production may be morphologic or endocrinologic.

*CNS Lesions*

Any anatomic lesion of the hypothalamus or pituitary can cause low gonadotropin production. These lesions can be congenital (e.g., stenosis of aqueduct, absence of sellar floor) or acquired (tumors). Many of these lesions, particularly pituitary adenomas, result in elevated PRL levels (see Chapter 37); however, non–PRL-secreting pituitary tumors (**chromophobe adenomas**) and craniopharyngiomas may not be associated with hyperprolactinemia and can rarely be the cause of primary amenorrhea with low gonadotropin levels. Thus all individuals with primary amenorrhea and low gonadotropin levels, with or without an elevated PRL level, should have computed tomography (CT) scanning or magnetic resonance imaging (MRI) of the hypothalamic-pituitary region to rule out the presence of a lesion.

*Inadequate GnRH Release (Hypogonadotropic Hypogonadism)*

Those without a demonstrable lesion and a low gonadotropin level were previously thought to have primary pituitary failure (**hypogonadotropic hypogonadism**); however, when they are stimulated with GnRH, there is an increase in FSH and LH levels, indicating that **the basic defect is primarily hypothalamic with insufficient GnRH synthesis or a CNS neurotransmitter defect**, resulting in inadequate GnRH synthesis, release, or both. This can also be the result of abnormal kisspeptin, as noted earlier. Although a single bolus of GnRH may not initially cause a rise in gonadotropin level in these individuals, after 4 days of GnRH administration (priming), the women will have a rise in gonadotropin levels after a single GnRH bolus. Because GnRH secretion occurs after migration of these specific cells from the olfactory lobe to the hypothesis during embryogenesis, anosmia may also occur in some patients with gonadotropin deficiency. This is caused by a specific defect of the *KAL* gene (Xp 22-3), which is responsible for neuronal migration. Other genetic defects resulting in gonadotropic deficiency may occur on the X chromosome or autosomes and include *FGFR1*, *PROKR2*, and *GNRHR* (Caronia, 2011) as well as loss of function mutations in the kisspeptin-1 receptor.

Females with Kallmann syndrome and related forms of gonadotropic deficiency have normal height and an increase in growth of long bones, resulting in a greater wingspan-to-height ratio. Men affected by gonadotropic deficiency have hypogonadism, an increased wingspan-to-height ratio, and altered spatial orientation abilities. Anosmia in Kallmann syndrome must be tested for by blinded testing of certain characteristic smells, such as coffee, cocoa, or orange. Not all women in this category of GnRH deficiency states will have anosmia, which is specific for some patients with Kallmann syndrome.

There is a tendency for GnRH deficiency to be familial/inherited through a variety of mechanisms, although the majority of cases, more than two-thirds, are sporadic.

*Isolated Gonadotropin Deficiency (Pituitary Disease)*

Rarely, individuals with primary amenorrhea and low gonadotropin levels do not respond to GnRH, even after 4 days of administration. This is known as **isolated gonadotropin deficiency**. They almost always have an associated disorder such as thalassemia major (with iron deposits in the pituitary) or retinitis pigmentosa. Occasionally this pituitary abnormality has been associated with prepubertal hypothyroidism, kernicterus, or mumps encephalitis.

*Estrogen Resistance*

This rare condition was first described in men and now has been described in a woman (breast absent, uterus present). A mutation in estrogen receptor alpha (ERα) does not allow estrogen signaling or a biologic response to estrogen action. Endogenous estrogen levels are high, gonadotropins are higher than the normal range (to try to provoke an estrogen response), and the ovaries are cystic. Exogenous estrogen does not normally induce changes except minimal changes with high pharmacologic doses (Quaynor, 2013).

## Breast Development Present and Uterus Absent

Two disorders present with primary amenorrhea associated with normal breast development and the absence of a uterus: androgen resistance and congenital absence of the uterus. The former is a genetically inherited disorder, whereas the latter is an accident of development and does not have an established pattern of inheritance.

### Androgen Resistance

**Androgen resistance syndrome**, originally termed testicular feminization, is a genetically transmitted disorder in which androgen receptor synthesis or action does not occur. It is rare, with an incidence of 1 in 60,000. The syndrome is caused by the absence of an X-chromosome gene responsible for cytoplasmic or nuclear testosterone receptor function. It is an X-linked recessive or sex-linked autosomal dominant disorder, with transmission through the mother. These individuals have an XY karyotype and normally functioning male gonads that produce normal male levels of testosterone and dihydrotestosterone; however, **because of a lack of receptors in target organs, there is lack of male differentiation**

**of the external and internal genitalia** (Gustafson, 1994). The external genitalia remain feminine, as occurs in the absence of sex steroids. Wolffian duct development, which normally occurs as a result of testosterone stimulation, fails to take place. Because müllerian duct regression is induced by antimüllerian hormone (AMH), also called *müllerian-inhibiting substance* (MIS, a glycoprotein synthesized by the Sertoli cells of the fetal testes), this process occurs normally in these individuals because steroid receptors are unnecessary for the action of glycoproteins. Thus women with this disorder have no female or male internal genitalia, normal female external genitalia, and a short or absent vagina. Pubic hair and axillary hair are absent or scanty as a result of a lack of androgenic receptors, but breast development is normal or enhanced. It is known that testosterone is responsible for inhibiting breast proliferation. Thus with androgen resistance, the absence of androgen action allows even low levels of estrogen to cause unabated breast stimulation. Estrogen levels here are in the normal male range, and LH is slightly elevated.

Testes that are intraabdominal or that occur in the inguinal canal have **an increased risk of developing a malignancy (gonadoblastoma or dysgerminoma)**, with an incidence reported to be approximately 20%; however, these malignancies rarely occur before age 20. Therefore it is usually recommended that the gonads be left in place until after puberty is completed to allow full breast development and epiphyseal closure to occur. After these events occur, which is typically around age 18, the gonads should be removed. It is recommended that those with androgen resistance be informed that they have an abnormal sex chromosome, without specifically mentioning a Y chromosome, because it is widely known that an XY karyotype indicates maleness; however, some families choose to have full disclosure and a complete understanding of the abnormality. In addition, because psychologically and phenotypically these individuals are female and have been raised as such, the term *gonads* should be used instead of *testes*. These individuals should also be informed that they can never become pregnant because they do not have a uterus and that their gonads must be removed after age 18 because of their high potential for malignancy.

#### Congenital Absence of the Uterus (Uterine Agenesis, Uterovaginal Agenesis, Mayer-Rokitansky-Küster-Hauser Syndrome)

The *Hox* genes are important for uterine development, and mutations (e.g., in *HOXA13*) have been found in genetic syndromes that include uterine abnormalities (e.g., hand-foot-genital and Guttmacher syndromes) and also in cases of bicornuate uterus. To date, however, no abnormalities have been found in cases of congenital absence of the uterus.

Congenital absence of the uterus is the **second most common cause of primary amenorrhea**. It occurs in 1 in 4000 to 5000 female births and accounts for approximately 15% of individuals with primary amenorrhea. Individuals with complete uterine agenesis have normal ovaries, with regular cyclic ovulation and normal endocrine function. Women with this disorder have normal breast and pubic and axillary hair development but have a shortened or absent vagina, in addition to absence of the uterus (Jones, 1971) (Fig. 36.7). Although often there are no bulbous structures, but merely streaklike tissue, in 7% to 10% of cases there are two nonfused rudimentary horns as in the figure. **On occasion one or both horns may have some functioning endometrium**. In this setting of obstructed outflow, cyclic pelvic pain, which may be severe at times, may be encountered. Congenital renal abnormalities occur in approximately one-third of these individuals and skeletal abnormalities in approximately 12%. Cardiac and other congenital abnormalities also occur with increased frequency. Occasional defects in the bones of the middle ear can also occur, resulting in some degree of deafness. The overwhelming majority of these disorders are caused by an isolated developmental defect, but on occasion the condition is genetically inherited. It is usually easy to differentiate these individuals from those with androgen resistance by the presence of normal pubic hair, but some with incomplete androgen resistance have some pubic hair.

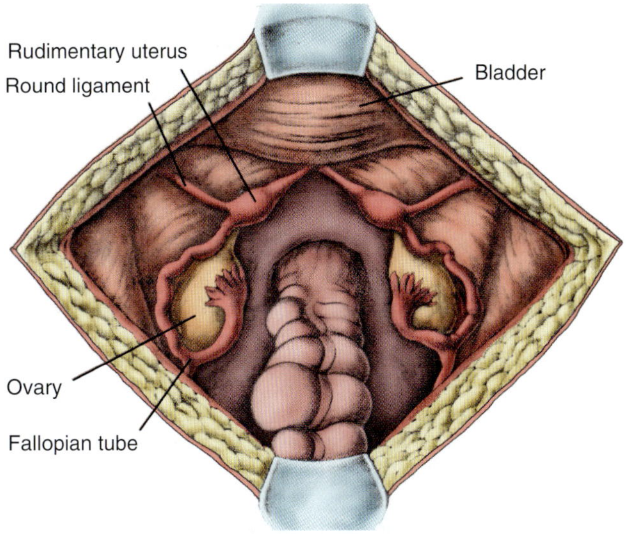


**Fig. 36.7** Congenital absence of vagina. Laparotomy revealed rudimentary uterus that showed evidence of failure of fusion of müllerian ducts. This is a common finding in this condition and indicates that the disorder is more extensive than simple anomaly of the vagina. (Modified from Jones HW Jr, Scott WW, eds. *Hermaphroditism, Genital Anomalies and Related Endocrine Disorders.* 2nd ed. Baltimore: Williams & Wilkins; 1971.)

Women in this category are normal endocrinologically and have been able to have children using a surrogate or gestational carrier. A woman underwent a uterine transplantation from a donated postmenopausal uterus and was able to have a live birth (Brännström, 2015).

### Absent Breast and Uterine Development

Individuals with no breast or uterine development are rare. They usually have a male karyotype, elevated gonadotropin levels, and testosterone levels in the normal or below-normal female range. The differential diagnosis for this phenotype includes deficiencies in CYP17 (17α-hydroxylase deficiency/17,20-desmolase deficiency) and agonadism (Mashchak, 1981). Individuals with predominant deficiency in ***17α***- hydroxlase activity have testes present but lack the enzyme necessary to synthesize sex steroids and thus have female external genitalia. Because they have testes, AMH is produced and the female internal genitalia regress; with low testosterone levels, the male internal genitalia do not develop. Insufficient estrogen is synthesized to develop breasts. A similar lack of sex steroid synthesis occurs in males with a ***17,20-desmolase*** deficiency.

Individuals with ***agonadism***, sometimes called the *vanishing testes syndrome*, have no gonads present, but because the female internal genitalia are also absent, it has been postulated that testicular AMH-MIS production occurred during fetal life but the gonadal tissue subsequently regressed.

### Secondary Sex Characteristics (Breasts) Present and Female Internal Genitalia (Uterus) Present

Individuals with secondary sex characteristics and female internal genitalia present are the second largest category of individuals with primary amenorrhea, accounting for approximately one-third of them. In the series reported by Mashchak, approximately 25% of these individuals had hyperprolactinemia and prolactinomas (Mashchak, 1981). The remaining women had profiles similar to those with secondary amenorrhea, including PCOS, and thus should be subcategorized and treated similarly as women with secondary amenorrhea, which will be discussed later.

### Primary Amenorrhea With Absent Endometrium

Primary amenorrhea with absent endometrium is a rare condition in this category of primary amenorrhea with uterus and breast present. Endocrine function is completely normal, as are the uterus, ovaries, and fallopian tubes; however, in two reported cases the endometrium was found to be absent, after repeated biopsies (Berker, 2008; Nigam, 2014). It is likely that some genetic defect is responsible for this rare finding, but the reported association of a translocation between chromosomes 4 and 20 (Nigam, 2014) is unlikely to be the cause.

## Differential Diagnosis and Management

After a history is obtained and a physical examination performed, including measurement of height, span, and weight, those with primary amenorrhea can be grouped into one of the four general categories listed in Box 36.1, depending on the presence or absence of breasts and a uterus. If breasts are absent but a uterus is present, the diagnostic evaluation should differentiate between CNS-hypothalamic-pituitary disorders and failure of normal gonadal development. Although individuals with both these disorders have similar phenotypes because of low $E_2$ levels, a single serum FSH assay can differentiate between these two major diagnostic categories (Mashchak, 1981) (Fig. 36.8). Women with hypergonadotropic hypogonadism (FSH > 40 mIU/mL), not those with hypogonadotropic hypogonadism, should have a peripheral white blood cell karyotype obtained to determine whether a Y chromosome is present. If a Y chromosome is present, the streak gonads should be excised. If a Y chromosome is absent, it is unnecessary to remove the gonads unless there are signs of hyperandrogenism. It is also unnecessary to perform a karyotype on the gonadal tissue to detect possible mosaicism with a Y chromosome in the gonad unless there is some evidence of hyperandrogenism.

All women with an elevated FSH level and an XX karyotype should have electrolyte and serum progesterone levels measured to rule out 17α-hydroxylase deficiency; a clue is if the patient is hypertensive. In addition to hypernatremia and hypokalemia, individuals with 17α-hydroxylase deficiency have an elevated serum progesterone level (>3 ng/mL), a low 17α-hydroxyprogesterone level (<0.2 ng/mL), and an elevated serum deoxycorticosterone level (>17 ng/100 mL) and usually have hypertension. Doses of conjugated equine estrogen (CEE) in the range of 0.625 mg or its equivalent are usually sufficient to cause breast proliferation. These rare individuals with 17α-hydroxylase deficiency need to have adequate cortisol replacement in addition to sex steroid treatment.

Women with ovarian failure or hypergonadotropic hypogonadism who wish to become pregnant may undergo egg donation. As long as the uterus is normal, which is usually the case, high pregnancy rates in the range of 60% to 70% per cycle may be expected. If the patient has Turner syndrome, cardiac evaluation is mandatory before pregnancy because of potential risks such as aortic dissection.

If the FSH level is low, the underlying disorder is in the CNS-hypothalamic-pituitary region and PRL should be determined. Even if the PRL level is not elevated, all women with hypogonadotropic hypogonadism should have a head CT scan or MRI to rule out a lesion. It is unnecessary to perform a karyotype because all those with hypogonadotropic hypogonadism are expected to be 46,XX. The use of GnRH testing is optional but is usually clinically unnecessary unless GnRH is going to be used

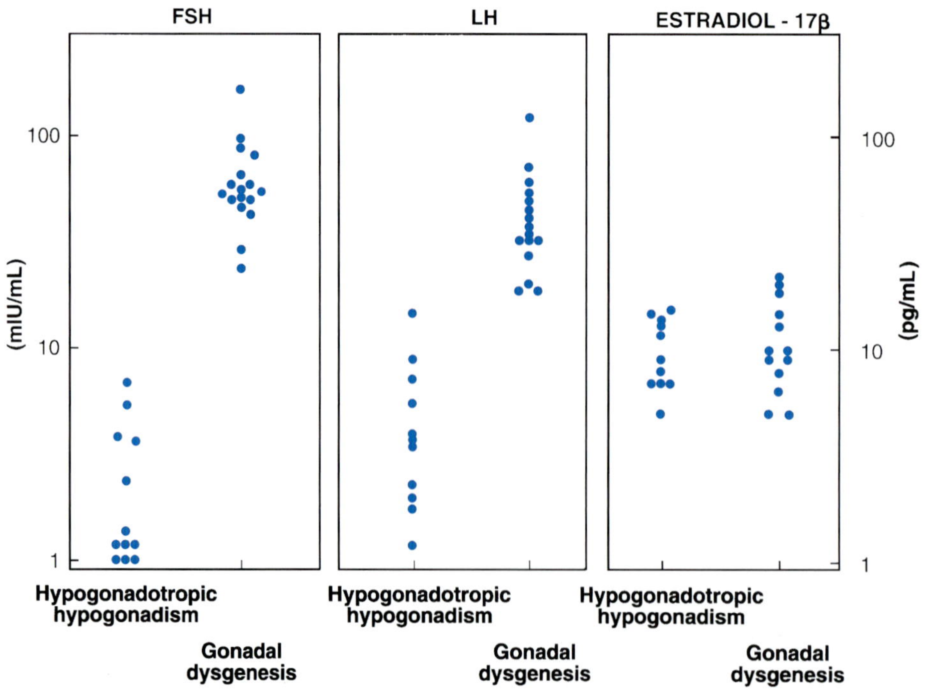


**Fig. 36.8** Levels of serum FSH, LH, and estradiol in patients with primary amenorrhea who have an intact uterus and no breast development. *FSH,* Follicle-stimulating hormone; *LH,* luteinizing hormone. (From Mashchak CA, Kletzky OA, Davajan V, et al. Clinical and laboratory evaluation of patients with primary amenorrhea. *Obstet Gynecol.* 1981;57:715.)

for ovulation induction. Ovulation can be induced in women with this disorder because their ovaries are normal. Initially they should receive estrogen-progestogen treatment to induce breast development and cause epiphyseal closure. When fertility is desired, human menopausal gonadotropins or pulsatile GnRH should be administered. Clomiphene citrate will be ineffective because of low endogenous $E_2$ levels.

The differential diagnosis of androgen resistance from uterine agenesis can easily be made by the presence in the latter condition of normal body hair, ovulatory and premenstrual-type symptoms, biphasic basal temperature, and a normal female testosterone level. Because women with uterine agenesis have normal female endocrine function, they do not require hormone therapy. A renal scan should be performed because of the high incidence of renal abnormalities. They may need surgical reconstruction of an absent vagina (McIndoe procedure), but progressive mechanical dilation with plastic dilators, as described by Frank, should be tried first and is usually successful in motivated individuals, particularly when using pressure from body weight, as with a bicycle seat. These women can now have their own genetic children. After ovarian stimulation and follicle aspiration, fertilized oocytes can be placed in the uterus of a surrogate recipient (gestational carrier). As noted earlier, a case report of a woman having a live birth after uterus transplantation has been reported (Brännström, 2015).

Individuals with androgen resistance have an XY karyotype and male levels of testosterone. After full breast development is attained and epiphyseal closure occurs, the gonads should be removed because of malignant potential. Thereafter, estrogen therapy should be administered. They do not need progestogen therapy in the absence of a uterus, and lower doses of estrogen are sufficient; typical menopause symptoms are usually not present.

The rare individuals without breast development and no internal genitalia should be referred to an endocrine center for the extensive evaluation necessary to establish the diagnosis. If gonads are present, they should be removed because a Y chromosome is present. Hormone therapy should be administered to these individuals.

## SECONDARY AMENORRHEA

### Causes

The symptom of amenorrhea associated with hyperprolactinemia or excessive androgen or cortisol production is not considered in this chapter because these disorders are discussed in Chapters 37, 38, and 39. If amenorrhea is present without galactorrhea, hyperprolactinemia, or hirsutism, the symptom can result from disorders in the CNS (hypothalamic-pituitary axis), ovary, or uterus. In a review of 262 patients presenting with secondary amenorrhea during a 20-year period at a tertiary medical center, Reindollar reported that 12% of cases resulted from a primary ovarian problem, 62% from a hypothalamic disorder, 16% from a pituitary problem (including prolactinomas), and 7% from a uterine disorder. The uterine cause of secondary amenorrhea is the only one in which normal endocrine function is present and is discussed first.

### Uterine Factor

**Intrauterine adhesions** (IUAs) or **synechiae** (Asherman syndrome) can obliterate the endometrial cavity and produce secondary amenorrhea. A pregnancy complication, prior instrumentation, or, rarely, endometrial tuberculosis can also cause endometrial damage with adhesion formation. **The most common antecedent factor of IUAs is endometrial curettage associated with pregnancy**—either evacuation of a live or dead fetus by mechanical means or postpartum or postabortal curettage. Curettage for a missed abortion results in a high incidence of IUA formation (30%). IUAs may also occur after diagnostic dilation and curettage

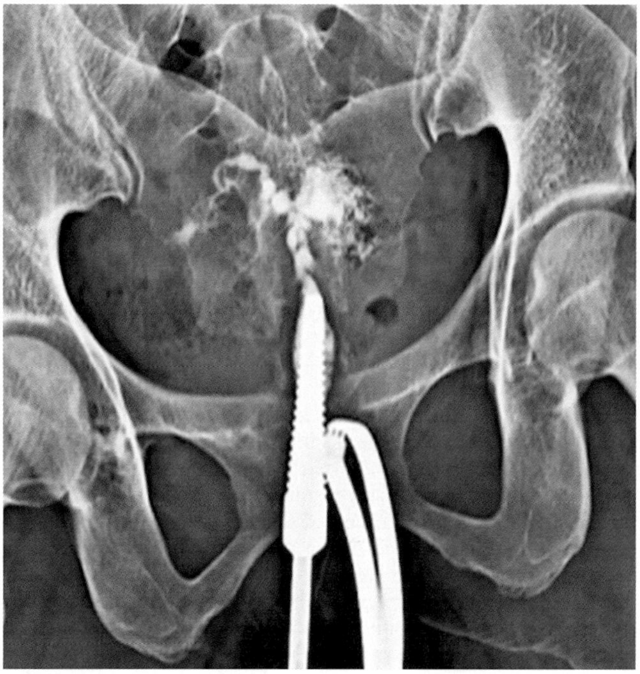

**Fig. 36.9** Hysterosalpingogram from a woman with infertility who had previously undergone a dilation and curettage procedure. Filling defects are noted throughout the cavity. (Courtesy Dr. MGK Murthy, Dr. Sumer Sethi, Dr. Srujana, and Mr. Verkat. From Sethi S. Asherman syndrome-HSG. Available at: https://www.indianradiology.com/.)

(D&C) in a nonpregnant woman, so this procedure should be performed only when indicated and not routinely at the time of other surgical procedures (e.g., diagnostic laparoscopy). A less common cause of IUA is severe endometritis or fibrosis after a myomectomy, metroplasty, or cesarean delivery. This cause of amenorrhea should be considered most likely if a temporal relationship exists between the onset of symptoms and uterine curettage.

Confirmation of the diagnosis is usually made by a hysterosalpingogram (Fig. 36.9) or another form of imaging including hysteroscopy. Although it has been suggested that sequential administration of estrogen-progestogen be used as the initial diagnostic procedure when IUA is suspected, withdrawal bleeding may occur after administration of the estrogen/progestogen in women with IUA and should not be relied on.

### CNS and Hypothalamic Causes

**CNS Structural Abnormalities**

The same anatomic lesions in the brainstem or hypothalamus, which have been discussed as causing primary amenorrhea (by interfering with GnRH release), can also cause secondary amenorrhea. Hypothalamic lesions include craniopharyngiomas, granulomatous disease (e.g., tuberculosis, sarcoidosis), and sequelae of encephalitis. When such uncommon lesions are present, circulating gonadotropins and $E_2$ levels are low and withdrawal uterine bleeding will not occur after progestogen administration.

**Drugs**

Phenothiazine derivatives, certain antihypertensive agents, and other drugs listed in Chapter 37 can also produce amenorrhea without hyperprolactinemia, although usually PRL is elevated. Therefore women with secondary amenorrhea should have a detailed medication history obtained, even if galactorrhea is not present. Oral contraceptive steroids inhibit ovulation by acting on the hypothalamus to suppress GnRH and directly on the pituitary to suppress FSH and LH. Occasionally this hypothalamic-pituitary suppression persists for several months after oral contraceptives are discontinued, producing the syndrome termed *postpill amenorrhea*. This oral contraception–induced suppression should not last longer than 6 months. It has been reported that the incidence of amenorrhea persisting more than 6 months after discontinuation of oral contraceptives (0.8%) is approximately the same as the incidence of secondary amenorrhea in the general population (0.7%). Thus the reason for amenorrhea persisting more than 6 months after discontinuation of oral contraceptives is probably unrelated to their use, except that the regular withdrawal bleeding produced by oral contraceptives masks the development of this symptom.

### Stress and Exercise

Stressful situations, including a sudden change in a normal routine, can produce amenorrhea. A high percentage of women who were in concentration camps or those sentenced for execution also became amenorrheic as a result of stress.

Feicht and colleagues reported that the incidence of secondary amenorrhea in runners has a positive correlation with the number of miles run per week (Feicht, 1978) (Fig. 36.10). In a comparison of amenorrheic and eumenorrheic athletes, they reported that physical parameters such as age, weight, lean body mass, and body fat were similar. The only significant difference between the two groups was the fact that the **amenorrheic athletes ran more miles weekly**. McArthur and associates have also reported there is no significant difference in the percentage of body fat in amenorrheic runners compared with runners who were menstruating. Both stress and exercise can increase brain-derived factors that can inhibit GnRH release (CRH, opioid peptides etc.) If the cause of GnRH inhibition is stress related, when the stressful situation abates, whether emotional in origin or related to strenuous exercise, normal cyclic ovarian function and regular menses usually resume in a few months.

### Weight Loss

Both male and female animals that are malnourished have decreased reproductive capacity. Weight loss is also associated with amenorrhea in women and has been classified into two groups: the moderately underweight group, which includes individuals whose weight is 15% to 25% less than ideal body weight, and severely underweight women, whose weight loss is more than 25% of ideal body weight. Weight loss can occur from excessive dietary restrictions and from malnutrition. An extreme form of this is **anorexia nervosa,** which is a psychiatric disorder. Vigersky demonstrated that women with amenorrhea associated with simple weight loss have direct and indirect evidence of **hypothalamic dysfunction**, but pituitary and end organ function is normal. Mason showed that in contrast to women with normal cycles, a group of women with weight loss amenorrhea had similar mean levels of LH and LH pulse amplitude, but they had a decreased frequency of LH pulses. Thus the amenorrhea associated with weight loss appears to be caused mainly by failure of normal GnRH release, with the lack of a pituitary response under extreme conditions. Hypoleptinemia, alterations in ghrelin, and GH and thyroid dysfunction contribute to these findings.

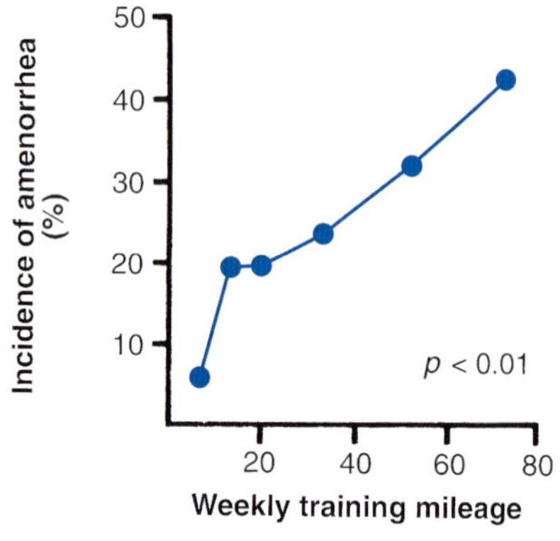


**Fig. 36.10** Correlation between training mileage and amenorrhea. Each point represents an average of 21 respondents. Statistical significance of relationship was obtained from point-biserial correlation (1 mile [1.6 km]). (From Feicht CB, Johnson TS, Martin BJ. Secondary amenorrhoea in athletes. *Lancet.* 1978;2:1145.)

### Polycystic Ovary Syndrome

PCOS is a heterogenous disorder that may present with prolonged periods of amenorrhea, although the more typical menstrual pattern is one of irregularity or oligomenorrhea. Women need not be overweight or obese, or have symptoms and signs of hyperandrogenism, which typically occurs. Although many women with PCOS have an elevated serum LH level, this level may be normal, particularly in women who are obese, and measurement of LH is not required as a diagnostic criterion. Nevertheless, the diagnosis of PCOS may be confirmed by visualizing polycystic ovaries on ultrasound, particularly in the absence of classic findings such as hyperandrogenism. According to the European Society of Human Reproduction and Embryology–American Society for Reproductive Medicine (ESHRE-ASRM) **Rotterdam criteria** for the diagnosis of PCOS, women may be diagnosed as having PCOS with only the menstrual disturbance (in this case amenorrhea) and polycystic ovaries seen with ultrasound. This subject is discussed in detail in Chapter 39. PCOS in a more severe form may present early and has been noted to be a cause of primary amenorrhea as well.

### Functional Hypothalamic Amenorrhea

Women with secondary amenorrhea who have no anatomic abnormalities, are not on drugs, and have no history of excessive exercise, stress, or large changes in body have an entity called **functional hypothalamic amenorrhea** (FHA). In the final analysis, these women have an alteration of hypothalamic GnRH release and do not exhibit characteristic cyclic alterations in LH pulsatility. They either have no pulses (Crowley, 1985) (Fig. 36.11) or have a persistent pattern of pulsatility that is normally found in only one portion of the ovulatory cycle, usually the slow frequency normally found in the luteal phase, despite having a steroid milieu similar to that in the follicular phase (see Fig. 36.11). As reported by Ferin and colleagues, administration of the opioid antagonists naloxone and naltrexone to women with FHA is followed by an increase in frequency of LH pulses and by induction of ovulation (Ferin, 1984).

Berga and associates measured several pituitary hormones at frequent intervals in a 24-hour period in 10 women with FHA and 10 women with normal cycles (Berga, 1989). As also reported by others, they found a 53% reduction in LH pulse frequency among the women with FHA; however, the LH pulse amplitude was similar in the two groups. In addition to reduced secretion of LH, there was reduced secretion of FSH, PRL, and thyroid-stimulating hormone (TSH), as well as altered rhythms of growth hormone (GH) and cortisol with elevated cortisol levels; however, the pituitary response to releasing hormones was unchanged. Thus a number of hormonal alterations occur in FHA as an adaptive central neuroendocrine event. Some data from Tschugguel and Berga have suggested that **in stress-induced hypothalamic amenorrhea, hypnotherapy and cognitive behavior therapy may be able to restore ovarian activity** (Tschugguel, 2003). Although this is a difficult approach that is not easy to duplicate, it is a logical approach from a physiologic perspective. Also, this method may be beneficial in that chronic stress reduction is generally beneficial for general health and can prevent cardiovascular

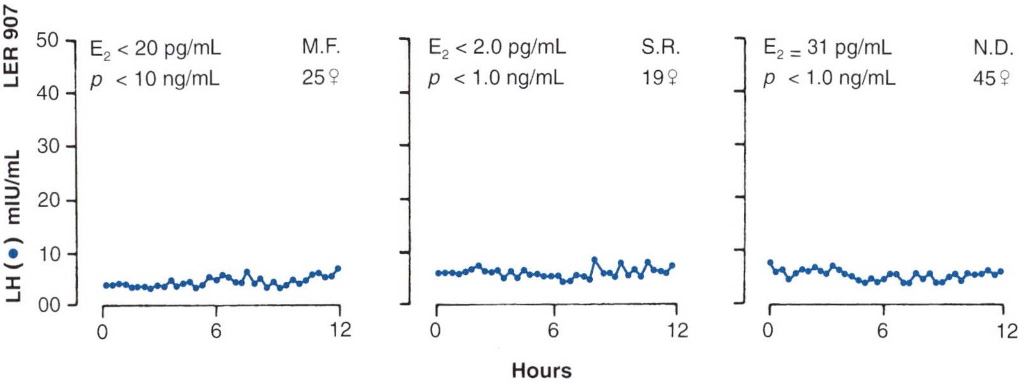


**Fig. 36.11** Pulsatile pattern of LH secretion in women with hypogonadotropic hypogonadism and hypothalamic amenorrhea. *E₂*, Estradiol; *LH,* luteinizing hormone. *M.F., S.R.,* and *N.D.* are the three patients' initials. (From Crowley WF Jr, Filicori M, Spratt DI, et al. The physiology of gonadotropin-releasing hormone [GnRH] secretion in men and women. *Rec Prog Hormone Res.* 1985;41:473.)

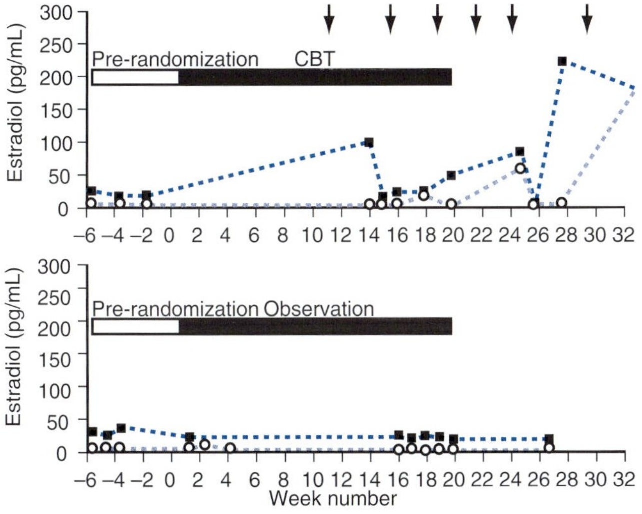


**Fig. 36.12** Estradiol *(dot)* and progesterone levels *(square)* in a woman with functional hypothalamic amenorrhea (FHA) who had a return of ovulatory menstrual cycles while undergoing cognitive behavioral therapy (CBT) *(top panel),* and estradiol and progesterone levels in a woman with FHA who remained anovulatory and amenorrheic during observation for 20 weeks *(bottom panel).* (From Berga, SL, Marcus MD, Loucks, et al. Recovery of ovarian activity in women with functional hypothalamic amenorrhea who were treated with cognitive behavior therapy. *Fertil Steril.* 2003;80:976.)

problems and immune compromise. In a controlled study over 20 weeks, normal ovarian activity was restored in approximately 80% of women (Berga, 2003) (Fig. 36.12).

The severity of the hypothalamic suppression can be assessed by a sensitive assay for $E_2$. Usually $E_2$ levels less than 30 pg/mL signify significant hypoestrogenism; typically levels are less than 20 pg/mL, as occurs after menopause. If endogenous $E_2$ has been sufficient to allow the endometrium to proliferate, then progestogen administration will result in withdrawal bleeding. This can also be determined by visualizing the endometrial stripe by ultrasound. If the thickness is less than 4 mm, hypoestrogenism is clearly present. The importance of knowing the estrogen status of these patients is that with severe hypoestrogenism caused by a severe hypothalamic suppression, bone loss occurs in these young women at a critical time, when attainment of peak bone mass should be occurring (up to age 30). In this setting, at least in the short term, estrogen should be prescribed.

**In up to 25% of women with FHA, polycystic ovaries may be seen on ultrasound,** creating a confusing differential diagnosis (Carmina, 2016). In some of these women, when the hypothalamic axis of these women with FHA recovers and estrogen levels rise, a PCOS-like picture emerges clinically (Wang, 2008). Although it is unclear if this situation arises only in women with PCOS who develop FHA or if some women with FHA have polycystic ovaries, it is likely both scenarios are possible. Importantly, however, when the women are hypoestrogenic and in the FHA state, they should be treated as such and not be considered to have PCOS.

## Pituitary Causes (Hypoestrogenic Amenorrhea)

### Neoplasms

Although most pituitary tumors secrete PRL, some do not and may be associated with the onset of secondary amenorrhea without hyperprolactinemia. Chromophobe adenomas are the most common non–PRL-secreting pituitary tumors; however, basophilic (ACTH-secreting) and acidophilic (GH-secreting) adenomas may not secrete PRL. Individuals with the latter types of tumor, although having secondary amenorrhea, commonly have other symptoms produced by these lesions and present to the clinician with symptoms of acromegaly or Cushing disease.

### Nonneoplastic Lesions

Pituitary cells can also become damaged or necrotic as a result of anoxia, thrombosis, or hemorrhage. When pituitary cell destruction occurs as a result of **a hypotensive episode during pregnancy, the disorder is called *Sheehan syndrome.*** When the disorder is unrelated to pregnancy, it is called ***Simmonds disease.*** It is important to diagnose this cause of secondary amenorrhea because, in contrast to the hypothalamic disorders, pituitary damage can be associated with decreased secretion of other pituitary hormones, particularly ACTH and TSH, in addition to LH and FSH. Specific stimulation studies are needed to characterize the different possible deficiencies.

## Ovarian Causes (Hypergonadotropic Hypogonadism)

The ovaries may fail to secrete sufficient estrogen to produce endometrial growth if the follicles are damaged as a result of infection, interference with blood supply, or depletion of follicles caused by bilateral cystectomies. These women may become amenorrheic after a variable time after medical treatment of a bilateral tubo-ovarian abscess, after bilateral cystectomy for benign ovarian neoplasms, or sometimes after a hysterectomy during which the vascular supply to the ovaries is compromised (also called *cystic degeneration of the ovaries*).

Occasionally the ovaries cease to produce sufficient estrogen to stimulate endometrial growth several years before the age of physiologic menopause. **When this condition occurs before the age of 40, the term *premature ovarian failure (POF)* or *premature ovarian insufficiency (POI)*** (Cooper, 2011) is used instead of *premature menopause* to best describe the clinical entity. A more in-depth discussion of POI may also be found in Chapter 14.

Coulam estimated that as many as 1% of women younger than 40 years have hypergonadotropic amenorrhea, with the incidence steadily increasing from ages 15 to 39. Commonly the condition of POI is transient before permanent ovarian failure occurs; occasionally, women with a diagnosis of POI may ovulate and conceive during this transition period. POI commonly occurs after gonadal irradiation or systemic chemotherapy and has also been reported in women with steroid hormonal enzyme deficiencies who menstruate temporarily and then have secondary amenorrhea. Approximately 16% of women who carry the premutation for fragile X may experience POI. Other genetic susceptibilities are also known to exist and are discussed in Chapter 14.

Histologically, women with POI have two types of ovarian pathologic findings. In most of them, there is generalized sclerosis similar to the findings of a normal postmenopausal ovary (Fig. 36.13), whereas in up to 30%, numerous primordial follicles with no progression past the early antrum stage are seen, which looks identical to a normal ovary (Fig. 36.14). The latter condition is caused by either an **autoimmune state,** which is more common (discussed later), or a gonadotropin receptor defect and is called **gonadotropin-resistant ovary syndrome.** Women with ovarian resistance syndrome often have primary amenorrhea, but usually sufficient estrogen is produced so that they menstruate for several months or even years. **More common are those individuals who have an autoimmune process with autoimmune diseases** such as hypoparathyroidism, Hashimoto thyroiditis, or Addison disease. Many women with POI who do not have clinical evidence of an autoimmune disease have antibodies to gonadotropins and several other endocrine organs, such as the thyroid and adrenal glands, which suggests an autoimmune origin. Although ovarian biopsies (which require a full-thickness section) are not recommended to make this diagnosis, the histologic findings often show lymphocytic infiltration along with the normal histologic characteristics as shown in Fig. 36.14.

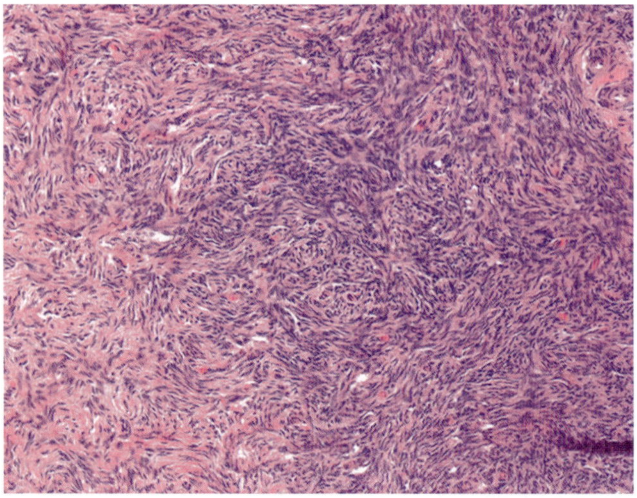

**Fig. 36.13** Histology of an ovarian section from a woman with premature ovarian insufficiency, devoid of follicles. (From Ramnani D. Ovarian failure. Available at: WebPathology.com.)

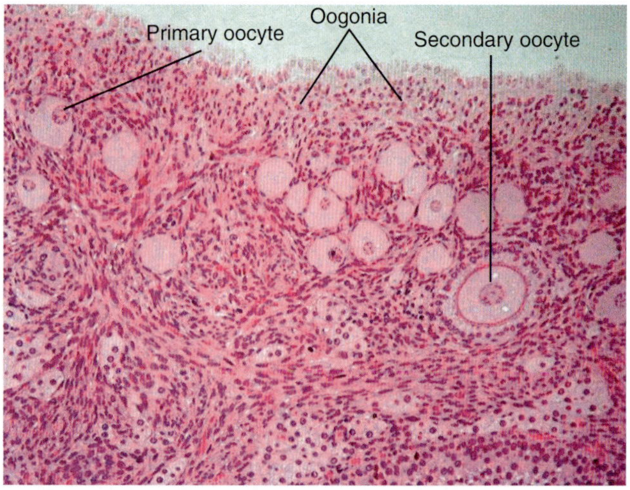


**Fig. 36.14** Histologic section of an ovary showing follicles up to the preantral stage, which is typical of a woman presenting with insensitive or "resistant" ovary syndrome. (From Shaco-Levy R, Robboy SJ. Normal ovaries, inflammatory and non-neoplastic conditions. In: Mutter GL, Prat J. *Pathology of the Female Reproductive Tract.* 3rd ed. Philadelphia: Elsevier; 2014.)

Alper estimated that approximately 30% to 50% of women with chromosomally normal POI without a history of irradiation or chemotherapy have an associated autoimmune disease, most commonly thyroid disease, which was present in 85% of the group with an autoimmune disorder (Alper, 1985). Using sophisticated immunofluorescence techniques, Mignot demonstrated that 92% of women with POI have laboratory evidence of autosensitization (Mignot, 1989). Approximately two-thirds of these were positive for non–organ-specific antibodies, mainly antinuclear antibodies and rheumatoid factors, and 50% had organ-specific antibodies. Although most of these women had no evidence of autoimmune disease, **it is recommended that immunologic screening be performed in young women with POI.** In the absence of symptoms, such as weakness, lethargy, or pain, which may suggest systemic disease, it is probably sufficient to obtain a complete blood cell count (CBC) and comprehensive metabolic panel, as well as TSH and antithyroid antibody levels. If adrenal failure (e.g., weakness) is suspected, adrenal antibodies (against 21-hydroxylase) and cortisol levels may be obtained; rarely, an ACTH stimulation test is warranted. It may be sufficient to obtain a general screen for adrenal function by obtaining levels of dehydroepiandrosterone sulfate (DHEAS). Some data point to lower (age-specific) levels of DHEAS in women with POI. Although available clinically, measurements of antiovarian antibodies have not been properly validated.

## Diagnostic Evaluation and Management

All women who consult a clinician for the symptom of **secondary amenorrhea** should have a diagnostic evaluation. The possibility of IUAs should be entertained initially. Any instrumentation of the endometrial cavity, particularly temporally related to pregnancy, should alert to the possibility of IUAs. If IUAs are ruled out, the history should disclose whether medications are currently being used or if oral contraceptives have been recently discontinued. In addition, questions regarding diet, weight loss, stress, and strenuous exercise are pertinent. A history of hot flushes, decreasing breast size, or vaginal dryness and physical examination are helpful in estimating the degree of estrogen deficiency. If the history and physical examination fail to reveal the cause of the amenorrhea, a CBC, urinalysis, and serum chemistries should be carried out to rule out systemic disease. A sensitive TSH assay, serum

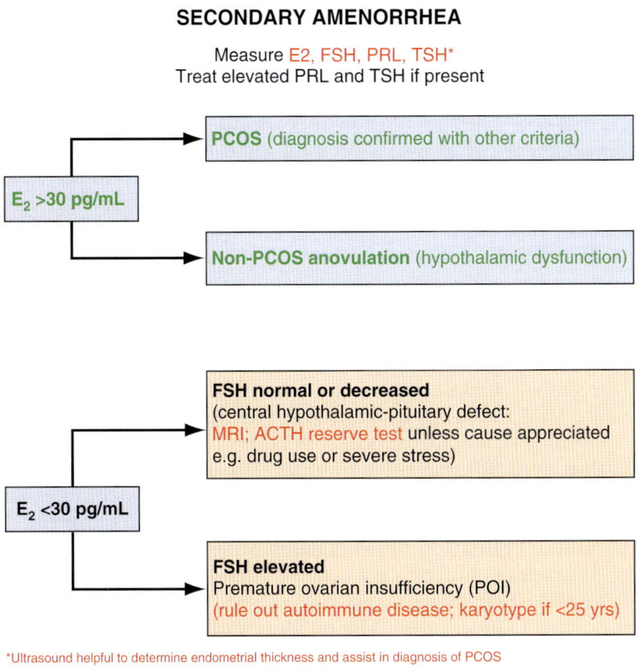


**Fig. 35.15** Diagnostic evaluation of secondary amenorrhea. Evaluation based on normal estradiol levels (>30 pg/mL) and low levels (<30 pg/mL). *ACTH,* Adrenocorticotropic hormone; *$E_2$,* estradiol; *FSH,* follicle-stimulating hormone; *MRI,* magnetic resonance imaging; *PCOS,* polycystic ovary syndrome; *PRL, prolactin; TSH,* thyroid-stimulating hormone.

$E_2$, FSH, and PRL should be measured (Fig. 36.15). If PRL levels are elevated, a diagnostic evaluation for the cause of this problem should be undertaken (see Chapter 37). Administration of injectable progesterone or oral progestogen is an indirect means of determining whether sufficient estrogen is present to produce endometrial growth that will slough after the progesterone levels fall (progesterone challenge test); however, it is preferable to order a sensitive $E_2$ assay to determine the true estrogen status. As noted, the thickness of the endometrial stripe on ultrasound is also beneficial. A cutoff value of 30 pg/mL is used here to differentiate between low and normal levels of E2. However, in recent years the sensitivity of assays has changed, particularly using mass spectrometry techniques. It is important to know the lab values of the assay the clinician is using. A cutoff value of 20 pg/mL may be more appropriate with newer assays.

Women who exercise or who have PCOS, moderate stress, weight loss, or hypothalamic-pituitary dysfunction will usually have $E_2$ levels of at least 30 pg/mL and withdrawal bleeding after progestogens usually occur. Those with pituitary tumors, ovarian failure, severe dietary weight loss or anorexia nervosa, severe stress, or the rare hypothalamic lesion will usually have very low $E_2$ levels, typically in the postmenopausal range.

If a sensitive serum $E_2$ value is more than 30 pg/mL and ultrasound confirms the presence of polycystic ovaries, the diagnosis of PCOS may be considered (see Chapter 39). If there is no sonographic evidence of polycystic ovaries and the woman has no history of drug use, stress, weight loss, or strenuous exercise, she should be told that hypothalamic-pituitary dysfunction is present and that the exact cause cannot be determined practically. She should also be informed that hypothalamic-pituitary dysfunction is usually a self-limiting disorder and not a serious threat to health or untreatable infertility.

Women with low $E_2$ and low FSH levels have a CNS lesion or severe hypothalamic-pituitary suppression. Women with low $E_2$ and elevated FSH levels (>30 mIU/mL) have POI. If severe weight loss, strenuous exercise, or severe stress is not present, and FSH and $E_2$ levels are low, MRI of the hypothalamic-pituitary region should be performed to rule out a lesion, even if the PRL level is normal. If a lesion is seen or if there is a history compatible with possible **pituitary destruction** (e.g., Sheehan syndrome), a test of ACTH reserve should be performed. An **insulin tolerance test** in which hypoglycemia is induced should normally cause a cortisol increase of 7 μg/100 mL within 120 minutes and is a satisfactory test of ACTH function. An alternative test is administration of CRH with or without other pituitary-releasing factors. Although many pituitary hormones can be assessed, the normal release of ACTH/cortisol is the major factor of interest and may require corticosteroid replacement.

If POI is diagnosed because of an elevated FSH level and no cause of ovarian destruction is elicited, the possibility of autoimmune disease should be considered, particularly in younger women. Therefore antithyroid and antinuclear antibody levels should be measured and other screening tests should be performed, as noted previously. Although commercially available tests for antiovarian and antiadrenal antibodies are available, they are not measured routinely.

To rule out mosaicism or a dysgenetic gonad, including the possibility of a Y cell line, a karyotype should be obtained in women with POF who are aged 25 years or younger. **Biopsy of the gonads by laparoscopy or laparotomy is not indicated.** Suppression of gonadotropin levels with estrogen, oral contraceptives, and GnRH analogs has been advocated to induce rebound ovulation after their withdrawal. Although these agents suppress gonadotropins, these techniques are usually ineffective for inducing ovulation. If ovulation occurs after such treatment, it is a sporadic event and not a result of the therapy. Most cases of spontaneous pregnancy have occurred during estrogen replacement.

The appropriate treatment depends on the diagnosis and on whether conception is desired. Women who have lost weight should be advised to gain weight. If strenuous exercise results in low estrogen levels (<30 pg/mL), the amount of exercise should be reduced or estrogen supplementation administered to prevent possible development of osteoporosis. Several investigators have shown that **amenorrheic and oligomenorrheic athletes with decreased E2** levels have decreased density of trabecular bone in the lumbar spine (Lloyd, 1988) (Fig. 36.16).

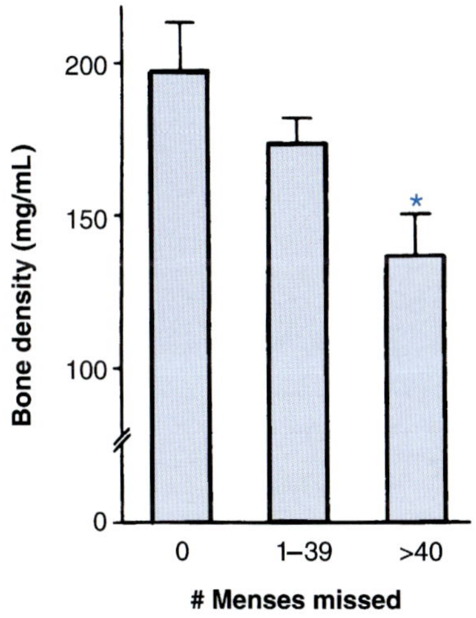


**Fig. 36.16** Relationship between bone density and number of missed menses in collegiate women athletes. For each subject, number of missed menses was determined from her menarche to age 19. *Asterisk* indicates a significant difference from the control group. (From Lloyd T, Myers C, Buchanan JR, et al. Collegiate women athletes with irregular menses during adolescence have decreased bone density. *Obstet Gynecol.* 1988;72:639.)

Klibanski showed that women with low $E_2$ levels caused by hypothalamic amenorrhea who have normal nutrition and activity levels have a profound reduction in spinal bone mineral density. The reduction in bone loss is independent of whether the PRL level is elevated or not. Bone loss has been found to be similar in hyperprolactinemic amenorrheic women with low estrogen levels and women with normal PRL and low estrogen levels.

Women with anovulation, including those with PCOS, who desire conception may be treated with **clomiphene citrate or letrozole, which are effective for inducing ovulation**. If pregnancy is not desired, periodic progestogen administration (medroxyprogesterone acetate, 10 mg/day or equivalent), for up to 10 days should be given to reduce the increased risk of endometrial proliferation associated with unopposed estrogen. It may be sufficient to administer the progestogen every 3 months. If a **woman with more severe hypothalamic-pituitary suppression (low estrogen levels) desires fertility, ovulation can be induced with exogenous gonadotropins or pulsatile GnRH**. Clomiphene is not successful if the estrogen levels are low. If pregnancy is not desired, estrogen-progestogen treatment is indicated for all amenorrheic women with low $E_2$ levels, including those with POI, to reduce the risk of osteoporosis. **Young women with POI and those with a chronic hypoestrogenic state are also vulnerable to accelerated atherosclerosis and diabetes and have been found to have increased all-cause mortality.** There is no increased cardiovascular risk in prescribing estrogen to these women. Women with POI may become pregnant with the use of donor oocytes and the priming of their endometrium with estrogen and progesterone for embryo transfer.

## PRECOCIOUS PUBERTY

The usual sequence of the physiologic events of puberty begins with breast development and the subsequent appearance of pubic and axillary hair, followed by the period of maximal growth velocity and, finally, menarche. Menarche may occur before the appearance of axillary or pubic hair in 10% of normal females. Normal puberty occurs over a wide range of ages. Fig. 36.17 gives the mean and ranges for pubertal onset and types of development in girls (Lee, 2003). The rate of growth is also of interest. Before breast development the growth velocity is close to 6 cm/year. At peak height velocity, around age 12, the velocity is around 8 cm/year; and by the completion of puberty, around age 14, the velocity is down to 1 cm/year, explained by closure of the epiphyses (Biro, 2006).

**Precocious puberty** is arbitrarily defined as the appearance of any signs of secondary sexual maturation at an early age. Puberty in girls is now recognized as occurring earlier than previously thought (Table 36.4). In an article by Kaplowitz and associates, it was suggested that girls with breast development or pubic hair should be evaluated when these signs occur before age 7 in white girls and age 6 in black girls (Kaplowitz, 1999). This has been somewhat controversial, and others have suggested that an evaluation is not warranted until age 8 in girls, because suggesting a diagnosis earlier may mask the ability to identify other diseases (Midyett, 2003). Accordingly, **we favor carrying out a complete evaluation of precocious puberty at age 8 years.**

Precocious puberty is associated with a wide range of disorders. It should be emphasized that regardless of the cause, precocious puberty is a rare disorder. **The incidence of this condition in the United States is estimated to be approximately 1 in 10,000 young girls.** When it is diagnosed, the physician should undertake a detailed investigation of the cause of the condition so as not to overlook a potentially correctable pathologic lesion. The two primary concerns of parents of children with precocious puberty are the social stigma associated with the child being physically different from her peers and the diminished ultimate height caused by the premature closure of epiphyseal growth centers.

Puberty is a time of accelerated growth, skeletal maturation, and resulting epiphyseal closure. Although precocious puberty may occur early in a child's life, it usually develops in the normal

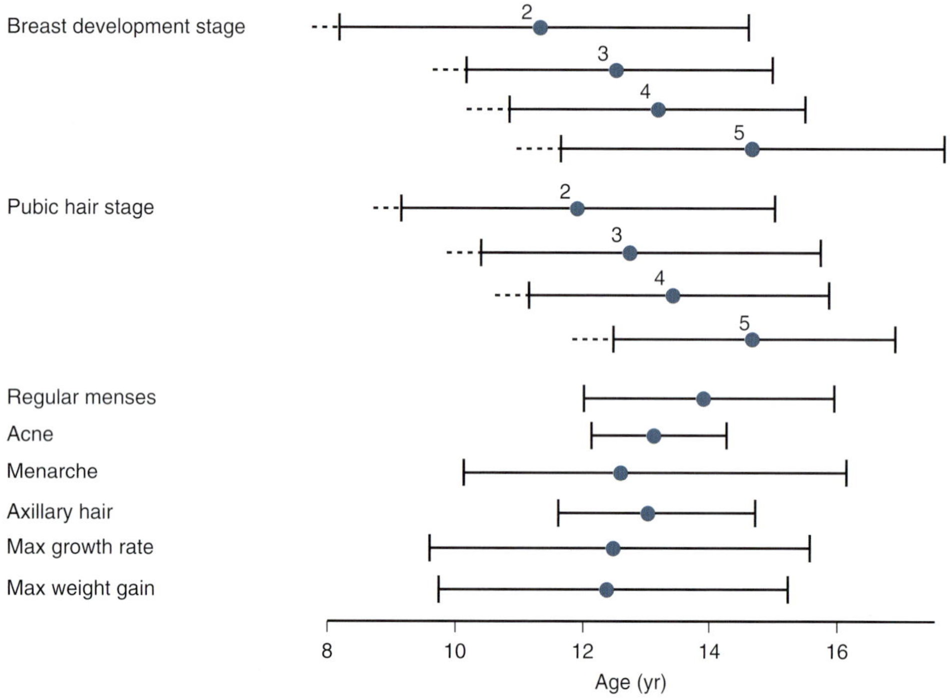


**Fig. 36.17** Mean ages *(dots)* and ranges *(horizontal lines)* of pubertal onset and development in girls. The numbers pertain to Tanner stages as depicted in Fig. 36.1. *Dashed lines* show the earlier limit for African American girls. *Max,* Maximum. (From Lee PA. Puberty and its disorders. In: Lifshitz F, ed. *Pediatric Endocrinology.* 4th ed. New York: Marcel Dekker; 2003:212.)

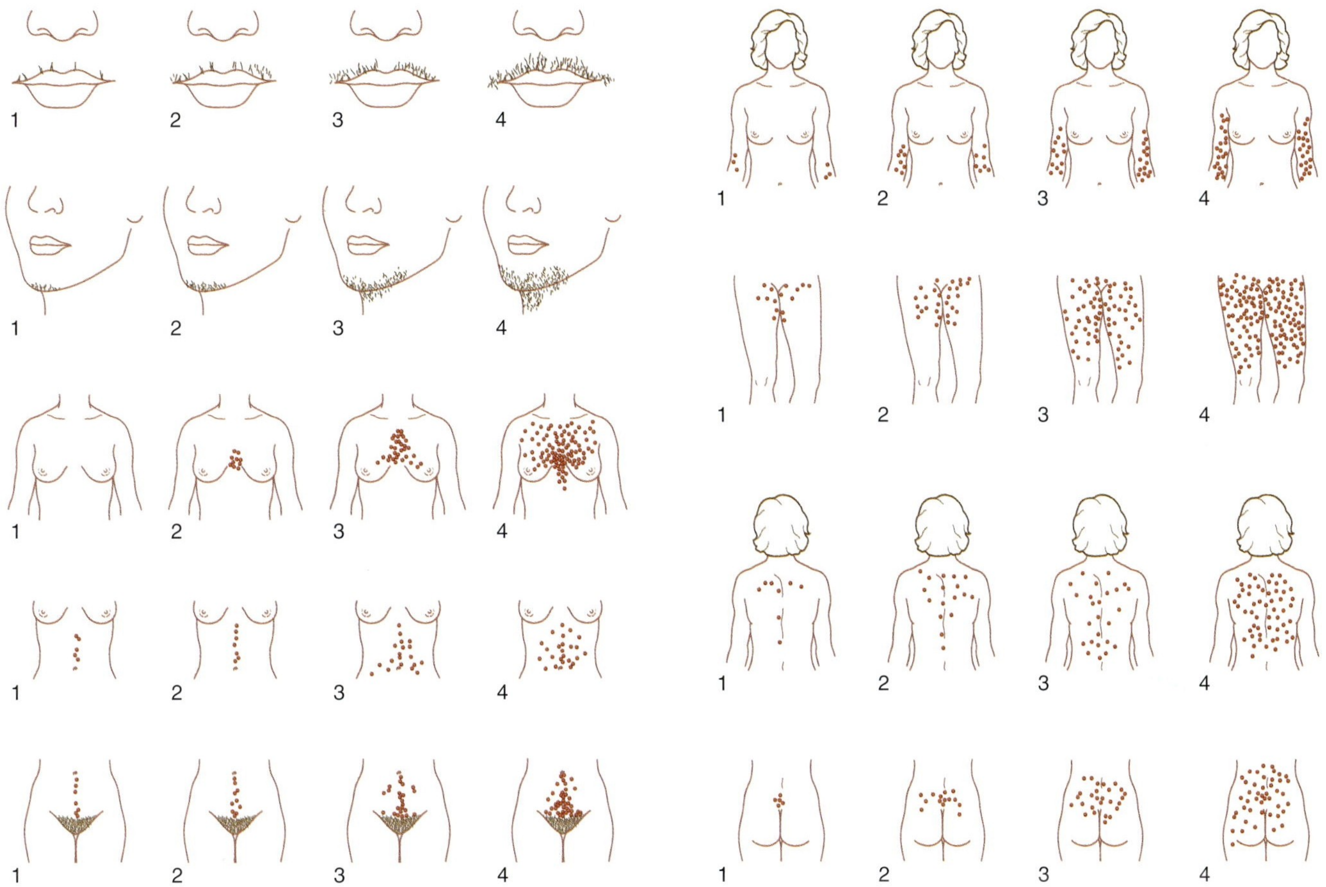

**Fig. 38.1** Modified Ferriman Gallwey score. (Modified from Hatch R, Rosenfield RL, Kim MH, et al. Hirsutism: implications, etiology and management. *Am J Obstet Gynecol.* 1981;140(7):815-830.)

**TABLE 38.1** Definition of Hair Gradings at 11 Sites*

| Site | Grade | Definition |
|---|---|---|
| Upper lip | 1 | Few hairs at outer margin |
| | 2 | Small mustache at outer margin |
| | 3 | Mustache extending halfway from outer margin |
| | 4 | Mustache extending to midline |
| Chin | 1 | Few scattered hairs |
| | 2 | Scattered hairs with small concentrations |
| | 3, 4 | Complete cover, light and heavy |
| Chest | 1 | Circumareolar hairs |
| | 2 | With midline hair in addition |
| | 3 | Fusion of these areas, with 75% cover |
| | 4 | Complete cover |
| Upper back | 1 | Few scattered hairs |
| | 2 | Rather more, still scattered |
| | 3, 4 | Complete cover, light and heavy |
| Lower back | 1 | Sacral tuft of hair |
| | 2 | With some lateral extension |
| | 3 | 75% cover |
| | 4 | Complete cover |
| Upper abdomen | 1 | Few midline hairs |
| | 2 | Rather more, still midline |
| | 3, 4 | Half- and full cover |
| Lower abdomen | 1 | Few midline hairs |
| | 2 | Midline streak of hair |
| | 3 | Midline band of hair |
| | 4 | Inverted V-shaped growth |
| Arm | 1 | Sparse growth affecting not more than 25% of limb surface |
| | 2 | More than this; cover still incomplete |
| | 3, 4 | Complete cover, light and heavy |
| Forearm | 1-4 | Complete cover of dorsal surface; two grades of light and two of heavy growth |
| Thigh | 1-4 | As for arm |
| Leg | 1-4 | As for arm |

From Ferriman D, Gallwey JD. Clinical assessment of body hair growth in women. *J Clin Endocrinol Metab.* 1961;21:1440-1447.
*Grade 0 at all sites indicates absence of terminal hair.

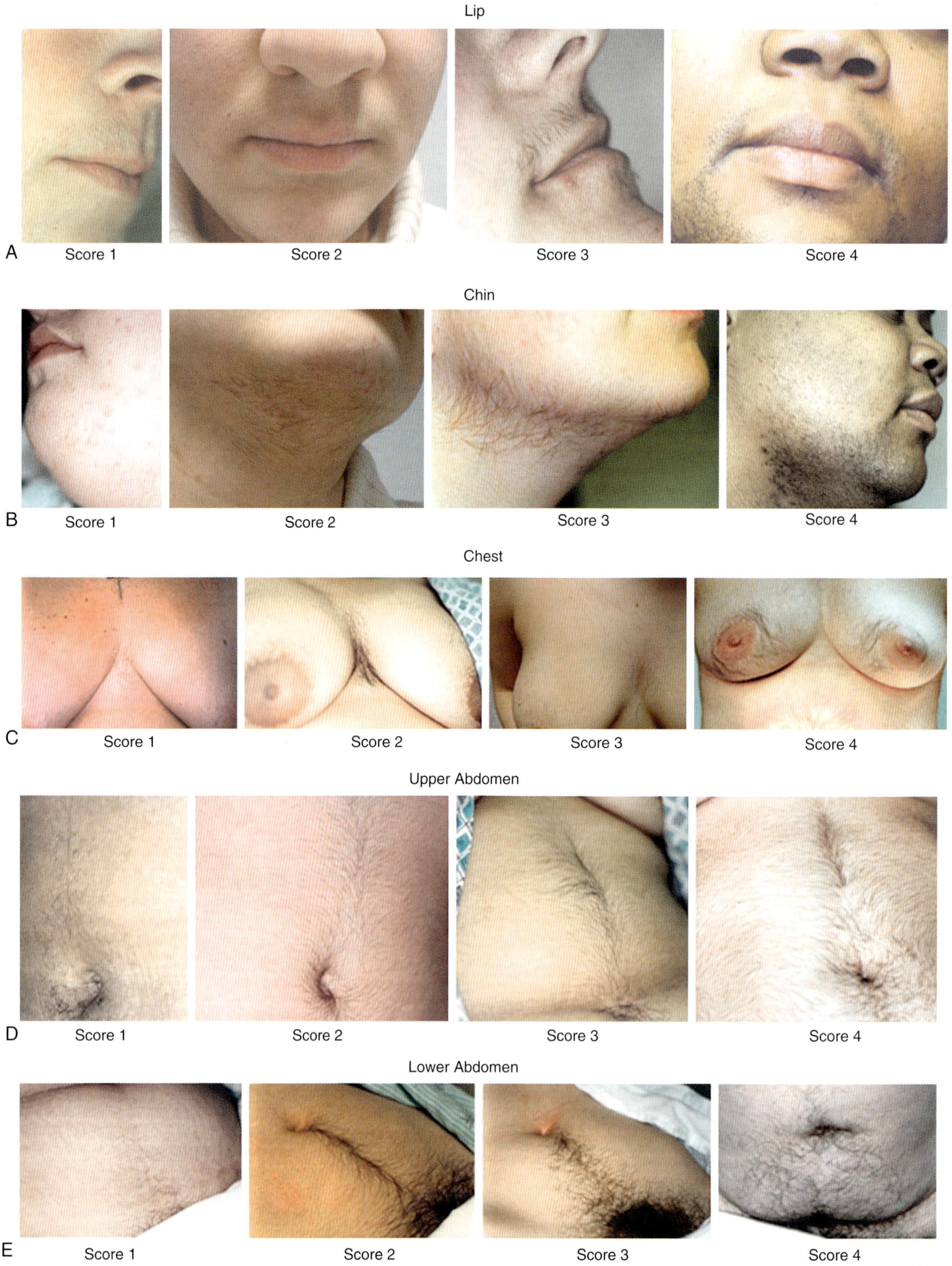


**Fig. 38.2** Examples of scoring for hirsutism using the Ferriman Gallwey method from Fig. 38.1. (Photographs of women without use of any method to remove body hair; obtained with personal confidentiality and institutional review board permission.) Panels **A-I** depict the nine different body areas as listed on each panel. (Modified from Yildiz BO, Bolour S, Woods K, et al. Visually scoring hirsutism. *Hum Reprod Update.* 2010;16(1):51-64.)

*Continued*

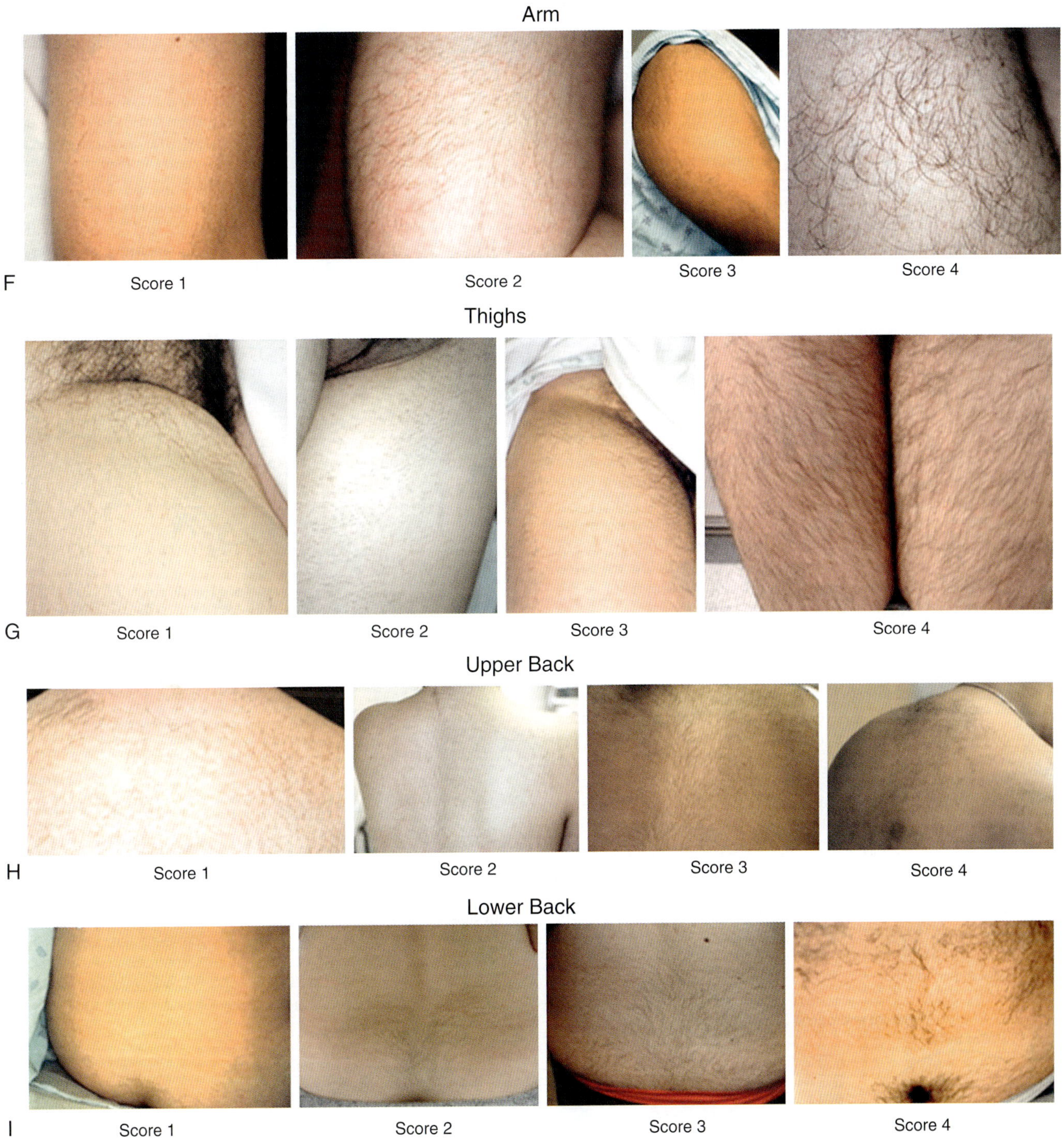


**Fig. 38.2, cont'd**

From a quantitative perspective, the major androgen produced by the ovaries is **testosterone** and that of the adrenal glands is **dehydroepiandrosterone sulfate (DHEAS)**. Measurement of the amount of these two steroids in the circulation provides clinically relevant information regarding the presence and source of increased androgen production. In addition to glandular production of androgens, conversion of androstenedione and dehydroepiandrosterone (DHEA) to testosterone occurs in peripheral tissues.

The ovaries secrete only approximately 0.1 mg of testosterone/day, mainly from the thecal and stroma cells. Other androgens secreted by the ovary are androstenedione (1 to 2 mg/day) and DHEA (<1 mg/day). The adrenal glands, in addition to secreting large quantities of DHEAS (6 to 24 mg/day), secrete approximately the same daily amount of androstenedione (1 mg/day) as the ovaries and less than 1 mg of DHEA/day. The normal adrenal gland secretes little testosterone, although some adrenal tumors have the ability to produce testosterone directly.

Androstenedione and DHEA do not have strong androgenic activity but are peripherally converted at a slow rate to the biologically active androgen, testosterone. Because the ovaries and adrenal gland secrete approximately equal amounts of androstenedione and DHEA, approximately two-thirds (0.22 mg) of the daily testosterone produced in a woman originates from the ovaries. Thus increased **circulating levels of testosterone usually indicate abnormal ovarian androgen production.** Clinical measurements of testosterone have not been sufficiently sensitive to differentiate normal from slightly elevated values; however, more laboratories are now moving toward using mass spectrometry and related methods, which are far more sensitive.

For practical purposes, circulatory levels of **DHEAS reflect an adrenal source of production**, and in women more than 95% is adrenal derived. Occasionally, in women who have increased production of ovarian DHEA, such as some with polycystic ovary syndrome (PCOS), the elevated levels of DHEAS might have an ovarian component because DHEA may be converted to DHEAS in the circulation. Another specific marker of adrenal androgen production, used for research purposes, is 11$\beta$-hydroxyandrostenedione, because the adrenal primarily has the ability to 11-hydroxylate androstenedione, whereas the ovary has a limited ability to do so.

Just in the last few years it has been realized using mass spectroscopy techniques that **11-oxygenated androgens produced by the adrenal circulate in blood in large quantities.** It has been suggested that these androgens are the predominant circulating androgens in women with PCOS (O'Reilly, 2017) Fig. 38.3. Some of these steroids such as 11-keto dihydrotestosterone are extremely potent and likely enhance androgen action. In the future it is likely that some of these androgens will be measured more routinely to have a better understanding of abnormal secretion and how they may be affected by treatment.

Although DHEAS serves as a good marker of adrenal hyperandrogenism, several guidelines for the evaluation of androgen excess in women omit this measurement, because DHEAS itself is a "weak" androgen and may not contribute much to the overall androgenicity. Nevertheless it is our perspective that the measurement of DHEAS gives a more complete picture of androgen production.

Most testosterone in the circulation (≈85%) is tightly bound to sex hormone–binding globulin (SHBG) and is believed to be biologically inactive. An additional 10% to 15% is loosely bound to albumin, with only approximately 1% to 2% not bound to any protein (**free testosterone**). **Both the free and albumin-bound fractions (often called *unbound* biologically active) are.** Serum testosterone can be measured as the total amount, the amount that is believed to be biologically active (unbound, or non-SHBG bound), and as the free form. As discussed later, because commercial laboratory measurements of "free" testosterone are not accurate, it may be useful to measure the ratio of testosterone and SHBG.

To exert a biologic effect, testosterone is metabolized peripherally in target tissues to the more potent androgen **5$\alpha$-dihydrotestosterone (DHT)** by the enzyme **5$\alpha$-reductase.** 5$\alpha$-reductase activity is important for testosterone action peripherally (as in the PSU) as well as in the genitalia (Serafini, 1985a). It is not necessary for testosterone action in other areas such as in muscle or bone. After further 3-keto reduction, DHT is converted to another metabolite, 5$\alpha$-androstane-3$\alpha$,17$\beta$-diol (3$\alpha$-diol). 3$\alpha$-Diol is conjugated to the sulfate or glucuronide. The glucuronide, **5$\alpha$-androstane-3$\alpha$,17$\beta$-diol glucuronide (3$\alpha$-diol-G)**, is a stable, irreversible product of intracellular 5$\alpha$-reductase activity and reflects this activity in blood (Fig. 38.4).

Even with normal circulatory levels of androgen, increased 5$\alpha$-reductase activity in the PSU results in increased androgenic activity, producing hirsutism (Paulson, 1986; Serafini, 1985a) (Fig. 38.5). Measurements of 5$\alpha$-reductase activity in skin biopsies have found that the level of activity correlated well with the degree of hirsutism present (Serafini, 1985b). The activity level is elevated in "idiopathic" hirsutism, where circulating levels of

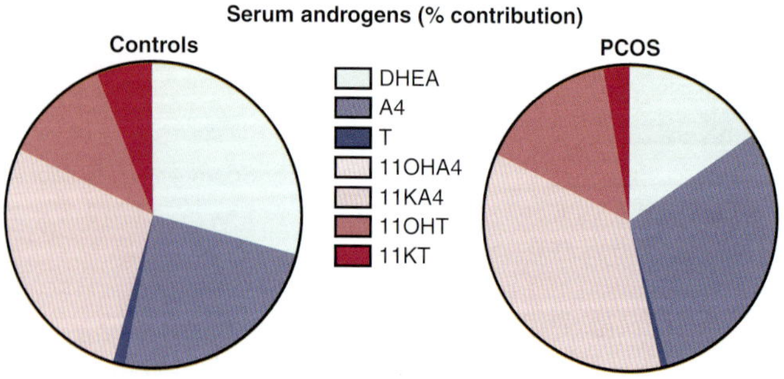


**Fig. 38.3** Proportion of circulating androgen is normal women (n = 49) and 114 women with polycystic ovary syndrome (PCOS). In blue are the classic androgens normally measured, and in red are the 11-oxygenated androgen thought to arise from the adrenal, and which are proportionately the largest group of circulating androgens in women with PCOS. *DHEA,* dehydroepiandrosterone. (From O'Reilly MW, Kempegowda P, Jaenkinson C, et al. 11-oxygenated C19 steroids are the predominant androgens in polycystic ovary syndrome. *J Clin Ebdocrinol Metab.* 2017;102:840-848.)

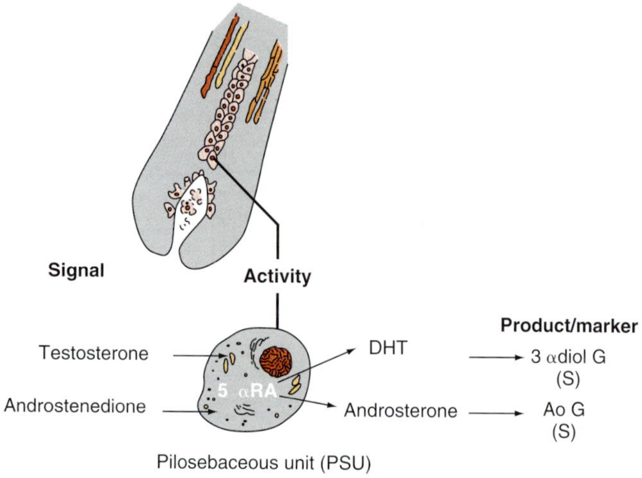


**Fig. 38.4** Peripheral androgen metabolism and markers of this activity. *Ao G,* Androsterone glucuronide; *DHT,* dihydrotestosterone; 3 αdiol G, 3α-androstanediol glucuronide; *(S),* serum. (From Lobo RA. Androgen excess. In: Mishell DR Jr, Davajan V, Lobo RA, eds. *Infertility, Contraception and Reproductive Endocrinology.* 3rd ed. Cambridge, MA: Blackwell Scientific; 1991.)

| Signal | | Activity | | Product |
|---|---|---|---|---|
| Normal | → | Normal 5α reductase | → | Normal DHT |
| Normal T | → | Increased 5α reductase | → | Increased DHT |
| Increased T | → | Normal 5α reductase | → | Increased DHT |

**Fig. 38.5** Influence of androgen substrate (signal; e.g., testosterone or androstenedione) and 5α-reductase activity (in pilosebaceous units) on local production of biologically active androgens. *T,* Testosterone; *DHT,* dihydrotestosterone. (From Lobo RA. Androgen excess. In: Mishell DR Jr, Davajan V, Lobo RA, eds. *Infertility, Contraception and Reproductive Endocrinology.* 3rd ed. Cambridge, MA: Blackwell Scientific; 1991.)

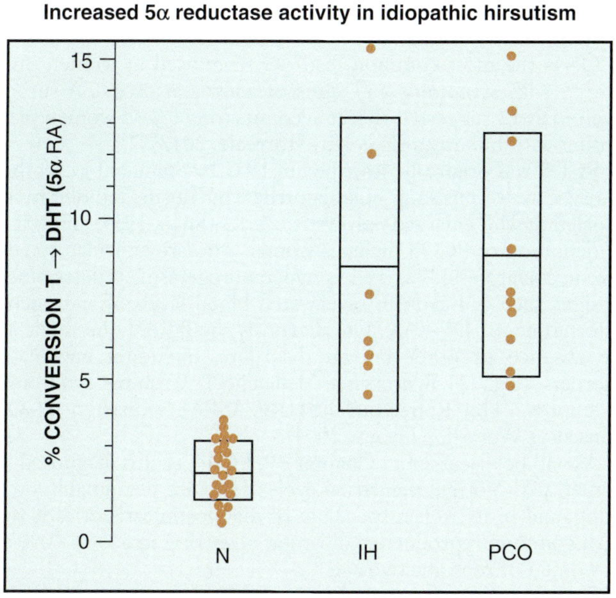


**Fig. 38.6** Levels of 5α-reductase activity in skin biopsies from normal women, women with idiopathic hirsutism and women with polycystic ovary syndrome (PCOS). Note that 5α-reductase activity is equally elevated in the hirsute groups compared with normal women, with almost no overlap in values between hirsute and normal women. (Modified from Serafini P, Lobo RA. Increased 5α reductase activity in idiopathic hirsutism. *Fertil Steril.* 1985;43:74-78.)

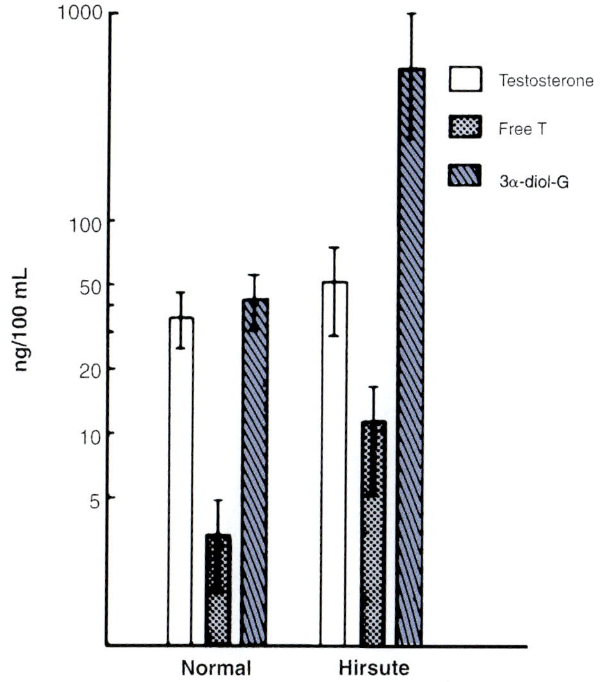


**Fig. 38.7** Plasma total testosterone, unbound testosterone (free T) and 5α-androstane-3α,17β-diol glucuronide (3α-diol-G) in normal and hirsute women. Note insignificant elevation with overlap for testosterone and free T testosterone and highly significant increase in 3α-diol-G without overlap between two groups of women. (From Horton R, Hawks D, Lobo RA. 3α,17β-androstanediol glucuronide in plasma: a marker of androgen action in idiopathic hirsutism. *J Clin Invest.* 1982;69:1203-1206.)

androgens are thought to be normal (Fig. 38.6). The degree of 5α-reductase activity can be measured in skin biopsy specimens by a variety of methods. This technique is only used for investigational purposes; if necessary for diagnostic reasons, 3α-diol-G levels can be directly measured in serum. We have found that the measurement of this metabolite is the most accurate indicator of the degree of peripheral androgen metabolism in women, as long as the level of glandular production (testosterone) is appreciated. Although serum levels of total testosterone are similar in normal and hirsute women, there are significant differences in 3α-diol-G (Lobo, 1983) (Fig. 38.7). In general, whereas non–SHBG-bound testosterone has been found to be elevated in approximately 60% to 70% of hirsute women, levels of 3α-diol-G have been found to be elevated in more than 80% of women in this setting.

In summary, there are three markers of androgen production in serum, one for each compartment in which androgens are produced (Table 38.2). These measurements best reflect the area of interest, although it is clear that each compartment also produces other hormones. Interpretation of levels of 3α-diol-G is controversial because these levels are highly dependent on circulating levels of precursor androgens, such as testosterone and also androstenedione. A reasonable argument may be that if testosterone and DHEAS are normal but there is significant hirsutism, then measuring 3α-diol-G may not be necessary and one may merely assume a peripheral source of androgen excess. As suggested earlier, it is envisioned that in the future the measurement of 11-oxygenated androgens will be part of our armamentarium.

**TABLE 38.2** Markers of Androgen Production

| Source | Marker |
|---|---|
| Ovary | Testosterone |
| Adrenal gland | DHEAS |
| Periphery | 3α-diol-G |

From Lobo RA. Androgen excess. In: Mishell DR Jr, Davajan V, Lobo RA, eds. *Infertility, Contraception and Reproductive Endocrinology.* 3rd ed. Cambridge, MA: Blackwell Scientific; 1991.
*DHEAS,* Dehydroepiandrosterone sulfate; *3α-diol-G,* 5α-androstane-3α,17β-diol glucuronide.

## CAUSES OF ANDROGEN EXCESS

Although most causes will result in hirsutism, each of the diagnostic categories can lead to any of the manifestations of androgen excess: acne, hirsutism, or alopecia. One common causative factor of signs of androgen excess is the administration of androgenic medication. In addition to testosterone itself, various anabolic steroids, 19-norprogestogens, and danazol have androgenic effects. Thus a careful history of medication intake is important for all women with hirsutism.

Hirsutism or virilization can also be associated with some forms of abnormal gonadal development. With this cause, individuals have signs of **external sexual ambiguity or primary amenorrhea,** in addition to findings of androgen excess, and a Y chromosome is often present.

Signs of androgen excess during pregnancy can be caused by increased ovarian testosterone production. This is usually caused by a **luteoma of pregnancy or hyperreactio luteinalis.** The former is a unilateral or bilateral solid ovarian enlargement; the latter is bilateral cystic ovarian enlargement. After pregnancy is completed, the excessive ovarian androgenic production resolves spontaneously and the androgenic signs regress.

A diagnosis of these three causes of androgen excess can usually easily be made by means of a careful history and physical examination. The remaining causes of androgen excess, together

**TABLE 38.3** Differential Diagnosis of Hirsutism and Virilization*

| Source | Diagnosis |
|---|---|
| Nonspecific | Exogenous, iatrogenic |
| | Abnormal gonadal or sexual development |
| Pregnancy | Androgen excess in pregnancy, luteoma or hyperreactio luteinalis |
| Periphery | Idiopathic hirsutism |
| Ovary | Polycystic ovary syndrome† |
| | Functional or idiopathic hyperandrogenism‡ |
| | Stromal hyperthecosis |
| | Ovarian tumors |
| Adrenal gland | Adrenal tumors |
| | Cushing syndrome |
| | Adult-onset congenital adrenal hyperplasia |

*Idiopathic hirsutism and polycystic ovary syndrome do not present with virilization.
†The hyperandrogenism in PCOS can also be of adrenal origin, at least in part.
‡Functional hyperandrogenism may well be a type of PCOS, but without clearly defined polycystic ovaries on ultrasound, and can also have an adrenal source of hyperandrogenism.
*PCOS,* Polycystic ovary syndrome.

with the origin of hyperandrogenism, are listed in Table 38.3. Details of each of these causes will be described. "Idiopathic" hirsutism and PCOS are the most common disorders, together making up more than 90% of cases. PCOS is the most common disorder, and because of its overall prevalence and importance among reproductive women, it is covered in detail in a separate chapter.

## Idiopathic Hirsutism (Peripheral Disorder of Androgen Metabolism)

Idiopathic hirsutism is diagnosed when there are signs of hirsutism and regular menstrual cycles in conjunction with normal circulating levels of androgens (both testosterone and DHEAS). Because this type of disorder is often present in certain families and ethnicities, it has also been called ***familial,* or *constitutional, hirsutism*.** Because neither ovarian nor adrenal androgen production is increased, the cause of the androgen excess has been called ***idiopathic hirsutism***. Several studies have been done, where it has been documented that some women so diagnosed have subtle increases in androgen production and metabolism; however, the more important way to characterize this disorder, where androgens are normal or very slightly increased, is that there is an enhancement of androgen action in the PSU (i.e., an increased androgen sensitivity), which also has a familial predisposition. We have found that approximately 80% of these women have increased levels of 3$\alpha$-diol-G, indirectly indicating that **the cause of hirsutism is largely the result of increased 5$\alpha$-reductase activity** (Paulson, 1986). Also, we have directly measured the percentage conversion of testosterone to DHT in genital skin as an assessment of the 5$\alpha$-reductase activity (5$\alpha$-RA level) in the skin of women with idiopathic hirsutism. The amount of 5$\alpha$-RA was increased in hirsute women compared with normal women and correlated well with the degree of hirsutism and levels of serum 3$\alpha$-diol-G (Serafini, 1985b). Thus idiopathic hirsutism is likely a disorder of the peripheral compartment and is possibly genetically determined, although it is also possible that early exposure to androgens can program increased 5$\alpha$-RA. **Antiandrogens that block peripheral testosterone action or interfere with 5$\alpha$-RA are effective therapeutic agents for this disorder.**

## Polycystic Ovary Syndrome

PCOS is the most common disorder diagnosed in women presenting with symptoms and signs of androgen excess. A survey taken in 2012 suggested that it accounts for 71% of women presenting with hirsutism (Escobar-Morreale, 2012).

PCOS was originally described in 1935 by Stein and Leventhal as a syndrome consisting of amenorrhea, hirsutism, and obesity in association with enlarged polycystic ovaries (Stein, 1935). The classic definition of PCOS includes women who are anovulatory and have irregular periods as well as hyperandrogenism, as determined by signs such as hirsutism or elevated blood levels of androgens, testosterone, or DHEAS. The diagnosis should only be made in the absence of other known disorders, including enzymatic disorders (e.g., 21-hydroxylase deficiency), Cushing syndrome, or tumors (The Rotterdam ESHRE/ASRM-Sponsored PCOS Consensus Workshop Group, 2004).

As will be discussed in Chapter 39, PCOS is also diagnosed in women with normal menstrual cycles, who are presumably ovulating, and in its widest spectrum of diagnostic categories is the most common reproductive disorder, occurring in 5% to 20% of all women of reproductive age.

For the purposes of understanding the interaction of androgen excess and PCOS, it should be appreciated that the most important feature of PCOS is that it is a hyperandrogenic disorder (Azziz, 2006). Although the majority of women will have an ovarian source of hyperandrogenism (i.e., an elevation in testosterone), adrenal hyperandrogenism (elevations in DHEAS) may be found in up to 50% of women (Carmina, 1992). In some women with PCOS and signs of hyperandrogenism (acne, hirsutism, or alopecia), blood levels of androgens may be "normal." This most likely relates to the lack of sensitivity of current assays.

Because there are important aspects of PCOS that are prevalent (metabolic disease, fertility concerns, cancer risk, etc.) and because this disorder is extremely common in women of reproductive age, even though it may not be accurately diagnosed, a separate chapter (Chapter 39) is devoted to this discussion.

Although most women with PCOS have elevated levels of circulating androgens, the presence or absence of hirsutism depends on whether those androgens are converted peripherally by 5$\alpha$-reductase to the more potent androgen, DHT, as reflected by increased circulating levels of 3$\alpha$-diol-G. Nonhirsute women with PCOS have elevated circulatory levels of testosterone, unbound testosterone, or DHEAS, but not 3$\alpha$-diol-G (Lobo, 1983).

## Functional or Idiopathic Hyperandrogenism

This category is included because it may be found in other reviews in the literature and is more commonly diagnosed by European clinicians; it is considered to occur in up to 15% of women presenting with hirsutism (Escobar-Morreale, 2012). It is diagnosed when androgens are elevated (either ovarian or adrenal) and menstrual cycles are regular and ovulatory. There is also no evidence on ultrasound for polycystic ovaries, making this an "idiopathic" state; however, it is our view that this category is really a variant of PCOS, in which women may be ovulatory, otherwise known as PCOS, phenotype C. Because ovarian morphologic type in women with PCOS is variable, this category may essentially be merged with PCOS.

## Stromal Hyperthecosis

**Stromal hyperthecosis** is an uncommon benign ovarian disorder in which the ovaries are typically bilaterally enlarged to approximately 5 to 7 cm in diameter. Histologically, there are nests of luteinized theca cells within the stroma (Fig. 38.8). The capsules of these ovaries are thick, similar to those found in PCOS,

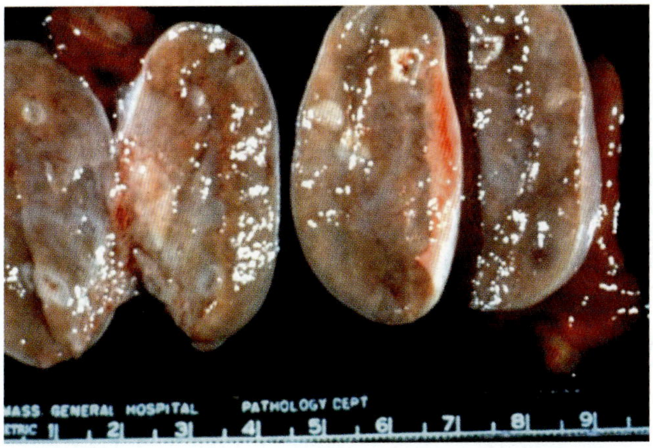


**Fig. 38.8** Surgical specimen of ovarian stromal hyperthecosis. Note fleshy appearance, without cystic activity.

but, unlike in PCOS, subcapsular cysts are uncommon. The theca cells produce large amounts of testosterone, as determined by retrograde ovarian vein catheterization. The ultrasound picture of stromal hyperthecosis may be variable (Brown, 2009). **Like PCOS, this disorder has a gradual onset and is initially associated with anovulation or amenorrhea and hirsutism; however**, unlike PCOS, **with increasing age the ovaries secrete steadily increasing amounts of testosterone.** Thus when women with this disorder reach the fourth decade of life, the severity of the hirsutism increases and signs of **virilization**, such as temporal balding, clitoral enlargement, deepening of the voice, and decreased breast size, appear and gradually increase in severity. By this time, serum testosterone levels are often in the range of 2 ng/mL, similar to levels found in ovarian and adrenal testosterone-producing tumors; however, with tumors, the symptoms of virilization appear and progress much more rapidly. Stromal hyperthecosis has also been found to be a cause of androgen excess in postmenopausal women. Here the ovaries are enlarged but not as large as in premenopausal women with the disorder; and testosterone levels are not as high.

## Androgen-Producing Tumors

Tumors are rare, occurring less than 1% of the time in women presenting with hyperandrogenism, but they represent the most important reason for evaluating women with androgen excess.

### Ovarian Neoplasms

It is possible for almost every type of ovarian neoplasm to have stromal cells that secrete excessive amounts of testosterone and cause signs of androgen excess. Thus on rare occasions, excess testosterone produced by benign and malignant cystadenomas, Brenner tumors, and Krukenberg tumors have caused hirsutism, virilization, or both. Certain germ cell tumors contain many testosterone-producing cells. The testosterone produced by two of these neoplasms, Sertoli-Leydig cell tumors and hilus cell tumors, almost always cause virilization. In addition, lipoid cell (adrenal rest) tumors can produce increased amounts of testosterone, DHEAS, or both. Rarely, granulosa/theca cell tumors can also produce testosterone in addition to increased levels of estradiol.

**Androgen-producing ovarian tumors usually produce rapidly progressive signs of virilization.** Sertoli-Leydig cell tumors usually develop during the reproductive years (second to fourth decades) and, by the time they produce detectable signs of androgen excess, the tumor is almost always (>85% of the time) palpable during bimanual examination. These tumors are uncommon. Less than 1% of solid ovarian neoplasms are Sertoli-Leydig cell tumors. Hilus cell tumors usually occur after menopause. They are usually small and not palpable during bimanual examination; however, the history of rapid development of signs of virilization and the presence of **markedly elevated levels of testosterone (more than 2.5 times the upper limits of the normal range),** with normal levels of DHEAS, usually facilitate the diagnosis.

### Adrenal Tumors

Almost all the androgen-producing adrenal tumors are adenomas or carcinomas that generate large amounts of the C19 steroids normally produced by the adrenal gland—DHEAS, DHEA, and androstenedione. Although these tumors do not usually secrete testosterone directly, testosterone is produced by extraglandular conversion of DHEA and androstenedione. Women with these tumors usually have markedly elevated serum levels of DHEAS (>8 $\mu$g/mL). Women with these laboratory findings and a history of rapid onset of signs of androgen excess should undergo a **computed tomography (CT) scan or magnetic resonance imaging (MRI) of the adrenal** to confirm the diagnosis. In addition to these uncommon tumors, a few testosterone-producing adrenal adenomas have been reported. The cellular patterns of these tumors resemble those of ovarian hilus cells, and the tumors secrete large amounts of testosterone. Because adrenal adenomas also secrete DHEAS, an adrenal adenoma is possible when DHEAS levels are greater than 8 $\mu$g/mL and testosterone levels are more than 1.5 ng/mL.

## Late or Adult-Onset 21-Hydroxylase Deficiency

**Congenital adrenal hyperplasia (CAH)** is an inherited disorder caused by an enzymatic defect (usually **21-hydroxylase [21-OHase]** or, less often, **11$\beta$-hydroxylase**), resulting in decreased cortisol biosynthesis. As a consequence, adrenocorticotropic hormone (ACTH) secretion increases and adrenal cortisol precursors produced proximal to the enzymatic block accumulate. The steroids involved are mainly to ***17-hydroxyprogesterone*** and ***androstenedione***, and androstenedione in turn is converted to testosterone, which produces signs of androgen excess. Late or adult onset CAH occurs in no more than 3% of women presenting with hirsutism (Escobar-Morreale, 2012).

Because the enzymatic defects are congenital, the classic severe form (complete block) of a mutated ***CYP21A2*** usually becomes clinically apparent in fetal life by producing masculinization of the female external genitalia. The severe form of CAH is the most common cause of sexual ambiguity in the newborn and is associated with only 0% to 2% of enzymatic activity. This leads to a deficiency of cortisol and aldosterone, which if untreated leads to shock and neonatal death.

The more attenuated (mild) block of 21-hydroxylase activity, where there is up to 50% of enzymatic activity, allows for sufficient cortisol production and usually does not produce the physical signs associated with increased androgen production until after puberty. Thus this condition, known as **late-onset 21-hydroxylase deficiency (LOHD)** or late-onset congenital adrenal hyperplasia (LOCAH), is associated with the development of signs of hyperandrogenism in a woman in the second or early third decade of life.

Although the incidence of classic CAH is only 1 in 14,500 live births worldwide, Speiser and coworkers, using histocompatibility locus antigen (HLA)–B genotyping of families with LOHD-affected individuals, have concluded that the incidence of LOHD varies among different ethnic groups but overall is probably the most common autosomal genetic disorder in humans. The incidence of LOCAH was estimated to be 0.1% in a diverse white population; in Yugoslavians, Hispanics, and Ashkenazi Jews, however, the incidence was 1.6%, 1.9%, and 3.7%, respectively (Speiser, 1985) (Fig. 38.9). **Both classic CAH and LOCAH are transmitted in an autosomal recessive manner at the *CYP21A2* locus in proximity to the HLA-B locus.**

The molecular basis of the disease is complex. In proximity to this gene are nonfunctional or pseudogenes *(CYP21A1)*. Depending on the population, 20% to 25% of individuals with classic CAH have a deletion of the *CYP21A2* locus or a rearrangement with the pseudogene *CYP21A1*. Current molecular techniques of genotyping can pick up well over 95% of these abnormalities, with most cases being 1 of 10 common mutations.

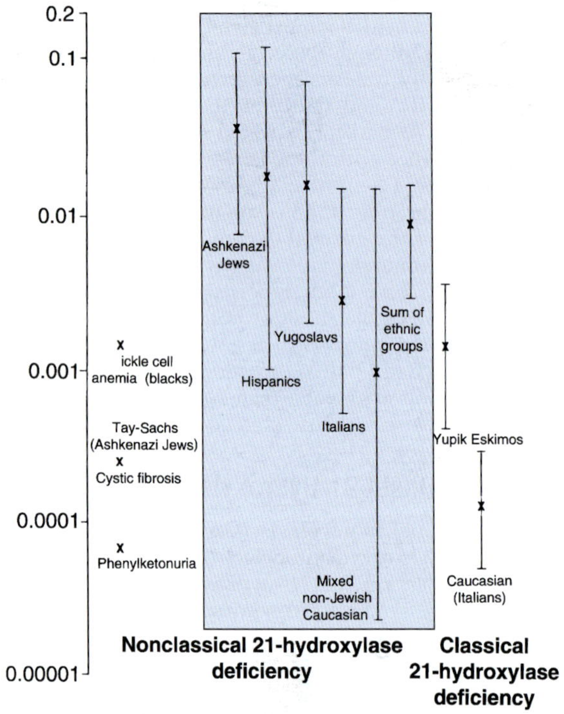


**Fig. 38.9** Relative frequencies of nonclassical 21-hydroxylase deficiency, classical 21-hydroxylase deficiency, and other autosomal recessive disorders. (From Speiser PW, Dupont B, Rubenstein P, et al. High frequency of nonclassical steroid 21-hydroxylase deficiency. *Am J Hum Genet.* 1985;37:650-657.)

A spectrum of mutations results in the enzymatic defects and clinical presentations shown in Table 38.4.

LOCAH is a phenotype that is symptomatic after adolescence and does not define the genotype. Affected individuals may be homozygous for alleles, yielding mildly abnormal enzymatic activity, or compound heterozygotes with a combination of defective alleles. The so-called *cryptic 21-hydroxylase deficiency*, on the other hand, represents mild or asymptomatic individuals with biochemically identified defects that, with the advent of molecular diagnostic techniques, have been redefined as belonging to several different clinical presentations.

New and coworkers have proposed a schema for identifying and classifying the clinical spectrum of disease shown in Table 38.4. Because there are three possible manifestations of *CYP21Y* alleles (normal, mildly defective, or severely defective), there are six possible genotypes representing three clinical phenotypes (asymptomatic, LOCAH, and classic CAH). Individuals with LOCAH may be compound heterozygotes, with one mildly and one severely defective allele, or homozygous, with two mildly defective alleles. **There is no perfect correlation between genotypes and phenotypes. Therefore because the genetics are complex, with many possible abnormalities, particularly in diverse populations, it has been recommended that for clinical purposes, the diagnosis and treatment of CAH should be based on biochemical findings.** In newborns, routine testing is carried out for levels of 17-hydroxyprogesterone such that affected neonates are identified immediately and all newborns are now screened. Carriers can be identified among family members who are heterozygous, with one normal allele. They have normal basal 17-hydroxyprogesterone levels; a mild degree of hirsutism, if present; and smaller increases of 17-hydroxyprogesterone after ACTH stimulation, usually between 3.5 and 10 ng/mL. **Molecular genotyping is primarily used for prenatal testing when there is a known severe mutation to determine the risk of having a severely affected child.** Genotyping in early fetal life, by chorionic villus sampling, is now carried out in potentially affected fetuses, which, along with the knowledge of the sex of the fetus, can help determine the need to treat with dexamethasone to prevent a female fetus from becoming virilized, although this is still a controversial topic.

LOCAH is also usually associated with menstrual irregularity. It has been hypothesized that the mechanism for anovulation is similar to that which occurs with PCOS. The increased levels of androgen lower SHBG levels, thus increasing the amount of biologically active circulating estradiol. The increased estradiol

**TABLE 38.4** Genotypic Characterization of the Forms of 21-Hydroxylase Deficiency

| Form of 21-Hydroxylase Deficiency | Clinical Phenotype | Hormonal Phenotype (in Response to ACTH) | Genotype |
|---|---|---|---|
| Classic (CAH) | Prenatal virilization, fully symptomatic | Marked elevation of precursors (serum 17-hydroxyprogesterone and Δ-androstenedione) | 21-OH-def$^{severe}$<br>21-OH-def$^{severe}$ |
| Nonclassic (LOHD) | Symptomatic: later development of virilization; milder symptoms<br>Asymptomatic: no virilization or other symptoms | Moderate elevation of precursors | 21-OH-def$^{severe}$<br>21-OH-def$^{mild}$<br>21-OH-def$^{mild}$<br>21-OH-def$^{mild}$ |
| Carrier | Asymptomatic | Precursor level greater than normal | 21-OH-def$^{severe}$<br>21-OHase (normal)<br>21-OH-def$^{mild}$<br>21-OHase (normal)<br>21-OHase (normal)<br>21-OHase (normal) |
| Normal | Asymptomatic | Lowest levels—some overlap seen with carriers | |

From New MI, White PC, Pang S, et al. The adrenal hyperplasias. In: Scriver CR, Beaudet AL, Sly S, Valle D, eds. *Metabolic Basis of Inherited Diseases.* 6th ed. New York: McGraw-Hill; 1989.
*ACTH,* Adrenocorticotropic hormone; *CAH,* congenital adrenal hyperplasia; *LOHD,* late-onset 21-hydroxylase deficiency.

stimulates tonic LH release, which increases ovarian androgen production and locally inhibits follicular growth and ovulation. Thus women with this disorder present with postpubertal onset of hirsutism and oligomenorrhea or amenorrhea, similar to women with PCOS; however, women with LOCAH, unlike those with PCOS, commonly have a history of prepubertal accelerated growth (at age 6 to 8 years), with later decreased growth and a short ultimate height. A history of this growth pattern, a family history of postpubertal onset of hirsutism, and findings of mild virilization are indicators of the presence of CAH.

To differentiate LOCAH from PCOS, measurement of basal (early morning) serum 17-hydroxyprogesterone levels should be performed. If basal levels are greater than 8 ng/mL, the diagnosis of LOCAH is established. If 17-hydroxyprogesterone is greater than normal (>2 ng/mL carried out in the early follicular phase or after menstruation) but less than 8 ng/mL, an ACTH stimulation test should be performed. A baseline 17-hydroxyprogesterone level should be measured and **0.25 mg of synthetic ACTH infused as a single bolus.** One hour later, another serum sample of 17-hydroxyprogesterone should be measured. **If the level increases more than 15 ng/mL, the diagnosis of LOCAH is established** (Fig. 38.10).

**Corticosteroid treatment is normally reserved for patients wishing to conceive to restore ovulatory function.** In other women, treatment is more efficient and safer using oral contraceptive (OC) pills, as in PCOS and other functional states described later.

It is important to measure ***11-desoxycortisol*** during the ACTH stimulation when the diagnosis is being evaluated, because of the possibility of 11-hydroxylase deficiency. This disorder is much rarer, but it also has an incomplete, adult form and may also be associated with **hypertension.** Women with this incomplete form also have increases in 17-hydroxyprogesterone and thus require the measurement of 11-desoxycortisol to differentiate it from 21-hydroxylase deficiency.

## Cushing Syndrome

Excessive adrenal production of glucocorticoids caused by increased ACTH secretion (Cushing disease) or adrenal tumors produces the signs and symptoms of Cushing syndrome. These findings include hirsutism and menstrual irregularity in addition to the classic findings of central obesity, dorsal neck fat pads, abdominal striae, and muscle wasting and weakness. The latter catabolic effect of glucocorticoid excess differs from the anabolic effects of testosterone excess, but some women with PCOS may have other clinical findings similar to those found with Cushing syndrome. Women with Cushing syndrome are more likely to present with other symptoms and signs of glucocorticoid excess, rather than because of hirsutism; but this has been found to occur in fewer than1% of cases.

**Cushing syndrome can be easily excluded by performing an overnight dexamethasone suppression test.** To perform this test, 1 mg of dexamethasone is ingested at 11 PM, and the plasma cortisol level is measured the following morning, at 8 AM. If the cortisol level is less than 5 $\mu$g/100 mL, Cushing syndrome is ruled out. If the cortisol level fails to suppress to this degree, the diagnosis of Cushing syndrome is not established. It is necessary to perform a complete dexamethasone suppression test (Liddle test) or measure the urinary free cortisol and plasma ACTH levels to determine whether Cushing syndrome exists.

Depression and other conditions can cause failure to suppress with the dexamethasone screening test just described. Accordingly, many endocrinologists prefer to depend on measurement of the 24-hour urinary free cortisol level or salivary cortisol. A creatinine level is also measured to gauge completeness of urine collection. Values more than 100 $\mu$g/24 hours in urine are abnormal, and values greater than 240 $\mu$g are almost diagnostic of Cushing syndrome. **Late-night salivary cortisol is now considered to be the most accurate method and is the primary method of choice.** Samples are usually obtained on two separate nights; values greater than 0.4 $\mu$g/dL are diagnostic for Cushing syndrome (Sakihara, 2010).

Cushing syndrome may result from a pituitary tumor producing ACTH (Cushing disease), an ectopic tumor in the body, adrenal neoplasms, or hyperplasia. Various algorithms have been developed for this differential diagnosis.

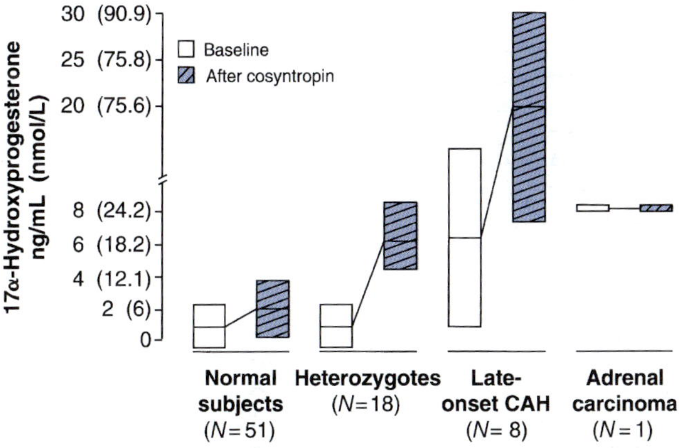


**Fig. 38.10** Means and ranges of 17α-hydroxyprogesterone levels before and after cosyntropin administered intramuscularly in normal subjects, suspected heterozygotes, patients with late-onset congenital adrenal hyperplasia (CAH), and one patient with adrenal carcinoma. (From Baskin HJ. Screening for late-onset congenital adrenal hyperplasia in hirsutism or amenorrhea. *Arch Intern Med.* 1987;147:847-848.)

## THE DIAGNOSTIC APPROACH FOR WOMEN WITH ANDROGEN EXCESS

Women with androgen excess present with acne, hirsutism, or alopecia, and some women have more than one of these three complaints. All women with these complaints should have a careful history encompassing a physical examination, laboratory assessment of circulating androgens, and often some sort of imaging.

Measurements of total testosterone, free (unbound) testosterone, or the free androgen index have all been advocated to assist in the diagnosis of androgen excess. In a clinical setting, commercial assays for testosterone are insensitive and cannot discriminate reliably between normal and abnormal values, unless values are very high (tumor or male range). Several organizations are addressing this issue, and now many laboratories are using a validated chromatography/mass spectrometry analysis. Clinicians should make themselves familiar with the particular lab assays they use, and their normal ranges. Although the free androgen index or non–SHBG-bound testosterone level is a better discriminator of hyperandrogenism than total testosterone, an accurate measurement of total testosterone may be all that is necessary. It is not clinically important whether a hirsute woman has a total testosterone level in the highest portion of the normal range or a mildly elevated level of non–SHBG-bound testosterone. Thus to determine the magnitude of elevated androgens and their source, measurement of total testosterone is more cost effective than the other assays and provides the clinician with the information necessary to establish the diagnosis. *To summarize, the laboratory* ***workup should include an accurate measure of testosterone (unbound testosterone or the free androgen index [testosterone/SHBG is optional]), DHEAS, and 17-hydroxyprogesterone when LOCAH is suspected (in younger individuals, those with a family history of androgen excess, and in those from***

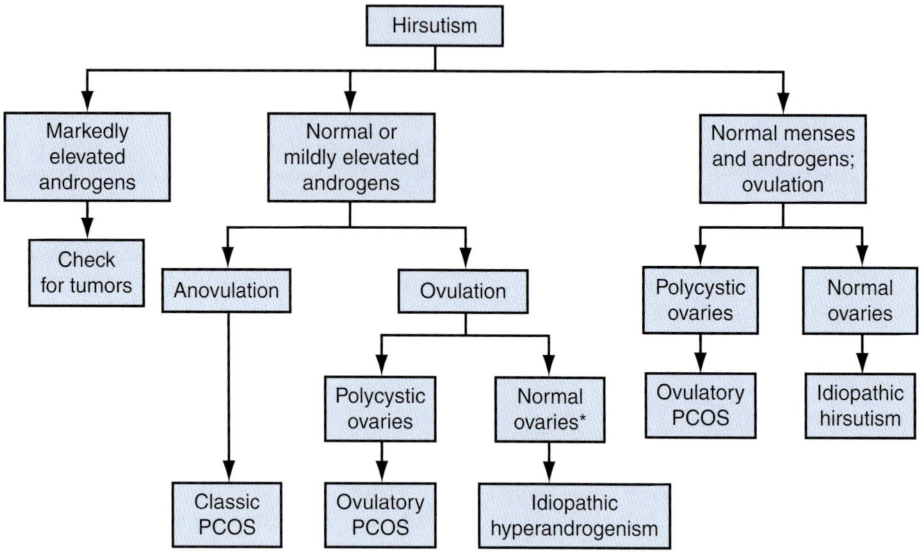


**Fig. 38.11** An algorithm for the diagnosis of hirsutism. Note that women with ovulatory polycystic ovary disease (PCOS) need only have hirsutism and can have "normal" androgen levels; also the ultrasound diagnosis of polycystic ovaries is not always accurate. (From Stanczyk CE, Lobo RA. Evaluation of hormonal status. In: Strauss JF, Barbieri RL, eds. *Yen and Jaffe's Reproductive Endocrinology.* 8th ed. Philadelphia: Elsevier; 2019:899.)

***ethnic groups with high prevalence).*** A practical algorithm for the differential diagnosis of women presenting with hirsutism is offered (Fig. 38.11).

As noted, androgen excess caused by iatrogenic causes, sexual ambiguity, or pregnancy-associated ovarian tumors usually can be easily determined by the history and physical examination.

***Masculinizing ovarian or adrenal tumors are associated with rapidly progressive signs of hirsutism and virilization.*** Serum testosterone levels higher than 2 ng/mL, with normal DHEAS levels, indicate the probable presence of an ovarian tumor. The diagnosis can be confirmed by bimanual pelvic examination and ultrasonography, CT, or MRI. Women with a rapid progression of virilization and DHEAS levels greater than 8 $\mu$g/mL most likely have an androgen-producing adrenal adenoma; CT or MRI can confirm the diagnosis. Values suggestive of an androgen-secreting tumor are lower in a postmenopausal woman; values of testosterone greater than 0.9 ng/mL (90 ng/dL) and DHEAS levels greater than 4 ug/mL are significant.

A long history of gradually increasing hirsutism, even if accompanied by virilization, is not consistent with the diagnosis of adrenal or ovarian tumors. The diagnosis of ovarian stromal hyperthecosis should be suspected for women with these signs and testosterone levels greater than 1.5 ng/mL. Women with physical findings consistent with Cushing syndrome should have the diagnosis ruled out. PCOS, LOHD, and idiopathic hirsutism or a diagnosis of functional hyperandrogenism may be associated with a similar history and findings at physical examination. Women with LOHD commonly have a family history of androgen excess and often belong to an ethnic group with a higher gene frequency for an abnormality. The diagnosis of LOHD is established by measurement of 17-hydroxyprogesterone, either by testing of an early morning serum sample or after ACTH stimulation.

Apart from tumors (requiring surgery), LOCAH, and Cushing syndrome (all of these being relatively rare disorders), the other disorders causing the androgen excess are functional disorders, in which the treatment is the same as discussed later. Women presenting with only acne or alopecia should still be evaluated as described previously, but each disorder will be discussed separately as well because of some of their unique features.

## TREATMENT OF ANDROGEN EXCESS

The success of treatment of hyperandrogenic disorders requires patience and persistence. The nature of the PSU and the hair cycle requires a longer time for improvement to be witnessed. In general, among the disorders, ***the most successful disorder to treat is acne with approximately 90% of women showing benefit; this is followed by hirsutism with an approximate 70% response rate, and finally alopecia, which only has a 30% response rate.***

### Specific Disorders

#### Ovarian and Adrenal Tumors

Tumors are best identified by high-grade imaging techniques. In the past, selective vein catheterization has been used, but this is seldom necessary today. Suppression and stimulation tests have not been beneficial because many tumors are LH responsive and androgens are suppressed somewhat with OCs and gonadotropin-releasing hormone (GnRH) agonists.

Almost all Sertoli-Leydig cell tumors are unilateral. If the woman has not completed her family and these tumors are well differentiated and confined to one ovary, the tumors may be treated by unilateral salpingo-oophorectomy. Because most hilus cell tumors occur after menopause, they are best treated by bilateral salpingo-oophorectomy and total abdominal hysterectomy. Adrenal adenomas and carcinomas should also be treated by operative removal. Adrenal carcinomas often have metastasized to the liver by the time the androgenic signs have developed. Despite chemotherapy, the prognosis is poor after metastases have occurred. Stromal hyperthecosis is also best treated by bilateral salpingo-oophorectomy in older women. After removal of the ovaries of women with stromal hyperthecosis or any of the androgen-producing tumors, the acne and oiliness of the skin disappear, breast size increases, and clitoral size decreases. The excess central hair becomes finer and grows less rapidly but does not disappear. Electrolysis or laser treatment can remove the body hair more effectively once the source of PSU stimulation has been removed.

## Late-Onset 21-Hydroxylase Deficiency (Congenital Adrenal Hyperplasia)

The treatment of women with LOCAH depends on their primary complaint. The androgen excess and menstrual irregularity can be treated as in women with PCOS, usually with an OC; however, if women wish to conceive, it is preferable to use glucocorticoids such as hydrocortisone (15 to 20 mg), prednisone (5 to 7.5 mg), or dexamethasone (0.5 to 0.75 mg) in divided doses. Doses as low as 2.5 mg of prednisone or 0.25 mg dexamethasone may be used initially. The aim of treatment is to suppress androstenedione and bring 17-hydroxyprogesterone and progesterone levels into the normal range. Ovulation usually resumes rapidly.

## Polycystic Ovary Syndrome

As is discussed in Chapter 39, because of the metabolic and other concerns in women with PCOS, lifestyle management has an important role in any treatment plan. It has been established that lifestyle measures and weight loss will assist in the treatment of hyperandrogenism in PCOS (Moran, 2011).

### Treatment of Skin Manifestations of Androgen Excess: Hirsutism

Although ovarian or adrenal androgen excess increases the likelihood of complaints, enhancement of these effects because of increased 5α-RA largely explains the abnormalities. Thus a successful strategy usually requires an antiandrogen added to suppression therapy, usually with an OC. Although it is reasonable to begin with monotherapy (OC), particularly if the disorder is relatively mild, in women with more significant complaints and findings, an antiandrogen can be used initially (Martin, 2018). It is important to use antiandrogens in conjunction with an OC because of the concerns of exposure during pregnancy.

In women who have "idiopathic" hirsutism and very mild and localized complaints, it is also reasonable not to use medical therapy and to use hair removal alone, as described later.

#### *Oral Contraceptives*

Oral contraceptives (OCs) (usually prescribed orally, but the effect would be similar with transdermal or vaginal preparations) suppress ovarian androgens by inhibiting LH stimulation of the ovary. They also decrease adrenal androgens (DHEAS) by about 30% (Klove, 1984) and inhibit 5α-RA (Cassidenti, 1991). In addition, the potency of ethinyl estradiol in OCs increases SHBG, which results in lower free or unbound testosterone.

Among the various preparations, it would seem logical to use a less androgenic progestogen (norgestimate, desogestrel, drospirenone) than more androgenic ones (levonorgestrel); however, there are no randomized trial data to support this assertion. There are some data to support the superiority of cyproterone acetate (CPA), which has significant antiandrogen activity, but CPA is not available in the United States. Randomized data have shown, however, that there is no difference in efficacy in using a 20 μg or 30/35 μg preparation and therefore OCs with a lower dose of estrogen should be used. Some evidence has suggested that the newer progestogens, which are less androgenic, as well as CPA, may increase the risk of thrombosis, compared with OCs containing levonorgestrel or norethindrone. Also it is known that women with PCOS, which represents many of the women with androgen excess complaints, have a higher risk of VTE versus women without PCOS, even after controlling for age and body mass index (BMI) (Okoroh, 2012). Nevertheless the increased risk with the less androgenic OCs is relatively small, and the absolute risk of thrombosis in young women is also rare and less than that of normal pregnancy. It is important, however, to use lower-dose estrogen products (20 μg). Also obesity is an additional risk factor for thrombosis, and thus lifestyle management is important, particularly in women with PCOS.

#### *Antiandrogens*

Peripheral androgen blockade with antiandrogens is dose related. Receptor blockade with **spironolactone** and **flutamide** and a specific 5α-2 inhibitor, **finasteride,** are the agents most commonly used. Cyproterone acetate (2 mg), which is a progestogen, is most often used in combination with ethinyl estradiol as an OC, although larger doses have been used as well. Drospirenone in the doses used in contraceptives (3 mg) does not have appreciable antiandrogenic activity and is estimated to have an equivalent effect of 10 mg of spironolactone.

Spironolactone has been used and studied extensively and should be considered the treatment of choice in the United States for women with idiopathic hirsutism, as well as many with PCOS (Lobo, 1985; Martin, 2018). In addition to being an androgen receptor blocker, it also decreases ovarian testosterone production and inhibits 5α-RA. Various dosages, from 50 to 200 mg daily, have been used. We have found that a dose of 200 mg/day of spironolactone is more effective than 100 mg/day (Lobo, 1985). Barth and associates have found a clinically evident response of decreased hair after 3 months of spironolactone, 200 mg/day (Barth, 1989). After 1 year of treatment, a 15% to 25% reduction was seen in hair shaft diameter and linear growth rate at all body sites. With the higher dose of spironolactone, liver function test results and plasma electrolyte levels are usually unchanged, and side effects occur infrequently, except for irregular uterine bleeding. The latter can be controlled with concomitant use of OCs. Electrolytes and blood pressure should be monitored for the first few weeks of therapy to ensure that hypotension and hyperkalemia do not occur.

Flutamide is a pure androgen blocker that has shown efficacy in the treatment of hirsutism. There is a dose-response relationship (250 to 750 mg/day), and even lower doses have some efficacy; however, the major concern is hepatic toxicity (Bruni, 2012). which may lead to death. Most guidelines have advised against the use of flutamide for this reason (Martin, 2018), and it should be used with caution at lower doses and with close monitoring of hepatic function. As with other antiandrogens, contraception should be used.

Finasteride, a 5α-reductase inhibitor (5 mg/day), is an effective treatment for hirsutism, and 5 mg has similar efficacy as 100 mg of spironolactone (Wong, 1995). Because finasteride is a specific 5α-2 inhibitor (there are two isoenzymes for 5α reductase: 1 and 2) and hirsutism is likely a combination of both types 1 and 2, a better inhibitor may be preferable. Dutasteride is an inhibitor of enzyme types 1 and 2 and is clinically available for use in men. Although on a theoretical basis it should be beneficial for the treatment of hirsutism in women, there are no data at hand. Finasteride is used currently as a second-line treatment when there are side effects or problems with using spironolactone.

#### *Other Agents for Treatment*

In severe cases, use of a **GnRH agonist** with estrogen or an OC add-back has been shown to be successful (Andreyko, 1986); however, this is expensive and cannot be used for long-term therapy. It has been used in women with high levels of circulating androgens.

**Ketoconazole**, which blocks adrenal and gonadal steroidogenesis by inhibiting cytochrome P450–dependent enzyme pathways, has been used in dosages of 200 mg, twice daily, to treat hyperandrogenism associated with PCOS and idiopathic hirsutism. This potent drug effectively decreases hair growth and acne, but major side effects and complications (including hepatitis) occur in most women so treated. These problems limit the use of ketoconazole to select women, who require careful monitoring.

In these severe cases it is probably preferable to use a GnRH agonist.

**Glucocorticoids** have been used for the treatment of androgen excess for many years. Although it is logical to suppress the adrenal gland in women who have adrenal androgen excess, and low doses have been used with some degree of success, the benefit is relatively modest compared with other agents such as antiandrogens. Because of its potential for serious side effects, glucocorticoids are not recommended for treating androgen excess but may be considered as an adjunct to ovulation induction in some women.

**Insulin sensitizers** have been proposed as agents to treat androgen excess and have been used in women with PCOS. Although some agents have shown some minor beneficial effects, they are not recommended as a primary therapy for manifestations of androgen excess.

**Eflornithine cream 13.9%** is a topical treatment that has been approved by the U.S. Food and Drug Administration (FDA) for facial hirsutism. Eflornithine is an inhibitor of ornithine decarboxylase, which is an enzyme necessary for the growth and development of the hair follicle. It was originally developed for the treatment of trypanosomal sleeping sickness. It is approved only for facial hirsutism and its mechanism is such that it affects all hair follicles and is not specific for hirsutism; it has been used for older women with nonterminal hair growth (Wolf, 2007). Its application twice a day results in a modest improvement in about 8 weeks. Thus for isolated facial hirsutism it may have an adjunctive role in that it can hasten the overall response, which takes much longer with traditional suppressive therapy. Side effects are minimal and include some local irritation; it is also expensive.

#### *Follow-up for Treatment of Hirsutism*

Because of the length of the hair growth cycle, responses to treatment should not be expected to occur within the first 3 months of therapy, and ***it usually takes about 6 months to see a response.*** Objective methods of assessing changes of hair growth, such as photographs, are useful. With the use of various therapies, a successful response for hirsutism should occur in approximately 70% of women within 1 year of therapy. Remaining excess hair can be removed by electrolysis or laser techniques. Treatment should be continued for 3 years and then stopped to determine whether hirsutism recurs. If so, therapy can be reinitiated.

#### *Hair Removal Techniques*

These cosmetic measures can be used as a primary treatment for mild isolated hirsutism or should be initiated after adequate suppressive therapy to remove unwanted hair once the growth rate has been inhibited by therapy.

Many depilatory methods have been used, but more definitive therapies are available such as the use of electrolysis and lasers, although these therapies may be expensive.

**Electrolysis** uses electrical energy through a wire electrode. Destruction of hair follicles results in its permanent removal. A "blended" technique has been thought to be more effective, although electrolysis is somewhat painful and can only be used for small areas at a given time.

**Photoepilation** uses lasers that apply heat to pigmented hair follicles. There are four types of lasers: Nd:YAG, diode, alexandrite, and ruby, and a meta-analysis suggested superiority of the diode laser. In general, long wavelength, long pulse duration lasers such as the Nd:YAG or diode are recommended for pigmented darker hair. For women with light or blond hair, electrolysis is recommended (Harris, 2014).

#### *Acne Vulgaris*

Acne vulgaris is considered to be a manifestation of androgen excess, although it need not be, and particularly in adolescents it merely reflects the physiologic responses of the PSU to the changing hormonal status and alterations in the bacteriologic flora. In general, however, ***androgens stimulate sebum production, and high doses of estrogen can inhibit it.*** There are many scoring systems for acne vulgaris, and the most common is the method presented by Cook, although it is primarily used for research purposes (Cook, 1979). Among hyperandrogenic disorders, acne vulgaris is the disorder that is most successfully treated, with response rates of close to 90%.

***Among women who present with acne, 52% can be found to have androgen excess,*** with increases in unbound testosterone being the most frequently encountered (Lucky, 1983). Thus in women who present with significant acne, particularly if they have not responded to routine dermatologic measures, an evaluation of androgen excess is warranted. An enhancement of $5\alpha$-reductase, mostly type 1, is a large part of the androgen abnormalities in acne (Carmina, 1991).

Treatment is usually with combination OCs (Arowojolu, 2012), which is at least as effective as chronic antibiotic therapy (Koo, 2014). Among OCs, less androgenic progestogens have been preferred, although there is limited evidence for superiority over androgenic progestogens (Kelly, 2010). The estrogen component of the contraceptive pill is particularly important for inhibiting sebum production, although it usually does not require increasing ethynyl estradiol greater than the 35-$\mu g$ dose. Although most antiandrogenic agents are effective (Fig. 38.12), OCs and pure antiandrogens are superior to finasteride. If OCs alone are not completely successful, as with hirsutism, the addition of antiandrogens are beneficial.

#### *Alopecia: Female Pattern Hair Loss*

Alopecia in women is a major source of stress and fear. Previously called androgenic alopecia, the preferred term currently is ***female pattern hair loss (FPHL)*** (Carmina, 2019). This may or may not be associated with androgen excess. Hair loss is usually on the frontal scalp and vertex, with relative sparing of the occipital scalp. It is important to rule out dermatologic diseases such as alopecia areata and specific scalp dermatologic diseases. Absent this, although it is important to rule out androgen excess, with hormonal evaluation as suggested previously, the prevalence of androgen abnormalities is low, with elevations occurring in only

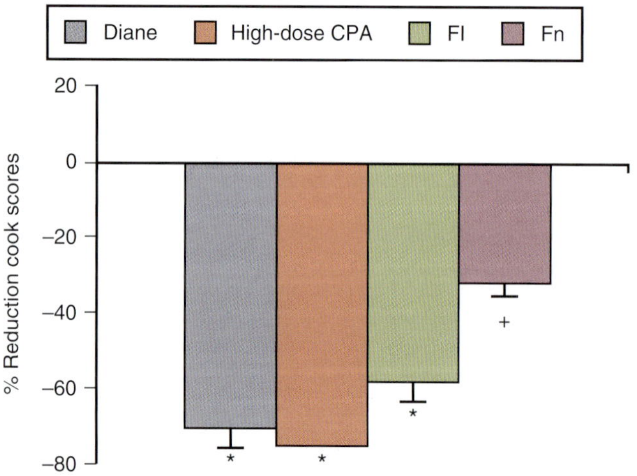


**Fig. 38.12** Percentage reduction in Cook scores after 1 year of treatment with either Diane (contraceptive pill with cyproterone acetate [CPA]/ethinyl estradiol [EE2]), high-dose CPA, flutamide 250 mg/day, or finasteride 5 mg/day. The asterisk signifies reduction at $P < .01$; the cross at $P < .05$. (Modified from Carmina E, Lobo RA. A comparison of the relative efficacy of antiandrogens for the treatment of acne in hyperandrogenic women. *Clin Endocrinol (Oxf).* 2002;57(2):231-234.)

39% of women (Futterweit, 1988). Androgen excess, perhaps estrogen abnormalities, and genetics play into the cause. With androgen excess, exaggerated 5$\alpha$-RA has been implicated in women with alopecia (Legro, 1994). There are several scoring systems for FHPL, with the method presented by Ludwig being the most commonly used, but mainly for research purposes (Ludwig, 1977).

Antiandrogen therapy is the mainstay of treatment. In women, spironolactone and flutamide (to be used with caution) have efficacy; however, finasteride, which is used widely in men, may not be effective in women, although there is some disagreement about this (Carmina, 2019). Many dermatologists advocate local injections and applications of various products to the scalp, but there are few data to support this strategy. Minoxidil is also used to stimulate hair growth. Consensus data from 2019 suggest that a combination of minoxidil with an antiandrogen is the most effective treatment for FPHL (Carmina, 2019). Ultimately, genetic manipulations and stem cell therapy may prove to be beneficial.

## REFERENCES


Arowojolu AO, Gallo MF, Lopez LM, et al. Combined oral contraceptive pills for treatment of acne. *Cochrane Database Syst Rev.* 2012;(7):CD004425.

Brown DL, Henrichsen TL, Clayton AC, et al. Ovarian stromal hyperthecosis: sonographic features and histologic associations. *J Ultrasound Med.* 2009;28(5):587–593.

Bruni V, Peruzzi E, Dei M, et al. Hepatotoxicity with low- and ultralow-dose flutamide: a surveillance study on 203 hyperandrogenic young females. *Fertil Steril.* 2012;98:1047–1052.

Carmina E, Koyama T, Chang L, et al. Does ethnicity influence the prevalence of adrenal hyperandrogenism and insulin resistance in polycystic ovary syndrome? *Am J Obstet Gynecol.* 1992;167:1807–1812.

Carmina E, Lobo RA. Peripheral androgen blockade versus glandular androgen suppression in the treatment of hirsutism. *Obstet Gynecol.* 1991;78:845–849.

Carmina E, Lobo RA. A comparison of the relative efficacy of antiandrogens for the treatment of acne in hyperandrogenic women. *Clin Endocrinol (Oxf).* 2002;57:231–234.

Carmina E, Azziz R, Bergfeld W, et al. Female pattern hair loss and androgen excess: a report from the multidisciplinary androgen excess and PCOS committee. *J Clin Endocrinol Metab.* 2019;104(7):2875–2891.

Cassidenti DL, Paulson RJ, Serafini P, et al. Effects of sex steroids on skin 5α-reductase activity in vitro. *Obstet Gynecol.* 1991;78:103–107.

Cook CH, Centner RL, Michaels SE. An acne grading method using photographic standards. *Arch Dermatol.* 1979;115(5):571–575.

Ebling FJ. The hair cycle and its regulation. *Clin Dermatol.* 1988;6:67–73.

Escobar-Morreale HF, Carmina E, Dewailly D, et al. Epidemiology, diagnosis and management of hirsutism: a consensus statement by the Androgen Excess and Polycystic Ovary Syndrome Society. *Hum Reprod Update.* 2012;18(2):146–170.

Ferriman D, Gallwey JD. Clinical assessment of body hair growth in women. *J Clin Endocrinol Metab.* 1961;21:1440–1447.

Futterweit W, Dunaif A, Yeh HC, et al. The prevalence of hyperandrogenism in 109 consecutive female patients with diffuse alopecia. *J Am Acad Dermatol.* 1988;19:831–836.

Harris K, Ferguson J, Hills S. A comparative study of hair removal at an NHS hospital: luminette intense pulsed light versus electrolysis. *J Dermatolog Treat.* 2014;25(2):169–173.

Hatch R, Rosenfield RL, Kim MH, et al. Hirsutism: implications, etiology, and management. *Am J Obstet Gynecol.* 1981;140:815–830.

Koo EB, Petersen TD, Kimball AB. Meta-analysis comparing efficacy of antibiotics versus oral contraceptives in acne vulgaris. *J Am Acad Dermatol.* 2014;71(3):450–459.

Legro RS, Carmina E, Stanczyk FZ, et al. Alterations in androgen conjugate levels in women and men with alopecia. *Fertil Steril.* 1994;62: 744–750.

Lobo RA, Goebelsmann U, Horton R. Evidence for the importance of peripheral tissue events in the development of hirsutism in polycystic ovary syndrome. *J Clin Endocrinol Metab.* 1983;57:393–397.

Lobo RA, Shoupe D, Serafini P, et al. The effects of two doses of spironolactone on serum androgens and anagen hair in hirsute women. *Fertil Steril.* 1985;43:200–205.

Lucky AW, McGuire J, Rosenfield RL, et al. Plasma androgens in women with acne vulgaris. *J Invest Dermatol.* 1983;81(1):70–74.

Ludwig E. Classification of the types of androgenic alopecia (common baldness occurring in the female sex). *Br J Dermatol.* 1977;97:247–254.

Martin KA, Rox Anderson R, Chang RJ et al. Evaluation and treatment of hirsutism in premenopausal women: An Endocrine Society Clinical Practice Guideline. *J Clin Endocrinol Metab.* 2018;103: 1233-1257.

Moran LJ, Hutchison SK, Norman RJ, et al. Lifestyle changes in women with polycystic ovary syndrome. *Cochrane Database Syst Rev.* 2011;(7):CD007506.

Okoroh EM, Hooper WC, Atrash HK, et al. Is polycystic ovary syndrome another risk factor for venous thromboembolism? United States, 2003-2008. *Am J Obstet Gynecol.* 2012;207:377.e1–e8.

O'Reilly MW, Kempegowda P, Jenkinson C, et al. 11-Oxygenated C19 steroids are the predominant androgens in Polycystic Ovary Syndrome. *J Clin Endocrinol Metab.* 2017;102:840–848.

Paulson RJ, Serafini PC, Catalino JA, et al. Measurements of 3α, 17β-androstanediol glucuronide in serum and urine and the correlation with skin 5α-reductase activity. *Fertil Steril.* 1986;46:222–226.

Sakihara S, Kageyama K, Oki Y, et al. Evaluation of plasma, salivary, and urinary cortisol levels for diagnosis of Cushing's syndrome. *Endocr J.* 2010;57(4):331–337.

Serafini P, Lobo RA. Increased 5α-reductase activity in idiopathic hirsutism. *Fertil Steril.* 1985a;43:74–78.

Serafini P, Ablan F, Lobo RA. 5α-Reductase activity in the genital skin of hirsute women. *J Clin Endocrinol Metab.* 1985b;60:349–355.

Speiser PW, Dupont B, Rubenstein P, et al. High frequency of nonclassical steroid 21-hydroxylase deficiency. *Am J Hum Genet.* 1985;37: 650–667.

The Rotterdam ESHRE/ASRM-sponsored PCOS consensus workshop group. Revised 2003 consensus on diagnostic criteria and long-term health risks related to polycystic ovary syndrome (PCOS). *Hum Reprod.* 2004;19:41–47.

Wolf Jr JE, Shander D, Huber F, et al. Randomized, double-blind clinical evaluation of the efficacy and safety of topical eflornithine HCl 13.9% cream in the treatment of women with facial hair. *Int J Dermatol.* 2007;46:94–98.

Wong IL, Morris RS, Chang L, et al. A prospective randomized trial comparing finasteride to spironolactone in the treatment of hirsute women. *J Clin Endocrinol Metab.* 1995;80:233–238.


**Suggested readings for this chapter can be found on ExpertConsult.com.**

# 39 Polycystic Ovary Syndrome

Roger A. Lobo

KEY POINTS

- Polycystic ovary syndrome (PCOS) is now diagnosed by the Rotterdam criteria, which are clinical end points, and is not a laboratory diagnosis. The diagnosis requires finding any two of the following: menstrual irregularity, hyperandrogenism (clinical or biochemical), or polycystic ovaries on ultrasound.
- The disorder is heterogeneous and is not a single-gene disorder, although several susceptibility genes have been identified; environmental influences are most likely involved as well.
- Treatment of women with PCOS should be directed at the specific complaint: menstrual function, skin disorders of androgen excess, or subfertility. Typically more than one complaint exists, and they can be dealt with concomitantly unless the woman is trying to conceive.
- Weight gain and metabolic concerns (particularly insulin resistance, prediabetes, etc.) are extremely common and should be treated aggressively (usually with lifestyle management), particularly before pregnancy. Evidence suggests that cardiovascular morbidity and mortality are not increased in PCOS unless the woman has obesity and/or diabetes.
- Long-term consequences of PCOS may include cardiovascular and metabolic concerns and the increased risks of endometrial and ovarian cancer, unless oral contraceptives have been used. With ovarian aging, cycles may become more regular, and some but not all the symptoms of PCOS may disappear as women approach menopause. The age of menopause may be later.

## POLYCYSTIC OVARY SYNDROME: DEFINITION

Polycystic ovary syndrome **(PCOS)** is the most common endocrine disorder in reproductive-age women. It is often misunderstood and may be underdiagnosed in the general population. PCOS, in its most classic sense, was first described in 1935 by Stein and Leventhal as a syndrome consisting of amenorrhea, hirsutism, and obesity in association with enlarged polycystic ovaries (Stein, 1935). The "classic" features include signs of elevated androgens, such as hirsutism, and oligomenorrhea or amenorrhea and occurs in 3% to 7% of the population**; however, using a broader, now more conventional definition, it is present in as many as 15% to 20% of reproductive-age women** (Fauser, 2012). Many of these women may go unddiagnosed because of lack of awareness on the part of a medical provider or because symptoms are relatively mild and are discounted as not being important. The diagnosis is usually made after the exclusion of other causes of irregular cycles and elevated androgens, such as enzymatic disorders (e.g., 21-hydroxylase deficiency), Cushing syndrome, or tumors.

In the United States the diagnosis does not require findings on ultrasound (US) of characteristic polycystic ovaries. This United States–based definition has been referred to as the National Institutes of Health (NIH) consensus definition because it followed an NIH conference in 1989; however, this was not a consensus conference, there was no true consensus among attendees (Zawadzki, 1992), and two other definitions have been used for PCOS.

In recognition that some women with PCOS may not have menstrual irregularity, and **stressing the importance of the US findings, the "Rotterdam" criteria emerged** after a European Society for Human Reproduction and Embryology/American Society for Reproductive Medicine (ESHRE/ASRM) conference in 2004 (Rotterdam ESHRE/ASRM-Sponsored PCOS Consensus Workshop Group, 2004). **Menstrual irregularity, symptoms or findings of hyperandrogenism, and polycystic ovaries on US are the three criteria used in the definition**, but only two of these three criteria are required for the definition. Thus several phenotypes are possible, including hyperandrogenism and polycystic ovaries in **ovulatory** women (so-called **phenotype C**) and irregular cycles and polycystic ovaries in the absence of documented hyperandrogenism (**phenotype D**). The latter is the most controversial phenotype, and it has been rejected by some investigators in the field. **Phenotype A** is the classic phenotype, which includes all three criteria with US findings of polycystic ovaries, and **phenotype B** denotes women with the NIH definition when there are no US findings. In some cases US has not been done, and in others US findings were considered to be normal.

Because hyperandrogenism is deemed to be an important feature of PCOS, the **Androgen Excess and Polycystic Ovary Syndrome (AEPCOS) Society** has offered a third definition of PCOS, which stresses hyperandrogenism as a key feature and then recognizes that women with PCOS can have polycystic ovaries on US or menstrual irregularity (anovulation) (Azziz, 2006).

A workshop at NIH in December 2012 attempted to draw a consensus among the various definitions. It was concluded among independent panelists that the Rotterdam criteria should be adopted for convention and familiarity (it is the most commonly used definition worldwide) but that it is not ideal and investigators should strive to find a more appropriate name for the disorder (NIH Evidence-based Methodology Workshop, 2012). Table 39.1 lists the four definitions with various phenotypes. More recently there was an international workshop for the diagnosis and management of PCOS (Teede, 2018) and indeed the Rotterdam criteria have now been universally accepted.

Clearly the diagnosis of PCOS is made on a clinical basis, and laboratory measurements can be supportive but are not necessary. For example, elevated luteinizing hormone (LH) levels are not a requirement, nor are elevated levels of testosterone or dehydroepiandrosterone sulfate (DHEAS), as long as there are clinical signs of hyperandrogenism such as hirsutism. Acne is much more variable as a complaint, and half the cases of acne are not caused by elevated androgens. Alopecia also is not a reliable manifestation of hyperandrogenism and could have a purely dermatologic cause. Laboratory assays for testosterone and free testosterone have been too insensitive, at least in the past, to be able to discriminate between slightly elevated levels and normal values; thus a normal testosterone level does not exclude the

**TABLE 39.1** Criteria for Diagnosis of Polycystic Ovary Syndrome

| Study* | Criteria |
|---|---|
| National Institute of Child Health and Human Development 1990 | Menstrual irregularity<br>Hyperandrogenism (clinical or biochemical) |
| ESHRE-ASRM 2003 Rotterdam criteria | Menstrual irregularity<br>Hyperandrogenism (clinical or biochemical)<br>Polycystic ovaries on ultrasound (two of three required) |
| AEPCOS Society 2006 | Hyperandrogenism (clinical or biochemical) and menstrual irregularity<br>Polycystic ovaries on ultrasound (either or both of the latter two) |
| NIH Workshop 2012 | Endorsement of Rotterdam criteria, acknowledging its limitations, and suggesting the name PCOS should be changed |

*All required the exclusion of other underlying hormonal disorders or tumors.

*AEPCOS,* Androgen Excess and PCOS; *ASRM,* American Society for Reproductive Medicine; *ESHRE,* European Society of Human Reproduction and Embryology; *NIH,* National Institutes of Health; *PCOS,* polycystic ovary syndrome.

hyperandrogenism criterion for the definition of PCOS as long as hirsutism is present. We now realize that we have not been measuring many of the important androgens in women with PCOS. A class of 11-oxygenated androgens, largely of adrenal origin, are extremely potent and make up more than 50% of circulating androgens but have not been measured until recently by more sophisticated analyses (O'Reilly, 2016).

## OVARIAN MORPHOLOGY

Another clinical variable is that of the US feature of polycystic ovaries. The classic definition required 12 or more peripherally oriented cystic structures (2 to 9 mm) in one sonographic plane, and typically the finding in one ovary is sufficient. Figs. 39.1 and 39.2 depict the typical polycystic ovary as seen at surgery and by US; however, the US definition has evolved particularly with the advent of greater resolution of vaginal US and 7- to 9-mHz transducers. Findings now suggest that **it is the total follicle count in each ovary that is most diagnostic** (Christ, 2014), and this is more important than the orientation of cystic structures in the ovary or ovarian volume, although ovarian volume is the second most valuable parameter, with **a volume of 10 mL or more** as being diagnostic. These criteria using follicle number per ovary (FNPO) also present a range for cutoff values. In the 2018 evidence-based guidelines on PCOS (Teede, 2018) it was suggested that the FNPO should be 19 to 20, whereas our own data have suggested using 22 and that of Christ suggested an FNPO of 28 (Christ, 2014). Although an antimüllerian hormone (AMH) value greater than 4.7 ng/mL has been useful as a surrogate marker of FNPO for the diagnosis of a polycystic ovary, it is not diagnostic or as valuable as US imaging, and the AMH level varies in different phenotypes, being lower in the milder phenotypes C and D.

It is also important to note that **10% to 25% of the normal reproductive-age population (no symptoms or signs of PCOS) may have polycystic ovaries found on US**. These ovaries have been called *polycystic-appearing ovaries (PAO)*, *polycystic ovarian morphology (PCOM)*, or simply *PCO* in the literature (Wong, 1995). This isolated finding should not be confused with the diagnosis of PCOS, but it may be a risk factor for other

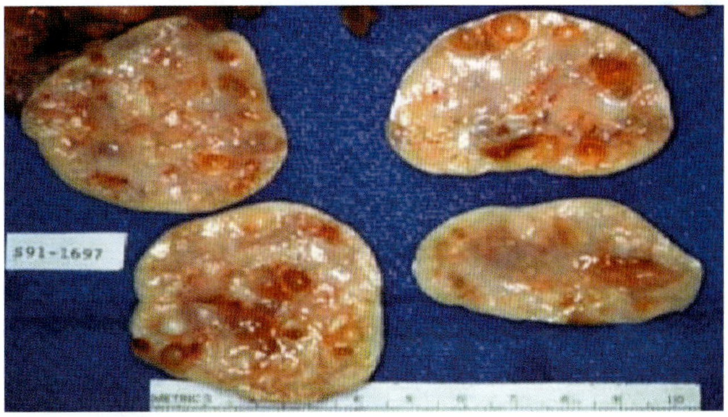


**Fig. 39.1** Surgical specimen of polycystic ovaries.

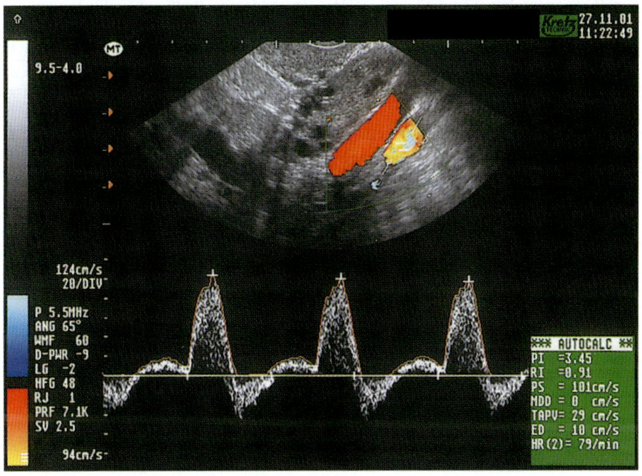


**Fig. 39.2** Typical color Doppler ultrasound of a polycystic ovary showing increased blood flow. (From Strauss JF, Barbieri RL, eds. *Yen and Jaffe's Reproductive Endocrinology.* 6th ed. Philadelphia: Elsevier; 2009:822.)

features of PCOS (e.g., insulin resistance, cardiovascular risk factors) discussed later.

## THE DIAGNOSIS IN ADOLESCENCE

A special category in the definition of PCOS is how it should, or should not, be diagnosed in adolescents. Clearly **Rotterdam criteria should not be used.** This is because all the three criteria for the diagnosis are in a state of flux and change during adolescents, including the evolution and disappearance of polycystic ovaries. Accordingly PCOS should not be diagnosed unless all three criteria are firmly in place (Carmina, 2010) and at a minimum of 3 years postmenarche (Teede, 2018). For the ovarian US criterion, because abdominal US is the mainstay, ovarian volumes of 10 mL or greater should be the criterion used; however, **it is not necessary to place a label on a teenaged girl who has some findings**. It should be suggested that with some features, t he teenager may be at risk and can be reassessed over time, around 8 years postmenarche (Teede, 2018). A firm diagnosis does not preclude treatment. For example, the provider may prescribe oral contraceptives or progestogens for menstrual irregularity.

## MENSTRUAL IRREGULARITY

Menstrual irregularity includes oligomenorrhea (cycles longer than 35 days) and a menstrual frequency of every few months and frank amenorrhea (longer than 6 months missed). Although the majority of women with PCOS have irregular cycles, signifying problems with ovulation, patients with the ovulatory phenotype (C) reporting regular cycles occurs with variable frequencies in different populations, from 3% in Korea to 30% in Italy among women diagnosed with PCOS (Carmina, 2007; Chae, 2008). The ovulatory phenotype may have fewer metabolic and cardiovascular risks, as will be discussed later. It has been reported that menstrual irregularity is the best correlate of insulin resistance in women with PCOS (Carmina, 2007; Chae, 2008). Additionally, although the subfertility of women with PCOS is predominantly caused by problems of anovulation, many women with PCOS with ovulatory function will present with subfertility as well.

## ANDROGEN EXCESS OR HYPERANDROGENISM

Often considered the cardinal feature of women with PCOS, **androgen excess may be difficult to diagnose**. As discussed in Chapter 38, production of androgens in excess may emanate from the ovary, the adrenal gland, or the periphery. Although symptoms of androgen excess, particularly of hirsutism, are sufficient for the inclusion of this parameter in the diagnosis of PCOS, blood measurements of testosterone may not always be accurate and often are normal in women with symptoms.

The androgen excess has been implicated in contributing to abnormalities in LH secretion, weight gain and adipose deposition, and the metabolic derangements of PCOS, discussed later. As discussed in Chapter 38, evidence suggests that 11-oxygenated androgens, derived principally from the adrenal, are quantitatively the most abundant androgens in women with PCOS and may explain many of the symptoms and derangements in metabolism. Adipose tissues also secrete androgen, and this intraadipose androgen source seems to contribute to lipid abnormalities and insulin resistance in women with PCOS (O'Reilly, 2017).

## CHARACTERISTIC ENDOCRINE FINDINGS IN POLYCYSTIC OVARY SYNDROME

Characteristic endocrinologic features include abnormal gonadotropin secretion caused **by increased gonadotropin-releasing hormone (GnRH) pulse amplitude or increased pituitary sensitivity to GnRH**. These abnormalities result in tonically elevated LH levels in approximately two-thirds of the women with this syndrome (Fig. 39.3). After a bolus of GnRH, there is usually an exaggerated response of LH but not of follicle-stimulating hormone (FSH; see Fig. 39.3). Because of issues of metabolic clearance, typically the **women with PCOS who are more obese will be found to have normal LH levels, whereas women with PCOS who are thin often have elevated levels.** The high tonic levels of LH, often referred to as "inappropriate gonadotropin secretion," are due to elevated androgen and unbound estradiol or hypothalamic/pituitary functional abnormalities related to neurotransmitters such as dopamine.

Because FSH levels in women with PCOS are normal or low, an elevated LH/FSH ratio has been used to diagnose PCOS; however, only 70% of women with a clinical diagnosis of PCOS have an elevated level of immunoreactive LH or an immunologic LH/FSH ratio greater than 3, although almost all women with PCOS had elevated serum levels of biologically active LH (Lobo, 1983) (Fig. 39.4). ***An elevated LH level or an elevated LH/FSH ratio is neither specific for nor required for the diagnosis of PCOS.*** These measurements should not be used as diagnostic tools.

In addition to increased levels of circulatory androgens, women with PCOS have increased levels of biologically active (non–sex hormone-binding globulin [SHBG]–bound) estradiol, although total circulating levels of estradiol are not increased

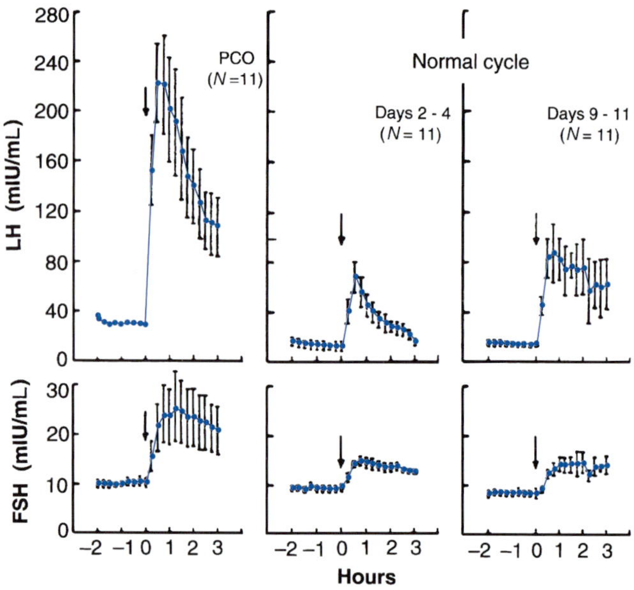


**Fig. 39.3** Comparison of quantitative luteinizing hormone (LH) and follicle-stimulating hormone (FSH) release in response to a single bolus of 150 μg of gonadotropin-releasing hormone (GnRH) in patients with polycystic ovarian syndrome (PCO) and in normal women during low-estrogen (early follicular) and high-estrogen (late follicular) phases of their cycles. (From Rebar R, Judd HL, Yen SSC, et al. Characterization of the inappropriate gonadotropin secretion in polycystic ovary syndrome. *J Clin Invest.* 1976;57(5):1320-1329.)

(Fig. 39.5). The increased amount of non–SHBG-bound estradiol is caused by a decrease in SHBG levels, which is brought about by the increased levels of androgens and obesity, with high insulin levels present in many of these women. Estrone is also increased because of increased peripheral (adipose) conversion of androgen. The tonically increased levels of biologically active estradiol may stimulate increased GnRH pulsatility and produce tonically elevated LH levels and anovulation. In addition, the lowered SHBG level increases the biologically active fractions of androgens in the circulation. This relative hyperestrogenism (elevated levels of estrone and non–SHBG-bound estradiol), which is often unopposed by progesterone because of anovulation, increases the risk of endometrial hyperplasia. The risk of hyperplasia or endometrial cancer is enhanced further in some women with PCOS who seem to have progesterone resistance (Savaris, 2011), meaning that progesterone does not work as well in downregulating the actions of estrogen on the endometrium.

**Androgens from a variety of sources are elevated in women with PCOS** (Fig. 39.6). Serum testosterone levels usually range from 0.55 to 1.2 ng/mL, and androstenedione levels are usually from 3 to 5 ng/mL. In addition, approximately 50% of women with this syndrome have elevated levels of DHEAS, suggesting adrenal androgen involvement. Note the data reviewed earlier and in Chapter 38 on the **abundant 11-oxygenated androgens, which are not measured clinically** at the present time. Although almost all women with PCOS have elevated levels of circulating androgens, the presence or absence of hirsutism depends on whether those androgens are converted peripherally by 5-alpha-reductase to the more potent androgen dihydrotestosterone (DHT), as reflected by increased circulating levels of 3-alpha-androstanediol glucuronide (3α-diol-G) (see Chapter 38). Women with PCOS who are not hirsute have elevated circulatory levels of testosterone, DHEAS, or both, but not 3α-diol-G (Lobo, 1983).

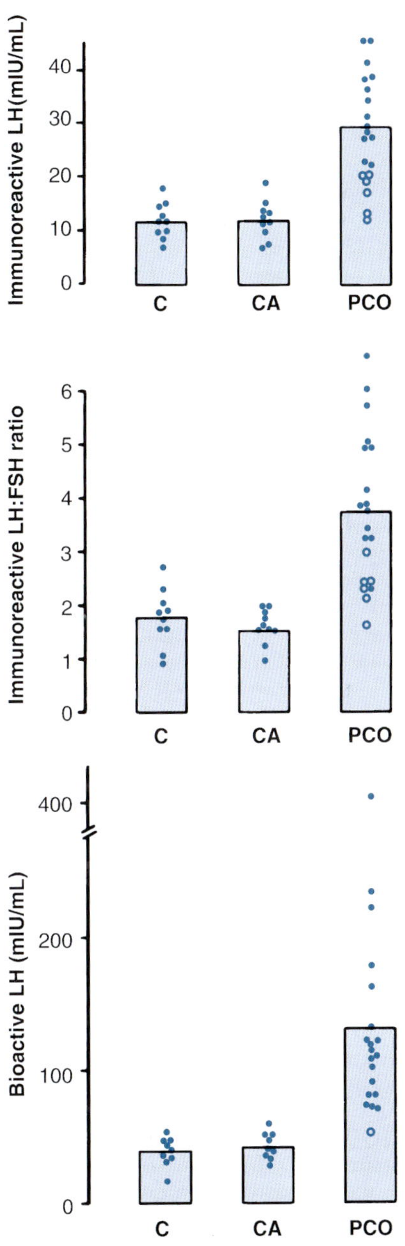


**Fig. 39.4** Serum measurements of immunoreactive luteinizing hormone (LH), immunoreactive LH–to–follicle-stimulating hormone (FSH) ratios, and bioactive LH in control subjects (C), women with chronic anovulation (CA), and women with polycystic ovary syndrome (PCO). Boxes represent the mean ± 3 standard deviation of control levels. (From Lobo RA, Kletzky OA, Campeau JD, et al. Elevated bioactive luteinizing hormone in women with the polycystic ovary syndrome. *Fertil Steril.* 1983;39(5):674-678.)

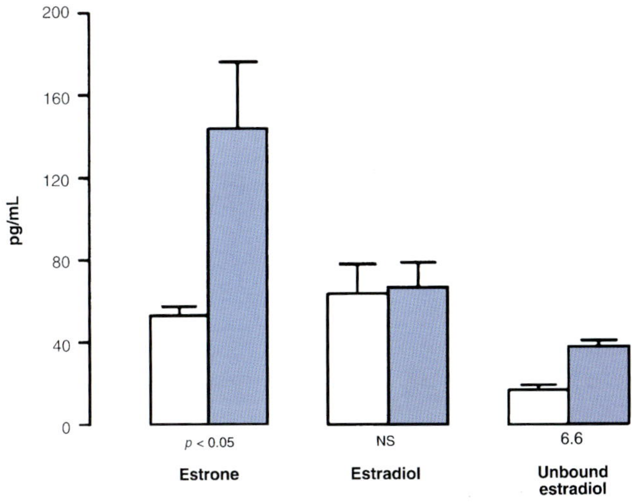


**Fig. 39.5** Serum estrogen concentrations in 13 patients without polycystic ovary syndrome (PCOS) and 22 patients with PCOS *(shaded areas).* (From Lobo RA, Granger L, Goebelsmann U, et al. Elevation in unbound serum estradiol as a possible mechanism for inappropriate gonadotropin secretion in women with PCOS. *J Clin Endocrinol Metab.* 1981;52(1):156-158.)

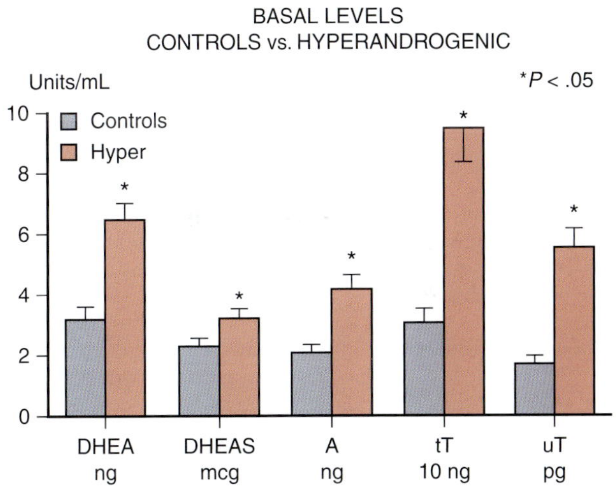


**Fig. 39.6** Basal levels of various androgens in hyperandrogenic women with polycystic ovary syndrome versus matched controls. All androgens, including dehydroepiandrosterone (DHEA), DHEA sulfate (DHEAS), androstenedione (A), total testosterone (tT), and unbound testosterone (uT), are significantly elevated.

**Approximately 20% to 30% of women with PCOS also have mildly elevated levels of prolactin (20 to 35 ng/mL),** possibly related to the increased pulsatility of GnRH, as a result of a relative dopamine deficiency or tonic stimulation from unopposed estrogen. In this setting, if the diagnosis of PCOS is clear, these mild elevations in prolactin level only should be followed.

## INSULIN RESISTANCE

It is well established that some degree of insulin resistance (IR) occurs in most women with PCOS, even in those of normal weight. Insulin and insulin-like growth factor 1 (IGF-1) enhance ovarian androgen production by potentiating the stimulatory action of LH on ovarian androstenedione and testosterone secretion. High levels of insulin bind to the receptor for IGF-1 because of the significant homology of the IGF-1 receptor with the insulin receptor. The granulosa cells also produce IGF-1 and IGF-binding proteins (IGFBPs). This local production of IGF-1 and IGFBP may result in paracrine control and enhancement of LH stimulation and production of androgens by the theca cells in women with PCOS. Because IGFBP levels are lower in women with PCOS, there is increased bioavailable IGF-1, which increases stimulation of the theca cells in combination with LH to produce higher levels of androgen production. In addition,

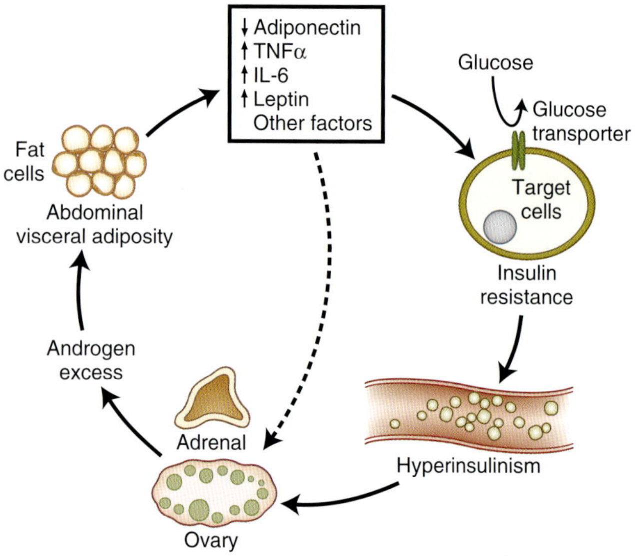


**Fig. 39.7** Diagrammatic depiction of the relationship among androgens, insulin, and body fat (release of adipokines). *IL-6,* Interleukin 6; *TNFα,* tumor necrosis factor alpha. (From Escobar-Morreale HF, San Milan JL. Abdominal adiposity and the polycystic ovary syndrome. *Trends Endocrinol Metab.* 2007;18(7):266-272.)

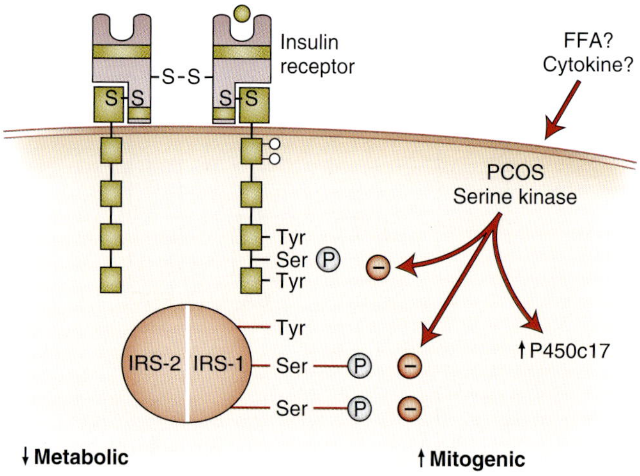


**Fig. 39.8** Mechanism of insulin resistance (IR) in women with polycystic ovary syndrome. At specific sites, IR is due to serine (Ser) phosphorylation affecting metabolic, but not mitogenic, actions of insulin. *PCOS,* polycystic ovary syndrome; *Tyr,* tyrosine. (From Sam S, Dunaif A. Polycystic ovary syndrome: syndrome XX? *Trends Endocrinol Metab.* 2003;14(8):365-370.)

elevated insulin levels (as well as androgen) stimulate adipocyte production of adipokines (adipocytokines), which interfere with the metabolism and breakdown of adipose tissue and further enhance IR (Fig. 39.7). **IR in PCOS is primarily characterized by an insulin resistance in peripheral tissues,** manifest primarily in muscle and adipose and minimally at the level of ovary or adrenal (Sam, 2003). Fig. 39.8 reflects these events with the less efficient serine phosphorylation (rather than tyrosine phosphorylation) resulting in less efficient insulin action (metabolic effect) but with no effects on the production of androgens (intact mitogenic effect) (Sam, 2003).

As part of this feedback loop as noted in Fig. 39.7, in addition to adipokines produced by adipose tissues, which enhance IR (see Fig. 39.8), we now know that androgen produced directly in adipose enhances this effect as well, intensifying the interaction (O'Reilly, 2017).

**The proximate cause of IR in PCOS is unknown**; it is not caused by insulin receptor defects but by signaling abnormalities as noted previously. It is likely that genetic factors contribute to these findings. **Most women with PCOS will be found to have euglycemia with peripheral IR; in more severe cases, there is also evidence of beta cell (secretory) dysfunction, which increases the risk of type 2 diabetes.** In a prospective evaluation of 254 women with PCOS who had an oral glucose tolerance test, it was found that 31% had impaired glucose tolerance and 7.5% had undiagnosed diabetes. In nonobese women with PCOS, 10% had impaired glucose tolerance and 1.5% had diabetes (Legro, 1999). Norman and coworkers have shown that over a mean follow-up period of 6.2 years, 9% of women with PCOS in Australia progressed to having impaired glucose tolerance and 8% developed diabetes (Norman, 2001). Thus the negative effects of obesity and PCOS on insulin resistance are additive. Although clinicians may assume most women with PCOS have some degree of IR, particularly those who are older and who are overweight or obese, it is recommended that testing should be directed at ruling out diabetes and glucose intolerance, rather than diagnosing IR (Fauser, 2012).

Fasting glucose levels are a poor predictor of diabetes in PCOS. A convenient way to assess glucose status is the measurement of the level of hemoglobin A1C. Values greater than 5.8% suggest prediabetes, and values greater than 6% suggest frank diabetes;, but there is still disagreement about the use of A1c as a screening test, and many still advocate performing an oral glucose tolerance test (Fauser, 2012).

Various techniques have been used to diagnose IR in women with PCOS, although it can be argued that women who are overweight or obese with PCOS have IR, and it is not necessary to confirm it. The methods include fairly complicated but more accurate measures used only in a research setting, such as the clamp test, intravenous frequent sampling glucose tolerance test, or insulin tolerance test. Using fasting glucose and insulin measurements and calculating the **quantitative insulin sensitivity check index (QUICKI) or homeostasis model assessment of insulin resistance (HOMA-IR)** have been useful and correlate well with the more invasive techniques (Table 39.2); however, as stated earlier, it may not be necessary to compute these parameters and clinicians should assume that women who are

**TABLE 39.2** Measurements of Insulin Sensitivity

| Test | Measurement | Normal Value* |
|---|---|---|
| Hyperinsulinemic clamp | M/1 (mean glucose use/mean plasma insulin concentration) | $>1.12 \times 10^{-4}$ |
| Homeostasis model assessment of insulin resistance (HOMA-IR) | (Fasting insulin [μU/mL] × fasting glucose [mmol/L])/ 22.5 | <2.77 |
| Glucose-to-insulin ratio | Fasting glucose (mg/dL)/ fasting insulin (μU/mL) | >4.5 |
| Quantitative insulin sensitivity check index (QUICKI) | 1/(log fasting insulin [μU/mL] + log + fasting glucose mg/dL]) | >0.357 |
| Fasting insulin | — | Assay dependent |

*Normal values may vary depending on the insulin assay used.

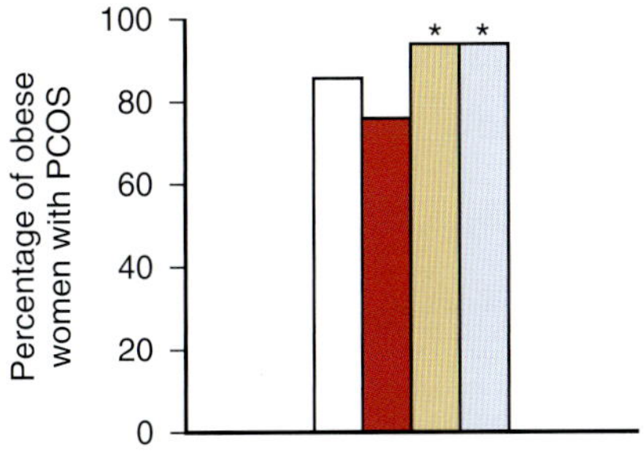


**Fig. 39.9** Percentage of 129 women with obesity and polycystic ovary syndrome (PCOS) with insulin resistance (IR) based on fasting basal insulin *(white)*, glucose/insulin (G/I) ratio *(red)*, homeostasis model assessment of insulin resistance (HOMA) *(yellow)*, or quantitative insulin sensitivity check index (QUICKI) *(light blue)*. *$P < .01$ compared with G/I ratio. (From Carmina E, Lobo RA. The use of fasting blood to assess the prevalence of insulin resistance in women with polycystic ovary syndrome. *Fertil Steril.* 2004;82(3):661-665.)

overweight or obese with PCOS are insulin resistant and an oral glucose tolerance test should be carried out to rule out impaired glucose tolerance or diabetes, which cannot be assumed or discounted. If fasting blood is obtained to detect IR, HOMA or QUICKI are the most valuable parameters (Fig. 39.9) (Carmina, 2004).

**Acanthosis nigricans** (AN) has been found in approximately 30% of hyperandrogenic women, and it is present in at least 50% of women with PCOS who are hyperandrogenic and obese . This velvety hyperpigmentation is usually found in the nape of the neck, axilla, and vulva regions and is often found if inspected for. The ***h***yper***a***ndrogenism, ***IR,*** and ***AN*** (the HAIR-AN syndrome) is a specific disorder associated with insulin receptor antibodies, and presents with very high insulin levels and severe IR. It is distinct from the common findings of most women with PCOS. The combination of increased insulin and IGF-1 in the face of overweight or obese status enhances the development of AN.

## ANTIMÜLLERIAN HORMONE IN PCOS

Müllerian-inhibiting substance (MIS) or AMH is a glycoprotein produced by the granulosa cells of preantral follicles. **Because of the larger number of preantral follicles in PCOS, the MIS or AMH level is significantly elevated in women with PCOS** (Dewailly, 2014). Physiologically, AMH attenuates a sensitivity of FSH in stimulating granulosa cells; the levels are higher in clomiphene-resistant women and in those who are chronically anovulatory compared with those with more regular cycles, even as they age (see Fig. 39.10) (Carmina, 2012a). AMH levels have also been positively correlated with LH levels. It has been suggested that **AMH is involved in the pathophysiology of anovulation in PCOS**, and recent data have suggested that it may explain some of the hereditary nature of women with PCOS. These data suggest that higher levels of AMH in amniotic fluid program the fetus in utero to have higher LH and androgens and dysregulate the hypothalamic-pituitary-ovarian axis, resulting in the development of PCOS (Tata, 2018).

Because AMH correlates with the number of ovarian preantral follicles, it has been suggested that AMH may be used as a blood test to substitute for US findings of a polycystic ovary. **A meta-analysis and our own review suggest a cutoff value of 4.7 ng/mL** (Iliodromiti, 2013), with values greater than this being consistent with PCOS; however, the degree of overlap in values of AMH between PCOS and normal women precludes its routine use (Casadei, 2013). Our data also suggest that the milder phenotypes such as C and D have lower levels of AMH.

## PATHOPHYSIOLOGIC CONSIDERATIONS

It is clear that there is a genetic predisposition to PCOS; however, it is likely that several genes are involved, and these are **susceptibility genes** that predispose the women affected to develop PCOS. A review by Kosova and Urbanek pointed out the many difficulties in finding a direct genetic linkage, which are related to the nature of the disorder, its heterogeneity, and the large sample size required to find meaningful associations (Kosova, 2013). There are also multiple family studies of sisters, brothers, and daughters of affected women all showing some traits associated with aspects of PCOS.

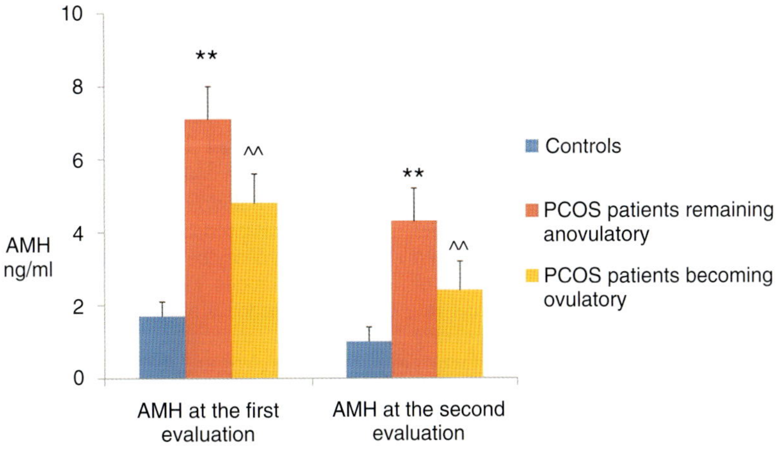


**Fig. 39.10** Elevated levels of antimüllerian hormone (AMH) in women with polycystic ovary syndrome (PCOS) decrease with time, and levels are lower in ovulatory women. Data are from a 20-year longitudinal study in women with PCOS. **, significant different from controls; [other symbol], significant difference between ovulatory and anovulatory PCOS. (From Carmina E, Campagna AM, Mansuet P, et al. Does the level of serum antimullerian hormone predict ovulatory function in women with polycystic ovary syndrome with aging? *Fertil Steril.* 2012;98(4):1043-1046.)

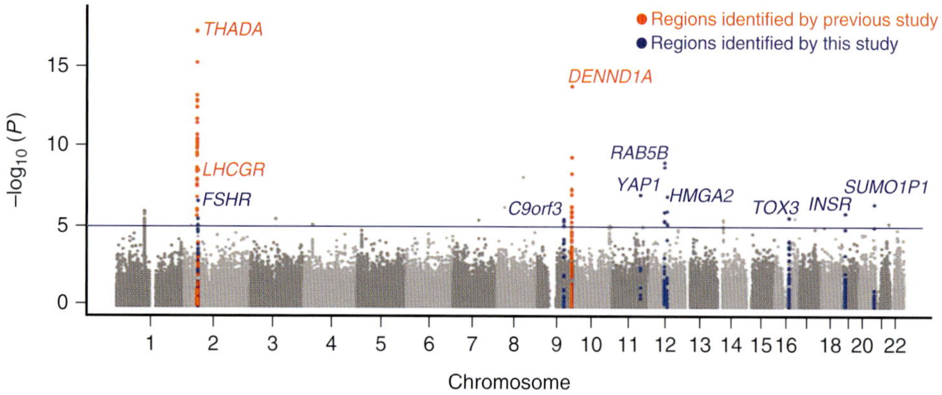


**Fig. 39.11** Genome-wide association studies in 8226 women with polycystic ovary syndrome (PCOS) diagnosed by Rotterdam criteria and 7578 controls, with several loci identified for susceptibility genes of interest. (From Shi Y, Zhao H, Shi Y, et al. Genome-wide association study identifies eight new risk loci for polycystic ovary syndrome. *Nat Genet.* 2012;44(9):1020-1027.)

**Environmental factors are clearly involved as well**, based on twin studies, in which PCOS is not always concordant on a genetic basis (Vink, 2006). Maternal exposure to androgen has been shown in a monkey model to contribute to the development of PCOS (Abbott, 2005). **Note the data of Tata and colleagues reviewed earlier, where the pregnancy environment, related to AMH, may also be implicated.**

Genome-wide association studies in Han Chinese and European families have pointed out certain susceptibility genes with some consistency. These include loci at 2p16.3, 2p21, and 9q 33.3, involving the LH/human chorionic gonadotropin (HCG) receptor, a thyroid adenoma locus, and *DENND1A*, potentially affecting function of the endoplasmic reticulum (Chen, 2010). This was confirmed in subsequent studies with the addition of other potential loci (Shi, 2012; Zhao, 2012) (Fig. 39.11). The 2p16.3 locus was confirmed in a U.S. study (Mutharasan, 2013). It has been long established that a vicious cycle propagates the disorder in PCOS, regardless of how it begins (Strauss, 2009) (Fig. 39.12). Thus it was attractive to postulate that dopamine deficiency in the hypothalamus might give rise to the exaggerated LH responses in PCOS, and there are several similar hypotheses, although it has been observed that morphologically identifiable polycystic ovaries are seen in children (Bridges, 1993); however, in the adolescent, ovarian morphology has been shown to be variable and can change from being polycystic to normal and vice-versa. This occurrence predicts puberty and other normal endocrinologic events, suggesting a central role for altered PCOM in the disorder.

Furthermore, not all women with isolated polycystic ovaries have PCOS, as stated earlier. Thus a pathophysiologic model can be put together as follows. An ovary is polycystic in up to 20% of girls, according to data from Bridges and colleagues. Thus the ovary transitions early in life from normal to polycystic appearing (PAO). This influence occurs in a specific way by genetic factors or environmental factors, or it is induced by other endocrine disturbances (Lobo, 1996) (Fig. 39.13). The woman who develops PAO may have normal menses, normal androgen levels, and normal ovulatory function and parity; however, if subjected to various susceptibility factors (likely genetic) or environmental or other challenges or insults, with varying degrees of severity, women with PAO may develop a full-blown syndrome (PCOS) (see Fig. 39.13). **The syndrome, if full-blown, exhibits the full extent of hyperandrogenism and anovulation, with the most**

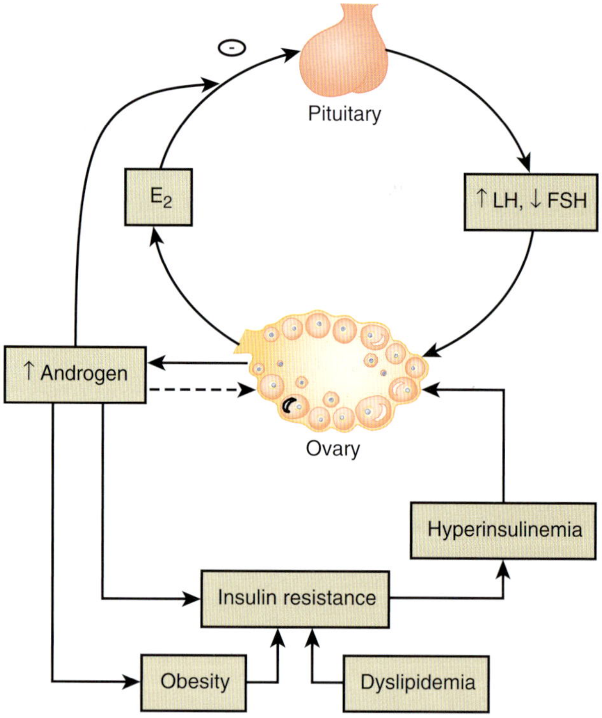


**Fig. 39.12** Pathophysiologic concept of polycystic ovary syndrome (PCOS). Increased luteinizing hormone (LH) secretion, together with enhanced theca cell responsiveness, drives the production of excess ovarian androgen. Increased androgen production may inhibit steroid negative feedback effects on hypothalamic gonadotropin-releasing hormone pulse generation to account for the rapid LH pulse frequency observed in women with PCOS. In addition, increased androgen levels are associated with android obesity, visceral fat deposition, and dyslipidemia, all of which may contribute to insulin resistance. Independently, hyperandrogenemia, obesity, and hyperinsulinemia may decrease sex hormone–binding globulin, thereby increasing bioactive testosterone. Finally, increased androgen may have direct effects on the ovary to increase follicle number and follicle size and possibly enhance granulosa cell responsiveness to follicle-stimulating hormone (FSH). $E_2$, Estradiol. (From Strauss JF, Barbieri RL, eds. *Yen and Jaffe's Reproductive Endocrinology.* 6th ed. Philadelphia: WB Saunders; 2009:509.)

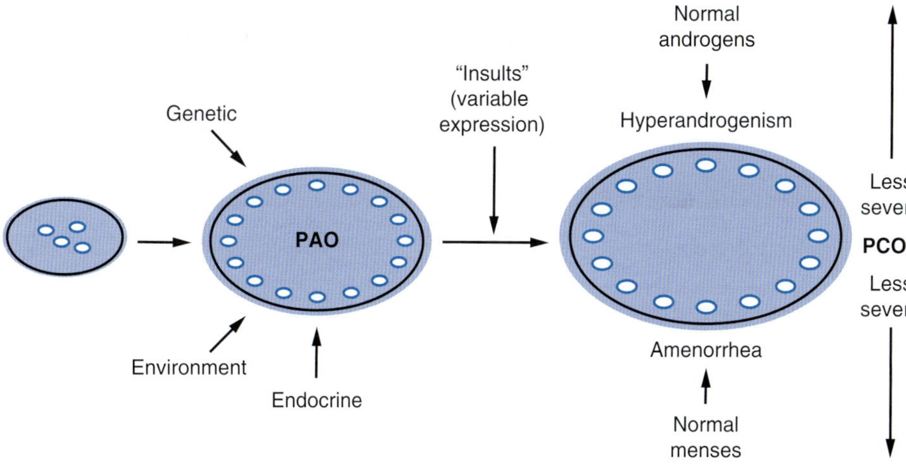


**Fig. 39.13** Pathophysiology of polycystic ovary syndrome (PCOS) showing differences in presentation. *PAO,* Polycystic-appearing ovaries.

**extreme form of this menstrual disturbance being amenorrhea (the type A or B phenotype according to Rotterdam criteria); however, in this spectrum of disorders, the androgen disturbances may also be near normal. Similarly, the menstrual disturbance may be mild.**

**This model requires that normal homeostatic factors may be able to ward off stressors or insults in some women** who can go through life without PCOS but have PAO, which does not change morphologically. Alternatively, with varying degrees of success, a woman's homeostatic mechanisms may at any time, early or later in reproductive life, allow symptoms of PCOS to emerge with varying degrees of severity. Two of the major insults are thought to be weight gain and psychological stress. Therefore the typical teenager born with PAO may develop PCOS fairly quickly, but a PCOS picture may only develop later in life in some women, even after having children, with weight gain, for example.

## Consequences of Polycystic Ovary Syndrome

The importance of diagnosing PCOS is that there are known long-term consequences of the diagnosis warranting lifelong surveillance. These include metabolic and cardiovascular risks as well as the risk of certain cancers with aging.

There have been several consensus meetings for the diagnosis and treatment of PCOS, as mentioned earlier. The first two dealt with the diagnosis of PCOS (Rotterdam ESHRE/ASRM-Sponsored PCOS Consensus Workshop Group, 2004) and the treatment of infertility (Thessaloniki ESHRE/ASRM-Sponsored PCOS Consensus Workshop Group, 2008). The third and most recent of these was held in Amsterdam and addressed the long-term consequences of PCOS (Fauser, 2012). Fig. 39.14 depicts the shift in emphasis with aging, requiring a multidisciplinary approach. With aging, concerns for cardiovascular disease, including hypertension, metabolic syndrome, diabetes, and cancer (endometrial and ovarian), become more prominent.

### WEIGHT GAIN/OBESITY AND METABOLIC SYNDROME

Weight gain as women age is a major predictor of abnormal metabolic findings and the emergence of cardiovascular (CV) disease risks; indeed all the symptoms of PCOS are worse with increasing body weight. The prevalence of obesity varies widely in different countries. It is lowest in countries such as China and Japan (<10%) and highest in the United States and some other Western countries (~70%). There is increased abdominal and visceral fat in women with PCOS, and this has been correlated to IR and metabolic dysfunction (Lord, 2006). Therefore lifestyle management has to be a priority for women with PCOS and must be maintained lifelong.

Metabolic syndrome, which is largely driven by obesity and leads to diabetes and CV disease (CVD), has a prevalence during the reproductive years. The prevalence of metabolic syndrome in the United States is approximately 60% in young (20 to 39 years) obese women with PCOS (Apridonidze, 2005). The diagnosis is made using Adult Treatment Panel III criteria (three of five of the following: waist circumference >88 cm, high-density lipoprotein <50 mg/dL, triglycerides >150 mg/dL; blood pressure >130/85 mm Hg, fasting blood sugar >110 mg/dL). In other countries in which obesity is less prevalent, the prevalence of metabolic syndrome in PCOS is still increased but is much lower (5% to 9%) (Carmina, 2006). **The constellation of risk factors that make up metabolic syndrome place women with PCOS at increased risk for CVD and diabetes,** but there is nothing specific of more significance regarding metabolic syndrome in PCOS.

### DIABETES

Type 2 diabetes mellitus is more prevalent (two to three times higher) in women with PCOS of reproductive age (Legro, 1999). This is driven by IR, which in turn is worsened by overweight status and menstrual irregularity. In prospective follow-up studies, there is a high conversion rate in women with PCOS from euglycemia toward impaired glucose tolerance, and in women followed for 6 years who had **impaired glucose tolerance the conversion rate to frank diabetes was 54%** (Norman, 2001). Thus it is extremely important to screen for diabetes in the overweight population with PCOS; it has been suggested that this is best done with an oral glucose tolerance test (Fauser, 2012). Lack of precision in the screening for diabetes with hemoglobin A1c measurements has precluded the recommendation of using hemoglobin A1c as a screening tool, although it has proven to be useful in the follow-up of women as they are being treated. **Diet and exercise remain the mainstays of treatment,** and metformin has a significant role to play. In at-risk women and those with glucose intolerance and prediabetes, metformin is often used with doses of 1500 mg/day. Doses are often higher in the presence of diabetes.

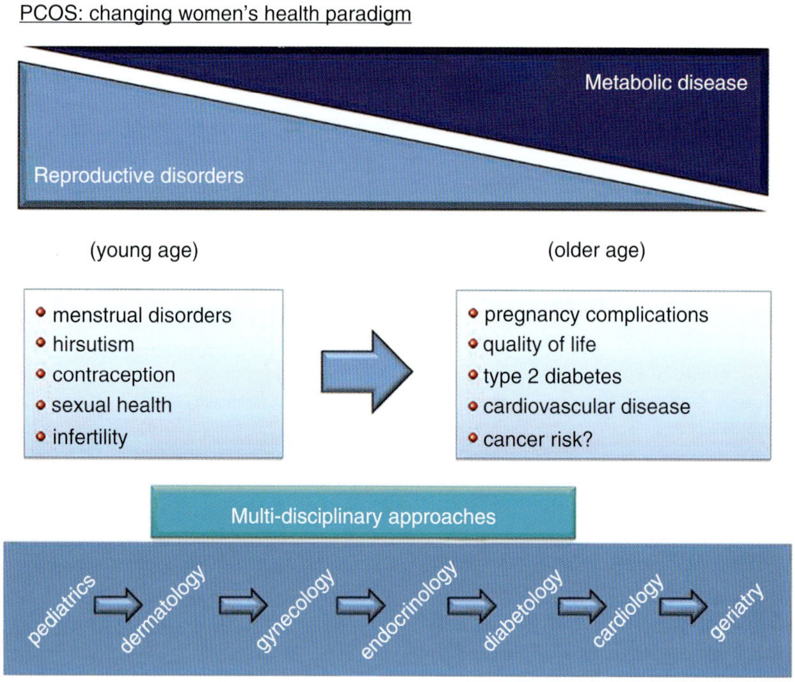


**Fig. 39.14** Schematic representation of the change in emphasis from early-age reproductive disorders to long-term metabolic and cardiovascular health. *PCOS,* Polycystic ovary syndrome. (From Fauser B, Tarlatzis B, Rebar RW, et al. Consensus on women's health aspects of polycystic ovary syndrome (PCOS): the Amsterdam ESHRE/ASRM-sponsored 3rd PCOS Consensus Workshop Group. *Fertil Steril.* 2012;97(1):28-38.e25.)

## QUALITY-OF-LIFE ISSUES

Although the data are not completely consistent, it is generally stated that there is poor quality of life among women with PCOS. This is most likely related to their burden of being overweight, having irregular cycles and decreased fertility, and having skin concerns such as acne and hirsutism, although not all women have the same number or degree of these symptoms. **Depression is a factor, which may play a major role in women with PCOS seeking care and being compliant with diet, lifestyle, and various treatments.** In a meta-analysis, Dokras found a fourfold increase in the prevalence of depression among women with PCOS (Dokras, 2011). Another meta-analysis showed that in addition to depression, **anxiety disorder** is also prevalent, with a two- to threefold increase (Brutocao, 2018). A strong argument has been made for **screening women** with PCOS for anxiety and depression. It has also been found that interventions, such as weight loss, are able to improve quality of life (Thomson, 2010).

## CARDIOVASCULAR CONCERNS

Women with PCOS have characteristic lipid and lipoprotein abnormalities (Wild, 1988) (Fig. 39.15). These older data have been replicated many times, and abnormal lipoprotein particles are also present, which adds to a long list of abnormalities that tend to increase CV risk. Table 39.3 depicts several CV risk factors, including the development of **hypertension and diabetes** as women approach menopause. Fig. 39.16 depicts data that have been generated from retrospective observations, and although it is yet not definitively established that these risks pertain to all women with PCOS, it provides evidence suggesting concern (Dahlgren, 1992). It is unlikely that these risks occur in women with "milder" phenotypes. Data have largely been obtained from women with more classic features of PCOS, particularly in conjunction with presence of obesity. There is evidence that women with the milder phenotypes diagnosed using the Rotterdam criteria have fewer CV risk factors. Fig. 39.17 depicts a hypothetical scheme for increasing CV risk in women with PCOS with various phenotypes (Jovanovic, 2010).

It is important to note, however, that there are no definitive data on whether PCOS increases CV mortality (Fauser, 2012). Although multiple risk factors are present (IR, lipids, adipocytokines, inflammatory markers, surrogate markers of atherosclerosis on imaging), (Fauser, 2012), **retrospective analyses have shown no increase in mortality, except among women** with diabetes (Fauser, 2012; Pierpoint, 1998; Wild, 2000). There has been some consideration that the older retrospective studies focused on a younger population of women and may not have been sufficiently rigorous to establish whether there is, or is not, an increased CV risk in PCOS. Although one study showed a lower CV event-free survival with time (greater CV mortality) in PCOS (Shaw, 2008), these data were subsequently retracted by the authors. A 2018 reassessment of this issue by us concluded that **unless a woman with PCOS has "classic" features of PCOS and has diabetes and obesity, there is no evidence for increased CV morbidity and mortality in women with PCOS** (Carmina, 2018). Because of the large constellation of risk factors and lack of adverse outcome data, it could be hypothesized that there may be some inherent protective factors in PCOS.

## CANCERS IN POLYCYSTIC OVARY SYNDROME

As depicted in Fig. 39.18, there is an **age-specific onset for some of the consequences of PCOS**. The risk for all cancers increases with aging, but endometrial cancer can begin at a younger age because of long-term anovulation and unopposed estrogen stimulation of the endometrium. It is likely that there

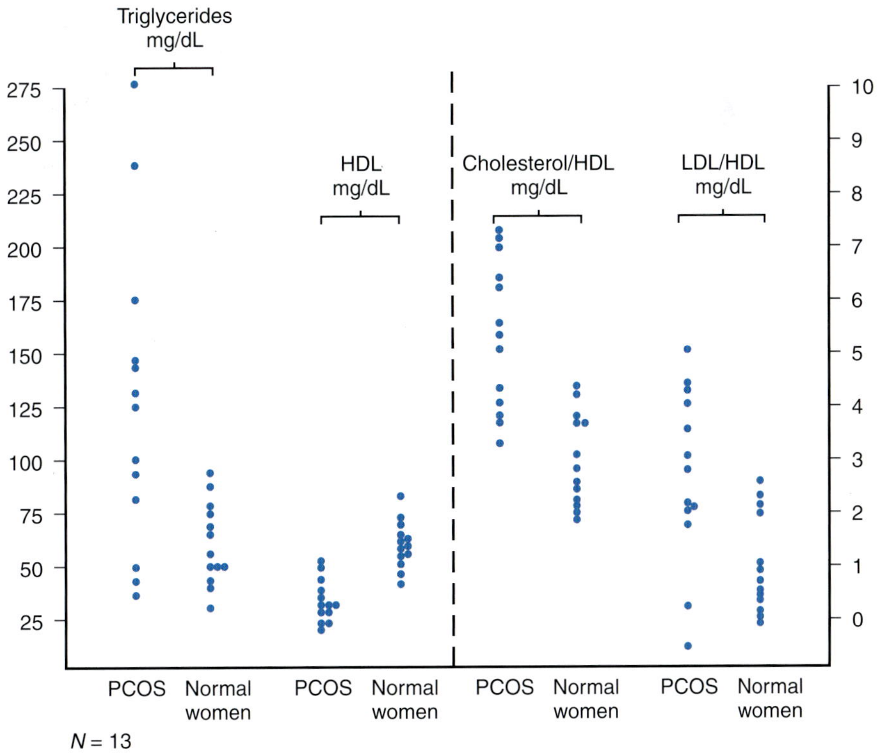


**Fig. 39.15** Lipid and lipoprotein profiles in 13 women with polycystic ovary syndrome (PCOS) versus control group when matched for percent ideal body weight. Differences are evident in all measures ($P < .01$). *HDL,* High-density lipoprotein; *LDL,* low-density lipoprotein; *PCOS,* polycystic ovary syndrome. (From Wild RA, Bartholomew MJ. The influence of body weight on lipoprotein lipids in patients with polycystic ovary syndrome. *Am J Obstet Gynecol.* 1988;159(2):423-427.)

**TABLE 39.3** Cardiovascular Risk Factors in Polycystic Ovary Syndrome

| Risk Factor | Features |
|---|---|
| Traditional risk factors | Obesity, insulin resistance, dyslipidemia, abnormal homocysteine, C-reactive protein, plasminogen activator inhibitor-1, increase in inflammatory adipocytokines such as TNF-α, decrease in adiponectin; higher prevalence of diabetes, hypertension |
| Atherosclerosis | Coronary catheterization studies, increase in carotid intima-media thickness, coronary calcium |
| Endothelial dysfunction by blood flow studies | All increased in classic PCOS; less of a concern with milder phenotypes using Rotterdam criteria |

*PCOS,* Polycystic ovary syndrome; *TNF-α,* tumor necrosis factor alpha.

are other susceptibilities as well, which contribute to the diagnosis of cancer at a younger age. Although breast cancer does not seem to be increased in women with PCOS (Chittenden, 2009), both endometrial and ovarian cancer are increased (Chittenden, 2009; Fauser, 2012). The data for these reports are negatively affected by the heterogeneity of the patient population and their retrospective nature. Most of the data pertain to women diagnosed with classic PCOS. It is likely that women with milder phenotypes may have little or no increased risk.

**Endometrial cancer is increased at least two- to threefold,** even when controlling for weight. Apart from unopposed estrogen

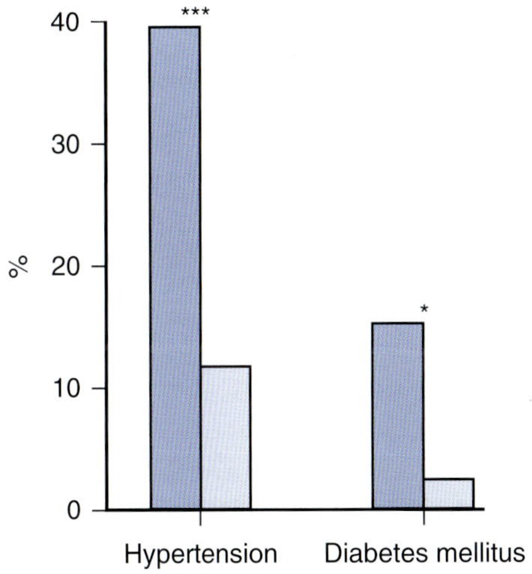


**Fig. 39.16** Prevalence of hypertension (medically treated) and manifest diabetes mellitus in 33 participants with polycystic ovary syndrome (PCOS) and 132 referents. The *dark-shaded bars* indicate the participants with PCOS. The *light-shaded bars* indicate the referents. Statistical comparisons were made between the women with PCOS and referents. Differences were considered significant at $^{*}P = .05$ and $^{***}P = .001$. (From Dahlgren E, Janson PO, Johansson S, et al. Women with polycystic ovary syndrome wedge resected in 1956 to 1965: a long-term follow-up focusing on natural history and circulating hormones. *Fertil Steril.* 199;57(3):505.)

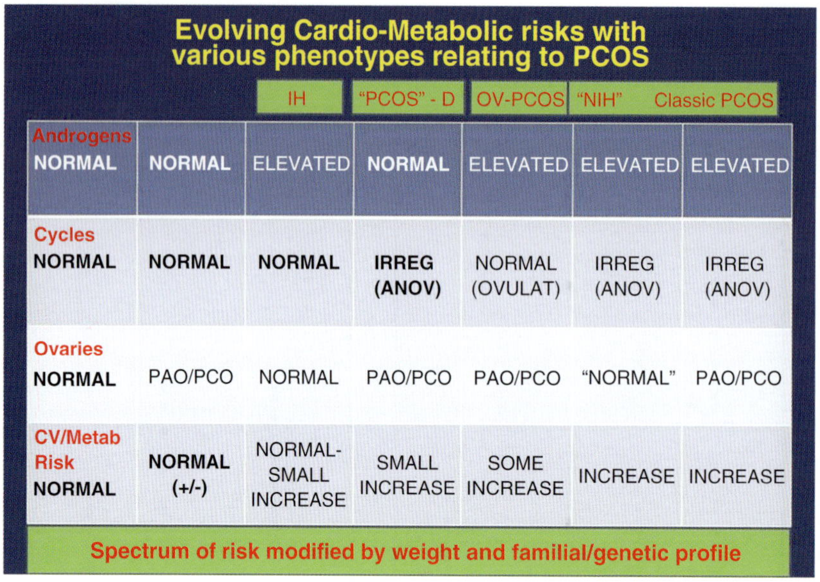

**Evolving Cardio-Metabolic risks with various phenotypes relating to PCOS**

| | | IH | "PCOS" - D | OV-PCOS | "NIH" | Classic PCOS |
|---|---|---|---|---|---|---|
| Androgens NORMAL | NORMAL | ELEVATED | NORMAL | ELEVATED | ELEVATED | ELEVATED |
| Cycles NORMAL | NORMAL | NORMAL | IRREG (ANOV) | NORMAL (OVULAT) | IRREG (ANOV) | IRREG (ANOV) |
| Ovaries NORMAL | PAO/PCO | NORMAL | PAO/PCO | PAO/PCO | "NORMAL" | PAO/PCO |
| CV/Metab Risk NORMAL | NORMAL (+/-) | NORMAL-SMALL INCREASE | SMALL INCREASE | SOME INCREASE | INCREASE | INCREASE |

Spectrum of risk modified by weight and familial/genetic profile

**Fig. 39.17** Evolving cardiometabolic risks with various phenotypes relating to polycystic ovary syndrome (PCOS). The spectrum of risk is modified by weight and familial and genetic profile. *Anov,* anovulatory; *CV/Metab,* cardiovascular/metabolic; *IH,* idiopathic hirsutism; *NIH,* National Institutes of Health; *OV-PCOS,* ovulatory PCOS; *Ovulat*, ovulatory; *PAO/PCO,* polycystic appearing ovary/polycystic ovary; *PCOS-D,* polycystic ovary syndrome phenotype D. (From Jovanovic VP, Carmina E, Lobo RA. Not all women diagnosed with PCOS share the same cardiovascular risk profiles. *Fertil Steril.* 2010;94(3):826-832.)

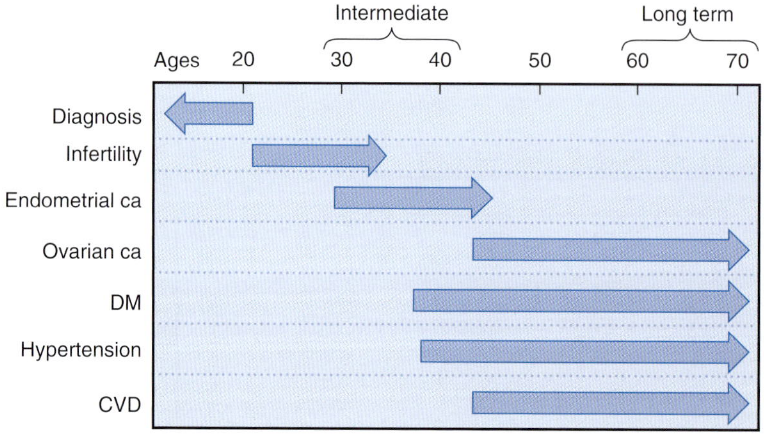


**Fig. 39.18** Consequences of polycystic ovary syndrome (PCOS) as a function of age. *ca,* Cancer; *CVD,* cardiovascular disease; *DM,* diabetes mellitus.

being a risk factor, there may also be a defect in progesterone signaling in the endometrium among cancer patients (Savaris, 2011). The data are less strong for **ovarian cancer, but the risk is thought to be about 2.5 times increased** (Chittenden, 2009).

This level of risk for endometrial and ovarian cancer can be brought down to a normal rate with the use of oral contraceptives (OCs). The decreased risk of these cancers with the use of OCs for about 5 years is well known (Grimbizis, 2010) and translates into a good strategy for normalizing cancer risk in women with PCOS, particularly because many women normally would be treated with OCs in any event for other symptoms. Also of interest, is that there is a growing body of evidence that **metformin, which may also be used for women with PCOS, has inhibitory effects on various cancers; the data are strongest for endometrial and breast cancer** (Col, 2012; Tan, 2011).

## OVARIAN AGING: POLYCYSTIC OVARY SYNDROME AND MENOPAUSE

As all women age, the ovaries decrease in size and androgen levels decrease; this is true for those with PCOS as well. It is logical to assume therefore that **at some juncture in time, the phenotype of PCOS may change or disappear.** An interesting phenomenon, which has been well documented, is that **as women with PCOS age, their menstrual cycles, if irregular when younger, become more regular and ovulatory** (Carmina, 2012b; Elting, 2003). This is because of a **decrease in the total follicular cohort** and subsequently **lower levels of AMH** (Carmina, 2012a). In our longitudinal studies of women with PCOS, followed for 20 years, by the fourth decade nearly half of the women had evidence of ovulatory function, and in 8% the diagnosis of PCOS could no longer be made (Carmina, 2012b).

Although with aging the follicular cohort is decreased, compared with other women of the same age, there are still more follicles and typically higher levels of AMH. This leads to the notion that there may be preserved fertility in women with PCOS as they age. This has been confirmed in one retrospective study in an *in vitro* fertilization (IVF) model, in which **the live birth rate was higher at an older age compared with women with tubal disease** (Mellembakken, 2011). As women enter menopause, which is likely to be at a later age (although not well documented [Fauser, 2012]), despite lowered androgen levels, **hirsutism may still be prevalent** (Schmidt, 2011). There is also evidence that there is a **persistence of the metabolic issues** that existed at an earlier age (Puurunen, 2011), thus requiring continued vigilance in managing and following these women.

## ISOLATED POLYCYSTIC OVARIES

We have found that women with normal ovulatory function and PAO or PCOM have a subtle form of ovarian hyperandrogenism when stimulated with gonadotropins or HCG (Wong, 1995). We have also found subtle changes in insulin sensitivity and altered lipoproteins (Chang, 2000). Therefore although many women with isolated PAO or PCOM may not have any problems, this finding may be considered as a risk factor for developing the consequences of PCOS.

## TREATMENT OF POLYCYSTIC OVARY SYNDROME

Treatment of women with PCOS should be directed at the **specific complaint**. These concerns fall into three main categories: **androgen excess and symptoms of hyperandrogenism; irregular bleeding** (in this setting often called dysfunctional uterine bleeding) and risks of endometrial disease as a result of unopposed estrogen stimulation from anovulation; **fertility concerns and subfertility**, mostly because of anovulation. In addition, a common complaint is weight gain or the inability to lose weight. This is also related to IR and metabolic concerns discussed previously. Accordingly, regardless of the complaint, **lifestyle management is an extremely important component of any treatment regimen.**

Androgen excess (acne, hirsutism, and alopecia) occurs in the majority of women with PCOS, but not in all women. At times the symptoms are sufficiently mild that the treatment focus is on other concerns such as subfertility. Specific treatment for androgen excess symptoms is covered in Chapter 40 and usually involves the use of an OC, with or without an antiandrogen.

Treatment of irregular bleeding should be directed at supplying the missing progesterone in anovulatory women. This potentially can lead to endometrial hyperplasia or cancer if not treated. Women who are overweight and older are a higher-risk group, and endometrial biopsy may be indicated, although there are no validated guidelines as to when a biopsy should be carried out (Fauser, 2012). It is important to remember that it is the women with PCOS along with menstrual irregularity who have IR and are more likely to have metabolic dysfunction. OCs are the most logical and effective treatment, particularly because it is known that they reduce the risk of endometrial cancer. OCs may also be indicated for treatment of symptoms of androgen excess. In other women, progestogen therapy alone may be used at 2- to 3-month intervals to shed the endometrium in chronically anovulatory women. Medroxyprogesterone acetate (5 to 10 mg) or norethindrone acetate (2.5 to 10 mg) may be used in this setting. More complicated cases of menometrorrhagia are treated, as would other patients.

**Treatment of subfertility in PCOS is predominantly a result of anovulation.** Even women with the ovulatory phenotype C may have subtle ovulatory disturbances, and it is known that some women have **endometrial defects in progesterone and insulin signaling** (DuQuesnay, 2009). Before treatment with ovulation induction, it is important to rule out other fertility factors, specifically male factors by obtaining a semen analysis (see Chapter 40).

## TREATMENT OF SUBFERTILITY IN POLYCYSTIC OVARY SYNDROME

Before ovulation induction, it is necessary to normalize overt abnormalities in glucose tolerance and to encourage weight loss for overweight women. Ovulation induction may be accomplished by a variety of agents, including metformin, clomiphene, letrozole, gonadotropins, and pulsatile GnRH, as well as ovarian diathermy or drilling. Adjunctive measures include the use of dexamethasone, dopamine agonists, thiazolidinediones, and various combinations of these options, although today these agents are rarely used. IVF (stimulated or unstimulated) may be indicated in difficult-to-manage cases or if other in fertility factors are present (Thessaloniki ESHRE/ASRM-Sponsored PCOS Consensus Workshop Group, 2008).

Although metformin had been used as a first-line treatment for infertility, with supportive evidence for some effectiveness including data from a Cochrane review (Tang, 2013), randomized trials with a focus on live births as an end point have suggested that clomiphene is superior to metformin for first-line therapy (Legro, 2007) (Fig. 39.19). Metformin should be used for women with overweight or obesity to achieve better metabolic control before pregnancy and for those who may have a more casual approach to their fertility, in that metformin takes longer to become effective and may not induce ovulation in some women. Even

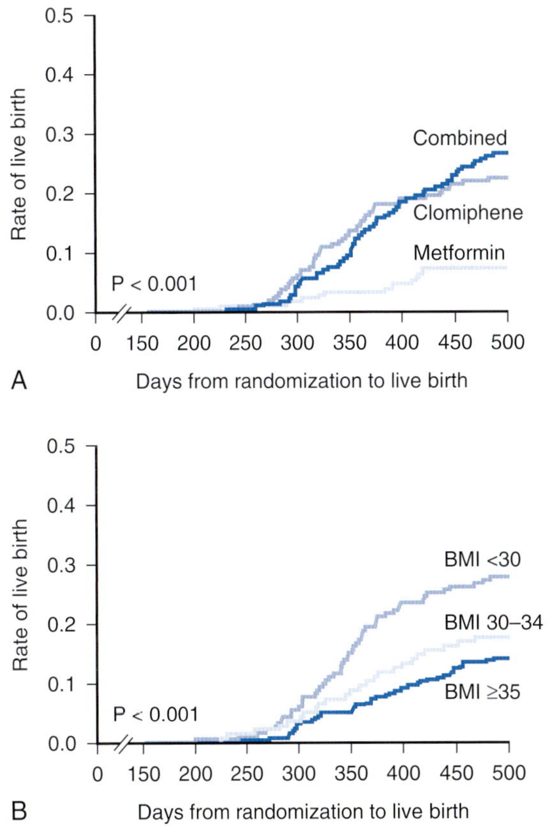


**Fig. 39.19** Kaplan-Meier curves for live birth, according to **(A)** study group or **(B)** body mass index (BMI). (From Legro RS, Barnhart HX, Schlaff WD, et al. Clomiphene, metformin, or both for infertility in the polycystic ovary syndrome. *N Engl J Med.* 2007;356(6):551-566.)

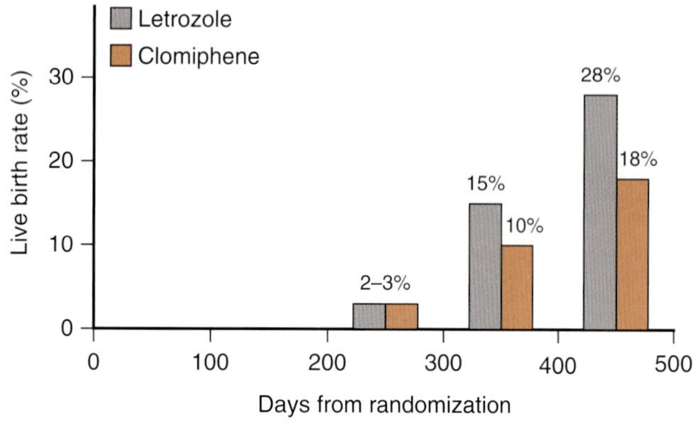


**Fig. 39.20** Results of a prospective randomized trial in women with polycystic ovary syndrome comparing the live-birth rates of the administration of letrozole versus clomiphene (Kaplan-Meier curves). Letrozole performed significantly better. (Data from Legro RS, Brzyski RG, Diamond MP, et al. Letrozole versus clomiphene for infertility in the polycystic ovary syndrome. *N Engl J Med.* 2014;371(2):119-129.)

when metformin cannot induce ovulation, its continued use may be beneficial when combined with clomiphene or gonadotropins. An improvement in oocyte quality with metformin has been suggested, but the effect has not been proved. It may decrease the risk of ovarian hyperstimulation syndrome (OHSS) in women with PCOS undergoing IVF (Tso, 2009; Palomba, 2011).

Clomiphene has been the mainstay for ovulation induction. Most pregnancies occur within the first few cycles. Accordingly, it is reasonable to use clomiphene, with or without metformin, as an initial approach, after obtaining a semen analysis, but not for more than three or four ovulatory cycles before a more comprehensive workup is undertaken. **Letrozole (2.5 to 5 mg/day, 5 days) has proved to be efficacious** as an alternative to clomiphene, and it is particularly suited for women who have side effects with clomiphene. **In a randomized head-to head comparison of clomiphene and letrozole in women with PCOS, letrozole was found to be superior** (Legro, 2014) (Fig. 39.20). **This was also confirmed in a Cochrane review** (Franik, 2015), and a cost analysis has shown letrozole to be more cost effective, thus establishing its place as first-line treatment for women with PCOS. Low-dose gonadotropin therapy is highly effective as a second-line treatment (for failure with oral agents and for the occasional patient who may have transitory low estrogen status); there is no evidence that any one gonadotropin preparation is better than another (Thessaloniki ESHRE/ASRM-sponsored PCOS Consensus Workshop Group, 2008).

Pulsatile GnRH therapy is rarely used, primarily because its use is cumbersome and less effective in PCOS compared with its use for hypothalamic amenorrhea. Ovarian drilling (diathermy) is a reasonable second-line therapy, particularly in clomiphene failures and when gonadotropin therapy has proved difficult. In randomized trials against standard gonadotropin therapy, ovarian drilling resulted in similar pregnancy rates but with a lower rate of multiple pregnancies (Thessaloniki ESHRE/ASRM-sponsored PCOS Consensus Workshop Group, 2008); however, in the United States, ovarian drilling or diathermy is rarely carried out, in part because of cost concerns.

For women who fail to conceive with ovulation induction over six cycles and in those with other infertility factors, IVF is the next step. Details of this treatment may be found in Chapter 41. ***The only caveat to IVF treatment in women with PCOS is the higher-than-normal risk of OHSS.*** This should always be kept in mind in treating women with PCOS, with significant dose adjustments in the treatment regimen, and using antagonist cycles, possibly metformin (when indicated), and the **GnRH agonist trigger** (see Chapter 41). Also, in the IVF model for women with PCOS, doing **frozen embryos transfer has been shown to be more successful than fresh embryo transfers**, because of an exaggerated endometrial response to medications used during IVF (Chen, 2016).

**TABLE 39.4** Treatment for Women with Polycystic Ovary Syndrome

| Complaint | Treatment Options |
|---|---|
| Infertility | Letrozole, clomiphene, with or without metformin, gonadotropins, ovarian cautery ("drilling") |
| Skin manifestations | Oral contraceptive + antiandrogen (spironolactone, finasteride), GnRH agonists |
| Abnormal bleeding | Cyclic progestogen, oral contraceptives |
| Weight, metabolic concerns | Diet/lifestyle management, metformin |

*GnRH,* Gonadotropin-releasing hormone.

## METABOLIC AND WEIGHT CONCERNS

The key management strategy should be directed at altering lifestyle variables. Exercise regimens, particularly when coordinated with a group of similar women, have been shown to be beneficial. Details of these approaches may be found elsewhere; however, this approach should be part of all therapies for PCOS, acknowledging that some women with PCOS who are thin or normal weight probably already have a healthy lifestyle.

Metabolic syndrome (MBS), driven largely by weight in the United States, is usually treated by a combination of diet and metformin. Six- to 12-month therapy has been shown to reduce weight by 5% to 7%, as well as to reduce insulin resistance and improve metabolic parameters. Positive results also have been reported with the use of bariatric surgery in women with PCOS and obesity, where most of the symptoms of PCOS were found to disappear after surgery (Escobar-Morreale, 2005). Nevertheless, this approach carries risks and should not be considered as first-line therapy.

Some data suggest that the use of antiandrogens (specifically flutamide) may also be efficacious for reducing body weight and visceral fat in women with PCOS (Gambineri, 2006). A combination of drospirenone and 17α-ethinylestradiol ($EE_2$) with flutamide and metformin also has been used successfully in adolescents (Ibanez, 2005); however, this multidrug regimen has not been tested in an adult population. Although therapy for women with PCOS should be directed at a woman's specific complaint, improvement of lifestyle variables, including weight reduction and fitness, should be the mainstay of all treatments. Metformin has an important role for metabolic concerns, particularly when MBS is present, and may aid in cases of subfertility.

A summary of various treatments for specific complaints in PCOS is provided in Table 39.4. Resources for patients may be found at the websites of the Australia AEPCOS Society (jeanhailes.org.au/health-a-z/pcos), Endo Society (www.ae-society.org), and ASRM (www.asrm.org).

## KEY REFERENCES

Abbott DH, Barnett DK, Bruns CM, et al. Androgen excess fetal programming of female reproduction: a developmental aetiology for polycystic ovary syndrome? *Hum Reprod Update.* 2005;11:357–374.

Azziz R, Carmina E, Dewailly D, et al. Positions statement: criteria for defining polycystic ovary syndrome. *Fertil Steril.* 2006;81:19–25.

Brutocao C, Zaiem F, Alsawas M. Psychiatric disorders in women with polycystic ovary syndrome: a systemic review and meta-analysis. *Endocrine.* 2018;62:318–325.

Carmina E, Campagna AM, Lobo RA. A 20-year follow-up of young women with polycystic ovary syndrome. *Obstet Gynecol.* 2012;119(2): 263–269.

Carmina E, Oberfield SE, Lobo RA. The diagnosis of polycystic ovary syndrome in adolescents. *Am J Obstet Gynecol.* 2010;203:201–205.

Carmina E, Lobo RA. Is there really increased cardiovascular morbidity in women with polycystic ovary syndrome? *J Womens Health.* 2018; 27:1385–1388.

Chang PL, Lindheim SR, Lowre C, et al. Normal ovulatory women with polycystic ovaries have hyperandrogenic pituitary-ovarian responses to gonadotropin-releasing hormone-agonist testing. *J Clin Endocrinol Metab.* 2000;85(3):995–1000.

Chen ZJ, Zhao H, He L, et al. Genome-wide association study identifies susceptibility loci for polycystic ovary syndrome on chromosome 2p16.3, 2p21 and 9q33.3. *Nat Genet.* 2010;43(1):55–60.

Chen ZJ, Shi J, Sun Y, et al. Fresh versus frozen embryos for infertility in the polycystic ovary syndrome. *N Engl J Med.* 2016;375:523–533.

Chittenden BG, Fullerton G, Maheshwari A, et al. Polycystic ovary syndrome and the risk of gynaecological cancer: a systematic review. *Reprod Biomed Online.* 2009;19:398–405.

Christ JP, Willis AD, Brooks ED, et al. Follicle number, not assessments of the ovarian stroma, represents the best ultrasonographic marker of polycystic ovary syndrome. *Fertil Steril.* 2014;101(1):280–287.

Dahlgren E, Janson PO, Johansson S, et al. Women with polycystic ovary syndrome wedge resected in 1956 to 1965: a long-term follow-up focusing on natural history and circulating hormones. *Fertil Steril.* 1992;57:505–513.

Dokras A, Clifton S, Futterweit W, et al. Increased risk for abnormal depression scores in women with polycystic ovary syndrome: a systematic review and meta-analysis. *Obstet Gynecol.* 2011;117(1):145–152.

Elting MW, Kwee J, Korsen TJ, et al. Aging women with polycystic ovary syndrome who achieve regular menstrual cycles have a smaller follicle cohort than those who continue to have irregular cycles. *Fertil Steril.* 2003;79:1154–1160.

Escobar-Morreale HF, Botella-Carretero JI, Alvarez-Blasco F, et al. The polycystic ovary syndrome associated with morbid obesity may resolve after weight loss induced by bariatric surgery. *J Clin Endocrinol Metab.* 2005;90:6364–6369.

Fauser B, Tarlatzis B, Rebar RW, et al. Consensus on women's health aspects of polycystic ovary syndrome (PCOS): the Amsterdam ESHRE/ASRM-sponsored 3rd PCOS Consensus Workshop Group. *Fertil Steril.* 2012;97(1):28–38.e25.

Franik S, Kremer JA, Nelen WL, et al. Aromatase inhibitors for subfertile women with polycystic ovary syndrome: summary of a Cochrane review. *Fertil Steril.* 2015;103(2):353–355.

Iliodromiti S, Kelsey TW, Anderson RA, et al. Can anti-mullerian hormone predict the diagnosis of polycystic ovary syndrome? A systematic review and meta-analysis of extracted data. *J Clin Endocrinol Metab.* 2013;98(8):3332–3340.

Jovanovic VP, Carmina E, Lobo RA. Not all women diagnosed with PCOS share the same cardiovascular risk profiles. *Fertil Steril.* 2010;94(3):826–832.

Kosova G, Urbanek M. Genetics of the polycystic ovary syndrome. *Mol Cell Endocrinol.* 2013;373(l-2):29–38.

Legro RS, Barnhart HX, Schlaff WD, et al. Clomiphene, metformin, or both for infertility in the polycystic ovary syndrome. *N Engl J Med.* 2007;356:551–566.

Legro RS, Brzyski RG, Diamond MP, et al. Letrozole versus clomiphene for infertility in the polycystic ovary syndrome. *N Engl J Med.* 2014;371(2):119–129.

Legro RS, Kunselman AR, Dodson WC, et al. Prevalence and predictors of risk for type 2 diabetes mellitus and impaired glucose tolerance in polycystic ovary syndrome: a prospective, controlled study in 254 affected women. *J Clin Endocrinol Metab.* 1999;84:165–169.

Lobo RA. A unifying concept for polycystic ovary syndrome. In: Jeffrey CR, ed. *Polycystic Ovary Syndrome.* Serono Symposia USA: Springer; 1996.

*NIH Evidence-based Methodology Workshop on Polycystic Ovary Syndrome (PCOS) Summary;* December, 2012. Available at https://prevention.nih.gov/research-priorities/research-needs-and-gaps/pathways-prevention/evidence-based-methodology-workshop-polycystic-ovary-syndrome-pcos.

O'Reilly MW, Kempegowda P, Jenkinson C, et al. 11-oxygenated C19 steroids are the predominant androgens in polycystic ovary syndrome. *J Clin Endocrinol Metab.* 2016;102:840–848.

O'Reilly MW, Kempegowda P, Walsh M. et al. AKR1C3-mediated adipose androgen generation drives lipotoxicity in women with polycystic ovary syndrome. *J Clin Endocrinol Metab.* 2017;102: 3327–3339.

Pierpoint T, McKeigue PM, Isaacs AJ, et al. Mortality of women with polycystic ovary syndrome at long-term follow-up. *J Clin Epidemiol.* 1998;51:581–586.

Rotterdam ESHRE/ASRM-Sponsored PCOS Consensus Workshop Group. Revised 2003 consensus on diagnostic criteria and long-term health risks related to polycystic ovary syndrome. *Fertil Steril.* 2004;81:19–25.

Sam S, Dunaif A. Polycystic ovary syndrome: syndrome XX? *Trends Endocrinol Metab.* 2003;14:365–370.

Savaris RF, Groll JM, Young SL, et al. Progesterone resistance in PCOS endometrium: a microarray analysis in clomiphene citrate-treated and artificial menstrual cycles. *J Clin Endocrinol Metab.* 2011;96:1737–1746.


**Full references and Suggested readings for this chapter can be found on ExpertConsult.com.**

# 40 Infertility

## Etiology, Diagnostic Evaluation, Management, Prognosis

Roger A. Lobo

### KEY POINTS

- Infertility is considered to be a disease and affects approximately 7% of all U.S. couples of reproductive age—more than 7 million women in the United States.
- A systematic evaluation of factors involved in infertility should be carried out rapidly, along with markers of ovarian reserve (antral follicle count, antimüllerian hormone); this will help frame the discussion with couples as to how best to proceed with treatment.
- The prognosis for fertility after tubal reconstruction depends on the amount of damage to the tube and the location of the obstruction. Mild abnormalities of the proximal tube may be treated with selective catheterization/cannulation under fluoroscopy. Large hydrosalpinges (distal disease) are best treated by salpingectomy and in vitro fertilization (IVF).
- In women with unexplained infertility, the use of controlled ovarian stimulation (COS) and intrauterine insemination (IUI) with clomiphene/IUI or gonadotropins/IUI yields monthly fecundity rates of approximately 8% to 10% (at least doubling the baseline rate) and should be the initial treatment for unexplained infertility. Use of gonadotropins does not offer a major advantage over clomiphene and carries more risks in terms of hyperstimulation and multiple pregnancies.
- After three to six cycles of COS/IUI, IVF should be offered as the next step, and IVF should be the primary therapy in women around age 40.

## INFERTILITY AND NATURAL CONCEPTION

The term ***infertility*** is generally used to indicate that a couple has a reduced capacity to conceive compared with the mean capacity of the general population. In a group of normally fertile couples, the monthly ability to get pregnant, or ***fecundability***, is approximately 20% (0.02). Analysis of data from presumably fertile couples who stop using contraception to conceive is depicted in Fig. 40.1, with both the actual and theoretical time trends. (Hull, 1985). **The 20% is an average number and can be as high as 25% for the first 3 months of trying to conceive, but then decreases** after that for the following months going forward (Leridon, 1984) (Table 40.1). As time goes on, during the fourth, fifth, and sixth years of attempting to conceive, only 48%, 42%, and 37% of nonpregnant women conceive without treatment. These data are highly influenced by age, which will be discussed later.

The definition of infertility is the inability of a couple to conceive after 1 year of trying. This timeline is relevant to help determine when an infertility investigation should begin. In women older than 35 years, this timeline should be after 6 months of trying. An early investigation is also warranted if any of the following is present: oligomenorrhea or amenorrhea; known tubal obstruction, uterine disease, or severe endometriosis; or known male factor infertility (Practice Committee ASRM, 2012a).

The World Health Organization (WHO) has defined infertility as a disease and a significant cause of disability (warranting evaluation and treatment) (see www.who.int/reproductivehealth/topics/infertility/definitions). Clearly, infertility is a cause of major distress for couples and should be assessed thoroughly and not neglected; and as with other disorders, counseling and support groups should be available in the clinical setting.

## INCIDENCE OF SUBFERTILITY AND INFERTILITY

**Approximately 6% to 7% of all reproductive-age women (15 to 44 years) in the United States are considered to be infertile** according to statistics from the Centers for Disease Control and Prevention (CDC). The number of women in this age group who have ever used infertility services has been estimated to be 12% or 7.3 million women in the United States.

## INFERTILITY AND AGE

Data from both older and more recent studies have indicated that **the percentage of infertile couples increases with increasing age of the female partner.** Analysis of data from three national surveys in the United States has revealed that the percentage of presumably fertile married women not using contraception who failed to conceive after 1 year of trying steadily increased from ages 25 to 44 years (Menken, 1986) (Table 40.2). Data from a study of presumably fertile nulliparous women married to husbands with azoospermia who underwent donor artificial insemination revealed that the percentage who conceived after 12 cycles of insemination declined substantially after age 30 (Schwartz, 1982) (Table 40.3). This older, classic study used fresh semen; currently, only frozen donor sperm is used, which does not achieve as favorable pregnancy rates. Decreasing fecundability with age is even more pressing in this context. With in vitro fertilization (IVF), data from the Society for Assisted Reproductive Technology (SART) in the United States indicate that the percentage of deliveries per oocyte retrieval procedure is 43.4% in women younger than 35, 25.4% by ages 38 to 40, 14% by ages 41 to 42 years, and only 5% in women older than 42 years (https://www.cdc.gov/art/artdata/index.html).

In general terms, approximately one in seven couples are infertile if the wife is 30 to 34, one in five is infertile if she is 35 to 40, and **one in four is infertile if she is aged 40 to 44 years.** Another way to interpret these data is to state that compared with women aged 20 to 24 years, fertility is reduced by 6% in the next 5 years, by 14% between ages 30 and 34, by 31% between ages 35 and 39, and to a much greater extent after age 40. Of interest is the finding that the most common diagnostic category among

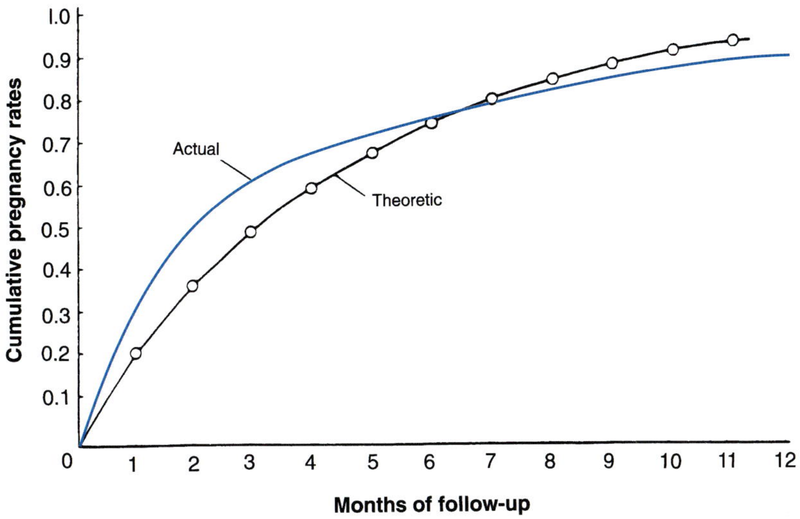


**Fig. 40.1** Curve of theoretic time to pregnancy in women with a monthly fecundability of 0.2 *(open circles)* and curve of actual time to pregnancy in fertile women discontinuing contraception *(solid line)*. (Open circle data from Hull MG, Glazener CM, Kelly NJ, et al. Population study of causes, treatment, and outcome of infertility. *Br Med J.* 1985;291(6510):1693-1697. Solid line data from Murray DL, Reich L, Adashi EY. Oral clomiphene citrate and vaginal progesterone suppositories in the treatment of luteal phase dysfunction: a comparative study. *Fertil Steril.* 1989;51(1):35-41.)

**TABLE 40.1** Incidence of Conception Over Time among Nonsterile Couples with Mean Fecundability of 0.2

| | Couples Not Yet Having Conceived | | |
|---|---|---|---|
| **Months without Conception** | **Proportion (%)** | **Mean Fecundability** | **Proportion (%) of Couples Who Will Conceive (within 12 mo)** |
| 0 | 100.0 | 0.20 | 86.0 |
| 6 | 31.9 | 0.14 | 77.0 |
| 12 | 14.0 | 0.11 | 69.2 |
| 24 | 4.3 | 0.08 | 57.0 |
| 36 | 1.9 | 0.06 | 48.2 |
| 48 | 1.0 | 0.05 | 41.7 |
| 60 | 0.6 | 0.04 | 36.7 |

Modified from Leridon H, Spira A. Problems in measuring the effectiveness of infertility therapy. *Fertil Steril.* 1984;41(4):580-586.

**TABLE 40.2** Married Women Who Are Infertile, by Age*

| Age (yr) | Infertile (%) |
|---|---|
| 20-24 | 7.0 |
| 25-29 | 8.9 |
| 30-34 | 14.6 |
| 35-39 | 21.9 |
| 40-44 | 28.7 |

*From three national U.S. surveys.
From Menken J, Trussell J, Larsen U. Age and infertility. *Science.* 1986;233:1389-1394.

**TABLE 40.3** Pregnancy Rates by Age at 1 Year in Normal Women with Azospermatic Husbands after Donor Insemination

| Age (yr) | Pregnancy Rate (%) |
|---|---|
| <25 | 73.0 |
| 26-30 | 74.1 |
| 31-35 | 61.5 |
| 36-40 | 55.8 |

From Schwartz D, Mayaux MJ. Female fecundity as a function of age: results of artificial insemination in 2193 nulliparous women with azoospermic husbands. *N Engl J Med.* 1982;306(7):404-406.

women undergoing IVF in the United States in the most recent survey cited previously is diminished ovarian reserve: 17% of cycles; which is a characteristic of older women undergoing treatment (https://www.cdc.gov/art/artdata/index.html).

## CAUSES OF INFERTILITY

The exact incidence of the various factors causing infertility varies among different populations and cannot be precisely determined. Collins reported that among 14,141 couples in 21 publications, ovulatory disorders occurred 27% of the time; male factor, 25%; tubal disorders, 22%; endometriosis, 5%; other, 4%; and unexplained factors, 17% (Collins, 1995a). It has not been shown that other abnormalities, such as antisperm antibodies, luteal phase deficiency, subclinical genital infection, or subclinical endocrine abnormalities such as hypothyroidism or hyperprolactinemia in ovulatory women, are true causes of infertility. No prospective randomized studies have demonstrated that treatment of these latter entities results in greater fecundability than without treatment. If any of these do cause infertility, they do so infrequently. With current techniques of investigation, it is **not possible to diagnose the cause of infertility in up to 20%** of couples, and they are considered to have **unexplained infertility**.

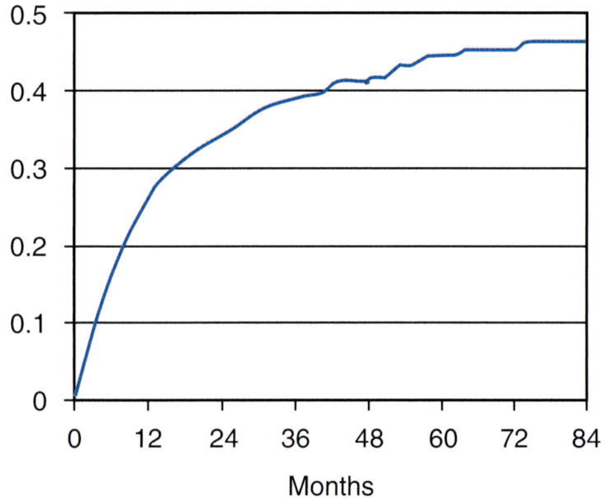


**Fig. 40.2** Cumulative rate of conceptions leading to live birth. Couples (873) remained untreated throughout follow-up; cumulative rate of live birth conception at 36 months was 38.2% (95% confidence interval, 34.2 to 42.3). (Modified from Collins JA, Burrows EA, Wilan AR. The prognosis for live birth among untreated infertile couples. *Fertil Steril.* 1995;64(1):22-28.)

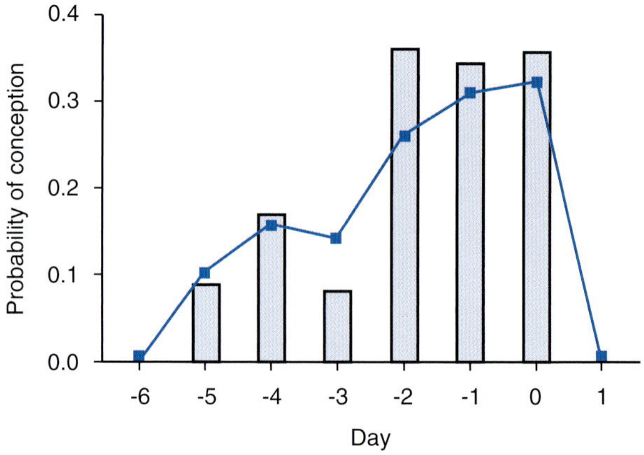


**Fig. 40.3** Probability of conception on specific days near the day of ovulation. The *bars* represent probabilities calculated from data on 129 menstrual cycles in which sexual intercourse was recorded to have occurred on only a single day during the 6-day interval ending on the day of ovulation (day 0). The *solid line* shows daily probabilities based on all 625 cycles, as estimated by the statistical model. (From Wilcox AJ, Weinberg CR, Baird DD. Timing of sexual intercourse in relation to ovulation: effects on the probability of conception, survival of the pregnancy, and sex of the baby. *N Engl J Med.* 1995;333:1517-1521.)

After a rigorous investigation, other reports have suggested this figure to be as low as 10%; however, it is unclear if subtle abnormalities, as noted, have much to do with infertility. Also, **most couples with unexplained infertility are subfertile rather than infertile, and some couples are able to conceive without treatment**, although it may take several years. A live birth rate among 873 infertile couples in several Canadian centers has been observed without treatment. The cumulative live conception rate was 38.2% at 3 years and 45% after 7 years (Collins, 1995b) (Fig. 40.2). Among the total group with the diagnosis of unexplained infertility who received no treatment, one-third had a live birth during the first 3 years of observation without treatment.

## DIAGNOSTIC EVALUATION

The diagnostic evaluation of infertility should be thorough and completed as rapidly as possible. During the initial interview, the couple should be informed about normal human fecundity and how these probabilities decrease with increasing age of the female partner and with the duration of infertility. The various tests in the diagnostic evaluation and why they are performed should be thoroughly explained. The available therapies and prognosis for treatment of the various causes of infertility should also be included in the dialogue. **The couple should be informed that after a complete diagnostic infertility evaluation, the cause for infertility cannot be determined in a large group of couples.** For many couples, the reduced fecundability can be suggested to be age related. Methods to increase the fecundity of couples with a normal diagnostic evaluation, such as *controlled ovarian stimulation* (COS) and intrauterine insemination, and the possibility of IVF should be covered.

Each couple should be instructed about the optimal time in the cycle for conception to occur and should be encouraged to have intercourse on the day before ovulation. Unless the husband has oligozoospermia (oligospermia), daily intercourse for 3 consecutive days at midcycle should be encouraged. When ovulation is more precisely determined, as with luteinizing hormone (LH) monitoring (discussed later), intercourse should occur for 2 consecutive days around the LH surge. Because the egg disintegrates less than 1 day after it reaches the ampulla of the tube, it is best that sperm be present in this area when the egg arrives so that fertilization can occur. Because normal sperm retain their fertilizing ability for up to 72 hours, it is preferable to have sperm in the tube before the arrival of the oocyte.

A study was performed by Wilcox and coworkers of fertile couples who stopped contraception to conceive and recorded the cycle day when they had sexual intercourse. Hormone analysis was performed to determine the day of ovulation. None of the women became pregnant in the group of couples who had intercourse after ovulation occurred. **The pregnancy rate was approximately 30% if intercourse occurred on the day of ovulation, as well as 1 and 2 days before ovulation.** The pregnancy rate was approximately 10% if coitus occurred 3, 4, or 5 days before ovulation. No pregnancies occurred when intercourse took place 6 days or more before ovulation (Wilcox, 1995) (Fig. 40.3). It is therefore considered optimal to perform insemination or have sexual intercourse on the day before ovulation.

Because peak levels of LH occur 1 day before ovulation, measurement of LH by urinary LH immunoassays is the best way to determine the optimal time to have intercourse or an insemination. Tests that measure LH in a random daily urine specimen are usually more convenient for planning natural or artificial insemination than tests that detect LH in the first morning urine specimen. **Ovulation most commonly occurs on the day after the detection of LH in a random specimen (12 to 24 hours later)**, and it occurs on the day when LH is detected in the first morning specimen, which contains urine formed during the prior night. Several types of commercial kits are available for determining peak LH, so women who find it difficult to determine a hormone change using one type can try another system or kit. Kits may vary in terms of sensitivity and variations may occur based on the dilution of the urine and hormonal conditions such as polycystic ovary syndrome (PCOS), which can give false positive tests. Basal body temperature (BBT) charts are not as precise for determining ovulation, with ovulation occurring over a span of several days of the thermogenic shift. In the last several years, multiple fertility apps have been launched, and a bracelet worn at night (Eva) has been advertised to provide information on a 5-day fertile window.

In some cases, women produce less than adequate amounts of vaginal lubricant. Various vaginal lubricants and chemicals, as well as saliva, used to improve coital satisfaction may interfere with sperm transport. Some men experience midcycle impotence because of the pressure of performing intercourse on demand. In such cases the intercourse schedule should be less rigorous. The couple should also be told that among fertile couples, there is only approximately a 20% chance of conceiving in each ovulatory cycle, even with optimally timed coitus, and that it takes time to become pregnant; thus the terms *time* and *timing* should be emphasized during the initial counseling session. Couples should also be advised to cease smoking cigarettes and drinking caffeinated beverages in excess. Cigarette smoking and caffeine consumption have been shown independently in several studies to decrease the chances of conception. The common practice of vaginal douching also reduces the chance of conception by approximately 30%.

All couples should have a complete history taken, including a sexual history, and a physical examination, which is often ultrasound based. After this initial evaluation, tests should be undertaken to determine whether the woman is ovulating and has patent fallopian tubes and if a semen sample of the male partner is normal.

## Documentation of Ovulation

Preliminary information that the woman is ovulatory is provided by a history of regular menstrual cycles. If the woman has regular menstrual cycles, a serum progesterone level should be measured in the midluteal phase to provide indirect evidence of ovulation and normal luteal function. Although serum progesterone levels vary in the normal luteal phase in a pulsatile manner, a serum progesterone level greater than 3 to 5 ng/mL suggests some ovulatory function; however, it cannot indicate the adequacy of normal ovulation. **Progesterone levels of 10 ng/mL or higher** are found during at least 1 day of the luteal phase of normal ovulatory cycles in which conception occurred (Hull, 1982). Measurement of the daily BBT provides indirect evidence that ovulation has taken place but does not give precise information about ovulation timing as does the LH kit. The quality of ovulation cannot be determined accurately but may be suggested by a well-timed progesterone level. With the number of other methods such as phone apps and the bracelet, the use of the BBT, which is difficult for many women to do, has appropriately decreased.

Women with oligomenorrhea (menses at intervals of 35 days or longer) or amenorrhea who wish to conceive should be treated with agents that induce ovulation, regardless of whether they have occasional ovulatory cycles. Therefore for these women, direct or indirect measurement of progesterone is unnecessary until after therapy is initiated.

The endometrial biopsy is sometimes considered as a diagnostic method for the adequacy of ovulation and luteal function. ***We feel that an endometrial biopsy is not indicated in this setting of assessing ovulatory function.*** It is invasive and painful, and it does not provide accurate information in terms of "endometrial dating" of the luteal phase, as was carried out in the past (Coutifaris, 2004); however, an endometrial biopsy may be indicated as a subsequent test when assessing for endometrial receptivity and ruling out chronic endometritis in the setting of repeated implantation failure or recurrent miscarriage, as will be discussed in other chapters.

## Semen Analysis

Although information about ovulation is being obtained, the male partner's reproductive system should be evaluated by means of a semen analysis. Most urologists dealing with male fertility issues require obtaining two semen analyses. Abnormalities in the semen analysis (male factor) **occurs in approximately 20% of couples with infertility as the sole factor and may be involved in 30% to 40% of cases overall**. The male partner should be advised to abstain from ejaculation for 2 to 3 days before collection of the semen sample. It is best to collect the specimen in a clean (not necessarily sterile) wide-mouthed jar after masturbation. It is important that the entire specimen be collected because the initial fraction contains the greatest density of sperm. Ideally, **collection should take place in the location where the analysis will be performed.** The degree of sperm motility should be determined as soon as possible after liquefaction, which usually occurs 15 to 20 minutes after ejaculation. Sperm motility begins to decline 2 hours after ejaculation, and it is best to examine the specimen within this period. Semen should not be exposed to marked changes in temperature and, if collected at home during cold weather, the specimen should be kept warm during transport to the laboratory.

Parameters used to evaluate the semen include volume, viscosity, sperm density, sperm morphology, and sperm motility. The last parameter should be evaluated in terms of percentage of total motile sperm and quality of motility (rapidity of movement and amount of progressive motility). Sperm morphology is an extremely important parameter and is correlated to fertilizing ability. Using strict criteria (Kruger), only approximately 4% or more of the sperm in an ejaculate may be considered normal according to the WHO criteria (Cooper, 2010). It should be remembered that the sperm analysis is a subjective test and that there is a fair degree of variability from test to test in the same man. Also, the semen profile reflects sperm production that occurred 3 months earlier, which is important to note if there was illness at that time. Table 40.4 lists the parameters that are generally considered normal for a semen analysis, according to the WHO study. It is beyond our scope here to discuss fully the causes and diagnostic evaluation of semen abnormalities. In broad terms, the various causes of semen abnormalities are cited in Table 40.5.

When semen analyses were performed on a group of men whose wives had conceived within the past 4 months, approximately 75% had at least one abnormal characteristic and 25% had two abnormalities. These results confirm that **there is normally a wide variability in the parameters used to characterize semen**. Because the characteristics of semen may vary over time and undergo normal biologic variability, it is best to repeat the test at least once if an abnormality is found. If abnormalities persist, **the male partner should have a urologic examination.** It is important not to miss a rare abnormality, such as a testicular tumor; in addition it has been appreciated that **male factor infertility is associated with other medical conditions** and subsequent problems (Eisenberg, 2015).

The comprehensive evaluation should include a history of physical examination (occasionally with ultrasound); hormonal evaluation (LH, follicle-stimulating hormone [FSH], testosterone, estradiol, prolactin [PRL], and thyroid-stimulating hormone [TSH]); and genetic abnormalities (karyotype and defects such as cystic fibrosis mutations and Y-chromosome microdeletions), particularly with severe sperm abnormalities (Practice Committee ASRM, 2012a).

**TABLE 40.4** Lower Fifth Percentile Values in Fertile Men*

| Parameter | Value |
|---|---|
| Semen volume (mL) | 1.5 |
| Sperm concentration (million/mL) | 15 |
| Total number (million/ejaculate) | 39 |
| Total motility (%) | 40 |
| Progressive motility (%) | 32 |
| Normal forms (%) | 4 |

Modified from Cooper TG, Noonan E, von Eckardstein S, et al. World Health Organization reference values for human semen characteristics. *Hum Reprod Update.* 2010;16(3):231-245.

*With time to pregnancy 12 months or less.

**TABLE 40.5** Causes of Semen Abnormalities

| Finding | Cause |
|---|---|
| **Abnormal Count** | |
| Azoospermia | Klinefelter's syndrome or other genetic disorder<br>Sertoli-cell–only syndrome<br>Seminiferous tubule or Leydig cell failure<br>Hypogonadotropic hypogonadism<br>Ductal obstruction, including Young syndrome<br>Varicocele<br>Exogenous factors |
| Oligozoospermia | Genetic disorder<br>Endocrinopathies, including androgen receptor defects<br>Varicocele and other anatomic disorders<br>Maturation arrest<br>Hypospermatogenesis<br>Exogenous factors |
| **Abnormal Volume** | |
| No ejaculate | Ductal obstruction<br>Retrograde ejaculation<br>Ejaculatory failure<br>Hypogonadism |
| Low volume | Obstruction of ejaculatory ducts<br>Absence of seminal vesicles and vas deferens<br>Partial retrograde ejaculation<br>Infection |
| High volume | Unknown factors |
| Abnormal motility | Immunologic factors<br>Infection<br>Varicocele<br>Defects in sperm structure<br>Metabolic or anatomic abnormalities of sperm<br>Poor liquefaction of semen |
| Abnormal viscosity | Cause unknown |
| Abnormal morphology | Varicocele<br>Stress<br>Infection<br>Exogenous factors<br>Unknown factors |
| Extraneous cells | Infection or inflammation<br>Shedding of immature sperm |

From Bernstein GS, Siegel MS. Male factor in infertility. In: Mishell DR Jr, Davajan V, Lobo RA, eds. *Infertility, Contraception and Reproductive Endocrinology.* 3rd ed. Cambridge, MA: Blackwell Scientific; 1991:629.

## Evaluation and Laboratory Tests

Aspects of the woman's medical history that should be highlighted include the following: any pregnancy complications if previously pregnant; previous pelvic surgery of any type; significant dysmenorrhea; dyspareunia or sexual dysfunction; abnormal cervical cytologic test results or procedures to treat cervical abnormalities; and use of medication, drugs, and tobacco. Family history should be explored for genetically related illnesses, birth defects, and, most importantly, the history of age of menopause in female family members. Finally, any symptoms suggestive of endocrine disorders should be solicited (e.g., weight changes, skin changes).

The physical examination should focus on extremes of body mass, skin changes, thyroid abnormalities, breast secretion, abnormal pain on abdominal or pelvic examination, and assessment of the vagina and cervix. In addition, if available, vaginal ultrasound performed at the same time may be extremely valuable in picking up abnormalities of the uterus (e.g., fibroids) endometrial thickness, pelvic masses, and ovarian morphology (e.g., polycystic appearance, unusually small). These may provide a guide for further testing.

In a healthy woman, a complete blood cell count (CBC), blood type, Rh factor, and rubella status are needed, together with the record of a Papanicolaou (Pap) test obtained within 3 years. Increasingly it is recommended (although not mandatory) to screen for genetic carrier status. Comprehensive screening for carrier status, including fragile X and other abnormalities such as cystic fibrosis, is easily carried out at the time of routine blood testing. Several laboratories can do such screening. Infectious disease screening (for chlamydia and gonorrhea) is carried out routinely in most practices at the time of the Pap test. Further infectious disease screening (e.g., syphilis, human immunodeficiency virus [HIV], hepatitis) is warranted, particularly for couples undergoing insemination or IVF.

In most women, and particularly in women older than 35 years, serum FSH and estradiol ($E_2$) levels should be obtained on cycle day 2 or 3. Elevated FSH values (>10 mIU/mL) suggest decreased ovarian reserve, which reflects the pool of viable oocytes remaining in the ovary. Levels greater than 20 mIU/mL afford a particularly poor prognosis; however, although FSH levels tend to fluctuate from cycle to cycle, once the FSH level has been elevated in a given cycle, the overall prognosis is reduced. $E_2$ levels, if elevated on days 2 and 3 (>70 pg/mL), do not allow for a valid interpretation of FSH values and may independently suggest a decreased prognosis regarding ovarian reserve.

**Antimüllerian hormone (AMH) has become a valuable standard for assessing ovarian reserve.** AMH, which is produced by the granulosa cells of small growing follicles, physiologically suppresses FSH stimulation of sustained follicular growth. Levels are highest in young women and lower with reproductive aging; various nomograms by age have been established (Seifer, 2011) (Fig. 40.4). Serum AMH decreases with aging, and when levels reach 0.05 ng/mL (essentially undetectable levels), menopause occurs within 4 to 5 years. Levels are higher in women with PCOS (Iliodromiti, 2013). The biggest concern with measurement of AMH is differences between assays because there is no international standard; however, in general, higher levels (>2 ng/mL) suggest a larger cohort of small available follicles and low levels (<0.5 ng/mL) suggest a decreased ovarian reserve. Values are of concern if they are less than 1 ng/mL. The level of AMH also reflects the sensitivity of the ovary to gonadotropic stimulation, and thus the choice of treatment when ovarian stimulation is desired. Unlike FSH, AMH values are fairly constant and stable throughout the menstrual cycle, particularly in the low ranges. Higher values, however, exhibit more variability in the early to midfollicular phase. It is now established that use of oral contraceptive pills decreases values by 15% to 20%.

### Use of Ultrasound in the Diagnostic Evaluation

It is most common to carry out a pelvic ultrasound evaluation as part of the investigation. By so doing, significant pathologic conditions such as fibroids, endometriosis, and other changes can be uncovered. In addition polycystic ovaries, which are prevalent, can be appreciated; and finally an **antral follicle count (AFC) can be obtained**, which is similar in value to the measurement of AMH, in the assessment of ovarian reserve. An age-related nomogram for AFCs has also been reported (Almog, 2011) (Fig. 40.5). For standardization it has been suggested that the AFC be obtained on cycle days 2 to 4, although an AFC can be obtained at other times in the cycle as long as all follicular structures over 10 mm are not counted.

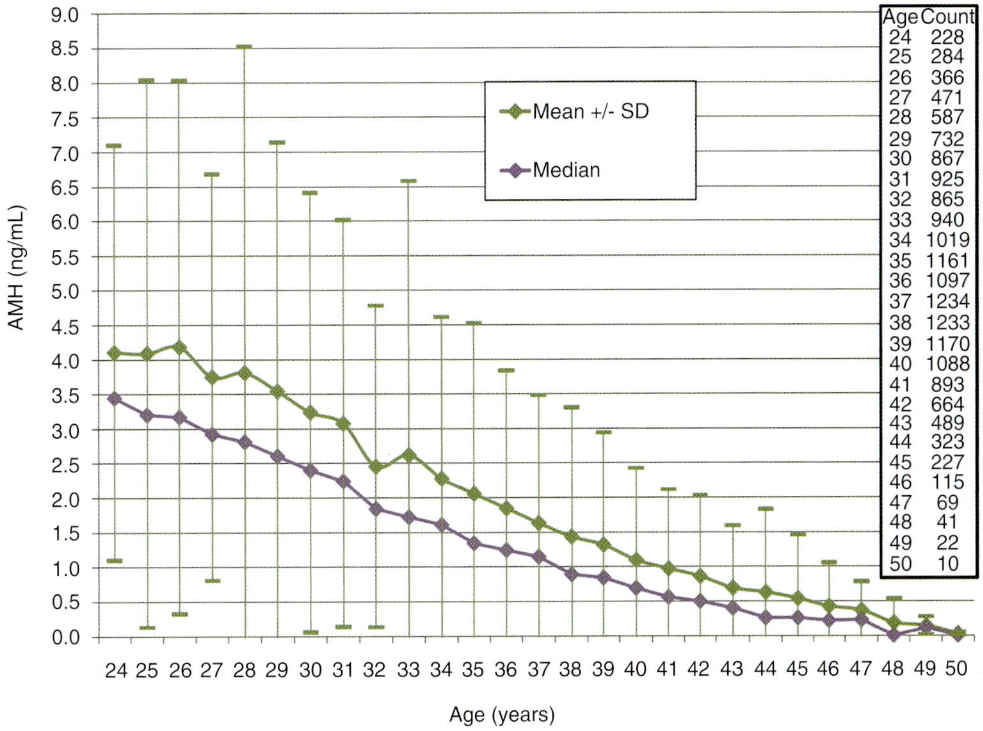


**Fig. 40.4** Antimüllerian hormone (AMH) age-specific median values with mean ± standard deviation values for women ages 24 to 50, n = 17,120, obtained at 1-year intervals. Note values are from a single laboratory using reagents from the older Beckman/Diagnostic Systems Laboratories (DSL) generation 1 assay; thus assays systems will vary for the absolute numbers but not for the trend of declining values with age. *SD,* Standard deviation. (From Seifer D, Baker VL, Leader B. Age specific serum AMH values for 17120 women presenting to fertility centers within the United States. *Fertil Steril.* 2011;95(2):747-750.)

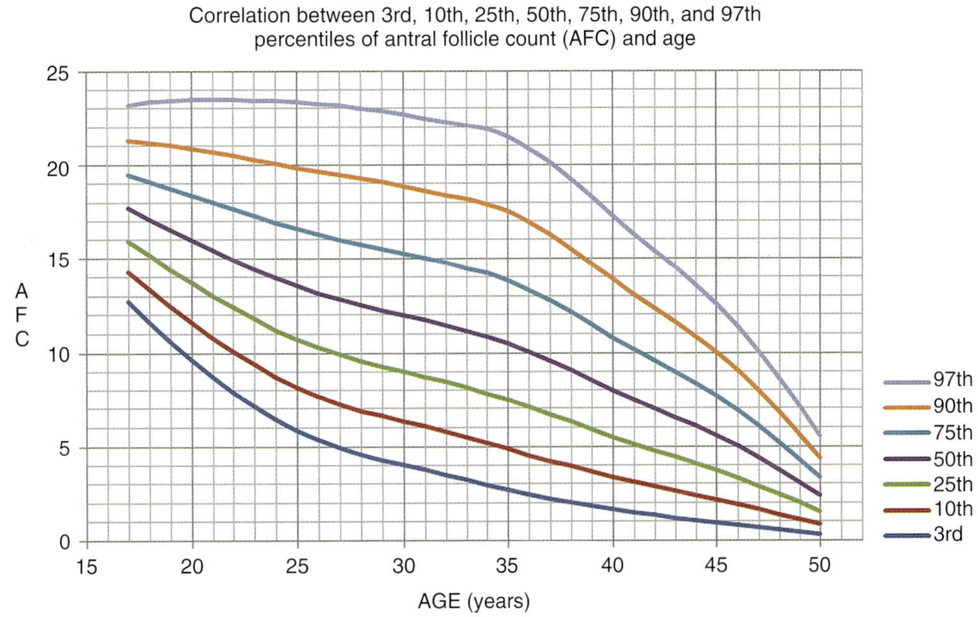


**Fig. 40.5** Age-related nomogram for antral follicle count depicted by various percentiles showing a biphasic decline and with a poor antral follicle count defined by a value under eight. (From Almog B, Shehata F, Shalom-Paz E, et al. Age-related nomogram for antral follicle count: McGill reference guide. *Fertil Steril.* 2011; 95(2):663-666.)

## Other Blood Testing

Some specialists obtain antibody titers for *Chlamydia trachomatis*, which if elevated may signify the possibility of tubal disease. It has been suggested that if the immunoglobulin G (IgG) antibody titer is greater than 1:32, 35% of patients have evidence of tubal damage. Whether this type of evaluation is routinely warranted as a focus for the infertility investigation continues to be debated.

Although not proven to be of major benefit in normal ovulatory women, most clinicians will measure TSH and PRL at the screening visit. TSH values in the normal range (<4.4 μU/mL), but higher than 2.5 mIU/mL are often considered to be abnormal in women presenting with infertility. This is because normal values in the first trimester of pregnancy should be less than 2.5 μU/mL; however, there is no evidence that values between 2.5 to 4 μU/mL affect fertility status or outcomes of pregnancy (Practice Committee ASRM, 2015). It is common to have slightly elevated PRL levels at the initial visit, which normalize when retested in the fasting state.

If an abnormality is found in one of the first two noninvasive diagnostic procedures (documentation of ovulation and semen analysis), it should be treated before proceeding with the more costly and invasive procedures, unless there is a history or findings suggestive of tubal disease. For example, if the woman has oligomenorrhea and does not ovulate each month, after a normal semen analysis is observed, ovulation should be induced with clomiphene citrate for two to three cycles before performing the other diagnostic measures. Provided that no other infertility factors are present, most anovulatory women (80%) conceive after induction of ovulation with therapeutic agents, and half the couples will conceive during the first three ovulatory cycles (Gysler, 1982).

If these initial diagnostic tests are normal, the more uncomfortable and costly hysterosalpingography (HSG) should be performed in the follicular phase of the next cycle.

## Hysterosalpingography

It is best to schedule the HSG during the week after the end of menses to avoid a possible pregnancy and also get better definition of the uterine cavity when the endometrium is still thin. The HSG should be avoided if there has been a history of salpingitis in the recent past or if there is tenderness on pelvic examination. As noted, most practices routinely screen for chlamydia and gonorrhea during the initial examination; however, we routinely prescribe prophylactic antibiotics at the time of HSG: doxycycline (100 mg twice daily for 3 days, starting 1 day before the procedure), but this recommendation is not universally followed. If a hydrosalpinx is seen with HSG, doxycycline should be continued for 1 week. The examination should be performed with use of a water-soluble contrast medium and image-intensified fluoroscopy. A water-soluble contrast medium enables better visualization of the tubal mucosal folds and vaginal markings than an oil-based medium. It is important to be able to evaluate the appearance of the intratubal architecture to determine the extent of damage to the tube (Fig. 40.6, *A* and *B*). Although it has

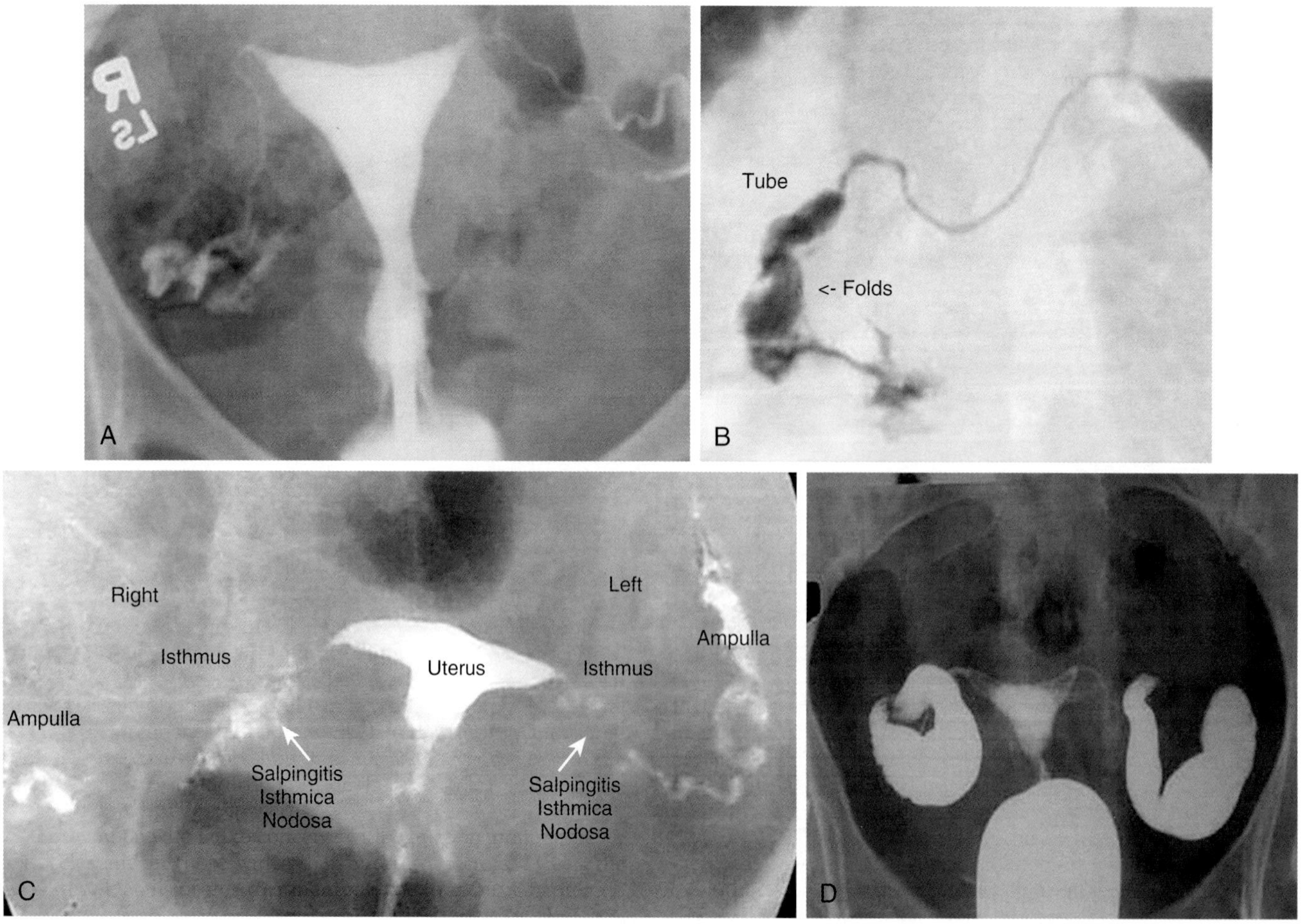


**Fig. 40.6** Representative hysterosalpingograms showing **(A)** a normal study, **(B)** normal ampullary folds, **(C)** bilateral salpingitis isthmica nodosa (proximal disease), and **(D)** bilateral hydrosalpinges (distal disease).

been debated for several years, **a large randomized trial in the Netherlands concluded that an oil-based contrast resulted in a higher ongoing pregnancy rate and live birth rate compared with water-based contrast** (Dreyer, 2017). An approach that has been advocated is to perform the test with a water-based medium, but to carry out tubal flushing with an oil base at the time of the procedure. It has been shown than flushing with oil contrast improves clinical pregnancy rates (Wang, 2019).

The diagnostic HSG provides important information about the magnitude of the disease process, if present, and provides information about the uterine cavity that cannot be obtained by laparoscopic visualization. The procedure can also determine whether salpingitis isthmica nodosa is present in the interstitial portion of the oviduct (Fig. 40.6, *C*). When an HSG shows lack of patency in one tube, this has been shown to be falsely positive, approximately 50% of the time at laparoscopy. Therefore it is not necessary to perform tubal reconstructive surgery on a woman with one patent tube. The finding of a normal endometrial cavity at the time of HSG obviates the need for hysteroscopy. If severe tubal disease, such as a large hydrosalpinx, is found at the time of HSG (Fig. 40.6, *D*), based on success rates, it is preferable for the couple to undergo IVF–embryo transfer (ET) than for the woman to have tubal surgery. If the hydrosalpinx is large and clearly visible on ultrasound, it is preferable to perform laparoscopic salpingectomy before IVF-ET because the pregnancy rate with IVF-ET may be decreased by as much as 40% (Zeyneloglu, 1998).

Quite often one or both tubes may show proximal obstruction. This may be the result of uterine spasm (contractions) caused by the discomfort of the procedure, or because of true obstruction; the latter may be only a mild obstruction caused by tubal debris. It has become common to attempt fluoroscopic-controlled selective cannulation of the proximal tube, either immediately or at a subsequent visit (Thurmond, 2008) (Fig. 40.7). This can be successful in up to 90% of cases, and if successful, it alleviates either unnecessary concern or the need for laparoscopy or IVF.

When the extent of tubal disease is unclear or the couple prefers not to undergo IVF-ET, diagnostic laparoscopy should be carried out in the follicular phase of the cycle. In general, the goal should be to have all tubal reconstruction carried out laparoscopically (discussed later).

## Postcoital Test (No Longer Routine)

Although important from a physiologic standpoint (cervical mucus being important for sperm transport), **the postcoital test (PCT) is now rarely indicated as a necessary part of the infertility investigation.** It is a very subjective test. A normal PCT is one in which at least five motile sperm are visible in normal cervical mucus obtained from the upper canal just before ovulation. A suboptimal test can be the result of technique, timing of the test, and problems with cervical mucus or with sperm. Although a good PCT has been correlated with a better prognosis for pregnancy, sperm have been recovered at laparoscopy when there was a poor PCT. Moreover, because the suggested treatment for a poor PCT is intrauterine insemination after ovarian stimulation, this is the exact next step taken, even if the PCT is normal, in the setting of unexplained infertility. Occasionally, as may happen with an orthodox Jewish couple, a semen analysis cannot be obtained. Here, a PCT provides a surrogate for visualizing motile, normal-appearing sperm.

## Laparoscopy: Is It a Routine Part of the Investigation?

In the past, this was an obligatory final step in the infertility investigation when all other test results were normal. Data have shown that in 20% to 40% of cases, some minor abnormalities may be found (e.g., endometriosis, adhesions), which may have a bearing on fecundability. Obviously, if there is something suspicious on ultrasound or examination, there has been prior pelvic surgery or appendicitis, or there is pelvic pain or dyspareunia, the index of suspicion is increased. The probability that peritubal adhesions of sufficient severity to cause infertility will be found at the time of laparoscopy is less than 5% in a woman with no history of salpingitis or symptoms of dysmenorrhea, a normal bimanual pelvic examination, and normal antibody titers (if obtained) (Fatum, 2002). Provided the woman is younger than

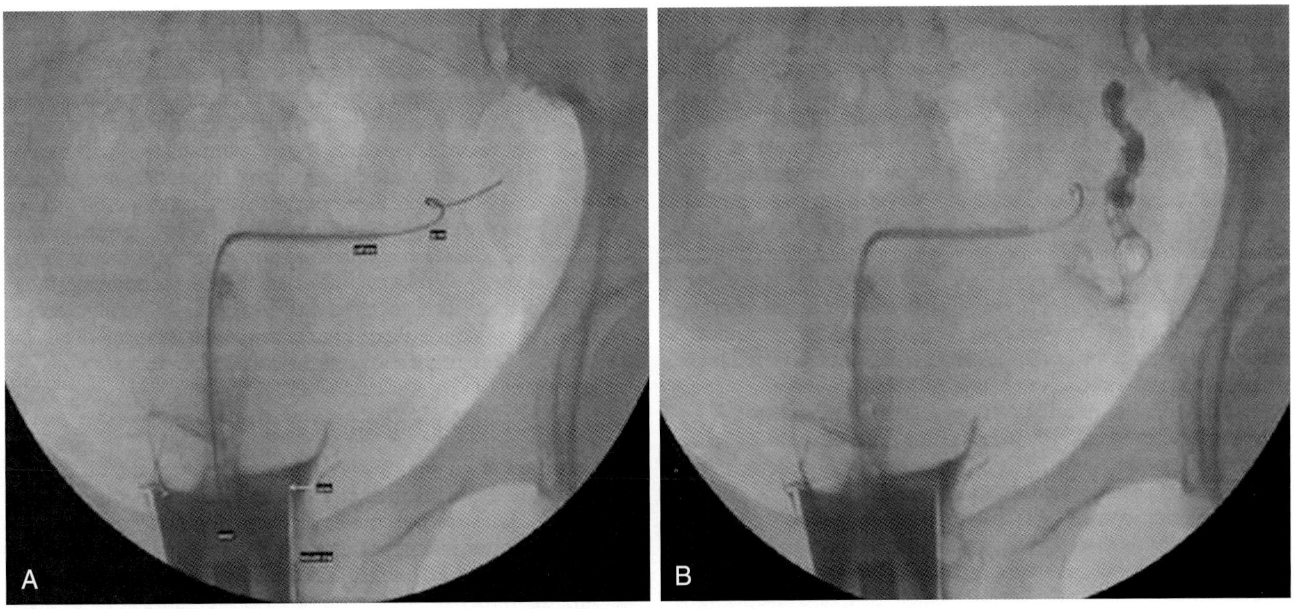


**Fig. 40.7** Technique of tubal cannulation using a vacuum cup on the cervix. **A,** Introduction of a 5.5-French catheter into the tubal ostium under fluoroscopy, by a 0.015-inch guidewire into the fallopian tube for dislodgement of debris. **B,** Injection of contrast through a 3-French catheter into the tube confirming successful cannulation and a normal-appearing patent tube. (From Thurmond AS. Fallopian tube catheterization. *Semin Intervent Radiol.* 2008;25(4):425-431.)

40 years and is having ovulatory cycles, and there is an acceptable semen analysis and an age-appropriate maker of ovarian reserve such as AMH, **several cycles of COS and intrauterine insemination may be undertaken before performing diagnostic laparoscopy or going directly to IVF-ET**. At this juncture, a decision can be revisited about whether performing a laparoscopy should be considered, although many couples usually prefer to proceed with IVF-ET, particularly if they have insurance coverage for IVF.

## Additional Testing for Couples Presenting With Infertility

### Significance of a Diagnosis of Luteal Deficiency (Is This a True Diagnosis?)

Although suggested for many years, it has never been established that luteal phase defects cause infertility. This pertains to women who are completely normal on evaluation and have regular cycles. Women who are oligoovulatory and have longer cycles and women with elevated PRL levels can have luteal inadequacy that is corrected by lowering of PRL levels and/or ovulation induction.

The diagnosis of luteal deficiency used to be made on finding serum progesterone levels consistently less than 10 ng/mL 1 week before menses or finding consistent evidence for a histologic delay (>3 days) in the pattern of the normal secretory endometrium, indicating an inadequate effect of progesterone on the endometrium. This endometrial defect had to be found in two consecutive cycles. Erroneous diagnoses of this entity occur because of cycle variability and the subjective interpretation of histologic dating criteria. There is at least a 10% disagreement of more than 2 days when the same observer dated the specimens on two separate occasions, and even more interobserver variability. As noted earlier, studies have confirmed the lack of efficacy of the endometrial biopsy (Coutifaris, 2004). ***Routine endometrial biopsies for the diagnosis of infertility should not be carried out.***

As noted regarding the PCT, ovarian stimulation with intrauterine insemination (IUI) is often the first empirical treatment for unexplained infertility. This essentially treats the luteal inadequacy, if it exists, preempting the need for invasive and imprecise endometrial biopsies.

### Immunologic Factors in Subfertility

Substantial evidence from animal studies has indicated that antibodies can be induced in females from antigens obtained from organs in the male reproductive tract and that these antibodies interfere with normal reproduction. Both sperm-agglutinating and sperm-immobilizing antibodies have been found in the serum of some infertile women, but also in the serum of fertile control subjects. Agglutinating antibodies are found more often than immobilizing antibodies in most series, and, in some reports, the incidence of sperm-agglutinating antibodies in infertile women is similar to that in the control group. Even with the finding of sperm agglutination or immobilization in interactions with serum (in vitro), it has not been demonstrated that a similar degree of sperm inactivation occurs in the lower genital tract. Thus there is **no definitive evidence that sperm agglutination or immobilization in the serum of infertile women is the cause of their infertility**. One of the reasons for this discrepancy is that both serum assays measure mainly immunoglobulin M (IgM) and IgG antibodies, whereas the antibodies locally produced in the genital tract are mainly IgA. Thus some investigators have measured antisperm antibodies in cervical mucus and found a correlation between their presence and infertility; however, no data have shown that the finding of antibodies against sperm in the male or female partner is a cause of infertility. In addition, corticosteroid treatment of the male or female partner does not significantly increase the pregnancy rate compared with no therapy.

Autoimmunity to sperm in semen and serum has been found in some infertile men, particularly those who have had testicular infection, injury, or a surgical procedure such as vasectomy reversal. Men with these antibodies have been treated with corticosteroid therapy and sperm-washing techniques. Nevertheless, the effectiveness of such treatment remains to be established.

Four prospective studies have reported the incidence of fertility occurring after a diagnostic infertility evaluation was performed in which the presence of antisperm antibodies was documented (Collins, 1993). These studies were performed in four different laboratories in three different countries. Several different techniques were used for the antibody tests. All four studies showed **no correlation between the presence of antisperm antibodies in either member of the couple and the chance of conception**. Pregnancy rates over time were similar in couples who had or did not have antisperm antibodies. Therefore tests to detect these antibodies as part of the diagnostic infertility evaluation are not justified because their presence does not affect fecundity.

### Significance of Infectious Diseases in Subfertility

Some researchers have suggested that asymptomatic, or occult, infection of the upper female genital tract and male genital tract is a cause of infertility. As early as 1973, it was suggested that infection with what was then called *T-mycoplasma* in the male could interfere with normal sperm function, and infection of the female reproductive tract could interfere with normal sperm transport. The current name now used for these organisms is *Ureaplasma urealyticum*. Two other microorganisms found in the female genital tract are *Mycoplasma hominis* and *M. fermentans*. These organisms have been found to colonize in the lower genital tract of some women and not to cause any problems making this a difficult issue in terms of pathology. Although it has been reported that treatment of infertile couples with antibiotics, such as tetracycline or doxycycline, that eradicate these organisms, may result in high pregnancy rates, **controlled studies have reported no difference in pregnancy rates between couples treated with antibiotics and those not treated**. Harrison and colleagues have studied 88 infertile couples with no demonstrable cause of infertility. One-third were treated with doxycycline, one-third received placebo, and one-third received no treatment. T-mycoplasma was isolated from approximately two-thirds of the couples in each group and was eradicated only in the group treated with doxycycline. Nevertheless, conception rates were similar in each group (Harrison, 1975), as was also reported by Matthews and coworkers (Matthews, 1978) Other investigators have suggested that asymptomatic *Chlamydia trachomatis* infection may also cause infertility, but the dosage of doxycycline used in the randomized studies cited earlier would also have eradicated these organisms. Thus there is no evidence that asymptomatic infection of the genital tract of the human male or female causes infertility.

### Are Other Tests of Sperm Function Indicated?

In that the semen analysis is subjective and variable, it has long been suggested that other more functional tests would improve the evaluation of the male partner (Oehninger, 2014).The zona-free hamster egg penetration test originally described by Yanagimachi and associates was a test developed to predict the fertilizing ability of sperm and provides an additional, perhaps more sensitive, parameter for assessing sperm function than routine semen analysis; however, many variables factors affect the test results. It has been shown that this test does not correlate well with IVF of human eggs. The sensitivity and specificity of the hamster egg penetration assay (sperm penetration assay) is considered to be too low to justify its routine use as part of the infertility investigation.

Some functional tests of sperm (such as the hypoosmotic swelling test) assess the integrity of the sperm cell membrane, and others (the zona pellucida binding test, acrosome reaction, and the hyaluronan binding assay) assess maturity and viability (Oehninger, 2014); however, there is **no evidence, at present, that these tests add information to the infertility investigation** or affects treatment. The **DNA fragmentation test** in sperm has become popular. This test, which is carried out by flow cytometry or direct microscopy, determines the rate of DNA fragments; a DNA fragmentation index of more than 30% has been suggested to indicate a poorer rate of fertilization and therefore suggests the need for IVF with intracytoplasmic sperm injection (ICSI); however, at present, **there is no evidence that this correlates with the success of IVF, and it cannot be advocated as a routine test** (Practice Committee ASRM, 2014).

## PROGNOSIS OF VARIOUS DIAGNOSES UNCOVERED BY THE INFERTILITY INVESTIGATION

Before discussing the specific treatments for abnormalities uncovered by the investigation, it is useful to frame a prognosis for the couple depending on what factor(s) have been found.

The highest probability of conception with treatment other than with IVF-ET occurs among couples in whom anovulation is the only abnormality, with substantially lower probabilities of pregnancy in couples with tubal disease and sperm abnormalities (Hull, 1985) (Fig. 40.8). Although these data are older, this information from Hull still provides the best available comparisons. Age is a major prognostic factor. Among a group of infertile couples with unexplained infertility who were followed for 2 years without treatment after the evaluation was completed, it was found that the chances of becoming pregnant were greater in women younger than 35 years (~75%) than in women older than 35 (50%) (Hull, 1985) (Fig. 40.9). The duration of infertility is also of prognostic significance. The cumulative conception rate at the end of 2 years without therapy for those couples was much greater for those who had tried to conceive for less than 3 years before evaluation (~75%) than those who had tried to conceive for more than 3 years (~30%) (Hull, 1994) (Fig. 40.10). In three of the four studies of infertile couples who received no therapy mentioned earlier, more than 50% of the couples who eventually conceived did so in the first year after completing the infertility evaluation.

In couples with no known factors, it has been suggested that couples have a better prognosis for spontaneous conception

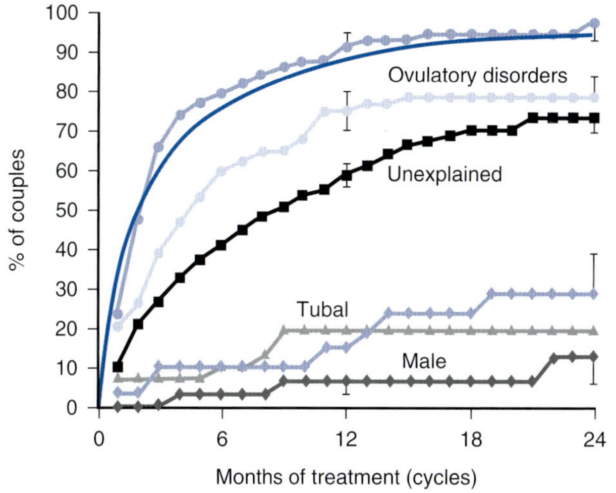


**Fig. 40.8** Effect of various treatments on fecundability: ovulatory, tubal, and male factors. (Modified from Hull MG, Glazener CM, Kelly NJ, et al. Population study of causes, treatment, and outcome of infertility. *Br Med J.* 1985;291(6510):1693-1697.)

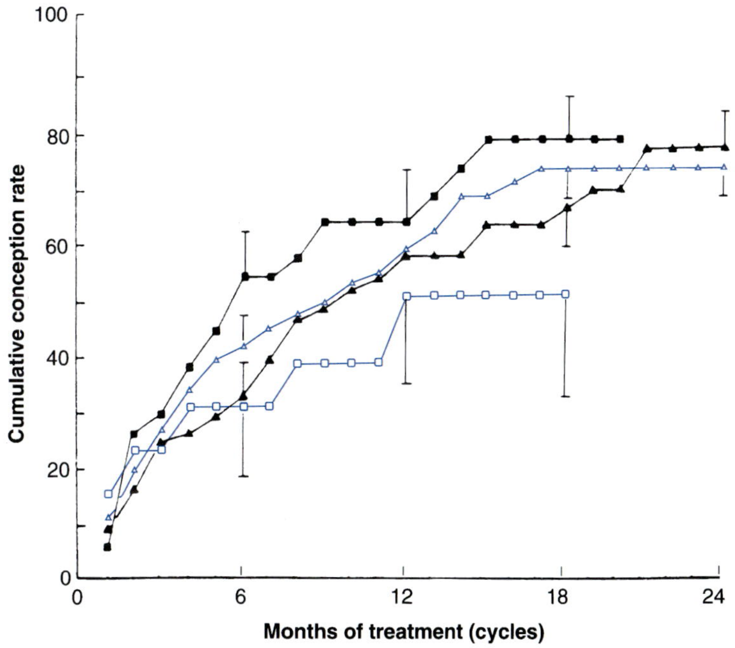


**Fig. 40.9** Cumulative rates of conception from first attendance at clinic in couples with unexplained infertility related to age of woman. Rates for each age group are shown: solid squares, younger than 25 years; blue triangles, 25 to 29 years; solid triangles, 30 to 34 years; blue squares, older than 35 years. Standard errors of proportions are given at 6, 12, 18, and 24 months. (From Hull MG, Glazener CM, Kelly NJ, et al. Population study of causes, treatment, and outcome of infertility. *Br Med J.* 1985;291(6510):1693-1697.)

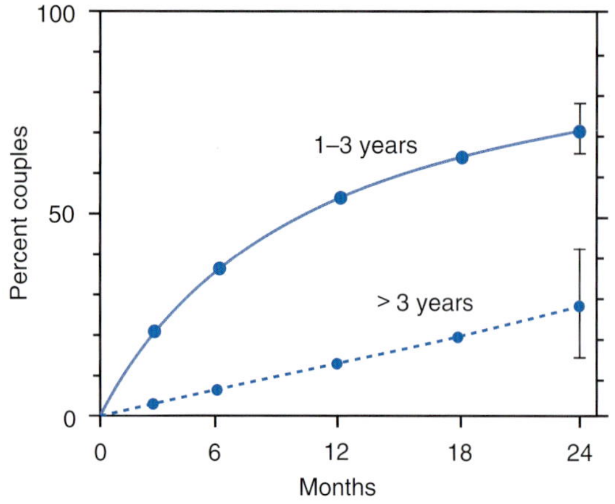


**Fig. 40.10** Cumulative pregnancy rates in unexplained infertility without treatment related to duration of infertility. (From Hull MG. Effectiveness of infertility treatments: choice and comparative analysis. *Int J Gynaecol Obstet.* 1994;47(2):99-108.)

based on their age and the time of trying to conceive. A prognostic score can be calculated (Hunault, 2004), and for those with a good prognosis, it has been suggested that these couples can just continue to try (**expectant management**) and it may not be necessary to start **empiric treatment** (discussed later). Generally, for couples presenting with the inability to conceive, even if no factors have been found (unexplained infertility), to increase their chances of conception or to shorten the time interval until conception takes place, various empiric treatments have been advocated. This generally increases the fecundity rate with unexplained infertility from a **baseline of around 4% to 9% to 10% per cycle,** as will be discussed later in the Unexplained Infertility section.

## TREATMENT OF VARIOUS CAUSES OF INFERTILITY

The management of the various causes of infertility will be presented here in the order generally followed in an infertility investigation.

### Medical Treatment for Anovulation and Subovulatory Function

At times it may be found that some women are oligoovulatory or may not have consistent normal ovulatory function based on cycle length and levels of progesterone. They should be treated as other women with anovulation as addressed here. Therapeutic agents currently available to induce ovulation are clomiphene citrate, letrozole, and urinary and recombinant gonadotropins. Adjunctive treatments include gonadotropin-releasing hormone (GnRH) agonist and antagonists, as well as human chorionic gonadotropin (HCG), which is used to trigger ovulation. In addition, as discussed in Chapter 39, if anovulation is caused by hyperprolactinemia, dopamine agonists are an effective means of inducing ovulation, although most women will also respond to clomiphene or letrozole. As noted in Chapter 38, ovulation may be induced by corticosteroid therapy in women with congenital adrenal hyperplasia, but here again in the adult-onset patient, clomiphene or letrozole can be used as well.

#### Clomiphene Citrate

Clomiphene citrate (CC) is the usual first-line pharmacologic agent for treating women with anovulation or subovulatory function as long as there is sufficient estrogen production. CC is a racemic mixture of en- and zu-clomiphene, which act as estrogen antagonists. The former has a shorter half-life and is more active than the zu-clomiphene isomer, which has a much longer half-life and is more estrogen agonistic than antagonistic. **CC acts by competing with endogenous circulating estrogens for estrogen receptor binding sites on the hypothalamus,** thereby blocking the negative feedback of endogenous estrogen. GnRH is then released in an enhanced manner, stimulating FSH and LH, which in turn cause oocyte maturation, with increased $E_2$ production. CC is usually given daily for 5 days, beginning 3 to 5 days after the onset of spontaneous menses or withdrawal bleeding induced with a progestogen.

During the days when CC is taken, serum levels of LH and FSH rise, accompanied by a steady increase in serum $E_2$ level. After CC is discontinued, $E_2$ levels continue to increase and the negative feedback on the hypothalamic-pituitary axis causes a decrease in FSH and LH levels, similar to the change seen in the late follicular phase of a normal ovulatory cycle. Approximately 5 to 9 days (mean, 7 days) after the last CC tablet, the exponentially rising level of $E_2$ from the dominant follicle has a positive feedback effect on the pituitary or hypothalamus, producing a surge in LH and FSH levels, which usually results in ovulation and luteinization of the follicle.

Timing of ovulation can be determined by using LH monitoring kits and serum progesterone can be measured 1 week after presumed ovulation. A rise in serum progesterone level greater than 3 ng/mL correlates well with the finding of a secretory endometrium, but it has been reported that the **maximal midluteal progesterone levels in CC-induced ovulatory conception cycles are consistently more than 15 ng/mL** (Hammond, 1983). These levels are higher than the 10 ng/mL level, which is the minimum concentration of progesterone found 7 days after ovulation in spontaneous ovulatory conception cycles (Hull, 1982). The level is higher with CC because more than one follicle usually matures and undergoes luteinization.

Various treatment regimens have been advocated for the use of CC. Most start with an initial dosage of 50 mg/day for 5 days, beginning on the third to fifth day of spontaneous or induced menses. If presumptive evidence of ovulation occurs with this dosage, the same dosage of CC is taken in subsequent cycles until conception occurs. If ovulation fails to occur with the initial dosage, a sequential, graduated, increasing dosage regimen has proven to be effective, with a minimum of side effects. With this regime, if ovulation does not occur with the 50-mg dose, the dosage of drug is increased in the next treatment cycle to 100 mg/day for 5 days. If ovulation does not occur with 100 mg/day in subsequent cycles, the dosage is sequentially increased to 150 mg. In the past we have used doses up to 250 mg, with and without HCG (Lobo, 1982). In the 10 years' experience with this treatment regimen as reported by Gysler and associates, approximately half of the women who ovulated and half of those who conceived did so after treatment with the 50-mg/day regimen, and an additional 20% ovulated with the 100-mg/day dosage (Gysler, 1982). Approximately 25% of all women who ovulated or conceived did so after treatment with a higher dosage regimen, indicating the value of the individualized sequential treatment regimen; however, from a practical standpoint, it is **unusual to use doses higher than 150 mg,** particularly when adjuncts are available, such as metformin in overweight women with PCOS or switching to letrozole. In the past, and still occasionally, dexamethasone has been used as an adjunct as well.

A newer regimen, the **stair-step regimen**, does not wait for menses after a failed response before moving to the next dose (Hurst, 2009); thus if there is no follicular development on ultrasound 5 days after the last clomiphene tablet, the patient is immediately placed on 100 mg for 5 days and subsequently to 150 mg for 5 days in the same cycle if follicular development does not occur. Although preliminary retrospective reports have shown that this is a reasonable approach to hasten therapy, prospective randomized trials are still in progress.

With the dosage regimen of CC up to 250 mg, more than 90% of women with oligomenorrhea and 66% with secondary amenorrhea and normal estrogen status will have presumptive evidence of ovulation. Although **only approximately 50% of patients who ovulate with this treatment will conceive,** (Gysler, 1982). The fecundability during several months of treatment with CC, if no other causes of infertility are present, are similar to those of a normal fertile population. Using life table analysis, the monthly pregnancy rate **(fecundability) of women treated with CC who had no other infertility factor was 22%** compared with a rate of 25% for women discontinuing diaphragm use. The monthly fecundability remained constant throughout almost 1 year of treatment. Almost all the anovulatory women without other infertility factors in this series, as well as other women with correctable infertility factors, had conceived after 10 cycles of treatment. This rate is also similar to the use of gonadotropins (Messinis, 1997) (Fig. 40.11).

These data indicate that discontinuation of therapy is the major reason for the reported difference in ovulation and conception rates in anovulatory women treated with CC; however, despite these data, many investigators believe that pregnancy rates are lower with CC than might be expected based on ovulation rates, and other factors (in some women), such as cervical mucus and endometrial problems, explain this discrepancy. In ovulatory women who respond to CC, **because as many as 80% of women will conceive by 3 months if there are no other factors,** additional testing should be done after 3 months if not carried out earlier. A HSG should be performed at this time. A semen analysis should be done before starting CC. When conception occurs after ovulation has been induced with CC, the incidence of multiple gestation is increased to approximately 8%, with almost all being twin gestations; however, when the drug is used in normally ovulating women with unexplained infertility, the rate increases to almost 20%. The incidence of **clinical spontaneous abortion ranges between 15% and 20%, similar to the rate in the general population**. The rates of intrauterine fetal death and congenital malformation are also not significantly increased. Animal data have shown that if the drug is given in high dosages during the time of embryogenesis, there is an increased incidence of fetal anomalies; however, limited human data have indicated that if the drug is ingested during the first 6 weeks after conception has occurred, the incidence of fetal malformation, although higher (5.1%) than in the normal non infertility population, it is not significantly increased. Women with infertility in general have been noted to have a higher anomaly rate, even when conceiving without medications. Although no definitive data have shown that the drug is teratogenic in humans, it is best that the woman be tested for pregnancy before each course of treatment.

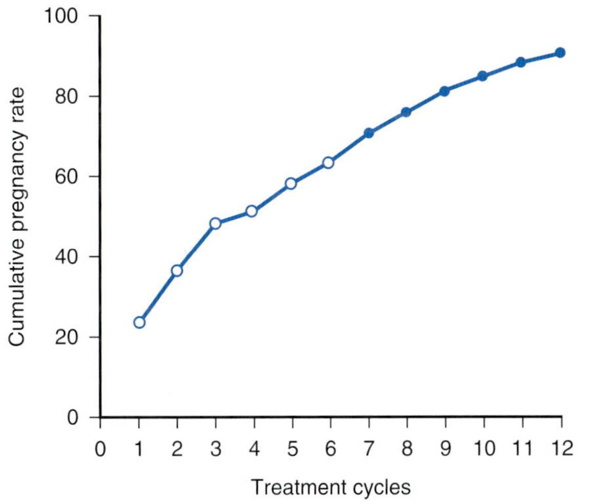


**Fig. 40.11** Cumulative pregnancy rate of 60% at 6 months with clomiphene. (From Messinis IE, Milingos SD. Current and future status of ovulation induction in polycystic ovary syndrome. *Hum Reprod Update.* 1997;3(3):235-253.)

Clinically palpable ovarian cysts occur in approximately 5% of women treated with CC but in less than 1% of treatment cycles. It is most efficient to carry out an ultrasound scan before prescribing CC, which is our current standard of practice. The cysts usually range in size from approximately 3 to 5 cm, do not require surgical excision, and usually regress spontaneously. On ultrasound smaller "cysts" are often encountered, but these should not preclude starting CC if they are less than 25 mm in diameter. Cysts can occur in any treatment cycle with any dosage, and the incidence is not increased with the higher dosages of drug. Recurrence of cyst formation with the same dosage is uncommon. Other side effects, which occur in less than 10% of women treated with CC, include vasomotor flushes, blurring of vision, abdominal pain or bloating, urticaria, and a slight degree of hair loss.

Up to 10% of women treated with CC fail to ovulate with the highest dosage. Older data have suggested that this so-called resistance is not caused by the inability of the hypothalamic-pituitary axis to respond, but to the lack of the ovarian response to raised gonadotropin levels. Contributors of **CC resistance include body mass index, free androgen, and insulin; higher values all contributing to this resistance**. Although various prediction models have been generated to determine the CC response, none has proven to be useful prospectively. Findings in women with PCOS also suggest that **higher levels of AMH may contribute to CC resistance** and affect the dosage required for gonadotropins in women with PCOS; AMH inhibits FSH action in the ovary (Mahran, 2013).

Some data suggest that in women with elevated levels of androgen, particularly dehydroepiandrosterone sulfate (DHEAS), the use of low doses of dexamethasone may enhance the ovulation-inducing effect of CC. This approach is less often used today. Other adjuncts that have been tested, but that lack validation, include adding a dopamine agonist such as bromocriptine and antiandrogens. Metformin and insulin sensitizers have also been used as adjunctive treatments.

## Metformin and Other Insulin Sensitizers

Metformin, a biguanide used to control blood sugar in diabetics, has a role in ovulation induction in women with PCOS and has been shown to be superior to placebo. Although not a true insulin sensitizer, it decreases hepatic glucose production and has some minor peripheral action, leading to some decrease in insulin resistance. It also has a direct role in inhibiting ovarian androgen steroidogenesis and acts on the endometrium.

Studies have confirmed the efficacy of metformin over placebo in inducing ovulation in women with PCOS; however, in direct comparisons with clomiphene, it was inferior to clomiphene in terms of live birth rates in women with PCOS (Legro, 2007) (Fig. 40.12). Therefore although not necessarily a first-line choice in women with PCOS, it is clearly an adjunct and may be helpful in women who exhibit some degree of insulin resistance; however, it should be considered as a preliminary option in heavy or obese women and for those with impaired glucose tolerance or significant insulin resistance before ovulation induction with other agents.

The typical dosage of metformin is 1500 mg/day. It is preferable to use long-acting tablets (extended release or extra strength) available in 500- and 750-mg tablets and to ingest them all at the same time during a meal, preferably at dinner; however, it should be initiated only at 500 mg and titrated up over several weeks. This is because of gastrointestinal effects (e.g., nausea, vomiting,

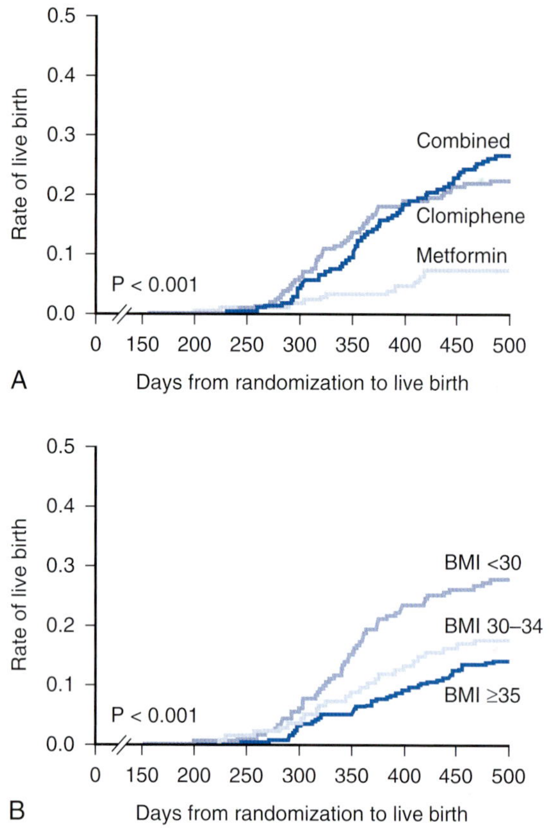


**Fig. 40.12** Kaplan-Meier curves for live birth, according to study group. **A,** All three groups. **B,** Groups divided by body mass index (BMI). (From Legro RS, Barnhart HX, Schlaff WD, et al. Clomiphene, metformin, or both for infertility in the polycystic ovary syndrome. *N Engl J Med. 2007;*356(6):551-566.)

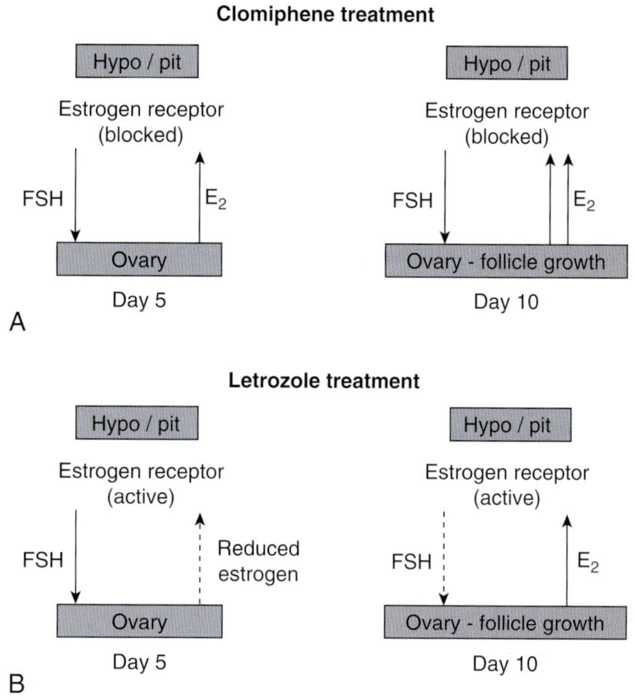


**Fig. 40.13** Clomiphene citrate **(A)** and letrozole treatment **(B).** *E*$_2$, Estradiol; *FSH,* follicle-stimulating hormone; Hypo/pit, hypothalamic-pituitary axis. (From Casper RF, Mitwally MF. Review: aromatase inhibitors for ovulation induction. *J Clin Endocrinol Metab.* 2006;91(3): 760-771.)

and diarrhea), which are the primary concern with metformin and preclude its use in up to 20% of women.

Lactic acidosis is a rare complication that occurs primarily in older individuals; however, checking chemistry blood levels after 3 months of metformin is good practice, and women also should be reminded not to drink alcohol heavily, although the occasional drink is acceptable. Minor elevations in liver enzymes, which often are caused by "fatty liver," are not a contraindication to using metformin. Many endocrinologists advocate a dose of 2000 mg/day for heavier women.

When metformin alone is prescribed for anovulatory women who wish to conceive, the ovulation rate is approximately 60% in adherent women. In CC-resistant patients, those who fail to ovulate with 150 mg/day (although the data are mixed), approximately 25% of women will respond to CC with metformin. Metformin is a category B substance for pregnancy and has been continued through the first trimester and beyond in some patients.

## Letrozole

**Aromatase inhibitors are efficacious as primary agents for ovulation induction.** Most of the experience is with letrozole. The mechanism of action is inhibition of $E_2$ production during the 5 days of administration, which results in negative feedback and an increase in FSH levels, much like the response to CC. Intraovarian androgen levels are also increased, which may enhance FSH sensitivity. Letrozole (2.5 or 5 mg) per day for 5 days is administered for 5 days, beginning on cycle days 3 to 5.

Because **letrozole is short acting**, the problems of thick cervical mucus or a thin endometrium associated with CC have not been reported with letrozole; however, $E_2$ levels are usually lower at ovulation. Pregnancy rates are comparable to those with CC alone, and there has been a suggestion for a reduced incidence of multiple pregnancies because of its shorter half-life and lack of stimulation of gonadotropins beyond the early follicular phase (Casper, 2006) (Fig. 40.13). A randomized trial comparing letrozole and CC in **women with PCOS showed the superiority of letrozole in terms of live births** (Legro, 2014) (Fig. 40.14). In this trial there were no differences in adverse effects or congenital anomalies, and the multiple pregnancy rates were comparable, which is at odds with the purported theoretical advantage of letrozole over CC. Including this trial, a meta-analysis from Cochrane also confirmed the superiority of letrozole (Franik, 2014). In that it has also been deemed to be cost effective, letrozole should be considered the first-line treatment (over CC) in women with PCOS, although to date it still has not been approved by the U.S. Food and Drug Administration (FDA) for ovulation induction; however, there is **no evidence of the superiority of letrozole over CC in women without PCOS**; indeed, CC performed better when used to enhance ovulation in women with unexplained infertility (discussed later).

There is little information about the effects of letrozole in CC-resistant patients, but anecdotally it has been found to be effective in this regard in many women. Letrozole with gonadotropins has also been used for ovarian stimulation. It has been suggested that it can reduce the gonadotropin dose needed when used as a sequential regimen (letrozole priming followed by gonadotropins), and it may be used in combination with gonadotropins in poor responders for IVF.

## Gonadotropins

Gonadotropin therapy is indicated for ovulation induction when estrogen levels are low and when there is no repose to CC or

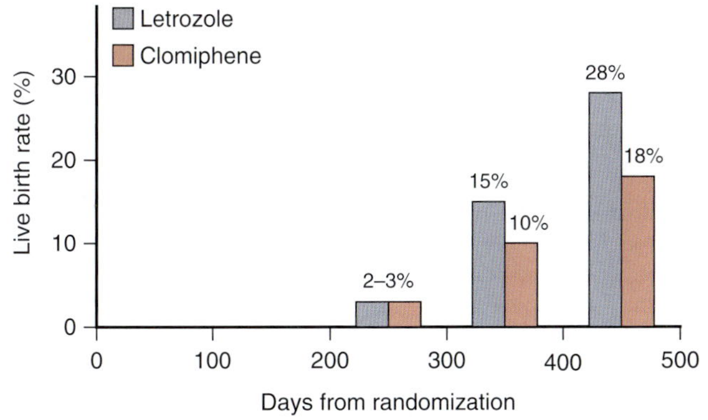


**Fig. 40.14** Live birth rates in a randomized trial of letrozole versus clomiphene in women with polycystic ovary syndrome. (Data from Legro RS, Brzyski RG, Diamond MP, et al. Letrozole versus clomiphene for infertility in the polycystic ovary syndrome. *N Engl J Med.* 2014;371(2):119-129.)

letrozole. Low serum $E_2$ levels (usually less than 20 to 30 pg/mL) or lack of withdrawal bleeding after progestogen administration signifies a state that will be unresponsive to oral therapies (CC, letrozole) that are dependent on a negative feedback system. Apart from this indication in usually amenorrheic women, it is appropriate to use gonadotropins when there is resistance to CC or letrozole. Gonadotropins have also been used when there has been the inability to conceive after several (four to six) cycles of CC or letrozole, although this indication is not as commonly applied today.

The original gonadotropin preparations were extracts of postmenopausal urine. Although purified, they contained large amounts of protein contaminants. These preparations are used less often today but are still available worldwide (Pergonal, Humegon). Newer preparations with additional purification have allowed them to be administered subcutaneously (SC) rather than intramuscularly (IM). These preparations (such as Menopur) are titrated to provide an equal quantity of LH (75 IU) and FSH (75 IU) in one ampule.

Further modifications of these urinary products have eliminated most of the LH activity and provided a relatively pure FSH urinary preparation (urofollitropin for injection [Bravelle or Metrodin], containing 75 IU FSH/ampule). All nonrecombinant preparations, because they are extracted from human sources, have batch to batch variability in terms of biologic activity.

Recombinant pure FSH preparations (from Chinese hamster ovarian cells) are currently available for subcutaneous administration (Gonal-F, Follistim, 75 IU FSH). Recombinant pure LH has also become available as a supplement (Luveris, 75 IU LH), although it is unclear if the addition of LH is really necessary in most cases.

Because each woman responds individually to the dosage of gonadotropins, even the same woman in different treatment cycles, it is essential to monitor treatment carefully with frequent measurements of estrogen levels and ovarian ultrasonography. **Close monitoring (ultrasound and $E_2$) is important to assess the adequacy of the response and to avoid ovarian hyperstimulation.**

There is a different concept regarding induction of ovulation with gonadotropins when the problem is anovulation or when gonadotropins are used in the setting of unexplained infertility or for the purposes of IVF (discussed later). Many practitioners often lose this concept, which then leads to a high rate of hyperstimulation and multiple pregnancies. It is for these reasons that gonadotropins are often avoided in the setting of failure to conceive after several ovulatory cycles of CC or letrozole, favoring an approach of going directly to IVF.

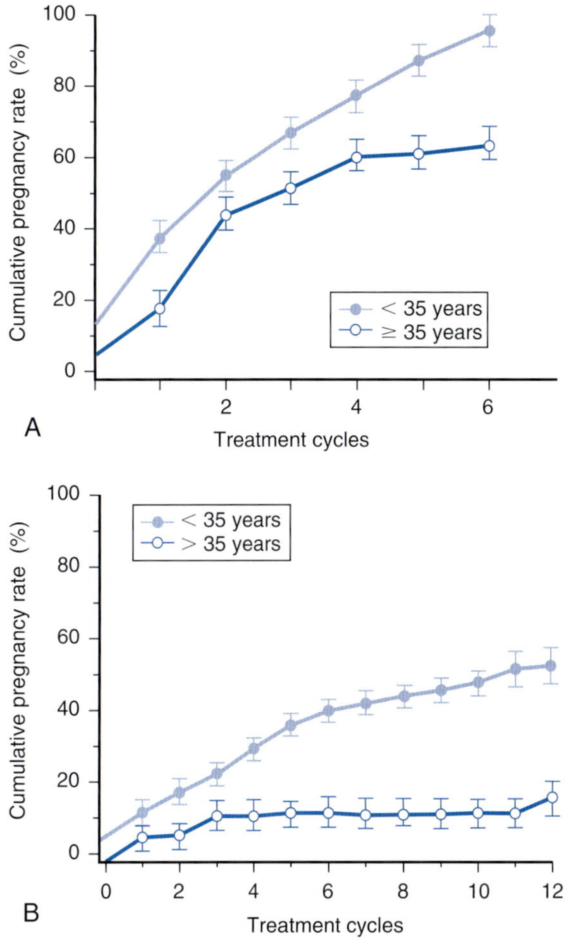


**Fig. 40.15 A,** Cumulative pregnancy rates for hypogonadotropic anovulatory women (World Health Organization [WHO] group I) treated with gonadotropins. *Solid circles* represent the cumulative pregnancy rate in women younger than 35 years. *Open circles* represent the cumulative pregnancy rate in women older than 35 years. **B,** Cumulative pregnancy rates after gonadotropin treatment for anovulatory women who did not respond to clomiphene induction of ovulation (WHO group II). *Solid circles* represent the cumulative pregnancy rate in women younger than 35 years. *Open circles* represent the cumulative pregnancy rate in women older than 35 years. (From Lunenfeld B, Insler V. Human gonadotropins. In: Wallach EE, Zacur HA, eds. *Reproductive Medicine and Surgery.* St. Louis: Mosby; 1995:617.)

The goal of therapy in anovulatory women is to produce one mature follicle, sometimes two. In women with low estrogen status, cycle fecundability approaches the ideal (~20%/cycle) if there are no other infertility factors. It is a little lower, however, in women who are CC failures or have PCOS (Lunenfeld, 1995) (Fig. 40.15). The risk of hyperstimulation is greatest in these patients, and great care has to be used when monitoring them (discussed later).

By injecting gonadotropins, the physiology behind this approach is to increase the serum FSH level to more than a critical threshold level, which is an unknown at the outset. The window for this therapeutic threshold is fairly wide in normal and hypoestrogenic women, but it is extremely narrow in PCOS, increasing the risk of hyperstimulation. A starting dose of 150 IU with FSH is used (as a recombinant preparation of pure FSH or a combination of LH and FSH in a urinary preparation). The $E_2$ level is determined and ultrasound is performed after approximately 5 days and then approximately every other day until a follicle

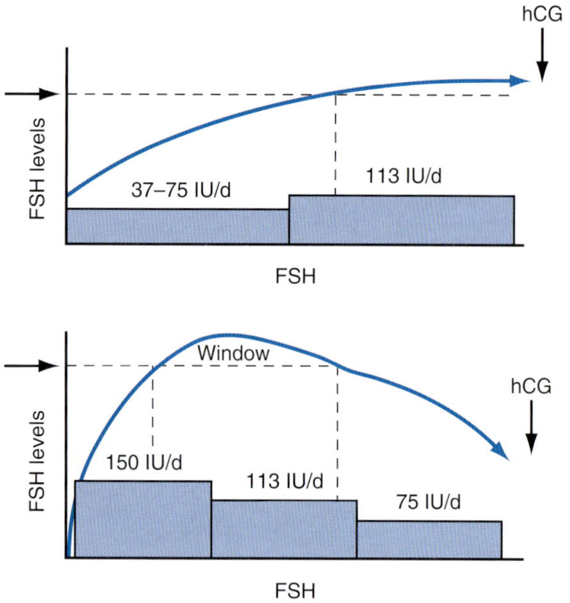


**Fig. 40.16** Schematic representation of serum follicle-stimulating hormone (FSH) levels and daily dose of exogenous FSH during low-dose step-up or step-down regimens for ovulation induction. *hCG,* Human chorionic gonadotropin. (From Macklon NS, Bart CJ. Medical approaches to ovarian stimulation for infertility. In: Strauss JF, Barbieri RL, eds. *Yen and Jaffe's Reproductive Endocrinology.* 6th ed. Philadelphia: WB Saunders; 2009:701.)

reaches a diameter of at least 18 mm. The **serum $E_2$ level should be at least in the range of 200 pg/mL for a mature follicle.** At this point, 5000 to 10,000 IU of HCG is administered IM (or pure recombinant HCG, Ovidrel, 250 µg SC) to trigger ovulation. Timed intercourse is usually advised if there is a normal semen analysis and good cervical mucus. **Ovulation should occur between 36 and 48 hours after the trigger of HCG.** Particularly in women with hypothalamic amenorrhea and low estrogen status, **vaginal progesterone supplementation (100 to 200 mg/day**) is usually prescribed, although this addition is not completely evidence-based.

In women with PCOS in whom the ovary is extremely sensitive to gonadotropin, a starting dose of only 50 to 75 IU is used. A slow step-up regimen is usually preferred, increasing the dose slowly only after 7 days (Macklon, 2009) (Fig. 40.16). Although there have been advocates for the use of a step-down approach (higher initial dose and then a rapid decrease), randomized trials in PCOS have suggested the preference for using the traditional step-up approach, which has better outcomes.

The pregnancy rate per cycle should be similar to that after CC therapy (~20%). With sufficient duration of treatment and no other infertility factors, cumulative pregnancy rates are excellent. It has been reported that the cumulative pregnancy rate after nine cycles of gonadotropin therapy is approximately 77%. These effects are influenced by age and type of anovulation as noted previously (see Fig. 40.15). The incidence of spontaneous abortion after gonadotropin therapy is higher than the normal rate (25% to 35%), and the overall multiple pregnancy rate (usually twins) is in the range of 15%, but there is a risk of this being much higher, particularly with inadequate monitoring.

## Ovarian Hyperstimulation Syndrome

Although enlarged ovaries are often encountered after gonadotropin administration, significant ovarian hyperstimulation syndrome (OHSS) occurs in **approximately 0.5% of women receiving gonadotropins; and can be as high as 10% in women with PCOS.** OHSS can be life threatening, causing massive fluid shifts, ascites, pleural effusion, electrolyte disturbances, and thromboembolism (Tan, 2013). The cause has not been completely elucidated but is related to the large cystic ovaries, high $E_2$ levels, and the ovarian elaboration of substances such as vascular endothelial growth factor (VEGF), which increases vascularity and vascular permeability. Several investigators have classified OHSS into mild, moderate, and severe forms. A representative categorization may be found in Box 40.1 (Navot, 1992). HCG triggers the syndrome, and blood levels of HCG continue to stimulate the ovaries in OHSS. Therefore the syndrome is worse if pregnancy occurs and abates within 1 week in the absence of pregnancy. For this reason, if severe OHSS is anticipated, HCG injection should be withheld. In IVF cycles, the embryos may be frozen rather than replaced to avoid pregnancy.

Treatment of OHSS is largely supportive, with judicious use of fluids (normal saline) and prevention of thrombosis. Correction of electrolyte disturbances and maintenance of urine output are of greatest importance. Occasionally, admission for intensive care unit (ICU) monitoring is necessary.

Avoidance of excessive stimulation is the primary approach for preventing OHSS. Lowering or withholding the dose of HCG is also advisable. An alternative approach is to use a GnRH agonist instead of HCG to trigger ovulation (as long as there is a normal pituitary able to release LH) because LH is much shorter acting

### BOX 40.1 Classification of Ovarian Hyperstimulation Syndrome

**MILD**

Ovarian enlargement (≤5 cm)
Abdominal discomfort

**MODERATE**

Ovarian enlargement (6-10 cm)
Nausea or gastrointestinal symptoms
Abdominal discomfort
Normal laboratory evaluation
Mild ascites, not clinically evident

**SEVERE**

Symptoms as above and other symptoms, such as respiratory distress
Ovarian enlargement
Severe ascites (clinically evident)
Hydrothorax
Elevated hematocrit (>45%)
Elevated WBC count (>15,000/µL)
Elevated creatinine
Electrolyte abnormalities (hyponatremia, hyperkalemia)
Elevated liver function tests

**Critical (as a subcategory of severe)**

Severe end organ dysfunction
  Oliguria, creatinine >1.6 mg/dL
  Severe respiratory distress
Thrombotic complications
Infection
Severe hemoconcentration
  Hematocrit >55%
  WBC count >25,000/µL

Modified from Navot D, Bergh PA, Laufer N. Ovarian hyperstimulation syndrome in novel reproductive technologies: prevention and treatment. *Fertil Steril.* 1992;58(2):249-261.
*WBC,* White blood cell.

and will clear from the circulation soon after ovulation. An approach to treat OHSS is the use of a dopamine agonist such as cabergoline, which interferes with the action of VEGF. Meta-analysis has shown this to be beneficial (Tang, 2012). Metformin use in women with PCOS, in the setting of IVF, has also been shown to decrease the risk of OHSS.

The majority of studies and meta-analyses have not shown a statistically significant increased risk of ovarian or breast cancer in women receiving gonadotropin therapy (Diergaarde, 2014).

### Gonadotropin-Releasing Hormone

An alternative to the administration of gonadotropins is GnRH treatment, particularly in estrogen-deficient women. Because continuous administration of GnRH will saturate the receptors and thus inhibit gonadotropin release to induce ovulation, GnRH must be administered in a pulsatile manner, as occurs normally, at intervals of 60 to 90 minutes. GnRH is a peptide, so it cannot be administered orally; the two methods of administration in current use are the intravenous (IV) and subcutaneous routes. More drug must be administered by the subcutaneous route than by the IV route; however, the subcutaneous route avoids use of an indwelling IV catheter, with its accompanying problems. The success rates, however, are better with IV delivery. The medication is given by means of a small portable pump, which is usually worn attached to an article of clothing. Ovulation rates of approximately 75% to 85% per treatment cycle have been reported; however, this approach is cumbersome, requiring a continuous line and a portable pump 24 hours a day. It is not often used.

## Other Therapeutic Modalities

### Weight and Lifestyle Management

Particularly in women who are clomiphene resistant, weight loss will often ameliorate the situation. In overweight women it is important to ensure that abnormalities in glucose and lipid metabolism are normalized as much as possible before induction of ovulation. There is evidence that lifestyle changes in diet and exercise may improve overall fitness and metabolic parameters, as well as ovulatory responses, even in the absence of true weight loss, although there could be a redistribution of body fat with lifestyle changes.

### Ovarian Electrocauterization

At a European Society of Human Reproduction and Embryology/American Society for Reproductive Medicine (ESHRE/ASRM) consensus meeting in Thessaloniki, Greece for the treatment of infertility in PCOS, it was concluded that a possible alternative to gonadotropin therapy in clomiphene-resistant women with PCOS is the use of ovarian electrocautery, which has similar efficacy (Thessaloniki ESHRE/ASRM–Sponsored PCOS Consensus Workshop Group, 2008).

Laparoscopic electrical or laser-generated burn holes through the ovarian cortex have been associated with improving ovulation rates, as was described many years ago with ovarian wedge resection, which is no longer performed. The major advantage of this more invasive method of ovarian electrocauterization is that it decreases the risk of hyperstimulation and multiple pregnancies. In addition to a concern of surgical complications, excessive destruction of the ovarian cortex can lead to premature ovarian failure. Only a limited number of burn holes (~10) should be made.

It has been reported that the endocrine changes may persist for at least 10 years (Gjonnaess, 1998). A Cochrane review has also reported an overall term pregnancy rate of 50% after surgery and a low multiple pregnancy rate (Farquhar, 2005).

Nevertheless, ovulation induction in women with PCOS should still be a medical treatment, particularly with the use of adjuncts if necessary. In our view, ovarian electrocauterization should be reserved for patients who have difficulties with gonadotropin stimulation (failure of dominant follicle selection or hyperstimulation risk) even in the setting of IVF, which is usually the next step in women who tend to have hyperstimulation with gonadotropin induction of ovulation.

## Male Factor Infertility

### The Male Evaluation

If the semen analysis is abnormal and has been repeated, it is important that the man be evaluated by an andrologist, usually a urologist. Important medical conditions must be ruled out, and occasionally an abnormality is found that can be treated. Blood should be obtained for hormone and other testing, as needed, and a careful urologic examination can diagnose problems such as testicular abnormalities and infection (Fig. 40.17). The more treatable conditions are hormonal abnormalities (apart from an elevated FSH level, signifying end organ seminiferous failure) and infection. **Varicocele** repair remains somewhat controversial, and the decision must be individualized based on the ages of the couple, other factors that may be involved, and whether the *varicocele is symptomatic, or at least clinically detected (palpable).* Although a varicocele has been **shown to correlate with poor sperm characteristics, there is often a variable response to surgery**. It is important to note that improvement may not be evident for 6 months, given that the cycle of spermatogenesis is approximately 3 months in length (Practice Committee ASRM, 2014).

In the most common findings of oligo-, astheno-, or teratospermia, it is important to know how the man should be evaluated. Fig. 40.18 provides a suggested algorithm (Bach, 2019).

If the evaluation is nondiagnostic or if no treatment is possible or indicated, the best therapy should be directed at improving the

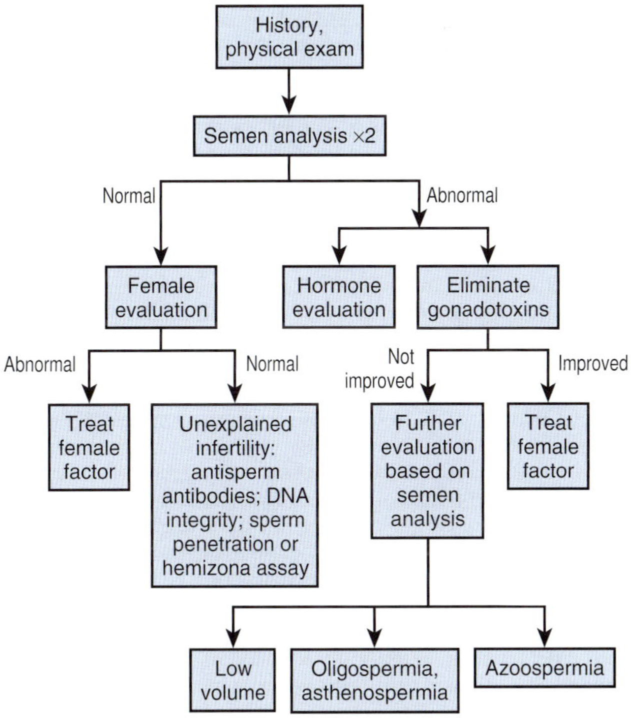


**Fig. 40.17** General algorithm for the diagnostic evaluation of male infertility. (From Turek PJ. Practical approaches to the diagnosis and management of male infertility. *Nat Clin Pract Urol.* 2005;2:226-238.)

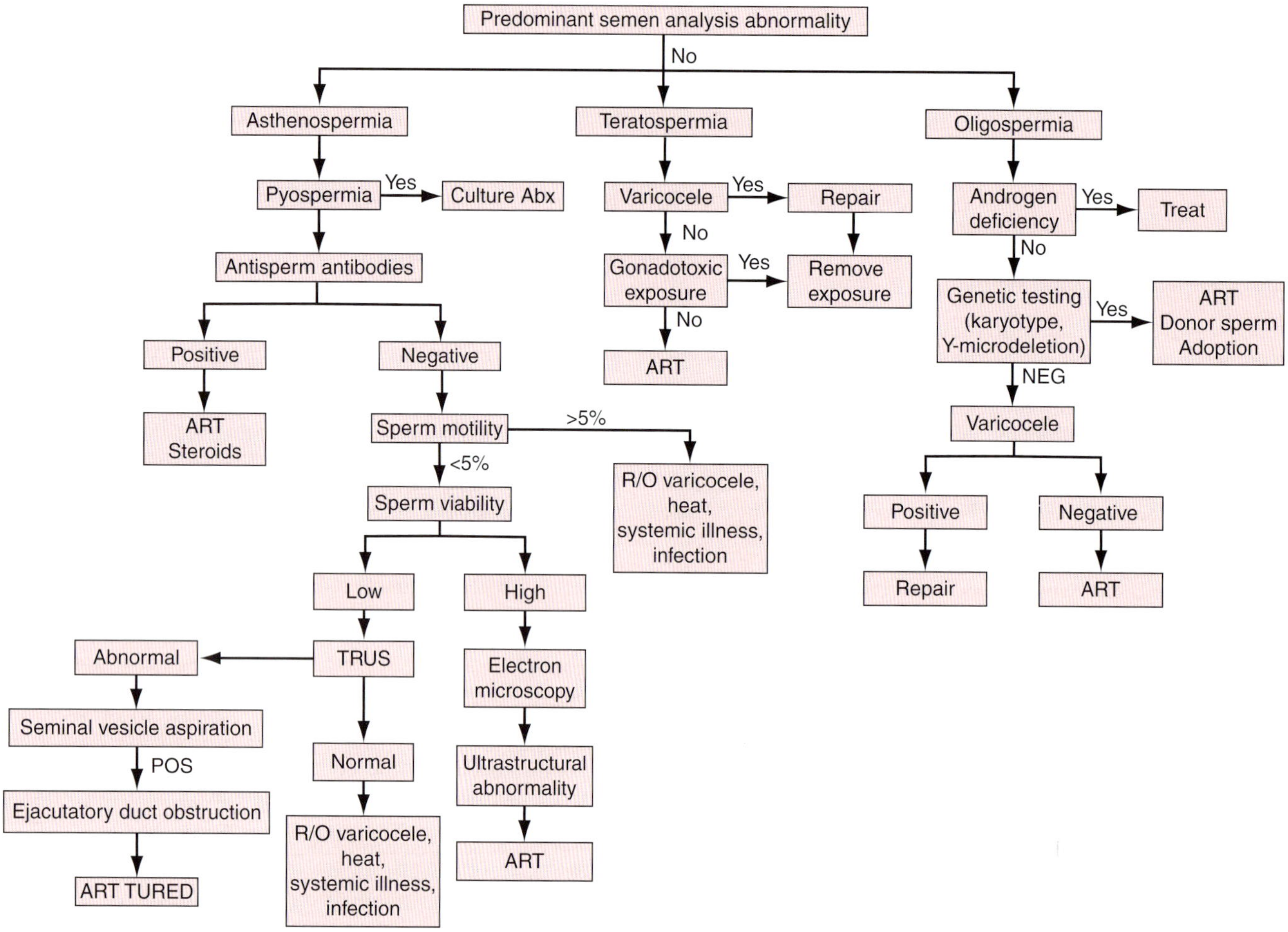


**Fig. 40.18** Algorithm for the evaluation and management of men with oligoasthenoteratospermia. *Abx,* Antibiotics; *ART,* assisted reproductive technology; *NEG,* negative; *POS,* positive; *R/O,* rule out; *TRUS,* transrectal ultrasound; *TURED,* transurethral resection of the ejaculatory ducts. (From Bach PV, Schlegel PN. Male infertility. In: *Yen and Jaffe's Reproductive Endocrinology.* 8th ed. Philadelphia: Elsevier; 2019:586.)

ejaculate for IUI or to carry out IVF with ICSI. IUI has been used to treat oligospermia and abnormalities of semen volume or viscosity to enhance fecundability. The limitation of successful IUI is when there is significant oligospermia or motility problems (less than 5 million motile sperm available) or with very poor morphology. Data, however, have suggested that abnormal morphology alone may not affect the success of IUI treatment (Deveneau, 2014), and abnormal morphology has been found often in previously fertile men.

The procedure of IUI (after washing and centrifugation of the ejaculate) is associated with higher pregnancy rates if combined with COS than when used in natural ovulatory cycles. IUI is also of benefit to women with variable degrees of cervical stenosis. Ideally insemination should take place on the day of or just before ovulation. It is advisable to use a urinary LH kit to determine the optimal date to perform insemination because the urinary LH peak occurs on the day before ovulation. Insemination should be scheduled for the morning after LH is initially detected in an afternoon urine specimen. In women who have difficulty with LH kits, or empirically, ovulation may be "triggered" with HCG injection (typically 250 μg of recombinant HCG Ovidrel SC), as long as follicular development is adequate (typically at least a 20-mm follicle on ultrasound).

Separation of sperm from the seminal fluid by double centrifugation, the swim-up technique, or use of a density gradient should be performed before IUI. This enhances sperm motility and is thought to increase capacitation (membrane changes in sperm that facilitate fertilization). IUI of unwashed seminal fluid should not be used because it may cause infection and can produce severe uterine cramps as a result of prostaglandin content in seminal fluid.

Until rather recently, if there were severe abnormalities in the semen analysis, the prognosis for fertility was less than that for any other cause of infertility (see Fig. 40.8), even with the use of IVF techniques. Attempts to enhance fertilization rates of aspirated oocytes with the technique of subzonal insemination of sperm were unsuccessful because fertilization rates remained low, approximately 15%. After Van Steirteghem and associates developed the technique of **ICSI**, fertilization rates of oocytes injected with a single normal sperm obtained from men with severe abnormalities in their semen analysis increased to more than 50% (Van Steirteghem, 1993). **Pregnancy rates per ET are now similar after ICSI compared with other indications for IVF.** When there is very low or no sperm in the ejaculate, IVF/ICSI can be carried out using testicular sperm (see Chapter 41).

Some couples, particularly those whose male partner has azoospermia, may choose to use donor sperm insemination. If they choose this option, the attitudes of both partners regarding the use of donor semen and the stability of the marriage must be thoroughly discussed before the procedure is performed. Donors from sperm banks are carefully screened for infectious diseases, and all semen samples are quarantined for at least 6 months because of the long time it takes for positive antibodies to HIV to appear after infection. ASRM has published a set of guidelines for semen donor insemination. These guidelines provide information regarding indications for donor insemination and suggested procedures for selection and screening of possible semen donors.

Freezing of sperm is the only way that donor insemination should be done because of the time necessary to quarantine samples to rule out infectious diseases, but freezing sperm affects fecundability. A cumulative pregnancy rate after insemination of approximately 50%, and a monthly fecundity rate of only 9% has been reported after 6 months of treatment; however, the range is variable and may be as high as a fecundity rate of 18%, with a 45% cumulative pregnancy rate at 3 months. There is a known variability of semen quality after thawing, even in normal fertile sperm donors.

## Uterine Causes of Infertility

In the evaluation of the uterus by HSG, a number of **filling defects** may be appreciated. These are usually polyps, submucous fibroids, or intrauterine adhesions. This imaging can also be assessed by saline sonography (SIS) and ultimately with hysteroscopy where findings can be treated.

### Intrauterine Adhesions/Synechiae

In addition to menstrual abnormalities and recurrent abortion, some women may not be able to conceive because of the presence of intrauterine adhesions (IUAs). Most women with IUAs have had a previous event affecting the uterus, typically a previous curettage of the uterine cavity, often during or shortly after a pregnancy. If the only abnormal finding in the infertility investigation is the presence of IUAs, the prognosis for conception after hysteroscopic lysis of the adhesions is good. March and Israel reported that of 69 infertile women with IUAs and no other infertility factors, 52 (75%) conceived after hysteroscopic treatment (March, 1981).

### Leiomyoma

Congenital uterine defects rarely cause infertility, and the uterine anomalies associated with maternal ingestion of diethylstilbestrol (DES) have not been shown in randomized studies to be a cause of infertility. It is also difficult to assess the effect of leiomyomas on conception because many women with leiomyomas have no difficulty conceiving; however, depending on their location, fibroids may decrease the chance of conception or increase the miscarriage rate. **Data indicate a global change in endometrial receptivity, even with intramural fibroids** (Rackow, 2010). If no other cause of infertility is found and myomas of moderate size and position are present, a myomectomy is justified. More recent data from the IVF literature point to a **decreased pregnancy rate with submucous fibroids, and larger intramural fibroids (>4 cm)**, but in those (intramural and subserosal fibroids) that do not distort the cavity, the pregnancy rate is not affected (Sunkara, 2010). *The overall pregnancy rate after myomectomy in women with no other causes of infertility has been found to be significantly improved in retrospective studies; surprisingly there are no prospective studies showing a benefit of myomectomy.*

### Tuberculosis

Although rare in the United States, genital tuberculosis should be kept in mind. If HSG reveals findings consistent with pelvic tuberculosis, endometrial biopsy and culture should be performed to confirm the diagnosis. The radiographic features of pelvic tuberculosis that are almost diagnostic include the following: (1) calcified lymph nodes or granulomas in the pelvis; (2) tubal obstruction in the distal isthmus or proximal ampulla, sometimes resulting in a pipe stem configuration of the tube proximal to the obstruction; (3) multiple strictures along the course of the tube; (4) irregularity to the contour of the ampulla; and (5) deformity or obliteration of the endometrial cavity without a previous curettage (Fig. 40.19). Appropriate antituberculosis medication should be initiated, but women with pelvic tuberculosis should be considered sterile because pregnancies after therapy are rare. Tubal reconstructive surgical procedures are therefore not indicated. If tuberculosis is present in the tube but not in the uterus, pregnancies have been reported after IVF.

### Tubal Causes of Infertility

Since the 1980s, the incidence of infertility caused by damage to the fallopian tube has increased because of an increased incidence of salpingitis. Obstructions occur at the distal or proximal portion of the tube and sometimes in both regions. Distal obstruction leading to a hydrosalpinx (Fig. 40.20) is much more common than proximal obstruction. The prognosis for fertility after surgical tubal reconstruction depends on the amount of damage to the tube and the location of the obstruction. If there

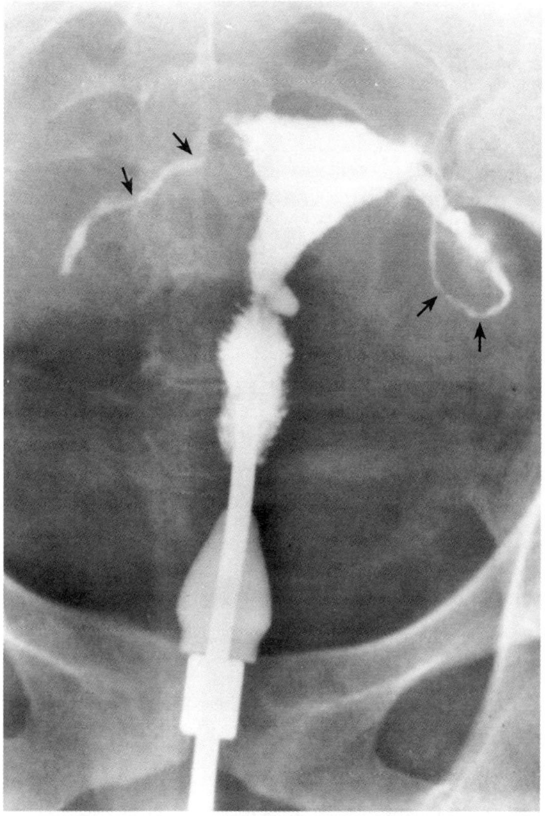

**Fig. 40.19** Tuberculous salpingitis in 37-year-old nulligravida with primary infertility for 15 years. Right tube is obstructed in the zone of transition between the isthmus and the ampulla. *Arrows* indicate multiple strictures in both tubes. Nodular contour of endometrial cavity may also be related to tuberculosis and is analogous to the pattern found in the ampulla in other cases. Small diverticulum near internal os probably represents adenomyosis. Diagnosis of tuberculosis was confirmed by endometrial culture. (From Richmond JA. Hysterosalpingography. In: Mishell DR Jr, Davajan V, Lobo RA, eds. *Infertility, Contraception and Reproductive Endocrinology.* 3rd ed. Cambridge, MA: Blackwell Scientific; 1991.)

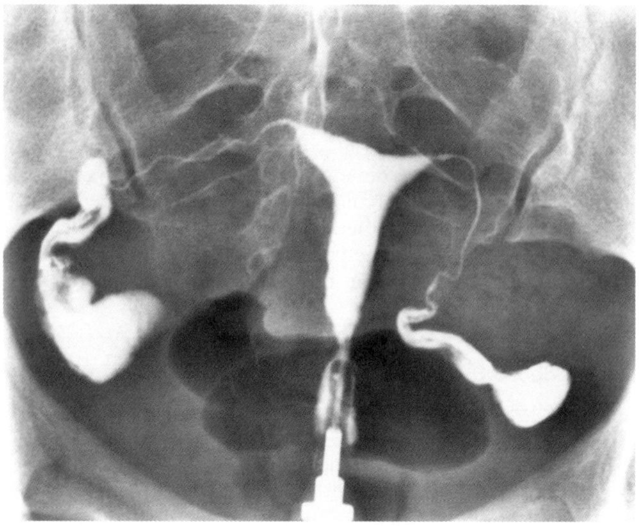

**Fig. 40.20** Hysterosalpingography showing bilateral hydrosalpinges with dilation, clubbing, and obstruction at fimbriated ends. Patient was 32-year-old woman with 10-year history of primary infertility. (From Richmond JA. Hysterosalpingography. In: Mishell DR Jr, Davajan V, Lobo RA, eds. *Infertility, Contraception and Reproductive Endocrinology.* 3rd ed. Cambridge, MA: Blackwell Scientific; 1991.)

is extensive damage, conception after tubal reconstruction is unlikely. Women with extensive tubal disease have a greater chance of conceiving with an IVF procedure, so the extent and location of the intrinsic and extrinsic tubal disease should be ascertained by HSG and possibly laparoscopy in an effort to determine whether tubal reconstruction or IVF offers the better prognosis (Practice Committee ASRM, 2012b). As noted, **if a large hydrosalpinx is seen at the time of HSG, it is best to suggest that the woman have IVF rather than undergo tubal reconstructive surgery. It is recommended that the hydrosalpinx be excised before IVF if it is large and visible by ultrasound**. If proximal and distal obstructions of the tube exist, the damage to the tube is usually so extensive that the tube cannot function normally. Therefore although it is possible to achieve tubal patency after surgical repair with proximal and distal blockage, subsequent intrauterine pregnancy is uncommon and surgical reconstruction should not be performed in such cases. In general, infertility surgery for tubal disease is a dying art—the pregnancy rates with IVF are far superior, and most women would prefer to avoid surgery as long as they have insurance coverage for IVF.

## Distal Tubal Disease

HSG can help determine whether the tubal obstruction is complete or partial, the size of the distal sacculation, and the appearance of the mucosal folds and rugal pattern of the endosalpinx (see Fig. 40.20). Laparoscopy will assist in determining the size of the hydrosalpinx, amount of muscularis, and thickness of the wall of the tube after distention with dye. Laparoscopic examination will determine whether pelvic adhesions are present and the extent of these adhesions. Women with fimbrial obstruction are not a homogeneous group, and the prognosis for intrauterine pregnancy after distal tubal reconstruction is related to the extent of the disease process. Therefore it is important to perform HSG and laparoscopy before surgical reconstruction to provide an individualized prognosis.

If the fimbriae of the distal end of the tube are relatively normal, with only partial occlusion by adhesions or fimbrial bridges, removal of these adhesions by means of a fimbrioplasty procedure will result in higher conception rates (~60%) than if the distal end is completely occluded and a cuff salpingostomy procedure is required. Overall conception rates after salpingostomy are in the 30% range, with a high percentage (~25%) being tubal pregnancies. Although microsurgical techniques had been used for all tubal infertility surgery, all procedures are carried out via laparoscopy. **The incidence of ectopic pregnancy after surgical reconstruction for distal tubal disease is directly related to the amount of tubal damage** existing before the operative procedure; however, **today less and less primary tubal reconstructive surgery is being done.**

The results of tubal reconstruction correlate with the degree of tubal damage according to the severity of five factors: (1) extent of adhesions, (2) nature of adhesions, (3) diameter of the hydrosalpinx, (4) appearance of the endosalpinx, and (5) thickness of the tubal wall, with the latter being the best correlated. Using these criteria, prognostic categories have been identified: good, with a cumulative pregnancy rate of approximately 75%; intermediate, approximately 20%; and poor, less than 5%. In the good category, only 1 of 22 pregnancies may be ectopic, but in the intermediate group, 50% of the pregnancies may be expected to be tubal. **In the poor prognostic group, most of the pregnancies will be ectopic**. Accordingly, in women with fixed adhesions, with absent rugal folds and a thick, fixed tubal wall, distal tubal reconstructive surgery probably should not be performed.

## Proximal Tubal Blockage

If no dye enters the tube during HSG, the diagnosis of proximal tubal blockage is likely; however, because spasm of the uterus during the procedure may occlude the intrauterine portion of the tube, the diagnosis cannot be confirmed. Here, at least half of the time, the tube will be found to be patent on subsequent testing or at laparoscopy. Laparoscopy also allows examination of the distal portion of the tube, which cannot be visualized radiographically if there is proximal blockage.

It is preferred to attempt selective catheterization of the proximal portion of a tube at HSG under fluoroscopy if it does not fill with dye (Thurmond, 2008) (see Fig. 42.7). Cannulation of the proximal portion is also possible under direct guidance at hysteroscopy. Cannulation to open the putative obstruction is possible as long as there is no gross disease visible, such as salpingitis isthmica nodosa (SIN). Proximal tubal blockage may be caused by debris or endometriosis, but a significant occlusion is usually explained by prior infection or SIN.

In the past, proximal obstructions were best handled by microsurgical cornual tubal reanastomosis, with pregnancy rates in the range of 50% and ectopic rates of only 10%. Although this approach may still be considered on a selective basis, ***most cases of obstruction not relieved by fluoroscopic or hysteroscopic selective cannulation are now treated by IVF.***

## Adjunctive Therapy After Tubal Surgery

Adjunctive procedures for surgical tubal reconstruction previously included prophylactic antibiotics, intraperitoneal corticosteroids, postoperative hydrotubation, and placement of tubal stents. Prospective studies have not demonstrated postoperative hydrotubation to have any benefit, and tubal stents should not be used because they may cause mucosal damage. Data from several studies have shown that **intraperitoneal adjuncts are not effective.**

The only barriers currently used with some efficacy are an absorbable adhesion barrier (Gynecare Interceed, Ethicon), to be used only in areas that are dry and not bleeding, and barriers impregnated with hyaluronic acid (Seprafilm, Genzyme). The latter can be used as a slurry at the end of laparoscopy. Gore-Tex requires suturing and removal; therefore it is rarely used and is not applicable for tubal disease.

If pregnancy does not occur within 6 to 12 months after tubal reconstruction, HSG should be performed. **If tubal obstruction has recurred, a repeat surgical procedure is not advised.** In this setting, the pregnancy rates are less than 10%.

## Endometriosis

Some investigators have estimated that as many as **40% of infertile women have endometriosis.** If endometriosis is found at the time of laparoscopy, the extent of the disease should be documented. The causes, diagnosis, and treatment of endometriosis are presented in detail in Chapter 19.

Although endometriosis is often encountered in an infertility population (20% to 40%), the diagnosis may be subtle and may only be realized if a laparoscopy is carried out. As noted, laparoscopy is often currently bypassed in the investigative workup. Thus unless there is a strong component of pain as a presenting complaint, or a large endometrioma is seen on ultrasound, the diagnosis may not be appreciated. The treatment for pain is somewhat different and is reviewed in Chapter 19.

If laparoscopy is carried out and mild lesions are seen, it makes sense to ablate them surgically by electrocauterization or laser. Although this may not have a major therapeutic value, the current thinking is that peritoneal endometriosis may release substances that could impair fertilization at various levels.

With endometriosis various structural factors, particularly adhesions, contribute to the infertility of endometriosis, and classification schemes have been used to take this into account, but classifications are not often used in a prospective manner. In general, **women with endometriosis have a reduced fecundability**. This **relates to inflammatory factors, reduction in ovarian reserve (lower AMH levels are common) and extensiveness of the disease, which relates to mechanical (obstructive) factors.**

Surgery in the setting of infertility is reserved for those patients with pain and if large endometriomas are present. Smaller, 2- to 4-cm endometriomas may be observed, particularly in older women, because of the concern of compromising ovarian reserve by ovarian cystectomy. Otherwise, women should be treated as if they have unexplained infertility (discussed later). Many women with unexplained infertility may have endometriosis that has not been diagnosed because laparoscopy was not performed. **The lowered cycle of fecundity in endometriosis is similar to that of women with unexplained infertility (~4%).** COS, generally with IUI, is the usual initial treatment. If pregnancy does not occur in three to six cycles, IVF is offered as the next step. When surgery has been offered as the primary treatment for moderate to severe disease, which is easily diagnosed, pregnancy rates of approximately 50% have been recorded with operative laparoscopy. This rate is similar to the rate after laparotomy (see Chapter 19).

IVF pregnancy rates have been suggested to be reduced, but this mainly occurs with severe disease. In select cases, prior suppression of known causes of endometriosis (e.g., using an oral contraceptive continuously or a GnRH agonist for 2 to 3 months) has been shown to improve IVF pregnancy rates. For COS, there also has been a preference for using letrozole (aromatase inhibitor), rather than CC, which results in lower estrogen levels during the cycle and may also be helpful as endometriosis lesions express aromatase.

## Unexplained Infertility

This diagnostic category is relatively arbitrary and is probably never truly unexplained. Nevertheless, it represents a large number of patients who are evaluated for infertility. Some patients **merely have reduced fecundability based on chronologic or biologic reproductive age.** Unexplained infertility is defined as couples with normal ovulation and pelvic evaluation with a normal uterus and patent tubes on hysterosalpingogram, as well as a normal semen analysis. In the past the diagnosis also required a normal PCT and a laparoscopy. Laparoscopy is no longer carried out routinely unless there are clues to significant pelvic abnormalities. The rationale for omitting laparoscopy in the required diagnostic workup is that it is invasive and costly, and it is unlikely that the subtle abnormalities will change the outcome of treatment. Some studies have included couples into the category of unexplained infertility with mild abnormalities in the semen analysis and the suggestion of mild endometriosis.

Using the broad definition of unexplained infertility, **approximately 20% of all couples will fall into this category.** If exhaustive meticulous testing is carried out, including laparoscopy, this figure has been reported to be less than 5%. Additional testing for defects in sperm function and for endometrial histologic and biochemical variables has not been validated for routine use in making the diagnosis. Subtle defects may be overcome by standard empirical treatment for unexplained infertility. **At the same time, it is likely that on more rare occasions that there are true defects at the level of sperm or oocyte.** Occult defects in sperm may only be known in the setting of IVF (Bungum, 2004), and the absence of sperm RNA elements has also been documented in normal-appearing sperm (Jodar, 2015). The finding of "defective" oocytes has also been documented (Ezra, 1992).

The routine empirical treatment of unexplained infertility is ovarian stimulation with CC or gonadotropins, coupled with IUI. Prospective studies have shown that CC alone or IUI alone is not efficacious (Bhattacharya, 2008). Several European studies have also suggested that patients with a good prognosis, based on age and shorter duration of infertility, should undergo "expectant management," meaning continued timed intercourse for another 6 months before proceeding to treatment. A prediction model for natural conception was constructed by Hunault in the Netherlands, which was based on data from three cohorts of women with subfertility. In women younger than 38 years, the prognosis was calculated based on PCT, age, duration of infertility, prior pregnancy, percentage of motile sperm, and the referral pattern. A score of 60% or more was considered to be "good" and one of 30% or lower was "poor." Patients with a good prognosis in the Netherlands have usually been assigned expectant management for 6 months. The criteria for the Humault model have been refined for greater precision and include more data, such as body mass index, FSH levels, and semen volume and morphology (Bensdor p, 2017).

This scenario is usually unacceptable for the U.S. population for social and economic reasons. Also, in Europe the standard management of unexplained infertility with CC/IUI results in a lower pregnancy rate per cycle (closer to an expectant group) because of a more conservative approach to ovarian stimulation (Custers, 2012). The efficiency of COS/IUI is highly age dependent. In women in their 30s, the expected fecundity rate is 8% to 9% and is not much different with the use of CC or gonadotropins, a conclusion that has been based on prospective data (Reindollar, 2010) (Table 40.6).

In 1998 Guzick and associates published a review of data from 45 published studies of various therapies of unexplained infertility,

**TABLE 40.6** Randomized Trial of Treatments for Unexplained Infertility

| Number of Initiated Cycles | CC/IUI | FSH/IUI | IVF |
|---|---|---|---|
| All subjects | 1294 | 700 | 622 |
| Live births per initiated cycle | 7.6% (6.2-9.2) | 9.8% (6.8-14) | 30.7% (27.1-34.5) |

Data from Reindollar RH, Regan MM, Neumann PJ, et al. A randomized clinical trial to evaluate optimal treatment for unexplained infertility: the fast track and standard treatment (FASTT) trial. *Fertil Steril.* 2010;94(3):888-899.

*CC,* Clomiphene citrate; *IUI,* intrauterine insemination; *FSH,* follicle-stimulating hormone; *IVF,* in vitro fertilization.

including mild endometriosis. After adjustment for study quality, pregnancy rates per initiated treatment cycle were 1.3% to 4.1% for no treatment, 8.3% for CC plus IUI, 17.1% for gonadotropins plus IUI, and 20.7% for IVF. Although the pregnancy rate in this analysis of nonrandomized studies was higher with gonadotropins/IUI than with CC/IUI, prospective data have shown that the rates are similar as noted previously (Reindollar, 2010). IVF pregnancy rates are also higher now than they were in 1998. Although **the rate of approximately 9% per cycle may seem low, the background rate for unexplained infertility is no more than 4%; thus the fecundity is more than doubled.** In terms of the choice of CC/IUI, whereas in a patient without PCOS and with unexplained infertility, letrozole/IUI may also be used, **it appears that CC/IUI may be more effective** (Fig. 40.21). In this National Institutes of Health (NIH)–sponsored trial coined **AMIGOS**, although gonadotropins resulted in a higher pregnancy and live birth rate, there was a **high multiple pregnancy rate of 32% compared with CC** and **letrozole**, which had similar rates

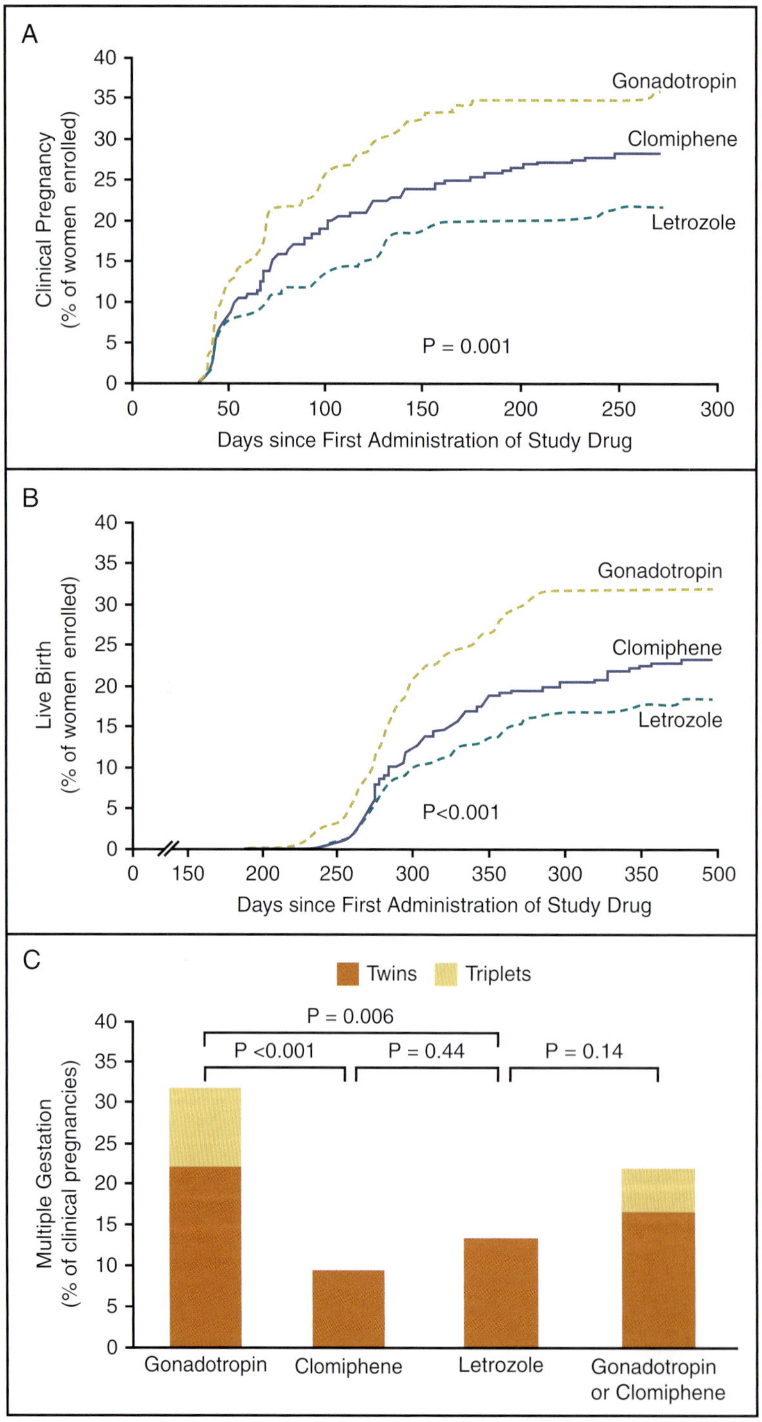


**Fig. 40.21** Pregnancy rates in the gonadotropin, clomiphene, and letrozole groups. **A,** Clinical pregnancy rates in the three groups, **B,** Live birth rates. **C,** Rates of multiple gestation. *P* values depict comparisons among the various groups. (From Diamond MP, Legro RS, Coutifaris C, et al. Letrozole, gonadotropin or clomiphene for unexplained infertility. *N Eng J Med.* 2015;373(13): 1230-1240.

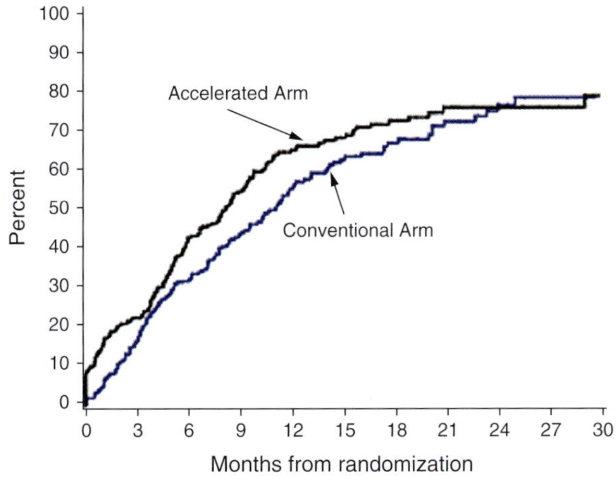


Number of couples

| | | | | | | | | | | | |
|---|---|---|---|---|---|---|---|---|---|---|---|
| Conventional | 247 | 199 | 154 | 118 | 79 | 50 | 36 | 23 | 14 | 11 | 8 |
| Accelerated | 256 | 195 | 135 | 98 | 63 | 47 | 31 | 19 | 14 | 10 | 5 |

| Time Period (m) | Hazard Ratio | 95% CI | | P-value |
|---|---|---|---|---|
| ≤3 | 1.52 | 1.02 | 2.28 | 0.04 |
| >3 to 11 | 1.40 | 1.03 | 1.90 | 0.03 |
| >11 | 0.60 | 0.34 | 1.06 | 0.08 |

**Fig. 40.22** Randomized clinical trial to evaluate optimal treatment for unexplained infertility: The Fast Track and Standard Treatment (FASTT) trial. *CI,* Confidence interval. (From Reindollar RH, Regan MM, Neumann PJ, et al. A randomized clinical trial to evaluate optimal treatment for unexplained infertility: The Fast Track and Standard Treatment [FASTT] trial. *Fertil Steril.* 2010;94(3):888-899.)

(9% and 13%); letrozole did not result in a lower multiple pregnancy rate as had been hypothesized (Diamond, 2015). For this reason, gonadotropin/IUI is less commonly used in couples with unexplained infertility.

A large prospective trial was carried out by Reindollar and colleagues to assess whether it was reasonable to skip gonadotropin/IUI therapy and proceed to IVF after three cycles of CC/IUI (called *fast track*). The logical next step after CC or gonadotropin/IUI therapy is still proceeding to IVF. One of the concerns with unexplained infertility is that there may be failure to fertilize, even if there are normal ovulation and semen characteristics. IVF also has a higher cycle fecundity rate (discussed later). In the prospective trial, as shown in Fig. 40.22, there was an increased pregnancy rate in the accelerated arm (100% to 156%; hazard ratio, 1.25). The median time to pregnancy was also shorter, 8 versus 11 months, and average charges per delivery were $9800 lower. Individual per cycle pregnancy rates for CC/IUI, gonadotropin/IUI, and IVF were 7.6%, 9.8%, and 30%, respectively (Reindollar, 2010). **The conclusion of these authors was that the gonadotropin/IUI step in the usual algorithm for unexplained infertility may be omitted.** Age is a significant factor in terms of efficacy of treatment. Table 40.7 shows the results of a large retrospective study of the success of CC/IUI according to age (Dovey, 2008). It is clear that in older women, because of reduced efficacy (**after age 42, cumulative pregnancy rates over 3 to 9 months are approximately 1.8%), couples should consider going directly to IVF.** In a follow-up study by Reindollar in a slightly older population (38 to 42 years), it was concluded that in

**TABLE 40.7** Realistic Chances of Pregnancy With Intrauterine Insemination: Age Dependency*

| Age of Woman (yr) | Pregnancy Rate per Cycle (%) |
|---|---|
| <35 | ≈10-11.5 |
| 35-37 | ≈8.2-9.2 |
| 38-40 | ≈6.5-7.3 |
| 40-41 | ≈3.6-4.3 |
| >42† | ≈0.8-1.0 |

From Dovey S, Sneeringer RM, Penzias AS. Clomiphene citrate and intrauterine insemination: analysis of more than 4100 cycles. *Fertil Steril.* 2008;90(6):2281-2286.
*Large cohort of 4100 cycles of CC IUI.
†In women older than 42 years, cumulative pregnancy rates = 1.8% (1 in 55).
*CC,* Clomiphene citrate; *IUI,* intrauterine insemination.

this group, going directly to IVF is probably a better option (Goldman, 2014).

Cycle fecundity may be reduced substantially, even in women younger than 40 years who have a low ovarian reserve. Accordingly, it is important to measure day 2 to 3 FSH levels as well as AMH and an AFC. Low parameters will help dictate how aggressive treatment should be, with many couples being directed toward IVF as a primary treatment. Because of the importance of IVF as a treatment option in current infertility management, a separate chapter is devoted to IVF and newer therapies (see Chapter 41).

## PREGNANCY OUTCOMES IN WOMEN TREATED FOR INFERTILITY

**Ovulation-inducing drugs and reconstructive tubal surgery** have independently been shown to be associated with an ***increased incidence of ectopic pregnancy*** compared with the normal population. Use of ovulation-inducing drugs alone has been shown to increase the incidence of multiple gestations. With IVF the chances of multiple gestations is better controlled based on the decision to transfer only one embryo (see Chapter 41); however, IVF does increase the risk of ectopic pregnancies, with a higher rate based on the number of embryos transferred (Perkins, 2015). There is also an increase in the risk of heterotopic pregnancies; therefore, if conception occurs after treatment with ovulation induction or tubal reconstructive surgery, monitoring of early gestation with serial HCG levels and ultrasonography assists in determining whether the pregnancy is intrauterine and how many gestational sacs are present; however, **infertile couples who conceive do not have a higher rate of spontaneous abortion or perinatal mortality than normal couples. Compared with the noninfertile population, the fetal malformation rate is slightly increased.** In all older women, there is a higher pregnancy loss rate because of aneuploidy.

## COUNSELING AND EMOTIONAL SUPPORT

The diagnosis of infertility can be a devastating and life-altering event that affects many aspects of a woman's life. Infertility and its treatment can affect a woman and her spouse or partner medically, financially, socially, emotionally, and psychologically. Feelings of anxiety, depression, isolation, and helplessness are not uncommon in women undergoing infertility treatment. Strained and stressful relationships with spouses, partners, and other loved ones occur among patients undergoing infertility treatment as treatment gets underway and progresses.

It is important that every program address the emotional and social needs of couples undergoing treatment. Individual counseling and support groups, as well as patient information sessions, should be part of every infertility practice. National support groups such as the National Infertility Association (RESOLVE, www.prnewswire.com) and the American Fertility Association (www.theafa.org) are also available to provide assistance and information. ASRM also has many educational resources, specifically designed for patients with a separate portal available at the society's website (www.asrm.org). Patient-oriented videos are available regarding various aspects of infertility at www.reproductivefacts.org.

## REFERENCES


Almog B, Shehata F, Suissa S, et al. Age-related normograms of serum antimullerian hormone levels in a population of infertile women: a multicenter study. *Fertil Steril.* 2011;95(7):2359–2363.

Bhattacharya S, Harrild K, Mollison J, et al. Clomiphene citrate or unstimulated intrauterine insemination compared with expectant management for unexplained infertility: pragmatic randomised controlled trial. *BMJ.* 2008;337:a716.

Casper RF, Mitwally MF. Review: aromatase inhibitors for ovulation induction. *J Clin Endocrinol Metab.* 2006;91(3):760–771.

Collins JA, Burrows EA, Wilan AR. The prognosis for live birth among untreated infertile couples. *Fertil Steril.* 1995;64:22–28.

Coutifaris C, Myers ER, Guzick DS, et al. Histological dating of timed endometrial biopsy tissue is not related to fertility status. *Fertil Steril.* 2004;82:1264–1272.

Custers IM, van Rumste MM, van der Steeg JW, et al. Long-term outcome in couples with unexplained subfertility and an intermediate prognosis initially randomized between expectant management and immediate treatment. *Hum Reprod.* 2012;27(2):444–450.

Deveneau NE, Sinno O, Krause M, et al. Impact of sperm morphology on the likelihood of pregnancy after intrauterine insemination. *Fertil Steril.* 2014;102(6):1584–1590.

Diamond MP, Legro RS, Coutifaris C, et al. Letrozole, Gonadotropin or clomiphene for unexplained infertility. *N Engl J Med.* 2015;373(13):1230–1240.

Dovey S, Sneeringer RM, Penzias AS. Clomiphene citrate and intrauterine insemination: analysis of more than 4100 cycles. *Fertil Steril.* 2008;90:2281–2286.

Dreyer K, van Rijswijk J, Mijatovic V, et al. Oil-based or water-based contrast for hysterosalpingography in infertile women. *N Engl J Med.* 2017;376(21):2043–2052.

Eisenberg ML, Shufeng Li, Behr B, et al. Relationship between semen production and medical comorbidity. *Fertil Steril.* 2015;103(1):66–71.

Gjonnaess H. Late endocrine effects of ovarian electrocautery in women with polycystic ovary syndrome. *Fertil Steril.* 1998;69:697–701.

Goldman MB, Thornton K, Ryley D, et al. A randomized clinical trial to determine optimal infertility treatment in older couples: the forty and over treatment trial (FORT-T). *Fertil Steril.* 2014;101:1574–1581.

Hull MG. Effectiveness of infertility treatments: choice and comparative analysis. *Int J Gynaecol Obstet.* 1994;47:99–108.

Hull MG, Glazener CM, Kelly NJ, et al. Population study of causes, treatment, and outcome of infertility. *Br Med J (Clin Res Ed).* 1985;291:1693–1697.

Hunault CC, Habbema JD, Eijkemans MJ, et al. Two new prediction rules for spontaneous pregnancy leading to live birth among subfertile couples, based on the synthesis of three previous models. *Hum Reprod.* 2004;19(9):2019–2026.

Hurst BS, Hickman JM, Matthews ML, et al. Novel clomiphene "stair-step" protocol reduces time to ovulation in women with polycystic ovarian syndrome. *Am J Obstet Gynecol.* 2009;200(5):510.e1–510.e4.

Legro RS, Barnhart HX, Schlaff WD, et al. Clomiphene, metformin, or both for infertility in the polycystic ovary syndrome. *N Engl J Med.* 2007;356(6):551–566.

Legro RS, Brzyski RG, Diamond MP, et al. Letrozole versus clomiphene for infertility in the polycystic ovary syndrome. *N Engl J Med.* 2014;371(2):119–129.

Leridon H, Spira A. Problems in measuring the effectiveness of infertility therapy. *Fertil Steril.* 1984;41:580–586.

Navot D, Bergh PA, Laufer N. Ovarian hyperstimulation syndrome in novel reproductive technologies: prevention and treatment. *Fertil Steril.* 1992;58(2):249–261.

Oehninger S, Franken DR, Ombelet W. Sperm functional tests. *Fertil Steril.* 2014;102(6):1528–1533.

Perkins KM, Boulet SL, Kissin DM, et al. Risk of ectopic pregnancy associated with assisted reproductive technology in the United States, 2001-2011. *Obstet Gynecol.* 2015;125(1):70–78.

Practice Committee of the American Society for Reproductive Medicine. Diagnostic evaluation of the infertile female: a committee opinion. *Fertil Steril.* 2012;98:302–307.

Practice Committee of American Society for Reproductive Medicine. Role of tubal reconstructive surgery in the era of assisted reproductive technology: a committee opinion. *Fertil Steril.* 2012;97:539–545.

Practice Committee of the American Society for Reproductive Medicine and the Society for Male Reproduction and Urology. Report on varicocele and infertility: a committee opinion. *Fertil Steril.* 2014;102(6):1556–1560.

Practice Committee of the American Society for Reproductive Medicine. Subclinical hypothyroidism in the infertile female population: a guideline. *Fertil Steril.* 2015;104(3):545–553.

Rackow BW, Taylor HS. Submucosal uterine leiomyomas have a global effect on molecular determinants of endometrial receptivity. *Fertil Steril.* 2010;93(6):2027–2034.

Reindollar RH, Regan MM, Neumann PJ, et al. A randomized clinical trial to evaluate optimal treatment for unexplained infertility: the fast track and standard treatment (FASTT) trial. *Fertil Steril.* 2010;94:888–899.

Seifer DB, Baker VL, Leader B. Age-specific serum antimullerian hormone values for 17,120 women presenting to fertility centers within the United States. *Fertil Steril.* 2011;95(2):747–750.

Tan BK, Mathur R. Management of ovarian hyperstimulation syndrome. Produced on behalf of the BFS Policy and Practice Committee. *Hum Fertil (Camb).* 2013;16(3):151–159.

Thessaloniki ESHRE/ASRM–Sponsored PCOS Consensus Workshop Group. Consensus on infertility in PCOS. *Fertil Steril.* 2008;89:505–522.

Thurmond AS. Fallopian tube catheterization. *Semin Intervent Radiol.* 2008;25(4):425–431.

Van Steirteghem AC, Liu J, Joris H, et al. Higher success rate by intracytoplasmic sperm injection than by subzonal insemination: report of a second series of 300 consecutive treatment cycles. *Hum Reprod.* 1993;8:1055–1060.

Wang R, van Welie N, van Rijswijk J, et al. Effectiveness on fertility outcome of tubal flushing with different contrast media: systematic review and network meta-analysis. *Ultrasound Obstet Gynecol.* 2019;54(2):172-181.

Wilcox AJ, Weinberg CR, Baird DD. Timing of sexual intercourse in relation to ovulation. Effects on the probability of conception, survival of the pregnancy, and sex of the baby. *N Engl J Med.* 1995;333:1517–1521.


**Suggested readings for this chapter can be found on ExpertConsult.com.**

# 41 In Vitro Fertilization

*Eric J. Forman, Roger A. Lobo*

## KEY POINTS

- For *in vitro* fertilization (IVF) with and without intracytoplasmic sperm injection, the delivery rate per cycle in which ova are retrieved is as high as 50%, depending on the age of the woman. The rate of pregnancy after IVF is directly related to the number of embryos placed in the uterine cavity.
- Strict guidelines set forth by American Society for Reproductive Medicine (ASRM), which limit the number of embryos transferred, has reduced the rate of high-order and twin multiple pregnancies in the United States.
- Preimplantation genetic testing of embryos for aneuploidy (PGT-A) or monogenetic disease before embryo transfer may help improve pregnancy rates, especially in older women. When PGT-A is performed, a single euploid embryo should be transferred at a time.
- Oocyte and embryo cryopreservation gives women the possibility of maintaining their future fertility potential even when faced with the possibility of premature menopause as a result of gonadotoxic medical treatments. Though still experimental, ovarian tissue freezing is another possible method of fertility preservation. Oocyte cryopreservation is available for healthy females who are interested in elective fertility preservation, but they need to be carefully counseled about the low pregnancy rates associated with cryopreserved oocytes.
- IVF technology has helped to expand research into stem cell therapy, which may further improve treatments for infertility and other medical conditions in the near future.

Because of the central importance of *in vitro* fertilization (IVF) in the treatment of infertility and its potential to answer fundamental questions in reproductive biology, a separate chapter has been devoted to this topic. *IVF* is often used interchangeably with the term *assisted reproductive technology (ART)*, which the American Society for Reproductive Medicine (ASRM) has defined as the manipulation of sperm and egg outside the body; however, some clinicians include ovarian stimulation cycles with the use of intrauterine insemination (IUI) in the definition of ART.

**In 2010, Robert Edwards was awarded the Nobel Prize for physiology and medicine** for his pioneering work in making IVF a reality (Steptoe, 1978). IVF has revolutionized the field of reproduction. Not only has it opened many avenues of research and broadened our understanding of basic human reproductive physiology, but its successful clinical use has allowed millions of couples to conceive who might otherwise have been unable to do so. **IVF has provided the ability to diagnose significant genetic defects before implantation and has led to the possibility of embryonic stem cell research.** IVF has also opened possibilities for fertility preservation (Lobo, 2005). Reproductive-age patients newly diagnosed with cancer can undergo ART to cryopreserve oocytes or embryos before embarking on their cancer therapy. Healthy reproductive-age women not yet ready to conceive but concerned about the normal age effect on their fecundity may pursue elective fertility preservation. Indications for IVF are listed in Box 41.1.

IVF was originally developed primary for women with tubal disease. This is still a major indication for IVF, and with the success of IVF, reconstructive tubal surgery is much less commonly performed, in favor of the more direct approach of IVF. As discussed in Chapter 40, a significantly dilated tube (hydrosalpinx) on ultrasound is an indication for salpingectomy before IVF because implantation rates are reduced in the presence of a communicating hydrosalpinx. Endometriosis is also a major indication for IVF, likely because of its impact on tubal function and oocyte pick up.

## SPECIFIC INDICATIONS FOR IN VITRO FERTILIZATION

### Male Factor Infertility

In the past, if there were severe abnormalities in the semen analysis, such as severe oligozoospermia (low sperm concentration), the prognosis for fertility was less than that for any other cause of infertility, even with the use of IVF. Attempts to enhance fertilization rates of aspirated oocytes with the technique of subzonal insemination of sperm were unsuccessful because fertilization rates remained low at approximately 15%. After Van Steirteghem and associates developed the technique of intracytoplasmic sperm injection (ICSI) (Palermo, 1992), fertilization rates of oocytes injected with a single normal sperm obtained from men with severe abnormalities in their semen analysis increased to more than 50%. **Pregnancy rates per embryo transfer are now similar after ICSI compared with other indications for IVF.** Fertilization rates of approximately 60% of the oocytes injected may be achieved with sperm from semen samples containing no motile sperm, few motile sperm, and high numbers of motile sperm (Tsirgotis, 1994). In addition, a fertilization rate of approximately 60% was attained whether the sperm were freshly obtained by masturbation or electroejaculation or were previously frozen. A fertilization rate of oocytes of almost 50% was also achieved when the sperm were aspirated directly from the epididymal fluid. In routine clinical use, a fertilization rate of greater than 80% can be achieved.

The excellent results obtained with ICSI by the group that originally described the technique have been replicated in other centers. By using this technique, the pregnancy rate of couples whose male partner has an extremely low concentration of motile sperm in semen samples (<100,000/mL) can reach a normal pregnancy rate for IVF, based on the age of the woman (discussed later). **Studies of pregnancies resulting from ICSI and standard IVF have revealed a similar rate of pregnancy loss and multiple gestation.** Therefore ICSI is now the treatment of choice for all causes of male infertility, as well as for couples with no known cause of infertility for whom fertilization has failed with standard IVF insemination procedures. At present, ICSI is used in 60% to 70% of all cases of IVF. The number of ICSI cases has increased because ICSI has been used even for minor sperm abnormalities and in other cases such as unexplained infertility and in older women where there is a concern about the rate of fertilization (Fig. 41.1). (Also see the video of an ICSI procedure [Video 41.1].)

The clinical pregnancy rate is higher when testicular or epididymal sperm is retrieved from men with obstruction of the vas

**BOX 41.1** Indications for In Vitro Fertilization

Blocked or absent fallopian tubes
Low sperm counts or absent sperm (azoospermia requiring TESE)
Advanced reproductive age
Endometriosis
Unexplained infertility unresponsive to IUI therapy
Screening for aneuploid embryos and/or genetic disease
Fertility preservation

*IUI,* Intrauterine insemination; *TESE,* testicular sperm extraction.

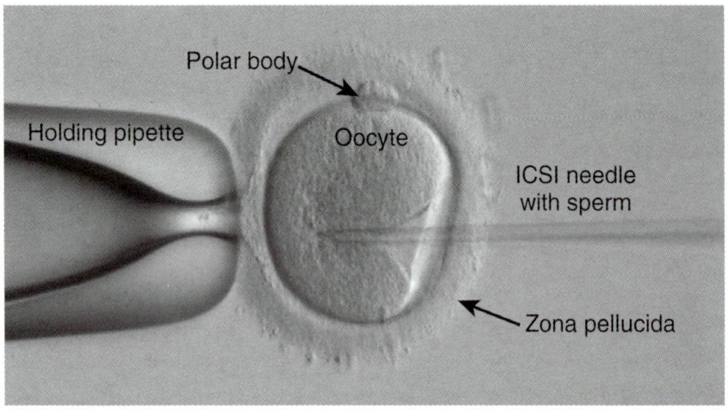


**Fig. 41.1** Intracytoplasmic sperm injection (ICSI). (Courtesy Center for Women's Reproductive Care at Columbia University.)

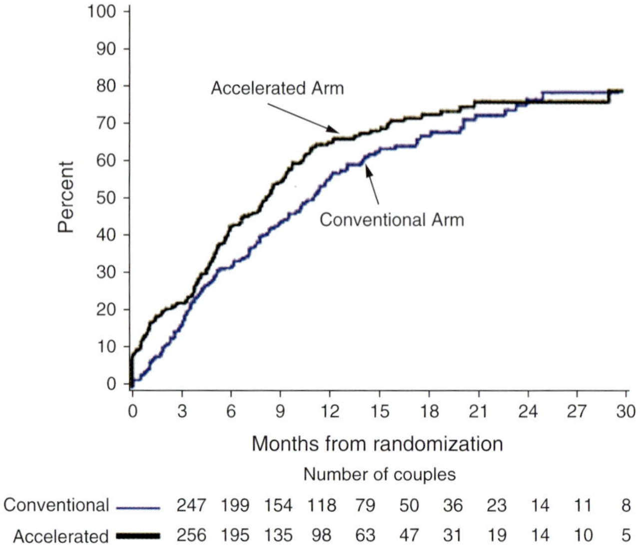


| Time Period (m) | Hazard Ratio | 95% CI | | P-value |
|---|---|---|---|---|
| ≤3 | 1.52 | 1.02 | 2.28 | 0.04 |
| >3 to 11 | 1.40 | 1.03 | 1.90 | 0.03 |
| >11 | 0.60 | 0.34 | 1.06 | 0.08 |

**Fig. 41.2** Randomized clinical trial to evaluate optimal treatment for unexplained infertility: the Fast Track And Standard Treatment (FASTT) trial. *CI,* Confidence interval. (From Reindollar RH, Regan MM, Neumann PJ, et al. A randomized clinical trial to evaluate optimal treatment for unexplained infertility: the fast track and standard treatment [FASTT] trial. *Fertil Steril.* 2010;94(3):888-899.)

deferens (obstructive azoospermia) than when testicular sperm is retrieved from men with azoospermia without reproductive tract obstruction (nonobstructive azoospermia) (Palermo, 1999). Even if the sperm retrieved from the testes remain immotile, the pregnancy rate after ICSI is acceptable at 15% or higher. The likelihood of retrieval of spermatozoa from testicular tissue of men with azoospermia and normal follicle-stimulating hormone (FSH) levels is almost 100%. Even if the man's FSH levels are markedly elevated, there is at least a 50% likelihood that spermatozoa can be retrieved from the testes and used to perform an ICSI procedure (Jezek, 1998). Thus the presence of a combination of azoospermia and an elevated FSH level is not a contraindication for performing a testicular sperm extraction (TESE) procedure, although it is advantageous to carry out a diagnostic TESE before an IVF cycle. Diligence is required with the aid of microscopy to select the best sperm for use in ICSI, and several groups have advocated a surgical microdissection of the testicular tubules to obtain viable sperm (Schlegel, 1999). Microdeletions in the azoospermia factor (AZF) region of the Y chromosome have been linked to nonobstructive azoospermia. Sperm has been successfully retrieved from men with AZFb and c microdeletions but not with the AZFa microdeletion, and extraction is not recommended in these cases.

## Unexplained Infertility/Advanced Reproductive Age

Patients with unexplained infertility may consider IVF treatment particularly if they fail to conceive after a few treatments with controlled ovarian stimulation and IUI. In fact, women of advanced reproductive age and infertility may be advised to consider moving directly to IVF, bypassing IUI therapy altogether (Donderwinkel, 2000).

A large prospective trial was carried out by Reindollar and colleagues to assess whether it was reasonable to skip gonadotropin and timed IUI therapy and proceed to IVF after three cycles of clomiphene-IUI (called "fast track") in women with unexplained infertility (Reindollar, 2010). **The logical next step after clomiphene or gonadotropin-IUI therapy is still IVF.** One of the concerns with unexplained infertility is that there may be failure to fertilize, even if there are normal ovulation and semen characteristics. IVF also has a higher cycle fecundity rate than IUI. In the prospective trial, which also included a cost analysis, conventional therapy included 3 months of clomiphene-IUI followed by three cycles of gonadotropin-IUI and then up to six cycles of IVF. The other arm of this randomized trial omitted the gonadotropin-IUI step and proceeded directly to IVF after clomiphene-IUI (Fig. 41.2).

As shown in Fig. 41.2, an increased pregnancy rate was reported in the accelerated arm (100% to 156%; hazard ratio, 1.25). The median time to pregnancy was also shorter, 8 versus 11 months, and average charges per delivery were $9800 lower. Individual per cycle pregnancy rates for clomiphene-IUI, gonadotropin-IUI, and IVF were 7.6%, 9.8%, and 30%, respectively. The authors concluded that the gonadotropin-IUI step in the usual algorithm for unexplained infertility may be omitted; however, this remains an area of controversy and may not be applicable to couples who do not have insurance coverage for IVF, unlike in Massachusetts (where the study was carried out) where IVF coverage is mandated.

The extension of this study (the Forty and Over Treatment Trial [FORT-T]) in older women, 38 to 42 years, strongly suggested that infertile women in this age category should consider going directly to IVF (Goldman, 2014). In this study, patients who proceeded directly to IVF achieved significantly higher clinical pregnancy rates compared with patients who tried two cycles of IUI treatment (with either clomiphene citrate or gonadotropin

**TABLE 41.1** Clinical Pregnancy and Live Birth Rates per Couple, by Randomization Assignment for the First Two Treatment Cycles and at the End of All Treatment

| | | First Two Treatment Cycles | | Duration of Study | |
|---|---|---|---|---|---|
| Randomized Treatment Arm | No. of Couples (%) | No. of Clinical Pregnancies*,† (%, 97.5% CI) | No. of Live Births‡ (%, 97.5% CI) | No. of Clinical Pregnancies§ (%, 97.5% CI) | No. of Live Births§ (%, 97.5% CI) |
| CC/IUI | 51 (33.1) | 11 (21.6, 10.2-37.3) | 8 (15.7, 6.2-30.5) | 38 (74.5, 58.4-86.9) | 25 (49.0, 32.9-65.2) |
| Gonadotropin (FSH)/IUI | 52 (33.8) | 9 (17.3, 7.3-32.2) | 7 (13.5, 4.9-27.6) | 34 (65.4, 49.0-79.5) | 22 (42.3, 27.1-58.7) |
| Immediate IVF | 51 (33.1) | 25 (49.0, 32.9-65.2) | 16 (31.4, 17.7-47.9) | 38 (74.5, 58.4-86.9) | 24 (47.1, 31.2-63.4) |
| Total¶ | 154 | 45 (29.2, 21.3-38.2) | 31 (20.1, 13.4-28.4) | 110 (71.4, 62.5-79.3) | 71 (46.1, 37.0-55.4) |

From Goldman MB, Thornton KL, Ryley D, et al. A randomized clinical trial to determine optimal infertility treatment in older couples: the Forty and Over Treatment Trial (FORT-T). *Fertil Steril.* 2014;101(6):1574-1581.
Note: Includes treatment-dependent pregnancies.
*CC,* Clomiphene citrate; *CI,* confidence interval; *FSH,* follicle-stimulating hormone; *IUI,* intrauterine insemination; *IVF,* in vitro fertilization.
*Number of clinical pregnancies includes all ultrasound confirmed pregnancies, including pregnancy losses.
†For clinical pregnancy rate after first two treatment cycles. $P = .0067$ for comparison between CC/IUI and immediate IVF; $P = .0007$ for comparison between FSH/IUI and immediate IVF.
‡For live-birth rate after first two treatment cycles. $P = .101$ for comparison between CC/IUI and immediate IVF; $P = .035$ for comparison between FSH/IUI and immediate IVF.
§For clinical pregnancy and live-birth rates after all treatment, there are no statistically significant differences, reflecting subsequent IVF, treatment in all arms.
¶Of these, there were 5, 2, and 4 clinical pregnancies and 5, 1, and 3 live births in the CC/IUI, FSH/IUI and immediate IVF arms, respectively, that occurred before treatment was initiated or between treatment cycles one and two. Over the duration of the study there were 11, 3, and 9 clinical pregnancies and 7, 1, and 6 live births in the CC/IUI, FSH, IUI, and immediate IVF arms, respectively, that occurred outside of treatment cycles.

therapy). Additionally, the ratio of treatment cycles to live birth rates was significantly lower in patients who went straight to IVF versus patients who started with conservative treatment (Table 41.1).

Table 41.2 shows the results of a large retrospective study of the success of clomiphene-IUI (Dovey, 2008). Because of the age-related decline in clomiphene-IUI pregnancy rates (after age 42, cumulative pregnancy rates over 3 to 9 months are approximately 1.8%), couples in which the female partner is older should consider going directly to IVF. This recommendation is particularly suited for women age 40 or older, those with a borderline elevated day 2 to day 3 FSH level, and women with decreased antral follicle counts and antimüllerian hormone levels.

## Oocyte/Embryo Cryopreservation for Fertility Preservation

Oocyte and embryo cryopreservation has been growing as indication for pursuing ART procedures. Not only is it an important method to **preserve fertility in young women with cancer about to undergo chemotherapy**, but increasingly it is being used in healthy young women who **electively wish to delay childbearing with the knowledge of the detrimental effects of aging on reproductive capacity**. When thawing previously frozen oocytes, ICSI is recommended because of premature hardening of the zona pellucida. **If the woman has a male partner and either is married or is in a stable relationship, use of sperm to fertilize the oocytes and then freeze embryos rather than oocytes is more successful in terms of ultimate pregnancy rates and therefore remains an option.** This topic is discussed in more detail later in the chapter.

**TABLE 41.2** Realistic Chances of Pregnancy With Intrauterine Insemination: Age Dependency*

| Age of Woman (years) | Pregnancy Rate per Cycle (%) |
|---|---|
| <35 | ≈10-11.5 |
| 35-37 | ≈8.2-9.2 |
| 38-40 | ≈6.5-7.3 |
| 40-41 | ≈3.6-4.3 |
| >42† | ≈0.8-1.0 |

From Dovey S, Sneeringer RM, Penzias AS. Clomiphene citrate and intrauterine insemination: analysis of more than 100 cycles. *Fertil Steril.* 2008;90(6):2281-2286.
*Large cohort of 4100 cycles of CC IUI.
†In women older than 42 years, cumulative pregnancy rates = 1.8% (1 in 55).

## Preconception Genetic Testing for Aneuploidy, Structural Rearrangements, and Monogenic Diseases

Another indication for IVF is to screen embryos for aneuploidy or genetic disease (see Preimplantation Genetic Testing later in the chapter). Couples suffering recurrent aneuploid pregnancy loss (as a result of a balanced translocation in a partner, for example) may consider IVF with preimplantation genetic testing for aneuploidy (PGT-A) as a means of screening their embryos before conceiving again and potentially suffering another miscarriage; however, the studies have not been able to demonstrate a statistical benefit, in part because of a relatively high rate of success with natural conception after two to three losses (Stray-Pedersen, 1984). The cost efficacy of this approach has also been questions. **This approach has also been increasingly used for couples with prior IVF failure or advanced reproductive age and to optimize selection for elective single embryo transfer.**

Couples who are found to carry mutations in life-threatening diseases (e.g., cystic fibrosis, Tay-Sachs disease) may opt to do IVF with preimplantation genetic testing for monogenic diseases (PGT-M) to eliminate the transmission of these diseases by excluding affected embryos. Specific probes are developed for each couple to improve accuracy by using linked markers on the chromosome with the mutation. Although controversial for ethical reasons, couples may also opt to undergo IVF/PGT for sex selection or "family balancing."

## IN VITRO FERTILIZATION PROCEDURE

The goal of a successful IVF treatment is the generation of good-quality embryos capable of implanting and resulting in a live birth. IVF can be carried out in a natural cycle, which was the original approach used by Steptoe and Edwards that led to the birth of Louise Brown; however, in this case usually only one oocyte and one embryo can be expected, and the success rate is far lower than with conventional IVF, in which gonadotropins are administered to increase the number of oocytes retrieved. Although unstimulated IVF remains an option on an individual basis, its use is limited because of the lower pregnancy rates and the expectations of couples to become pregnant as efficiently as possible. Improvement in embryo cryopreservation has provided more opportunities for pregnancy from supernumerary frozen embryos.

With conventional IVF, gonadotropin stimulation with recombinant FSH and/or purified human menopausal gonadotropin (HMG) is administered, usually subcutaneously, for approximately 8 to 10 days. The starting daily dose typically ranges from 150 to 450 IU of FSH and/or HMG. HMG preparations contain both 75 IU of FSH and 75 IU of luteinizing hormone (LH) in the form of human chorionic gonadotropin (HCG). The starting dose is chiefly determined by the patient's ovarian reserve and age, with higher doses used for older patients with decreased ovarian reserve and lower doses for patients with a more robust reserve and for women with polycystic ovary syndrome (PCOS). The traditional long cycle protocol begins with downregulation using a gonadotropin-releasing hormone (GnRH) agonist for 2 weeks before gonadotropin administration. Once downregulation is evidenced with estradiol levels less than 50 pg/mL, the patient is started on gonadotropin stimulation while maintaining ovulation suppression with the daily use of the GnRH agonist. Increasingly, however, a GnRH antagonist is used to block spontaneous ovulation from occurring once follicular development occurs. With this "short protocol," gonadotropins are begun on cycle day 2 or 3, without prior downregulation, and the antagonist is added around day 6 of stimulation. Data support an equal efficacy of the two approaches (Al-Inany, 2011).

When criteria for progression to oocyte retrieval are reached—for example, at least two mature follicles on ultrasound (18 mm) with an appropriate rise of serum estradiol ($E_2$), a bolus of HCG is administered (5000 to 10,000 IU). **Vaginal ultrasound aspiration of the follicles is typically performed 34 to 36 hours later** (Fig. 41.3). This procedure is usually performed with the patient sedated, although it can be performed with local anesthetic use. **Complications include infection, torsion, and internal bleeding, though rates are low (<0.25%)** (Roest, 1996).

The harvested oocytes are then combined with a sperm sample from a male partner or from donor sperm. One of two methods is used to fertilize the oocytes: insemination (where tens of thousands of highly motile sperm are placed in a microdroplet with one or two oocytes) or ICSI. On average, about 60% to 70% of the mature oocytes should fertilize with insemination and normal-functioning sperm and oocytes. With ICSI, embryologists can select individual sperm and microinject a sperm into each mature, metaphase II (MII) oocyte. Approximately 12 to 18 hours later the oocytes are inspected for evidence of fertilization (Fig. 41.4). **ICSI does not yield better fertilization rates than in the normal situation; rather, it helps to produce normal fertilization rates in situations where fertilization may not occur or will occur at a low rate.**

**The embryology laboratory environment is the key factor in the success of IVF.** Typically, 3 days after oocyte aspiration,

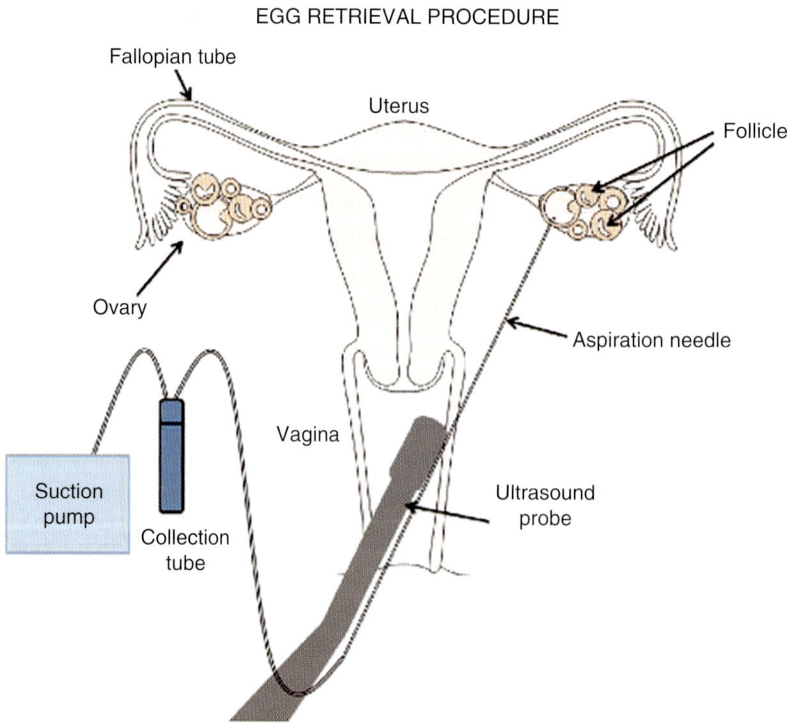


**Fig. 41.3** Diagram of oocyte retrieval. (Modified from American Society for Reproductive Medicine: *Assisted reproductive technologies: a guide for patients.* American Society for Reproductive Medicine, Birmingham, AL: 2015.)

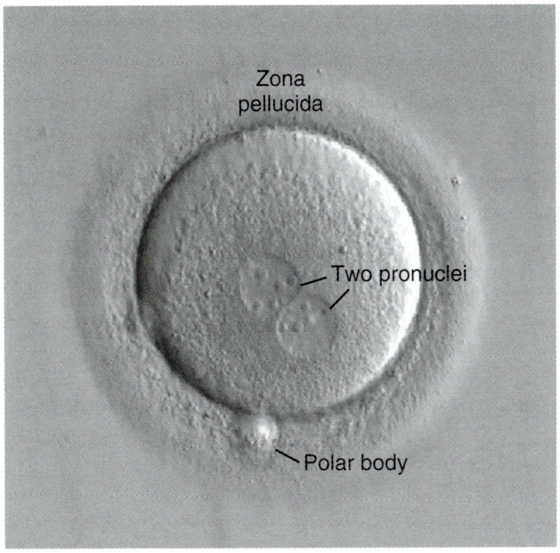


**Fig. 41.4** Evidence of normal fertilization: two pronuclei. (Courtesy Center for Women's Reproductive Care at Columbia University.)

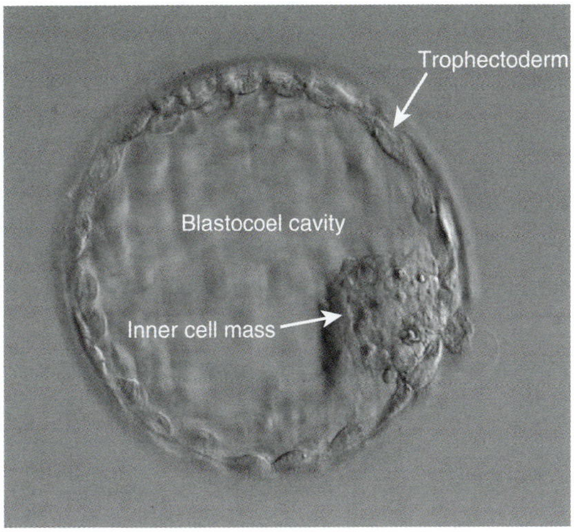


**Fig. 41.6** Blastocyst (day 5 or 6 embryo).

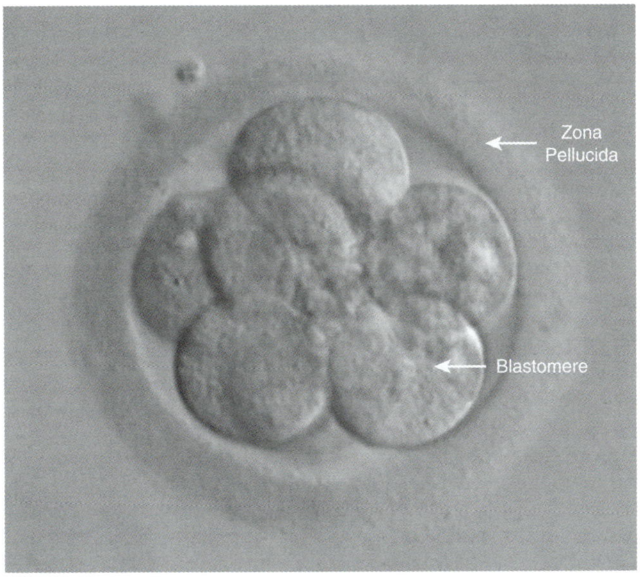


**Fig. 41.5** Day 3 embryo.

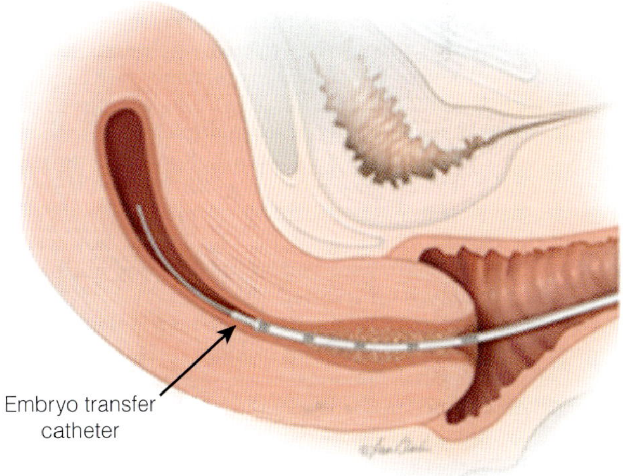


**Fig. 41.7** Embryo transfer with catheter. (Copyright Lisa Clark, Courtesy Cook Medical, 2010.)

cleavage stage embryos with six to eight cells are obtained. Three-day-old embryos can be assessed for potential transfer using criteria assessing the blastomere morphology and symmetry as well as the degree of embryo fragmentation (Fig. 41.5). Fragmentation is felt to be the extracellular debris created by the dividing embryonic cells, and embryos with a high degree of fragmentation (i.e., >10% of the embryo) are associated with lower implantation and pregnancy rates (Luke, 2014).

**At the time of a day 3 transfer, the embryologist may opt to use assisted hatching (AH).** Using acid or a laser, the embryologist can make a small breech in the zona pellucida of the embryo. A meta-analysis suggested improved implantation and clinical pregnancy rates with AH use but concluded that live birth rates were not improved (Carney, 2012). The authors concluded that AH may be most useful in older women (i.e., >37 years old) and in women with previously unexplained IVF failures. One downside to the use of AH is the slightly increased potential for monozygotic twinning (1% to 2%) (Hershlag, 1999).

Increasingly, with improved quality of sequential culture media, embryo culture is continued to days 5 to 6, when a blastocyst has developed (Fig. 41.6). **Fertilized oocytes that can be cultured on day 5 or 6 are usually of better quality and afford a higher pregnancy rate compared with day 3 embryos** (Glujovsky, 2012).

Typically, patients are awake for the embryo transfer, which is carried out with one of several specialized catheters (similar to those used for IUI) under ultrasound guidance (Fig. 41.7). A major initiative by the ASRM has begun, teaching the techniques of successful embryo transfer using simulated models, with certification offered for successful completion of the course.

The decision regarding the number of embryos to transfer is key to optimizing success and reducing the chance of multiple pregnancies. ASRM has published firm guidelines to assist in this decision-making process (Practice Committee ASRM, 2017) (Table 41.3). Implementation of these guidelines has proved to be successful in reducing the rate of high-order multiple pregnancies, with far less than 1% of live births after IVF being triplets or higher. The rate of twins has begun to decrease substantially

**TABLE 41.3** American Society for Reproductive Medicine's Recommended Limits on the Numbers of Embryos to Transfer

| | Age (years) | | | |
|---|---|---|---|---|
| **Prognosis** | **<35** | **35-37** | **38-40** | **41-42** |
| **CLEAVAGE-STAGE EMBRYOS*** | | | | |
| Favorable† | 1-2 | 2 | 3 | 5 |
| All others | 2 | 3 | 4 | 5 |
| **BLASTOCYSTS*** | | | | |
| Favorable† | 1 | 2 | 2 | 3 |
| All others | 2 | 2 | 3 | 3 |

From Practice Committees of the American Society for Reproductive Medicine and the Practice Committee of the Society for Assisted Reproductive Technology. Criteria for number of embryos to transfer: a committee opinion. *Fertil Steril.* 2013;99(1):44-46.

with the increased use of single embryo transfer. In 2013, the Society for Assisted Reproductive Technology (SART) reported a nearly 30% twin rate in patients younger than 35; in 2016, that rate declined to 16%. In women with a good overall prognosis for pregnancy—such as women younger than 35 or women with a history of a prior live pregnancy—elective single embryo transfer (eSET) can still lead to an acceptable pregnancy rate while minimizing the risk of multiples (Luke, 2015). Single embryo transfer does not totally eliminate the risk for multiples because there is a nearly 2% risk for monozygotic twinning after blastocyst transfer (Kanter, 2015). Transferring embryos on day 5 when the embryos are more developed and proportionately more "normal" is becoming the trend for all IVF cycles. This means, however, that some women who have poor embryo quality may not have any good-quality embryos for transfer.

Several methods have been suggested to help in the selection of a normal embryo for transfer. This includes an analysis of the culture media for metabolic parameters and secreted proteins, as well as an analysis of time-lapse videos of the cultured embryos for normal developmental parameters (Kirkegaard, 2015; Krisher, 2015); however, none of these methods is currently the standard of practice in IVF.

**Excess embryos of good quality that are not transferred may be cryopreserved. Vitrification** is a method of ultrarapid freezing using high concentrations of cryoprotectants has largely replaced slow cooling as the preferred cryopreservation technique for oocytes and embryos. The pregnancy rates from thawed, good-quality embryos may exceed the rate of fresh cycles in some instances. A large randomized trial performed in China showed that women with PCOS had a higher chance of live birth after frozen embryo transfer versus fresh (49% vs. 42%) (Chen, 2016). Another trial performed in China showed that ovulatory women planning single embryo transfer also had a higher live birth rate after frozen embryo transfer than fresh (50% vs. 40%) (Wei, 2019). No known increased fetal risks are associated with embryo cryopreservation; in fact, there may be a reduced risk of preterm delivery and a fetus that is small for gestational age.

## In Vitro Fertilization Success Rates

What is important to couples is their overall chance of pregnancy resulting in a live birth. The most current clinical data published by SART (2016) may be found in Table 41.4. These rates are influenced by age and far less so by diagnosis of treatment. **Live birth rates per transfer range from 45.7% in women younger than 35 years to 7.8% at age older than 42.** When a larger number of cycles have been studied over time, the overall optimistic chance of pregnancy after six cycles of IVF is 72% (95% confidence interval [CI], 70% to 74%) (Dor, 1996).

*Optimistic* means continuous treatment without any dropouts; the conservative cumulative pregnancy rate, which includes some dropouts, is 51% (CI, 49% to 52%) (Malizia, 2009) (Fig. 41.8); however, this is influenced by age, as noted previously (Fig. 41.9).

Pregnancy rates over six cycles are fairly constant over time and may continue to increase at the same rate, although some data suggest a plateau effect after six cycles (Fig. 41.10). This latter point is unclear because few IVF patients (<10%) exceed six cycles of treatment.

Patients can estimate their chance for IVF success using SART's interactive calculator, called **"Predict My Success,"** which can be found on the organization's home page (www.sart.org). **This patient predictor is based on data obtained from nearly 500,000 treatment cycles performed in the United States and on the experience of all SART clinics.** This calculator therefore gives an average expectation for success with cycles one, two, and so on, and for the number of embryos replaced. Patients merely enter demographic data and their infertility diagnosis to calculate their chance for IVF pregnancy.

## Gamete Intrafallopian Transfer and Other Alternatives to Traditional In Vitro Fertilization

A modification of IVF, called *gamete intrafallopian transfer* **(GIFT)**, can be used if the infertile woman has functional fallopian tubes. With this technique, both oocytes and sperm are placed into the tube through a catheter at the time of laparoscopy. Although IVF, embryo culturing, and embryo transfer into the uterus are avoided by this technique, controlled ovarian hyperstimulation and laparoscopy are still required. Because this technique requires laparoscopy, GIFT is rarely done at present because pregnancy rates are similar or lower to those of routine IVF and embryo transfer (IVF-ET) when matched for age and diagnosis (Leeton, 1987; Ranieri, 1995). Modifications of GIFT include pronuclear stage tubal transfer (**PROST**), or zygote intrafallopian transfer (**ZIFT**), and tubal embryo stage transfer (**TEST**). With ZIFT, the oocytes are fertilized *in vitro* and transferred 24 hours later. Tubal embryo transfer (TET) is similar to ZIFT except that the embryos are transferred 8 to 72 hours after fertilization. Again, because laparoscopy is required, these procedures are rarely performed today.

**Another option for IVF is to aspirate immature eggs in a natural cycle,** usually in anovulatory women with PCOS. No or minimal gonadotropin stimulation is used before oocyte aspiration. ***In vitro* maturation (IVM) of the oocytes** is then carried out, followed by ICSI. IVM may be most reasonable in women with PCOS because their larger ovaries with multiple small follicles allow for easier aspiration of immature oocytes (vs. women with decreased ovarian reserve, for instance) (Walls, 2015). The main advantage of IVM is the elimination of hyperstimulation risk; however, even in specialized centers, **the success rate for IVM is significantly lower than the rates seen with conventional IVF-ET, and it is not recommended for routine use** (Chian, 2009; Practice Committees ASRM and SART, 2013).

# RISKS OF IN VITRO FERTILIZATION

## Ovarian Hyperstimulation Syndrome

Ovarian hyperstimulation syndrome **(OHSS)** is typically an iatrogenic complication of gonadotropin stimulation. Patients at highest risk of OHSS are those with PCOS, normo-ovulatory patients with a high ovarian reserve, and patients who experienced OHSS in a prior IVF cycle. OHSS is discussed in Chapter 40.

**Avoidance of excessive stimulation is the primary approach for preventing OHSS**; however, even with careful

**TABLE 41.4** Society for Assisted Reproductive Technology (SART)–Clinic Outcome Reporting System (CORS) IVF Clinic Success Rate, 2016*

| **2016 ART Cycle Profile Type of ART and Procedural Factors†** | | | | **Patient Diagnosis†,‡** | | | | | |
|---|---|---|---|---|---|---|---|---|---|
| IVF | >99% | With ICSI | 66% | Tubal Factor | 12% | Uterine factor | 6% | Multiple Factors: | |
| Unstimulated | 1% | PGD/PGS | 22% | Ovulatory dysfunction | 16% | Male factor | 32% | Female factors only | 13% |
| Used gestational carrier | 3% | | | Diminished ovarian reserve | 31% | Other factor | 21% | Female & male factors | 17% |
| | | | | Endometriosis | 8% | Unknown factor | 13% | | |

**2016 ART Success Rates§,‖**

| | **Total number of cycles‖: 263,577 (includes 934 cycles using fresh embryos from frozen nondonor eggs)** | | | | |
|---|---|---|---|---|---|
| | **Age of Patient** | | | | |
| **Type of Cycle Fresh Embryos from Fresh Nondonor Eggs** | **<35** | **35-37** | **38-40** | **41-42** | **>42** |
| Number of cycles | 36,625 | 18,278 | 16,109 | 8,264 | 6,961 |
| Cancelations before retrieval (%) | 6.2 | 10.9 | 16.3 | 20.0 | 22.6 |
| Number of transfers | 24,878 | 11,672 | 9,149 | 4,093 | 2,894 |
| Average number of embryos transferred | 1.5 | 1.7 | 2.0 | 2.4 | 2.4 |
| Percentage of elective single embryo transfers (eSET) (%) | 42.7 | 25.2 | 9.0 | 3.7 | 2.8 |
| **Outcomes Per Cycle** | | | | | |
| Cycles resulting in pregnancies (%) | 35.9 | 29.5 | 21.7 | 12.6 | 6.3 |
| Cycles resulting in live births (%) | 31.0 | 24.0 | 15.5 | 8.0 | 3.2 |
| Cycles resulting in singleton live births (%) | 24.9 | 19.0 | 12.7 | 7.0 | 2.9 |
| Cycles resulting in twin live births (%) | 5.9 | 4.8 | 2.8 | 1.0 | 0.4 |
| Cycles resulting in term, normal weight, and singleton live births¶ (%) | 21.0 | 15.8 | 10.4 | 5.6 | 2.2 |
| **Outcomes Per Transfer** | | | | | |
| Embryos transferred resulting in implantation (%) | 41.8 | 32.6 | 22.0 | 11.7 | 5.9 |
| Transfers resulting in pregnancies (%) | 52.9 | 46.2 | 38.3 | 25.5 | 15.2 |
| Transfers resulting in live births (%) | 45.7 | 37.6 | 27.4 | 16.1 | 7.8 |
| Transfers resulting in singleton live births (%) | 36.7 | 29.8 | 22.3 | 14.1 | 6.9 |
| Transfers resulting in twin live births (%) | 8.7 | 7.6 | 4.8 | 2.0 | 0.9 |
| Transfers resulting in term, normal weight, and singleton live births¶ (%) | 30.9 | 24.7 | 18.3 | 11.3 | 5.3 |
| **Frozen Embryos From Nondonor Eggs** | | | | | |
| Number of cycles | 39,894 | 21,400 | 15,529 | 5,749 | 3,694 |
| Number of transfers | 37,461 | 19,913 | 14,200 | 5,142 | 3,194 |
| Estimated average number of transfers per retrieval | 1.2 | 1.0 | 0.8 | 0.6 | 0.4 |
| Average number of embryos transferred | 1.4 | 1.4 | 1.4 | 1.4 | 1.6 |
| Embryos transferred resulting in implantation (%) | 49.6 | 46.7 | 42.6 | 35.5 | 23.9 |
| Transfers resulting in pregnancies (%) | 59.3 | 57.1 | 54.1 | 48.6 | 38.1 |
| Transfers resulting in live births (%) | 49.4 | 46.5 | 42.7 | 37.9 | 27.7 |
| Transfers resulting in singleton live births (%) | 41.5 | 40.3 | 37.9 | 34.5 | 25.2 |
| Transfers resulting in twin live births (%) | 7.8 | 6.1 | 4.7 | 3.3 | 2.5 |
| Transfers resulting in term, normal weight, and singleton live births¶ (%) | 35.4 | 34.2 | 32.0 | 28.9 | 20.9 |
| **Number of egg or embryo banking cycles** | 20,949 | 14,556 | 14,913 | 7,661 | 7,761 |
| Number of fertility preservation cycles | 4,273 | 3,941 | 3,286 | 1,258 | 1,174 |

*Continued*

**TABLE 41.4** Society for Assisted Reproductive Technology (SART)–Clinic Outcome Reporting System (CORS) IVF Clinic Success Rate, 2016*—cont'd

| Donor Eggs# | Fresh Eggs | Frozen Eggs | Frozen Embryos | Donated Embryos |
|---|---|---|---|---|
| Number of cycles | 5,644 | 3,329 | 13,458 | 1,869 |
| Number of transfers | 4,446 | 2,723 | 12,391 | 1,758 |
| Average number of embryos transferred | 1.5 | 1.5 | 1.4 | 1.7 |
| Embryos transferred resulting in implantation (%) | 53.9 | 41.9 | 46.1 | 38.4 |
| Transfers resulting in pregnancies (%) | 65.0 | 54.7 | 55.8 | 53.1 |
| Transfers resulting in live births (%) | 54.6 | 44.9 | 44.8 | 42.7 |
| Transfers resulting in singleton live births (%) | 41.7 | 36.2 | 37.7 | 33.9 |
| Transfers resulting in twin live births (%) | 12.7 | 8.4 | 6.9 | 8.5 |
| Transfers resulting in term, normal weight, and singleton live births¶ (%) | 32.5 | 28.1 | 29.4 | 26.8 |

| Current Services & Profile | | | | Number of Reporting Clinics: 463 | |
|---|---|---|---|---|---|
| Percentage of clinics that allow cycles involving: | | | | Clinic profile: | |
| Donor eggs | 88% | Single women | 99% | SART member | 82% |
| Donor embryos | 63% | Gestational carriers | 88% | Verified lab accreditation | |
| Embryo cryopreservation | >99% | | | Yes | 92% |
| Egg cryopreservation | 97% | | | No | 5% |
| | | | | Pending | 2% |

Data from Society for Assisted Reproductive Technology. SART national summary: clinic summary report: all SART member clinics, 2016. Available at www.sart.org.

*Comparison of success rates across clinics may not be meaningful. Patient medical characteristics and treatment approaches vary.

†Excludes cycles evaluating new procedures and banking cycles: unstimulated percentage includes fresh egg cycles only.

‡Total patient diagnosis percentages may be greater than 100% because more than one diagnosis can be reported for each ART cycle.

§Multiple-infant births (for example, twins) with at least one live infant are counted as one live birth.

‖Total cycle number and success rates exclude two cycle(s) evaluating new procedures. Success rates exclude cycles using fresh embryos from frozen nondonor eggs.

¶In this report, births are defined as term if at least 37 full weeks gestation and normal birth weight if at least 2,500 grams (approximately 5 pounds, 8 ounces).

#All ages are reported together because previous data show that patient age does not materially affect success with donor eggs.

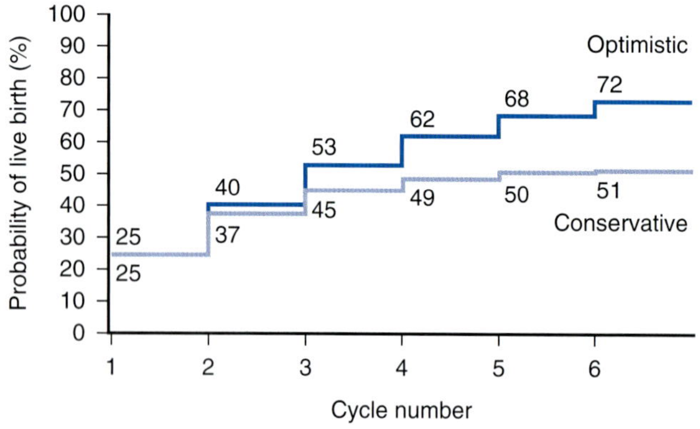


**Fig. 41.8** Expectations of live birth with *in vitro* fertilization–embryo transfer. (From Malizia BA, Hacker MR, Penzias AS. Cumulative live-birth rates after in vitro fertilization. *N Engl J Med.* 2009;360(3): 236-243.)

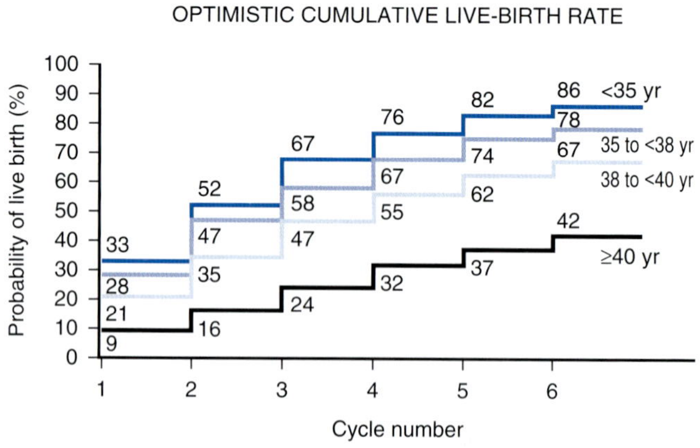


**Fig. 41.9** Expectations of live birth with *in vitro* fertilization–embryo transfer by age. (From Malizia BA, Hacker MR, Penzias AS. Cumulative live-birth rates after in vitro fertilization. *N Engl J Med.* 2009;360(3):236-243.)

monitoring of gonadotropin dosage and follicular response, OHSS can still develop. Coasting (withholding daily gonadotropin treatment while monitoring follicular development toward the end of the IVF cycle) may help decrease OHSS risk, although suboptimal pregnancy rates have been noted with more than 3 days of coasting (Nardo, 2006). GnRH antagonist cycles have been associated with lower OHSS rates as opposed to GnRH agonist "long" cycles (Xiao, 2014). **Deferring ET immediately after retrieval and cryopreserving the embryos for a future frozen ET cycle helps decrease the duration of OHSS by (temporarily) avoiding pregnancy.**

Administration of a daily dopamine agonist for starting immediately after HCG trigger administration and continuing for up to 8 days after the HCG trigger has been shown in some studies to decrease OHSS development (Leitao, 2014).

**To date the most effective means of decreasing OHSS risks with conventional IVF is using a GnRH agonist trigger.** Using doses of 1 to 4 mg of GnRH agonist in lieu of HCG has

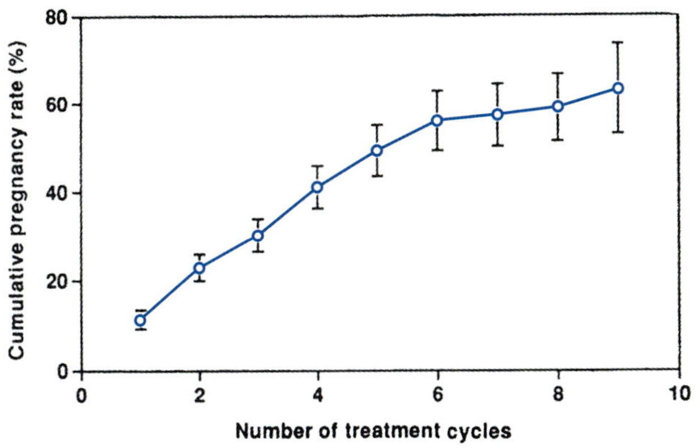


**Fig. 41.10** Overall cumulative pregnancy rate in *in vitro* fertilization treatment (95% confidence interval). (From Dor J, Seidman DS, Ben-Shlomo I, et al. Cumulative pregnancy rate following in vitro fertilization: the significance of age and infertility aetiology. *Hum Reprod.* 1996;11(2):425-428.)

dramatically (though not entirely) reduced OHSS development in the most high-risk patients. Lower pregnancy rates, likely as a result of luteal phase insufficiency, limited the use of this method in the past. This defect likely occurs for the same reason that the GnRH agonist trigger successfully limits OHSS risks—the shorter half-life of the GnRH agonist versus HCG minimizes the cascade of events leading to prolonged OHSS. **By combining the agonist trigger with a greatly reduced dose of HCG (i.e., 1000 IU or 1500 IU) and with the addition of supplemental estrogen and progesterone in the luteal phase, pregnancy rates are similar to those found with the conventional HCG trigger** (Griffin, 2012).

## In Vitro Fertilization Pregnancy Complications

**The major pregnancy concerns after IVF are related to multiple gestations resulting in prematurity and other sequelae** (Schieve, 1999). Because of the risks of prematurity with high-order multiples, couples may elect to undergo selective fetal reduction early in pregnancy. This is considered a safe procedure but carries an overall risk of pregnancy loss of approximately 1%.

However, some pregnancy-related risks do occur, even with singletons (Table 41.5); therefore careful obstetric care is extremely important. Congenital anomaly risks in IVF pregnancies may be slightly increased (3% to 4%) compared with the natural rate of birth defects in the normal population (2% to 3%) but not compared with an infertility population not undergoing IVF.

Although controversial, there may be a slightly increased risk of chromosomal structural defects in children born after ICSI. In a study of 8319 live births, Van Steirteghem and coworkers found a rate of sex chromosomal aneuploidy of 0.6% in the ICSI offspring versus 0.2% in the general neonatal population and structural autosomal abnormalities in 0.4% versus 0.07%, as well as an increase in structural aberrations related to the infertile fathers (Van Steirteghem, 2002). **Increasingly data have suggested that although there may be a slightly increased rate of birth defects with IVF compared with the general population, it is not increased compared with an infertile population that did not use IVF to conceive** (Rimm, 2011). Similarly a meta-analysis has suggested no difference in risk between IVF with and without ICSI (Wen, 2012). In addition, there is no direct evidence of ICSI increasing the risk of imprinting disorders, which was suggested previously (Vermeiden, 2013). Follow-up of the children, however, does suggest an increased rate of urogenital abnormalities,

**TABLE 41.5** Potential Risks in Singleton IVF Pregnancies

| Perinatal Risks | Absolute Risk in IVF Pregnancies (%) | Relative Risk (vs. Non-IVF Pregnancies) |
|---|---|---|
| Preterm birth | 11.5 | 2.0 (1.7-2.2) |
| Low birth weight (<2500 g) | 9.5 | 1.8 (1.4-2.2) |
| Very low birth weight (<1500 g) | 2.5 | 2.7 (2.3-3.1) |
| Small for gestational age | 14.6 | 1.6 (1.3-2.0) |
| Neonatal ICU admission | 17.8 | 1.6 (1.3-2.0) |
| Stillbirth | 1.2 | 2.6 (1.8-3.6) |
| Neonatal mortality | 0.6 | 2.0 (1.2-3.4) |
| Cerebral palsy | 0.4 | 2.8 (1.3-5.8) |
| **Genetic Risks** | | |
| Imprinting disorder | 0.03 | 17.8 (1.8-432.9) |
| Major birth defect | 4.3 | 1.5% (1.3-1.8) |
| **Chromosomal Abnormalities (after ICSI)** | | |
| Of a sex chromosome | 0.6 | 3.0 |
| Of another chromosome | 0.4 | 5.7 |

Modified from Reddy UM, Wapner RJ, Rebar RW, et al. Infertility, assisted reproductive technology, and adverse pregnancy outcomes. Executive Summary of a National Institute of Child Health and Human Development Workshop. *Obstet Gynecol.* 2007;109(4):967-977.

In this table, the absolute risk is the percentage of IVF pregnancies in which the risk occurred. The relative risk is the risk in IVF versus the risk in non-IVF pregnancies; for example, a relative risk of 2.0 indicates that twice as many IVF pregnancies experience this risk compared with non-IVF pregnancies. The numbers in parentheses (confidence interval) indicate the range in which the actual relative risk lies.

*ICSI*, Intracytoplasmic sperm injection; *ICU*, intensive care unit; *IVF*, in vitro fertilization.

which may be related to the male subfertility. Counseling of patients about these findings before ICSI is important. The uncertainty surrounding these issues is that it is likely that the infertile population also carries some risks (independent of IVF) compared with the normal fertile population (Simpson, 2014).

## Ovarian and Breast Cancer Risks After In Vitro Fertilization

Most studies do not show an increased risk for ovarian and breast cancer in patients previously exposed to IVF treatment (Brinton, 2013). **Overall, IVF complication rates are low, with a survey of ART complications (i.e., OHSS, hospitalizations, infections, maternal deaths) in the United States revealing rates far less than 1%** (Kawwass, 2015).

## Preimplantation Genetic Testing

A variety of genetic tests can help clinicians screen for heritable diseases or aneuploidy before ET. PGT-M, previously known as preimplantation genetic diagnosis (PGD), identifies specific genetic mutations that are known to cause disease. A common use of PGT-M is to screen for the presence of autosomal recessive diseases such as cystic fibrosis (CF). If both prospective parents are CF carriers, PGT-M can identify embryos that are homozygous for CF genes. Parents may elect to use PGT-M to avoid transferring these embryos. PGT-A, previously known as preimplantation genetic selection (PGS), refers to screening embryos for aneuploidy. Because aneuploid pregnancy rates increase with maternal age, PGT-A may be most beneficial for older women (older than age 37) to select for euploid embryos. Because of the higher implantation potential of euploid embryos, PGT-A may be used to achieve similar delivery rates to double ET, without the high risk of twins and obstetric complications (Forman, 2014). Although ethically controversial (ASRM Ethics Committee, 2004), PGT-A can be used for sex selection and family balancing.

PGT can be conducted on the polar body of unfertilized oocyte, blastomeres from cleavage stage (day 3) embryos or the trophectoderm of day 5 or 6 blastocysts. Because polar body biopsy cannot detect genetic errors occurring postfertilization, PGT is most commonly conducted on embryos. Until recently, PGT most commonly occurred with day 3 embryos with the removal of one to two blastomeres per embryo. Fluorescence in situ hybridization (FISH) was then conducted on the biopsied cells. Results could return within 24 to 48 hours, at which point only the euploid or unaffected embryos could be selected for transfer as blastocysts (embryo day 5 or 6). Because of false-positive and false-negative test risks (Hanson, 2009) and the risk of embryonic mosaicism leading to incomplete biopsy results, researchers sought more sensitive screening tests. **With the development of array comprehensive genetic hybridization (aCGH) and blastocyst biopsy techniques, more accurate results could be obtained with trophectoderm biopsy of day 5 or 6 blastocysts** (Fig. 41.11). Biopsy at the later blastocyst stage does not seem to impair embryonic survival in contrast to embryos biopsied on day 3 (Scott, 2013).

A variety of genetic screening techniques can be used to test embryonic cells: FISH, single-nucleotide polymorphism microarray, aCGH, real-time polymerase chain reaction, and next-generation sequencing. Multiple randomized trials clearly demonstrated that FISH-based PGT-A was not effective at improving outcomes after IVF. Randomized trials have shown benefit of PGT-A using aCGH and real-time polymerase chain reaction (PCR) (Dahdouh, 2015). With advances in genetic technology, next-generation sequencing has become the predominant method used for PGT-A, but prospective trials showing benefit are still lacking.

Studies (Franasiak, 2014) of PGT-A show an age-related increase in aneuploidy that parallels the increased risk of aneuploidy miscarriage and ongoing aneuploidy pregnancy with increasing maternal age. **The transfer of euploid embryos may help maintain consistently high live birth rates across age groups for those patients who are able to produce a euploid embryo** (Harton, 2013).

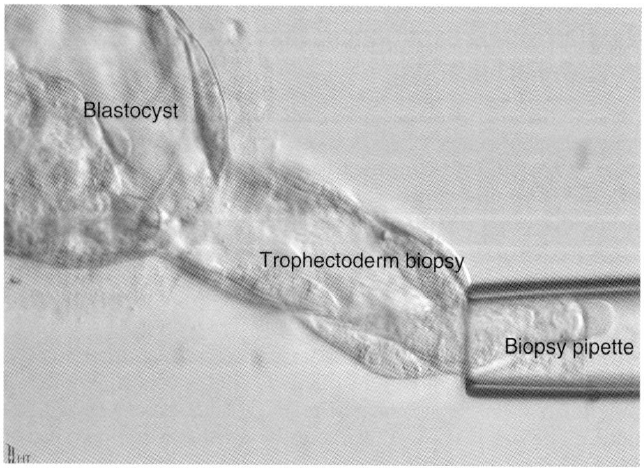


**Fig. 41.11** Trophectoderm biopsy. (Courtesy Center for Women's Reproductive Care at Columbia University.)

## Risks of Preimplantation Genetic Testing

False-positive results may stem from mosaicism within the biopsied embryo, leading to the discarding of a potentially normal embryo. False-negative results can lead to the transfer of an affected embryo and the conception of a disease-affected pregnancy. Because of this small risk (1% to 2%), patients are still advised to undergo antenatal genetic testing (i.e., chorionic villus sampling or amniocentesis) even after PGS. Compared with standard IVF, PGT does not seem to be associated with an increased risk for obstetric complications or congenital anomalies in resultant offspring (Beukers, 2013; Eldar-Geva, 2014). Limited data are available regarding the outcomes from transfer of embryos with a predicted mosaic biopsy result. It appears these embryos result in a lower chance of live birth and higher risk of miscarriage than euploid embryos (Munne, 2017), but healthy newborns without evidence of mosaicism have been born. Whether this is because of a technical error of the PGT-A technology or embryonic self-correction remains a subject of debate in the field.

## Donor In Vitro Fertilization

Donor IVF enables pregnancy in patients who are unable to conceive using their own oocytes as a result of decreased ovarian reserve or menopausal changes occurring naturally or after gonadotoxic therapy for cancer. A known or anonymous oocyte donor undergoes controlled ovarian stimulation. Once her oocytes are retrieved, they can then be fertilized with sperm (patient's partner or donor sperm). Resultant embryos are then transferred into the recipient patient's uterus after estrogen and progesterone priming to promote endometrial receptivity (see the Frozen Embryo Transfer section later in this chapter). Because of age-related effects on declining oocyte quality, **pregnancy rates using oocytes from younger oocyte donors (20 to 30) are typically in the 60% to 70% rate.** The rate is relatively independent of the age of the recipient as long as her uterus is normal. Egg donation cycles can safely be carried out in healthy women into their 50s. Pregnancy rates may slightly decline in recipients older than 40, but live birth rates of close to 50% per donor cycle can be expected in women into their 50s. **Obstetric complication rates increase, however, in the extremes of advanced maternal age, with higher incidences of gestational diabetes and preeclampsia** (Kort, 2012, Paulson, 2002).

## Frozen Embryo Transfer

Estrogen therapy (administered via oral, transdermal, or intramuscular routes) is administered typically over a 2-week period to "prime" or proliferate the endometrium, readying it for ET. Alternatively, a frozen transfer can be done in a natural ovulatory cycle, without estrogen priming, but this approach requires more intensive ultrasound monitoring. Monitoring of patient response to the hormone therapy can be done with vaginal ultrasound measurement of endometrial thickness and blood measurements of $E_2$. Once an endometrial thickness of 6 to 8 mm or more is attained, progesterone supplementation (via either vaginal or intramuscular injection route) is begun 4 to 6 days before the scheduled ET.

**Embryos are thawed on the day of the scheduled transfer.** Survival rates of frozen embryos vary from clinic to clinic. The freezing method (most commonly vitrification at the present time) and the baseline quality of the embryos before cryopreservation affect embryo survival rates. **With vitrification, survival**

**of more than 95% is standard in IVF laboratories.** Thawed embryos are then transferred into the patient's uterus, typically using ultrasound guidance and a soft catheter.

**The number of thawed embryos to transfer depends on the age of the woman at the time of freezing and on ASRM guidelines.** Because implantation and pregnancy rates decline with female age and oocyte quality, the recommended number to transfer will increase with the age of the woman at the time of freeze. For instance, women who froze embryos before turning age 35 would be counseled to transfer just one embryo if it was a blastocyst. Women freezing embryos at age 40 and older might be permitted to transfer two or three embryos. As with fresh IVF transfer, there is an increasing trend toward transferring exclusively at the blastocyst (day 5/6) stage over the day 3 stage. When PGT-A has been performed, single ET is advised across age groups.

## Recurrent Implantation Failure

Despite the improving efficacy of IVF, there are still patients who fail to conceive despite multiple attempts. Recurrent implantation failure is generally diagnosed after the inability to conceive after three or more transfers of one to two good-quality embryos (Coughlan, 2014). With the higher implantation of euploid embryos, this diagnosis may also be considered after two failed transfers with euploid blastocysts. A thorough evaluation for potential causes of failed transfer should include a thorough anatomic evaluation including imaging of the uterus (saline sonohysterography and/or hysteroscopy). If not previously performed, a hysterosalpingography should be ordered to rule out hydrosalpinges communicating with the uterine cavity. Close attention should be paid to the quality of the embryos because earlier stage embryos and untested embryos from older reproductive-age women have a lower chance of implantation. Although some clinicians perform a recurrent miscarriage evaluation, evidence does not support testing for inherited or acquired thrombophilia or parental karyotypes in the evaluation of recurrent implantation failure.

A newer concept regarding recurrent implantation failure relates to the timing of ET. Implantation is complex process requiring a cross-talk between a viable embryo and a receptive endometrium. The embryo thaw for a frozen ET is aimed to be in the middle of the receptive window, typically 5 days after the initiation of vaginal or intramuscular progesterone in programmed cycles, or 5 days after ovulation in natural cycles. **The endometrial receptivity analysis (ERA)** relies on **gene expression analysis of an endometrial sample** take by biopsy at the time during the implantation window, when a frozen ET would have been performed (Diaz-Gimeno, 2013). These gene profiles in the biopsy are read as being receptive, prereceptive, or postreceptive, and a greater proportion of women with recurrent implantation failure have been found to have nonreceptive ERA (Ruiz-Alonso, 2013). When there is a suspected displaced window of implantation, a recommendation is made to perform a subsequent ET using a longer or shorter duration of progesterone exposure. Prospective validation studies proving the benefit of the ERA are still lacking, and it is not the standard of care at present. Also to be considered at the time of biopsy is a histologic reading of **chronic endometritis,** which has also been considered to result in implantation failure and/or recurrent loss, as well as a putative marker for endometriosis and progesterone resistance, ***BCL6*** (Lessey, 2019), which also has not been completely validated as a cause of recurrent implantation failure.

## Fertility Preservation

Patients at risk for future infertility because of gonadotoxic therapy for cancer or an immunologic disorder have several fertility preservation (FP) options. ART to harvest and cryopreserve mature oocytes or embryos is the most well-established method of fertility preservation. Oocyte biology explains why there is a generally lower pregnancy rate with cryopreserved oocytes compared with embryos. Improvements in oocyte cryopreservation methods have led to improved freeze/thaw survival rates of oocytes and hence pregnancy rates. Nevertheless, even in younger (i.e., younger than 37 years) women, the pregnancy rate per frozen oocyte has ranged from 4% to 12%, with a rapid decline occurring with older patients (Practice Committee ASRM, 2013). To date, only a few thousand live births have been reported from cryopreserved/thawed oocytes, whereas millions of pregnancies have resulted from cryopreserved embryos (Noyes, 2009).

ASRM has long stated that FP should be discussed with any reproductive-age woman at risk for iatrogenic premature ovarian failure. **It was not until 2013 that ASRM finally reversed its opinion that elective fertility preservation be considered "experimental"; however, ASRM has still not endorsed its routine use for storing or "banking" embryos for the purpose of delaying pregnancy** (Practice Committee ASRM, 2013). Although IVF and embryo cryopreservation has led to millions of pregnancies in infertile populations of women, few studies exist demonstrating cryopreservation pregnancy rates in women undergoing FP electively. Concern that the ART process may endanger a woman's future fertility potential—for instance, because of a postprocedure infection leading to pelvic adhesions—is an area of concern and for discussion when counseling women seeking to electively freeze oocytes/embryos; however, the risk of complication after IVF is extremely low. Additionally, concern remains that a woman might receive false hope through a FP cycle, leading her to further delay childbearing to an age when ART may no longer be able to assist her should she develop infertility.

## Ovarian Tissue Cryopreservation

Research is ongoing in the area of ovarian tissue cryopreservation. For patients unable to go through an ART procedure, surgical removal of a whole or part of an ovary for cryopreservation may offer another way to preserve future fertility potential. The frozen tissue can then be thawed and orthotopically or heterotopically transplanted back into the patient's body at a future date if the need arises. To date, few live births (Donnez, 2013) have been reported after this process. Ovarian tissue cryopreservation is available at a limited number of centers in the United States and requires Institutional Review Board (IRB) approval. Ovarian tissue cryopreservation is not advised for patients suffering from hematologic cancers such as leukemia. Metastatic sites have been found in ovarian tissue harvested from patients with leukemia, leading to concern that transplantation of such tissue may lead to reseeding of malignant cells (Bastings, 2013).

**GnRH agonist use may confer some ovarian protection against the gonadotoxic effect of certain chemotherapeutic agents** (Del Mastro, 2014). GnRH agonists may work in one of several possible ways to protect the ovaries: suppression of the hypothalamic-pituitary gonadal axis leading to decreased blood flow to the ovaries, thereby minimizing ovarian exposure to chemotherapy; suppression of FSH-driven follicular recruitment; and activation of factors within the ovaries that might work directly to protect ovarian reserve (Blumenfeld, 2007). GnRH agonist administration initially leads to a transient increase in endogenous gonadotropin secretion, potentially stimulating the maturation of a "wave" of oocytes and thereby exposing more oocytes to the gonadotoxic agent. Because of this flare effect, it is important to administer the agonist 7 to 10 days prechemotherapy exposure. This sequence allows for the flare effect to fade and the agonist's suppressive/protective effect to come to the forefront. A study in reproductive-age breast cancer patients showed that GnRH agonist administration before and during chemotherapy significantly improved ovarian function and pregnancy potential after cancer therapy compared with the control patients who received no agonist (Moore, 2015).

**Patients facing impending pelvic radiation therapy may consider ovarian transposition** via laparoscopy or laparotomy; the ovaries can be lifted above the pelvic brim and fixed to the anterior abdominal wall. Fixing the ovaries out of the field of radiation may help shield them from injury, thus helping patients to maintain their ovarian function (Gubbala, 2014).

## FUTURE DEVELOPMENTS

IVF and PGS have opened opportunities for **stem cell research**. Somatic cell nuclear transfer into oocytes has led to the development of pluripotent stem cell lines. Research into inducing somatic cells transformation into pluripotent stem cells may allow for **tissue development for organ transplantation and repair of injured tissue**. This technology may translate into repairing injured cardiac myocytes after an infarction, repairing damaged retinal tissue, or possibly generating oocytes for patients diagnosed with ovarian failure. **Nuclear transfer into an enucleated donor cell has paved the way for treating rare mitochondrial diseases** (Paul, 2013). All these areas are still experimental, conducted under IRB approval where appropriate (Trounson, 2013). Future areas of research may involve *in vitro* gametogenesis to produce new oocytes or sperm for those with ovarian or testicular failure.

To date, more than 8 million babies have resulted from IVF since Louise Brown was conceived via IVF in 1978. In the United States 1% of babies are conceived via IVF, whereas in Europe, up to 3% are conceived with IVF. With improvements in PGT and IVF technology, goals include improving pregnancy rates particularly in women of advanced reproductive age while minimizing the risk for multiple pregnancies. In the future, advances in stem cell research may allow for innovative treatments for rare genetic and more common medical disorders while also offering possibilities for extending reproductive opportunities for patients with gonadal failure.

### REFERENCES


Al-Inany HG, Youssef MA, Aboulghar M, et al. Gonadotropin-releasing hormone antagonists for assisted reproductive technology. *Cochrane Database Syst Rev.* 2011;(5):CD001750.

Chen ZJ, Shi Y, Sun Y, et al. Fresh versus frozen embryos for infertility in the polycystic ovary syndrome. *N Engl J Med.* 2016;375:523–533.

Coughlan C, Ledger W, Wang Q, et al. Recurrent implantation failure: definition and management. *Reprod Biomed Online.* 2014;28:14–38.

Dahdouh EM, Balayla J, Garcia-Velasco JA, et al. Comprehensive chromosome screening improves embryo selection: a meta-analysis. *Fertil Steril.* 2015;104:1503–1512.

Diaz-Gimeno P, Ruiz-Alonso M, Blesa D, et al. The accuracy and reproducibility of the endometrial receptivity array is superior to histology as a diagnostic method for endometrial receptivity. *Fertil Steril.* 2013; 99:508–517.

Donnez J, Dolmans MM, Pellicer A, et al. Restoration of ovarian activity and pregnancy after transplantation of cryopreserved ovarian tissue: a review of 60 cases of reimplantation. *Fertil Steril.* 2013;99(6): 1503–1513.

Eldar-Geva T, Srebnik N, Altarescu G, et al. Neonatal outcome after preimplantation genetic diagnosis. *Fertil Steril.* 2014;102(4):1016–1021.

Forman EJ, Hong KH, Franasiak JM, et al. Obstetrical and neonatal outcomes from the BEST Trial: single embryo transfer with aneuploidy screening improves outcomes after in vitro fertilization without compromising delivery rates. *Am J Obstet Gynecol.* 2014;210(2):157. e1–157.e6.

Franasiak JM, Forman EJ, Hong KH. The nature of aneuploidy with increasing age of the female partner: a review of 15,169 consecutive trophectoderm biopsies evaluated with comprehensive chromosomal screening. *Fertil Steril.* 2014;101(3):656–663.

Goldman MB, Thornton KL, Ryley D, et al. A randomized clinical trial to determine optimal infertility treatment in older couples: the Forty and Over Treatment Trial (FORT-T). *Fertil Steril.* 2014;101(6): 1574–1581.

Harton GL, Munne S. Surrey M, et al. Diminished effect of maternal age on implantation after preimplantation genetic diagnosis with array comparative genomic hybridization. *Fertil Steril.* 2013;100:1695–1703.

Kawwass JF, Kissin DM, Kulkarni AD, et al. Safety of assisted reproductive technology in the United States, 2000-2011. *JAMA.* 2015;313(1): 88–90.

Kirkegaard K, Ahlstrom A, Infersley HJ, et al. Choosing the best embryo by time lapse versus standard morphology. *Fertil Steril.* 2015;103(2): 323–332.

Kort DH, Gosselin J, Choi JM, et al. Pregnancy after age 50: defining risks for mother and child. *Am J Perinatol.* 2012;29(4):245–250.

Lessey BA, Young SL. What exactly is endometrial receptivity? *Fertil Steril.* 2019;111;611–617.

Lobo RA. Potential options for preservation of fertility in women. *N Engl J Med.* 2005;353(1):64–73.

Luke B, Brown MB, Stern JE, et al. Using the Society for Assisted Reproductive Technology Clinic Outcome System morphological measures to predict live birth after assisted reproductive technology. *Fertil Steril.* 2014;102(5):1338–1344.

Luke B, Brown MB, Wantman E, et al. Application of a validated prediction model for in vitro fertilization: comparison of live birth rates and multiple birth rates with 1 embryo transferred over 2 cycles vs 2 embryos in 1 cycle. *Am J Obstet Gynecol.* 2015;212(5):676.e1–676.e7.

Munne S, Blazek J, Large M, et al. Detailed investigation into the cytogenetic constitution and pregnancy outcome of replacing mosaic blastocysts detected with the use of high-resolution next-generation sequencing. *Fertil Steril.* 2017;108:62–71.

Palermo G, Joris H, Devroey P, Van Steirteghem AC. Pregnancies after intracytoplasmic injection of single spermatozoon into an oocyte. *Lancet.* 1992;340(8810):17–18.

Practice Committee of the American Society for Reproductive Medicine. Guidance on the limits to the number of embryos to transfer: a committee opinion. *Fertil Steril.* 2017;107:901–903.

Ruiz-Alonso M, Blessa D, Diaz-Gimeno P, et al. The endometrial receptivity array for diagnosis and personalized embryo transfer as a treatment for patients with repeated implantation failure. *Fertil Steril.* 2013;100:818–824.

Scott RT, Upham KM, Forman EJ, et al. Cleavage-stage biopsy significantly impairs human embryonic implantation potential while blastocyst biopsy does not: a randomized and paired clinical trial. *Fertil Steril.* 2013; 100(3):624–630.

Simpson JL. Birth defects and assisted reproductive technologies. *Semin Fetal Neonatal Med.* 2014;19(3):177–182.

Steptoe PC, Edwards RG. Birth after the reimplantation of a human embryo. *Lancet.* 1978;2(8085):366.

Wei D, Liu JY, Sun Y, et al. Frozen versus fresh single blastocyst transfer in ovulatory women: a multicentre randomized controlled trial. *Lancet.* 2019; 393:1310–1318.


**Suggested readings for this chapter can be found on ExpertConsult.com.**

# INDEX

*Note:* Page numbers followed by *f* indicate figures, *t* indicate tables, and *b* indicate boxes.


## A

Abdominal exam, 132, 132*f*. *see also* Physical examinations
Abdominal leak point pressure (ALPP), 468
Abdominal pregnancy, 346–347
  management of, 355
Abdominal wall hernias, 428–431, 429*f*, 430*f*
  diagnosis of, 430–431
  etiology of, 429–430
  management of, 431
    incisional hernia, 431
    umbilical hernia repair, 431
  signs of, 430–431
  symptoms of, 430–431
Abnormal uterine bleeding, 594–605
  approaches to treatment, 604–605
  causes of, 594–598, 595*f*
    adenomyosis, 595, 595*f*, 596*f*
    coagulopathy, 596–597
    endometrial bleeding, 598, 598*f*
    endometrial polyps, 595
    iatrogenic bleeding, 598
    leiomyoma, 595–596, 597*f*
    malignancy, 596
    ovulatory dysfunction, 597–598
  diagnostic approach, 599–600, 599*f*, 600*f*
  management of, 602–605
    androgen for, 603
    dilation and curettage for, 603
    endometrial ablation for, 603–604
    estrogens for, 602–603
    hysterectomy for, 604
    pharmacologic agents for, 602–603
    progestogens for, 603
    selective progesterone receptor modulators, 603–604
  transabdominal ultrasound, 598, 598*f*
  treatment of, 600–602
    endometrial, 600–601, 601*f*
    nonsteroidal antiinflammatory drugs, 601–602, 601*t*
    ovulatory dysfunction, 600
Abortion
  aspiration method, 252
  dilation and evacuation method, 252–253
  induced, 252, 252*f*
  medication method, 253
  septic, 339–340
Abuse, 123, 182–185
  domestic violence, 182
  elderly, 185
  female circumcision as, 181–182, 181*f*
  intimate partner violence (IPV), 182–185, 183*b*, 184*b*
  posttraumatic stress disorder (PTSD), 158–162
Abuse *(Continued)*
  rape, 176–182. *see also* Rape.
  sexual, 233–235
Acanthosis nigricans, PCOS and, 829
Accessory nipples, 292
Accessory ovary, abnormalities of, 219
Accidental genital trauma, 232–237
  sexual abuse, 233–235, 235*f*
  vulvar hematomas, 233, 233*f*
  vulvar trauma, lacerations and straddle injury, 232–233
Acne vulgaris, in androgen excess, 822, 822*f*
ACOG. *see* American College of Obstetricians and Gynecologists (ACOG)
ACS. *see* American Cancer Society (ACS)
*Actinomyces* infection, 541
*Actinomyces israelii*, 541
Actinomycin D, 630–631
Activin, 91
Acupuncture, for menopause, 287
Acute grief, 185
Adaptive immunity, 608–609
  B cells and immunoglobulins, humoral immunity, 608, 608*f*
  T cells, cellular immunity, 608–609, 609*f*
Adenoacanthoma, 696
Adenocarcinomas, 674–675, 675*b*
Adenofibroma, 406
Adenohypophysis, 81
Adenoid cystic carcinomas, 676
Adenoma malignum, 676, 676*f*
Adenomatoid tumors, 395, 395*f*
Adenomyosis, 393–395, 595, 595*f*, 596*f*, 773–774
  clinical diagnosis of, 394–395, 394*f*
  management of, 395
  pathology of, 393–394, 393*f*, 394*f*
Adenosquamous carcinoma, 696
Adhesive vulvitis, 228
Adjuvant systemic therapy, for early stage endometrioid endometrial cancer, 701
Adnexa
  in adolescent patient, 235–237
  in pediatric patient, 235–237
Adnexal mass and ovarian cancer, 714–741, 714*b*
  evaluation of, 714–715
Adolescence, obesity in, 157
Adolescent patients, 221–237
  office visit and examination, 224–226, 225*b*
  ovarian cysts in, 236
  ovarian tumors in, 236–237
  ovary and adnexa in, 235–237
Adrenal hyperplasia, 796*t*
Adrenal tumors, 796*t*, 817
Adult, vaginal tumors of, 668–672
  clear cell adenocarcinoma, 670, 670*t*, 671*f*
  malignant melanoma, 670–671
  squamous cell carcinoma, 665–666*f*, 668–670, 669*f*
  vaginal adenocarcinomas arising in endometriosis, 671–672
Alcohol, 334, 335*t*
Alkylating agents, 632
Allele, 24
Allergic disease, 141–142, 141*b*, 142*t*, 143*t*
Alloimmune disorders, 332
Alopecia, in androgen excess, 822–823
ALPP. *see* Abdominal leak point pressure (ALPP)
Altretamine, 631*t*, 633
Amastia, 292
Ambiguous genitalia, 207–212, 208*b*, 208*f*
Amenorrhea, 594, 781
  primary, 781–800
    absent breast and uterine development, 787
    breast development present and uterus absent, 786–787, 787*f*
    breasts absent and uterus present, 783–786, 785*f*
    causes of, 783–788, 785*b*
    differential diagnosis and management, 788–789, 788*f*
    primary amenorrhea with absent endometrium, 788
    secondary sex characteristics present and female internal genitalia present, 787–788
  secondary, 781–800
    causes of, 789–792, 789*f*, 790*f*, 791*f*
    CNS and hypothalamic causes, 789–791
    diagnostic evaluation and management of, 792–794, 793*f*
    ovarian causes, 791–792, 792*f*
    pituitary causes, 791
    uterine factor, 789
American Cancer Society (ACS), 305–306
American College of Obstetricians and Gynecologists (ACOG), 298
American Society of Anesthesiologists (ASA) Physical Status Classification, 548*t*
American Society of Clinical Oncology (ASCO), 115, 306
AMH. *see* Antimüllerian hormone (AMH)
Amikacin, 9–12*t*
Aminoglycosides, 9–12*t*
Amoxicillin, 9–12*t*
Amphotericin B, 9–12*t*
Ampicillin, 9–12*t*

Anal incontinence, 495–514
causes and pathophysiology of, 497–498, 497*b*
diagnosis and assessment of, 498–505, 500*f*, 502*f*, 503*t*
diagnostic procedure in, 501–505
anal manometry, 501–502, 504*f*, 505*f*
colonoscopy for, 501
defecography, 504–505, 505*f*
electromyography for, 502–504
endoanal ultrasound, 501, 503*f*, 504*f*
magnetic resonance imaging, of anal sphincters, 501
pudendal nerve terminal motor latency, 504
transit study, 505, 506*f*
electrical stimulation therapy for, 509–510
anal plugs, 510
devices, 510
percutaneous tibial nerve stimulation, 510
stem cells, 510
epidemiology, 495–512, 496*b*
evaluation of, 498–500, 498*b*, 499*f*, 499*t*, 500*f*, 500*t*
medications for, 510, 510*t*
physical examination, 500–501, 500*f*
physiology of, 495–496, 496*t*, 497*f*
rectovaginal fistulas, 512–513, 513*t*
sacral nerve stimulation, 512
neosphincters, 512
stoma creation, 512
surgery in, 510–512
anterior sphincteroplasty, 511–512, 511*f*
injectables, 510
SECCA procedure, 510–511
testing in, 501, 502*f*, 503*t*
treatment of, 505–512, 507–508*t*, 509*t*
biofeedback, 506–509
education, diet, and lifestyle interventions, 506
Anal manometry, for anal incontinence, 501–502, 504*f*, 505*f*
Androgen excess, in women, 810–823
causes of, 815–819, 816*t*
androgen-producing tumors, 817
Cushing syndrome, 819
functional/idiopathic hyperandrogenism, 816
idiopathic hirsutism, 816
late-onset 21-hydroxylase deficiency, 817–819, 818*f*, 818*t*, 819*f*
polycystic ovary syndrome, 816
stromal hyperthecosis, 816–817, 817*f*
diagnostic approach, 819–820, 820*f*
genetic disorders with, 786
PCOS and, 826
treatment of, 820–823
late-onset 21-hydroxylase deficiency, 821
ovarian and adrenal tumors, 820
polycystic ovary syndrome, 821–823, 822*f*
in women, 810, 811*f*, 811*t*, 812*f*
physiology of, 810–815, 814*f*, 815*f*, 815*t*
Androgen insensitivity, 213–214
Androgen resistance syndrome, 786–787
Androgen therapy, 285
Androgen-producing tumors, 817
Androgens, for acute bleeding, 603
Androstenedione, 84
Angiogenesis and VEGF, 612
Aneuploidy, 30
Angelman syndrome (AS), 28
Anorexia nervosa, 151, 790
Anovaginal fistula, 512–513
Anovulation, medical treatment for, 848–853
Anovulatory cycles, 128
Anterior vaginal wall prolapse, 441–443, 442*f*
anterior colporrhaphy, 443, 444*f*
concomitant antiincontinence surgery, 443
concomitant apical support procedure, 443
diagnosis of, 442–443, 442*f*
mesh-augmented surgery, 445, 446*f*
postoperative restrictions on, 445
postoperative voiding dysfunction on, 443–445
recurrent, 445
surgical treatment, 443
symptoms, 441–442
Antiadrenergic agents, for postoperative ileus, 580*t*
Antiandrogens, 821
Antibiotic-associated diarrhea, 582–583, 582*t*
Antibiotics, for postoperative infections, 593.e8
Anticancer hormone therapy, 634
Anticipation, 27
Antidepressants, for menopause, 286
Antifibrinolytic agents, 601–602
Antihypertensives, for menopause, 286
Antimetabolites, 632
Antimüllerian hormone (AMH), 13, 829, 829*f*, 842
Antiphospholipid syndrome, 332–333
diagnosis of, 332*b*
Antitumor antibiotics, 630–631
Antral follicles, 92
cohort of, recruitment of, 92, 94*f*
maturing, 93–94, 95*f*, 96*f*, 97*f*
Antrum, 94
Anxiety disorders, 158–162
Aortic nodes, 66
Apical prolapse, after hysterectomy, 456–459
Arcuate nucleus, 48
Arias-Stella reaction, 349
Aromatase deficiency syndrome, 86
Aromatase enzyme, 86, 88*f*
Aromatase inhibitors (AIs), 703
for breast cancer, 307
for endometriosis, 422
Arteries, 62–63
common iliac, 63
hypogastric artery, 63
inferior mesenteric, 62–63
ovarian, 63
uterine, 63, 64*f*
vaginal, 63
Arthritis, degenerative, 271
AS. *see* Angelman syndrome (AS)
ASCO. *see* American Society of Clinical Oncology (ASCO)
Asherman syndrome, 329–330, 329*f*, 329*t*, 789
Aspiration method, abortion, 252
Assay markers, choice of, 103
Assisted reproductive technologies, 861
Atelectasis, 561, 562–564, 563*b*, 563*f*
Athelia, 292
Atomic number (Z), 619
Attachment style, preoccupied, 167
Atypical glandular cells, 641
Autoimmune state, 792
Autosomal dominant inheritance pattern, 25, 25*f*
Autosomal recessive inheritance pattern, 25–26, 26*f*
Aztreonam, 9–12*t*

## B

Bacterial vaginosis, 526–528, 528*f*, 529*t*
Bartholin gland carcinoma, of vulva, 663
Bartholin glands, 50, 51*f*
infections of, 516, 517*f*, 518*f*
Basal body temperature (BBT), 98
Basal cell carcinoma, of vulva, 663
Basic science
anatomy, reproductive, 47–75
embryogenesis, 1–20
epidemiology, clinical, 106–115
evidence-based medicine, 106–115
fertilization, 1–20
risk management, medical-legal, 116–126
Battered woman, 182
BBT. *see* Basal body temperature (BBT)
Behçet disease, 372
Benign breast disorders, 293–295, 294*t*
Benign cystic teratomas, 401–403, 401*f*, 402*f*, 403*f*, 743–744, 744*f*
Benign gynecologic lesions, 362–408
adenomyosis, 393–395, 393*f*, 394*f*
cervix, 378–380
endocervical and cervical polyps, 378–379, 378*f*, 379*f*
lacerations, 379
myomas, 379–380, 379*f*, 380*f*
nabothian cysts, 379
stenosis, 380
dermatologic diseases, 369–375
Behçet disease, 372
contact dermatitis, 369–370, 369*f*, 370*f*
edema, 373–375, 374*b*, 374*f*
hidradenitis suppurativa, 372–373, 373*f*
lichen planus, 371, 372*f*
pruritus, 369
psoriasis, 370–371, 371*f*
seborrheic dermatitis, 371
ovary, 397–407
benign neoplasms, 401–407
functional cysts, 397–401
oviduct, 395–397
adenomatoid tumors, 395, 395*f*
leiomyomas, 395
paratubal cysts, 395–396, 396*f*
torsion, 396–397, 396*f*
uterus, 380–393
endometrial polyps, 381–383, 384*f*
hematometra, 383–384
leiomyomas, 384–393, 385*f*, 386*f*, 387*f*, 388*f*, 391*f*, 391*t*, 392*f*, 393*f*
ultrasound, 380–381, 382*f*, 383*f*
vagina, 375–378
dysontogenetic cysts, 376–377, 376*f*, 377*f*
inclusion cysts, 376
local trauma, 378
tampon problems, 377–378
urethral diverticulum, 375–376, 375*t*, 376*f*
vulva, 363–369
abnormal tissues presenting vulvar masses, 368

Benign gynecologic lesions *(Continued)*
cysts, 364–365, 364*f*
endometriosis, 367–368
fibroma, 366, 366*f*
granular cell myoblastoma, 368
hemangioma, 366
hematomas, 368–369, 368*f*
hidradenoma, 367, 367*f*
lipoma, 366–367, 367*f*
nevus, 365–366, 365*f*
syringoma, 367
urethral caruncle, 363–364, 363*f*
urethral prolapse, 363–364, 364*f*
von Recklinghausen disease, 368
Bethesda system, 640, 640*f*
Amsterdam II criteria, 614*b*
Bevacizumab, 631*t*, 633, 633*f*
Bilateral ligation, 567, 567*f*
Bimanual examination, 135–136, 136*f*
Binge eating disorder, 151
"Bioidentical" therapy, 285–286
Biologic and targeted agents, 420–421
Biosynthesis, ovarian steroids, 84–86, 86*f*, 87*f*
Bisphosphonates, for osteoporosis, 270
Bladder
anatomy and function of, 462–465, 465*f*, 466*f*
development of, 11, 12*f*
diary, 466, 467*f*
overactive, 483*t*, 486–493
diagnosis, 488
etiology, 488
mixed urinary incontinence, 491–493
other types, urinary incontinence, 493
treatment, 488–489, 489*t*, 490*f*, 491*f*, 491*t*, 492*f*
Blastula stage, 5–8, 8*f*
Bleeding, in spontaneous early pregnancy loss, 338
Bleomycin, 631, 631*t*
Bone, health, menopause and, 268–271, 268*f*, 269*f*, 269*t*, 270*f*, 270*t*
Borderline ovarian tumors, treatment of, 711*f*, 711*t*, 712*f*, 720–722, 721*f*, 722*f*
Borderline personality disorder, 167
Bowel resection, 727
Brachytherapy, 623–626
BRCA1 and BRCA2, 613
Breast
abnormalities, congenital developmental, 292–299
benign breast disorders, 293–295, 294*t*
breast tissue, 292–293
fat necrosis, 299
fibroadenomas, 294, 295*f*
fibrocystic change, 295–297, 296*f*, 297*f*
inflammatory disease, 298
intraductal papilloma, 298–299
mastalgia (breast pain), 297, 297*b*
mastitis, 298
nipple, 292
nipple discharge, 298, 299*f*
phyllodes tumors, 295, 295*f*
anatomy/embryology, 290–292, 291*f*, 292*f*, 293*f*
clinical examination of, 308, 309*f*
lactating, 290*f*
pain in, 297*b*
Breast *(Continued)*
self-examination of, 308
structures of, 291*f*
Breast carcinoma/cancer, 299–300
assessment and prevention on, 303–306, 304*t*, 305*t*, 306*t*
chemoprophylaxis and chemotherapeutic risk reduction, 306–307, 307*t*
chemotherapy for, 321
classification of, 313, 314*t*
computed tomography, 312
core needle biopsy, 313
demographic associations, 300, 301*t*
detection and diagnosis of, 307–313
digital mammography, 311
ductal carcinoma in situ of, 313–314
epidemiology and risk for, 300, 300*t*, 301*t*
estrogen-related exposure risks of, 300–301
with estrogen use, risk of, 277–280, 279*f*, 280*t*, 281*f*
excisional biopsy, 313
fine-needle aspiration, 313
genomic profiling, 315–316, 316*t*
HER2-directed therapy for, 320–321
history and characteristics of, 302, 302*f*
hormonal therapy for, 320
infiltrating/invasive ductal carcinoma, 314, 314*f*
infiltrating lobular carcinoma, 314, 315*f*
inflammatory, 314–315, 315*f*
inherited and familial risks of, 302–303, 303*t*
lifestyle and dietary risk factors of, 301–302
lobular carcinoma in situ of, 314
magnetic resonance imaging, 311–312, 312*f*
mammography, 308–311, 310*f*, 311*f*
management of, 316–321, 316*t*
medical therapy for, 320
Paget disease, 315, 315*f*
during pregnancy, 321
radiation exposure and, 303
radiation therapy for, 319–320
surgical therapy for, 317–319, 317*t*, 318*f*, 319*f*
surveillance, 321–322
tissue sampling, 313
tomosynthesis, 312–313
ultrasound, 312, 312*f*
Breast diseases, 289–322
Breast exam, 131–132, 132*b*
Breast growth, classification of, 782*t*
Breast tissue
congenital developmental abnormalities of, 292–293
sampling, in breast cancer, 313
Bremsstrahlung, 620
Brenner tumors, 405–406, 405*f*, 713, 713*f*
Broad ligaments, 69–70, 71*f*
Bromocriptine, 780
for prolactinomas, 804–806
Bulimia nervosa, 151
Bupropion, for depression, 150–151
Burch procedure, 483, 484*f*

## C

Cabergoline, for prolactinomas, 806*f*, 807, 807*t*
Caffeine, 334
CAH. *see* Congenital adrenal hyperplasia (CAH)
Calcitonin, for vertebral fractures, 271
*Camptotheca acuminata*, 631–632
Cancer, 146–147
risk, in postmenopausal women, 275–280, 279*f*
Cancer antigen 125 (CA-125), 714, 714*b*
surveillance, after primary therapy, 733
*Candida vaginitis*, 530–532, 530*f*
fungal vulvovaginitis, 531–532, 531*f*, 532*b*
Cannabis abuse, 163
CAP strategy, 124, 124*f*
Capecitabine, 631*t*
Caprini Score Risk Assessment Model for Venous Thromboembolism, 555*t*
Carbapenems, 9–12*t*
Carbon dioxide laser, 656
Carboplatin, 631*t*, 633
Carcinoma in situ, of vulva, 651, 652*f*
Carcinomas, 717–720
breast, 299–300
diagnosis, staging, spread, preoperative evaluation, and prognostic factors, 717–720, 717*t*, 718*f*, 719*f*, 719*t*, 720*f*, 721*f*
Carcinosarcoma, 704*b*, 705, 742
Cardinal ligaments, 70
Cardiopulmonary comorbidities, assessment of, 557
Cardiovascular problems, 565
deep vein thrombosis, 569–572, 569*b*, 570*f*, 570*t*, 571*t*
hematomas, 568
hemorrhagic shock, 565–568, 566*b*, 567*f*, 567*t*, 568*f*
pulmonary embolism, 568–575, 572*t*, 573*f*, 574*f*
retained foreign body, 568
superficial thrombophlebitis, 569
thrombophlebitis and pulmonary embolus, 568–575
Cardiovascular system, estrogen and estrogen/progestogen, current data on, 275, 277*f*, 278*f*, 279*f*
Case reports, 107–108
Case series, 107–108
Case-control studies, 108–109, 108*f*
Caspofungin, 9–12*t*
CCs. *see* Combined contraceptives (CCs)
Cefamandole, 9–12*t*
Cefazolin, 9–12*t*
Cefepime, 9–12*t*
Cefmetazole, 9–12*t*
Cefonicid, 9–12*t*
Ceforanide, 9–12*t*
Cefotaxime, 9–12*t*
Cefotetan, 9–12*t*
Cefoxitin, 9–12*t*
Ceftizoxime, 9–12*t*
Cefuroxime, 9–12*t*
Celiac disease, 333
Cell cycle dependency, of cell kill
in chemotherapy, 628
in radiation therapy, 619
Cell survival curves, 622*f*
Central nervous system (CNS)
disease, 145–146
disorders, 804

Central nervous system (CNS) *(Continued)*
lesions, 786
menopause effects on, 263–266, 264*b*, 264*f*, 265*f*, 266*f*, 267*f*
metastases, 765
tumor, 796*t*
Central nervous system-hypothalamic-pituitary disorders, 786
Cephalosporins, 9–12*t*
Cephalothin, 9–12*t*
Cephapirin, 9–12*t*
CER. *see* Comparative effectiveness research (CER)
Cervical cancer, 616, 637
colposcopy for, 641–643, 643*f*
cervical dysplasia in pregnancy, 642
cervical intraepithelial neoplasia, natural history of, 642–643
etiology of, 637
prevention in low- and middle-income countries, 637
primary prevention of, 638
risk factors of, 637–638, 638*f*
screening guidelines, 639
secondary prevention of, 638–641
abnormal cervical screening tests management, 640
atypical glandular cells, 641
atypical squamous cells, 640
Bethesda system, 640, 640*f*
cervical cancer screening guidelines, 639
cervical cytology testing, 638, 639*f*
high-grade squamous intraepithelial lesion, 641, 642*f*
low-grade squamous intraepithelial lesion, 640–641, 641*f*
primary human papillomavirus testing, 639
in vaginal intraepithelial neoplasia, 646
in vulvar intraepithelial neoplasia, 646, 646*f*
Cervical cytology testing, 638, 639*f*
Cervical dysplasia
in pregnancy, 642
treatment of, 643–646
ablative method for, 644–645
CIN 1, 643–644
CIN 2/3, 644
cold knife conisation, 645
$CO_2$ laser ablation, 644
cryotherapy for, 644
excisional methods for, 645, 645*f*
follow-up after of, 645
thermal ablation, 644–645
Cervical glands, menstrual cycle and, 102–104
Cervical incompetence, 330, 330*f*, 331*f*
Cervical myomas, 379–380, 379*f*, 380*f*
Cervical polyps, 378–379, 378*f*, 379*f*
Cervical pregnancy, 347
management of, 355
Cervical stenosis, 380, 773–774, 774*f*
Cervical stump tumors, 686
Cervicitis, 532–534
Cervix, 53–54, 55*f*, 56*f*, 532
abnormalities in, 215
benign gynecologic lesions, 378–380
endocervical and cervical polyps, 378–379, 378*f*, 379*f*
lacerations, 379
myomas, 379–380, 379*f*, 380*f*
Cervix *(Continued)*
nabothian cysts, 379
stenosis, 380
carcinoma of, 677–687
clinical considerations of, 677
inadvertently removed at simple hysterectomy, 686–687
natural history and spread, 677–678, 679*f*
in pregnancy, 687
prognostic factors, 678–680, 679*t*
staging of, 677, 678*t*, 679*f*
clinical correlations for, 55–58, 56*f*
malignant diseases of, 674–690, 675*b*
considerations, 686–687
histologic types of, 675–677, 675*f*, 676*f*, 677*f*
recurrence in, 687–689
treatment of, 680–686, 682*f*
Cesarean scar ectopic pregnancy, 347
Cesarean scar pregnancy, management of, 356
Chancroid, 522
Chemoradiation, 684–685
Chemotherapeutic agents, 629–634, 630*f*
Chemotherapy, 627–635, 628*b*
alkylating agents, 632
altretamine, 633
anticancer hormone therapy, 634
antimetabolites, 632
antitumor antibiotics, 630–631, 631*t*
approaches to treatment, 628–629, 629*t*
biologic and targeted agents, 633–634, 633*f*
chemotherapeutic agents, 629–634, 630*f*
drug resistance, 634
in gynecologic cancer, principles of, 618–636
new agents, evaluation of, 634–635, 635*t*
PARP inhibitors, 634
platinum analogues, 629–630
principles and guidelines of, 628
regimens, for intermediate- and high-risk gestational trophoblastic disease, 765*t*
results, evaluation of, 732
taxanes, 630
topoisomerase I and II inhibitors, 631–632
vinca alkaloids, 632–633
Chief complaint, 127
Children, vaginal tumors of, 672–673
endodermal sinus tumor, 672
pseudosarcoma botryoides, 673
sarcoma botryoides, 672, 672*f*
*Chlamydia trachomatis*, 534, 534*b*
Chloramphenicol, 9–12*t*
Cholinergic agents, for postoperative ileus, 580*t*
Choriocarcinoma, 745
Chorionic gonadotropin, 83
Chromophobe adenomas, 786
Chromosomal abnormalities, 30–34
numerical, 30–34, 31*f*, 32*t*
pregnancy outcome and, 34
structural, 32–34
contiguous gene syndromes, 34, 34*t*
microdeletion, 34, 34*t*
microduplication, 34
translocations, balanced reciprocal, 32–34, 33*f*
Chromosomal microarray, 40–41
Chronic anticoagulation and bleeding disorders, 555–558
cardiopulmonary comorbidities, assessment of, 557
cardiovascular disease, 557
pulmonary disease, 557
stress-dose steroids, 556, 556*t*
Chronic ectopic pregnancy, 348
Ciprofloxacin, 9–12*t*
Circumcision, female, 181–182, 181*f*
Cisapride, for postoperative ileus, 580*t*
Claim, 122–123, 123*b*
Clavulanic acid plus, 9–12*t*
Clear cell adenocarcinoma, 676
of vagina, 666*t*, 668*t*, 670, 671*f*
Clear cell carcinoma, 741
Clear cell tumors, 712, 713*f*
Cleavage, early, 3–8, 5*f*, 6*f*, 7*f*
Clindamycin, 9–12*t*
Clinical epidemiology, evidence-based medicine and, 106–115
Clitoral anomalies, 209, 209*f*, 210*f*
Clitoris, 49–50, 50*f*
Clomiphene citrate, for oligomenorrhea, 848–849, 849*f*
CNV. *see* Copy number variants (CNV)
$CO_2$ laser ablation, 644
Coagulopathy, 596–597
Cognitive behavior therapy, for menopause, 287
Coherent scattering, 620
Cohort studies, 109
Coitus-related methods, 251
Cold knife conization, 645
Collagen, menopause effects on, 266–267
Colonoscopy, for anal incontinence, 501
Colorectal cancer, 248, 280
Colpocleisis, 453–454
Colporrhaphy
anterior, 443, 444*f*, 445
posterior, 447
Colposcopy, 641–643, 643*f*
Combined contraceptives (CCs), 771
Common iliac artery, 63
Common iliac nodes, 65
Communication, 124, 125*b*
with patient, 118–119, 118*b*
through medical records, 121, 121*b*
Comparative effectiveness research (CER), 111–113, 112*f*
Complex atypical hyperplasia, 693, 693*f*
Complex hyperplasia, 693*f*
Complicated grief, 185
Comprehensive evaluations
aspectsadditional considerations, gynecologic care, 148–187
endoscopy, 188–206
examinations, physical, 127–139
histories, 127–139
hysteroscopy, 188–206
laparoscopy, 188–206
medical disease-physiology interaction, 140–147
preventive health care, 127–139
Compton effect, 620, 621*f*
Computed tomography, for breast cancer, 312
Condoms, male and female, 250, 250*f*

Congenital abnormalities, of reproductive tract, 207–220
cervix, 215
ovarian, 219
perineal and hymenal anomalies, 209–212
androgen insensitivity, 213–214
clitoral, 209, 209*f*, 210*f*
congenital adrenal hyperplasia, 210–211, 210*f*, 211*f*
embryology, 212
hymenal anomalies, 211–212, 211*f*, 212*f*
labial fusion, 209–212
Müllerian, 212–219
transverse vaginal septum, 214–215, 214*f*
vaginal adenosis, 215
vaginal agenesis, 213–214, 213*f*
uterus, 215–219, 215*f*, 216*f*, 217*f*
diagnosis, 218–219
imaging, 216, 218*f*
management, 219
symptoms and signs, 216–218
Congenital absence of uterus, 787, 787*f*
Congenital adrenal hyperplasia (CAH), 210–211, 210*f*, 211*f*, 817, 821
Congenital nipple inversion, 292
Congenital obstructive anomalies, 775
Consultation, with anesthesiologist, 548, 548*t*
Contact dermatitis, 369–370, 369*f*, 370*f*
Contiguous gene syndromes, 34, 34*t*
Continuous combined hormone treatment, endometrial cancer with, 277
Continuous urinary incontinence, 493
Contraception, 238–254, 239*t*
barrier methods, 249–250, 249*f*
birth control method apps, 250
breast cancer, 247–248
breastfeeding, 251–252
cancer prevention, 242
cervical cancer, 247
coagulation parameters, 248
coitus interruptus, 251
coitus-related methods, 251
colorectal cancer, 248
complications, 244
contraceptive patch, 248, 249*f*
counseling, 238
drug interactions, 244–245
effectiveness, 238–251, 240*t*, 241*f*
fertility awareness, 250
hormonal contraceptives, 244
infection, 244
initiation method, 239
injectable suspensions, 245–246, 246*f*
intrauterine devices, 242–245, 243*f*
lactational amenorrhea method, 250
liver adenoma, 248
long-acting reversible (LARC) methods, 242
male and female condoms, 250, 250*f*
mechanisms of action, 242–243
medical eligibility criteria, 238
neoplastic risks and benefits, 247
noncontraceptive health benefits, 245
oral contraceptives, 246–247
contraindications, 248
pain, 243
postpartum, 251
progestin-only pills, 248
safety, 244
Contraception *(Continued)*
spermicides, 251
sterilization, 239–242
subdermal implants, 244–245
surgical approach, 241–242, 242*f*
tubal sterilization, 239–242
uterine bleeding, 243
uterine perforation, 243
vaginal ring, 248–249, 249*f*
vasectomy, 239
Conventional external beam radiation, 624–625, 625*f*
Copy number variants (CNV), 24
Core needle biopsy, in breast cancer, 313
Cornual pregnancy, 346
Corpus luteum, 96
endocrine factors and, 96–98
Corpus luteum cysts, 399–400, 399*f*, 400*t*
Corpus luteum regression (luteolysis), 98
Cortical bone, 268
Cost-effectiveness analysis, 114–115
Cough stress test, 467–468
Crab louse, 516
Craniopharyngioma, 804
Cross-sectional studies, 108
Cryotherapy, 644
Cul-de-sac of Douglas, 71*f*, 74
clinical correlations, 75
Culdocentesis, 348–349
Cushing syndrome, 819
Cyclophosphamide, 631*t*
Cystadenofibroma, 406
Cystitis, 469–473
acute bacterial, 469–473, 472*f*
interstitial, 473–477, 474*t*, 475*f*, 476*b*
urethral diverticulum, 477–479, 478*f*
Cystocele, 441–443, 442*f*
*Cystosarcoma phyllodes*, 295
Cystourethroscopy, 468–469, 470*b*
Cysts, 364–365, 364*f*
Cytokines, 609–610
adaptive immunity, 610
chemokines, 609
colony-stimulating factors, 610
hematopoiesis, 610
innate immunity, 609–610
interferons, 609–610
interleukins, 609
Cytoreduction, secondary, 734–735


## D


Dactinomycin, 631*t*
Danazol
administration route of, 422
for endometriosis, 420
for fibrocystic change, 297
Data registry studies, 113–114
“Date rape,” 177
DCIS. *see* Ductal carcinoma in situ (DCIS)
Death and dying, 186–187
Decidual cast, 349, 349*f*
Decidualization, 9–10
Deep femoral nodes, 66
Deep vein thrombosis, 569–572, 569*b*, 570*f*, 570*t*, 571*t*
Defecography, for anal incontinence, 504–505
Degenerative arthritis, menopause and, 271
Dehiscence and evisceration, 584–586, 585*f*, 585*t*, 586*t*, 587*f*
Delayed menarche, 781–783, 782*f*, 782*t*, 783*f*, 784*f*, 785*f*
Denosumab, for osteoporosis, 271
Department of Justice, 182
“Dependent clingers,” 166
Depression, 148–151, 149*b*, 149*t*, 150*t*
Dermatologic diseases, 369–375
Behçet disease, 372
contact dermatitis, 369–370, 369*f*, 370*f*
edema, 373–375, 374*b*, 374*f*
hidradenitis suppurativa, 372–373, 373*f*
lichen planus, 371, 372*f*
pruritus, 369
psoriasis, 370–371, 371*f*
seborrheic dermatitis, 371
DES. *see* Diethylstilbestrol (DES)
Descensus, 443
Desensitization, GnRH receptor, 81–82, 82*f*
Detrusor hyperactivity with impaired contractile function (DHIC), 488
Detrusor instability, 488
DHIC. *see* Detrusor hyperactivity with impaired contractile function (DHIC)
DHT. *see* 5α-Dihydrotestosterone (DHT)
Diabetes
mellitus, 331
PCOS and, 831
*Diagnostic and Statistical Manual*, Fifth Edition (DSM-5), for eating disorders, 151
Diaphragm, 68–70
clinical correlations of, 71–72
Diaphragmatic stripping/resection, 726–727
Diethylstilbestrol (DES)
exposure, leading to ectopic pregnancy, 345
“Difficult” patients, 166–168
Digital mammography, 311
5α-Dihydrotestosterone (DHT), 814
Dilation and curettage, for ectopic pregnancy, 352
Dilation and evacuation method, abortion, 252–253
Direct observations, before speaking to patient, 127
Discharge instructions and postoperative visits, 592
Disorder of sexual development (DSD), 207–208
Diuretics, 780
DNA mismatch repair genes, 613–614
Docetaxel, 630, 631*t*
Domestic violence, 182
Dominant follicle
growth of, 93–94, 95*f*, 96*f*, 97*f*
selection of, 93, 94*f*
Donor in vitro fertilization, 870
Donovanosis, 520–521, 521*f*
Dose intensity, in chemotherapy, 628
Dose-dense chemotherapy, 731–732
Doxorubicin, 629
Doxycycline, 9–12*t*
Drug resistance, 634
in chemotherapy, 628
DSD. *see* Disorder of sexual development (DSD)
Dual-energy x-ray absorptiometry (DEXA) scans, for osteopenia, 268

DUB. *see* Dysfunctional uterine bleeding (DUB)
Ductal carcinoma in situ (DCIS), 313–314
Duloxetine, for stress urinary incontinence, 482
Dysesthetic vulvodynia, 373–375
Dysfunction, sexual, 170–171, 174*f*
Dysfunctional uterine bleeding (DUB), 594
Dysgerminomas, 744–745, 744*f*
Dysmenorrhea, 768
  incidence and epidemiology, 768–769, 769*t*
  menstruation and menstrual cycle, relationship to, 769
  primary, 769–773, 769*f*, 770*f*, 771*t*, 772*f*
  secondary, 773–774, 773*b*, 774*f*
Dysontogenetic cysts, 376–377, 376*f*, 377*f*
Dyspareunia, 173, 173*b*, 173*f*
Dysthymic disorder, 150

## E

Early cleavage, 3–8, 5*f*, 6*f*, 7*f*
Early mobilization, for postoperative ileus, 580*t*
"Easy" Gram-negative ampicillin, 9–12*t*
Eating disorders, 151–154, 152–153*b*, 152*b*
Ebb phase, 562
Ectopic endometrial tissue, 773–774
Ectopic pregnancy, 342–361
  contraception failure and, 345
    intrauterine device, 345
    in vitro fertilization, 346
    ovarian stimulation, 345–346
    tubal sterilization, 345, 345*f*
  differential diagnosis of, 350
  epidemiology of, 342–343
  etiology of, 343–346
  factor contributing to, 343, 343*t*
  histopathology of, 348–349, 349*f*
  hormonal alterations and, 345
  infertility, 360
  management of, 353–360
    abdominal pregnancy, 355
    cervical pregnancy, 355
    cesarean scar pregnancy, 356
    interstitial pregnancy, 355, 356*f*
    ovarian pregnancy, 355
    persistent, 356–360, 357*f*, 357*t*, 358*b*, 358*t*, 359*f*
    tubal pregnancy, 353–355, 355*f*, 356*f*
  mortality of, 343
  procedures used for diagnostic evaluation of, 350–353, 353*f*, 354*f*
    dilation and curettage, 352
    human chorionic gonadotropin, 350–351, 350*f*
    progesterone, 351, 351*f*
    ultrasonography, 351–352, 351*f*, 352*f*
  ruptured, 348–349
  signs of, 350–353
  sites of, 346–348, 346*f*, 347*f*, 348*f*
  subsequent fertility, 360–361, 360*f*
  symptoms of, 349, 349*f*
  tubal pathology leading to, 344–345, 344*f*
    diethylstilbestrol exposure, 345
    endometriosis, 344*f*
    ectopic pregnancy, history of, 345
    salpingitis isthmica nodosa, 344*f*
    surgery, 344–345
Ectropion, 135
Edema, 373–375, 374*b*, 374*f*
Eflornithine cream 13.9%, 822
Electrical stimulation therapy, for anal incontinence, 509–510
  anal plugs, 510
  devices, 510
  percutaneous tibial nerve stimulation, 510
  stem cells, 510
Electrolysis, 822
Electromyography, for anal incontinence, 502–504
Embryo-endometrial communication, 10
Embryogenesis and fertilization, 1–20
  blastula stage, 5–8, 8*f*
  crossover and female aneuploidy, 3
  early cleavage, 3–8, 5*f*, 6*f*, 7*f*
  early organogenesis, 10–11
  genitourinary system, development of, 11
    bladder and urethra development, 11, 12*f*
    genital development, 13*f*, 14*f*, 15*f*
    renal development, 11
  implantation, 8–11, 9*t*
    decidualization, 9–10, 10*f*
    embryo-endometrial communication, 10
    immunology of, 10
  morula stage, 5–8, 8*f*
  oocyte and meiosis, 1–3, 2*f*, 3*b*, 3*f*, 4*f*
  sex differentiation, 13–18
    external genitalia, 16–18, 18*f*, 19*f*
    genital development, 13–14, 13*f*, 14*f*, 15*f*
    genital duct system, 14–16, 16*t*, 17*f*
Embryology, 212
Embryonal carcinomas, 745
Embryonal rhabdomyosarcoma, of vagina, 672, 672*f*
Emergency contraception, 251
Empty sella syndrome, 804, 804*f*
Endoanal ultrasound, for anal incontinence, 501, 503*f*, 504*f*
Endocervical polyps, 378–379, 378*f*, 379*f*
Endocrine disease, 144–145
Endocrinology and infertility
  adenomas, pituitary, 803
  amenorrhea, primary *vs.* secondary, 781, 810–823
  androgen excess, 810–823
  dysmenorrhea, primary *vs.* secondary, 768–780
  galactorrhea, 802–803, 802*f*
  hyperprolactinemia, 801–809
  infertility, 838–860
Endodermal sinus tumor, of vagina, 232, 672
Endometrial adhesions, 329*f*
Endometrial bleeding, 598, 598*f*
  treatment of, 600–601
Endometrial cancer, 276–277
  immunotherapy and, 615
  oncogenes, 615
  tumor suppressor genes, 614–615
Endometrial carcinoma, 691, 694–704
  chemotherapy, 703
  clinical factors, 696
  evaluation of, 698
  histologic types, 694–696, 694*b*, 695*f*, 696*f*
  hormone therapy, 703
  immunotherapy, 703–704
  management of, 699–700, 701*t*
Endometrial carcinoma *(Continued)*
  pathologic factors, 696–698, 697*f*, 697*t*, 698*t*, 699*f*, 699*t*, 700*t*
  prognostic factors, 696–698
  risk factors, 692*b*
  spread of, patterns of, 698
  staging of, 696, 696*t*
  symptoms, signs, and diagnosis, 694
  targeted therapy, 703
Endometrial hyperplasia, 693–694
  diagnosis and endometrial sampling, 694
  hyperplasia with atypia, 693*f*
  hyperplasia without atypia, 693, 693*f*
  management of, 694
  natural history of, 694
Endometrial polyps, 328–329, 381–383, 384*f*, 595
Endometrial stromal sarcoma, 705
Endometrioid tumors, 712, 712*f*, 742
Endometriomas, 423–424
  of ovary, 403–404, 404*f*
Endometriosis, 344*f*, 367–368, 409–427, 773
  associated with ovarian cancer, 418–419
  clinical diagnosis of, 416–418
  clinical findings of, 417–418
  diagnostic laparoscopy of, 417–418, 418*f*
  endometrial biopsy, 417
  etiology of, 410–416
  extra pelvic, 427, 427*f*
  gastrointestinal tract, 425–426, 425*f*
  genetic predisposition of, 413, 414*b*
  gonadotropin-releasing hormone agonists, 420–421, 421*f*
  iatrogenic dissemination of, 411
  imaging of, 417, 417*f*
  immunologic changes of, 411–413, 411*b*, 412*f*, 413*f*, 414*f*
  lymphatic and vascular metastasis and, 411
  markers of, 418–419
  medical therapies for, 420
  metaplasia and, 410–411, 411*f*
  nonsteroidal antiinflammatory drugs, 422
  oral contraceptives, 421–422
  at other sites, 422, 425–426
  pathology of, 413–416, 414*f*, 415*f*, 415*t*, 416*f*
  retrograde menstruation and, 410, 410*f*
  route of administration, 422
  subfertility, therapy for, 424–425, 424*f*, 425*f*
  surgical management, 423
    endometriomas, 423–424, 423*f*
    fertility, 423–424
  surgical therapy for, 422–423
  symptoms of, 416–417
  treatment of, 419–425, 419*f*
    hormonal, 422
  urinary tract, 426, 426*f*
  vaginal adenocarcinomas in, 671–672
Endometritis, 534
Endometrium
  menstrual cycle and, 99–102, 99*f*
  in proliferative (follicular) phase, 99–100, 100*f*
  in secretory (luteal) phase, 100–101, 101*f*
β-Endorphin, 80
Endoscopy, 188–206
  adnexal pathology, 202
    risk-reducing, 202

Endoscopy *(Continued)*
gynecologic laparoscopy, 197–200
accessory port placement, 200
enhanced recovery after surgery, 198
indications for, 197
operating room setup, 198
port placement, 198–200, 198*f*, 199*f*
preparation for, 197–198
single-site surgery and vnotes, 200
surgical site infection, 198
gynecologic surgery, triple aim, 205, 205*b*
hand-assisted laparoscopy, 200–202
anesthesia, 200
endometriosis, 201–202, 202*f*
hysterectomy, 201, 201*f*
myomectomy, 201
procedures, 201–202
surgical management, ectopic pregnancy, 202
surgical principles, 200, 200*f*
hysteroscopy, 190–197
cervical stenosis, 195
complications, 196–197, 196*t*
endometrial ablation, 195–196, 196*b*
equipment, 191–192, 192*f*, 193*f*
fluid management, 192
indications, 190–191, 190*f*, 191*b*, 191*f*
International Federation of Gynecology and Obstetrics, 196*f*
intrauterine polyp, 194*f*
minimal impact technique, 192–195
myomectomy, 195
office-based hysteroscopy, 192–195, 194*b*
paracervical block, 194–195
polypectomy, 195
procedures, 195–196
smaller caliber hysteroscopes, 194
uterine perforation, 195
vaginoscopy, 195
laparoscopy
in pregnancy, 203–204, 204*f*
robotics in, 204–205
oncology, 203
pelvic inflammatory disease, 202–203
pelvic prolapse, 203
preoperative decision making, 189–190
imaging options, 189–190, 190*f*
ultrasound, 189
simulation, 205
specimen removal, 203–205, 203*f*
sterilization, 202
Enhanced recovery, 548–550, 549*t*
Enteral nutrition, early, for postoperative ileus, 580*t*
Enterocele, 450–451
diagnosis of, 450, 450*f*, 451*f*
management of, 450
McCall culdoplasty, 451
recurrent enterocele, 451
surgical enterocele repair, 450, 451, 452*f*
"Entitled demanders," 166
Ephrin family, ligands and receptors, 612
Epidemiology, clinical, 106–115
Epidermal growth factor receptor family, 611
Epidural anesthesia, for postoperative ileus, 580*t*
Epigenetic variation, 24
Epithelial ovarian neoplasms, 710–713, 711*f*, 711*t*, 712*f*, 713*f*, 713*t*
adnexal mass and ovarian cancer, 714–741, 714*b*
carcinomas, 717–720
diagnosis, staging, spread, preoperative evaluation, and prognostic factors, 717–720, 717*t*, 718*f*, 719*f*, 719*t*, 720*f*, 721*f*
complications and other considerations, 740–741
ovarian cancer screening, 715–717, 716*t*
treatment of, 720–741
advanced-stage ovarian cancer, 725
borderline ovarian tumors, 711*f*, 711*t*, 712*f*, 720–722, 721*f*, 722*f*
early-stage ovarian carcinomas, 723–725
frontline treatment strategies, alterations in, 728–733
invasive epithelial carcinomas, 722–723
platinum-refractory disease, 733–740
postoperative therapy for advanced epithelial carcinomas, 728
primary cytoreductive surgery, 725–728
Epithelial ovarian tumors, 710, 711*t*
EROS-CTD, 172
Ertapenem, 9–12*t*
Erythromycin, for postoperative ileus, 580*t*
Estradiol, 89
positive feedback loop, 90–91
Estradiol-17β, 90
Estrogen
for acute bleeding, 602–603
GnRH receptor and, 81
lower urinary tract and, 482
resistance, 786
use of, breast cancer and, 277–280, 279*f*, 280*t*, 281*f*
Etoposide, 631*t*, 632
Evaluations, comprehensive
additional considerations, gynecologic care, 148–187
endoscopy, 188–206
examinations, physical, 127–139
histories, 127–139
hysteroscopy, 188–206
laparoscopy, 188–206
medical disease-physiology interaction, 140–147
preventive health care, 127–139
Evidence-Based Enhanced Recovery after Surgery (ERAS) Protocol for Gynecologic Surgery Patients, 549*t*
Evidence-based medicine
clinical epidemiology and, 106–115
comparative effectiveness research, 111–113, 112*f*
evidence-based guideline development, 111–112
meta-analyses, 111–112
patient-centered outcomes research institute, 113
pragmatic clinical trials, 112–113
systematic reviews, 111–112
health services research, 113–115
cost-effectiveness analysis, 114–115
data registry studies, 113–114
quality improvement, 114
Evidence-based medicine *(Continued)*
statistical interpretation, 110–111, 111*f*
traditional clinical study design, 107–111, 107*t*
case-control studies, 108–109, 108*f*
case reports, 107–108
case series, 107–108
cohort studies, 109
cross-sectional studies, 108
experimental studies, 109–110
observational studies, 107–109
randomized controlled trials, 109–110
value in health care, 115
Examinations, physical, 127–139, 128*b*, 545–546
abdominal, 132, 132*f*
breast, 131–132, 132*b*
components of, 130–137, 131*t*
histories and, 127–139
family, 130, 130*f*
general health, 129–130
gynecologic history, pertinent, 128–129, 129*b*, 129*t*
occupational, 130
of present illness, 127–128, 128*b*
social, 130
for special populations, 139
pelvic, 132–137
bimanual, 135–136, 136*f*
inspection, 132, 133*f*
palpation, 132–134, 133*f*, 134*f*
Papanicolaou smear, 135, 135*t*, 136*f*
rectal, 137
rectovaginal, 136, 137*f*
speculum, 134–135, 134*f*
physical, 130–131
Excisional biopsy, in breast cancer, 313
Exercise, 156
Expanded-spectrum carbenicillin, 9–12*t*
Experimental studies, 109–110
External genitalia, 16–18, 18*f*, 48–50
Bartholin glands, 50, 51*f*
clinical correlations for, 50–51, 51*f*
clitoris, 49–50, 50*f*
hymen, 49
labia majora, 49
labia minora, 48, 49*f*
mons pubis, 48
pelvis innervation, 68, 68*f*
Skene glands, 50
urethra, 50
vestibular bulbs, 50
vestibule, 50
vulva, 48, 49*f*
External iliac nodes, 65, 65*f*
Extra pelvic endometriosis, 427, 427*f*

# F

Factor V Leiden, 333
Falling hemoglobin, management of, 562
Fallopian tube, and peritoneal carcinoma, 750–752
causes of, 750
clinical findings of, 750–751
diagnosis of, 750–751
CA-125 level, 751
imaging modalities in, 751
ultrasound for, 750

Fallopian tube, and peritoneal carcinoma
*(Continued)*
pathologic findings of, 751–752, 751*f*
prognosis in, 752
staging, 750–751
treatment of, 752
Fallopian tube carcinoma, 751, 751*f*
cause of, 750
clinical findings of, 751
pathologic findings of, 751–752
Familial ovarian cancer, 709–710
Family history, 130, 130*f*
Fat necrosis, of breast, 299
Fecal incontinence (FI), 495, 496*b*
Fecundability, 838, 839*f*, 839*t*, 840, 845–846, 847*f*, 849
Female circumcision, 181–182, 181*f*
Female genital ducts, 14–16, 16*t*, 17*f*. *see also* Genital duct system
Female pattern hair loss (FPHL), 822–823
Female reproductive concepts
basic science
anatomy, reproductive, 47–75
embryogenesis, 1–20
epidemiology, clinical, 106–115
evidence-based medicine, 106–115
fertilization, 1–20
risk management, medical-legal, 116–126
endocrinology and infertility
adenomas, pituitary, 803
amenorrhea, primary *vs.* secondary, 781–800
androgen excess, 810–823
dysmenorrhea, primary *vs.* secondary, 768–780
galactorrhea, 802–803, 802*f*
hyperprolactinemia, 801–809
infertility, 838–860
evaluations, comprehensive
additional considerations, gynecologic care, 148–187
endoscopy, 188–206
examinations, physical, 127–139
histories, 127–139
hysteroscopy, 188–206
laparoscopy, 188–206
medical disease-physiology interaction, 140–147
preventive health care, 127–139
general gynecology
adolescent patients, 221–237
anal incontinence, 495–514
benign gynecologic lesions, 362–408
breast diseases, 289–322
ectopic pregnancy, 342–361
endometriosis, 409–427
genital tract infections, 515–542
lower urinary tract, function and disorders of, 461–494
mature woman, care of, 255–288
menopause, 255–288
pediatric patients, 221–237
pelvic organ prolapse, 428–460
preoperative counseling and management, 543–558
reproductive tract, congenital abnormalities of, 207–220
Female reproductive concepts *(Continued)*
oncology
fallopian tube, and peritoneal carcinoma, 750–752
gestational trophoblastic disease, 754–767
lower genital tract, intraepithelial neoplasia of, 637–647
malignant diseases of cervix, 674–690
malignant diseases of ovary, 707–753
malignant diseases of uterus, 691–706
malignant diseases of vagina, 648–673
neoplastic diseases of vulva, 648–673
radiation therapy, principles of, in gynecologic cancer, 618–636
Femoral hernia, 430
Femoral nerve, 588
Fertility, subsequent, prognosis for, 360–361, 360*f*
Fertility preservation, 871
Fertility-sparing surgery, 682–683
Fertilization and embryogenesis, 1–20
blastula stage, 5–8, 8*f*
crossover and female aneuploidy, 3
early cleavage, 3–8, 5*f*, 6*f*, 7*f*
early organogenesis, 10–11
genitourinary system, development of, 11
bladder and urethra development, 11, 12*f*
genital development, 13*f*, 14*f*, 15*f*
renal development, 11
implantation, 8–11, 9*t*
decidualization, 9–10, 10*f*
embryo-endometrial communication, 10
immunology of, 10
morula stage, 5–8, 8*f*
oocyte and meiosis, 1–3, 2*f*, 3*b*, 3*f*, 4*f*
sex differentiation, 13–18
external genitalia, 16–18, 18*f*, 19*f*
genital development, 13–14, 13*f*, 14*f*, 15*f*
genital duct system, 14–16, 16*t*, 17*f*
Fetal aneuploidy, 327
Fever, 561
FHA. *see* Functional hypothalamic amenorrhea (FHA)
Fibroadenomas, 294, 295*f*
Fibrocystic change, 295–297, 296*f*, 297*f*
Fibroids, 328. *see also* Leiomyomas
Fibroma, 366, 366*f*, 748
FIGO. *see* International Federation of Gynecology and Obstetrics (FIGO)
Figure eight rash, 227
Finasteride, 821
Fine-needle aspiration (FNA), in breast cancer, 313
Fistulas, rectovaginal, 512–513, 513*t*
Fletcher-suit applicator, 623
Fluconazole, 9–12*t*
Fluoride, for osteoporosis, 271
5-Fluorouracil (5-FU), 631*t*, 632, 656
Flutamide, 821
FMR1. *see* Fragile X mental retardation 1 (FMR1)
Follicle-stimulating hormone (FSH), 83
Follicular cysts, 397–399, 398*f*
Follicular phase, of menstrual cycle, 92–94
Folliculogenesis, ovarian, 83, 84*f*
Foreign bodies, in prepubertal children, 231–232
46 XY gonadal dysgenesis, 785
FPHL. *see* Female pattern hair loss (FPHL)
Fractional cell kill
in chemotherapy, 628
in radiation, 619
Fragile X mental retardation 1 (FMR1), 27
Fragile X syndrome, 27–28
Fraud, 123
Frozen embryo transfer, 870–871
FSH. *see* Follicle-stimulating hormone (FSH)
Functional bowel disease, relation to, in secondary dysmenorrhea, 775
Functional hyperprolactinemia, 804
Functional hypothalamic amenorrhea (FHA), 790–791, 791*f*
Functional/idiopathic hyperandrogenism, 816
Functional test, for sperm, 847

## G

Gabapentin, for menopause, 286
GAD. *see* Generalized anxiety disorder (GAD)
Galactorrhea, 802–803, 802*f*
Gametogenesis, ovarian, 83
Gastrointestinal complications, 576–583
antibiotic-associated diarrhea, 582–583, 582*t*
ileus, 578–579, 579*t*, 580*t*, 581*t*
intestinal obstruction and adhesions, 579–582, 581*t*
postoperative diet, 576–577
postoperative nausea and gastrointestinal function, 577–578, 577*t*, 578*t*
rectovaginal fistula, 582
Gastrointestinal disease, 143–144
Gastrointestinal tract considerations, 550
Gastrointestinal tract endometriosis, 425–426, 425*f*
Gatifloxacin, 9–12*t*
Gemcitabine, 631*t*, 632
Gene therapy, for ovarian cancer, 740
General gynecology
adolescent patients, 221–237
anal incontinence, 495–514
benign gynecologic lesions, 362–408
breast diseases, 289–322
ectopic pregnancy, 342–361
endometriosis, 409–427
genital tract infections, 515–542
lower urinary tract, function and disorders of, 461–494
mature woman, care of, 255–288
menopause, 255–288
pediatric patients, 221–237
pelvic organ prolapse, 428–460
preoperative counseling and management, 543–558
reproductive tract, congenital abnormalities of, 207–220
General health history, 129–130
Generalized anxiety disorder (GAD), 158
Genetic abnormalities, diagnostic techniques for, 38–44
chromosomal microarray, 40–41, 43*t*
invasive prenatal diagnostic tests, 38–39, 39*f*, 40*f*
molecular genetic analysis techniques, 39–40, 41*f*, 42*f*, 43*f*
preimplantation genetic testing, 43
sequencing, 43–44

Genetic predisposition, of endometriosis, 413, 414*b*
Genetic variation, 24
Genetics, reproductive, 44–45, 44*t*
building blocks of, 22–24
epigenetic variation, 24
genomic variation, 24
mitosis/meiosis, 22
molecular, 22, 23*f*
cancer genome sequencing, 45
diagnosis, ethical considerations of, 45–46
disease basis of, 22, 23*t*
malignancies of, 44–45
pathology of, 24–34, 24*f*
chromosomal abnormalities, 30–34
mendelian inheritance patterns, 25–27
multifactorial inheritance, 29–30, 29*t*
nonmendelian inheritance patterns, 27–29, 27*t*
single gene disorders, 25–30, 25*f*
perinatal, 34–44
abnormalities, diagnostic techniques for, 38–44
biochemical and sonographic screening, 37
cell-free DNA screening, 37–38, 38*t*
common diseases, carrier screening, 35–37
counseling and risk assessment, 35, 35*t*
testing of, 37–38
Genital development, 13*f*, 14*f*, 15*f*
Genital duct system, 14–16, 16*t*, 17*f*
Genital herpes, 519–520, 519*t*, 520*f*, 521*t*
Genital tract infections, 515–542
*Actinomyces* infection, 541
Bartholin glands, 516, 517*f*, 518*f*
cervicitis, 532–534
*Chlamydia Trachomatis*, 534, 534*b*
etiology, 533
mucopurulent cervicitis, 532–533, 532*f*, 533*f*
*Neisseria gonorrhoeae*, 533–534, 534*b*
treatment, 533
endometritis, 534
genital ulcers, 519–525
infections of vulva, 515–525
molluscum contagiosum, 517–519, 518*f*
pediculosis pubis and scabies, 516–517, 518*f*
pelvic inflammatory disease, 535–541
diagnosis, 536–538, 538*b*, 538*t*, 539*f*
etiology, 535–536, 535*f*, 536*t*
risk factors, 538–539
sequelae, 536, 536*f*, 536*t*, 537*t*
treatment, 539–541, 539*b*, 540*b*, 541*f*
toxic shock syndrome, 532
tuberculosis, 541
vaginitis, 525–532, 526*t*, 527*t*
bacterial vaginosis, 526–528, 528*f*, 529*t*
*Candida vaginalis*, 530–532, 530*f*, 531*f*, 532*b*
*Trichomonas* vaginal infection, 528–530, 529*f*
Genital ulcers, 519–525, 519*t*
chancroid, 522
genital herpes, 519–520, 519*t*, 520*f*, 521*t*
granuloma inguinale, 520–521, 521*f*
lymphogranuloma venereum, 521–522, 521*f*
syphilis, 522–525, 522*f*, 523*t*
follow-up, 524–525
latent-stage, 523
Genital ulcers *(Continued)*
primary, 523, 523*f*
secondary, 523, 524*f*
tertiary, 524, 525*f*
treatment, 524, 525*b*
Genital warts, 234–235, 235*f*
Genitalia
ambiguous, 207–212, 208*b*, 208*f*
external, 16–18, 18*f*, 48–50
Bartholin glands, 50, 51*f*
clinical correlations for, 50–51, 51*f*
clitoris, 49–50, 50*f*
hymen, 49
labia majora, 49
labia minora, 48, 49*f*
mons pubis, 48
Skene glands, 50
urethra, 50
vestibular bulbs, 50
vestibule, 50
vulva, 48, 49*f*
internal, 51–53
cervix, 53–58, 54*f*, 55*f*, 56*f*
ovaries, 61–62, 61*f*, 62*f*
oviducts, 58–60, 60*f*, 61*f*
uterus, 56–59, 57*f*, 58*f*, 59*f*
vagina, 51–53, 52*f*, 53*f*
Genitourinary system, development of, 11
bladder and urethra development, 11, 12*f*
genital development, 13*f*, 14*f*, 15*f*
renal development, 11
Genomic imprinting and uniparental disomy, 28
Genomic variation, 24
Gentamicin, 9–12*t*
Germ cell tumors, 710, 713*t*, 742–747, 743*f*
granulosa-theca cell tumors, 747–748, 747*f*
specialized, 747
teratomas, 743–745, 743*b*
treatment, 745–747
Germline mosaicism, 28
Gestational trophoblastic disease, 754–767, 755*b*
gestational trophoblastic neoplasia, 760–767
hydatidiform mole, 755–760, 756*f*, 757*f*, 757*t*, 758*f*, 759*f*
Gestational trophoblastic neoplasia, 760–767
characteristics of, 760–761
clinical features of, 761, 761*b*
histopathology and cytogenetic features, 760–761
classification and staging of, 761–762, 762*t*
diagnosis of, 762–763
malignant, 761
treatment of, 763–764
centralization of care, 766–767
high-risk gestational trophoblastic neoplasia, 764, 764*b*, 765*t*
low-risk gestational trophoblastic neoplasia, 763, 764*b*
placental site trophoblastic tumor and epithelioid trophoblastic tumor, 766
pregnancy after, 766
psychosocial considerations, 766
resistant/recurrence, 765–766
surveillance after, 766
ultra-high-risk gestational trophoblastic neoplasia, 765
Glassy cell carcinoma, 676–677, 677*f*
Glucocorticoids, 822
Glycopeptides, 9–12*t*
GnRH agonists, 82
GnRH analogues, GnRH receptor and, 82
GnRH antagonists, 82
GnRH-R. *see* Gonadotropin-releasing hormone receptor (GnRH-R)
Gonadal failure, 783–784
Gonadal streak, 784, 785–786, 785*f*
Gonadoblastomas, 747
gynandroblastomas, 749
Leydig cell tumors, 749
Sertoli-Leydig cell tumors, 748–749, 749*f*
sex cord tumors with annular tubules, 749
thecomas and fibromas, 748
Gonadotrophin-releasing hormone agonist, 602
Gonadotropin receptors, 83–84, 85*f*
Gonadotropin-releasing hormone (GnRH), 76–81, 77*f*, 848
neuronal system of, 77, 78*f*
olfactory system and, in early fetal life, 76
pulsatility
mechanisms responsible for, 77–79, 79*f*
modulatory influences on, 79–80
pulse generator of, 77, 79*f*
release of
metabolic influences and, 80–81
pulse frequency and, 80
transport of, to anterior pituitary, 77, 78*f*
Gonadotropin-releasing hormone agonists, 780
for endometriosis, 420–421, 421*f*
Gonadotropin-releasing hormone receptor (GnRH-R), 81–82
activation of, 81
desensitization, 81–82
estrogens and, 81
GnRH analogs and, 82, 83*b*
GnRH pulse frequency and gonadotropin release, 81
Gonadotropin-resistant ovary syndrome, 792
Gonadotropins, 83
for infertility, 201*f*, 850–853, 851*f*
structure of, 83
Goodall-Power modification, of Le Fort operation, 454
Granular cell myoblastoma, 368
of vulva, 664–665
Granulation tissue, 588
Granuloma inguinale, 520–521, 521*f*
Granulosa-theca cell tumors, 747–748, 747*f*
Great dermatologic imitator, 516
Grief, 185–186
Gynandroblastomas, 749
Gynecologic cancer, 606–617
adaptive immunity, 608–609
B cells and immunoglobulins, humoral immunity, 608, 608*f*
T cells, cellular immunity, 608–609, 609*f*
cervical cancer, 616
cytokines, 609–610
adaptive immunity, 610
chemokines, 609
colony-stimulating factors, 610
hematopoiesis, 610
innate immunity, 609–610
interferons, 609–610
interleukins, 609

Gynecologic cancer *(Continued)*
endometrial cancer
immunotherapy and, 615
oncogenes, 615
tumor suppressor genes, 614–615
immunologic response, 606–611
immunotherapy, 610–611
innate immunity, 607, 607*f*
molecular oncology, 611–614
oncogenes, 611–614, 611*t*
peptide growth factors, 611–614
ovarian cancer
immunotherapy, 616
oncogenes, 616
tumor suppressor genes, 615–616
tumor cell killing, 610–611
Gynecologic care, 148–187
abuse, 182–185
elderly, 185
intimate partner violence, 182–185, 183*b*, 184*b*
anxiety disorders, 158–162
death and dying, 186–187
depression, 148–151, 149*b*, 149*t*, 150*t*
Patient Health Questionnaire (PHQ-9), 148–149
psychotherapies for, 151
suicide and, 151
treatment goal for, 150–151
"difficult" patients, 166–168
eating disorders, 151–154, 152–153*b*, 152*b*
female circumcision, 181–182, 181*f*
grief and loss, 185–186
lesbian, gay, bisexual, and transgender (LGBT) health care, 175–176, 176*b*
obesity, 154–155*t*, 154–158, 155*t*, 156*f*
additional considerations, 157–158
in adolescents, 157
bariatric surgery, 157
diet, 155–156
exercise, 156
management, 155
pharmacologic interventions, 156–157, 157*t*
obsessive-compulsive disorder, 158–162
oral contraceptives, 162
posttraumatic stress disorder, 158–162
psychotropic medications, 162
rape, 176–182
date, 177
emotional support of, 180–181
medical responsibility, 177–179, 178*f*, 179*b*
medicolegal, 180, 180*t*
physician's responsibility in, 177–180, 177*b*
pregnancy, 179–180
sexual assault, 176–185
sexual function, 168–174, 168*b*, 168*f*, 169*f*, 170*f*
and dysfunction, 170–171, 174*f*
dyspareunia, 173, 173*b*, 173*f*
genito-pelvic pain penetration disorders, 172–174
menopause, 170
orgasmic disorders, 174, 175*t*
sexual interest/arousal disorders, 171–172, 171*f*
sexual response, 170
substance use disorders, 162–166, 163*b*, 164*b*, 165*b*
Gynecologic history, essence of, 127–130
chief complaint, 127
family, 130, 130*f*
general health, 129–130
history of present illness (HPI), 127–128, 128*b*
nutritional/dietary assessment, 130
occupational, 130
pertinent, 128–129
cervical cancer screening, 129
contraception, 129
gynecologic infections, 128–129, 129*t*
menstrual, 128
pelvic pain, 129
pregnancy, 128
sexual history, 129, 129*b*
surgical procedures, 129
review of systems (ROS), 130
safety issues, 130
social, 130
Gynecologic laparoscopy, 197–200
accessory port placement, 200
enhanced recovery after surgery, 198
indications for, 197
operating room setup, 198
port placement, 198–200, 198*f*, 199*f*
preparation for, 197–198
single-site surgery and vnotes, 200
surgical site infection, 198
Gynecologic Oncology Group Performance Status Scale, 635*t*
Gynecologic surgery, triple aim, 205, 205*b*
Gynecological concepts
basic science
anatomy, reproductive, 47–75
embryogenesis, 1–20
epidemiology, clinical, 106–115
evidence-based medicine, 106–115
fertilization, 1–20
risk management, medical-legal, 116–126
endocrinology and infertility
amenorrhea, primary *vs.* secondary, 781–800
androgen excess, 810–823
dysmenorrhea, primary *vs.* secondary, 768–780
galactorrhea, 802–803, 802*f*
hyperprolactinemia, 801–809
infertility, 838–860
evaluations, comprehensive
additional considerations, gynecologic care, 148–187
endoscopy, 188–206
examinations, physical, 127–139
histories, 127–139
hysteroscopy, 188–206
laparoscopy, 188–206
medical disease-physiology interaction, 140–147
preventive health care, 127–139
general gynecology
adolescent patients, 221–237
anal incontinence, 495–514
benign gynecologic lesions, 362–408
breast diseases, 289–322
ectopic pregnancy, 342–361
endometriosis, 409–427
Gynecological concepts *(Continued)*
genital tract infections, 515–542
lower urinary tract, function and disorders of, 461–494
mature woman, care of, 255–288
menopause, 255–288
pediatric patients, 221–237
pelvic organ prolapse, 428–460
preoperative counseling and management, 543–558
reproductive tract, congenital abnormalities of, 207–220
oncology
fallopian tube, and peritoneal carcinoma, 750–752
gestational trophoblastic disease, 754–767
lower genital tract, intraepithelial neoplasia of, 637–647
malignant diseases of cervix, 674–690
malignant diseases of ovary, 707–753
malignant diseases of uterus, 691–706
malignant diseases of vagina, 648–673
neoplastic diseases of vulva, 648–673
radiation therapy, principles of, in gynecologic cancer, 618–636
Gynecology
additional considerations, 148–187
adolescent, 221–237
office visit and examination, 224–226
ovary and adnexa in, 235–237
pediatric, 221–237
general approach, 222
hymen, normal findings of, 224
ovary and adnexa in, 235–237
performance exam, 222–224, 223*f*, 224*f*
vagina, normal findings of, 224
visit and examination, 222–232


## H


Hair removal techniques, in androgen excess, 822
Hamster egg penetration assay, 846–847
Hand-assisted laparoscopy, 200–202
anesthesia, 200
endometriosis, 201–202, 202*f*
hysterectomy, 201, 201*f*
myomectomy, 201
procedures, 201–202
surgical management, ectopic pregnancy, 202
surgical principles, 200, 200*f*
"Hateful patients," 166
Health services research (HSR), 113–115
"Heartsink" patients, 166
Hemangioma, 366
Hematologic diseases, 144–145
Hematomas, 368–369, 368*f*, 568
Hematometra, 383–384
Hemoperitoneum, 346
Hemorrhagic shock, 565–568, 566*b*, 567*f*, 567*t*, 568*f*
Hepatic resection, 727
Hermaphrodite, 209
Hernias, abdominal wall, 428–431, 429*f*, 430*f*
diagnosis of, 430–431
etiology of, 429–430
management of, 431
incisional hernia, 431
umbilical hernia repair, 431

Hernias, abdominal wall *(Continued)*
signs of, 430–431
symptoms of, 430–431
Herpes, genital, 519–520, 519*t*, 520*f*, 521*t*
Heterosexual/virilizing precocious puberty, 797
Heterotopic pregnancy, 347–348
H-hCG. *see* Hyperglycosylated hCG (H-hCG)
Hidradenitis suppurativa, 372–373, 373*f*
Hidradenoma, 367, 367*f*
High-grade squamous intraepithelial lesion, 641, 642*f*
High-risk gestational trophoblastic neoplasia, 764, 764*b*, 765*t*
Hilus cell tumors, 820
Hirsutism, follow-up for treatment of, 822
Histories, 127–139
family, 130, 130*f*
general health, 129–130
gynecologic
essence of, 127–130
pertinent, 128–129, 129*b*, 129*t*
occupational, 130
of present illness, 127–128, 128*b*
social, 130
for special populations, 139
History of present illness (HPI), 127–128, 128*b*
Hobnail cells, 712, 713*f*
Hormonal suppression, 779–780
Hormone responsive element (HRE), 88
Hot flushes, 286
Hourglass rash, 227
Hox genes, 787
HPI. *see* History of present illness (HPI)
HRE. *see* Hormone responsive element (HRE)
HSR. *see* Health services research (HSR)
Human chorionic gonadotropin, 758
for ectopic pregnancy, 350–351, 350*f*
Human papillomavirus, 637
Human papillomavirus therapy, 649, 651*f*
*Human Sexual Response*, 168
Hydatidiform mole, 755–760
clinical features of, 757–758, 757*t*
diagnosis of, 758, 758*f*
epidemiology of, 755
histopathology and cytogenetic features, 755–757, 756*f*, 757*f*, 757*t*
risk factors of, 755
age, 755
diet, 755
genetics, 755
reproductive history, 755
treatment of, 758–760
hysterectomy for, 758–759
phantom β-HCG, 760
pituitary β-HCG, 760
prophylactic chemotherapy for, 759–760, 759*f*
quiescent GTD, 760
suction dilation and curettage for, 758
surveillance following hydatidiform mole evacuation, 760
Hydrops tubae profluens, 751
17α-hydroxylase deficiency, with 46, XX karyotype, 788
Hymen, 49
in evaluation of sexual abuse, 234, 235*f*
prepubertal child, normal findings of, 224
Hymenal anomalies, 211–212, 211*f*, 212*f*
Hyperglycosylated hCG (H-hCG), 9
Hyperplastic dystrophy, of vulva, 651*f*
Hyperprolactinemia, 331, 801–809
causes of, 803–806, 803*b*
central nervous system disorders, 804
hypothalamic causes, 804
pituitary causes, 804, 804*f*, 805*f*
prolactinomas, 804–806
Hypertensive diseases, 143–144
Hyperthermic intraperitoneal chemotherapy (HIPEC), 729–730
Hypertrichosis, 810
Hypoactive sexual desire disorder, 171
Hypogastric artery (internal iliac artery), 63
Hypogonadotropic hypogonadism, 786
Hypophyseal portal vessels, 77
Hypothalamic dysfunction, 790
Hypothalamic-pituitary dysfunction, 793
Hypothalamic-pituitary-ovarian endocrine axis, communication with, 88–91
Hypothalamus, 76–81
anatomy of, 76–77
nuclear organization of, 78*f*
physiology of, 77–81
Hysterectomy, 568
apical prolapse after, 456–459
Hysteroscopy, 190–197
cervical stenosis, 195
complications, 196–197, 196*t*
endometrial ablation, 195–196, 196*b*
equipment, 191–192, 192*f*, 193*f*
fluid management, 192
indications, 190–191, 190*f*, 191*b*, 191*f*
International Federation of Gynecology and Obstetrics, 196*f*
intrauterine polyp, 194*f*
minimal impact technique, 192–195
myomectomy, 195
office-based hysteroscopy, 192–195, 194*b*
paracervical block, 194–195
polypectomy, 195
procedures, 195–196
smaller caliber hysteroscopes, 194
uterine perforation, 195
vaginoscopy, 195

## I

Iatrogenic bleeding, 598
Iatrogenic dissemination, endometriosis and, 411
Iatrogenic/factitious precocious puberty, 797
ICSI. *see* Intracytoplasmic sperm injection (ICSI)
Idiopathic detrusor overactivity, 488
Idiopathic granulomatous lobular mastitis (IGLM), 298
Idiopathic granulomatous mastitis (IGM), 298
Idiopathic hirsutism, 815*f*, 816
IDSA. *see* Infectious Disease Society of America (IDSA)
IGLM. *see* Idiopathic granulomatous lobular mastitis (IGLM)
IGM. *see* Idiopathic granulomatous mastitis (IGM)
Ileus, 578–579, 579*t*, 580*t*, 581*t*
Imipenem, cilastatin, 9–12*t*
Immature teratomas, 744
Immune disease, 141–142, 141*b*, 142*t*, 143*t*
Immunology, of implantation, 10
Immunotherapy, 610–611
for ovarian cancer, 738–740
Implantation, 8–11, 9*t*
decidualization, 9–10, 10*f*
early organogenesis, 10–11
embryo-endometrial communication, 10
immunology of, 10
Induced abortion, 252, 252*f*
Innate immunity, 607, 607*f*
In vitro fertilization, 861–872, 862*b*
future developments, 872
indication for, 861–864
male factor infertility, 861–862, 862*f*
oocyte/embryo cryopreservation for fertility preservation, 863
preconception genetic screening and diagnosis, 863–864
unexplained infertility/reproductive aging, 862–863, 862*f*, 863*t*
procedure in, 864–866, 864*f*, 865*f*, 866*t*
gamete intrafallopian transfer and other alternatives to "traditional," 866
success rate, 866, 867–868*t*, 868*f*, 869*f*
risk of, 866–872
donor, 870
fertility preservation, 871
frozen embryo transfer, 870–871
ovarian and breast cancer risk after, 869
ovarian hyperstimulation syndrome, 866–869
ovarian tissue cryopreservation, 871–872
pregnancy complications, 869, 869*t*
preimplantation genetic diagnosis/screening, 869–870, 870*f*
preimplantation genetic testing, 870
recurrent implantation failure, 871
Inability to void, 575
Incarcerated hernia, 429
Incisional hernia, 430, 431, 588
Inclusion cysts, 376
Indian hedgehog (Ihh) protein, 10
Inevitable abortion, 323
Infants, vaginal tumors of, 672–673
endodermal sinus tumor, 672
pseudosarcoma botryoides, 673
sarcoma botryoides, 672, 672*f*
Infection, 334, 583–584, 583*b*, 584*f*
contraception, 244
of lower urinary tract, 469–479
Infectious Disease Society of America (IDSA), 471
Inferior gluteal nodes, 65–66
Inferior mesenteric arteries, 62–63
Infertility, 838–860
additional testing, for couples presenting with, 846–847
immunologic factors in subfertility, 846
luteal deficiency, significance of, diagnosis of, 846
significance of infectious diseases in subfertility, 846
sperm, test of, 846–847
and age, 838–839, 839*t*

Infertility *(Continued)*
causes of, 839–840, 840*f*
counseling and emotional support, 859–860
diagnostic evaluation of, 840–847, 840*f*
documentation of ovulation, 841
endometriosis, 857
evaluation and laboratory tests, 842–846, 843*f*
blood testing for, 844
hysterosalpingography, 844–845, 844*f*, 845*f*
laparoscopy for, 845–846
postcoital test, 845
ultrasound in, 842, 843*f*
fecundability, 838, 839*f*, 839*t*, 840, 845–846, 847*f*, 849
history of, diagnosis in, 360
incidence of subfertility and, 838
male factor of, 853–855
male evaluation, 853–855, 853*f*, 854*f*
metformin and other insulin sensitizers, 849–850, 850*f*
gonadotropin-releasing hormone, 853
gonadotropins, 850–853, 851*f*, 852*f*
letrozole, 850, 850*f*, 851*f*
natural conception, 838, 839*f*, 839*t*
ovarian hyperstimulation syndrome, 852–853, 852*b*
pregnancy in women undergoing various treatments, outcomes of, 859
prognosis of various diagnoses uncovered by, 847–848, 847*f*, 848*f*
semen analysis, 841, 841*t*
therapeutic modalities, 853
ovarian electrocauterization, 853
weight and lifestyle management, 853
treatment of, causes of, 848–859
anovulation and subovulatory function, medical treatment for, 848–853
clomiphene citrate, 848–849, 849*f*
unexplained, 857–859, 857*t*, 858*f*, 859*f*, 859*t*
uterine cause of, 855–857
adjunctive therapy, 856–857
distal tubal disease, 856
intrauterine adhesions/synechiae, 855
leiomyoma, 855
proximal tubal blockage, 856
tubal causes of infertility, 855–856, 856*f*
tuberculosis, 855, 855*f*
Infiltrating lobular carcinoma, 314, 315*f*
Inflammatory breast cancer, 314–315, 315*f*
Inflammatory disease, of breast, 298
Inguinal hernia, 428
Inherited thrombophilias, 333–334, 334*b*
Inhibins, 91
Injectable suspensions, 245–246, 246*f*
Innervation, of pelvis, 66–68
clinical correlations of, 68
Inspection, pelvic examination, 132, 133*f*
Insulin resistance, 331
PCOS and, 827–829, 828*f*, 828*t*, 829*f*
Insulin sensitizers, 822
Insulin tolerance test, 793
Intermittent parathyroid hormone (PTH), for osteoporosis, 271
Internal anal sphincter (IAS), 496*t*, 504*f*
Internal endometriosis, 409
Internal genitalia, 51–53
cervix, 53–58, 54*f*, 55*f*, 56*f*
ovaries, 61–62, 61*f*, 62*f*
oviducts, 58–60, 60*f*, 61*f*
uterus, 56–59, 57*f*, 58*f*, 59*f*
vagina, 51–53, 52*f*, 53*f*
Internal iliac nodes, 65
Internal pudendal artery, 63
International Federation of Gynecology and Obstetrics (FIGO)
Classification for Gestational Trophoblastic Neoplasia, 762*t*
Criteria for Diagnosis of Gestational Trophoblastic Neoplasia, 761*b*
Staging and Nodal Metastasis, 699*t*
staging system, 677, 678*t*
*International Statistical Classification of Diseases and Related Health Problems*, 296
Interstitial cystitis, 473–477, 474*t*, 475*f*, 476*b*
Interstitial pregnancy, management of, 355, 356*f*
Interval cytoreduction, 729
Intestinal obstruction and adhesions, 579–582, 581*t*
Intimate partner violence (IPV), 182–185, 183*b*, 184*b*
Intracellular molecular oxygen, 621–622
Intracytoplasmic sperm injection (ICSI), 847
Intraductal papilloma, 298–299
Intraepithelial neoplasia
of lower genital tract, 637–647
natural history of, 642–643
of vulva, 649–650, 650*f*, 651*f*
Intraperitoneal therapy, 730–731
Intrauterine adhesions (IUAs), 329–330, 789
causes of, 329*t*
in infertility, 855
sonohysterography of, 329*f*
Intravenous leiomyomatosis, 392, 392*f*
Intrinsic sphincter deficiency (ISD), 468, 486
Invasive ductal carcinoma, 314, 314*f*
Invasive prenatal diagnostic tests, 38–39
Inverse square law, 620*f*
IPV. *see* Intimate partner violence (IPV)
ISD. *see* Intrinsic sphincter deficiency (ISD)
Isodose curve, 626, 626*f*
Isolated gonadotropin deficiency, 786
Isolated polycystic ovaries, PCOS and, 835
IUAs. *see* Intrauterine adhesions (IUAs)


## J


Joint Commission, medical-legal risk management and, 124


## K


Kallmann syndrome, 76
Karnofsky Performance Status Scale, 634, 635*t*
Ketoconazole, 821–822
Keyes punch biopsy, 653, 653*f*
Kisspeptin, 77–79


## L


Labia majora, 49
Labia minora, 48, 49*f*
Labial adhesions, prepubertal children, 228–229, 228*f*
Labial fusion, 209–212
Laboratory and preoperative diagnostic procedures, 546–547, 546*f*
Lacerations, cervical, 379
β-Lactamase inhibitor combination, 9–12*t*
Lactating breast, 290*f*
Lactational amenorrhea method, 250
*Lactobacillus*, 526
Laparoscopic extraperitoneal paraaortic lymphadenectomy, 680
Laparoscopic radical surgery, 682
Laparoscopic surgery, for postoperative ileus, 580*t*
Laparoscopy. *see also* Gynecologic laparoscopy
in pregnancy, 203–204, 204*f*
robotics in, 204–205
Late-onset 21-hydroxylase deficiency, 817–819, 818*f*, 818*t*, 819*f*
treatment of, 821
Late-onset congenital adrenal hyperplasia (LOCAH), 817
Laxatives, for postoperative ileus, 580*t*
Le Fort – type colpocleisis, 459
Leber hereditary optic neuropathy (LHON), 29
Leiomyomas, 329, 384–393, 385*f*, 386*f*, 387*f*, 388*f*, 595–596, 597*f*
heavy menstrual bleeding, therapies for, 390
in infertility, 855
medical treatment, future options for, 390, 391*t*
minimally invasive interventions for, 392–393, 392*f*, 393*f*
uterine artery embolization, 390–392, 391*f*
Leiomyomatosis peritonealis disseminata (LPD), 392
Leiomyosarcoma, 704–705, 704*f*
Leptin, 781–782
Lesbian, gay, bisexual, and transgender (LGBT) health care, 175–176, 176*b*
Letrozole, 631*t*
Leukemia inhibitory factor (LIF), 9–10
Leukoplakia, of vulva, 651–652
Leuprolide acetate, 631*t*
Levofloxacin, 9–12*t*
Levonorgestrel-releasing intrauterine system (LNG-IUS), 600, 601*f*
Leydig cell tumors, 749
LGBT health care. *see* Lesbian, gay, bisexual, and transgender (LGBT) health care
LGV. *see* Lymphogranuloma venereum (LGV)
LH. *see* Luteinizing hormone (LH)
LHON. *see* Leber hereditary optic neuropathy (LHON)
Lichen planus, 371, 372*f*
*Lichen sclerosus*
in prepubertal children, 229–230, 230*f*
of vulva, 649–650, 650*f*
LIF. *see* Leukemia inhibitory factor (LIF)
Ligaments, 69–70
clinical correlations of, 71–72
Linezolid, 9–12*t*
Lipid tumors, 749
Lipoma, 366–367, 367*f*
Liposomal doxorubicin, 631, 631*t*
Liver metastases, 765

Lobular carcinoma in situ (LCIS), 314
LOCAH. *see* Late-onset congenital adrenal hyperplasia (LOCAH)
Local progestogen exposure, 600–601, 601*f*
Local trauma, 378
Locus, 24
Long-acting reversible (LARC) methods, 242
Lower genital tract, intraepithelial neoplasia of, 637–647
Lower urinary tract
 anatomy and physiology (female continence), 462–465, 465*f*, 466*f*
 diagnostic procedures, 465–469
  bladder diary, 466, 467*f*
  cough stress test and pad weight test, 467–468
  cystourethroscopy, 468–469, 470*b*, 470*f*
  office cystometrics, 466–467
  residual urine/postvoid residual, 466
  urinalysis and culture, 465–466
  urodynamics, 468, 469*f*
 function and disorders of, 461–494
 infections of, 469–479
  acute bacterial cystitis, 469–473, 472*f*
  bladder pain syndrome (interstitial cystitis), 473–477, 474*t*, 475*f*, 476*b*
  urethral diverticulum, 477–479, 478*f*
 micturition, physiology of, 461–465
  neurophysiology, 461–462, 462*f*, 463*f*, 463*t*, 464*t*
 urgency urinary incontinence/overactive bladder, 483*t*, 486–493
 urinary incontinence, 479–486
  evaluation of, 481–485
  intrinsic sphincter deficiency, 486
  mesh risks, 485–486
  postoperative voiding trial, 486
  risk factors, 479*b*, 480*f*
  stress, 480
  surgical management, autologous fascia pubovaginal sling, 486, 487*f*
  surgical procedure selection, 486
  treatment, 481–485, 482*f*, 483*f*, 483*t*, 484*f*, 485*f*
Low-grade serous carcinoma, 741–742
Low-grade squamous intraepithelial lesion, 640–641, 641*f*
Low-risk gestational trophoblastic neoplasia, 763, 764*b*
LPD. *see* Leiomyomatosis peritonealis disseminata (LPD)
Lupus anticoagulant, 333
Luteal deficiency, significance of, diagnosis of, 846
Luteal phase, menstrual cycle, 96–98
Luteal-follicular transition, menstrual cycle, 99
Luteinizing hormone (LH), 3
Luteolysis, 98
Lymphadenectomy, 700
Lymphatic system, 65–66
 clinical correlations of, 66
Lymphocyst, 588
Lymphogranuloma venereum (LGV), 521–522, 521*f*
Lynch syndrome, 692–693
 malignancy and, 596

## M

Macroadenoma, 806
 radiation therapy for, 808
Macrolides, 9–12*t*
Magnetic resonance imaging (MRI)
 of anal sphincters, for anal incontinence, 501
 in breast cancer, 311–312, 312*f*
Major depression, 148–149. *see also* Depression
Major histocompatibility complex (MHC) class I molecules, 607
Male genital ducts, 14. *see also* Genital duct system
Molecular oncology, gynecologic cancer, 606–617
Malignancy, 596
Malignant bowel obstruction, 740–741
Malignant diseases, of vagina, 665–666*f*, 665–666, 666*t*
 detection and diagnosis, 666–667, 667*f*
 symptoms and diagnosis, 667–668, 668*f*, 668*t*
 treatment of, 667
Malignant effusions, 740
Malignant melanoma, of vagina, 670–671
Malignant mixed müllerian tumors, 704*b*, 705
Malpractice, 116
Mammary-like gland adenoma, 367, 367*f*
Mammography, 308–311, 310*f*, 311*f*
Manchester, 453
"Manipulative help-rejecters," 166
MAS. *see* McCune-Albright syndrome (MAS)
Mass spectrometry assays, 104
Mastalgia (breast pain), 297, 297*b*
Mastitis, 298
Matter, 619
Mature woman, care of, 255–288
McCall culdoplasty, 451
McCall stitch, 451
McCune-Albright syndrome (MAS), 796*t*, 797, 798*f*
 in prepubertal children, 230–231
Median eminence, 77
Medical disease-physiology interaction, 140–147
 allergic disease, 141–142, 141*b*, 142*t*, 143*t*
 cancer, 146–147
 central nervous system disease, 145–146
 endocrine disease, 144–145
 gastrointestinal disease, 143–144
 hematologic diseases, 144–145
 hypertensive diseases, 143–144
 immune disease, 141–142, 141*b*, 142*t*, 143*t*
 mental health issues, 146, 146*b*
 migraine headaches, 146
 pulmonary disease, 140–142, 141*b*
 renal disease, 144
 seizure disorders, 145–146, 145*t*
 thrombotic diseases, 144–145
 vascular diseases, 143–144
Medical-legal risk management, 116–126, 125*f*
 alteration of records, 121–122
 anticipation, 124
 cancellations and "no shows," 120
 CAP strategy, 124, 124*f*
 claim, 122–123, 123*b*
 communication, 124, 125*b*
Medical-legal risk management *(Continued)*
  consistent, with institutional policies, 122, 122*b*
  informed consent, 119
  informed refusal of care, 119
  with patient, 118–119, 118*b*
  postoperative care, 119
  surgical documentation, 119
  through medical records, 121, 121*b*
 coverage arrangements, 120
 fraud and abuse, 123
 historical perspective of, 117–118
 laboratory tests, 123–124
 malpractice, 116, 117*b*, 117*f*
 medication errors, 120–121
 patient reviews, responding to, 122
 poor outcome, 119–120, 120*b*
 practical insight of, 118–124
 preparation, 125
 procedures, closed claims, 116, 117*f*
 reproductive medicine and, 118
Medical records, 121, 121*b*
 alteration of, 121–122
Medication errors, 120–121
Medication method, abortion, 253
Medicolegal, 180, 180*t*
Meiosis and oocyte, 1–3, 2*f*, 3*b*, 3*f*, 4*f*
Meiosis/mitosis, 22
Melanoma
 of vagina, 666*t*
  malignant, 670–671
 of vulva, 663–664, 663*f*
Menarche, delayed, 781–783, 782*f*, 782*t*, 783*f*, 784*f*, 785*f*
Mendelian inheritance patterns
 autosomal dominant, 25, 25*f*
 autosomal recessive, 25–26, 26*f*
 non, 27–29, 27*t*
 X-linked trait, 26–27
Menopausal transition (perimenopause), 257–263, 258*f*, 259*f*
 types of ovarian changes during, 258–263, 259*f*, 260*f*, 261*f*
  hormonal changes, 260–263, 262*f*, 263*f*
Menopause, 170, 255–288, 256*t*
 alternative therapies for, 286–287, 286*b*
  acupuncture, 287
  antidepressants, 286
  antihypertensives, 286
  cognitive behavior therapy, 287
  gabapentin, 286
  phytoestrogens, 286, 287*f*
  stellate ganglion blockade, 287
 cardiovascular effects on, 271–275, 272*f*, 273*f*, 273*t*, 274*f*, 276*f*, 277*f*, 278*f*, 279*f*
 disease prevention after, 280–286, 282*t*, 283*f*
  androgen therapy, 285
  "bioidentical" therapy, 285–286
  hormone regimens, 282–285, 284*b*, 284*t*
  progestogen, use of, 285
  side effects and, 285
  TSEC concept, 286
 definition of, 255
 degenerative arthritis and, 271
 effects of, on various organ systems, 263–271
  bone health, 268–271, 268*f*, 269*f*, 269*t*, 270*f*, 270*t*

Menopause *(Continued)*
central nervous system, 263–266, 264b, 264f, 265f, 266f, 267f
collagen and other tissues, 266–267
genitourinary syndrome of menopause, 267, 267t
vulvovaginal atrophy, 267
hormonal changes with established, 260–263, 262f, 263f
PCOS and, 834–835
postmenopausal women, cancer risks, 275–280, 279f
breast cancer risk, with estrogen use, 277–280, 279f, 280t, 281f
colorectal cancer, 280
ovarian cancer, 280
premature ovarian insufficiency, 256–257, 256b
management, 257, 257f
Menstrual bleeding, therapies for, 390
Menstrual cycle, 91–99
cervical glands and, 102–104
endometrium and, 99–102
follicular phase, 92–94
luteal-follicular transition, 99
luteal phase, 96–98
ovulation, 94–96
ovulatory gonadotropin surge, 94–96
Menstrual irregularity, 818–819
Mental health conditions, in secondary dysmenorrhea, 775
Mental health issues, 146, 146b
Mental status changes, 591–592, 591b
Meropenem, 9–12t
Mesh, risk of, 485–486
Meta-analyses, 111–112
Metabolic syndrome, PCOS and, 831
Metabolism, of blood, ovarian steroids, 86–88
Metaplasia, 134–135
endometriosis and, 410–411, 411f
Metastases, ultra-high-risk sites of, 765
Metastatic ovarian tumors, 749–752, 749f
Metformin, for infertility, 849–850, 850f
gonadotropin-releasing hormone, 853
gonadotropins, 850–853, 851f, 852f
letrozole, 850, 850f, 851f
Methicillin, 9–12t
Methotrexate, 629, 631t, 632
Metoclopramide, for postoperative ileus, 580t
Metronidazole, 9–12t
Microadenoma, 804, 804f
Microdeletion, 83–88
Microduplication, 83–88
Microinvasion, 680
Micturition, physiology of, 461–465, 462f, 463f, 463t, 464t
Midurethral slings, 484–485, 484f, 485f
Migraine headaches, 146
Minimal deviation adenocarcinoma, 676
Minimally invasive surgery, 683
Minimally invasive gynecologic surgery, 188–206
adnexal pathology, 202
risk-reducing, 202
gynecologic laparoscopy, 197–200
accessory port placement, 200
enhanced recovery after surgery, 198
indications for, 197
Minimally invasive gynecologic surgery *(Continued)*
operating room setup, 198
port placement, 198–200, 198f, 199f
preparation for, 197–198
single-site surgery and vnotes, 200
surgical site infection, 198
gynecologic surgery, triple aim, 205, 205b
hand-assisted laparoscopy, 200–202
anesthesia, 200
endometriosis, 201–202, 202f
hysterectomy, 201, 201f
myomectomy, 201
procedures, 201–202
surgical management, ectopic pregnancy, 202
surgical principles, 200, 200f
hysteroscopy, 190–197
cervical stenosis, 195
complications, 196–197, 196t
endometrial ablation, 195–196, 196b
equipment, 191–192, 192f, 193f
fluid management, 192
indications, 190–191, 190f, 191b, 191f
International Federation of Gynecology and Obstetrics, 196f
intrauterine polyp, 194f
minimal impact technique, 192–195
myomectomy, 195
office-based hysteroscopy, 192–195, 194b
paracervical block, 194–195
polypectomy, 195
procedures, 195–196
smaller caliber hysteroscopes, 194
uterine perforation, 195
vaginoscopy, 195
laparoscopy
in pregnancy, 203–204, 204f
robotics in, 204–205
oncology, 203
pelvic inflammatory disease, 202–203
pelvic prolapse, 203
preoperative decision making, 189–190
imaging options, 189–190, 190f
ultrasound, 189
simulation, 205
specimen removal, 203–205, 203f
sterilization, 202
Mirtazapine, for depression, 150–151
Missed abortion, 323
Mitochondrial inheritance, 28–29
Mitogen-activated protein kinase (ERK), 81
Mitosis/meiosis, 22
Mixed carcinomas, 675b
Mixed germ cell tumors, 745
specialized, 743b
treatment of, 745–747
Mixed urinary incontinence, 491–493
Miyazaki hook ligature carrier, 457
Modified Classification of Uterine Sarcomas, 704b
Modified radical hysterectomy, 681
Mole, 365
Molecular building blocks, 22, 23t
Molecular genetic analysis techniques, 39–40, 42f
Molluscum contagiosum, 517–519, 518f
Monobactams, 9–12t
Mons pubis, 48
Morula stage, 5–8, 8f
Mosaicism, definition of, 28
Moxifloxacin, 9–12t
Mucinous borderline tumors, 712f, 722
Mucinous carcinoma, 742
Mucinous tumors, 711–712, 712f
Mucopurulent cervicitis, 532–533, 532f, 533f
Müllerian adenosarcoma, 705
Müllerian anomalies, 212–219
duct development, 212–215
Müllerian tubercle, 212
Multifactorial inheritance, 29–30
Multimodality therapy, for postoperative ileus, 580t
Mutation, 86
*Mycoplasma genitalium*, 532
Myelosuppression, 629
Myolysis, 392

## N

NAAT. *see* Nucleic acid amplification testing (NAAT)
Nabothian cysts, 134–135, 379
Nafcillin, 9–12t
Nasogastric tube, for postoperative ileus, 577t
NASPAG. *see* North American Society of Pediatric and Adolescent Gynecology (NASPAG)
Natural killer cells, 332
Negative steroid feedback loop, 89–90
*Neisseria gonorrhoeae*, 533–534, 534b
Neoadjuvant chemotherapy, 685, 728–729
Neonatal ovarian cysts, 236
Malignant diseases of uterus, 691–706
endometrial carcinoma, 691, 694–704
endometrial hyperplasia, 693–694
epidemiology of, 691–693, 692b, 692f
sarcomas, 704–705, 704b
of vulva, 649
malignant conditions, 657–665, 657b, 657f, 658b, 658f, 659f, 659t, 660f, 661f, 663f, 664f
vulvar atypias, 649–656, 649b, 650f, 651f, 652f, 653f, 654f
Neosphincters, 512
Nerve-sparing radical hysterectomy, 682
Netilmicin, 9–12t
Neurogenic detrusor overactivity, 488
Nevus, 365–366, 365f
Nipple
congenital developmental abnormalities of, 292
discharge in, 298, 299f
Nocturnal enuresis, 493
Nongenital pelvic organs, 72–74
Nongynecologic causes, pelvic pain, 775
Non-Mendelian inheritance patterns, 27–29, 27t
fragile X syndrome, 27–28
genomic imprinting and uniparental disomy, 28
germline mosaicism, 28
mitochondrial inheritance, 28–29
trinucleotide-repeat disorders, 27
Nonpelvic recurrence, 688

Non-steroidal anti-inflammatory drugs (NSAIDs), 335, 601–602, 601*t*, 770–771, 771*t*
for endometriosis, 422
for postoperative ileus, 580*t*
Nonverbal clues, 127, 128*b*
Norfloxacin, 9–12*t*
North American Society of Pediatric and Adolescent Gynecology (NASPAG), 230
NovaSure radiofrequency electricity system, 604
NSAIDs. *see* Non-steroidal anti-inflammatory drugs (NSAIDs)
Nucleic acid amplification testing (NAAT), 134, 528
Numerical chromosomal abnormalities, 30–32, 31*f*

## O

OAB. *see* Overactive bladder (OAB)
Obesity, 154–155*t*, 154–158, 155*t*, 156*f*, 335
in adolescence, 157
malignancy and, 596
PCOS and, 831
urinary incontinence and, 479
Observational studies, 107–109
Obsessive-compulsive disorder (OCD), 158–162
OCD. *see* Obsessive-compulsive disorder (OCD)
Office cystometrics, 466–467
Office of Victims of Crime, 180
Ofloxacin, 9–12*t*
Olfactory system, GnRH system and, 76
Oligomenorrhea, 594
Omphalocele, 430
Oncology
fallopian tube, and peritoneal carcinoma, 750–752
gestational trophoblastic disease, 754–767
lower genital tract, intraepithelial neoplasia of, 637–647
malignant diseases of cervix, 674–690
malignant diseases of ovary, 707–753
malignant diseases of uterus, 691–706
malignant diseases of vagina, 648–673
neoplastic diseases of vulva, 648–673
radiation therapy, principles of, in gynecologic cancer, 618–636
Oocyte and meiosis, 1–3, 2*f*, 3*b*, 3*f*, 4*f*
Oogenesis, 1
Oogonia, 1
Operative site complications, 586
granulation tissue, 588
incisional hernia, 588
lymphocyst, 588
pelvic cellulitis and abscess, 586
postoperative neuropathy, 588–589, 589*f*
prolapsed fallopian tube, 588
Opiate antagonists, for postoperative ileus, 580*t*
Optimistic, 866
Oral contraceptives, 162, 246–247
contraindications, 248
steroids, 821
Orgasmic disorders, 174, 175*t*
Osteopenia, dual-energy x-ray absorptiometry scans for, 268
Osteoporosis, menopause and, 266–267
Ovarian abnormalities, 219
Ovarian and adrenal tumors, 820
Ovarian and breast cancer risk, after in vitro fertilization, 869
Ovarian artery, 63
Ovarian cancer, 280, 708, 709*f*, 709*t*
endometriosis associated with, 418–419
immunotherapy, 616, 739*t*
oncogenes, 616
screening, 715–717, 716*t*
tumor suppressor genes, 615–616
Ovarian cysts
in children and adolescents, 236
neonatal, 236
prenatal, 235–236
Ovarian folliculogenesis, 83
Ovarian gametogenesis (oogenesis), 83
Ovarian hyperstimulation syndrome, 852–853, 852*b*, 866–869
Ovarian morphology, 811*f*, 812*f*, 814*f*, 815–819
Ovarian neoplasms, 817
classification of, 710, 710*t*
epithelial, 710–713, 711*f*, 711*t*, 712*f*, 713*f*, 713*t*
adnexal mass and ovarian cancer, 714–741, 714*b*
carcinomas, 717–720, 717*t*, 718*f*, 719*f*, 719*t*, 720*f*, 721*f*
complications and other considerations, 740–741
ovarian cancer screening, 715–717, 716*t*
treatment of, 720–741
Ovarian pregnancy, 345–346
management of, 355
Ovarian remnant syndrome, 407, 407*f*
Ovarian reserve, 92
Ovarian steroids, 84–86
Ovarian tissue cryopreservation, 871–872
Ovarian torsion, 236
Ovarian tumors, 796*t*
in children and adolescents, 236–237
Ovarian-hypothalamic-pituitary feedback loops, 88–91
Ovary, 61–62, 61*f*, 62*f*
in adolescent patient, 235–237
anatomy of, 83
benign gynecologic lesions, 397–407
benign neoplasms, 401–407
functional cysts, 397–401
malignant diseases of, 707–753, 710*t*
epithelial ovarian neoplasms, 710–713, 711*f*, 711*t*, 712*f*, 713*f*, 713*t*
familial ovarian cancer, 709–710
germ cell tumors, 710, 713*t*, 742–747, 743*f*
gonadoblastomas, 747
lipid tumors, 749
metastatic ovarian tumors, 749–752, 749*f*
sex cord-stromal tumors, 747–749
small cell carcinoma, 742
in pediatric patient, 235–237
physiology of, 83–88
Overactive bladder (OAB), 483*t*, 486–493
diagnosis of, 488
etiology, 488
mixed urinary incontinence, 491–493
other types, urinary incontinence, 493
treatment of
Overactive bladder (OAB) *(Continued)*
behavioral, 488
pharmacologic, 488–489, 489*t*
procedures, 489–491, 490*f*, 491*f*, 491*t*
Overflow incontinence, 493
Oviducts, 58–60, 60*f*, 61*f*
benign gynecologic lesions, 395–397
adenomatoid tumors, 395, 395*f*
leiomyomas, 395
paratubal cysts, 395–396, 396*f*
torsion, 396–397, 396*f*
Ovulation, 94–96
Ovulatory dysfunction, 597–598
treatment of, 600
Ovulatory gonadotropin surge, 94–96
Oxacillin, 9–12*t*

## P

Paclitaxel, 628, 630, 631*t*
carboplatin backbone and, 730, 730*f*, 731*t*
Pad weight test, 467–468
Paget disease, 315, 315*f*
of vulva, 651, 652*f*
Pain control protocols, 593.e13
Pain relief, 589–590, 589*f*, 590*f*, 590*t*
Pair production, 620–621
PALM-COEIN Classification System, 594, 595*f*
Panic disorder, 158, 159
Papanicolaou smear, 135, 135*t*, 136*f*
Papillary, 715
Paraaortic node involvement, 686
Parametria, 74
Pararectal spaces, 74–75
Paratubal cysts, 395–396, 396*f*
Parauterine nodes, 66
Paravesical spaces, 74–75
Partner abuse, 182
Paternal uniparental disomy, 28
Patient-Centered Outcomes Research Institute (PCORI), 113
Patient education and informed consent, 547–548
Patient Health Questionnaire (PHQ-9), 148–149
PCORI. *see* Patient-Centered Outcomes Research Institute (PCORI)
PCOS. *see* Polycystic ovary syndrome (PCOS)
PCS. *see* Pelvic congestion syndrome (PCS)
Pediatric patients, 221–237
general approach for, 222
hymen, normal findings of, 224
ovarian cysts in, 236
ovarian tumors in, 236–237
ovary and adnexa in, 235–237
performance exam, 222–224, 223*f*, 224*f*
vagina, normal findings of, 224
visit and examination, 222–232
Pediculosis pubis, 516–517, 518*f*
Pelvic cellulitis and abscess, 586
Pelvic congestion syndrome (PCS), 774
Pelvic diaphragm, 68–69
Pelvic examination, 132–137
bimanual, 135–136, 136*f*
inspection, 132, 133*f*
palpation, 132–134, 133*f*, 134*f*
Papanicolaou smear, 135, 135*t*, 136*f*

Pelvic examination *(Continued)*
rectal, 137
rectovaginal, 136, 137*f*
speculum, 134–135, 134*f*
Pelvic exenteration, 688
Pelvic floor muscle strengthening, for stress urinary incontinence, 481–482, 481*b*
Pelvic inflammation, 774
Pelvic inflammatory disease, 535–541
diagnosis of, 536–538, 538*b*, 538*t*, 539*f*
etiology of, 535–536, 535*f*, 536*t*
risk factors of, 538–539
sequelae, 536, 536*f*, 536*t*, 537*t*
treatment of, 539–541, 539*b*, 540*b*, 541*f*
Pelvic node dissection, 681–683
Pelvic organ prolapse (POP), 431–445, 433*f*
anterior vaginal wall prolapse, 441–443, 442*f*
anatomy, 434–435, 435*f*, 436*f*
conservative management of, 440–441
complications, 441
expectant management, 440
pelvic floor strengthening, 440
pessaries, 440–441, 440*f*
pregnancy, 441
surgery, 441
topical vaginal estrogen, 440
enterocele, 450–451
epidemiology, 431–434, 434*b*, 434*f*
measurement, 437–438, 438*f*
pathophysiology, 435, 436*f*, 437*f*
posterior vaginal wall prolapse (rectocele), 445–446
diagnosis, 445–447, 447*f*
management, 446
perineorrhaphy, 447–449, 449*f*
posterior colporrhaphy, 447, 448*f*
posterior repairs, 446–447
recurrent, 449
site-specific posterior repair, 447, 449*f*
symptoms and signs, 445
quantification of, 438–439, 439*f*, 440*b*
rectal prolapse, 459
symptoms, 435–437, 437*b*
uterine prolapse, 451–456, 452*f*
cervical elongation, 453
fertility-sparing surgery, 454–456, 455*f*
management, 451
obliterative prolapse procedures, 453–454, 453*f*, 454*f*
surgery for, 451–453
symptoms and signs, 451
vaginal vault prolapse (apical prolapse after hysterectomy), 456–459, 456*f*, 458*f*, 459*f*
Pelvic organ prolapse quantitative, 438–439, 439*f*, 440*b*
Pelvic recurrence, 687–688
Pelvic tuberculosis, 541
Pelvis
innervation of, 66–68
vascular system of, 62–64
Penicillin G, 9–12*t*
Peptides, ovarian feedback loops, 91
Perimenopause, 257–263, 258*f*, 259*f*
types of ovarian changes during, 258–263, 259*f*, 260*f*, 261*f*
hormonal changes, 260–263, 262*f*, 263*f*
Perineal anomalies, 209–212
Perineal scars, surgical correction of, 654*f*
Perineorrhaphy, 447–449, 449*f*
Perioperative management, of complications, 559–593, 560*f*
cardiovascular problems, 565
deep vein thrombosis, 569–572, 569*b*, 570*f*, 570*t*, 571*t*
hematomas, 568
hemorrhagic shock, 565–568, 566*b*, 567*f*, 567*t*, 568*f*
pulmonary embolism, 568–575, 572*t*, 573*f*, 574*f*
retained foreign body, 568
superficial thrombophlebitis, 569
thrombophlebitis and pulmonary embolus, 568–575
discharge instructions and postoperative visits, 592
falling hemoglobin, management of, 562
gastrointestinal complications, 576–583
antibiotic-associated diarrhea, 582–583, 582*t*
ileus, 578–579, 579*t*, 580*t*, 581*t*
intestinal obstruction and adhesions, 579–582, 581*t*
postoperative diet, 576–577
postoperative nausea and gastrointestinal function, 577–578, 577*t*, 578*t*
rectovaginal fistula, 582
operative site complications, 586
granulation tissue, 588
incisional hernia, 588
lymphocyst, 588
pelvic cellulitis and abscess, 586
postoperative neuropathy, 588–589, 589*f*
prolapsed fallopian tube, 588
postoperative fever, 561–562, 561*t*
psychological sequelae, 589–592
mental status changes, 591–592, 591*b*
pain relief, 589–590, 589*f*, 590*f*, 590*t*
postoperative concerns, in older surgical patients, 591, 591*b*
psychosexual problems and depression, 591
respiratory complications, 562
atelectasis, 562–564, 563*f*, 563*b*
pneumonia, 564–565, 564*b*
sleep apnea, 565
urinary tract problems, 575–576
inability to void, 575
ureteral injury and urinary fistula, 575–576, 576*f*
urinary tract infection, 575
wound complications, 583–586
dehiscence and evisceration, 584–586, 585*f*, 585*t*, 586*t*, 587*f*
infection, 583–584, 583*b*, 584*f*, 587*f*, 587*t*
obesity, 586, 587*b*
Peritoneal carcinoma
cause of, 750
clinical findings of, 750–751
pathologic findings of, 752
Persistent depressive disorder, 150
Persistent ectopic pregnancy
management of, 356–360, 357*f*
expectant, 359–360, 359*f*
medical treatment for, 357–359, 357*t*, 358*b*, 358*t*, 359*f*
Pertinent gynecologic history, 128–129, 129*b*, 129*t*
Pessaries, 440–441, 440*f*
for stress urinary incontinence, 480
PGD. *see* Preimplantation genetic diagnosis (PGD)
Phantom β-human chorionic gonadotropin, 760
Phosphoinositide 3-kinase pathway, 612
Photodisintegration, 621
Photoelectric effect, 620
Photoepilation, 822
PHQ-9. *see* Patient Health Questionnaire (PHQ-9)
Phyllodes tumors, 295, 295*f*
Physical examinations, 127–139, 128*b*, 545–546
abdominal, 132, 132*f*
breast, 131–132, 132*b*
components of, 130–137, 131*t*
histories and, 127–139
family, 130, 130*f*
general health, 129–130
gynecologic history, pertinent, 128–129, 129*b*, 129*t*
occupational, 130
of present illness, 127–128, 128*b*
social, 130
for special populations, 139
pelvic, 132–137
bimanual, 135–136, 136*f*
inspection, 132, 133*f*
palpation, 132–134, 133*f*, 134*f*
Papanicolaou smear, 135, 135*t*, 136*f*
rectal, 137
rectovaginal, 136, 137*f*
speculum, 134–135, 134*f*
Physiologic discharge, prepubertal children, 229
Phytoestrogens, for menopause, 286, 287*f*
Pilosebaceous unit, 810
Piperacillin, 9–12*t*
Pituitary adenomas, 803
Pituitary destruction, 793
Pituitary gland, anterior, 81–83
anatomy of, 81
physiology of, 81–83
PKC. *see* Protein kinase C (PKC)
Platelets, disorders of, 596
Platinum analogs, 629–630
Platinum sensitivity, 634
Platinum-refractory disease, 733–740
Platinum-resistant disease, 733, 734*t*
Platinum-sensitive disease, 733–734, 735*t*
Pleural effusions, 740
PMDD. *see* Premenstrual dysphoric disorder (PMDD)
Pneumonia, 564–565
POF. *see* Premature ovarian failure (POF)
Poly (ADP-ribose) polymerase inhibitors, 737–738, 739*t*
Polycystic ovary syndrome (PCOS), 331, 790, 816, 824–837
antimüllerian hormone, 829, 829*f*
cancers in, 832–834, 834*f*
cardiovascular concerns, 832, 833*f*, 833*t*, 834*f*
characteristic endocrine findings in, 826–827, 826*f*, 827*f*

Polycystic ovary syndrome (PCOS) *(Continued)*
consequences of, 831, 832*f*
definition of, 824–825, 825*t*
diabetes, 831
diagnosis of, in adolescents, 825
Doppler ultrasound, 825*f*
hyperandrogenism/androgen excess, 826
insulin resistance, 827–829, 828*f*, 828*t*, 829*f*
isolated, 835
menopause and, 834–835
menstrual irregularity, 825–826
metabolic and weight concerns, 836, 836*t*
ovarian morphology of, 825, 825*f*
pathophysiologic considerations, 829–831, 830*f*, 831*f*
quality-of-life issues, 832
subfertility in, treatment of, 835–836, 835*f*, 836*f*
treatment of, 821–823, 835
weight gain/obesity and metabolic syndrome, 831
Polyembryomas, 745
Polymastia, 292–293
Polyploidy, 30
POP. *see* Pelvic organ prolapse (POP)
Portio vaginalis, 134–135
Portland Continuous Intravenous Insulin Protocol (Version 2001), 593.e7
Postcoital test, 845
Postdischarge nausea and vomiting, 578
Posterior vaginal wall prolapse (rectocele), 445–446
diagnosis of, 445–447, 447*f*
management of, 446
perineorrhaphy, 447–449, 449*f*
posterior colporrhaphy, 447, 448*f*
posterior repairs, 446–447
recurrent, 449
site-specific posterior repair, 447, 449*f*
symptoms and signs of, 445
Postmenopausal women, cancer risk in, 275–280, 279*f*
breast cancer risk, with estrogen use, 277–280, 279*f*, 280*t*, 281*f*
colorectal cancer, 280
ovarian cancer, 280
Postoperative concerns, in older surgical patients, 591
Postoperative diet, 576–577
Postoperative fever, 561–562, 561*t*
workup for, 561
Postoperative nausea and gastrointestinal function, 577–578, 577*t*
Postoperative neuropathy, 588–589, 589*f*
Postoperative voiding trial, 486
Postpill amenorrhea, 789–790
Posttraumatic stress disorder (PTSD), 158–162
Prader-Willi syndrome (PWS), 38
Pragmatic clinical trials, 112–113
Precocious puberty, 781–800, 794*f*, 795*t*
diagnostic evaluation, 797, 798*f*, 799*t*
gonadotropin-releasing hormone-dependent precocious puberty, 796–797
CNS lesions, 797
idiopathic, 796–797
primary hypothyroidism, 797
Precocious puberty *(Continued)*
gonadotropin-releasing hormone-independent precocious puberty, 797, 798*f*
premature pubarche/adrenarche, 795–796
premature thelarche, 795, 796*f*
treatment of, 798–799, 799*f*
types of disorders, 795–797, 796*t*
Predecidual stromal cells, 101
Pregnancy, complications related to, adverse effects of IUD, 244
Preimplantation genetic diagnosis (PGD), 8
risk of, 869–870, 870*f*
Premature adrenarche, 796*t*
Premature ovarian failure (POF), 256–257, 256*b*, 784, 792
management of, 257, 257*f*
Premature thelarche, 795, 796*f*
Premenstrual dysphoric disorder (PMDD), 768–780
causes of, 776–777, 777*f*
cognitive behavioral therapy for, 779
definition of, 775
diagnosis of, 777–778, 778*b*
diet, supplements, exercise, and lifestyle changes, 778–779
incidence and epidemiology of, 775
pharmacologic agents for, 779–780, 779*t*
surgical treatment in, 780
symptoms of, 776, 776*b*
treatment of, 778–780
vitamin $B_6$ deficiency in, 778
Premenstrual syndrome, 768–780
causes of, 776–777, 777*f*
cognitive behavioral therapy for, 779
definition of, 775
diagnosis of, 777–778, 778*b*
diet, supplements, exercise, and lifestyle changes, 778–779
incidence and epidemiology of, 775
pharmacologic agents for, 779–780, 779*t*
surgical treatment in, 780
symptoms of, 776, 776*b*
treatment of, 778–780
vitamin $B_6$ deficiency in, 778
Prenatal ovarian cysts, 235–236
Preoperative counseling and management, 543–558
chlorhexidine/alcohol skin preparation, 552
chronic anticoagulation and bleeding disorders, 555–558
cardiopulmonary comorbidities, assessment of, 557
cardiovascular disease, 557
prophylaxis against infective endocarditis, 557–558
pulmonary disease, 557
stress-dose steroids, 556, 556*t*
complications, 550–555
consultation with anesthesiologist, 548, 548*t*
enhanced recovery, 548–550, 549*t*
evaluation of, 545
gastrointestinal tract considerations, 550
glucose control in diabetic and nondiabetic, 552–554
hair removal, 552
history of, 545
Preoperative counseling and management *(Continued)*
laboratory and, diagnostic procedures, 546–547, 546*f*, 547*f*
minimally invasive surgery, 552
normothermia, 552
patient education and informed consent, 547–548
physical examination, 545–546
preparation for, 548
preoperative briefing, 550
prophylactic antibiotics, 551–552
site marking and universal protocol in, 550
surgery, positioning for, 550
surgical site infection prevention, 550–551, 551*f*, 552*b*
surgical site infection reduction bundles, 551, 553*f*
smoking, 552
*Staphylococcus aureus*, screening for, 554
venous thromboembolism prevention, 554–555, 555*t*
Preoperative prolapse reduction standing stress test, 442–443
Prepubertal children
bleeding
vaginal, 230–231
vaginoscopy for, 232
without secondary signs of puberty, 230–232, 231*b*
endodermal sinus tumors of vagina, 232
foreign bodies, 231–232
hymen and vagina of, normal findings of, 224
McCune-Albright syndrome, 232
problems in, 226–227
labial adhesions, 228–229, 228*f*
lichen sclerosus, 229–230, 230*f*, 231*f*
physiologic discharge of puberty, 229
urethral prolapse, 229, 229*f*
vulvovaginitis, 226–227, 226*t*, 227*b*, 228*f*
sarcoma botryoides, 232
vaginal tumors, 232
Prevalence, definition of, 108
Prevalence of Female Sexual Problems Associated with Distress and Determinants of Seeking Treatment (PRESIDE) study, 170
Preventive health care, 127–139
absent breast and uterine development, 787
advocacy, screening, interventions, and referral, Primary amenorrhea, 137–139, 138*t*, 139*t*, 781–800
breast development present and uterus absent, 786–787, 787*f*
breasts absent and uterus present, 783–786, 785*f*
causes of, 783–788, 785*b*
differential diagnosis and management, 788–789, 788*f*
primary amenorrhea with absent endometrium, 788
secondary sex characteristics present and female internal genitalia present, 787–788
Primary dysmenorrhea, 769–773
behavioral interventions, 770
diagnosis of, 770, 770*f*

Primary dysmenorrhea *(Continued)*
medications for, 770–772, 771*t*, 772*f*
nonpharmacologic interventions, 770
exercise, 770
heat, 770
other treatments, 772–773
pathogenesis of, 769–770, 769*f*
severity of, 769*t*
treatment of, 770
vitamins and diet for, 770
Primary empty sella syndrome, 804
Primary human papillomavirus testing, 639
Primary oocytes, 83
Primary syphilis, 523, 523*f*
Primordial follicle, 83
Procidentia, 459
Progesterone, 9–10
in ectopic pregnancy, 349
negative feedback loop, 89
Progesterone deficiency, 330
Progestin-only formulations, 772
Progestin-only pills, 248
Progestins, for advanced/recurrent disease, 703
Progestogen
for acute bleeding, 603
use of, 285
Prolactin, 101, 801
concentrations, pharmacologic agents affecting, 803*b*
diagnostic techniques of, 806
diagnostic evaluation in, 806
imaging studies for, 806
measurement of, 802
physiology of, 801–803, 802*f*
pregnancy and treatment, of prolactinomas, 808–809
women with hyperprolactinemia who do not wish to conceive, 809
prolactinoma, operative approaches for, 808, 808*f*
radiation therapy, for macroadenomas, 808
treatment of, 806–809
bromocriptine, 806–807, 806*f*
cabergoline, 807, 807*t*
expectant treatment, 806
prolactinomas, medical treatment of, 806–808
women with prolactinomas, outcomes of treatment in, 807–808, 807*f*
Prolactinomas, 804–806
medical treatment of, 806–808
operative approaches for, 808, 808*f*
outcomes of treatment in women with, 807–808, 807*f*
pregnancy and treatment of, 808–809
Prolapse
anterior vaginal wall, 441–443, 442*f*
anterior colporrhaphy, 443, 444*f*
concomitant antiincontinence surgery, 443
concomitant apical support procedure, 443
diagnosis of, 442–443, 442*f*
mesh-augmented surgery, 445, 446*f*
postoperative restrictions on, 445
postoperative voiding dysfunction on, 443–445
recurrent, 445
surgical treatment, 443
symptoms, 441–442
Prolapse *(Continued)*
posterior vaginal wall, 445–446
diagnosis, 445–447, 447*f*
management, 446
perineorrhaphy, 447–449, 449*f*
posterior colporrhaphy, 447, 448*f*
posterior repairs, 446–447
recurrent, 449
site-specific posterior repair, 447, 449*f*
symptoms and signs, 445
rectal, 459
uterine, 451–456, 452*f*
cervical elongation, 453
fertility-sparing surgery, 454–456, 455*f*
management, 451
obliterative prolapse procedures, 453–454, 453*f*, 454*f*
surgery for, 451–453
symptoms and signs, 451
vaginal vault, 456–459, 456*f*, 458*f*, 459*f*
Prolapsed fallopian tube, 588
Prophylactic antibiotics, 551–552
Prophylaxis, for infective endocarditis, 557–558
Prostaglandins, 88
Protein kinase C (PKC), 81
Prozone phenomenon, 522
Pruritus, 369
Pseudosarcoma botryoides, 673
Psoriasis, 370–371, 371*f*
Psychoactive drugs, 779
Psychological preoperative preparation, for postoperative ileus, 580*t*
Psychological sequelae, 589–592
mental status changes, 591–592, 591*b*
pain relief, 589–590, 589*f*, 590*f*, 590*t*
postoperative concerns, in older surgical patients, 591, 591*b*
psychosexual problems and depression, 591
Psychosexual problems and depression, 591
Psychotropic medications, 153
PTSD. *see* Posttraumatic stress disorder (PTSD)
Puberty
physiologic discharge of, 229
precocious, 781–800, 794*f*, 795*t*
diagnostic evaluation, 797, 798*f*, 799*t*
gonadotropin-releasing hormone-dependent precocious puberty, 796–797
gonadotropin-releasing hormone-independent precocious puberty, 797, 798*f*
premature pubarche/adrenarche, 795–796
premature thelarche, 795, 796*f*
treatment of, 798–799, 799*f*
types of disorders, 795–797, 796*t*
secondary signs of, prepubertal bleeding without, 230–232, 231*b*
Pubic hair growth, classification of, 782*t*
Pubic louse, 518*f*
Puborectalis muscle, 496, 503*f*
Pubovaginal slings, 486, 487*f*
Pudendal nerve terminal motor latency, for anal incontinence, 504
Pudendum, 48
Pulmonary disease, 140–142, 141*b*
Pulmonary embolism, 572–575, 572*t*, 573*f*, 574*f*
Pulmonary metastases, 765
Pure gonadal dysgenesis, 783–786
PWS. *see* Prader-Willi syndrome (PWS)


## Q


Quality improvement, 114
Quiescent gestational trophoblastic disease, 760
Quinupristin-dalfopristin, 9–12*t*


## R


Radiation biology, 621–623
Radiation complications, 686
Radiation dose rate, 619
Radiation physics, basic, 619–620, 620*f*
Radiation resistance, 619
Radiation therapy
for ovarian cancer, 740
principles of, in gynecologic cancer, 618–627, 619*f*
basic radiation physics, 619–620, 620*f*
brachytherapy and teletherapy, 623–626, 624*f*, 624*t*, 625*f*, 626*f*
therapeutic radiation production, 620–623, 621*f*, 622*f*, 623*f*
therapeutic ratio, 619*f*
tissue tolerance and radiation complications, 626–627, 627*t*
Radiation treatment, 623–626, 624*f*, 624*t*, 625*f*, 626*f*
Radical hysterectomy, 680
Raloxifene
in bone health, 270
for breast cancer, 307
Randomized controlled trials (RCTs), 109–110
Rape, 176–182
date, 177
emotional support of, 180–181
medical responsibilities, 177–179, 178*f*, 179*b*
medicolegal, 180, 180*t*
physician's responsibility in, 177–180, 177*b*
pregnancy, 179–180
RCTs. *see* Randomized controlled trials (RCTs)
Records, medical, 121, 121*b*
alteration of, 121–122
Rectal examination, 137
Rectal nodes, 66
Rectal prolapse, 459
Rectocele, 445–446
Rectovaginal examination, 136, 137*f*
Rectovaginal fistulas, 512–513, 513*t*, 582
Rectum, 74
Rectus diastasis, 429
Recurrence, 687–689
chemotherapy as treatment for, 688–689
pelvic recurrence, 687–688
Recurrent endometrial cancer, 702
Recurrent pregnancy loss (RPL), 323–341, 325*t*, 326*t*
chromosomal, 325–327, 327*f*, 328*t*
endocrine factors, 330–331
diabetes mellitus, 331
hyperprolactinemia, 331

Recurrent pregnancy loss (RPL) *(Continued)*
insulin resistance, 331
luteal phase deficiency, 330
polycystic ovary syndrome, 331
thyroid disease, 330–331
environmental factors
alcohol, 334, 335*t*
caffeine, 334
maternal weight, 335
nonsteroidal antiinflammatory drugs, 335
smoking, 334
stress, 335
etiology, 325
evaluation, 324–325
immunologic factors, 331–333
alloimmune disorders, 332
antiphospholipid syndrome, 332–333, 332*b*
celiac disease, 333
infections, 334
inherited thrombophilia, 333–334, 334*b*
male factors, 335–336
unexplained loss, 336
uterine anomalies, 327–330
Recurrent uterine serous carcinoma, chemotherapy for advanced and, 703
Recurrent vulvovaginal candidiasis (RVVC), 531
Renal development, 11
Renal disease, 144
Reproductive anatomy, 47–75
external, 16–18, 18*f*, 48–50
Bartholin glands, 50, 51*f*
clinical correlations for, 50–51, 51*f*
clitoris, 49–50, 50*f*
hymen, 49
labia majora, 49
labia minora, 48, 49*f*
mons pubis, 48
Skene glands, 50
urethra, 50
vestibular bulbs, 50
vestibule, 50
vulva, 48, 49*f*
internal genitalia, 51–53
cervix, 53–58, 54*f*, 55*f*, 56*f*
ovaries, 61–62, 61*f*, 62*f*
oviducts, 58–60, 60*f*, 61*f*
uterus, 56–59, 57*f*, 58*f*, 59*f*
vagina, 51–53, 52*f*, 53*f*
vascular system, of pelvis, 62–64, 63*f*
arteries, 62–63
Reproductive concepts
basic science
anatomy, reproductive, 47–75
embryogenesis, 1–20
epidemiology, clinical, 106–115
evidence-based medicine, 106–115
fertilization, 1–20
risk management, medical-legal, 116–126
endocrinology and infertility
adenomas, pituitary, 803
amenorrhea, primary *vs.* secondary, 781–800
androgen excess, 810–823
dysmenorrhea, primary *vs.* secondary, 768–780
galactorrhea, 802–803, 802*f*
Reproductive concepts *(Continued)*
hyperprolactinemia, 801–809
infertility, 838–860
evaluations, comprehensive
additional considerations, gynecologic care, 148–187
endoscopy, 188–206
examinations, physical, 127–139
histories, 127–139
hysteroscopy, 188–206
laparoscopy, 188–206
medical disease-physiology interaction, 140–147
preventive health care, 127–139
general gynecology
adolescent patients, 221–237
anal incontinence, 495–514
benign gynecologic lesions, 362–408
breast diseases, 289–322
ectopic pregnancy, 342–361
endometriosis, 409–427
genital tract infections, 515–542
lower urinary tract, function and disorders of, 461–494
mature woman, care of, 255–288
menopause, 255–288
pediatric patients, 221–237
pelvic organ prolapse, 428–460
preoperative counseling and management, 543–558
reproductive tract, congenital abnormalities of, 207–220
oncology
fallopian tube, and peritoneal carcinoma, 750–752
gestational trophoblastic disease, 754–767
lower genital tract, intraepithelial neoplasia of, 637–647
malignant diseases of cervix, 674–690
malignant diseases of ovary, 707–753
malignant diseases of uterus, 691–706
malignant diseases of vagina, 648–673
neoplastic diseases of vulva, 648–673
radiation therapy, principles of, in gynecologic cancer, 618–636
Reproductive endocrinology, 76–105
anterior pituitary gland, 81–83
assay evaluation of, 104
gonadotropin-releasing hormone (GnRH), 76–81, 77*f*
gonadotropins, 81–83
hormone assay techniques, 103–104
antibodies, preparation of, 103
assay markers, choice of, 103
bound and unbound antigen, separation of, 103
immunoassay reaction, 103
immunoassays, 103–104
standard curve, 103–104
hypothalamic-pituitary-ovarian endocrine axis, communication within, 88–91
hypothalamus, 76–81
menstrual cycle, 91–99
cervical glands, 102–104
endometrium and, 99–102
ovaries, 83–88
Reproductive genetics, 21–46
Reproductive tract, structural abnormalities, 774, 774*f*
pelvic congestion syndrome, 774
Residual urine, test for, 466
Respiratory complications, 562
atelectasis, 562–564, 563*b*, 563*f*
pneumonia, 564–565, 564*b*
Retained foreign body, 568
Retrograde menstruation, endometriosis and, 410, 410*f*
Retroperitoneal lymphadenectomy, 727–728
Revised FIGO Staging, for endometrial cancer, 696*t*
Risk management, medical-legal, 116–126
alteration of records, 121–122
anticipation, 124
cancellations and "no shows," 120
CAP strategy, 124, 124*f*
claim, 122–123, 123*b*
communication, 124, 125*b*
consistent, with institutional policies, 122, 122*b*
informed consent, 119
informed refusal of care, 119
with patient, 118–119, 118*b*
postoperative care, 119
surgical documentation, 119
through medical records, 121, 121*b*
coverage arrangements, 120
fraud and abuse, 123
historical perspective of, 117–118
laboratory tests, 123–124
malpractice, 116, 117*b*, 117*f*
medication errors, 120–121
patient reviews, responding to, 122
poor outcome, 119–120, 120*b*
practical insight of, 118–124
preparation, 125
procedures, closed claims, 116, 117*f*
reproductive medicine and, 118
Rokitansky-Küster-Hauser syndrome. *see* Uterus, congenital absence of
Ruptured ectopic pregnancy, 348–349
RVVC. *see* Recurrent vulvovaginal candidiasis (RVVC)

## S

Sacral nerve stimulation, for anal incontinence, 512
neosphincters, 512
stoma creation, 512
Sacral nodes, 66
Sacrospinous ligament suspension, 456
Salpingitis, 343, 535
Salpingitis isthmica nodosa (SIN), 344, 344*f*
SANE. *see* Sexual Assault Nurse Evaluation (SANE)
Sarcoma botryoides, 232, 672, 672*f*
Sarcomas, 704–705, 704*b*
carcinosarcoma, 705
endometrial stromal sarcoma, 705
leiomyosarcoma, 704–705, 704*f*
Müllerian adenosarcoma, 705
of vulva, 664
SARTs. *see* Sexual Assault Response Teams (SARTs)
Scabies, 516–517, 518*f*

Schwannoma, 368
Seborrheic dermatitis, 371
SECCA procedure, for anal incontinence, 510–511
Secondary amenorrhea, 781–800
causes of, 789–792, 789*f*, 790*f*, 791*f*
CNS and hypothalamic causes, 789–791
CNS structural abnormalities, 789
drugs, 789–790
functional hypothalamic amenorrhea, 790–791, 791*f*
polycystic ovary syndrome, 790
stress and exercise, 790, 790*f*
weight loss, 790
diagnostic evaluation and management of, 792–794, 793*f*
ovarian causes, 791–792, 792*f*
pituitary causes, 791
neoplasms, 791
neoplastic lesions, 791
uterine factor, 789
Secondary dysmenorrhea, 768–780
causes and management, 773–774, 773*b*
cervical stenosis, 773–774, 774*f*
ectopic endometrial tissue, 773–774
functional bowel disease, relation to, 775
mental health conditions in, 775
other causes of, 775
pelvic congestion syndrome, 774
pelvic inflammation, 774
Secondary syphilis, 523, 524*f*
Seizure disorders, 145–146, 145*t*
Selective estrogen receptor modulators (SERMs), 703
in bone health, 267
for fibrocystic change, 297
Selective serotonin reuptake inhibitors (SSRIs), for menopause, 286
"Self-destructive deniers," 166
Semen analysis, 841, 841*t*
Sentinel lymph nodes, 317–318
Sentinel node biopsy, 683
Septic abortion, 339–340
SERMs. *see* Selective estrogen receptor modulators (SERMs)
Serotonin, 574, 577
Serotonin norepinephrine reuptake inhibitors (SNRIs)
for depression, 150–151
for menopause, 286
Serous tubal intraepithelial carcinoma, cause of, 750
Sertoli-Leydig cell tumors, 748–749, 749*f*, 817
Sex cord-stromal tumors, 747–749
with annular tubules, 749
Sex differentiation, molecular basis of, 13–18
external genitalia, 16–18, 18*f*, 19*f*
genital development, 13–14, 13*f*, 14*f*, 15*f*
Sex hormone-binding globulin (SHBG), 86
Sexual abuse, 233–235
genital warts, 234–235, 235*f*
history in, 233–234
hymens in evaluation of, 234, 235*f*
legal issues in reporting possible, 234
physical examination, 234
scope of problem, 233
sexually transmitted infections, 234
Sexual arousal disorders, 171–172, 171*f*
Sexual Assault Nurse Evaluation (SANE), 180
Sexual Assault Response Teams (SARTs), 180
Sexual function, 168–174, 168*b*, 168*f*, 169*f*, 170*f*
and dysfunction, 170–171, 174*f*
dyspareunia, 173, 173*b*, 173*f*
genito-pelvic pain penetration disorders, 172–174
menopause, 170
orgasmic disorders, 174, 175*t*
sexual interest/arousal disorders, 171–172, 171*f*
sexual response, 170
Sexual pain disorders, 173–174
Sexual response, 170
Sexually transmitted infections (STIs), 515
physical examination and evaluation for, 234
Sham feeding, for postoperative ileus, 580*t*
SHBG. *see* Sex hormone-binding globulin (SHBG)
*Shigella vaginitis*, 232
Shock, 565
Single gene disorders, 25–30
Single nucleotide polymorphisms (SNPs), 24
Sinovaginal bulbs, 212
Site marking and universal protocol, in preoperative counseling and management, 550
positioning for surgery, 550
preoperative briefing, 550
prophylactic antibiotics, 551–552
surgical site infection prevention, 550–551, 551*f*, 552*b*
surgical site infection reduction bundles, 551, 553*f*
Skene glands, 50
Sleep apnea, 565
Sliding scale insulin treatments, 577
Small cell carcinoma, 742
of cervix, 677
Smoking, environmental factors, 334
SNPs. *see* Single nucleotide polymorphisms (SNPs)
Social anxiety disorder, 159
Social phobia, 159
Sonohysterography, of intrauterine adhesion, 329*f*
Southern blot procedure, 39–40, 42*f*
Speculum examination, 134–135, 134*f*
Sperm, functional tests of, 846–847
Spermicides, 251
Sphincteroplasty, anterior, for anal incontinence, 511–512, 511*f*
Spigelian hernia, 428
Spironolactone, 821
Splenectomy, 727
Spontaneous early pregnancy loss
alloimmunization prevention, 339
bleeding in, 338
clinical presentation, 336
diagnostic evaluation, 336–338
epidemiology, 323–324, 324*f*, 325*f*
follow-up care, 340
laboratory evaluation, 336–337
management, 338–340
expectant, 338–339
medical, 339
second-trimester, 340
surgical, 339
ultrasound, 337, 337*f*, 337*t*, 338*b*
Spouse abuse, 182
Squamous cell carcinoma, 675*b*
of vagina, 665–666*f*, 668–670, 669*f*
survival of, 670
treatment of, 669
of vulva, 649, 657–660, 657*b*, 657*f*, 658*b*, 658*f*, 659*f*, 659*t*, 660*f*
Stellate ganglion blockade, for menopause, 287
Steroid receptors, 88–89
STIs. *see* Sexually transmitted infections (STIs)
Strangulated hernia, 429
Stress, 335
Stress urinary incontinence, 480
Stress urinary incontinence, on prolapse reduction, 442–443
Stress-dose steroids, 556, 556*t*
Stromal hyperthecosis, 816–817, 817*f*
Structural chromosome abnormalities, 32–34
Subfertility
immunologic factors in, 838
therapy for, 424–425, 424*f*, 425*f*
Substance use disorders, 162–166, 163*b*, 164*b*, 165*b*
Suicide, and depression, 151
Sulbactam plus, 9–12*t*
Superficial femoral nodes, 66
Superficial thrombophlebitis, 569
Superior gluteal nodes, 66
Supernumerary ovary, abnormalities of, 219
Swyer syndrome, 785
Synechiae, 789
Synthetic mesh, 483
Syphilis, 522–525, 522*f*, 523*t*
Syringoma, 367
Systematic reviews, 111–112


## T


Tamoxifen, 631*t*, 692
for fibrocystic change, 297
Tampon problems, 377–378
Tanycytes, 77
Targeted therapy, for ovarian cancer, 735–737, 736*t*, 737*t*
Taxanes, 630
Tazobactam plus, 9–12*t*
Teletherapy, 623–626, 626*f*
Tension-free vaginal tape (TVT) sling, 484, 484*f*
Teratomas, 743–745, 743*b*
benign cystic teratomas, 743–744, 744*f*
choriocarcinomas, 745
dysgerminomas, 744–745, 744*f*
embryonal carcinomas, 745
immature teratomas, 744
mixed germ cell tumors, 745
polyembryomas, 745
yolk sac tumors, 745, 745*f*
Tertiary syphilis, 524, 525*f*
Testicular feminization, 786–787
Testicular feminization syndrome, 213–214
TET. *see* Tubal embryo transfer (TET)
Tetracycline, 9–12*t*
Theca lutein cysts, 400–401, 400*f*
Thecoma, 748
Therapeutic radiation production, 620–623, 621*f*, 622*f*, 623*f*

Threatened abortion, 323
Thrombophlebitis and pulmonary embolus, 568–575
Thrombotic diseases, 144–145
Thyroid disease, 330–331
Tibolone, for osteoporosis, 270
Ticarcillin, 9–12*t*
amoxicillin and, 9–12*t*
Tigecycline, 9–12*t*
Time and timing, 840–841
Tissue Selective Estrogen Complex (TSEC) concept, 286
Tissue tolerance, and radiation complications, 626–627, 627*t*
TKIs. *see* Tyrosine kinase inhibitors (TKIs)
Tocolytics, 772
Toll-like receptors (TLRs), 607, 607*f*
Tomosynthesis, for breast cancer, 312–313
Topoisomerase I and II inhibitors, 631–632
Topotecan, 631–632, 631*t*
Torsion
of ovary, 406–407, 407*f*
of oviduct, 396–397, 396*f*
Toxic shock syndrome, 532
Trabecular bone, 268
Transit study, for anal incontinence, 505, 506*f*
Transitional cell carcinoma, 719
Transitional cell tumors, 405–406, 405*f*, 406*f*
Translocations, balanced reciprocal, 32–34, 33*f*
Transobturator (TOT) tape sling, 485
Transverse vaginal septum, 214–215, 214*f*
Trazodone, for depression, 150–151
*Treponema pallidum*, 522, 522*f*
*Trichomonas* vaginal infection, 528–530, 529*f*
Trichomoniasis, 533
Trinucleotide-repeat disorders (unstable mutations), 27
Tubal abortion, 346–347
Tubal embryo transfer (TET), 866
Tubal pregnancy, 344–345
management of, 353–355, 355*f*, 356*f*
Tubal surgery, 344–345
Tuberculosis, 541
in infertility, 855, 855*f*
Tuberculous salpingitis, 541
Tubulocystic cell pattern, 670, 671*f*
Tumor suppressor genes, 612–613
Tumor thickness, 664
Turner syndrome, 784
Typical adenocarcinoma, 676*f*
Tyrosine kinase inhibitors (TKIs), 633–634

## U

UAE. *see* Uterine artery embolization (UAE)
Ultrasonography, for ectopic pregnancy, 351–352, 351*f*, 352*f*
Ultrasound
for breast cancer, 312, 312*f*
in early pregnancy, 323, 326*t*
endoanal, for anal incontinence, 501, 503*f*, 504*f*
spontaneous early pregnancy loss, 337, 337*f*, 337*t*, 338*b*
transvaginal, 330*f*
uterus, 380–381, 382*f*, 383*f*
Umbilical hernias, 429, 430*f*
repair of, 431, 432*f*
Uncomplicated grief, 185
Unopposed estrogen therapy, endometrial cancer and, 276–277
Unstable bladder, 488
*Ureaplasma urealyticum*, 536
Ureteral injury and urinary fistula, 575–576, 576*f*
Ureters, 72–73
Urethra, 50
anatomy and function of, 462–465, 465*f*, 466*f*
Urethral caruncle, 363–364, 363*f*
Urethral diverticulum, 375–376, 375*t*, 376*f*, 477–479, 478*f*
complications, 478–479
diagnosis, 477, 478*f*
etiology, 477
symptoms and signs, 477
treatment, 477–478
Urethral mucosa, prolapse of, 229, 229*f*
Urethral prolapse, 363–364, 364*f*
Urethrocele, 442
Urinalysis, 465–466
Urinary bladder, 73–74
Urinary incontinence, 479–486
evaluation of, 481–485
intrinsic sphincter deficiency, 486
mesh risks, 485–486
postoperative voiding trial, 486
risk factors, 479*b*, 480*f*
stress, 480
surgical management, autologous fascia pubovaginal sling, 486, 487*f*
surgical procedure selection, 486
treatment, 481–485, 482*f*, 483*f*, 483*t*, 484*f*, 485*f*
Urinary tract endometriosis, 424–425, 424*f*, 425*f*
Urinary tract infections (UTIs), 469–470, 575
Urinary tract problems, 575–576
inability to void, 575
ureteral injury and urinary fistula, 575–576, 576*f*
urinary tract infection, 575
Urine culture, 465–466
Urodynamics, 468, 469*f*
Urogenital diaphragm, 69
Uterine adhesions, 789, 789*f*
Uterine agenesis. *see* Uterus, congenital absence of
Uterine anomalies, 327–330
acquired
cervical incompetence (cervical insufficiency), 330, 330*f*, 331*f*
endometrial polyps, 328–329
fibroids, 328
intrauterine adhesions (Asherman syndrome), 329–330, 329*f*, 329*t*
development of, 327–328
Uterine artery, 63, 64*f*
Uterine artery embolization (UAE), 390–392, 391*f*
Uterine bleeding, 243
abnormal, 594–605
approaches to treatment, 604–605
causes of, 594–598, 595*f*
diagnostic approach, 599–600, 599*f*, 600*f*
management of, 602–605
treatment of, 600–602
Uterine perforation, 243
Uterine prolapse, 451–456, 452*f*
cervical elongation, 453
fertility-sparing surgery, 454–456, 455*f*
management, 451
obliterative prolapse procedures, 453–454, 453*f*, 454*f*
surgery for, 451–453
symptoms and signs, 451
Uterine serous carcinoma, 701
Uterosacral ligaments, 70
suspension, 451–452
Uterovaginal agenesis. *see* Uterus, congenital absence of
Uterus, 56–59, 57*f*, 58*f*, 59*f*
abnormalities of, 215–219, 215*f*, 216*f*, 217*f*
diagnosis, 218–219
imaging, 216, 218*f*
management, 219
symptoms and signs, benign gynecologic lesions, 216–218, 380–393
endometrial polyps, 381–383, 384*f*
hematometra, 383–384
leiomyomas, 384–393, 385*f*, 386*f*, 387*f*, 388*f*, 391*f*, 391*t*, 392*f*, 393*f*
congenital absence of, 787, 787*f*
malignant diseases of, 691–706
epidemiology of, 691–693, 692*b*, 692*f*
ultrasound of, 380–381, 382*f*, 383*f*
UTIs. *see* Urinary tract infections (UTIs)

## V

Vagina, 51–53, 52*f*, 53*f*
benign gynecologic lesions, 375–378
dysontogenetic cysts, 376–377, 376*f*, 377*f*
inclusion cysts, 376
local trauma, 378
tampon problems, 377–378
urethral diverticulum, 375–376, 375*t*, 376*f*
endodermal sinus tumors of, 232
malignant diseases of, 665–666*f*, 665–666, 666*t*
detection and diagnosis, 666–667, 667*f*
symptoms and diagnosis, 667–668, 668*f*, 668*t*
treatment of, 667
premalignant disease of, 666–667, 667*f*
prepubertal child, normal findings of, 224
tumors of
adult, 668–672
infants and children, 672–673
Vaginal adenocarcinomas, in endometriosis, 671–672
Vaginal adenosis, 215
Vaginal agenesis, 213–214, 213*f*
treatment of, 214
Vaginal bleeding, in pubertal children, 230–231
Vaginal intraepithelial neoplasia, 646
Vaginal metastases, 765
Vaginal septum, transverse, 214–215, 214*f*
Vaginal tumors, in prepubertal children, 232
Vaginal vault prolapse, 456–459, 456*f*, 458*f*, 459*f*
Vaginismus, 172–173, 173*f*

Vaginitis, 525–532, 526*t*, 527*t*
bacterial vaginosis, 526–528, 528*f*, 529*t*
*Candida vaginalis*, 530–532, 530*f*, 531*f*, 532*b*
*Trichomonas* vaginal infection, 528–530, 529*f*
Vaginoscopy, for prepubertal bleeding without signs of puberty, 232
Vancomycin, 9–12*t*
Vascular diseases, 143–144
Vascular system, of pelvis, 62–64, 63*f*
Vasectomy, 239
Veins, 63–64
Venlafaxine, for depression, 150–151
Ventral hernia, 428
Verrucous carcinoma, 663, 676, 676*f*
Very advanced spectrum mezlocillin, 9–12*t*
Vestibular bulbs, 50
Vestibule, 50
Vestibulodynia, 373–375
Video-assisted thoracoscopy, utility of, 726
Vinca alkaloids, 632–633
*Vinca rosea*, 632–633
Vincristine, 631*t*, 632–633
Vinorelbine, 631*t*
Violence. *see also* Abuse
domestic, 182
intimate partner, 182–185, 183*b*, 184*b*
Virginal hypertrophy (breast), 293
Virilization, 810
Visceral peritoneum, 57
Vitamin D, 139, 139*t*
Vitelline membrane, 94
von Recklinghausen disease, 368
Voriconazole, 9–12*t*
V/Q scan, 574
Vulva, 48, 649, 650*f*
advanced vulvar tumors, 662–663
lymphatic mapping and sentinel lymph node biopsy, 662–663
quality of life and vulvar carcinoma, 662
radiation therapy and recurrences, 662
benign gynecologic lesions, 363–369
abnormal tissues presenting vulvar masses, 368
cysts, 364–365, 364*f*
endometriosis, 367–368
fibroma, 366, 366*f*
granular cell myoblastoma, 368
hemangioma, 366
hematomas, 368–369, 368*f*
Vulva *(Continued)*
hidradenoma, 367, 367*f*
lipoma, 366–367, 367*f*
nevus, 365–366, 365*f*
syringoma, 367
urethral caruncle, 363–364, 363*f*
urethral prolapse, 363–364, 364*f*
von Recklinghausen disease, 368
carcinoma of, 658–660
definition and clinicopathologic relationships, 658–660, 660*f*
treatment of, 660
infections of, 515–525
Bartholin glands infection, 516, 517*f*, 518*f*
genital ulcers, 519–525, 519*t*
molluscum contagiosum, 517–519, 518*f*
pediculosis pubis, 516–517, 518*f*
scabies, 516–517, 518*f*
invasive carcinoma of, 657*f*, 660–662, 661*f*
malignancies of, 663–665
microinvasive carcinoma of, 658–660
neoplastic diseases of, 648–673
Vulvar atypias, 649–656
classification of, 649*b*
diagnosis of, 651–653, 652*f*, 653*f*
specific conditions of, 649–651
carcinoma in situ, 651, 652*f*
intraepithelial neoplasia, 649–650, 650*f*, 651*f*
Paget disease, 651, 652*f*
treatment of, 653–656, 654*f*
Paget disease of vulva in, 656
vulvar intraepithelial neoplasia in, 655–656
Vulvar hematomas, 233, 233*f*
Vulvar intraepithelial neoplasia, 646, 646*f*
treatment of, 655–656
Vulvar lymph drainage, 658*f*
Vulvar pain syndromes, 373–375, 374*b*
Vulvar trauma, lacerations and straddle injury, 232–233
Vulvar tumors, 662–663
Vulvar vestibulitis, 373–375, 374*f*
Vulvectomy, 657*f*
Vulvodynia, 173–174
Vulvovaginal atrophy, 267
Vulvovaginitis, in prepubertal children, 226–227, 226*t*, 227*b*
treatment of, 227, 228*f*


## W


Warnings, black box, 150–151
Washout, 567
Weight changes, associated with injectable suspensions, 245–246
Weight gain, PCOS and, 831
Weight loss, for stress urinary incontinence, 482
Weight Watchers, 155
Well-differentiated adenosquamous carcinoma, 676, 677*f*
Withdrawal bleeding, 247
World Health Organization
female circumcision, 181–182, 181*f*
obesity, 154
World Health Organization Classification of Gestational Trophoblastic Disease, 755*b*
Wound complications, 583–586
dehiscence and evisceration, 584–586, 585*f*, 585*t*, 586*t*, 587*f*
infection, 583–584, 583*b*, 584*f*, 587*f*, 587*t*
obesity, 586, 587*b*


## X


X chromosome, structurally abnormal, 784–786
X-inactive specific transcript (XIST), 26
X-linked trait, of Mendelian inheritance patterns, 26–27


## Y


Y chromosomes, 26
Yew, Pacific/Western *vs.* English, 630
Yolk sac tumors, 745, 745*f*
of vagina, 672


## Z


Z. *see* Atomic number (Z)
Zona pellucida, 94
Zygote, 5–8
Zygotene substage, 2–3